Textbook of Clinical
Gastroenterology
and Hepatology

Companion website

This book is accompanied by a website:

www.textbookclinicalgastrohep.com

The website includes:
- Over 85 high-definition surgical videos of diagnostic and therapeutic endoscopic procedures
- 300+ MCQs written to mirror the American College of Gastroenterology postgraduate course exams
- More than 35 management protocol charts for different diseases, all fully downloadable and editable, to help clinicians tailor the management programs for different patients
- All 850+ illustrations, available as downloadable digital files for use in scientific presentations.

Textbook of Clinical Gastroenterology and Hepatology

SECOND EDITION

EDITORS

C. J. Hawkey FMedSci
Professor of Gastroenterology
Nottingham Digestive Diseases Centre
University of Nottingham and Nottingham University Hospitals
Nottingham, UK

Jaime Bosch MD, PhD
Chair of Medicine
Head, Hepatic Hemodynamic Laboratory, Liver Unit
Hospital Clínic-IDIBAPS, University of Barcelona;
Director, Biomedical Research Centre Network of Hepatic and Digestive
Diseases (CIBERehd), National Institute of Health Carlos III
Ministry of Science and Innovation
Barcelona, Spain

Joel E. Richter MD, FACP, MACG
Hugh Culverhouse Professor of Medicine
Director, Division of Gastroenterology and Nutrition
Director, Joy M. Culverhouse Center for Esophageal Diseases
University of South Florida
Tampa, FL, USA

Guadalupe Garcia-Tsao MD
Professor of Medicine
Section of Digestive Diseases
Yale University, School of Medicine
New Haven;
Veterans Affairs Connecticut Healthcare System
West Haven, CT, USA

Francis K. L. Chan MD
Professor of Medicine
Chief of Gastroenterology & Hepatology
Associate Dean (Clinical)
Department of Medicine & Therapeutics
The Chinese University of Hong Kong
Hong Kong SAR, China

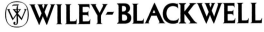

WILEY-BLACKWELL

A John Wiley & Sons, Ltd., Publication

This edition first published 2012 © 2012 by Blackwell Publishing Ltd
First edition published 2005, © 2005 Elsevier, Inc.

Blackwell Publishing was acquired by John Wiley & Sons in February 2007. Blackwell's publishing program has been merged with Wiley's global Scientific, Technical and Medical business to form Wiley-Blackwell.

Registered office: John Wiley & Sons, Ltd, The Atrium, Southern Gate, Chichester, West Sussex, PO19 8SQ, UK

Editorial offices: 9600 Garsington Road, Oxford, OX4 2DQ, UK

The Atrium, Southern Gate, Chichester, West Sussex, PO19 8SQ, UK

350 Main Street, Malden, MA 02148-5020, USA

For details of our global editorial offices, for customer services and for information about how to apply for permission to reuse the copyright material in this book please see our website at www.wiley.com/wiley-blackwell

Library of Congress Cataloging-in-Publication Data

Textbook of clinical gastroenterology and hepatology / editors, C.J. Hawkey . . . [et al.]. – 2nd ed.
        p. ; cm.
    Rev. ed. of: Clinical gastroenterology and hepatology / editors, Wilfred M. Weinstein, C.J. Hawkey, Jaime Bosch. 2005.
    Includes bibliographical references and index.
    ISBN-13: 978-1-4051-9182-1 (hardcover : alk. paper)
    ISBN-10: 1-4051-9182-1 (hardcover : alk. paper)
    I. Hawkey, C. J. II. Clinical gastroenterology and hepatology.
    [DNLM: 1. Digestive System Diseases–diagnosis. 2. Digestive System Diseases–therapy. 3. Liver Diseases–diagnosis. 4. Liver Diseases–therapy. WI 141]
    LC classification not assigned
    616.3'3–dc23
                                    2011029724

A catalogue record for this book is available from the British Library.

Wiley also publishes its books in a variety of electronic formats. Some content that appears in print may not be available in electronic books.

Set in 8.75/12 pt Palatino by Toppan Best-set Premedia Limited
Printed and bound in Singapore by Markono Print Media Pte Ltd

1 2012

Contents

Companion website

This book is accompanied by a website:

www.textbookclinicalgastrohep.com

The website includes:
- Over 85 high-definition surgical videos of diagnostic and therapeutic endoscopic procedures
- 300+ MCQs written to mirror the American College of Gastroenterology postgraduate course exams
- More than 35 management protocol charts for different diseases, all fully downloadable and editable, to help clinicians tailor the management programs for different patients
- All 850+ illustrations, available as downloadable digital files for use in scientific presentations.

List of contributors

Juan G. Abraldes MD, MMSc
Hepatic Hemodynamic Laboratory
Liver Unit, Institut de Malalties Digestives i Metaboliques
University of Barcelona, CIBERehd
Barcelona, Spain

Ahmed Abu Shanab MD
Alimentary Pharmabiotic Centre
Department of Medicine
University College Cork
Cork, Ireland

Austin G. Acheson MB, Bch, MD, FRCS
Division of GI Surgery
Nottingham University Hospitals
Nottingham, UK

Feras T. Alissa MBBS, MD
Department of Pediatrics
University of Pittsburgh School of Medicine
Children's Hospital of Pittsburgh of UPMC
Pittsburgh, PA, USA

Majid Almadi MBBS, FRCPC, MSc (Epi)
Department of Gastroenterology
King Khalid University Hospital
King Saud University
Riyadh, Saudi Arabia

Haitham M. Al-Salama MD
Director of Research Programmes
Qatar Foundation
Doha, Qatar

Bhupinder Anand MD, PhD
Professor of Medicine
Baylor College of Medicine;
Staff Physician
Michael E. DeBakey VA Medical Center
Houston, TX, USA

Jervoise Andreyev MA, PhD, FRCP
Consultant Gastroenterologist in Pelvic Radiation Disease
The GI Unit
The Royal Marsden NHS Foundation Trust
London, UK

Nadir Arber MD, MSc, MHA
Professor of Medicine and Gastroenterology
Yeichel and Helen Lieber Professor for Cancer Research
Head, Department of Cancer Prevention
The Integrated Cancer Prevention Center
Gastroenterology and Liver Institute
Tel-Aviv Sourasky Medical Center;
Sackler Faculty of Medicine
Tel-Aviv University
Tel-Aviv, Israel

Christian Arnold MD
Department of Gastroenterology
Klinikum Friedrichshafen
Friedrichshafen, Germany

Tarik Asselah MD, PhD
Service d'Hépatologie
Hôpital Beaujon
University of Paris
Clichy, France

John C. Atherton MD
Professor of Gastroenterology and Head of School of Clinical Sciences
Nottingham Digestive Diseases Centre
University of Nottingham and Nottingham University Hospitals
Nottingham, UK

Ashok Attaluri MD
Division of Gastroenterology and Hepatology
Department of Internal Medicine
University of Iowa Carver College of Medicine
Iowa City, IA, USA

Kiran Bambha MD, MSc
Assistant Professor of Medicine
Hepatology and Liver Transplantation
University of Colorado Anschutz Medical Campus
Aurora, CO, USA

Rafael Bañares MD
Professor of Medicine
Hepatology and Liver Unit
Hospital General Universitario Gregorio Marañón
Universidad Complutense
CIBERehd
Madrid, Spain

Matthew R. Banks BSc, PhD, FRCP
Division of Gastroenterology
University College London Hospitals
London, UK

Heike Bantel MD
Department of Gastroenterology, Hepatology and Endocrinology
Hannover Medical School
Hannover, Germany

Alan Barkun MDCM, FRCPC, MSc(Epi)
Division of Gastroenterology
McGill University and the McGill University Health Centre (MUHC)
Montreal, QC, Canada

M. Beaugrand MD
Liver Unit
Hôpital Jean Verdier
Université Paris XIII
Bondy, France

Cristina Bellarosa MD
Centro Studi Fegato
Fondazione Italiana Fegato
University of Trieste
Trieste, Italy

Pascal O. Berberat MD
Department of Surgery
Klinikum rechts der Isar
Technische Universität München
Munich, Germany

Nora V. Bergasa MD
Chief of Medicine
Metropolitan Hospital Center
New York, NY, USA

Annalisa Berzigotti MD, PhD
Hepatic Hemodynamic Laboratory
Liver Unit, Institut de Malalties Digestives i Metaboliques
University of Barcelona, CIBERehd
Barcelona, Spain

Rakesh Bhardwaj MD, FRCS (Gen Surg)
Consultant Colorectal Surgeon
Darent Valley Hospital
Dartford, UK

Adil E. Bharucha MD
Professor of Medicine
Division of Gastroenterology and Hepatology
Clinical Enteric Neuroscience Translational and Epidemiological Research Program
Mayo Clinic
Rochester, MN, USA

Juliane Bingener MD
Associate Professor of Surgery
Division of Gastroenterologic and General Surgery
Mayo Clinic
Rochester, MN, USA

Stephan C. Bischoff MD
Professor of Medicine
Director, Department of Nutritional Medicine and Immunology
University of Hohenheim
Stuttgart, Germany

Ingvar Bjarnason MD, MSc
Professor of Digestive Diseases
Department of Gastroenterology
King's College Hospital
London, UK

Jaime Bosch MD, PhD
Chair of Medicine
Head, Hepatic Hemodynamic Laboratory, Liver Unit
Hospital Clínic-IDIBAPS, University of Barcelona;
Director, Biomedical Research Centre Network of Hepatic and Digestive Diseases (CIBERehd), National Institute of Health Carlos III
Ministry of Science and Innovation
Barcelona, Spain

Gerd Bouma MD, PhD
Department of Gastroenterology
Vrije Universiteit Medical Center
Amsterdam, The Netherlands

T. E. Bowling MD, FRCP
Consultant in Gastroenterology and Clinical Nutrition
Nottingham University Hospitals
Nottingham, UK

Thomas A. Brown MD
MetroHealth Medical Center;
Division of Gastroenterology and Hepatology
Case Western Reserve University
Cleveland, OH, USA

William R. Brugge MD
Director, Gastrointestinal Endoscopy
Massachusetts General Hospital;
Professor of Medicine
Harvard Medical School
Boston, MA, USA

Miquel Bruguera Cortada MD
Liver Unit, Hospital Clinic, and Department of Medicine
University of Barcelona
Barcelona, Spain

Jordi Bruix MD
Senior Consultant
Professor of Medicine
BCLC Group, Liver Unit
Hospital Clinic
Biomedical Research Centre
Network of Hepatic and Digestive Diseases (CIBERehd)
University of Barcelona
Barcelona, Spain

Markus W. Büchler MD
Professor and Chairman
Department of General Surgery
University of Heidelberg
Heidelberg, Germany

Alan L. Buchman MD, MSPH
Professor of Medicine and Surgery
Division of Gastroenterology
Feinberg School of Medicine
Northwestern University
Chicago, IL, USA

Nicola E. Burch MBChB, MRCP (UK) (*Gastro*), MSc (Hons)
Consultant Gastroenterologist
University Hospitals Coventry and Warwickshire NHS Trust
Coventry, UK

Christophe Bureau MD
Service d'Hépato-Gastro-Entérologie et INSERM
Université de Toulouse
Toulouse, France

Andrés Cárdenas MD, MMSc
Institut Clinic de Malalties Digestives i Metaboliques
Hospital Clinic
University of Barcelona
Barcelona, Spain

Anna Casburn-Jones MB, MRCP
Consultant Gastroenterologist
St Mary's Hospital
London, UK

Güralp O. Ceyhan MD
Department of Surgery
Klinikum rechts der Isar
Technische Universität München
Munich, Germany

Francis K.L. Chan MD
Professor of Medicine
Chief of Gastroenterology & Hepatology
Associate Dean (Clinical)
Department of Medicine & Therapeutics
The Chinese University of Hong Kong
Hong Kong SAR, China

Kenneth J. Chang MD
Chief, Division of Gastroenterology
Professor of Clinical Medicine
University of California
Irvine, CA, USA

Daniel Cherqui MD
Professor of Surgery
New York Presbyterian / Weill Cornell Medical College
New York, NY, USA

Runjan Chetty MB BCh, FFPath, FRCPA, FCAP, FRCPath, DPhil (Oxon)
Professor and Director of Translational Pathology and Consultant GI / Pancreatic Pathologist
Department of Cellular Pathology
Nuffield Department of Clinical
Laboratory Sciences and Oxford Biomedical Research Centre
Oxford University Hospitals Trust
University of Oxford
Oxford, UK

Winnie C.W. Chu MBChB, FRCR
Professor
Department of Diagnostic Radiology & Organ Imaging
Chinese University of Hong Kong
Hong Kong SAR, China

Guido Costamagna MD
Director, Gastrointestinal Endoscopy
Catholic University of the Sacred Heart
"A. Gemelli" Hospital
Rome, Italy

John Croese FRACP, MD
Department of Gastroenterology
The Townsville Hospital
Townsville, QLD, Australia

Abraham H. Dachman MD
Department of Radiology
The University of Chicago Medical Center
Chicago, IL, USA

Zilvinas Dambrauskas MD
Department of Surgery
Kaunas University of Medicine Hospital
Kaunas, Lithuania

Gennaro D'Amico MD
Chief of Gastroenterology
Department of Gastroenterology
Ospedale V Cervello
Palermo, Italy

Srinivasan Dasarathy MD
Departments of Gastroenterology, Hepatology and Pathobiology
Cleveland Clinic Lerner College of Medicine
Case Western Reserve University
Cleveland, OH, USA

Mark Davenport ChM FRCS (Eng), FRCS (Paeds)
Professor of Paediatric Surgery
Department of Paediatric Surgery
King's College Hospital
London, UK

Andrea De Gottardi MD, PhD
Visiting Hepatologist
Hepatic Hemodynamic Laboratory, Liver Unit
Hospital Clinic
Barcelona, Spain

Amar R. Deshpande MD
Assistant Professor of Medicine
Department of Medicine, Division of Gastroenterology
University of Miami Miller School of Medicine
Miami, FL, USA

Jean-Charles Deybach MD, PhD
Professor of Medicine
Head of Department of Biochemistry and Molecular Genetics
Centre Français des Porhpyries
Hôpital Louis Mourier
Colombes, France

Daniel Dhumeaux MD
Henri Mondor Hospital
Créteil, France

Elizabeth Drewe MD
Department Clinical Immunology and Allergy
Nottingham University Hospitals
Nottingham, UK

Franz Ludwig Dumoulin MD
Head of Department of Medicine
Gemeinschaftskrankenhaus Bonn;
Associate Professor of Medicine
University of Bonn
Bonn, Germany

Andrew W. DuPont MD, MSPH
The University of Texas Health Science Center at Houston
Houston, TX, USA

Herbert L. DuPont MD
Director, Center for Infectious Diseases
Professor of Epidemiology
The University of Texas-Houston School of Public Health;
Chief, Internal Medicine Service
St. Luke's Episcopal Hospital;
Vice Chairman, Department of Medicine
Baylor College of Medicine
Houston, TX, USA

Luca Fabris MD, PhD
Assistant Professor of Gastroenterology
Department of Surgical, Oncological and Gastroenterological Sciences
University of Padua, Padua, Italy;
Liver Center and Section of Digestive Diseases
Yale University
New Haven, CT, USA

Michael B. Fallon MD
Division Director and Professor of Medicine
Division of Gastroenterology, Hepatology and Nutrition
The University of Texas Health Science Center at Houston
Houston, TX, USA

Dai-ming Fan MD, PhD
Xijing Hospital of Digestive Diseases
State Key Laboratory of Cancer Biology
Fourth Military Medical University
Xi'an, China

Patrizia Farci MD
Chief, Hepatic Pathogenesis Section
Laboratory of Infectious Diseases
National Institute of Allergy and Infectious Diseases
National Institutes of Health
Bethesda, MD, USA

Michael J.G. Farthing MD, FRCP
Vice Chancellor and Professor of Medicine
University of Sussex
Brighton, UK

Ronnie Fass MD
Professor of Medicine
University of Arizona College of Medicine;
Chief of Gastroenterology
Head, Neuroenteric Clinical Research Group
Southern Arizona VA Health Care System
Tucson, AZ, USA

Peter Ferenci MD
Professor of Medicine
Department of Internal Medicine
Gastroenterology and Hepatology
Medical University of Vienna
Vienna, Austria

Katrin Feuser PhD
Department of Nutritional Medicine
University of Hohenheim
Stuttgart, Germany

Martin H. Floch MD, MACG, AGAF, FACP
Clinical Professor of Medicine
Yale University School of Medicine
New Haven, CT, USA

Evan L. Fogel MD
Professor of Clinical Medicine
Division of Gastroenterology / Hepatology
Indiana University Health
Indianapolis, IN, USA

Alexander C. Ford MBChB, MD
Department of Academic Medicine
St. James's University Hospital
Leeds, UK

Alejandro Forner MD
Clinical Research Associate
BCLC Group, Liver Unit
ICMDM, Hospital Clinic
Biomedical Research Centre Network of Hepatic and
Digestive Diseases (CIBERehd)
University of Barcelona
Barcelona, Spain

Xavier Forns MD, PhD
Consultant in Liver Diseases
Hospital Clinic, CIBERehd, IDIBAPS
Barcelona, Spain

Paul J. Fortun BM, MRCP, FRACP
Consultant Gastroenterologist
Department of Gastroenterology
Royal Cornwall Hospitals NHS Trust
Truro, UK

Bruce M. Fox MBBS, MRCP, FRCR, PGCE
Consultant GI Radiologist
Honorary University Fellow
Derriford Hospital
Plymouth, UK

Juan Miguel Abdo Francis MD
Division of Medicine
Hospital General de México
Mexico City, Mexico

Helmut Friess MD
Professor and Chairman
Department of Surgery
Klinikum rechts der Isar
Technische Universität München
Munich, Germany

James Frith MB ChB MRCP, PhD
Academic Clinical Lecturer
UK NIHR Biomedical Research Centre in Ageing
Institute for Ageing and Health
Newcastle University
Newcastle upon Tyne, UK

Juan Carlos García-Pagán MD
Senior Consultant in Hepatology
Hepatic Hemodynamic Laboratory
Liver Unit, Hospital Clínic, CIBERehd
Barcelona, Spain

Guadalupe Garcia-Tsao MD
Professor of Medicine
Section of Digestive Diseases
Yale University, School of Medicine
New Haven;
Veterans Affairs Connecticut Healthcare System
West Haven, CT, USA

Robert H. Geelkerken MD PhD
Consultant Vascular Surgeon
Department of Vascular Surgery
Medisch Spectrum Twente
Enschede, The Netherlands

Robert M. Genta MD
Chief for Academic Affairs
Caris Diagnostics / Miraca;
Clinical Professor of Pathology and Medicine (Gastroenterology)
University of Texas Southwestern Medical Center
Irving, TX, USA

Paula Ghaneh MBChB, MD, FRCS
Reader in Surgery
Department of Molecular and Clinical Cancer Medicine
Institute of Translational Medicine
University of Liverpool
Liverpool, UK

Kevin A. Ghassemi MD
Division of Digestive Diseases
David Geffen School of Medicine at UCLA
Los Angeles, CA, USA

Alexander Gimson FRCP
Clinical Director, Division of Medicine
Consultant Physician and Hepatologist
Liver Transplantation Unit
Cambridge University Hospitals NHS Foundation Trust
Cambridge, UK

Pere Ginès MD
Chairman, Liver Unit
Professor of Medicine
Hospital Clinic
University of Barcelona
Barcelona, Spain

Ajay Goel PhD
Director, Epigenetics and Cancer Prevention
Baylor Research Institute and Charles A Sammons Cancer Center
Baylor University Medical Center
Dallas, TX, USA

Martin Goetz MD, PhD
Internist, Gastroenterologe
I. Medizinische Klinik und Poliklinik
Universitätsmedizin Mainz
Mainz, Germany

Tamas A. Gonda MD
Assistant Professor of Medicine
Division of Digestive and Liver Diseases
Columbia University Medical Center
New York, NY, USA

Gregory J. Gores MD
Reuben R. Eisenberg Professor of Medicine
Chair, Division of Gastroenterology and Hepatology
Center for Basic Research in Digestive Diseases
Mayo Clinic
Rochester, MN, USA

Penny A. Gowland PhD
Sir Peter Mansfield Magnetic Resonance Centre
School of Physics and Astronomy
University of Nottingham
Nottingham, UK

Andrea Grin MD, FRCPC
Resident in Pathology
Department of Laboratory Medicine and Pathobiology
University of Toronto
Toronto, ON, Canada

Roberto J. Groszmann MD
Department of Internal Medicine
Digestive Diseases Section
Yale University School of Medicine
New Haven, CT, USA

Madhusudan Grover MBBS
Mayo Clinic
Rochester, MN, USA

Sushovan Guha MD, PhD
Assistant Professor
Department of Gastroenterology, Hepatology, and Nutrition
The University of Texas MD Anderson Cancer Center
Houston, TX, USA

Neil Gupta MD, MPH
Fellow
Division of Gastroenterology / Hepatology
University of Kansas Medical Center
Kansas City Veterans Administration
Kansas City, MO, USA

Aliya G. Hasan MD
Assistant Professor of Medicine
Division of Gastroenterology and Hepatology
University of Colorado Denver
Aurora, CO, USA

C. J. Hawkey FMedSci
Professor of Gastroenterology
Nottingham Digestive Diseases Centre
University of Nottingham and Nottingham University Hospitals
Nottingham, UK

Philip N. Hawkins PhD, FRCP

National Amyloidosis Centre
Centre for Amyloidosis and Acute Phase Proteins
Division of Medicine
University College London Medical School
London, UK

J. Eileen Hay MB, ChB

Professor of Medicine
Consultant in Gastroenterology and Hepatology
Mayo Clinic
Rochester, MN, USA

J. Michael Henderson MD

Chief Quality Officer and Staff Surgeon
Cleveland Clinic
Cleveland, OH, USA

Karin Herrmann MD

Associate Professor of Radiology
Institute of Clinical Radiology
Ludwig-Maximilians-University of Munich
Munich, Germany

Tiberiu Hershcovici MD

Research Fellow
Neuroenteric Clinical Research Group
Southern Arizona VA Health Care System
Tucson, AZ, USA

Frank Hoentjen MD, PhD

Assistant Professor in Medicine
Department of Gastroenterology
Radboud University Medical Center
Nijmegen, The Netherlands

Joyce Wai Yi Hui MBChB, FRCR

Department of Diagnostic Radiology and Organ Imaging
Prince of Wales Hospital
The Chinese University of Hong Kong
Shatin, Hong Kong SAR, China

David J. Humes BSc MBBS MRCS PhD

NIHR Lecturer in Surgery
Nottingham Digestive Diseases Centre
Nottingham University Hospitals
Nottingham, UK

Haruhiro Inoue MD

Professor
Faculty of Medicine
Showa University;
Showa University International Training Center for Endoscopy (SUITE)
Digestive Disease Center
Showa University Northern Yokohama Hospital
Yokohama, Japan

Christian S. Jackson MD

Chief, Section of Gastroenterology
Loma Linda VA Healthcare System;
Assistant Professor
Loma Linda University Medical Center
Loma Linda, CA, USA

Simon A. Jackson MBBS, FRCS, FRCR

Consultant GI Radiologist
Imaging Directorate
Derriford Hospital
Plymouth, UK

Janusz A. Jankowski MD, PhD, FRCP, FACG

Consultant Gastroenterologist
Digestive Diseases Centre UHL Trust
Leicester;
James Black Senior Fellow and Professor
University of Oxford
Oxford;
Fellow and Professor
Cancer Research UK and Queen Mary, University of London
London, UK

Dennis M. Jensen MD

CURE / Digestive Disease Research Center
David Geffen School of Medicine at UCLA
Los Angeles, CA, USA

Robert T. Jensen MD

Chief, Cell Biology Section
Digestive Diseases Branch
National Institute of Diabetes and Kidney Diseases
National Institutes of Health
Bethesda, MD, USA

Michael D. Johnson MD

Hepato-Pancreato-Biliary and Transplant Surgery
Cleveland Clinic
Cleveland, OH, USA

Rome Jutabha MD

Director, UCLA Center for Small Bowel Diseases
Division of Digestive Diseases
David Geffen School of Medicine at UCLA
Los Angeles, CA, USA

Peter J. Kahrilas MD

Gilbert H. Marquardt Professor of Medicine
Department of Medicine
Division of Gastroenterology
Feinberg School of Medicine
Northwestern University
Chicago, IL, USA

Anthony N. Kalloo MD

The Moses and Helen Golden Paulson Professor of Gastroenterology
The Johns Hopkins University School of Medicine;
Chief, Division of Gastroenterology and Hepatology
Johns Hopkins Hospital
Baltimore, MD, USA

Patrick S. Kamath MD

Professor of Medicine
Consultant and Vice Chair (Education)
Division of Gastroenterology and Hepatology
Mayo Clinic
Rochester, MN, USA

Philip O. Katz MD
Clinical Professor of Medicine
Jefferson Medical College
Thomas Jefferson University;
Chairman, Division of Gastroenterology
Albert Einstein Medical Center
Philadelphia, PA, USA

Ciarán P. Kelly MD
Professor of Medicine
Harvard Medical School;
Director of the Celiac Center
Beth Israel Deaconess Medical Center
Boston, MA, USA

David J. Kerr CBE, MA, MD, DSc, FRCP(Glas,Lon & Edin), FRCGP(Hon), FMedSci
Professor of Cancer Medicine
Nuffield Department of Clinical and Laboratory Sciences
University of Oxford
Oxford, UK;
Adjunct Professor of Medicine
Professor of Cancer Therapeutics
Weill-Cornell College of Medicine
New York, NY, USA

David Kershenobich MD, PhD
Department of Experimental Medicine
Faculty of Medicine, UNAM
Hospital General de México
Mexico City, Mexico

Arjun Khosla MD
University Hospitals Case Medical Center
Cleveland, OH, USA

Ralf Kiesslich MD, PhD
Head of Endoscopy Department
I. Medizinische Klinik und Poliklinik
Universitätsmedizin Mainz
Mainz, Germany

Kazufumi Kimura MD, PhD
Research Fellow
Microbiology and Immunology
School of Biomedical, Biomolecular and Chemical Sciences
University of Western Australia
Perth, WA, Australia

Michael S. Kipper MD
Clinical Professor of Radiology
University of California at San Diego
San Diego, CA, USA

Rajan Kochar MD, MPH
Assistant Professor of Medicine
Division of Gastroenterology, Hepatology and Nutrition
The University of Texas Health Science Center at Houston
Houston, TX, USA

Jeroen J. Kolkman MD
Consultant Gastroenterologist
Medisch Spectrum Twente
Enschede, The Netherlands

Ayman Koteish MD
Assistant Professor of Medicine
Division of Gastroenterology
The Johns Hopkins University School of Medicine
Baltimore, MD, USA

Thomas O.G. Kovacs MD
Professor of Medicine
CURE / Digestive Disease Research Center
David Geffen School of Medicine at UCLA
Los Angeles, CA, USA

Benjamin Krevsky MD, MPH
Professor of Medicine
Temple University School of Medicine
Philadelphia, PA, USA

Olivier Lada PhD
Service d'Hépatologie
Hôpital Beaujon
University of Paris
Clichy, France

Maria Eliana Lai MD
Professor of Medicine
Department of Medical Sciences
University of Cagliari
Policlinico Universitario
Monserrato, Cagliari, Italy

Richard H. Lash MD
Chief Medical Officer
Caris Diagnostics / Miraca;
Clinical Associate Professor
University of Texas Southwestern Medical Center
Irving, TX, USA

James Y.W. Lau FRCS (Edin)
Department of Surgery
Chinese University of Hong Kong
Hong Kong SAR, China

Konstantinos N. Lazaridis MD
Division of Gastroenterology and Hepatology
Center for Basic Research in Digestive Diseases
Mayo Clinic
Rochester, MN, USA

Philippe Lefere MD
Department of Radiology
Stedelijk Ziekenhuis
Roeselare, Belgium

Daniel A. Leffler MD
Assistant Professor of Medicine
Division of Gastroenterology and Hepatology;
Director of Clinical Research at the Celiac Center
Beth Israel Deaconess Medical Center
Harvard Medical School
Boston, MA, USA

Keith Leiper MD (deceased)
Consultant Gastroenterologist
Department of Gastroenterology
Royal Liverpool University Hospital
Liverpool, UK

Vivian Y.F. Leung PDDR, PhD
Senior Radiographer
Department of Diagnostic Radiology & Organ Imaging
Chinese University of Hong Kong
Hong Kong SAR, China

Joel S. Levine MD
Professor of Medicine
Division of Gastroenterology and Hepatology
University of Colorado Denver
Aurora, CO, USA

Blair S. Lewis MD, PC
Clinical Professor of Medicine
Mount Sinai School of Medicine
New York, NY, USA

Charles J. Lightdale MD
Professor of Clinical Medicine
Division of Digestive and Liver Diseases
Columbia University Medical Center
New York, NY, USA

Keith D. Lindor MD
Executive Vice Provost Health Solutions
Arizona State University
Tempe, AZ, USA

Dileep N. Lobo MS, DM, FRCS, FACS
Professor of Gastrointestinal Surgery
Division of Gastrointestinal Surgery
Nottingham Digestive Diseases Centre NIHR Biomedical Research Unit
Nottingham University Hospitals
Nottingham, UK

Alain Luciani MD, PhD
Henri Mondor Hospital
Créteil, France

Michael R. Lucey MD
Professor of Medicine
Chief, Section of Gastroenterology and Hepatology
University of Wisconsin School of Medicine and Public Health
Madison, WI, USA

Ryan D. Madanick MD
Assistant Professor of Medicine
Department of Medicine, Division of Gastroenterology and Hepatology
University of North Carolina School of Medicine
Chapel Hill, NC, USA

Yashwant R. Mahida MD
Professor of Medicine
Institute of Infection, Immunity and Inflammation
Nottingham University Hospitals
Nottingham, UK

Erica Makin MSc, FRCS(Paeds)
Specialist Registrar
King's College Hospital
London, UK

Giuseppe Malizia MD
Consultant in Gastroenterology
Department of Gastroenterology
Ospedale V Cervello
Palermo, Italy

Jayan Mannath MD, MRCP
Research Fellow
Nottingham Digestive Diseases Centre and Biomedical Research Unit
University of Nottingham and Nottingham University Hospitals
Nottingham, UK

Michael P. Manns MD
Professor and Chairman
Department of Gastroenterology, Hepatology and Endocrinology
Hannover Medical School
Hannover, Germany

Magnus J. Mansard MS
Senior Registrar
Department of Surgical Gastroenterology
Asian Institute of Gastroenterology
Hyderabad, India

Patrick Marcellin MD, PhD
Service d'Hépatologie
Hôpital Beaujon
University of Paris
Clichy, France

Luca Marciani PhD
Lecturer in GI MRI
Nottingham Digestive Diseases Centre and NIHR Biomedical Research Unit
School of Clinical Sciences
University of Nottingham and Nottingham University Hospitals
Nottingham, UK

Michele Marchese MD
Gastrointestinal Endoscopy Unit
Catholic University of the Sacred Heart
"A. Gemelli" Hospital
Rome, Italy

Barry J. Marshall MD, FRACP
Clinical Professor
Microbiology and Immunology
School of Biomedical, Biomolecular and Chemical Sciences
University of Western Australia
Perth, WA, Australia

Cindy Matsen MD
Resident, General Surgery
University of Utah
Salt Lake City, UT, USA

Catherine McCrann MD
Gastroenterology Fellow
Yale University
New Haven, CT, USA

Arthur J. McCullough MD
Professor of Medicine
Cleveland Clinic Lerner College of Medicine
Case Western Reserve University
Digestive Diseases Institute
Cleveland, OH, USA

George B. McDonald MD
Professor of Medicine
University of Washington;
Gastroenterology / Hepatology Section
Fred Hutchinson Cancer Research Center
Seattle, WA, USA

Dermot McGovern MD, PhD
Cedars-Sinai IBD Center
Los Angeles, CA, USA

Donald P. McManus BSc(Hons), PhD, DSc
National Health and Medical Research Council of Australia Senior
Principal Research Fellow
Professor and Laboratory Head
Queensland Institute of Medical Research
Brisbane, QLD, Australia

A. Merrie MBChB, PhD, FRACS
Consultant Surgeon
Discipline of Oncology
Faculty of Medical and Health Sciences
University of Auckland
Auckland, New Zealand

Rachel S. Midgley MD, BSc(Hons) MB ChB(Hons) FRCP, PhD
Consultant Medical Oncologist and DH / HEFCE Clinical Senior Lecturer
Department of Oncology
University of Oxford
Oxford, UK

Giorgina Mieli-Vergani MD, PhD
Alex Mowat Professor of Paediatric Hepatology
Department of Child Health and Institute of Liver Studies
King's College Hospital
London, UK

Hitomi Minami MD
Faculty of Medicine, Showa University
Showa University
Showa University International Training Center for Endoscopy (SUITE)
Digestive Disease Center
Showa University Northern Yokohama Hospital
Yokohama, Japan

Paul Moayyedi BSc, MB ChB, PhD, MPH, FRCP (London), FRCPC, FACG, AGAF
Director, Division of Gastroenterology
Department of Medicine
Health Sciences Centre
McMaster University
Hamilton, ON, Canada

Dana C. Moffatt MD
Division of Gastroenterology / Hepatology
Indiana University Health
Indianapolis, IN, USA

Tanya M. Monaghan BSc (Hons), BSc (Hons), BM, MRCP
Specialist Registrar in Gastroenterology
Institute of Infection, Immunity and Inflammation
Nottingham University Hospitals
Nottingham, UK

Andrew R. Moore MBChB, MRCP
Specialist Registrar in Gastroenterology
Royal Liverpool University Hospital
Clinical Research Fellow
Institute of Translational Medicine
University of Liverpool
Liverpool, UK

Rosa Miquel Morera MD
Pathology Department
Hospital Clinic and University of Barcelona
Barcelona, Spain

Koenraad J. Mortele MD
Department of Radiology
Beth Israel Deaconess Medical Center
Harvard Medical School
Boston, MA, USA

N. Mortensen MD, FRCS
Professor of Surgery
Nuffield Department of Surgery
University of Oxford
Oxford, UK

Menachem Moshkowitz MD
The Integrated Cancer Prevention Center
Gastroenterology and Liver Institute
Tel-Aviv Medical Center;
Sackler Faculty of Medicine
Tel-Aviv University
Tel-Aviv, Israel

Rami Moucari MD, PhD
Service d'Hépatologie
Hôpital Beaujon
University of Paris
Clichy, France

Chris Mulder MD, PhD
Department of Gastroenterology
Vrije Universiteit Medical Center
Amsterdam, The Netherlands

Kevin D. Mullen MD
MetroHealth Medical Center;
Division of Gastroenterology and Hepatology
Case Western Reserve University
Cleveland, OH, USA

Ulf Müller-Ladner MD
Chair, Department for Internal Medicine and Rheumatology
Justus-Liebig University Giessen;
Department for Rheumatology and Clinical Immunology
Kerckhoff Clinic
Bad Nauheim, Germany

Simon Murch PhD, FRCP, FRCPCH
Professor of Paediatrics and Child Health
Division of Metabolic and Vascular Health
Warwick Medical School
The University of Warwick
Coventry, UK

V. Raman Muthusamy MD
Director, Gastroenterology Fellowship Program, Health Sciences Associate
Clinical Professor of Medicine
H.H. Chao Comprehensive Digestive Disease Center
Division of Gastroenterology
Department of Medicine
University of California
Irvine, CA, USA

John P. Neoptolemos FMedSci
The Owen and Ellen Evans Chair of Surgery
Director Liverpool Cancer Research UK Centre
Department of Molecular and Clinical Cancer Medicine
Institute of Translational Medicine
University of Liverpool
Liverpool, UK

Leigh Neumayer MD
Professor of Surgery
University of Utah
Salt Lake City, UT, USA

Julia L. Newton MBBS, FRCP, PhD
Professor of Ageing – Medicine
UK NIHR Biomedical Research Centre in Ageing
Institute for Ageing and Health
Newcastle University
Newcastle upon Tyne, UK

Timothy T. Nostrant MD
Professor
Department of Internal Medicine
University of Michigan Health Center
Ann Arbor, MI, USA

Kjell Öberg MD, PhD
Professor of Endocrine Oncology
Department of Medical Sciences
Endocrine Oncology
Uppsala University Hospital
Uppsala, Sweden

Sebastian Obrzut MD
Assistant Professor of Radiology
University of California at San Diego
San Diego, CA, USA

John G. O'Grady MD, FRCPI
Consultant Hepatologist
Institute of Liver Studies
King's College School of Medicine
London, UK

Philippe Otal MD
Service de Radiologie
Université de Toulouse
Toulouse, France

Bergein F. Overholt MD
Center of Excellence for Treatment of Barrett's Esophagus
Thomson Cancer Survival Center
Knoxville, TN, USA

Masoud Panjehpour PhD
Center of Excellence for Treatment of Barrett's Esophagus
Thomson Cancer Survival Center
Knoxville, TN, USA

Georgios Papachristou MD
Division of Gastroenterology, Hepatology and Nutrition
Departments of Medicine
University of Pittsburgh
Pittsburgh, PA, USA

Michael C. Parker BSc, MS, FRCS, FRCS (Ed)
Fawkham Manor Hospital
Fawkham, UK

Henry P. Parkman MD
Professor of Medicine
Director, GI Motility Laboratory;
Gastroenterology Section
Department of Medicine
Temple University School of Medicine
Philadelphia, PA, USA

Stephen P. Pereira BSc, PhD, FRCP, FRCPE
Reader in Hepatology and Gastroenterology
University College London Hospitals
London, UK

David H. Perlmutter MD
Vira I. Heinz Professor and Chair
Department of Pediatrics
Professor of Cell Biology and Physiology
University of Pittsburgh School of Medicine;
Physician-in-Chief and Scientific Director
Children's Hospital of Pittsburgh of UPMC
Pittsburgh, PA, USA

Lucio Petruzziello MD
Gastrointestinal Endoscopy Unit
Catholic University of the Sacred Heart
"A. Gemelli" Hospital
Rome, Italy

Patrick R. Pfau MD
Associate Professor of Medicine
Chief of Clinical Gastroenterology
Section of Gastroenterology and Hepatology
University of Wisconsin School of Medicine and Public Health
Madison, WI, USA

Antonello Pietrangelo MD, PhD
Professor of Medicine
Head, Division of Internal Medicine
and "Mario Coppo" Liver Research Center
University Hospital of Modena
Modena, Italy

Jeffrey L. Ponsky MD
Chairman, Department of Surgery
University Hospitals of Cleveland
Cleveland, OH, USA

Todd A. Ponsky MD
Associate Professor
Division of Pediatric Surgery
Rainbow Babies & Children's Hospital
University Hospitals Case Medical Center
Cleveland, OH, USA

John J. Poterucha MD
Professor of Medicine
Division of Gastroenterology and Hepatology
Mayo Clinic
Rochester, MN, USA

Benjamin K. Poulose MD, MPH
Assistant Professor
Department of Surgery
Vanderbilt University Medical Center
Nashville, TN, USA

Raoul Poupon MD
Université Pierre et Marie Curie
AP-Hôpitaux de Paris
Service d'Hepatologie
Hôpital Saint-Antoine
Paris, France

Hervé Puy MD, PhD
Professor of Medicine
Centre Français des Porhpyries
Hôpital Louis Mourier
Colombes, France

Rodrigo M. Quera MD
Gastroenterologist
Clinica Las Condes
Santiago, Chile

Eamonn M. M. Quigley MD, FRCP, FACP, FACG, FRCPI
Professor of Medicine and Human Physiology
Alimentary Pharmabiotic Centre
University College Cork
Cork, Ireland

Krish Ragunath MD, DNB, MPhil, FRCP
Associate Professor and Reader in GI Endoscopy
Nottingham Digestive Diseases Centre and Biomedical Research Unit
University of Nottingham and Nottingham University Hospitals
Nottingham, UK

G. V. Rao MS, MAMS
Director and Chief of Gastrointestinal and Minimally Invasive Surgery
Department of Surgical Gastroenterology
Asian Institute of Gastroenterology
Hyderabad, India

Satish S. C. Rao MD, FRCP (Lon), PhD
Professor of Medicine
Chief, Gastroenterology / Hepatology
Director, Digestive Health Center
Medical College of Georgia
Georgia Health Sciences University
Augusta, GA;
President
American Neurogastroenterology & Motility Society / FBG
Belleville, MI, USA

D. Nageshwar Reddy MD, DM, FAMS, FRCP
Chairman and Chief Gastroenterologist
Department of Gastroenterology
Asian Institute of Gastroenterology
Hyderabad, India

Jürg Reichen MD
Professor Emeritus of Medicine
University Clinic of Visceral Surgery and Medicine
University of Berne
Berne, Switzerland

María Reig MD
Clinical Research Associate, BCLC Group
Liver Unit, ICMDM, Hospital Clinic
Biomedical Research Centre
Network of Hepatic and Digestive Diseases (CIBERehd)
University of Barcelona
Barcelona, Spain

Adrian Reuben MBBS, FRCP, FACG
Director of Liver Service
Division of Gastroenterology and Hepatology
Department of Medicine
College of Medicine
Medical University of South Carolina
Charleston, SC, USA

Melanie L. Richards MD, MHPE
Associate Professor of Surgery
Department of Gastroenterology and General Surgery
Mayo Clinic
Rochester, MN, USA

Joel E. Richter MD, FACP, MACG
Hugh Culverhouse Professor of Medicine
Director, Division of Gastroenterology and Nutrition
Director, Joy M. Culverhouse Center for Esophageal Diseases
University of South Florida
Tampa, FL, USA

Kinan Rifai MD
Department of Gastroenterology, Hepatology and Endocrinology
Hannover Medical School
Hannover, Germany

Cristina Ripoll MD
Hepatology and Liver Unit
Hospital General Universitario Gregorio Marañón
CIBERehd
Madrid, Spain

Guillermo Robles-Diaz MD
Professor of Medicine
Department of Experimental Medicine
Facultad de Medicina
Universidad Nacional Autonoma
de Hospital General de México
Mexico City, Mexico

Carlos Rodriguez de Lope MD
Clinical Research Associate, BCLC Group
Liver Unit, ICMDM, Hospital Clinic
Biomedical Research Centre Network of Hepatic and Digestive
Diseases (CIBERehd)
University of Barcelona
Barcelona, Spain

Arvey I. Rogers MD, FACP, MACG
Professor Emeritus
Department of Medicine
Division of Gastroenterology
University of Miami Miller School of Medicine
Miami, FL, USA

Pablo R. Ros MD, MPH, PhD
Theodore J. Castele University Professor and Chairman
Department of Radiology
Case Western Reserve University
University Hospitals Case Medical Center;
Radiologist-in-Chief
University Hospitals Health System
Cleveland, OH, USA

Simon Rushbrook MBBS, MRCP, PhD
Senior Clinical Fellow in Hepatology
Liver Transplantation Unit
Cambridge University Hospitals NHS Foundation Trust
Cambridge, UK

Paul Rutgeerts MD, PhD, FRCP
Division of Gastroenterology
University of Leuven
Leuven, Belgium

Priyanka Sachdeva MD, MRCP
Gastroenterology Section
Department of Medicine
Temple University School of Medicine
Philadelphia, PA, USA

V. Anik Sahni MD
Division of Abdominal Imaging and Intervention
Department of Radiology
Brigham and Women's Hospital
Harvard Medical School
Boston, MA, USA

Jose M. Sánchez-Tapias MD
Senior Consultant
Liver Unit
Hospital Clinic, CIBERehd, IDIBAPS
Barcelona, Spain

Arun J. Sanyal MD
National Amyloidosis Centre
Department of Medicine
Royal Free and University College London Medical School
Royal Free Hospital
London, UK

Prayman T. Sattianayagam MA, MRCP
Clinical Research Fellow
National Amyloidosis Centre
Centre for Amyloidosis and Acute Phase Proteins
Division of Medicine
University College London Medical School
London, UK

Tilman Sauerbruch MD
Professor of Medicine and Director
Department of Medicine I
University of Bonn
Bonn, Germany

Jürgen Schölmerich MD
Professor of Medicine
Medical Director
University Clinic Frankfurt
Frankfurt, Germany

John H. Scholefield ChM, FRCS
Professor of Surgery
Division of GI Surgery
Nottingham University Hospitals
Nottingham, UK

Ila Sethi DMRD
Department of Radiology
The University of Chicago Medical Center
Chicago, IL, USA

Fergus Shanahan MD
Alimentary Pharmabiotic Centre and Department of Medicine
University College Cork
Cork, Ireland

Prateek Sharma MD
Division of Gastroenterology / Hepatology
University of Kansas Medical Center
Kansas City Veterans Administration
Kansas City, MO, USA

Varun Sharma MD
Division of Gastroenterology, Hepatology and Nutrition
Department of Internal Medicine
Virginia Commonwealth University School of Medicine
Richmond, VA, USA

Stuart Sherman MD
Division of Gastroenterology / Hepatology
Indiana University Health
Indianapolis, IN, USA

Anish A. Sheth MD
Assistant Professor of Medicine
Yale University School of Medicine
New Haven, CT, USA

Tomas J. Silber MD, MASS
Director, Adolescent Medicine Fellowship Program
Medical Director
Don Delaney Eating Disorders Program
Division of Adolescent and Young Adult Medicine;
Director, Pediatric Ethics Program
Research Subject Advocate
Children's National Medical Center;
Professor of Pediatrics
Professor of Global Health
George Washington University
Washington, DC, USA

Giovanna M. da Silva MD
Colorectal Fellow
Cleveland Clinic Florida
Weston, FL, USA

John Simpson PhD, FRCS
Associate Professor / Consultant Pancreaticobiliary Surgeon
Department of General Surgery
Nottingham University Hospitals
Nottingham, UK

Vijay Singh MD
Division of Gastroenterology, Hepatology and Nutrition
Departments of Medicine
University of Pittsburgh
Pittsburgh, PA, USA

Kenneth R. Sirinek MD, PhD
Professor and Division Head
General and Laparoscopic Surgery
Department of Surgery
University of Texas Health Science Center at San Antonio
San Antonio, TX, USA

Guy Sisson MD
Research Specialist Registrar in Gastroenterology
Department of Gastroenterology
King's College Hospital
London, UK

Maria H. Sjogren MD
Gastroenterology Service
Walter Reed Army Medical Center
Washington, DC, USA

Amer Skopic DO
Staff Gastroenterologist
National Naval Medical Center
Bethesda, MD, USA

Robin C. Spiller MD
Nottingham Digestive Diseases Centre and NIHR Biomedical Research Unit
University of Nottingham and Nottingham University Hospitals
Nottingham, UK

Matthew P. Spinn MD
Division of Gastroenterology, Hepatology, and Nutrition
University of Texas Health Science Center Houston – Medical School
Houston, TX, USA

Robert J. C. Steele MD
Professor and Head of Academic Surgery
University of Dundee
Dundee, Scotland

Guido Stirnimann MD
Institute of Clinical Pharmacology and Visceral Research
University of Berne
Berne, Switzerland

Mario Strazzabosco MD, PhD
Professor of Gastroenterology
Department of Clinical Medicine and Prevention
University of Milan-Bicocca
Milan, Italy;
Liver Center and Section of Digestive Diseases
Yale University
New Haven, CT, USA

Lisa Swize MD
Gastroenterology Fellow
Section of Gastroenterology and Hepatology
University of Wisconsin School of Medicine and Public Health
Madison, WI, USA

Jan Tack MD PhD
Professor of Medicine
Translational Research Center for Gastrointestinal Disorders (TARGID)
University of Leuven;
Head, Department of Pathophysiology
University of Leuven;
Head of Clinic
Department of Gastroenterology
University Hospital Gasthuisberg
Leuven, Belgium

Stephan R. Targan MD
Cedars-Sinai IBD Center
Los Angeles, CA, USA

Shari L. Taylor MD
Medical Director
Caris Diagnostics / Miraca
Irving, TX, USA

Christina A. Tennyson MD
Columbia University College of Physicians and Surgeons
New York, NY, USA

Anthony Y. B. Teoh FRCSEd (Gen)
Specialist Surgeon
Division of Upper Gastrointestinal Surgery
Department of Surgery
Chinese University of Hong Kong
Hong Kong SAR, China

Norah A. Terrault MD, MPH
Professor of Medicine
University of California San Francisco
San Francisco, CA, USA

Richard Thompson MRCP, MRCPCH
Senior Lecturer in Paediatric Hepatology
Institute of Liver Studies
King's College Hospital
London, UK

Peter D. Thurley FRCR
Radiology
Derby Hospitals
Derby, UK

Eva Tiensuu Janson MD, PhD
Professor of Medicine
Department of Medical Sciences
Endocrine Oncology
Uppsala University Hospital
Uppsala, Sweden

Claudio Tiribelli MD, PhD
Centro Studi Fegato
Fondazione Italiana Fegato
University of Trieste
Trieste, Italy

Sombat Treeprasertsuk MD, MSc
Associate Professor
Division of Gastroenterology
Faculty of Medicine
Chulalongkorn University
Bangkok, Thailand

Brian G. Turner MD
Gastroenterology Associates
Massachusetts General Hospital
Boston, MA, USA

Dominique-Charles Valla MD
Professor of Hepatology
Head of Liver Unit
Hôpital Beaujon
Clichy, France

Gert Van Assche MD, PhD, FRCP
Division of Gastroenterology
University of Leuven
Leuven, Belgium

J. Hajo van Bockel MD
Department of Surgery
Leiden University Medical Center
Leiden, The Netherlands

Jon A. Vanderhoof MD
Attending Gastroenterologist
Children's Hospital;
Lecturer in Pediatrics
Harvard Medical School
Boston, MA, USA

Hendrikus S. Vanderveldt MD, MBA
Assistant Professor of Clinical Medicine
Division of Gastroenterology
University of Miami Miller School of Medicine
Miami, FL, USA

Séverine Vermeire MD, PhD
Division of Gastroenterology
University Hospital Gasthuisberg
Leuven, Belgium

Jean-Pierre Vinel MD
Service d'Hépato-Gastro-Entérologie et INSERM
Université de Toulouse
Toulouse, France

Jerome D. Waye MD
Clinical Professor of Medicine, Mount Sinai Medical Center
Director of Endoscopic Education, Mount Sinai Hospital
President, World Endoscopy Organization
Mount Sinai Hospital
New York, NY, USA

George J. M. Webster BSc, MD, FRCP
Consultant Gastroenterologist
Department of Gastroenterology
University College London Hospitals
London, UK

Linda Wedlake RD, MSc, MMedSc
Research Dietitian
The Royal Marsden NHS Foundation Trust
London, UK

Jennifer T. Wells MD
Division of Hepatology
Department of Internal Medicine
Baylor University Medical Center
Dallas, TX, USA

Julia Wendon MD, FRCP
Institute of Liver Studies
King's College School of Medicine
London, UK

Steven D. Wexner MD, FACS, FRCS, FRCS(Ed)
Professor and Chairman
Department of Colorectal Surgery
Cleveland Clinic Florida
Weston, FL, USA

David C. Whitcomb MD, PhD
Giant Eagle Professor of Cancer Genetics
Professor of Medicine, Cell Biology & Physiology, and Human Genetics
Chief, Division of Gastroenterology, Hepatology and Nutrition
University of Pittsburgh & UPMC
Pittsburgh, PA, USA

C. Mel Wilcox MD
Professor
Department of Medicine
Division of Gastroenterology and Hepatology
University of Alabama at Birmingham
Birmingham, AL, USA

Helen M. Windsor PhD
Research Fellow
Microbiology and Immunology
School of Biomedical, Biomolecular and Chemical Sciences
University of Western Australia
Perth, WA, Australia

Louis-Michel Wong Kee Song MD
Associate Professor
Division of Gastroenterology and Hepatology
Mayo Clinic
Rochester, MN, USA

Kai-chun Wu MD, PhD
Xijing Hospital of Digestive Diseases
State Key Laboratory of Cancer Biology
Fourth Military Medical University
Xi'an, China

Hironori Yamamoto MD, PhD
Department of Internal Medicine
Division of Gastroenterology
Jichi Medical University
Tochigi, Japan

Tomonori Yano MD
Department of Internal Medicine
Division of Gastroenterology
Jichi Medical University
Tochigi, Japan

Chong-Meng Yeo
Yale School of Medicine
New Haven, CT, USA

Neville D. Yeomans MBBS, MD, FRACP, AGAF, FACG
School of Medicine
University of Western Sydney
Penrith, NSW, Australia

Rosemary J. Young APRN
Pediatric GI Nurse Practitioner
Boys Town National Research Hospital
Boys Town, NE, USA

Simon Chun-Ho Yu MD
Professor
Department of Diagnostic Radiology and Organ Imaging
Prince of Wales Hospital
The Chinese University of Hong Kong
Shatin, Hong Kong SAR, China

Elie Serge Zafrani
Henri Mondor Hospital
Créteil, France

Stacey R. Zavala MD
Attending Gastroenterologist
Albert Einstein Medical Center
Philadelphia, PA, USA

Zeino Zeino MD
Specialist Registrar in Gastroenterology
Department of Gastroenterology
King's College Hospital
London, UK

Preface

With this book we have asked an international team of editors and authors from all continents who have worldwide reputations and are at the height of their career to produce something that is both informative about gastrointestinal and liver disease and extremely practical for patient management. On the practical side, each chapter starts with text boxes summarizing essential features in a short, pithy, and easy to find way. In the Disease sections there are three boxes for each chapter, "Essential facts about Causation," "Essentials of Diagnosis," and "Essentials of Treatment." The idea is that at a glance you can be on top of a subject that you know little about.

Another practical feature is the inclusion of downloadable didactic management protocols, accessed via the book's companion website. These are not guidelines that state broad generalities, but highly didactic instruction sheets that can be put in the notes of each patient for which they are appropriate to ensure timely, focused, and comprehensive management by juniors and staff unfamiliar with the patient. Everyone has their own individual variation on how to deliver the essentials of care so these protocols are adaptable to your own unit and situation.

Other online features include over 85 high-quality videos showing how to do it for many procedures, all 850 figures in a downloadable digital format and, finally, specimen multiple-choice questions to help you prepare for professional exams.

However, the modern medical world in which management is distilled into cookery book instructions tends to be drab and unrewarding. Our book, therefore, contains up to date and relevant background information about pathogenesis, epidemiology, and prognosis as well as descriptive text about patient investigation and management. We have asked authors to avoid text and concepts that are no longer relevant, which often persist in other textbooks only to confuse, and specifically to include up to date information that may be starting to impinge on management with, for example, a specific request to cover information about genetic susceptibility.

In short, some textbooks are practical but with little explanation, while others are detailed but not easily translatable into real patient management. We believe that we have produced a book that achieves both.

C. J. Hawkey

PART 1

Symptoms, Syndromes, and Scenarios

CHAPTER 1

Heartburn and noncardiac chest pain

Tiberiu Hershcovici[1] and Ronnie Fass[1,2]

[1]Neuroenteric Clinical Research Group, Southern Arizona VA Health Care System, Tucson, AZ, USA
[2]University of Arizona College of Medicine, Tucson, AZ, USA

KEY POINTS

- Heartburn is described as a retrosternal burning sensation that moves orad from behind the xiphoid bone upward to the neck and is the cardinal symptom of patients with gastroesophageal reflux disease (GERD)
- Non-cardiac chest pain (NCCP) is defined as recurring, angina-like, retrosternal chest pain of non-cardiac origin. NCCP may be a manifestation of a gastrointestinal (GI) or non-GI-related disorder. GERD is the most common esophageal cause of NCCP
- The typical reflux syndrome can be diagnosed on the basis of symptoms characteristic without diagnostic testing. Symptom response to antireflux treatment is used to further cement the diagnosis of GERD prior entertaining any invasive investigation
- Patient's history and characteristics do not reliably distinguish between cardiac and esophageal causes of chest pain

Introduction

In this chapter, heartburn and non-cardiac chest pain are discussed in tandem for each subsection. The objective is to provide comparisons and contrasts in each category discussed. Noncardiac chest pain (NCCP) is a different symptom complex from heartburn, yet, as discussed subsequently, gastroesophageal reflux is the most common cause of NCCP. In other words, reflux may result in typical heartburn or, in more atypical discomfort, NCCP. Heartburn is the cardinal symptom of patients with gastroesophageal reflux disease (GERD). In patients with heartburn as the predominant symptom, GERD is the likely cause in at least 75% of individuals [1]. In a US population-based study, the prevalence of at least one episode of heartburn over 1 year was 42% and weekly episodes of heartburn was 20% [2]. However, the majority of patients with heartburn will never seek medical attention and treat their symptom with over-the counter medications.

NCCP is defined as recurrent chest pain that is indistinguishable from ischemic heart pain after a reasonable work-up has excluded a cardiac cause. Sir William Osler, in 1892, described "esophagismus," or pain secondary to spasms of the esophagus, which may have initiated the clinical concept that esophageal pain can mimic cardiac angina. It has been estimated that the US prevalence of NCCP is 23% [2]. NCCP is a benign condition, although the associated morbidity, and the economic burden resulting from inability to work and healthcare utilization, are significant.

What is it?
Heartburn

Heartburn is described as a retrosternal burning sensation that moves orad from behind the xiphoid bone upward to the neck. It most often occurs within 1 to 2 hours after a meal, particularly a large volume or fatty meal, exacerbated by bending over or assuming the recumbent position, and is typically relieved by antacids.

Heartburn may be associated with other GERD symptoms such as water brash and sour or bitter taste in the mouth. Additionally, heartburn often disturbs the sleep of affected individuals and significantly impairs patients' quality of life. Neither heartburn frequency nor severity is predictive of the presence or absence of erosive esophagitis in the individual patient [3,4].

The word "heartburn" does not translate literally between most languages. Consequently, different words for the same condition are used by patients and physicians in many countries [5]. It is important during history-taking to ensure that the patient and physician alike have similar understanding of the term "heartburn".

NCCP Patients may report squeezing or burning substernal chest pain that may radiate to the back, neck, arms, and jaws. There are many causes for NCCP, which are not limited to the esophagus, and these include musculoskeletal, pulmonary, cardiovascular, infectious, drug-related, and psychological as well as other gastrointestinal disorders (Table 1.1) [6].

Rome III Criteria do not specifically address NCCP but rather a subset of patients with NCCP termed "functional chest pain of presumed esophageal origin" [7]. These are patients with recurrent episodes of substernal chest pain of visceral quality with no apparent explanation using currently available tests. As with all other functional esophageal disorders, GERD and esophageal dysmotility should be ruled out before the diagnosis is established.

A patient's history and characteristics do not reliably distinguish between cardiac and esophageal causes of chest pain [8]. Therefore, all patients who present with chest pain, regardless of its character, should initially undergo a proper cardiac evaluation before being referred to a gastroenterologist. The cardiologist's first priority is to exclude any acute life-threatening

Textbook of Clinical Gastroenterology and Hepatology, Second Edition. Edited by C. J. Hawkey, Jaime Bosch, Joel E. Richter, Guadalupe Garcia-Tsao, Francis K. L. Chan.

Table 1.1 Different causes of noncardiac chest pain

1. Musculoskeletal
   - Costochondritis
   - Fibromyalgia
   - Precordial catch syndrome
   - Slipping rib syndrome
   - Xiphoditis
   - Thoracic outlet syndrome
   - Cervical or thoracic spinal disease
2. Gastrointestinal
   - Gastroesophageal reflux disease
   - Esophageal dysmotility
   - Peptic ulcer disease
   - Biliary disease
   - Pancreatitis
   - Intra-abdominal masses (benign and malignant)
3. Pulmonary or intrathoracic
   - Pneumonia
   - Pleurisy
   - Pulmonary embolus
   - Lung cancer
   - Sarcoidosis
   - Pneumothorax or pneumomediastinum
   - Pleural effusions
   - Mediastinitis
   - Aortic aneurysm
   - Pericarditis or myocarditis
   - Pulmonary hypertension
   - Intrathoracic masses (benign and malignant)
4. Psychiatric causes
   - Panic disorder
   - Anxiety
   - Depression
   - Somatization
   - Hypochondriasis
   - Munchausen's syndrome
5. Miscellaneous
   - Herpes zoster
   - Drug-induced pain
   - Sickle cell crisis

Table 1.2 Risk factors for gastroesophageal reflux disease

Risk factor	Underlying mechanisms
Smoking	Decreases LES pressure and alters esophageal defense mechanisms
Alcohol	Direct mucosal damage
Obesity	Increases intragastric pressure
High-fat diet	Decreases LES pressure, increases TLESR, increases esophageal sensitivity to acid and delays gastric emptying
Chocolate, peppermint, caffeine	Decreases LES pressure
Drugs (calcium channel blockers, tricyclics, nitrates, benzodiazepines, aspirin, NSAIDs, etc.)	Decreases LES pressure or cause direct mucosal damage
Abdominal trauma	Disrupts diaphragmatic sphincter function
Nasogastric tubes	Direct trauma to the esophageal mucosa and LES interruption
Exercise	Increases intra-abdominal pressure
Systemic disorders	• Scleroderma – decreases or abolishes LES pressure, decreases esophageal peristalsis • Diabetes mellitus – autonomic neuropathy and reduced esophageal peristalsis
Asthma	• Increases pressure gradient between thorax and abdomen • Increases incidence of hiatal hernia and effects of medications used to treat asthma
Sleep apnea	Large negative intrapleural pressure during apnea
Stress	Increases perception of intraesophageal stimuli
Poor sleep	Increases perception of intraesophageal stimuli

LES, lower esophageal sphincter; NSAID, nonsteroidal anti-inflammatory drug; TLESR, transient lower esophageal sphincter relaxation.

cardiovascular condition. The extent of cardiac workup is individually determined and does not include cardiac angiography in all subjects [9].

How common is it?

GERD Population-based studies suggest that GERD is a common condition with a prevalence of 10–30% in Western Europe and North America [10]. In the Asia-Pacific region, the prevalence of GERD in the general population is around 2–5% [11]. All phenotypic presentations of GERD appear to affect Caucasians more often than African Americans or Native Americans. GERD without esophageal mucosal damage (nonerosive reflux disease-NERD) is more common in females. In contrast, erosive esophagitis, peptic stricture, and Barrett's esophagus are more common in males. The prevalence of GERD increases with age, and several risk factors for GERD have been identified (Table 1.2).

NCCP The incidence and prevalence of NCCP have scarcely been studied. Several population-based studies have demonstrated that the prevalence of NCCP ranged between 20 and 25% [2,12]. It appears that NCCP is a very common disorder, regardless of gender or ethnicity. While most tertiary referral-based studies report a female predominance, a population-based study showed no gender predilection [2]. However, women with NCCP tend to consult healthcare providers more often than men and are more likely to present to hospital emergency departments [13,14]. Whilst there are no gender differences regarding chest pain intensity, women tend to use terms like "burning" and "frightening" more often than men [15,16].

Information about risk factors that are associated with NCCP is scarce. Patients with GERD-related NCCP are likely to share the same risk factors as the general GERD population (Table 1.2). Otherwise, psychological factors such as anxiety, panic disorder, major depression, and somatoform disorders have all been demonstrated to be closely associated with NCCP.

Pathophysiology
Pathophysiology of heartburn
The mechanisms responsible for the development of heartburn remain poorly understood. It has been postulated that sensitization of esophageal chemoreceptors, either directly by exposure to acidic or weakly acidic reflux or indirectly through release of inflammatory mediators, is responsible for the generation of heartburn [17]. Both animal models and human studies have demonstrated dilatation of intercellular spaces in acidic or weakly acidic exposed tissues, and this might permit an increase in paracellular permeability, allowing acid to reach sensory nerve endings that are located within the esophageal mucosa [18]. However, this prevailing hypothesis does not fully explain symptoms in patients with heartburn, primarily because more than 95% of acid reflux events are never perceived by patients with GERD.

Several luminal mechanisms have been identified to facilitate perception of a reflux event: proximal migration, lower pH nadir, larger pH drops, larger volume and longer acid clearance time, and preceding higher esophageal cumulative acid exposure time. Overall, acidic reflux (pH < 4) is more commonly the cause of heartburn than nonacidic reflux (pH ≥ 4). Central factors such as psychological co-morbidity, anxiety and poor sleep have all been demonstrated to also facilitate perception of reflux events.

Triggers
Physiologically, the most common trigger for GERD symptoms is a meal, particularly if it contains a large amount of fat. However, the mechanisms by which luminal fat and possibly other nutrients modulate the perception of esophageal stimuli remain to be elucidated. Fat causes a reduction in lower esophageal sphincter (LES) basal pressure and delay in gastric emptying. Additionally, fat may also exacerbate symptoms of GERD by heightening perception of intraesophageal acid. Enteric hormones such as cholecystokinin or other gut neurotransmitters and enzymes are believed to mediate the effect of fat on the lower esophageal sphincter and sensory afferents. Furthermore, non-reflux-related intraesophageal stimuli may also lead to the development of heartburn. For example, esophageal

balloon distensions have been shown to induce heartburn symptoms in a subset of normal subjects and reproduce typical heartburn in half of the patients with GERD [19], suggesting that mechanical distension of the esophagus *per se*, may also result in heartburn even in the absence of actual acid reflux.

This suggests that heartburn is not stimulus specific, and that non-reflux-related intraesophageal events may lead to this type of symptom as well. These poorly understood events are likely the causes of functional heartburn. Simultaneous intraesophageal impedance and pH measurements have demonstrated that nonacidic reflux (weakly acidic or weakly alkaline that is a pure liquid or a mixture of gas and liquid) also plays a role in the pathophysiology of heartburn, more commonly in patients who failed proton pump inhibitor (PPI) treatment. Central factors, such as psychological comorbidity (anxiety, depression, etc.,), stress, and poor sleep have all been shown to modulate esophageal sensitization and thus cause patients to perceive low-intensity esophageal stimuli as being painful (Figure 1.1).

Pathophysiology of NCCP
GERD is the most common esophageal cause of NCCP, as abnormal 24-hour esophageal pH monitoring and/or positive endoscopic findings are present in up to 60% of the patients [20]. This is further supported by the efficacy of acid suppressive therapy in relieving patients' symptoms and the reproducibility of chest pain by esophageal acid perfusion studies. Acid perfusion into the distal esophagus has been demonstrated to alter the perception of painful stimuli in the distal

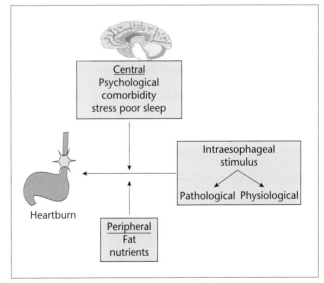

Figure 1.1 The "Fass & Tougas" conceptual model for esophageal symptom generation in nonerosive reflux disease (NERD). Proposed causes of heartburn – interactions between intraesophageal stimuli and the brain. (Reproduced from Fass R, Tougas G. Functional heartburn – the stimulus, the pain and the brain. *Gut.* 2002;51:885–892, with permission from BMJ Publishing Group Ltd.)

portion of the esophagus (primary hyperalgesia) as well as the proximal portion of the esophagus (secondary hyperalgesia) in patients with NCCP.

Motility
The increased prevalence of esophageal motility disorders in patients with NCCP suggests that chest pain may also result from stimulation of mechanoreceptors within the esophageal wall. Approximately 30% of patients with NCCP demonstrate some type of esophageal dysmotility. The motility abnormalities include diffuse esophageal spasm, nutcracker esophagus, achalasia, nonspecific esophageal motor disorder, hypotensive and hypertensive lower esophageal sphincter [21]. However, there is a poor temporal correlation between esophageal motility disorders and episodes of chest pain, suggesting that the presence of esophageal dysmotility during esophageal manometry may be a marker for an underlying motor disorder rather than the direct cause responsible for the patient's symptoms. Furthermore, in NCCP patients who underwent simultaneous esophageal manometry and pH testing, chest pain was more commonly associated with acid reflux events than motility abnormalities [22]. High-frequency intraesophageal ultrasonography has revealed a strong correlation between spontaneous and edrophonium-induced chest pain and sustained esophageal contractions (SECs).These contractions are caused by shortening of the longitudinal muscle of the esophagus and thus are not readily detected by traditional esophageal manometry. SECs have been suggested to be the motor corollary for esophageal chest pain. However, it is still unclear whether SECs are the direct cause of chest pain or simply an epiphenomenon.

Esophageal hypersensitivity
Cerebral-evoked potential studies in patients with NCCP using esophageal balloon distention protocols demonstrated abnormal cerebral processing of esophageal stimuli. The recorded cerebral-evoked potentials (marker of central nociceptive processing) were of lower quality and amplitude and with longer latency compared with those of control subjects. Peripheral and central sensitization of esophageal sensory afferents and spinal cord neurons has been suggested to cause increased responses to innocuous and noxious intraesophageal stimuli. It has been postulated that inflammation or other injuries to the esophageal mucosa set off a cascade of events that leads to the up-regulation of receptors and induces the development of esophageal hypersensitivity through peripheral and central sensitization. Patients with NCCP appear to have decreased thresholds for sensation, discomfort and pain for various esophageal stimulations.

Psychological factors
Up to 75% of NCCP patients have been observed to have an increased association with psychological disorders, including depression, anxiety, somatization and panic disorder [23]. These patients often report chest pain or tightness under stress,

possibly due to sympathetic nervous system arousal. Studies have been inconsistent when the frequency of panic disorder, anxiety, and depression were compared between NCCP patients and those with coronary artery disease (CAD). Some studies reported increase in the prevalence of psychological disorders in NCCP patients, while others found no significant difference between the two groups [24,25].

For many NCCP patients, psychological co-morbidity may contribute to the emergence of chest pain by heightening the perception of intraesophageal events [26]. In addition, psychological comorbidity may affect patients' personal attitude towards the disease, response to treatment, and relapse.

Causes/differential diagnosis
In addition to GERD, functional heartburn, eosinophilic esophagitis, achalasia, peptic ulcer disease or esophageal/gastric malignancy can lead to heartburn symptoms. Furthermore, a sudden and isolated attack of heartburn may be caused by pill-induced esophageal injury, or even caustic injury to the esophageal mucosa. The most important diagnosis to be excluded during the evaluation of a patient with chest pain is ischemic heart disease (Figure 1.2). The potential causes of NCCP (besides esophageal disorders) include gastric and gallbladder disorders, musculoskeletal abnormalities, pulmonary and pericardial disorders, and psychiatric abnormalities (primarily panic disorder) (Table 1.1).

Symptom complexes
Heartburn, as the predominant symptom, is highly specific for the diagnosis of GERD. However, other symptoms are also commonly found in patients with GERD and are outlined below.

Regurgitation
Regurgitation is defined as the perception of flow of refluxed gastric content into the mouth or hypopharynx [5]. Although regurgitation is less prevalent than heartburn in patients with GERD, in some it may be the sole presentation of the disorder. Regurgitation is particularly severe at night, when patients are recumbent, or when bending over. Among patients with regurgitation, abnormally low LES basal pressure, gastroparesis, and esophagitis are more common. For these reasons regurgitation appears to be more difficult to control medically than heartburn. It should be emphasized that regurgitation may also be a presentation of a pharyngeal pouch, esophageal obstruction, or gastric outlet obstruction.

Water brash
Water brash is the sudden filling of the mouth with clear, slightly salty fluid due to secretions of the salivary glands in response to intraesophageal acid reflux events.

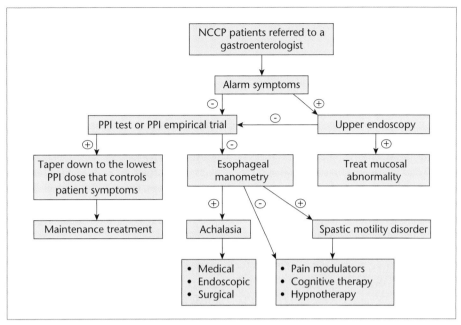

Figure 1.2 Suggested algorithm for the diagnosis and treatment of patients with noncardiac chest pain (NCCP). PPI, proton pump inhibitor. (Reproduced from Fass R, Navarro-Rodriguez T. Noncardiac chest pain. *J Clin Gastroenterol.* 2008;42:636–646, with permission from Wolters Kluwer Health.)

Globus sensation

Globus is the constant sensation of a lump or fullness in the throat, which improves transiently during swallowing. Globus usually occurs in the absence of dysphagia.

Dysphagia

The term dysphagia refers to the sensation that food is being hindered in its normal passage from the oral cavity to the stomach. In patients with GERD, sensation of dysphagia may be perceived below the breast bone anywhere up to the sternal notch. The latter is commonly referred sensation from a lesion in the distal part of the esophagus. Dysphagia may be referred cephalad to the site of the obstruction but never caudad. Dysphagia in a patient with heartburn may suggest the presence of erosive esophagitis, peptic stricture, ulceration, or malignant tumor of the esophagus.

Dyspepsia

Many patients with predominantly heartburn symptoms may also complain of dyspeptic symptoms, such as epigastric pain or discomfort, bloating, early satiety, nausea, and even vomiting. These symptoms are reported at a similar frequency by patients with or without esophageal mucosal injury. It is unclear whether these symptoms represent an overlap with functional dyspepsia or are part of the GERD symptom complex.

Odynophagia

Odynophagia is pain during swallowing. It occurs occasionally in patients with severe erosive esophagitis. However its presence should raise suspicion for an alternative esophageal cause, especially infections (Candida, herpes) or corrosive (pills) induced injury. A milder variant is a sensation that the patient can feel solids and liquids passing down the esophagus without pain.

Diagnosis

The typical reflux syndrome can be diagnosed on the basis of the characteristic symptoms without diagnostic testing. Symptom response to antireflux treatment should be used to further cement the diagnosis of GERD prior entertaining any invasive investigation [5]. Tools that are currently available for diagnosing GERD include the PPI test, barium esophagram, upper endoscopy, esophageal pH monitoring, and multichannel intraluminal impedance with pH sensor (MII-pH). In contrast, clinical history does not help to distinguish esophageal from cardiac chest pain. Both esophageal and cardiac chest pain can produce a pressure-like squeezing or burning substernal chest pain. Both may improve with nitrates or calcium channel blockers. Additionally, both may be exertional in nature. The presence of heartburn, regurgitation and pain relieved with antacids may suggest an esophageal etiology in patients with NCCP.

The proton pump inhibitor (PPI) test

GERD The PPI test is a simple, noninvasive diagnostic tool for GERD that is widely available to community-based physicians [27]. The test is a short course (1–4 weeks) of high-dose

PPI given two to three times daily for the diagnosis of GERD. If symptoms disappear or markedly improve with therapy and then return when medication is discontinued, then GERD could be assumed as the diagnosis, and no further testing is required. Several trials in patients with typical symptoms of GERD have demonstrated that the sensitivity of the PPI test ranges from 66% to 89% and the specificity from 35% to 73%. However, there is still no consensus about the desired level of symptom response (cut-off level), optimal dose, frequency, or duration of the PPI test for GERD. In the absence of warning signs, the PPI test is a safe and reasonable first step in diagnosing and treating GERD.

NCCP The PPI test is recommended for diagnosing GERD-related NCCP prior to any invasive or noninvasive testing. In a meta-analysis, the overall sensitivity, specificity, and diagnostic odds ratio for the PPI test vs. endoscopy and 24-hour esophageal pH monitoring in diagnosing GERD in NCCP patients were 80%, 74% and 19.35, respectively [28]. The PPI test is a cost-effective diagnostic strategy for GERD-related NCCP primarily due to significant reduction in the usage of invasive diagnostic tools [29].

Barium esophagram

Barium esophagram should not serve as the primary test for the evaluation of patients with heartburn. The test is considered positive for GERD diagnosis if reflux is witnessed during examination or if there is morphologic evidence of reflux esophagitis. However, the test has a low sensitivity and specificity for the diagnosis of GERD. The presence of barium reflux does not necessarily denote GERD, as 20% of normal subjects may demonstrate similar abnormality during esophagram. Barium esophagram may be helpful and should be considered as the first diagnostic tool in patients with GERD who develop dysphagia. In patients with NCCP without alarm symptom, barium esophagram has never been shown to be of value.

Upper endoscopy

GERD According to most guidelines and consensus statements, upper endoscopy is recommended for GERD patients who do not respond to therapy, those with recurrent or alarm symptoms and to exclude Barrett's esophagus [30]. Endoscopy is the gold standard for diagnosing erosive esophagitis, Barrett's esophagus, peptic stricture, and adenocarcinoma of the esophagus. Furthermore, the test allows assessment of the degree of esophageal mucosal injury, provides an opportunity for histopathologic diagnosis, and allows assessment of response to antireflux therapy. Upper endoscopy has a low sensitivity for diagnosing GERD, because 50–70% of reflux patients do not demonstrate any evidence of esophageal mucosal injury. The clinical roles of new endoscopic technologies including narrow band imaging, chromoendoscopy, confocal endomicroscopy, magnification and high-resolution endoscopy, capsule endoscopy and ultrathin unsedated transnasal endoscopy are under investigation. However, early studies have suggested that these techniques may increase the sensitivity for diagnosing GERD in patients with normal endoscopy.

NCCP Upper endoscopy in the absence of alarm symptoms, while commonly performed in clinical practice, has been shown to provide little useful information in the initial evaluation of NCCP. In the largest study thus far addressing the role of upper endoscopy in NCCP, 44% of the NCCP patients had a normal endoscopy. Endoscopic findings in those with abnormal endoscopy were GERD-related and included hiatal hernia (28.6%), erosive esophagitis (19.4%), Barrett's esophagus (4.4%), esophageal stricture or stenosis (3.6%), and peptic ulcer (2%) [31].

pH testing

GERD Twenty-four-hour esophageal pH monitoring or the wireless pH capsule are sensitive tests for the diagnosis of GERD but should not be considered as the gold standard. The wireless pH capsule has extended the duration of the test to 48 hours and has somewhat improved its sensitivity. The original role of esophageal pH testing was to objectively diagnose GERD in patients with heartburn but normal endoscopy. However the empiric use of PPIs in this group of patients has altered its role. Presently, pH monitoring use is limited to patients who have not responded to at least a double dose of PPI, patients with normal endoscopy who are candidates for antireflux surgery, and patients who have had antireflux surgery but report recurrence of GERD symptoms. In patients with atypical or extraesophageal manifestations of GERD, pH monitoring should be performed in those who have failed treatment on at least double-dose PPI given over a period of at least 3 months (the test is done on treatment) [30]. The pH test may be uncomfortable to patients (because of the pH probe), costly, and may not be readily available to community-based physicians.

NCCP The use of 24-hour esophageal pH monitoring in NCCP has been transformed in the past decade, primarily owing to increased usage of empiric PPI therapy or the PPI test. Presently, the test has been reserved for NCCP patients in whom objective evidence of GERD is required (off therapy) or in whom response to a therapeutic PPI trial is equivocal or negative (on therapy). In patients with NCCP, 24-hour esophageal pH monitoring on therapy has a therapeutic predictive value in addition to its diagnostic merit. Patients with greater esophageal acid exposure appear to have a greater response to antireflux treatment [32]. Extending pH monitoring to 48 hours by using the wireless pH capsule improves detection of reflux-associated chest pain symptoms.

The sensitivity of pH monitoring in NCCP is unknown, but approximately 50–60% of patients with untreated NCCP demonstrated increased distal esophageal acid exposure and/or a positive symptom index alone.

Esophageal manometry

GERD Esophageal manometry should not be used to establish the diagnosis of GERD. It may identify manometric abnormalities commonly found in GERD (for example ineffective esophageal motility and reduced LES basal pressure). However, these findings are absent in the majority of GERD patients. The role of esophageal manometry in patients with reflux symptoms is primarily to assist in the placement of a pH measuring device and to exclude achalasia.

NCCP Esophageal motility abnormalities have been identified in 30% of patients with NCCP. Hypotensive lower esophageal sphincter (61%) is the most common motility abnormality diagnosed, followed by hypertensive lower esophageal sphincter, nonspecific esophageal motor disorder, and nutcracker esophagus (10% each). Achalasia and diffuse esophageal spasm are very uncommon in NCCP [21]. The presence of a motility abnormality during esophageal manometry is rarely associated with reports of chest pain, raising a question about the exact relationship between the aforementioned motility findings and chest pain.

Multichannel intraluminal impedance (MII)

The MII + pH sensor can determine the nature (liquid, gas, or mixed), proximal extent, and acidity of a reflux event. The technique has been shown to be primarily useful in identifying weakly acid or alkaline reflux in GERD patients who failed PPI twice daily [33]. MII + pH sensor has not been evaluated in NCCP patients, and thus its value in this condition remains unknown.

Provocative tests

Provocative tests for NCCP include the Bernstein or acid perfusion test (reproducing chest pain by infusing acid into the mid esophagus), the Tensilon test (reproducing chest pain by inducing augmented esophageal contractions using intravenous edrophonium, an acetylcholine esterase antagonist), and the balloon distention test (reproducing chest pain by using graded esophageal balloon distensions). At present, provocative tests are rarely used in clinical practice, due to low sensitivity, discomfort and potential adverse events.

Future directions

Despite current advances in the understanding of the pathophysiology, diagnosis, and treatment of patients with heartburn and NCCP, the exact underlying mechanisms for these symptoms remain poorly understood. The lack of association between symptom severity and anatomical as well as pathophysiological findings remains perplexing. Future investigation should bring further understanding of the peripheral and central factors that may modulate perception of heartburn or NCCP. New or refined imaging techniques will be introduced and their value in diagnosing GERD will be determined. Further focus of investigation will be on non reflux causes for

heartburn and the underlying mechanisms for functional chest pain. The value of multichannel intraluminal impedance as well as other new diagnostic techniques will be assessed in special GERD groups and patients with NCCP.

SOURCES OF INFORMATION FOR PATIENTS AND DOCTORS

http://www.patient.co.uk/showdoc/345/
http://www.iffgd.org/
http://www.motilitysociety.org/

References

1. Dent J, Brun J, Fendrick A, *et al.* An evidence-based appraisal of reflux disease management - the Genval Workshop Report. *Gut.* 1999;44:S1–S16.
2. Locke GR, Talley NJ, Fett SL, *et al.* Prevalence and clinical spectrum of gastroesophageal reflux: a population-based study in Olmsted County, Minnesota. *Gastroenterology.* 1997;112(5):1448–1456.
3. Avidan B, Sonnenberg A, Schnell TG, *et al.* There are no reliable symptoms for erosive oesophagitis and Barrett's oesophagus: endoscopic diagnosis is still essential. *Alimentary Pharmacology & Therapeutics.* 2002;16(4):735–742.
4. El-Serag HB, Johanson JF. Risk factors for the severity of erosive esophagitis in Helicobacter pylori-negative patients with gastroesophageal reflux disease. *Scand J Gastroenterol.* 2002;37(8):899–904.
5. Vakil N, van Zanten SV, Kahrilas P, *et al.* The Montreal definition and classification of gastroesophageal reflux disease: a global evidence-based consensus. *Am J Gastroenterol.* 2006;101(8):1900–1920; quiz 43.
6. Faybush EM, Fass R. Gastroesophageal reflux disease in noncardiac chest pain. *Gastroenterol Clin North Am.* 2004;33(1):41–54.
7. Galmiche JP, Clouse RE, Balint A, *et al.* Functional Esophageal Disorders. In: Drossman DA, Corazziari E, Delvaux M, Spiller RC, Talley NJ, Thompson WG, *et al.*, editors. *Rome III: The Functional Gastrointestinal Disorders.* Third Edition. McLean, VA: Degnon Associates, Inc.; 2006.
8. Jerlock M, Welin C, Rosengren A, *et al.* Pain characteristics in patients with unexplained chest pain and patients with ischemic heart disease. *Eur J Cardiovasc Nurs.* 2007;6:130–6.
9. Fenster PE. Evaluation of chest pain: a cardiology perspective for gastroenterologists. *Gastroenterol Clin N Am.* 2004;33(1):35–40.
10. Dent J, El-Serag HB, Wallander MA, *et al.* Epidemiology of gastro-oesophageal reflux disease: a systematic review. *Gut.* 2005;54(5):710–717.
11. Wong WM, Lai KC, Lam KF, *et al.* Prevalence, clinical spectrum and health care utilization of gastro-oesophageal reflux disease in a Chinese population: a population-based study. *Aliment Pharmacol Ther.* 2003;18(6):595–604.
12. Wong WM, Risner-Adler S, Beeler J, *et al.* Noncardiac chest pain: the role of the cardiologist – a national survey. *J Clin Gastroenterol.* 2005;39:858–862.
13. Eslick GD. Noncardiac chest pain: epidemiology, natural history, health care seeking, and quality of life. *Gastroenterol Clin North Am.* 2004;33(1):1–23.

14. Chiocca JC, Olmos JA, Salis GB, *et al.* Prevalence, clinical spectrum and atypical symptoms of gastro-oesophageal reflux in Argentina: a nationwide population-based study. *Aliment Pharmacol Ther.* 2005;22(4):331–342.

15. Kennedy JW, Killip T, Fisher LD, *et al.* The clinical spectrum of coronary artery disease and its surgical and medical management, 1974–1979. The Coronary Artery Surgery study. *Circulation.* 1985;66(5, Pt 2):III16–III23.

16. Mousavi S, Tosi J, Eskandarian R, *et al.* Role of clinical presentation in diagnosing reflux-related non-cardiac chest pain. *J Gastroenterol Hepatol.* 2007;22:218–221.

17. Fass R, Tougas G. Functional heartburn: the stimulus, the pain, and the brain. *Gut.* 2002;51:885–892.

18. Barlow WJ, Orlando RC. The pathogenesis of heartburn in non-erosive reflux disease: a unifying hypothesis. *Gastroenterology.* 2005;128(3):771–778.

19. Fass R, Naliboff B, Higa L, *et al.* Differential effect of long-term esophageal acid exposure on mechanosensitivity and chemosensitivity in humans. *Gastroenterology.* 1998;115(6):1363–1373.

20. Fass R, Navarro-Rodriguez T. Noncardiac chest pain. *J Clin Gastroenterol.* 2008;42(5):636–646.

21. Dekel R, Pearson T, Wendel C, *et al.* Assessment of oesophageal motor function in patients with dyspepsia or chest pain – the Clinical Outcomes Research Initiative experience. *Aliment Pharmacol Ther.* 2003;18(11–12):1083–1089.

22. Peters L, Maas L, Petty D, *et al.* Spontaneous noncardiac chest pain. Evaluation by 24-hour ambulatory esophageal motility and pH monitoring. *Gastroenterology.* 1988;94:878–886.

23. Bass C, Wade C, Hand D, *et al.* Patients with angina with normal and near normal coronary arteries: clinical and psychosocial state 12 months after angiography. *Br Med J (Clin Res Ed)* 1983;287(6404):1505–1508.

24. Dammen T, Arnesen H, Ekeberg O, *et al.* Psychological factors, pain attribution and medical morbidity in chest-pain patients with and without coronary artery disease. *Gen Hosp Psychiatry.* 2004;l26(6):463–469.

25. Katon W, Hall ML, Russo J, *et al.* Chest pain: relationship to psychiatric illness to coronary arteriographic results. *Am J Med* 1988;84(1):1–9.

26. Fass R, Malagon I, Schmulson M. Chest pain of esophageal origin. *Curr Opin Gastroenterol.* 2001;17:376–380.

27. Gasiorowska A, Fass R. The proton pump inhibitor (PPI) test in GERD: does it still have a role? *J Clin Gastroenterol* 2008 Sep;42(8):867–874.

28. Wang W, Huang J, Zheng G, *et al.* Is proton pump inhibitor testing an effective approach to diagnose gastroesophageal reflux disease in patients with noncardiac chest pain? *Arch Intern Med.* 2005;165(11):1222–1228.

29. Fass R, Fennerty MB, Ofman JJ, *et al.* The clinical and economic value of a short course of omeprazole in patients with noncardiac chest pain. *Gastroenterology.* 1998;115(1):42–9.

30. Hirano I, Richter JE. Practice Parameters Committee of the American College of Gastroenterology. ACG practice guidelines: esophageal reflux testing. *Am J Gastroenterol* 2007;102(3): 668–685.

31. Dickman R, Mattek N, Holub J, *et al.* Prevalence of upper gastrointestinal tract findings in patients with noncardiac chest pain versus those with gastroesophageal reflux disease (GERD)-related symptoms: results from a national endoscopic database. *Am J Gastroenterol.* 2007;102:1173–9.

32. Fass R, Fennerty MB, Johnson C, *et al.* Correlation of ambulatory 24-hour esophageal pH monitoring results with symptom improvement in patients with noncardiac chest pain due to gastroesophageal reflux disease. *J Clin Gastroenterol.* 1999;28(1): 36–39.

33. Kahrilas PJ, Sifrim D. High-resolution manometry and impedance-pH/manometry: valuable tools in clinical and investigational esophagology. *Gastroenterology.* 2008;135(3):756–769.

CHAPTER 2
Dysphagia and odynophagia

Stacey R. Zavala[1] and Philip O. Katz[1,2]
[1]Albert Einstein Medical Center, Philadelphia, PA, USA
[2]Jefferson Medical College, Thomas Jefferson University, Philadelphia, PA, USA

KEY POINTS

- Distinguishing oropharyngeal from esophageal dysphagia is key to guiding the work-up
- Barium swallow and endoscopy are complementary in evaluation of dysphagia
- A solid bolus (e.g., 13 mm pill) should be given when a barium swallow is performed to evaluate dysphagia
- Odynophagia (pain, often retrosternal during a swallow) should prompt a search for infectious or medication induced injury
- Endoscopy is the procedure of choice to evaluate odynophagia
- Manometry should be used to aid in diagnosis of non structural dysphagia

Introduction

Dysphagia is defined as difficulty or delay in preparation and/or passage of a liquid or solid food bolus that is sensed by the patient within seconds of initiation of a swallow attempt. Difficulty initiating the swallow is known as oropharyngeal dysphagia. This is not to be confused with globus, which is a constant sensation of a lump in the throat or neck, that may improve with swallowing. Complaints of food "sticking" or "hanging up" in the center of the chest, suggests esophageal dysphagia. In contrast, odynophagia may be described as a burning or retrosternal pain as food or liquid moves down the esophagus. These are important distinctions to make, as the history will guide appropriate diagnostic tests.

Prevalence

Dysphagia is a common complaint. In 2008, Eslick *et al.* conducted a study in which a questionnaire was given to 672 random individuals. Sixteen percent reported dysphagia at some time in their life [1]. The problem is becoming even more prevalent in the elderly as the baby boomer population ages. The number of people over 65 years old is projected to increase from 39 million in 2010 to 69 million in 2030 [2]. Chen *et al.* found an overall prevalence of dysphagia in 15% of subjects over the age of 65. Over half with dysphagia reported substantial impairment in quality of life [3].

Pathogenesis

Deglutination involves a coordinated sequence of events to move a bolus from the mouth, into the hypopharnyx and down the esophagus. A swallow is broken up into 3 different phases and any perturbation in these events can result in dysphagia. The first phase is the oral phase; the only voluntary event in a swallow. Food enters the oral cavity where mastication and bolus formation occur. In the pharyngeal phase, the tongue elevates and propels the bolus to the pharynx. The soft palate elevates to seal the nasopharynx to prevent backwards flow of contents (nasopharyngeal regurgitation). The larynx and hyoid bone move anterior and upward while the epiglottis moves posterior and downward to close, converting this region from a respiratory system to a swallowing system. The pharynx shortens and the upper esophageal sphincter (UES) relaxes to allow passage of a bolus into the esophagus beginning the esophageal phase. The swallow stimulates primary peristalsis which is controlled by preganglionic neurons in the dorsal motor nucleus of the vagus that project onto inhibitory and excitatory neurons in the esophageal myenteric plexus. This results in coordinated contractions down the esophagus and lower esophageal sphincter (LES) relaxation. Contraction duration is usually 2–4 seconds and total time for a contraction to traverse the entire esophageal length is typically 6–8 seconds. Secondary peristalsis (a reflex distal contraction) may occur to clear the esophagus of any residual food [4,5].

Dysphagia, either oropharyngeal or esophageal, can result from one of two mechanisms: 1) mechanical obstruction and/or structural abnormality or 2) neuromotor defect. Table 2.1 lists the common causes of dysphagia and odynophagia.

Symptom complexes

Helpful symptom complexes can aid in making the distinction between esophageal and oropharyngeal dysphagia. For example, cough or choking within a second of initiation of a swallow is suggestive of oropharyngeal dysphagia. In contrast, patients with esophageal dysphagia have a sensation of food "hanging up" in the center of the chest, heartburn, or

Table 2.1 Causes of dysphagia and odynophagia

Oropharyngeal dysphagia	Esophageal dysphagia	Odynophagia
Structural	**Structural**	Gastroesophageal reflux disease (unusual)
Poor dentition	*Intraluminal*	Medication induced esophagitis
Xerostomia	Stricture	Infectious esophagitis
Intraluminal	Schatzki's ring	(Candida, herpes, CMV)
Zenker's diverticulum	Cancer	Radiation injury
Cervical web	Hiatal hernia	Caustic ingestion
Oropharyngeal tumor	Eosinophilic esophagitis	
Extraluminal	*Extraluminal*	
Cervical osteophytes	Mediastinal tumors (lymphoma, lung cancer)	
Thyromegaly	Vascular structures	
Lymphadenopathy	(dysphagia lusoria, dysphagia aortica)	
	Duplication cyst	
	Postsurgical changes (fundoplication)	
Myogenic	**Motility abnormalities**	
Myasthenia gravis	*Primary*	
Dermatomyositis	Achalasia	
Polymyositis	Distal esophageal spasm	
Alcoholic myopathy	Hypercontractile motility	
Amyloidosis	Hypertensive LES	
Hypo/hyperthyroidism	Nutcracker esophagus	
Cushing's syndrome	Hypocontractile motility	
	Hypotensive LES	
	Ineffective esophageal motility	
	Secondary	
	Secondary achalasia from tumor, infiltrative	
	disorders (sarcoidosis, amyloidosis, eosinophilic esophagitis)	
	Diabetes mellitus	
	Collagen vascular diseases	
Nervous system	Drugs	
Head injury		
Brainstem tumors		
Amyotrophic lateral sclerosis		
Cerebrovascular accident		
Alzheimer's disease		
Parkinson's disease		
Multiple sclerosis		
Extrapyramidal syndromes		
Guillain-Barré		

regurgitation. Table 2.2 lists symptoms to help differentiate between esophageal and oropharyngeal dysphagia.

Diagnosis

Medical history

A detailed history of the patient with dysphagia will provide a presumptive diagnosis most of the time. The history should include questions regarding dysphagia to solids, liquids or both, location of dysphagia, duration of symptoms and whether they are progressive or intermittent, associated medical conditions (e.g., HIV patients), prior surgery or radiation treatment, (e.g., Nissen fundoplication) and associated weight loss. In addition to the above, for patients with odynophagia (with or without dysphagia) a detailed history of current and recently used medication should be elicited.

Table 2.2 Symptom complexes

Oropharyngeal dysphagia	Esophageal dysphagia
Dysphagia within 1 sec of swallowing	Dysphagia delayed until mid chest
Choking, cough with initiation of eating	Heartburn
Nasal regurgitation	Regurgitation
Dysarthria and diplopia	Chest pain
Facial muscle weakness (ptosis, facial droop)	Cough
Dysphonia/nasal speech	
Halitosis/gurgling noise	

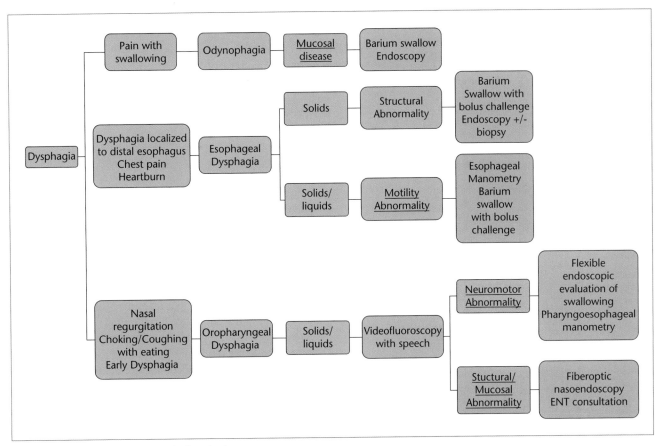

Figure 2.1 Algorithm for dysphagia and odynophagia.

These questions will help guide appropriate testing to confirm the suspected diagnosis (Figure 2.1 and Table 2.2).

The accuracy of localization of dysphagia is variable. Patients localizing the sticking of food to the cervical area or mid-chest often do not have a cause in this area. However, those that complain of distal dysphagia are accurate in 80% of cases [6].

Dysphagia only to solids suggests a mechanical obstruction. Combined solid and liquid dysphagia is suggestive of an esophageal motility abnormality such as achalasia. Solid dysphagia that progresses to liquid dysphagia may be due to a high-grade obstruction.

Dysphagia may be intermittent. For example, patients with a peptic stricture may complain of food getting stuck when eating quickly or only with certain foods. Progressive solid food dysphagia with weight loss may be indicative of a malignancy.

Patients may have another medical condition in which dysphagia is a part of the constellation of symptoms of their underlying disease. For example in a recent study, patients with Sjögren's syndrome complain of dysphagia more than controls [7]. Pharyngeal and esophageal dysmotility was found in 15% and 40% of patients respectively, suggesting

other mechanisms such as xerostomia and esophageal webs may play a role. Other systemic diseases include polymyositis, rheumatoid arthritis, thyrotoxicosis, diabetes mellitus, myasthenia gravis and Parkinson's disease. Patients with a history of cancer and radiation to the oral cavity and neck can lead to dysphagia due to a stricture. If the history of radiation of exposure is recent and the patient is suffering from odynophagia, esophagitis should also be considered.

A detailed medication list (Table 2.3) is equally important as many drugs can act either centrally or peripherally to impair neuromuscular transmission, neural function, muscle function, or salivary secretion to cause dysphagia [8,9]. For example centrally acting drugs such as dopamine antagonists (for example phenothiazine and metoclopramide) can cause extrapyramidal symptoms leading to dysphagia. Antibacterials, nonsteroidal anti-inflammatory drugs, bisphosphonates, and ferrous sulfate can cause direct damage to the esophageal mucosa leading to odynophagia [10].

Physical examination
Careful examination of the oral cavity, head and neck, lymph nodes and thyroid as well as a detailed neurological exam, should be performed. Signs of a systemic disease such as

Table 2.3 Medications implicated in esophageal injury and dysphagia

Drugs implicated in esophageal injury	Drugs and dysphagia
Antibacterials	**Effects on striated muscle function**
Doxycycline	Sedatives
Tetracycline	Narcotics
Amoxicillin	Antipsychotics
Penicillin	Neuroleptic therapy (extrapyramidal
Clindamycin	motor disturbances)
Rifampin	**Effects on smooth muscle function**
Nonsteroidal anti-	*Inhibitory*
inflammatory drugs	Alcohol
Aspirin	Tricyclic antidepressants
Ibuprofen	Theophylline
Naproxen	Calcium channel blockers
Diclofenac	Alcohol
Indomethacin	*Excitatory*
Bisphosphonates	Cholinergic agonists
Alendronate	Prokinetics
Pamidronate	**Decrease lower esophageal pressure**
Etidronate	Progesterone
Risedronate	Calcium channel blockers
Others	Nitrates
Ascorbic acid	Alcohol
Ferrous sulfate	**Xerostomia**
Prednisone	Anticholinergics
Potassium chloride	Antiemetics
Quinidine	Antihypertensives
Theophylline	ACE inhibitors
	Antihistamines
	Diuretics
	Opiates
	Antipsychotics

connective tissue disease or metabolic diseases may also be apparent on exam.

A bedside water swallow evaluation may also be conducted when oropharyngeal dysphagia is suspected [11]. Patients are given 30 ml of water while in the upright position. Observations of delayed swallowing, drooling, and cough during or within 1 min of swallow and dysphonia are suggestive of a neurological cause of dysphagia.

Imaging

Barium swallow is useful in evaluating patients with dysphagia and should measure esophageal emptying, type of hiatal hernia, strictures, rings, and esophagitis as well as evaluate esophageal motility and the presence of reflux. A solid-bolus phase, such as a 13 mm barium tablet, a marshmallow , or a food bolus challenge with something the patient complains gets stuck (such as meat, chicken) should be given to assess the size of the esophageal lumen as well as identify subtle rings, strictures or vascular anomalies that can be missed by other modalities [12].

Videofluoroscopy is the best test to evaluate suspected oropharyngeal dysphagia. Patients are given different consistencies

to swallow and videotaped from both the anteroposterior and lateral directions. This test assesses excessive delay in initiation of pharyngeal swallowing, aspiration, nasopharyngeal regurgitation, and residue of test material in the pharyngeal space after swallowing. Additionally, the test allows for the efficacy of compensatory swallowing maneuvers, postures, or dietary modifications, under direct observation by a speech therapist [13].

Manometry is useful in assessing those with both non-obstructive oropharyngeal and esophageal dysphagia. After placing a motility catheter, patients are given a series liquid swallows to assess lower esophageal relaxation and esophageal contractions. This test will reveal motility abnormalities (Table 2.1). The motility catheter may be positioned in the upper esophageal sphincter to assess abnormalities in pharyngeal contraction and UES relaxation.

Impedance is a technique that measures differences in resistance to alternating current of intraluminal contents allowing detection of bolus movement during a swallow. Impedance can be combined with pH monitoring or manometry to help clarify esophageal function abnormalities. Tutuian *et al.* studied 350 patients with a variety of symptoms and manometric diagnoses and found that those with achalasia and scleroderma had no bolus movement while approximately 50% of those with IEM and DES had normal bolus movement. Patients with normal manometry, nutcracker esophagus, or hyper/hypotensive LES, had normal bolus transit. Finally those with dysphagia were more likely to have incomplete bolus transit on MII testing [14]. The clinical utility of impedance testing is unclear.

High-resolution manometry (HRM) provides a topographic analysis of esophageal peristalsis. Multiple transducers are placed 1 cm apart to allow for testing with the catheter in one position. Simply it is a combination of classic manometry and impedance. HRM has been useful in sub-classifying achalasia [15] as well as evaluating patients with globus and UES abnormalities [16]. For those who do manometry infrequently, this technology simplifies the performance of the manometry study.

Endoscopy is indicated for evaluating patients for structural or mucosal etiologies. This is the procedure of choice in evaluating a patient with odynophagia, to assess for the presence of esophageal ulceration. Pill induced lesions most typically occur at the level of the aortic arch or indentation of the left atrial appendage. Biopsies for eosinophilic esophagitis should include at least five total samples from the distal, mid and proximal esophagus to maximize sensitivity of diagnosis [17]. This may be done even in those in which the esophageal mucosa appears normal but the clinical suspicion is high [18]. Fiberoptic endoscopic examination of swallowing (FEES) involves passing a small-diameter endoscope transnasally to visualize the laryngeal and pharyngeal structures under direct vision while patients swallow liquid and solid food boluses.

Conclusion

A detailed history and judicious use of diagnostic testing as outlined above will almost always provide a diagnosis of dysphagia and/or odynophagia (see Figure 2.1).

References

1. Eslick GD, Talley NJ. Dysphagia: Epidemiology, risk factors and impact on quality of life — a population-based study. *Aliment Pharmacol Ther.* 2008; 27(10):971–979.
2. US Census Bureau. *Current Population Reports: Population Projections of the United States by Age, Sex, Race, and Hispanic Origin – 1995 to 2050.* US Census Bureau, 1996. p. 25–1130.
3. Chen P, Golub JS, Hapner ER. Prevalence of perceived dysphagia and quality-of-life impairment in a geriatric population. *Dysphagia.* 2009;24(1):1–6.
4. Lind CD. Dysphagia: evaluation and treatment. *Gastroenterol Clin N Am.* 2003;32(2):553–575.
5. Malagelada JR, Bazzoli F, Elewaut A. Dysphagia. *World Gastroenterology Organization Practice Guidelines: Dysphagia.* World Gastroenterology Organization; 2007.
6. Roeder BE, Murray JA, Diekhising RA. Patient localization of esophageal dysphagia. *Dig Dis Sci.* 2004;49(4):697–701.
7. Mandl T, Ekberg O, Wollmer P, *et al.* Dysphagia and dysmotility of the pharynx and oesophagus in patients with primary Sjögren's syndrome. *Scand J Rheumatol.* 2007;36:394–401.
8. Cook IJ. Disorders causing oropharyngeal dysphagia. In: Castell DO, Richter JE editors. *The Esophagus,* 4th Edition. New York: Lippincott Williams and Wilkins; 2004.
9. Stoschus B. Allescher HD. Drug-induced dysphagia. *Dysphagia.* 1993;8(2):154–159.
10. Jaspersen D. Drug-Induced oesophageal disorders. Pathogenesis, incidence, prevention and management. *Drug Saf.* 2000; 22(3):237–249.
11. Bours GJ, Speyer R, Lemmens J. Bedside screening tests vs. videofluoroscopy or fiberoptic evaluation of swallowing to detect dysphagia in patients with neurological disorders: systematic review. *J Adv Nurs.* 2009;65(3):477–493.
12. Allen B., Baker M., Falk G. Role of barium esophagography in evaluating dysphagia. *Cleve Clin J Med.* 2009;76(2):105–111.
13. Cook IJ, Kahrilas PG. AGA technical review on management of oropharyngeal dysphagia. *Gastroenterology.* 1999;116(2):455–478.
14. Tutuian R, Castell DO. Combined multichannel intraluminal impedance and manometry clarifies esophageal function abnormalities. Study in 350 patients. *Am J Gastroenterol.* 2004;99(6): 1011–1019.
15. Pandolfino JE, Kwiatek MA, Nealis T. Achalasia: A new clinically relevant classification by high-resolution manometry. *Gastroenterology.* 2008;135(5):1526–1533.
16. Kwiatek MA, Mirza F, Kahrilas PJ, *et al.* Hyperdynamic upper esophageal sphincter pressure: a manometric observation in patients reporting globus sensation. *Am J Gastroenterol* 2009; 104(2):289–298.
17. Gonsalves N, Policarpio-Nicolas M, Zhang Q, *et al.* Histopathologic variability and endoscopic correlates in adults with eosinophilic esophagitis. *Gastrointest Endosc.* 2006;64(3):313–319.
18. Liacouras CA, Spergel JM, Ruchelli E, *et al.* Eosinophilic esophagitis: a 10-year experience in 381 children. *Clin Gastroenterol Hepatol.* 2005;3(12): 1198–1206.

CHAPTER 3

Chronic or recurrent abdominal pain

Ayman Koteish[1] and Anthony N. Kalloo[1,2]
[1]The Johns Hopkins University – School of Medicine, Baltimore, MD, USA
[2]Johns Hopkins Hospital, Baltimore, MD, USA

KEY POINTS

- Chronic abdominal pain is a common complaint, and the vast majority of patients will have a functional disorder (i.e., IBS). Initial work-up is therefore focused on differentiating benign functional illness from organic pathology
- Care must be given to chronic lower abdominal pain (pelvic pain) in women (discussed separately)
- Although abdominal pain in IBS can vary, however, it should not be associated with weight loss, rectal bleeding, or anemia, nor should it be nocturnal or progressive
- Features that suggest organic illness include unstable vital signs, weight loss, fever, dehydration, electrolyte abnormalities, symptoms or signs of gastrointestinal blood loss, anemia, or signs of malnutrition
- The bowel habit is an important part of the history for chronic abdominal pain. While many organic conditions can result in chronic diarrhea, IBS often presents with alternations between diarrhea and constipation, a less likely pattern with organic disease
- Physical examination must be complete, since many multisystem illnesses could contribute to a nonspecific abdominal complaint. Specifically, one should identify any focus of abdominal tenderness that may require further investigation. Weight should be followed over time, and evidence of dehydration should be sought

Introduction

Whether acute or chronic, abdominal pain remains the most common chief complaint in gastroenterology and family medicine practices. The reporting of pain by patients, however, is highly subjective. Moreover, numerous psychosocial, neurophysiologic, anatomic, and pathologic factors influence the patient's presentation, thus accounting for a wide range of variability in the perception and reporting of pain [1]. See Chapter 19 for a discussion of acute abdominal pain.

What is it?

When referring to abdominal pain or discomfort, several terminologies are worth defining as they are widely used and may have different implications. **Recurrent abdominal pain** (or chronic intermittent abdominal pain) refers to situations where the patient has episodic attacks of pain and is entirely asymptomatic between attacks. **Chronic persistent abdomi-**

nal pain can be attributed to conditions that can be positively diagnosed and to others where the diagnosis is one of exclusion. The latter includes *chronic intractable pain*, defined as undiagnosed abdominal pain of at least 6 months' duration despite adequate medical evaluation.

Most of this chapter is focused on diagnosable causes of abdominal pain. *Dyspepsia* is one of the most commonly reported symptoms, yet is nonspecific. In fact, dyspepsia is better considered as a symptom complex, because it encompasses a wide spectrum of individual symptoms, namely indigestion, heartburn, pain, or generalized abdominal discomfort. When reported as a symptom, dyspepsia refers to **persistent or recurrent abdominal pain** or **discomfort located in the upper abdomen**. Dyspepsia can be caused by a variety of disorders, and has been defined by several international and national expert committees (for example the Rome III and the American Gastroenterology Association (AGA) guidelines). See Chapter 4 for a more detailed discussion of dyspepsia.

Pathophysiology
Neurologic basis of pain

Two types of nerve fiber are involved in mediating pain (that is, nociception): unmyelinated C fibers and myelinated A fibers. The majority of fibers are C fibers, located within the mucosa and muscularis of the gastrointestinal tract, on the serosal surface, and in the mesentery, that mediate mechanical, chemical, and thermal stimuli. C fibers transmit most of the painful stimuli from abdominal viscera, and relay sensation that is poorly localized, dull, gradual in onset, and longer in duration.

The other group of fibers consists of A fibers, which are mainly located in the mucosa (as well as skin and muscle, and respond to mechanical and heat stimuli, hence the name Amechano–heat).These fibers relay sharp, sudden, and localized pain after an acute injury. Cell bodies of these **first-order** C or A neurons lie in the dorsal ganglia. **Second-order** neurons transmit information from the dorsal horn via the contralateral spinothalamic tract up to the thalamic nuclei, and to the reticular formation in the pons and medulla. *Third-order* neurons project from the pons to the somatosensory cortex,

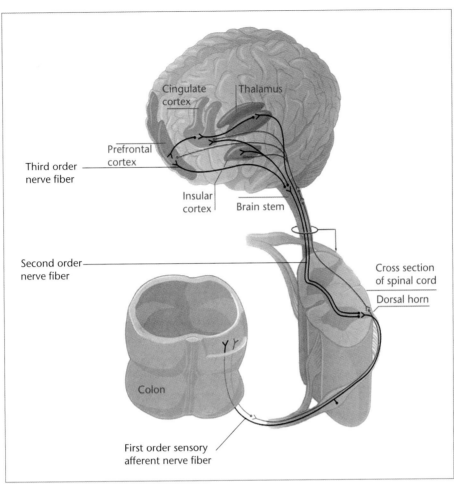

Figure 3.1 Neuronal visceral sensory pathway. Schematic representation of first, second, and third order neurons. (Reproduced with permission from www.hopkins-gi.org)

and from the medulla to the limbic system and frontal cortex (Figure 3.1).

Anatomic basis of pain (localization of pain)

Localization of abdominal pain may be quite frustrating to patients. The difficulty is due to the fact that relatively few visceral sensory afferents enter the spinal cord at a given level. Moreover, one splanchnic afferent neuron may originate from multiple sites in the viscera. More importantly, however, a single first-order afferent may activate a large number of second order neurons at the level of the dorsal horn, hence activating a large number of spinothalamic tract neurons and resulting in poor pain localization. Despite the imprecise location of visceral pain, a few facts are worth highlighting when evaluating a patient at the bedside:

- Because of the bilateral symmetric innervation of the gastrointestinal tract, visceral pain is most commonly located to the midline. When felt laterally, the ipsilateral kidney, ureter, ovary, or somatic structures may be the source, as they have unilateral sensory innervation.
- The site of perceived visceral pain corresponds to the spinal level of entry of the visceral afferent into the spinal cord. For example, afferents from the liver, biliary tree, pancreas, distal esophagus, stomach, and proximal duodenum enter the spinal cord between segments T5–T6 and T8–T11, resulting in pain between the xiphoid and the umbilicus [2–5].

Somatoparietal pain

Contrary to visceral pain, which is dull and vague, **somatoparietal pain** is more intense and more precisely located, in part because innervation of different parts of the parietal peritoneum is unilateral. This type of pain is aggravated by movement and is caused by noxious stimuli to the parietal peritoneum. An example of the difference between the two types of pain is appendicitis pain. At first this tends to be

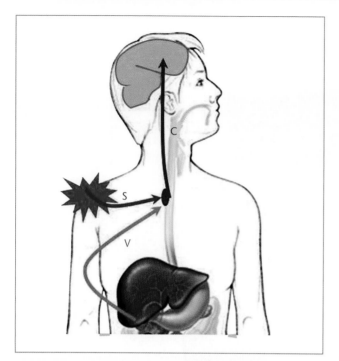

Figure 3.2 Basis of referred pain. This figure illustrates the example of cholecystitis: visceral (first order) neuron afferents synapse with second-order neurons in the spinal cord at the same level as somatic afferent neurons from the shoulder (C3–C5). The cortex perceives the pain as if originating from the right shoulder. V, visceral first-order neuron afferents; C, second-order neurons in the spinal cord; S, somatic afferent neurons. (Reproduced with permission from www.hopkins-gi.org)

many entities or conditions may present differently depending on severity or stage of the illness (for example vasculitides, inflammatory bowel disease, early versus late malignancy) [6,7]. Not uncommonly, however, the physician may fail to define an organic etiology for the pain despite adequate and extensive testing; this in fact characterizes functional disorders.

Chronic recurrent abdominal pain

CAUSES AND DIFFERENTIAL DIAGNOSIS

Causes of chronic recurrent abdominal pain
Irritable bowel syndrome (IBS); Nonulcer dyspepsia (NUD); Acute relapsing pancreatitis; Sphincter of Oddi dysfunction; Cholelithiasis; Diabetic gastroparesis; Radiculopathy; Intermittent intestinal obstruction; Inflammatory bowel disease; Chronic mesenteric ischemia; Musculoskeletal syndromes; Endometriosis; Familial Mediterranean fever; Acute intermittent porphyria; Nerve entrapment syndromes; Functional abdominal pain syndromes (FAPS).

Causes of chronic persistent abdominal pain
Chronic pancreatitis; Malignancy; Intra-abdominal abscess(es); Somatoform disorders.

Causes of chronic persistent undiagnosable abdominal pain
Irritable bowel syndrome (IBS); Nonulcer dyspepsia (NUD); Functional abdominal pain syndromes (FAPS).

---

vague and periumbilical [1] as a result of visceral inflammation, but is followed by a more intense pain, localized at McBurney's point, as a result of the inflammation extending to the overlying peritoneum.

Referred pain

Not only is abdominal pain poorly localized, it may also tend to be reported at sites far distant from the affected organ, thus giving rise to the concept of **referred pain** (Figure 3.2). Referred visceral pain most commonly involves cutaneous dermatomes that share the same spinal entry level as the sensory visceral afferents. For example, gallbladder nociceptive stimuli enter the cord between T5 and T10; hence, cholecystitis pain may be perceived in the back, right shoulder, or right scapula.

Causes/differential diagnosis

The differential diagnosis pertaining to chronic abdominal pain is wide [2]. One must therefore start by taking a good history and review of systems as well as performing a complete physical examination in order to identify the correct diagnosis. Categorization of chronic abdominal pain as intermittent or recurrent, or as persistent helps to orient the clinical investigation. These categories are not mutually exclusive as

Chronic persistent abdominal pain

Certain conditions can cause persistent abdominal pain for several months or more. The most common causes are malignancies, neuromuscular degenerative disorders, autoimmune or connective tissue diseases, infiltrative disorders, chronic pancreatitis, severe inflammatory bowel disease, history of abdominal trauma, and iatrogenic postsurgical complications [8,9]. In many patients the underlying cause of the pain is not curable. Treatment should therefore be aimed at decreasing the patient's suffering [10]. To improve patient survival, it is important, however, to make the distinction between malignant and nonmalignant processes.

Chronic undiagnosed abdominal pain: the functional abdominal pain syndrome (FAPS)

This entity is also referred to as chronic intractable abdominal pain. The International Working Team Committee has recently defined criteria to help diagnose FAPS. There is overlap between the definition of FAPS and that of irritable bowel syndrome (IBS) and nonulcer dyspepsia (NUD) [11–15]. In fact, these entities may coexist in the same patient. It is important to note, however, that in contrast to the pain of IBS and NUD, which is intermittent, the pain of FAPS is constant and persistent. Although FAPS may occur in bouts lasting for hours to days to weeks, it is characterized by persistent

Table 3.1 Management guidelines in functional abdominal pain syndromes

- Gain the patient's trust
- Frequent visits
- Acknowledge existence of real disorder
- Minimize testing and focus on therapy
- Set goals of therapy
- Absence of cure
- Symptomatic therapy
- Encourage patient to cope and get back to functional social life
- Consider consultatory help from psychiatry, physical therapy, pain management clinic

Table 3.2 Localization of abdominal pain

- *Right upper quadrant* Biliary colic; Slipping rib syndrome
- *Left upper quadrant* Splenic abscess or infarct
- *Right lower quadrant* Ileitis; Renal disorders; Sacroileitis; Iliopsoas syndrome
- *Left lower quadrant* Tubo-ovarian disorders; Colitis; Sacroileitis; Iliopsoas syndrome
- *Epigastric* Peptic ulcer disease; Pancreatitis
- *Diffuse* Inflammatory bowel disease; Familial Mediterranean fever; Acute intermittent porphyria; Irritable bowel syndrome; Nonulcer dyspepsia; Functional abdominal pain syndromes

residual pain between attacks. Patients do appear to have a higher prevalence of psychosocial disturbance, and frequently emotional disturbance. Pain is a central feature of the patients' lives and is usually described in vague, nonspecific terms. It tends to be exacerbated by psychologic or social stressors, and is associated with a multitude of somatic complaints.

FAPS does appear to be less common than IBS, but is nevertheless important to consider, as these patients utilize significant medical resources, are unresponsive to standard medical therapy, and have a high morbidity. Women constitute 70% of this patient population, and a history of physical and sexual abuse is not uncommon. Lack of weight loss and fever, in the absence of major or significant depression, is supportive of a diagnosis of FAPS. Table 3.1 gives management guidelines for patients with FAPS.

Extra-abdominal causes of abdominal pain

This subgroup is more relevant to acute abdominal pain, which is covered in detail in Chapter 22. An example would be a herpes zoster attack [16] involving lower thoracic dermatomes that may be confounded with an acute cholecystitis attack.

Diagnosis
History

The history remains the most important clue to the etiology of abdominal pain. Consequently, several features of the pain are worth identifying to home in on the diagnosis.

Location

In chronic pain disorders, location tends to be less well characterized except in defined pathologies, e.g., sphincter of Oddi dysfunction. Examples of diseases according to the location of the pain are, for **right upper quadrant syndromes**, biliary disease (for example cholelithiasis, sphincter of Oddi dysfunction, cholecystitis, cholangitis, and gallstone pancreatitis); similarly, diaphragmatic, pulmonary (e.g., right lower lobe pneumonia) gastric, pancreatic, and intestinal disorders may also present with right upper quadrant pain. **Left upper quadrant pain** may indicate peptic ulcer disease, splenic rupture (more acute than chronic) or abscess (Table 3.2).

Pain quality

Certain conditions are associated with rather specific pain qualities. Whereas "sharp" or "cutting" pain is characteristic of pancreatitis, "crampy" or "rhythmically squeezing pain" is more typical of intestinal obstruction. Although renal and biliary pain is described as typically colicky, obstruction of either organ may yield a rather constant pain. The pain of appendicitis, on the other hand, may be gnawing and dull.

Pain severity

It is easy to classify acute abdominal pain as severe, moderate, or mild. Chronic pain, on the other hand, is much more difficult to assess, as psychological factors play an important role in modifying pain perception. One must therefore resort to an indirect assessment of pain severity, that is., whether the pain interferes with sleep or daily activities.

Aggravating and alleviating factors

The identification of pain-modifying factors may further help in the diagnosis and management of abdominal pain. For example, pain relieved by acid suppression indicates reflux esophagitis, or peptic ulcer disease. Pain from pancreatitis, intestinal obstruction, mesenteric ischemia, and gastric ulcer is almost always exacerbated by food intake. Meal intake, on the other hand, may relieve duodenal ulcer pain. Body position may also impact abdominal pain: spinal hyperextension relieves irritable bowel pain, but exacerbates pancreatic pain, which is relieved by leaning forward in the sitting position. Moreover, the supine position exacerbates heartburn, which is relieved by an upright position.

Pain chronology

Changes in the nature of the pain (e.g., from intermittent to constant), in the time to reach peak intensity, as well as diurnal variation, provide valuable information that may assist in reaching a diagnosis. For example, pelvic pain at regular monthly intervals suggests endometriosis.

Associated symptoms

Nausea and/or vomiting commonly accompany abdominal pain. The temporal relation to pain may hint to the etiology: pain precedes nausea in patients with a disorder requiring surgery, but tends to follow nausea in nonsurgical disorders. When occurring early in the disease course, a fever may suggest cholangitis or a urinary infection. On the other hand, fevers that develop late in the disease course may implicate diverticulitis, cholecystitis, or appendicitis. Patients with familial Mediterranean fever, and those with connective tissue diseases, may have arthritis and/or pleuritis. Accompanying jaundice should suggest pancreatobiliary disorders. If anorexia and weight loss are prominent, one should suspect a malignant process. Fever may suggest intra-abdominal abscesses, autoimmune disorders, or malignancies such as lymphoma.

Physical examination

The examination should start by noting the general appearance and well-being of the patient. Severe pain is invariably reflected in the face, although this may be less apparent or nonexistent in patients with chronic pain. Moreover, restlessness with diaphoresis point to a more severe illness. Patients with peritonitis usually lie motionless. A complete physical examination is mandatory with special attention to abdominal, rectal, pelvic, and genitourinary regions. On abdominal examination, the presence of bowel sounds should be elicited to look for evidence of ileus, or bowel obstruction. This should be followed by gentle percussion for peritoneal signs, distention, or the presence of ascites. Muscular guarding (or abdominal rigidity) is an early indication of the presence of peritoneal inflammation. The "Carnett's" sign refers to increased local tenderness during muscle tensing. While supine, the patient is asked to simultaneously raise both legs off the table (at the same time) while the examining finger is on the painful site. Another maneuver is to raise only the head while in the supine position, which can serve the same purpose. These maneuvers cause the rectus abdominis muscles to tighten, thus increasing the pain from the entrapped nerve. An important point to remember with this test is that a pure visceral source of the pain is associated with less tenderness when abdominal muscles are tense.

The sensitivity and specificity of the Carnett's sign have not been well established. The largest study included 33 patients with chronic abdominal wall pain who were compared with 62 patients with visceral pain. The sensitivity and specificity of the Carnett's sign were 78 and 88 percent, respectively. However, inter-observer agreement was only 76 percent. Of note, the Carnett's sign may not be interpretable in patients who cannot adequately comply with performing the maneuver. Moreover, a false positive test may occur from visceral causes of pain that involve the local parietal peritoneum.

Palpation is also important to detect enlarged organs or masses, and identify any focal points of tenderness, which if present may warrant further investigation. Weight should be followed over time, and evidence of dehydration (such as orthostatic changes in vital signs) should be sought further. Focal pain that worsens when the patient flexes their abdominal muscles is suggestive of abdominal wall pain.

Other parts of the examination are also indispensable, as any finding may provide valuable diagnostic information. For instance, scleral icterus and jaundice suggest hepatic, pancreaticobiliary, or hemolytic disease. Adenopathy with hepatomegaly may point to malignancy. Perianal fissures or fistulae may suggest Crohn's disease. Skin findings such as purpura may suggest vasculitis or an autoimmune process.

Initial diagnostic testing

The following lab tests constitute a reasonable initial evaluation for patients with chronic abdominal pain:

* Complete blood count with differential
* Electrolytes, BUN, creatinine, glucose and calcium
* Liver panel including a bilirubin
* Lipase
* Iron studies including ferritin.

The above lab studies should be normal in patients with functional abdominal pain. However, they are important to rule out anemia, and signs of inflammation (elevated white blood cell count, and/or elevated platelet counts). A low ferritin suggests iron deficiency, which should raise the suspicion of conditions such as celiac disease or inflammatory bowel disease. Although abdominal pain is not a common presentation of hyper- or hypothyroidism, when symptoms suggest abnormalities of thyroid function, a thyroid stimulating hormone (TSH) should be measured.

C-reactive protein and ESR are nonspecific, yet sensitive markers that may point to an occult organic disease, and may have some utility in ruling out an organic cause of chronic abdominal pain and diarrhea.

Future perspectives

Our understanding of the exact pathophysiology of chronic abdominal pain syndromes remains limited; hence, current therapeutic interventions remain modest at best. Despite the fact that our approach to these disorders should remain multidisciplinary, the ongoing trials for the development of drugs with multiple yet more specific sites of action in the pain pathway are quite promising. Newer drugs have been studied for the treatment of IBS, the newest being 5-HT3 antagonists and 5-HT4 agonists. These drugs have been shown effective in decreasing visceral sensitivity and pain. One would speculate that expansion of this work to target specific receptor types at one or multiple synapse levels (primary, secondary, or tertiary neurons, and/or centrally) may yield more pain relief with minimal side effects (for example alteration in bowel motility, or sedation, in the case of centrally acting drugs). Lubiprostone, a locally acting chloride channel activator, enhances chloride-rich intestinal fluid secretion. It received initial approval from the United States Food and Drug Administration for treatment of chronic idiopathic constipation but later also received approval for treatment of irritable bowel syndrome with constipation in women 18 years and older [17]. On a different level, alternative therapies are gaining more attention. For example, hypnotism has been shown in randomized controlled trials to enhance coping mechanisms and reduce pain in patients with IBS. Therefore, an integrated multidisciplinary approach to manage chronic abdominal pain syndromes seems indispensable, and should inform the development of future therapeutic strategies.

SOURCES OF INFORMATION FOR PATIENTS AND DOCTORS

http://www.nlm.nih.gov/medlineplus/abdominalpain.html
Children: http://www.aafp.org/afp/990401ap/1823.html

References

1. Melzack R, Wall PD. Pain mechanisms: a new theory. *Science.* 1965;150:971–979.
2. Kalloo AN. Overview of differential diagnoses of abdominal pain. *Gastrointest Endosc.* 2002;56:675–680.
3. Leek B. Abdominal visceral receptors. In: Neil E, ed. *Enteroceptors: handbook of sensory physiology*, vol. 3. New York: Springer; 1972,113.
4. Yamamoto W, Kono H, Maekawa H, *et al.* The relationship between abdominal pain regions and specific diseases: an epidemiologic approach to clinical practice. *J Epidemiol.* 1997;7:27–32.
5. Fields H. *Pain. New* York: McGraw-Hill, 1987.
6. Moawad J, Gewertz BL. Chronic mesenteric ischemia. Clinical presentation and diagnosis. *Surg Clin North Am.* 1997;77:357–369.
7. Poole JW, Sammartano RJ, Boley SJ. Hemodynamic basis of the pain of chronic mesenteric ischemia. *Am J Surg.* 1987;153:171–176.
8. Lankisch PG. The problem of diagnosing chronic pancreatitis. *Dig Liver Dis.* 2003;35:131–134.
9. Evans JP, Cooper J, Roediger WE. Diverticular colitis—therapeutic and etiological considerations. *Colorectal Dis.* 2002;4:208–212.
10. Chambers PC. Coeliac plexus block for upper abdominal cancer pain. *Br J Nursing.* 2003;12:838–844.
11. Schwetz I, Bradesi S, Mayer EA. Current insights into the pathophysiology of irritable bowel syndrome. *Curr Gastroenterol Rep.* 2003;5:331–336.
12. Hoogerwerf WA, Pasricha PJ, Kalloo AN, *et al.* Pain: the overlooked symptom in gastroparesis. *Am J Gastroenterol.* 1999;94:1029–1033.
13. Vakil N. Epigastric pain in dyspepsia and reflux disease. *Rev Gastroenterol Disord.* 2003;3(Suppl 4):S16–S21.
14. Kurata JH, Nogawa AN, Everhart JE. A prospective study of dyspepsia in primary care. *Dig Dis Sci.* 2002;47:797–803.
15. Westbrook JI, McIntosh JH, Duggan JM. Accuracy of provisional diagnoses of dyspepsia in patients undergoing first endoscopy. *Gastrointes Endosc.* 2001;53:283–288.
16. Au WY, Ma SY, Cheng VC, *et al.* Disseminated zoster, hyponatremia, severe abdominal pain and leukemia relapse: recognition of a new clinical quartet after bone marrow transplantation. *Br J Dermatol.* 2003;149:862–886.
17. Drossman DA, Chey WD, Johanson JF, *et al.* Clinical trial: lubiprostone in patients with constipation-associated irritable bowel syndrome – results of two randomized, placebo-controlled studies. *Aliment Pharmacol Ther.* 2009;29(3):329–341.

CHAPTER 4

Dyspepsia: ulcer and non-ulcer/bloating and early satiety/belching and rumination

Alexander C. Ford[1] and Paul Moayyedi[2]

[1]St. James's University Hospital, Leeds, UK
[2]Health Sciences Centre, McMaster University, Hamilton, ON, Canada

---

KEY POINTS

- Dyspepsia is common
- The commonest clinically significant finding encountered at upper gastrointestinal endoscopy is gastro-esophageal reflux disease
- Most peptic ulcers are caused by either *Helicobacter pylori* or non-steroidal anti-inflammatory drugs
- Most patients will have no structural cause for their symptoms; these individuals have functional dyspepsia
- The chronic, relapsing and remitting course of functional dyspepsia should be explained to the patient at the earliest opportunity
- Repeated investigation to reassure the patient with functional dyspepsia is inadvisable

Introduction

Dyspepsia is a hybrid word, derived from Latin and Greek, meaning bad (*dys*) digestion (*pepsis*). The term was coined a few centuries ago, but symptoms consistent with the condition were described over 2000 years ago. Diagnosis and treatment of the underlying cause for dyspepsia remained empirical until the advent of radiology in the early part of the twentieth century, and the development of fiberoptic endoscopy in the late 1960s allowed further advances in management. The absence of any structural pathology to account for the symptoms of dyspepsia following examination of the upper gastrointestinal (GI) tract by either of these techniques led to the description of a new condition, non-ulcer dyspepsia. This term has, however, been superseded in the last 10–15 years by the phrase **functional dyspepsia**.

What is it?

Dyspepsia is a complex of symptoms referable to the upper GI tract. Beyond this there is no consistent agreement as to which particular symptoms make up the condition. As a result there are various definitions of dyspepsia in existence. In 1988 a working party met and proposed in their report that a broad definition of dyspepsia, which included symptoms such as

heartburn and reflux, be used [1]. The Rome committee met for the first time in 1991, and the definition of dyspepsia was restricted to a feeling of **pain and discomfort centered in the upper abdomen** [2]. Heartburn and reflux were considered to be cardinal symptoms of gastro-esophageal reflux disease, and were therefore excluded from the symptom complex. The Rome criteria have been revised on two subsequent occasions and the latest iteration, the **Rome III** criteria, now divide dyspepsia into two distinct syndromes: **epigastric pain** and **postprandial distress** [3].

The exclusion of symptoms suggestive of gastro-esophageal reflux disease from the definition of organic and functional dyspepsia is very useful for research purposes, where the aim is to recruit individuals with homogeneous symptoms into clinical trials of therapies for these conditions in secondary or tertiary care, but it may not be generalizable to primary care, where individuals often present with numerous overlapping symptoms [4], which are not necessarily predictive of underlying pathology [5]. In fact, there is recent evidence to suggest that even when individuals with Rome-defined dyspepsia do undergo upper GI endoscopy, the commonest organic finding encountered is erosive esophagitis [6].

How common is it?

There have been numerous cross-sectional surveys reporting the prevalence of dyspepsia in the general population, which varies according to the criteria used to define its presence. The **prevalence** is between 30% and 40% if a broad definition is used [7,8], but if the Rome criteria are used it is between 10% and 25% [9,10].

In terms of the prevalence of underlying clinically significant findings encountered at upper GI endoscopy in individuals with dyspepsia, a recent systematic review and meta-analysis that pooled data from studies performing upper GI endoscopy in unselected individuals with dyspepsia reported a prevalence of 13% for erosive esophagitis, 8% for peptic ulcer

---

disease, and less than 1% for upper GI malignancy, whilst almost 80% of individuals had a structurally normal upper GI tract [11].

Pathophysiology
Ulcer and non-ulcer epigastric pain
The normal gastric mucosal defence mechanisms, which include adherent mucous gel, mucosal bicarbonate secretion, and paracellular junctions between gastric mucosal cells, all serve to create a pH gradient between the lumen of the stomach and the epithelial cells of the mucosa. In peptic ulcer disease these defences become compromised, leading to damage of the mucosa by acid and pepsin. The commonest causes of mucosal compromise are *Helicobacter pylori* (*H. pylori*) and non-steroidal anti-inflammatory drugs (NSAIDs). Subjects infected with *H. pylori* demonstrate either antral or corpus-predominant gastritis on gastric biopsy [12]. Which of these develops may depend upon parietal cell mass of the individual at the time of infection [13]. In duodenal ulcer, antral gastritis occurs [14], leading to hypergastrinemia [15] and hypersecretion of acid by the corpus [16].

Excess acid entering the duodenal bulb causes gastric metaplasia in the duodenum, allowing colonisation by *H. pylori*. The bacterium then promotes focal ulceration through a combination of induction of an inflammatory response, epithelial injury, and reduced duodenal bicarbonate excretion. In gastric ulcer, on the other hand, *H. pylori* infection usually promotes a pangastritis, with subsequent gastric atrophy and, as a result, total acid secretion is reduced [12]. However the compromise of the mucosal defence, and the inflammatory response to infection that results, can lead to gastric ulceration even in a relatively hypochlorhydric environment.

Non-steroidal anti-inflammatory drugs exert their harmful effects on the gastric mucosa through a combination of inhibition of local prostaglandin synthesis, activation of circulating neutrophils, and alterations in the integrity of the vascular endothelium [17]. This impairs the integrity of the mucosal defence mechanisms, allowing ulceration to occur.

Postprandial distress
The pathogenesis of **functional dyspepsia** remains poorly understood, and it is unlikely that there is a single unifying explanation for the symptoms that sufferers experience. Although there is no convincing evidence that patients with functional dyspepsia have a higher acid output than normal individuals, some investigators have reported that direct instillation of acid into the duodenum reproduces their symptoms suggesting hypersensitivity to low pH [18]. **Abnormal pain processing** has also been implicated. Subjects with functional dyspepsia demonstrate increased visceral perception to mechanical distension of the stomach [19], and activation of the central nervous system in response to this type of stimulus occurs at a lower threshold than in healthy controls [20]. **Gastric motility** is also thought to be impaired in a subset of

individuals with functional dyspepsia. A meta-analysis of case-control studies reported that delayed gastric emptying was present in almost 40% of functional dyspepsia patients, and that gastric emptying was, on average, 1.5 times slower than in normal individuals [21]. Functional dyspepsia may be exacerbated by **psychological co-morbidity**. A recent study conducted in tertiary care demonstrated that symptoms in patients with functional dyspepsia were significantly more severe in those with a history of depression, childhood sexual abuse, or somatisation [22].

Causes
Despite a declining prevalence of infection in the developed world, *H. pylori* is still the main cause of most **duodenal and gastric ulcers** worldwide. Of the reminder, the majority are caused by NSAIDs, with more rare diagnoses such as Zollinger-Ellison syndrome and Crohn's disease of the upper GI tract accounting for less than 1% of total ulcer burden. Stress ulcers are an important pathological phenomenon in the critically ill patient in intensive care, and these occur due to acute injury arising from compromised mucosal defences as described earlier.

In **functional dyspepsia**, etiological factors are less well-defined. Some investigators have reported that the prevalence of *H. pylori* is higher in individuals with functional dyspepsia than in healthy asymptomatic individuals [23], and eradication of the infection appears to be of modest benefit in terms of symptom improvement [24]. In addition, as with irritable bowel syndrome, there appears to be a **post-infectious form of dyspepsia**. In a case-control study the odds ratio for dyspepsia in cases with bacterial gastroenteritis, confirmed by a positive stool culture, compared with non-exposed individuals was 2.9 at 6 months post-infection [25]. In a series of dyspeptic patients undergoing investigation, 17% reported an acute onset of symptoms accompanied by other symptoms suggestive of an infective process, such as fever, myalgia, diarrhea, or vomiting [26]. The authors of this study demonstrated that there was a defect in gastric accommodation at the level of intrinsic nitrergic neurons in the stomach, and postulated that this impairment of function arose as a consequence of transient GI inflammation induced during an acute infection.

Symptom complexes
The original report from the Working Party in 1988 divided dyspepsia into categories, according to the predominant symptom reported by the patient [1]. These included dyspepsia which was ulcer-like, reflux-like, dysmotility-like, and idiopathic (where symptom overlap prevented clear division into one of the first three categories). With the advent of the Rome process [2] and the exclusion of symptoms suggestive of gastro-esophageal reflux disease from the definition, subgroups of symptom complexes have become increasingly well-defined

and discrete. The current Rome III criteria describe two distinct entities, epigastric pain syndrome and post-prandial distress syndrome [3]. **Epigastric pain syndrome** is defined as intermittent pain or burning localised to the epigastrium, which does not generalise to other abdominal or chest regions, does not fulfil criteria for other functional GI disorders such as irritable bowel syndrome, is of moderate severity, and has occurred once per week or more for at least the last 3 months. Post-prandial distress syndrome consists of fullness or early satiety, which interferes with the consumption of a normal-sized meal, and has occurred several times per week for at least the last 3 months. The rationale for the creation of these entities was primarily for therapeutic and pathophysiological research purposes. At the present time, there have been few prospective validation studies conducted to confirm the utility of this approach in clinical practice.

Despite attempts to classify dyspepsia, gastro-esophageal reflux disease, and irritable bowel syndrome separately, there is evidence that these symptom complexes demonstrate a lack of stability over time, particularly over extended periods of follow-up [27,28], as well as a significant degree of overlap. A recent systematic review and meta-analysis reported that the prevalence of irritable bowel syndrome in individuals with dyspepsia was 8-fold that of asymptomatic individuals [29].

Diagnosis

The ability of the clinician to distinguish between organic causes of dyspepsia and functional dyspepsia on clinical grounds alone is poor. Perhaps as a result of this, computer models have been developed by researchers in an attempt to differentiate between the two more accurately. These models incorporate patient demographics, risk factors, and items from the clinical history and use statistical techniques including logistic regression and discriminant analysis. A systematic review and meta-analysis, that examined the accuracy of both a physician's opinion and statistical models in discriminating between organic and functional dyspepsia in symptomatic individuals referred for upper GI endoscopy, found that both these techniques performed only modestly in predicting an organic cause of dyspepsia accurately [30].

According to the Rome definition of **functional dyspepsia**, the diagnosis is one of exclusion, and requires that any structural abnormality that could explain the patient's symptoms be excluded by upper GI investigation. In practice dyspepsia is so common that many patients' management will be pragmatic on the basis of a clinical history. In some patients, particularly where there is new onset in older patients or alarm features, upper GI endoscopy will be the investigation of choice. The accuracy of endoscopy at diagnosing peptic ulcer disease is not well-reported, but it appears that the sensitivity and specificity are in excess of 95%. Once a peptic ulcer has been detected at upper GI endoscopy, exclusion of *H. pylori* infection is warranted, and this will usually be done at the time of the examination by obtaining gastric biopsies for either

rapid urease testing or histological examination. Eradication of the organism in this situation is effective in both facilitating ulcer healing and preventing ulcer relapse [31]. In the absence of *H. pylori* infection, it is important to question the patient about NSAID use, particularly in over-the-counter preparations. In the absence of NSAID use, rarer causes of peptic ulcer need to be considered and excluded.

As the diagnosis of functional dyspepsia is one of exclusion, and individuals may present with multiple abdominal symptoms, other conditions such as endoscopy-negative reflux disease, gallstones, celiac disease, and small bowel or pancreatic pathology may need to be ruled out using 24-hour pH studies, abdominal ultrasound, serological testing, or cross-sectional abdominal imaging, before the diagnosis can be reached with confidence. However, there is little evidence that the reassurance value of a negative test will allay the patient's fears of underlying organic illness for any significant length of time [32] and the use of repeated testing in an attempt to ameliorate this anxiety is inadvisable. It is preferable to explain the diagnosis and natural history of the condition to the patient at the earliest opportunity, in an attempt to reduce future healthcare-seeking behavior.

References

1. Colin-Jones DG, Bloom B, Bodemar G, *et al.* Management of dyspepsia: report of a working party. *Lancet.* 1988;331:576–579.
2. Talley NJ, Colin-Jones DG, Koch KL, *et al.* Functional dyspepsia: a classification with guidelines for diagnosis and management. *Gastroenterology Intl.* 1991;4:145–160.
3. Tack J, Talley NJ, Camilleri M, *et al.* Functional gastroduodenal disorders. *Gastroenterology.* 2006;130:1466–1479.
4. Tougas G, Chen MS, Hwang P, *et al.* Prevalence and impact of upper gastrointestinal symptoms in the Canadian population: Findings from the DIGEST study. *Am J Gastroenterol.* 1999;94(10): 2845–2854.
5. Johnsen R, Bernersen B, Straume B, *et al.* Prevalence of endoscopic and histological findings in subjects with and without dyspepsia. *Br Med J.* 1991;302:749–752.
6. Vakil N, Talley NJ, Veldhuyzen van Zanten S, *et al.* Cost of detecting malignant lesions by endoscopy in 2741 primary care dyspeptic patients without alarm symptoms. *Clin Gastroenterol Hepatol.* 2009;7:756–761.
7. Jones R, Lydeard S. Prevalence of symptoms of dyspepsia in the community. *Br Med J.* 1989;298:30–32.
8. Moayyedi P, Forman D, Braunholtz D, *et al.* The proportion of upper gastrointestinal symptoms in the community associated with *Helicobacter pylori*, lifestyle factors, and nonsteroidal anti-inflammatory drugs. *Am J Gastroenterol.* 2000;95(6):1448–1455.
9. Talley NJ, Fett SL, Zinsmeister AR, *et al.* Gastrointestinal tract symptoms and self-reported abuse: a population- based study. *Gastroenterology.* 1994;107:1040–1049.
10. Talley NJ, Boyce PM, Jones M. Dyspepsia and health care seeking in a community: how important are psychological factors? *Dig Dis Sci.* 1998;43:1016–1022.
11. Ford AC, Marwaha A, Lim A, *et al.* What is the prevalence of clinically significant endoscopic findings in subjects with dyspepsia? Systematic review and meta-analysis. *Clin Gastroenterol Hepatol.* 2010;8:830–837.

12. Schultze V, Hackelsberger A, Gunther T, *et al.* Differing patterns of *Helicobacter pylori* gastritis in patients with duodenal, prepyloric, and gastric ulcer disease. *Scand J Gastroenterol.* 1998;33: 137–142.

13. Blaser MJ, Chyou P-H, Nomura A. Age at establishment of *Helicobacter pylori* infection and gastric carcinoma, gastric ulcer, and duodenal ulcer risk. *Cancer Res.* 1995;55:562–565.

14. Wyatt JI, Rathbone BJ, Dixon MF, *et al. Campylobacter pyloridis* and acid induced gastric metaplasia in the pathogenesis of duodenitis. *J Clin Pathol.* 1987;40:841–848.

15. McColl KE, Fullarton GM, Chittajalu R, *et al.* Plasma gastrin, daytime intragastric pH, and nocturnal acid output before and at 1 and 7 months after eradication of *Helicobacter pylori* in duodenal ulcer subjects. *Scand J Gastroenterol.* 1991;26:339–346.

16. El-Omar EM, Penman ID, Ardill JE, *et al. Helicobacter pylori* infection and abnormalities of acid secretion in patients with duodenal ulcer disease. *Gastroenterology.* 1995;109:681–691.

17. Wallace JL, Keenan CM, Granger DM. Gastric ulceration induced by nonsteroidal anti-inflammatory drugs is a neutrophil-dependent process. *Am J Physiol.* 1990;259:G462–G467.

18. Samsom M, Verhagen MA, van Berge Henegouwen GP, *et al.* Abnormal clearance of exogenous acid and increased acid sensitivity of the proximal duodenum in dyspeptic patients. *Gastroenterology.* 1999;116:515–520.

19. Salet GA, Samsom F, Roelofs JM, *et al.* Responses to gastric distension in functional dyspepsia. *Gut.* 1998;42:823–829.

20. Vandenberghe J, Dupont P, van Oudenhove L, *et al.* Regional cerebral blood flow during gastric balloon distension in functional dyspepsia. *Gastroenterology.* 2007;132:1684–1693.

21. Quartero AO, de Wit NJ, Lodder AC, *et al.* Disturbed solid-phase gastric emptying in functional dyspepsia: A meta-analysis. *Dig Dis Sci.* 1998;43:2028–2033.

22. van Oudenhove L, Vandenberghe J, Geeraerts B, *et al.* Determinants of symptoms in functional dyspepsia: Gastric sensorimotor function, psychosocial factors or somatisation? *Gut.* 2008;57:1666–1673.

23. Bernersen B, Johnsen R, Bostad L, *et al.* Is *Helicobacter pylori* the cause of dyspepsia? *Br Med J.* 1992;304:1276–1279.

24. Moayyedi P, Deeks J, Talley NJ, *et al.* An update of the Cochrane systematic review of *Helicobacter pylori* eradication therapy in non-ulcer dyspepsia: resolving the discrepancy between systematic reviews. *Am J Gastroenterol.* 2003;98:2621–2626.

25. Parry SD, Stansfield R, Jelley D, *et al.* Does bacterial gastroenteritis predispose people to functional gastrointestinal disorders? A prospective, community-based, case-control study. *Am J Gastroenterol.* 2003;98:1970–1975.

26. Tack J, Demedts I, Dehondt G, *et al.* Clinical and pathophysiological characteristics of acute-onset functional dyspepsia. *Gastroenterology.* 2002;122:1738–1747.

27. Agreus L, Svardsudd K, Talley NJ, *et al.* Natural history of gastroesophageal reflux disease and functional abdominal disorders. *Am J Gastroenterol.* 2001;96:2905–2914.

28. Ford AC, Forman D, Bailey AG, *et al.* Fluctuation of gastrointestinal symptoms in the community: a 10-year longitudinal follow-up study. *Aliment Pharmacol Ther.* 2008;28:1013–1020.

29. Ford AC, Marwaha A, Lim A, *et al.* Systematic review and meta-analysis of the prevalence of irritable bowel syndrome in individuals with dyspepsia. *Clin Gastroenterol Hepatol.* 2010;8: 401–409.

30. Moayyedi P, Talley NJ, Fennerty MB, *et al.* Can the clinical history distinguish between organic and functional dyspepsia? *JAMA.* 2006;295:1566–1576.

31. Ford AC, Delaney BC, Forman D, *et al.* Eradication therapy in *Helicobacter pylori* positive peptic ulcer disease: systematic review and economic analysis. *Am J Gastroenterol.* 2004;99:1833–1855.

32. Lucock MP, Morley S, White C, *et al.* Responses of consecutive patients to reassurance after gastroscopy: results of self administered questionnaire survey. *Br Med J.* 1997;315:572–575.

CHAPTER 5
Nausea and vomiting

Jan Tack

Translational Research Center for Gastrointestinal Diseases (TARGID), University of Leuven; University Hospital Gasthuisberg, Leuven, Belgium

---

KEY POINTS

- Nausea is the sensation of the imminent need to vomit, while vomiting is the forceful oral expulsion of gastric contents
- Most causes can be easily diagnosed on routine clinical grounds
- Functional gastroduodenal disorders and gastroparesis are frequently associated with nausea and vomiting
- If severe and/or prolonged, loss of water and electrolytes may lead to dehydration and hypokalaemic metabolic acidosis
- Gastric motor disorders may be considered in refractory cases and investigated by measurement of gastric emptying
- Antiemetics are often given as symptomatic treatment, regardless of the underlying cause

---

Introduction

Nausea and vomiting are commonly reported symptoms in the general population, as well as in consultations with general practitioners and gastroenterologists. **Nausea** is the unpleasant sensation of the imminent need to vomit. The symptoms usually comprise epigastric discomfort as well as a generalized feeling of sickness. **Vomiting** is the forceful oral expulsion of gastric contents associated with contraction of the abdominal and chest wall muscles. Vomiting is usually preceded by and associated with **retching**, repetitive contractions of the abdominal wall without expulsion of gastric contents.

Vomiting needs to be distinguished from **regurgitation**, which is characterized by the effortless return of food back into the mouth, in the absence of contraction of the abdominal and chest wall muscles. Regurgitation is not preceded by nausea or retching and results from esophageal disorders like achalasia or severe reflux disease.

Rumination is another entity that needs to be distinguished from vomiting. Rumination is characterized by the effortless regurgitation of undigested food after every meal. Although the mechanism is a transient voluntary increase in abdominal pressure, occurring during or soon after finishing a meal, this is usually not a conscious act. Rumination is not preceded by nausea or retching and the food does not have an acidic taste. Depending on the circumstances, the patient may spit out or reswallow the food.

Two classes of disorders frequently associated with nausea and vomiting are the functional gastroduodenal disorders and gastroparesis [1,2]. **Gastroparesis** is characterized by delayed gastric emptying in the absence of mechanical obstruction [2]. A large number of patients seen in gastroenterology practice have chronic symptoms that are not readily explained by underlying organic disease and are attributable to the gastroduodenal region [1]. This group with functional gastroduodenal disorders includes patients who experience dyspeptic symptoms (early satiation, postprandial fullness, epigastric pain or burning), excessive belching, or recurrent unexplained nausea or vomiting without underlying organic disease. According to the Rome III consensus, the functional gastroduodenal disorders are subdivided into functional dyspepsia, belching disorders, nausea and vomiting disorders, and rumination syndrome [1].

Differential diagnosis

Nausea and vomiting are controlled by the vomiting center in the medulla oblongata in the brainstem. A variety of stimuli can activate the vomiting center: the vagal sensory pathways from chemo- or mechano-receptors in the gastrointestinal tract, neural pathways from the labyrinth of higher centers of the cortex, intracranial baroreceptors, and the chemoreceptor trigger zone (CTZ), which is activated by a variety of drugs and toxins (Figure 5.1).

Nausea and vomiting may occur as a result of many systemic and gastroenterological disorders (Table 5.1). In spite of the long and varied list of potentially involved disorders, most causes of nausea and vomiting can be readily diagnosed on routine clinical grounds.

Gastrointestinal as well as extraintestinal infections may be associated with acute nausea and vomiting. Gastric or intestinal obstruction as well as a number of acute abdominal disorders may present with or may be associated with nausea and vomiting. A number of chemical substances, either given as drug therapy or accidentally ingested, may stimulate the CTZ. Extensive lists of drugs that may induce nausea and vomiting are available in the literature [3]. Postoperative nausea and vomiting may be in part related to the use of drugs in the perioperative setting, and in part to the associated derangement in gastrointestinal motor function. Several metabolic and

---

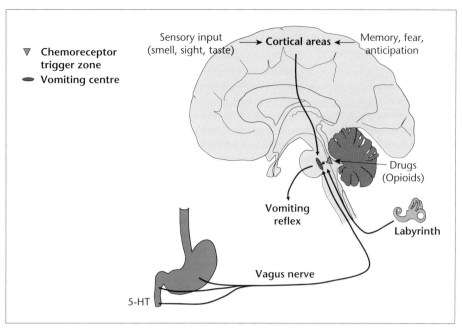

Figure 5.1 Pathways involved in triggering nausea and vomiting. (This figure was published in *Clinical Gastroenterology and Hepatology*, Wilfred M. Weinstein, Christopher J. Hawkey, Jaime Bosch, Nausea and vomiting, Pages 1–5, Copyright Elsevier, 2005.)

endocrine disorders may also be associated with nausea and vomiting, which are occasionally the presenting symptoms [1].

Functional and motor disorders are important causes of nausea and vomiting, to be considered once organic disease has been ruled out. Gastroparesis and functional nausea and vomiting disorders are the most important causes, but less frequent conditions like pseudo-obstruction syndrome or the so-called cyclic nausea and vomiting syndrome (a relatively rare idiopathic disorder characterized by acute episodes of nausea and vomiting separated by intervening asymptomatic periods), should also be considered.

Finally, a number of central nervous system disorders and primary psychiatric syndromes may present with or be complicated by nausea and vomiting.

Complications

Loss of water and electrolytes, caused by severe and/or prolonged vomiting episodes, may lead to dehydration and hypokalemic metabolic alkalosis, mainly due to the loss of hydrochloric acid-containing gastric secretions. Profound hypokalemia may induce abnormalities of cardiac rhythm and of skeletal muscle control.

Clinical approach

History taking should identify the principal and associated symptoms, their course of onset, frequency, and duration. Careful history taking will allow vomiting to be differentiated from regurgitation and rumination, and will identify associ-

ated symptoms suggestive of reflux disease, peptic ulcer, obstruction, etc. A practical approach to diagnosis and treatment is outlined in Figure 5.2.

The timing and duration of the symptoms may help to indicate the most likely etiology. Nausea and vomiting of recent onset is most suggestive of an infectious cause (gastroenteritis), acute abdominal event (pancreatitis, obstruction) or drug-induced vomiting. The timing of vomiting may also provide clues to the underlying disorder. Early morning vomiting, before breakfast, is most suggestive of pregnancy, intracranial hypertension or uremia, or may be alcohol related. Late postprandial vomiting is most compatible with gastroparesis or obstruction, whereas vomiting that occurs during or immediately after food ingestion is more suggestive of a psychogenic cause, and should raise suspicion of rumination. Projectile vomiting, that is, forceful and not preceded by nausea, is a sign of intracranial hypertension. Conditioned, "learned" vomiting may lead to persistent symptoms once the acute cause has regressed, as seen in late chemotherapy-induced vomiting and after a transient organic disorder [4].

The physical examination should look for signs that reveal the etiology of nausea and vomiting, and assess signs suggestive of complications of nausea and vomiting. In addition, a neurologic examination is indispensable as it may provide clues to a central nervous system cause for the symptoms [5].

Initial diagnostic evaluations will be aimed at identifying underlying causes suspected from the clinical evaluation, and ruling out peptic ulcer and obstruction. Routine laboratory testing should be done in all patients to assess the influence on blood electrolytes, and in women of childbearing potential,

Table 5.1 Causes of nausea and vomiting

Organic gastrointestinal diseases	Gastrointestinal motor and functional disorders
• Peptic ulcer • Mechanical obstruction • Biliary colic • Pancreatic tumors • Secondary gastroparesis (diabetes, vagotomy, scleroderma, etc.) • Peritonitis (cholecystitis, pancreatitis, appendicitis, etc.) • Hepatitis • Gastrointestinal ischemia	• Functional dyspepsia • Idiopathic gastroparesis • Chronic idiopathic intestinal pseudo-obstruction • Idiopathic nausea and vomiting syndrome • Roux-en-Y syndrome • Cyclic nausea and vomiting disorder

Toxic or drug-induced	Postoperative nausea and vomiting

• Ethanol
• Cancer chemotherapy
• Radiotherapy
• Miscellaneous drugs (analgesics, antibiotics, cardiovascular drugs, etc.)
• Miscellaneous intoxications
	• Central nervous system disorders:
	  – Migraine
	  – Increased intracranial pressure (tumor, hemorrhage, infection, etc.)
	  – Seizure disorders
	  – Labyrinthine disorders (motion sickness, labyrinthitis', Ménière's disease, etc.)
	• Psychiatric disorders:
	  – Psychogenic nausea and vomiting
	  – Bulimia nervosa

Endocrine/metabolic disorders
• Pregnancy • Diabetic ketoacidosis • Hyperthyroidism • Uremia • Addison's disease • Parathyroid disorders

a pregnancy test is added. An electrocardiogram may provide additional information on the impact of electrolyte imbalance. The laboratory tests should include a screening thyroid-stimulating hormone measurement. The presence of hyponatremia may suggest a possible Addison's disease. Serum drug levels for patients on digoxin or theophylline may rule out or confirm drug toxicity-related symptoms.

Patients with suspected severe underlying disease (e.g., obstruction) or complications (e.g., dehydration, electrolyte imbalance) will need to be hospitalized. In the absence of these urgent considerations, additional investigations like endoscopy and barium X-rays may be performed on an outpatient basis. In case of a readily identifiable treatable or self-limited cause (e.g., drug adverse effect or viral gastroenteritis), removal of the cause and symptomatic treatment may be the only interventions necessary. In more complex cases, additional examinations are performed to rule out gastrointestinal obstruction

[abdominal computed tomography (CT), small bowel X-ray], metabolic disorders (thyroid function, cortisol, pregnancy test) and central nervous system disorders [CT scan or magnetic resonance imaging (MRI)]. A psychiatric work-up is required for refractory and unexplained cases [5].

If there are no identifiable organic disorders and underlying psychopathology, functional or motor disorders can be considered. The benefit of performing motility studies is controversial, as the diagnostic yield and therapeutic impact of, for instance, finding delayed gastric emptying, is limited.

Assessment of gastric motor function

Gastric motor disorders are often considered in refractory cases. The most popular test is measurement of gastric emptying. Antroduodenojejunal manometry can be performed in cases of suspected generalized motor dysfunction, but its yield is likely to be low. Electrogastrography should be considered an experimental investigation.

Radionuclide gastric emptying is still the standard method to assess gastric emptying rate [6]. Solid and liquid emptying can be assessed separately or simultaneously. The solid and/or liquid meal fractions are each labeled with a (different) radioisotope, usually ^{99}Tc or ^{111}In. The number of counts in a given region of interest (total, proximal or distal stomach, small intestine) is measured during a certain period of time after ingestion of a meal, using a gamma camera. Correction factors for distance to the camera and decay of the isotope are taken into consideration. Mathematical processing with curve fitting allows the half-emptying time, lag phase, and percentage retention at different time points after a meal to be calculated. Although not routinely used, the radioisotope technique also provides information on distribution within the stomach (proximal versus distal). This test is disadvantaged by its use of radioactive labels, high costs, and poor standardization of meal composition and measuring times between different laboratories [6].

The ^{13}C breath test is increasingly considered a valid and practical alternative to the scintigraphic emptying test. The solid or liquid phase of a meal includes a ^{13}C-labeled substrate (octanoic acid, acetic acid, glycin or spirulina) [7–10]. As soon as the labeled substrate leaves the stomach, it is rapidly absorbed and metabolized in the liver to generate $^{13}CO_2$, which appears in the breath [9]. Breath sampling at regular intervals and mathematical processing of its $^{13}CO_2$ content over time allows a gastric emptying curve to be defined. The advantages of this test are its non-radioactive nature and the ability to perform the test outside a hospital setting. Disadvantages are the lack of standardization of meal and substrate. In spite of its merits, the gastric emptying breath test still has not gained worldwide acceptance [11].

Antropyloroduodenal manometry allows investigation of the mechanisms that are involved in the regulation of normal and abnormal gastric emptying. This is mainly a research tool,

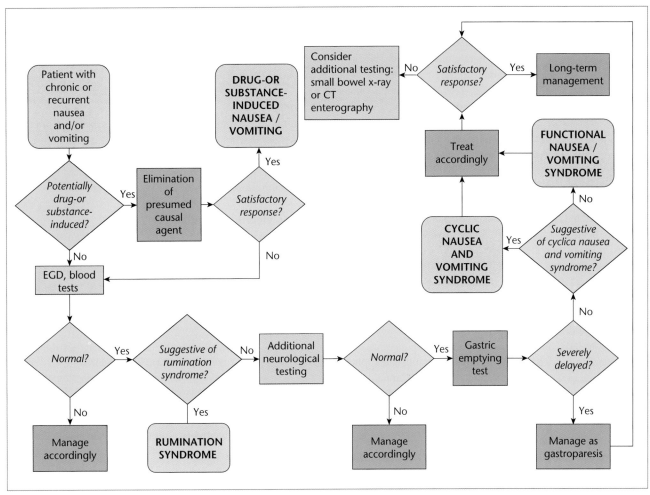

Figure 5.2 Algorithm for a clinical approach to patients with nausea and vomiting. CT, computed tomography; EGD, esophagogastroduodenoscopy.

with clinical application in the investigation of generalized motility disorders, including chronic idiopathic intestinal pseudo-obstruction (CIIP).

Cutaneous electrodes allow the electrical activity of the stomach to be measured. This so-called electrogastrography (EGG) provides information on frequency and regularity of gastric pacemaker activity, as well as changes in power of the signal after meal ingestion. EGG is an experimental tool [12].

Treatment

Figure 5.2 summarizes a diagnostic and therapeutic management algorithm for the patient who presents with nausea and vomiting. Antiemetic agents are often administered as a symptomatic treatment, regardless of the underlying cause. The principal antiemetic drugs are dopamine receptor antagonists, antihistamines, and anticholinergic drugs [1,5].

Dopamine receptors in the area postrema are the target for antiemetic drugs like chlorpromazine, promethazine haloperi-

dol, metoclopramide and domperidone. Older dopamine antagonists of the phenothiazine class (chlorpromazine, promethazine) and butyrophenone class (haloperidol, droperidol). have important central nervous system side effects like sedation, drowsiness, orthostatic hypotension, and extrapyramidal symptoms. Metoclopramide and domperidone are dopamine antagonists with gastroprokinetic properties and are therefore often used in gastroparesis or in functional nausea and vomiting. They have fewer sedative side effects than the older dopamine antagonists. However, metoclopramide may induce extrapyramidal symptoms and orofacial dyskinesia, which make it an unattractive drug to use [13]. Domperidone, which crosses the blood–brain barrier poorly, is almost free from these adverse events, but it has been associated with QT prolongation [14]. All dopamine receptor antagonists may induce hyperprolactinemia and galactorrhea.

Histamine 1 receptor antagonists have central antiemetic effects, but are often associated with drowsiness. Drugs like dramamine or cinnarizine are mainly used in the treatment of motion sickness. Anticholinergics are not widely used in the treatment of nausea and vomiting because of lack of specificity and the occurrence of anticholinergic side effects. The only exception is the use of scopolamine in the treatment of motion sickness.

Serotonin 3 receptor antagonists, developed for the treatment of chemotherapy-induced nausea and vomiting, are more expensive and can be used as second-line drugs. They act on serotonin 3 receptors on the CTZ and on vagal afferents. Examples of this class of drugs are ondansetron, granisetron, and tropisetron. 5-HT$_3$ receptor antagonists have also shown efficacy in postoperative nausea and vomiting [15–17]. Their use in functional or gastroparesis-associated nausea and vomiting has been poorly studied, and available reports do not suggest a major beneficial effect [18]. Neurokinin-1 receptor antagonists are also used for late vomiting associated with chemotherapy [19]. Their role in functional nausea and vomiting or in gastroparesis-associated vomiting has not been explored, but there is emerging data of efficacy in postoperative nausea and vomiting [20].

Corticosteroids and benzodiazepines, both also used in chemotherapy-induced vomiting, have no established application in other causes of nausea and vomiting. Cannabinoids have occasionally been used in refractory nausea and vomiting or chemotherapy-induced nausea and vomiting [21].

Prokinetic agents are mainly used for the treatment of chronic nausea and vomiting resulting from gastroparesis or dyspepsia. Cholinomimetics like bethanechol have been abandoned for lack of specificity and cholinergic side effects. As described above, dopamine antagonists like domperidone and metoclopramide have gastroprokinetic properties and studies have established their efficacy in gastroparesis and dyspepsia [22–24].

Several studies have reported on the successful use of cisapride, a 5-HT$_4$ receptor agonist, in gastroparesis and dyspepsia [25,26], but the drug has been withdrawn because of an enhanced risk of QT prolongation with cardiac arrhythmias [27]. Tegaserod, a 5-HT$_4$ agonist from a different class, has been evaluated in functional dyspepsia and gastroparesis [28,29]. The drug was originally marketed for chronic constipation and irritable bowel syndrome with constipation, but it has been withdrawn because of an increased incidence of cardiovascular ischemic events [30].

Short-term studies in diabetic and postsurgical gastroparesis have reported beneficial effects of treatment with erythromycin (3 x 250–500 mg) [31]. This macrolide antibiotic acts as a motilin receptor agonist and it has prokinetic properties. Attempts to develop macrolide prokinetics devoid of antibiotic properties have been disappointing [32,33].

Botulinum toxin binds to the synaptosomal-associated protein 25 to block acetylcholine release from excitatory nerve endings. Uncontrolled studies suggest benefit from intrapyloric injection of botulinum toxin in gastroparesis, but two controlled studies showed no benefit over saline [34–36].

Nutritional intervention

Endoscopic placement of a percutaneous endoscopic feeding gastrostomy or jejunostomy may provide adequate calorie intake and some symptom relief, but is not devoid of complications [37].

Surgery

Although there are selected reports of favorable outcome, surgical treatment for refractory symptoms of gastroparesis and motility disorders has proven unpredictable and often disappointing [37]. Completion gastrectomy appears to provide benefit in refractory postoperative gastroparesis.

Gastric electrical stimulation

Studies have reported that gastric electrical stimulation may relieve symptoms in patients with intractable nausea and vomiting, and gastroparesis [38,39]. However, controlled trials of this treatment approach have not shown convincing evidence of efficacy [39,40].

References

1. Tack J, Talley NJ, Camilleri M, *et al.* Functional gastroduodenal disorders. *Gastroenterology.* 2006;130:1466–1479.
2. Parkman HP, Camilleri M, Farrugia G, *et al.* Gastroparesis and functional dyspepsia: excerpts from the AGA/ANMS meeting. *Neurogastroenterol Motil.* 2010;22:113–133.
3. Quigley EEM, Hasler WL, Parkman HP. American Gastroenterology Association Technical Review on Nausea and Vomiting. *Gastroenterology.* 2001;120:263–286.
4. Muraoka M, Mine K, Nakai Y, Nakagawa T. Psychogenic vomiting: the relation between patterns of vomiting and psychiatric diagnoses. *Gut.* 1990;31:526–528.
5. Tack J, Talley NJ. Gastroduodenal disorders. *Am J Gastroenterol.* 2010;105:757–763.
6. Abell TL, Camilleri M, Donohoe K, *et al.* American Neurogastroenterology and Motility Society and the Society of Nuclear Medicine. Consensus recommendations for gastric emptying scintigraphy: a joint report of the American Neurogastroenterology and Motility Society and the Society of Nuclear Medicine. *Am J Gastroenterol.* 2008;103:753–763.
7. Ghoos YF, Maes BD, Geypens BJ, *et al.* Measurement of gastric emptying rate of solids by means of a carbon-labeled octanoic acid breath test. *Gastroenterology.* 1993;104:1640–1647.
8. Maes BD, Ghoos YF, Geypens BJ, *et al.* Combined carbon-13-glycine/carbon-14-octanoic acid breath test to monitor gastric emptying rates of liquids and solids. *J Nucl Med.* 1994;35:824–831.
9. Braden B, Adams S, Duan LP, *et al.* The [13C]acetate breath test accurately reflects gastric emptying of liquids in both liquid and semisolid test meals. *Gastroenterology.* 1995;108:1048–1055.
10. Lee JS, Camilleri M, Zinsmeister AR, *et al.* A valid, accurate, office based non-radioactive test for gastric emptying of solids. *Gut.* 2000;46:768–773.
11. Verbeke K. Will the 13C-octanoic acid breath test ever replace scintigraphy as the gold standard to assess gastric emptying? *Neurogastroenterol Motil.* 2009;21:1013–1016.
12. Tack J. Mandatory and optional function tests in gastroduodenal disorders. *Best Pract Res Clin Gastroenterol.* 2009;23:387–393.

13. Rao AS, Camilleri M. Review article: metoclopramide and tardive dyskinesia. *Aliment Pharmacol Ther.* 2010;31:11–19.

14. Rocha CM, Barbosa MM. QT interval prolongation associated with the oral use of domperidone in an infant. *Pediatr Cardiol.* 2005;26:720–723.

15. Tramèr MR, Reynolds DJ, Moore RA, *et al.* Efficacy, dose-response, and safety of ondansetron in prevention of postoperative nausea and vomiting: a quantitative systematic review of randomized placebo-controlled trials. *Anesthesiology.* 1997;87: 1277–1289.

16. Tramèr MR, Moore RA, Reynolds DJ, *et al.* A quantitative systematic review of ondansetron in treatment of established postoperative nausea and vomiting. *BMJ.* 1997;314:1088–1092.

17. Carlisle JB, Stevenson CA. Drugs for preventing postoperative nausea and vomiting. *Cochrane Database Syst Rev.* 2006;3:CD004125.

18. Nielsen OH, Hvid-Jacobsen K, Lund P, *et al.* Gastric emptying and subjective symptoms of nausea: lack of effects of a 5-hydroxytryptamine-3 antagonist ondansetron on gastric emptying in patients with gastric stasis syndrome. *Digestion.* 1990; 46:89–96.

19. Curran MP, Robinson DM. Aprepitant: a review of its use in the prevention of nausea and vomiting. *Drugs.* 2009;69:1853–1878.

20. Apfel CC, Malhotra A, Leslie JB. The role of neurokinin-1 receptor antagonists for the management of postoperative nausea and vomiting. *Curr Opin Anaesthesiol.* 2008;21:427–432.

21. Tramer MR, Carroll D, Campbell FA, *et al.* Cannibinoids for control of chemotherapy induced nausea and vomiting: quantitative systemic review. *BMJ.* 2001;323:16–21.

22. Soo S, Moayyedi P, Deeks J, *et al.* Pharmacological interventions for non-ulcer dyspepsia. *Cochrane Database Syst. Rev* 2000;2: CD001960.

23. Sturm A, Holtmann G, Goebell H, *et al.* Prokinetics in patients with gastroparesis: a systematic analysis. *Digestion.* 1999;60: 422–427.

24. Finney JS, Kinnersley N, Hughes M, *et al.* Meta-analysis of antisecretory and gastrokinetic compounds in functional dyspepsia. *J Clin Gastroenterol.* 1998;26:312–320.

25. Veldhuyzen van Zanten SJ, Jones MJ, Verlinden M, *et al.* Efficacy of cisapride and domperidone in functional dyspepsia: a meta-analysis. *Am J Gastroenterol.* 2001;96:689–696.

26. Corinaldesi R, Stanghellini V, Raiti C, *et al.* Effect of chronic administration of cisapride on gastric emptying of a solid meal and on dyspeptic symptoms in patients with idiopathic gastroparesis. *Gut.* 1987;28:300–305.

27. Enger C, Cali C, Walker AM. Serious ventricular arrhythmias among users of cisapride and other QT-prolonging agents in the United States. *Pharmacoepidemiol Drug Saf.* 2002;11:477–486.

28. Vakil N, Laine L, Talley NJ, *et al.* Tegaserod treatment for dysmotility-like functional dyspepsia: results of two randomized, controlled trials. *Am J Gastroenterol.* 2008;103:1906–1919.

29. Degen L, Matzinger D, Merz M, *et al.* Tegaserod, a 5-HT4 receptor partial agonist, accelerates gastric emptying and gastrointestinal transit in healthy male subjects. *Aliment Pharmacol Ther.* 2001;15:1745–1751.

30. Pasricha PJ. Desperately seeking serotonin…A commentary on the withdrawal of tegaserod and the state of drug development for functional and motility disorders. *Gastroenterology.* 2007; 132:2287–2290.

31. Janssens J, Peeters TL, Vantrappen G, *et al.* Improvement of gastric emptying in diabetic gastroparesis by erythromycin. *N Engl J Med.* 1990;332:1028–1031.

32. Talley NJ, Verlinden M, Snape W, *et al.* Failure of a motilin receptor agonist (ABT-229) to relieve the symptoms of functional dyspepsia in patients with and without delayed gastric emptying: a randomized double-blind placebo-controlled trial. *Aliment Pharmacol Ther.* 2000;14:1653–1661.

33. Talley NJ, Verlinden M, Geenen DJ, *et al.* Effects of a motilin receptor agonist (ABT-229) on upper gastrointestinal symptoms in type 1 diabetes mellitus: a randomised, double blind, placebo controlled trial. *Gut.* 2001;49:395–401.

34. Arts J, van Gool S, Caenepeel P, *et al.* Influence of intrapyloric botulinum toxin injection on gastric emptying and meal-related symptoms in gastroparesis patients. *Aliment Pharmacol Ther.* 2006;24:661–667.

35. Arts J, Holvoet L, Caenepeel P, *et al.* Clinical trial: a randomized-controlled crossover study of intrapyloric injection of botulinum toxin in gastroparesis. *Aliment Pharmacol Ther.* 2007;26:1251–1258.

36. Friedenberg FK, Palit A, Parkman HP, *et al.* Botulinum toxin A for the treatment of delayed gastric emptying. *Am J Gastroenterol.* 2008;103:416–423.

37. Jones MP, Maganiti P. A systematic review of surgical therapy for gastroparesis. *Am J Gastroenterol.* 2003;98:2122–2129.

38. Abell TL, Van Cutsem E., Abrahamsson H, *et al.* Gastric electrical stimulation in intractable symptomatic gastroparesis. *Digestion.* 2002;66:204–212.

39. Abell T, McCallum R, Hocking M, *et al.* Gastric electrical stimulation for medically refractory gastroparesis. *Gastroenterology.* 2003;125:421–428.

40. McCallum RW, Snape W, Brody F, *et al.* Gastric electrical stimulation with Enterra improves symptoms from diabetic gastroparesis in a prospective study. *Clin Gastroenterol Hepatol.* 2010;8: 947–954.

CHAPTER 6

Diarrhea

Matthew R. Banks[1] and Michael J. G. Farthing[2]

[1]University College London Hospitals, London, UK
[2]University of Sussex, Brighton, UK

KEY POINTS

- The definition of diarrhea requires that the daily stool output exceeds 200 g for adults in the developed world and up to 400 g in the developing world
- The pathophysiology of diarrhea can be considered in terms of factors that promote secretion or attenuate absorption, favoring a net increase in fluid and electrolyte movement into the intestinal lumen
- When considering the etiology of diarrhea factors involved include those that induce active secretion, those that inhibit active absorption, osmotic agents, and factors that stimulate intestinal motility
- Differentiating osmotic from secretory diarrhea can be simply achieved by starving the patient of food for 24 hours and measuring stool output, which will decrease substantially in osmotic diarrhea
- Acute diarrhea is defined as that limited to 2 weeks and is generally the result of infection
- Chronic diarrhea, with the exception of *Entamoeba histolytica* and *Giardia intestinalis*, is mostly non-infective and has a far broader etiology

Introduction

Diarrhea is responsible for the deaths of several million people each year worldwide and thus remains a significant clinical problem. Although acute infectious diarrhea is by far the most common clinical problem, chronic diarrhea presents the clinician with complex diagnostic and therapeutic challenges. This chapter will describe the pathophysiology and etiology of diarrhea, giving the reader a "first principle" approach to diagnosis.

What is it

The term "diarrhea" is often used to describe an increase in frequency of defecation or a change in the consistency of stool to that with a greater liquid content. However, the precise definition of this condition requires that the daily stool output exceeds 200 g for adults in the developed world and up to 400 g in the developing world. For the purposes of research and ease

of measurement in clinical practice, two or more loose stools per day appear to be used most often to define diarrhea. Fecal urgency is often the most frequent symptom wrongly ascribed as "diarrhea" and is often a reflection of abnormal rectal physiology or sensation (see Chapter 10). The differentiation between acute, and chronic diarrhea is often arbitrary, but experts generally refer to acute diarrhea as that lasting less than 14 days, and chronic lasting more than 14 days.

How common

In the developing world diarrhea is one of the principal causes of morbidity and mortality among children. Although there has been a decline in the mortality rates from diarrhea over the last 40 years, 2.5 million children still died from diarrheal disease each year in the 1990s [1]. The incidence of diarrhea is highest among children aged 6–11 months, who experience a median of 4.8 episodes of diarrhea per year, with the incidence falling progressively to 1.4 episodes per year in 4 year olds.

Although far less common in affluent countries, diarrhea still remains one of the two most common reasons for emergency attendance. Estimates of the incidence of diarrhea vary from 1 to 45 cases per 100 person years, the range largely a result of variations in reporting of symptoms and isolation of pathogens.

Pathophysiology

Understanding the physiology of fluid and electrolyte movement within the gastrointestinal tract is of paramount importance in gaining insight into processes responsible for diarrheal disease and for making management decisions. The intestine functions as both a secretory and absorptive organ, where 10 liters of fluid enter the small intestine each day from ingestion and secretions from the salivary glands, stomach, pancreas, bile ducts and small intestine. Approximately 7.5 liters are absorbed in the small intestine and the remainder is absorbed by the colon, with less than 200 milliliters constituting stool volume. Broadly speaking the majority of intestinal fluid

---

secretion occurs in the crypts, while absorption occurs in the villi (Figure 6.1).

The pathophysiology of diarrhea can therefore be considered in terms of factors that promote secretion or attenuate absorption, favoring a net increase in fluid and electrolyte movement into the intestinal lumen. These factors fall into four categories: those that induce active secretion, those that inhibit active absorption, osmotic agents, and factors that stimulate intestinal motility. Most diarrhea is, however, multifactorial, with overlap of these four different pathophysiological processes. It is also important to understand that although diarrhea is a result of increased stool fluid, the movement of fluid is dependent upon, and secondary to, the movement of solutes.

Active secretion

Stimulation of active intestinal secretion occurs as a result of secretogogues which bind to the enterocyte and activate three principal second messengers: cyclic AMP, cyclic GMP and calcium. These then promote the active secretion of chloride ions into the intestinal lumen by opening apical (luminal) chloride channels, following the induction of a phosphorylation cascade. Chloride ions are followed passively by sodium and subsequently water into the intestinal lumen. Examples of such pro-secretory secretogogues include bacterial enterotoxins, hormones such as serotonin, many inflammatory mediators including histamine and prostaglandin E2, and bile acids (Figure 6.1). Alternatively, active secretion can be induced indirectly through the activation of the enteric nervous system and the subsequent release of secretory neurotransmitters into the mucosa (Figure 6.1). An example of this process is typified by *Vibrio cholerae*, which produces an enterotoxin that causes diarrhea by direct actions on enterocytes and also through activation of the enteric nervous system [2]. Once bound to the enterocytes, cholera toxin activates sensory neurons through the release of mucosal serotonin. When activated, the sensory

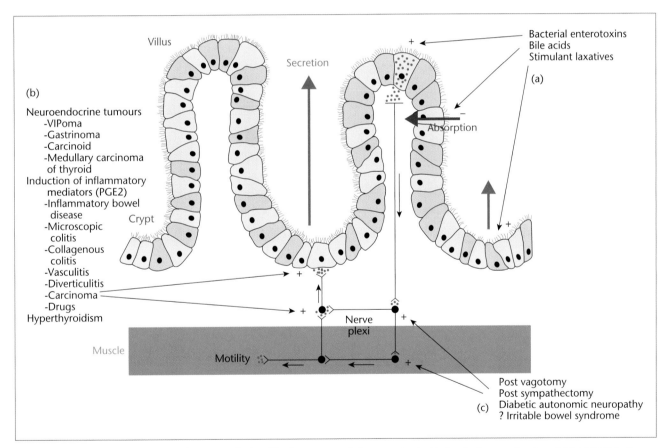

Figure 6.1 Causes and pathophysiology of secretory diarrhea. The figure demonstrates the intestinal mucosa with the villi projecting into the intestinal lumen. The muscle layers represent the lamina propria and the nerves represent the afferent, efferent and interneurons of the enteric nervous system with arrows indicating direction of stimulation. Secretion occurs in the crypts and absorption into the villi. Secretion is induced by three basic mechanisms. (a) Luminal secretagogues bind to the epithelium and either induce secretion and inhibit absorption directly, or indirectly through the activation of nerve circuits. (b) Mural secretogogues may induce secretion by binding to the serosal surface of the epithelium or activating the secretomotor nerves. These include intestinal hormones such as vasoactive intestinal peptide (VIP) and inflammatory mediators such as prostaglandin E2 and histamine. (c) The function of the enteric nervous system can be influenced by surgery, neuropathies and, possibly, irritable bowel syndrome (IBS), such that secretion is augmented and motility altered. (This figure was published in *Clinical Gastroenterology and Hepatology*, Wilfred M. Weinstein, Christopher J. Hawkey, Jaime Bosch, Diarrhea, Pages 1–8, Copyright Elsevier, 2005.)

neurons initiate an excitatory neural cascade culminating in the release of secretomotor neuropeptides such as vasoactive intestinal peptide and acetylcholine [3] onto the enterocytes, to induce intestinal secretion.

Inhibition of absorption

Many secretogogues in addition to stimulating active secretion also directly inhibit the enterocyte s ability to absorb fluid. Furthermore, the activation of inhibitory neural secretory reflexes also downregulates absorption. Other factors that attenuate absorption include disease processes that reduce the absorptive surface area of the intestine such as the villous atrophy induced by celiac disease or infection with *Giardia lamblia* (Figure 6.2). The absorptive capacity of the intestine is also reduced following intestinal resection, such that patients with less than 100 centimeters of small intestine experience persistent diarrhea. Rotavirus, in addition to invading the enterocytes, produces a calcium-dependent enterotoxin (NSP4), which inhibits brush-border disaccharides and the glucose-dependent absorption of sodium. Enterotoxigenic *Escherichia coli* has been shown to inhibit Na–H exchange and Cl–OH/HCO_3 exchange, and norovirus is likely to have a similar mechanism.

Osmotic diarrhea

Non-absorbed or poorly absorbed aqueous solutes increase the osmotic potential of the intestinal lumen (Figure 6.3). This high luminal osmolality attenuates the absorptive capacity of the intestine and promotes the passive inward movement of fluid and electrolytes. This may simply be the result of ingested non-absorbable substances such as lactulose and sorbitol. Alternatively, conditions such as villous atrophy or lactase deficiency lead to carbohydrate malabsorption.

Altered intestinal motility

Increasing intestinal transit with pro-motility agents such as erythromycin reduces the intestinal capacity to absorb thus leading to diarrhea. Alternatively, ineffective peristalsis due to

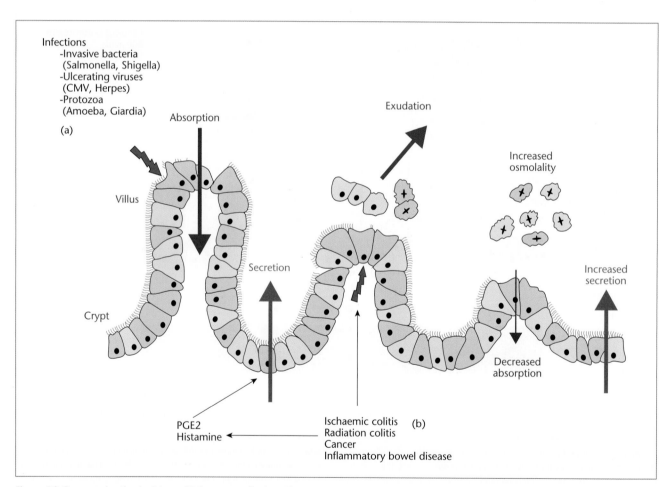

Figure 6.2 Causes and pathophysiology of inflammatory diarrhea. The figure demonstrates the destruction of the intestinal mucosa, with a loss of villi. Luminal invasive infections (a) and intrinsic causes of intestinal inflammation (b) result in cell apoptosis. This process favors secretion through three mechanisms: 1. villus destruction reduces the absorptive capacity of the intestine and causes malabsorption and an increase in luminal osmolality; 2. cell exudation further increases the luminal osmolality; 3. immune recruitment of inflammatory mediators such as prostaglandin E2 and histamine induce active secretion directly and through intermediate neural and cellular pathways. (This figure was published in *Clinical Gastroenterology and Hepatology*, Wilfred M. Weinstein, Christopher J. Hawkey, Jaime Bosch, Diarrhea, Pages 1–8, Copyright Elsevier, 2005.)

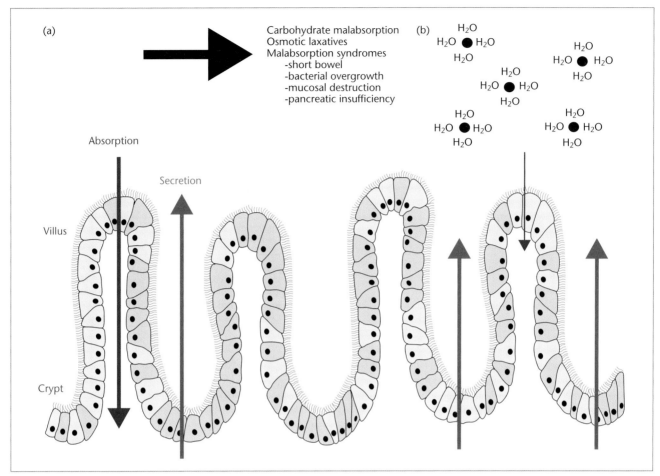

(a)

Carbohydrate malabsorption
Osmotic laxatives
Malabsorption syndromes
  -short bowel
  -bacterial overgrowth
  -mucosal destruction
  -pancreatic insufficiency

(b)

Absorption

Secretion

Villus

Crypt

Figure 6.3 Causes and pathophysiology of osmotic diarrhea. The figure demonstrates the pro-secretory effects of osmotic agents on intestinal fluid movement. (a) represents the normal luminal environment and (b) represents the effects of osmotic agents such as non-absorbed carbohydrates. (This figure was published in *Clinical Gastroenterology and Hepatology*, Wilfred M. Weinstein, Christopher J. Hawkey, Jaime Bosch, Diarrhea, Pages 1–8, Copyright Elsevier, 2005.)

autonomic neuropathy or systemic sclerosis promotes bacterial overgrowth leading to bile salt deconjugation and fat malabsorption.

Causes

A complete list of the causes of diarrhea is in Table 6.1; however, a few specific etiological agents are described below.

Infection

Infections are responsible for the vast majority of acute diarrhea illnesses and will be covered in more detail in the section "Intestinal infections and infestations". Common viruses are listed in Table 6.1, all of which induce a self limiting, although occasionally severe, diarrheal illness, often associated with nausea and vomiting. Viruses induce diarrhea through epithelial invasion, causing inflammation and cell destruction, which impairs absorption (Figure 6.2).

Most bacteria cause diarrhea by direct invasion, inducing an inflammatory response, and through the production of secretory toxins. Some bacteria produce cytolytic toxins which destroy epithelial cells causing inflammation and impairing absorption, such as *Shigella dysenteriae* (shiga toxin).

Dilutional diarrhea

In rare instances patients have been known to dilute stools with fluids such as urine, water and tea. Management of patients with factitious diarrhea is complex and often requires inpatient assessment [4].

Surgery

Surgery induces diarrhea by a variety of different mechanisms. Vagotomy and sympathectomy appear to alter intestinal secretion and motility resulting in diarrhea. Furthermore, any major distortion in anatomy such as the construction of blind loops, may result in bacterial overgrowth.

HIV-associated diarrhea

Diarrhea associated with HIV is frequently attributed to opportunistic infections and is dependent upon the degree

Table 6.1 The causes of diarrhea

Etiology	Examples	Mechanism	Symptom complexes
Bacterial infection	*Shigella* spp. *Escherichia coli* spp. *Campylobacter* spp. *Salmonella* spp. *Clostridium difficile*	Inflammation-induced secretion and reduced absorption	Acute diarrhea Inflammatory diarrhea
	Enterotoxigenic *Escherichia coli* Cholera	Stimulation of secretion	Acute diarrhea Watery diarrhea
Viral infection	Rotavirus, norovirus, enteric adenovirus (types 40, 41), caliciviruses and astroviruses	Inflammation and inhibition of secretion (rota- and noroviruses)	Acute diarrhea
Protozoa	*Giardia*	Generalized malabsorption	Fatty diarrhea Chronic diarrhea
	Cyclospora and isospora *Entamoeba histolytica*	Inflammation-induced secretion and reduced absorption	Acute or chronic diarrhea Inflammatory diarrhea
Inflammatory bowel disease	Crohn's disease	Impaired absorption Inflammation-induced secretion Secondary bile salt malabsorption	Chronic diarrhea Inflammatory diarrhea Watery diarrhea
	Ulcerative colitis	Inflammation-induced secretion and reduced absorption	Chronic diarrhea Inflammatory diarrhea
Drugs			
Antibiotics	Pseudomembranous colitis	—	Acute, inflammatory diarrhea
	Erythromycin	Enhanced motility	—
Laxatives	Senna	Enhanced motility	—
	Docusate sodium	Increased secretion	—
	Magnesium salts	Osmotic diarrhea	—
Protease inhibitors	—	—	—
Metformin	—	—	—
Sorbitol	—	Osmotic diarrhea	—
Neuroendocrine syndromes	VIPoma [12]	Secretory diarrhea	Chronic, watery diarrhea
	Gastrinoma	Secretory diarrhea	Chronic, watery diarrhea
	Carcinoid syndrome	Secretory diarrhea	Chronic, watery diarrhea
	Medullary carcinoma of the thyroid	Secretory diarrhea	Chronic, watery diarrhea
	Thyrotoxicosis	Enhanced motility	Chronic, watery diarrhea
	Diabetes mellitus	Autonomic neuropathy with altered motility and fluid transport	Chronic diarrhea
Inherited diarrhea	Sucrase–isomaltase deficiency	Carbohydrate malabsorption	Chronic diarrhea Osmotic diarrhea
	Glucose–galactose malabsorption	Carbohydrate malabsorption	Chronic diarrhea Osmotic diarrhea
	Na/H and Cl/HCO$_3$ exchange proteins	Impaired solute absorption	Chronic diarrhea
Bile salt malabsorption [13]	Crohn's disease Terminal ileal resection Congenital Vagotomy Cholecystectomy	Bile salt-induced colonic solute and fluid secretion	Chronic, watery diarrhea
Colorectal cancer	—	Inflammatory, mucous secretion	Acute or chronic
Small intestinal bacterial overgrowth	Jejunal diverticulosis Post surgical blind loops	Bile acid deconjugation and fat malabsorption	Chronic, fatty diarrhea
HIV-associated diarrhea	Microsporidia Cytomegalovirus Cryptosporidia *Mycobacterium avium* complex	Inflammatory-induced secretion and impaired absorption	Inflammatory, chronic diarrhea
IBS	Post-infectious IBS	Upregulation of serotonin pathways	Chronic diarrhea
	Diarrhea-predominant IBS	—	Chronic diarrhea
Intestinal lymphangiectasia	Congenital Neoplastic	Increased intestinal permeability	Chronic diarrhea

IBS, inflammatory bowel syndrome.

of immune suppression. Typical causative organisms include microsporidia, cytomegalovirus, cryptosporidia and *Mycobacterium avium* complex. The other most common cause is the use of protease inhibitors, which has been found to induce diarrhea in 12–56% of patients [5].

Intestinal lymphangiectasia

Cancer is a common cause of intestinal lymphagiectasia, although many cases appear to be congenital. Obstruction of the lymphatics results in an increase in the interstitial hydrostatic pressure. This results in the disruption of cellular tight junctions with an increase in epithelial permeability to solutes, water and larger molecules such as proteins. The consumption of fat increases the pressure in the lymphatics, thereby inducing further fluid and electrolyte loss resulting in diarrhea.

Symptom complexes
Acute diarrhea

Rapid onset diarrhea lasting several days to weeks in the developed world is most commonly due to viruses, and bacteria such as *Campylobacter jejuni* or *Salmonella* spp. (see Chapter 45). Viral diarrhea, such as that due to the small round- structured viruses (e.g., norovirus) is often associated with outbreaks notably on cruise ships or in residential homes or hospitals. Traveler's diarrhea affects visitors to resource-poor regions and is usually due to enterotoxigenic *Escherichia coli* (ETEC), which produces two secretory enterotoxins, heat labile and heat stable toxins (see Chapter 46). Cholera is classically related to poor sanitation, the source of infection typically being contaminated water supplies. Protozoa such as *Entamoeba histolytica* and *Giardia intestinalis* may present as acute diarrhea.

Chronic diarrhea

Any diarrhea persisting for more than 2 weeks is termed chronic and is a useful classification when investigating diarrhea. The most common causes are infection and inflammatory bowel disease (IBD). Most bacteria may cause persistent symptoms; however, typical examples include *Shigella* spp., *Mycobacterium tuberculosis, Salmonella* spp., *Yersinia enterocolitica* and *Tropheryma whippelii* (the cause of Whipple disease). More commonly, protozoa such as *Giardia intestinalis, Entamoeba histolytica* and *Cyclospora cyatanensis* give rise to diarrhea lasting many months if untreated (see Chapter 45). Rarer causes of persistent diarrhea include hormone-secreting tumors (see Chapter 112), pancreatic insufficiency (see Chapter 70), and autonomic neuropathies.

A useful diagnostic approach to chronic diarrhea is to consider the characteristics of the diarrhea in terms of three categories: watery (secretory or osmotic), inflammatory, and fatty diarrhea. However, as discussed in the section on pathophysiology the aetiologies with complex mechanisms may overlap different categories.

Watery diarrhea

Large volume watery diarrhea is generally due to either the promotion of active intestinal secretion or to an osmotic load (Figures 6.1 and 6.3). Secretory diarrhea, such as that due to cholera, bears no relationship to the ingestion of foodstuffs and will persist on fasting. Conversely, osmotic diarrhea only occurs following the ingestion of specific or general unabsorbed foodstuffs.

Inflammatory diarrhea

Characteristics of inflammatory diarrhea (Figure 6.2), such as that due to ulcerative colitis or an infective colitis, may include abdominal pain, pyrexia and bloody diarrhea. Peripheral leukocytosis and raised inflammatory markers are useful indicators and examination of the stool may reveal blood and leukocytes.

Fatty diarrhea

Fatty stools typically are described at pale stools with an oily texture which float in the toilet pan and are difficult to wash away. The most common cause is pancreatic insufficiency (see Chapter 70) with reduction of pancreatic lipases,; however, loss of small intestinal absorptive capacity following *Giardia* infection or celiac disease may also lead to fat malabsorption.

Diagnosis
History and examination

A careful history may be sufficient to suggest a likely diagnosis and is likely to direct and focus investigations. For example, a history of bloody diarrhea will suggest colitis, whereas profuse large volume diarrhea suggests small intestinal etiology. The general examination may illicit systemic manifestations of diarrheal illnesses such as rashes associated with IBD and arthritis associated with vasculitis. Furthermore, the examination is important as an assessment of the patient's nutritional status and fluid balance.

A range of laboratory investigations have been listed in Table 6.2, although some are described in more detail below.

Stool examination

Confirmation of loose stools and the general appearance such as fatty (fat malabsorption), pale (biliary obstruction) or bloody stools can be demonstrated, simply by inspection of a stool specimen. Quantitative stool collection over 48–72 hours can be accomplished at home or in hospital and confirms the presence of a true diarrhea (>200 grams/24 hours), in addition to providing an assessment of magnitude of diarrhea. During the collection period, all drugs influencing stool output such as opiates should be stopped, and a normal diet should be adhered to. If factitious diarrhea is suspected, stool collection should ideally be supervised as an inpatient.

Table 6.2 Investigations for the diagnosis of diarrhea

Investigation	Abnormality	Possible etiology
Full blood count	Microcytic anemia	IBD, celiac disease, colorectal cancer
	Leukocytosis	Infection, IBD
	Leukopenia	HIV
C-reactive protein	Raised	Infectious or inflammatory diarrhea
Vitamin B$_{12}$	Deficiency	Crohn's disease, terminal ileal resection, malabsorption
Red cell folate	Deficiency	Malabsorption (celiac, *Giardia*)
Serological markers	Positive	Amebiasis, strongyloidiasis, celiac disease
Stool microscopy and culture	Leukocytes	Infection or IBD
	Entamoeba histolytica, Giardia intestinalis, Salmonella spp., *Shigella* spp., *Campylobacter* spp. and *E. coli* spp., cryptosporidium, cyclospora and *Isospora belli*	—
Stool *Giardia*-antigen	*Giardia intestinalis*	—
Stool toxin assay	*Clostridium difficile* toxin A and B	*Clostridium difficile*
Stool osmotic gap 290 − 2([Na$^+$] + [K$^+$])	>50 mOsm/kg	Osmotic diarrhea
	<50 mOsm/kg	Secretory diarrhea
Stool pH	<5	Carbohydrate malabsorption
Stool Clinitest® for reducing sugars	Positive	Glucose, galactose, fructose, maltose or lactose malabsorption
Stool fat collection	>14 g/day	Pancreatic insufficiency, bile salt disorders, small intestinal enteropathies
Fecal lactoferrin and fecal calprotectin	Raised levels	IBD, cancer, infection
Gut hormone blood assay	Raised levels	Neuroendocrine tumors
Urinary 5-hydroxyindole acetic acid	Raised	Carcinoid tumor
Gastroscopy and duodenal biopsies	Increased intra-epithelial lymphocytes, crypt hyperplasia and villous atrophy	Celiac disease, *Giardia*
Flexible sigmoidoscopy or colonoscopy	Colitis or terminal ileitis	IBD, infection, cancer
H$_2$ breath tests		
Lactulose	Rise > 20 ppm H$_2$	Small intestinal bacterial overgrowth
100 g oral glucose	Rise > 20 ppm H$_2$	Small intestinal bacterial overgrowth
25 g oral lactose	Rise > 20 ppm H$_2$	Lactase deficiency
^{75}Se-homocholic-acid taurine	<5% retention of oral dose	Bile salt malabsorption [14]

IBD, inflammatory bowel disease.

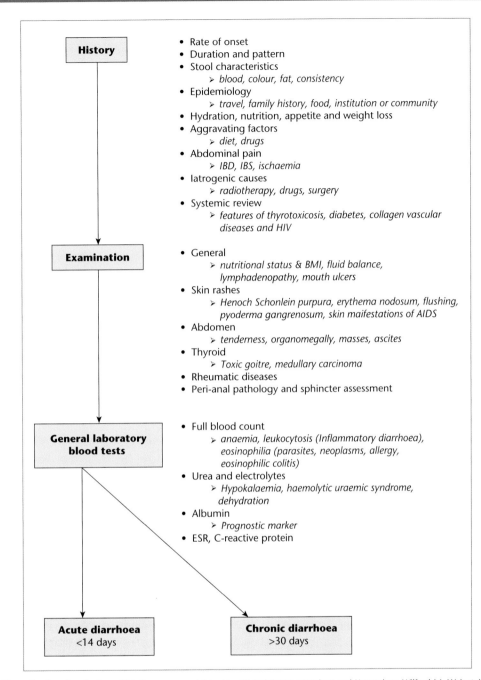

Figure 6.4 General investigations for diarrhea. (This figure was published in *Clinical Gastroenterology and Hepatology*, Wilfred M. Weinstein, Christopher J. Hawkey, Jaime Bosch, Diarrhea, Pages 1–8, Copyright Elsevier, 2005.)

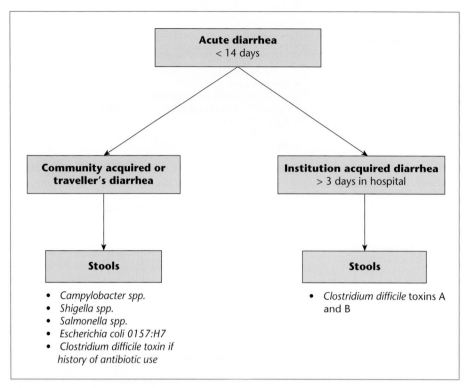

Figure 6.5 Specific investigations for acute diarrhea. (This figure was published in *Clinical Gastroenterology and Hepatology*, Wilfred M. Weinstein, Christopher J. Hawkey, Jaime Bosch, Diarrhea, Pages 1–8, Copyright Elsevier, 2005.)

Stool microscopy is useful for the diagnosis of infections; however, in hospital-acquired diarrhea (developing after 3 days in hospital), the yield for most pathogens is very low and unless there is significant co-morbidity, such as neutropenia or HIV infection (see Chapter 114), examination should be limited to *Clostridium difficile* toxins A and B [6,7] (Table 6.2).

Endoscopy

Endoscopic inspection of the colon is indicated in acute diarrhea where a non-infectious etiology is suspected such as IBD, and in chronic diarrhea (see Chapter 124). We would suggest flexible sigmoidoscopy and biopsy as a primary investigation as the additional yield from colonoscopy is small [8], given the additional cost and risk. If there are features suggestive of malignancy such as weight loss, a possibility of a right-sided colitis or disease affecting the terminal ileum, such as Crohn's disease or tuberculosis, then full colonoscopy would be indicated (Table 6.2)

Radiology

Barium studies of the small intestine may be useful in defining abnormal anatomy of the small intestine in chronic diarrhea.

A barium follow-through is the most commonly used investigation and appears to have no major disadvantage compared to a "small-bowel enema" or enteroclysis, in which barium is infused into the small intestine via a nasogastric tube [9]. (see Chapter 132). Typical diseases found following barium studies include Crohn s disease, lymphoma, jejunum diverticulosis and systemic sclerosis. Similarly, computed tomography will diagnose abdominal lymph nodes associated with tuberculosis or lymphoma and any structural intestinal abnormalities as described for barium studies (see Chapter 133). There have, however, been no investigations assessing the diagnostic yield of either computed tomography or barium studies in the evaluation of chronic diarrhea.

Diagnostic approach to diarrhea

Figure 6.4 is a suggested algorithm for a diagnostic approach for all presentations of diarrhea. Having characterized the diarrhea to a particular disease pattern such as acute [10], chronic [11] or HIV associated [5], the specific investigation pathways can be followed in Figures 6.5, 6.6, and 6.7.

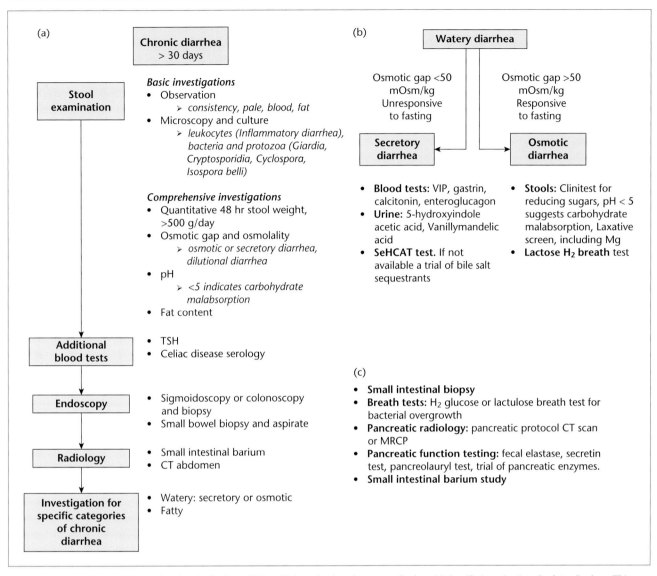

Figure 6.6 (a) Specific investigations for chronic diarrhea. (b) Specific investigations for watery diarrhea. (c) Specific investigations for fatty diarrhea. (This figure was published in *Clinical Gastroenterology and Hepatology*, Wilfred M. Weinstein, Christopher J. Hawkey, Jaime Bosch, Diarrhea, Pages 1–8, Copyright Elsevier, 2005.)

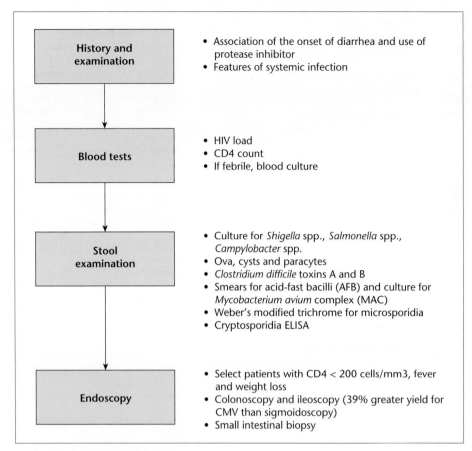

Figure 6.7 Specific investigations for HIV-associated diarrhea. (This figure was published in *Clinical Gastroenterology and Hepatology*, Wilfred M. Weinstein, Christopher J. Hawkey, Jaime Bosch, Diarrhea, Pages 1–8, Copyright Elsevier, 2005.)

References

1. Kosek M, Bern C, Guerrant RL. The global burden of diarrhoeal disease, as estimated from studies published between 1992 and 2000. *Bull World Health Org.* 2003;81:197–204.

2. Turvill JL, Connor P, Farthing MJ. The inhibition of cholera toxin-induced 5-HT release by the 5-HT(3) receptor antagonist, granisetron, in the rat. *Br J Pharmacol.* 2000;130:1031–1036.

3. Banks MR, Golder M, Farthing MGJ, *et al.* Intracellular potentiation between two second messenger systems may contribute to cholera toxin-induced intestinal secretion in humans. *Gut.* 2004;53:50–57.

4. Pollock RCG, Banks MR, Fairclough PD, *et al.* Dilutional diarrhoea – underdiagnosed and over-investigated. *Eur J Gastroenterol Hepatol.* 2000;12:1–3.

5. Oldfield EC. Evaluation of chronic diarrhea in patients with human immunodeficiency virus infection. *Rev Gastroenterol Disord.* 2002;2:176–188.

6. Hines J, Nachamkin I. Effective use of the clinical microbiology laboratory for diagnosing diarrhoeal diseases. *Clin Infect Dis.* 1996;23:1292–1301.

7. Bauer TM, Lalvani A, Fahrenbach J. Derivation and validation of guidelines for stool cultures for enteropathogenic bacteria other than *Clostridium difficile* in hospitalized adults. *JAMA* 2001;285:313–319.

8. Marshall JB, Singh R, Diaz-Arias AA. Chronic, unexplained diarrhea: are biopsies necessary if colonoscopy is normal? *Am J Gastroenterol.* 1995;90:372–376.

9. Ott DJ, Chen YM, Gelfand DW, *et al.* Detailed per-oral small bowel examination vs. enteroclysis. *Radiology.* 1985;155:29–31.

10. Guerrant RL, Van Gilder T, Steiner TS, *et al.* Practice guidelines for the management of infectious diarrhoea. *Clin Infect Dis.* 2001;32:331–351.

11. AGA technical review on the evaluation and management of chronic diarrhea. *Gastroenterology.* 1999;116:1464–1486.

12. Bloom SR, Polak JM, Pearse AG. Vasoactive intestinal peptide and watery-diarrhoea syndrome. *Lancet.* 1973;2:14–16.

13. Smith MJ, Cherian P, Raju GS, *et al.* Bile acid malabsorption in persistent diarrhoea. *J R Coll Physicians Lond.* 2003;34:448–451.

14. Wildt S, Norby Rasmussen S, Lysgard Madsen J, *et al.* Bile acid malabsorption in patients with diarrhoea: Clinical value of SeHCAT test. *Scand J Gastroenterol.* 2003;38:826–830.

CHAPTER 7
Fecal incontinence

Ashok Attaluri[1] and Satish S. C. Rao[2]

[1]University of Iowa Carver College of Medicine, Iowa City, IA, USA
[2]Georgia Health Sciences University, Augusta, GA; American Neurogastroenterology & Motility Society / FBG, Belleville, MI, USA

KEY POINTS

- Fecal incontinence, the involuntary discharge of bowel contents, is a common problem that significantly impairs quality of life
- Manometric and imaging modalities together with detailed history will provide good insights regarding pathophysiology and characterize the bowel dysfunction
- One or more of the following – antidiarrheal drugs such as loperamide, biofeedback therapy, anal sphincteroplasty and sacral nerve stimulation – should help most patients with incontinence

---

Introduction

Fecal incontinence (FI) is defined as the involuntary discharge of, or the inability to control, stool output [1]. The prevalence estimates vary from 2.2% to 18.4% depending on the definition of incontinence, the frequency of occurrence, and the clinical setting [2,3]. Its prevalence is disproportionately higher in women, in nursing home residents, and the elderly [2] and more than 1 in 10 adult women have FI [3].

Pathophysiology

Three subgroups are recognized: a) **passive incontinence** – the involuntary discharge of stool or gas without awareness; b) **urge incontinence** – the discharge of fecal matter in spite of active attempts to retain bowel contents, and c) **fecal seepage** – the involuntary leakage of small volumes of stool after normal evacuation [4]. Disruption of the normal structure or function of the anorectal unit leads to FI and the majority of patients have more than one abnormality [1].

Structural abnormalities

Muscular The most common cause of anal sphincter disruption is obstetric trauma and may involve the external anal sphincter (EAS) or internal anal sphincter (IAS), or pudendal nerves. Other causes include anorectal surgery for hemorrhoids, fistula and fissures; accidental perineal trauma, or pelvic fracture [1]. Weakness of puborectalis muscle or puborectalis atrophy can be associated with idiopathic FI [5] (Figure 7.1).

Rectum Hypersensitivity, impaired rectal wall compliance and abnormal rectal accommodation may also lead to incontinence. Radiation-induced colitis, as well as ulcerative colitis or Crohn's disease, radical hysterectomy, and spinal cord injury may reduce rectal compliance and cause FI [1].

Neurological impairment Sphincter degeneration secondary to pudendal neuropathy and obstetric trauma may cause FI [1]. Damage to the pelvic nerves may lead to impaired accommodation and rapid transit through the rectosigmoid region, overwhelming the continence barrier mechanisms.

Functional abnormalities

Perception of sensory stimuli from the rectal wall, pelvic floor and anal canal are essential for maintaining normal continence and defecation [1]. Impaired rectal sensation may lead to excessive accumulation of stool, causing fecal impaction, mega-rectum (extreme dilation of the rectum), and fecal overflow.

Stool characteristics and miscellaneous

The consistency, volume, and frequency of stool and the presence or absence of irritants in stool may also play a role in the pathogenesis of incontinence [1].

Diagnosis

The first step in diagnosis of fecal incontinence is a detailed history with an assessment of its nature (that is, incontinence of flatus, liquid or solid stool), the timing and duration, and its impact on the quality of life. The use of pads or other devices and the ability to discriminate between formed or unformed stool and gas should be documented. A detailed inquiry of obstetric history and coexisting problems such as diabetes mellitus, pelvic radiation, neurological problems, spinal cord injury, dietary history, and urinary incontinence is useful. A prospective stool diary may also be helpful. Based on clinical features, grading systems such as the St. Marks score have been proposed. These provide an objective method of quantifying the degree of incontinence. A detailed

---

Textbook of Clinical Gastroenterology and Hepatology, Second Edition. Edited by C. J. Hawkey, Jaime Bosch, Joel E. Richter, Guadalupe Garcia-Tsao, Francis K. L. Chan.
© 2012 Blackwell Publishing Ltd. Published 2012 by Blackwell Publishing Ltd.

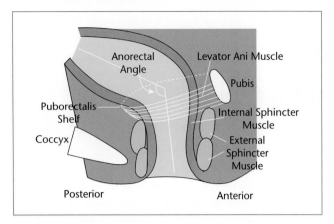

Figure 7.1 Sagittal diagrammatic view of the structure of the anorectum. (Reproduced with permission from Rao SS. Pathophysiology of adult fecal incontinence. *Gastroenterology.* 2004;126(Suppl 1):S14–S22.)

examination should be performed to rule out a systemic or neurological disorder. A digital rectal examination should assess the resting sphincter tone, length of anal canal, integrity of the puborectalis sling, acuteness of the anorectal angle, and the strength of the anal muscle during voluntary squeeze [4] (Figure 7.2).

Endoscopic evaluation

A flexible sigmoidoscopy or colonoscopy may not be necessary if not required for other reasons, e.g., colon cancer screening.

Anorectal manometry

Anorectal manometry provides an assessment of sphincter pressures and reflexes (Figure 7.3). Two large studies have reported that maximum squeeze pressure has the greatest

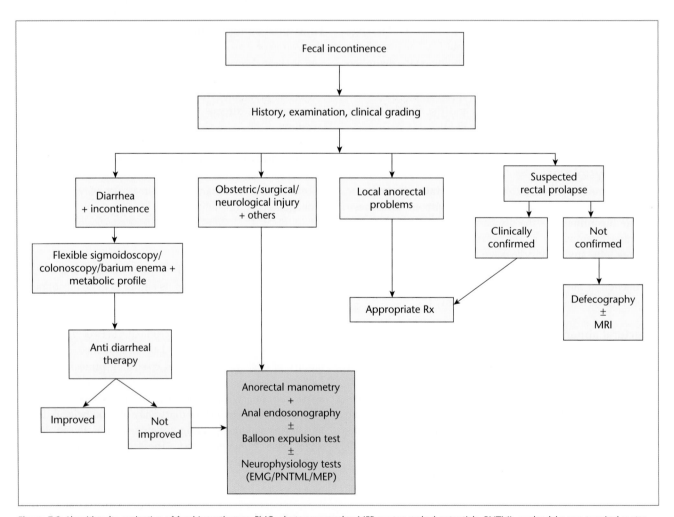

Figure 7.2 Algorithm for evaluation of fecal incontinence. EMG, electromyography; MEP, motor-evoked potentials; PNTML, pudendal nerve terminal motor latency.

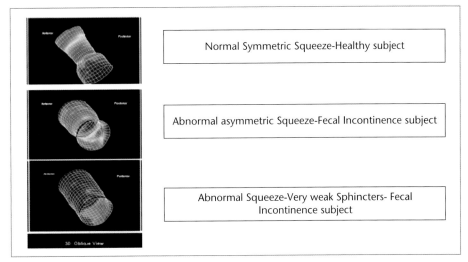

Normal Symmetric Squeeze-Healthy subject

Abnormal asymmetric Squeeze-Fecal Incontinence subject

Abnormal Squeeze-Very weak Sphincters- Fecal Incontinence subject

30 Oblique View

Figure 7.3 High definition anorectal manometry with topographic images of the anal sphincter as depicted in a three-dimensional profile. The sphincter is shown axially, that is, the upper portion is superior. The color blue shows low pressure, similar to atmospheric pressures 0–10 mm Hg, and red shows high pressures 150–300 mm Hg, and the green and yellow are in between these ranges of pressures. The top panel shows three-dimensional changes during a squeeze maneuver in a normal healthy subject with a symmetric increase in anal pressure. The lower two panels show variable degrees of weakness and asymmetry of the anal sphincter during squeeze in subjects with fecal incontinence. (Reproduced with permission from Rao SS. Pathophysiology of adult fecal incontinence. *Gastroenterology.* 2004;126(Suppl 1):S14–S22.)

sensitivity and specificity for discriminating incontinent patients. The ability of the external anal sphincter to contract by reflex is assessed by having the subject cough. This reflex response is absent in patients with lesions of the cauda equina or sacral plexus. Anorectal manometry is also useful in evaluating the responses to biofeedback training or surgery [4].

Rectal sensory testing and compliance
Rectal sensation and compliance are commonly measured by incremental balloon distention. A higher threshold for rectal sensory perception is associated with autonomic neuropathy, or congenital neurogenic anorectal malformation [1]. Rectal compliance reflects both the distensibility and the ability of the rectum to accommodate. Patients with incontinence often have lower rectal compliance.

Anal endosonography
Anal endosonography provides an assessment of the thickness and structural integrity of the anal sphincter muscle and the presence of scarring. Anal endosonography is a simple and inexpensive method of imaging the anal sphincters [4].

Defecography
This radiographic test is used to assess anorectal angle, pelvic floor descent, length of anal canal, presence of rectocele, rectal prolapse, or mucosal intussusception.

Magnetic resonance imaging (MRI)
MRI and endosonography have been compared for the evaluation of anal sphincters. The internal anal sphincter is seen more clearly on anal endosonography, whereas the external anal sphincter is seen more clearly on MRI [4]. Disadvantages of MRI defecography include limited availability and lack of data comparing symptomatic with normal volunteers.

Pudendal nerve terminal motor latency (PNTML)
The pudendal nerve terminal motor latency measures the functional integrity of the terminal portion of the pudendal nerve and helps to distinguish whether a weak sphincter muscle is due to muscle or nerve injury [4]. A prolonged nerve latency time suggests pudendal neuropathy and this may occur following obstetric or surgical trauma, excessive perineal descent, or idiopathic fecal incontinence [4]. A normal PNTML does not exclude pudendal neuropathy. Translumbar and transsacral motor evoked potentials may offer a novel and objective method of evaluating peripheral neuropathy causing fecal incontinence [6].

Clinical utility of tests for fecal incontinence
History and physical examination alone detected an underlying cause in only 9 of 80 patients (11%), whereas anorectal physiologic tests revealed an abnormality in 66% of patients [1]. In another prospective study, physiological testing confirmed clinical impression and management was altered in 76% of patients [1].

Management
The goal of treatment is to restore continence and to improve the quality of life. The following strategies may be useful.

Supportive measures

The underlying predisposing condition(s) such as fecal impaction, dementia, neurological problems, and inflammatory bowel disease should be treated. Hygienic measures such as changing undergarments, cleaning the perianal skin immediately following a soiling episode, and the use of moist tissue paper (baby wipes) rather than dry toilet paper and barrier creams such as zinc oxide and calamine lotion may be useful [4].

Pharmacologic therapy

Loperamide 4 mg tid, diphenoxylate/atropine 5 mg qid cal helps temporarily by decreasing stool frequency and increasing sphincter tone [4]. Other agents that have been tried include cholestyramine that binds bile salts and amitriptyline through anticholinergic effects [4].

Biofeedback therapy

The goals of biofeedback therapy are: (1) to improve the strength of the anal sphincter muscles; (2) to improve coordination during voluntary squeeze and following rectal perception; and (3) to enhance the anorectal sensory perception. Biofeedback training is often performed using either visual, auditory, or verbal feedback techniques [7,8]. One prospective study showed that one year after starting therapy there was a significant increase in squeeze pressure, rectal sensation, and capacity [7]. In a randomized controlled trial of biofeedback therapy with standard care, Kegel exercises, and home treatment, similar improvement was seen in all four groups [7]. However, a recent RCT showed that 70% of subjects who had biofeedback had adequate relief of symptoms versus 30% for subjects who had Kegel exercises [9].

Surgery

In 80% of patients with obstetrical damage, anal sphincter repair resolves symptoms, at least temporarily. In patients with incontinence due to a weak but intact anal sphincter, post-anal repair has been tried but success rates are low. Over time, the success of sphincter repair seems to wear off and less than one-third of patients remain continent after five years [4].

Sacral nerve stimulation

In this technique, electrodes are placed percutaneously through the sacral foramina and a stimulator is implanted. In a multicenter, double-blinded study, 89% improved during one month's active treatment compared to placebo (63%) [10], especially their ability to postpone defecation; symptom severity and quality of life also improved.

References

1. Rao SS. Pathophysiology of adult fecal incontinence. *Gastroenterology*. 2004;126(Suppl 1):S14–S22.
2. Perry S, Shaw C, McGrother C, *et al*. Prevalence of faecal incontinence in adults aged 40 years or more living in the community. *Gut*. 2002;50:480–484.
3. Bharucha AE, Zinsmeister AR, Locke GR, *et al*. Prevalence and burden of fecal incontinence: a population-based study in women. *Gastroenterology*. 2005;129:42–49.
4. Rao SS, American College of Gastroenterology Practice Parameters Committee. Diagnosis and management of fecal incontinence. *Am J Gastroenterol*. 2004;99:1585–1604.
5. Bharucha AE, Fletcher JG, Harper CM, *et al*. Relationship between symptoms and disordered continence mechanisms in women with idiopathic faecal incontinence. *Gut*. 2005;54: 546–555.
6. Rao SS, Tantiphlachiva K, Attaluri, A, *et al*. Translumbar and Transsacral Magnetic Stimulation: A Novel Test of Assessing Anorectal Neuropathy in Fecal Incontinence. *Gastroenterology*. 2008;S1826:A278.
7. Norton C, Chelvanayagam S, Wilson-Barnett J, *et al*. Randomized controlled trial of biofeedback for fecal incontinence. *Gastroenterology*. 2003;125:1320–1329.
8. Rao SS, Welcher KD, Happel J. Can biofeedback therapy improve anorectal function in fecal incontinence? *Am J Gastroenterol*. 1996;91:2360–2366.
9. Heymen S, Scarlett Y, Jones K, *et al*. Randomized, controlled trial shows biofeedback to be superior to alternative treatments for patients with pelvic floor dyssynergia-type constipation. *Dis Colon Rectum*. 2007;50(4):428–441.
10. Leroi AM, Parc Y, Lehur PA, *et al*. Sacral nerve stimulation for fecal incontinence. Results of a multicenter double-blind crossover study. *Ann Surg*. 2005;242:662–669.

CHAPTER 8
Rectal bleeding

Benjamin Krevsky

Temple University School of Medicine, Philadelphia, PA, USA

KEY POINTS

- Determining the severity of hemorrhage is an essential first step in the evaluation of rectal bleeding
- Do not forget that rectal bleeding can have an upper gastrointestinal origin
- A systems approach to thinking about the differential diagnosis will keep the clinician's mind open to the many possible causes of lower gastrointestinal bleeding
- Colonoscopy is the mainstay of both the diagnosis and treatment of rectal bleeding. In an emergent situation, it can be performed within 4 hours of a patient's arrival at hospital
- While colonoscopy is important, other testing can be complementary. These tests include upper endoscopy (EGD), enteroscopy, angiography, red blood cell bleeding scans, computed tomography (CT) enteroscopy, and CT enteroclysis

---

Introduction

Rectal bleeding is a common complaint among adults presenting to gastroenterologists, primary care physicians, and emergency room staff [1]. While the severity of the bleeding can vary greatly from patient to patient, the fact that there is bleeding at all is usually of great concern to the patient and their family. Cancer is usually high on the patient's own list of potential causes but fortunately, this feared diagnosis is actually low in the differential diagnosis.

The severity of rectal bleeding can range from microscopic (e.g., in the patient referred for a positive fecal occult blood test) all the way to massive rectal bleeding. The initial evaluation is therefore aimed at differentiating the severe bleed from the minor one. Triage and resuscitation – if needed – occur next. After this has been accomplished, the next step is to determine the etiology of the bleeding. Finally, therapy can be initiated.

Colonoscopy has evolved as the mainstay of both diagnosis and therapy for serious rectal bleeding. Jensen and Machicado in 1988, demonstrated the utility of rapidly administering a prep and then performing colonoscopy within 4 hours [2,3]. At the same time, therapy can be initiated if the bleeding site is identified [4]. However, colonoscopy should be just one of many tools in the armamentarium of the gastroenterologist. Scintigraphic bleeding scans, angiography, double balloon enteroscopy, and wireless capsule enteroscopy are just a few of the techniques that may be needed in the evaluation of rectal bleeding.

This chapter reviews the epidemiology, etiology, and evaluation of the various causes of rectal bleeding. The therapeutic approaches are left to the chapters on specific diseases elsewhere in this book.

What is it?

There is a spectrum of rectal bleeding that ranges from occult to massive. **Occult rectal bleeding** is when blood that is not visible to an observer is found by a test to be present in the stool. The most common method of detection is the fecal occult blood test (FOBT) or guaiac test. This test consists of placing a specimen of feces on a paper slide containing guaiac – an indicator. When peroxide is added to the feces, the peroxidase in red blood cells reacts with the peroxide, and the indicator turns blue. There are other tests for occult blood that are becoming more popular because of their improved performance, such as the fecal immunochemical test (FIT). Because it is based on the immune characteristics of human red cells, it is not as prone to false positives (e.g., from animal blood or radishes) or false negatives (e.g., from vitamin C). External sources of rectal bleeding, such as from external hemorrhoids or localized skin abrasions, are usually noted on the toilet paper, but can be severe enough to drip into the toilet or stain the patient's garments. Small volume bleeding is usually identified by the patient as bright red blood on the toilet paper, but can also be noted as blood in the toilet bowl, admixed with feces or alone. This can be confused by the patient as being much more severe than it really is, because even a little blood mixed in the toilet bowel water appears to be much more serious than it really is.

Melena (jet black, tarry bowel movements) or large volumes of maroon stool usually are from an upper gastrointestinal (GI) source (proximal to the ligament of Treitz), and connote a serious hemorrhage. While this form of bleeding may be from a lower GI tract source, the upper source must be ruled out [5,6]. **Large volume rectal bleeding** is a medical emergency and mandates hospitalization, resuscitation, and a rapid

---

Textbook of Clinical Gastroenterology and Hepatology, Second Edition. Edited by C. J. Hawkey, Jaime Bosch, Joel E. Richter, Guadalupe Garcia-Tsao, Francis K. L. Chan.
© 2012 Blackwell Publishing Ltd. Published 2012 by Blackwell Publishing Ltd.

approach to evaluation and treatment. Finally, **massive rectal bleeding**, while fortunately rare, requires intensive care and possibly surgical intervention.

How common is it?

Occult rectal bleeding is a common phenomenon. While it depends on the method of testing, approximately 2–10% of adults over 50 who are screened for colon cancer will be positive by one of the occult blood tests [7]. Even a single positive test cannot be ignored and warrants a work-up to rule out colon cancer.

Bleeding from an external (perianal) source or small volume rectal source is both common and distressing to patients. Talley and Jones reported that 13% of their study population had small volume bleeding [1]. **Hemorrhoids** (internal and external) are a common cause of this type of bleeding – accounting for 3.2 million physician visits in the USA in 2004 [8]. While the differentiation of internal and external hemorrhoids is often confusing to patients and practitioners alike, this combined diagnosis is in the top five leading outpatient digestive system diagnoses. The true prevalence of hemorrhoidal bleeding is underestimated by studies, as many patients do not seek medical attention. Fortunately hospitalizations (for surgery) and mortality (6 in 100 000) are rare [8].

Significant rectal bleeding can be either from upper GI or lower GI tract sources. Once the upper GI source has been ruled out (e.g., by nasogastric lavage), the most common cause of active bleeding is **diverticulosis** (33%) [9]. Other sources include neoplasia (19%), colitis/ulcers (18%), unknown (18%), angioectasias (8%), miscellaneous – such as post-polypectomy, anastomotic ulcers, etc. (8%), and anorectal (4%) [9]. Of course, age plays a role in this distribution. It has been reported that angioectasias are the most common cause of lower GI bleeding in individuals over 65 years of age [10].

In a study by Longstreth, 20.5 patients/100 000 had lower GI bleeding severe enough to warrant hospitalization [11]. Among these patients, the mortality was 2.4%. Again, the most common diagnosis was diverticulosis (41.6%) [11].

Pathophysiology: causes and differential diagnosis

Rectal bleeding can be categorized either by the severity of the bleeding, or by the etiology of the bleeding. Table 8.1 lists the major causes of rectal bleeding based on the severity. This type of approach should be useful to the clinician faced with a patient who has rectal bleeding. Typically, the occult, external, and small volume categories are chronic in nature, do not present an immediately life-threatening situation, and may have been present for months. In contrast, the melena or maroon stool, large volume, and massive lower GI bleeding categories are acute, require hospitalization, and carry a significant mortality.

Table 8.1 Clinical levels of rectal bleeding and associated etiologies

- Occult:
  - Benign or malignant neoplasms
  - Angioectasias
  - Upper GI bleeding
  - Mucosal inflammation
- External:
  - Perianal fistula
  - External hemorrhoids
  - Excoriated skin and local infections
- Small volume:
  - Internal hemorrhoids
  - Anal fissure
  - Radiation proctopathy
  - Rectosigmoid cancer
  - Inflammatory bowel disease
  - Infection
- Melena or maroon stool:
  - Upper GI bleeding
  - Meckel's diverticulum
  - Right colonic angioectasias
  - Right colonic diverticulosis
  - Inflammatory bowel disease (IBD)
- Large volume:
  - Diverticulosis
  - Angioectasias
  - Colitis (IBD, infection, ischemia, etc.)
  - Post-polypectomy bleeding
  - Trauma to rectum
  - Anticoagulation
  - NSAIDs
- Massive lower GI bleeding:
  - Arterial-enteric fistula
  - Post-polypectomy bleeding
  - Diverticulosis
  - Dieulafoy lesion

A systems approach to the causes (Table 8.2) will keep the clinician's mind open to the many possible causes of lower GI bleeding. Unfortunately, the cause is not identified in all patients.

A systems approach shows that "anatomical" causes of bleeding contain some of the most common – and rarest – of etiologies. While diverticulosis with bleeding is common, bleeding from a Meckel's diverticulum is rare. **Vascular etiologies** are common causes of occult or small volume bleeds, but may be responsible for profound anemia due to ongoing bleeding. This category includes angioectasias, radiation proctopathy, ischemia, and hemorrhoids. **Inflammatory conditions** such as inflammatory bowel disease, infection, and exposure to toxins may cause bleeding. While a common cause of occult bleeding, **neoplasms** can also cause small volume bleeding – but rarely do they leak enough blood to cause large volume or massive bleeding. **Trauma** to the anorectum should be evident from the history, as should a prior colonoscopic polypectomy or bowel surgery. These can all cause small or large volume bleeding. **Medications** such as non-steroidal anti-inflammatory drugs (NSAIDs) or aspirin can cause

Table 8.2 Differential diagnosis by system

- Anatomic:
  - Diverticulosis
  - Anal fissure
  - Meckel's diverticulum
- Inflammatory:
  - Infection
  - Inflammatory bowel disease
  - Idiopathic
  - Toxic
  - NSAIDs and rectal ulcers
- Neoplastic
  - Advanced benign neoplasms
  - Cancer
- Post-polypectomy and post-surgical
- Trauma
- Unknown
- Vascular:
  - Angioectasias
  - Ischemia
  - Radiation proctopathy
  - Hemorrhoids (internal and external)
  - Rectal varices
  - Dieulafoy lesion

mucosal inflammation or frank ulceration anywhere from the esophagus to the rectum. Likewise, the bleeding caused by medications can range from occult to massive.

Diagnosis of the cause

In all cases, a thorough history and physical examination is crucial to making the diagnosis. The history will determine the severity, chronicity, and important co-morbidities, and yield important clues that will lead to a determination of the etiology. Vital signs, including the orthostatic pressure and pulse evaluation, and the rectal examination remain important parts of the evaluation, reflecting the severity of the bleeding. External and anal causes of bleeding, such as fissures, perianal excoriation, and external hemorrhoids, will be evident. If there is any doubt about an upper versus lower source – especially in an active bleed – nasogastric lavage is helpful. The presence of bile in an otherwise negative lavage indicates that there is no active bleeding above the ligament of Treitz. The absence of bile may be due to pyloric outlet obstruction and therefore, a duodenal bleed cannot be ruled out. There is no utility to testing the lavage fluid for blood: it is either grossly evident or not. At this point the clinician will know whether hospitalization is needed, whether the bleeding is likely to be from an upper or lower GI source, and be able to map out a diagnostic and therapeutic plan.

Occult rectal bleeding requires an **endoscopic approach** [5,12] . In the absence of upper GI symptoms, the source is usually colonic. Colonoscopy would be the test of choice. However, there should be a low threshold to performing an

esophagogastroduodenoscopy (EGD). Any upper GI symptoms or a negative colonoscopy would lead in that direction. If these tests are negative, wireless capsule enteroscopy is a sensitive and specific test for the detection of small bowel bleeding [13]. This technique is not therapeutic, though, so if a source is found, push enteroscopy [14], single balloon enteroscopy [15] or double balloon enteroscopy [16] may be needed to effect therapy. While push enteroscopy is limited to the proximal jejunum, it is widely available and may be useful in some cases. Single balloon enteroscopy can reach further than push enteroscopy. The entire small bowel can be evaluated in most patients with double balloon enterosocopy, utilizing both a per oral and per rectal approach. In the absence of other technologies, an intraoperative enteroscopy can be performed with the surgeon sleeving a pediatric colonoscope or dedicated push enteroscope manually though the entire small bowel.

Flexible sigmoidoscopy should be limited to the evaluation of small volume bleeding considered to be originating from the anus or rectum in adults younger than 35 years of age, or when a colitis is suspected. Sigmoidoscopy, because of its limited extent of examination, could easily miss lesions more proximal than the sigmoid colon. Because of its limited reach, patient discomfort, and the lack of experienced practitioners, the use of rigid sigmoidoscopy is now only of historical interest.

Colonoscopy is an essential tool for the evaluation of large volume and massive GI bleeding [5,6,17]. Not only can this study be performed within 4 hours of arrival at hospital, but the definitive therapy can often be achieved at that time [2,3]. Rapid lavage with a polyethylene glycol-based electrolyte solution can be accomplished with the patient drinking the solution or having it administered via a thin silicone nasogastric tube at a pump rate of 1 L every 30–45 minutes.

Radiographic studies are sometimes useful in making a diagnosis. Barium enemas should not be used because of low sensitivity, inability to image mucosal abnormalities, and intereference with imaging by colonoscopy and CT by residual barium. Red blood cell (RBC) scintigraphic scans can detect bleeding at a rate of 0.1 mL/min [18]. Using dynamic imaging techniques, excellent localization of bleeding sites can be accomplished [19]. Since the radionuclide binds to the red cell, imaging can be performed for at least 12 hours after injection. If the initial scan is negative, the patient can be brought back for a repeat scan later without the need for re-injection. Because of its sensitivity, an RBC scan should precede the higher risk angiography [20]. If the RBC scan is negative, the angiography will also be negative and need not be performed at that time. In unusual circumstances, a CT enteroclysis or CT enteroscopy [21] may be helpful. These radiographic techniques give exquisite images of the small bowel. In CT enteroclysis a catheter is placed into the small bowel fluoroscopically or endoscopically and a special barium mixture is injected prior to CT imaging. In CT enteroscopy, the patient drinks a large volume of special contrast prior to the CT.

SOURCES OF INFORMATION FOR PATIENTS AND DOCTORS

Patients

Preparing for a colonoscopy
  http://www.gastro.org/wmspage.cfm?parm1=858
Hemorrhoids
  http://www.gastro.org/wmspage.cfm?parm1=858
Colorectal cancer
  http://www.gastro.org/wmspage.cfm?parm1=5724
Bleeding in the digestive tract
  http://digestive.niddk.nih.gov/ddiseases/pubs/bleeding/index.htm
Small bowel bleeding and capsule endoscopy
  http://www.acg.gi.org/patients/gihealth/smallbowel.asp

Doctors

Obscure bleeding
  http://www.gastro.org/user-assets/Documents/02_Clinical_Practice/medical_position_statments/obscure_bleeding_mps.pdf
Endoscopy and lower GI bleeding
  http://www.asge.org/WorkArea/showcontent.aspx?id=3336

References

1. Talley NJ, Jones M. Self-reported rectal bleeding in a United States community: prevalence, risk factors, and health care seeking. *Am J Gastroenterol.* 1998;93:2179–2183.

2. Jensen DM, Machicado GA. Diagnosis and treatment of severe hematochezia. The role of urgent colonoscopy after purge. *Gastroenterology.* 1988;95:1569–1574.

3. Jensen DM, Machicado GA, Jutabha R, Kovacs TO. Urgent colonoscopy for the diagnosis and treatment of severe diverticular hemorrhage. *N Engl J Med.* 2000;342:78–82.

4. Machicado GA, Jensen DM. Endoscopic diagnosis and treatment of severe lower gastrointestinal bleeding. *Ind J Gastroenterol.* 2006;25 (Suppl 1):S43–51.

5. Davila RE, Rajan E, Adler DG, *et al.* ASGE Guideline: the role of endoscopy in the patient with lower-GI bleeding. *Gastrointest Endosc.* 2005;62:656–660.

6. Eisen GM, Dominitz JA, Faigel DO, *et al.* An annotated algorithmic approach to acute lower gastrointestinal bleeding. *Gastrointest Endosc.* 2001;53:859–863.

7. Bond JH. Fecal occult blood test screening for colorectal cancer. *Gastrointest Endosc Clin North Am.* 2002;12:11–21.

8. Everhart JE, editor. *The Burden of Digestive Diseases in the United States.* Washington, DC: US Department of Health and Human Services, Public Health Service, National Institutes of Health, National Institute of Diabetes and Digestive and Kidney Diseases. US Government Printing Office, 2008.

9. Zuckerman GR, Prakash C. Acute lower intestinal bleeding. Part II: etiology, therapy, and outcomes. *Gastrointest Endosc.* 1999;49:228–238.

10. Boley SJ, DiBiase A, Brandt LJ, Sammartano RJ. Lower intestinal bleeding in the elderly. *Am J Surg.* 1979;137:57–64.

11. Longstreth GF. Epidemiology and outcome of patients hospitalized with acute lower gastrointestinal hemorrhage: a population-based study. *Am J Gastroenterol.* 1997;92:419–424.

12. Raju GS, Gerson L, Das A, Lewis B, American Gastroenterological Association. American Gastroenterological Association (AGA) Institute medical position statement on obscure gastrointestinal bleeding. *Gastroenterology.* 2007;133:1694–1696.

13. Sidhu R, Sanders DS, Kapur K, Hurlstone DP, McAlindon ME. Capsule endoscopy changes patient management in routine clinical practice. *Dig Dis Sci.* 2007;52:1382–1386.

14. Adrain AL, Dabezies MA, Krevsky B. Enteroscopy improves the clinical outcome in patients with obscure gastrointestinal bleeding. *J Laparoendosc Adv Surg Tech Part A.* 1998;8:279–284.

15. Tsujikawa T, Saitoh Y, Andoh A, Imaeda H, Hata K, Minematsu H, et al. Novel single-balloon enteroscopy for diagnosis and treatment of the small intestine: preliminary experiences. *Endoscopy* 2008;40:11–15.

16. Suzuki T, Matsushima M, Okita I, *et al.* Clinical utility of double-balloon enteroscopy for small intestinal bleeding. *Dig Dis Sci.* 2007;52:1914–1918.

17. Jensen DM, Machicado GA. Colonoscopy for diagnosis and treatment of severe lower gastrointestinal bleeding. Routine outcomes and cost analysis. *Gastrointest Endosc Clin North Am.* 1997;7:477–498.

18. Smith R, Copely DJ, Bolen FH. 99mTc RBC scintigraphy: correlation of gastrointestinal bleeding rates with scintigraphic findings. *AJR Am J Roentgenol.* 1987;148:869–874.

19. Maurer AH, Rodman MS, Vitti RA, Revez G, Krevsky B. Gastrointestinal bleeding: improved localization with cine scintigraphy. *Radiology* 1992;185:187–192.

20. Krevsky B. Detection and treatment of angiodysplasia. *Gastrointest Endosc Clin North Am.* 1997;7:509–524.

21. Huprich JE, Fletcher JG, Alexander JA, Fidler JL, Burton SS, McCullough CH. Obscure gastrointestinal bleeding: evaluation with 64-section multiphase CT enterography – initial experience. *Radiology.* 2008;246:562–571.

CHAPTER 9
Anorectal pain and pruritus ani

Steven D. Wexner and Giovanna M. da Silva
Cleveland Clinic Florida, Weston, FL, USA

Anorectal pain

KEY POINTS

- Anorectal pain may be of urological, gynecological or proctological origin, or may be functional when no specific cause is identified
- Organic causes include fissure, abscess, fistulas and thrombosed hemorrhoids
- Functional causes include proctalgia fugax and levator ani syndrome
- A careful history of the pain pattern and its relation with bowel movements often leads to the correct diagnosis

Introduction

Anorectal pain is a very common complaint. Organic causes are common while functional pain is estimated to occur in 6–19% of patients with anal pain, with a slightly higher prevalence in women from 30 to 60 years of age [1]. Although effective treatment exists for many of the organic causes, management of functional anorectal pain is challenging.

Pathophysiology

The anal region is richly supplied with free nerve endings of C fibers, which are activated by a laceration, burn, tear or swelling. The afferent nerves of the viscera and pelvic floor musculature cannot localize noxious stimuli as precisely as nerves from the skin. As a result, pain related to the pelvic floor muscles may not be perceived as originating in the pelvic musculature. Conversely, patients may have symptoms from surrounding visceral structures attached to the pelvic floor (urinary urgency, rectal pain, dyspareunia). Neural pathways lead to the limbic centers and therefore patients may also experience varying degrees of emotional distress [2].

Causes/differential diagnosis

The most common causes of functional pain are levator ani syndrome and proctalgia fugax. Levator ani syndrome is a vague, dull ache or pressure sensation in the rectum that usually worsens when supine or sitting and may last for 20min or longer. Proctalgia fugax is characterized by sudden onset of

severe sharp, stabbing, or crampy rectal pain that lasts for seconds to minutes and then disappears. Sometimes it awakens the patient from sleep. It may occur in clusters as often as three to four times weekly, several times a year.

Symptom complexes

Pain associated with bleeding is usually secondary to anal fissure and thrombosed hemorrhoids. The presence of fever suggests an abscess while diarrhea indicates bowel inflammation such as radiation proctitis and inflammatory bowel disease.

Patients with functional pain usually have associated functional gastrointestinal complaints. In a study of 60 consecutive patients with chronic intractable rectal pain, 95% had one or more associated factors, the most common of which was constipation or dyschezia (57%)[3].

Diagnosis

The evaluation of anorectal pain includes a detailed history and physical examination. The quality of pain and its relationship to bowel movements frequently helps in determining the etiology. Proctological examination reveals the most common anorectal pathologies. Colonoscopy may be indicated in selected patients, especially in the presence of bleeding and change in bowel habits. If no source of the pain is identified or the patient cannot tolerate office examination, an examination under anesthesia is warranted. Diagnostic imaging including computed tomography (CT), magnetic resonance imaging (MRI), and endorectal ultrasonography may be helpful to rule out a tumor or abscess.

A diagnosis of functional pain is made after all organic causes have been excluded. In patients with levator ani syndrome, the pain may be elicited by rectal massage. The diagnosis of proctalgia fugax is obtained from the patient's history as there are no physical findings or tests for diagnosing this condition. A complete work-up including anorectal physiology studies, CT, colonoscopy, and MRI may be required in addition to gastroenterologic, gynecologic, pain management, neurologic, and psychologic evaluation. Multiple negative testing may be needed to provide reassurance.

Textbook of Clinical Gastroenterology and Hepatology, Second Edition. Edited by C. J. Hawkey, Jaime Bosch, Joel E. Richter, Guadalupe Garcia-Tsao, Francis K. L. Chan.
© 2012 Blackwell Publishing Ltd. Published 2012 by Blackwell Publishing Ltd.

Pruritus ani

Introduction

Pruritus ani is a common symptom that occurs in approximately 1–5% of the general population, with a greater incidence in males than in females (4:1) in the fifth and sixth decades of life.

Pathophysiology

Although pruritus ani and pain share a common neurologic pathway, studies show that pruritus is mediated by a distinct subset of afferent C fibers that are insensitive to mechanical stimuli but responsive to histamine and other pruritogens. These are elicited by local irritation from excoriation, alkaline secretions, and chemical irritants [4]. The complex interactions between pain and itch may explain the antipruritic effect of scratching, which may turn into a chronic cycle, resulting in significant skin excoriation and soreness.

Causes/differential diagnosis

Pruritus ani is classified as primary or idiopathic, and secondary, when a specific cause is identified. In a study evaluating 209 patients with pruritus, 75% of patients were found to have coexisting anal or colorectal pathology [5]. Causes include:

1) Benign anorectal diseases: hemorrhoids, fissures, fistulas, etc.
2) Inadequate hygiene.
3) Diarrhea: due to stool contact and frequent cleaning.
4) Diet: tomatoes, citrus, spicy foods, caffeine, milk products, and alcohol.
5) Dermatoses: seborrhea, atopic eczema, lichen sclerosis, and psoriasis (Figure 9.1).
6) Infection: viral (herpes), bacterial, fungal, parasites such as scabies and pinworm (especially in children).
7) Neoplasm: Bowen's disease (Figure 9.2), Paget's disease and squamous cell carcinoma. Anal and rectal tumors may result in excessive seepage.
8) Systemic diseases: jaundice, chronic renal failure, vitamin deficiency (A, C, and D), polycythemia vera (secondary to histamine release), thyrotoxicosis, myxedema, diabetes mellitus (candida infection), and Hodgkin's disease.
9) Drugs: quinidine, colchicines, oral mineral oil, tetracycline, and hydrocortisone.
10) Contact dermatitis: topical ointment, toilet paper, wet wipes and perfumes.
11) Psychogenic.

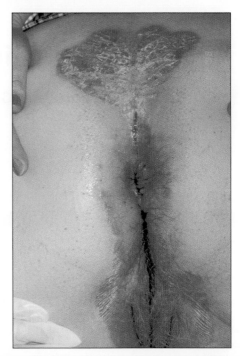

Figure 9.1 Psoriasis. Psoriasis often appears atypical in the cleft and around the labia, lacking the silvery scale that is so characteristic. Isolated areas of involvement in the cleft occur and require biopsy confirmation by a competent skin pathologist. (Figure courtesy of ASCRS Textbook (Chapter 16): The ASCRS Textbook of Colon and Rectal Surgery Wolff, B.G., Fleshman, J.W., Beck, D.E., Pemberton, J.H., Wexner, S.D. (Eds.), 2007, ISBN 978-0-387-36374-5.)

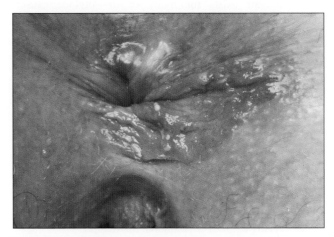

Figure 9.2 Anal Bowen's. Anal Bowen's disease or squamous cell carcinoma in situ may have a varied appearance and be indistinguishable from Paget's disease by clinical examination. The white pearls on the red background are often present and are a clue to the diagnosis. Despite sharp-appearing edges, the process often involves normal-looking skin and requires frozen section to confirm negative margins. (Figure courtesy of ASCRS Textbook (Chapter 16): The ASCRS Textbook of Colon and Rectal Surgery Wolff, B.G., Fleshman, J.W., Beck, D.E., Pemberton, J.H., Wexner, S.D. (Eds.), 2007, ISBN 978-0-387-36374-5.)

Symptom complexes

Pruritus associated with a lump, or other local abnormality suggests the local condition as the causative factor. Pruritus secondary to systemic disease may be associated with features of a specific disease. Pruritus is common in patients undergoing hemodialysis for chronic renal failure. Evidence of concomitant anemia may suggest iron deficiency as a causative factor of the pruritus, although anemia may be absent. A history of pruritus exacerbated by alcohol may be indicative of Hodgkin's disease, whereas pruritus aggravated by bathing may suggest polycythemia vera. Patients with diet-induced pruritus often associate the onset of the symptom with ingestion of a specific food or drink.

Diagnosis

Idiopathic pruritus is a diagnosis of exclusion. The history should consider diet, clothing habits, medication use, diarrheal states, hygiene practices, sexual activity, anorectal pathologies, previous surgery, and systemic illnesses such as diabetes, chronic renal failure. Vaginal discharge and other gynecologic conditions should also be evaluated in females. Stress and anxiety should be investigated.

Physical examination begins with evaluation of the entire body to identify psoriasis, seborrheic dermatitis, fungal or other infections. The perianal area is examined for signs of moisture, soiling, excoriation, skin maceration, or dermatoses. Severe pruritus is marked by lichenification, accentuation of folds, fissuring of the skin and indistinct border (Figure 9.3). Patch testing, cultures, biopsies or scraping of lesions may be indicated. The anal tonus is assessed by digital examination. Endoscopy may be useful to rule out proctitis, inflammatory bowel disease, rectal lesions, or infections. Laboratory tests should include blood count and stool examination for ova and parasites. Manometry may indicate low sphincter tone causing minor leakage. A combined evaluation with a dermatologist may be greatly beneficial in the diagnosis and treatment of these patients.

> **SOURCES OF INFORMATION FOR PATIENTS AND DOCTORS**
>
> http://www.fascrs.org/

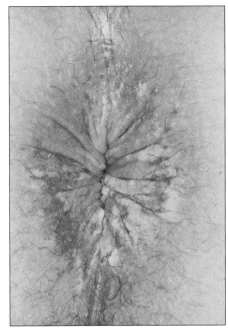

Figure 9.3 Severe pruritus. Classic severe pruritus ani is marked by lichenification (leathery thickening of the skin), accentuation of folds, fissuring of the skin, and erosions and an indistinct border. Changes this severe require short-term aggressive therapy with high-potency steroids for 4–8 weeks which then are rapidly tapered to a maintenance program, if possible without steroids. It is important to rule out secondary infection, which requires specific treatment. (Figure courtesy of ASCRS Textbook (Chapter 16): The ASCRS Textbook of Colon and Rectal Surgery Wolff, B.G., Fleshman, J.W., Beck, D.E., Pemberton, J.H., Wexner, S.D. (Eds.), 2007, ISBN 978-0-387-36374-5.)

References

1. Wald A. Functional anorectal and rectal pain. *Gastroenterol Clin N Am.* 2001;30:243–251.
2. Weiss J. Chronic pelvic pain and myofascial trigger points. *Pain Clinic.* 2000;2:13–18.
3. Ger GC, Wexner SD, Jorge JM, *et al.* Evaluation and treatment of chronic intractable rectal pain — a frustrating endeavor. *Dis Colon Rectum.* 1993;36:247–248.
4. Ikoma A, Rukwied R, Stander S, *et al.* Neurophysiology of pruritus. Interaction of itch and pain. *Arch Dermatol.* 2003;139:1475–1478.
5. Daniel GL, Longo WE, Vernava AM III. Pruritus ani. Causes and concerns. *Dis Colon Rectum.* 1994;37(7):670–674.

CHAPTER 10

Functional gastrointestinal disease

C. J. Hawkey,[1] Jaime Bosch,[2] Joel E. Richter,[3] Guadalupe Garcia-Tsao,[4] and Francis K. L. Chan[5]

[1]Nottingham Digestive Diseases Centre, University of Nottingham and Nottingham University Hospitals, Nottingham, UK
[2]Liver Unit, Hospital Cliníc-IDIBAPS, University of Barcelona, Barcelona, Spain
[3]University of South Florida, Tampa, FL, USA
[4]Department of Internal Medicine, Yale University, School of Medicine, New Haven, CT, USA
[5]The Chinese University of Hong Kong, Hong Kong SAR, China

A high proportion of gastrointestinal disorders are functional. Functional disorders are those in which significant gastrointestinal symptoms are not associated with organic disease but are due to metabolic, infectious, neoplastic, or other structural abnormalities. A number of functional symptoms have been recognized, based on clusters of symptoms. There have been a number of attempts to define these as precisely as possible, of which the Rome III criteria are the most recent and best developed [1] (Tables 10.1–10.9). These criteria have been found to be useful in clinical trials. In clinical practice there is a dilemma in that the more precise the definition, the lower the proportion of patients that are encompassed by it [2] so

text continues on p. 60

Table 10.1 Functional gastrointestinal disorders

A. Functional esophageal disorders
  A1. Functional heartburn
  A2. Functional chest pain of presumed esophageal origin
  A3. Functional dysphagia
  A4. Globus
B. Functional gastroduodenal disorders
  B1. Functional dyspepsia
    B1a. Postprandial distress syndrome
    B1b. Epigastric pain syndrome
  B2. Belching disorders
    B2a. Aerophagia
    B2b. Unspecified excessive belching
  B3. Nausea and vomiting disorders
    B3a. Chronic idiopathic nausea
    B3b. Functional vomiting
    B3c. Cyclic vomiting syndrome
  B4. Rumination syndrome in adults
C. Functional bowel disorders
  C1. Irritable bowel syndrome
  C2. Functional bloating
  C3. Functional constipation
  C4. Functional diarrhea
  C5. Unspecified functional bowel disorder
D. Functional abdominal pain syndrome
  D. Functional abdominal pain syndrome
E. Functional gallbladder and sphincter of Oddi disorders
  E. Functional gallbladder and sphincter of Oddi disorders
    E1. Functional gallbladder disorder
    E2. Functional biliary sphincter of Oddi disorder
    E3. Functional pancreatic sphincter of Oddi disorder

F. Functional anorectal disorders
  F1. Functional fecal incontinence
  F2. Functional anorectal pain
    F2a. Chronic proctalgia
      F2a.1. Levator ani syndrome
      F2a.2. Unspecified functional anorectal pain
    F2b. Proctalgia fugax
  F3. Functional defecation disorders
    F3a. Dyssynergic defecation
    F3b. Inadequate defecatory propulsion
G. Childhood functional GI disorders: infant/toddler
  G1. Infant regurgitation
  G2. Infant rumination syndrome
  G3. Cyclic vomiting syndrome
  G4. Infant colic
  G5. Functional diarrhea
  G6. Infant dyschezia
  G7. Functional constipation
H. Childhood functional GI disorders: child/adolescent
  H1. Vomiting and aerophagea
    H1a. Adolescent rumination syndrome
    H1b. Cyclic vomiting syndrome
    H1c. Aerophagia
  H2. Abdominal pain-related functional GI disorders
    H2a. Functional dyspepsia
    H2b. Irritable bowel syndrome
    H2c. Abdominal migraine
    H2d. Childhood functional abdominal pain
      H2d1. Childhood functional abdominal pain syndrome
  H3. Constipation and incontinence
    H3a. Functional constipation
    H3b. Nonretentive fecal incontinence

Textbook of Clinical Gastroenterology and Hepatology, Second Edition. Edited by C. J. Hawkey, Jaime Bosch, Joel E. Richter, Guadalupe Garcia-Tsao, Francis K. L. Chan.

Table 10.2 A. Functional esophageal disorders

A1. Functional heartburn
Diagnostic criteria* must include **all** of the following:
1. Burning retrosternal discomfort or pain
2. Absence of evidence that gastroesophageal acid reflux is the cause of the symptom
3. Absence of histopathology-based esophageal motility disorders

* Criteria fulfilled for the last 3 months with symptom onset at least 6 months prior to diagnosis

A2. Functional chest pain of presumed esophageal origin
Diagnostic criteria* must include **all** of the following:
1. Midline chest pain or discomfort that is not of burning quality
2. Absence of evidence that gastroesophageal reflux is the cause of the symptom
3. Absence of histopathology-based esophageal motility disorders

* Criteria fulfilled for the last 3 months with symptom onset at least 6 months prior to diagnosis

A3. Functional dysphagia
Diagnostic criteria* must include **all** of the following:
1. Sense of solid and/or liquid foods sticking, lodging, or passing abnormally through the esophagus
2. Absence of evidence that gastroesophageal reflux is the cause of the symptom
3. Absence of histopathology-based esophageal motility disorders

* Criteria fulfilled for the last 3 months with symptom onset at least 6 months prior to diagnosis

A4. Globus
Diagnostic criteria* must include **all** of the following:
1. Persistent or intermittent, nonpainful sensation of a lump or foreign body in the throat
2. Occurrence of the sensation between meals
3. Absence of dysphagia or odynophagia
4. Absence of evidence that gastroesophageal reflux is the cause of the symptom
5. Absence of histopathology-based esophageal motility disorders

* Criteria fulfilled for the last 3 months with symptom onset at least 6months prior to diagnosis

Table 10.3 B. Functional gastroduodenal disorders

B1. Functional dyspepsia
Diagnostic criteria* must include:
1. **One or more** of the following:
   a. Bothersome postprandial fullness
   b. Early satiation
   c. Epigastric pain
   d. Epigastric burning
AND
2. No evidence of structural disease (including at upper endoscopy) that is likely to explain the symptoms

* Criteria fulfilled for the last 3 months with symptom onset at least 6 months prior to diagnosis

B1a. Postprandial distress syndrome
Diagnostic criteria* must include **one or both** of the following:
1. Bothersome postprandial fullness, occurring after ordinary-sized meals, at least several times per week
2. Early satiation that prevents finishing a regular meal, at least several times per week

* Criteria fulfilled for the last 3 months with symptom onset at least 6 months prior to diagnosis

Supportive criteria:
1. Upper abdominal bloating or postprandial nausea or excessive belching can be present
2. Epigastric pain syndrome may coexist

B1b. Epigastric pain syndrome
Diagnostic criteria* must include **all** of the following:
1. Pain or burning localized to the epigastrium of at least moderate severity, at least once per week
2. The pain is intermittent
3. Not generalized or localized to other abdominal or chest regions
4. Not relieved by defecation or passage of flatus
5. Not fulfilling criteria for gallbladder and sphincter of Oddi disorders

* Criteria fulfilled for the last 3 months with symptom onset at least 6 months prior to diagnosis

Supportive criteria:
1. The pain may be of a burning quality, but without a retrosternal component
2. The pain is commonly induced or relieved by ingestion of a meal, but may occur while fasting
3. Postprandial distress syndrome may coexist

B2. Belching disorders
B2a. Aerophagia
Diagnostic criteria* must include **all** of the following:

1. Troublesome repetitive belching at least several times a week
2. Air swallowing that is objectively observed or measured

* Criteria fulfilled for the last 3 months with symptom onset at least 6 months prior to diagnosis

B2b. Unspecified excessive belching
Diagnostic criteria* must include **all** of the following:
1. Troublesome repetitive belching at least several times a week
2. No evidence that excessive air swallowing underlies the symptom

* Criteria fulfilled for the last 3 months with symptom onset at least 6 months prior to diagnosis

Table 10.3 (*Continued*)

B3. Nausea and vomiting disorders
B3a. Chronic idiopathic nausea
Diagnostic criteria* must include **all** of the following:
1. Bothersome nausea occurring at least several times per week
2. Not usually associated with vomiting
3. Absence of abnormalities at upper endoscopy or metabolic disease that explains the nausea

* Criteria fulfilled for the last 3 months with symptom onset at least 6 months prior to diagnosis

B3b. Functional vomiting
Diagnostic criteria* must include **all** of the following:
1. On average one or more episodes of vomiting per week
2. Absence of criteria for an eating disorder, rumination, or major psychiatric disease according to the *Diagnostic and Statistical Manual of Mental Disorders* (DSM-IV)
3. Absence of self-induced vomiting and chronic cannabinoid use and absence of abnormalities in the central nervous system or metabolic diseases to explain the recurrent vomiting

* Criteria fulfilled for the last 3 months with symptom onset at least 6 months prior to diagnosis

B3c. Cyclic vomiting syndrome
Diagnostic criteria must include **all** of the following:
1. Stereotypical episodes of vomiting regarding onset (acute) and duration (less than one week)
2. Three or more discrete episodes in the prior year
3. Absence of nausea and vomiting between episodes

Supportive criterion:
History or family history of migraine headaches

B4. Rumination syndrome in adults
Diagnostic criteria must include **both** of the following:
1. Persistent or recurrent regurgitation of recently ingested food into the mouth with subsequent spitting or remastication and swallowing
2. Regurgitation is not preceded by retching

Supportive criteria:
1. Regurgitation events are usually not preceded by nausea
2. Cessation of the process when the regurgitated material becomes acidic
3. Regurgitant contains recognizable food with a pleasant taste

Table 10.4 C. Functional bowel disorders

C1. Irritable bowel syndrome
Diagnostic criterion:*
Recurrent abdominal pain or discomfort** at least 3 days/month in the last months associated with **two or more** of the following:
1. Improvement with defecation
2. Onset associated with a change in frequency of stool
3. Onset associated with a change in form (appearance) of stool

* Criterion fulfilled for the last 3 months with symptom onset at least 6 months prior to diagnosis
** "Discomfort" means an uncomfortable sensation not described as pain
In pathophysiology research and clinical trials, a pain/discomfort frequency of at least 2 days a week during screening evaluation is recommended for subject eligibility

C2. Functional bloating
Diagnostic criteria* must include **both** of the following:
1. Recurrent feeling of bloating or visible distension at least 3 days/month in the last 3 months
2. Insufficient criteria for a diagnosis of functional dyspepsia, irritable bowel syndrome, or other functional gastrointestinal disorder

* Criteria fulfilled for the last 3 months with symptom onset at least 6 months prior to diagnosis

C3. Functional constipation
Diagnostic criteria:*
1. Must include **two or more** of the following:
   a. Straining during at least 25% of defecations
   b. Lumpy or hard stools in at least 25% of defecations
   c. Sensation of incomplete evacuation for at least 25% of defecations
   d. Sensation of anorectal obstruction/blockage for at least 25% of defecations
   e. Manual maneuvers to facilitate at least 25% of defecations (for example, digital evacuation, support of the pelvic floor)
   f. Fewer than three defecations per week
2. Loose stools are rarely present without the use of laxatives
3. Insufficient criteria for irritable bowel syndrome

* Criteria fulfilled for the last 3 months with symptom onset at least 6months prior to diagnosis

C4. Functional diarrhea
Diagnostic criterion:*
Loose (mushy) or watery stools without pain occurring in at least 75% of stools

* Criterion fulfilled for the last 3months with symptom onset at least 6 months prior to diagnosis

C5. Unspecified functional bowel disorder
Diagnostic criterion:*
Bowel symptoms not attributable to an organic etiology that do not meet criteria for the previously defined categories

* Criterion fulfilled for the last 3 months with symptom onset at least 6 months prior to diagnosis

Table 10.5 D. Functional abdominal pain syndrome

D. Functional abdominal pain syndrome
Diagnostic criteria* must include **all** of the following:
1. Continuous or nearly continuous abdominal pain
2. None or only occasional relationship of pain with physiological events (for example, eating, defecation, or menses)
3. Some loss of daily functioning
4. The pain is not feigned (e.g., malingering)
5. Insufficient symptoms to meet criteria for another functional gastrointestinal disorder that would explain the pain

* Criteria fulfilled for the last 3 months with symptom onset at least 6 months prior to diagnosis

Table 10.6 E. Functional gallbladder and sphincter of Oddi disorders

E. Functional gallbladder and sphincter of Oddi disorders
Diagnostic criteria must include episodes of pain located in the epigastrium and/or right upper quadrant and **all** of the following:
1. Episodes lasting 30 minutes or longer
2. Recurrent symptoms occurring at different intervals (not daily)
3. The pain builds up to a steady level
4. The pain is moderate to severe enough to interrupt the patient's daily activities or lead to an emergency department visit
5. The pain is not relieved by bowel movements
6. The pain is not relieved by postural change
7. The pain is not relieved by antacids
8. Exclusion of other structural disease that would explain the symptoms

Supportive criteria:
The pain may present with one or more of the following:
1. Associated with nausea and vomiting
2. Radiates to the back and/or right infra subscapular region
3. Awakens from sleep in the middle of the night

E1. Functional gallbladder disorder
Diagnostic criteria must include **all** of the following:
1. Criteria for functional gallbladder and sphincter of Oddi disorder
2. Gallbladder is present
3. Normal liver enzymes, conjugated bilirubin, and amylase/lipase

E2. Functional biliary sphincter of Oddi isorder
Diagnostic criteria must include **both** of the following:
1. Criteria for functional gallbladder and sphincter of Oddi disorder
2. Normal amylase/lipase

Supportive criterion:
Elevated serum transaminases, alkaline phosphatase, or conjugated bilirubin temporarily related to at least two pain episodes

E3. Functional pancreatic sphincter of Oddi disorder
Diagnostic criteria must include **both** of the following:
1. Criteria for functional gallbladder and sphincter of Oddi disorder and
2. Elevated amylase/lipase

Table 10.7 F. Functional anorectal disorders

F1. Functional fecal incontinence
Diagnostic criteria:*
1. Recurrent uncontrolled passage of fecal material in an individual with a developmental age of at least 4 years and **one or more** of the following:
   a. Abnormal functioning of normally innervated and structurally intact muscles
   b. Minor abnormalities of sphincter structure and/or innervation
   c. Normal or disordered bowel habits, (i.e., fecal retention or diarrhea)
   d. Psychological causes
AND
2. Exclusion of **all** the following:
   a. Abnormal innervation caused by lesion(s) within the brain (e.g., dementia), spinal cord, or sacral nerve roots, or mixed lesions (e.g., multiple sclerosis), or as part of a generalized peripheral or autonomic neuropathy (e.g., due to diabetes)
   b. Anal sphincter abnormalities associated with a multisystem disease (e.g., scleroderma)
   c. Structural or neurogenic abnormalities believed to be the major or primary cause of fecal incontinence

* Criteria fulfilled for the last 3 months

F2. Functional anorectal pain
F2a. Chronic proctalgia
Diagnostic criteria* must include **all** of the following:
1. Chronic or recurrent rectal pain or aching
2. Episodes last 20 minutes or longer
3. Exclusion of other causes of rectal pain such as ischemia, inflammatory bowel disease, cryptitis, intramuscular abscess, anal fissure, hemorrhoids, prostatitis, and coccygodynia

* Criteria fulfilled for the last 3 months with symptom onset at least 6 months prior to diagnosis
Chronic proctalgia may be further characterized into levator ani syndrome or unspecified anorectal pain based on digital rectal examination

F2a.1. Levator ani syndrome
Diagnostic criterion:
Symptom criteria for chronic proctalgia and tenderness during posterior traction on the puborectalis

F2a.2. Unspecified functional anorectal pain
Diagnostic criterion:
Symptom criteria for chronic proctalgia but no tenderness during posterior traction on the puborectalis

F2b. Proctalgia fugax
Diagnostic criteria must include **all** of the following:
1. Recurrent episodes of pain localized to the anus or lower rectum
2. Episodes last from seconds to minutes
3. There is no anorectal pain between episodes

For research purposes criteria must be fulfilled for 3 months; however, clinical diagnosis and evaluation may be made prior to 3 months

(Continued)

Table 10.7 (*Continued*)

F3. Functional defecation disorders

Diagnostic criteria:*

1. The patient must satisfy diagnostic criteria for functional constipation**
2. During repeated attempts to defecate must have **at least two** of the following:
   a. Evidence of impaired evacuation, based on balloon expulsion test or imaging
   b. Inappropriate contraction of the pelvic floor muscles (that is, anal sphincter or puborectalis) or less than 20% relaxation of basal resting sphincter pressure by manometry, imaging, or EMG
   c. Inadequate propulsive forces assessed by manometry or imaging

* Criteria fulfilled for the last 3 months with symptom onset at least 6 months prior to diagnosis
** Diagnostic criteria for functional constipation:

1. Must include **two or more** of the following:
   (a) Straining during at least 25% of defecations
   (b) Lumpy or hard stools in at least 25% of defecations
   (c) Sensation of incomplete evacuation for at least 25% of defecations
   (d) Sensation of anorectal obstruction/blockage for at least 25% of defecations
   (e) Manual maneuvers to facilitate at least 25% of defecations (for example, digital evacuation, support of the pelvic floor)
   (f) Fewer than three defecations per week
2. Loose stools are rarely present without the use of laxatives.
3. Insufficient criteria for irritable bowel syndrome.

F3a. Dyssynergic defecation

Diagnostic criterion:

Inappropriate contraction of the pelvic floor or less than 20% relaxation of basal resting sphincter pressure with adequate propulsive forces during attempted defecation

F3b. Inadequate defecatory propulsion

Diagnostic criterion:

Inadequate propulsive forces with or without inappropriate contraction or less than 20% relaxation of the anal sphincter during attempted defecation

Table 10.8 G. Childhood functional GI disorders: infant/toddler

G1. Infant regurgitation

Diagnostic criteria must include **both** of the following in otherwise healthy infants

3 weeks to 12 months of age:

1. Regurgitation two or more times per day for 3 or more weeks
2. No retching, hematemesis, aspiration, apnea, failure to thrive, feeding or swallowing difficulties, or abnormal posturing

G2. Infant rumination syndrome

Diagnostic criteria must include **all** of the following for at least 3 months:

1. Repetitive contractions of the abdominal muscles, diaphragm, and tongue
2. Regurgitation of gastric content into the mouth, which is either expectorated or rechewed and reswallowed
3. Three or more of the following:
   a. Onset between 3 and 8 months
   b. Does not respond to management for gastroesophageal reflux disease, or to anticholinergic drugs, hand restraints, formula changes, and gavage or gastrostomy feedings
   c. Unaccompanied by signs of nausea or distress
   d. Does not occur during sleep and when the infant is interacting with individuals in the environment

G3. Cyclic vomiting syndrome

Diagnostic criteria must include **both** of the following:

1. Two or more periods of intense nausea and unremitting vomiting or retching lasting hours to days
2. Return to usual state of health lasting weeks to months

G4. Infant colic

Diagnostic criteria must include **all** of the following in infants from birth to 4 months of age:

1. Paroxysms of irritability, fussing or crying that starts and stops without obvious cause
2. Episodes lasting 3 or more hours/day and occurring at least 3 days/ wk for at least 1 week
3. No failure to thrive

G5. Functional diarrhea

Diagnostic criteria must include **all** of the following:

1. Daily painless, recurrent passage of three or more large, unformed stools
2. Symptoms that last more than 4 weeks
3. Onset of symptoms that begins between 6 and 36 months of age
4. Passage of stools that occurs during waking hours
5. There is no failure-to-thrive if caloric intake is adequate

G6. Infant dyschezia

Diagnostic criteria must include **both** of the following in an infant less than 6 months of age:

1. At least 10 minutes of straining and crying before successful passage of soft stools
2. No other health problems

G7. Functional constipation

Diagnostic criteria must include one month of **at least two** of the following in infants up to 4 years of age:

1. Two or fewer defecations per week
2. At least one episode/week of incontinence after the acquisition of toileting skills
3. History of excessive stool retention
4. History of painful or hard bowel movements
5. Presence of a large fecal mass in the rectum
6. History of large diameter stools which may obstruct the toilet

Accompanying symptoms may include irritability, decreased appetite, and/or early satiety. The accompanying symptoms disappear immediately following passage of a large stool.

Table 10.9 H. Childhood functional GI disorders: child/adolescent

H1. Vomiting and aerophagea
H1a. Adolescent rumination syndrome
Diagnostic criteria* must include **all** of the following:
1. Repeated painless regurgitation and rechewing or expulsion of food that
   a. begin soon after ingestion of a meal
   b. do not occur during sleep
   c. do not respond to standard treatment for gastroesophageal reflux
2. No retching
3. No evidence of an inflammatory, anatomic, metabolic, or neoplastic process that explains the subject's symptoms

* Criteria fulfilled for the last 3 months with symptom onset at least 6 months prior to diagnosis

H1b. Cyclic vomiting syndrome
Diagnostic criteria must include **both** of the following:
1. Two or more periods of intense nausea and unremitting vomiting or retching lasting hours to days
2. Return to usual state of health lasting weeks to months

H1c. Aerophagia
Diagnostic criteria* must include **at least two** of the following:
1. Air swallowing
2. Abdominal distention due to intraluminal air
3. Repetitive belching and/or increased flatus

* Criteria fulfilled at least once per week for at least 2 months prior to diagnosis

H2. Abdominal pain-related functional GI disorders
H2a. Functional dyspepsia
Diagnostic criteria* must include **all** of the following:
1. Persistent or recurrent pain or discomfort centered in the upper abdomen (above the umbilicus)
2. Not relieved by defecation or associated with the onset of a change in stool frequency or stool form (that is, not irritable bowel syndrome)
3. No evidence of an inflammatory, anatomic, metabolic or neoplastic process that explains the subject's symptoms

* Criteria fulfilled at least once per week for at least 2 months prior to diagnosis

H2b. Irritable bowel syndrome
Diagnostic criteria* must include **both** of the following:
1. Abdominal discomfort** or pain associated with **two or more** of the following at least 25% of the time:
   a. Improvement with defecation
   b. Onset associated with a change in frequency of stool
   c. Onset associated with a change in form (appearance) of stool
2. No evidence of an inflammatory, anatomic, metabolic, or neoplastic process that explains the subject's symptoms

* Criteria fulfilled at least once per week for at least 2 months prior to diagnosis
** "Discomfort" means an uncomfortable sensation not described as pain.

H2c. Abdominal migraine
Diagnostic criteria* must include **all** of the following:
1. Paroxysmal episodes of intense, acute periumbilical pain that lasts for an hour or more
2. Intervening periods of usual health lasting weeks to months
3. The pain interferes with normal activities
4. The pain is associated with 2 of the following:
   a. Anorexia
   b. Nausea
   c. Vomiting
   d. Headache
   e. Photophobia
   f. Pallor
5. No evidence of an inflammatory, anatomic, metabolic, or neoplastic process considered that explains the subject's symptoms

* Criteria fulfilled two or more times in the preceding 12 months

H2d. Childhood functional abdominal pain
Diagnostic criteria* must include **all** of the following:
1. Episodic or continuous abdominal pain
2. Insufficient criteria for other functional gastrointestinal disorders
3. No evidence of an inflammatory, anatomic, metabolic, or neoplastic process that explains the subject's symptoms

* Criteria fulfilled at least once per week for at least 2 months prior to diagnosis

H2d1. Childhood functional abdominal pain syndrome
Diagnostic criteria* must satisfy criteria for childhood functional abdominal pain and have for 25% of the time at least **one or more** of the following:
1. Some loss of daily functioning
2. Additional somatic symptoms such as headache, limb pain, or difficulty sleeping

* Criteria fulfilled at least once per week for at least 2 months prior to diagnosis

H3. Constipation and incontinence
H3a. Functional constipation
Diagnostic criteria* must include **two or more** of the following in a child with a developmental age of at least 4 years with insufficient criteria for diagnosis of IBS:
1. Two or fewer defecations in the toilet per week
2. At least one episode of fecal incontinence per week
3. History of retentive posturing or excessive volitional stool retention
4. History of painful or hard bowel movements
5. Presence of a large fecal mass in the rectum
6. History of large diameter stools which may obstruct the toilet

* Criteria fulfilled at least once per week for at least 2 months prior to diagnosis

H3b. Nonretentive fecal incontinence
Diagnostic criteria* must include **all** of the following in a child with a developmental age at least 4 years:
1. Defecation into places inappropriate to the social context at least once per month
2. No evidence of an inflammatory, anatomic, metabolic, or neoplastic process that explains the subject's symptoms
3. No evidence of fecal retention

* Criteria fulfilled for at least 2 months prior to diagnosis

that many of the Rome III criteria exclude patients who might attract a particular "label" in more informal clinical practice. Whether the current criteria are too narrow, whether informal approaches adopted in practice are too lax, and whether a symptom- rather than a syndrome-based approach to functional gastrointestinal disorders would be more productive are all unanswered questions. To assist readers in considering these issues, the editors have reproduced here the overall classification of functional gastrointestinal disorders and the formal diagnostic criteria for establishing them [1].

References

1. Rome Foundation. *Rome III Diagnostic Criteria for Functional Gastrointestinal Disorders*, Third Edition 2006. Further details at: http://www.romecriteria.org/edproducts/romeiii.cfm http://www.romecriteria.org/assets/pdf/19_RomeIII_apA_885-898.pdf.
2. Hungin AF,Whorwell PJ,Tack J, Mearin F. The prevalence, patterns and impact of irritable bowel syndrome: an international survey of 4000 subjects. *Aliment Pharmacol Ther.* 2003;17:643–650.

CHAPTER 11
Anorexia nervosa and bulimia nervosa

Tomas J. Silber
Don Delaney Eating Disorders Program, Division of Adolescent and Young Adult Medicine; Children's National Medical Center; George Washington University, Washington, DC, USA

KEY POINTS

- Malnutrition caused by restrictive eating induces delayed gastric emptying, impaired intestinal motility and ketosis , which in turn make it more difficult to eat
- Laboratory evaluation may be normal. Typical abnormal laboratory findings are: leukopenia; low T3; elevated liver enzymes (AN); hypochloremic, hyponatremic, hypokalemic alkalosis; and elevated amylase (salivary) in bulimia
- The morbidity from anorexia nervosa includes severe constipation, superior mesenteric artery syndrome, liver steatosis, renal isostenuria, amenorrhea, osteopenia, brain changes, bradycardia, prolongation of the QT interval, and arrhythmia
- The morbidity from bulimia includes parotid hypertrophy, dental loss, esophagitis, electrolyte imbalance, dehydration
- Mortality is due to starvation, suicide, sudden cardiac death, liver failure, renal failure and electrolyte imbalance
- Treatment needs to be alert to the possibility of a refeeding syndrome, the induction of hypophosphatemia, which can result in edema, cardiac insufficiency, severe bone pain, psychosis and death

---

Introduction

Eating disorders are usually considered as belonging to the field of mental health. However, the reality is that there are serious medical complications, including death, that require patients to be monitored and treated by physicians. This chapter has been written to facilitate a clinician's ability to:

- Diagnose anorexia nervosa, bulimia nervosa, and eating disorders, not otherwise specified;
- Consider a differential diagnosis;
- Select the appropriate laboratory assessments;
- Understand the physiopathology of starvation and electrolyte imbalance;
- Anticipate and detect potential medical complications;
- Recognize water loading;
- Identify and prevent the refeeding syndrome;
- Make judicious use of medication.

What are they?

Anorexia nervosa is a condition that is usually suspected whenever a young person, who is otherwise healthy, is found to have marked weight loss, or to be malnourished. Characteristically they refuse to maintain body weight above the minimal normal weight for age and height, have an intense fear of weight gain (recovery), of getting fat, experience a body image disorder, and have become amenorrheic (unless on hormonal replacement). Patients with anorexia nervosa often consider themselves fit and resist the idea that they have a medical problem. "There is nothing wrong with me," goes the typical comment, "I always eat healthy." The distinguishing features are: a fanatical pursuit of thinness, loss of 15% or more of bodyweight, amenorrhea, phobic fear of weight gain or fatness, body image distortion, and denial of the seriousness of the condition. Patients may or may not purge.

Bulimia nervosa is a condition characterized by binge eating followed by purging. This usually consists of self-induced vomiting (manually, with instruments or with ipecac), but purging may also be done by laxatives, diuretics, and/or compulsive exercising. Purging is a solitary and secretive activity practiced by patients who mostly are of normal weight. Therefore it may be difficult to detect unless the patient self-reports, is "caught in the act," or medical complications ensue.

Eating disorders, NOS (not otherwise specified) There are an even greater number of people who have subthreshold presentations, whose eating habits are clearly disordered, who may engage in frequent fasting, binging, and purging, but who do not fit the criteria for either anorexia nervosa or bulimia. They are often malnourished and in need of treatment, and are all subsumed under the diagnosis of eating disorders, NOS.

The psychiatric diagnosis of an eating disorder is confirmed following the criteria established in the *Diagnostic and Statistical Manual of Medical Disorders* (DSM-IV TR), criteria [1].

How common are they?

The lifetime prevalence of anorexia nervosa is approximately 0.5%; close to half of individuals with anorexia nervosa will eventually develop bulimia nervosa. Moreover, the lifetime prevalence for the latter is estimated to be between 1% and 3%. The incidence of eating disorders, NOS is unknown, but certainly much higher. The ratio of female to male patients with eating disorders ranges from 10:1 to 20:1. These conditions can begin in childhood, almost always arise during adolescence

---

Textbook of Clinical Gastroenterology and Hepatology, Second Edition. Edited by C. J. Hawkey, Jaime Bosch, Joel E. Richter, Guadalupe Garcia-Tsao, Francis K. L. Chan.
© 2012 Blackwell Publishing Ltd. Published 2012 by Blackwell Publishing Ltd.

Table 11.1 Physiopathology of human starvation, purging, water intoxication, and refeeding starvation

---

Starvation
- Initial phase – accelerated hepatic gluconeogenesis
- Final phase – ketosis, reduction of protein catabolism
- Glycogen depletion, hypoglycemia, low T3 levels, hypercholesterolemia, hypercarotenemia
- Hypometabolic state – amenorrhea, bradycardia, hypotension, orthostasis, hypothermia, lanugo, organic brain syndrome, confusion, lethargy, coma, death

---

Purging, water intoxication, and refeeding starvation
- Hypokalemic alkalosis, hypochloremia, hyponatremia (secondary hyperaldosteronism)
- Acidosis (laxative abuse)
- Hyponatremia, dilutional ("water loading")
- Hypomagnesemia, hypocalcemia, zinc deficiency (starvation)
- Hypophosphatemia, hypomagnesemia ("refeeding syndrome," extracellular phosphorus level falls abruptly as it becomes intracellular)
- Seizures, delirium, arrhythmias, sudden death

---

and young adulthood, and seldom develop after the age of 40 years. There is an increased risk of anorexia nervosa among first-degree biologic relatives. The concordance rate for monozygotic twins is significantly higher than for dizygotic twins. The long-term mortality rate was close to 20% for anorexia nervosa and is currently declining substantially, and is unknown for bulimia nervosa [2].

Pathophysiology

Patients with anorexia nervosa who are pure food restrictors develop severe malnutrition, whereas anorexic patients who purge, patients with bulimia nervosa, and in general all those who self-induce vomiting or abuse laxatives, tend to have complications relating to electrolyte imbalances. Dramatic and dangerous physiologic changes may take place during refeeding attempts [2–6] (Table 11.1).

Malnutrition eventually results in emaciation, amenorrhea, hypothermia, bradycardia, hypotension, orthostasis, and chronic depression. It is useful to understand the physiology of starvation. The organism's attempts at adaptation to lack of food take place at a metabolic and neuroendocrine level. These metabolic changes can be understood as an attempt to maintain glucose homeostasis (initial phase) and to conserve protein (final phase). Initially there is an acceleration of hepatic gluconeogenesis (alanine produced by the muscles is its main substrate).When starvation is prolonged, the organism responds to the depletion of protein with a metabolic shift to the burning of fat and production of ketone bodies, thus giving priority to protein conservation.

Ketonemia has a special significance. Acetone gradually replaces glucose as fuel for the brain. In addition, ketones send signals to the muscles to reduce their catabolic rate. However this attempt of adaptation to starvation fails if malnutrition is

allowed to progress, and gives way to a persistent hypometabolic state, with amenorrhea, hypothermia, marked bradycardia, hypotension, and orthostasis. As starvation continues unabated, the patient subsequently develops an organic brain syndrome that progresses to obtundation, lethargy, coma, and death.

Hypophosphatemia in its protean manifestations, more commonly occurs when hospitalized patients receive an excessive nutritional treatment (**refeeding syndrome**). Hypophosphatemia is rare in the untreated anorexic because phosphorus is found in nearly all foods. During the phase of starvation, phosphorus is not much needed for fat metabolism. By contrast, metabolism of glucose requires the presence of phosphate. With the arrival of food, the extracellular phosphorus enters the cells and hypophosphatemia ensues. Hypophosphatemia is characterised by:

- nausea and vomiting
- weakness
- anorexia.

In severe cases there may be:

- hemolytic anemia
- rhabdomyolysis
- cardiomyopathy
- respiratory insufficiency.

The central nervous system is sensitive to hypophosphatemia, responding with:

- confusion
- delirium
- psychosis
- convulsions.

Death may even result. Therefore, rapid loading of parenteral glucose or brisk realimentation should be avoided and phosphorus given with increased nourishment.

Waterloading Occasionally, anorectic patients drink large amounts of water to conceal weight loss. This can cause dilutional hyponatremia, with weakness, irritability, and confusion, progressing to brain edema, seizures and even death.

Purgation leads to reduced blood volume, compensatory hyperaldosteronism and hypochloremic alkalosis. Patients who abuse laxatives tend to become acidotic.

Gastrointestinal manifestations Eating disorders in which malnutrition predominates show delayed gastric emptying and impaired intestinal motility and constipation, which conspire against nutritional rehabilitation. Malnutrition can also induce fatty infiltrate of the liver and, rarely, liver failure. When a significant amount of omentum is lost, the aortic-mesenteric compass can collapse resulting in intermittent obstruction of the third portion of the duodenum. Self induced vomiting can cause Mallory–Weiss tears or esophageal rupture. Acute dilatation from severe binging is recognised.

Causes and differential diagnosis

The eating disorders have been described for centuries, ranging from behaviors manifested in the Roman "vomitoriums" to the feats of the starving saints. Leading researchers declare themselves "agnostic" in relationship to the cause of eating disorders [7]. The causes of these psychiatric illnesses are more than likely multifactorial in that there is:

- A strong genetic component (probably relating to traits such as perfectionism and obsessiveness),
- An important sociocultural component (influencing the role of body image),
- A significant psychological component, manifest as:
  o emotional avoidance
  o perfectionism
  o set shifting difficulties
  o alexithymia in anorexia nervosa
  o impulsivity and addictive tendencies in bulimia nervosa.

Triggering factors have been described often, such as losses and stress (a move, a sibling going to college, a death in the family) or critical remarks about the young person's body. Past episodes of sexual abuse do not occur more often than in the general psychiatric population.

Biological factors such as hypothalamic malfunction, hormonal abnormalities and alterations of the function of serotonin and other neuronal systems, have also been implicated. Currently there are attempts to link eating disorders to hormones involved in appetite control such as leptin and peptide yy [8].

Not every young person with weight loss and amenorrhea has anorexia nervosa, nor does everybody with weight concerns and recurrent vomiting have bulimia nervosa. The reason for this is that dissatisfaction with body image and dieting are almost universal preoccupations, and therefore may simply coincide with another illness. There is a long list of differential diagnoses to consider, including other psychiatric pathology, particularly depression. A not infrequent pitfall is to overdiagnose as an eating disorder what is actually a **gastrointestinal pathology**. The most common cause of error is overlooking Crohn's disease (see Chapter 50). The same holds true for celiac disease (see Chapter 40) and achalasia (see Chapter 36).

Psychiatric conditions may lead to emaciation. Patients with major depression may suffer psychomotor retardation, insomnia and profound lack of appetite. On the other hand, severe malnutrition can result in marked depression. Schizophrenia or other psychotic conditions may manifest with bizarre ideas, such as the fear of being poisoned, with the resulting food refusal. Social phobias may incline to the avoidance of being seen eating. Obsessive compulsive disorder may involve unusual eating rituals. An episode of choking can lead to a swallowing phobia.

DIFFERENTIAL DIAGNOSIS OF THE EATING DISORDERS

Behavioral or psychiatric pathology
Major depression, psychosis, or schizophrenia
Substance abuse (cocaine, amphetamines)
Social phobia

Gastrointestinal pathology
Inflammatory bowel disease
Celiac and other malabsorption syndromes
Achalasia
Superior mesenteric artery syndrome

Endocrine pathology
Hyperthyroidism
Diabetes mellitus type 1
Addison's disease
Hypothalamic tumors
Sheehan's syndrome
Obsessive compulsive disorder
Dysmorphophobia
Swallowing phobia

Miscellaneous
Hyperemesis gravidarum
Emaciating diseases (AIDS, tuberculosis, metastatic cancer)

Crohn's disease can be overlooked, especially when it follows an indolent course, with scant if any GI symptoms such as a very slow progression of puberty, weight loss, and growth deceleration.

Celiac disease and other malabsorption syndromes may also mimic anorexia nervosa. Weight loss may occur years after the initial diagnosis has been forgotten; typically, with the beginning of adolescence and the desire to be "like everybody else," the gluten-free diet is abandoned and the malnutrition ensues.

Achalasia can lead to severe weight loss and amenorrhea as a result of dysphagia, which may be ignored as "typical manipulation of patients with eating disorders," unless a barium swallow demonstrates the condition.

Superior mesenteric artery syndrome may induce remarkable weight loss secondary to recurrent vomiting. It is caused by intermittent compression of the second portion of the duodenum, clamped between the superior mesenteric artery and the aorta, in patients who have experienced rapid weight loss (e.g., following bariatric surgery). The patients assume a typical position when eating: they bend forward. This syndrome can be a complication of anorexia nervosa.

Endocrine disorders can also result in marked weight loss and amenorrhea. Hyperthyroidism can present with rapid and progressive malnutrition, but is easily differentiated from anorexia nervosa because of tachycardia, hypertension, and a hypermetabolic state. Often the simple observation of the hyperphagic, hyperthyroid adolescent is sufficient to rule out anorexia nervosa.

Diabetes type 1 can also present with rapid weight loss. However, these patients are polydipsic, polyphagic, and polyuric, and deteriorate rapidly into ketoacidosis.

Addison's disease manifests with fatigue, anorexia, recurrent vomiting, and hypotension. The patient is very weak and develops brownish skin pigmentation. The diagnosis is suspected by electrolyte abnormalities and confirmed by endocrine testing.

Sheehan's syndrome occurs in young women following a hypothalamic injury as the result of a massive postpartum hemorrhage, resulting in weight loss, weakness, and amenorrhea due to panhypopituitarism.

A variety of tumors and hypothalamic lesions can induce abnormal eating behaviors and weight loss, which is not surprising because the hypothalamus regulates appetite. However, these lesions are associated with findings suggestive of a central nervous system disorder, such as headaches, abnormal thirst, diplopia, papilledema, and/or spontaneous projectile vomiting.

Systemic conditions such as severe infections (tuberculosis), immunologic disorders (AIDS), chronic conditions (cystic fibrosis), and malignancies may lead to emaciation and amenorrhea, but these patients appear much sicker than those with eating disorders and appropriate tests easily confirm their diagnosis.

Pregnancy may be confused with bulimia nervosa in secretive adolescents developing hyperemesis gravidarum. A complete sexual history and pregnancy testing should always be part of the evaluation.

Substance abuse can cause malnutrition, especially if it involves powerful appetite suppressors (cocaine or amphetamines). Patients with bulimia nervosa, who often have an impulse disorder, may also harbor drug addictions and alcoholism.

Symptom complexes

Symptoms vary depending on whether starving or purging predominate [1–6] (Figure 11.1).

Anorexia nervosa Semistarvation leads to constipation, abdominal pain, and postprandial discomfort. Most patients develop delayed gastric emptying and impaired intestinal motility. They suffer from cold intolerance, become hypothermic, and develop acrocyanosis and lanugo. Dehydration and orthostasis are common. Peripheral edema on cessation of the use of laxatives and diuretics can be dramatic. Edema can also occur upon refeeding. The skin may look yellow due to raised levels of carotene. Many develop normochromic, normocytic anemia. Impaired renal function can manifest with

isosthenuria. Cardiovascular symptoms are due to impaired myocardial contractility, mitral valve prolapse, and arrhythmias. Prolonged amenorrhea and reduced estrogen secretion may result in osteopenia, osteoporosis, and fractures.

Bulimia nervosa Exposure to gastric contents leads to loss of dental enamel. The teeth become chipped and appear "motheaten," with increased dental cavities. Patients also develop marked parotid hypertrophy and conjunctival hemorrhage. Those that stimulate the gag reflex manually develop calluses on the dorsal surface of their hand (Russell's sign).

Deadly cardiomyopathy and muscle injury may result from the use of ipecac to induce emesis. Recurrent vomiting can induce chest pain (see Chapter 1), esophagitis, and Barrett's esophagus (see Chapter 29). Many become laxative dependent and develop melanosis coli, cathartic colon, rectal prolapse, and melena. Electrolyte changes stemming from purging can result in fatal arrhythmias. Other potentially fatal complications include esophageal tears, gastric rupture, and acute dilatation of the stomach (see Chapters 19 and 20).

It always needs to be remembered that psychiatric comorbidity is common in patients with eating disorders, including mood disorders, anxiety disorders, obsessive compulsive disorder, personality disorders, and addictive disorders. Suicide is a leading cause of death in patients with eating disorders.

Diagnosis

The term anorexia is a misnomer because patients with anorexia nervosa initially do not suffer from loss of appetite. After recovery from the illness, many confess to have suffered from chronic hunger. Patients with bulimia nervosa who binge and purge keep this shrouded in secrecy and usually admit to it only when "caught in the act."

A **diagnosis** needs to be based on more than malnutrition and amenorrhea, requiring the presence of positive data, such as distorted body image, fanatic pursuit of thinness, binge eating followed by purging, etc. A series of screening questions may help to elicit the data necessary to fulfil DSM-IV criteria [1–6]. They include inquiry about eating patterns, bingeing, purging, exercise, degree of satisfaction with the body, undue influence of shape and weight on self-evaluation, fear of being or becoming fat (in an underweight individual), refusal to reach or maintain a medically recommended bodyweight, and denial of the seriousness of the condition. A mental health provider can confirm the diagnosis with an eating disorders evaluation.

Many patients are not forthcoming with their symptoms. The **physical examination** may detect elements of a hypometabolic states (being cold all the time). The characteristic dental changes of loss of enamel should always raise the question of bulimia with vomiting, as should Russell's sign (Figure 11.1). Anthropometric measurements should include an assessment of height and weight for calculation of the body mass index

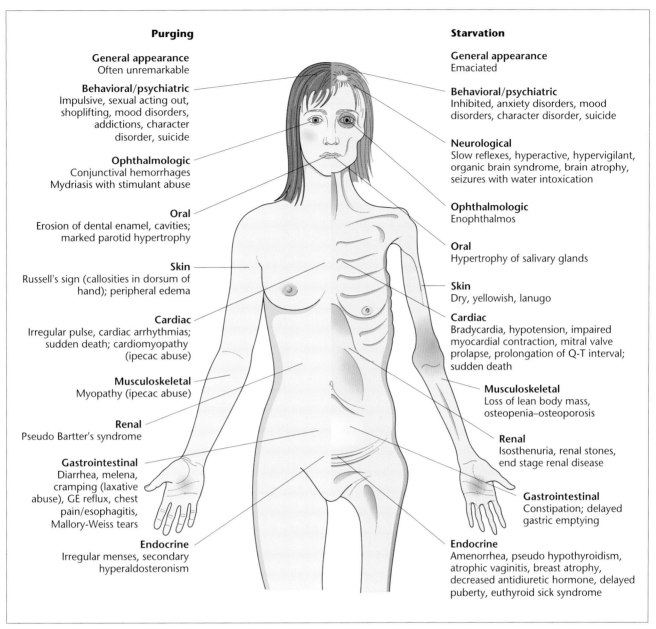

Purging

General appearance
Often unremarkable

Behavioral/psychiatric
Impulsive, sexual acting out, shoplifting, mood disorders, addictions, character disorder, suicide

Ophthalmologic
Conjunctival hemorrhages
Mydriasis with stimulant abuse

Oral
Erosion of dental enamel, cavities; marked parotid hypertrophy

Skin
Russell's sign (callosities in dorsum of hand); peripheral edema

Cardiac
Irregular pulse, cardiac arrhythmias; sudden death; cardiomyopathy (ipecac abuse)

Musculoskeletal
Myopathy (ipecac abuse)

Renal
Pseudo Bartter's syndrome

Gastrointestinal
Diarrhea, melena, cramping (laxative abuse), GE reflux, chest pain/esophagitis, Mallory-Weiss tears

Endocrine
Irregular menses, secondary hyperaldosteronism

Starvation

General appearance
Emaciated

Behavioral/psychiatric
Inhibited, anxiety disorders, mood disorders, character disorder, suicide

Neurological
Slow reflexes, hyperactive, hypervigilant, organic brain syndrome, brain atrophy, seizures with water intoxication

Ophthalmologic
Enophthalmos

Oral
Hypertrophy of salivary glands

Skin
Dry, yellowish, lanugo

Cardiac
Bradycardia, hypotension, impaired myocardial contraction, mitral valve prolapse, prolongation of Q-T interval; sudden death

Musculoskeletal
Loss of lean body mass, osteopenia–osteoporosis

Renal
Isosthenuria, renal stones, end stage renal disease

Gastrointestinal
Constipation; delayed gastric emptying

Endocrine
Amenorrhea, pseudo hypothyroidism, atrophic vaginitis, breast atrophy, decreased antidiuretic hormone, delayed puberty, euthyroid sick syndrome

Figure 11.1 Symptom complexes in patients with eating disorders. The right side shows the general appearances in patients who starve themselves, and the left side shows appearances in those who purge. Symptoms may overlap as patients with anorexia nervosa who purge will develop complications associated with purging, and patients with bulimia nervosa may also fast or diet, becoming malnourished. (This figure was published in *Clinical Gastroenterology and Hepatology*, Wilfred M. Weinstein, Christopher J. Hawkey, Jaime Bosch, Anorexia nervosa and bulimia nervosa, Pages 1–6, Copyright Elsevier, 2005.)

(BMI). This is obtained by dividing weight in kilograms by height in meters squared. A BMI of $16\,\mathrm{kg/m^2}$ or less is characteristic of anorexia nervosa. This measurement has less utility in children, where the trajectory along the percentiles is of more significance, especially for following the patient's growth, as this can be stunted by malnutrition.

Laboratory assessment
Laboratory findings can be falsely reassuring, as many patients have been known to die with "normal lab values" [4].

Baseline laboratory testing A full blood count may show hemoconcentration, as well as a malfunctioning bone marrow, with leukopenia with low total lymphocyte count. A comprehensive metabolic panel may suggest fatty liver infiltrate when there are raised liver enzyme levels (see Chapter 18), dehydration (pre-renal azotemia), and acute starvation (low prealbumin and transferrin may be useful markers for fasting, as their half-life is much shorter than that of albumin).

Patients who vomit frequently may demonstrate hypochloremic, hypokalemic, hyponatremic metabolic alkalosis as well as increased levels of amylase (salivary). Persistent hypoglycemia is an ominous sign. Hormonal profiles in amenorrheic patients, show prepubertal gonadotropins and low estradiol levels. Triiodothyronine (T3), is low in starvation with a normal thyroid stimulating hormone ruling out hypothyroidism. Urinalysis may show proteinuria (increased exercise), ketonuria (fasting), isosthenuria (renal impairment), low specific gravity (waterloading) or abnormal microscopy findings (dehydration).

Bone density by dexa-scan may reveal osteopenia or osteoporosis.

Neuroradiology can demonstrate brain atrophy, mostly of white matter but also of some gray matter, which may be only partially reversible. Arterial flow alterations through the brain have also been observed. These are usually research studies. However those few patients with atypical eating disorders, who complain of headaches or explosive vomiting without nausea require imaging to rule out a brain tumor.

Electrocardiogram can rapidly detect hypokalemia, prolongation of the QT interval, and arrhythmia. Hospitalized patients require cardiac monitors. If mitral valve prolapse or diminished contractility is suspected, an echocardiogram can be indicated.

Treatment approaches and current developments

The eating disorders are considered psychiatric illnesses and there is still ongoing debate as to the best treatment. **Practice guidelines** have been proposed by the American Psychiatric Association [3], the American Academy of Pediatrics [4], the Society for Adolescent Medicine [5], the American Dietetic Association [6], and most recently by the UK National Institute for Clinical Excellence [2–5].

Currently there is consensus that specialized multidisciplinary treatment teams might offer the best possibility for recovery [1–7]. **Nutritional rehabilitation** is at the heart of recovery (see Chapter 144). **Family therapy** is the most helpful treatment for children and adolescents, with individual therapy for young adults. The **Maudsley approach** trains parents on how to best help their child by taking care of the nutritional rehabilitation first, and only once this is achieved, is there follow-up with adolescent and family issues [7]. **Cognitive behavioral therapy** seems to be of great help to patients with bulimia. Treatments based on standard protocols are gaining ascendance [6–9].

Hospitalization is recommended when there is severe malnutrition or out-of-control purging, not only because these situations are dangerous, but also because therapy is not possible with a starved brain [2–7]. Various behavioral therapeutic inpatient programs have been successful in the acute care treatment phase, including nocturnal nasogastric pump

refeeding as the initial approach to nutritional rehabilitation rather than as a treatment of last resort [9]. The degree of nutritional rehabilitation is a crucial variable: patients discharged before reaching 90% of ideal bodyweight have a higher incidence of rehospitalization [10].

Medications are of limited help in the treatment of anorexia nervosa. **Chlorpropamide** given 20 min before meals can alleviate delayed gastric emptying. However this medication has been implicated in the development of tardive dyskinesia. **Phosphorus** is essential during refeeding. The treatment of **osteopenia** is controversial: multivitamins and calcium need to be supplemented, birth control pills seem not to be helpful. Nasal **calcitonin**, oral **alendronate**, and **dehydroepiandrosterone (DHEA)** are experimental. Psychopharmacologic treatment is indicated for psychiatric co-morbidity. **Fluoxetine** has been used to stabilize the weight of chronically ill anorexics. Patients with bulimia nervosa often respond to treatment with selective **serotonin reuptake inhibitors (SSRIs)**. Risperidone and olanzapine (atypical antipsychotic) have shown benefit but risk excessive weight gain with hypertriglyceridemia. **Ondansetron** and **topotecan** are being investigated.

Prognosis

Contrary to general belief, most patients receiving consistent treatment will recover. Patients diagnosed early may respond to brief interventions. A minority of seriously ill or chronically ill patients will require care in specialized programs and even Residential Treatment Centers. Anorexia nervosa, however, has had a disturbingly high long-term mortality rate, as high as 20%. Though this death rate seems to be having an important decline, death is still mostly due to starvation and suicide. Nevertheless many patients with the various eating disorders die from arrhythmias, renal failure, liver failure, and ipecac abuse. The effectiveness of pharmacologic and non-pharmacologic treatment has not been firmly established [11]. The limited data point to the Maudsley method as the most promising one for children and adolescents [12]. The prognosis is more guarded for those who develop their illness later in life, nevertheless even among those who have been seriously ill for many years, recovery is still possible [2–6].

SOURCES OF INFORMATION FOR PATIENTS AND DOCTORS

http://www.patient.co.uk/showdoc/23069106/
http://www.aafp.org/afp/20040401/1729ph.html
http://www.mentalhealth.com/dis/p20-et02.html

Eating disorders – general:
http://www.edauk.com
www.somethingfishy.org
http://www.Feast-ed.org
http://www.maudsleyparents.org

References

1. American Psychiatric Association. *Diagnostic and statistical manual of mental disorders*. 4th edn, text revision. Washington, DC: American Psychiatric Association; 2000.
2. American Psychiatric Association. Practice guideline for the treatment of patients with eating disorders. *Am J Psychiatry.* Suppl 2000;157:1–39.
3. American Academy of Pediatrics. Committee on Adolescence. Policy statement. Identifying and treating eating disorders. *Pediatrics.* 2003;111:204–211.
4. Society for Adolescent Medicine. Eating disorders in adolescents. Position paper of the Society for Adolescent Medicine. *J Adol Health.* 2003;33:496–503.
5. American Dietetic Association. Nutrition intervention in the treatment of anorexia nervosa, bulimia nervosa, and eating disorder not otherwise specified (EDNOS). Position paper. *J Am Diet Assoc.* 2001;101:810–819.
6. Silber TJ. Anorexia nervosa Among Children and Adolescents. *Adv Pediatr.* 2005;52:49–76.
7. Lock J, Le Grange D, Agras WS, *et al. Treatment manual for anorexia nervosa. A family based approach.* New York: Guilford Press; 2001.
8. Kaye W, Frank GK, Bailer UF, *et al.* Neurobiology of Anorexia Nervosa; clinical implications of alterations of the function of serotonin and other neuronal systems. *Int J Eat Disord.* 2005;37: S15–S19.
9. Robb AS, Silber TJ, Orrell-Valente JK, *et al.* Supplemental nocturnal nasogastric refeeding for better short-term outcome in hospitalized adolescent girls with anorexia nervosa. *Am J Psychiatry.* 2002;159:1347–1353.
10. Baran SA, Weltsin TE, Kaye WH. Low discharge weight and outcome in anorexia nervosa. *Am J Psychiatry.* 1995;152: 1070–1072.
11. Gowers SG, Clark C, Roberts A, *et al.* Clinical effectiveness of treatment for anorexia nervosa in adolescence: randomized controlled trial. *Br J Psychiatry.* 2007;191:427–433.
12. National Institute for Clinical Excellence website (www. nice.org.uk). *Quick reference guide; NICE guidelines – full guidelines.* 2004.

CHAPTER 12
Weight loss

Arvey I. Rogers, Hendrikus S. Vanderveldt and Amar R. Deshpande
University of Miami Miller School of Medicine, Miami, FL, USA

ESSENTIAL FACTS ABOUT CAUSATION

The most common causes of involuntary weight loss are malignancy (GI and other), psychological (specific eating disturbances and depression) and benign disorders of the GI tract

Weight loss occurs if intake is inadequate or metabolic demand is increased. It occurs when energy expenditure exceeds energy available through supplied calories. It may also occur when caloric intake is reduced or remains unchanged

Anorexia, mechanical difficulties, sitophobia → reduced intake

Hypermetabolism, catabolism, ↑activity, gut or urine losses may cause weight loss when caloric intake is unchanged

---

ESSENTIALS OF DIAGNOSIS

Evaluation varies with presentation: previous diagnosis; accompanying symptoms; asymptomatic state

Careful history, physical examination, selective laboratory tests focusing on factors → reduced caloric intake and factors → excessive caloric expenditure with normal intake

Use of selective diagnostic procedures for confirmatory purposes

---

ESSENTIALS OF TREATMENT

Identify and correct when possible underlying pathophysiology responsible for reduced caloric intake or excessive caloric losses

Utilize gastrointestinal tract when possible to replace calculated nutritional deficits, i.e., oral or gastroenteric

Parenteral nutrition should be considered when gut cannot be utilized, as a supplement and for short terms; consider appetite stimulants

---

Introduction

Weight loss is a common reason for referral to a Gastroenterologist and is the result of many causes of which cancers, psychological factors (particularly depression) and benign gastrointestinal disorders are the most common. This chapter provides guidelines for effective diagnosis of involuntary weight loss that:

- is accompanied by symptoms of a gastrointestinal disorder
- occurs in the course of an established gastrointestinal disorder
- occurs de novo as the primary presenting symptom.

Definition, prevalence and confirmation

Definition Involuntary weight loss is an umbrella term used to define any clinically significant unintentional or involuntary loss of weight. As such, involuntary weight loss encompasses all other more specific descriptors of weight loss (such as cachexia, wasting and sarcopenia). Clinically significant weight loss is defined as a greater than 5% loss in baseline body weight over a period of 6–12 months [1].

Prevalence The reported prevalence of unintentional weight loss varies greatly by author; however, in the general adult population the prevalence has been reported to be between 1.3% and 10% [2,3]. Unintentional weight loss is more prevalent in older patients as it has been reported in between 13% and 19% of selected elderly outpatient populations [1,2].

Confirmation Many patients don't follow their own weight and only notice significant weight loss as a result of ill-fitting clothes or because of comments made by friends or family. Therefore, the initial stages of weight loss can be easily overlooked. Assessment can be greatly facilitated if weight is recorded at every hospital visit and used to calculate the Body Mass Index (BMI) – weight in kilograms/height in m². At presentation, the extent of weight loss is not always apparent, whilst it also is not uncommon for patients to think they have lost weight when they have not.

In order to uncover and document involuntary weight loss, it is important to develop a practice whereby each patient's weight is recorded with the rest of the patient's vital signs, in essence creating a "fifth vital sign."

An equally important factor useful in the evaluation of a patient's weight is the Body Mass Index (BMI). This number, which can easily be calculated using available on line calculators, is used to standardize a patient's weight by the patient's height. Although it has traditionally been used to track or analyze obesity, the BMI can also give the physician an idea of whether a patient is, at any given time, underweight for his/her size relative to standardized charts.

Differential diagnosis

Unintentional weight loss is due to:

- Caloric intake insufficient to sustain basic metabolic demands.
- Increased metabolic demands.
- A combination of both.

Reduced caloric intake. As well as anorexia and mechanical difficulties, patients may reduce intake in order to avoid symptoms of coughing, pyrosis, chest pain, dysphagia/odynophagia, postprandial fullness, nausea/vomiting, abdominal pain, or diarrhea. An example would be sitophobia (fear of eating) to avoid the abdominal pain that occurs with mesenteric ischemia. For patients dependent on a caretaker, it is important to check that sufficient calories are offered. Important causes of malabsorption resulting in weight loss include celiac disease (Chapter 40), intestinal short gut syndrome (Chapter 41), and bacterial overgrowth (Chapter 42).

Caloric intake unchanged. Weight loss occurring when caloric intake is unchanged suggests a loss of body caloric resources secondary to increased metabolic demands. Its pathophysiology may be the result of: **catabolic states** i.e., inflammation, neoplasm; **hypermetabolic states** i.e., hyperthyroidism; increased losses (gut, urine); or an increase in caloric needs secondary to heightened levels of activity (Table 12.1).

Unintentional weight loss often occurs because of a combination of decreased intake and increased caloric demand. For example, a septic patient may be anorexic as well having enhanced body catabolism.

Diagnostic investigation

Problem solving weight loss (Figure 12.1). Effective identification of the cause of weight loss depends on assessing associated symptoms, considering possible complications of already diagnosed gastrointestinal disorders, and when necessary adopting an approach appropriate to a patient with no overt accompanying symptomatology.

Evaluating associated symptoms. The question to be addressed is:

Do the symptoms (such as nausea and vomiting) explain or suggest a reason for the weight loss or did the symptoms develop secondary to the progression of the weight loss? Once it has been determined that the symptom(s) are a likely explanation for the weight loss, then do these symptoms relate to

an already established medical problem (GI or non-GI-related) or do the symptoms represent the initial presentation of an undiagnosed disease process? (Table 12.2).

If the weight loss and associated symptoms are presenting in a patient without related medical issues, then an in depth work-up of the symptoms themselves is required. One way to

Table 12.1 Etiology of weight loss

Reduced caloric intake
- Anorexia
  - Specific eating disorders
  - Depression
  - Drug side effects
  - Neoplasia
- Mechanical difficulties
  - Oropharynx
    - Dental
    - Mucosal
    - Neuromuscular
  - Esophagus
    - Dysphagia
    - Odynophagia
  - Stomach
    - Early satiety
    - Nausea/vomiting
- Sitophobia
- Reduced feeding by a carer

Unchanged caloric intake
- Hypermetabolism
- Hyperthyroidism
- Catabolism
  - Inflammation
  - Neoplasm
- Increased losses
  - Gut
    - Malassimilation
  - Urinary loss
    - Diabetes mellitus
- Increased physical activity

Table 12.2 Important symptoms in patients with involuntary weight loss

• Anorexia	• Insomnia
• Sitophobia	• Palpitations
• Dysphagia/odynophagia	• Depression
• Early satiety[1]	• Claudication[2]
• Abdominal/back pain[1,2]	• Dyspnea[5]
• Nausea/vomiting	• Cough
• Diarrhea[3]	• Bone pain
• Change in bowel habits[3,4]	• Night sweats[6]
• Polyuria	• Pruritus[7]
• Polydipsia	
• Heat intolerance	

1, gastric/pancreas neoplasm; 2, mesenteric vascular disease; 3, IBD, malabsorption; 4, colonic neoplasm; 5, cardiopulmonary insufficiency, anemia, pulmonary neoplasm, emboli; 6, neoplasm (lymphoma), tuberculosis; 7, neoplasm (lymphoma), bile salt retention, iron deficiency.

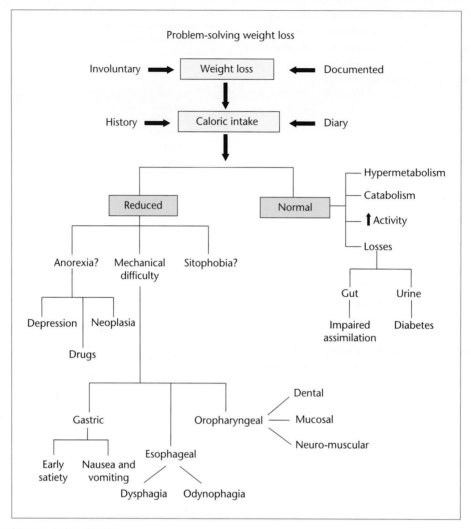

Figure 12.1 Problem-solving weight loss algorithm.

start would be to consider whether any associated symptoms (such as nausea and vomiting) relate primarily to the gastrointestinal tract. If the symptoms do relate to the gastrointestinal tract then the next step in our algorithm would be to decide if the symptoms result from a disorder of structure or function. Based on these assumptions, order the appropriate confirmatory tests. If the symptoms are not related to the gastrointestinal tract but are still considered part of the primary cause, for example severe shortness of breath, then diagnostics should be directed at elucidating the cause of the non-gastrointestinal symptomatology.

Assessing the contribution of already diagnosed gastrointestinal disorder. When there is an established illness, one should consider whether the symptoms might have resulted from the illness itself, a complication of the illness, a consequence of therapy, related in some way to a diagnostic procedure, or having nothing to do with the illness itself. An example would be weight loss accompanied by nausea and vomiting in a patient with a history of stricturing small intestinal Crohn's

disease who is on immunomodulation therapy. In this patient, the diagnostic dilemma is to determine whether the weight loss and vomiting have occurred because the Crohn's disease is poorly controlled, the result of a stricture (either through obstruction or associated bacterial overgrowth), or a consequence of the medical therapy. In resolving this dilemma, one should look for clues in the patient's history. For example, if the patient has experienced a previous exacerbation of his or her Crohn's disease, was weight loss present and reversed when the patient recovered? Additionally, if a medication is suspected, when was the medication started in relation to the onset of symptoms? (Tables 12.3, 12.4).

Approach in the absence of accompanying symptomatology. If the cause of a patient's weight loss is not apparent because of a lack of symptoms and/or related disease, then the physician investigator should next screen the patient for occult disease. Following a complete history and physical, a good place to start would be a basic laboratory work-up. This work-up should include complete blood count, comprehensive metabolic panel, thyroid stimulating hormone level, HIV

Table 12.3 Clinical evaluation of weight loss in a patient with an established diagnosis

---

Example: inflammatory bowel disease

Is the weight loss due to:
- The disorder itself?
  - Active inflammation
    - Diarrhea/fluid depletion
    - Catabolism
    - Anorexia
  - Depression → anorexia
  - Sitophobia
- A complication of the disorder?
  - Neoplasm
  - Stricture → obstruction → sitophobia
  - Stricture → obstruction → bacterial overgrowth
  - Fistula → bacterial overgrowth
- The result of a treatment for the disorder?
  - Anorexia secondary to medication
  - Drug-induced immunocompromise → infection
  - Reduction in edema 2° diuretics
- A complication of a diagnostic procedure?
  - Occult perforation following endoscopy
  or
- Unrelated to the disorder?

Table 12.4 Reasons for weight loss in the patient with diagnosed gastrointestinal disorder

---

Selected examples:
- Chronic pancreatitis
  - Enzyme replacement inadequate
    - None provided
    - Insufficient dose
    - Inactivated preparation
  - Sitophobia
    - Pain exacerbated by meals
  - Reduced fat intake to ↓ diarrhea
  - Diabetes (poorly controlled)
  - malignant change
- Peptic ulcer
  - Outlet obstruction
    - Early satiety → sitophobia
    - Dyspepsia and heartburn →↓ intake; odynophagia
    - Emesis
  - Bacterial overgrowth
    - Fistula complicating perforation
    - Secondary to acid suppression
    - Gastric stasis
- Inflammatory bowel disease
  - Ulcerative colitis
    - Active inflammation
    - Neoplasm/immunocompromise
    - Sclerosing cholangitis
  - Crohn's disease
    - Active inflammation
    - Neoplasm
    - Stricture
      Bacterial overgrowth
      Obstruction → sitophobia
    - Fistulae
      Bacterial overgrowth
- Celiac disease
  - Relapse secondary to dietary indiscretion
  - Malignant change (lymphoma)
- Chronic hepatitis
  - Hepatocellular carcinoma

---

test, stool examination for fat and blood, and urinalysis for blood, sugar, thyroid stimulating hormone level, and HIV test. Consideration should be given to obtaining selective tumor markers (e.g. CA 19-9 in a patient with elevated liver chemistries) with a plan for follow-up if abnormalities are revealed. In addition the physician should tailor further orders concerning labs, imaging, or procedures based on leads generated from the patient interview and physical or secondary to factors such as the patient's age, gender, family history, past medical history, and risk factors (Table 12.5).

Treatment

Once unintentional weight loss has been detected and a diagnostic workup has been initiated, the next step is correcting the weight loss and treating the underlying etiology. Treatment directed to the weight loss itself should be guided by the amount of weight loss, current nutritional status, as well as the patient's ability to maintain enteral nutrition.

There are many options available to the physician ranging from nutritional supplements to total parenteral nutrition. As a basic guideline, if the gut works and the patient is able to tolerate oral intake, one should use the enteral route. This is important because it helps maintain the integrity of the GI tract and lessens exposure and susceptibility to infection. At its simplest, this involves changing the diet to remove or eliminate foods causing complicating symptoms and ensuring that caloric demands are met. In general, most hospitalized patients will require between 25 and 35 kcal/kg/day [4]. (Chapter 144).

When dietary changes are insufficient or not tolerated there are **enteral supplements** available in a variety of formulations designed to meet the specific needs of patients. Although most formulations are available on-line for review, the physician should be aware of potential personnel resources that can be of assistance in selecting a supplement. Pharmacists and registered dieticians can provide a wealth of information about specific product choices.

In those patients unable to tolerate oral intake, consideration should be given to the use of nasogastric or nasoenteric versus percutaneous gastrostomy/jejunostomy tubes.

Finally, in those unable to meet caloric needs despite diet and supplementation, the physician can consider medications (if appetite is the issue) versus parenteral feeds (if the patient has primary gut dysfunction or is severely nutritionally deteriorated).

Prognosis with and without treatment

As indicated previously, clinically significant involuntary weight loss is often a harbinger of a serious underlying

Table 12.5 Evaluating weight loss – searching for occult disease

Physical findings
- Adenopathy
- Clubbing
- Abdominal bruit (non-specific)
- Abdominal mass
- Mass in rectal wall or pouch of Douglas
- Jaundice
- Blumer shelf (rectal)
- Prominent ovary (pelvic)
- Breast lump
- Edema

- Skin changes consistent with neoplasia
- Findings suggesting malabsorption
  - Vitamin deficiency features
  - Muscle spasm/tetany (hypocalcemia, hypomagnesemia)
  - Symptoms of hypokalemia

Laboratory evaluation
- CBC
  - Anemia
  - ↑ platelets
  - ↑ WBCs
- Stool
  - Fat
  - Blood
  - Ova and parasites
- Biochemical profile
  - Liver enzymes
  - Na, K, Ca
  - Fasting blood glucose (consider hemoglobin A1c)
  - Pancreatic enzymes
- Thyroid function
- Urinalysis
- Tumor markers?

Diagnostic procedures
- Carefully selected
- Based on clinical findings
- Avoid "shotgun" battery of tests
- Have a plan to react to results

condition. Not only does the underlying medical reason for the weight loss create a significant health, and sometimes cosmetic, impact on the patient, but the weight loss itself can result in a reduced capacity for the patient to ward off infection or to heal normally. Wallace *et al.* reported that as many as 25% of patients with involuntary weight loss may die within 1 year [5,6]. While weight loss alone may contribute to increased mortality, the underlying cause of the loss of weight is usually responsible. That being said, it has been suggested that at least in those with HIV, mortality may be more closely related to body mass depletion than to the disease itself [7].

References

1. Lankisch PG, Gerzmann M, Gerzmann JF *et al.* Unintentional weight loss: diagnosis and prognosis. The first prospective follow up study from a secondary referral centre. *J Intern Med.* 2001;249: 41–46.
2. Graham MG, Knight B. The many causes of involuntary weight loss: a three step approach to the diagnosis. *Resid Staff Physician.* 2006;52(10):8–15, online, accessed 28 Jun 2009. <http://www.residentandstaff.com/issues/articles/2006-11_04.asp>.
3. Metalidis C, Knockaert DC. Involuntary weight loss. Does a negative baseline evaluation provide adequate reassurance? *Eu J Intern Med.* 2008;19:345–349.
4. Alpers DH, Stenson WF, Taylor BE, Bier DM. Protein and Calories: Requirements, Intake, and Assessment In: *Manual of Nutritional Therapeutics* 5th edition. Philadelphia: Lippincott Williams & Wilkins. 2008, 86.
5. Wallace JI, Schwartz RS, LaCroix AZ *et al.* Involuntary weight loss in older outpatients: incidence and clinical significance. *J Am Geriatr Soc.* 1995;43:329–337.
6. Marton KI, Sox HC, Krupp JR. Involuntary weight loss: diagnostic and prognostic significance. *Ann Intern Med.* 1981;95: 568–574.
7. Kotler DP, Tierney AR, Wang J, *et al.* Magnitude of body-cell-mass depletion and the timing of death from wasting in AIDS. *AM J Clin Nutr.* 1989;50:444.

CHAPTER 13

Gastrointestinal causes of anemia and occult bleeding

Kevin A. Ghassemi, Dennis M. Jensen and Rome Jutabha

David Geffen School of Medicine at UCLA, Los Angeles, CA, USA

KEY POINTS

- Occult gastrointestinal (GI) bleeding is the most common cause of iron deficiency anemia
- Initial endoscopic evaluation of obscure/occult GI bleeding should include colonoscopy and upper endoscopy (push enteroscopy)
- If initial endoscopic evaluation is negative, capsule endoscopy should be used to investigate for small intestinal causes of bleeding
- New modalities for small intestinal evaluation, which have therapeutic potential, include double-balloon, single-balloon and spiral enteroscopy

Introduction

Iron deficiency anemia and gastrointestinal (GI) bleeding are common sources of referral to Gastroenterologists. Good evidence exists to support a standardized approach to evaluating these clinical syndromes. The majority of these patients will improve with empiric or targeted therapy based on the results of a limited initial evaluation. A small subset of patients presenting with occult GI bleeding, and a fraction of those presenting with overt GI bleeding without a source identified on initial evaluation, will have recurrent bleeding and warrant further diagnostic evaluation. These patients fall into the category of GI bleeding of obscure origin.

In this chapter, we present a rational approach to the evaluation of patients with anemia due to a suspected GI source, including iron deficiency anemia, as well as occult and/or obscure GI bleeding.

What is it?

Iron deficiency anemia, occult GI bleeding, and obscure GI bleeding may have significant overlap and are often confused. These interrelated syndromes have distinct diagnostic and therapeutic implications. Thus, it is essential to offer a clear definition of terms.

The World Health Organization uses the following thresholds to define anemia: 13 g/dL for adult men, 12 g/dL for adult non-pregnant women and 11 g/dL for pregnant women. Iron deficiency is most readily diagnosed by measuring the serum ferritin level, and it is best defined as the depletion of iron stores in the bone marrow, liver, and spleen as a result of chronic negative iron balance from bleeding, inadequate dietary intake, increased requirements, malabsorption, or infection.

Occult bleeding refers to the detection of fecal occult blood test (FOBT)-positive stool, with or without iron deficiency anemia or GI symptoms, in a patient without a history of overt GI bleeding (i.e., passage of visible blood from the mouth or rectum). The amount of luminal GI blood loss required for visual detection of blood in the stool may depend on the location of the lesion, the rate of bleeding, the degree of heme degradation, the transit time, and observer perception. Patients with as much as 100 mL of gastroduodenal blood loss per day may have normal-appearing stools, whereas blood may be seen with much smaller volumes that are lost distally, such as the anorectum.

Obscure GI bleeding is persistent or recurrent bleeding, despite negative initial GI evaluation, including upper panendoscopy, colonoscopy and radiologic evaluation of the small bowel such as small bowel follow-through [1]. This is characterized further as overt (visible blood) or occult (FOBT-positive only).

Not all gastrointestinal cases of anemia are the result of bleeding or manifest as iron deficiency. Cobalamin (vitamin B12) and folate deficiencies present classically with a megaloblastic anemia (higher than normal mean corpuscular volume), and are frequently seen in patients who have undergone gastrectomy or gastric bypass surgery. The classic cause of cobalamin deficiency is pernicious anemia, an autoimmune disease that leads to the destruction of gastric mucosa and loss of intrinsic factor production, which is necessary for cobalamin absorption [2].

Textbook of Clinical Gastroenterology and Hepatology, Second Edition. Edited by C. J. Hawkey, Jaime Bosch, Joel E. Richter, Guadalupe Garcia-Tsao, Francis K. L. Chan.
© 2012 Blackwell Publishing Ltd. Published 2012 by Blackwell Publishing Ltd.

How common is it?

Iron deficiency anemia is the most common cause of anemia. The prevalence is approximately 1–2% among adults in the USA [3], but it rises to as high as 5% in patients older than 65 years, with the most common etiology being chronic GI bleeding.

The majority of cases of occult bleeding are found in the course of colorectal cancer screening or during the evaluation of iron deficiency anemia. Colorectal cancer screening studies have demonstrated that 2–16% of average-risk patients older than 50 years test positive with FOBT. However, false-positive results (associated with red meat consumption, dietary peroxidases, and sample rehydration) and false-negative results (associated with hemoglobin degradation, storage, and vitamin C consumption) are not uncommon [4].

The prevalence of recurrent, obscure GI bleeding is rare [5]. In up to half of all patients with occult GI bleeding, the source will not be found on initial endoscopic evaluation. However, a very small number of these patients will develop clinically significant bleeding. Similarly, the proportion of patients with recurrent GI bleeding after a negative initial evaluation is very small.

The prevalence of cobalamin deficiency is about 20% in industrialized countries. Pernicious anemia is one of the most frequent causes of vitamin B12 deficiency [6]. In gastric bypass patients, cobalamin deficiency may appear 1–9 years after surgery, with a prevalence of about 12–33% [7].

Pathophysiology

The amount of blood normally lost from the gastrointestinal tract (0.5–1.5 mL per day) is not typically detected by FOBT, nor is it substantial enough to cause iron deficiency anemia. A steady blood loss of 3–4 mL per day is sufficient to cause a negative iron balance. This degree of blood loss is usually assumed to originate from the bowel unless otherwise dictated by the history [8].

In addition to blood loss, iron deficiency can occur through malabsorption. Iron is absorbed in the proximal small intestine, and absorption is dependent on an intact mucosal surface and gastric acidity. Celiac disease, with its villous atrophy, is the most common cause of iron malabsorption [9]. Dietary iron is found predominantly in the ferric (Fe^{3+}) form, which is insoluble at pH values above 3, but gastric acid renders it more available for absorption. Patients with a gastrectomy/vagotomy or gastric bypass do not have the necessary acidity to augment iron absorption in the small intestine [10]. This may be overcome, at least in part, with the concurrent administration of ascorbic acid (vitamin C) and iron supplements, as the vitamin chelates the iron, making it more soluble over a wide pH range [11].

There appears to be an association between *Helicobacter pylori* and iron deficiency anemia. Although the exact mechanism is not known, possible explanations include gastrointestinal blood loss, gastric acid suppression, and competition for the iron between bacteria and host [12].

Causes

The causes of iron deficiency anemia, occult, and obscure GI bleeding are summarized in Tables 13.1–13.3. Occult GI bleeding is by far the most common source of iron deficiency anemia. A broad range of lesions can lead to occult GI bleeding, with or without iron deficiency. The upper GI tract is the more common source than the lower GI tract for both occult bleeding and iron deficiency anemia [13].

Table 13.1 Gastrointestinal causes of iron deficiency anemia

Iron loss/bleeding
  Cancer/polyp
  Ulcers
  Esophagitis
  NSAID gastropathy/enteropathy/colopathy
  IBD
  Intestinal parasites
  Hemorrhoids
  Cameron's lesions
  Portal hypertensive gastropathy
  Vascular ectasias
  Meckel's diverticulum
Impaired iron absorption
  Atrophic gastritis
  Celiac disease
  Partial/total gastrectomy
  Gastric bypass
Dietary deficiency

Adapted with permission from Bemejo F, Garcia-Lopez S. A guide to diagnosis of iron deficiency and iron deficiency anemia in digestive diseases. *World J Gastroenterol.* 2009;15(37):4638–4643. IBD, inflammatory bowel disease.

Table 13.2 Causes of occult GI bleeding

Upper GI lesions	Colonic lesions
Esophagitis	Colorectal polyps/cancer
Ulcers	Vascular ectasia
Gastritis/erosions	Ulcer
Duodenitis	Colitis/IBD
Vascular ectasias (including GAVE)	Parasitic infections
Portal hypertensive gastropathy	Hemorrhoids
Esophageal/gastric cancer	Diverticula
Celiac disease	
Gastric/duodenal polyps	
Crohn's disease	
Lymphoma	
Partial gastrectomy	

Adapted with permission from Zuckerman GR, Prakash C, Askin MP, Lewis BS. AGA technical review on the evaluation and management of occult and obscure gastrointestinal bleeding. *Gastroenterology.* 2000;118(1):201–221. GAVE, gastric antral vascular ectasia; IBD, inflammatory bowel disease.

Table 13.3 Causes of obscure GI bleeding

Within reach of endoscope/ colonoscope	Mid-GI
Cameron's lesions	Aortoenteric fistula
Dieulafoy's lesion	Crohn's disease
Fundic varices	Dieulafoy's lesion
Neoplasm	Hemobilia
Ulcers	Hemosuccus pancreaticus
Vascular ectasia (including GAVE)	Meckel's diverticulum NSAID enteropathy Neoplasm Vascular ectasia

Adapted with permission from Raju GS, Gerson L, Das A, Lewis B. American Gastroenterological Association (AGA) Institute technical review on obscure gastrointestinal bleeding. *Gastroenterology.* 2007;133(5):1697–1717. GAVE, gastric antral vascular ectasia.

Causes of obscure bleeding can be grouped into those that are within reach of traditional endoscopes, and small intestinal lesions beyond the reach of an endoscope. In the evaluation of obscure bleeding, common causes that have been missed on a previous endoscopy may be found upon re-examination. Commonly missed upper GI sources include Cameron's lesions (erosions or linear ulcers within large hiatal hernias), gastric antral vascular ectasia (Watermelon stomach), and Dieulafoy's lesion (aberrant submucosal vessel in the absence of a primary ulcer). Missed colonic sources include vascular ectasias and internal hemorrhoids. The latter may be noted on prior examination, but their significance may have been underestimated.

Vascular ectasias are the most common cause of bleeding from the small intestine. Mainly as a result of increased aspirin/NSAID use, erosions and ulcers in the small bowel are being detected with increased frequency on capsule endoscopy [14]. Two uncommon extra-luminal causes of GI bleeding include hemosuccus pancreaticus (bleeding from the pancreatic duct, usually due to a neoplasm, trauma/surgery, or ruptured pseudoaneurysm) and hemobilia (bleeding from the bile duct from a hepatobiliary tumor or after a liver biopsy).

Diagnosis
Patient history
A focused history is essential to help guide the diagnostic approach to anemia from occult and obscure bleeding. Age may be the most important and readily defined variable, especially in the evaluation of obscure GI bleeding. Medications, including NSAIDs, steroids, bisphosphonates, and tetracycline, as well as over-the counter supplements and herbal preparations, may cause mucosal erosions and ulcers. Chronic anticoagulation with warfarin, within the therapeutic range,

has not been shown to increase the risk of bleeding secondary to insignificant lesions [15]. Instead, it induces bleeding from pre-existing lesions before they would have bled if anticoagulation had not been given.

The past medical history may provide some clues. Patients with aortic valve replacements, as well as those with end-stage renal disease, are more likely to have intestinal vascular ectasias. Other previous surgical procedures that may lead to GI bleeding are: aortic aneurysm repair (aorto-enteric fistula), bowel resection (anastomotic ulcer), and liver biopsy (hemobilia). In patients with HIV, neoplasms such as lymphoma and Kaposi's sarcoma should be considered. A family history of an inherited polyposis syndrome, hereditary bleeding disorder, hereditary telangiectasia, or neurofibromatosis may be relevant. In addition to these unique associations, it is necessary to query about prior GI malignancy (recurrence), extraintestinal malignancy (metastasis), inflammatory bowel disease (erosion, ulcer, tumor), alcohol abuse (erosive gastritis or varices), gastroesophageal reflux disease (esophagitis), and liver disease (portal hypertensive gastropathy).

Iron deficiency anemia and occult bleeding
GI evaluation of iron deficiency anemia is indicated in adult men, regardless of age, and post-menopausal women. Women who have not reached menopause may warrant a GI evaluation after obvious or potential causes of iron deficiency/blood loss have been excluded [16]. Other tests – peripheral smear, bilirubin, lactate dehydrogenase, and haptoglobin to evaluate for hemolysis; anti-endomysial and anti-tissue transglutaminase antibody assays to test for celiac disease; and blood eosinophil percentage with stool ova/parasite exams for possible parasitic infections – may be useful in detecting sources of anemia not due to GI bleeding.

Endoscopy is the crux of initial investigation for occult GI blood loss. Determining which procedure to perform first depends mainly on findings from the medical history. If a significant lesion consistent with bleeding is found, treatment should be performed without further investigations as multiple lesions are rare. However, patients over 50 years of age should undergo a colonoscopy, even if initial upper endoscopy detected a lesion that was treated, because of the increased risk of colorectal cancer. In this context, upper and lower examinations on the same day are appropriate.

If bi-directional endoscopic evaluation dose not reveal a source of bleeding/iron deficiency anemia, push enteroscopy (PE) with a small bowel enteroscope or pediatric colonoscope should be considered. This examination facilitates evaluation of the proximal small intestine, but also allows for a second-look evaluation for any missed lesions in the upper GI tract. Biopsies of the small intestine should be taken to look for villous atrophy if celiac disease serology tests were not obtained, or to confirm the disease if the tests were positive. Wireless capsule enteroscopy (capsule endoscopy, CE) should be performed, either as an alternative to PE or if PE is negative. CE has the advantage over PE of being able to visualize the entire length of the small bowel. Compared with PE, CE increased the diagnostic yield by approximately 40% [1]. In occult GI bleeding, CE has a diagnostic yield of about 50% [17].

Obscure bleeding

Obscure bleeding is a significant source of morbidity for patients, and often poses a diagnostic challenge. The first step in the evaluation of obscure GI bleeding is to determine if the bleeding is best described as obscure-occult or obscure-overt. Obscure-occult bleeding is best investigated using the same algorithm described in the previous section.

In the case of obscure-overt bleeding, repeat bi-directional endoscopy is indicated because the cause of bleeding frequently can be missed on initial evaluation (Figures 13.1–13.2). However, the repeat upper examination should be carried out as a PE to look for proximal small bowel lesions as well. If these exams are normal, CE should be performed to evaluate for more distal small bowel lesions (Video 13.1).

In recent years, three new endoscopic modalities have emerged to better evaluate the small intestine, collectively known as deep enteroscopy: double-balloon enteroscopy (DBE), single-balloon enteroscopy (SBE) and spiral enteroscopy (SE). DBE and SBE employ an overtube balloon and, in the case of DBE, an enteroscope balloon to slide the small intestine over the enteroscope. Either from the mouth (uni-directionally) or from both mouth and anus (bi-directionally), DBE and SBE can visualize the entire length of the small bowel. Their major advantage over CE is that they offer

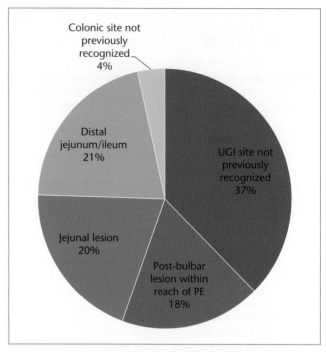

Figure 13.1 Location of obscure GI bleeding based on a cohort of 206 patients. In 41% of patients, the source of bleed was within reach of traditional endoscopes. (Reproduced with permission from Jensen DM. Current diagnosis and treatment of severe obscure GI hemorrhage. *Gastrointest Endosc.* 2003;58(2):256.66.) PE, push enteroscopy; UGI, upper gastrointestinal.

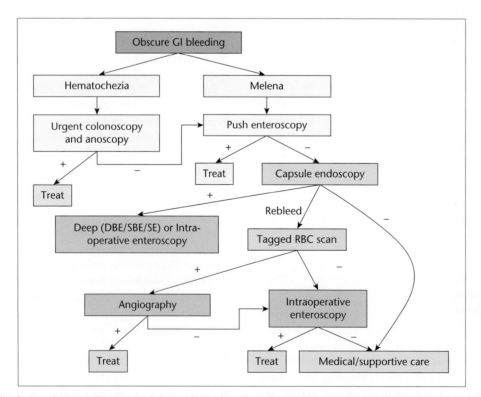

Figure 13.2 Algorithm for investigation and treatment of obscure GI bleeding. (Reproduced with permission from Dulai GS, Jensen DM. Severe gastrointestinal bleeding of obscure origin. *Gastrointest Endosc Clin N Am.* 2004;14(1):101–113.) DBE, double-balloon enteroscopy; RBC, red blood cell; SBE, single-balloon enteroscopy; SE, spiral enteroscopy.

diagnostic and therapeutic options. DBE has been shown to have a high diagnostic yield and therapeutic impact in patients with obscure GI bleeding [18,19]. SBE may be easier to operate than DBE. It has a diagnostic yield similar to that of DBE [20]. SE, the newest of the three modalities uses an enteroscope with a spiral overtube to advance in an anterograde fashion through the small intestine. Although only evaluated in preliminary safety studies, it has been shown to be an effective technique for visualizing the small intestine in patients with obscure GI bleeding [21].

For overt bleeding, a technetium-99m-labeled red blood cell (RBC) scan may be useful, but it requires an active bleeding rate of at least 0.1–0.4 mL/min for a positive result. The sensitivity of localizing the bleeding site is greater if the scan becomes positive earlier, as late positive scans may indicate pooled blood that has moved distally, rather than the actual site of bleeding. Angiography is usually required to confirm the location, but requires a bleeding rate of more than 0.5 mL/min for detection. If the RBC scan is positive, but angiography is not confirmatory, intraoperative enteroscopy may be necessary. However, given the high yield of balloon enteroscopy, it usually is more appropriate to refer such a patient to a tertiary care center where DBE/SBE is available.

SOURCES OF INFORMATION FOR PATIENTS AND DOCTORS

http://www.patient.co.uk/health/Rectal-Bleeding-Blood-in-Faeces.htm
http://www.patient.co.uk/doctor/Upper-Gastrointestinal-Bleeding.htm
http://www.medicinenet.com/balloon_endoscopy/article.htm

References

1. Raju GS, Gerson L, Das A, *et al.* American Gastroenterological Association (AGA) Institute technical review on obscure gastrointestinal bleeding. *Gastroenterology.* 2007;133(5):1697–1717.
2. Gisbert JP, Gomollón F. A short review of malabsorption and anemia. *World J Gastroenterol.* 2009;15(37):4644–4652.
3. Looker AC, Dallman PR, Carroll MD, *et al.* Prevalence of iron deficiency in the United States. *JAMA.* 1997;277(12):973–976.
4. Mandel JS, Bond JH, Church TR, *et al.* Reducing mortality from colorectal cancer by screening for fecal occult blood. *N Engl J Med.* 1993;328(19):1365–1371.
5. Dulai GS, Jensen DM. Severe gastrointestinal bleeding of obscure origin. *Gastrointest Endosc Clin N Am.* 2004;14(1):101–113.
6. Andrès E, Loukili NH, Noel E, *et al.* Vitamin B12 (cobalamin) deficiency in elderly patients. *CMAJ.* 2004;171(3):251–259.
7. Toh SY, Zarshenas N, Jorgensen J. Prevalence of nutrient deficiencies in bariatric patients. *Nutrition.* 2009;25(11–12):1150–1156.
8. Kandel GP, Rasul I. An approach to iron deficiency anemia. *Can J Gastroenterol.* 2001;15(11):739–747.
9. Halfdanarson TR, Litzow MR, Murray JA. Hematologic manifestations of celiac disease. *Blood.* 2007;109(2):412–421.
10. Farrell JJ. Digestion and absorption of nutrients and vitamins. In: Feldman M, Friedman LS, Brandt LJ, editors. *Gastrointestinal and Liver Disease.* 8th ed. Philadelphia: Saunders; 2006. p 2147–2197.
11. Lynch SR. Interaction of iron with other nutrients. *Nutr Rev.* 1997;55(4):102–110.
12. Muhsen K, Cohen D. Helicobacter pylori infection and iron stores: a systematic review and meta-analysis. *Helicobacter.* 2008;13(5):323–340.
13. Rockey DC, Koch J, Cello JP, *et al.* Relative frequency of upper gastrointestinal and colonic lesions in patients with positive fecal occult blood tests. *N Engl J Med.* 1998;339(3):153–159.
14. Estévez E, González-Conde B, Vázquez-Iglesias JL, *et al.* Diagnostic yield and clinical outcomes after capsule endoscopy in 100 consecutive patients with obscure gastrointestinal bleeding. *Eur J Gastroenterol Hepatol.* 2006;18(8):881–888.
15. Greenberg PD, Cello JP, Rockey DC. Asymptomatic chronic gastrointestinal blood loss in patients taking aspirin or warfarin for cardiovascular disease. *Am J Med.* 1996;100(6):598–604.
16. Annibale B, Capurso G, Chistolini A, *et al.* Gastrointestinal causes of refractory iron deficiency anemia in patients without gastrointestinal symptoms. *Am J Med.* 2001;111(6):439–445.
17. Carey EJ, Leighton JA, Heigh RI, *et al.* A single-center experience of 206 consecutive patients undergoing capsule endoscopy for obscure gastrointestinal bleeding. *Am J Gastroenterol.* 2007;102(1):89–95.
18. Sun, B, Rajan E, Cheng S, *et al.* Diagnostic yield and therapeutic impact of double-balloon enteroscopy in a large cohort of patients with obscure gastrointestinal bleeding. *Am J Gastroenterol.* 2006;101(9):2011–2015.
19. Manabe N, Tanaka S, Fukumoto A, *et al.* Double-balloon enteroscopy in patients with GI bleeding of obscure origin. *Gastrointest Endosc.* 2006;64(1):135–140.
20. Ramchandani M, Reddy DN, Gupta R, *et al.* Diagnostic yield and therapeutic impact of single-balloon enteroscopy: series of 106 cases. *J Gastroenterol Hepatol.* 2009;24(10):1631–1638.
21. Akerman PA, Agrawal D, Chen W, *et al.* Spiral enteroscopy: a novel method of enteroscopy by using the Endo-Ease Discover SB overtube and a pediatric colonoscope. *Gastrointest Endosc.* 2009;69(2):327–332.
22. Bemejo F, Garcia-Lopez S. A guide to diagnosis of iron deficiency and iron deficiency anemia in digestive diseases. *World J Gastroenterol.* 2009;15(37):4638–4643.
23. Zuckerman GR, Prakash C, Askin MP, *et al.* AGA technical review on the evaluation and management of occult and obscure gastrointestinal bleeding. *Gastroenterology.* 2000;118(1):201–221.
24. Jensen DM. Current diagnosis and treatment of severe obscure GI hemorrhage. *Gastrointest Endosc.* 2003;58(2):256–266.
25. Dulai GS, Jensen DM. Severe gastrointestinal bleeding of obscure origin. *Gastrointest Endosc Clin N Am.* 2004;14(1):101–113.

CHAPTER 14
Pruritus

Nora V. Bergasa

Metropolitan Hospital Center, New York, NY, USA

KEY POINTS

- Pruritus is a complication of liver diseases, especially those characterized by cholestasis, as measured by blood tests
- Increased opioidergic tone contributes to the pruritus of cholestasis; a central mechanism is proposed
- Opiate antagonists ameliorate the pruritus of cholestasis, including its behavioral manifestation: scratching activity
- Imaging methodology that explores neurotransmission may offer insight into the pathophysiology of pruritus
- The placebo effect of therapeutic interventions to ameliorate pruritus is substantial
- Clinical studies on pruritus should include measurements of behavioral methodology, degree of expectations for relief of this symptoms, and quality of life measures

---

Introduction

Pruritus or itch, is one of the symptoms associated with liver disease. It can have a marked negative impact on the quality of life of patients and it may lead to suicidal ideations. Severe pruritus is an indication for liver transplantation.

What is it?

Hafenreffer, in 1660, defined pruritus as an unpleasant sensation that elicits the need to scratch. Scratching is the behavior that universally results from pruritus; it appears to have evolved as a protective reflex.

How common?

The reported percentage range of patients with primary biliary cirrhosis (PBC) that present with pruritus is 25 to 70 [1]. A survey conducted via the Internet through the website of the "PBCers" organization revealed that 68% of the 242 patients who responded to the survey experienced pruritus. In 75% of the patients with pruritus, the symptom had been present from two to five years prior to the diagnosis of PBC [2]. The percentage range of pruritus prevalence in primary sclerosing cholangitis has been reported to be from 5 to 23 in some clinical trials. Retrospective studies report the prevalence of pruritus in liver disease secondary to chronic hepatitis C to be around 5%.

Pathophysiology

The pathogenesis of the pruritus of liver disease is unknown. It has been considered that the pruritus results from the accumulation of substances that are excreted in bile, and as a result of decreased bile flow they accumulate in tissues. The pruritogenic substances have not been identified. Bile acids accumulate in tissues in cholestasis and have been considered pruritogens. Arguments proposed in support of this idea include: (i) the reported pruritogenic effect of bile acids when injected into the skin of normal volunteers; however, this experiment is not a model of the pruritus of cholestasis, and (ii) the reported amelioration of the pruritus associated with interventions aimed at the decrease in the enterohepatic circulation of bile acids, including the intake of cholestyramine (a non-absorbable resin that binds anions in the small intestine), and ileal and partial bile external diversions [1 and references cited]. Cholestyramine, however, may exert effects different from decreasing the enterohepatic circulation of bile acids including the release of endogenous antiopiates (e.g., cholecystokinin) that may result in a decrease in the perception of pruritus. The surgical interventions stated above may remove, in addition to bile acids, other substances that may be involved in the pruritus. In the context of bile acids, not all patients with cholestasis and elevated serum levels of these compounds report pruritus; the pruritus of cholestasis may spontaneously remit, not in association with changes in serum bile acids, and some patients with liver disease and pruritus do not have increased concentration of bile acids in serum. It may be that a certain profile of bile acids is necessary for these substances to mediate pruritus but, based on current data, a role for bile acids in the mediation of the pruritus of cholestasis has not been proven.

Pruritus can also be of central origin. In 1990 the hypothesis that the pruritus of cholestasis was mediated in the brain by increased opioidergic tone was proposed [3]. A link between opioid receptors and pruritus and scratching of central origin is well established [1]: (i) the pharmacological increase in opioidergic tone (for example, central administration of morphine) is associated with pruritus and scratching in human beings and in laboratory animals, and (ii) this type of pruritus, and scratching are ameliorated and/or prevented by opiate antagonists, suggesting that the pruritus is opioid-receptor

---

Textbook of Clinical Gastroenterology and Hepatology, Second Edition. Edited by C. J. Hawkey, Jaime Bosch, Joel E. Richter, Guadalupe Garcia-Tsao, Francis K. L. Chan.

mediated; in this context, behavioral experimental data from laboratory animals including primates have revealed that the morphine induced scratching behavior is mediated by activation of the mu opioid receptor, and that stimulation of the kappa receptor prevents morphine induced scratching [4]. That cholestasis is associated with increased central opioidergic tone in human beings is suggested by the opiate withdrawal-like syndrome that patients with cholestasis can experience at the administration of opiate antagonists [5]. The reason for increased opioidergic tone in cholestasis is unknown; however, increased availability of opioid ligands from peripheral sources may be an explanation, as suggested by the increased serum concentration of some of the opioid peptides in patients with cholestasis [5]. The origin of opioid peptides in cholestasis is unknown but the liver is a possible source [1]. In this context, periphery-derived endogenous opioids may reach itch-mediating centers including the medullary dorsal horn in the central nervous system [1 and references cited].

Positron emission tomography and functional magnetic resonance imaging (fMRI) methodology have identified activation of brain areas by pruritogenic stimuli including histamine and allergens. The findings have been interpreted as defining sensory and motor components of the itch scratch connection [1 and references cited]. A recent study reported the results of brain scans by single photon emission computed tomography and fMRI methodology in patients with pruritus of cholestasis during periods of itch and no itch. Itch was reported not to be associated with sensory cortex activation; increasing itch severity was reported to correlate with activity in the prefrontal cortex, orbital frontal cortex, putamen, globus pallidus, insular cortex, and orbital anterior and posterior cingulate cortices. Based on the pattern of activation, the authors concluded that the limbic system is the primary central nervous system pathway involved in the perception of itch, and state that the findings support a central origin for this type of pruritus or itch [6]. These preliminary studies support the hypothesis that the pruritus of cholestasis is mediated in the brain [3].

The subjective nature of pruritus has been recognized as a research challenge by investigators in the field. Instruments that recorded limb movements as an index of "scratching" were developed in the 1970s [3 and references cited]. These pioneer efforts were followed by the ground breaking work of Talbot, Schmidt and Walker who applied piezoelectric technology to develop a scratching activity monitoring system (SAMS) [3,7]. This system uses a piezo film sensor attached to a finger and the supporting electronics to amplify, transmit, and process the signals generated by the piezo film. The signals are derived from the vibration of the fingernail as it traverses the skin in the act of scratching, and are independent from gross body movements. The piezo film acts as a contact microphone on the fingernail of the individual from whom scratching behavior is being recorded. The SAMS has been used in clinical trials of therapeutic interventions for the pruritus of cholestasis that had a well-defined end-point, change in scratching activity. The SAMS has been adapted for ambulatory use; thus, clinical trials that record scratching behavior from participating subjects in their living environment are now possible.

Complete resolution of biliary obstruction results in relief of pruritus; this observation suggests that the pruritogen(s) is excreted in bile. Liver transplantation also results in the relief of the pruritus of cholestasis; this observation supports the idea that the pruritogens(s) or co-factors required for pruritus to be perceived are synthesized in the liver. The pruritus of cholestasis, however, does not consistently respond to treatments directed to the liver disease. Accordingly, it requires treatment directed to the symptom. The therapies for pruritus adopted by the American Association for the Study of Liver Disease are listed in Table 14. 1 [1 and references cited].

The hypothesis that the endogenous opioid system contributes to the pruritus of cholestasis was tested in controlled clinical trials in which the SAMS was used to collect behavioral data. In these studies, the administration of the opiate antagonists naloxone and nalmefene was associated with a decrease in scratching activity [7,1]) (Figure 14.1). The use of opiate antagonists to treat this type of pruritus can be accompanied by an opiate withdrawal-like syndrome, originally described by Thornton and Loswosky [5]. The introduction of opiate antagonists at low doses tends to decrease or avoid the reaction as treatment with this type of drugs is initiated [1 and references cited]. The identification of opiate antagonists as a therapeutic alternative to treat the pruritus of liver disease changed the treatment from empirical to specific. Furthermore, it focused attention to other neurotransmission systems including that of serotoninergic and cannabinoidergic neurotransmissions. In this context, in a clinical study of patients with pruritus secondary to liver disease, the serotonin reuptake inhibitor, sertraline, was reported to be associated with decrease in pruritus [1 and references cited]. Increases in cannabinoidergic neurotransmission with dronabinol, was reported to decrease intractable pruritus in a small group of patients [1 and references cited] but this has not been confirmed in controlled studies.

Increased opioidergic tone, a feature of cholestasis, activates mechanisms that promote pain, in part, through the NK-1 receptor, through which substance P acts. In this context, substance P is an excitatory neurotransmitter synthesized by primary afferent nociceptors, which is released into the spinal cord after noxious stimuli, and that participates in the central sensitization associated with hyperalgesia. The serum concentration of substance P is significantly higher in patients with chronic liver disease and pruritus than in patients with chronic liver disease without this symptom, and higher than in a group of control subjects. As pruritus can be considered a noxious stimulus, substance P may contribute to the pathogenesis of the pruritus of cholestasis. This possibility provides a rationale for the study of substance P antagonists to treat this type of pruritus [1 and references cited].

Autotaxin is the enzyme that activates lipophosphatidic acid (LPA). It was reported that its serum activity was higher in

Table 14.1 Selected publications on the treatment of pruritus on cholestasis

Medication	Aim	Dose /mode of administration/ frequency	Type of study/ duration	n	End-points	Results
Cholestyramine	Removal of pruritogen(s)	3.3–12 g/PO/day	Single blind, open label/ placebo controlled crossover [1]/ 6–32 months	27	Not reported	23 patients experienced relief of pruritus [1]
Rifampicin	Unknown; the drug stimulates the pregnane-X-receptor, which mediates the induction of enzymes involved in steroid metabolism and xenobiotic detoxification	150 mg PO/BID if serum bilirubin >3 mg/dL; 150 mg PO/TID if serum bilirubin <3	Double blind, randomized placebo controlled crossover/ 4 weeks [2]	9	Change in VAS[1]	Highly significant decrease in the 7-day summed VAS [2]
Naloxone	To decrease opioidergic tone	0.2 μg/kg/min IV continuous infusions preceded by 0.4 mg IV bolus	Double blind, placebo controlled, randomized crossover/ 4 consecutive days	29	Change in HSA	Geometric mean HSA 34% lower on naloxone than on placebo
Naltrexone	To decrease opioidergic tone	25 mg PO/BID on day 1 followed by 50 mg PO daily	Randomized placebo controlled/ 4 weeks[3]	16	Change in VAS	Daytime and nighttime VAS down by 54% and 44%, respectively

N, total number of patients.

[1]Compared to an observational control group that did not receive cholestyramine but that received norethandrolone or no treatment.

[2]Patients were allowed to continue taking cholestyramine; during the study, the number of cholestyramine packs per day was counted. Mean change in VAS not reported; VAS graphed per patient.

[3]Concomitant use of antipruritic medications were allowed. VAS, mean visual analog score; HAS, hourly scratching activity.

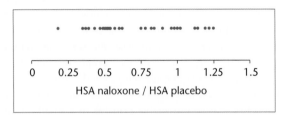

0   0.25   0.5   0.75   1   1.25   1.5

HSA naloxone / HSA placebo

Figure 14.1 Effect of naloxone on hourly scratching activity (HAS). The data are expressed are ratios of HAS on naloxone over HAS on placebo infusions. Each dot represents a patient; dots to the left of 1 indicate that HAS was less on naloxone than on placebo. Most patients scratched less on naloxone than on placebo infusions. (Reproduced with permission from Bergasa NV, Alling DW, Talbot TL, Swain MG, Yurdaydin C, Schmitt JM, Walker EC, *et al.* Naloxone ameliorates the pruritus of cholestasis: results of a double-blind randomized placebo-controlled trial. *Annals of Internal Medicine.* 1995;123:161–167.)

pregnant women with cholestasis and pruritus than in those without, that it correlated with the intensity of the pruritus as assessed by a visual analogue scale, and that it decreased in association with relief of pruritus from nasobiliary drainage in patients with PBC [10]. A role of autotaxin and LPA on the neurophysiology of itch has not been provided; however, the reported associated scratching in association with the intradermal administration of LPA in mice is not evidence of its role in the pathogenesis of the pruritus of cholestasis, as the model used is not a model of pruritus in cholestasis [10].

The drug gabapentin, which changes the threshold to nociception, of which pruritus has been defined as a second order, was studied in a double-blind, randomized, placebo-controlled clinical trial in which scratching activity was continuously recorded for at least 24 hours at baseline, and after four weeks of treatment with a study medication (i.e., gabapentin or its placebo) [8]. The most remarkable results of this study can be appreciated in Figures 14.2a and b. Patients on placebo scratched less (Figure 14.2b) than they had scratched at baseline (Figure 14.2a), and less than those on gabapentin (data not shown); these results indicate that the placebo effect resulted not only in a subjective improvement, but also in a change in behavior. The results of this study have further underscored the importance of including quantitative behavioral methodology in clinical trials of pruritus, including the pruritus of cholestasis. In this context, the use of objective methodology revealed a 24-hour rhythm in the scratching behavior of some patients with cholestasis and pruritus in a clinic trial [7] (Figure 14.3). This finding highlights the uncertainty of data on the intensity of pruritus collected randomly, as it appears that the perception of this symptom has spontaneous variability that can be misinterpreted as improvement of the symptom in association with a study intervention.

The 24-hour rhythm in scratching behavior led to the idea of exploring the effect of light, which regulates biological rhythms via retinothalamic pathways, on scratching behavior

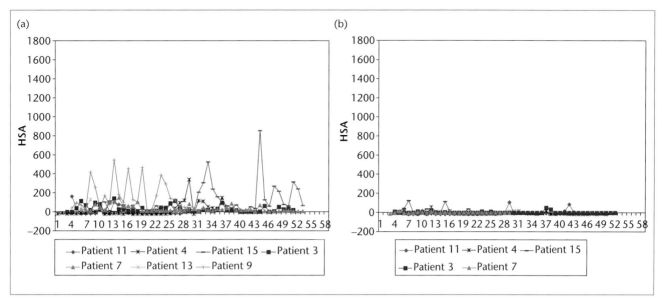

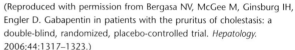

Figures 14.2 (a, b)The figures depict the mean hourly scratching activity (HSA) of patients with liver disease and pruritus at baseline (a), and after randomization to the placebo medication, which they had been taking for at least four weeks (b). Scratching activity on placebo was near zero.

(Reproduced with permission from Bergasa NV, McGee M, Ginsburg IH, Engler D. Gabapentin in patients with the pruritus of cholestasis: a double-blind, randomized, placebo-controlled trial. *Hepatology.* 2006;44:1317–1323.)

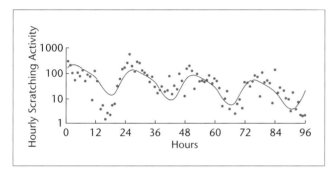

Figure 14.3 Mean hourly scratching activity (HAS) during the 96-hour study period of a patient with benign recurrent intrahepatic cholestasis who participated in a study of naloxone infusions for the pruritus of cholestasis. The continuous line indicates the 24-hour rhythm that best fits the observation. The line has a significant downward trend, which is consistent with the sequence of infusion (placebo, placebo, naloxone, naloxone) indicating that the patient scratched less on the study drug. (Reproduced with permission from Bergasa NV, McGee M, Ginsburg IH, Engler D. Gabapentin in patients with the pruritus of cholestasis: a double-blind, randomized, placebo-controlled trial. *Hepatology.* 2006;44:1317–1323.)

in a controlled open label pilot study in patients with chronic liver disease and pruritus. Hourly scratching activity was lower after eight weeks of treatment with bright light therapy than at baseline, in seven of the eight study participants; furthermore, the outbursts of scratching behavior were significantly decreased in all [1 and references cited].

Procedures to remove pruritogens from the circulation and from the bile have been performed in patients with severe pruritus including anion adsorption and plasma separation, and the extracorporeal liver support systems (Molecular Adsorbent Recirculating System (MARS ™), and Prometheus,™ [1 and

references cited]. Nasobiliary drainage in patients with pruritus secondary to PBC and in patients with benign recurrent intrahepatic cholestasis have also been used to relieve severe pruritus [1]. The placebo effect of these interventions may be substantial but, in patients with intractable pruritus, they are considered in an effort to provide relief, even if temporary. Risk versus benefits must be considered, as these interventions have not been tested in clinical trials, and the probabilities of being studied in controlled studies are low based on the nature of the procedures.

Causes and differential diagnosis

Many liver diseases, some of which are included in Table 14.2, can be associated with pruritus, irrespective of the serum liver profile, and the degree of cholestasis, as measured by current available tests (e.g., fasting or two hour postprandial bile acids).

Pruritus or itch is a symptom associated with diseases in the discipline of internal medicine, including hemato-oncological conditions such as polycythemia vera, and lymphoma, neurological disorders such as multiple sclerosis and cerebrovascular accidents, and chronic kidney and liver disease; pruritus is also the most common symptom from skin disorders. Chronic pruritus has a marked negative impact on the quality of life of patients and it may lead to suicidal ideations.

In the context of liver disease, pruritus is experienced more frequently by patients with conditions characterized by cholestasis, although it can also be experienced by patients with liver diseases in which hepatocellular injury predominates. The skin of patients with the pruritus of cholestasis may display excoriations, prurigo nodularis, and marked

Table 14.2 Liver diseases that can be associated with pruritus

Childhood	Adulthood
Progressive familial intrahepatic cholestasis	Primary biliary cirrhosis
Allagille's syndrome	Primary sclerosing cholangitis
Biliary atresia	Chronic viral hepatitis
Primary sclerosing cholangitis	Drug-induced cholestasis with and without ductopenia
Drug-induced cholestasis with and without ductopenia	Biliary obstruction
Cystic fibrosis[1]	Pregnancy
Biliary obstruction	Hepatic sarcoidosis[2]
Alpha-1-antitrypsin deficiency	Cirrhosis secondary to alcohol Alpha-1-antitrypsin deficiency

[1]Pruritus was reported in one publication of patients with cholestasis and cystic fibrosis.
[2]Ductopenia may be associated with hepatic sarcoidosis. Pruritus secondary to cholestasis in sarcoidosis is well documented in adults but not in children.

destructive lesions secondary to scratching . Hyperpigmentation is a clue to the presence of some cholestatic conditions such as PBC and primary sclerosing cholangitis.

The pruritus associated with morphine and opiate drugs is mediated by the mu opioid receptor; thus, mutations that change the function of the mu opioid receptors may be relevant to understanding why not all patients with liver disease experience pruritus. In this context, the single nucleotide polymorphism (SNP) A118G in Exon1 of the opioid receptor mu 1 (OPRM1) gene predicts an Asn-to-Asp change in amino acid residue 40 in the extracellular domain of the receptor, at a putative N-linked glycosylation site [1 and references cited]. A118G has been associated with alterations in functions mediated by the endogenous opioid system, of which the pruritus of cholestasis is considered to be one [3]. A118G was found in heterozygosity 1.5 times more frequently in the DNA samples from patients with PBC living in the United States and who had not reported pruritus than in the rest of the study samples, which were from Italian patients [1 and references cited]. These findings may suggest that A118G in the OPRM1 of patients with PBC protects them from pruritus. In another study, a SNP characterized by the substitution of valine for glutamate (V1188E) in exon 25 of the multidrug resistance protein (MRP)2 gene was found in heterozygosity in a significantly higher number of patients with PBC and pruritus than in those without pruritus [1 and references cited]. MRP2 (ABCC2) is a member of the family of ATP-binding cassette (ABC) transporters expressed in various organs including the liver and the blood brain barrier [1 and references cited]. In

the hepatocyte, MRP2 mediates the transport of several organic anions, and interestingly, in the context of the pruritus of cholestasis, opioid ligands have been reported to be MRP2 substrates [1 and references cited]. In regards to the pruritus of cholestasis, V1188E in MRP2 may alter the pruritogen(s) or its cofactors from being transported from the hepatocyte into bile or into the central nervous system. It has been reported that the intact skin of patients with atopic dermatitis, a condition characterized by chronic pruritus, allows for the enhanced penetration of chemical solutes [9]. This observation has suggested that mutations in the gene that codes for filaggrin, a protein necessary for the formation of the stratum corneum, and hence pivotal in the maintenance of the skin as a barrier, may be relevant in the pathogenesis of this disease. Skin permeability may also be relevant in the vulnerability of patients with liver disease to experience pruritus, in light of the fact that not all patients do. Thus, genetic studies to identify mutations in the gene that codes for filaggrin merit consideration [9]. Thus, large population studies exploring combinations of SNP in potentially relevant genes (e.g., those that code for transport proteins in the hepatobiliary system and CNS, and those involved in sensory neurotransmission, and skin permeability) may provide some insight into the pathogenesis of pruritus.

When the cause of pruritus is not apparent (e.g., absence of a diagnostic rash) diagnostic investigations must include a thorough review of systems and appropriate radiographic and laboratory tests, including those designed to diagnose liver disease.

Symptom complexes

In general, patients with liver disease and pruritus describe their symptom as "irritation", "pins and needles", or "crawling" [2]. Twenty five percent of the patients with PBC who participated in the Internet survey conducted via the "PBCers" organization reported that the degree of pruritus increased prior to menstruation [2]. The majority of patients with liver disease and pruritus report that it is worse in the afternoon and at night, when they return home from their daily activities, than at other times. This characteristic tends to suggest that activities that require mental engagement may suppress the sensation of pruritus to some degree.

Diagnosis

The diagnosis of pruritus is made by taking a history. Pruritus can precede the diagnosis of liver disease by years.

Current controversies and their future resolution

It is necessary to develop methodology to study the neurophysiology and pathophysiology of the itch sensation and the resulting protective scratching reflex in human beings, and to develop quality of life measures sufficiently sensitive to detect the impact of a given therapeutic intervention on patients' well-being.

The endogenous opioid system may be relevant in the mediation of pruritus from various conditions including kidney and dermatological diseases in addition to liver disease. Experimental data indicating that stimulation of the kappa receptor can prevent opiate-induced pruritus allows for the development of drugs with specific antipruritic effects; in this context, nalfurafine, a kappa receptor agonist, has been associated with a decrease in pruritus in patients with kidney disease [1 and references cited]. The effect of this drug in the pruritus of cholestasis secondary to PBC is being studied.

The use of brain imaging technology offers the opportunity to explore neural pathways activated in association with the perception of itch and its behavioral manifestation, scratching.

Anecdotal observations on the ameliorating effect of the pruritus of cholestasis by reasonable interventions should be followed by controlled clinical trials that include objective methodology that can be used, ideally, in the ambulatory setting. Objective data obtained via quantitative methodology can be standardized and generalized with the final aim of developing effective and specific therapies for pruritus in cholestasis.

References

1. Bergasa NV. Pruritus in primary biliary cirrhosis: pathogenesis and therapy. *Clin Liver Dis*. 2008;12:385–406; x.

2. Rishe E, Azarm A, Bergasa NV. Itch in primary biliary cirrhosis: a patients' perspective. *Acta Derm Venereol*. 2008;88:34–37.

3. Jones EA, Bergasa NV. The pruritus of cholestasis: from bile acids to opiate agonists. *Hepatology*. 1990;11:884–887.

4. Ko MC, Lee H, Song MS, *et al*. Activation of kappa-opioid receptors inhibits pruritus evoked by subcutaneous or intrathecal administration of morphine in monkeys. *J Pharmacol Exp Ther*. 2003;305:173–179.

5. Thornton JR, Losowsky MS. Opioid peptides and primary biliary cirrhosis. *BMJ*. 1988;297:1501–1504.

6. Barnes LB, Devous MD, Harris TS, *et al*. The central nervous system activity profile of cholestatic pruritus. *Hepatology*. 2009;50:375, Abstract 153.

7. Bergasa NV, Alling DW, Talbot TL, *et al*. Naloxone ameliorates the pruritus of cholestasis: results of a double-blind randomized placebo-controlled trial. *Ann Intern Med*. 1995;123:161–167.

8. Bergasa NV, McGee M, Ginsburg IH, *et al*. Gabapentin in patients with the pruritus of cholestasis: a double-blind, randomized, placebo-controlled trial. *Hepatology*. 2006;44:1317–1323.

9. McLean WH, Hull PR. Breach delivery: increased solute uptake points to a defective skin barrier in atopic dermatitis. *J Invest Dermatol*. 2007;127:8–10.

10. Kremer, A. E., Martens, J. J., Kulik, *et al*. Lysophosphatidic acid is a potential mediator of cholestatic pruritus. *Gastroenterology*. 2010;139:1008–18.

CHAPTER 15

Jaundice

Adrian Reuben

Medical University of South Carolina, Charleston, SC, USA

KEY POINTS

- Jaundice and icterus are interchangeable terms that describe the visible yellowing of the sclerae of the eyes, skin and mucous membranes that occurs when serum bilirubin levels rise above 3 mg/dL (51 μmole/L)
- Hyperbilirubinemia occurs when the bilirubin load presented to the liver exceeds hepatic clearance capacity and/or when hepatic uptake, hepatocellular processing or biliary excretion of bilirubin are impaired by hepatobiliary disease, xenobiotics, hereditary defects in conjugation and transport, or extrahepatic diseases that adversely influence influence liver function
- The diagnosis of jaundice relies on a good history, thorough physical examination, interpretation of standard laboratory tests that include blood count, hepatic panel, disease-specific serology and newly available genetic testing for hereditary cholestatic disorders, cross-sectional imaging of the liver and biliary tree, and where necessary direct cholangiography and sometimes liver biopsy

Introduction

The term jaundice denotes yellowness that is seen in the sclerae, skin, and mucous membranes when circulating bilirubin levels rise approximately 3-fold or more above normal, that is, when serum bilirubin levels exceed ~3 mg/dL (51 μmol/L). Hyperbilirubinemia can occur either when too great a load of bilirubin is presented to the normal liver or, more commonly, when any hepatobiliary condition causes defects in hepatic uptake , hepatocellular processing and/or biliary excretion of bilirubin. The word jaundice comes from the Middle English *jaunice* (*jaunisse*) that was adapted from *jaune* – the French word for yellow – as far back as the 12th century CE; the letter "d" in *jaundice* was acquired a couple of hundred years later, by so-called phonetic accretion. *Icterus* means exactly the same as jaundice, namely yellowness. The alternative term icterus is derived from the Greek *ikteros* for oriole, the yellow-breasted bird that many Greeks kept as pets, the mere sight of which was thought to cure jaundice [1].

What is it?

Jaundice refers to an abnormally yellow hue to tissues that are ordinarily white (or near-white) but become visibly stained with bilirubin (and possibly biliverdin also), which binds to them after diffusing from the blood. Jaundice does not cause any unusual sensation in the skin or the eyes apart from the extremely rare experience of *xanopsia* (seeing yellow). Jaundice is first detected visibly in the sclerae of the eyes, where there is abundant elastic tissue to which bilirubin readily binds. This is followed by yellowing of the skin and mucous membranes, being particularly noticeable in the frenulum of the tongue. Scars, edematous areas, and parts that are paralyzed are usually spared. Jaundice also affects bodily secretions and fluids (especially those that are protein-rich), such as tears, sweat, semen, milk, sputum, and ascites; even cerebrospinal fluid may be yellow in jaundiced patients, so that xanthochromia may be misdiagnosed. Jaundice may also be misdiagnosed when yellow discoloration of the skin is caused not by staining with bilirubin but by xenobiotics, such as quinacrine (mepacrine), or carotenes in individuals who consume large amounts of tomatoes, carrots, and papaya; in neither case are the sclerae yellow. In Victorian times, jaundice was often mistaken for the yellow-green countenance of the severe anemic state known then as chlorosis [2]. Other conditions that were confused with jaundice were the grayish-yellow of the cancer patient, the dusky yellow of the chronic malaria sufferer, and the bronzing of hemochromatosis and Addisonian hypoadrenalism. Finally, it may be difficult to tell whether jaundice is present in the eyes of non-Caucasians, whose natural pigmentation may give an appearance to the sclerae that is often described as being "muddy," making any yellowness there difficult to discern.

How common is it?

Jaundice is a defining feature of any disorder that interferes with the handling of bilirubin sufficiently to raise its serum level above 3 mg/dL. It follows that jaundice is common in hepatobiliary diseases that impede the metabolism and transport of bilirubin, its excretion into bile and its passage into the duodenum. Hematologic and other conditions in which heightened degradation of heme and/or other hemoproteins

---

yields an increased bilirubin load for excretion by the liver, also cause jaundice. Jaundice can complicate extrahepatic conditions that impair bilirubin metabolism and/or hepatic clearance without causing biliary obstruction or structural liver injury *per se*, such as sepsis, pregnancy, or the use of drugs that inhibit hepatic bilirubin transport like C_{17}^- alkylated steroids. Drugs, such as aspirin, sulfonamides and warfarin, can displace unconjugated bilirubin from binding with albumin and from other extrahepatic sites, thereby increasing the load for the liver to process. Increased circulating levels of unconjugated bilirubin can cause cerebral toxicity (kernicterus) especially in neonates, because of binding to brain tissue. Moderate to severe necroinflammatory liver injury is often characterized by jaundice; this is seen especially in alcoholic, viral and idiosyncratic drug-induced liver injury, but not usually in acetaminophen hepatotoxicity [3]. The prevalence of jaundice in viral hepatitis is greater in older patients, who also fare less well than younger patients. In idiosyncratic drug reactions, the outcome (namely spontaneous recovery, transplantation, or death), can be related to the height of the bilirubin level [4,5]. Cholestatic disorders [6,7] are more likely to show jaundice earlier than later in the course of the disease, whether the lesion is: (i) at the level of the hepatocyte and canalicular membrane transport systems; (ii) in injured bile ductules and intrahepatic bile ducts, for example in primary biliary cirrhosis (PBC), chronic liver allograft rejection, etc., and with drug-induced bile ductular and ductal inflammation caused by

amoxicillin–clavulanic acid, and other drugs [8]; or (iii) due to mechanical obstruction of the extrahepatic biliary tree. Paradoxically, some patients with cholestatic disorders do not present with jaundice initially, but they do complain of pruritus. About a third of patients who develop cholestasis due to sepsis become jaundiced before the infection is apparent [9], whereas jaundice does not occur where there is unilateral hepatic duct obstruction, as seen with a Klatskin tumor. With so many different etiologies of jaundice, the distribution of causes varies between populations, depending on the age of the patient, lifestyle, geography, and socioeconomics [10].

Metabolism and transport of bilirubin: normal physiology

The best insight into the pathophysiology of jaundice comes from understanding the normal physiology of bilirubin metabolism and transport (Figure 15.1).

A. Bilirubin is the end-product of heme degradation. Eighty percent comes from senescent red cell hemoglobin released in the reticuloendothelial system, and the rest is derived from the turnover of other hemoproteins, (myoglobin, cytochromes, catalase). There is a small pool of free heme in hepatocytes and some newly-synthesized heme is degraded in the bone marrow as a result of "ineffective erythropoiesis." Heme, the iron atom-containing heterocyclic tetrapyrrole ring, ferroprotoporphyrin

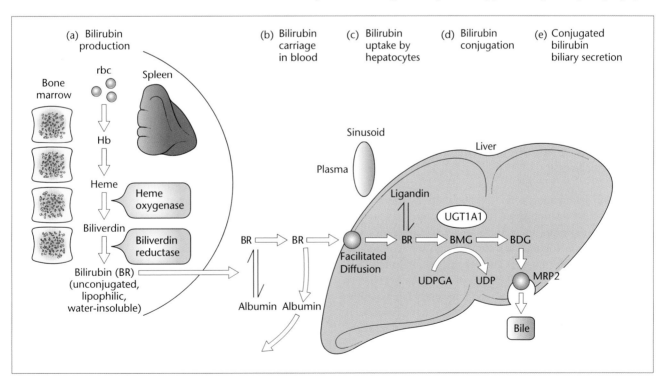

Figure 15.1 Overview of bilirubin production, transport in blood, hepatocyte uptake, conjugation, and biliary secretion. BDG, bilirubin diglucuronide; BMG, bilirubin monoglucuronide; BR, bilirubin; Hb, hemoglobin; MRP2, multidrug resistance-associated protein 2; rbc, red blood cells; UDP, uridine diphosphate; UDPGA, uridine disphosphoglucuronic acid;

UGT1A1, 1A1 (bilirubin-specific) uridine diphosphoglucuronosyltransferase enzyme. (This figure was published in *Clinical Gastroenterology and Hepatology*, Wilfred M. Weinstein, Christopher J. Hawkey, Jaime Bosch, Jaundice, Pages 1–8, Copyright Elsevier, 2005.)

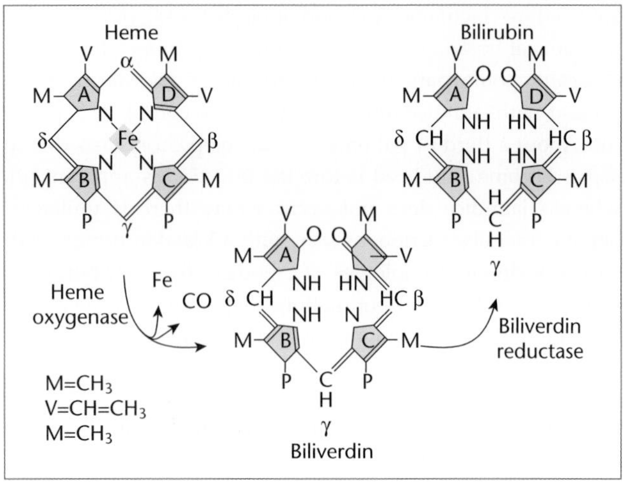

Figure 15.2 Bilirubin synthesis. Conversion of heme to biliverdin and then to bilirubin. Heme ring-opening at the α-carbon bridge of heme is catalyzed by heme oxygenase, resulting in the formation of biliverdin and release of the iron atom and carbon monoxide. This is followed by reduction of biliverdin to bilirubin in a reaction catalyzed by biliverdin reductase. (Adapted from Chowdhury NR, Chowdhury JR. *Bilirubin metabolism.* Up To Date Online www.uptodate.com18.2, (accessed March 3, 2010).)

IX, is catalytically cleaved to the water-soluble linear tetrapyr-role biliverdin, by microsomal heme oxygenase that oxidizes and opens the α-carbon bridge, with the loss of iron and carbon monoxide (Figure 15.2). The green pigment biliverdin is reduced by cytosolic biliverdin reductase to generate 250–400 mg of water-insoluble orange-yellow bilirubin each day. Bilirubin is an antioxidant of likely physiologic importance that also acts as a major physiologic cytoprotectant [11].

B. Transporting water-insoluble bilirubin in the circulation is done by reversible binding to albumin that carries it in the plasma to the liver.

C. Bilirubin elimination from the body via bile and urine is carried out by conjugation with glucuronic acid, which converts bilirubin to its water-soluble glucuronides. The bilirubin-albumin complex diffuses through the fenestrae of the endothelial cells, towards the hepatocytes. Bilirubin then dissociates from albumin, to be taken up at the hepatocyte sinusoidal (basolateral) plasma membrane by facilitated diffusion. It is still unclear which carrier protein in the basolateral membrane mediates this transfer. Bilirubin is then trapped in the hepatocyte cytosol by binding to glutathione-S-transferases (originally identified as ligandin) and possibly to fatty acid-binding protein too, which retards bilirubin reflux back into the blood. Unconjugated bilirubin moves intracellularly by membrane-to-membrane transfer towards membranes with a high cholesterol/phospholipid ratio, that is, the endoplasmic reticulum.

D. Conjugation of bilirubin occurs in the endoplasmic reticulum, mediated by the bilirubin-specific isoform (UGT1A1) of the uridine diphosphoglucuronosyltransferase family of enzymes that uses uridine diphosphoglucuronic acid (UDPGA) to form bilirubin monoglucuronide first, and then the major conjugate, bilirubin diglucuronide.

E. Conjugated bilirubin is secreted into bile by an ATP-dependent active transport mechanism, mediated by the canalicular isoform of the multidrug resistance-associated protein 2 (MRP2, formerly known as the canalicular multispe-cific organic anion transporter cMOAT) [7]. Finally, bile flows from the canaliculi into the canals of Hering, and thence successively to the bile ductules (cholangioles), intralobular and interlobular bile ducts, and the conducting area and segmental bile ducts. Bile enters the gallbladder for temporary storage and/or traverses the common bile duct to enter the second part of the duodenum through the papilla of Vater.

Potential sites of interference with hepatobiliary bilirubin metabolism, transport and flow into the duodenum are shown in Figure 15.3. There is always some bile flow into the duodenum; the proportion directed into the gallbladder is determined by the tone of the sphincter of Oddi, according to the feeding/fasting status of the individual. Approximately half of the bilirubin in the intestine may be metabolized by bacteria to the colorless compound urobilinogen, which can be absorbed from the intestine into portal blood, taken up and re-excreted by the liver, while ~20% is excreted in the urine. Intestinal bacterial metabolism of urobilinogen yields stercobilin that together with other biliary pigments imparts the normal color to stools. Urinary urobilinogen excretion increases with over-production of bilirubin and in the early stages of liver injury that impair hepatic urobilinogen uptake. In contrast, in chole-static jaundice, urobilinogen disappears from the urine because of the absence of bilirubin in the intestine and, in parallel, stercobilin disappears from the stools that acquire the typical clay or light color of cholestatic jaundice, in contrast to the dark color of bilirubin in the urine. In cholestatic jaundice, some conjugated bilirubin forms an irreversible complex with albumin, which is not excreted by the kidneys unless there is proteinuria.

Abnormal metabolism and transport of bilirubin: pathophysiology and causes

The pathophysiology of many causes of jaundice is now explicable in terms of inherited or acquired molecular defects in one or more of the steps in the physiology of bilirubin, and/or macroscopic changes along the pathway of bile formation and entry into the duodenum (Figure 15.3). Primary molecular defects in bilirubin handling are often hereditary. The main pathologic processes of injury, inflammation, fibrosis and obstruction, have secondary effects on bile formation that are being unraveled at the cellular and molecular levels [7,12]. The different mechanisms that lead to jaundice are classified below.

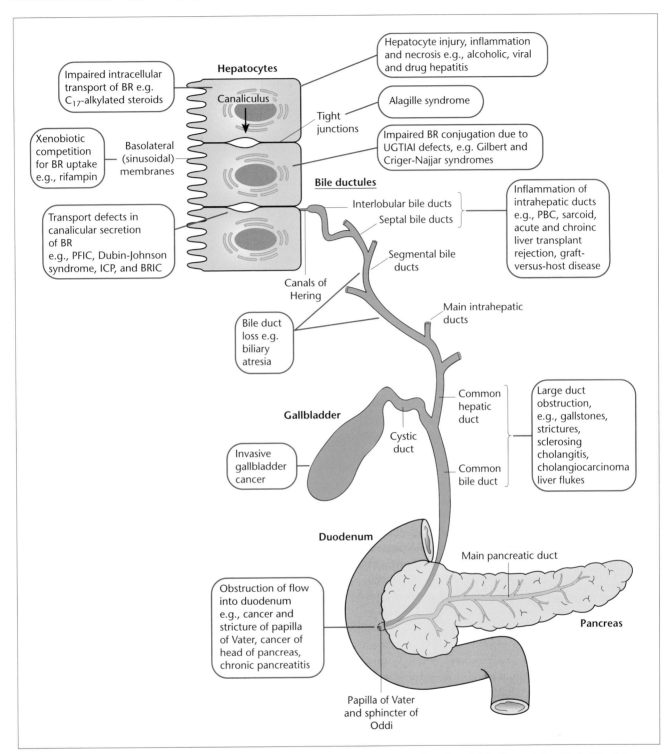

Figure 15.3 Potential sites of interference with the hepatobiliary metabolism and transport of bilirubin from hepatocyte to duodenum (with examples). BR, bilirubin; BRIC, benign recurrent intrahepatic cholestasis; ICP, intrahepatic cholestasis of pregnancy; PBC, primary biliary cirrhosis; PFIC, progressive familial intrahepatic cholestasis; UGT1A1, 1A1 (bilirubin-specific) isoform of uridine diphosphoglucuronosyltransferase enzyme. (Adapted from Chowdhury NR, Chowdhury JR. *Bilirubin metabolism.* Up To Date Online www.uptodate.com 18.2, (accessed March 3, 2010). See also Roskams TA, Theisen D, Balabaud C, *et al.* Nomenclature of the finer branches of the biliary tree: canals, ductules, and ductular reactions in human livers. *Hepatology.* 2004;39:1739–1745.)

CAUSES AND DIFFERENTIAL DIAGNOSIS

Causes of jaundice

Bilirubin overproduction
- Excessive red cell breakdown (hemolysis, hematomas, etc.)
- Ineffective erythropoiesis
- Nonhemoglobin hemoprotein degradation (myoglobin)

Disordered plasma transport of bilirubin
- Intravenous albumin infusion
- Conjugated bilirubin–albumin, irreversibly bound

Impaired uptake of bilirubin by hepatocytes
- Disruption of sinusoid–hepatocyte interface (cirrhosis)
- Reduced or bypassed hepatic blood flow
- Xenobiotic competition for bilirubin uptake (e.g., by rifampin)

Reduced intrahepatic bilirubin conjugation
- Immature UGT1A1 enzyme (physiologic jaundice of the newborn)
- Defective UGT1A1 enzyme biosynthesis (Gilbert and Crigler-Najjar syndromes)
- Xenobiotic competition for UGT1A1 activity (indinavir)

Nonobstructive cholestatic syndromes
- Hereditary and acquired transport defects

Obstructive cholestasis
- Inflammation, fibrosis, injury, malignant and non-malignant obstruction of the microscopic and macroscopic biliary tree

Bilirubin overproduction is usually caused by an excessive and/or premature breakdown of red cells. Consequently, hepatic uptake of unconjugated bilirubin becomes saturated and leads to a rise in serum unconjugated bilirubin concentration that rarely exceeds 4 mg/dL, unless there is coexisting hepatobiliary disease. Although only 4% of bilirubin in normal plasma is conjugated, the diazo assay used in clinical laboratories overestimates this component at 10–15%, which is therefore the maximum so-called "direct" bilirubin fraction that is seen in conditions of isolated bilirubin overproduction, or impairment of hepatic uptake and/or conjugation. Almost all circulating bilirubin, in this setting, is unconjugated, and therefore not executed in the urine. Hemolysis may be due to: (i) abnormal red cell morphology, as occurs in sickle cell disease and hereditary spherocytosis; (ii) mechanical red cell damage due to prosthetic heart valves and other intravascular devices; disseminated intravascular coagulation; hemolytic-uremic syndrome, etc.; and (iii) immune and drug-induced red cell injury. When there is ineffective erythropoiesis, as occurs in thalassemia, pernicious anemia etc., hemoglobin incorporation into red cells is impaired and its heme is degraded. Increased breakdown of myoglobin that occurs when there is extensive muscle damage (rhabdomyolysis), can add to the bilirubin load, as can hemoglobin degradation in hematomas and gastrointestinal bleeding. Certain drugs, such as rifampin, probenecid and others, can compete with unconjugated bilirubin for hepatic uptake, leading to an increase in serum level. When liver perfusion is poor, as may occur in heart failure and shock, bilirubin delivery to the liver is slowed. In portal hypertension, in which there is extensive portosystemic collateralization, unconjugated bilirubin and drugs may

circumvent the liver at the "first pass." In both cases, reduced or delayed hepatic uptake contributes further to unconjugated hyperbilirubinemia. A barrier for unconjugated bilirubin uptake by hepatocytes also occurs in cirrhosis as the sinusoid-hepatocyte interface is disrupted by loss of microvilli, closure of endothelial fenestrae, and fibrosis.

Defective bilirubin conjugation maybe due to a variety of hereditary and acquired anomalies of UGT1A1 [13]. The commonest hereditary anomaly of UGT1A1 lies in its upstream promotor and is responsible for the benign autosomal recessive partial defect of bilirubin conjugation known as Gilbert syndrome, which affects up to 10% of Western populations and, in a subset of individuals, may be associated with reduced red cell survival and/or hepatocyte uptake of bilirubin [14]. In the severe familial unconjugated hyperbilirubinemia known as the Crigler-Najjar syndrome, UGT1A1 activity is abolished in the lethal type I variant, or reduced to less than 10% (albeit, still phenobarbitone-inducible) in the type II variant, due to a variety of UGT1A1 gene defects. Immaturity of normal UGT1A1 is common in neonates, causing so-called physiological jaundice of the newborn. In premature infants, especially, serum unconjugated bilirubin levels can rise sufficiently high (above 20 mg/dL) to cause kernicterus. Exposure of the infant to ultraviolet light produces water-soluble photoisomerization of unconjugated bilirubin in the skin, which, though unstable, lasts long enough to permit biliary excretion that reduces serum bilirubin to safe levels. Finally UGT1A1 activity can be inhibited by a factor present in maternal milk that causes "breast milk jaundice." Indinavir, a viral protease inhibitor that is used to treat HIV infection, causes unconjugated hyperbilirubinemia partly from UGT1A1 inhibition and partly from hemolysis.

Cholestatic liver disease represents a very large group of overlapping disorders in adults and children, in which the common theme is failure or impairment of bile secretion. For many of these disorders, precise molecular abnormalities of the normal bile secretory transport apparatus (Figure 15.4) have been identified, particularly those that are hereditary diseases of childhood [15]. Some of these hereditary diseases are represented in adults too, although with less severe phenotypes. In adults, however, most cases of cholestasis are acquired, of which a few may be due to inhibition of bile secretion without overt liver injury, such as seen in cholestasis of sepsis [9]. Even in the more common acquired forms of cholestasis, in which there are microscopic or macroscopic lesions of the biliary tree, secondary changes can be identified in the molecular biliary secretory apparatus that may contribute to the cholestatic syndrome, or even ameliorate it to some extent [7,12].

Hereditary, familial, and related cholestatic syndromes

Bile formation and the transport of solutes into bile are mediated by an array of channels, exchangers, and transporters that are embedded in the canalicular membrane (Figure 15.4). Genetic defects have been reported that are responsible for

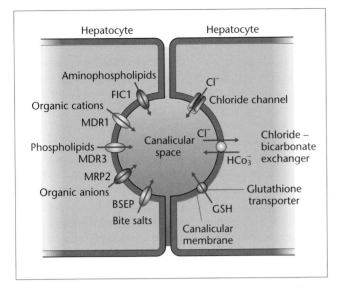

Figure 15.4 Canalicular membrane transporters – a selection. A canaliculus between two neighboring hepatocytes is represented. The canalicular membranes contain several ATP-dependent export pumps: the multidrug resistance-1 P-glycoprotein (MDR1) that transports organic cations into bile; the phospholipid transporter multidrug resistance-3 P-glycoprotein (MDR3). The multidrug resistance-associated protein 2 (MRP2, previously termed the canalicular multispecific organic anion transporter, cMOAT); and the canalicular bile salt export pump (BSEP). The canalicular membrane also contains ATP-dependent transport systems for chloride extrusion into bile, chloride–bicarbonate exchange, glutathione (GSH) transport, and the product of the *FIC1* (Familial Intrahepatic Cholestasis type 1) gene, which has been redesignated *ATP8B1*, a P-type ATPase that transports aminophospholipids. (This figure was published in *Clinical Gastroenterology and Hepatology*, Wilfred M. Weinstein, Christopher J. Hawkey, Jaime Bosch, Jaundice, Pages 1–8, Copyright Elsevier, 2005.)

several rare homozygous recessive disorders of infancy, originally known as Progressive Familial Intrahepatic Cholestasis (PFIC). PFIC can now be subdivided according to the mutation of genes that encode for specific canalicular transporters and their corresponding phenotypic expression. PFIC-1 was previously recognized as Byler disease and is due to a mutation in the ATP8B1 gene that codes for an aminophospholipid transporter (flippase), FIC1, which results in progressive cholestasis, malabsorption, and pancreatitis. This genetic defect is thought to be related to the rare syndrome in adults of Benign Recurrent Intrahepatic Cholestasis (BRIC). A defect in the gene ABCB11 of the bile salt export pump, BSEP, is responsible for PFIC-2 (Byler syndrome), which causes jaundice in infancy associated with a nonspecific giant cell hepatitis. Mutations of the gene (ABCB4) for the multidrug resistance transporter MDR3, abolish phospholipid secretion into bile and this leads to liver damage with extensive bile ductular proliferation, pruritus, and cirrhosis (PFIC-3) in childhood. The same MDR3 defect may be associated with intrahepatic cholestasis of pregnancy (ICP). Additionally, some cases of BRIC are MDR3-related, and some cases of ICP are due to FIC1 defects. Mutation of the canalicular organic anion transporter, the multidrug resistance-associated protein 2 (MRP-2) (coded for by ABCC2

is responsible for the benign conjugated hyperbilirubinemia syndrome known as Dubin-Johnson syndrome. The defect responsible for the Rotor syndrome, a conjugated hyperbilirubinemia that is benign, appears to be a fault in intrahepatic storage of conjugated organic anions that then reflux into plasma. Hepatobiliary transport systems are regulated at both the transcriptional and post-translational level, including the participation of nuclear receptors that also have genetic defects [7]. Bile formation requires the integrity of tight junctions between hepatocytes and normal bile duct development. In this context, the syndromic form of familial paucity of intrahepatic bile ducts, known as Alagille syndrome or arteriohepatic dysplasia, is not due to a primary canalicular transport abnormality but to an autosomal dominant mutation of the Jagged 1 gene, which encodes a ligand of Notch I (one of four members of a family of transmembrane receptor proteins) that is required for normal bile duct genesis. Alagille syndrome and the PFIC transporter defects can now be diagnosed by microarray chip assay on peripheral blood.

Extrahepatic causes of cholestasis

Among the most frequent extrahepatic causes of cholestasis are choledocholithiasis, and inflammation, injury and disappearance of bile ducts. Hepatic changes that are secondary to cholestasis itself (even if caused by diseases extrinsic to the hepatobiliary system) may be visible histologically as bile retention in hepatocytes, bile canaliculi, and other parenchymal elements. In addition, a feathery rarified and frothy appearance is imparted to the hepatocyte cytoplasm (pseudoxanthomatous change); it is sometimes referred to as *cholatestasis,* which implies that liver cell injury is due to the toxic effect of retained bile salts. Cholestasis is also the histologic picture seen in heart failure, sickle cell disease, functional bile flow impairment after liver transplantation, and in the early stage of some of the hereditary canalicular transport defects. Several drugs can inhibit canalicular transporters to cause jaundice [16]. Estrogens cause cholestasis, via a combination of a dose-related effect and genetic susceptibility. Androgens, cyclosporin, and synthetic progestogens cause dose-related cholestasis. Rarer associations occur with some antimicrobials and nonsteroidal anti-inflammatory drugs.

Sepsis, septic shock, and the hemodynamic, metabolic, and immune alterations that occur in major trauma, have been characterized as the "systemic inflammatory response syndrome" (SIRS), which is a potent cause of cholestasis [9]. The mechanism of cholestasis in sepsis is complex, involving infiltration with many inflammatory cell types, impairment of bile formation by endotoxin-mediated tumor necrosis factor alpha (TNFα) and proinflammatory cytokines. Cholestasis of sepsis is seen with *Escherichia coli* but also with *Staphylococcus* and other Gram-positive organisms. The primary site of infection may be intra-abdominal, but it can also be pneumonia, endocarditis, pyelonephritis, cellulitis, and abscesses. Recently, a secondary sclerosing cholangitis syndrome has been described in patients in intensive care units who have severe sepsis or SIRS [17].

Secondary changes in hepatocyte transport in acquired cholestatic liver disease

In general, the cellular and molecular pattern of response to cholestasis from any cause is to protect hepatocytes from the accumulation of toxic compounds, notably bile salts. There is downregulation of the normal sinusoidal membrane transporters by which bile salts and other organic anions enter hepatocytes from sinusoidal blood. Bile salt export pumps continue to be expressed and, in some cases, upregulated at the canalicular pole. Upregulation of the expression of exporters on the sinusoidal membrane [18] may provide a compensatory efflux pump for hepatocytes that cannot export into the canalicular space. It remains to be seen whether adaptive responses of bile salt transport on cholangiocytes, in the kidney and the intestine, may help rid the body of potentially toxic compounds that the liver can no longer expel [19].

Diagnosis of the cause of jaundice

All the usual modalities of clinical investigation are used to diagnose the cause of jaundice, including standard and special laboratory blood tests, some form of hepatobiliary imaging, and frequently liver biopsy. Nonetheless, the importance of acquiring an exhaustive clinical history and of performing a careful and thorough physical examination cannot be overemphasized.

History

The age and gender of the patient should be taken into account because of the relationship between these variables and different causes of jaundice, especially cholestasis. The duration of jaundice, the patient's age at onset and a persistent or relapsing nature all relate to different causes. Contemporary events should be ascertained, such as pain, intercurrent illness, all medications used (both current and over the past 6 months to 3 years), fever, and other comorbid events, such as pregnancy, heart failure, anemia, episodes of hypotension or hypoxemia, surgery (especially abdominal), abdominal injury, blood transfusions, weight loss, gastrointestinal bleeding, and injury with hematoma formation. Alcohol use should be quantified and psychological evidence sought for alcohol and/or other substance dependency. The family history should seek liver disease and jaundice in close relatives, with questions about cholestasis of pregnancy and with oral contraceptive steroid use, connective tissue disorders, and other autoimmune processes, as well as any history of unusual anemia.

Physical examination

A detailed discussion of the physical signs of liver disease can be found in Chapter 16. Jaundice should be confirmed in good light by careful examination of the accessible sclera of the eyes, the mucous membranes (especially the frenulum), and the skin, including the palms of the hands and soles of the feet. The jaundice in hemolytic anemia is said to be lemon-yellow, in contrast to the orange-yellow of hepatocellular jaundice,

and the green-yellow pigmentation seen in obstructive or cholestatic jaundice (Figure 15.5). These color differences are subtle and may be difficult to distinguish in practice. When cholestasis is prolonged, the skin becomes hyperpigmented with melanin, and lipid deposits may appear around the eyes (xanthelasmas) and at pressure points in the skin (xanthomas). Spider nevi, palmar erythema, "paper money" skin, petechiae or ecchymoses, finger clubbing, and abdominal wall veins, should be sought. Skin excoriations, especially the papular lesions of *prurigo nodularis*, corroborate the severity of itching. Signs of heart failure and other causes of raised systemic venous pressure must be checked. The characteristic facies of Alagille syndrome, the size of the liver, presence of splenomegaly, ascites, other abdominal masses, lymphadenopathy, and peripheral edema should be noted, in addition to the patient's level of consciousness, cognitive function, asterixis, and other neurologic abnormalities.

Laboratory tests

Red cell indices, red cell morphology (especially to look for causes of hemolytic anemia, such as spherocytosis, sickling, and spur cells), white cell count and differential (including eosinophils), and platelet count, should be examined. Aspartate (AST) and alanine (ALT) aminotransferases, alkaline phosphatase, both total and direct bilirubin, total protein, and albumin are measured. Gammaglutamyltransferase (transpeptidase) is occasionally useful in identifying a liver origin for raised alkaline phosphatase levels, and also helps to distinguish between the different forms of PFIC. Urine testing for bilirubin (which must be conjugated to be excreted by the kidneys) and urobilinogen is often overlooked. Acholuria, the urinary absence of bilirubin, is characteristic of indirect (unconjugated) hyperbilirubinemia due to hemolysis and/or bilirubin overproduction. Urinary urobilinogen excretion is increased in indirect hyperbilirubinemic states, but the urine is not dark unless it is left to stand long enough for brown urobilin to be formed from colorless urobilinogen. Urine is very dark (tea-colored) in obstructive jaundice whereas the stools are typically clay-colored because of the absence of stercobilin. Urinary urobilinogen is absent in biliary obstruction because no bilirubin enters the bowel. In cholestasis, conjugated bilirubin that is covalently bound to albumin is not excreted in the urine but lingers in the plasma with the half-life of the albumin moiety. Thus jaundice can persist in recovering cholestasis long after the urine color has normalized.

More specialized hematologic testing may be needed to look for specific hemolytic syndromes, as well as for causes of ineffective erythropoiesis. Testing for specific causes of liver disease is guided by the history and physical examination, and the results of standard liver tests.

Hepatobiliary imaging

This is used in almost all cases of jaundice unless bilirubin overproduction is the obvious diagnosis from the clinical evaluation and tests of urine and blood. The choice between

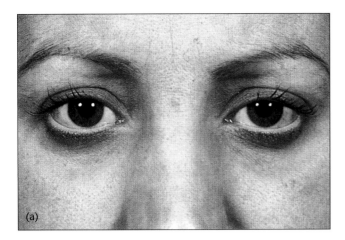

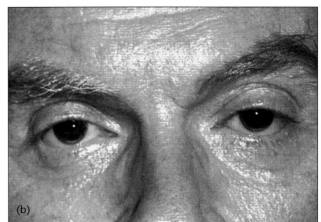

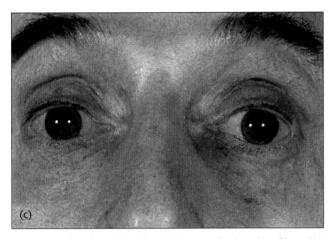

Figure 15.5 Three faces of jaundice. (a) Lemon-yellow jaundice of hemolytic anemia. (b) Orange-yellow jaundice of hepatitis. (c) Green-yellow jaundice of cholestasis, showing skin hyperpigmentation. (Reproduced with permission from Sherlock S, Summerfield JA. *A colour atlas of liver disease.* London: Wolfe Medical Publications; 1979.)

ultrasonography, computed tomography and magnetic resonance imaging, is considered elsewhere in this book. Direct biliary imaging, by endoscopic retrograde cholangiopancreatography (ERCP) or percutaneous transhepatic cholangiography (PTHC), is used to verify and define biliary anatomic abnormalities, allowing both tissue sampling for histologic diagnosis and therapy to relieve obstruction, at the same time.

Liver biopsy

Liver biopsy is not usually necessary in acute jaundice but is used to make the diagnosis of chronic hepatitis or cirrhosis, to find evidence for and possible causes of prolonged drug reactions, to distinguish among various cholestatic syndromes (especially those of bile duct injury and loss), and is the modality of choice for the diagnosis of liver graft dysfunction, including acute and chronic rejection, infection with herpes family viruses, alcohol recidivism, recurrence of pre-transplant liver disease and the occurrence of *de novo* diseases, like alloimmune hepatitis that may not be diagnosable by other means.

References

1. Reuben A. By indirections find directions out. *Hepatology.* 2002;35:1287–1290.
2. Murchison C. Spurious jaundice. Lecture IX. Jaundice. In: *Clinical lectures and disease of the liver.* Jaundice and abdominal dropsy, including the Croonian Lectures on functional derangements of the liver delivered at the Royal College of Physicians in 1874. 2nd edn. London: Longmans, Green; 1877: 310–313.
3. Larson AM, Polson J, Fontana RJ, *et al.* Acetaminophen-induced acute liver failure: results of a United States multi-center prospective study. *Hepatology.* 2005;42:1364–1372.
4. Reuben A. Hy's law. *Hepatology.* 2004;39:574–578.
5. Reuben A, Koch DG, Lee WM. Drug-induced acute liver failure. Results of a United States multicenter, prospective study. *Hepatology.* 2010;52;2065–2076
6. Hirschfield GM, Heathcote EJ. Cholestasis and cholestasis syndromes. *Curr Opin Gastroenterol.* 2009;25:175–179.
7. Wagner M, Zollner G, Trauner M. New molecular insights into the mechanisms of cholestasis. *J Hepatol.* 2007;5:776–782.
8. Desmet VJ. Vanishing bile duct syndromes in drug-induced liver disease. *J Hepatol.* 1997;20(Suppl 1):31–35.

9. Fuchs M, Sanyal AJ. Sepsis and cholestasis. *Clin Liver Dis.* 2008;12:151–172.

10. Reisman Y, Gips CH, Lavelle SM, *et al.* Clinical presentation of (subclinical) jaundice – the Euricterus product in the Netherlands. United Dutch Hospitals and Euricterus Project Management Group. *Hepatogastroenterology.* 1996;43:1190–1195.

11. Baranano DE, Rao M, Ferris CD, *et al.* Bilirubin reductase: a major physiologic cytoprotectant. *Proc Natl Acad Sci USA.* 2002;99:16093–16098.

12. Jansen PLM, Roskams T. Why are patients with liver disease jaundiced? ATP-binding cassette transporter expression in human liver disease. *J Hepatol.* 2001;35:811–813.

13. Bogma PJ. Inherited disorders of bilirubin metabolism. *J Hepatol.* 2003;38:107–117.

14. Innocenti F, Undevia SD, Tyer L *et al.* Genetic variants in the *UDPglucuronosyltransferase1A1* gene predict the risk of severe neutropenia of irinotecan. *J Clin Oncol.* 2004;22:1382–1388.

15. Karlsen TH, Hov JR. Genetics of cholestatic disease. *Curr Opin Gastroenterol.* 2010;26:251–258.

16. Bohan A, Boyer JL. Mechanism of hepatic transport of drugs; implications of cholestatic drug reactions. *Semin Liver Dis.* 2002;22:123–136.

17. Ruemmele P, Hofstaedter Gelbman CM. Secondary sclerosing cholangitis. *Nat Rev Gastroenterol Hepatol.* 2009;6:287–295.

18. Soroka CJ, Ballatori N, Boyer JL. Organ solute transporter OSTα-OSTβ: Its role in bile acid transport and cholestasis. *Semin Liver Dis.* 2010;30:178–185.

19. Dawson PA, Lan T, Rao A. Bile acid transporters. *J Lipid Res.* 2009;50:2340–2357.

CHAPTER 16
Spotting and dealing with signs of chronic liver disease: a guided tour

Adrian Reuben
College of Medicine, Medical University of South Carolina, Charleston, SC, USA

KEY POINTS

- Liver disease has global effects on health that show as protein-calorie malnutrition, deconditioning, muscle wasting and peripheral edema, in addition to specific abnormal physical signs in many organ systems
- Dermatological signs in advanced liver disease, besides jaundice, include spider nevi and other forms of telangiectasias, palmar erythema, finger clubbing and other nail changes. Gynecomastia also results from the estrogen–androgen imbalance that causes the aforementioned cutaneous abnormalities
- Cutaneous signs are also associated with (i) the cause of liver disease, like the vasculitic rash of cryglobulinemia and porphyria cutanea tarda, or (ii) its effects, e.g., the lipid deposits, excoriations and prurigo nodularis, of cholestasis
- Abdominal distension from ascites, is often accompanied with abdominal wall venous dilatations and umbilical herniation that can rupture
- Liver disease causes or is associated with many neurological abnormalities, including asterixis, fine tremors, cognitive deficits and decreased consciousness of encephalopathy, and the consequences of alcohol excess in the form of cerebral and cerebellar degeneration and peripheral neuropathy

Introduction

Clinical hepatology is a treasure trove of physical signs, which, though not necessarily pathognomonic, can indicate the presence of liver disease, gauge its severity and, together with the history, give insight into its cause. The classical armamentarium of inspection, percussion, palpation, auscultation and even olfaction, is put to good use in the evaluation of the liver patient and, together with the findings of a comprehensive history and results of preliminary blood tests, can provide a rational basis for choosing laboratory, imaging, and invasive tests for patient investigation. A reasonable scheme for classifying physical signs would be to catalog them by organ system; however, a more practical approach is to categorize signs by their bodily location during the conduct of the physical examination, starting with an overall assessment of the patient, followed by specific examinations of the face, head and neck, limbs, chest, and so forth.

General appearance

For the patient who is lethargic, jaundiced, gaunt and edematous, with prominent spider nevi and an abdomen grossly distended with ascites, a single glance confirms the presence of liver disease and judges its severity. In general, however, one begins by noting if the patient looks well or ill, is alert or drowsy, and well-nurtured or not. **The nutritional state** can give clues to the nature and severity of liver disease and its outcome [1] . Most useful is the so-called Global Subjective Assessment [1] that includes components of history – weight change, appetite, etc; physical appearance – muscle wasting, fat stores; and a rating of the degree of nurture. **Obesity**, which is quantified by calculating the body mass index (making allowances for fluid retention), may be associated with nonalcoholic fatty liver disease and impair survival from liver disease and liver transplantation [1,2].

Regional physical signs
Face, head, and neck

Face: Muscle loss in advanced cirrhosis or cancer is evident as temporal wasting and sunken cheeks (Figure 16.1); occasionally, the characteristic facies of a **childhood storage disorder**, or the widely set eyes, flat forehead, and small pointed chin of **Alagille syndrome** give a clue to the diagnosis. **Jaundice** is seen first in the sclerae and later in the skin and mucous membranes, especially beneath the tongue; hyperpigmentation of the skin due to melanin deposition complicates longstanding cholestasis. In prolonged cholestasis, lipids are deposited in the skin as creamy yellow excrescences called **xanthelasmas** when they occur around the eyes and xanthomas when they are elsewhere) (Figure 16.2), usually in areas that are exposed or subject to trauma or pressure. **Petechiae** and **ecchymoses** localize to sites of trauma in patients with thrombocytopenia, but periorbital bruising suggests amyloidosis. **Telangiectasias** are common in liver cell failure, particularly spider angiomas or spider nevi [3] (Figure 16.3 and Video 16.1); infrequently there are mat-shaped telangiectasias, white spots, and fine

Textbook of Clinical Gastroenterology and Hepatology, Second Edition. Edited by C. J. Hawkey, Jaime Bosch, Joel E. Richter, Guadalupe Garcia-Tsao, Francis K. L. Chan.
© 2012 Blackwell Publishing Ltd. Published 2012 by Blackwell Publishing Ltd.

threadlike vessels in the skin reminiscent of the silk threads in paper US dollar bills (**paper money skin**) (Figure 16.4a). Spider nevi, the surface manifestation of enlarged coiled skin arterioles (Figure 16.3d) occur predominantly on the face (Figure 16.3b), neck, shoulders, and chest, with fewer on the arms

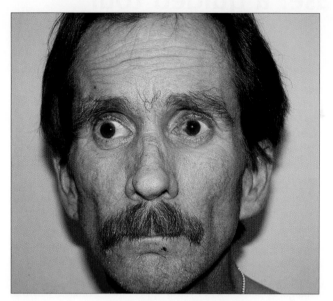

Figure 16.1 Temporal wasting and sunken cheeks in patient with advanced cirrhosis.

(Figure 16.3a) , hands and abdomen, rarely on the legs, but sometimes even on mucous membranes (Figure 16.3c). As the arteriole reaches the surface and numerous branches radiate to form the spider's "legs," its terminus is seen as a central red spot that pulsates under light pressure; heavy pressure blanches the whole spider. Spider nevi occur in pregnancy, estrogen treatment, and in some normal individuals, and must be distinguished from telangiectasias seen in sun-exposed areas and in hereditary hemorrhagic telangiectasia (Osler-Weber-Rendu syndrome). Spider nevi are especially common in alcoholic liver disease and are associated with palmar erythema, digital clubbing, esophageal varices, and a poor outcome of cirrhosis [3]. Spider number greater than 20, size greater than 15 mm and an atypical location, correlate with an increased risk of esophageal variceal rupture [3]. **Parotid gland enlargement** is typical of alcoholism (Figure 16.4b), but though flushing in rosacea (Figure 16.5) is exacerbated by alcohol, it is unclear if this skin disease *per se* or rhinophyma are alcohol-induced. The skin of the face may be **bronzed** in patients with hemochromatosis, tight and thickened in scleroderma, or marked with acne in alcohol abuse, autoimmune hepatitis and steroid treatment.

Feminization: The **soft skin, fine hair** and **sparse beard** of feminization, occur predominantly in men with alcoholic

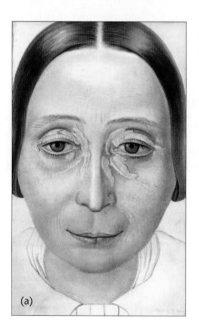

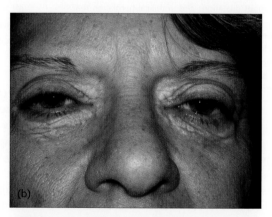

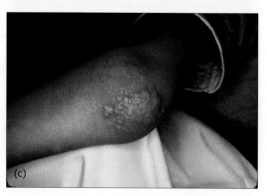

Figure 16.2 Xanthelasmas and xanthomas. (a) Xanthelasmas around the eyes.
(Reproduced from the color plates of J. L. Tupper in: Addison T, Gull W. On a certain affection of the skin, Vitiligoidea – α plana, β tuberosa. With remarks and plates. *Guys Hosp Rep*. 1851; 7:265–276. Images courtesy of Information Services and Systems Department of GKT, Kings College London.) (b) Xanthelasmas in patient with clarithromycin-induced cholestasis. (c) Xanthomas on elbow of patient in 16.2b.

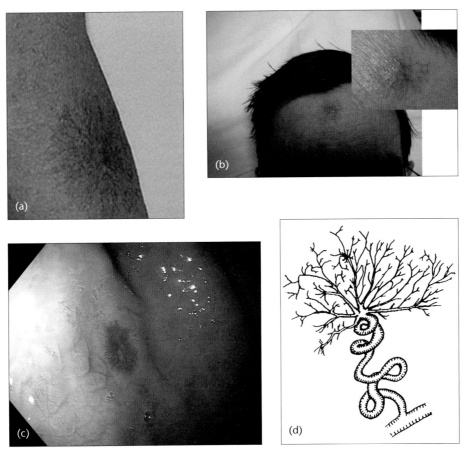

Figure 16.3 Spider nevi. (a) Upper arm; (b) forehead, with close-up; (c) gastric antral mucosa at esophagogastroduodenoscopy; (d) drawing of coiled skin arteriole.
(Figure 16.3d reproduced from Bean WB. *Vascular Spiders and Related Lesions of the Skin.* Springfield: Charles C. Thomas 1958;1–372.)

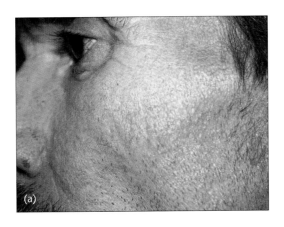

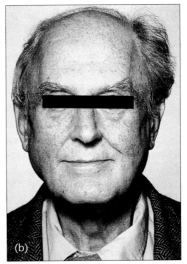

Figure 16.4 Signs – face, head, and neck.
(a) Paper money skin. Fine thread-like superficial veins on the face of a patient with alcoholic cirrhosis, resembling the finely chopped red and blue silk threads embedded in US dollar bills. (b) Parotid gland enlargement in an alcoholic patient. Patient also has paper money skin. (Reproduced with permission from Misiewicz JJ *et al.* A slide atlas of gastroenterology: Unit 18. Produced and published by Gower Medical Publishing Ltd, London UK for Glaxo, Research Triangle Park, Durham, North Carolina 27709. 1987.)

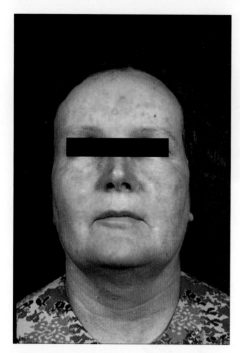

Figure 16.5 Rosacea in a patient with alcoholic liver disease.

cirrhosis. To this can be added, exacerbation of acne and psoriasis, the presence of various dermatitides, or the characteristic skin fragility and blistering of porphyria cutanea tarda [4].

Eyes: Aside from jaundice, the eyes may show the characteristic **Kayser-Fleischer rings** of Wilson disease (see Chapter 92). These rings, which are often complete, nearly always bilateral and most intense and wide at the superior and inferior aspects of the cornea, constitute the single most important diagnostic sign of Wilson disease and should be confirmed by slit-lamp examination. Kayser-Fleischer rings are seen occasionally in non-Wilsonian liver disease and sometimes in patients with prolonged cholestasis. The eyes in Wilson's disease may also show characteristic sunflower cataracts. The deformity of the anterior chamber of the eye known as posterior embryotoxon is characteristic of Alagille syndrome.

The mouth: should be inspected for lesions that occur in systemic disorders, e.g., **glossitis** and **angular stomatitis** are common in vitamin B-deficient alcoholics, telangiectasias decorate the lips in Osler-Weber-Rendu syndrome, and lichen planus may be associated with chronic hepatitis C infection and primary biliary cirrhosis. The dental hygiene of the liver transplant candidate must be checked when screening for risks of perioperative infection. In children, prolonged cholestasis discolors the growing teeth (**chlorodontia**). Central **cyanosis**, a blue discoloration of the lips, tongue, and other mucous membranes, points to hypoxemia that may be due to hepatopulmonary syndrome or other lung disorders. Cyanosis may be inapparent, if the patient is anemic. Finally, once whiffed, the characteristic "mousey" odor of the breath of patients with liver failure, the fetor hepaticus, is hard to forget.

Jugular veins: One cannot overstate the importance of looking for jugular venous pressure elevation, especially if it is exacerbated by deep inspiration, as its presence should make the examiner suspicious that a patient's ascites is due to constrictive pericarditis and not cirrhosis. Jugular venous pressure elevation may also be caused by fluid overload, tricuspid regurgitation, systolic or diastolic dysfunction, and pulmonary hypertension. These cardiac abnormalities can explain or aggravate hepatomegaly and adversely affect patient outcome and transplant candidacy. When eliciting the "**hepatojugular reflux**" **sign**, which relies on increasing venous return through the inferior vena cava, abdominal pressure should be applied anywhere but over a liver that is enlarged, congested, and tender.

Arms and hands

Characteristic, albeit nonspecific, signs of liver disease are seen in the hands, but examining the rest of the upper limbs is rewarding too. The arms should be inspected for the loss of **muscle bulk** of advanced cirrhosis, for excoriations and prurigo nodularis that indirectly indicate the severity of a patient's pruritus, and for axillary hair loss in men that is further evidence of **feminization**. **Tattoos** and **needle marks** may indicate a lifestyle that is conducive to viral hepatitis acquisition. Hypotension, which is not usually thought of as a physical sign, is a predictor of reduced survival in cirrhosis [5], and is common in patients with advanced liver disease because systemic arterial vasodilatation is a consequence of portal hypertension. Common too are warm hands and a bounding pulse, which are peripheral signs of the hyperdynamic circulation of advanced cirrhosis. Measurement of postural changes in pulse and blood pressure are important when evaluating a patient for reduced blood volume due to bleeding or fluid loss, since supine blood pressure may be normal in this setting. Reduced skin turgor may help in the diagnosis of fluid depletion too. **Petechiae** may appear on the arm following blood pressure measurement in patients with thrombocytopenia, platelet dysfunction, or capillary fragility if the cuff is held inflated between venous and arterial pressure for more than a few moments.

The arms and hands of chronic liver disease patients may show the same skin changes that affect the face and neck, especially lesions that are exacerbated by sunlight exposure. **Vitiligo** may accompany autoimmune liver diseases, e.g., primary biliary cirrhosis. The particular form of palmar erythema that localizes to the thenar and hypothenar eminences (Figure 16.6a), which can also involve both palmar and dorsal surfaces of the distal phalanges, is typical of cirrhosis but it can also occur in rheumatoid arthritis, thyrotoxicosis, pregnancy, bronchogenic carcinoma, and some normal individuals. Similarly, the Hippocratic sign of **finger clubbing** (Figure 16. 6a and b) occurs not only in cirrhosis but also in heart disease (cyanotic congenital deformities, spontaneous bacterial

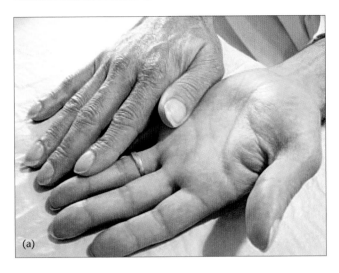

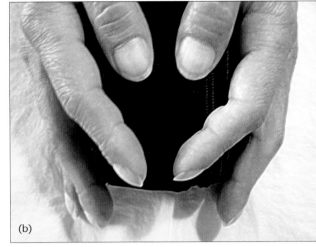

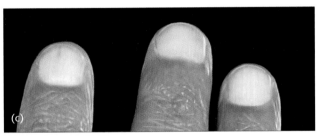

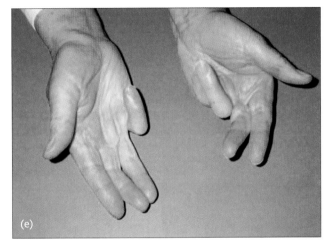

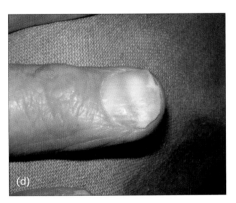

Figure 16.6 Signs – hands.
(a, b) Palmar erythema and finger clubbing, together with the proximal leukonychia and distal dark pigmentation of Terry nails, in a patient with hepatitis C cirrhosis and hepatocellular carcinoma. (c) Leukonychia involving the whole nail. (d) Muehrcke lines. (e) Dupuytren contracture of the palmar fascia causing flexion of the fingers. (Reproduced with permission from Gudmundsson KG, Jonsson T and Arngrimsson R. Guillaume Dupuytren and finger contractures. *Lancet* 2003;362:165–168.)

endocarditis, and atrial myxoma), lung disease (pyogenic abscess, bronchiectasis, bronchogenic carcinoma, interstitial fibrosis, and mesothelioma), and inflammatory bowel disease (especially Crohn's disease). If hypoxemia complicates cirrhosis, clubbing may be noticeable but disappears with successful liver transplantation. When finger clubbing coincides with **palmar erythema** and **spider nevi,** cirrhosis is virtually assured, yet it must be admitted that there is considerable interobserver variation and a lack of objective diagnostic criteria in the diagnosis of clubbing.

Besides clubbing and hypertrophic osteoarthropathy, the hands may show other disfigurements. The **nails** in cirrhosis may be thickened, ridged, brittle, flat, or even concave. Nail discoloration includes reddened lunulae in alcoholism (without cirrhosis), blue lunulae in Wilson disease, and streaks of green that bear witness to prior cholestasis. Whitening (**leukonychia**), which occurs in hypoalbuminemia, cirrhosis, heart failure, renal failure and diabetes, may involve the whole nail (Figure 16.6c) or occur in bands only (**Muehrcke lines**, Figure 16.6d), or may be associated with distal reddening (**Terry nails**, Figure 16.6b) that is probably due to telangiectasias (Figure 16.6a). A curious deformity of the hand and fingers described by Felix Platter in seventeenth century Basel, was popularized by French surgeon Baron Guillaume Dupuytren

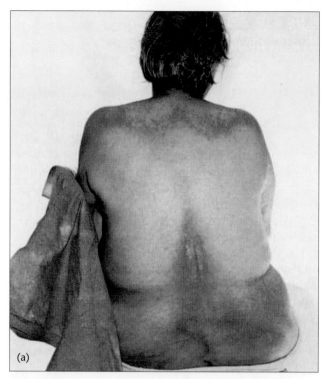

(a)

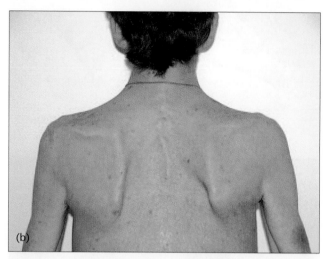

(b)

Figure 16.7 Signs – back. (a) The back of a patient with severe pruritus showing a pigmented peripheral region that has been repeatedly scratched, and a pale "butterfly" area of skin that the patient could not reach with the fingernails. (b) Prominent muscle wasting of the back in a patient with alcoholic cirrhosis, revealing the spines of vertebrae and the bony outlines of

the scapulae. A very large spider nevus is also visible on the patient's right upper arm (same patient as in figures 16.1, 16.3(a), 16.4(a), and 16.9(a)). (Figure 16.7a reproduced with permission from Reynolds TB. The "butterfly" sign in patients with chronic jaundice and pruritus. *Ann Int Med.* 1973;78:595–596.)

in the nineteenth century, and was recognized by him as a fibrotic contracture of the palmar fascia that involves the digits, usually beginning with flexion of the ring and/or little finger (Figure 16.6e). **Dupuytren contracture** occurs in both genders and all ethnic groups, but it is predominantly a disease of older men of northern European ancestry and, by repute, it originated with the Vikings [6]. Dupuytren contracture, which is a feature of alcoholism rather than liver disease as such, also complicates diabetes, seizure disorders, cigarette smoking, and probably vibration-induced hand injury, especially in genetically susceptible individuals. Finally, testing for the flapping irregular tremor of asterixis (Video 16.2) is usually done during examination of the hands.

Chest

Telangiectasias that occur in sunlight-exposed skin must be distinguished from spider nevi. **Extensive scratching** because of pruritus causes hyperpigmentation of the skin, whereas there is sparing of the unreachable central area of the back that remains pale in a characteristic "butterfly" configuration (Figure 16.7a). **Loss of muscle** may be conspicuous in the pectoral girdle and especially the back, where the vertebrae and bony outlines of the scapulae may be prominent (Figure 16.7b). **Gynecomastia** (Figure 16.8) is another feature of

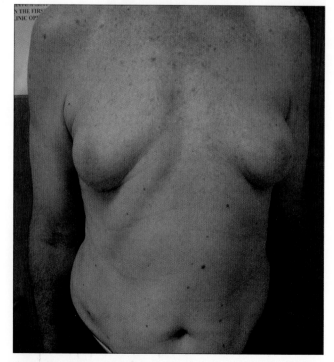

Figure 16.8 Gynecomastia (with spider nevi restricted to upper trunk) in a male patient with alcoholic cirrhosis.

feminization, but it may also be caused by spironolactone therapy (in which the breasts are often tender) and can be a presenting sign of fibrolamellar carcinoma. Gynecomastia should be investigated further by breast imaging or biopsy, if there is doubt. The **heart** should be examined for signs of a hyperdynamic circulation and for pulmonary hypertension. The **respiratory examination** may show pleural effusion, usually but not invariably associated with ascites, i.e., a hepatic hydrothorax, most commonly right-sided.

Abdomen

Spider nevi are infrequent on the abdomen, and are sometimes mistaken for cherry angiomas (Campbell de Morgan spots), benign flat or slightly raised, bright red or purple circular angiokeratoses that appear with advancing years and do not blanch with pressure. **Dilated superficial abdominal wall**

veins with cephalad blood flow are often seen in the upper abdomen in cirrhosis (Figure 16.9a and b). These cutaneous veins carry blood from a recanalized umbilical vein or paraumbilical veins in portal hypertension, or bypass an obstructed inferior vena cava that is either compressed by an enlarged liver (usually the caudate lobe) or is constricted. However, it is rare to see a fully-fledged caput Medusae, the radiating system of hepatofugal veins that emanate from the umbilicus, supplied through a patent umbilical vein (Figures 16.9c). **Ascites** is a hallmark of decompensation in cirrhosis [5]. Until 1–2 L of fluid collect, however, ascites is only detected reliably by imaging, i.e., ultrasonography, computed tomography, or magnetic resonance imaging. As ascites increases, the flanks and abdomen bulge and fluid collects in the pelvis to form a U-shaped region of dullness to percussion. That abdominal distention is due to free fluid in the peritoneal cavity is best

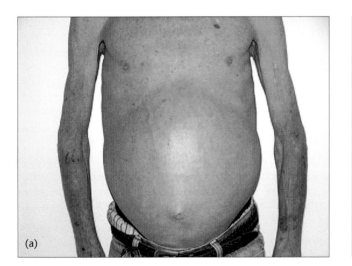

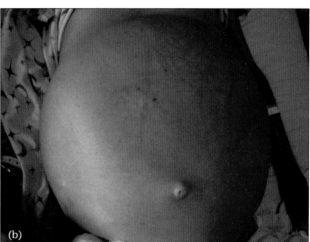

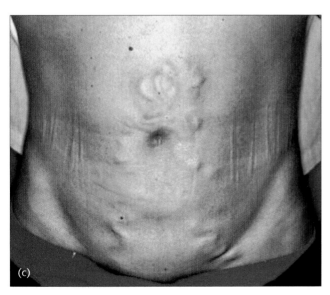

Figure 16.9 Signs – abdomen.
(a, b) Abdomen distended with ascites and superficial veins that have cephalad flow. (c) Caput Medusae. (Figure 16.9c reproduced with permission from Yang PM, Chen DS., Images in clinical medicine. Caput medusae., *N Engl J Med* 2005:353;(21). Copyright Massachusetts Medical Society.)

KEY PHYSICAL SIGNS IN CHRONIC LIVER DISEASE

Signs	Comments
Face, head and neck	
Jaundice (icterus)	• First seen in sclerae, then in mucous membranes and skin • Distinguish from exogenous yellow pigment that does not color sclerae, e.g., carotene
Spider nevi (spider angiomas)	• Also seen on chest, back, and arms; very uncommon on abdomen and legs • Distinguish from other telangiectasias (e.g., solar telangiectasias and Osler-Weber-Rendu syndrome) and cherry angiomas • Also seen in pregnancy and estrogen therapy • Due to relative estrogen to androgen excess, caused by liver cell failure
Temporal wasting	• Part of generalized muscle loss in cirrhosis, due to impaired protein metabolism • Also affects the muscles of the back, arms, shoulders, and legs,
Xanthelasmas	• Lipid deposits in periocular skin, secondary to hyperlipidemia of cholestasis • Associated with cutaneous lipid deposits (xanthomas) on areas exposed or subject to trauma • Also occurs in disorders of severe hyperlipidemia or dyslipidemia
Paper money skin	• Fine thread-like telangiectasias on face due to relative estrogen to androgen excess, caused by liver cell failure • Also occurs on chest
Feminization	• Soft skin and sparse beard • Associated with sparse hair in axillae and elsewhere, and with gynecomastia
Kayser-Fleischer rings	• Typical brown-green pigmentation of cornea in Wilson disease; due to copper deposition in Descemet membrane • Also occurs in cholestatic and occasionally non-cholestatic chronic liver disease
Sunflower cataracts	• Typical of Wilson disease
Central cyanosis	• Indicates hypoxemia that may be due to hepatopulmonary syndrome or other cardiopulmonary disease
Elevated jugular venous pressure	• May indicate pulmonary hypertension due to cirrhosis, but can result from other cardiac dysfunction
Hands and arms	
Finger clubbing	• Especially likely in cirrhosis if patient is hypoxemic • Also seen in certain cardiac, respiratory, and bowel disorders • May be accompanied by hypertrophic osteoarthropathy
Nail discoloration	• White nails (leukonychia), also seen in diabetes, hypoalbuminemia, heart failure, and renal failure • White nail color may be uniform or show lines (Muehrcke) or bands (Beau), or distal dusky redness (Terry nails) • Green streaks from previous cholestasis
Nail disfigurement	• Brittle, ridged, concave, or convex nails
Dupuytren contracture	• Thickening and nodularity of palmar fascia • Causes flexion deformities of digits, especially ring and little fingers • Occurs infrequently in feet • A feature of alcoholism rather than liver disease per se, also seen in diabetes, epilepsy, cigarette smoking, and vibration injury; genetic predisposition
Chest and back	
Muscle wasting	• Especially of shoulders, back, and upper arms
Gynecomastia	• May be bilateral or unilateral • Breasts tender with spironolactone use • Due to relative estrogen to androgen excess, caused by liver cell failure • Can occur with fibrolamellar carcinoma

Signs	Comments
Pleural effusion (hepatic hydrothorax)	• Derived from ascites that may or may not be apparent • Almost always right-sided
Cardiac signs of pulmonary hypertension	• Tricuspid regurgitation may follow
Abdomen Ascites	• Detectable clinically when more than 1–2L fluid present • Confirmed by demonstrating shifting dullness • Diarrhea and fat pannus can also give shifting dullness
Dilated superficial abdominal wall veins	• Flow is cephalad or caudal in obstruction of inferior or superior vena cava, respectively • Caput Medusae rarely seen • Associated with recanalization of umbilical vein or inferior vena cava compression
Abdominal wall striae	• Secondary to prior or current abdominal distention of any cause
Umbilical hernia	• Secondary to increased intra-abdominal pressure • Erosion and leakage creates medical emergency with high mortality • Can lead to bowel and omental incarceration
Legs and feet Clubbing of toes, plantar erythema, plantar Dupuytren contracture	• All uncommon compared to finger clubbing, but carry same implications
Edema	• Check near Achilles tendon and sacrum for gravity-dependent edema during recumbency

corroborated by demonstrating "shifting" of the dullness when the patient turns from one side to the other. Shifting dullness may also be found in the occasional patient with diarrhea or a large fat pannus. With gross ascites it is possible to elicit a "fluid wave" in the supine patient, by tapping one flank and feeling the percussion ripple at the other. An assistant must immobilize the abdominal wall, with hand pressure. Massive ascites can cause umbilical herniation that can lead to bowel or omental incarceration, or rupture with its attendant morbidity and high mortality [7].

Abdominal examination for the diagnosis of cirrhosis, has been found wanting [8]. Clinical estimates of liver size, splenic enlargement, and ascites have been inadequate by comparison with imaging results. Between-observer agreement and, within-observer variability have been found to be at fault. Yet, for all that, physical examination of the abdomen is of value. Some investigators have stressed the value of percussion over palpation of the liver and spleen, but both are used together to assess liver span, and palpation best assesses liver consistency and nodularity, detects the pulsatile hepatomegaly of tricuspid regurgitation, and finds the enlarged left lobe of cirrhosis in the epigastrium. Dullness to percussion of Traube's space [9], the crescent-shaped region of gastric resonance above the left costal margin, is an early finding in splenomegaly before the spleen is palpable. A right subcostal mass may

be a distended gallbladder in malignant jaundice due to distal biliary obstruction or occasionally in acute cholecystitis, a Reidel lobe, or even the lower pole of an anteriorly placed right kidney. The abdominal examination includes the inguinal regions and the genitalia, where edema and ascites may collect, and mimic an inguinal hernia. Auscultation of the abdomen may disclose the arterial bruit of a liver tumor or a venous hum from the dilated umbilical vein in portal hypertension (Cruveilhier-Baumgarten syndrome).

Legs and feet

Plantar erythema, clubbing of the toes (Figure 16.10) and **plantar fascia contractures** are the infrequent pedal counterparts of respective signs in the hands, and have the same clinical significance. **Loss of muscle bulk** in the thighs may be less noticeable than in the arms and shoulders; in contrast, **edema** is much more common in the legs and feet. There is no generally agreed grading scheme or scale for edema, so we suggest the terms trace, mild, moderate, and severe be applied to describe the depth and compressibility of the edema, and describe its distribution in the feet, legs, sacral region, and abdominal wall. When patients have been recumbent for more than 12 hours, it is important to press near the Achilles tendons and in the sacral region, otherwise redistributed dependent edema might be neglected. Other physical signs that are common in the legs

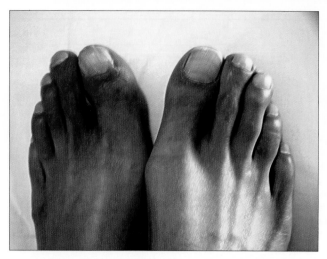

Figure 16.10 Clubbing and erythema of toes – same patient as in Figures 16.6a and 16.6b.

and feet of patients with liver disease are **petechiae** due to thrombocytopenia, and the petechial rash, palpable purpura, and ulceration associated with **cryoglobulinemic vasculitis**, which afflicts those with chronic hepatitis C.

SOURCES OF INFORMATION FOR PATIENTS AND DOCTORS

http://www.patient.co.uk/showdoc/23068925/
http://patients.uptodate.com/topic.asp?file=livr_dis/4490

References

1. Stephenson GR, Moretti EW, El-Moalem H, *et al*. Malnutrition in liver transplant patients: preoperative subjective global assessment is predictive of outcome after liver transplantation. *Transplantation*. 2001;72:666–670.
2. Nair S, Verma S, Tuluvath PH. Obesity and its effect on survival in patients undergoing orthotopic liver transplantation in the United States. *Hepatology*. 2002;35:105–109.
3. Reuben A. Along came a spider. *Hepatology*. 2002;35:735–756.
4. Higgins EM, du Vivier AWP. Cutaneous disease and alcohol misuse. *Br Med Bull*. 1994;50:85–98.
5. Fernandez-Esparrach G, Sanchez-Fueyo A, Gines P, *et al*. A prognostic model for predicting survival in cirrhosis with ascites. *J Hepatol*. 2001;34:46–52.
6. Flatt AE. The Vikings and Baron Dupuytren's disease. *Baylor Uni Med Center Proc* 2001;14:378–384.
7. Maniatis AG, Hunt CM. Therapy for spontaneous umbilical hernia rupture. *Am J Gastroenterol*. 1995;90:310–312.
8. de Bruyn G, Graviss EA. A systematic review of the diagnostic accuracy of physical examination for the detection of cirrhosis. *BMC Med Inform Decis Mak*. 2001;1:6.
9. Castell DO, Frank BB. Abdominal examination: role of percussion and auscultation. *Postgrad Med*. 1977;62:131–134.

CHAPTER 17

Ascites

Guadalupe Garcia-Tsao

Yale University, School of Medicine, New Haven; Veterans Affairs Connecticut Healthcare System, West Haven, CT, USA

KEY POINTS

- Ascites is a pathological condition characterized by the accumulation of fluid in the peritoneal cavity
- The main causes of ascites are cirrhosis, right heart failure, and peritoneal malignancy
- The presence of ascites can be confirmed by abdominal ultrasonography
- A diagnostic paracentesis should always be performed in a patient with new-onset ascites in order to establish the cause of ascites
- Initial testing should include determination of the serum–ascites albumin gradient and ascites total protein

Introduction

Ascites (from the Greek *askos*, meaning a leather bag used to carry wine, water or oil) is the pathological accumulation of fluid in the peritoneal cavity. Cirrhosis is the most common cause of ascites, accounting for more than 75% of patients with ascites. Less common causes are peritoneal malignancy (12%), cardiac failure (5%), and peritoneal tuberculosis (2%) [1]. Ascites secondary to severe ovarian hyperstimulation syndrome (as a result of follicle stimulation for *in vitro* fertilization) is increasingly recognized.

Data are lacking regarding the prevalence and incidence of ascites, and the distribution of its different etiologies worldwide. For instance, while ascites secondary to tuberculous peritonitis is extremely rare in developed countries, it is still an important cause of ascites in many developing countries. There is more information regarding the most common type, cirrhotic ascites. It is present in 20–60% of patients with cirrhosis at the time of diagnosis [2]. The cumulative probability of developing ascites ranges from 35% to 50% over 5 years [2,3] and it is the most common cause of cirrhosis decompensation.

Pathophysiology and causes

Ascites can be classified according to its pathophysiology/source into the following types.

Hepatic sinusoidal ascites

This type of ascites is due to leakage of lymph from hypertensive hepatic sinusoids. The main cause is **cirrhosis** in which increased intrahepatic resistance due to fibrosis, regenerative nodules, and hepatic venular vasoconstriction leads to sinusoidal hypertension. Ascites formation is maintained because of sodium retention secondary to splanchnic and systemic vasodilatation that leads to a decreased effective arterial blood volume and activation of sodium-retaining systems (renin–angiotensin–aldosterone, sympathetic nervous system) (see Chapter 99). Other causes of ascites secondary to sinusoidal hypertension are intrahepatic (sinusoidal obstruction syndrome) or extrahepatic (Budd–Chiari syndrome, congestive heart failure, constrictive pericarditis).

Peritoneal ascites

This type of ascites is due to leakage of mesenteric lymph from obliterated peritoneal lymphatics and/or from an inflamed peritoneal surface. The main cause is **peritoneal carcinomatosis**. It is important to distinguish malignant ascites from ascites secondary to massive liver metastases or to "pseudo-cirrhosis" (secondary to profound desmoplastic response to infiltrating breast cancer or secondary to nodular regenerative hyperplasia related to chemotherapy), in which case the source is sinusoidal. Another cause of peritoneal ascites is **tuberculous peritonitis** [4].

Miscellaneous types of ascites

In other rare causes of ascites the source is variable. **Chylous ascites** is a milky-appearing ascites rich in triglycerides due to disruption of intra-abdominal lymphatics from trauma or obstruction (benign or malignant) [5]. **Pancreatic ascites** is related to the disruption of the pancreatic duct or leakage from a pseudocyst, which may occur during acute or chronic pancreatitis [6]. **Bile ascites** is due to disruption of the biliary tree and typically occurs after biliary tract surgery and trauma to the abdomen or, more rarely, as a complication of percutaneous liver biopsy and transhepatic cholangiography. **Myxedema ascites** is due to increased extravasation of plasma proteins because of abnormal capillary permeability and relatively slow lymphatic drainage [7].

Textbook of Clinical Gastroenterology and Hepatology, Second Edition. Edited by C. J. Hawkey, Jaime Bosch, Joel E. Richter, Guadalupe Garcia-Tsao, Francis K. L. Chan.
© 2012 Blackwell Publishing Ltd. Published 2012 by Blackwell Publishing Ltd.

Symptom complexes

The most frequent symptoms are increased abdominal girth (tightness of a belt or garments around the waist) and weight gain. The rapid onset of symptoms in a matter of weeks helps to distinguish ascites from obesity, which usually develops over a period of months to years. Dyspnea may occur as a consequence of increasing abdominal distension and/or the concomitant presence of pleural effusions.

A detailed history of cardiac disease or malignancy, or ongoing symptoms of cancer (such as lymphadenopathy and weight loss) or other diseases (kidney, thyroid, infectious, ovarian, autoimmune) should be obtained. In patients with known cirrhosis, the presence of precipitants such as hepatocellular carcinoma or portal vein thrombosis should be investigated.

Physical examination is relatively insensitive for detecting ascitic fluid, particularly when the amount is small and/or the patient is obese. Amounts >1500 mL can be identified on examination by bulging flanks, flank dullness, and shifting dullness (the most sensitive finding) [8].

Several aspects on examination require attention. The presence of spider angiomas, palmar erythema, and muscle wasting, as well as jaundice and/or signs of portal hypertension, such as splenomegaly and abdominal wall collaterals, suggest cirrhosis. Finding a palpable (or ballotable) left lobe of the liver (in the epigastric area) is almost pathognomonic of cirrhosis. Tender hepatomegaly in the presence of ascites is characteristic of acute alcoholic hepatitis or Budd–Chiari syndrome. Distended neck veins, an S3 gallop, uniform hepatomegaly with hepatojugular reflux or peripheral edema suggests congestive heart failure. Presence of a small nodule at the umbilicus (Sister Joseph Mary nodule) or an enlarged supraclavicular lymph node (Virchow's node) suggests malignant ascites.

The initial, least invasive, and most cost-effective method to confirm the presence of ascites is **abdominal ultrasonography**. It can detect amounts as small as 100 mL and is considered the gold standard for the diagnosis of ascites. Abdominal ultrasound is also useful in locating the optimal site to perform a paracentesis, particularly in patients with a small amount of ascites or in those with loculated ascites. Additionally, findings on ultrasound (nodular surface, splenomegaly) can indicate the presence of cirrhosis and Doppler examination of the hepatic venous system is an important initial test to rule out the presence of hepatic vein obstruction, a frequently overlooked cause of ascites [9].

Differential diagnosis

A diagnostic paracentesis should be the first test performed in a patient with new-onset ascites (see Chapter 154). In a diagnostic paracentesis, 20–50 mL of ascitic fluid is obtained and routinely evaluated for gross appearance, albumin (with simultaneous estimation of serum albumin), total protein, white blood cell count, and differential. Other tests are performed depending on individual circumstances: bacteriological cultures (if infection is suspected); glucose and lactic dehydrogenase (if secondary peritonitis is suspected) [10]; amylase (if pancreatic ascites is suspected); cytology (to exclude malignant ascites); acid-fast bacilli smear and culture, and adenosine deaminase determination (to exclude peritoneal tuberculosis) in high prevalence areas [11,12]; triglycerides (if the fluid has a milky appearance, i.e., chylous ascites) [5]; and red blood cell count when the fluid is unusually bloody.

Gross appearance

Ascites is usually a transparent and yellow/amber-colored fluid. A cloudy ascitic fluid suggests the presence of a large number (>5000/mm^3) of white blood cells. Milky-appearing fluid suggests increased triglycerides (i.e., chylous ascites). Bloody ascites (red blood cell count >20000/mm^3) may be caused by a traumatic tap (blood will clot) or may suggest malignancy (blood will not clot as it has already clotted intraperitoneally and the clot has lysed). A tea- or black-colored fluid can be seen in pancreatic ascites and is due to breakdown of ascitic fluid red cells. Bile ascites is green.

Ascites total protein and serum–ascites albumin gradient

These are two inexpensive tests that, taken **together**, are most useful in determining the etiology of ascites and therefore in guiding the work-up of patients with ascites. The **ascites total protein** is high (>2.5 g/dL) in peritoneal ascites and in cases of post-sinusoidal or post-hepatic sinusoidal hypertension when sinusoids are normal and protein-rich lymph leaks into the peritoneal cavity. In cirrhosis, ascites total protein is low (<2.5 g/dL) because deposition of fibrous tissue in the sinusoids ("capillarization of the sinusoid") renders them less leaky to protein. **Serum–ascites albumin gradient (SAAG)** correlates with hepatic sinusoidal pressure [13] and therefore it is high (>1.1 g/dL) in hepatic sinusoidal causes of ascites and low (<1.1 g/dL) in all other causes of ascites [14]. As shown in Table 17.1, the three main causes of ascites – cirrhosis, peritoneal pathology (malignancy or tuberculosis), and heart failure – can be distinguished by combining the results of both the SAAG and the ascites total protein content, and the work-up of the patient with ascites can thus be further refined (Figure 17.1). In patients with mixed ascites (e.g., cirrhosis with superimposed peritoneal malignancy), findings of ascites due to cirrhosis predominate [15]. The definitive test to determine whether ascites is the result of sinusoidal hypertension is hepatic vein catheterization with hepatic venous pressure gradient (HVPG) measurement (Table 17.2) (see Chapter 140).

Leukocyte count and differential

It is useful to determine the presence of infection in ascites. In uninfected ascites, the white blood cell count is generally

Table 17.1 Most common causes of ascites (accounting for >95%) and differential diagnosis by serum–ascites albumin gradient (SAAG), ascites protein, and confirmatory tests

	SAAG*	Ascites protein**	Confirmatory tests
Cirrhosis and/or alcoholic hepatitis	High	Low	HVPG (with TJLB)[+]
Congestive heart failure	High	High	Cardiac echo, HVPG[++]
Peritoneal malignancy	Low	High	CT scan, peritoneal biopsy
Peritoneal tuberculosis	Low	High	Ascites ADA, peritoneal biopsy

*Cut-off for low/high SAAG is 1.1 g/dL.
**Cut-off for low/high ascites protein is 2.5 g/dL.
ADA, adenosine deaminase; CT, computed tomography; HVPG, hepatic venous pressure gradient; TJLB, transjugular liver biopsy.
[+]An HVPG >12 mmHg confirms an hepatic sinusoidal source of ascites.
[++]A normal HVPG (3–5 mmHg) with a high free hepatic venous pressure confirms congestive heart failure as cause of ascites.

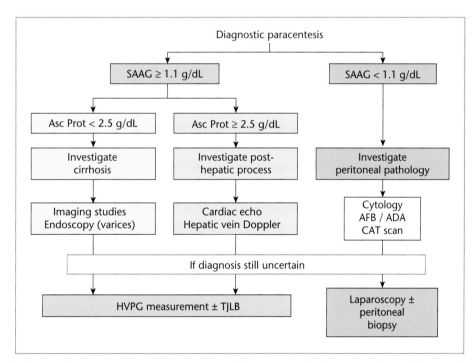

Figure 17.1 Approach to the patient with new-onset ascites. SAAG, serum–ascites albumin gradient; Asc Prot, ascites protein; HVPG, hepatic venous pressure gradient; TJLB, transjugular liver biopsy; AFB, acid-fast bacilli.

Table 17.2 Less common causes of ascites (accounting for <2% of all cases) and results (mostly theoretical) of serum–ascites albumin gradient (SAAG) and ascites protein

	SAAG*	Ascites protein**
Massive hepatic metastases	High	Low
Nodular regenerative hyperplasia	High	Low?
Fulminant liver failure	High	Low?
Budd–Chiari syndrome (late)	High	Low
Budd–Chiari syndrome (early)	High	High
Constrictive pericarditis	High	High
Veno-occlusive disease	High	High
Nephrogenous (dialysis) ascites	High	High
Mixed ascites (cirrhosis + peritoneal)	High	Variable
Myxedema	Variable	High
Pancreatic ascites	Low	High
Serositis (connective tissue disease)	Low	High
Chlamydial/gonococcal	Low	High
Biliary	Low	High?
Ovarian hyperstimulation syndrome	Low?	High
Nephrotic syndrome	Low	Low?
Protein-losing enteropathy/ malnutrition	Low	Low?
Disruption of thoracic duct/ lymphatics (chylous ascites)	Low	High

*Cut-off for low/high SAAG is 1.1 g/dL.
**Cut-off for low/high ascites protein is 2.5 g/dL.

fewer than 500/mm^3, with predominance of mononuclear cells (>75%). The diagnosis of spontaneous bacterial peritonitis (SBP) is made when the fluid sample has a polymorphonuclear (PMN) count >250/mm^3 (see Chapter 100). A high proportion (>80%) of mononuclear leukocytes (lymphocytes and monocytes) should suggest tuberculous peritonitis [12].

SOURCES OF INFORMATION FOR PATIENTS AND DOCTORS

http://patients.uptodate.com/topic.asp?file=livr_dis/4490
http://www.patient.co.uk/showdoc/40002410/

References

1. Runyon BA. Care of patients with ascites. *N Engl J Med.* 1994;330:337–342.
2. D'Amico G, Morabito A, Pagliaro L, *et al.* Survival and prognostic indicators in compensated and decompensated cirrhosis. *Dig Dis Sci.* 1986;31:468–475.
3. Gines P, Quintero E, Arroyo V. Compensated cirrhosis: natural history and prognosis. *Hepatology.* 1987;7:122–128.
4. Manohar A, Simjee AE, Haffejee AA, *et al.* Symptoms and investigative findings in 145 patients with tuberculous peritonitis diagnosed by peritoneoscopy and biopsy over a five year period. *Gut.* 1990;31:1130–1132.
5. Cardenas A, Chopra S. Chylous ascites. *Am J Gastroenterol.* 2002;97:1896–1900.
6. Gomez-Cerezo J, Barbado CA, Suarez I, *et al.* Pancreatic ascites: study of therapeutic options by analysis of case reports and case series between the years 1975 and 2000. *Am J Gastroenterol.* 2003;98:568–577.
7. de Castro F, Bonacini M, Walden JM, *et al.* Myxedema ascites. Report of two cases and review of the literature. *J Clin Gastroenterol.* 1991;13:411–414.
8. Cummings S, Papadakis M, Melnick J, *et al.* The predictive value of physical examinations for ascites. *West J Med.* 1985;142:633–636.
9. Black M, Friedman AC. Ultrasound examination in the patient with ascites. *Ann Intern Med.* 1989;110:253–255.
10. Soriano G, Castellote J, Alvarez C, *et al.* Secondary bacterial peritonitis in cirrhosis: A retrospective study of clinical and analytical characteristics, diagnosis and management. *J Hepatol.* 2010;5239–5244.
11. Dwivedi M, Misra SP, Misra V, *et al.* Value of adenosine deaminase estimation in the diagnosis of tuberculous ascites. *Am J Gastroenterol.* 1990;85:1123–1125.
12. Kim NJ, Choo EJ, Kwak YG, *et al.* Tuberculous peritonitis in cirrhotic patients: comparison of spontaneous bacterial peritonitis caused by *Escherichia coli* with tuberculous peritonitis. *Scand J Infect Dis* 2009;41:852–856.
13. Hoefs JC. Serum protein concentration and portal pressure determine the ascitic fluid protein concentration in patients with chronic liver disease. *J Lab Clin Med.* 1983;102:260–273.
14. Henriksen JH. Colloid osmotic pressure in decompensated cirrhosis. A 'mirror image' of portal venous hypertension. *Scand J Gastroenterol.* 1985;20:170–174.
15. Runyon BA, Montano AA, Akriviadis EA, *et al.* The serum-ascites albumin gradient is superior to the exudate-transudate concept in the differential diagnosis of ascites. *Ann Intern Med.* 1992;117:215–220.

CHAPTER 18
Abnormal liver function tests

Varun Sharma[1] and Arun J. Sanyal[2]
[1]Virginia Commonwealth University School of Medicine, Richmond, VA, USA
[2]Royal Free and University College Medical School, Royal Free Hospital, London, UK

KEY POINTS

Laboratory test for the evaluation of liver injury
- AST and ALT
  - Markers of hepatocyte injury
- Alkaline Phosphatase, gamma glutamyl transferase
  - Markers of cholestatic disease

Laboratory test for the evaluation of liver function
- Bilirubin
- INR
- Albumin

Introduction

Liver function tests (LFTs) are tests that are commonly used to diagnose the presence of liver disease and evaluate its severity. They are a non-invasive method to assess (1) liver injury and (2) liver function. While they play an important role in the evaluation of liver disease, the information obtained from these tests must be considered in the appropriate clinical context in order for this information to be meaningful. The nature, limitations and use of LFTs are discussed below.

Epidemiology and clinical features

The prevalence of abnormally elevated LFTs in the US population is close to 8.9% [1]. This percentage includes those who consume excessive amounts of alcohol or have hepatitis C; however, while new cases of hepatitis C have plateaued, the prevalence of elevated LFTs have continued to rise over the last decade. This may be related to a concurrent rise in the rates of obesity and Non-Alcoholic Fatty Liver Disease (NAFLD). The clinical features associated with abnormal LFTs depend on their cause, mode of presentation (acute vs. chronic), etiology and the severity of injury. Clinical features can vary from non-specific symptoms to the stigmata of chronic liver disease.

Types of liver function tests
Markers of liver Injury

Aspartate aminotransferase (AST), also known as serum glutamate-oxaloacetate transaminase, (SGOT), and alanine aminotransfersase, (ALT), also known as serum glutamate-pyruvate transaminase (SGPT), are common markers of hepatocellular injury. These enzymes catalyze the transfer of amino groups between amino acids and carboxylic acids during gluconeogenesis. While both enzymes are found in the cytoplasm of hepatocytes, AST is also found within the mitochondria [2]. Both enzymes are most highly concentrated within the liver; however, AST is also found in significant amounts in other tissues such as cardiac and striated muscle. This makes AST less sensitive and specific to the liver and an isolated or disproportionate elevation of AST should prompt an investigation for pathology outside the liver (see Table 18.1).

The upper limit of normal for the aminotransferases is generally accepted to be 40 IU/L although there remains some debate if this number truly reflects the normal range. The reference range of AST and ALT was based on values obtained from self-reported normal individuals. Many of these individuals may have had underlying hepatitis C or NAFLD. It is now recognized that even in those with AST and ALT values below 40 IU/L, clinically significant liver pathology may exist and that those with "high" normal values are at greater risk of liver related mortality than those with "low" normal values. Males, nonwhites and individuals with a larger body mass have a tendency to have higher levels of aminotransferases. Increased serum lipid levels may also correlate with increased aminostransferase levels. Based on these considerations, it has been proposed that the upper limits of normal should be 19 IU/L for women and 30 IU/L for men [3]. This improves the sensitivity for detection of liver disease but is associated with a loss of specificity. Due to the potential implications of unnecessary testing that would be generated if these norms were applied to the general population, there is a lack of consensus on the utility of decreasing the upper limits of normal. In cases of individuals with end stage renal disease on dialysis, lower values of normal increase the sensitivity of LFTs. The mechanism for this is not yet understood [4].

Textbook of Clinical Gastroenterology and Hepatology, Second Edition. Edited by C. J. Hawkey, Jaime Bosch, Joel E. Richter, Guadalupe Garcia-Tsao, Francis K. L. Chan.

Table 18.1 Non-hepatic sources of elevated AST levels

Heart
Acute myocardial infarction
Pericarditis

Skeletal muscle
Acute skeletal muscle injury
Muscle inflammation
Muscular dystrophy
Recent surgery
Delirium tremens

Kidney
Acute renal injury or damage
Renal infarct

Other
Intestinal infarction
Shock
Cholecystitis
Acute pancreatitis
Pancreatic carcinoma
Lymphoma
Hypothyroidism
Heparin therapy (60–80% of cases)

Table 18.2 Non-hepatic sources of elevated AP levels

Bone
Physiologic infant and adolescent bone growth
Metastatic tumor with osteoblastic reaction
Fracture healing
Paget's disease of bone

Capillary endothelial
Granulation tissue formation

Pregnancy
Placental production (3rd trimester)

Other
Thyrotoxicosis
Benign transient hyperphosphatemia
Primary hyperparathyroidism
Sepsis
Chronic renal failure
Drugs

Markers of cholestasis
Alkaline phosphatase (AP)

This enzyme catalyzes the hydrolysis of phosphate esters and is present in the liver and epithelium cells of the bile duct. AP is also found in bones, intestine, placenta and kidney (Table 18.2) [5]. Cholestatic disorders increase levels of AP in the serum. The plasma concentration of AP ranges from 25 to 85 IU/L, however the normal physiologic range may vary during an individual's lifetime. Periods of increased osteoblastic activity seen during bone growth in children and adolescents may elevate AP levels to three times the level of a healthy adult. There is also a gradual increase in baseline serum levels seen with aging, particularly in elderly women.

Gamma glutamyl transferase (GGT)

This is a microsomal enzyme found in many tissues including the liver. GGT levels are extremely sensitive to minor degrees of liver injury, limiting its specificity and diagnostic utility. In addition to serving as a marker of liver injury in cases of isolated AP elevation, an isolated persistent elevation of GGT may be seen with alcohol abuse [6].

Tests of liver function
Serum Bilirubin

Bilirubin is a breakdown product of hemoglobin and is derived from destroyed red blood cells. It is water insoluble and cannot be excreted in the urine; instead it is transported to the liver loosely bound to albumin. Hepatocyte basolateral membrane transporters take up the bilirubin from the sinusoidal circulation by a process that has not yet been fully characterized. Within hepatocytes, it is conjugated to water soluble bilirubin mono- and diglucuronides, which are excreted into bile by the canalicular multiple organic anion transporter (MRP2). This is the rate-limiting step in bilirubin excretion. Once in the intestinal lumen, bilirubin is degraded mainly to urobilinogen, which is reabsorbed and excreted by the kidneys.

Serum bilirubin is measured by a colorimetric assay where a purple color is produced by the reaction of a diazo reagent with bilirubin in the presence (total bilirubin) or absence (conjugated or direct bilirubin) of an accelerator, (e.g., alcohol). Indirect bilirubin is the difference between total and direct bilirubin levels and reflects unconjugated bilirubin. The normal range of serum bilirubin is between 3 and 15 μmol/L (0.2–0.8 mg/dL). Hyperbilirubinemia and jaundice result from the increased production or the decreased clearance of bilirubin. Serum bilirubin is normally in an unconjugated form. Unconjugated hyperbilirubinemia (>85% of total bilirubin) results from an increase in production (e.g., hemolysis) or a disruption in hepatic uptake and conjugation of bilirubin (e.g., Gilbert syndrome, Crigler-Najjar syndrome). Conjugated hyperbilirubinemia (>50% of total bilirubin is conjugated) results from either parenchymal liver injury or cholestatis (Table 18.3).

Albumin

Albumin is a plasma protein that is produced by the liver. Approximately 10 grams of albumin are synthesized and excreted everyday with normal plasma concentrations ranging from 3.5–5.0 g/dL. A decrease in serum albumin levels may reflect a decreased production secondary to hepatocellular injury, increased clearance (for example renal losses in nephrotic syndrome, burns, protein-losing enteropathy) or decreased delivery of amino acids to the liver secondary to malnutrition (Table 18.4). Differentiation between the latter and liver failure may be difficult because they frequently coexist. The degree of hypoalbuminemia correlates with

Table 18.3 Differential diagnosis of hyperbilirubinemia

Unconjugated hyperbilirubinemia
Increased bilirubin production
Hemolysis
Dyserythropoiesis
Blood transfusion
Extravasation
Decreased hepatocellular uptake
Drugs (e.g., rifampicin)
Gilbert's syndrome
Decreased conjugation
Gilbert's syndrome
Crigler-Najjar syndrome
Physiologic jaundice of the newborn

Conjugated hyperbilirubinemia
Parenchymal
Hepatocellular Injury
Viral hepatitis
Hepatotoxins (e.g., acetaminophen)
Drugs (e.g., isoniazid)
Alcoholic hepatitis
Sepsis or ischemia
Metabolic disorders (e.g., Wilson's disease, Reye's syndrome)
Pregnancy-related (e.g., acute fatty liver of pregnancy, preeclampsia)
Autoimmune hepatitis
Metabolic (hemochromatosis, nonalcoholic steatohepatitis)
Cholestasis
Infiltrative disorders
Granulomatous diseases (e.g., mycobacterial infections, lymphoma)
Amyloidosis
Malignancy
Obstruction or inflammation of the bile ducts
Gallstones
Primary sclerosing cholangitis
AIDS cholangiopathy
Postsurgical strictures
Neoplasms
Extrinsic compression of the biliary tree
Neoplasms
Pancreatitis
Vascular enlargement (e.g., aneurysm)

Table 18.4 Diseases associated with hypoalbuminemia

Decreased synthesis
Liver dysfunction
Malnutrition

Increased catabolism
Stress
Sepsis
Trauma
Surgery

Increased loss
Renal disease
Protein- losing enteropathy
Burns
Lymphatic lockage or intestinal mucosal disease (e.g., inflammatory bowel disease, bacterial overgrowth)
Gastrointestinal bleeding

Redistribution
Hemodilution (e.g., congestive heart failure, ascites)

Table 18.5 Diseases associated with elevated prothrombin time

Bone
Afibrinogenemia
Anticoagulants
Disseminated intravascular coagulation
Drugs (e.g., raloxifene)
Dysfibrinogenemia
Liver disease
Vitamin K deficiency

outcomes and is part of the Child-Pugh scoring system to assess prognosis of advanced liver disease [7].

Prothrombin time/International normalized ratio

The synthesis of coagulation factors (except factor VIII) is an important function of the liver. The prothrombin time (PT) is a direct measurement of the conversion rate of prothrombin to thrombin and the activity of coagulation factors II, V, VII and X. The normal prothrombin time is 11–15 seconds. Coagulation factors II, V, VII and X are vitamin K dependent; thus when vitamin K deficiency occurs, (such as in malnutrition, altered gut flora or cholestasis) the PT is prolonged (Table 18.5). In such cases, vitamin K administration should correct the PT within 24 hours. In the absence of vitamin K deficiency, prolonged PT is a reliable marker of liver dysfunction.

However, it is not a sensitive measure of liver function and over 80% of the hepatic functional reserve has to be compromised before the PT becomes abnormal [8]. Acute liver failure is associated with the highest PT levels and correlates with mortality.

Inter-laboratory variability in PT has led to the increased use of International Normalized Ratio (INR), which divides an individual's PT by a mean control PT. The normal range of INR is 0.8–1.2. The interpretation of the INR is otherwise similar to the interpretation of the prothrombin time. The INR is a component of the Model for End-State Liver Disease (MELD) scoring system, implemented in 2002 for assessing the severity of chronic liver disease and prioritizing allocation of liver transplants [9].

Diagnosis
An integrated approach to evaluation of abnormal LFTs

There are three fundamental steps in the assessment of a patient with liver disease: (1) to determine the nature of the

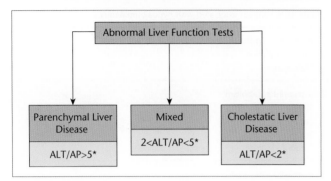

Figure 18.1 Etiology of abnormal liver function tests. ALT/AP is expressed as the fold elevation above the upper limit of normal. (This figure was published in *Clinical Gastroenterology and Hepatology*, Wilfred M. Weinstein, Christopher J. Hawkey, Jaime Bosch, Abnormal liver function tests, Pages 1–6, Copyright Elsevier, 2005.)

liver disease (that is, parenchymal vs. cholestatic vs. mixed pattern); (2) to determine the etiology of liver disease; and (3) to assess the prognosis of the patient.

Identification of the nature of liver disease

Elevations in AST and ALT are associated with hepatocyte injury in parenchymal liver disease. Elevations in AP are more closely associated with cholestatic diseases. The ALT/AP (both expressed as the fold elevation above upper limit of normal) ratio is typically >5 in parenchymal diseases and <2 in cholestatic disorders (Figure 18.1) [10]. An ALT/AP ratio between 2 and 5 may present in a mixed pattern of LFT abnormality in which both parenchymal and cholestatic disease components are present (for example drug toxicity; cholestatic diseases with ongoing hepatocellular toxicity).

Identification of the etiology of liver disease
Parenchymal liver disease

The degree of AST and ALT elevation may provide insight into the disease process affecting the liver. A 10-fold or greater elevation of aminotransferases is a specific finding of active hepatocellular necrosis, although the extent of elevation does not histologically correlate with the extent of necrosis. A greater than 10-fold increase in AST and ALT is associated with viral hepatitis, drug or toxin-mediated injury (e.g., acetaminophen toxicity), ischemia, autoimmune hepatitis and Wilson's disease. Hepatitis A, B, C, D and E can all cause acute hepatitis and active hepatocellular necrosis. A greater than 50-fold increase (>2000 IU/L) is associated with ischemic and toxic liver injury. Extrahepatic biliary obstruction rarely produces an elevation in aminotransferase greater than 1000 IU/L but the passage of a gallstone may cause a marked increased in AST that is followed by a rapid return to baseline values once the stone has passed.

AST and ALT values that are <10-fold, the upper limit of normal, can be seen in those with lesser degrees of hepatocellular necrosis, (such as chronic liver diseases or milder forms of acute liver injury). Acute microvesicular steatosis (e.g.,

Reye's syndrome) is usually associated with a modest ALT elevation. Hepatitis B, C and D are common causes of chronic viral hepatitis. The ratio of AST/ALT may also provide insight into the underlying disease process. Alcoholic liver injury is commonly associated with non- specific AST and ALT values below 300–400 IU/L but an AST/ALT ratio greater than 2 is very suggestive of alcoholic liver disease [11]. An AST/ALT ratio between 1 and 2 is often seen in cirrhosis and Wilson's disease. Other common causes of AST and ALT elevations <10-fold should be assessed by the appropriate laboratory tests listed in Figure 18.2. When common causes of AST and ALT elevations have been excluded, the presence of underlying NAFLD must be considered, especially in those with obesity, diabetes and other features of the metabolic syndrome [12]. Fatty liver can usually be detected by ultrasonography but a liver biopsy is needed for the definitive diagnosis of steatohepatitis.

AST and ALT levels can also be followed to provide information into the course of disease. In the setting of ischemic liver, the return of AST and ALT to baseline levels may occur over several days with the resolution of the underlying etiology (e.g., hypotension). In contrast, return of values to baseline may take several months in acute viral hepatitis or drug-induced liver damage. In the case of acute fulminant hepatitis however, a rapid decline in AST and ALT levels with a concomitant rise in serum bilirubin and PT is suggestive of a poor prognosis.

Cholestatic liver diseases

In asymptomatic individuals with an isolated elevation of AP, the presence of a cholestatic disorder can be verified by checking for an elevated GGT value or the AP isoforms. Cholestatic disorders can be broadly categorized as those due to mechanical biliary obstruction versus those due to medical cholestasis. A large number of conditions can cause mechanical biliary obstruction (Figure 18.3). The presence of Charcot's triad (fever, right upper quadrant pain and jaundice) suggests gallstone disease with cholangitis, while a firm, palpable gallbladder with jaundice (Courvoisier's sign) suggests the presence of pancreatic cancer. The level of biliary obstruction and its cause is best evaluated by an imaging study (sonography, magnetic resonance cholangiopancreatography (MRCP) where the presence of ductal dilation above the level of obstruction is sought. The obstruction can be confirmed, and often treated, using endoscopic retrograde cholangiography (ERCP). Choledocholithiasis is the most common cause of mechanical biliary obstruction and ERCP is the gold standard in its diagnosis.

Medical cholestasis refers to conditions where cholestasis is due to diseases of intrahepatic microscopic bile ducts, (e.g., primary biliary cirrhosis), infiltrative conditions (e.g., lymphoma), or hepatocellular diseases (e.g., drug induced, estrogen toxicity). Primary sclerosing cholangitis (PSC) may present with fibrosis and destruction of only intrahepatic ducts, but in 65% of individuals there is both intra- and

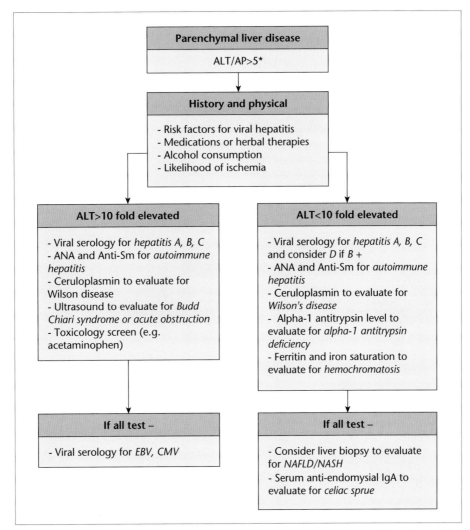

Figure 18.2 Diagnosis and approach to the parenchymal liver diseases. ALT/AP is expressed as the fold elevation above the upper limit of normal. (This figure was published in *Clinical Gastroenterology and Hepatology*, Wilfred M. Weinstein, Christopher J. Hawkey, Jaime Bosch, Abnormal liver function tests, Pages 1–6, Copyright Elsevier, 2005.)

extrahepatic duct involvement. Once the presence of biliary obstruction and a hepatic space-occupying lesion are excluded by an imaging test, the diagnosis is established by the appropriate laboratory tests (for example antimitochondrial antibody in primary biliary cirrhosis) and liver biopsy (Figure 18.3).

Mixed pattern (ALT/APratio 2 < R5)

The most important cause of this pattern of injury is drug-induced liver injury. This includes herbal therapies. Iatrogenic liver disease is one of the major causes of liver failure in North America. After excluding other common causes of parenchymal liver injury, diagnosis of iatrogenic liver disease can be made from the pattern of enzyme elevation along with the clinical history. When more than one pathologic process is suspected, the appropriate laboratory tests along with liver biopsy are required to make the diagnosis.

Prognosis

The prognosis of patients with liver disease depends on the degree of liver failure and the presence of complications from liver disease. Although the serum levels of aminotransferases reflect hepatocyte injury, their levels do not necessarily correlate with the extent of liver disease. Measurements of liver function (e.g., serum bilirubin, albumin levels and PT) are a reliable reflection of liver disease. The presence of complications, (e.g., ascites, spontaneous bacterial peritonitis, variceal hemorrhage, encephalopathy) further contribute to mortality and thus are important determinants of prognosis. The presence of renal failure is an ominous sign in those with advanced liver disease. The Child-Pugh and MELD scores are algorithms that have been developed to assess prognosis in acute and chronic liver disease. The Child-Pugh score factors the liver function as well as the presence of complications into a patient's prognosis. The MELD score, which includes bilirubin,

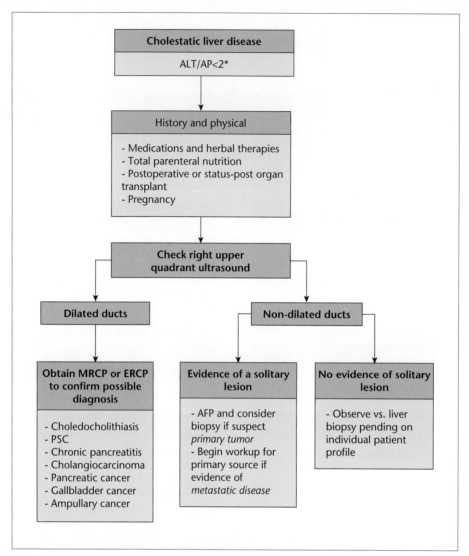

Figure 18.3 Diagnosis and approach to cholestatic liver diseases. ALT/AP is expressed as the fold elevation above the upper limit of normal. (This figure was published in *Clinical Gastroenterology and Hepatology*, Wilfred M. Weinstein, Christopher J. Hawkey, Jaime Bosch, Abnormal liver function tests, Pages 1–6, Copyright Elsevier, 2005.)

INR and creatinine, reflects not only liver function but renal function as well.

Summary

A medical misnomer, LFTs not only provide information on liver biosynthetic function but are also markers of liver injury. In the context of a patient's history and clinical evaluation, they can be useful in directing the diagnostic evaluation of patients with liver disease. LFTs can also provide insight into the prognosis and course of liver disease. However, it is important to keep in mind the factors that limit the diagnostic utility of individual tests. It is the clinical picture along with the nature of liver enzyme abnormalities that ultimately dictate the optimal sequence of tests.

References

1. Ioannou GN, B. E., Lee SP. The prevalence and predictors of elevated serum aminotransferase activity in the United States in 1999–2002. *Am J Gastroenterol.* 2006;101(1):76–82.
2. R., R. Aspartate aminotransferase activity and isoenzyme proportions in human liver tissues. *Clin Chem.* 1978 ;24: 1971–1979.
3. Manolio TA, B. G., Savage PJ, *et al.* Sex- and race-related differences in liver associated serum chemistry tests in young adults in the CARDIA study. *Clin Chem.* 1992;38:1853–1859.

4. Hung KY, L. K., Yen CJ, Wu KD, *et al.* Revised cutoff values of serum aminotransferase in detecting viral hepatitis among CAPD patients: experience from Taiwan, an endemic area for hepatitis B. *Nephrol Dial Transplant.* 1997;12(1):180–183.

5. Kaplan MM. Alkaline phosphatase. *Gastroenterology.* 1972;62: 452–468.

6. Whitehead TP, Clarke CA, Whitfield AG. Biochemical and haematological markers of alcohol intake. *Lancet.* 1978;1:978–981.

7. Pugh RN, Murray-Lyon IM, Dawson JL, et al. Transection of the oesophagus for bleeding oesophageal varices. *Br J Surg.* 1973; 60:646–649.

8. Johnston DE, Special considerations in interpretating liver function tests. *Am Fam Physician.* 1999;59:2223–2230.

9. Kamath PS, Wiesner RH, Malinchoc M, *et al.* A model to predict survival in patients with end-stage liver disease. *Hepatology.* 2001;33(2):464–470.

10. Bussiers JF, H. M. Application of International Consensus Meeting Criteria for classifying drug-induced liver disorders. *Ann Pharmacother.* 1995;29:875–878.

11. Cohen JA, K. M. The SGOT/SGPT ratio – an indicator of alcoholic liver disease. *Dig Dis Sci.* 1979;24:835–838.

12. Skelly MM, J. P., Ryder SD. Findings on liver biopsy to investigate abnormal liver function tests in the absence of diagnostic serology. *J Hepatol.* 2001;35:195–199.

CHAPTER 19

Acute abdominal pain

Dileep N. Lobo

Nottingham Digestive Diseases Centre NIHR Biomedical Research Unit, Nottingham University Hospitals, Nottingham, UK

KEY POINTS

- Acute abdominal pain accounts for 5% of visits to the emergency department, with 18–25% of patients admitted and 10% needing surgery
- Common gastrointestinal causes include:
  - luminal obstruction
  - inflammation
  - perforation
  - volvulus or torsion
  - intestinal ischemia.
- Extra-abdominal causes must not be forgotten, whilst a cause is not found in up to 40% of admitted patients
- The immediate goals of diagnosis are to decide if the patient needs:
  - admission to hospital
  - urgent or emergency surgery
- Resuscitation may be needed prior to investigation or sometimes simultaneously
- Many patients require substantial analgesia, which should be given as soon as possible
- Appropriate investigation and treatment are dependent on astute clinical acumen for optimal selection

Introduction

Sir William Osler once wrote "Medicine is a science of uncertainty and an art of probability." Acute abdominal pain, which accounts for a large proportion of gastrointestinal emergency work, poses problems of uncertainty where probability is an important component of management. Acute abdominal pain usually results from gastrointestinal disorders but other causes, which include a spectrum of medical and surgical conditions, must not be forgotten.

What is it?

Acute pain

Acute pain arises from **nociceptor activation** at sites of stimulation or injury [1,2]. The local injury alters the response characteristics of the nociceptors, their central connections, and the autonomic nervous system in the region. Therefore acute pain can be considered to be the initial phase of an extensive, persistent nociceptive and behavioral cascade triggered by **tissue injury** [2,3]. However, in malignant diseases, the invasion of body tissues can produce continuous acute pain. Acute abdominal pain has loosely been described as pain occurring in the abdomen with an onset of less than 6–8 hours. However, a more pragmatic definition is that of previously undiagnosed abdominal pain that arises suddenly and is of less than 7 days and usually less than 48 hours duration. The likelihood of surgical intervention is greater if acute abdominal pain lasts for more than 6 hours.

Visceral pain

Visceral pain, in contrast to somatic pain, is diffuse, difficult to localize, and is referred to cutaneous dermatomes. Patterns of referred sensations overlap considerably and can cause problems with differential diagnosis. Distension of hollow viscera, such as the bowel and bladder, can produce pain in the absence of injury. Visceral pain can also be associated with motor and autonomic reflexes, such as nausea and vomiting [4].

Referred pain

Pain as a result of irritation of an abdominal organ is usually not felt in the viscus, but in a somatic structure that may be at a considerable distance from it. This is known as referred pain and when visceral pain is both local and referred, it may seem to radiate from the local to the distant site. When pain is referred, it is usually to a structure that developed from the same embryonic segment or dermatome as the organ the pain originates from. Thus, pain that originates from the **foregut is referred to the epigastrium** (T8), that from the **mid gut to the umbilical region** (T10), and that from the **hindgut to the hypogastrium** (T12). A more dramatic form of referred pain is that from the **diaphragm** (innervated by the phrenic nerve C3–5) to the shoulder tip, which receives its cutaneous innervation from the same spinal segments.

How common is it?

Acute abdominal pain is relatively common and accounts for **5% of visits to the emergency department** [5]. Although most patients presenting with acute abdominal pain have minor

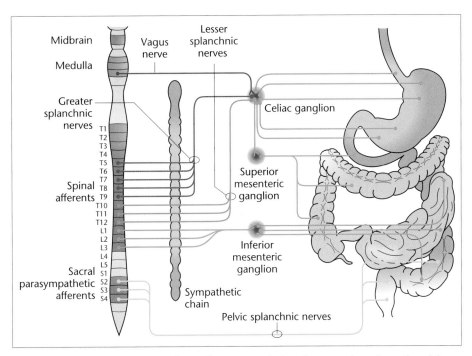

Figure 19.1 Efferent autonomic pathways of the gastrointestinal tract. The parasympathetic pathways are shown in purple and the sympathetic pathways in red. (Reproduced from Mertz HR, Mayer EA. Functional gastrointestinal syndromes. In: Zinner MJ, Schwartz SI, Ellis H, eds. *Maingot's abdominal operations.* vol. 1, 10th ed. Stamford: Appleton & Lange; 1997: 361–378, with permission from McGraw Hill.)

problems, about **18–25% of patients** have a serious enough condition to warrant hospital admission for investigation and treatment [5,6] and about 10% of patients need emergency or urgent surgery [5]. A large audit from the UK has shown that up to 50% of all general surgical admissions are emergencies, half of which are due to acute abdominal pain [7]. Missing the diagnosis in patients with acute abdominal pain can lead to delayed treatment, major morbidity, mortality, and ensuing litigation.

Pathophysiology

The abdominal viscera are connected to the cerebral cortex by three levels of sensory neurons (Figures 19.1 and 19.2). Nociceptive stimuli are detected by specialized transducers attached to A and C fibers and are transmitted almost exclusively by the sympathetic nervous system. The first-order neurons link the viscera to the spinal cord and pass through autonomic plexuses usually associated with a major artery supplying the organs such as the celiac, superior mesenteric, and inferior mesenteric arteries.

Pain can be elicited by a **wide variety of insults**, which include mechanical, chemical, and thermal stimuli. Damaged tissue can release **neurotransmitter-like substances** such as substance P, potassium, histamine, prostaglandins, serotonin, bradykinin, gaba-aminobutyric acid, neuropeptide Y, adenosine, noradrenaline, capsaicin, and a host of others [2–4]. **Nociceptive nerve endings** themselves may release substance P and other mediators, via axon reflexes originating in other branches, causing additional inflammation and edema. Signalling via **second- and third-order neurons** activates the **limbic system** thalamus and cingulate gyrus, giving pain its unpleasant nature.

Second-order or postsynaptic neurons begin in the dorsal horn and cross at the midline to the contralateral side and then travel within the ventrolateral quadrant of the spinal cord upward toward the brainstem via pathways such as the **spinothalamic tracts**. Third-order neurons travel from the spinoreticular tracts to the frontal cortex and limbic system. Third-order neurons that ascend from the thalamus to the **post central gyrus** of the cerebral cortex form the pathway for the localization of pain and those that ascend from the intralaminar nuclei to **cingulate gyrus** (in association with the limbic cortex) form the pathway related to the unpleasantness of pain.

Nausea and diaphoresis are examples of autonomic responses provoked by visceral pain. Referred visceral pain is thought to be the result of convergence of somatic and visceral afferents on the same spinal cord neurons. There is also evidence that single distal processes of dorsal root ganglia branch, with one branch going to body surface and one to viscera. This convergence-projection theory explains the features of referred pain.

Causes

Acute pain in the abdomen is usually due to luminal obstruction, inflammation, perforation, volvulus or torsion, and

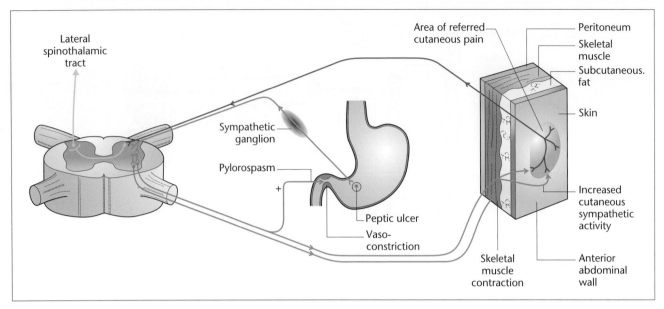

Figure 19.2 Visceral pain pathway from the gastrointestinal tract. (This figure was published in *Clinical Gastroenterology and Hepatology*, Wilfred M. Weinstein, Christopher J. Hawkey, Jaime Bosch, Acute abdominal pain, Pages 1–10, Copyright Elsevier, 2005.)

intestinal ischemia. The common causes of acute abdominal pain are listed in Tables 19.1 and 19.2 and depicted in Figure 19.3.

Symptom complexes
Luminal obstruction

Luminal obstruction usually starts with **abdominal colic** that is referred to the dermatomes supplying the part of the gut proximal to the obstruction. **Vomiting** is a prominent feature of gastric outlet obstruction and small bowel obstruction. If the ileocecal valve is competent, patients with large bowel obstruction may not vomit. **Abdominal distension** is more pronounced in patients with large bowel obstruction and this condition is usually associated with absolute constipation. Patients with small bowel obstruction may continue to pass small amounts of flatus and feces. **Visible peristalsis** may be observed and bowel sounds are usually hyperdynamic.

Hernial orifices must be examined meticulously. If untreated, luminal obstruction may lead to adynamic ileus, strangulation, and perforation. Intestinal obstruction in patients who have had previous surgery is usually due to adhesions and it is worthwhile instituting a trial of **nasogastric aspiration** and intravenous fluids for 24–48 hours. **Surgery** is indicated if the patient's condition fails to resolve, or at the first sign of deterioration (e.g., tachycardia, increasing white cell count, increasing pain and distension, feculent aspiration). Patients with large bowel obstruction should ideally undergo an unprepared lower gastrointestinal contrast study to rule out pseudo-obstruction.

Inflammation

Intraperitoneal inflammation usually arises from **intraabdominal organs** such as the appendix, gallbladder, pancreas, small and large bowel (inflammatory bowel disease, diverticulitis), and pelvic organs. **Primary peritonitis** occurs rarely, in young girls and in patients with ascites (cirrhosis, nephrotic syndrome). Vomiting may be a vagal response to the pain. In most instances, the inflammation is secondary to infection or ischemia. Initially, the inflammation is confined to the organ of origin and the physical signs will be localized to the area of peritoneal inflammation, characterized by local tenderness with exacerbation on rebound. A large proportion of patients with inflammatory conditions respond to nonoperative management, but untreated and progressive inflammation will eventually lead to gangrene and necrosis, with consequent perforation of the viscus and resultant generalized peritonitis.

Peritonitis

Generalized peritonitis usually manifests with the classic signs of **tenderness, guarding, rebound tenderness, and rigidity** (see Table 19.4).The abdomen may be distended and bowel sounds may be absent if the condition is established. Bowel contents, bile, urine, and blood are irritant to the peritoneum and generalized peritonitis can be due to

- a **perforated viscus**
- **mesenteric ischemia**
- **strangulation** of the bowel secondary to an internal or external hernia, or a volvulus

Table 19.1 Causes of acute abdominal pain

Main pain location	Organ	Additional localization	Pathology
RUQ	Liver	Epigastrium Also referred to tip of shoulder	Hepatitis, abscess, infarction, bleed into tumor, expanding hematoma, congestive cardiac failure
	Biliary tract	May radiate to back along rib cage	Stones in gall bladder/cystic duct: colic, cholecystitis Stones in common bile duct: colic, ascending cholangitis Mucocele, empyema, gallbladder perforation
Epigastric	Pancreas	R & L hypochondria Radiates to back May be relieved by leaning forward	Acute pancreatitis or exacerbation of chronic pancreatitis Complications of pancreatitis, pancreatic cancer, obstruction (pancreas divisum and sphincter of Oddi dysfunction)
	Stomach	R and L upper quadrants[a]	Ulcer, volvulus, perforation, cancer acute dilatation Gastric outlet obstruction, hiatus hernia
	Duodenum Esophagus	R and L upper quadrants[a] Retrosternal	Ulcer, perforation, obstruction Esophagitis, spasm, rupture, hiatus hernia
LUQ	Spleen	May radiate to flank	Splenomegaly, infarction, rupture, expanding splenic hematoma Sickle cell crisis
Central	Aorta	Epigastrium/periumbilical/flank /back/may become generalized	Ruptured/dissecting aneurysm
	Small bowel	May later localize to area of inflammation of parietal peritoneum[a]	Obstruction (adhesions, herniae, volvulus, tumor, stricture, gallstone ileus, bezoars, intussusception, tuberculosis) Perforation, ischemia Crohn's disease, Meckel's diverticulum, mesenteric adenitis, gastroenteritis, motility disorders/IBS
	Appendix R colon	Later lacalizes to R lower quadrant[a] May later localize to area of inflammation of parietal peritoneum[a]	Acute appendicitis, appendicular abscess Obstruction (malignant/benign strictures, volvulus) Perforation, ischemia, acute diverticulitis and its complications Inflammatory bowel disease
Hypogastrium	L colon	May then localize to area of inflammation of parietal peritoneum or become generalized	Obstruction (malignant/benign strictures, volvulus) Perforation, ischemia, acute diverticulitis and its complications Constipation/fecal impaction Inflammatory bowel disease, amoebic colitis
	Urinary bladder	May radiate to base of penis	Cystitis, bladder calculus, acute urinary retention, obstructing bladder tumors
	Uterus, ovaries	R and L lower quadrants	Ectopic pregnancy, ovarian torsion, uterine perforation
	Fallopian tubes	May be referred to the inner thighs May be generalized	Pelvic inflammatory disease, acute salpingitis, ovarian cysts Endometriosis, mittelschmerz, dysmenorrhea
Loin to groin	Kidneys/ureters	May radiate to testes or labia	Calculi, infection, pyelonephritis, obstruction (e.g., tumor)
Scrotum	Testes	Hypogastrium, R and L lower quadrant	Torsion, trauma, epididymoorchitis
Other	Abdominal wall		Herniae, muscular contusions/hematoma, abdominal wall abscess, herpes zoster, entrapment neuropathy
	Abdominal trauma		Trauma to abdominal wall, hemoperitoneum, rupture of solid or hollow viscus Retroperitoneal hematoma
	Postoperative		Intra-abdominal bleeding, anastomotic dehiscence, Intra-abdominal abscess Abdominal compartment syndrome

[a]Generalized in perforation.

Table 19.2 Extra-abdominal/systemic causes of acute abdominal pain

Lungs	Lobar pneumonia
	Pleurisy
	Pulmonary embolism
Heart	Acute myocardial infarction
	Congestive cardiac failure
	Myocarditis
Metabolic/endocrine	Porphyrias
	Diabetic ketoacidosis
	Lead poisoning
	Hypercalcemia
	Adrenal insufficiency
Vasculitis	Henoch-Schonlein purpura
	Systemic lupus
	Polyarteritis nodosa
	Familial Mediterranean fever

- an **intraperitoneal bleed**
- **rupture of a localized abscess** into the general peritoneal cavity.

Free intraperitoneal gas is not always present on chest X-ray and this is particularly true of appendicular and gallbladder perforations. A **laparotomy** is usually necessary after adequate resuscitation and although a preoperative diagnosis of the etiology is desirable, time must not be wasted in overinvestigating a critically ill patient.

Nonspecific abdominal pain

It has been estimated that a cause for acute abdominal pain is not discovered in up to 40% of patients who are admitted to hospital [8,9]. Although no cause for the pain is found, these patients may have very real and distressing symptoms and it is important to reassure the patients that the diagnosis of nonspecific abdominal pain does not necessarily mean that there is no pain or no cause for it. Some of these patients may have tenderness in addition to the pain, but the signs are usually not enough to make a diagnosis of peritonitis.

Most patients are young and almost two-thirds are female. The diagnosis is one of exclusion and patients must be observed for 24–48 hours in order to ensure that there is no progression of the symptoms and signs. The pain usually subsides spontaneously. Undiagnosed causes of nonspecific abdominal pain include:

- viral infections
- parasitic infestations
- gastroenteritis
- mesenteric adenitis
- ovulatory pain
- torsion of the appendices epiploicae of the colon.

Some patients may have irritable bowel syndrome (see Chapter 62).

Munchausen's syndrome (spurious abdominal pain)

Globally there are a few patients who seek admission to hospital in the absence of genuine symptoms prompted by the need for a bed, drugs, attention, or help. Such patients usually present to the accident and emergency department with a dramatic history of an acute abdominal event. They can usually simulate appropriate physical signs and often appear to be in a great deal of distress. Many of these patients may be admitted for observation for several days before the true diagnosis is revealed.

Patients may visit hospitals some distance from their area of domicile, and other clues include a very meticulous history, early and repeated demands for opiate analgesia, and many previous admissions to hospital. In the classical case of Munchausen's syndrome, there are also multiple abdominal scars [10]. Even when the diagnosis is suspected it is difficult to confront the patient and it is prudent to investigate the background by contacting doctors who have treated the patient in the past. Demands for pain relief should be met by the offer of nonopiate analgesics. Most patients leave the hospital, often without informing the staff, once this process of enquiry starts or when they fail to obtain the treatment sought.

Diagnosis
History and examination

The two immediate goals in the diagnosis of acute abdominal pain are to decide if the patient needs admission to hospital and to ascertain whether the patient needs urgent or emergency surgery. Resuscitation may be needed prior to investigation or sometimes simultaneously, for example in patients who have pain secondary to trauma, an intra-abdominal hemorrhage or peritonitis. A careful clinical history and examination then helps narrow down the diagnosis. The clinician should have a mental picture of the topography of the abdomen and correlate the symptoms and signs with the underlying anatomical structures and possible pathological diagnoses.

Questions that should be asked whilst taking the history are outlined in Table 19.3. The age of the patient must also be considered when making a differential diagnosis. However, it must be remembered, for example, that even the elderly can get acute appendicitis, albeit rarely. Patients with acute abdominal pain may manifest the **systemic inflammatory response syndrome** [11] and the initial step in the clinical examination is to document the vital signs that include pulse rate and rhythm, blood pressure, respiratory rate, temperature, and the Glasgow Coma Score. The general physical examination must document the presence or absence of pallor, cyanosis, jaundice, edema, and lymphadenopathy.

The abdomen should be examined with the patient lying supine with the arms at the side and the legs flat. The usual sequence of inspection, palpation, percussion, and auscultation must be followed with the abdomen exposed from nipples to mid thigh and the genitals covered. Common clinical signs and their possible significance are listed in Table 19.4. The

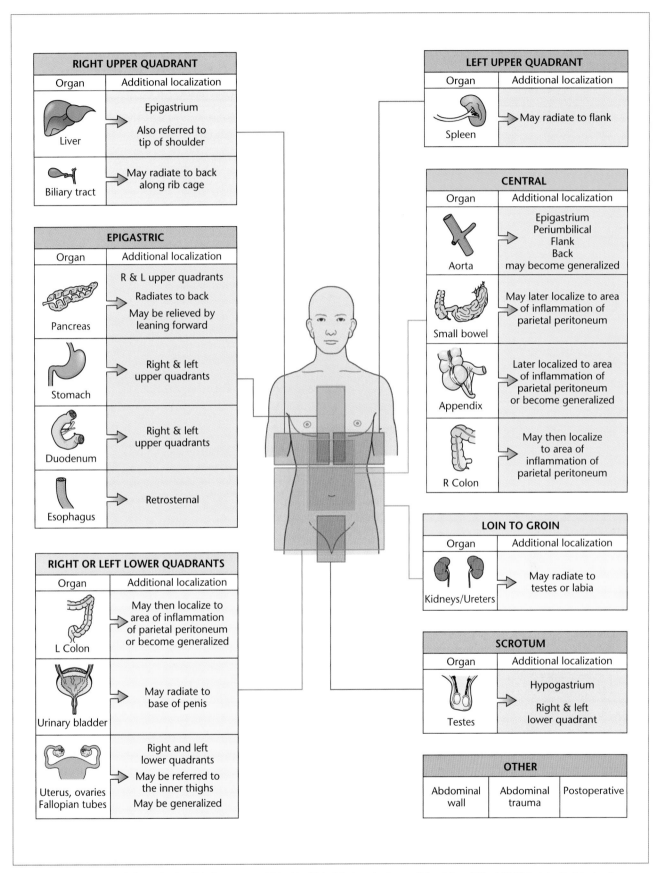

Figure 19.3 Sites of acute abdominal pain. (This figure was published in *Clinical Gastroenterology and Hepatology*, Wilfred M. Weinstein, Christopher J. Hawkey, Jaime Bosch, Acute abdominal pain, Pages 1–10, Copyright Elsevier, 2005.)

Table 19.3 Clinical examination of the acute abdomen

Sign	Definition/cautions	Implication
INSPECTION		
Distention		Ascites, obstruction, pseudo-obstruction, ileus, toxic dilatation, trauma, peritonitis, ovarian cyst
Bruising	Around umbilicus: Cullen's sign In flank: Grey-Turner's sign	Either can Indicate: ruptured aortic aneurysm, acute pancreatitis Grey-Turner also: retroperitoneal hemorrhage/inflammation
Visible peristalsis	May not be visible in the obese	Bowel obstruction
Regional fullness/asymmetry		Organomegaly/mass
Hernia		Obstructed/strangulated hernia
Skin lesions	Scratch marks Pyoderma gangrenosum Sr. Joseph's nodule Acanthosis nigricans	Obstructive jaundice Inflammatory bowel disease Advanced cancer Advanced cancer
Superficial veins	Caput medusae Caudal-cephalad flow	Cirrhosis IVC obstruction
Surgical scars		Adhesions, recurrence of malignancy, incisional herniae
PALPATION		
Tenderness	Usually from parietal peritoneum	Patients can often accurately localize the site of most intense pain
Guarding	Voluntary	Peritoneal irritation
Rigidity	Involuntary, varies from minor to board-like	Established peritonitis
Rebound tenderness	Pain on rapid removal of hand, abdominal pain with coughing, Rovsing's sign (see Chapter 69)	Peritoneal irritation or peritonitis
Loin or costovertebral angle tenderness	Make the patient sit forward	Renal pathology, e.g., pyelonephritis
PERCUSSION		
Tympanic	Gaseous distention	Gas-filled bowel loops in obstruction Pneumoperitoneum
Dull	Usually fluid	Ascites, ovarian cyst, fluid-filled bowel loops
Shifting dullness, fluid thrill	Free fluid	Ascites, intraperitoneal bleed
AUSCULTATION		
Bowel sounds	Listen for at least a minute Increased Tinkling Absent	Intestinal obstruction Paralytic ileus Paralytic ileus/peritonitis
Succussion splash	Shake patient with stethoscope on abdomen to elicit sloshing sound	Gas and fluid in an obstructed hollow organ (stomach or colon)
Bruit	Listen over aorta and renal vessels	Aneurysm or renal artery stenosis
Peritoneal rub	Similar to a pleural rub	Peritoneal irritation
OTHER TESTS		
Male genitalia		Hernias, hydroceles, torsions, and epididymoorchitis
Rectal examination	Feel the rectum, rectovesical (uterine) pouch and prostate. Inspect the stool on the glove	Rectal tumors, constipation, pelvic abscesses, rectal bleeding, and prostatic enlargement
Vaginal examination	In women with pelvic pain	Cervix, uterine and adnexal (ovarian, tubal) pathology
Psoas spasm	Inability to extend the hip completely	Psoas abscess, acute appendicitis (retrocecal)

Table 19.4 Questions to ask when taking the patient history

- When and where did the pain start?
- Was the onset sudden and what brought the pain on?
- Where is it now?
- What is the character of the pain?
- How severe is it?
- Does the pain radiate elsewhere?
- Are there any aggravating or relieving factors?
- Has this happened before?
- Are there any associated symptoms? (e.g., distention, nausea, vomiting, fever, diarrhea, absolute constipation, anorexia, jaundice, prutitus, gastrointestinal bleeding, dysuria, oliguria, chest pain)
- When was your last period and is there any chance of you being pregnant?
- History of alcohol intake
- Drug (medicinal and recreational) history
- History of ingestion of toxins, poisons or foreign bodies
- History of previous surgery
- History of pre-existing disease
- History of travel, especially foreign travel
- Family history

signs must be interpreted in conjunction with the history and the general condition, age, gender, and potential risk factors of the patient. The individual conditions listed in Tables 19.1 and 19.4 are described in more detail elsewhere in this textbook.

Initial management

The patient with acute abdominal pain may need resuscitation or emergency surgery, and it is sensible to keep the patient nil by mouth and insert two large-bore venous cannulae at first contact. Intravenous fluids should be administered at an appropriate rate. Blood should be sampled at the time of insertion of the cannulae and sent to the laboratory for the investigations listed in Table 19.5. Arterial blood gas analysis should be performed if indicated. Laboratory tests may also help with the diagnosis of medical conditions such as diabetic ketoacidosis and adrenal crisis. Patients who are hemodynamically unstable and those with copious vomiting or peritonitis will benefit from the insertion of a nasogastric tube and urinary catheter.

Table 19.5 Investigations for acute abdominal pain

Investigations	Subcategory/comment	Interpretation/usefulness
Full blood count	Hemoglobin ↓ Hemoglobin ↑ Leukocytes ↑ Leukocytes ↓ Platelets ↑ Platelets ↓	Blood loss Dehydration/hemoconcentration/polycythemia Inflammation or infection Overwhelming inflammation Active inflammatory bowel disease Overwhelming sepsis
Clinical chemistry	Creatinine ↑ Urea ↑ Electrolytes	Renal failure Dehydration/hemoconcentration
Serum amylase	Fourfold increase Lesser increases	Acute pancreatitis (but may be normal) Almost any acute abdominal condition
Liver function tests	Biliary enzymes Transaminases/mixed	Obstructive jaundice(but alkaline phosphatase slow to rise with acute obstruction) Acute liver injury sepsis, cholangitis
Calcium	Calcium ↑	Medical cause of abdominal pain
Blood glucose	Glucose ↑	Ketoacidosis can cause abdominal pain
Culture	Urine/blood	Prelude to antibiotics
Group/cross mach		Prelude to surgery, transfusion
Arterial blood gases	Acidosis and elevated lactate PO_2	?Mesenteric ischemia, illnesses severity, e.g., in acute pancreatitis Latent hypoxia
Urinalysis	Stick tests Microscopy Culture	Blood and proteinurla (? infection) Ketones (starvation or ketoacidosis) Red cells, casts(? tubular necrosis), white cells(? infection) Infection

(Continued)

Table 19.5 (*Continued*)

Investigations	Subcategory/comment	Interpretation/usefulness
Pregnancy test		Ruptured ectopic
Electrocardiogram		Myocardial infarction as cause of abdominal pain. Preoperative investigation for patients over the age of 50 years
Supine abdominal	Intestinal lumen and pattern	Obstruction, ileus, IBD
X-ray	Calcification Pneumobilia Foreign bodies Skeletal abnormalities Soft tissue masses	Gallstones(10%), renal stones, pancreatic calcification, aortic rim Ascending cholangitis
Erect chest x-ray	Detection of free subdiaphragmatic air	Perforation. Also look at lung fields and cardiac contour
Lateral decubitus film	≥1 mL of free peritoneal gas can be visualized	Perforation
Abdominal ultrasound	Percutaneous ultrasound Transvaginal ultrasound	Bile duct dilatation, gallstones, fluid collections, aortic aneurysms Gynecological causes
Abdominal CT scan	Value high especially with intravenous and intraluminal contrast enhancement	Multiple diagnoses Provides both anatomical and etiological diagnosis
Intravenous urography/CT kideny, ureters and bladder (KUB)	Important if blood in urine	Urological causes Useful in urological trauma
Magnetic resonance imaging	Not as popular as CT for the acute abdomen. MRCP	Excellent images of biliary tract pathology
Gastrointestinal contrast studies	Lower GI	Large bowel obstruction vs. pseudo-obstruction (may be therapeutic)
	Upper GI	Cryptic perforation or obstruction
Visceral angiography	Diagnostic	Intestinal ischemia, obscure bleeding
	Therapeutic	Embolization in gastrointestinal bleeding
Endoscopy	Upper and lower GI endoscopy	Helpful in selected cases
	Sigmoidoscopy	May be therapeutic for sigmoid volvulus
	ERCP	Therapeutic in biliary obstruction, especially ascending cholangitis
Laparoscopy	Increasingly popular, especially for the diagnosis of obscure acute abdominal pain	Therapeutic in duodenal ulcer perforations, acute cholecystitis, acute appendictis, and gynecological conditions
Laparotomy	Ultimate arbiter in difficult cases	Also therapeutic

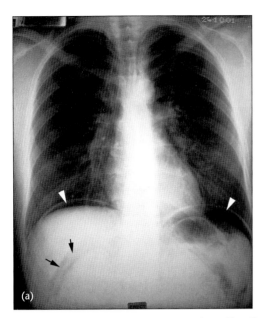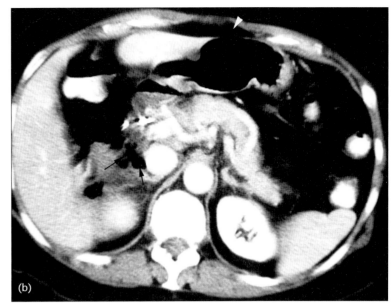

Figure 19.4 Intraperitoneal and retroperitoneal gas. Chest X-ray **(a)** and abdominal CT scan **(b)** demonstrating both intraperitoneal (white arrowheads) and retroperitoneal (black arrows) gas. The patient had a duodenal perforation secondary to an endoscopic sphincterotomy.

Pain relief

Many patients require substantial analgesia, which should be given as soon as possible. A recent controlled trial [12] found no evidence that use of morphine affects diagnostic accuracy. Thus, establishing effective analgesia does not compromise investigation and treatment and probably facilitates the process.

Investigations and definitive management

The usual initial investigation is an **erect chest and a supine abdominal X-ray** (Table 19.5 and Figures 19.4–19.6). The widespread availability of high-quality **ultrasonography** (US) and helical/multi-detector **computed tomography** (CT) has revolutionized the management of patients with acute abdominal pain. In one study ultrasonography was shown to increase the rate of correct diagnosis from 70% to 83% [13,14]. CT scanning is very helpful in the stable patient (Figures 19.4, 19.6–19.8) and two recent prospective, randomized trials have demonstrated that its routine early use can identify unforeseen conditions and reduce length of hospital stay and overall mortality in patients with acute abdominal pain of unknown etiology [15,16]. The "early" use of CT has been shown to improve the accuracy of diagnosis in the acute abdomen from 50% to 75% [15]. It has also been demonstrated recently that if US abdomen is used first, followed by CT only in those patients in whom US has been negative, the number of requests for CT would be reduced by half without a diminution in the quality of care [17]. However, more complex investigations such as US and CT may not add very much to information obtained using simpler investigations (e.g., gas under the diaphragm on erect

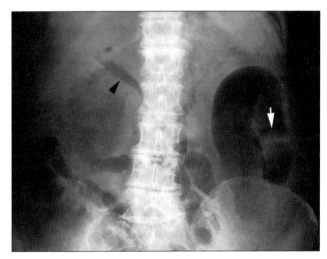

Figure 19.5 Gallstone ileus. Supine abdominal X-ray demonstrating pneumobilia (black arrowhead) and a radiopaque gallstone obstructing the small bowel (white arrow).

chest X-ray) and the desire to obtain an accurate preoperative diagnosis should not be allowed to delay therapeutic intervention in the critically ill or unstable patient.

Magnetic resonance imaging is a promising alternative to CT in the evaluation of acute abdominal pain and does not involve the use of ionizing radiation. However, data on the use of magnetic **resonance** imaging for acute abdominal pain are presently sparse [18]. Gastrointestinal **contrast studies** and **endoscopy** can be helpful in selected cases (Table 19.5) and

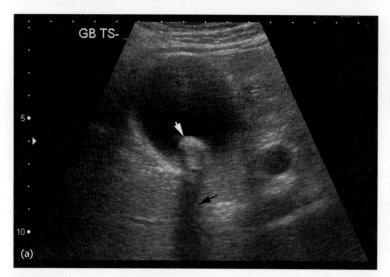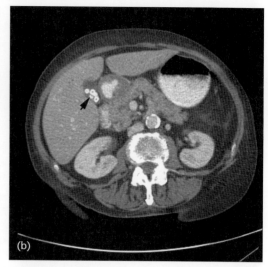

Figure 19.6 Gallstones. Abdominal ultrasound **(a)** showing a sonodense gallstone (white arrow) within the gallbladder with posterior acoustic shadowing (black arrow). Contrast-enhanced CT scan **(b)** of another patient with multiple radio-opaque gallstones (black arrow).

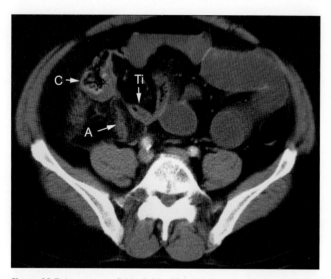

Figure 19.7 Acute appendicitis. Pelvic CT scan of a patient with acute appendicitis. A, inflamed appendix; C, cecum; Ti, terminal ileum.

early laparoscopy can provide a higher diagnostic accuracy and improved quality of life in patients with acute abdominal pain of uncertain etiology [19]. However, although there is no evidence of harm, currently there is insufficient evidence to recommend routine use of early laparoscopy as the gold standard in patients with undifferentiated acute abdominal pain [20]. Finally, a **laparotomy** can be the ultimate diagnostic investigation in difficult cases, in addition to it being of therapeutic benefit.

Conclusions

Over the past few decades there have been major advances in imaging modalities and laparoscopic techniques to facilitate the diagnosis of acute abdominal pain. Computer programs based on Bayesian reasoning and neural networks have been developed to help increase the diagnostic accuracy in this condition. However, despite the giant strides forward, only an astute clinician can obtain the information that is needed from a patient with acute abdominal pain, choose the best investigations, and plan appropriate treatment.

The doctor who first sees a patient with acute abdominal pain in hospital makes a correct diagnosis in 45% of cases. A combination of review of the patient by a senior clinician, analysis of the results of the investigations, and regular reassessment of the patient can improve the diagnostic accuracy to 75–80%. This leads to optimum treatment of the patient, with interventions planned at the appropriate time and a lower rate of negative surgical explorations. If the patient deteriorates or fails to make progress after institution of treatment, the working diagnosis must be reassessed and the possibility of another coexisting condition must be entertained. Further investigations, and even the possibility of a diagnostic laparotomy must be considered in this situation. The acute abdomen has been likened to Pandora's box, containing all the evils of the world. Sometimes, it is necessary to open this box and let the evils out!

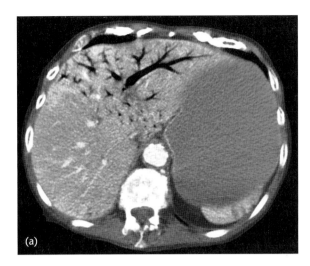

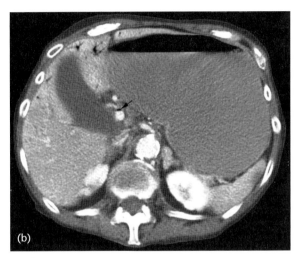

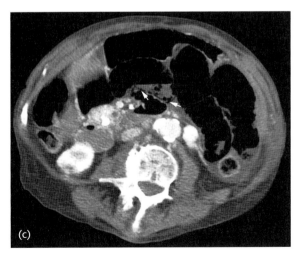

Figure 19.8 Acute mesenteric ischemia. Abdominal CT scans done at admission showing **(a)** gas in the intrahepatic branches of the left portal vein, **(b)** intravenous contrast and gas (arrow) in the main portal vein and **(c)** intramural bowel gas (arrows).

References

1. Merskey H, Bogduk N. *Classification of chronic pain: descriptions of chronic pain syndromes and definition of pain terms.* Report by the International Association for the Study of Pain Task Force on Taxonomy, 2nd edn. Seattle: IASP Press; 1994.
2. Basbaum AI, Bautista DM, Scherrer G, *et al.* Cellular and molecular mechanisms of pain. *Cell.* 2009;139:267–284.
3. Carr DB, Goudas LC. Acute pain. *Lancet.* 1999;353:2051–2058.
4. Sengupta JN. Visceral pain: the neurophysiological mechanism. *Handb Exp Pharmacol.* 2009;194:31–74.
5. Kamin RA, Nowicki TA, Courtney DS, *et al.* Pearls and pitfalls in the emergency department evaluation of abdominal pain. *Emerg Med Clin North Am.* 2003;21:61–72.
6. Graff IV LG, Robinson D. Abdominal pain and emergency department evaluation. *Emerg Med Clin North Am.* 2001;19: 123–136.
7. Ellis BW, Rivett RC, Dudley HA. Extending the use of clinical audit data: a resource planning model. *BMJ.* 1990;301:159–162.
8. Gray DW, Collin J. Non-specific abdominal pain as a cause of acute admission to hospital. *Br J Surg.* 1987;74:239–242.
9. Irvin TT. Abdominal pain: a surgical audit of 1190 emergency admissions. *Br J Surg.* 1989;76:1121–1125.
10. Huffman JC, Stern TA. The diagnosis and treatment of Munchausen's syndrome. *Gen Hosp Psychiatry.* 2003;25:358–363.
11. Bone RC. Sir Isaac Newton, sepsis, SIRS and CARS. *Crit Care Med.* 1996;24:1125–1128.
12. Thomas SH, Silen W, Cheema F, *et al.* Effects of morphine analgesia on diagnostic accuracy in Emergency Department patients with abdominal pain: a prospective, randomized trial. *J Am Coll Surg.* 2003;196:18–31.
13. Allemann F, Cassina P, Rothlin M, *et al.* Ultrasound scans done by surgeons for patients with acute abdominal pain: a prospective study. *Eur J Surg.* 1999;165:966–970.
14. Lindelius A, Törngren S, Sondén A, *et al.* Impact of surgeon-performed ultrasound on diagnosis of abdominal pain. *Emerg Med J.* 2008;25:486–491.
15. Ng CS, Watson CJ, Palmer CR, *et al.* Evaluation of early abdominopelvic computed tomography in patients with acute abdominal pain of unknown cause: prospective randomised study. *BMJ.* 2002;325:1387.
16. Tsushima Y, Yamada S, Aoki J, *et al.* Effect of contrast-enhanced computed tomography on diagnosis and management of acute abdomen in adults. *Clin Radiol.* 2002;57:507–513.
17. Laméris W, van Randen A, van Es HW, *et al.* Imaging strategies for detection of urgent conditions in patients with acute abdominal pain: diagnostic accuracy study. *BMJ.* 2009;338:b2431.
18. Stoker J, van Randen A, Laméris W, *et al.* Imaging patients with acute abdominal pain. *Radiology.* 2009;253:31–46.
19. Decadt B, Sussman L, Lewis MP, *et al.* Randomized clinical trial of early laparoscopy in the management of acute non-specific abdominal pain. *Br J Surg.* 1999;86:1383–1386.
20. Maggio AQ, Reece-Smith AM, Tang TY, *et al.* Early laparoscopy versus active observation in acute abdominal pain: systematic review and meta-analysis. *Int J Surg.* 2008;6:400–403.

CHAPTER 20

Hematemesis and melena

Anthony Y. B. Teoh and James Y. W. Lau

Chinese University of Hong Kong, Hong Kong SAR, China

ESSENTIAL FACTS ABOUT CAUSATION

Diagnosis	Number of patients (%) 2007[16]	Mortality (%)
Ulcer	1826 (27)	162 (8.9)
Erosive disease (gastric and duodenum)	1731 (26)	195 (14.1)
Esophagitis	1177 (17)	65 (5.5)
Varices and portal hypertensive gastropathy	819 (12)	87 (14)
Malignancy	187 (3)	31 (17)
Mallory-Weiss syndrome	213 (3)	10 (4.7)
Other diagnosis	797 (12)	125 (16)
Total	6750	675 (10)

Data adapted from The United Kingdom National Audit in Upper Gastrointestinal Bleeding 2007 [16].

ESSENTIALS OF DIAGNOSIS

- Symptoms: Coffee ground vomiting, hematemesis, melena, hematochezia, anemic symptoms
- Past medical history: Liver cirrhosis, use of non-steroidal anti-inflammatory drugs
- Signs: Hypotension, tachycardia, pallor, altered mental status, melena or blood per rectum, decreased urine output
- Bloods: Anemia, raised urea, high urea to creatinine ratio
- Endoscopy: Ulcers, varices, Mallory-Weiss tear, erosive disease, neoplasms, vascular ectasia, and vascular malformations

ESSENTIALS OF TREATMENT

Algorithm for management of acute GI bleeding

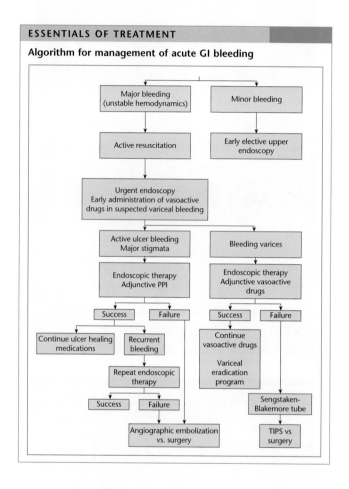

and therapeutic tool in managing these patients. Stratification of the patients into low- or high-risk groups aids in formulating a clinical management plan and early endoscopy with aggressive post-hemostasis care should be provided in high-risk patients.

Introduction

Upper gastrointestinal bleeding (UGIB) is a common medical emergency that carries substantial mortality. Despite advances in medical management, the mortality rate still ranges from 15% to 50% [1–3]. Upper endoscopy is the standard diagnostic

What are the signs and symptoms?

Hematemesis and melena are signs of upper gastrointestinal bleeding. Hematemesis is defined as vomiting of blood or blood clots, whereas melena is defined as passage of dark, tarry stool with a characteristic pungent smell. Fresh hematemesis is often a reliable sign signifying ongoing or active bleeding. Occasionally, vomiting of swallowed blood from hemoptysis or bleeding from the upper aero-digestive tract, e.g., nasopharynx, can confuse the diagnosis. Coffee ground vomiting is also a classic sign of upper gastrointestinal bleeding. The sign usually indicates a less severe bleed. The vomitus looks like ground coffee as a result of oxidized iron within heme molecules of red blood cells after their exposure to gastric acid. Melena occurs when hemoglobin is converted to hematin or other hemochromes by bacterial degradation. This can be produced experimentally by the ingestion of as little as 100–200 mL of blood. Blood is absorbed by the small intestine causing raised blood urea. A raised blood urea (BUN): creatinine ratio can therefore aid the diagnosis of UGIB. Some of this azotemia is probably secondary to hypovolemia. If the volume of an upper GI bleed is large, the patient may present with hematochezia (passage of fresh blood per rectum). Conversely, if the volume of bleeding is small but sufficient to supply enough hemoglobin for degradation, and if colonic motility is sufficiently slow, bleeding from the small bowel or proximal colon may cause melena. Small bowel bleeding is however uncommon. Bleeding from colonic sources, e.g. tumors, is either slow, leading to anemia or hemoccult positive stool; or rapid, such as in diverticular disease leading to hematochezia.

How common is upper gastrointestinal bleeding?

Upper gastrointestinal bleeding (UGIB) is a common medical emergency. The annual incidence in United Kingdom varies from 103 to 172 per 100 000 population [1,4]. In a recent United Kingdom national audit, the median age of patients who presented with upper gastrointestinal bleeding was 68 years [5]. Eighty-two percent of these patients were new admissions and 16% were patients who developed bleeding while hospitalized for other illnesses. The proportion of patients aged over 60 and 80 was 63% and 80% respectively. The overall mortality was 10%. Deaths occur mostly in elderly patients with co-morbid illnesses.

Initial management

It is mandatory that patients who develop acute gastrointestinal bleeding are assessed urgently. The aim of initial patient assessment is to stratify them into low- or high-risk groups for bleeding and mortality. This aids in formulating a clinical management plan [6,7]. In 80% of patients, bleeding has already stopped at their presentations. There are several risk scoring systems. The Rockall score is a composite score combining pre- and post-endoscopy clinical data with the aim to predict mortality. A score greater than 8 is associated with a 41% mortality and a rebleeding rate of 42.1%. The Glasgow-Blatchford Bleeding Score (GBS) is calculated using clinical

Table 20.1 Glasgow Blatchford bleeding score – admission risk markers and score values

Admission risk markers	Score value
Blood urea (mmol/L)	
6.5–7.9	2
8.0–9.9	3
10.0–24.9	4
≥25	6
Hemoglobin for men (g/L)	
120–129	1
100–119	3
<100	6
Hemoglobin for women (g/L)	
100–119	1
<100	6
Systolic blood pressure (mmHg)	
100–109	1
90–99	2
<90	3
Other markers	
Pulse ≥ 100/min	1
Presentation with melaena	1
Presentation with syncope	2
Hepatic disease	2
Cardiac failure	2

and laboratory data on admission (Table 20.1 and Chapter 146) [8]. It has been found to accurately predict the need for intervention and also deaths. A score of 0 is classified as low risk for intervention or death. In these patients, outpatient management could be considered and this has been shown to be safe and may reduce hospital admissions [9]. Those judged to be of high risk should be admitted to high dependency areas and considered for urgent endoscopy.

Resuscitation is the first priority in the management of patients with UGIB. Table 20.2 provides a schema on the assessment of volume deficit. Large-bore intravenous cannulae should be inserted for rapid fluid administration. Circulating volume should be restored initially using crystalloid or

Table 20.2 Hypovolemic shock: symptoms, signs and fluid replacement

Blood loss (mL)	<750	750–1500	1500–2000	>2000
Blood loss (%)	<15	15–30	30–40	>40
Pulse rate	<100	>100	>120	>140
Blood pressure	Normal	Normal	Decreased	Decreased
Pulse pressure	Normal or increased	Decreased	Decreased	Decreased
Respiratory rate	14–20	20–30	30–40	>35
Urine output (mL)	>30	20–30	5–15	Negligible
Mental status	Slightly anxious	Mildly anxious	Anxious and confused	Confused and lethargic
Fluid replacement	Crystalloid	Crystalloid	Crystalloid and blood	Crystalloid and blood

colloid solutions. Red blood cells should be transfused when hemodynamics are unstable and/or hemoglobin is less than 10 g/dL at the time of presentation. In those with impaired mental status, their airways should be protected and often orotracheal intubation is required prior to endoscopy. A urinary catheter is useful, especially in those with hemodynamic compromise, to detect oliguria. A central venous catheter is useful for monitoring volume replacement, particularly in those with incipient heart failure. Physical examination may reveal stigmata of chronic liver disease that may call for specific treatments such as vasoactive drugs, antibiotics, and drugs to prevent encephalopathy.

Endoscopy

Endoscopy defines the cause of bleeding and provides prognostic information, and more importantly, therapies carried out during endoscopy can improve patients' outcomes. In pooled analyses of randomized controlled trials, endoscopic therapy reduces recurrent bleeding, hospitalization, transfusion, need for surgery, and deaths. Early endoscopy within 24 hours is recommended in most patients [10]. In selected patients with signs of ongoing bleeding and hypotension, urgent endoscopy with therapy may be lifesaving. Endoscopic procedures should be performed by medical or surgical gastroenterologists with expertise in therapeutic endoscopy. This should be performed in a unit supported by appropriate staff, monitoring and resuscitation equipment.

Causes of bleeding and their treatment

For practical management, UGIB can also be categorized into variceal and non-variceal bleeding. The Essential Facts about Causation box shows the endoscopic diagnoses in patients from the National Audit in 2007 [5]. Peptic ulcers remain the commonest cause accounting for 27% of cases. *Helicobacter pylori* infection is less prevalent in bleeding peptic ulcers when

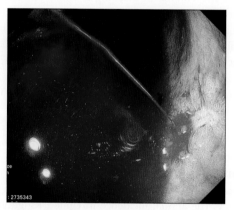

Figure 20.1 Ulcer with spurting hemorrhage.

compared to uncomplicated peptic ulcers. Non-steroidal anti-inflammatory drugs or aspirin use are common in the elderly. Patients suffering from variceal bleeding have increased over the past decade accounting for 8% of those presenting with acute upper GIB.

Peptic ulcer bleeding

The endoscopic appearances of bleeding peptic ulcers can be categorized into those that are actively bleeding (Forrest I), ulcers that exhibit stigmata of recent bleeding (nonbleeding visible vessel defined as protuberant discoloration (II a), an adherent clot (II b), and flat pigmentations (II c)), and a clean base ulcer (Forrest III) (Figures 20.1–20.3). Their prevalence, risks of further bleeding, and need for surgery is summarized in Table 20.3 [11]. Endoscopic therapy is indicated in ulcers that are actively bleeding or with a non-bleeding visible vessel, which is defined as a protuberant discoloration in an ulcer base (Figures 20.4–20.5) (Videos 20.1 and 20.2). It is controversial whether clots overlying ulcer craters should be removed. Ulcers with flat pigmentations or a clean base are associated with small or negligible risk of recurrent bleeding. No

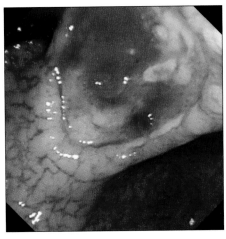

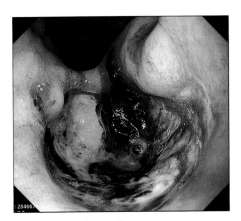

Figure 20.3 Ulcer with an adherent clot.

Figure 20.2 Blood oozing from a visible vessel.

Table 20.3 Bleeding ulcers: prevalence, risk, and need for surgery

Endoscopic characteristics	Prevalence (%)	Further bleeding (%)	Surgery (%)	Mortality (%)
Clean base	42	5	0.5	2
Flat spot	20	10	6	3
Adherent clot	17	22	10	7
Nonbleeding visible vessel	17	43	34	11
Active bleeding	18	55	35	11

Data are from patients in prospective trials that did not receive endoscopic therapy. (Modified from Laine L and Peterson WL. *N Engl J Med.* 1994; 331:717–727.5. © 1994 Massachusetts Medical Society. All rights reserved.)

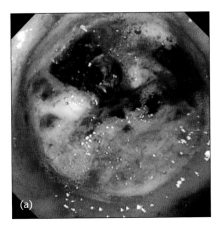
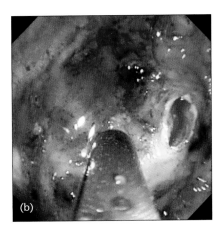
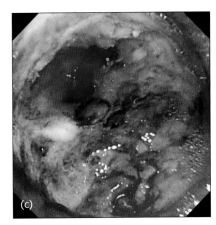

Figure 20.4 Heater probe application to a visible vessel.

endoscopic therapy is indicated. After endoscopic hemostasis to bleeding peptic ulcers, the use of high-dose proton pump inhibitor (PPI) up to 72 hours has been shown to reduce recurrent bleeding (Chapter 146).

Large ulcers in the bulbar duodenum and lesser curve of the stomach can erode into branches of the gastroduodenal artery complex and the left gastric artery. Endoscopic treatment often

fails to stop bleeding from these arteries. Factors that have consistently been identified to predict failure of endoscopic therapy include: hemodynamic instability, comorbid illnesses, active bleeding, large ulcer size of greater than 2 cm, posterior bulbar or lesser curve ulcer [12].

In the management of patients with recurrent bleeding after initial endoscopic control, further endoscopic control can often

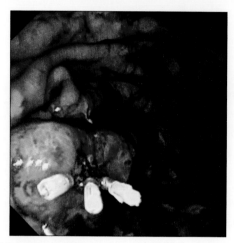

Figure 20.5 Hemoclip application to a visible vessel.

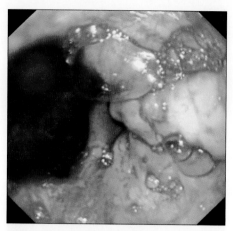

Figure 20.7 Bleeding esophageal varices.

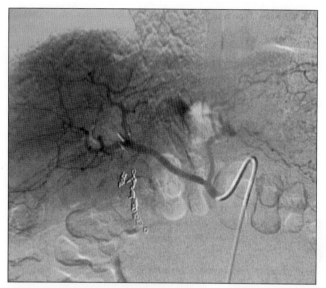

Figure 20.6 Transarterial embolization of the gastroduodenal artery. Hemoclips placed endoscopically are still visible.

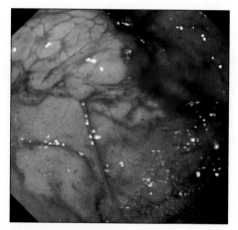

Figure 20.8 Bleeding gastric varices.

Variceal bleeding

Bleeding from esophago-gastric varices is often severe and mortality from the first bleeding is often high (Figures 20.7, 20.8). The overall prognosis is often dependent on the severity of liver disease as indicated by the Child-Pugh grading. The presence of features suggesting chronic liver disease e.g. alcohol use, ascites and jaundice should alert the possibility of a variceal bleed. It calls for specific treatments of prophylactic broad spectrum antibiotics and vasoactive drugs. Emergency endoscopic treatment is often associated with transient bacteremia. The administration of prophylactic antibiotics decreases the incidence of sepsis such as bacterial peritonitis and has been shown to improve survival [7]. Early administration of a vaso-active drug such as vasopressin or its analog or somatostatin or its analogs reduces portal venous blood flow and variceal pressure. This makes subsequent endoscopic treatment easier. Vasoactive drugs should be continued 2–5 days after endoscopic control to prevent recurrent bleeding [15]. Occasionally with massive bleeding, passage of a Sengstaken-Blakemore tube (with orotracheal protection of the airway) is

be successful. More definitive methods of ulcer hemostasis either in the form of surgery or angiographic embolization should however be offered to patients with episodes of hypotension and large ulcers [13]. Traditionally, surgery is considered the most definitive method of controlling bleeding. However, postoperative mortality occurs in around 20–25% of patients. When the expertise is available, angiographic embolization is an attractive alternative in those who fail endoscopic haemostasis [14] (Figure 20.6). Major ischemic complications are uncommon and ranged from 0% to 16%. A retrospective comparison between surgery and angiographic embolization favors the latter treatment in managing massive bleeding from ulcers that fail endoscopic treatment.

necessary. In up to 30% of cirrhotic patients presenting with UGIB, the bleeding source is non-variceal. In those with massive bleeding and often obtunded mental state from shock or encephalopathy, an orotracheal tube is required prior to endoscopy. Band ligation is the endoscopic treatment of choice for esophageal varices. When compared to endoscopic sclerotherapy, band ligation is associated with less local complications such as mediastinitis, esophageal strictures and leads to faster eradication of esophageal varices (Video 20.3).

Gastric varices can be divided into those in continuity with esophageal varices and those that occur in isolation. Isolated fundal varices are associated with high risk of recurrent bleeding and death. In the control of acute bleeding from isolated fundal varices, histoacryl glue injection appears to be the only effective method. Many would consider a transjugular intrahepatic portosystemic shunt (TIPS) or early shunt surgery as an alternative, especially after initial control with glue injection. In those patients where endoscopic therapy fails, a Sengstaken-Blakemore tube can tamponade bleeding in about 90% of cases; however, following deflation of the balloons, recurrent bleeding occurs in about 50% of cases.

Miscellaneous causes of upper GI bleeding

Other causes of upper GI bleeding are uncommon. Fresh hematemesis that occurs after emesis is typical of a Mallory-Weiss tear. The condition is often self-limiting and carries an excellent prognosis. Gastric vascular ectasia or "watermelon stomach" is characterized by the presence of linear red streaks radiating from the pylorus. Treatment is often difficult. The use of thermal ablative techniques appears to be the most effective option, although repeated sessions may be required [16]. Other causes include neoplasms and vascular malformations.

Prognosis

Despite advances in medical management, the mortality rate of patients suffering from upper gastrointestinal bleeding remains high and depends on the underlying pathology. In patients with non-variceal bleeding, a mortality rate up to 15% has been reported [1]. A number of studies have identified independent predictors for mortality and these include age, comorbidities, shock at presentation, in-hospital bleeders and presence of rebleeding [1,2]. In acute variceal hemorrhage, the risk of mortality can be up to 50% and the risk of mortality is strongly dependent on pre-existing liver function and the severity of cirrhosis [3]. The recognition of these predictors may help select patients who are most at risk and may benefit from intensive post-hemostasis care.

References

1. Blatchford O, Davidson LA, Murray WR, *et al*. Acute upper gastrointestinal hemorrhage in west of Scotland: case ascertainment study. *BMJ*. 1997;315:510–514.
2. Chiu PW, Ng EK, Cheung FK, *et al*. Predicting mortality in patients with bleeding peptic ulcers after therapeutic endoscopy. *Clin Gastroenterol Hepatol*. 2009;7:311–316.
3. Gatta A, Merket C, Amodio P, *et al*. Development and validation of a prognostic index predicting death after upper gastrointestinal bleeding in patients with liver cirrhosis: a multicenter study. *Am J Gastroenterol*. 1994;89:1528–1536.
4. Rockall TA, Logan RFA, Devlin HB, *et al*. Incidence of and mortality from acute upper gastrointestinal haemorrhage in the United Kingdom. *BMJ*.1995;311:222–226.
5. Hearnshaw SA, Logan RF, Lowe D, et al. Acute upper gastrointestinal bleeding in the UK: patient characteristics, diagnoses and outcomes in the 2007 UK audit. Gut. 2011 Jun 10. [Epub ahead of print]
6. British Society of Gastroenterology Endoscopy Committee. Non-variceal upper gastrointestinal haemorrhage: guidelines. *Gut*. 2002;51(Suppl 4):iv1–iv6.
7. Jalan R, Hayes PC. UK guidelines on the management of variceal haemorrhage in cirrhotic patients. *Gut*. 2000;46(Suppl 3): iii1–iii15.
8. Blatchford O, Murray WR, Blatchford M. A risk score to predict need for treatment for upper-gastrointestinal haemorrhage. *Lancet*. 2000;356:1318–1321.
9. Stanley AJ, Ashley D, Dalton HR, *et al*. Outpatient management of patients with low-risk upper-gastrointestinal haemorrhage: multicentre validation and prospective evaluation. *Lancet*. 2009;373:42–47.
10. Spiegel BM, Vakil NB, Ofman JJ. Endoscopy for acute non-variceal upper gastrointestinal tract hemorrhage: is sooner better? A systematic review. *Arch Intern Med*. 2001;161: 1393–1404.
11. Laine L, Peterson WL. Bleeding peptic ulcer. *N Engl J Med*. 1994;331:717–727.
12. Elmunzer BJ, Young SD, Inadomi JM, *et al*. Systematic review of the predictors of recurrent hemorrhage after endoscopic hemostatic therapy for bleeding peptic ulcers. *Am J Gastroenterol*. 2008; 103:2625–2632.
13. Lau JY, Sung JJ, Lam YH, *et al*. Endoscopic retreatment compared with surgery in patients with recurrent bleeding after initial endoscopic control of bleeding ulcers. *N Engl J Med*. 1999;340 :751–756.
14. Loffroy R, Guiu B, Cercueil JP, *et al*. Refractory bleeding from gastroduodenal ulcers: arterial embolization in high-operative-risk patients. *J Clin Gastroenterol*. 2008;42:361–367.
15. Ioannou G, Doust J, Rockey DC. Terlipressin for acute esophageal variceal hemorrhage. *Cochrane Database Syst Rev*. 2003;(1): CD002147.
16. Pavey DA, Craig PI. Endoscopic therapy for upper-GI vascular ectasias. *Gastrointest Endosc*. 2004;59:233–238.

CHAPTER 21
Acute lower gastrointestinal bleeding

Thomas O. G. Kovacs and Dennis M. Jensen
David Geffen School of Medicine at UCLA, Los Angeles, CA, USA

KEY POINTS

1 Severe hematochezia is the most common presentation of acute lower gastrointestinal bleeding.
2 15–20% of patients hospitalized with severe hematochezia have a forgut source of the bleeding.
3 After initial resuscitation, urgent colonoscopy is the diagnostic test of choice.
4 The most common colonic cause of hemorrhage is diverticulosis, followed by internal hemorrhoids, ischemic colitis, rectal ulcers, post-polypectomy ulcers, polyps or cancer, and angiomas.
5 Therapeutic hemostasis of focal lesions includes epinephrine-saline injection, hemoclips and multipolar electrocoagulation.
6 Effective management results in improved patient outcomes such as decreased rebleeding rates as well as reduced transfusion requirements, median hospital stays and direct costs of medical care.

CAUSES OF SEVERE HEMATOCHEZIA

Colonic source
Diverticulosis
Internal hemorrhoids
Ischemic colitis
Rectal ulcers
Other colitis
Post-polypectomy ulcer
Polyp/cancer
Angiomas

UGI source
Ulcer
Varices
Angiomas

Small bowel source
Angiomas

ESSENTIALS OF DIAGNOSIS OF SEVERE HEMATOCHEZIA

- **Nasogastric lavage** to determine whether UGI bleeding is present
- If no UGI source, rapid **oral lavage** to cleanse the colon
- **Urgent colonoscopy** is the diagnostic test of choice
- If colonoscopy not diagnostic, do **anoscopy and push enteroscopy** If colonoscopy, anoscopy and enteroscopy are not diagnostic, then:
- **Scintiography** (threshold GI bleeding rate ≥0.1 mL/min)
- **Angiography** (threshold GI bleeding rate ≥0.5 mL/min)
- **Capsule endoscopy** may have a role in selected patients with recurrent hematochezia and negative diagnostic evaluation

ESSENTIALS OF TREATMENT OF SEVERE HEMATOCHEZIA

- Initial resuscitation in a monitored care setting
- Colonoscopy to provide both diagnosis and therapeutic hemostasis of focal lesions (with epinephrine-saline injection, hemoclips, multipolar electrocoagulation), angiomas (with MPEC) and internal hemorrhoids (with band ligation)
- Angiography with transcatheter embolization
- Emergency surgery when bleeding not controlled by endoscopic hemostasis and angiography

Introduction and epidemiology

Acute lower gastrointestinal (LGI) bleeding, defined as bleeding from a site distal to the duodenum (most commonly the colon), has an annual hospitalization rate of about 20 per 100,000 adults [1] and has been increasing substantially over the past decade. If the patient presents with severe hematochezia, clinicians cannot determine the site of the lesion clinically as foregut, midgut or colon. Even without a history of, or signs of, upper gastrointestinal (UGI) lesions, approximately 15–20% of patients hospitalized with severe hematochezia have a foregut (UGI or proximal jejunum) source of the severe hematochezia. Based upon these data, we prefer the term "severe hematochezia" instead of "acute lower GI bleeding," because the latter can confuse clinicians. In most ambulatory patients with hematochezia, the bleeding stops spontaneously (in about 80% of cases), allowing elective diagnostic evaluation. However, 10–40% of patients with colonic sources of bleeding have recurrent hemorrhage, usually within 48 hours of the initial bleed, and these patients with continued and recurrent severe hematochezia require urgent attention to minimize further bleeding and complications. Mortality rates still range between 3–5% because the incidence of LGI bleeding increases markedly in the elderly (typically >65 yrs of age) and these patients frequently have significant comorbidity [1]. A recent US study reported that the all-cause in-hospital mortality rate in LGI hemorrhage was 3.9%. The strongest predictors of mortality included advanced age, intestinal ischemia and comorbid illness [2].

What is it?

For patients who present with severe hematochezia, the diagnostic and therapeutic approach is not standardized in most medical centers. However, we have evaluated a standardized approach and found it to be effective, safe, and cost-effective. During the resuscitation of patients with severe hematochezia, we recommend nasogastric (NG) aspiration to exclude a potential UGI source. If this is negative (bile present, no blood), then a rapid oral lavage to cleanse the colon is recommended, followed by urgent colonoscopy. Urgent colonoscopy provides an accurate diagnosis and if required, an opportunity for hemostasis during the same examination. If urgent colonoscopy is not diagnostic for a bleeding site, a slotted anoscopy examination is indicated to exclude anal canal bleeding sources (such as internal hemorrhoids or anal fissures) and if that is negative, a push enteroscopy is recommended to exclude foregut lesions. This approach improves the diagnostic and therapeutic efficacy while reducing direct costs of patient care [3,4] (Figure 21.1).

Our primary criterion for proving (i.e., classifying as "definitive source") that a lesion caused the bleeding is to identify stigmata of recent hemorrhage – SRH – (such as active bleeding, non-bleeding visible vessel, an adherent clot or flat spots for colonic lesions) on a focal lesion. A lesion is classified as the "presumptive cause" of the bleeding when fresh blood is in that location (such as the colon) or a lesion is found there without stigmata and no other likely bleeding sites are identified on colonoscopy, anoscopy, and push enteroscopy. A lesion (such as diverticulosis found during the colonoscopy) is classified as "incidental" when more than one type of lesion is found, but another lesion is the bleeding site based upon

stigmata of recent hemorrhage or other endoscopic evidence, such as its extent, ulceration, or number of lesions.

The most common colonic cause of hemorrhage was diverticulosis (either presumed or definitive) and other common causes were internal hemorrhoids, ischemic colitis, rectal ulcers, delayed bleeding from post-polypectomy ulcers, colon polyps or cancer, and colon angiomas or radiation telangiectasia [3]. The findings at urgent colonoscopy also permitted triage of patients. High risk patients were treated with colonoscopic hemostasis after a diagnosis of focal definitive lesions (with SRH) was made. This usually included combination therapy with dilute epinephrine injection (1:20,000 dilution in saline) and hemoclipping. Coagulation (usually with multipolar probe – MPEC) was used for some focal lesions or angioma syndromes causing bleeding. Low risk patients (without SRH and/or severe comorbidity) were allocated to less intensive and less expensive care, which often facilitated early discharge.

Causes

Diverticulosis

Diverticular bleeding is the most common colonic cause for patients hospitalized with severe hematochezia. It originates frequently (about 50%) from the right half of the colon (at or proximal to the splenic flexure). Actively bleeding colonic diverticula have been treated with epinephrine injection, multipolar probe coagulation (MPEC) and metallic clips. Reported rebleeding rates range from 7.1% to 38% in 30 days [5].

We treat active bleeding (Figure 21.2) or adherent clots (Figure 21.3) with a 1:20 000 epinephrine/saline solution in

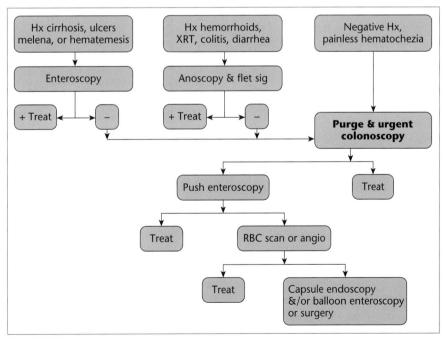

Figure 21.1 Algorithm for severe hematochezia.

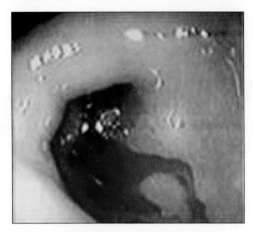

Figure 21.2 Bleeding diverticulum.

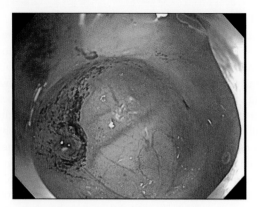

Figure 21.4 Diverticulum with non-bleeding visible vessel.

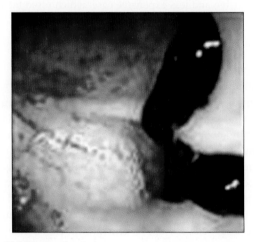

Figure 21.3 Clot on diverticulum.

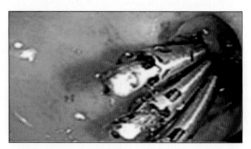

Figure 21.5 Hemoclips on non-bleeding visible vessel shown in Figure 21.4.

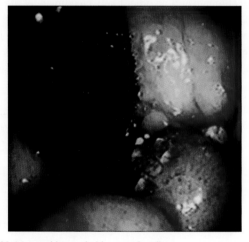

Figure 21.6 Internal hemorrhoids – post-banding.

1–2 mL aliquots [5,6]. After epinephrine injection, adherent clots can be safely guillotined off with a snare. After the bleeding stops and for non-bleeding visible vessels – NBVV – (Figure 21.4), endoclips are applied across the NBVV on either side to occlude the underlying feeding artery (Figure 21.5). This usually provides definitive hemostasis. The hemoclips may also be useful as radiologic targets for angiography if hemostasis fails or severe rebleeding occurs. We also advocate India ink labeling of the diverticulum with SRH after successful endoscopic hemostasis. This facilitates localization and follow-up of the bleeding site, endoscopic retreatment (if necessary), surgery in case of early rebleeding, and histopathologic correlation. In our series, 4.8% of patients required surgery or interventional radiology (IR) embolization.

Internal hemorrhoids

Internal hemorrhoids are the most common cause of colonic bleeding in ambulatory outpatient adults. Most internal hemorrhoid bleeding is self-limited, and manifested by bright red blood on the toilet tissue. Medical therapy consists of fiber supplementation, stool softeners, rectal suppositories and sitz baths. Internal hemorrhoids are also the second most common cause of severe hematochezia in patients hospitalized with presumed colonic hemorrhage (Figure 21.6) [4].

Prior to assuming that severe hematochezia is from more proximal lesions, the anal canal should always be examined by rigid slotted anoscope. If that is not diagnostic, try turn-around in the rectum with a flexible sigmoidoscope to identify internal hemorrhoids. We usually use rubberband ligation for emergency hemostasis of bleeding internal hemorrhoids (Figure 21.6) [7]. Emergency colonoscopy can be obviated in such cases, although an elective colonoscopy might still be considered in patients at risk for concomitant polyps or colorectal cancer. Hemorrhoidal surgery is required for patients with continued severe bleeding not responding to medical and anoscopic treatment.

Focal ulcers or colitis

Focal ulcers proximal to the sigmoid colon are an uncommon cause of severe colonic hemorrhage. In one large series, these accounted for the bleeding site in 8% of patients [8] (Table 21.1). Bleeding colonic ulcers were caused by: recent polypectomy with ulceration (Figure 21.7), inflammatory bowel disease (IBD), ischemic ulcers (Figure 21.8), or infectious colitis (such as pseudomembranous colitis or cytomegalovirus – CMV – ulcers). In our recent experience, the most common cause was delayed bleeding from a post-polypectomy-induced ulcer. The median time to severe colonic bleeding was 8 days (range 3–10) after initial polypectomy of colonic polyps (Figure 21.7). The majority of these patients resumed taking over-the-counter (OTC) aspirin, NSAIDs, anticoagulants, or gingko after

polypectomy, and most cases were large sessile polyps removed by piecemeal polypectomy. For patients with severe hematochezia after recent polypectomy, we recommend an oral purge prior to colonoscopy.

Focal, discrete colonic ulcers secondary to infection, ischemia, or IBD are much less common causes of severe colonic hemorrhage. Urgent colonoscopy usually shows a diffuse mucosal process and patients do not usually benefit from endoscopic hemostasis (Figure 21.8).

Rectal ulcers

Rectal ulcers (Figure 21.9) may be a cause of severe lower GI hemorrhage, especially in elderly or debilitated patients with constipation, who are often confined to bed. The ulcers may be either solitary or multiple, and associated with fecal impaction, rectal prolapse, ischemia or trauma [9].

Colonic tumors

Colonic tumors, either cancer or stromal tumors, occasionally present with hematochezia and may occur anywhere in the rectum or colon. Overt bleeding suggests that the lesion has ulcerated into underlying vessels, usually an artery. Although endoscopic therapy with thermal devices, injection,

Table 21.1 Eight most common colonic sources of severe hematochezia (486 cases)[1]

Diagnosed lesion	Frequency (%)[2]
1. Diverticulosis	31.9
2. Internal hemorrhoids	12.8
3. Ischemic colitis	11.9
4. Rectal ulcers	7.6
5. Colon angiomas or radiation telangiectasia	7.0
6. Ulcerative colitis, Crohn's disease, other colitis	6.2
7. Other LGI diagnoses	5.6
8. Post-polypectomy ulcer	4.7

[1]Personal communications DM Jensen, CURE Hemostasis Research Group 2010.
[2]Expressed as percent of colorectal sources.

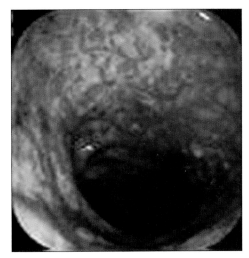

Figure 21.8 Ischemic colitis.

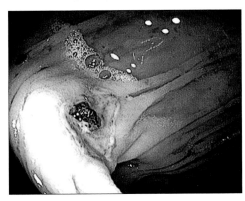

Figure 21.7 Clot on post-polypectomy ulcer.

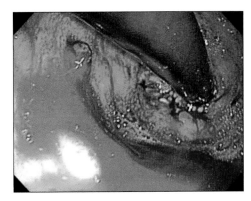

Figure 21.9 Rectal ulcer – bleeding visible vessel.

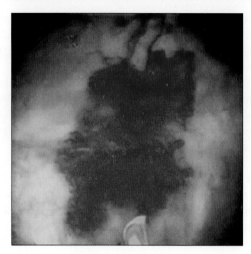

Figure 21.10 Ascending colon large angioma.

or a combination of both usually produces temporary hemostasis, surgical resection is the best long-term treatment [4,8].

Colonic angiodysplasia

Bleeding colonic angiodysplasias most often occur in the right colon and are usually multiple or diffuse (Figure 21.10). They may be associated with advanced age and medical conditions such as chronic renal insufficiency, cirrhosis, valvular heart disease, and collagen vascular disorders. Bleeding from angiodysplasia is usually mild to moderate and is self-limited. Such bleeding is usually intermittent and usually presents with slow GI bleeding and chronic iron deficiency anemia. The main risk of endoscopic coagulation of angiodysplasia is severe, delayed bleeding and post-coagulation syndrome [10]. Perforations have been reported more often than with MPEC for hot biopsy forceps, monopolar electrocoagulation, Nd-YAG laser, or argon plasma coagulator (APC) hemostasis of right colon angiodysplasia. This relates to deeper coagulation and the potential for transmural coagulation with these non-MPEC thermal devices.

Radiation telangiectasia

Radiation telangiectasia can occasionally cause severe hematochezia, although these are most often associated with mild to moderate chronic rectal bleeding. Chronic radiation injury develops 6 to 18 months after radiation therapy for prostatic, gynecologic, rectal or bladder tumors. The radiation damage is caused by altered vascularity and ensuing mucosal ischemia. Rectal telangiectasia and friability are the endoscopic features of radiation proctitis. Endoscopic hemostasis with thermal treatment has been effective and safe for patients with chronic or recurrent acute bleeding despite medical therapies [10].

General measures and diagnosis

Risk factors including abnormal vital signs 1 hour after initial medical assessment (suggesting hemodynamic instability),

gross blood on initial rectal examination, (suggesting continued bleeding), initial hematocrit ≤35%, and significant comorbidity were reported to be independent predictors of severe lower GI bleeding and adverse outcomes [11,12]. Patients with these high-risk factors should have urgent diagnosis and receive focused therapy with the aim of improving outcomes.

The first concern in patients with persistent, severe hematochezia should be to start aggressive resuscitative measures in a monitored care setting [8]. A consultation with a general or GI surgeon should be obtained at an early stage to follow the patients and to consider emergency surgery, in case bleeding cannot be controlled medically, endoscopically, or angiographically. Subsequently, an orogastric or nasogastric tube is recommended to determine whether evidence of UGI bleeding (coffee grounds, blood clots) is present. If there is bile without blood or coffee grounds in the nasogastric aspirate, a lesion proximal to the ligament of Treitz is unlikely when ongoing hematochezia is documented. In patients with severe hematochezia, return of clear fluid without bile should not be considered a negative NG aspirate. Since continuity has not been established between the NG tube in the stomach and the duodenum, the patient may have a duodenal ulcer or other duodenal lesions.

Colonoscopy

Prior to preparation for emergency colonoscopy, tap water enemas are recommended to clear the distal colon and permit examination of the rectosigmoid colon and anal canal with anoscopy followed by flexible sigmoidoscopy with retroflexion in the rectum in selected patients (Figure 21.1). This is particularly indicated in patients with a history of bleeding internal hemorrhoids, anorectal disease, or distal colitis. A rigid sigmoidoscopy is not adequate because there may be lesions in the blind area of the rectum. However, with flexible sigmoidoscopy, an examination of the sigmoid and descending colon and retroflexed view of the distal colon lesions, are all feasible.

If no evidence of UGI bleeding is found and the flexible sigmoidoscopy and anoscopy do not reveal a rectosigmoid source of hemorrhage, cleansing the colon with an oral purge is recommended, followed by urgent colonoscopy in the monitored bed area or ICU when the colon is clear of stool and clots by the purge. Urgent colonoscopy is a safe diagnostic test, which also provides potential therapeutic intervention. Several factors determine the "yield" including timing of colonoscopy, thoroughness of colonic preparation, and definition of what is the source of bleeding.

A randomized controlled trial of urgent colonoscopy versus standard care (tagged red blood cell scan, followed by angiography, if positive, with elective colonoscopy) showed a significant diagnostic advantage in finding a definitive bleeding site for urgent colonoscopy but failed to reveal any other statistically significant benefit in other important outcomes [13].

Subsequently, several trials have demonstrated that urgent colonoscopy does benefit outcomes such as hospital stay and direct costs [3]. In a retrospective study comparing early colonoscopy to angiography for severe lower intestinal hemorrhage, the likelihood of post-polypectomy bleeding, and logistical factors such as admission on a weekday or late in the day, predicted early colonoscopy, while signs and symptoms of severe bleeding predicted angiography use [14].

Should the colonoscopy, anoscopy and push enteroscopy not be diagnostic, then scintigraphy and angiography are warranted in patients with recurrent hematochezia. For those patients who stop bleeding or present with less severe bleeding, colonoscopy within 24 hours of presentation should still be considered the initial diagnostic and therapeutic procedure of choice (Table 21.1).

Scintigraphy

The threshold rate of GI bleeding for localization with radio-isotope scanning is about 0.1 mL/min or more. Scintigraphy may be particularly useful for identification of small bowel or colonic bleeding sites that are actively bleeding and at least moderately severe [3]. Two different types of scintigrams are available: (a) sulfur colloid with technetium and (b) autologous red blood cells (RBCs) tagged with technetium. Sulfur colloid is rapidly cleared from the circulation after intravenous (IV) injection but tagged RBCs stay in the vascular space for about 24 hours. Technetium-tagged RBC scans are more commonly used than sulfur colloid scans. Injection of labeled RBCs and early scanning (at least 30 minutes, 60 minutes, and 4 hours) is recommended to identify and localize actively bleeding sites. Since specific localization and etiologic diagnosis are not possible with RBC scanning, confirmatory examinations such as angiography and/or endoscopy or enteroscopy are recommended prior to surgical exploration. Delayed scans (12 to 24 hours) are not reliable for localization in the gut, particularly as a guide for surgical exploration, because blood in the gut (with the radionucleotide) moves between scans and localization on delayed scans can be misleading.

Angiography, magnetic resonance imaging (MRI), computed tomography (CT) and barium X-rays

If the rate of ongoing arterial bleeding is at least 0.5 mL/min, selective visceral angiography may show extravasation of contrast into the lumen to identify a bleeding site [8]. Emergency visceral angiography can be useful for diagnosis and treatment of colonic, small bowel, or UGI lesions.

If extravasation of contrast into the gut lumen was identified, angiographic therapy was often effective, with relatively low rebleeding (20%) and ischemic complication (10%) rates [15]. However, in one study, 65% of patients with LGI hemorrhage who had failed endoscopic therapy had a negative angiographic study [15]; only 47% of patients with LGI bleeding

had angiography showing a source of hemorrhage; and 57% of patients continued to bleed after angiography.

Major advancements in radiology, such as helical computed tomography (CT) or magnetic resonance imaging (MRI) angiography, are being used in some centers instead of standard visceral angiography in the diagnosis of patients with severe hematochezia.

Barium studies (barium enema or small bowel follow-through) have no role in the emergency assessment of severe hematochezia since they cannot demonstrate active bleeding or SRH. Barium also takes several days to clear the colon or small bowel and this interferes with subsequent evaluation or treatment by colonoscopy, angiography, or surgery.

Small bowel evaluation

As an emergency examination, a small bowel evaluation with push enteroscopy is indicated for those patients with negative colonoscopy and upper endoscopy. Standard push enteroscopy provides examination of the proximal 60–80 cm of the jejunum [8]. Capsule endoscopy may have a role in selected patients with recurrent hematochezia, and when no diagnosis or localization has been made by urgent colonoscopy, anoscopy, push enteroscopy, or RBC scanning. Deep enteroscopy is now possible with newer techniques such as balloon enteroscopy or overtubes. This may be indicated in selected patients with small bowel lesions, documented or suspected after positive RBC scan or capsule endoscopy.

Emergency surgery

Emergency surgery should be considered for patients with: (1) hypotension or shock, despite resuscitative efforts; (2) continued bleeding with transfusion of six or more units of blood and no diagnosis by emergency endoscopy (push enteroscopy, colonoscopy, and anoscopy); and (3) when severe active bleeding cannot be controlled by colonoscopy or angiography. Segmental resection after the bleeding site has been identified is the definitive treatment with mortality rates of about 7%. "Blind" segmental resection or subtotal colectomy is associated with much higher mortality rates, ranging from 25–57%.

Summary

Severe hematochezia remains a challenging medical, surgical, and interventional radiology problem. There are at present insufficient prognostic criteria to identify patients with severe hematochezia; we would need better clinical prognostic criteria to predict who is at high and low risk of recurrent bleeding. For patients whose bleeding persists, identification of the cause and localization of the bleeding are essential for patient management. Urgent colonoscopy should be performed by experienced endoscopists skilled in the recognition of stigmata of hemorrhage and use of hemostasis techniques in the colon. With this approach, patients can be effectively managed with decreased rebleeding rates as well as reduced transfusion requirements, median hospital stays, and direct costs of medical care.

References

1. Longstreth GF. Epidemiology and outcome of patients hospitalized with acute lower gastrointestinal hemorrhage. A population-based study. *Am J Gastroenterol.* 1997;92:419–424.
2. Strate LL, Ayanian JZ, Kotler G, *et al.* Risk Factors for mortality in lower intestinal bleeding. *Clin Gastroenterol Hepatol.* 2008;6: 1004–1010.
3. Jensen DM, Machicado GA. Colonoscopy for diagnosis and treatment of severe lower gastrointestinal bleeding. Routine outcomes and cost analysis. *Gastroenterol Cl of NA.* 1997;7:477–498.
4. Savides TJ, Jensen DM. Evaluation and endoscopic treatment of severe lower gastrointestinal bleeding. *Tech Gastrointest Endosc.* 2003;5:148–154.
5. Jensen DM. Diverticular bleeding. An appraisal based on stigmata of recent hemorrhage. *Tech Gastrointest Endosc.* 2001;3: 192–198.
6. Jensen DM, Machicado GA, Jutabha R, *et al.* Urgent endoscopy for the diagnosis and treatment of severe diverticular hemorrhage. *New Engl J Med.* 2000;342:38–382.
7. Jutabha R, Miura-Jutabha C, Jensen DM. Current medical, anoscopic, endoscopic and surgical treatment for bleeding internal hemorrhoids. *Tech Gastrointest Endosc.* 2001;3:199–120.
8. Kovacs TOG, Jensen DM. Recent advances in the endoscopic diagnosis and therapy of upper gastrointestinal, small intestinal and colonic bleeding. *Med Clin N Am.* 2002;86:1319–1356.
9. Kanwal F, Dulai G, Jensen DM, *et al.* Major stigmata of recent hemorrhage on rectal ulcers in patients with severe hematochezia: endoscopic diagnosis, treatment and outcomes. *Gastrointest Endosc.* 2003;57:462–468.
10. Machicado GA, Jensen DM. Bleeding colonic agiomas and radiation telangiectasias: Endoscopic diagnosis and treatment. *Tech Gastrointest Endosc.* 2001;3:185–191.
11. Velayos FS, Williamson A, Sousa KH, *et al.* Early predictors of severe lower gastrointestinal bleeding and adverse outcomes: A prospective study. *Clin Gastroenterol Hepatol.* 2004;2:485–490.
12. Strate LL, Saltzman JR, Ookubo R, *et al.* Validation of a clinical prediction rule for severe acute lower intestinal bleeding. *Am J Gastroenterol.* 2005;100:1821–1827.
13. Jensen DM. Management of patients with severe hematochezia – with all current evidence available. *Am J Gastroenterol.* 2005;100:2403–2406.
14. Strate LL, Syngal S. Predictors of utilization of early colonoscopy vs radiography for severe lower intestinal bleeding. *Gastrointest Endosc.* 2005;61:46–52.
15. Maleux G, Roeflaer F, Heye S, *et al.* Long-term outcome of transcatheter embolotherapy for acute lower gastrointestinal hemorrhage. *Am J Gastroenterol.* 2009;104:2042–2046.

CHAPTER 22

H. pylori: its diseases and management

Barry J. Marshall, Helen M. Windsor and Kazufumi Kimura

University of Western Australia, Perth, WA, Australia

KEY POINTS

- *Helicobacter pylori* is a Gram-negative spiral bacterium adapted to survive in the mucus layer of the stomach
- It induces an inflammatory response which is more vigorous when toxins are present
- This results in a range of illnesses from acute gastritis through to mucosal ulceration, and chronic gastritis associated with gastric cancers and lymphomas
- Essentials of diagnosis are IgG antibody serology, urea breath test or histology at endoscopy
- In dyspepsia, test and treat if *H. pylori* prevalence is high and risk of gastric cancer low
- Standard initial therapy: proton pump inhibitor (e.g. omeprazole 20 mg), amoxicillin 1 g (or metronidazole 500 mg), and clarithromycin 500 mg all given bd for 7–14 days
- Resistant cases require endoscopy and culture to define antibiotic sensitivies

---

Introduction

Helicobacter pylori (Video 22.1) is the type strain of the genus *Helicobacter*, a group of microaerophilic spiral flagellated organisms adapted to colonisation of the gut, especially the stomach. The survival of this organism in the stomach is made possible by its production of **urease enzyme** which splits urea to form ammonia and carbon dioxide, thus protecting the organism from gastric acid (Figures 22.1 and 22.2). *H. pylori* colonizes the mucus secreting cells which line the stomach thereby activating the innate and adaptive immune systems to cause active chronic gastritis.

History and discovery

Gastric bacteria have been observed in the mucosa of cats, dogs and various animals since 1892 [1]. With the advent of endoscopy, the common association between gastritis, peptic ulcer and gastric cancer was studied in humans but the presence of *Helicobacter pylori* was either missed or ignored because it was known that the acidic gastric juice was sterile [2]. In 1979, Robin Warren in Perth, Western Australia observed **spiral bacteria** in association with **gastritis** and, following

clinical studies starting in 1981 with colleague Barry Marshall, the two were able to culture the bacteria and connect it with gastritis, peptic ulcer, and gastric cancer [3].

Microbiology

H. pylori is a **Gram-negative spiral shaped bacterium** with 2 to 7 polar sheathed **flagella** which allow it to move in the viscous environment of the gastric mucus. A new genus, *Helicobacter*, was created for these organisms which are usually isolated from the gastrointestinal tracts of mammals and birds. There are now at least 30 different *Helicobacter* species (Figure 22.3). *H. pylori* is **cultivated** from gastric biopsy samples on blood agar plates at 37°C under microaerobic conditions. *H. pylori* colonies are urease, catalase and oxidase positive and show characteristic Gram negative spiral morphology (Figure 22.4). The genome of *H. pylori* is compact with only 1500 (no space) genes because it lives only in the human stomach and it does not possess enzymatic pathways to survive in other environments.

Epidemiology and transmission

Most humans are colonised by *H. pylori*, acquiring the infection in **early childhood** and carrying it throughout their lives unless it is specifically eradicated with antibiotics. In the 19th century nearly all individuals were infected with *H. pylori* but in the 20th century, because of smaller family size, improved standards of living and clean drinking water, the **prevalence of *H. pylori* has decreased** in Western countries. In the United States and Australia the prevalence is 15 to 25% depending on socioeconomic status and country of birth. Figure 22.5 shows the approximate prevalence of *H. pylori* throughout the world. In every country it can vary depending upon cultural group, socioeconomic status, city versus rural habitation and water supply.

Transmission of *H. pylori* is thought to be via **saliva transfer** from mother to child [4], or within family groups and between children by **fecal-oral route** or via **vomitus** [5]; and by fecal contamination of the water supply in developing countries [6].

Textbook of Clinical Gastroenterology and Hepatology, Second Edition. Edited by C. J. Hawkey, Jaime Bosch, Joel E. Richter, Guadalupe Garcia-Tsao, Francis K. L. Chan.
© 2012 Blackwell Publishing Ltd. Published 2012 by Blackwell Publishing Ltd.

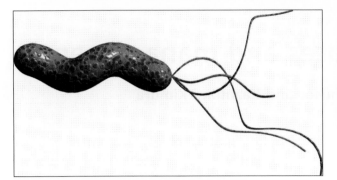

Figure 22.1 *H. pylori*, a spiral shaped organism with 2–7 polar sheathed flagella.

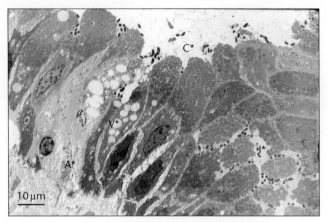

Figure 22.2 *H. pylori* associated with gastric epithelium (×3000). The bacteria are visible in the gastric mucus layer and adherent to the cells. Some cells separate and *H. pylori* invade these spaces [I*] and other cells show vacuoles [V*].

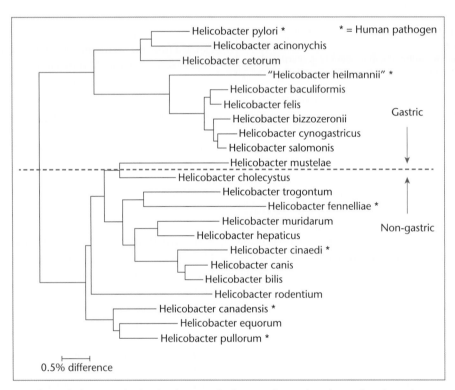

Figure 22.3 Phylogenetic tree of 22 *Helicobacter* species showing the separation between the gastric and enterohepatic species.

Acquisition **in adulthood** is uncommon although transfer between spouses can occur. After eradication of *H. pylori*, re-infection is uncommon in developed countries (1 to 2% p.a.) but quite common in developing countries (30% p.a.)[7].

Pathogenesis and disease associations

In the acute phase *H. pylori* colonises the entire gastric mucosa and liberates cytokines particularly **interleukins IL8 and IL1β** Acid secretion is impaired so that the acute phase is called "gastritis with **hypochlorhydria**". Peptic ulcers do not usually occur in the acute phase, although a mild vomiting illness can occur, and within two weeks the gastric mucosa is infiltrated with **polymorphs and mononuclear cells**. A transient IgM **antibody response** is seen but after three weeks IgG (almost 100% of cases) and IgA (about 80% of cases) can be detected in serum.

In Western countries 60% of *H. pylori* strains secrete **cytotoxins (CagA and VacA)** which increase the risk of **peptic ulcer** or, in later life, **gastric cancer**. The diseases caused by *H. pylori* are related to the presence of a more vigorous inflammatory response when the toxins are present (Table 22.1).

Adenocarcinoma of the stomach occurs in 1–5% of individuals who have lifelong *H. pylori*, usually starting after the fifth decade of life. The etiology is probably related to lifelong chronic gastritis which leads to atrophy and intestinal metaplasia followed by malignant transformation of **bone marrow-derived stem cells** [8].

B cell lymphoma of the stomach is a rare malignancy which affects the mucosa associated lymphoid tissue (MALT-lymphoma). This tumour goes into clinical remission in 60% of cases when *H. pylori* is eradicated.

Causes and differential diagnosis

H. pylori is most commonly diagnosed non-invasively with **IgG antibody serology**. However serology should not be used

for confirmation of cure after treatment as IgG levels decline slowly. The **urea breath test** (UBT) is a highly accurate diagnostic test whereby the patient swallows urea labelled with C^{13} or C^{14}. If *H. pylori* is present, the urea is split into CO_2 and NH_3 and labelled CO_2 appears in the breath. The UBT only detects urease from live *H. pylori* organisms so it can be used for initial diagnosis and screening, confirmation of serology or of eradication after treatment. The UBT should be performed at least 4 weeks after completing antibiotic therapy. It is important that the patient does not take a **proton pump inhibitor** (PPI) prior to the test as they can cause a negative UBT in about 30% of patients. The detection of *H. pylori* antigens in feces is useful for diagnosing *H. pylori* infection, especially in pediatric populations.

The **sensitivity and specificity** of the various diagnostic tests is given in Table 22.2.

If an endoscopy is being performed, *H. pylori* can easily be diagnosed invasively by studying at least two gastric antral biopsy specimens. Histology stained with hematoxylin and eosin (H&E) stain usually shows **chronic gastritis**

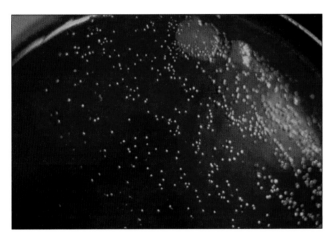

Figure 22.4 *H. pylori* colonies on the surface of a blood agar plate.

Table 22.1 Bacterial and host factors affecting gastroduodenal pathogenesis

H. pylori		Host
Conserved:	Urease	Acid secretion
	Flagella	Mucus production
	Adhesins	Epithelial barrier
Variable:	Cag A toxin	Lewis antigens (blood group)
	VacA toxin	Cytokine polymorphisms
	Bab A adhesin	

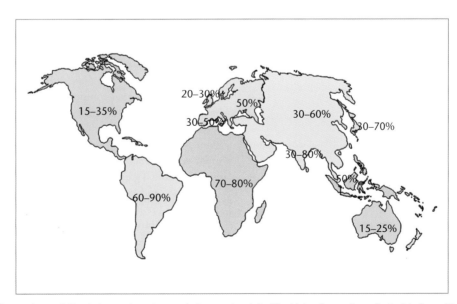

Figure 22.5 Worldwide prevalence of *H. pylori* – numbers show typical ranges in adults. The higher figure often reflects data from elderly people, immigrants or lower socioeconomic groups.

Table 22.2 The sensitivity and specificity of diagnostic tests for *H. pylori*

Diagnostic method	Sensitivity (%)	Specificity (%)	Notes
Non-invasive			
IgG serology	95	85	
Urea breath test	95	98	
Fecal antigen test	93	95	
Invasive			
Histology	93	99	Requires expert histopathologist
Rapid urease test	92	98	
Bacterial culture	80	100	Allows antimicrobial susceptibility testing

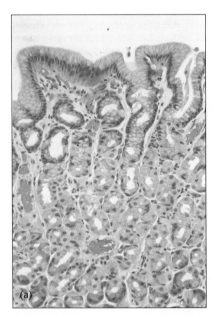 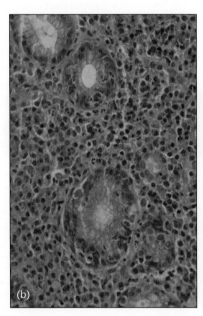 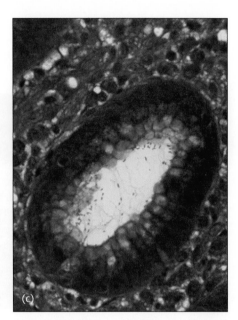

Figure 22.6 Histology of (a) normal gastric mucosa, (b) active gastritis and (c) *H. pylori*-infected gastric mucosa. (Reproduced from Talley NJ *et al.* (ed), *Practical Gastroenterology and Hepatology*, Esophagus and Stomach. Oxford: Wiley-Blackwell, 2010.)

(Figure 22.6). A second biopsy sample can be tested with a **rapid urease test** whereby the tissue is placed into a reactive test, e.g. a gel containing urea, and a colour change is noted as ammonia is generated and the pH rises allowing an immediate diagnosis in the endoscopy room [9].

Culture of *H. pylori* is of value when patients have failed one or more eradication therapies and antibiotic susceptibilities can be determined.

Therapy

H. pylori is **almost universally sensitive** to amoxicillin, tetracycline or bismuth (e.g. bismuth-subsalicylate (Pepto-Bismol) or bismuth subcitrate (DeNol)). As such, these compounds form the basis of most treatments (see Table 22.3). Even when treatments fail, *H. pylori* does not usually develop resistance to these antibacterial agents, therefore they can be reused repeatedly in combination with other antimicrobials.

H. pylori is **initially susceptible t**o metronidazole, clarithromycin, quinolones and rifamycins although, when treatment fails, the post-treatment isolate of *H. pylori* is found to be resistant. PPIs are essential components of treatment because antibiotics are more effective at neutral pH.

Eradication of *H. pylori* usually consists of a 7–14 day treatment with a PPI plus two antibiotics given concurrently. The **most widely used treatment** is twice daily doses of 20 mg esomeprazole, 1 g amoxicillin, and 500 mg clarithromycin [10]. In Australia and Europe this treatment is given for 7 days and in the USA for 10–14 days. In countries with a high usage of macrolides, the cure rate of the standard *H. pylori* "triple therapy" has declined in recent years to 75%.

In order to raise cure rates without increasing side effects, **sequential therapy** can be used, whereby a PPI is given for 10 days but in the first 5 days of therapy only amoxicillin is given, switching to a combination of clarithromycin and tinidazole from day 6 to 10 [11].

Table 22.3 Treatment for *H. pylori*

Treatment			Duration	Cure rate
Standard initial therapy				
PPI (e.g., esomeprazole)	20 mg	bid		
Amoxicillin	1 g	bid		
Clarithromycin	500 mg	bid		
Penicillin allergic patients:				
Substitute amoxicillin with Metronidazole	500 mg	bid	7–14 days	<80%
Bismuth-based therapy				
Bismuth subsalicylate/subcitrate	120 mg	qid		
Tetracycline	500 mg	qid		
Metronidazole	250 mg	qid		
PPI	20 mg	bid		
OR Ranitidine	150 mg	bid	10–14 days	>80%
Sequential therapy				
PPI (e.g., pantoprazole)	40 mg	bid		
Amoxicillin	1 g	bid		
Clarithromycin	500 mg	bid		
Tinidazole	500 mg	bid		89% [11]
Salvage therapy				
PPI		bid		
Amoxicillin	1 g	bid		
Quinolone (e.g., levofloxacin)	500 mg	bid	10 days	87% [13]
OR				
PPI (e.g. rabeprazole)	20 mg	bid		
Quinolone (e.g., levofloxacin)	500 mg	daily		
Rifabutin	300 mg	daily	7 days	91% [12]

Treatment failures can be retreated with higher doses of amoxicillin and PPI supplemented by quinolones and rifabutin [12,13] and/or furazolidone.

Who to diagnose and treat

For dyspepsia in young patients who do not have a significant risk of gastric cancer (such as persons less than 50 years in Western countries) a "**test and treat**" strategy is used. Typically, the patient has diagnosis with serology and/or UBT. If the test is positive, the general practitioner prescribes *H. pylori* eradication therapy. One month after treatment the patient undergoes a follow-up UBT to confirm absence of *H. pylori* [14,15].

When treatment has failed on two occasions or if a patient continues to have chronic or worsening symptoms after *H. pylori* treatment, further management is best done by a gastroenterologist who can perform an endoscopy or prescribe specialist *H. pylori* treatment. **Relatives of patients with gastric cancer** should be screened for *H. pylori* since cancer is more common in this group. There are also non-GI diseases possibly related to *H. pylori* [16]. In the author's opinion any chronic illness for which the etiology is uncertain and for which a simple treatment or cure is not possible, could be influenced by *H. pylori* infection.

References

1. Figura N, Bianciardi L. Helicobacters were discovered in Italy in 1892. An episode in the scientific life of an eclectic pathologist, Giulio Bizzozero. In: Marshall B, editor. *Helicobacter pioneers: Firsthand accounts from the scientists who discovered Helicobacters, 1892–1982.* Melbourne: Blackwell Science Asia; 2002. p. 1–13.

2. Steer HW, Colin-Jones DG. Mucosal changes in gastric ulceration and their response to carbenoxolone sodium. *Gut.* 1975; 16(8):590–597.

3. Marshall BJ, Warren JR. Unidentified curved bacilli in the stomach of patients with gastritis and peptic ulceration. *Lancet.* 1984;323(8390):1311–1315.

4. Weyermann M, Adler G, Brenner H, Rothenbacher D. The mother as source of *Helicobacter pylori* infection. *Epidemiology.* 2006;17(3):332–334.

5. Perry S, de la Luz Sanchez M, Yang S, Haggerty TD, Hurst P, Perez-Perez G, et al. Gastroenteritis and transmission of *Helicobacter pylori* infection in households. *Emerg Infect Dis.* 2006;12(11): 1701–1708.

6. Ahmed KS, Khan AA, Ahmed I, Tiwari SK, Habeeb A, Ahi JD, et al. Impact of household hygiene and water source on the prevalence and transmission of *Helicobacter pylori*: a South Indian perspective. *Singapore Med J.* 2007;48(6):543–549.

7. Soto G, Bautista CT, Roth DE, Gilman RH, Velapatino B, Ogura M, et al. *Helicobacter pylori* reinfection is common in Peruvian

adults after antibiotic eradication therapy. *J Infect Dis*. 2003; 188(9):1263–1275.

8. Houghton J, Stoicov C, Nomura S, Rogers AB, Carlson J, Li H, *et al*. Gastric cancer originating from bone marrow-derived cells. *Science*. 2004;306(5701):1568–1571.

9. Marshall BJ, Warren JR, Francis GJ, Langton SR, Goodwin CS, Blincow ED. Rapid urease test in the management of *Campylobacter pyloridis*-associated gastritis. *Am J Gastroenterol*. 1987; 82(3):200–210.

10. Lind T, Megraud F, Unge P, Bayerdorffer E, O'Morain C, Spiller R, *et al*. The MACH2 study: role of omeprazole in eradication of *Helicobacter pylori* with 1-week triple therapies. *Gastroenterology*. 1999;116(2):248–253.

11. Vaira D, Zullo A, Vakil N, Gatta L, Ricci C, Perna F, *et al*. Sequential therapy versus standard triple-drug therapy for *Helicobacter pylori* eradication: a randomized trial. *Ann Intern Med*. 2007; 146(8):556–563.

12. Wong WM, Gu Q, Lam SK, Fung FM, Lai KC, Hu WH, *et al*. Randomized controlled study of rabeprazole, levofloxacin and rifabutin triple therapy vs. quadruple therapy as second-line treatment for *Helicobacter pylori* infection. *Aliment Pharmacol Ther*. 2003;17(4):553–560.

13. Saad RJ, Schoenfeld P, Kim HM, Chey WD. Levofloxacin-based triple therapy versus bismuth-based quadruple therapy for persistent *Helicobacter pylori* infection: a meta-analysis. *Am J Gastroenterol*. 2006;101(3):488–496.

14. Chey WD, Wong BC. American College of Gastroenterology guideline on the management of *Helicobacter pylori* infection. *Am J Gastroenterol*. 2007;102(8):1808–1825.

15. Malfertheiner P, Megraud F, O'Morain C, Bazzoli F, El-Omar E, Graham D, *et al*. Current concepts in the management of *Helicobacter pylori* infection: the Maastricht III Consensus Report. *Gut*. 2007 Jun;56(6):772–781.

16. Suzuki H, Marshall BJ, Hibi T. Overview: *Helicobacter pylori* and extragastric disease. *Int J Hematol*. 2006 Nov;84(4):291–300.

CHAPTER 23

Being on nonsteroidal anti-inflammatory drugs

Neville D. Yeomans[1] and Francis K. L. Chan[2]

[1]University of Western Sydney, Penrith, NSW, Australia
[2]The Chinese University of Hong Kong, Hong Kong SAR, China

KEY POINTS

- Erosions and ulcers are very common in patients on NSAIDs, including low-dose aspirin
- The damage mainly affects the stomach and duodenum, but enteric, colonic and esophageal injury is also quite frequent
- Dyspepsia occurs in many patients, but most often is unrelated to the presence of ulcers
- COX-2 selective NSAIDs produce *less* ulceration and ulcer complications, but whether they cause *more* cardiovascular adverse events than traditional NSAIDs is currently a "hot topic"

Introduction

Nonsteroidal anti-inflammatory drugs (NSAIDs) have been used for several thousand years, ever since the therapeutic properties of the salicylate-containing willow bark were recognized. Recently, their use has reached unprecedented levels – as the greater longevity of populations increases the burden of painful degenerative joint disease, and as the recognition of the anti-platelet and anti-cancer properties of aspirin creates new uses for this old drug.

This chapter deals with the features, causation and epidemiology of the adverse effects of NSAIDs on the GI tract. It does not discuss their treatment, which is dealt with elsewhere in this book under each individual disease.

What symptoms and disorders do NSAIDs cause?

The problems NSAIDs cause in the gastrointestinal (GI) tract are listed in Table 23.1.

Erosions are shallow abrasions that do not extend deeper in the wall than the mucosa. Some are only visible with microscopy, but many are seen at endoscopy as areas of denuded surface a millimeter or so in size (Figure 23.1a). They normally do not cause symptoms and heal in a matter of days without ever having come to clinical attention.

Ulcers (Figure 23.1b) are deeper and larger lesions that arise when one or more erosions enlarges instead of healing, and extends down to the submucosa or muscularis of the gastric or duodenal wall. The more common site for NSAID-induced ulcers is the stomach, although they also occur in the duodenum.

Dyspepsia (epigastric discomfort or pain) is another common consequence of NSAID treatment and is also experienced (but less frequently) when patients take cyclooxygenase (COX)-2 selective NSAIDs.

Imaging of the small intestine with either capsule endoscopy (Chapter 128) or enteroscopy (Chapter 127) shows that erosions and ulceration are also common in the small bowel mucosa [1]. An example of an intestinal ulcer is shown in Figure 23.2.

There is some evidence that NSAIDs may also aggravate gastrointestinal reflux disease, based on a case-control study of patients with heartburn and one prospective cohort study [2,3].

NSAIDs may also exacerbate colitis, as shown in case-control studies as well as anecdotal case reports. There is some uncertainty about whether this also occurs with selective COX-2 inhibitors.

Hepatitic reactions have been described uncommonly with a number of NSAIDs, including COX-2 inhibitors. These have rarely been serious.

How common are these problems?

Table 23.2 sets out prevalences and incidences for ulcers, erosions and their complications, together with estimates of relative risk for some of the other GI adverse consequences of NSAIDs. The prevalence of small intestinal lesions given in the table represents a composite prevalence for large erosions plus frank ulcers, since these cannot be reliably distinguished from each other at present by capsule endoscopy.

Textbook of Clinical Gastroenterology and Hepatology, Second Edition. Edited by C. J. Hawkey, Jaime Bosch, Joel E. Richter, Guadalupe Garcia-Tsao, Francis K. L. Chan.
© 2012 Blackwell Publishing Ltd. Published 2012 by Blackwell Publishing Ltd.

Table 23.1 Adverse gastrointestinal effects of NSAIDs

- Gastric and duodenal erosions
- Gastric and duodenal ulcers
- NSAID dyspepsia
- Small bowel erosions and ulcers
- Exacerbation/induction of GERD?
- Exacerbation of colitis
- Drug-induced hepatitis

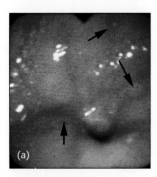 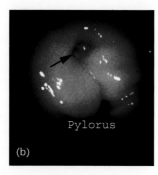

Figure 23.1 (a) Antral erosions in vicinity of pylorus in a patient taking aspirin for several days (arrows). (b) Prepyloric ulcer (arrow) in a patient who had been taking a nonselective NSAID for several months.

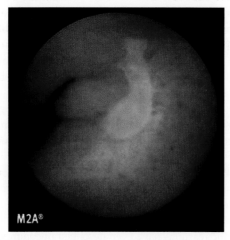

Figure 23.2 Ulcer in small intestine, visualized by M2A™ capsule endoscopy, in a patient taking nonselective NSAIDs. (Photo by courtesy of Given Imaging Ltd.)

Pathophysiology

The mechanism of NSAID injury is probably multifactorial, but inhibition of prostaglandin synthesis via blockade of cyclooxygenase (COX) is a major contributor. Constitutive production of prostaglandins in the gastric mucosa is mainly due to the COX-1 isoenzyme, and this was the rationale for developing highly selective COX-2 inhibitors in order to spare the COX-1 generation of gastric prostaglandins. The story is a little more complicated, though, since animal studies indicate a need to block both COX-1 and COX-2 before substantial gastric damage results [4]. There is also some evidence for direct damage to gastric cells by some NSAIDs, especially aspirin, as they

Table 23.2 Frequency of gastrointestinal (GI) events in patients taking NSAIDs

GI event	Prevalence, incidence or relative risk	Comments
Gastric erosions	50–90% point prevalence (including low-dose aspirin) [17,18]	Much less common with COX-2 inhibitors
Gastric or duodenal ulcers	12–30% point prevalence [19]	Reduced by >70% with COX-2 inhibitors [13]
Ulcer complications (hemorrhage, perforation)	1–2 per 100 patient years [20]	Much higher if prior ulcer complication. Reduced by median of about 60% with COX-2 inhibitors [13]
Small intestinal erosions/ulcers	~25% significant damage	Based on capsule endoscopy data [21]. Substantially less frequent with a COX-2 inhibitor [22]
Dyspepsia	10–35%	Controlled trials and observational studies [23,24]
Gastroesophageal reflux disease (GERD)	Relative risk ~2	Based on case-control study [2]
Exacerbation of colitis	Relative risk ~2	From case-control studies and case reports [25]
Hepatitic reactions	<1% clinically significant LFT elevations for most NSAIDs; severe liver injury in <1 per 10 000	

traverse the lumen. For most NSAIDs this is a minor component of damage, since rectal and even transcutaneous administration still produce gastroduodenal erosions and ulcers.

The low pH of the gastric lumen appears to play an important part in gastric and probably duodenal injury [5], and the success of proton pump inhibitors in reducing NSAID gastric and duodenal ulcers in humans is presumably a manifestation of this [6]. The mechanisms of damage to the small intestine and colon are rather less well understood; however, inhibition of COX enzymes appears to still play a part but gastric acid is presumably of no importance.

The life-threatening complication of ulcer hemorrhage may be aggravated by impaired platelet aggregation when dual COX-inhibitors are used. This is likely to be most important with aspirin, because of its long-lasting antiplatelet effect.

The mechanism of NSAID dyspepsia is poorly understood. There is only a weak correlation with the macroscopic damage, although some suggestion that acid diffusing back into the mucosa as the result of the widespread microscopic damage activates nociceptive nerves in some people [7].

Contributing causes (risk factors) for NSAID ulcers and erosions

A number of factors are now known to contribute to the risk of NSAID gastric and duodenal ulcers and their complications. Much less is known about risk factors for the other GI adverse events of NSAIDs. It is useful to divide these risk factors into those that relate to the NSAID itself, and those that are intrinsic to the particular patient.

NSAID-related risk factors

The class of NSAID is one important determinant. Although there has been some debate about how much safer are the COX-2 inhibitors (see the section "Current Controversies" below), there is little doubt that overall there are fewer ulcers and fewer complications produced by the coxibs than the classical NSAIDs, so long as low-dose aspirin is not added in as well (to essentially reconstitute a dual COX inhibitor) [8].

Dose of NSAID is the second important determinant of risk. This has been particularly well shown for ibuprofen, where the very low end of the marketed dosage scale carries little more risk than placebo. Aspirin damage is also broadly dose related, but doses even as low as 75 mg daily still carry a significant ulcer and ulcer-bleeding risk [9].

Risk factors in the individual patient
Age

Older patients are at increased risk of NSAID ulcers, and also at increased risk of succumbing to an ulcer bleed. The increase with age is curvilinear upwards but there is no particular age at which a sudden step up in risk occurs, so it is not practicable to define one particular age as the dividing point between low and high risk.

Past ulcer history

A history of previous peptic ulcer increases the risk of an NSAID ulcer and ulcer hemorrhage several fold. The risk is particularly high if the patient recently had a **bleeding** ulcer whilst on NSAIDs – amounting to almost 20% recurrent bleeding in 6 months in one important study [10].

Helicobacter pylori

There has been controversy about whether coexistent *H. pylori* infection is a risk factor for NSAID gastric ulcers, but the evidence does support an interaction between *H. pylori* and NSAIDs in causing duodenal ulcers.

Other co-administered drugs

Corticosteroids modestly increase the risk of NSAID ulcer complications. Aspirin can be thought of as effectively increasing the total NSAID dose (and hence ulcer risk), whereas other anticoagulants and antiplatelet agents increase the risk of NSAID ulcers bleeding without increasing the underlying rate of ulceration. In the case of warfarin-like anticoagulants, the relative risk for bleeding in patients taking these in combination with an NSAID can be as high as 20-fold compared with those taking neither of these therapies.

Symptom complexes

Dyspepsia – described as burning, discomfort or pain in the upper abdomen – is common during NSAID therapy. Several studies have shown that it is less common during treatment with COX-2 inhibitors. There is nothing very specific about these symptoms, which are similar to those described by some patients with peptic ulcer and by patients not taking NSAIDs who are labeled as having non-ulcer dyspepsia.

These symptoms are a poor predictor of whether the patient has visible injury in the stomach or duodenum. Erosions are usually asymptomatic, as indeed are many frank ulcers in NSAID users. However new dyspepsia, arising after patients have been taking NSAIDs for some time, does give some indication (albeit with sensitivity and specificity of only about 50%) that an ulcer may have developed.

The symptoms of **hematemesis** or **melena** in patients taking NSAIDs will be readily recognized, and point to the likelihood of a gastric, duodenal or small intestinal ulcer in roughly that order of frequency. Similarly, the development of sudden, severe epigastric pain, with features of shock and signs of peritonismus, will immediately raise the suspicion of peptic ulcer perforation.

Symptoms of **anemia** developing in patients taking NSAIDs should raise the possibility of chronic blood loss, which can occur from erosions as well as ulcers, and again may originate from the upper gut or mid gut or both. Of course more sinister causes such as bleeding from a colonic neoplasm normally need to be ruled out.

Diagnosis

The investigation of NSAID dyspepsia rationally depends on when the dyspepsia develops, and whether there are any associated features such as overt bleeding or anemia to point to ulcer development. Dyspepsia that begins **immediately** with the commencement of an NSAID is very unlikely to be due to development of a new ulcer. Investigation of such patients is therefore usually not needed. In practice, clinicians will often stop or switch NSAIDs in such patients, and recent data show that treatment with a proton pump inhibitor can also be effective in reducing dyspepsia [11].

On the other hand, it is important to remember that ulcers can develop quickly – even a week is sufficient – so dyspepsia developing a little after the onset of NSAID treatment may warrant gastroscopy, and the onset of bleeding **certainly** warrants upper gastrointestinal endoscopy. Figure 23.3 illustrates the endoscopic appearance of an ulcer with active bleeding.

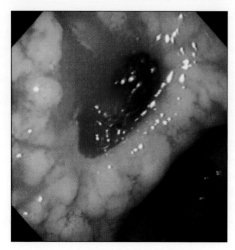

Figure 23.3 Bleeding ulcer in a patient taking NSAIDs.

Capsule endoscopy (Chapter 128) can be useful for investigating the patient with NSAID-associated anemia who has had negative upper and lower gastrointestinal endoscopy.

Current controversies and their future resolution

The main area of recent controversy has been about the benefits and safety of the COX-2 inhibitors. Initial randomized controlled trials (RCTs) comparing COX-2 selective with conventional NSAIDs showed many less ulcers developing over the first month or two in those randomized to the former. However, one large RCT failed to show a significant reduction in the incidence of ulcer complications among patients receiving celecoxib compared with patients receiving diclofenac [12]. This may have been partly due to many patients also taking low dose aspirin. A recent meta-analysis has found that the majority of studies confirm a lower (by about 60%) risk of ulcer complications in patients taking a COX-2 inhibitor [13].

The major area of uncertainty now is whether COX-2 selective NSAIDs carry a higher risk of cardiovascular events than nonselective NSAIDs. In one large trial, a subgroup analysis found a higher incidence of myocardial infarction in those receiving rofecoxib compared with naproxen [14]. A lively debate ensued about whether this was due to an imbalance ensuing between pro- and anti-thrombotic mechanisms at the level of the vascular endothelium, or a protective effect of naproxen, or simply chance. Negative findings in some other studies appeared to indicate one of the latter. However, rofecoxib was withdrawn by the manufacturer when a long-term study of rofecoxib versus placebo for preventing precancerous colonic polyp development showed a near doubling of the rate of myocardial infarction after about 18 months [15]. Although very similar results occurred in one near identical study with celecoxib, that coxib remains on the market. A flurry of case-control data then emerged showing that conventional NSAIDS appear to also increase the risk of myocardial infarction, to a broadly similar extent. One large cardiovascular outcome RCT is currently underway to try to settle the question of whether a coxib carries the same or different cardiovascular risk compared to two commonly used nonselective NSAIDs [16].

References
1. Graham D, Qureshi WA, Willingham K, *et al*. A controlled study of NSAID-induced small bowel injury using video capsule endoscopy. *Gastroenterology*. 2003;124(Suppl 1):A19.
2. Kotzan J, Wade W, Yu HH. Assessing NSAID prescription use as a predisposing factor for gastroesophageal reflux disease in a Medicaid population. *Pharm Res*. 2001;18(9):1367–1372.
3. Kulig M, Leodolter A, Vieth M, *et al*. Quality of life in relation to symptoms in patients with gastro-oesophageal reflux disease – an analysis based on the ProGERD initiative. *Aliment Pharmacol Ther*. 2003;18:767–776.
4. Wallace JL, McKnight W, Reuter BK, *et al*. NSAID-induced gastric damage in rats: requirement for inhibition of both cyclooxygenase 1 and 2. *Gastroenterology*. 2000;119:706–714.
5. Elliott SL, Ferris RJ, Giraud AS, *et al*. Indomethacin damage to rat gastric mucosa is markedly dependent on luminal pH. *Clin Exper Pharmacol Physiol*. 1996;23:432–434.
6. Yeomans ND, Tulassay Z, Juhász L, *et al*. A comparison of omeprazole with ranitidine for ulcers associated with nonsteroidal antiinflammatory drugs. *N Engl J Med*. 1998;338:719–726.
7. Holtmann G, Gschossmann J, Buenger L, *et al*. Do changes in visceral sensory function determine the development of dyspepsia during treatment with aspirin? *Gastroenterology*. 2002;123:1451–1458.
8. Rostom A, Moayyedi P, Hunt R, Canadian Association of Gastroenterology Consensus Group. Canadian consensus guidelines on long-term nonsteroidal anti-inflammatory drug therapy and the need for gastroprotection: benefits versus risks. *Aliment Pharmacol Ther*. 2009;29:481–496.
9. Weil J, Colin-Jones D, Langman M, *et al*. Prophylactic aspirin and risk of peptic ulcer bleeding. *Br Med J*. 1995;310:827–830.
10. Chan FKL, Chung SCS, Suen BY, *et al*. Preventing recurrent upper gastrointestinal bleeding in patients with *Helicobacter pylori* infection who are taking low-dose aspirin or naproxen. *N Engl J Med*. 2001;344:967–973.
11. Hawkey CJ, Talley NJ, Yeomans ND, *et al*. Improvements with esomeprazole in upper gastrointestinal symptoms in patients taking non-steroidal anti-inflammatory drugs, including selective COX-2 inhibitors. *Am J Gastroenterol*. 2005;100:1028–1036.
12. Silverstein FE, Faich G, Goldstein JL, *et al*. Gastrointestinal toxicity with celecoxib vs nonsteroidal anti-inflammatory drugs for osteoarthritis and rheumatoid arthritis: the CLASS study: A randomized controlled trial. Celecoxib long-term arthritis safety study. *JAMA*. 2000;284:1247–1255.
13. Rostom A, Muir K, Dube C, *et al*. Gastrointestinal safety of cyclooxygenase-2 inhibitors: a Cochrane Collaboration systematic review. *Clin Gastroenterol Hepatol*. 2007;5:818–828.
14. Bombardier C, Laine L, Reicin A, *et al*. Comparison of upper gastrointestinal toxicity of rofecoxib and naproxen in patients with rheumatoid arthritis. *N Engl J Med*. 2000;343:1520–1528.
15. Baron JA, Sandler RS, Bresalier RS, *et al*. Cardiovascular events associated with rofecoxib: final analysis of the APPROVe trial. *Lancet*. 2008;372:1756–1764.

16. Becker MC, Wang TH, Wisniewski L, *et al*. Rationale, design, and governance of Rationale, design and governance of prospective randomized evaluation of celecoxib integrated safety versus ibuprofen or naproxen (PRECISION), a cardiovascular endpoint trial of non-steroidal anti-inflammatory agents in patients with arthritis. *Am Heart J.* 2009;157:606–612.

17. Elliott SL, Yeomans ND, Buchanan RRC, *et al*. Efficacy of 12 months' misoprostol as prophylaxis against NSAID- induced gastric ulcers: a placebo controlled trial. *Scand J Gastroenterol.* 1994;23:171–176.

18. Hart J, Hawkey CJ, Lanas A, *et al*. Predictors of gastroduodenal erosions in patients taking low-dose aspirin. *Aliment Pharm Ther.* 2010;31:143–149.

19. Raskin JB. Gastrointestinal effects of nonsteroidal anti-inflammatory therapy. *Am J Med.* 1999;106:3S–12S.

20. Fries JF, Williams CA, Bloch DA, *et al*. Nonsteroidal anti-inflammatory drug-associated gastropathy: incidence and risk factor models. *Am J Med.* 1991;91:213–222.

21. Qureshi WA, Wu J, Demarco D, *et al*. Visible small-intestinal mucosal injury in chronic NSAID users. *Clin Gastroenterol Hepatol.* 2005;3:55–59.

22. Goldstein JL, Eisen GM, Lewis B, *et al*. Small bowel mucosal injury is reduced in healthy subjects treated with celecoxib compared with ibuprofen plus omeprazole, as assessed by video capsule endoscopy. *Aliment Pharmacol Ther.* 2007;25:1211–1222.

23. Emery P, Zeidler H, Kvien TK, *et al*. Celecoxib versus diclofenac in long-term management of rheumatoid arthritis: randomised double-blind comparison. *Lancet.* 1999;354:2106–2111.

24. Hollenz M, Stolte M, Leodolter A, *et al*. NSAID-associated dyspepsia and ulcers: a prospective cohort study in primary care. *Dig Dis.* 2006;24:189–194.

25. Evans JMM, McMahon AD, Murray FE *et al*. Non-steroidal anti-inflammatory drugs are associated with emergency admission to hospital for colitis due to inflammatory bowel disease. *Gut.* 1997;40:619–622.

CHAPTER 24
Gastrointestinal problems in the elderly

James Frith and Julia L. Newton
Newcastle University, Newcastle upon Tyne, UK

KEY POINTS

- Gastrointestinal problems are very common in the elderly, including:
  - Dysphagia
  - Gastroesophageal reflux disease (GERD)
  - Esophageal dysmotility
  - Esophageal and gastric cancer
  - Peptic ulcer disease
  - Gastric atrophy
  - Small bowel bacterial overgrowth (due to dysmotility)
  - Colonic cancer
  - Constipation
  - Diarrhea
  - Diverticular disease
  - *Clostridium difficile* diarrhea
- Irritable bowel rarely presents in old age – exclude colorectal cancer
- Bleeding peptic ulcer remains common and has a high mortality in the elderly
- Reasons for gastrointestinal disease in the elderly include:
  - Impaired mucosal defences and repair mechanisms
  - Increased prevalence of *Helicobacter pylori*
  - Use of non-steroidal anti-inflammatory drugs
- Undernutrition in older people is common. Reasons are not fully understood but include:
  - Decreased food intake
  - Gastrointestinal diseases
  - Maldigestion
  - Malabsorption
  - Hypermetabolism

Introduction

Older people are an increasing proportion of the population and, although there are no gastrointestinal diseases specific to older people, many symptoms and diseases become more common in older age groups. As the population ages, the number of older people consulting with gastrointestinal symptoms will increase. The challenges of managing gastrointestinal disease in older people are outlined in Table 24.1. Evidence-based studies examining the management of gastrointestinal problems in older people are rare, and in most of the current literature older people are specifically excluded from studies. As a result, a great deal of clinical practice in the elderly is extrapolated from studies in the young. In this chapter changes in gastrointestinal physiology in the elderly are reviewed and details specific to the diagnosis, investigation, and management of gastrointestinal symptoms and diseases in older people are discussed. Further details of individual conditions should be sought in relevant chapters.

Prevalence

Nearly 50% of older people suffer from gastrointestinal symptoms. The elderly are more likely to consult a doctor about their symptoms, which has implications as those with gastrointestinal symptoms have significant healthcare utilization and poorer quality of life. Abdominal symptoms in the majority of older people are self-limiting and frequently relapsing. Despite this, the prognosis of all symptoms appears good [1].

Investigations

Taking a **history** from an elderly patient can be challenging and examination requires an open mind [2]. In terms of **investigation**, older people tolerate upper gastrointestinal endoscopy and colonoscopy well (see Chapter 119) and should not be denied the benefits of diagnostic investigation [3]. It might sometimes be felt that seeking a diagnosis is not appropriate if ultimately little can be offered in the way of treatment. However, older people also tolerate **surgery** well; even when extensive curative surgery is not appropriate, palliation of symptoms might be possible.

Nutrition

Older people are at increased risk of **impaired nutrition** and nutritional deficiency, although the absolute prevalence depends on the population studied and definitions used. It is unclear whether aging alone results in dysfunction of the gastrointestinal tract leading to undernutrition, or whether undernutrition in older people points to another disease or simply

---

Textbook of Clinical Gastroenterology and Hepatology, Second Edition. Edited by C. J. Hawkey, Jaime Bosch, Joel E. Richter, Guadalupe Garcia-Tsao, Francis K. L. Chan.
© 2012 Blackwell Publishing Ltd. Published 2012 by Blackwell Publishing Ltd.

Table 24.1 Why gastroenterology in an aging population is more difficult

- Young people with gastrointestinal diseases become old
- Many gastrointestinal diseases increase in prevalence in the elderly
- Gastrointestinal diseases can present for the first time in older people
- Older people can present nonspecifically
- The elderly may not be suitable for investigations that are routine in younger patients
- Polypharmacy is common in older people
- Older people are more sensitive to the effect of drugs
- Older people may not be considered suitable for surgery
- Older people have a high prevalence of co-morbidity
- Diseases in older people frequently have a different clinical course

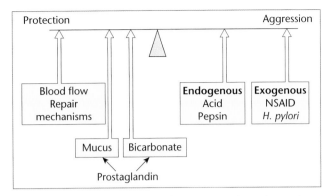

Figure 24.2 Disruption of the balance between aggressive and protective mechanisms in the human stomach leads to pathology. (This figure was published in *Clinical Gastroenterology and Hepatology*, Wilfred M. Weinstein, Christopher J. Hawkey, Jaime Bosch, Gastrointestinal problems in the elderly, Pages 1–6, Copyright Elsevier, 2005.)

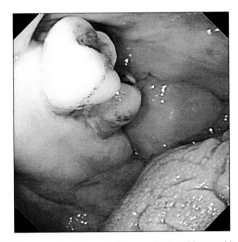

Figure 24.1 Poor oral health. Inside the mouth of an 89-year-old man with some of his own teeth remaining.

reflects social or physical conditions such as inability to chew, poverty, and social isolation. Poor **oral health** (Figure 24.1) has been consistently correlated with malnutrition and, although the prevalence of edentulousness among older independent adults is projected to decrease, because of demographic changes the absolute number of edentulous elderly will remain high [4]. (See also Chapters 1, 15, and 138.)

Gastrointestinal mucosal protection

In the human gastrointestinal tract there is a balance between aggressive factors and mucosal protective mechanisms; when this equilibrium is disrupted, pathology results (Figure 24.2). There are no age-related increases in the endogenous aggressors: acid and pepsin. Therefore, the imbalance that leads to diseases seen more commonly in older people, such as cancer or ulceration, is due to an age-associated impairment of mucosal protective mechanisms (see Figure 24.3).

Prostaglandins Prostaglandins are molecules involved in mucosal protection, via mucus, bicarbonate secretion, and blood flow. One study has suggested that their concentration may be reduced with advancing age [5]. Medications such as nonsteroidal anti-inflammatory drugs (NSAIDs), which also

inhibit the production of prostaglandins, are used widely by older people, making them particularly vulnerable (see Chapter 32).

Mucus Mucus covers the gastrointestinal tract with an adherent gel, with some barrier properties and a "sloppy" luminal layer, which acts as a lubricant (Figure 24.3).The amount of mucus, its quality, and the number of mucus-producing cells in the stomach are reduced with age and *H. pylori* infection [6], and may contribute to the risk of ulcer development in older people.

Bicarbonate Bicarbonate neutralizes gastric acid and inactivates pepsin by increasing pH. Bicarbonate secretion may be lower in the elderly, and hence the ability of the gastric mucosa to produce bicarbonate in response to prostaglandins is impaired [7].

Repair mechanisms In animals aging is associated with decreased reparative ability in the gastric mucosa, and with delays in both resolution of mucosal injury and regeneration of injured gastric mucosa. It is unclear whether this also occurs in the human stomach. Blood flow to an injured area is important during repair, to bring nutrients and remove waste. Reduction in blood flow alone is sufficient to cause ulceration in the mucosa and likely to contribute to human disease. In aged rats, basal gastric blood flow and flow in response to injury is reduced.

Histology and structure in the gastrointestinal tract

Changes in gastrointestinal physiology with age are summarized in Figure 24.2. **Inflammation** in the upper gastrointestinal tract increases with age, and the prevalence of gastric atrophy is commoner in older people partly, but not entirely, due to the increased prevalence of *Helicobacter pylori* in older people. Gastrointestinal **transit time** is slower in older

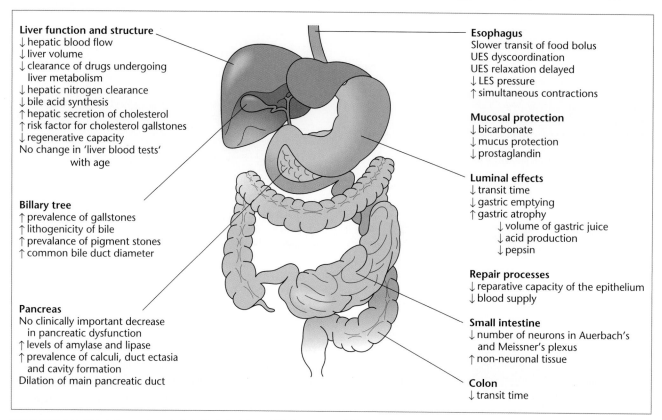

Liver function and structure
↓ hepatic blood flow
↓ liver volume
↓ clearance of drugs undergoing
    liver metabolism
↓ hepatic nitrogen clearance
↓ bile acid synthesis
↑ hepatic secretion of cholesterol
↑ risk factor for cholesterol gallstones
↓ regenerative capacity
No change in 'liver blood tests'
            with age

Billary tree
↑ prevalence of gallstones
↑ lithogenicity of bile
↑ prevalance of pigment stones
↑ common bile duct diameter

Pancreas
No clinically important decrease
    in pancreatic dysfunction
↑ levels of amylase and lipase
↑ prevalence of calculi, duct ectasia
    and cavity formation
Dilation of main pancreatic duct

Esophagus
Slower transit of food bolus
UES dyscoordination
UES relaxation delayed
↓ LES pressure
↑ simultaneous contractions

Mucosal protection
↓ bicarbonate
↓ mucus protection
↓ prostaglandin

Luminal effects
↓ transit time
↓ gastric emptying
↑ gastric atrophy
        ↓ volume of gastric juice
        ↓ acid production
        ↓ pepsin

Repair processes
↓ reparative capacity of the epithelium
↓ blood supply

Small intestine
↓ number of neurons in Auerbach's
    and Meissner's plexus
↑ non-neuronal tissue

Colon
↓ transit time

Figure 24.3 Age-related changes in gastrointestinal physiology. (This figure was published in *Clinical Gastroenterology and Hepatology*, Wilfred M. Weinstein, Christopher J. Hawkey, Jaime Bosch, Gastrointestinal problems in the elderly, Pages 1–6, Copyright Elsevier, 2005.)

people owing to age-related changes in the innervation and composition of neuronal tissue in the gut wall. This reduced transit can lead to conditions that include:

- esophageal dysmotility
- decreased gastric emptying
- diverticular disease
- constipation.

(See also Chapter 138.)

Managing common upper gastrointestinal problems in older people
Gastroesophageal reflux disease and heartburn
Gastroesophageal reflux disease (GERD) becomes more prevalent with age, peaking in the seventh decade [8]. A **non-specific presentation** is more common with regurgitation, dysphagia, respiratory problems and vomiting as well as heartburn [9]. Despite there being no increase in the severity of symptoms with advancing age [10], mucosal injury is more severe and complications are more common [9]. Many self-medicate in the community, presenting for the first time with the complications of longstanding reflux, such as **benign esophageal stricture**.

Studies specific to the **treatment** of older people are rare. In one small study patients over the age of 60 years were less likely to receive advice regarding lifestyle modification compared to those aged less than 60 years [11]. There is no evidence to recommend whether stepping up treatment according to symptoms or stepping down when symptoms have resolved, or the use of empiric treatment without endoscopy, is most appropriate in older people. In view of the tendency for atypical presentation in older people, caution suggests referral for endoscopy to exclude malignancy. (See also Chapter 27).

Peptic ulceration
Peptic ulceration is more common in the elderly (Figure 24.4). Increased **NSAID use** in older age groups is in part responsible for this. Older people with ulcers are more likely to suffer **complications** of perforation and bleeding, and, although admissions have decreased overall, in those over the age of 75 years admission rates have actually increased. Death from peptic ulceration is predominantly attributable to co-morbid disease, and so it is not surprising that the mortality rate is highest amongst older people. **Death rates** due to duodenal ulcers are higher in older men than in older women, but comparable for gastric ulcers. On average, death from peptic ulceration is 20 times greater in people over 75 years of age than in those aged 45–64 years [12]. (See also Chapter 32).

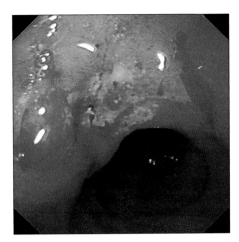

Figure 24.4 Peptic ulcer in a 67-year-old presenting with iron deficiency anemia.

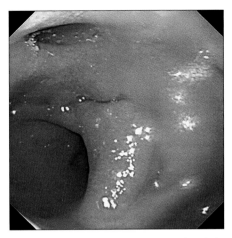

Figure 24.5 Small bowel bacterial overgrowth. View taken during gastroscopy in a 93-year-old woman with malnutrition showing a duodenal diverticulum that is causing small bowel overgrowth.

Dyspepsia

Older people report **fewer symptoms** despite having higher rates of pathology and often present atypically. Despite an increased risk of malignancy in this older group, controversy exists as to whether investigation with endoscopy should precede empirical treatment [13]. Clinical judgement may be more appropriate; in the frail elderly considered unfit for investigation, the adoption of an empiric treatment approach may be appropriate. However, age alone should not be used as a contraindication to further investigation. (See also Chapters 3 and 4).

Helicobacter pylori

There is a particularly high prevalence of *H. pylori* in older people but investigation and treatment rates are low. Some studies suggest lower success rates and increased side effects of triple therapy. However more recent studies show high success rates and a low incidence of side effects, with a sequential treatment regime [14]. Ulcer recurrence and complications are more common in older people, therefore investigation and treatment should not be denied. Moreover, successful eradication of *H. pylori* should be confirmed by a follow-up breath test. (See also Chapter 22).

Small bowel bacterial overgrowth

Risk factors for small bowel bacterial overgrowth are more common in older people (reduced motility, diverticulosis, previous surgery). **Presentation** is typically nonspecific with weight loss, weakness and lethargy, but a significant proportion of healthy older people will demonstrate bacterial overgrowth on investigation [15]. It is an under-recognized cause of **malnutrition** in older people resulting in malabsorption of nutrients and vitamins (Figure 24.5). Treatment with antibiotics should be directed to older adults demonstrating bacterial overgrowth with evidence of malabsorption [15]. (See also Chapter 42).

Managing common lower gastrointestinal problems in older people
Colonic cancer

Approximately one third of cases with colorectal cancer are aged over 80 years. Older people with colorectal cancer present with a different profile of symptoms to younger groups [16], and 1 in 5 older patients present acutely. **Irritable bowel syndrome** rarely presents for the first time in the elderly and should be a diagnosis of exclusion. **Screening** of older people by fecal occult blood (FOB) and particularly sigmoidoscopy reduces mortality [17]. Despite this, these tools are used inappropriately in those over the age of 65 years, with an overuse of FOB and underuse of sigmoidscopy.

Survival following surgery for colorectal cancer in older people is reduced. This is partly explained by the existence of more co-morbidities and a later stage at presentation. However, mortality following surgery is no greater with advancing age as a result of cancer [18]. Although treatment is generally surgical, older people are more often referred to medical or geriatric units. **Chemotherapy**, used as an adjunct to surgery (see Chapter 59), is just as successful in the older person as in the young, with up to 70% 5-year survival in selected patients over the age of 65 years [19]. Mortality from colorectal cancer remains high in those over the age of 65 years; those considered unsuitable to undergo treatment should be offered **palliation** such as stenting and radiotherapy, if appropriate, as these are successful in older people. (See also Chapters 57, 58 and 59).

Functional constipation

Functional constipation is common for many reasons including:

- dehydration
- poor diet

- inactivity
- effect of medications.

The importance of constipation should not be underestimated; it can have significant impact on physical function and quality of life. Once serious pathology has been ruled out, management generally involves the use of laxatives. This increases frequency of bowel movement, softens the stool and improves symptoms but can contribute to fecal incontinence if used inappropriately. There is currently little evidence for marked differences in effectiveness between laxatives. Further good quality trial evidence is required in the management of constipation in older people. (See also Chapters 6, 66, 68 and 69).

Clostridium difficile

Clostridium difficile causes gastrointestinal infections ranging from asymptomatic colonization to severe diarrhea, pseudomembranous colitis, and toxic megacolon. Infection with C. difficile increased 4-fold in all age groups between 1994 and 1997; however, reports in over 65-year-olds increased 6-fold over the same period, with more than 80% of cases in those aged over 65 years.

The **incidence and mortality** is highest amongst older people, who can present atypically. A history of antibiotic treatment is identifiable in virtually all patients. Once acquired, the infection may be more severe in the elderly. Older age and frailty are predictors for **recurrent disease**. The use of probiotics in this group may be restricted by the increased prevalence of heart valve abnormalities. **Colectomy** is reserved for severe cases; the outcome in the older person is controversial with conflicting results, therefore decisions should be made on an individual basis. (See also Chapters 45 and 55).

Chronic diarrhea

Chronic diarrhea is one of the most common reasons for referral to gastroenterologists. It is commoner in older people, with prevalence rates of 7–14% [20]. **Causes** of chronic diarrhea to consider in older people are shown in Table 24.2, and signs and symptoms that should initiate prompt further **investigation** are shown in Table 24.3. Mortality is greater in this group, irrespective of *clostridium difficile* infection [21]. (See also Chapter 6).

Age-related changes in the pancreas, liver, and biliary tree

Liver disease is increasing in older people, in part because of the increase in systemic diseases that affect the liver and also due to improved management of liver diseases, which enables those with liver disease to live into older age. There appear to be no liver diseases specific to older age. **Presentation and clinical course** can be more subtle, but vigilance should remain when interpreting abnormal investigations. **Serum transaminases** show no age related changes and there is no age-associated increase in mortality for people undergoing liver

Table 24.2 Differential diagnosis of diarrhea in older people

- Previous gastrointestinal surgery, particularly of the ileum and right colon
- Lack of absorptive surface – fat and carbohydrate malabsorption
- Decreased transit time
- Malabsorption of bile acids
- Bacterial overgrowth
- Previous pancreatic disease
- Systemic disease
- Thyrotoxicosis
- Parathyroid disease
- Diabetes mellitus
- Alcohol
- Drugs
- Recent overseas travel or other potential sources of infectious gastrointestinal pathogens
- Recent antibiotic use and C. *difficile* infection
- Lactase deficiency

Table 24.3 Reasons for further investigation of diarrhea in the elderly

- History of diarrhea of >3 months
- Predominantly nocturnal diarrhea
- Continuous rather than intermittent diarrhea
- Weight loss
- Steatorrhea
- Passage of malodorous pale stools
- Mucus
- Blood
- Family history – neoplastic, inflammatory bowel or celiac disease

biopsy [22]. On the whole, management of liver disease is similar in older people as in younger age groups, with a few special considerations, such as polypharmacy and an increase in side effects. Age-related changes in the pancreas, liver, and biliary tree are summarized in Figure 24.2. (See also Chapter 27.)

Summary

- The demographics of the population are changing as the proportion of older people increases.
- Gastrointestinal symptoms and diseases are a major cause of morbidity and mortality in older people and impact hugely upon quality of life.
- Age alone should not be used to deny investigations or treatments to older people.
- Research needs to be directed towards a better understanding of the underlying changes that occur in the gastrointestinal tract with aging, to help explain why older people are more susceptible to diseases such as peptic ulcer.
- Clinical studies carried out specifically in older people are required to confirm that management of common gastrointestinal syndromes is effective and efficient in older people.
- An examination of why older people are more likely to suffer from malnutrition is high on the research agenda.

References

1. Chaplin A, Curless R, Thomson R, *et al.* Prevalence of lower gastrointestinal symptoms and associated consultation behaviour in a British elderly population determined by face-to-face interview. *Br J Gen Pract.* 2000;50:798–802.

2. Barry PP, Barry PP. An overview of special considerations in the evaluation and management of the geriatric patient. *Am J Gastroenterol.* 2000;95:8–10.

3. National Institute of Clinical Excellence. Clinical Guideline 17: *Dyspepsia- management of dyspepsia in adults in primary care.* 2005. Available from: http://www.nice.org.uk/nicemedia/pdf/CG017quickrefguide.pdf.

4. Budtz-Jorgensen E, Chung JP, Rapin CH, *et al.* Nutrition and oral health. *Baillieres Best Pract Res Clin Gastroenterol.* 2001;15:885–896.

5. Lee A, Veldhuyzen van Zanten S, Lee A, *et al.* The aging stomach or the stomachs of the ages (comment). *Gut.* 1997;41:575–576.

6. Allen A, Newton J, Oliver L, *et al.* Mucus and H. pylori. *J Physiol Pharmacol.* 1997;48:297–305.

7. Guslandi M, Pellegrini A, Sorghi M, *et al.* Gastric mucosal defences in the elderly. *Gerontology.* 1999;45:206–208.

8. Fass R, Pulliam G, Johnson C, *et al.* Symptom severity and oesophageal chemosensitivity to acid in older and young patients with gastro-oesophageal reflux. *Age Ageing.* 2000;29:125–130.

9. Raiha I, Hietanen E, Sourander L, *et al.* Symptoms of gastro-oesophageal reflux disease in elderly people. *Age Ageing.* 1991;20:365–370.

10. Triadafilopoulos G, Sharma R, Triadafilopoulos G, *et al.* Features of symptomatic gastroesophageal reflux disease in elderly patients. *Am J Gastroenterol.* 1997;92:2007–2011.

11. Blair DI, Kaplan B, Spiegler J, *et al.* Patient characteristics and lifestyle recommendations in the treatment of gastroesophageal reflux disease. *J Fam Pract.* 1997;44:266–272.

12. Rockall TA, Logan RF, Devlin HB, *et al.* Incidence of and mortality from acute upper gastrointestinal haemorrhage in the United Kingdom. Steering Committee and Members of the National Audit of Acute Upper Gastrointestinal Haemorrhage (see comment). *BMJ.* 1995;311:222–226.

13. Zagari RM, Fuccio L, Bazzoli F, *et al.* Investigating dyspepsia (see comment). *BMJ.* 2008;337:a1400.

14. Zullo A, Gatta L, De Francesco V, *et al.* High rate of Helicobacter pylori eradication with sequential therapy in elderly patients with peptic ulcer: a prospective controlled study *Aliment Pharmacol Ther.* 2005;21:1419–1424.

15. Lewis SJ, Potts LF, Malhotra R, *et al.* Small bowel bacterial overgrowth in subjects living in residential care homes. *Age Ageing.* 1999;28:181–185.

16. Curless R, French J, Williams GV, *et al.* Comparison of gastrointestinal symptoms in colorectal carcinoma patients and community controls with respect to age. *Gut.* 1994;35:1267–1270.

17. Au HJ, Mulder KE, Fields AL, *et al.* Systematic review of management of colorectal cancer in elderly patients (see comment). *Clin Colorectal Cancer.* 2003;3:165–171.

18. Anonymous. Surgery for colorectal cancer in elderly patients: a systematic review. Colorectal Cancer Collaborative Group (see comment). *Lancet.* 2000;356:968–974.

19. Fata F, Mirza A, Craig G, *et al.* Efficacy and toxicity of adjuvant chemotherapy in elderly patients with colon carcinoma: a 10-year experience of the Geisinger Medical Center. *Cancer.* 2002;94:1931–1938.

20. Thomas PD, Forbes A, Green J, *et al.* Guidelines for the investigation of chronic diarrhoea, 2nd edition (see comment). *Gut.* 2003;52 Suppl 5:v1–v15.

21. Ryan MJ, Wall PG, Adak GK, *et al.* Outbreaks of infectious intestinal disease in residential institutions in England and Wales 1992–1994. *J Infect.* 1997;34:49–54.

22. Gilmore I, Burroughs A, Murray-Lyon I, *et al.* Indications, methods and outcomes of percutaneous liver biopsy in England and Wales: an audit by the British Society of Gastroenterology and the Royal College of Physicians of London. *Gut.* 1995;36:437–441.

CHAPTER 25
Preventing GI cancer in those at risk

Nicola E. Burch[1] and Janusz A. Jankowski[2]
[1]University Hospitals Coventry and Warwickshire NHS Trust, Coventry, UK
[2]Cancer Research UK and Queen Mary, University of London, London, UK

KEY POINTS

- GI cancer incidence continues to rise
- Current cancer prevention strategies are inadequate
- New techniques may improve endoscopic surveillance
- Targeted endotherapy may be safer and more effective than traditional surgical approaches
- Robust chemoprevention trials are required to evaluate promising agents

Introduction

Gastrointestinal (GI) cancer is common, with approximately 25% of all cancers being of GI origin and accounting for up to 9% of worldwide cancer-related deaths. More concerning is that despite more advanced techniques for diagnosis and management, incidence continues to increase with newer management strategies making no apparent impact on long-term survival [1]. Incidence of esophageal adenocarcinoma, for example, has rapidly increased over the past 20 years, with 5-year survival remaining disappointing at just 5–10% [4]. High incidences of GI cancer coupled with significant associated world-wide morbidity and mortality has increased the drive over the past 20 years for better screening and surveillance, and research into chemoprevention. Generalized population strategies may have a role, but the key to cancer prevention is identification and management of those particularly at risk. Although not an exhaustive list this chapter will discuss the main at-risk groups for GI cancer including Barrett's esophagus (BE), colorectal polyps, and inflammatory bowel disease (IBD). Mechanisms by which we can attempt to prevent cancer in those at risk include dietary manipulation, health education, screening, surveillance, and chemoprevention strategies (see Figure 25.1).

Upper GI cancers

This section focuses on the most common risk factors for upper GI malignancy and includes some practical guidance on potential screening, surveillance, and possible chemoprevention strategies. Whilst not an exhaustive text, the main categories are discussed including: Barrett's esophagus and reflux esophagitis; *Helicobacter pylori*; pernicious anaemia; gastric polyps and familial cancer syndromes; and celiac disease.

Barrett's esophagus and reflux esophagitis

BARRETT'S KEY LEARNING POINTS

- Consider BE in all Grade C/D reflux disease
- Intestinal metaplasia (IM) may not be present in all BE
- Aspirin is a potential agent for chemoprevention – awaiting analysis in AspECT trial
- Surveillance unproven – await BOSS trial outcome
- Consider targeted endotherapy in all who are unfit for surgery

Background

Barrett's esophagus is an acquired pre-malignant condition of the esophagus with an increasing incidence. British Society of Gastroenterology (BSG) guidelines define Barrett's as the presence of characteristic changes above the gastroesophageal junction on endoscopy, confirmed with biopsies demonstrating presence of columnar lined esophagus [2]. The American College of Gastroenterology guidelines however emphasize the importance of finding intestinal metaplasia (IM) on histology in addition to columnar lined esophagus [3]. Barrett's associated esophageal adenocarcinoma is known to occur in segments where there is IM. Despite this the BSG currently feel that inconsistency in current surveillance practice may mean some at-risk individuals could be missed due to sampling error if IM is included in the definition of Barrett's [4].

Overall risk of adenocarcinoma in BE is approximately 0.5–1% per year. This can be further sub-stratified according to the level of dysplasia [5–9] (Table 25.1). It is thought that there is gradual phenotypic progression through IM, LGD, HGD, and eventual AC in BE; however some studies show regression of dysplasia on sequential sampling [6]. This may reflect sampling error, thus current guidelines suggest ongoing surveillance strategies appropriate to the highest level of dysplasia found in that segment [3].

Screening

Screening for BE in those with gastroesophageal reflux (GERD) is contentious and currently not widely practiced. Although

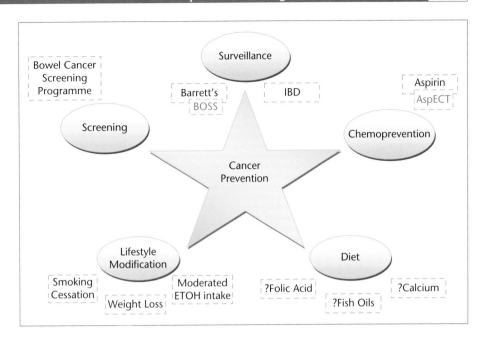

Figure 25.1 Cancer prevention principles. ETOH, ethyl alcohol; IBD, inflammatory bowel disease.

Table 25.1 Risk of progression to adenocarcinoma in Barrett's esophagus

Stage	Research evidence	Results
All Barrett's: AC 0.5–1%/year		
LGD	25 patients with LGD; 26 months follow-up[a]	Persistent LGD: 12–25%
	48 patients with LGD; 41 months follow-up[b]	Regression to IM: 62–65% HGD/AC in-situ: 10–28%
HGD	76 patients with HGD; 5 yr follow-up[c]	AC Risk: 1yr 38%
	79 patients with HGD; 7 yr mean follow-up[d]	3yrs 56% 5yrs 20–60%

NB: Focal HGD may have lower risk of progression to AC with figures suggesting 7% at 1 yr, 14% at 3 yrs[e]

[a]Skacel *et al.* (2000) [5];
[b]Weston *et al.* (2001) [6];
[c]Reid *et al.* (2000) [7];
[d]Schnell *et al.* (2001) [8];
[e]Buttar *et al.* (2001) [9].

GERD has a known association with BE, as many as 6–10% of patients with no reflux symptoms have BE. Indeed postmortem evaluation has shown a 20-fold increased prevalence compared to predicted incidence, suggesting that a significant proportion of BE remains undiagnosed [10]. Thus screening only GERD patients would miss a significant percentage of BE. Mode of screening is also important to consider, since some "worried well" may consider standard endoscopy unacceptable in the absence of symptoms. This has produced interest in the possibility of capsule endoscopy for Barrett's screening.

Initial small pilot studies suggest a high sensitivity in diagnosis [3]. Overall cost issues currently remain prohibitive for general population screening in Barrett's. Additionally recent studies have suggested that diagnostic sensitivity may not be as impressive as initially thought [11].

Surveillance

The surveillance protocol in BE varies according to level of dysplasia found (see Figure 25.2). Current guidelines suggest four-quadrant biopsies every 2 cm, but it is vital to appreciate that this method will only allow evaluation of approximately 3.5% of the area being investigated [12]. Multiple retrospective studies have shown an overall survival benefit if cancers are detected early with endoscopic surveillance, and there is indirect evidence that current surveillance strategies are beneficial [3]. Overall risk of carcinoma development in Barrett's remains very low but it is of concern that approximately 50% of those identified with HGD or AC on surveillance have no evidence of any dysplasia on their preceding two endoscopies [13]. It is pertinent that 5% of diagnosed esophageal cancers were Barrett's-related but not previously identified for surveillance, and thus the benefit of screening has been called into question [14]. The forthcoming prospective multi-centre BOSS trial (Barrett's Oesophagus Surveillance versus no Surveillance) will hopefully answer these questions regarding the effect of surveillance versus no surveillance in Barrett's, as well as assessing cost-effectiveness.

Targeted screening

New endoscopic techniques enable targeted biopsies to be taken aiming to increase sensitivity and specificity of dysplasia detection. Older techniques such as chromoendoscopy can be utilized in addition to newer modalities including narrow

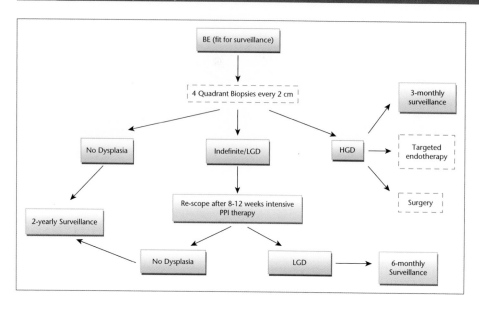

Figure 25.2 Surveillance in Barrett's esophagus. HGD, high grade dysplasia; LGD, low grade dysplasia, PPI, proton pump inhibitor.

band imaging, autofluorescence imaging, optical coherence tomography, and laser confocal microscopy.

Chromoendoscopy

Available for over 20 years, various stains have been evaluated with respect to Barrett's including methylene blue, crystal violet, indigo carmine, and acetic acid. The majority of stains provide superior dysplasia detection when compared to standard white light endoscopy. Lack of standardization, however, coupled with increased procedure time and decreased patient tolerability mean that newer techniques such as narrow band imaging may be more practical long-term.

Narrow band imaging (NBI)

This uses filters to exclude red light from standard white light endoscopes, in order that just blue and green light waves are emitted. This narrowed wavelength only penetrates tissue superficially enabling greater enhancement of superficial mucosal features, and when coupled with high magnification endoscopy has been shown to be highly effective at identification of high-grade dysplasia within Barrett's. Although one study suggested a sensitivity of 100% and specificity of 98.7% [13], studies evaluating inter-observer agreement for diagnosis have yet to be undertaken. Clearly further evaluation is required prior to recommendation of NBI in all BE surveillance programmes.

Autofluorescence imaging

This uses blue light illumination to detect degree of fluorescence from tissues at a cellular level. Dysplastic areas show less fluorescence than healthy segments, and show up as dark red areas. This enables focused biopsies from potentially dysplastic areas, and can be used to image entire Barrett's segments. Again initial results appear promising, with one study

suggesting 100% sensitivity for identification of HGD although specificity was poor [15].

Laser confocal microscopy and optical coherence tomography

More detailed evaluation of small areas of mucosa is possible with these techniques. They could be used in conjunction with the above methods enabling in-depth evaluation of areas identified as likely to represent dysplasia. Mucosa can be evaluated at a cellular level in real time, and negates the need for delay in diagnosis of HGD while awaiting microscopy of biopsy specimens. Clearly these technologies are not yet widely available, and are time- and labour-intensive. Cost effectiveness and practicalities of application need to be formally evaluated, but these are exciting techniques that could revolutionize the future management of BE.

Targeted endotherapy versus surgery

Targeted endotherapy is a very exciting prospect particularly when considering that standard management of HGD until recently involved esophagectomy in all except those with greatest operative risk. This practice was based on early figures suggesting that 43% with HGD may have an occult cancer missed by surveillance biopsies [16]. Recent post-operative data however suggests only 17% of esophagectomy specimens contain an occult focus of adenocarcinoma [17]. Moreover metastatic potential from these lesions is very low (<4%), with the majority representing very early stage tumours [8]. Minimally invasive esophagectomy via laparoscopy and thoracoscopy is now available; however major complication rates remain high at more than 30% [18].

Targeted endotherapy has increasingly therefore been utilized in order to locally destroy areas of dysplasia promoting re-epithelialization with squamous mucosa. Techniques include mucosal ablation and photodynamic therapy [19–22]

Table 25.2 Targeted endotherapy techniques

	Mechanism	Evidence in Barrett's
Photodynamic therapy	Uses photosensitizing agent: absorbs into all cells, but retained longer in abnormal cells Esophageal mucosa then exposed to certain wavelength light after pre-specified time Produces cell death in all cells still retaining sensitizing agent (e.g., dysplastic and malignant)	Significant initial risk reduction in cancer and HGD[a] Long term cancer incidence not affected[b]
Thermal ablation	Argon plasma coagulation Multi-polar thermal coagulation Laser therapy Radiofrequency ablation Complications[d] • Post procedural chest pain • Upper GI bleed (1.2%) • Esophageal stricture (6%)	Ablation of entire Barrett's segment in 80–90% following repeated applications[c] Eradication of LGD in 90.5%, and HGD in 81% in recent prospective RCT[d] Less disease progression following ablation compared to control[d]

[a]Overholt et al. (2005) [19];
[b]Pech et al. (2005) [20];
[c]Wang&Sampliner (2008) [21];
[d]Shaheen et al. (2009) [22].

(see Table 25.2). Data regarding effectiveness of these techniques compared to traditional surgical therapies are limited, with a recent Cochrane review demonstrating no randomized-controlled trials (RCT) evaluating this at the time of search [23].

Radiofrequency ablation (RFA) has however recently been evaluated [22]. In this study RFA resulted in complete eradication of LGD in 90.5%, and HGD in 81% [22]. Additionally disease progression was reduced in the RFA arm, with a decreased overall cancer incidence. Perhaps of concern may be the complications associated with RFA, with 1.2% having a post-procedural GI bleed, and 6% subsequently developing an esophageal stricture [22]. Despite this, overall morbidity and mortality associated with targeted endotherapy are significantly lower than traditional surgical techniques.

Chemoprevention

Since surveillance has not had a huge impact, chemoprevention seems an attractive alternative. There is a wealth of data suggesting potential chemopreventative agents, but long-term prospective data for their role in esophageal AC chemoprevention are lacking. The AspECT Trial (Aspirin Esomeprazole Chemoprevention Trial) is a large UK multi-center, randomized, open label trial, which began recruitment in 2005.

Table 25.3 The AspECT Trial

	Low-dose PPI	High-dose PPI
No aspirin	Nexium 20 mg (n = 625)	Nexium 80 mg (n = 625)
Aspirin	Nexium 20 mg + 300 mg aspirin (n = 625)	Nexium 80 mg + aspirin 300 mg (n = 625)

Already the largest Barrett's RCT world-wide, there will be a minimum 8-year follow-up (see Table 25.3). It aims to evaluate both the effect of aspirin on all-cause mortality in Barrett's patient's, in addition to any potential effect of aspirin with or without esomeprazole in the prevention of adenocarcinoma development in BE. Although some animal studies have suggested increased risk of progression of Barrett's in those on prolonged PPI therapy, it is reassuring to note that a recent large prospective analysis of gastrin biology in BE failed to demonstrate clonal expansion of Barrett's [24].

Gastric polyps and familial cancer syndromes

The frequency of polypoid lesions found at upper GI endoscopy is difficult to estimate, with wide ranging variation in the literature depending upon whether studies are retrospective reviews of endoscopic data or pathology-based studies. A recent large-scale population study estimated that gastric polyps are found in 3.75% of all upper GI endoscopies, with 77.2% of these fundic gland polyps, 14.4% hyperplastic polyps, and 0.7% gastric adenomas [25]. Identification and determination of underlying type of polyp is essential, since dysplastic potential and surveillance guidelines vary depending upon type and number of polyp identified. A summary of the associations, risks for dysplasia, and suggested management guidance is listed in Table 25.4 [26–32].

Helicobacter pylori infection

It is well known that infection with H. pylori is associated with an increased risk of development of gastric carcinoma. Studies suggest an increased risk of gastric cancer development between 2 to 16-fold with H. pylori infection [33]. Additionally a large prospective Japanese cohort demonstrated a 2.9% gastric cancer incidence in H. pylori-infected patients compared to 0% in the sero-negative population [34].

Gastric cancer is not universally increased with H. pylori infection however. Non-cardia (distal) gastric cancer incidence is increased with H. pylori infection, whereas it is protective and associated with decreased incidence of esophageal and cardia cancers. As such, widespread eradication of H. pylori as a means of chemoprevention is somewhat controversial. Interestingly, recent data have suggested that eradication of H. pylori is not always associated with an increased incidence of esophageal and gastric cardia carcinoma [33], and therefore further research needs to undertaken to formally establish whether there is a role for H. pylori eradication in primary

Table 25.4 Quick reference guide for management of gastric polyps

Polyp type	Associations	Dysplastic potential	Suggested management[b]
Fundic gland polyp (FGP)	• Rare in *H. pylori* • Increased incidence with PPI • May regress upon PPI cessation • Multiple FGPs seen in familial adenomatous polyposis (FAP)	• Low malignant potential • 30–50% are dysplastic in FAP patients[a]	Small (<0.5 cm): Biopsy 1 polyp Medium (0.5–1 cm): Biopsy all polyps this size Large (>1 cm): – Consider polypectomy – ?Stop PPI • All patients with FAP should have screening OGD • Consider colonoscopy in patients with multiple FGPs (? Attenuated FAP)
Hyperplastic	*H. pylori* in 25%	• Overall dysplasia risk <3% • Increased dysplasia risk in polyps >2 cm • Increased cancer risk if associated extensive gastric atrophy/ metaplasia[c]	• Excise all polyps >2 cm • Gastric mapping – ideally biopsy polyps **and** adjacent tissue • Eradicate *H. pylori* • ?Re-scope in 4–6/12 to evaluate HP status and evaluate for polyp recurrence
Adenoma	Chronic atrophic gastritis	• Increased dysplasia risk in polyps >2 cm • Synchronous gastric adenocarcinoma at distant site in 30% with gastric adenoma[d] • 50% polyps >2 cm contain dysplastic focus	• Gastric mapping – ideally biopsy polyps **and** adjacent tissue • ASGE suggest annual surveillance OGD if adenoma with co-existent atrophic metaplastic gastritis[e]

Gastric polyposis syndromes	a) FAP
	b) Peutz-Jeghers syndrome
	c) Juvenile polyposis
		• Associated with FGPs: 30–50% dysplasia incidence[b]
		• Lifetime risk gastric Ca approx 30%[f]
		• Also increased risk of colonic, breast, pancreatic, small intestinal, ovarian, uterine, and testicular Ca
		• Rare. Limited data
		• Lifetime gastric Ca risk approx 15–20%
		• Also increased risk CRC
			• 3-yearly OGDs after 30 yrs
			• If multiple polyps / presence of dysplasia: Annual OGD
			• Screen all >18 yrs[b]. Investigate 2–3 yearly with:
			  - OGD
			  - Small bowel imaging
			1–2 yearly OGD and colonoscopy[g]

[a]Bertoni G *et al.* (1999) [26];
[b]Carmack SW *et al.* (2009) [27];
[c]Hattori T (1985) [28];
[d]Abraham SC *et al.* (2003) [29];
[e]Hirota WK *et al.* (2006) [30];
[f]Giardiello FM *et al.* (2000) [31];
[g]Dunlop MG (2002) [32].

cancer prevention. Secondary prevention with antibiotics in *H. pylori*-positive patients following a diagnosis of gastric metaplasia or early gastric cancer has been shown to be efficacious, however, with a lower recurrence rate in eradicated patients [35].

Celiac disease

The association between celiac disease and GI cancer risk has been well documented. Long-standing celiac disease and poor compliance with gluten-free diet are the two main risk factors associated with development. Predominant cancer types associated with celiac disease include small bowel lymphoma, and adenocarcinoma of the oro-pharynx, esophagus and small intestine.

Overall the risk of lymphoma is increased by a factor of 3 in celiac disease [36]. The most serious of these is the aggressive non-Hodgkin Lymphoma (NHL) subtype Enteropathy-associated T-cell lymphoma (EATL). This carries a very poor prognosis with many patients having metastatic disease at the time of diagnosis [36]. Extra-intestinal deposits may be found throughout the body including brain, liver, spleen, skin, nasal cavity, and thyroid gland. Unfortunately EATL responds very poorly to treatment, with the only effective chemoprevention strategy thus far being strict adherence to a gluten-free diet.

Pernicious anemia

Pernicious anemia is a consequence of progressive atrophic gastritis within the fundus and body of the stomach which causes achloryhdria. The resulting loss of feedback inhibition on gastric antral G-cells produces sustained gastrin release and hypergastrinaemia. It is well documented that pernicious anemia is associated with increased risk of GI cancer development, particularly esophageal and gastric tumours. Reassuringly overall incidence remains low and issues surrounding potential surveillance in these patients have been long debated.

Cancer risk

Overall it is estimated that approximately 1–3% of patients with pernicious anemia develop gastric adenocarcinoma, with pernicious anemia associated gastric adenocarcinoma accounting for just 2% of total gastric adenocarcinoma incidence [37]. Gastric carcinoid tumours are more frequently associated with pernicious anemia than adenocarcinoma, with studies suggesting a 1–7% incidence in those undergoing endoscopic surveillance [37].

Standardized incidence ratio (SIR) for all-type gastric cancer distal to the cardia is 2.4 in pernicious anemia, and 3.3 for squamous cell carcinoma of the esophagus [38]. Interestingly there is no apparent increased risk of either esophageal adenocarcinoma or gastric cardia cancer, possibly reflecting the underlying pathophysiology of carcinogenesis in pernicious anemia. There appears to be no difference in cancer risk between male and female populations [38]. Overall risk of cancer development in pernicious anemia appears decreased with increased age at time of diagnosis of pernicious anemia [38]. This may be a reflection of a slow carcinogenesis sequence but it is interesting to note that many patients have atrophic gastritis for 20–30 years prior to diagnosis; indeed 32% of patients are over 70 years of age at the time of diagnosis, and 64% are over 60 years [37].

Issues regarding screening

Currently there are no universal guidelines on surveillance in pernicious anemia, and regular endoscopic surveillance remains controversial. The ASGE guidelines suggest a single upper GI endoscopy at the index diagnosis of pernicious anemia to exclude any pre-existing lesions, but do not recommend regular surveillance thereafter unless symptoms develop [39].

Colorectal cancer

CRC KEY LEARNING POINTS

- Most CRC arises following dysplasia in an adenomatous polyp
- Larger polyps have higher dysplastic potential
- Dysplasia in IBD is often flat and multi-focal
- Current surveillance in IBD is sub-optimal
- Targeted biopsies with emerging endoscopic techniques may be a better approach
- Chemoprevention trials in CRC are currently disappointing

Background

Colorectal cancer (CRC) is the third commonest UK cancer, with an approximate 1 in 20 lifetime risk. It accounts for approximately 677 000 deaths world-wide according to World Health Organization statistics [40]. At-risk groups for CRC include those with adenomatous polyps, long-standing inflammatory bowel disease (IBD), primary sclerosing cholangitis, and inherited polyposis coli syndromes. Cancer prevention strategies focus on these groups, although it is important to realize that a significant number of cases occur outside these cohorts. Approaches to CRC prevention include diet, screening, surveillance, and chemoprevention.

Polyps
Screening and surveillance

Most CRC occurs following development of dysplasia within an adenomatous polyp. Therefore much emphasis is placed on screening and surveillance for polyps. The absolute cancer potential of colonic adenomas is unknown, however increased size is associated with greater likelihood of dysplasia [41]. Development of dysplasia occurs over many years, thus allowing opportunity for identification and removal of polyps prior to development of advanced dysplasia and cancer. This principle is the basis for the National Bowel Cancer Screening Programme. Population screening in the UK utilizes fecal occult blood testing (FOBT) to identify those at risk who may benefit from screening. FOBT-based bowel cancer screening decreases risk of emergency admission due to CRC and improves post-operative outcomes [42].

Colonic evaluation may be via flexible sigmoidoscopy, colonoscopy, double-contrast barium enema, or CT colonoscopy [43,44] (see Table 25.5). Despite growing evidence suggesting the effectiveness of screening and surveillance in CRC, the potential miss-rate of lesions, risk of radiation exposure with imaging, and patient acceptance of invasive imaging modalities are all cause for concern. As a result there is a drive towards research evaluating alternative non-invasive imaging technologies, application of technologies to enhance standard white-light endoscopy, and chemopreventative strategies which may obviate the need for population screening.

Inflammatory bowel disease
Screening and surveillance

Both long-standing ulcerative colitis (UC) and Crohn's disease are thought to increase risk of CRC development by a factor of 2–3 compared to the general population [45]. Risk of cancer significantly increases with duration, extent and activity of colitis [46]. Initial meta-analysis data suggested a 2% cancer incidence after 10 years of UC, compared to an 18% incidence after 30 years [47]. Recent re-evaluation however suggests cancer risk may be lower, with incidence of 2.5% at 20 years and 7.6% at 30 years [46]. Data regarding Crohn's disease are slightly less clear cut, with early studies often concluding a lack of increased colorectal cancer risk. Further meta-analysis

Table 25.5 Quick reference guide to colonic imaging

	Advantages	Disadvantages
Colonoscopy	Therapeutic potential Higher detection rate than CT/barium enema for lesions <6 mm, and flat lesion[a] Histology attainable	Up to 20% polyp miss-rate (even with expert operator)[b] Risk of perforation (0.1%) Patient discomfort
Barium enema	Non-invasive Cheap Quick to report	Significant miss-rate Unpleasant Radiation exposure
CT colonogram	Non-invasive Equivalent polyp detection to colonoscopy in lesions >6 mm[a] Better detection rate than barium enema	Radiation dose (equivalent to 350 x-rays) Less effective than colonoscopy for detection of lesions <6 mm[a] Risk of contrast reactions (0.04%) Reporting takes time (40 mins if novice/ 20 mins if expert)

[a]Rosman AS, Korsten MA (2007) [43];
[b]Heresbach D, Barrioz T, Lapalus MG, *et al.* (2008) [44].

of data has shown that risk for CRC development in Crohn's is strongly influenced by location of disease, with extensive colonic disease conveying a relative risk of 4.5 for CRC compared to 1.1 for small bowel disease [48]. Although accounting for a smaller percentage of all GI cancers (approximately 1–5% only) it is important to note that the relative risk of small bowel neoplasm in Crohn's is 33.2 [48].

Up until recently colonic surveillance in IBD relied upon regular colonic examination of the bowel with multiple random biopsies throughout the colon [49] (see Figure 25.3). In 2010 BSG Guidelines changed in accordance with new data suggesting that degree of inflammation is a more accurate predictor of subsequent dysplasia risk than simply duration of colitis alone [50]. Moreover there is emerging data to suggest the benefit of targeted biopsies over random colonic sampling for the detection of dysplasia. A summary of the 2010 BSG surveillance guidelines can be seen in Figure 25.4.

The aim of surveillance is to detect dysplasia early in order to stratify risk and consider prophylactic colectomy [50]. Even with surveillance, however, it is known that areas of dysplasia may be undetected [45]. This may reflect the fact that UC-associated dysplasia is often multi-focal and arises in non-polypoid lesions which are harder to detect [51].

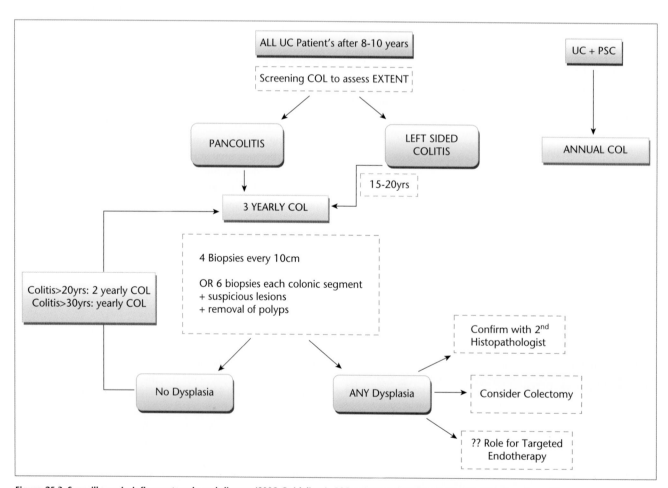

Figure 25.3 Surveillance in inflammatory bowel disease (2002 Guidelines). PSC, primary sclerosing cholangitis; UC, ulcerative colitis.

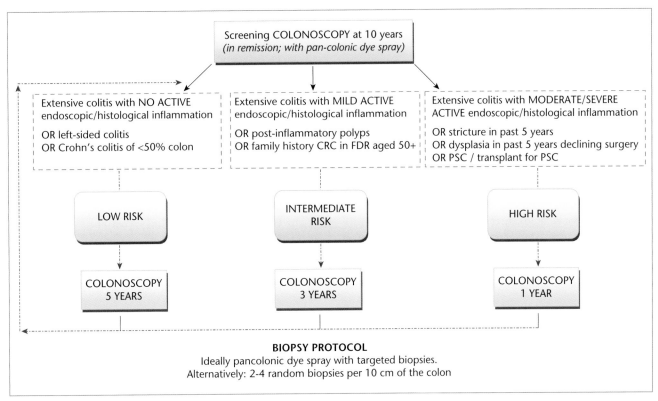

Figure 25.4 Surveillance in inflammatory bowel disease (2010 Guidelines). FDR, first degree relative; PSC, primary sclerosing cholangitis.

As previously discussed, emerging technologies may allow enhanced endoscopy with clearer identification of dysplastic tissue. Certainly chromoendoscopy has been shown to increase identification of dysplastic areas on colonoscopy, and future research will further evaluate the use of NBI, autofluorescence imaging and laser confocal endoscopy.

Chemoprevention

Several recent trials have focused on polyp recurrence and dysplasia incidence as surrogate markers for subsequent CRC risk. Good quality prospective human trials remain limited.

Aspirin reduced CRC incidence by 22% in cohort studies [40]. A recent large prospective trial of aspirin 300mg post-polypectomy resulted in a 21% overall polyp reduction, and a 37% reduction in advanced adenomas at follow-up endoscopy [52]. Chemopreventative properties increase with dose, but higher doses are associated with increased risk of major GI complications [53]. Currently the risk of GI side-effects and lack of long-term substantive data mean it is not possible to recommend aspirin for widespread use as chemoprevention.

Nonsteroidal inflammatory drugs (NSAIDs) have been shown to be equally promising for CRC chemoprevention, but again associated with significant GI upset. Recent trials of COX-2 inhibitors have shown a safer GI side-effect profile, but unfor-

tunately have been linked to significant cardiovascular morbidity [54].

Statins appear to have conflicting results with regards to CRC chemoprevention [55].

5-ASAs are the mainstay of treatment in IBD and have been shown to have a concurrent chemotherapeutic effect [56]. Prospective evidence is awaited with regards to the most efficacious dosing regimen.

PSC and PSC-IBD

Primary sclerosing cholangitis (PSC) is a chronic idiopathic condition which involves progressive hepatic fibrosis and liver failure (see Chapter 76). It is associated with an increased risk of many GI malignancies including colorectal cancer, cholangiocarcinoma, hepatocellular, gallbladder and pancreatic cancers [57].

Approximately 70–80% of patients PSC have co-existent IBD. In contrast, patients with chronic IBD only have co-existent PSC in 2–7.5% cases [58]. PSC-IBD could be considered as a separate phenotype of chronic IBD since it has several notable features including pan-colitis with rectal sparing and backwash ileitis, possibly a reflection of activity of inflammation. The most common associated colonic disease is chronic ulcerative colitis (87%), with Crohn's colitis and indeterminate colitis being the minority of cases (7% each) [59]. Although associated with extensive colitis, patients often have relatively few bowel symptoms, and so the colitis may remain undiagnosed for a significant length of time.

Cancer screening and surveillance

Overall the lifetime risk of colorectal cancer development in PSC-IBD is 10 times greater than the background population [60], and therefore it is vital to provide a comprehensive screening program for these patients. Additionally, the rate of development of dysplasia in this cohort appears more rapid than the general chronic IBD cohort, hence annual screening is offered to these patients following diagnosis. There is much debate surrounding whether concomitant PSC is an independent risk factor for colonic cancer development in the presence of IBD, with much conflicting data [59]. Since the bowel involvement in PSC-IBD is often relatively asymptomatic, and thus often diagnosed at a later stage compared to chronic IBD alone, it is proposed that the earlier development of dysplasia post-diagnosis may simply reflect duration of colonic disease. Additionally the colonic involvement in PSC-IBD is usually extensive (87% pan-colitis) versus chronic ulcerative colitis (54% pan-colitis) [59].

PSC is also associated with risk of bile duct cancer, with cholangiocarcinoma development in 7% cases [59]. This accounts for a significant morbidity and mortality burden. Currently screening for cholangiocarcinoma in PSC is not routine, with most centers monitoring for signs of deterioration and evaluation for biliary obstruction with annual ultrasound in the first instance. Subsequent more detailed evaluation uses a combination of imaging such as MRI, CT, ERCP/ MRCP, or PET in addition to biochemical markers in an attempt to diagnose and stage cholangiocarcinoma early. Gallbladder disease and hepatocellular surveillance is achieved by annual USS in all patients and 6-monthly alfafetoprotein measurement. Patients with identified gallbladder polyps should be referred for surgery, since a significant proportion of these will be hiding a malignant focus.

Chemoprevention

Pathophysiology of cancer development in PSC-IBD is poorly understood, but bile acid metabolism is thought to play a role. Frequently ursodeoxycholic acid (URSO) is used for the treatment of cholestasis in PSC, and it is interesting to note that in these patients there is a subsequent decline in incidence of colorectal neoplasia [61]. Whether there is any direct chemopreventative effect of URSO on incidence of either sporadic colonic cancer development or IBD-associated dysplasia is yet to be evaluated in randomised controlled trials. Although known to be chemoprotective in IBD, 5-ASAs have not been shown to reduce cancer incidence or dysplasia in PSC-IBD [57].

Family history of CRC and inherited cancer syndromes

Colorectal cancer is a common diagnosis and as such it can often be difficult to evaluate the significance of family history.

Between 4 and 7% of individuals have at least one affected relative in control cohorts [62]. Concerned relatives often present following the diagnosis of CRC within their family wanting to know if they are at increased risk, and it must be decided whether or not to arrange colonic evaluation. Various guidelines have been produced recommending screening strategies for both family history of CRC and specific cancer syndromes, and are summarized in Table 25.6 [62–64].

Dietary considerations

The association between dietary intake and CRC is well recognized, with much research surrounding potential causative or preventative aspects. There are six key areas of diet associated with CRC including fruit and vegetable intake, folate or folic acid, red meat and fish, dietary fat, vitamins, and probiotics.

Fruit, vegetables, and folate

There is much epidemiological evidence regarding decreased CRC risk with high fruit and fibre intake, particularly distal lesions [65]. This is thought to relate to the folate content of such a diet. Much research has confirmed the inverse relationship between ingestion of dietary folate and CRC incidence [66,67]. Prospective trials evaluating folic acid supplementation for polyp prevention, however, have shown conflicting results [52,68,69].

Red meat, fish, and dietary fat

Red meat ingestion is associated with a 9–55% increased risk of CRC with 100 g/day increase in consumption [70,71]. Some hypothesize that this may relate to dietary fat intake, although direct evaluation of dietary fat showed no correlation [72]. High intake of fish has been associated with a relative reduction of 30% in CRC incidence [70].

Vitamins and probiotics

Voluntary ingestion of dietary supplements has significantly increased over the past decade, with more than 35% taking at least one supplement [73]. The effect this may have on CRC and polyp incidence is unknown. Folic acid is still an unknown entity regarding chemoprevention, but emerging evidence regarding other supplements may be important.

Calcium supplementation has been shown to decrease polyp recurrence post-polypectomy [74]. Antioxidants such as Vitamin E have been suggested as potential agents for reducing inflammatory pathways in a number of diseases, but as yet data for gastrointestinal malignancy are conflicting [75]. There are also some promising results regarding probiotics in colon cancer, but data are inconsistent [76].

Discussion

It is clear that despite improvements in diagnosis and management, GI cancer still represents a significant burden in terms

Table 25.6 To screen or not to screen – a quick reference guide

Family history or cancer syndrome	Estimated cancer risk	Recommendations
1 × 1st degree relative <45[a] or >2 × 1st degree relatives >45[a]	3–4 × background pop. risk[a]	• Colonoscopy age 35–40 yrs (or at index consultation if older) • Repeat colonoscopy at 55 – If NAD: revert to standard population screening • Consider referral to Clinical Genetics
1 × 1st degree relative >45	2–3 × background pop. risk[a]	• Standard population screening • Consider starting at earlier age
2nd or 3rd degree relative of any age	1.5 × background pop. risk[a]	• Standard population screening
FAP[b] – Patient – At-risk family member	• 100% Risk CRC (69% in attenuated FAP) • 7% Risk gastric Ca if gastric polyposis (fundic gland polyps) • 12–29% risk rectal Ca in retained stump post colectomy	• FAP families register with regional clinical genetics centre • Colectomy before 25 yrs: – Subsequent annual rectal stump review for life • Annual FOS from 13–15yrs until 30 yrs • Once >30 yrs: 3–5 yrly FOS until 60 yrs
HNPCC[b] Diagnostic criteria: – Gene carrier or – >3 relatives with CRC in 2 sequential generations (1<50yrs) or – >2 relatives with CRC and 1 endometrial Ca in 2 sequential generations (1>50yrs)	• 80% Risk CRC • 13–20% Risk gastric Ca (50% risk of being a gene carrier if have 1 HNPCC affected parent)[c]	• Refer to Clinical Genetics • 6-monthly colonic surveillance age 25yrs onwards (or 5 yrs earlier than index relative diagnosis) • Continue surveillance until 75yrs

Peutz-Jeghers syndrome[b]	• 10–20% Risk CRC
	• Mutation identified in 20–63%[c]
		• Surveillance protocol not proven (small numbers of affected patients)
		• BSG suggest colonic surveillance 3 yearly after age 18 years with either:
		  – Colonoscopy or
		  – Sigmoidoscopy and barium enema

Juvenile polyposis syndrome[b]	• 10–38% Risk CRC • 21% Risk gastric Ca • Mutation identified in approx 50%[c]	• 1–2 yearly colonic surveillance from 15–18 yrs onwards • ? increase to every 3 years after age 35 • Survey until age 70 • Discuss potential for prophylactic surgery

[a]Dunlop MG (2002) [62];
[b]Dunlop MG (2002) [63];
[c]Durt RW (2009) [64].

of cancer-related mortality worldwide. While there may be some population strategies which may convey some cancer prevention benefit, it is clearly important to focus on identification and management of those particularly at risk. Newer imaging modalities and endoscopic techniques have provided a new level in terms of potential for accurate diagnosis of those with early dysplasia. Additionally, emerging targeted endotherapy options may provide the key to management of pre-cancerous lesions, with resultant decreased morbidity and mortality. Therefore it is likely that future surveillance programmes may incorporate a combination of these techniques. Undoubtedly it is an exciting time in GI cancer prevention, and results of forthcoming large scale randomized control trials such as AspECT will hopefully go some way to answering key questions regarding whether chemoprevention

agents are a realistic adjunct to cancer prevention in those at risk.

References

1. Jankowski JA, Hawk ET. A methodologic analysis of chemoprevention and cancer prevention strategies for gastrointestinal cancer. *Nature Clin Pract Gastroenterol.* 2006;3(2):101–111.

2. Playford RJ. New British Society of Gastroenterology (BSG) guidelines for the diagnosis and management of Barrett's esophagus. *Gut.* 2004;55:442–443.

3. Wang KK, Sampliner RE. Updated Guidelines 2008 for the diagnosis, surveillance and therapy of Barrett's Esophagus. *Am J Gastroenterol.* 2008;103:788–797.

4. Singh R, Ragunath K, Jankowski JA. Barrett's Esophagus: Diagnosis, Screening, Surveillance, and Controversies. *Gut and Liver.* 2007;1(2):93–100.

5. Skacel M, Petras RE, Gramlich TL, *et al.* The diagnosis of low-grade dysplasia in Barrett's esophagus and its implications for disease progression. *Am J Gastroenterol.* 2000;95:3383–3387.

6. Weston AP, Banarjee SK, Sharma P, *et al.* p53 overexpression in low grade dysplasia (LGD) in Barrett's esophagus: immunohistochemical marker predictive of progression. *Am J Gastroenterol.* 2001;96:1355–1362.

7. Reid BJ, Blount PL, Feng Z, & Levine DS. Optimizing endoscopic biopsy detection of early cancers in Barrett's high-grade dysplasia. *Am J Gastroenterol.* 2000;95:3089–3096.

8. Schnell TG, Sontag SJ, Chejfec G, *et al.* Long-term non-surgical management of Barrett's esophagus with high-grade dysplasia. *Gastroenterology.* 2001;120:1607–1619.

9. Buttar NS, Wang KK, Sebo TJ, *et al.* Extent of high grade dysplasia in Barrett's esophagus correlates with risk of adenocarcinoma. *Gastroenterology.* 2001;120:1630–1639.

10. Cameron AJ, Zinsmeister AR, Ballard DJ, *et al.* Prevalence of columnar lined (Barrett's) esophagus: comparison of population-based clinical and autopsy findings. *Gastroenterology.* 1990;99:918–922.

11. Lin O, Schembre DB, KM, *et al.* Blinded comparison of esophageal capsule endoscopy for diagnosis of Barrett's esophagus versus conventional endoscopy for diagnosis of Barrett's esophagus in patients with chronic esophageal reflux. *Gastrointest Endosc.* 2007;65(4):577–583.

12. Tschanz ER. Do 40% of patients resected for Barrett's esophagus with high grade dysplasia have unsuspected adenocarcinoma? *Arch Pathol Lab Med.* 2005;129:177–180.

13. Sharma P, Falk GW, Weston AP, *et al.* Dysplasia and Cancer in a large multicentere cohort of patients with Barrett's Esophagus. *Clin Gastr & Hepatol.* 2006;4(5):566–572.

14. Corley DA, Levin TR, Habel LA, *et al.* Surveillance and survival in Barrett's adenocarcinomas: a population-based study. *Gastroenterology.* 2002;122(3):633–640.

15. Kara MA, Peters FP, Fockens P, *et al.* Endoscopic video-autofluorescence imaging followed by narrow band imaging for detecting early neoplasia in Barrett's esophagus. *Gastrointest Endosc.* 2006;64(2):176–185.

16. Nigro JJ, Hagen JA, DeMeester TR, *et al.* Occult esophageal adenocarcinoma. Extent of disease and implications for effective therapy. *Ann Surg.* 1999;230:433–444.

17. Tseng EE, Wu TT, Yeo CF, *et al.* Barrett's esophagus with high grade dysplasia: surgical results and long-term outcome – an update. *J Gastrointest Surg.* 2003;7:164–171.

18. Luketich JD, Landreneau RJ. Minimally invasive resection and mechanical cervical esophagogastric anastamotic techniques in the management of esophageal cancer. *J Gastrointest Surg.* 2004;8:927–929.

19. Overholt BF, Lightdale CJ, Wang KK, *et al.* Photodynamic therapy with porfimer sodium for ablation of high-grade dysplasia in Barrett's esophagus: international, partially blinded, randomized phase III trial. *Gastrointest Endosc.* 2005;62:488–498.

20. Pech O, Gossner L, May A, *et al.* Long-term results of photodynamic therapy with 5-aminolevulinic acid for superficial Barrett's cancer and high-grade intraepithelial neoplasia. *Gastrointest Endosc.* 2005;62:24–30.

21. Wang KK, Sampliner RE. Updated guidelines 2008 for the diagnosis, surveillance and therapy of Barrett's esophagus. *Am J Gastroenterol.* 2008;103:788–797.

22. Shaheen NJ, Sharma P, Overholt BF *et al.* Radiofrequency ablation in Barrett's Esophagus with Dysplasia. *N Engl J Med.* 2009;360(22):2277–2288.

23. Green S, Tawil A, Barr H *et al.* Surgery versus radical endotherapies for early cancer and high grade dysplasia in Barrett's Oesophagus. *Cochrane Database Syst Rev.* 2009; Issue 2. Art. No: CD007334. DOI: 10.1002/14651858.CD007334.pub2.

24. Obszynska JA, Atherfold PA, Nanji M, *et al.* Long-term proton pump induced hypergastrinaemia does induce lineage-specific restitution but not clonal expansion in benign Barrett's oesophagus in vivo. *Gut* 2010;59(2):156–163.

25. Carmack SW, Genta RM, Schuler CM, *et al.* The current spectrum of gastric polyps: A 1-Year National Study of over 120,000 Patients. *Am J Gastro.* 2009;04:1524–1532.

26. Bertoni G, Sassatelli R, Nigrisoli E, *et al.* Dysplastic changes in gastric fundic gland polyps of patients with familial adenomatous polyposis. *Ital J Gastroenterol Hepatol.* 1999;31:192–197.

27. Carmack SW *et al.* Management of gastric polyps: a pathology-based guide for gastroenterologists. *Nat Rev Gastroenterol Hepatol.* 2009;6:331–341.

28. Hattori T. Morphological range of hyperplastic polyps and carcinomas arising in hyperplastic polyps of the stomach. *J Clin Pathol.* 1985;38:662–630.

29. Abraham SC, Park SJ, Lee JH, *et al.* Genetic alterations in gastric adenomas of intestinal and foveolar phenotypes. *Mod. Pathol.* 2003;16:786–795.

30. Hirota WK, Zuckerman MJ, Adler DG, *et al.* ASGE Guideline: the role of endoscopy in the surveillance of premalignant conditions of the upper GI tract. *GI Endoscopy.* 2006;63:570–580.

31. Giardiello FM, Brensinger JD, Tersmette AC, *et al.* Very high risk of cancer in familial Peutz-Jeghers syndrome. *Gastroenterology.* 2000;119:1447–1453.

32. Dunlop MG. Guidance on GI surveillance for hereditary non-polyposis colorectal cancer, familial adenomatous polyposis, juvenile polyposis, and Peutz-Jeghers syndrome. *GUT.* 2002; Suppl.5:V21–V27.

33. Crew KD, Neugut AI. Epidemiology of Gastric Cancer. *World J Gastro.* 2006;12(3):354–362.

34. Uemura N, Okamoto S, Yamamoto S, *et al.* Helicobacter pylori infection and the development of gastric cancer. *N Engl J Med.* 2001;345:784–789.

35. Uemura N, Mukai T, Okamoto S, *et al.* Effect of *H. pylori* eradication on subsequent development of cancer after endoscopic resection of early gastric cancer. *Cancer Epidemiol Biomarkers Prev.* 1997;6:639–642.

36. Catassi C, Bearzi I, Holmes GKT. Association of celiac disease and intestinal lymphomas and other cancers. *Gastroenterology.* 2005;128(4):S79–S86.

37. Sjoblom SM, Sipponen P, Jarvinen H. Gastroscopic follow-up of pernicious anaemia patients. *Gut.* 1993;34:28–32.

38. Ye W, Nyren O. Risk of cancers of the oesophagus and stomach by histology or subsite in patients hospitalised for pernicious anaemia. *Gut.* 2003;52:938–941.

39. Hirota WK, Zuckerman MJ, Adler DG *et al.* Standards of Practice Committee, American Society for Gastrointestinal endoscopy. ASGE guideline: the role of endoscopy in the surveillance of pre-malignant conditions of the upper GI tract. *Gastrointest Endosc.* 2006;63(4):570–580.

40. Das D, Jankowski J. Prevention of Colorectal Cancer by combining early detection and chemoprevention. *Curr Colorectal Cancer Rep.* 2009;5:48–54.

41. Butterly L, Chase M, Pohl H, *et al.* Prevalence of Clinically Important Histology in Small Adenomas. *Clin Gastroenterol Hepatol.* 2006;4(3):343–348.

42. Goodyear SJ, Leung E, Menon A, *et al.* The effect of population-based faecal occult blood test screening upon emergency colorectal cancer admissions in Coventry and north Warwickshire. *Gut.* 2008;57:218–222.

43. Rosman AS, Korsten MA. Meta-analysis comparing CT Colonography, air contrast barium enema, and colonoscopy. *Am J Med.* 2007;120:203–210.

44. Heresbach D, Barrioz T, Lapalus MG, et al. Miss rate for colorectal neoplastic polyps: a prospective multicentre study of back-to-back video colonoscopies. *Endoscopy.* 2008;40:284–290.

45. Bernstein NC, Shanahan F, Weinstein MW. Are we telling the truth about surveillance colonoscopy in ulcerative colitis? *Lancet.* 1994;343:71–74.

46. Rutter MD, Saunders BP, Wilkinson KH, *et al.* Thirty-year analysis of a colonoscopic surveillance program for neoplasia in ulcerative colitis. *Gastroenterology.* 2006;130:1030–1038.

47. Eaden JA, Abrams KR, Mayberry JF. The risk of colorectal cancer in ulcerative colitis: a meta-analysis. *Gut.* 2001;48:526–535.

48. Canavan C, Abrams KR, Mayberry J. Meta-analysis: colorectal and small bowel cancer risk in patients with Crohn's disease. *Aliment Pharm & Therapeutics.* 2006;23:1097–1104.

49. Eaden JA, Mayberry JF. Guidelines for screening and surveillance of asymptomatic colorectal cancer in patients with inflammatory bowel disease. *Gut.* 2002;51(v):v10–v12.

50. Cairns SR, Scholefield JH, Steele RJ, et al. Guidelines for colorectal cancer screening and surveillance in moderate and high risk groups (update from 2002). *Gut.* 2010;59:666–690.

51. Xie J, Itzkowitz SH. Cancer in Inflammatory Bowel Disease. *World J Gastroenterol.* 2008;14(2):378–389.

52. Logan RFA, Grainge MJ, Shepherd VC, *et al.* Aspirin and folic acid for the prevention of recurrent colorectal adenomas. *Gastroenterology.* 2008;134:29–38.

53. Dube C, Rostom A, Lewin G, *et al.* The use of aspirin for primary prevention of colorectal cancer: a systematic review prepared for the US Preventative services task force. *Ann Intern Med.* 2007;146:365–375.

54. Baron JA, Sandler RS, Bresalier RS, *et al.* A randomised trial of Rofecoxib for the chemoprevention of colorectal adenomas. *Gastroenterology.* 2006;131:1674–1682.

55. Bonovas S, Filioussi K, Flordellis CS, *et al.* Statins and the risk of colorectal cancer: a meta-analysis of 18 studies involving more then 1.5 million patients. *J Clin Oncol.* 2007;25:3462–3468.

56. Velayos FS, Terdiman JP, Walsh JM. Effect of 5-aminosalicylate use on colorectal cancer and dysplasia risk: a systematic review and meta-analysis of observational studies. *Am J Gastroenterol.* 2005;100:1345–1353.

57. Kitiyakara T, Chapman RW. Chemoprevention and screening in primary sclerosing cholangitis. *Postgrad Med Journal.* 2008;84:228–237.

58. Loftus EV, Sandborn WJ, Lindor KD, *et al.* Interactions between chronic liver disease and inflammatory bowel disease. *Inflammatory Bowel Disease.* 1997;3:288–302.

59. Loftus EV, Harewood GC, Loftus CG, *et al.* PSC-IBD: a unique form of inflammatory bowel disease associated with primary sclerosing cholangitis. *Gut.* 2005;54:91–96.

60. Bergquist A, Ekbom A, Olsson R, *et al.* Hepatic and extra-hepatic malignancies in Primary Sclerosing Cholangitis. *J Hepatol.* 2002;36:321–327.

61. Pardi DS, Loftus EV, Kremers WK, *et al.* Ursodeoxycholic acid as chemopreventative agent in patients with ulcerative colitis and primary sclerosing cholangitis. *Gastroenterology.* 2003;124:889–893.

62. Dunlop MG. Guidance on large bowel surveillance for people with two first degree relatives with colorectal cancer or one first degree relative diagnosed with colorectal cancer under 45years. *Gut.* 2002;51:v17–v20.

63. Dunlop MG. Guidance on gastrointestinal surveillance for hereditary non-polyposis colorectal cancer, familial adenomatous polyposis, juvenile polyposis, and Peutz-Jeghers syndrome. *Gut.* 2002;51:v21–v27.

64. Burt RW. Genetics and inherited syndromes of colorectal cancer. *Gastroenterology & Hepatology.* 2009;5(2):119–130.

65. Koushik A, Hunter DJ, Spiegelman D, *et al.* Fruits, vegetables, and colon cancer risk in a pooled analysis of 14 cohort studies. *J Natl Cancer Inst.* 2007;99:1471–1483.

66. Giovannucci E. Epidemiologic studies of folate and colorectal neoplasia: a review. *J Nutr.* 2002;132(s):2350s–2355s.

67. Hamack L, Jacobs DR, Nicodemus K, *et al.* Relationship of folate vitamin B-6, vitamin B-12, and methionine intake to the incidence of colorectal cancers. *Nutr Cancer.* 2002;43:152–158.

68. Jaszewski R, Misra S, Tobi M, *et al.* Folic acid supplementation inhibits recurrence of colorectal adenomas: a randomised chemoprevention trial. *World J Gastroenterol.* 2008;14(28):4492–4498.

69. Cole BF, Baron JA, Sandler RS, *et al.* Folic acid for the prevention of colorectal adenomas: a randomised clinical trial. *JAMA.* 2007;297:2351–2359.

70. Norat T, Bingham S, Ferrari P, *et al.* Meat, fish, and colorectal cancer risk: the European Prospective Investigation into cancer and nutrition. *J Natl Cancer Inst.* 2005;97(12):906–916.

71. Larsson SC, Wolk A. Meat consumption and risk of colorectal cancer: a meta-analysis of prospective studies. *IJC.* 2006;119(11):2657–2664.

72. Giovannucci E, Rimm EB, Stampfer MJ, *et al.* Intake of fat, meat and fibre in relation to risk of colon cancer in men. *Cancer Research.* 1994;54:2390–2397.

73. Harrison RA, Holt D, Pattison DJ, *et al.* Are those in need taking dietary supplements? A survey of 21 923 adults. *British J Nutr.* 2004;91:617–623.

74. Weingarten MA, Zalmanovici A, Yaphe J. Dietary calcium supplementation for preventing colorectal cancer and adenomatous polyps. *Cochrane Database Syst Rev.* 2008;Issue 1. Article number: CD003548.

75. Bjelakovic G, Nikolova D, Simonetti RG, *et al.* Systematic review and meta-analysis: primary and secondary prevention of gastrointestinal cancers with anti-oxidant supplements. *Aliment Pharmacol Ther.* 2008;83:23–34.

76. Capurso G, Marignani M, Delle FG. Probiotics and the incidence of colorectal cancer: when evidence is not evident. *Dig Liver Dis.* 2006;38(2):s277–s282.

CHAPTER 26
Problems in pediatrics

Simon Murch

Warwick Medical School, Coventry, UK

Introduction

The nutritional requirements of infants and young children are relatively higher than for adults, because of the requirements for growth. There is also relative functional immaturity of the immune system in early life, and an increased tendency for sensitization to dietary components. The spectrum of gastrointestinal problems in children is therefore different to adults, and conditions which may have relatively minor significance for the adult patient may compromise growth and weight gain. In young infants presenting with gastrointestinal disease, there is an increased chance compared to older patients of detecting underlying inherited abnormality such as immunodeficiency.

Gastroenterological problems in infancy
Congenital GI abnormalities

Congenital GI abnormalities may present in the first hours or days of life with symptoms of obstruction. The initial features may be non-specific, and there may be similar symptoms in infants with sepsis, which may also mimic congenital metabolic disorders or cause neonatal jaundice.

Jaundice

Jaundice is common in newborn infants and it is important to differentiate physiological from pathological causes and to determine whether bilirubin is conjugated. Pathological jaundice may be caused by increased red cell breakdown (commonly feto-maternal blood group incompatibility) or decreased clearance. Conjugated hyperbilirubinemia mandates early further investigation to exclude hepatic disease (often infectious or metabolic) or extrahepatic obstruction (e.g. biliary atresia). Causes of jaundice are discussed in Chapter 15.

Hirschsprung disease

This important cause of constipation, due to defective innervation of the rectum, is the manifestation of several genes, the principal ones being the RET (rearranged during transfection) gene and components of the endothelin signalling pathways [1]. Hirschsprung disease may present initially with delayed passage. Diagnosis requires full thickness rectal biopsy. Long-term management is required, and many children have significant problems despite surgical resection of the aganglionic segment.

Necrotizing enterocolitis (NEC)

This is a severe and frequently life-threatening intestinal disease, which may result in fatal intestinal perforation. NEC is characterized by diffuse or patchy ischemic lesions of the small and/or large intestine (Figure 26.1), causing ulceration and frequently progressing to necrosis and perforation [2].

Causes Early reports of NEC were in relatively mature infants, usually in association with factors such as birth asphyxia, umbilical catheterization, polycythemia or sepsis. With modern neonatal care NEC is now usually associated with extreme prematurity, often without other recognized predisposing factors (Table 26.1). NEC frequently affects the terminal ileum, a vascular "watershed" area, suggesting that mesenteric blood flow is an important determinant.

Other risk factors include dysmotility, hypoxia, ischemia with reperfusion, luminal bacteria and formula feeding. Certain bacteria, particularly *Clostridia*, have been implicated

Textbook of Clinical Gastroenterology and Hepatology, Second Edition. Edited by C. J. Hawkey, Jaime Bosch, Joel E. Richter, Guadalupe Garcia-Tsao, Francis K. L. Chan.
© 2012 Blackwell Publishing Ltd. Published 2012 by Blackwell Publishing Ltd.

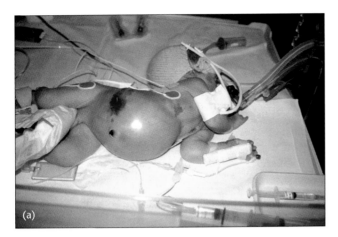

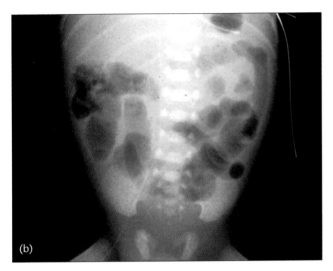

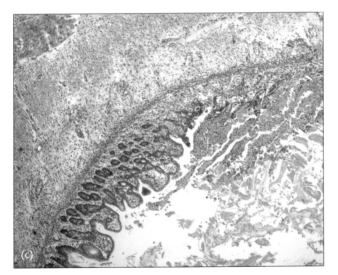

Table 26.1 Risk factors for the development of necrotizing enterocolitis

Factors affecting epithelial integrity
Prematurity (particularly extreme prematurity)
Systemic infection
Hypoxia

Factors affecting mesenteric blood supply
Placental insufficiency
Polycythemia
Cyanotic congenital heart disease
Indomethacin treatment (patent ductus arteriosus)
Maternal cocaine abuse

Luminal factors
Formula feeds (breastfeeding is protective)
Intestinal obstruction
Intestinal bacteria

Figure 26.1 Neonatal necrotizing enterocolitis. (a) A preterm infant with acute NEC, showing a grossly distended and dark-colored abdomen. (b) Plain abdominal X-ray of an infant with acute NEC, showing loops of distended small bowel and colon, with bowel wall thickening. (c) Full thickness resection specimen shows focal mucosal ulceration, with relatively minor inflammatory infiltrate.

in localized outbreaks, but most cases are sporadic. Probiotics are emerging as potential preventative agents.

Management is then based on stopping enteric feeds and commencing antibiotics, and many cases are self-limiting. The disease may progress, with increasing distension and signs of perforation or sepsis. Characteristic X-ray findings include distended bowel loops with wall thickening, and free gas in the peritoneum or biliary tree (Figure 26.1). Laparotomy is often required, and affected bowel may appear ischemic or frankly gangrenous. Late consequences include stricturing and short bowel syndrome.

Neonatal diarrhea

It is uncommon for neonates to present with diarrhea, and this may herald an underlying inherited abnormality (Table 26.2). It is important to differentiate between osmotic and secretory diarrhea. Two rare conditions, **chloridorrhea** and **sodium diarrhea,** present with profuse secretory diarrhea. Early recognition is important to prevent CNS and renal complications, but subsequent treatment is straightforward and dependent on electrolyte replacement. By contrast, in **glucose–galactose malabsorption**, due to mutations in the sodium–glucose co-transporter (SGLT-1), the diarrhea is entirely osmotic. An important clinical clue is perianal burning due to carbohydrate malabsorption. Treatment is based on fructose-based milk formulae, as fructose is absorbed by a separate transporter (Glut 5).

Less frequently, the onset of persistent diarrhea in infancy is a manifestation of one of the **intractable diarrhea syndromes** [3], which usually present in the first few days of life with intestinal failure, requiring long-term TPN therapy. **Microvillous inclusion disease** is caused by mutation in a myosin motor protein and characterized by abnormal microvilli and glycocalyx, with characteristic ultrastructural findings of vesicles containing microvilli (Figure 26.2). In **tufting enteropathy**,

Table 26.2 Potential causes of persistent diarrhea in infants and young children

Misdiagnosis or poor treatment of recognized food-sensitive enteropathy

Unrecognized immunodeficiency and/or infection

Inflammatory enteropathy or colitis

Anatomical abnormalities or dysmotility syndromes (pseudo-obstruction)

Primary specific absorption failures (e.g., chloridorrhea)

Enteropathy associated with primary metabolic diseases (e.g., mitochondrial cytopathy abetalipoproteinemia, congenital disorders of glycosylation)

True intractable diarrhea syndromes:

a) Epithelial – microvillous inclusion disease, tufting enteropathy, heparan sulfate deficiency

b) Autoimmune enteropathy syndromes, e.g. IPEX syndrome

caused by mutation in epithelial cell adhesion molecules, there are tufts of extruding epithelium. Both disorders are lethal unless long TPN is maintained, and small bowel transplantation is increasingly attempted. Hopes for the future include gene transfer.

Infant protein-losing enteropathy

Infant protein-losing enteropathy is most frequently due to lymphangiectasia, but rare causes include enterocyte heparan sulfate deficiency. Similar presentations may occur as a rare manifestation of other primary disorders, including mitochondrial cytopathies, immunodeficies and congenital disorders of glycosylation.

Autoimmune enteropathy

This is an uncommon, but important cause of severe persistent diarrhea in infancy [4], due to an autoimmune response to the gut epithelium (Figure 26.3). Inflammation may be confined to the intestine or be part of a multisystem process, often in association with endocrinopathy. There have been important recent advances in the molecular basis of autoimmune enteropathy syndromes. The immune polyendocrinopathy X-linked (IPEX) syndrome is due to mutation in the transcription factor FOXP3, a master regulator of regulatory lymphocyte generation [4]. Affected infants cannot generate normal regulatory lymphocytes, and thus present with a multifocal autoimmune disease, characterized by hyper-IgE, intractable diarrhea, eczema and a variety of endocrinopathies. The disease is of major conceptual interest and bone marrow transplantation is potentially curative.

Gastroesophageal reflux

Gastroesophageal reflux (GOR) is common in infancy, due largely to the relatively straight gastroesophageal alignment at that age. Neural immaturity makes reflux almost universal in very preterm infants, and neurological abnormalities of any kind predispose to later reflux. Symptoms are variable, with some infants showing vomiting or pain, while others present more insidiously with aspiration or feed refusal.

Treatment Treatment has classically been based on posture control and feed thickening, with medical therapy a combination of acid suppressing agents and prokinetics, with the surgical option of Nissen's fundoplication a last resort [5]. Impedance monitoring has shown that the great majority of reflux episodes are non-acid, and thus missed on pH testing. Gastroesophageal reflux clasically improves as the infant grows. However the consequences of inadequate treatment may include later feeding difficulty.

Recently, a second important cause of GOR has been recognized. In **allergic dysmotility,** GOR is precipitated by ingested dietary antigen, most commonly milk. Multiple food antigens have now been implicated, and induced mast cell and eosinophil degranulation is thought to be the likely mechanism of the induced dysmotility [6]. Thus antigen exclusion may need to be combined with conventional therapy in the management of infants with reflux, and empirical antigen restriction is attempted in most cases resistant to classic therapy. This disorder overlaps with **eosinophilic esophagitis**, in which transmural infiltration of eosinophils occurs, inducing dysmotility and subsequent fibrosis. This disorder is diagnosed on the basis of characteristic endoscopic findings of ridged edematous mucosa that is easily traumatized. Histological findings are more patchy than might be expected from such a striking macroscopic appearance, as penetration of eosinophils into the epithelium from the deeper layers where they are recruited is variable. Thus findings of more than 15 eosinophils per high power field in one single biopsy is diagnostic. The disorder shows significant ovelap to the pathology seen in asthma, and is rising significantly in incidence.

Food allergies

Food allergies now affect 5% or more of children in most developed countries [7] and previously uncommon allergies have become much more prevalent [8]. Current theories include changing antigen intake in infancy, and reduced infectious exposures [9]. IgE-mediated allergies generally present soon after ingestion, and the diagnosis is usually supported by positive skinprick and specific-IgE tests. Non-IgE-mediated allergies usually present later after ingestion, and the causative antigen may be more difficult to detect. In IgE-mediated reactions, children may complain of tingling of the tongue or lips, or simply appear apprehensive. This may be followed rapidly by skin rash, urticaria or wheezing. Angioneurotic edema can follow, and in more severe cases anaphylactic shock. Some children manifest a biphasic response, with a relatively modest initial reaction followed several hours later by a potentially life-threatening response. Severe food allergic reactions require urgent assessment, and adrenaline therapy is required if there is any evidence of airway obstruction or systemic hypotension [10]. Late onset symptoms of non-IgE-mediated food allergy are often insidious. Potential symptoms include failure to thrive or chronic diarrhea, eczema, rhinitis, or rectal bleeding. These symptoms are mediated by T cells or eosinophils in a delayed hypersensitive reaction, and may not be recognized

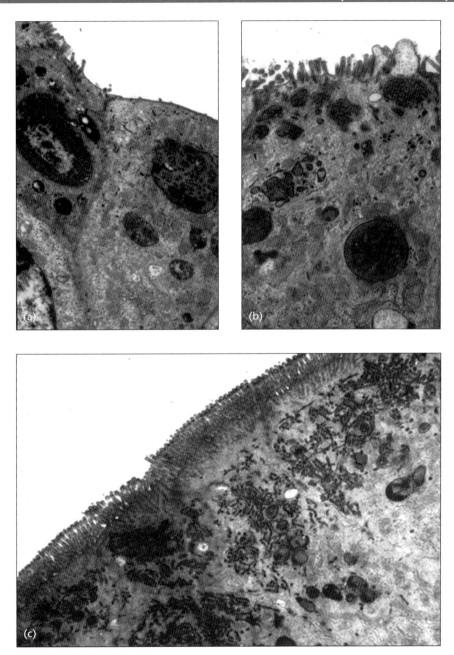

Figure 26.2 Electron microscopic features of microvillous inclusion disease/ microvillous atrophy (courtesy of Prof Alan Phillips). (a) and (b) show the characteristic findings of disrupted surface microvilli on villous epithelium, with intracellular vesicles containing microvillous components. (c) shows crypt epithelium, with intact surface microvilli, but the presence of intracellular secretory granules. The molecular basis has yet to be determined.

as due to food ingestion. They may also occur in exclusively breastfed infants in response to maternally ingested antigen. Although intestinal biopsy may show enteropathy or mucosal eosinophilia, skin prick tests and specific IgE tests may be negative.

Food sensitive enteropathy

The major mucosal manifestation of food allergy is food sensitive enteropathy, charaterized by lymphocyte infiltration, epithelial abnormality or architectural disturbance. This may impair absorption, causing micronutrient deficiency or frank malabsorption. Diagnosis is based on histological features at biopsy and clinical response to antigen exclusion and challenge. By contrast to celiac disease, such enteropathies are usually restricted to early life, and later challenge is usually tolerated. The mucosal lesion is classically patchy, and less severe than in celiac disease.

Food protein-induced enterocolitis syndrome (FPIES) is a severe and sometimes life-threatening form of mucosal food hypersensitivity. It is classically associated with cow's milk or

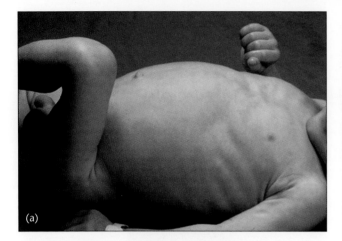

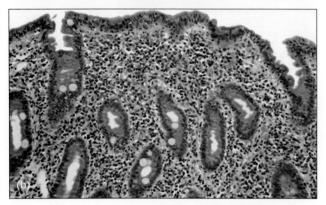

Figure 26.3 A case of autoimmune enteropathy, due to IPEX syndrome. (a) shows the characteristic abdominal distension and buttock wasting. (b) shows histological features in the duodenum, with crypt hyperplastic villous atrophy. Unlike celiac disease, the intraepithelial lymphocyte density is often normal.

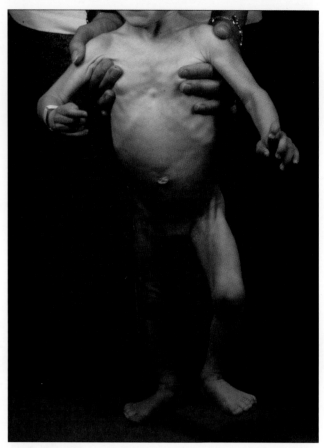

Figure 26.4 The classical appearance of celiac disease, with abdominal distension and wasting of the buttocks and thighs. Many current cases show less florid features, and celiac serology is being performed increasingly readily in pediatric practice (e.g. in Down syndrome, unexplained epilepsy, diabetes).

soya ingestion in infants, but has recently been reported in older children in response to several foods of usually low antigenicity [11]. It is also common for such symptoms to occur in exclusively breastfed infants, triggered by milk protein in the mother's diet. Negative skin prick tests do not exclude this diagnosis. Mild cases present with loose stools containing mucus or blood and respond rapidly to exclusion of cow's milk from the diet (cow's milk colitis). More severe cases present with vomiting and diarrhea or melena, dehydration or shock.

Constipation

Constipation is a relatively common problem in children, with prevalence in otherwise normal children up to 8%. Development of severe constipation in infancy raises the possibility of structural or neurological abnormality, and makes neurological assessment and rectal examination important. Most cases do not have a clear structural basis, and are labelled functional constipation. Two major groups can be differentiated by transit studies, either due to slow transit throughout the colon, or outflow obstruction (rectal impaction) due to local dysmotility of the sphincter mechanisms. The majority of cases are

managed by general pediatricians, and referral to pediatric gastroenterologists is usually reserved for severe or treatment-resistant cases. Some cases of apparently intractable constipation may be relieved by exclusion diets [12], but many remain resistant to medical therapy.

Celiac disease

The incidence of celiac disease in childhood is higher than previously recognized. It is important to recognize that the classical presentation, with steatorrhea, abdominal distension, poor growth and anemia is actually quite uncommon in childhood celiac disease (Figure 26.4). Estimates of incidence have increased since the 1970s from 1 in 2000 children to more than 1 in 100 [13]. This is because of better detection by specific serology, and population-based serological studies have demonstrated that silent or atypical celiac disease is far more common than usually appreciated [13].

The early feeding of infants has an important influence on presentation of celiac disease. In Sweden there was a major increase in infant presentation when a high wheat-containing weaning diet was recommended, and a dramatic fall when recommendations changed [14]. It is not known whether this will lead to a truly lowered incidence or an increase in the numbers of children presenting late and atypically.

Pathogenesis of celiac disease in childhood is similar to adult celiac disease (Chapter 40). However, in contrast to adult celiac disease, in which there are clearly a very few immuno-dominant peptide sequences in the gliadin molecule, responses in children may be directed to a large number of peptide sequences in both gliadin and glutenin [15].

As in adult celiac disease, the only current treatment is a lifelong strict gluten-free diet. There are a very small number of children who develop apparent celiac disease in the first two years of life, who then recover on a gluten-free diet and never relapse subsequently (**Transient Gluten Intolerance of Infancy**). Such early onset makes advisable a later formal gluten challenge, including serial biopsies on and off gluten. However, for all children diagnosed after two years, current ESPGHAN recommendations suggest that a single abnormal biopsy is diagnostic if specific serology is positive [16]. Forth-coming ESPGHAN guidelines will allow diagnosis without biopsy in certain specific circumstances (high titre screening serology, confirmed on second blood test with appropriate HLA-DQ status).

Inflammatory bowel disease

True IBD is uncommon in infants under 2, and many such cases represent inherited immunological conditions. Histo-logical findings of granulomata in such cases make exclusion of chronic granulomatous disease important. Other conditions to exclude in the very young child with apparent IBD include Behçet's disease and autoimmune enteropathy. However there has been undoubted increase in true inflammatory bowel disease in younger children in the 0–4 and 5–9 years age groups, which contributes to an overall increase in the inci-dence of pediatric IBD [17,18]. It is not clear why there is such a trend towards the younger development of pediatric IBD. Changing early life infectious exposures is one potential con-tributory factor, although no single change has so far emerged.

In older children, classic IBD occurs, with manifestations broadly similar to adult disease, but with additional effects on growth and puberty. Cases may present without classic fea-tures of diarrhea, weight loss and pain, but with unexplained poor growth or pubertal delay [18]. There is now international consensus on investigation, designed to minimize diagnostic delay [19]. For initial diagnosis, it is important to perform full ileocolonoscopy, with upper endoscopy [20].

The essential lesion of IBD is similar in children to that seen in adults (Figure 26.5). However the disease is often of rela-tively recent onset in young people, which offers increased potential opportunities for treatment. There is now a trend towards early aggressive therapy with immunosuppressive treatment to try to alter the course of disease [21]. The ideal aim of therapy is to induce and maintain clinical and histologi-cal remission, rather than just symptomatic improvement. Suc-cessful treatment should allow children to achieve their full potential for growth and educational attainment. Treatment

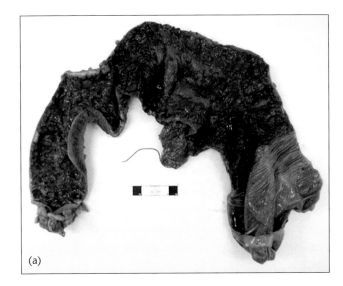

(a)

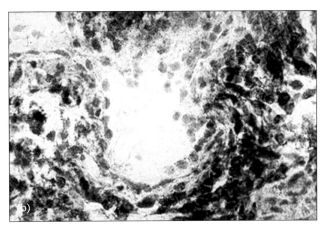

(b)

Figure 26.5 (a). Severe ulcerative colitis in a 12-year-old, requiring emergency resection. There is a sharp demarcation between severely affected and relatively normal colon. (Photograph courtesy of Dr Alan Bates.) (b). A submucosal vessel from the ileum of a 14-year-old with Crohn's disease, causing growth failure and pubertal delay. The vessel is surrounded by multiple TNF-α immunoreactive cells (stained red.)

modalities are similar to those used in adult patients, although therapies for children should not interfere with growth and pubertal development. Thus there is an increased use of enteral nutrition therapy and reduced use of corticosteroids in chil-dren with Crohn's disease [22].

Current developments and controversies

The significant rise in the childhood incidence of established disorders such as IBD, together with the emergence of newly recognized disorders such as eosinophilic esophagitis, FPIES and multiple food allergy in exclusively breastfed infants raises the question of commonality of underlying mechanism. In particular, the emerging data on the role of gut colonization in the development of regulatory immune responses in the gut has led to speculation whether the dramatic changes that have occurred in the colonization of the intestine of infants during the last half century (modified by elective cesarean section and perinatal antibiotic use) may have affected evolutionarily conserved mechanisms of immune imprinting [23]. The focus is thus beginning to shift towards study of the factors determining the establishment of immune regulatory networks in early life.

SOURCES OF INFORMATION FOR PATIENTS AND DOCTORS

British Society of Paediatric Gastroenterology, Hepatology and Nutrition www.bspghan.org.uk
European Society of Paediatric Gastroenterology, Hepatology and Nutrition http://espghan.med.up.pt/joomla
North American Society of Paediatric Gastroenterology, Hepatology and Nutrition www.naspghan.org
Crohn's in Childhood Research Association www.cicra.org/index.asp
National Association for Crohn's and Colitis www.nacc.org.uk/content/home.asp British Society for Allergy and Clinical Immunology www.bsaci.org

---

References

1. Amiel J, Sproat-Emison E, Garcia-Barcelo M, *et al.* Hirschsprung disease, associated syndromes and genetics: a review. *J Med Genet.* 2008;45:1–14.
2. Thompson AM, Bizzarro MJ. Necrotising enterocolitis in newborns: – pathogenesis, prevention and management. *Drugs.* 2008;68:1227–1238.
3. Murch SH. Protracted diarrhea. In: Wyllie R, Hyams JS. editors. *Pediatric Gastrointestinal and Liver Disease, 3rd edn.* Elsevier; 2006. p. 491–505.
4. Murch S. Advances in the understanding and management of autoimmune enteropathy. *Current Paediatrics.* 2006;305–316.
5. Salvatore S, Vandenplas Y. Gastro-oesophageal reflux disease and motility disorders. *Best Pract Res Clin Gastroenterol.* 2003;17:163–179.
6. Murch S. Allergy and intestinal dysmotility – evidence of genuine causal linkage? *Curr Opin Gastroenterol.* 2006;22: 664–668.
7. Wood RA. The natural history of food allergy. *Pediatrics.* 2003;111:1631–1637.
8. Hourihane JO. Peanut allergy – current status and future challenges. *Clin Exp Allergy.* 1997;27:1240–1246.
9. Murch SH. The immunologic basis for intestinal food allergy. *Curr Opin Gastroenterol.* 2000;16:552–557.
10. Sampson HA. Anaphylaxis and emergency treatment. *Pediatrics.* 2003;111:1601–1608.
11. Nowak-Wegrzyn A, Sampson HA, Wood RA, *et al.* Food protein-induced enterocolitis syndrome caused by solid food proteins. *Pediatrics.* 2003;111:829–835.
12. Iacono G, Cavataio F, Montalto G, *et al.* Intolerance of cow's milk and chronic constipation in children. *N Engl J Med.* 1998;339: 1100–1104.
13. Maki M, Mustalahti K, Kokkonen J, *et al.* Prevalence of Celiac disease among children in Finland. *N Engl J Med.* 2003;348: 2517–2524.
14. Hernell O, Ivarsson A, Persson LA. Coeliac disease: effect of early feeding on the incidence of the disease. *Early Hum Devel.* 2001;65:S153–S160.
15. Vader W, Kooy Y, van Veelen P *et al.* The gluten response in children with celiac disease is directed toward multiple gliadin and glutenin peptides. *Gastroenterology.* 2002;122:1729–1737.
16. Walker-Smith JA, Guandalini S, Schmitz J, *et al.* Revised criteria for diagnosis of coeliac disease. Report of Working Group of European Society of Paediatric Gastroenterology and Nutrition. *Arch Dis Child.* 1990;65:909–911.
17. Benchimol EI, Guttmann A, Griffiths AM, *et al.* Increasing incidence of paediatric inflammatory bowel disease in Ontario, Canada: evidence from health administrative data. *Gut.* 2009;58:1490–1497.
18. Buller H, Chin S, Kirschner B, *et al.* Inflammatory bowel disease in children and adolescents: working group report of the first world congress of pediatric gastroenterology, hepatology, and nutrition. *J Pediatr Gastroenterol Nutr.* 2002;35:S151–S158.
19. Sawczenko A, Sandhu BK. Presenting features of inflammatory bowel disease in Great Britain and Ireland. *Arch Dis Child.* 2003;88:995–1000.
20. Escher JC *et al.* Inflammatory Bowel Disease in Children and Adolescents: Recommendations for Diagnosis – The Porto Criteria. *J Pediatr Gastroenterol Nutr.* 2005;41:1–7.
21. Markowitz J, Grancher K, Kohn N, *et al.* A multicenter trial of 6-mercaptopurine and prednisone in children with newly diagnosed Crohn's disease. *Gastroenterology.* 2000;119:895–902.
22. Heuschkel RB, Menache CC, Megerian JT, *et al.* Enteral nutrition and corticosteroids in the treatment of acute Crohn's disease in children. *J Pediatr Gastroenterol Nutr.* 2001;31:8–15.
23. Bedford Russell AR, Murch SH. Could peripartum antibiotics have delayed health consequences for the infant? *Br J Obstetr Gynaecol.* 2006;113:758–765.

PART 2

Diseases of the Gut and Liver

CHAPTER 27

Gastroesophageal reflux disease

Tiberiu Hershcovici and Ronnie Fass

Southern Arizona VA Health Care System, Tucson, AZ, USA

Upper GI Tract

ESSENTIAL FACTS ABOUT PATHOGENESIS

- GERD is a sensory-motor disorder
- Anatomical abnormalities, such as hiatal hernia, can aggravate esophageal reflux
- Patients with GERD fall into three categories:
  1. nonerosive reflux disease (NERD),
  2. erosive esophagitis
  3. Barrett's esophagus
- Residual reflux (nonacidic, acidic, or bile), functional heartburn, psychological comorbidity, and concomitant functional bowel disorder are common causes of treatment failure with a proton pump inhibitor (PPI)

ESSENTIALS OF DIAGNOSIS

- Treatment with a PPI is highly sensitive but not specific for diagnosing GERD
- Upper endoscopy is primarily performed in GERD patients to identify Barrett's esophagus and other complications of GERD (such as peptic stricture)
- Ambulatory 24-hour pH esophageal monitoring is indicated in NERD patients who are candidates for antireflux surgery or patients reporting symptoms post antireflux surgery
- Multichannel intraluminal impedance is most useful in GERD patients who failed PPI twice daily

ESSENTIALS OF TREATMENT AND PROGNOSIS

- Treatment in GERD is primarily directed to control symptoms but also to provide mucosal healing and prevent relapse of both
- PPIs are the most effective class of drugs in controlling GERD symptoms, healing erosive esophagitis, and preventing relapse or GERD complications
- Antacids and histamine 2-receptor antagonists are more effective than PPIs in relieving acute postprandial heartburn
- Antireflux surgery could be considered in carefully selected GERD patients who are responsive or nonresponsive to PPIs

---

Introduction and definition

Gastroesophageal reflux disease (GERD) is a very common disorder affecting between 10% and 30% of the Western population (Figure 27.1). GERD is the digestive disease with the highest annual direct cost in the United States (US$9.3 billion) [1].

According to the Montreal International Consensus Group [2], GERD is defined as a condition that develops when the reflux of stomach contents causes troublesome reflux-associated symptoms. While GERD is commonly diagnosed in clinical practice based on symptoms alone, it has been demonstrated that esophageal symptoms are not stimulus-specific and thus heartburn could result from non-reflux related stimuli. Based on upper endoscopy results, patients with GERD are further classified into erosive esophagitis, if visible mucosal breaks in the distal esophagus are present, and non-erosive reflux disease (NERD) if the mucosal breaks are absent. Esophageal complications of GERD are ulceration, stricture, Barrett's esophagus and adenocarcinoma of the esophagus. Barrett's esophagus is a change in the distal esophageal epithelium of any length that can be recognized as columnar type mucosa at endoscopy and is confirmed to have intestinal metaplasia by biopsy of the tubular esophagus [3].

Natural course studies revealed that most patients with GERD remain within their phenotypic presentation over the years [4]. It has been estimated that approximately 10% of NERD patients will progress over time to develop primarily low grade erosive esophagitis [5]. However the durability of these new mucosal lesions remains unknown. Presently we are still lacking prospective evidence that patients with NERD or erosive esophagitis progress over time to develop Barrett's esophagus.

The Los Angeles classification is a validated and reproducible standardized classification to describe the extent of esophageal mucosal injury (Figure 27.2). It has a good correlation with the degree of esophageal acid exposure as measured by ambulatory 24-hour esophageal pH monitoring and severity of heartburn symptoms [6]. However, in response to proton

---

Textbook of Clinical Gastroenterology and Hepatology, Second Edition. Edited by C. J. Hawkey, Jaime Bosch, Joel E. Richter, Guadalupe Garcia-Tsao, Francis K. L. Chan.
© 2012 Blackwell Publishing Ltd. Published 2012 by Blackwell Publishing Ltd.

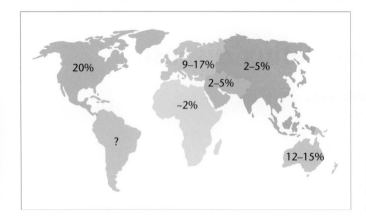

Figure 27.1 Prevalence of GERD in the world. (This figure was published in *Clinical Gastroenterology and Hepatology*, Wilfred M. Weinstein, Christopher J. Hawkey, Jaime Bosch, Gastroesophageal reflux disease, Pages 157–166, Copyright Elsevier, 2005.)

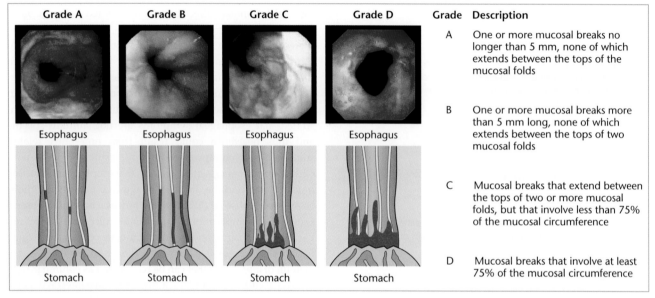

Grade A	Grade B	Grade C	Grade D	Grade	Description
				A	One or more mucosal breaks no longer than 5 mm, none of which extends between the tops of the mucosal folds
				B	One or more mucosal breaks more than 5 mm long, none of which extends between the tops of two mucosal folds
				C	Mucosal breaks that extend between the tops of two or more mucosal folds, but that involve less than 75% of the mucosal circumference
				D	Mucosal breaks that involve at least 75% of the mucosal circumference

Figure 27.2 The Los Angeles classification of esophageal mucosal injury. (This figure was published in *Clinical Gastroenterology and Hepatology*, Wilfred M. Weinstein, Christopher J. Hawkey, Jaime Bosch, Gastroesophageal reflux disease, Pages 157–166, Copyright Elsevier, 2005.)

pump inhibitor (PPI) treatment, Los Angeles Grade A demonstrates almost similar healing rate as Grade B, and healing rates of esophagitis Grade C and D are lower than those of esophagitis Grade A and B [7].

The complications of GERD such as esophageal stricture and Barrett's esophagus are discussed in Chapters 30 and 31.

Epidemiology

Population-based studies suggest that GERD is a common condition with a prevalence of 10–30% in Western Europe and North America [8]. In the United States, 42% of the adult population experience GERD-related symptoms annually and 20% weekly [9]. GERD is less commonly seen in the Asia-Pacific region [10]. The prevalence of GERD in other parts of

the world, such as Africa or South America, is largely unknown. An estimated prevalence of weekly reports of heartburn in different parts of the world is presented in Figure 27.1.

The prevalence of erosive esophagitis is more difficult to determine. Studies have suggested that 7% of the US adult population has erosive esophagitis whereas in Europe and Asia the prevalence has been estimated to range between 2–10% [8]. Furthermore, erosive esophagitis is usually milder in Asia (predominantly Los Angeles grade A and B) and complications such as esophageal stricture, Barrett's esophagus, and esophageal adenocarcinoma are relatively uncommon [11].

The prevalence of GERD and related disorders has been steadily increasing in the US, western Europe, Australia and Asia [8]. An opposing trend was observed between 1970 and

1995 in the prevalence of peptic ulcer disease and GERD in the USA. The rates of peptic ulcer and gastric cancer fell while at the same time the rates of GERD and esophageal adenocarcinoma rose significantly [12]. Possible explanations for the increase in prevalence of GERD include increase in food consumption, BMI and sedentary lifestyle, decrease in the prevalence of *H. pylori* infection, and habits such as smoking and alcohol consumption.

Most patients with GERD-related symptoms never seek medical attention. Therefore, those who do seek medical attention represent just the tip of the GERD "iceberg." GERD is associated with considerable morbidity and various complications. However, in a population-based study with over 50,000 person-years of follow-up, reflux symptoms were not associated with worse survival [13].

Patients with NERD are more commonly females, usually leaner, report a shorter symptom duration and have a lower incidence of hiatus hernia compared to patients with erosive esophagitis. Furthermore, complicated GERD is more commonly seen in Caucasian men, and is associated with increased age. Of all ethnic groups, Caucasians demonstrate the highest rates of GERD, Barrett's esophagus and esophageal adenocarcinoma.

The prevalence of hiatus hernia varies between 29% and 96% in patients with GERD [14], and the prevalence is much lower in patients with no reflux symptoms, indicating the importance of hiatus hernia in the pathophysiology of GERD. It has been demonstrated that 96% of the patients with long segment (≥3 cm) Barrett's esophagus, 72% with short-segment (<3 cm) Barrett's esophagus, 71% with erosive esophagitis, and 29% with NERD have hiatus hernia [14].

Causes, risk factors and disease associations

Risk factors purported to be associated with GERD include cigarette smoking, alcohol, coffee, obesity, high fat diet, food products such as chocolate, peppermint, and citrus juices; as well as a slew of medications (narcotics, calcium channel blockers etc.) A recent systematic review of the currently available literature demonstrated that there is no direct evidence that carbonated beverages promote or exacerbate GERD [15].

Obesity is associated with a 1.5- to 2-fold increase in the risk for GERD symptoms and erosive esophagitis, as well as a 2- to 2.5-fold increase risk for esophageal adenocarcinoma as compared to individuals with normal BMI. There was also a dose-dependent relationship between BMI and the previously mentioned GERD-related disorders [16]. Increased waist circumference rather than BMI *per se* appears to explain a considerable part of this association. Several underlying mechanisms have been proposed to explain the close relationship between increased BMI and GERD, including increased gastroesophageal pressure gradient, increased prevalence of hiatal hernia, increased prevalence of transient lower esophageal sphincter relaxations (TLESR), as well as others [17].

GERD is more common in pregnant women due to increased intra-abdominal pressure and the relaxing effect of progesterone on the lower esophageal sphincter. The prevalence of GERD increases with age, and older patients are more likely to develop severe disease [18]. Systemic diseases such as scleroderma-CREST syndrome (cutaneous calcinosis, Raynaud's phenomenon, esophageal dysfunction, sclerodactyly, and telangiectasia), Sjögren's syndrome, and diabetes mellitus are associated with a higher incidence of GERD.

Table 27.1 lists the conditions associated with erosive esophagitis. Depending on the clinical presentation, several of these clinical entities should be considered before labeling the patient as having GERD. For example, in the immunocompromised patient, infectious causes should be considered. In young males with history of esophageal dysphagia and possible history of food impaction, eosinophilic esophagitis should be entertained. In patients of all ages with new-onset apparent GERD, pill-induced esophagitis should be excluded.

The relationship between *Helicobacter pylori* and GERD has been controversial. Some studies suggested that *H. pylori* infection conferred protection from GERD and its eradication was associated with an increased risk of developing the disorder. However, a post hoc analysis of eight double blind prospective

Table 27.1 Causes of erosive esophagitis

- **Gastroesophageal reflux disease**
- **Infections**
  Candida
  Viral (cytomegalovirus, herpes virus, human immunodeficiency virus)
  Bacterial (*Nocardia*, syphilis)
  Mycobacterium (tuberculosis, atypical mycobacteria)
  Parasitic (Chagas' disease)

- **Systemic disease**
  Skin pathology (epidermolysis bullosa, pemphigus, drug induced)
  Behçet's disease
  Graft versus host disease
  Inflammatory bowel disease
  Sarcoidosis
  Metastatic cancer
  Collagen vascular disease (scleroderma, CREST syndrome, Sjögren's syndrome)

- **Iatrogenic**
  Pill-induced esophagitis (tetracycline, potassium chloride, alendronate, NSAIDs)
  Radiation-induced esophagitis
  Chemotherapy-induced esophagitis
  Sclerotherapy-induced erosions/ulcerations

- **Nasogastric tube (Ryle's tube) induced trauma**

- **Zollinger-Ellison syndrome**

(Adapted with permission from Oviedo J *et al.* Erosive esophagitis. In: Fass R, editor *GERD/dyspepsia.* Philadelphia: Hanley & Belfus; 2004. p. 83–99.)

trials revealed that eradication of *H. pylori* in patients with duodenal ulcer was not associated with the development of erosive esophagitis, new symptomatic GERD, or worsening of symptoms in patients with pre-existing GERD [19]. A more recent meta-analysis of twelve trials revealed no association between *H. pylori* eradication and the development of new cases of GERD in dyspeptic patients [20]. However, in cohort studies, there was a two–fold increase in the risk of developing erosive GERD in patients with peptic ulcer disease. The latter findings were not supported by randomized clinical trials.

Pathogenesis

The pathogenesis of heartburn was discussed in Chapter 1. GERD is believed to be caused by the effect of refluxed gastric acid on esophageal epithelial cells. Several factors have been proposed as important in the pathophysiology of GERD. They include dysfunction of the lower esophageal sphincter, hiatal hernia, esophageal dysmotility, impaired esophageal defense mechanisms, gastric acid hypersecretion, duodenogastro-esophageal reflux, esophageal hypersensitivity, delayed gastric emptying and genetic factors (Figure 27.3).

Dysfunction of the LES and hiatal hernia

It is presently accepted that the major elements that compose the antireflux barrier are the lower esophageal sphincter (LES) and the crural diaphragm. The LES is a thickened ring of circular smooth muscle located at the distal 2–3 cm of the esophagus and serves as a mechanical barrier between the stomach and the esophagus. The right crus of the diaphragm encircle the LES and thus provide additional mechanical support. The

variations in LES pressure are usually coupled with esophageal and gastric contractions, whereas the pressure contributed by the crural diaphragm is in response to physical activity such as inspiration, coughing, Valsalva maneuver, abdominal compression, and others. Traditionally, gastroesophageal reflux is thought to occur across a hypotensive LES in the presence of hiatal hernia. However, the LES basal pressure in GERD patients is within normal limits. In fact, for most patients with GERD, the predominant mechanism of gastroesophageal reflux is transient lower esophageal sphincter relaxation (TLESR), in which spontaneous (not preceded by a swallow), prolonged relaxations of the LES (>10 sec) are triggered primarily by fundic relaxation and mediated by a vasovagal reflex. TLESRs have been established as the primary mechanism for gastroesophageal reflux in normal subjects and patients with GERD, as well as the underlying mechanism for belching [21]. Although recent trials found no increased rate of TLESR's in patients with GERD, a TLESR was more likely to be associated with an acid reflux event in patients with GERD as compared to healthy controls [22]. This may be caused by the increase in compliance of the esophagogastric junction in GERD patients which leads to an increase in luminal cross-sectional area during opening. Conversely, this results in greater volume of the refluxate and a reduced ability to limit the refluxate to gas.

The presence of a hiatal hernia, particularly if it is large (≥5 cm) is associated with increased severity of GERD (Figure 27.4). Displacement of LES from the crural diaphragm into the chest reduces its basal pressure and shortens the length of the high pressure zone because of the loss of the intra-abdominal LES segment.

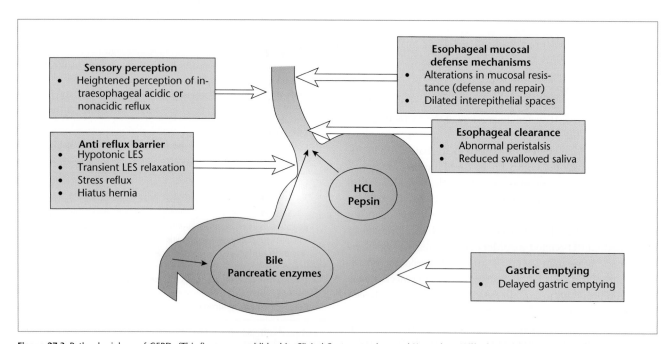

Figure 27.3 Pathophysiology of GERD. (This figure was published in *Clinical Gastroenterology and Hepatology*, Wilfred M. Weinstein, Christopher J. Hawkey, Jaime Bosch, Gastroesophageal reflux disease, Pages 157–166, Copyright Elsevier, 2005.)

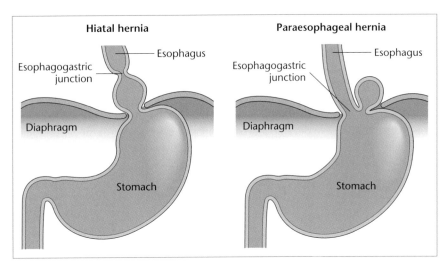

Figure 27.4 Schematic representation of hiatus hernia and paraesophageal hernia. Note the proximal displacement of the esophagogastric junction in hiatus hernia, whereas in paraesophageal hernia the anatomic location of the esophagogastric junction is preserved. (This figure was published in *Clinical Gastroenterology and Hepatology*, Wilfred M. Weinstein, Christopher J. Hawkey, Jaime Bosch, Gastroesophageal reflux disease, Pages 157–166, Copyright Elsevier, 2005.)

The prevalence of hiatal hernia increases with the severity of esophageal mucosal involvement. Patients with NERD demonstrated the lowest prevalence (20–30%), and those with long segment Barrett's esophagus the highest, prevalence (95%).

The presence of hiatal hernia disrupts the integrity of the sphincter mechanism and prolongs esophageal clearance, leading to an increase in esophageal acid exposure and acid reflux events. Severity of erosive esophagitis appears to correlate with the size of the hernia [23]. The presence of hiatal hernia is associated with a reduced threshold for TLESR in response to gastric distension [24]. Patients with hiatal hernia have acid reflux associated with low LES pressure; swallow associated normal LES relaxations and straining during periods with low LES pressure [25].

Esophageal mucosal defense mechanisms

Esophageal mucous and bicarbonate layer, cell membranes, intercellular junctional complexes, and an adequate mucosal blood flow are important defense mechanisms against injury by gastroesophageal reflux. Exchangers at the basolateral membrane can restore intracellular pH by exchanging intracellular H^+ for extracellular Na^+ or intracellular Cl^- for extracellular HCO_3^-. Increased esophageal permeability and reduced mucin production improve after antisecretory therapy, suggesting that these abnormalities are caused by gastroesophageal reflux.

Esophageal clearance

The most common physiologic aberration causing increased acid contact time is ineffective refluxate clearance. Impairment of acid clearance can be secondary to either peristaltic dysfunction and/or re-reflux (the to-and-fro movement of reflux fluid), which is seen in association with hiatus hernia.

Esophageal peristaltic dysfunction in GERD is well documented [26,27], and is increasingly observed with more severe grades of erosive esophagitis. There has been a longstanding argument as to whether the dysmotility precedes or is caused by GERD [26]. Elimination of reflux does not result in normalization of motility, but it may be that severe reflux has permanently damaged the distal esophageal "pump."

Non-transmitted swallows or simultaneous esophageal contractions are ineffective in clearing the volume of the refluxate. Ineffective esophageal motility, defined by the presence of abnormally low amplitude (<3 mm Hg) contractions in the distal esophagus (30% or moee of wet swallows), was also found to be associated with prolonged esophageal acid clearance in both the upright and recumbent positions [27].

Gastric acid secretion

There is no strong evidence to suggest that hypersecretion of gastric acid plays an important role in the pathogenesis of GERD [14,22]. However, Zollinger-Ellison syndrome, which is characterized by gastric acid hypersecretion, is associated with increased risk of having GERD and specifically esophageal mucosal injury.

Duodenogastroesophageal (bile) reflux

It has been suggested that duodenogastroesophageal reflux (DGER) by itself does not cause significant damage to the esophageal mucosa but may act synergistically with acid reflux to produce erosive esophagitis. Studies have demonstrated that a combination of acid and bile reflux is the most common reflux pattern in patients with GERD [28]. DGER occurs in 50% of the NERD patients, 79% of those with erosive esophagitis, and 95% of the patients with long segment Barrett's esophagus. Recent studies have demonstrated that bile reflux can cause heartburn symptoms.

Acid pocket

The presence of an "acid pocket" (an area of highly acidic gastric juice) in the proximal gastric cardia that escapes buffering by food has been suggested to aggravate the re-reflux phenomenon which has been described in association with hiatal hernia [29]. The "acid pocket" may extend longer, both cranially in the high pressure zone and caudally in the stomach, in GERD patients as compared with normal controls [30,31]. This has been suggested to explain the much greater acid exposure just above the esophagogastric junction (EGJ) and thus the propensity of this area to develop mucosal damage. However, while subcardial pH has been confirmed to be highly acidic early after meals, there is no difference in the pH of this region between healthy subjects and GERD patients with or without hiatal hernia, during both the supine and postprandial periods [32].

Gastric dysmotility

Approximately 20% of the patients with GERD have delayed gastric emptying, but there is no direct correlation between the degree of the delay and severity of GERD [14,33]. However, slow proximal gastric emptying in patients with GERD has been shown to correlate with increased 24-hour esophageal pH monitoring, number of reflux episodes per hour, and postprandial acid exposure.

Genetic factors

A genetic predisposition for GERD was suggested based on the results of several family and twin studies. Reflux symptoms were more frequent among parents and siblings of those with either Barrett's or adenocarcinoma of the esophagus as compared to spouses and control relatives [34]. A large twin study has shown an increased concordance for GERD in monozygotic pairs, compared with dizygotic pairs, suggesting that genetic factors accounted for 31% of the risk of developing GERD [35]. A novel study by deVries *et al.* found that C825T polymorphism in the G-protein Beta-3 subunit (GNB3) was more prevalent in GERD patients compared with normal controls [36]. The authors suggested that the increased signal transduction upon GPCR activation associated with the 825T allele may be responsible for increased perception of reflux events. Further studies are needed to verify their findings.

Pathology

Figure 27.2 depicts the different grading of erosive esophagitis according to the Los Angeles classification [6]. In this classification, the histopathologic term – erosive esophagitis – is replaced by a descriptive term – mucosal break. An endoscopic mucosal break is defined as "an area of slough or erythema with a discrete line of demarcation from the adjacent, more normal looking mucosa." Documenting mucosal breaks on endoscopy is an indication for the presence of erosive esophagitis, but minor changes such as erythema, edema, and friability are not.

It has been widely accepted that reflux esophagitis develops from a caustic, chemical injury that starts at the luminal surface of the squamous epithelium, and progresses through the epithelium and lamina propria into the submucosa. The

acid-induced death of surface cells is assumed to stimulate a proliferative response in the basal cells that renew the squamous epithelium [37]. This has been presumed to result in hyperplasia of the basal cell layer and the papillae, histologic findings that are considered characteristic of reflux esophagitis. Finally, acid-induced epithelial injury and cell death is assumed to promote an inflammatory response, which is manifested histologically by inflammatory cells infiltrating the damaged squamous epithelium [38].

Various histologic findings have been described in patients with NERD including the presence of inflammatory cells (neutrophils and eosinophils), epithelial hyperplasia (basal cell hyperplasia and elongated papillae), and dilated vessels in the papillae.

Dilation of intercellular space (DIS) is the most consistently reported histologic finding in patients with NERD or erosive esophagitis [39]. The mean intercellular space width is at least two times greater in patients than in controls, irrespective of the level of esophageal acid exposure. New basal cell hyperplasia and papillary elongation are more common in NERD patients as compared with controls. Both of these features are more prevalent in patients with abnormal esophageal acid exposure. All histologic changes reversed during acid-suppressive therapy.

Clinical presentation

Heartburn and regurgitation are the hallmark symptoms of reflux disease (see Chapter 1). Heartburn describes a sensation of discomfort or burning behind the sternum rising up to the neck, made worse after meals and eased by antacids. Regurgitation is defined as the perception of flow of refluxed gastric content into the mouth or hypopharynx. The sensitivity of reflux symptoms in diagnosing endoscopically erosive esophagitis is in the range of 30–76% and the specificity is 62–92% [40].

Angina-like chest pain, globus sensation, chronic cough, hoarseness, and asthma are considered atypical manifestations of GERD (see Chapter 1). The reported odds ratios for these symptoms in GERD patients range from 1.2 to 3 with nocturnal cough and chest pain having the strongest association. Dysphagia and odynophagia usually suggest the presence of esophageal mucosal injury. GERD symptom frequency or severity doe not correlate with the extent of esophageal mucosal involvement in patients with erosive esophagitis. Clinical studies have demonstrated that heartburn severity and intensity are similar in patients with erosive esophagitis and NERD [41].

In the elderly patient with GERD, heartburn is less frequent (54%) than in younger subjects with GERD and acid regurgitation is present in less than 25% of the patients [42,43]. In contrast, atypical symptoms such as vomiting, anorexia, dysphagia, respiratory symptoms, belching, dyspepsia, hoarseness, and postprandial fullness are more common presentations of GERD in the elderly. One of the explanations for the pronounced decrease in severity and frequency of GERD-related symptoms, despite increase in the degree of esophageal inflammation in the elderly, is altered esophageal pain perception to chemical and mechanical stimuli [18].

Irritable bowel syndrome (IBS) like symptoms as well as dyspeptic symptoms are common in GERD patients [44]. Approximately 50% of both NERD and erosive esophagitis patients report dyspeptic and IBS-like symptoms. In NERD patients, these symptoms were shown to determine reflux symptom severity independently [45].

Natural history of GERD

The retrospective studies that evaluated the natural course of GERD revealed limited progression (~10%) from NERD to erosive esophagitis (mostly low-grade) and no evidence to support progression of NERD to Barrett's esophagus [46]. There is no evidence that erosive esophagitis may progress over time to Barrett's esophagus or that Barrett's esophagus may regress in length or regress completely over time. There is limited evidence, from a retrospective study, that patients with erosive esophagitis may regress over time to NERD, although the durability of this regression has never been determined [47]. Overall, there appears to be very limited movement in between the different GERD groups (NERD, erosive esophagitis, and Barrett's esophagus) [48].

Differential diagnosis

Although heartburn is strongly associated with the diagnosis of GERD, studies have demonstrated that esophageal symptoms are not stimulus specific. Patients with functional heartburn, peptic ulcer disease, gastric cancer, and delayed gastric emptying may present with heartburn. Furthermore, sudden and isolated attacks of heartburn may be caused by pill-induced esophagitis, or caustic or radiation injury to the esophageal mucosa. Patients with achalasia may also report heartburn. In patients with heartburn who also present with alarm symptoms such as anorexia, weight loss, anemia, dysphagia, and hematemesis, early upper endoscopy is indicated. The presence of erosive esophagitis in patients undergoing upper endoscopy is usually indicative of GERD, but other etiologies have been identified and should be considered (see Table 27.2).

Diagnostic methods

The diagnostic methods available for GERD (see Table 27.3) include clinical evaluation, barium esophagogram, upper endoscopy, esophageal pH monitoring, esophageal manometry, multichannel intraluminal impedance and pH monitoring, and the use of the PPI test.

Table 27.2 Diagnostic methods for GERD

DIAGNOSTIC METHODS

COMMONLY USED METHODS FOR THE DIAGNOSIS OF GERD

Test	Advantages	Disadvantages	Recommended use
Barium swallow	Noninvasive Widely available	Poor sensitivity and specificity	For patients with GERD who present with dysphagia
Upper endoscopy	Highly sensitive for the diagnosis of erosive GERD and GERD complications Obtain tissue biopsies Treat peptic strictures	Limited sensitivity for general GERD Invasive Expensive Not always readily available	GERD with alarm symptoms Detection of Barrett's esophagus
24-h esophageal pH monitoring Conventional catheter	Assesses esophageal acid exposure Correlation of symptoms with acid reflux events	Transnasal intubation is not well tolerated by patients Limitation in everyday activities during the study may effect accuracy	Failure of PPI therapy (twice daily) Before antireflux surgery (NERD) Following antireflux surgery after symptom recurrence
Bravo capsule	Avoids the need for nasal intubation	Endoscopy may be required for placement of capsule	
PPI test	Widely available Noninvasive Cost effective	Subjective outcome Limited specificity in GERD	Atypical symptoms of GERD

Modified with permission from Sunil J *et al.* Gastroesophageal reflux disease: diagnosis of GERD. In: Fass R, ed. GERD/dyspepsia. Philadelphia: Hanley & Belfus; 2004:41–54.

Table 27.3 Alarm symptoms in GERD patients

- Dysphagia
- Odynophagia
- Anorexia
- Weight loss
- Anemia
- Hematemesis/coffee ground emesis

Clinical evaluation

The clustering of symptoms in the postprandial period and rapid relief by antacids are useful positive diagnostic criteria. Several validated GERD symptom questionnaires have been developed, but their usage has been limited to clinical trials [49].

The proton pump inhibitor (PPI) test

The PPI test is a simple non-invasive diagnostic as well as a therapeutic tool for GERD that is widely available to community-based physicians [50]. The PPI test is the usage of a short course (1–4 weeks) of high-dose PPI given twice daily for the diagnosis of GERD in patients with typical, atypical, or extraesophageal manifestations of GERD. If symptoms disappear with therapy and then return when medication is stopped, GERD can be assumed and no further testing is required. Several trials in patients with typical symptoms of GERD have demonstrated that the sensitivity of the PPI test ranges from 66% to 89%, and the specificity from 35% to 73%. However, there is still no consensus about the desired level of symptom response (cut-off level), optimal dose, frequency, or duration of the empiric PPI test for GERD.

Barium esophagogram

Barium esophagogram has shown a low sensitivity (20%) in the diagnosis of GERD. However, the sensitivity of this test improves when assessing for anatomic abnormalities associated with GERD such as severe erosive esophagitis and complicated GERD (stricture and ulceration) [51]. The test is not sensitive for Barrett's esophagus but may help in determining the presence and size of hiatus hernia as well as the length of the esophagus.

Upper endoscopy

Upper endoscopy is the gold standard procedure for diagnosing erosive esophagitis, GERD complications, and Barrett's esophagus. Additionally, endoscopy allows an assessment of the degree of esophageal mucosal injury, and tissue sampling can be performed if necessary. Endoscopy has a sensitivity of about 30–50% in patients with typical symptoms of GERD, as most patients with GERD have NERD; however it has an excellent specificity (90–95%). The value of histopathologic examination of normal-appearing esophageal mucosa to confirm or exclude pathologic acid reflux remains

controversial. In accordance with the current guidelines and recommendations, patients with uncomplicated GERD should undergo acid suppressive treatment prior to endoscopic evaluation. However this treatment can heal esophagitis and may significantly limit the sensitivity of endoscopy as a diagnostic tool.

Upper endoscopy is indicated in patients with GERD and alarm symptoms (Table 27.3) and to exclude Barrett's esophagus in long term sufferers. In patients who failed PPI therapy, upper endoscopy is a low yield procedure and is commonly normal [52].

It has been proposed that better visualization of minute changes of the esophageal mucosa of GERD patients with normal endoscopy can be obtained by narrow-band imaging (NBI). This technique utilizes spectral narrow band filters and enables imaging of superficial tissue structures such as capillary and mucosal patterns without the use of dye. It was recently demonstrated that the best predictor for GERD diagnosis when using NBI is an increase in number and dilatation of intra-papillary capillary loops [53].

Ambulatory 24-hour esophageal pH monitoring

This test involves the transnasal placement of a flexible pH recording probe into the distal esophagus. The tip of the probe is positioned 5 cm above the proximal margin of the LES. The test allows assessment of 24-hour esophageal acid exposure and the temporal relationship between patient symptoms and acid reflux events. Esophageal pH monitoring is normal in 25% of patients with erosive esophagitis and in up to 50% of those with NERD [49]. Because of nasal and pharyngeal discomfort, patients often limit their daily activity during pH monitoring, which may decrease the accuracy of the test [54]. Migration of the pH probe into the stomach during the test may lead to erroneous results.

Despite these drawbacks, ambulatory 24-hour esophageal pH monitoring should be considered in the following circumstances:

- patients with NERD being considered for antireflux surgery;
- patients after antireflux surgery who continue to be symptomatic;
- patients with GERD-related symptoms despite PPI treatment (including symptoms of noncardiac chest pain, suspected otolaryngologic manifestations of GERD, adult-onset refractory asthma).

Patients who failed the PPI test (see above) should undergo 24-hour pH monitoring while continuing to take the treatment. Recent studies suggest that impedance-pH sensor is a more sensitive tool for GERD patients who failed PPI treatment than pH testing alone, primarily because weakly acidic or alkaline reflux, which are not detected by a regular pH test, are important causes for symptoms in this patient population (Figure 27.5).

Upper GI Tract

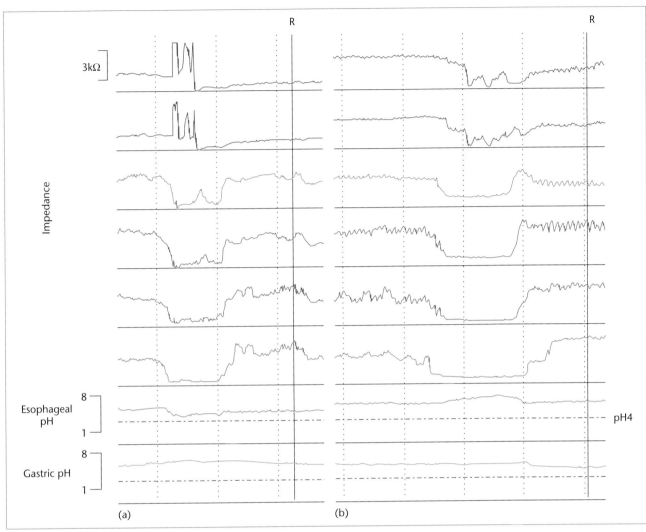

Figure 27.5 Examples of symptomatic reflux events detected with esophageal impedance-pH monitoring in a patient during treatment with a proton pump inhibitor (A, weakly acidic reflux; B, weakly alkaline reflux). (Reproduced from Fass R, Sifrim D. Management of heartburn not responding to proton pump inhibitors. *Gut.* 2009 Feb;58(2):295–309, with permission from the BMJ Publishing Group Ltd.)

The wireless pH capsule

The wireless pH capsule is a radio-transmitter pH system that was introduced as a more patient-friendly pH monitoring system [55]. The capsule is attached to the distal esophageal mucosa using a delivery system after either endoscopy or esophageal manometry. The capsule transmits pH changes via radio signals to a receiver worn by the patient around the waist. Therefore, pH recordings using the wireless pH system improve patients' ability to perform their daily activities and thus provide a more accurate picture of their acid exposure profile as well as improve their compliance with the study [56]. Unlike the pH probe procedure, the wireless capsule provides an extended 48 hours of pH recording. This technique is better tolerated by patients and provides improved assessment of the relationship between symptoms and acid reflux events.

Esophageal manometry

While esophageal manometry has no role in the diagnosis of GERD (since it does not measure acid reflux), it is routinely performed to determine the proper location of the LES prior to placement of a pH probe. Additionally, esophageal manometry is commonly used to evaluate patients with GERD who are candidates for antireflux surgery, in order to exclude esophageal motility abnormalities [57].

Multichannel intraluminal impedance

While esophageal pH monitoring is considered a valuable tool for gastroesophageal reflux detection, it may not accurately detect GERD when weakly acidic or alkaline reflux are present. Esophageal impedance monitoring is a technique that can be used to detect all types of reflux (acidic, weakly acidic and weakly alkaline). This technique is based on the measurement of electrical impedance between closely arranged electrodes mounted on a thin intraluminal probe. Air has a low conductivity and yields an increase in impedance, while swallowed or refluxed material has a high conductivity and thus yields a drop in impedance.

Changes in temporal–spatial patterns in impedance are identified at various levels within the esophagus allowing differentiation between antegrade (i.e., swallow) and retrograde (i.e., reflux) bolus movement. In this way, impedance can be used to evaluate intra-esophageal liquid movements (bolus transit tests and reflux monitoring) or gas movement (aerophagia and belching). However, impedance is unable to quantify the volume of gastroesophageal reflux. In healthy adults, the total rate of reflux episodes measured with impedance–pH is about 40–70 per 24 hours with one-third being acidic and two-thirds being weakly acidic and weakly alkaline. Impedance–pH monitoring should be analyzed in a quantitative fashion, similar to 24-hour esophageal pH monitoring, by searching for increased numbers of reflux episodes, prolonged acid or volume exposures, or increased numbers of proximal reflux events. In addition, qualitative analysis of the reflux–symptom association, using symptom index (SI) or symptom association probability (SAP), is essential.

It is currently suggested that impedance–pH monitoring is useful in reaching a diagnosis in patients with refractory GERD. Approximately 10% of refractory GERD patients on twice daily PPI have a positive SI for acid reflux, and 37% have a positive SI for non-acid reflux [58]. A European multicenter study found similar results and showed that adding impedance to pH monitoring improves the diagnostic yield by 15–20% and allows better symptom analysis than pH monitoring alone [59]. Because impedance–pH monitoring is currently the most sensitive tool for detecting reflux, a negative study (normal number of total reflux events and negative symptom association analysis) rules out GERD as a cause of persistent heartburn symptoms. It is important to recall that patients with refractory GERD have similar number of reflux events as those off treatment and have similar pattern of reflux as GERD patients, who are responders to PPI [60]. Consequently, symptoms related to weakly or alkaline reflux are likely to occur due to esophageal hypersensitivity.

Treatment

The aims of GERD management include: (1) confirmation of the diagnosis of GERD; (2) adequate relief of GERD symptoms; (3) healing of erosive esophagitis, if present; (4) maintenance of mucosal healing and (5) improvement of patient-reported quality of life. For patients with mild and infrequent reflux symptoms, antacids and lifestyle modifications (weight loss, cessation of smoking, elevation of head of the bed, and avoidance of aggravating foods) may provide adequate treatment. In a recent systematic review of all publications that evaluated

the value of lifestyle modifications in GERD patients, the authors determined that only weight loss and elevation of head of the bed are effective in improving GERD [61]. There were no sufficient data to support any of the other commonly practiced lifestyle modifications.

Most gastroenterologists either no longer prescribe antacids or provide them to patients with only occasional symptoms. The vast majority will start with an H2-receptor antagonist or PPI. The use of any type of anti-reflux treatment does not obviate the need to adopt lifestyle modifications [49]. A suggested algorithm for the management of patients with GERD is provided in Figure 27.6.

PPIs allow an effective control of reflux symptoms and a high rate of healing of erosive esophagitis. In a meta-analysis of 7,635 patients with erosive esophagitis, complete relief of heartburn was the highest with PPIs (77%), versus 48% with H2-receptor antagonists. Furthermore, PPIs provided the highest healing rate of erosive esophagitis (84%), when compared with H2-receptor antagonists (52%), sucralfate (39%), or placebo (28%) [62]. Failure of a 4-week course of initial therapy with a PPI should prompt a review of the diagnosis. A once-daily morning dosing of PPI, half an hour before a meal, is generally the most appropriate initial therapy, but may fail in up to 30% of patients.

In general, the proportion of NERD patients responding to a standard dose of PPI is approximately 20–30% lower than what has been documented in patients with erosive esophagitis. In a systematic review of the literature, the PPI symptomatic response pooled rate was 36.7 (95% CI: 34.1–39.3) in NERD patients and 55.5 (95% CI: 51.5–59.5) in those with erosive esophagitis [63].

Multiple approaches have been used to enhance acid suppression with PPIs. The immediate-release omeprazole (IR-OME) contains non-enteric coated omeprazole, and an antacid buffer that protects the omeprazole from gastric acid degradation in the stomach and allows for rapid absorption. IR-OME has demonstrated effective control of gastric acidity when dosed on an empty stomach at bedtime. IR-OME has been shown to provide more rapid control of night-time gastric pH and nocturnal acid breakthrough as compared with esomeprazole or lansoprazole [64].

Dexlansoprazole MR contains the dual delayed release technology. The drug is the R-enantiomer of lansoprazole, with two distinct drug release periods that prolong the plasma concentration–time profile and thus extend the duration of acid suppression [65–67].

Treatment for GERD may follow three different clinical strategies: step-up, step-down or step-in. The step-up approach initiates patients on the least effective antireflux modality and upgrades treatment if satisfactory control of symptoms is not achieved. The step-down approach initiates patients on the most potent antireflux modality and downgrades patients to a therapeutic modality that still controls their symptoms effectively. The step-in approach initiates and maintains patients on the most potent antireflux modality [68,69]. The latter

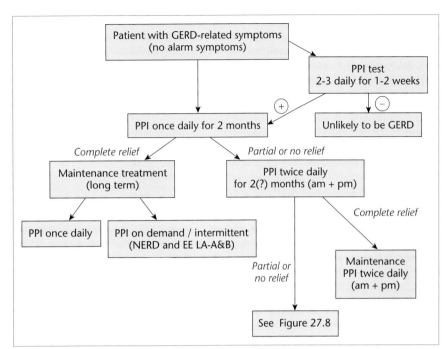

Figure 27.6 Management algorithm for patients with symptoms of gastroesophageal reflux but without alarm symptoms. GERD, gastroesophageal reflux disease; NERD, non erosive reflux disease; EE, erosive esophagitis; PPI, proton pump inhibitor; LA Los Angeles classification.

Upper GI Tract

approach has become the most popular therapeutic strategy in clinical practice.

Because GERD is mostly a non-progressive disorder, treatment of these patients can be symptom driven. On-demand or intermittent PPI therapy is an attractive therapeutic strategy in patients with NERD and potentially in those with mild erosive esophagitis. This therapeutic approach is convenient, cost effective, and decreases the likelihood of rebound of acid secretion. Studies have demonstrated that intermittent or on-demand PPI therapy in NERD is associated with improved quality of life and reduced cost [70].

Antacids and alginates

Antacids are basic compounds composed of different combinations of acid-neutralizing agents such as aluminum and magnesium hydroxide, calcium carbonate, sodium citrate, and sodium bicarbonate. They provide transient symptom relief but do not contribute to the healing or prevention of GERD complications [71,72].

Histamine type 2 receptor antagonists

Histamine type 2 receptor antagonists (H2RAs) are still widely used for the treatment of GERD. This class of drugs reduces gastric acid output by competitive inhibition of histamine at H2 receptors on the parietal cells. Standard doses have been proven to be effective in controlling symptoms and in healing mild to moderate erosive esophagitis. The potential effect of H2RAs on night-time histamine driven surge of gastric acid secretion led to the popular use of these drugs at bedtime by patients who continued to be symptomatic on a standard or double-dose PPI therapy [73]. However, tachyphylaxis

develops quickly with H2RAs, limiting their regular use in clinical practice [74]. The main appeal of H2RAs is their rapid effect on GERD symptoms, unsurpassed by any of the currently available PPIs.

Promotility and prokinetic drugs

Motility-modulating drugs may improve gastroesophageal reflux by increasing LES basal pressure, restoring esophageal peristalsis and thus acid clearance, and facilitating gastric emptying. However, the benefit of these compounds in controlling heartburn and in healing erosive esophagitis has been very modest, primarily because of lack of effect on TLESR.

Metoclopramide is a dopamine antagonist and cholinomimetic that crosses the blood–brain barrier and neutralizes the inhibitory effect of dopamine in the central nervous system and on the gastrointestinal smooth muscle. Its therapeutic efficacy in GERD is limited because of multiple adverse effects of a neurologic and psychotropic nature, including lethargy, mental status changes, and extrapyramidal abnormalities, which may not be reversible after discontinuation of the drug.

Domperidone is a potent peripheral dopamine antagonist whose properties are similar to those of metoclopramide. Unlike metoclopramide, however, it does not readily cross the blood–brain barrier. Domperidone is commonly used to treat GERD in patients who have delayed gastric emptying, primarily to improve gastric motility.

TLESR reducers

Baclofen – a gamma-aminobutyric acid β receptor agonist – is used as an add-on treatment for patients who failed PPI treatment (once or twice daily). The drug reduces TLESR rate by

40 to 60% and reflux episodes by 43%, increases lower esophageal sphincter basal pressure, and accelerates gastric emptying. Baclofen was found to significantly reduce weakly acidic and bile reflux as well as gastroesophageal reflux-related symptoms [75]. In patients with persistent heartburn despite PPI treatment, doses of up to 20 mg three times daily have been used [76]. Because the drug crosses the blood-brain barrier, a variety of central nervous system (CNS)-related side effects may occur. They primarily include somnolence, confusion, dizziness, lightheadedness, drowsiness, weakness, and trembling. The side effects are an important limiting factor in the routine usage of baclofen in clinical practice. However, several baclofen-like prototypes with better clinical and side-effect profiles are currently in development.

Antireflux surgery

Antireflux surgery is offered to patients in the hope of obviating the need for continuous medical therapy, which may result in the patient's inconvenience, increased costs, and concerns about safety. Nissen fundoplication remains the most commonly performed operation and consists of a 360° wrap of the gastric fundus around the distal esophagus, which results in augmentation of LES basal pressure and a decrease in the rate of TLESR. At this time fundoplication is commonly done laparoscopically (see Chapters 156 and 157). Complications due to antireflux surgery are determined by the expertise of the surgeon, which has been shown to correlate closely with the number of procedures performed. Offering surgery to young patients because of the prospect of long-term medical therapy should be individualized and discussed in an unbiased way. Ultimately, the success of antireflux surgery depends on selecting the appropriate patients and surgeon. Presurgical evaluation includes esophageal manometry, primarily to exclude achalasia and ineffective peristalsis, upper endoscopy, and 24-hour esophageal pH monitoring in those patients without erosive esophagitis. As discussed in Chapter 157, a positive response to medical therapy is the best predictor of successful surgical outcome.

Antireflux surgery relieves reflux symptoms and heals erosive esophagitis. However Barrett's esophagus does not regress and there is no evidence that antireflux surgery reduces the risk for the development of adenocarcinoma of esophagus [77]. A multicenter, prospective, randomized comparative trial between medical treatment (omeprazole) and antireflux surgery for GERD, revealed that after 12 years follow up period, the proportion of patients in continuous remission was significantly higher in the surgical group (53%) than in the medical group (40–45%) [78]. During the follow-up period, 36% of the patients who had a fundoplication were subsequently treated with a PPI, whereas 14% of the patients randomized to the medical group were subsequently referred for fundoplication. However, the surgical therapeutic strategy was affected by postoperative adverse events resulting in similar scores for quality of life as the medical treatment group. In an ongoing similar study comparing a PPI with standardized laparoscopic antireflux surgery, the proportion of patients who remained in remission after three years were similar for both groups (93% vs. 90%) [79].

Refractory GERD

Approximately 10 to 40% of patients with GERD fail to respond symptomatically, either partially or completely, to a standard dose PPI. Failure of the PPI treatment to resolve GERD-related symptoms has become the most common presentation of GERD in clinical practice [80]. Most patients with GERD who do not respond to a PPI originate from the nonerosive reflux (NERD) and functional heartburn groups, primarily due to their relative large size among the heartburn patient population (up to 70%) and low response rate to PPI once daily. In contrast, patients with erosive esophagitis that account for only 30 to 40% of the GERD population are more likely to respond to PPIs than patients with NERD (pooled symptomatic response rate to PPI once daily at four weeks of 56 versus 37%, respectively) [81].

Various underlying mechanisms have been suggested to contribute to the failure of PPI treatment. They include weakly acidic reflux, duodenogastroesophageal reflux, residual acidic reflux, functional bowel disorders, psychological co-morbidity and esophageal hypersensitivity (Figure 27.7).

Evaluation of proper compliance and adequate dosing time should be the first management step when assessing patients with heartburn who are not responding to PPI before instituting any other intervention. Further diagnostic evaluation of refractory GERD may include an upper endoscopy, pH testing and esophageal impedance with pH monitoring.

For those who do not respond adequately to once-daily PPI, the addition of a second daily dose before the evening meal is commonly prescribed [49].

Two main therapeutic strategies are available in patients who failed twice daily PPI therapy. The proper strategy may be determined by utilizing esophageal impedance + pH testing, which detects whether residual reflux (acidic or nonacidic) is the underlying cause of the patient's symptoms. If residual reflux is present, then a transient lower esophageal sphincter relaxation reducer should be considered. However, if there is no evidence that residual reflux is the direct cause of symptoms, then esophageal pain modulators, either peripherally or centrally, should be entertained. Anti-reflux surgery may be suitable for a subset of patients with clear evidence of residual reflux (acidic or non-acidic) despite PPI treatment [82]. A suggested algorithm for the management of patients with refractory GERD is provided in Figure 27.8.

Complications and their management

Complications of GERD include upper gastrointestinal bleeding (due to erosive esophagitis or bleeding esophageal ulcers), esophageal stricture (see Chapter 28), and Barrett's esophagus (see Chapter 29), which increases the risk of developing

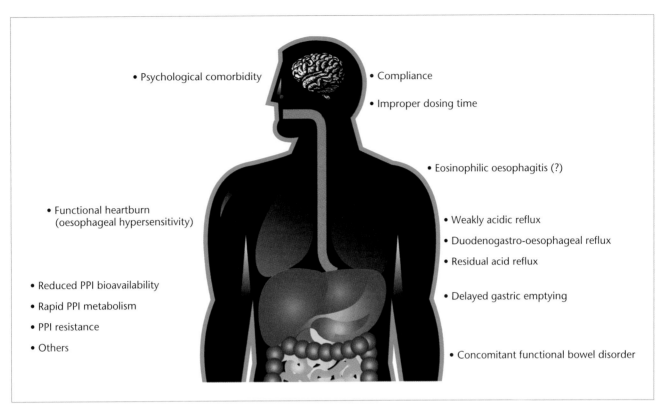

- Psychological comorbidity

- Compliance

- Improper dosing time

- Eosinophilic oesophagitis (?)

- Functional heartburn
  (oesophageal hypersensitivity)

- Weakly acidic reflux

- Duodenogastro-oesophageal reflux

- Residual acid reflux

- Reduced PPI bioavailability

- Rapid PPI metabolism

- PPI resistance

- Others

- Delayed gastric emptying

- Concomitant functional bowel disorder

Figure 27.7 Proposed mechanisms for refractory GERD (persistent heartburn despite PPI treatment). (Reproduced from Fass R, Sifrim D. Management of heartburn not responding to proton pump inhibitors. *Gut.* 2009 Feb;58(2):295–309, with permission from the BMJ Publishing Group Ltd.)

adenocarcinoma of the esophagus. Other complications include involvement of the oropharynx, larynx, and respiratory system, resulting in symptoms and signs termed extraesophageal manifestations of GERD (hoarseness, chronic cough, asthma, etc.) Other complications may include sleep disturbances, obstructive sleep apnea and linked cardiac angina.

Prognosis with and without treatment

In patients with erosive esophagitis, the disease will invariably relapse after cessation of therapy. Similarly, for patients with NERD, only 25% of those who initially achieved complete symptom resolution while taking PPIs remain asymptomatic after six months of not receiving any antireflux treatment [48,83]. For patients with complicated GERD, such as esophageal stricture and Barrett's esophagus, long-term lifelong maintenance treatment with PPIs is needed.

Harmful consequences of medical treatment

The safety of long-term use of PPIs has been of potential concern for many physicians and patients alike. Initial reports suggested that long-term acid suppression with a PPI may potentially lead to metaplastic changes in the gastric mucosa and subsequently to the development of gastric cancer. However, with more than 20 years of extensive global

experience with PPIs, studies thus far have failed to document malignant transformation in long-term users. Studies of patients who are infected with *H. pylori* and require long-term PPI therapy have suggested that gastric atrophy and potential intestinal metaplasia (the precursor for adenocarcinoma of the stomach) may develop. Consequently, some authorities have recommended testing for the presence of *H. pylori* infection and eradication of infection prior to commencement of long-term PPI therapy in patients with GERD [84].

Long term treatment with PPIs may result in decrease in intragastric concentration of vitamin C and consequently a decrease in circulating vitamin C. Similarly, there is also evidence for a decrease in circulating levels of vitamin B12. Those at risk for decrease in serum B12 are the slow metabolizers of PPIs and patients with atrophic gastritis. The reduction in both serum vitamin levels is not associated with significant clinical consequences. Presently, there is very little support for the development of iron deficiency in patients receiving long term PPI treatment.

Chronic PPIs or H2RA treatment has been associated with various enteric infections such as gastroenteritis, traveler's diarrhea, salmonella, campylobacter and cholera [85]. Furthermore, both PPIs and H2RAs have been shown to increase the risk for *Clostridium difficile* associated diarrhea [86]. Moreover, PPIs have also been associated with small bowel bacterial overgrowth (SIBO).

Upper GI Tract

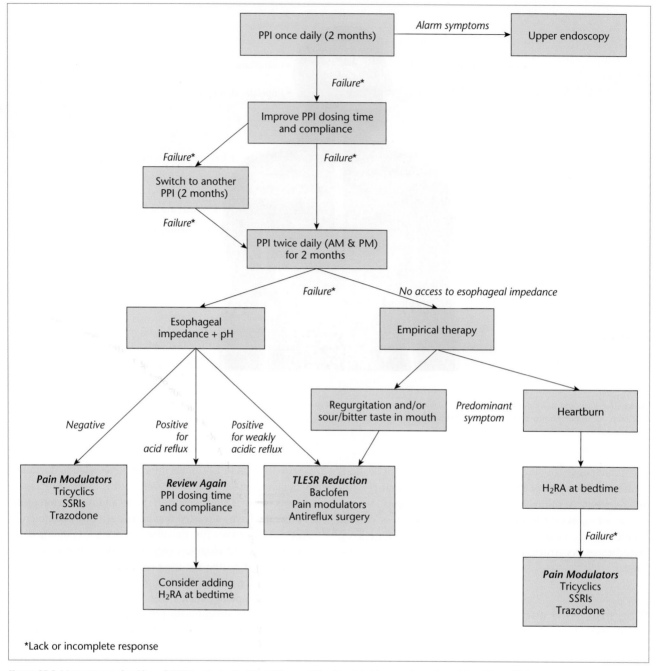

Figure 27.8 Management algorithm of GERD patient who failed PPI once daily. (Reprinted by permission from Macmillan Publishers Ltd: Ronnie Fass, Proton Pump Inhibitor Failure – What Are the Therapeutic Options? *Am J Gastroenterol.* 104:S33–S38.)

Several population-based studies have shown that chronic PPI treatment increases the risk for community acquired pneumonia (27–50%) [87,88]. The risk is particularly high in patients with co-morbidities, the elderly and those on more than once daily PPI. In addition, population-based studies have revealed that chronic PPI treatment is associated with increased risk for osteoporosis and hip fracture.

The safety of PPIs has not been fully established in pregnant women. This class of drugs has been assigned category B (except omeprazole – category C), suggesting that proper human studies substantiating the safety of these compounds have not been conducted in pregnant women. Nevertheless, there is no increase in major congenital abnormalities in pregnant women treated with PPIs.

Data from recent observational studies have suggested that PPI use might attenuate the antiplatelet effect of clopidogrel in patients with coronary artery disease who receive the drug [89–92]. Recently, the FDA specifically recommended avoiding usage of clopidogrel with either omeprazole or esomeprazole.

Patients should be advised not to stop PPIs abruptly if they have been taking a PPI for several months or more. When chronic PPI therapy is discontinued, acid production rebounds due to increase in serum gastrin levels and in parietal-cell mass during therapy. The rebound acid secretion can last for at least four weeks [93]. There is no defined regimen for PPI withdrawal, for example prior to performing 24-hour esophageal pH monitoring. One approach is to taper down the PPI dose from twice daily to once daily for two weeks, and then one PPI every other day for 2–3 weeks before stopping treatment. During the withdrawal, H2 receptor antagonists can be used on an as-needed basis for breakthrough symptoms.

SOURCES OF INFORMATION FOR PATIENTS AND DOCTORS

Reassurance of patients about the benign nature of the disease is important and relieves anxiety associated with the fear of cancer. Patients should be instructed to report any change in their symptoms over time, primarily the development of alarm symptoms such as dysphagia, odynophagia, anorexia, and weight loss. Some websites helpful for patient education are listed below.
- American College of Gastroenterology: www.acg.gi.org
- American Gastroenterological Association: www.gastro.org
- National Library of Medicine: www.nlm.nih.gov/medlineplus
- National Institute of Diabetes & Digestive & Kidney Diseases: www.niddk.nih.gov
- Heartburn-help: http://heartburn-help.com
- National Digestive Diseases Information Clearinghouse (NDDIC): http://digestive.niddk.nih.gov

References

1. Sandler RS, Everhart JE, Donowitz M, et al. The burden of selected digestive diseases in the United States. Gastroenterology. 2002;122(5):1500–1511.
2. Vakil N, van Zanten SV, Kahrilas P, et al. The Montreal definition and classification of gastroesophageal reflux disease: a global evidence-based consensus. Am J Gastroenterol. 2006;101(8):1900–1920; quiz 43.
3. Wang KK, Sampliner RE. Updated guidelines 2008 for the diagnosis, surveillance and therapy of Barrett's esophagus. Am J Gastroenterol. 2008;103(3):788–797.
4. Fass R, Fennerty MB, Vakil N. Nonerosive reflux disease – current concepts and dilemmas. Am J Gastroenterol. 2001;96(2):303–314.
5. Fass R. Erosive Esophagitis and Nonerosive Reflux Disease (NERD): Comparison of Epidemiologic, Physiologic, and Therapeutic Characteristics. J Clin Gastroenterol. 2007;41(2):131–137.
6. Lundell LR, Dent J, Bennett JR, et al. Endoscopic assessment of oesophagitis: clinical and functional correlates and further validation of the Los Angeles classification. Gut. 1999;45(2):172–180.
7. Richter JE, Kahrilas PJ, Johanson J, et al. Efficacy and safety of esomeprazole compared with omeprazole in GERD patients with erosive esophagitis: a randomized controlled trial. Am J Gastroenterol. 2001;96(3):656–665.
8. Dent J, El-Serag HB, Wallander MA, et al. Epidemiology of gastro-oesophageal reflux disease: a systematic review. Gut. 2005;54(5):710–717.
9. Locke GR, 3rd, Talley NJ, Fett SL, et al. Prevalence and clinical spectrum of gastroesophageal reflux: a population-based study in Olmsted County, Minnesota. Gastroenterology. 1997;112(5):1448–1456.
10. Fock KM, Talley N, Hunt R, et al. Report of the Asia-Pacific consensus on the management of gastroesophageal reflux disease. J Gastroenterol Hepatol. 2004;19(4):357–367.
11. Wong WM, Lam SK, Hui WM, et al. Long-term prospective follow-up of endoscopic oesophagitis in southern Chinese – prevalence and spectrum of the disease. Aliment Pharmacol Ther. 2002;16(12):2037–2042.
12. el-Serag HB, Sonnenberg A. Opposing time trends of peptic ulcer and reflux disease. Gut. 1998;43(3):327–333.
13. Talley NJ, Locke GR, 3rd, McNally M, et al. Impact of gastro-esophageal reflux on survival in the community. Am J Gastroenterol. 2008;103(1):12–19.
14. Cameron AJ. Barrett's esophagus: prevalence and size of hiatal hernia. Am J Gastroenterol. 1999;94(8):2054–2059.
15. Johnson T, Gerson L, Hershcovici T, et al. Systematic review: the effects of carbonated beverages on gastro-oesophageal reflux disease. Aliment Pharmacol Ther. 2010;31(6):607–614.
16. Hampel H, Abraham NS, El-Serag HB. Meta-analysis: obesity and the risk for gastroesophageal reflux disease and its complications. Ann Intern Med. 2005;143(3):199–211.
17. Fass R. The pathophysiological mechanisms of GERD in the obese patient. Dig Dis Sci. 2008;53(9):2300–2306.
18. Poh CH, Navarro-Rodriguez T, Fass R. Treatment of GERD in the Elderly. Am J Med. 2010;123:496–501.
19. Laine L, Sugg J. Effect of Helicobacter pylori eradication on development of erosive esophagitis and gastroesophageal reflux disease symptoms: a post hoc analysis of eight double blind prospective studies. Am J Gastroenterol. 200297(12):2992–2997.
20. Yaghoobi M, Farrokhyar F, Yuan Y, et al. Is There an Increased Risk of GERD After Helicobacter pylori Eradication?: A Meta-Analysis. Am J Gastroenterol. 2010;105(5):1007–1013.
21. Dodds WJ, Dent J, Hogan WJ, et al. Mechanisms of gastroesophageal reflux in patients with reflux esophagitis. N Engl J Med. 1982;307(25):1547–1552.
22. Penagini R, Carmagnola S, Cantu P. Review article: gastro-oesophageal reflux disease – pathophysiological issues of clinical relevance. Aliment Pharmacol Ther. 2002;(16 Suppl 4):65–71.
23. Jones MP, Sloan SS, Rabine JC, et al. Hiatal hernia size is the dominant determinant of esophagitis presence and severity in gastroesophageal reflux disease. Am J Gastroenterol. 2001;96(6):1711–1717.
24. van Herwaarden MA, Samsom M, Smout AJ. Excess gastroesophageal reflux in patients with hiatus hernia is caused by mechanisms other than transient LES relaxations. Gastroenterology. 2000;119(6):1439–1446.
25. Kahrilas PJ, Shi G, Manka M, et al. Increased frequency of transient lower esophageal sphincter relaxation induced by gastric distention in reflux patients with hiatal hernia. Gastroenterology. 2000;118(4):688–695.
26. Singh P, Adamopoulos A, Taylor RH, et al. Oesophageal motor function before and after healing of oesophagitis. Gut. 1992;33(12):1590–1596.

27. Lin S, Ke M, Xu J, *et al.* Impaired esophageal emptying in reflux disease. *Am J Gastroenterol.* 1994;89(7):1003–1006.

28. Vaezi MF, Richter JE. Role of acid and duodenogastroesophageal reflux in gastroesophageal reflux disease. *Gastroenterology.* 1996;111(5):1192–1199.

29. Sloan S, Kahrilas PJ. Impairment of esophageal emptying with hiatal hernia. *Gastroenterology.* 1991;100(3):596–605.

30. Clarke AT, Wirz AA, Manning JJ, *et al.* Severe reflux disease is associated with an enlarged unbuffered proximal gastric acid pocket. *Gut.* 2008;57(3):292–297.

31. Pandolfino JE, Zhang Q, Ghosh SK, *et al.* Acidity surrounding the squamocolumnar junction in GERD patients: "acid pocket" versus "acid film". *Am J Gastroenterol.* 2007;102(12):2633–2641.

32. Grigolon A, Cantu P, Bravi I, *et al.* Subcardial 24-h wireless pH monitoring in gastroesophageal reflux disease patients with and without hiatal hernia compared with healthy subjects. *Am J Gastroenterol.* 2009;104(11):2714–2720.

33. Helm JF, Dodds WJ, Pelc LR, *et al.* Effect of esophageal emptying and saliva on clearance of acid from the esophagus. *N Engl J Med.* 1984;310(5):284–288.

34. Romero Y, Cameron AJ, Locke GR, 3rd, *et al.* Familial aggregation of gastroesophageal reflux in patients with Barrett's esophagus and esophageal adenocarcinoma. *Gastroenterology.* 1997;113(5):1449–1456.

35. Cameron A, Lagergren J, Henriksson C, *et al.* Gastroesophageal reflux disease in monozygotic and dizygotic twins. *Gastroenterol.* 2002;122:55–59.

36. de Vries DR, ter Linde JJ, van Herwaarden MA, *et al.* Gastro-esophageal reflux disease is associated with the C825T polymorphism in the G-protein beta3 subunit gene (GNB3). *Am J Gastroenterol.* 2009;104(2):281–285.

37. Ismail-Beigi F, Horton PF, Pope CE. Histological consequences of gastroesophageal reflux in man. *Gastroenterology.* 1970;58(2):163–174.

38. Zentilin P, Savarino V, Mastracci L, *et al.* Reassessment of the diagnostic value of histology in patients with GERD, using multiple biopsy sites and an appropriate control group. *Am J Gastroenterol.* 2005;100(10):2299–2306.

39. Dent J. Microscopic esophageal mucosal injury in nonerosive reflux disease. *Clin Gastroenterol Hepatol.* 2007;5(1):4–16.

40. Moayyedi P, Talley NJ, Fennerty MB, *et al.* Can the clinical history distinguish between organic and functional dyspepsia? *JAMA.* 2006;295(13):1566–1576.

41. Smout AJPM. Endoscopy-negative acid reflux disease. *Aliment Pharmacol Ther.* 1997;11(Suppl 2):81–85.

42. Mold JW, Reed LE, Davis AB, *et al.* Prevalence for gastroesophageal reflux in elderly patients in a primary care setting. *Am J Gastroenterol.* 1991;86(8):965–970.

43. Räihä I, Hietanen E, Sourander L. Symptoms of gastro-oesophageal reflux disease in elderly people. *Age Ageing.* 1991;20(5):365–370.

44. Wu JC, Cheung CM, Wong VW, *et al.* Distinct clinical characteristics between patients with nonerosive reflux disease and those with reflux esophagitis. *Clin Gastroenterol Hepatol.* 2007;5(6):690–695.

45. Zimmerman J, Hershcovici T. Bowel symptoms in nonerosive gastroesophageal reflux disease: nature, prevalence, and relation to acid reflux. *J Clin Gastroenterol.* 2008;42(3):261–265.

46. Fass R. Non-erosive reflux disease (NERD) and erosive esophagitis – a spectrum of disease or special entities? *Zeitschrift fur Gastroenterologie.* 2007;45(11):1156–1163.

47. Labenz J, Nocon M, Lind T, *et al.* Prospective follow-up data from the ProGERD study suggest that GERD is not a categorial disease. *Am J Gastroenterol.* 2006;101(11):2457–2462.

48. Fass R. Gastroesophageal reflux disease revisited. *Gastroenterol Clin North Am.* 2002;31:S1–S10.

49. Dent J. Management of reflux disease. *Gut.* 2002;(50 Suppl 4):iv67–iv71.

50. Fass R. Empirical trials in treatment of gastroesophageal reflux disease. *Dig dis* (Basel, Switzerland). 2000;18(1):20–26.

51. Thompson JK, Koehler RE, Richter JE. Detection of gastro-esophageal reflux: value of barium studies compared with 24-hr pH monitoring. *AJR Am J Roentgenol.* 1994;162(3):621–626.

52. Poh CH, Gasiorowska A, Navarro-Rodriguez T, *et al.* Upper GI tract findings in patients with heartburn in whom proton pump inhibitor treatment failed versus those not receiving antireflux treatment. *Gastrointest Endosc.* 2010;71(1):28–34.

53. Sharma P, Wani S, Bansal A, *et al.* A feasibility trial of narrow band imaging endoscopy in patients with gastroesophageal reflux disease. *Gastroenterology.* 2007;133(2):454–464; quiz 674.

54. Fass R, Hell R, Sampliner RE, *et al.* Effect of ambulatory 24-hour esophageal pH monitoring on reflux-provoking activities. *Dig Dis Sci.* 1999;44(11):2263–2269.

55. Wong WM, Bautista J, Dekel R, *et al.* Feasibility and tolerability of transnasal/per-oral placement of the wireless pH capsule vs. traditional 24-h oesophageal pH monitoring – a randomized trial. *Aliment Pharmacol Ther.* 2005;21(2):155–163.

56. Hirano I, Richter JE. ACG practice guidelines: esophageal reflux testing. *Am J Gastroenterol.* 2007;102(3):668–685.

57. Waring JP, Hunter JG, Oddsdottir M, *et al.* The preoperative evaluation of patients considered for laparoscopic antireflux surgery. *Am J Gastroenterol.* 1995;90(1):35–38.

58. Mainie I, Tutuian R, Shay S, *et al.* Acid and non-acid reflux in patients with persistent symptoms despite acid suppressive therapy: a multicentre study using combined ambulatory impedance-pH monitoring. *Gut.* 2006;55(10):1398–1402.

59. Zerbib F, Roman S, Ropert A, *et al.* Esophageal pH-impedance monitoring and symptom analysis in GERD: a study in patients off and on therapy. *Am J Gastroenterol.* 2006;101(9):1956–1963.

60. Katz P, Gideon RM, Tutuian R. Reflux symptoms on twice daily (BID) proton pump inhibitor (PPI) associated with non acid reflux; a manifestation of hypersensitive esophagus? (abstract). *Am J Gastroenterol.* 2005;128(4 Suppl 2):925, A-130.

61. Kaltenbach T, Crockett S, Gerson LB. Are lifestyle measures effective in patients with gastroesophageal reflux disease? An evidence-based approach. *Arch Intern Med.* 2006;166(9):965–971.

62. Chiba N, De Gara C, Wilkinson J, *et al.* Speed of healing and symptom relief in grade II to IV gastroesophageal reflux disease: a meta-analysis. *Gastroenterol.* 1997;117:1798–1810.

63. Dean BB, Gano AD, Jr., Knight K, *et al.* Effectiveness of proton pump inhibitors in nonerosive reflux disease. *Clin Gastroenterol Hepatol.* 2004;2(8):656–664.

64. Katz PO, Koch FK, Ballard ED, *et al.* Comparison of the effects of immediate-release omeprazole oral suspension, delayed-release lansoprazole capsules and delayed-release esomeprazole capsules on nocturnal gastric acidity after bedtime dosing in patients with night-time GERD symptoms. *Aliment Pharmacol Ther.* 2007;25(2):197–205.

65. Metz DC, Vakily M, Dixit T, *et al.* Review article: dual delayed release formulation of dexlansoprazole MR, a novel approach to overcome the limitations of conventional single release proton

pump inhibitor therapy. *Aliment Pharmacol Ther*. 2009;29(9): 928–937.

66. Sharma P, Shaheen NJ, Perez MC, *et al*. Clinical trials: healing of erosive oesophagitis with dexlansoprazole MR, a proton pump inhibitor with a novel dual delayed-release formulation – results from two randomized controlled studies. *Aliment Pharmacol Ther*. 2009;29(7):731–741.

67. Fass R, Chey WD, Zakko SF, *et al*. Clinical trial: the effects of the proton pump inhibitor dexlansoprazole MR on daytime and nighttime heartburn in patients with non-erosive reflux disease. *Aliment Pharmacol Ther*. 2009;29(12):1261–1272.

68. Howden CW, Henning JM, Huang B, *et al*. Management of heart-burn in a large, randomized, community-based study: compari-son of four therapeutic strategies. *Am J Gastroenterol*. 2001;96(6): 1704–1710.

69. Inadomi JM, Jamal R, Murata GH, *et al*. Step-down management of gastroesophageal reflux disease. *Gastroenterology*. 2001;121 (5):1095–1100.

70. Gerson L, Robbins A, Garbert A, *et al*. A cost-effectiveness analy-sis of prescribing strategies in the management of gastroesopha-geal reflux disease. *Gastroenterology*. 2000;95:395–407.

71. Weberg R, Berstad A. Symptomatic effect of a low-dose antacid regimen in reflux oesophagitis. *Scand J Gastroenterol*. 1989;24 (4):401–406.

72. Grove O, Bekker C, Jeppe-Hansen MG, *et al*. Ranitidine and high-dose antacid in reflux oesophagitis. A randomized, placebo-controlled trial. *Scand J Gastroenterol*. 1985;20(4):457–461.

73. Peghini PL, Katz PO, Castell DO. Ranitidine controls nocturnal gastric acid breakthrough on omeprazole: a controlled study in normal subjects. *Gastroenterology*. 1998;115(6):1335–1339.

74. Fackler WK, Ours TM, Vaezi MF, *et al*. Long-term effect of H2RA therapy on nocturnal gastric acid breakthrough. *Gastroenterol-ogy*. 2002;122(3):625–632.

75. Lidums I, Lehmann A, Checklin H, *et al*. Control of transient lower esophageal sphincter relaxations and reflux by the GABA(B) agonist baclofen in normal subjects. *Gastroenterology*. 2000;118(1):7–13.

76. Koek GH, Sifrim D, Lerut T, *et al*. Effect of the GABA(B) agonist baclofen in patients with symptoms and duodeno-gastro-oesophageal reflux refractory to proton pump inhibitors. *Gut*. 2003;52(10):1397–1402.

77. Tran T, Spechler SJ, Richardson P, *et al*. Fundoplication and the risk of esophageal cancer in gastroesophageal reflux disease: a Veterans Affairs cohort study. *Am J Gastroenterol*. 2005;100(5): 1002–1008.

78. Lundell L, Miettinen P, Myrvold HE, *et al*. Comparison of out-comes twelve years after antireflux surgery or omeprazole main-tenance therapy for reflux esophagitis. *Clin Gastroenterol Hepatol*. 2009;7(12):1292–1298; quiz 60.

79. Lundell L, Attwood S, Ell C, *et al*. Comparing laparoscopic antireflux surgery with esomeprazole in the management of

patients with chronic gastro-oesophageal reflux disease: a 3-year interim analysis of the LOTUS trial. *Gut*. 2008;57(9):1207–1213.

80. Fass R, Gasiorowska A. Refractory GERD: what is it? *Curr Gas-troenterol Rep*. 2008;10(3):252–257.

81. Dean BB, Gano AD, Jr., Knight K, *et al*. Effectiveness of proton pump inhibitors in nonerosive reflux disease. *Clin Gastroenterol Hepatol*. 2004;2(8):656–664.

82. Fass R, Sifrim D. Management of heartburn not responding to proton pump inhibitors. *Gut*. 2009;58(2):295–309.

83. Fass R. Epidemiology and pathophysiology of symptomatic gastroesophageal reflux disease. *Am J Gastroenterol*. 2003;98(3 Suppl):S2–7.

84. Malfertheiner P, Megraud F, O'Morain C, *et al*. Current concepts in the management of Helicobacter pylori infection – the Maas-tricht 2-2000 Consensus Report. *Aliment Pharmacol Ther*. 2002;16 (2):167–180.

85. Ali T, Roberts DN, Tierney WM. Long-term safety concerns with proton pump inhibitors. *Am J Med*. 2009;122(10):896–903.

86. Aseeri M, Schroeder T, Kramer J, *et al*. Gastric acid suppression by proton pump inhibitors as a risk factor for clostridium difficile-associated diarrhea in hospitalized patients. *Am J Gas-troenterol*. 2008;103(9):2308–2313.

87. Sarkar M, Hennessy S, Yang YX. Proton-pump inhibitor use and the risk for community-acquired pneumonia. *Ann Intern Med*. 2008;149(6):391–398.

88. Herzig SJ, Howell MD, Ngo LH, *et al*. Acid-suppressive medica-tion use and the risk for hospital-acquired pneumonia. *JAMA*. 2009;301(20):2120–2128.

89. Ho PM, Maddox TM, Wang L, *et al*. Risk of adverse outcomes associated with concomitant use of clopidogrel and proton pump inhibitors following acute coronary syndrome. *JAMA*. 2009;301(9):937–944.

90. O'Donoghue ML, Braunwald E, Antman EM, *et al*. Pharmacody-namic effect and clinical efficacy of clopidogrel and prasugrel with or without a proton-pump inhibitor: an analysis of two randomised trials. *Lancet*. 2009;374(9694):989–997.

91. Wiviott SD, Braunwald E, McCabe CH, *et al*. Prasugrel versus clopidogrel in patients with acute coronary syndromes. *N Engl J Med*. 2007;357(20):2001–2015.

92. Wiviott SD, Trenk D, Frelinger AL, *et al*. Prasugrel compared with high loading- and maintenance-dose clopidogrel in patients with planned percutaneous coronary intervention: the Prasugrel in Comparison to Clopidogrel for Inhibition of Platelet Activa-tion and Aggregation-Thrombolysis in Myocardial Infarction 44 trial. *Circulation*. 2007;116(25):2923–2932.

93. Reimer C, Sondergaard B, Hilsted L, *et al*. Proton-pump inhibitor therapy induces acid-related symptoms in healthy volunteers after withdrawal of therapy. *Gastroenterology*. 2009;137(1):80–87.

Upper GI Tract

Upper GI Tract

CHAPTER 28

Benign esophageal strictures and caustic esophageal injury

Timothy T. Nostrant

University of Michigan Health Center, Ann Arbor, MI, USA

ESSENTIAL FACTS ABOUT PATHOGENESIS

- Acid is still the predominant cause of strictures but other causes of strictures increasing
- Eosinophils cause tissue remodeling (fibrosis)
- Both drug concentration and pH are important for caustic/pill injury
- Obesity, poor medication usage, and rising malignancy rate are major causes

ESSENTIALS OF DIAGNOSIS

- The first test is endoscopy (especially in caustic injury)
- Endoscopy determines simple/complex strictures
- Biopsy is critical, especially eosinophilic esophagitis (EoE)
- Proximal and distal biopsies should be taken for EoE
- Barium should be used for complex strictures

ESSENTIALS OF TREATMENT

- Dilation is key
- Savary dilation is the most cost-effective
- Cautious dilation early
- Dilate early in caustic injury
- Steroids/PPIs may reduce dilation episodes
- Novel therapies (incisions, stents) are promising

Causes

Eighty percent of strictures are acid peptic (including Schatzki rings). Eosinophilic esophagitis (EoE), radiation and caustic injury, and pill-induced strictures are increasing in percentage terms as better/earlier acid control reduces acid peptic strictures. EoE may account for 70% of chronic esophageal strictures. Increasing radiation usage, Barrett's esophagus, and gastroesophageal junction adenocarcinoma are increasing causes of esophageal strictures [1].

Benign esophageal strictures

These strictures can be divided into simple and complex [2]. **Simple strictures** are short (<2 cm), straight, usually distal, acid peptic in origin, and respond to dilation with low recurrence (≤25%). **Complex strictures** are longer (>3–5 cm), frequently tortuous, do not admit standard endoscopes [27–29 Fr

(8–9 mm)], and are resistant to dilation (>50% recur). Complex acid peptic strictures are seen in patients with high continuous acid exposure, Zollinger–Ellison syndrome, gastroparesis, tissue injury, and fibrosis (caustic, radiation), and in patients who are mentally challenged or have prolonged recumbancy.

Eosinophilic esophagitis

Eosinophilic esophagitis (EoE) is increasing in both adults and children [5% of gastroesophageal reflux disease (GERD), 25% of dysphagia, 70% of chronic stenoses] [3]. Early symptoms are frequently ignored until diagnosis after age 30 years. Solid food dysphagia/impaction is the usual presentation. Sixty to 70% have atopic histories. Concentric rings, longitudinal furrows, white spots, and a small caliber esophagus are endoscopic signs. A normal endoscopy is seen in 10%. Eosinophil by-products (eotaxin, interleukin-5) cause fibrosis in animals. High eosinophil concentrations (>20 eosinophils/HPF in five or more fields) are diagnostic. Both proximal (most specific) and distal biopsies are required.

Caustic injury

About 25 000 cases of caustic esophageal injury occur annually in the USA [4]. Most are accidents in children under 4 years of age (17 000) or suicide attempts. Drug concentration and pH are critical. Only high concentrations for strong alkalis (pH 9–11; including sodium hydroxide – lye, drain, oven, dishwashing cleaners) cause injury. Even small amounts of alkalis with a pH of 11 or greater cause injury [5]. Granules are more adherent than liquids, but injury may be limited to the mouth/pharynx. Liquids are tasteless and odorless and thus more may be ingested, causing more severe esophageal injury. Liquefactive necrosis and deep injury are common mechanisms. Worse injury and poor repair occurs if neutralization is attempted because of heat injury.

Acid injury occurs in 15% of ingestions. The rapid transit to the stomach causes coagulative gastric injury predominately. Early gastric perforation or late pre-pyloric strictures are the usual findings. Drain (sulfuric acid) and toilet bowl (hydrochloric acid, sodium bisulfate) cleaners cause the most severe

Textbook of Clinical Gastroenterology and Hepatology, Second Edition. Edited by C. J. Hawkey, Jaime Bosch, Joel E. Richter, Guadalupe Garcia-Tsao, Francis K. L. Chan.
© 2012 Blackwell Publishing Ltd. Published 2012 by Blackwell Publishing Ltd.

injuries. Swimming pool and tile cleaners are toxic even in small amounts as they are highly concentrated.

Pill-induced esophagitis

More than 70 medications produce injury [6]. Antibacterial agents produce more than 50% of injuries. Biphosphonate injury is increasing in the elderly because of lack of knowledge of risk factors.

Esophageal retention of capsules/tablets is universal if taken supine and without water. Medication absorption and high pH are critical. Acid reflux may increase injury. Motility disorders (collagen vascular disease, Parkinson disease, achalasia), tumors, and strictures may increase contact time. Most injury occurs in the mid-esophagus near the aortic arch where there is a transition between skeletal and smooth muscle.

Radiation injury

Radiation treatment for neck, lung, breast, mediastinal, and esophageal tumors is common. Achalasia, caustic injury, and Barrett's adenocarcinoma are increasing. Radiation doses >4500 mGy or radiation enhancers (gemcytobine) with low-dose radiation cause almost universal injury. Fibrosis, microischemia, and dysmotility are proposed mechanisms.

Miscellaneous causes [1,2]

Newer treatments for Barrett's esophageal dysplasia, such as photodynamic therapy, endoscopic mucosal resection, and radiofrequency ablation (BARRX), cause strictures in 5–30% of cases. Bullous squamous disease (pemphigoid, pemphigus, lichen planus) causes submucosal fibrosis, reducing esophageal compliance. Similar changes can be seen in Crohn's disease and amyloidosis.

Clinical presentation

Solid food dysphagia is the usual complaint [4]. Moldable foods (bread, rice, chicken, steak) are common offenders. Food impaction produces spastic pain, hypersalivation, and mucus regurgitation. Spontaneous bolus passage to complete obstruction can be seen. Suprasternal (50%) and chest location predict an esophageal source in most cases (>90%).

Acid peptic disease [1,2,6–8]

Onset is usually gradual with relief with liquids. Esophagitis and pills may speed progression. Schatzki rings are forme fruste of GERD (70%). Rapid progression suggests cancer. Symptoms may be absent, particularly with Barrett's esophagus.

Eosinophilic esophagitis [3]

Lifelong symptoms of dysphagia with food impaction are common. Atopy (60–80%) is suggestive. Longitudinal furrows and white spots are most specific, although concentric rings at endoscopy are most commonly seen. Biopsies in both the distal and proximal esophagus are diagnostic if more than 20 eosinophils/HPF are seen in five or more fields. Post-dilation pain is seen in most cases, but full perforation is rare. Conservative treatment for post-procedure pain is all that is needed usually.

Caustic injury

Drooling, odynophagia, and chest pain are the most common complaints. Symptoms cannot predict injury severity and endoscopy is mandated after perforation is ruled out. Complete absence of symptoms has a low rate of injury (2–3%). Airway symptoms, disseminated intravascular coagulation, and organ failure usually require surgical intervention.

Malignancy/radiation

Known Barrett's esophagus and rapid weight loss with dysphagia or radiation (with or without enhancers) are the usual presentations and mimic acid peptic injury.

Differential diagnosis

GERD-associated dysphagia secondary to acid-induced dysmotility is a major differential diagnosis. This will usually respond to acid reduction therapy. Achalasia and scleroderma mimic acid reflux, but regurgitation is usually of undigested food. Raynaud's disease, skin changes, and arthritis usually predict scleroderma with or without acid reflux.

Diagnostic testing [7,8]

Endoscopy is the best single test. Endoscopy allows stricture detection, evaluation of complexity, biopsy for malignancy and EoE, and dilation for treatment. Both proximal and distal biopsies are required for EoE.

Treatment/prevention [1,2,7,8]

Esophageal dilation is the first-line treatment. Three types of dilators are used: Maloney (Medovations, Inc., Germantown, WI, USA), Savary-Gilliard (Wilson-Cook Medical, Bloomington, IN, USA), and through the scope (TTS; CRE dilation balloons; Boston Scientific, Natick, MA, USA). No dilating system has a clear advantage but Savary dilators are reusable. Full-length esophageal dilation is another advantage of Savary dilation. Longitudinal shear in EoE is a minor disadvantage of Savary dilation. Proton pump inhibitor (PPI) therapy should be given post procedure to reduce post-dilation acid damage (especially Schatzki rings).

The dilation strategy is based on stricture size and length. If standard endoscopic passage is possible but moderate resistance is felt, then dilation should go from 32 to 38 Fr on initial dilation and repeated in 1–2 weeks to allow mucosal healing. Dilation size can be increased up to 60 Fr if only moderate resistance is felt on subsequent dilation. If a stricture cannot be passed even with an 18-Fr scope, then a barium esophogram to assess stricture complexity is necessary. If straight, then dilation can proceed as above. Balloon dilation under radiological control rarely may be necessary. Complex strictures, particularly caustic/radiation injuries, have a high recurrence rate (>50%).

Special attention should be given to EoE patients. Mucosal tearing and pain post procedure occurs in most patients. Since resistance to dilator passage may not be easily felt, visualization after dilation and early termination for severe damage may be prudent. Chest pain responds to topical anesthetics (one-third donnatal, one-third Maalox, one-third viscous lidocaine) if perforation is excluded.

Proximal radiation strictures may require a team approach. Since most unpassable strictures are closed short membranes, the proximal side can be approached antegrade and the distal side approached retrograde through scope passage into a mature gastrostomy site (≥24 F). A wire can be placed through the membrane antegrade and retrieved retrograde. Dilation can then be done as outlined above.

Steroid injections may reduce dilation sessions. One randomized controlled trial compared balloon dilation alone to balloon and four-quadrant triamcinolone injections [0.5 mL (40 mg/cm^3)] [9]. In acid peptic strictures repeat dilation was needed in 13% of steroid-treated patients compared to 60% of controls.

Completely covered (Polyflex) stents have had anecdotal success. Migration and granulation ingrowth are problems. Pre-stent dilation is usually needed. The long-term efficacy of these stents has been as low as 6% at 6 months and they have been difficult to remove. Devices for stent removal are in development.

Incisional therapy with a naked cautery wire (sphinterotomy) or endoscopic scissors are in development for resistant anastomatic strictures and Schatzki rings. Results are promising.

Complications [1,2,7,8]

Perforation, bleeding, and bacteremia at rates between 0.3% and 0.5% have been reported. Complex strictures are most at risk. Ascites and mechanical valves can be infected post dilation and antibiotic prophylaxis should be given.

References

1. Nostrant TT, Rabine JC. Esophageal dilation. In: Shackelford RT, editor. *Shackelford's Surgery of the Alimentary Tract*, 6th edition. Philadelphia: WB Saunders, 2002:167.
2. Siersema PD. Treatment options for esophageal strictures. *Nat Clin Pract Gastroenterol Hepatol.* 2008;5:142–152.
3. Furuta GT, Liacouras CA, Collins MH, et al. Eosinophilic esophagitis in children and adults: a systematic review and consensus recommendations for diagnosis and treatment. *Gastroenterology.* 2007;133:1342–1363.
4. Kay M, Wyllie R. Caustic ingestions in children. *Curr Opin Pediatr* 2009;21:651–654.
5. Atug O, Dobrucali A, Orlando RC. Critical pH level of lye (NaOH) for esophageal injury. *Dig Dis Sci.* 2009;54:980–987.
6. Zografos GN, Georgiadou D, Thomas D, et al. Drug-induced esophagitis. *Dis Esophagus* 2009;22:633–637.
7. Piotet E, Escher A, Monnier P. Esophageal and pharyngeal strictures: report on 1,862 endoscopic dilations using the Savary-Gilliard technique. *Eur Arch Otorhinolaryngol.* 2008;265:357–364.
8. Spechler SJ. AGA technical review on treatment of patients with dysphagia caused by benign disorders of the distal esophagus. *Gastroenterology.* 1999;117:233.
9. Ramage JI Jr, Rumalla A, Baron TH, et al. A prospective, randomized, double-blind, placebo-controlled trial of endoscopic steroid injection therapy for recalcitrant esophageal peptic strictures. *Am J Gastroenterol.* 2005;100:2419–2425.

Upper GI Tract

CHAPTER 29
Barrett's esophagus

Neil Gupta and Prateek Sharma

University of Kansas Medical Center, Kansas City Veterans Administration, Kansas City, MO, USA

ESSENTIAL FACTS ABOUT PATHOGENESIS

- Barrett's esophagus is a consequence of chronic GERD
- Other environmental and genetic factors may play a role. In symptomatic patients risk factors include age, male gender, Caucasian race, obesity, hiatus hernia and use of tobacco and alcohol

---

ESSENTIALS OF DIAGNOSIS

- Classically presents in Caucasian males with chronic GERD and advanced age
- Usually detected as a result of endoscopy for reflux symptoms
- Predicting the presence/absence of Barrett's esophagus prior to endoscopy remains a clinical challenge
- Endoscopy is required for diagnosis although the requirements for diagnosing Barrett's esophagus remains controversial
- The Prague criteria should be used for the endoscopic grading of Barrett's esophagus
- Histology shows columnar epithelium +/− intestinal metaplasia (international consensus on criteria is lacking)

ESSENTIALS OF MANAGEMENT

- Acid suppression therapy to control GERD symptoms and heal any erosive esophagitis
- Endoscopic surveillance with systematic biopsy protocol +/− enhanced imaging techniques for detection of dysplasia
- Multiple forms of endoscopic eradication therapy are effective at restoring squamous mucosa including radiofrequency ablation, photodynamic therapy, and endoscopic mucosal resection
- Focal lesions (dysplastic areas or intramucosal cancers) should be removed by endoscopic mucosal resection

---

Introduction

Barrett's esophagus is a **metaplastic change** of the esophageal mucosa that results in replacement of the normal squamous lined epithelium with a columnar lined epithelium containing goblet cells. It is the **pre-malignant condition** for esophageal adenocarcinoma. It occurs as a complication of **chronic gastroesophageal reflux disease** (GERD), however many patients with Barrett's esophagus may be asymptomatic [1, 2]. Upper endoscopy with tissue biopsy is required for diagnosis. Despite the controversies, surveillance remains the cornerstone of Barrett's esophagus management. However, endoscopic therapies are beginning to show effectiveness for select patients, specifically those at high risk for malignant transformation.

Epidemiology

In unselected Caucasian populations **prevalence** varies between 1.6% (Sweden) [2] and 6.8% (USA) [1]. Higher prevalence rates have been found in select patient populations including those with **chronic GERD** (13.2%), the **elderly** (16.7%), and **veterans** (25%). Lower prevalence rates have been found in other populations including the general **Korean** (0.84%) and **Chinese** (0.06%) population [3–7].

Barrett's esophagus is the pre-malignant condition for **esophageal adenocarcinoma**. The majority of esophageal and gastroesophageal junction adenocarcinoma patients have underlying Barrett's esophagus, with estimates ranging between 75–97% [8]. One study reported that patients with longer segments of Barrett's esophagus were estimated at having a 30–125 times increased risk for developing esophageal adenocarcinoma when compared to those without Barrett's esophagus [9]. While the incidence of esophageal adenocarcinoma in the United States has been substantially increasing, the exact reason for this trend is unknown [10]. It is speculated that the rising incidence of esophageal adenocarcinoma may be a result of increasing incidence and prevalence of Barrett's esophagus as a result of **obesity** and consquent GERD, but others factors such as diet are likely involved.

Risk factors

The presence of longstanding GERD symptoms increases the risk for having Barrett's esophagus [11]. When evaluating

---

GERD symptoms, duration and frequency have been found to be reliable predictors, while severity has not had similar results [12]. Additional risk factors include:

- advanced age
- male gender
- Caucasian race
- presence of a hiatal hernia
- history of tobacco use
- obesity
- history of alcohol use [12,13].

However, the majority of Barrett's esophagus patients are thought to be asymptomatic, and these risk factors have not been found to be reliable for detecting Barrett's esophagus in the asymptomatic population [4].

Pathogenesis

The **metaplastic change** of Barrett's esophagus is thought to be a response to longstanding GERD, where bile and acid cause inflammation of the esophageal mucosa. Consequently, the normal squamous cell mucosa is replaced by columnar mucosa. However, only about 10–15% of patients with GERD have Barrett's esophagus [1,3,5]. Epidemiological studies have found a higher prevalence in Caucasians, males, the obese, and individuals with a family history of Barrett's esophagus; a lower prevalence has been found in patients with *H. pylori* [13–17]. As a result, it is speculated that other environmental and genetic factors may play a role in the pathogenesis of Barrett's esophagus.

The exact **molecular changes** of Barrett's esophagus are being identified, and multiple polymorphisms in inflammatory response genes are associated with both the presence and progression of Barrett's esophagus. Several **biomarkers** have been created to help identify those at high risk for Barrett's esophagus progression including p53 mutations, aneuploidy, The **Ki-67** protein, cylcin A immunopositivity, and alpha-methylacyl coenzyme A racemase [18–21]. However, none of these have been found to be reliable markers of disease progression, and they are not routinely used at this time.

Clinical presentation

The majority of patients diagnosed with Barrett's esophagus have reflux symptoms; however Barrett's esophagus can be an asymptomatic disease. Some cohorts have found that up to 55% of Barrett's esophagus patients are asymptomatic [1,2] Despite the identification of many risk factors, predicting which patients will have Barrett's esophagus prior to endoscopy remains a major challenge. In addition, the cost effectiveness of **screening programs** have been limited due to the costs of endoscopy, lack of reliable Barrett's esophagus predictors in the asymptomatic population, and failure to show a reduction in esophageal adenocarcinoma mortality. Consequently,

screening the general population is not currently recommended. The current American College of Gastroenterology guidelines recommend an **individualized approach** to screening with an attempt to focus on high risk individuals: male patients over the age of 40 with long standing GERD appear to be the highest risk group [22] (Table 29.1). However, additional research is required to identify which specific patient populations should undergo screening for Barrett's esophagus.

Diagnosis

Barrett's esophagus is most commonly diagnosed during endoscopy, often carried out for the symptoms of reflux. **Intestinal metaplasia** is the presumed precursor lesion for esophageal adenocarcinoma, and its presence on biopsies confers an increased risk for the development of cancer [8] (Figure 29.1). However, it is unknown whether the presence of columnar lined epithelium proximal to the GEJ without histologically confirmed intestinal metaplasia also carries an increased risk for neoplasia development.

Table 29.1 Summary of American College of Gastroenterology recommendations for Barrett's esophagus surveillance

Dysplasia	Surveillance interval
No dysplasia	Endoscopy every year until two exams with no dysplasia, then every 3 years.
Low-grade dysplasia	Repeat endoscopy in 6 months. If no dysplasia progression found, then repeat every year until no dysplasia on two consecutive endoscopies. Can then increase interval.
High-grade dysplasia	Referral for endoscopic or surgical therapy. Endoscopy every 3 months if unable to perform therapy.

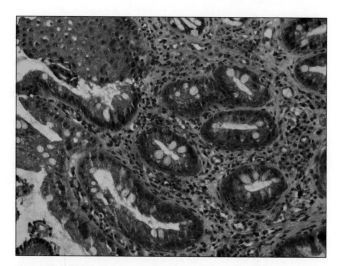

Figure 29.1 A biopsy of the esophagus revealing intestinal metaplasia.

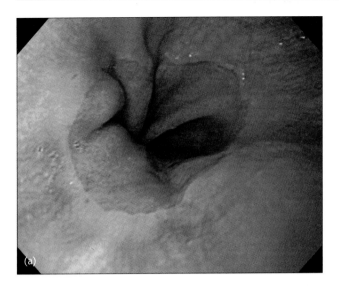

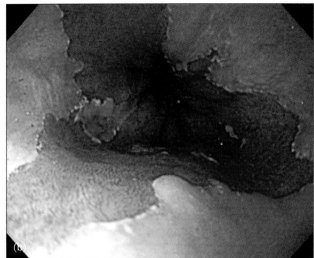

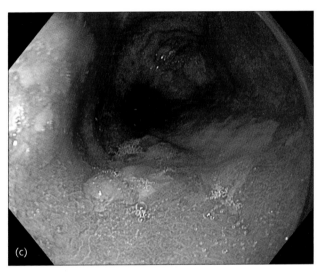

Figure 29.2 An example of a normal squamocolumnar junction, Barrett's esophagus, and esophageal adenocarcinoma seen using white light endoscopy. (a) The normal squamocolumnar junction. (b) Columnar lined epithelium seen proximal to the GEJ consistent with Barrett's esophagus. (c) An area of nodular mucosa seen within a segment of Barrett's esophagus. EMR confirmed the presence of adenocarcinoma.

Debate continues regarding the criteria needed to diagnose Barrett's esophagus: using only endoscopic recognition versus requiring histological confirmation of intestinal metaplasia. Upper endoscopy is the primary method for visually inspecting the esophagus and obtaining biopsies. Endoscopically, Barrett's esophagus appears as columnar lined epithelium with a pink/salmon color that results in displacement of the squamocolumnar junction proximal to the GEJ (Figure 29.2). When columnar lined epithelium is seen above the GEJ, multiple biopsies should be taken to evaluate for intestinal metaplasia and dysplasia, which confirm an increased of esophageal cancer [8] (Figure 29.1). At this time, US guidelines recommend that only those patients with biopsy confirmed intestinal metaplasia be diagnosed with Barrett's esophagus [22], although in other countries the presence of intestinal metaplasia is not required.

Endoscopic recognition of columnar lined epithelium proximal to the GEJ can be difficult if the endoscopist is unable to clearly identify the GEJ and the squamocolumnar junction. The presence of a hiatal hernia, esophagitis, or a patulous lower esophageal sphincter may distort these landmarks and make identification difficult. When columnar lined epithelium is seen proximal to the GEJ, it should be graded using a standardized system. There is interest in using enhanced imaging techniques to increase detection of Barrett's esophagus but it is unclear whether they improve accuracy compared to high resolution white light endoscopy [24–26]. The longitudinal extent of disease should be measured using the Prague Classification System which records the length (in centimeters of the circumferential (C) columnar lined epithelium and the maximum length (M) of the highest columnar lined epithelium [23].

Surveillance

Most European and North American endoscopists practice surveillance [36-37], although evidence is divided about

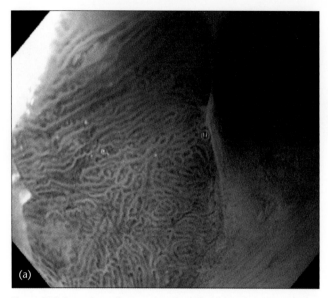
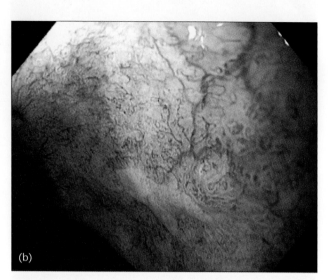

Figure 29.3 Barrett's esophagus seen using NBI. (a) Regular mucosal and vascular patterns. Biopsies confirmed the presence of non-dysplastic Barrett's esophagus. (b) Flat mucosal pattern and irregular vascular pattern. Biopsies confirmed the presence of HGD.

survival bracket [27–32] and cost effectiveness [33–35]. Patients should be told the risks and benefits of surveillance prior to enrollment in such a program. Surveillance endoscopy should be performed when symptoms are controlled and erosive esophagitis healed with proton pump inhibitor treatment because inflammation can inhibit detection and histological assessment of dysplasia [38].

A systematic approach should be taken to the detection of dysplasia with two main complementary approaches.

Systematic biopsy

Current guidelines recommend **four quadrant biopsies every 2 cm** of the Barrett's esophagus along with additional biopsies of any visible lesions (Seattle Protocol) [39] (Video 29.1). Patients with high-grade dysplasia (HGD) should have four quadrant biopsies taken every 1 cm; obtaining fewer biopsies has been associated with a cancer miss rate of up to 50% [40]. Biopsies should be obtained using large capacity forceps and using the turn-and-suck technique [41,42]. Specimens from each segment should be submitted for histopathological assessment in **separate jars** so that future targeted biopsies could be obtained if any dysplasia is detected. Although treatment decisions are based on the degree of dysplasia, there is significant **interobserver variability in dysplasia grading**, even amongst expert gastrointestinal pathologists [43,44]. Biopsies with dysplasia should be reviewed by at least two expert gastrointestinal pathologists, since there is significant inter observer variability in grading [43,44].

Enhanced imaging techniques

Several image enhancement techniques, particularly auto-fluorescence imaging, narrow band imaging and appear to improve the endoscopist's ability to detect dysplastic areas (Figure 29.3).

After illumination by blue light (390–470 nm), there is **fluorescence** of normal and dysplastic **tissue** with different wavelines, returning a light green color for normal and dark violet purple color for dysplastic tissue. This results in improved detection of dysplasia and cancer but there is a high false positive rate compared to white light high resolution endoscopy [46].

Use of narrow band imaging to enhance visualization of mucosal and blood vessel patterns improves the detection of dysplastic areas (Figure 29.3), and improves the endoscopist's ability to select appropriate sites for biopsy [45], and can reduce false positives when used in combination with autofluorescence.

Confocal laser endomicroscopy

Confocal laser endomicroscopy allows the endoscopist to obtain in vivo microscopic analysis of the esophageal mucosa. Initial studies have been promising with a high sensitivity (93%) and specificity (98%) for detecting Barrett's associated neoplasia [47] but may have to be coupled with broad surface imaging as only a small area can be inspected. See Chapter 129.

Treatment
Acid suppression

Patients should receive proton pump inhibitors with dose titration until reflux symptoms are controlled and/or erosive esophagitis healed. While studies have revealed that PPI therapy can decrease markers of proliferation and perhaps development of dysplasia, there has been no proven decrease in overall cancer risk [48,49].

Anti-reflux surgery

Anti-reflux surgery can be considered as an option for the management of gastroesophageal reflux symptoms, however up to 20% of patients may develop symptom recurrence during long-term follow up [50]. While there are some reports of regression of Barrett's esophagus and dysplasia after anti-reflux surgery, this has not been a consistent finding and there has been no firm documented reduction in cancer risk [51].

Endoscopic eradication therapy

A variety of endoscopic therapies is available for patients with HGD and mucosal cancer. The following techniques have been found to be effective.

 ### Endoscopic muscosal resection (EMR) (Video 29.2)

EMR can achieve dysplasia and cancer eradication rates in over 95% of patients with HGD or intra-mucosal adenocarcinoma [56–58]. The technique has the advantage over RFA and PDT in that it generates a sample that can be assessed histologically. Consequently, EMR should be used as a partially diagnostic technique in any patients with focal lesions. Some cohort studies have reported a change in diagnosis of as much as 50% of cases [52]. Major complications include post-procedure bleeding (19%) and stricture formation (12%), although these can be managed endoscopically in most cases [56–58].

 ### Radiofrequency ablation (RFA) (Video 29.3)

Repeated application of radiofrequency treatment to the columnar mucosa can result in complete eradication of the columnar mucosa with replacement by squamous mucosa in approximately 77% of cases and complete eradication of dysplasia in 86% [55]. Major side effects can include chest pain for up to one week after the procedure and a 6% risk of stricture formation.

Photodynamic therapy

Photo sensitization with Photophrin™ and laser light treatment in a classic trial nearly doubled the rate of eradication of high grade dysplasia and led to a 50% reduction in cancer [53]. However, its use is associated with an approximately 23% risk of stricture formation [54]. See Chapter 147.

Complications

The major complication of Barrett's esophagus is the development of esophageal adenocarcinoma. Increasingly, early lesions detected as part of surveillance are managed endoscopically. The management and prognosis of more advanced lesions is dependent on accurate staging using endoscopic ultrasound and CT scanning as discussed in Chapter 30.

Prognosis

While patients with Barrett's esophagus are at an increased risk of developing esophageal adenocarcinoma, the absolute risk is very low and most patients die with Barrett's esophagus and not from it.

> **SOURCES OF INFORMATION FOR PATIENTS AND DOCTORS**
>
> Patients need to know the natural history and neoplastic risk of Barrett's esophagus. The overall risk of progression to esophageal cancer is low, but select patients (such as those with HGD) have a considerable cancer risk. These issues along with procedure risks and costs, patient life expectancy, and patient preferences should be discussed before proceeding with Barrett's surveillance. The following links are helpful resources:
>
> www.acg.gi.org/patients/gihealth/barretts.asp
> http://digestive.niddk.nih.gov/ddiseases/pubs/barretts/index.htm
> www.mayoclinic.com/health/barretts-esophagus/HQ00312

Current controversies and future resolution

Identifying predictors for Barrett's esophagus in the asymptomatic population or **minimally invasive techniques** will be needed to improve the value of screening programs. The natural history of columnar lined epithelium without histologic evidence of intestinal metaplasia needs to be further defined in order to develop surveillance recommendations. Continued development of **biomarkers** may augment traditional risk factors and help identify patients at high risk of neoplastic progression in Barrett's esophagus. As the options for advanced imaging continue to increase, additional **clinical trials** will be needed to create the optimal surveillance strategy. The same holds true for endoscopic therapies in Barrett's esophagus patients with HGD and intramucosal adenocarcinoma.

References

1. Rex DK, Cummings OW, Shaw M, *et al.* Screening for Barrett's esophagus in colonoscopy patients with and without heartburn. *Gastroenterology.* 2003;125(6):1670–1677.
2. Ronkainen J, Aro P, Storskrubb T, Johansson *et al.* Prevalence of Barrett's esophagus in the general population: an endoscopic study. *Gastroenterology.* 2005;129(6):1825–1831.
3. Ward EM, Wolfsen HC, Achem SR, *et al.* Barrett's esophagus is common in older men and women undergoing screening colonoscopy regardless of reflux symptoms. *Am J Gastroenterol.* 2006;101(1):12–17.
4. Gerson LB, Shetler K, Triadafilopoulos G. Prevalence of Barrett's esophagus in asymptomatic individuals. *Gastroenterology.* 2002; 123(2):461–467.
5. Westhoff B, Brotze S, Weston A, *et al.* The frequency of Barrett's esophagus in high-risk patients with chronic GERD. *Gastrointest Endosc.* 2005;61(2):226–231.
6. Tseng PH, Lee YC, Chiu HM, *et al.* Prevalence and clinical characteristics of Barrett's esophagus in a Chinese general population. *J Clin Gastroenterol.* 2008;42(10):1074–1079.

7. Park JJ, Kim JW, Kim HJ, *et al.* The Prevalence of and Risk Factors for Barrett Esophagus in a Korean Population: A Nationwide Multicenter Prospective Study. *J Clin Gastroenterol.* 2009;43(10): 907–914.

8. Theisen J, Stein HJ, Dittler HJ, *et al.* Preoperative chemotherapy unmasks underlying Barrett's mucosa in patients with adenocarcinoma of the distal esophagus. *Surg Endosc.* 2002;16(4): 671–673.

9. Cameron AJ, Ott BJ, Payne WS. The incidence of adenocarcinoma in columnar-lined (Barrett's) esophagus. *N Engl J Med.* 1985;313(14):857–859.

10. Trivers KF, Sabatino SA, Stewart SL. Trends in esophageal cancer incidence by histology, United States, 1998–2003. *Int J Cancer.* 2008;123(6):1422–1428.

11. Conio M, Filiberti R, Blanchi S, *et al.* Risk factors for Barrett's esophagus: a case-control study. *Int J Cancer.* 2002; 97(2):225–229.

12. Eloubeidi MA, Provenzale D. Clinical and demographic predictors of Barrett's esophagus among patients with gastroesophageal reflux disease: a multivariable analysis in veterans. *J Clin Gastroenterol.* 2001;33(4):306–309.

13. Edelstein ZR, Bronner MP, Rosen SN, *et al.* Risk factors for Barrett's esophagus among patients with gastroesophageal reflux disease: a community clinic-based case-control study. *Am J Gastroenterol.* 2009;104(4):834–842.

14. Romero Y, Cameron AJ, Schaid DJ, *et al.* Barrett's esophagus: prevalence in symptomatic relatives. *Am J Gastroenterol.* 2002; 97(5):1127–1132.

15. Vaezi MF, Falk GW, Peek RM, *et al.* CagA-positive strains of Helicobacter pylori may protect against Barrett's esophagus. *Am J Gastroenterol.* 2000;95(9):2206–2211.

16. El-Serag HB, Kvapil P, Hacken-Bitar J, *et al.* Abdominal obesity and the risk of Barrett's esophagus. *Am J Gastroenterol.* 2005; 100(10):2151–2156.

17. Wang A, Mattek NC, Holub JL, *et al.* Prevalence of complicated gastroesophageal reflux disease and Barrett's esophagus among racial groups in a multi-center consortium. *Dig Dis Sci.* 2009; 54(5):964–971.

18. Reid BJ, Prevo LJ, Galipeau PC, *et al.* Predictors of progression in Barrett's esophagus II: baseline 17p (p53) loss of heterogosity identifies a patient subset at increased risk for neoplastic progression. *Am J Gastroenterol.* 2001;96(10):2839–2848.

19. Sikkema M, Kerkhof M, Steyerberg EW, *et al.* Aneuploidy and Overexpression of Ki67 and p53 as Markers for Neoplastic Progression in Barrett's Esophagus: A Case-Control Study. *Am J Gastroenterol.* 2009;104:2673–2680.

20. Lao-Sirieix P, Lovat L, Fitzgerald RC. Cyclin A immunocytology as a risk stratification tool for Barrett's esophagus surveillance. *Clin Cancer Res.* 2007;13(2 Pt 1):659–665.

21. Scheil-Bertram S, Lorenz D, Ell C, *et al.* Expression of alpha-methylacyl coenzyme A racemase in the dysplasia carcinoma sequence associated with Barrett's esophagus. *Mod Pathol.* 2008;21(8):961–967.

22. Wang KK, Sampliner RE. Updated guidelines 2008 for the diagnosis, surveillance and therapy of Barrett's esophagus. *Am J Gastroenterol.* 2008;103(3):788–797.

23. Sharma P, Dent J, Armstrong D, *et al.* The development and validation of an endoscopic grading system for Barrett's esophagus: the Prague C & M criteria. *Gastroenterology.* 2006; 131(5):1392–1399.

24. Kara MA, Peters FP, Rosmolen WD, *et al.* High-resolution endoscopy plus chromoendoscopy or narrow-band imaging in Barrett's esophagus: a prospective randomized crossover study. *Endoscopy.* 2005;37(10):929–936.

25. Ferguson DD, DeVault KR, Krishna M, *et al.* Enhanced magnification-directed biopsies do not increase the detection of intestinal metaplasia in patients with GERD. *Am J Gastroenterol.* 2006;101(7):1611–1616.

26. Ngamruengphong S, Sharma VK, Das A. Diagnostic yield of methylene blue chromoendoscopy for detecting specialized intestinal metaplasia and dysplasia in Barrett's esophagus: a meta-analysis. *Gastrointest Endosc.* 2009;69(6):1021–1028.

27. Corley DA, Levin TR, Habel LA, *et al.* Surveillance and survival in Barrett's adenocarcinomas: a population-based study. *Gastroenterology.* 2002;122(3):633–640.

28. Bani-Hani K, Sue-Ling H, Johnston D, *et al.* Barrett's oesophagus: results from a 13-year surveillance programme. *Eur J Gastroenterol Hepatol.* 2000;12(6):649–654.

29. Cooper GS, Yuan Z, Chak A, *et al.* Association of prediagnosis endoscopy with stage and survival in adenocarcinoma of the esophagus and gastric cardia. *Cancer.* 2002;95(1):32–38.

30. Kearney DJ, Crump C, Maynard C, *et al.* A case-control study of endoscopy and mortality from adenocarcinoma of the esophagus or gastric cardia in persons with GERD. *Gastrointest Endosc.* 2003;57(7):823–829.

31. Conio M, Blanchi S, Lapertosa G, *et al.* Long-term endoscopic surveillance of patients with Barrett's esophagus. Incidence of dysplasia and adenocarcinoma: a prospective study. *Am J Gastroenterol.* 2003;98(9):1931–1939.

32. Dulai GS, Shekelle PG, Jensen DM, *et al.* Dysplasia and risk of further neoplastic progression in a regional Veterans Administration Barrett's cohort. *Am J Gastroenterol.* 2005;100(4):775–783.

33. Inadomi JM, Sampliner R, Lagergren J, *et al.* Screening and surveillance for Barrett esophagus in high-risk groups: a cost-utility analysis. *Ann Intern Med.* 2003;138(3):176–186.

34. Gerson LB, Groeneveld PW, Triadafilopoulos G. Cost-effectiveness model of endoscopic screening and surveillance in patients with gastroesophageal reflux disease. *Clin Gastroenterol Hepatol.* 2004;2(10):868–879.

35. Provenzale D, Schmitt C, Wong JB. Barrett's esophagus: a new look at surveillance based on emerging estimates of cancer risk. *Am J Gastroenterol.* 1999;94(8):2043–2053.

36. Falk GW, Ours TM, Richter JE. Practice patterns for surveillance of Barrett's esophagus in the united states. *Gastrointest Endosc.* 2000;52(2):197–203.

37. Gross CP, Canto MI, Hixson J, *et al.* Management of Barrett's esophagus: a national study of practice patterns and their cost implications. *Am J Gastroenterol.* 1999;94(12):3440–3447.

38. Hanna S, Rastogi A, Weston AP, *et al.* Detection of Barrett's esophagus after endoscopic healing of erosive esophagitis. *Am J Gastroenterol.* 2006;101(7):1416–1420.

39. Reid BJ, Weinstein WM, Lewin KJ, *et al.* Endoscopic biopsy can detect high-grade dysplasia or early adenocarcinoma in Barrett's esophagus without grossly recognizable neoplastic lesions. *Gastroenterology.* 1988;94(1):81–90.

40. Reid BJ, Blount PL, Feng Z, Levine DS. Optimizing endoscopic biopsy detection of early cancers in Barrett's high-grade dysplasia. *Am J Gastroenterol.* 2000;95(11):3089–3096.

41. Schafer TW, Hollis-Perry KM, Mondragon RM, Brann OS. An observer-blinded, prospective, randomized comparison of

forceps for endoscopic esophageal biopsy. *Gastrointest Endosc.* 2002;55(2):192–196.

42. Levine DS, Reid BJ. Endoscopic biopsy technique for acquiring larger mucosal samples. *Gastrointest Endosc.* 1991;37(3):332–337.

43. Downs-Kelly E, Mendelin JE, Bennett AE, *et al.* Poor interobserver agreement in the distinction of high-grade dysplasia and adenocarcinoma in pretreatment Barrett's esophagus biopsies. *Am J Gastroenterol.* 2008;103(9):2333–2340; quiz 41.

44. Kerkhof M, van Dekken H, Steyerberg EW, *et al.* Grading of dysplasia in Barrett's oesophagus: substantial interobserver variation between general and gastrointestinal pathologists. *Histopathology.* 2007;50(7):920–927.

45. Sharma P, Bansal A, Hawes RH, *et al.* Detection of Metaplasia (IM) and Neoplasia in Patients with Barrett's Esophagus (BE) Using High-Definition White Light Endoscopy (HD-WLE) Versus Narrow Band Imaging (NBI): A Prospective, Multi-Center, Randomized, Crossover Trial. *Gastrointest Endosc.* 2009;69(5):AB135.

46. Borovicka J, Fischer J, Neuweiler J, *et al.* Autofluorescence endoscopy in surveillance of Barrett's esophagus: a multicenter randomized trial on diagnostic efficacy. *Endoscopy.* 2006;38(9):867–872.

47. Kiesslich R, Gossner L, Goetz M, *et al.* In vivo histology of Barrett's esophagus and associated neoplasia by confocal laser endomicroscopy. *Clin Gastroenterol Hepatol.* 2006;4(8):979–987.

48. Ouatu-Lascar R, Fitzgerald RC, Triadafilopoulos G. Differentiation and proliferation in Barrett's esophagus and the effects of acid suppression. *Gastroenterology.* 1999;117(2):327–335.

49. El-Serag HB, Aguirre TV, Davis S, *et al.* Proton pump inhibitors are associated with reduced incidence of dysplasia in Barrett's esophagus. *Am J Gastroenterol.* 2004;99(10):1877–1883.

50. Hofstetter WL, Peters JH, DeMeester TR, *et al.* Long-term outcome of antireflux surgery in patients with Barrett's esophagus. *Ann Surg.* 2001;234(4):532–538; discussion 8–9.

51. Chang EY, Morris CD, Seltman AK, *et al.* The effect of antireflux surgery on esophageal carcinogenesis in patients with barrett esophagus: a systematic review. *Ann Surg.* 2007;246(1):11–21.

52. Peters FP, Brakenhoff KP, Curvers WL, *et al.* Histologic evaluation of resection specimens obtained at 293 endoscopic resections in Barrett's esophagus. *Gastrointest Endosc.* 2008;67(4):604–609.

53. Overholt BF, Wang KK, Burdick JS, *et al.* Five-year efficacy and safety of photodynamic therapy with Photofrin in Barrett's high-grade dysplasia. *Gastrointest Endosc.* 2007;66(3):460–468.

54. Yachimski P, Puricelli WP, Nishioka NS. Patient predictors of esophageal stricture development after photodynamic therapy. *Clin Gastroenterol Hepatol.* 2008;6(3):302–308.

55. Shaheen NJ, Sharma P, Overholt BF, *et al.* Radiofrequency ablation in Barrett's esophagus with dysplasia. *N Engl J Med.* 2009;360(22):2277–2288.

56. Larghi A, Lightdale CJ, Ross AS, *et al.* Long-term follow-up of complete Barrett's eradication endoscopic mucosal resection (CBE-EMR) for the treatment of high grade dysplasia and intramucosal carcinoma. *Endoscopy.* 2007;39(12):1086–1091.

57. Lopes CV, Hela M, Pesenti C, *et al.* Circumferential endoscopic resection of Barrett's esophagus with high-grade dysplasia or early adenocarcinoma. *Surg Endosc.* 2007;21(5):820–824.

58. Giovannini M, Bories E, Pesenti C, *et al.* Circumferential endoscopic mucosal resection in Barrett's esophagus with high-grade intraepithelial neoplasia or mucosal cancer. Preliminary results in 21 patients. *Endoscopy.* 2004;36(9):782–787.

CHAPTER 30

Esophageal cancer

Tamas A. Gonda and Charles J. Lightdale

Columbia University Medical Center, New York, NY, USA

ESSENTIAL FACTS ABOUT PATHOGENESIS

- The majority of esophageal cancers are squamous cell carcinomas and adenocarcinomas
- Risk factors for SCC and ACA are different
- The most important risk factors for SCC are smoking and alcohol consumption, while GERD, Barrett's esophagus and obesity are most important for ACA
- The incidence of squamous cell carcinoma varies widely by geographic region and the incidence is steady or decreasing
- Adenocarcinoma is more common in developed countries, where the incidence has at least doubled over the past 30 years
- Genetic and epigenetic changes of both the epithelial and tumor stromal cells are being recognized as key to the pathogenesis of esophageal cancers

---

ESSENTIAL FACTS ABOUT DIAGNOSIS

- Most common presentation: dysphagia, weight loss
- Distal disease is usually ACA, whereas SCC is usually proximal
- 50% of patients are incurable at diagnosis
- Initial diagnostic modalities include: CT, EUS and PET

ESSENTIAL FACTS ABOUT THERAPY

- Endoscopic mucosal resection is emerging as an alternative to esophagectomy in T1m disease
- Surgical resection is recommended for stage II and T3 stage III disease
- Chemoradiation with curative intent may also be considered in stage II–III disease in patients who are not surgical candidates
- Brachytherapy and esophageal stenting should be considered in unresectable disease

---

CLINICAL TIPS

- Ask patients what they can and can't eat. Patients will often unconsciously modify their diet and deny dysphagia
- Endoscopic biopsy usually leads to the diagnosis. In some cases, malignant cells may be submucosal, and repeated deep biopsies or EUS/fine-needle aspiration cytology may be necessary
- Respiratory problems with esophageal cancer may be related to esophagorespiratory fistulae, aspiration, or tracheal invasion
- Staging is the key to management of esophageal cancer. It is the key to treatment and the key to prognosis
- Differences in management of SCC and ACA are a result of different locations. With distal tumors (usually ACA), stent placement violates the gastroesophageal junction and may exacerbate gastroesophageal reflux. High cervical tumors (usually SCC) pose a technical challenge for stenting
- Esophageal cancer usually recurs after initial therapy
- Palliative measures (stenting, percutaneous endoscopic gastrostomy, analgesia, hospice care) are extremely important in minimizing suffering in the late stages of the disease

---

Introduction

Approximately 400000 new cases of esophageal cancer occur each year, and esophageal cancer remains the sixth leading cause of cancer death worldwide. Despite significant advances in screening, early diagnosis and treatment, the mortality of esophageal cancers remains very high. The two most common types of cancers, squamous cell carcinoma (SCC) and adenocarcinoma (ACA) have similar clinical presentations but their epidemiology, pathogenesis and therefore the therapeutic approaches are somewhat different. In this chapter we emphasize both these similarities and differences and highlight recent advances in their management.

Epidemiology and disease burden

The incidence of esophageal cancer shows important geographic and ethnic variation. In the United States, as in several other Western countries, the incidence of SCC has declined by >25% as ACA has increased by 4–5 fold over the last 25 years. In contrast to the overall relatively low incidence of SCC of 3–5 per 100000 in the U.S.A., in certain Asian countries the incidence is over 100 per 100000. The "hot spot" of SCC is seen in countries of the Asian Belt, spanning from North-Central China to Iran [1]. In the U.S.A., African Americans and Hispanic males have the highest incidence, albeit the largest reduction over the past 25 years has also been seen in the incidence of SCA among African Americans. This is in sharp contrast to the epidemiology of ACA, which shows a predominance of cases among white males. Men are 6–8-fold more

---

Textbook of Clinical Gastroenterology and Hepatology, Second Edition. Edited by C. J. Hawkey, Jaime Bosch, Joel E. Richter, Guadalupe Garcia-Tsao, Francis K. L. Chan.

Table 30.1 Risk factors of esophageal cancer

	SCC	ACA
GERD		++
BE		+++
Bile reflux		+
Tobacco	+++	+
Alcohol (beer, liquor>wine)	++	
Obesity	(−)	++
HPV	+	
Dietary contaminants	+	+
Dietary deficiencies (vitamins and oligo-elements)	+	+
Achalasia	+	
Caustic injury	+++	
Thermal injury (repeated exposure)	+	
Helicobacter pylori	?+	?−

likely than women to suffer from esophageal ACA, and caucasians are 3–4-fold more likely than African Americans [2]. Esophageal cancer is the third most common digestive system cancer (after colorectal and pancreatic cancer). There are >15 000 deaths per year in the USA. The mortality from esophageal cancer has plateaued since 2004. The combined cost of esophageal cancers per year is estimated at over 2.5 billion dollars, and ranks third among GI cancers [3].

Causes and pathogenesis
Risk factors of SCC
Although the pathogenesis of SCC and ACA share similarities, the most significant risk factors that predispose to the development of these lesions are distinct (Table 30.1). The two major carcinogens are tobacco and alcohol, and combined exposure may result in synergy. Analogous to the situation in lung cancer, the risk following smoking cessation begins to decline after 10 years.

Dietary and nutritional factors also play an important role in SCC carcinogenesis. Both the direct carcinogenic effect of certain compounds (polycyclic aromatic hydrocarbons in fat-cooked meals; nitrosamines; toxic alkaloids or mycotoxins), deficiencies in oligo-elements such as zinc, selenium, vitamin A, folate, and direct thermal trauma (repeated consumption of hot beverages) has been linked to SCC [4,5,6]. However, obesity was not associated with SCC and may even be protective.

Although the association of head and neck squamous cell cancers (HNCa) with high-risk HPV types (i.e., HPV 16, 18) has been shown, such an association remains somewhat controversial in SCC of the esophagus [7]. On the other hand studies have shown an association of synchronous and metachronous SCC in 2–10 % of patients with HNCa or other cancers of the aero-digestive tract [8]. This likely represents a field effect, potentially mediated by oncogenic HPV. Screening endoscopy is recommended in these patients.

Plummer-Vinson syndrome (also known as the Patterson-Kelly syndrome) is a rare syndrome of esophageal webs, iron deficiency anemia, and epithelial lesions, and patients with this disorder have a 3–15% risk of developing esophageal cancer. Tylosis, an autosomal dominant disorder resulting in hyperkeratosis of the palms and the soles, is associated with SCC of the esophagus and oropharyngeal leukoplakia. Caustic injury also increases the risk of SCC, although the prognosis (potentially due to lead time bias) is better then in sporadic SCC.

Risk factors of ACA
Although GERD and obesity are the major risk factor for ACA, it is important to recognize that smoking and several of the dietary factors associated with SCC also contribute to ACA, albeit to a lesser degree. The role of *Helicobacter pylori* infection remains debated. Eradication of *H. pylori* has been suggested as a force behind the change in SCC:ACA incidence ratios.

Although GERD is the major risk factor for Barrett's esophagus (BE), up to 40% of patients with BE do not report reflux symptoms. In addition, the majority of patients with reflux esophagitis heal with regeneration of squamous cells, and only a minority (10%) develop columnar epithelium with intestinal metaplasia as part of the histological healing. The role of inflammation appears central to the process. Long term use of NSAIDs was associated with a decreased risk of ACA, but a prospective study did not find a benefit of COX-2 inhibitors in preventing the progression of BE [9].

The histological changes that precede ACA are intestinal metaplasia without dysplasia (non-dysplastic BE), low and high-grade dysplasia. Probably less than 10% of patients with BE develop either high grade dysplasia or cancer. The annual risk of progression from non-dysplastic BE to ACA is 0.5–1% per patient-year, whereas as many as 10% of patients with high-grade dysplasia develop ACA per patient-year.

Obesity is a strong risk factor for ACA. Although an association of obesity with GERD has also been shown, the role of obesity in the development of BE remains less straightforward (ref 11). It appears that the risk of BE is not increased by an elevated BMI among GERD patients, and it has been suggested that an elevated BMI should not be considered a predictor of progression from GERD to BE [10,11].

Pathogenesis
Central to the pathogenesis of BE and ACA are mechanical and molecular alterations. As GERD is a significant risk factor,

mechanical and physiologic factors that contribute to GERD may increase the risk of BE and ACA. One of the mechanistic links between elevated BMI and ACA can also be due to an increased prevalence of hiatal hernias among this population. Acid is believed to induce inflammation like esophagitis and might be sufficient to induce metaplastic or even neoplastic changes, although it does appear that bile acids play a more important role in the development of intestinal metaplasia. However, as the majority of patients with even severe reflux esophagitis never develop BE or ACA, additional molecular and cellular changes must occur at both the squamous to columnar and metaplasia to dysplasia transformation. Chronic inflammation that accompanies reflux esophagitis may have an important role in not only the transdifferentiation of cells (intestinal metaplasia) and transformation of neoplastic cells (via paracrine signalling), but as increasingly recognized, in the recruitment of bone marrow-derived cells. In multiple inflammation-related cancers an emerging role has been suggested for bone marrow-derived cells to contribute to both the tumor epithelium and the supporting stromal cells that surround it. There is increasing evidence that this happens in early Barrett's metaplasia.

Since the majority, if not all, of ACA arise in the background of BE, an important focus has become the mechanism of metaplasia, or transformation from squamous epithelium to columnar epithelium. CDX1 and CDX2, members of the homeobox class of genes that are responsible for intestinal epithelial development have been shown to be over-expressed in all stages of BE and their expression appears to be induced by acid or bile exposure [12]. The subsequent transformation that leads from metaplasia to dysplasia and carcinoma is associated with both genetic alterations (i.e., loss of heterozygosity or chromosomal instability) and epigenetic changes (i.e., DNA methylation, histone acetylation). Many of these genetic and epigenetic changes are seen in both SCC and ACA. Some of the genes that show an early increase in expression are Cyclin D1EGFR, whereas decreased expression of key tumor suppressor genes (i.e., p53, p16) is seen as well. Loss of p16 expression, caused by mutation, LOH or in a very significant number of cases to hyperemthylation of CpG islands in the promoter region is an especially important and early feature of BE/ ACA. Finally, increased expression of matrix metalloproteinases (i.e., MMP7 and 9) and BMP-4 in the stromal component of tumors has underlined the importance of the role of the tumor microenvironment in regulating tumor progression and especially invasion. Gene methylation and chromosomal aneuploidy are currently being investigated as both biomarkers of disease progression and therapeutic targets.

Pathology

ACA and SCC comprise more than 90% of esophageal cancers. ACA usually develops in the distal esophagus, whereas SCC may arise at any location in the esophagus (Figures 30.1 and 30.2). Invasion of the submucosa occurs early in SCC, with

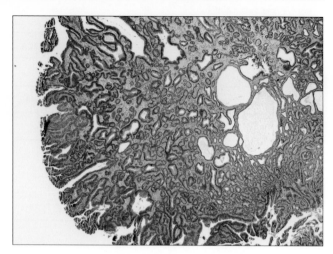

Figure 30.1 Adenocarcinoma. Low-power (×40) view of invasive adenocarcinoma showing neoplastic glands throughout the field extending deep in the wall of the esophagus.

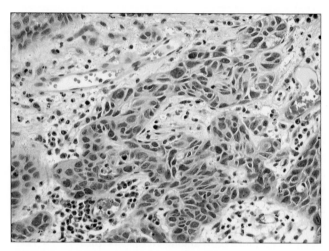

Figure 30.2 Squamous cell carcinoma. High-power view (×400) of invasive squamous cell carcinoma with infiltrating sheets of neoplastic cells.

proximal extension of tumor along the mucosal surface. Invasion of the lymphatic system is another early event in SCC due to the superficial location of lymph nodes in the mid-esophagus. After involvement of the regional nodes, spread to the celiac and periaortic lymph nodes occurs. Distant metastases occur in 30% of patients, most commonly to the liver, bone, and lung.

Clinical presentation

Most patients with esophageal cancer do not develop symptoms until the tumor is large enough to cause mechanical obstruction. At presentation, the most common symptoms are dysphagia, odynophagia, and weight loss or anorexia. Chest pain may indicate invasion into the mediastinum. Cough and recurrent pneumonia may indicate an esophagorespiratory fistula, compression of the trachea, or aspiration. Hoarseness may occur if there is involvement of the recurrent laryngeal nerve. Gastrointestinal bleeding as a presentation is rare.

Differential diagnosis

Rare causes of esophageal cancer include verrucous carcinoma, spindle cell carcinoma, small cell carcinoma, leiomyosarcoma, Kaposi's sarcoma, lymphoma, and malignant melanoma. Cancers that may metastasize to the esophagus include melanoma, breast, lung, germ cell tumor, and renal cell carcinomas. Although benign lesions rarely cause dysphagia, they include squamous papilloma, leiomyomas, fibrovascular polyps, lymphangiomas, and lipomas.

Diagnostic methods

Upon presentation, a thorough history of gastroesophageal reflux symptoms (including duration and severity), tobacco and alcohol use, and residence in an endemic area is of importance. On physical examination, lymphadenopathy, cachexia, presence of fecal occult blood, or hepatomegaly should be noted. Laboratory studies may reveal iron deficiency anemia or signs of malnutrition such as hypoalbuminemia or prolonged prothrombin time. Although patients presenting with dysphagia may undergo barium esophagography (Figure 30.3), it is now more common to perform endoscopy, with

tissue biopsy and, if appropriate, treatment (Figure 30.4). Early cancers may appear as a superficial plaque or ulcer. Advanced cancerous lesions appear as polypoid, friable, often ulcerated, eccentric, or circumferential masses. Biopsies are essential and the diagnostic accuracy increases with the number of biopsies taken. On rare occasions, tumor infiltration may involve only the submucosa, resulting in a normal-appearing esophagus on endoscopy. In such cases, superficial endoscopic biopsies may be nondiagnostic. Lugol's iodine solution and toluidine blue can be used for the detection of endoscopically non-distinct SCC lesions (Figure 30.5). Malignant squamous cells are depleted of glycogen and therefore the stain is not taken up by these cells. Absent staining is indicative of SCC. Although not routinely used, it should be considered as an adjunct to screening patients from endemic areas or with a personal history of squamous cancers of the head and neck.

Advanced imaging techniques can aid not only the diagnosis or target sampling but may also help in defining the extent of lesions. Chromoendoscopy, the use of dyes to evaluate the mucosa, is increasingly being replaced by techniques such as narrow band imaging, auto-fluorescence and endomicroscopy. High resolution narrow band imaging has been valuable in the early detection of squamous intraepithelial neoplasia, predicting SCC tumor depth, identifying foci of HGD or carcinoma-in-site in BE segments and defining the precise extent of lesions [13]. Autofluorescence imaging and confocal endomicroscopy have so far shown promise primarily in the diagnosis of pre-neoplastic lesions. A combination of these techniques will likely enhance the ability to diagnose early cancers and when appropriate achieve complete endoscopic resections.

Treatment of both SCC and ACA is influenced by depth of invasion (T stage), the presence of spread to lymph nodes (N stage) and distant metastasis (M stage). Commonly used modality to accurately stage esophageal cancers include endoscopic ultrasound (EUS), computer tomography (CT) and 18F-fluoro-2-deoxy-D-glucose positron emission tomography

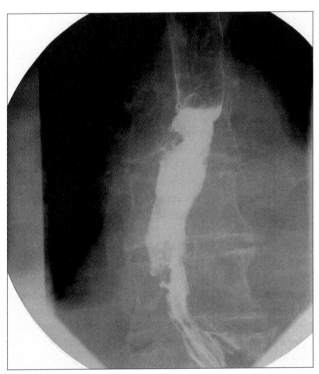

Figure 30.3 Barium esophagogram of a patient with adenocarcinoma. There is a markedly irregular area of ulceration and mucosal irregularity in the distal esophagus extending for a distance of approximately 6 cm, almost to the gastroesophageal junction.

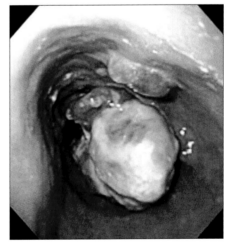

Figure 30.4 Endoscopic image of invasive adenocarcinoma in the distal esophagus. A friable exophytic mass partially obstructs the lumen.

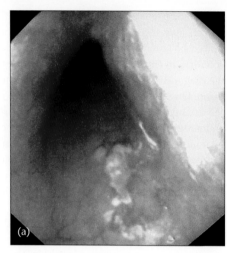 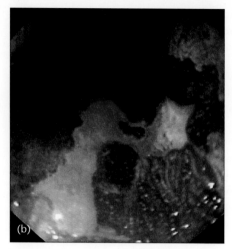

Figure 30.5 Chromoendoscopy images. (a) White plaque represents biopsy-proven squamous cell carcinoma. (b) After staining with Lugol's iodine, the lesion is more precisely defined.

Table 30.2 Sensitivity and specificity of EUS (±FNA), FDG PET and CT for nodal and distant metastasis staging in esophageal cancer (adopted from EPM van Vilet et al., *Br J Cancer*. 2008)

Imaging method	Sensitivity (95% confidence interval)	Specificity (95% confidence interval)
Regional LN staging		
EUS	0.80(0.75–0.84)	0.70(0.65–0.75)
FDG-PET	0.57(0.43–0.70)	0.85(0.76–0.95)
CT	0.50(0.41–0.60)	0.83(0.77–0.89)
Staging of distant metastasis		
FDG-PET	0.71(0.62–0.79)	0.93(0.89–0.97)
CT	0.52(0.33–0.71)	0.91(0.86–0.96)

(FDG-PET) [14]. EUS is the most sensitive method for local and lymph node staging, and the specificity when combined with FNA is comparable to PET or CT scans (Table 30.2). However, the sensitivity of these modalities may not be sufficient to exclude the presence of LN metastasis in endoscopically resected lesions. For this reason, recent works have suggested that correlation with depth of mucosal invasion in EMR specimens should also be used to assess the risk of LN involvement. This is an important concept that suggests that in individuals staged by EUS or other modalities as having T1 lesions but EMR specimens demonstrating submucosal invasion, the risk of LN metastasis may be too high and esophagectomy should be considered [15,16]. It has recently been proposed that T1a and T1b lesions should be subdivided based on the depth of invasion as this may correlate with lymphatic spread (Table 30.3). These sub-classifications may be especially important when deciding between endoscopic resection (which may be appropriate for lesions with the lowest chance of lymphatic invasion) versus surgical resection [17].

For distant metastasis PET and CT are similar in performance characteristics (Figure 30.6 and Figure 30.7). In patients with endoscopically resectable disease (T1), it is paramount to perform accurate lymph node staging and exclude LN involvement prior to proceeding with endoscopic resection. For more advanced lesions, the focus of staging is to exclude distant metastasis, which can be done by either PET or CT. Current practice is to perform EUS (with FNA when indicated) and either PET or CT.

Treatment and prevention
Treatment
The treatment of esophageal cancer is dependent on the stage of disease (Table 30.4) Unfortunately, esophageal cancer is rarely detected in the early stages and over half of patients have unresectable disease at the time of diagnosis. The overall 5-year survival rate is 13% (Table 30.5).

Stage 0–I disease
The goal of therapy for stage 0–I disease (Barrett's esophagus with high-grade dysplasia (carcinoma in situ) and stage I esophageal cancer) is surgical resection with intent to cure. In Barrett's esophagus, high-grade dysplasia and carcinoma in situ are synonymous. The convention is to use high-grade dysplasia (HGD) as the preferred term. High-grade dysplasia (carcinoma in situ) is rarely detected outside of surveillance programs, but outcomes are excellent when cancer is detected at an early stage. Despite the conventional teaching that an esophagectomy is indicated there is an increasing role for endoscopic therapy and less morbid surgical approaches.

Table 30.3 Sub-classification of T1 stage in esophageal cancer. Depth of invasion correlates with LN metastasis and lymphovascular invasion. These features are predictive of recurrence and in several reports of disease-free 5-year survival

T stage	M/SM stage	Maximal depth of invasion	Lymph node metastasis (%) EAC and SCC	Vascular invasion (%) EAC and SCC
T1a	M1	Epithelial layer	0–5	0–5
	M2	Lamina propria		
T1b	M3	Muscularis mucosae	0–12	0–18
T1c	SM1	Upper 1/3	17–37	25–72
	SM2	Intermediate 1/3		
T1d	SM3	Lower 1/3	49–67	48–91

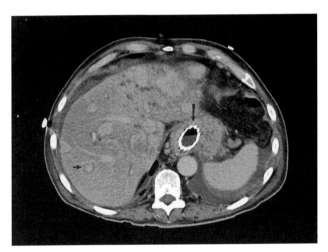

Figure 30.6 Computed tomogram showing metastatic adenocarcinoma of the distal esophagus. A metal stent is located in the distal esophagus and there is diffuse and irregular mucosal thickening of this area (long arrow). Multiple metastatic lesions are seen in the liver (short arrow).

Lesions confined to the lamina propria have a minimal risk of lymph node or distant metastasis (0–5%) so an effective means of local resection could obviate the risks of surgery for patients with mucosal disease. Endoscopic mucosal resection (EMR) has demonstrated feasibility and efficacy for the resection of T1m lesions. Complication rates associated with EMR have been low and include perforation, bleeding, stricture formation and pain (0–7% depending on the extent of EMR). Most importantly, recurrence rates in correctly staged T1m lesions have been similar to post-surgical recurrences for both SCA [18] and ACA [19], albeit no prospective studies have been performed. EMR is generally limited to lesions <20 mm. Emerging studies suggest that endoscopic submucosal dissection (ESD) may have a role in select patients with larger lesions. Although the spectrum of Barrett's ablation techniques are described in greater detail in Chapter 29, it is important to note

that focal resection by EMR is often combined with ablation of residual BE (Figure 30.8).

There are also multiple acceptable surgical options. Transthoracic esophagectomy, using a combined abdominal incision and gastric conduit (an Ivor-Lewis esophagectomy) and the transhiatal esophagectomy performed through an abdominal incision are increasingly being replaced by minimally invasive esophagectomy. Although early studies have reported lower complication rates and post-operative mortality, randomized trials have not been performed and open esophagectomy may still be preferred for higher thoracic lesions and larger bulky tumors.

Post-operative (adjuvant) chemoradiation is not indicated for node-negative disease, although aggressive tumor characteristics (poorly differentiated histology, vascular invasion) and younger patients with adenocarcinoma may be recommended to receive adjuvant treatment.

Stage II–III disease
Surgical resection with intent to cure or long-term remission is recommended for operative candidates with stage II and T3 stage III lesions. Although survival decreases with increasing tumor stage, some patients with stage II–III disease have good long-term outcomes.

Radiation alone The superior results of combined therapy, have minimized the role of radiotherapy alone.

Chemoradiation without surgery Unlike surgery, chemoradiation has the advantage of treating both local disease and distant micrometastases. Chemoradiation alone may result in similar outcomes without subjecting patients to the morbidity and mortality of esophagectomy. Chemoradiation is superior to radiation alone and is the standard of care for patients who are not surgical candidates. Tumor location may also impact on this choice of therapy. Esophageal cancer of the cervical esophagus may be particularly amenable to chemoradiation

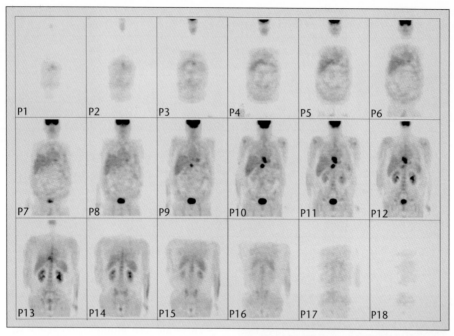

Figure 30.7 Metastatic adenocarcinoma of the esophagus. Positron emission tomogram from a patient with metastatic adenocarcinoma of the esophagus. Abnormal [18F]fluorodeoxyglucose accumulation is seen at the site of the distal esophageal carcinoma. There is also intense abnormal accumulation at an enlarged supraceliac lymph node, the smaller adjacent gastrohepatic ligament, and distal paraesophageal lymph nodes.

Table 30.4 Options for treating esophageal cancer

AJCC stage group	Primary treatment
Stage 0–I	Surgery Endoscopic mucosal resection Photodynamic therapy
Stage II	Surgery Chemoradiation ± surgery
Stage III	Surgery Chemoradiation ± surgery Palliation
Stage IV	Endoscopic therapy Palliation Chemoradiation

AJCC, American Joint Commission on Cancer.
Adapted from the National Comprehensive Cancer Network Clinical Practice Guidelines.

Table 30.5 Five-year survival by stage at diagnosis (adopted from the American Cancer Society Factsheet 2007)

Stage	5-year survival (%)
0	>95%
I	50–80%
IIA	30–40%
IIB	10–30%
III	10–15%
IV	<5%

alone, especially given the high morbidity associated with surgery. A combination of cisplatin and 5-fluorouracil (5-FU) is the mainstay for treatment of esophageal cancer, although paclitaxel, carboplatin, and irinotecan may also be used.

Neoadjuvant chemoradiation The frequent occurrence of distant metastases after surgical resection has prompted the investigation of multimodality therapy for localized esophageal cancer. Neoadjuvant chemoradiation compared to surgery

alone has been the subject of a number of trials and meta-analyses. These have shown a trend towards benefit of neoadjuvant treatment, although the impact seems more significant for ACA then for SCA. Chemoradiation therapy may be superior to neo-adjuvant chemotherapy alone [20]. Preoperative chemoradiation was associated with a higher likelihood of achieving complete resection at the time of surgery. National guidelines currently support either surgery alone or surgery with neoadjuvant chemoradiation for patients with operable T1–T3 tumors.

Stage III–IV disease

The goal of T4 stage III and stage IV disease is nonsurgical palliation. Patients may benefit from radiation, chemotherapy,

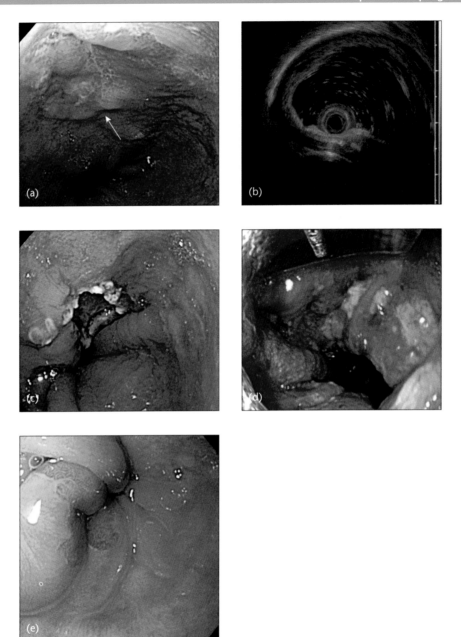

Figure 30.8 (a) Short segment Barrett's esophagus with nodular area (arrow). (b) Endoscopic ultrasound showing absence of invasion into the submucosa or deeper layers. (c) Endoscopic mucosal resection. Pathology revealed focus of intramucosal carcinoma and absence of carcinoma at the resection margin. Circumferential biopsies showed Barrett's esophagus with low grade dysplasia. (d) Radiofrequency ablation of the residual Barrett's segments. (e) Six months after diagnosis there is no macroscopic evidence of Barrett's. Biopsies did not show residual intestinal metaplasia.

or endoscopic therapy. Surgical resection for palliation is not usually considered because of the morbidity of the operation, but may be an appropriate option in selected patients. Palliation of local disease is primarily aimed at alleviating dysphagia and complications related to fistula formation.

Radiation Radiation is well tolerated and very effective for maintenance of local disease control and for palliation of dysphagia. Radiation improves dysphagia in 71% of patients and provides adequate control of symptoms until death in 54%.

Unfortunately, radiation rarely results in sustained remission and the 5-year survival rate ranges from 0% to 10%.

Brachytherapy Brachytherapy delivers a constant dose of localized radiation via an intraluminally implanted radioactive source. The exact role of brachytherapy in the management of esophageal cancer remains to be defined, but current recommendations discourage use of concurrent brachytherapy and chemotherapy(due to severe toxicity) or the use of brachytherapy in the setting of local recurrence(due to high risk of fistula formation). Brachytherapy may also be an alternative to endoscopic stenting in the palliative treatment of dysphagia. Consideration between stenting and brachytherapy depend on the balance between the rapidity of symptom relief, side effect profile and durability of response. Randomized trials have found that stenting results in quicker onset of symptom relief, but side effects (hemorrhage) and durability of response were better after brachytherapy. Advances in stent technologies may impact these outcomes.

Chemoradaition Although survival benefits have not been demonstrated, combination modality treatment was very effective in ameliorating symptoms of dysphagia. Symptom relief was noted by two weeks and maximal benefit was achieved at four weeks.

Endoscopic therapy A number of endoscopically performed therapies are effective for palliation of symptoms. These include dilatation, neodymium-doped yttrium–aluminum–garnet (Nd:YAG) laser therapy, injection therapy, photodynamic therapy (PDT), electrocautery, cryotherapy and stent placement. The choice of modality is tailored to specific patient clinical characteristics. Endoscopic dilatation can temporarily relieve dysphagia and perforation rates are low (1%) but symptom recurrence is universal unless repeated procedures are performed. Tumor ablation with Nd:YAG laser is associated with a high success rate; over 75% of patients with inoperable cancer have functional swallowing after laser therapy. In several studies, PDT was found to be of comparable or superior efficacy to laser therapy. The choice of endoscopic ablation therapy will likely be determined by efficacy, availability and toxicity.

Endoscopic stenting has become the standard of care for palliation of malignant dysphagia and for management of esophagorespiratory fistulae [21]. Self-expanding metal stents (SEMSs) are effective, easy to insert, associated with few complications, and well tolerated by patients. Stent characteristics should be individualized to the location and length of the tumor. Some stents include features that are helpful in specific situations, such as proximal or distal release systems when precise deployment is essential, or a distal valve to prevent reflux when the stent crosses the gastroesophageal junction. The choice of stents has expanded, and now considerations may include covered stents (for lower risk of tumor-ingrowth) and removability. These improvements may come at a cost of higher stent migration rates. The final diameter of the stent, and therefore the efficacy of symptom relief, depends on the radial force of the stent and the tumor characteristics. Late complications are not uncommon, occurring in 20–40% of patients. Complications include stent migration, tumor ingrowth, tissue hyperplasia, chest pain, hemorrhage, fistulization, gastroesophageal reflux, (aspiration) pneumonia [22].

Supportive care Percutaneous endoscopic gastrostomy (PEG) and hospice care play important roles in the management of patients with endstage esophageal cancer. Not all patients will be interested in PEG feeding, but the option should be presented to patients with severe anorexia or dysphagia resistant to therapy. Hospice care is an invaluable aid to comfort patients and their families at the end of life.

Prevention

Lifestyle modifications, primarily the minimization of tobacco and alcohol use, are the first line of prevention against SCC. Dietary changes may modify the risk for SCC in high-incidence areas. Diets rich in fresh fruits and vegetables may help to prevent SCC.

In developed nations, the incidence of SCC is low enough that routine screening is not cost-effective, except in the highest risk groups, such as those with head and neck cancer, achalasia, or tylosis. In high-incidence regions, an effective screening method could have a dramatic impact on public health. The primary risk factor for ACA is longstanding gastroesophageal reflux and Barrett's esophagus, so routine endoscopic screening is recommended for these patients. Medical therapy with proton pump inhibitors heals esophagitis but rarely reverses Barrett's esophagus. The frequency of screening depends on the presence of Barrett's esophagus and/or dysplasia. The use of endoscopic ablative therapy to halt the progression of Barrett's esophagus to ACA is an area of active investigation.

Chemoprevention may also play a role in the prevention of esophageal cancer, however thus far no single agent has shown sufficient efficacy to recommend clinical use.

SOURCES OF INFORMATION FOR PATIENTS AND DOCTORS

The following websites are maintained by either the National Cancer Institute or medical societies and provide information on diagnosis, treatment and clinical trials. Most sites have both patient and health professional tailored sections.

http://digestive.niddk.nih.gov/ddiseases/pubs/barretts
www.cancerhelp.org.uk/help
www.cancer.gov/cancerinfo/types/esophageal

References

1. Anon. Esophageal cancer: epidemiology, pathogenesis and prevention. *Nat Clin Pract Gastroenterol Hepatol.* 2008;5:517–526.
2. Kubo A, Corley DA. Marked multi-ethnic variation of esophageal and gastric cardia carcinomas within the United States. *Am J Gastroenterol.* 2004;99:582–588.
3. Everhart JE, Ruhl CE. Burden of digestive diseases in the United States part I: overall and upper gastrointestinal diseases. *Gastroenterology.* 2009;136:376–386.
4. Freedman ND, Abnet CC, Leitzmann MF, *et al.* A prospective study of tobacco, alcohol, and the risk of esophageal and gastric cancer subtypes. *Am J Epidemiol.* 2007;165:1424–1433.
5. Brooks PJ, Enoch MA, Goldman D, *et al.* The alcohol flushing response: an unrecognized risk factor for esophageal cancer from alcohol consumption. *PLoS Med.* 2009;6:e50.

6. Lambert R, Hainaut P. The multidisciplinary management of gastrointestinal cancer. Epidemiology of oesophagogastric cancer. *Best Pract Res Clin Gastroenterol.* 2007;21:921–945.

7. Gao GF, Roth MJ, Wei WQ, *et al.* No association between HPV infection and the neoplastic progression of esophageal squamous cell carcinoma: result from a cross-sectional study in a high-risk region of China. *Int J Cancer.* 2006;119:1354–1359.

8. Muto M, Hironaka S, Nakane M, *et al.* Association of multiple Lugol-voiding lesions with synchronous and metachronous esophageal squamous cell carcinoma in patients with head and neck cancer. *Gastrointest Endosc.* 2002;56:517–521.

9. Heath EI, Canto MI, Piantadosi S, *et al.* Secondary chemoprevention of Barrett's esophagus with celecoxib: results of a randomized trial. *J Natl Cancer Inst.* 2007;99:545–557.

10. Cook MB, Greenwood DC, Hardie LJ, *et al.* A systematic review and meta-analysis of the risk of increasing adiposity on Barrett's esophagus. *Am J Gastroenterol.* 2008;103:292–300.

11. Edelstein ZR, Farrow DC, Bronner MP, *et al.* Central adiposity and risk of Barrett's esophagus. *Gastroenterology.* 2007;133:403–411.

12. Souza RF, Krishnan K, Spechler SJ. Acid, bile, and CDX: the ABCs of making Barrett's metaplasia. *Am J Physiol Gastrointest Liver Physiol.* 2008;295:G211–G218.

13. Larghi A, Lecca PG, Costamagna G. High-resolution narrow band imaging endoscopy. *Gut.* 2008;57:976–986.

14. van Vliet EP, Heijenbrok-Kal MH, Hunink MG, *et al.* Staging investigations for oesophageal cancer: a meta-analysis. *Br J Cancer.* 2008;98:547–557.

15. Kim DU, Lee JH, Min BH, *et al.* Risk factors of lymph node metastasis in T1 esophageal squamous cell carcinoma. *J Gastroenterol Hepatol.* 2008;23:619–625.

16. Liu L, Hofstetter WL, Rashid A, *et al.* Significance of the depth of tumor invasion and lymph node metastasis in superficially invasive (T1) esophageal adenocarcinoma. *Am J Surg Pathol.* 2005;29:1079–1085.

17. Shimada H, Nabeya Y, Matsubara H, *et al.* Prediction of lymph node status in patients with superficial esophageal carcinoma: analysis of 160 surgically resected cancers. *Am J Surg.* 2006;191:250–254.

18. Das A, Singh V, Fleischer DE, *et al.* A comparison of endoscopic treatment and surgery in early esophageal cancer: an analysis of surveillance epidemiology and end results data. *Am J Gastroenterol.* 2008;103:1340–1345.

19. Kim JH, Chung HS, Youn YH, *et al.* Treatment outcomes of 70 cases of early esophageal carcinoma: 12 years of experience. *Dis Esophagus.* 2007;20:297–300.

20. Stahl M, Walz MK, Stuschke M, *et al.* Phase III comparison of preoperative chemotherapy compared with chemoradiotherapy in patients with locally advanced adenocarcinoma of the esophagogastric junction. *J Clin Oncol.* 2009;27:851–856.

21. Tietjen TG, Pasricha PJ, Kalloo AN. Management of malignant esophageal stricture with esophageal dilation and esophageal stents. *Gastrointest Endosc Clin N Am.* 1994;4:851–862.

22. Simmons DT, Baron TH. Endoluminal palliation. *Gastrointest Endosc Clin N Am.* 2005;15:467–484, viii.

Upper GI Tract

Upper GI Tract

CHAPTER 31

Infections of the esophagus and stomach

George B. McDonald

University of Washington; Fred Hutchinson Cancer Research Center, Seattle, WA, USA

ESSENTIAL FACTS ABOUT PATHOGENESIS

- Esophageal and stomach infections can occur in reasonably healthy people, but they are much more common and severe when patients have evidence of immune impairment
- Infections in the esophagus in apparently healthy people are usually caused by *Candida albicans*, but HSV and EBV esophagitis can be seen. In immune compromised patients, esophagitis caused by *Candida* species and by herpesviruses is common

ESSENTIALS OF DIAGNOSIS

- Diagnosis of *Candida* esophagitis should include esophageal brushings, but in patients with HIV-AIDS, fluconazole can be given empirically when there is oral thrush and esophageal symptoms
- Apart from *Helicobacter pylori* and community-acquired viruses, gastric infections are uncommon in healthy people. Unusual infections caused by Anisakis worms, *M. tuberculosis*, syphilis may be seen in endemic areas
- Cytomegalovirus is the most common cause of gastric infection in immune compromised patients, but other virus, fungi, bacteria, and parasites can cause infection
- Achlorhydria or proton pump inhibitor (PPI) treatment usually result in asymptomatic colonization

ESSENTIALS OF TREATMENT

- *Candida albicans:* Fluconazole 100–200 mg daily for most patients. Many alternatives available
- HSV esophagitis: Intravenous acyclovir (250 mg per m² tds) then oral valacyclovir (1000 mg tds) or foscarnet (40 mg/kg tds)
- CMV esophagitis: Ganciclovir (5 mg/kg bd) or foscarnet (90 mg/kg iv bd)

Introduction

In the settings of immunologic impairment, motility disorders, and gastric acid suppression, the esophagus and stomach may become infected with bacteria, fungi, viruses, and parasites, but normal people are commonly infected only by *H. pylori* and community-acquired viruses that cause vomiting and diarrhea (Rotavirus, Norovirus, Astrovirus, Sapovirus).

Infection is defined as the presence of organisms that invade or elicit an inflammatory response in the mucosa, in contrast to colonization. Nonspecific complaints may be the only clinical manifestations of infection in immunosuppressed patients. Effective treatment is available for most esophageal and gastric infections.

Epidemiology

Aside from *H. pylori* (see Chapter 22, "H. pylori: its diseases and management" and Chapter 35), the only common organisms that infect completely healthy people are community-acquired viruses and rarely, *Herpes simplex* virus, varicella zoster virus (VZV), Epstein-Barr virus, and Anasikis worms. *Candida albicans* may cause esophagitis in apparently healthy patients with subtle immune defects, for example, patients who are elderly, diabetic, or receiving antibiotics. In immune suppressed patients, these same organisms may cause more severe infection, and different organisms can infect the esophagus and stomach, for example, Cytomegalovirus (CMV) and molds. HIV infection is associated with idiopathic esophageal ulcers. Human papilloma virus (HPV) may cause esophageal condylomata and possibly contribute to carcinoma.

Causes, risk factors and disease associations

Antibiotics disrupt the balance among bacteria and fungi; this permits *Candida* overgrowth. Immune deficiency involving T cells or granulocytes, whether genetic or acquired, increases the risk of infection. Fungal infections are common in HIV-AIDS patients not receiving highly active antiretroviral therapy (HAART) and in those with hematologic malignancy and those receiving immune suppressive medicines, including chemotherapy. Predisposing illnesses include diabetes mellitus, esophageal motility disorders, alcoholism, and advanced age. Corticosteroids, including corticosteroid inhalers, predispose to fungal esophagitis.

Textbook of Clinical Gastroenterology and Hepatology, Second Edition. Edited by C. J. Hawkey, Jaime Bosch, Joel E. Richter, Guadalupe Garcia-Tsao, Francis K. L. Chan.
© 2012 Blackwell Publishing Ltd. Published 2012 by Blackwell Publishing Ltd.

Table 31.1 organisms causing esophageal infections

Reasonably healthy people	Immunocompromised patients
Common	**Common**
Candida species	Candida species
	Cytomegalovirus (CMV)
	Herpes simplex virus (HSV)
Uncommon	**Uncommon**
Herpes simplex virus	HIV-associated ulcers
Epstein-Barr virus (mononucleosis)	Varicella zoster virus (VZV)
	Aspergillus species
	Bacteria from the oral flora
Rare	**Rare**
Varicella zoster virus (disseminated)	Parasitic infection
Human papilloma virus (HPV)	
Mycobacterium tuberculosis	
Histoplasma	
Other fungal organisms	

Esophageal infections (Table 31.1)

Fungal esophagitis

Pathology

Candida species colonize by superficial adherence. Invasion into epithelia requires a defect in cellular immunity. Infection is distinguished from colonization by adherent plaques at endoscopy and budding yeast on histology. Other fungi such as Aspergillus, Histoplasma, Cryptococcus, and Blastomyces are rare causes of esophagitis.

Clinical presentation

Most patients have dysphagia or odynophagia; associated symptoms may include retrosternal discomfort, heartburn, and nausea [1]. In granulocytopenic patients, fever, sepsis, and abdominal pain suggest disseminated candidiasis as a consequence of swallowed yeast forms traversing the normal small intestine [2]. Patients with subtle T-cell defects may be without esophageal symptoms despite chronic infection.

Differential diagnosis

The differential diagnosis includes esophagitis caused by viruses, pills, and acid-peptic reflux and strictures leading to dysphagia.

Diagnostic methods

Endoscopic brushing and biopsy should be performed unless there is obvious oropharyngeal Candida infection [1,3]. Candida plaques are white/yellow and if dislodged show a raw surface (Figure 31.1). Brushings should be spread onto slides, air dried, and stained. Cultures are rarely helpful unless an unusual fungus or resistant Candida species is suspected. Radiographs are of limited value.

Treatment and prevention

Most patients with Candida albicans infection should receive oral **fluconazole** or a topical agent. Fluconazole (100–200 mg p.o. daily) is convenient and the choice for immunodeficient patients, but **clotrimazole** or **nystatin troches** (pastilles retained in the mouth for local delivery) are effective and lack side effects and drug–drug interactions. In HIV infection, oral thrush with esophageal symptoms predicts Candida esophagitis, and empiric treatment with fluconazole is recommended, with endoscopy reserved for patients without a clinical response within 3–5 days (to exclude resistant Candida and viral infection). **Itraconazole** 200 mg daily is an effective alternative.

For **granulocytopenic patients fluconazole** and **itraconazole** are effective for local mucosal infection. Liposomal amphotericin (3–5 mg/kg/day) or an echinocandin such as caspofungin or micafungin should be used in febrile patients with disseminated infection. Risk factors should be sought and eliminated.

For **HIV-infected patients**, prophylaxis with fluconazole is effective, but a better strategy is HAART. In patients with **hematologic disorders**, fluconazole or oral amphotericin B reduces recurrences.

Complications and their management

Yeast forms of Candida may disseminate in granulocytopenic patients [2]. Rarely, esophageal ulcers penetrate into the mediastinum.

Viral esophagitis

Pathology

HSV esophagitis usually occurs after reactivation of latent virus. Histology reveals multinucleated giant cells, ballooning degeneration, and "ground glass" intranuclear inclusions (Figure 31.1).

CMV infection is identified by large cells with intranuclear and cytoplasmic inclusions and a halo surrounding the nuclear inclusions.

VZV shows ballooning degeneration and multinucleated giant cells with intranuclear eosinophilic inclusions [2].

Clinical presentation

CMV infection Fever, nausea, and vomiting often dominate the clinical picture.

HSV causes odynophagia and nausea [4].

VZV infection Esophageal manifestations are often of minor significance compared to encephalitis, pneumonia, and hepatitis.

HIV-associated idiopathic ulcerations range from small aphthoid lesions to giant, deep ulcers [5].

HPV lesions present as erythematous plaques or nodules and are usually asymptomatic.

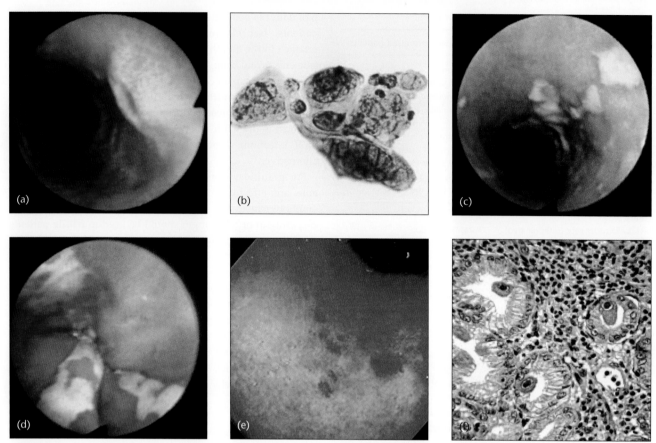

Figure 31.1 Endoscopic and histologic features of esophageal and gastric infections. **(a)** Endoscopy photograph of a volcano-like lesion caused by HSV in the esophagus. The crater of the volcano represents sloughed squamous epithelium, forming an ulcer. A diagnosis can be made by biopsy or brushing an edge of the ulcer. **(b)** Photomicrograph of a cluster of multinucleate giant cells, typical of HSV infection of squamous epithelium. The specimen was obtained at endoscopy using a brush. **(c)** Endoscopy photograph of adherent white plaques with reddened edges, typical of *Candida* esophagitis. **(d)** Endoscopy photograph of linear ulcerations in the esophagus caused by CMV. This endoscopic appearance can be confused with *Candida* esophagitis. **(e)** Endoscopy photograph of gastric mucosa, showing small punctate bleeding sites (overlying erosions), caused by CMV infection. **(f)** Photomicrograph of a gastric biopsy, showing typical findings of CMV infection – three megaloid cells within crypt epithelium, each containing an inclusion surrounded by a light-colored rim. Lymphoid cells are increased in the lamina propria.

Differential diagnosis

The differential diagnosis includes fungal esophagitis, reflux esophagitis, pill esophagitis, and, less likely, malignancy.

Diagnostic methods

Viral esophagitis is diagnosed by endoscopy [1]. Radiographs are not accurate.

HSV infection causes vesicles, erosions, or large superficial ulcers (Figure 31.1).

CMV infection results in erosions or ulcers (Figure 31.1). Specimens from ulcer bases lack epithelial cells and are inadequate to exclude HSV, whereas CMV-infected fibroblasts and endothelial cells reside in the ulcer base (Figure 31.2). Biopsy samples for viral culture and histology should be obtained from ulcer margins, ulcer base, and surrounding mucosa. Immunohistology, PCR, and viral culture are more accurate than histology alone [6].

VZV esophagitis occurs with dermatologic VZV and results in vesicles and ulcers. HIV-associated idiopathic ulceration is a diagnosis of exclusion.

Treatment and prevention

HSV esophagitis is treated with intravenous acyclovir, 250 mg/m² every 8 hours, then oral valacyclovir (1000 mg t.i.d.) for a total duration of treatment of 14–21 days. **Foscarnet** (40 mg/kg t.i.d.) is effective for acyclovir-resistant HSV. Prophylaxis with oral acyclovir or **valacyclovir** prevents recurrences.

CMV esophagitis is treated with **ganciclovir** (5 mg/kg every 12 hours for 2 weeks) or **foscarnet** (90 mg/kg intravenously every 12 hours for 2–3 weeks). Maintenance therapy with ganciclovir or foscarnet for 3 additional weeks is indicated. Recurrence is common if immunodeficiency persists (as in HIV). Screening of blood products prevents CMV disease among CMV-naïve transplant recipients.

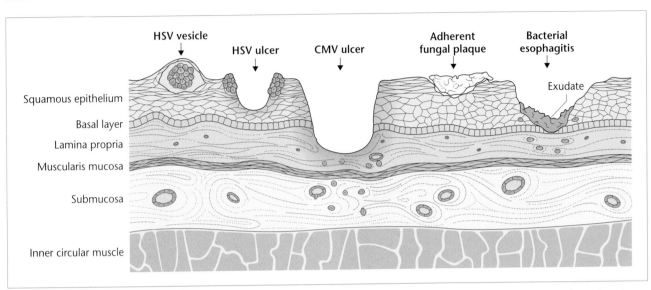

Figure 31.2 Location of organisms causing esophageal infection. Schematic diagram of the esophageal mucosa showing the location of organisms that cause infection. HSV infects squamous epithelium whereas CMV infects only subepithelial cells (endothelial cells, fibroblasts). Fungal and bacterial esophagitis infect superficial layers of the mucosa but may extend more deeply. (This figure was published in *Clinical Gastroenterology and Hepatology*, Wilfred M. Weinstein, Christopher J. Hawkey, Jaime Bosch, Infections of the esophagus and stomach, Pages 1–4, Copyright Elsevier, 2005.)

VZV infection is treated with intravenous **acyclovir. Foscarnet** is effective for acyclovir-resistant VZV.

Idiopathic HIV-associated ulcers respond to prednisone (40 mg/ day for 2 weeks, then a one month taper). Another option is thalidomide (200 mg/day for 4 weeks).

Complications
Complications can include extensive mucosal necrosis, super-infection, Boerhaave syndrome, hemorrhage, strictures, HSV or VZV pneumonia, tracheoesophageal fistula formation, and disseminated infection.

Bacterial infections of the esophagus Tuberculosis of the esophagus may occur via mediastinal extension. In granulocytopenic patients, bacteria from the oral flora may infiltrate esophageal tissues.

Infections of the stomach (Table 31.2)
In reasonably healthy people, gastric infections are rare except for *Helicobacter pylori* infection (see Chapters 22 and 35) and community-acquired viruses such as Rotavirus, Norovirus, Astrovirus, and Sapovirus, where vomiting is a prominent feature of illness along with diarrhea. Ingestion of raw fish can lead to acute gastric infection with Anisakis worms.

In immunodeficient patients, gastric infections occur more commonly.

CMV and VZV can cause and ulceration and inflammation in the stomach (Figure 31.2) [6,7] as well as in the esophagus.

Bacterial overgrowth also occurs with achlorhydria or treatment with proton pump inhibitors, but manifests only as

Table 31.2 Organisms causing gastric infections

Reasonably healthy people	Immunocompromised patients
Common	**Common**
H. pylori (Chapters 22, 35)	*Cytomegalovirus* (CMV)
Community-acquired viruses (Norovirus, Rotavirus, Astrovirus, Sapovirus)	
Uncommon	**Uncommon**
Anisakis worms	*Varicella zoster virus* (VZV)
	Fungal infection (especially molds)
	Cryptosporidium
Rare	**Rare**
Other spiral bacteria (*H. heilmannii*)	Phlegmonous gastritis
Mycobacterium tuberculosis	*Epstein-Barr virus* lymphoproliferative disease (EBV-LPD)
Treponema pallidum (syphilis)	
Cytomegalovirus	

asymptomatic colonization. However, **phlegmonous gastritis**, a rare infection of the submucosa of the stomach caused by bacteria, has been described in the setting of alcoholism, trauma, and granulocytopenia. It presents as an acute abdomen, usually with peritoneal signs, and endoscopy reveals erythematous or purple mucosa, cobblestoning, and sometimes frank pus. CT X-rays showing air in the gastric wall are diagnostic (Figure 31.3). Gastrectomy may be required but prompt antibiotic treatment can effect resolution [8].

Gastritis can also rarely be caused by **spiral-shaped bacteria** (*Helicobacter heilmannii, H. felis*) other than *H. pylori*; symptoms and low-grade MALT lymphoma respond to treatment [9,10].

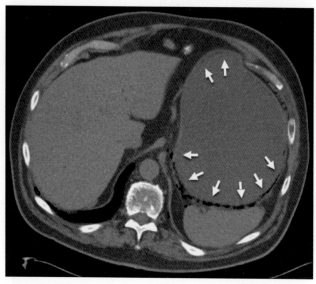

Figure 31.3 CT X-ray of the abdomen demonstrating phlegmonous gastritis. CT image of a distended stomach with gas in the gastric wall (arrows). The patient was an 82-year-old diabetic who presented with nausea, vomiting and abdominal distension. She recovered with antibiotic treatment. (Courtesy of Dr. P. Rajvanshi)

Gastric syphilis is characterized by an inflammatory infiltrate, erosions, ulcerations, and thickened folds, sometimes resembling malignancy but responding to treatment for secondary syphilis [11].

Gastric tuberculosis is usually secondary to pulmonary infection but primary gastric infection presenting as a mass lesion can be seen [12].

CMV infection has also been associated with marked gastric rugal hypertrophy and transient protein-losing enteropathy, similar to Ménétrier's disease.

Fungal gastric infections including *Candida*, *Histoplasma* and *Zygomycetes* can occur in granulocytopenic patients.

Cryptosporidium oocysts can be found in gastric mucosa in HIV+ and transplant recipients receiving immune suppressive drugs; only restoration of immunity can effect clearance.

References

1. Baehr PH, McDonald GB. Esophageal infections: risk factors, presentation, diagnosis and treatment. *Gastroenterology.* 1994;106:509–532.
2. Krause W, Matheis H, Wulf F. Fungaemia and funguria after oral administration of Candida albicans. *Lancet.* 1969;1:598–599.
3. Greenson JK. Infections of the esophagus. *Pathol Case Rev.* 2002;7:19–26.
4. Ramanathan, J, Rammouni M, Baran J, *et al.* Herpes simplex virus esophagitis in the immunocompetent host: an overview. *Am J Gastroenterol.* 2000;95:2171–2176.
5. Wilcox CM, Schwartz DA. Comparison of two corticosteroid regimens for the treatment of HIV-associated idiopathic esophageal ulcer. *Am J Gastroenterol.* 1994; 89:2163.
6. Hackman RC, Wolford JL, Gleaves CA, *et al.* Recognition and rapid diagnosis of upper gastrointestinal cytomegalovirus infection in marrow transplant recipients. A comparison of seven virologic methods. *Transplantation.* 1994;57:231–237.
7. Steinbach G, McDonald GB. Gastrointestinal infections after solid organ or hemopoietic cell transplantation. In: Bowden RA, Ljungman P, Snydman DR editors. *Transplant Infections.* 3rd ed. Philadelphia, PA, Lippincott Williams & Wilkens, 2010, Chapter 18.
8. Rajendran S, Baban C, Lee G, *et al.* Rapid resolution of phlegmonous gastritis using antibiotics alone. *BMJ Case Reports.* 2009;261:bcr0220091541.
9. Morgner A, Lehn N, Andersen LP, *et al.* Helicobacter heilmannii-associated primary gastric low grade MALT lymphoma: complete remission after curing the infection. *Gastroenterology.* 2000;118:821–828.
10. Fox JG. The non-*H. pylori* helicobacters: their role in gastrointestinal and systemic diseases. *Gut.* 2002;50:273–283.
11. Long BW, Johnston JH, Wetzel W, *et al.* Gastric syphilis: endoscopic and histologic features mimicking lymphoma. *Amer J Gastroenterol.* 2008;90:1504–1507.
12. Amarapurkar DN, Patel ND, Amarapurkar AD. Primary gastric tuberculosis – report of 5 cases. *BMC Gastroenterology.* 2003;3:6.

CHAPTER 32

Peptic ulcer

C. J. Hawkey and John C. Atherton

Nottingham Digestive Diseases Centre, University of Nottingham and Nottingham University Hospitals, Nottingham, UK

ESSENTIALS OF PATHOGENESIS

- *Helicobacter pylori* and NSAIDs are the commonest causes of peptic ulceration
- Most duodenal ulcers are caused by *H. pylori*
- Most gastric ulcers in developed countries are caused by NSAIDs
- Smoking is an important cofactor particularly for *H. pylori*-induced ulcers
- Virulence factors (CagA, VacA and others) influence whether *H. pylori* colonization leads to ulceration
- NSAIDs inhibit the synthesis of gastroprotective prostaglandins

---

ESSENTIALS OF DIAGNOSIS

- Typical ulcer symptoms are localized epigastric pain occurring overnight or pre-prandially and relieved by milk or antacids
- Symptoms are however often atypical, especially with gastric ulcers and/or NSAID use
- Many ulcers are now treated without a formal diagnosis
  - In younger patients without alarm features, *H. pylori* infection is usually detected and eradicated in the community
  - For NSAID patients, prophylactic measures in at risk patients rather than diagnosis is key to management
- Where formal diagnosis is needed endoscopy is the method of choice
- Biopsy of gastric ulcers is traditionally recommended to detect gastric cancer or lymphoma but duodenal ulcers should also be biopsied if there is a possibility of Crohn's disease (e.g., *H. pylori* and NSAID negative)

ESSENTIALS OF TREATMENT AND PROGNOSIS

- Successful *H. pylori* eradication results in permanent ulcer healing in the vast majority of patients if there are no other risk factors (including NSAID use)
- *H. pylori* eradication prior to NSAID initiation may reduce ulcer risk. Risk can be further reduced by co-prescription of PPIs.
- Ulcers and ulcer complications are much less likely if patients take selective COX-2 inhibitors

---

Introduction and definition

Peptic ulcers are localized breaches of the gastric or duodenal mucosa with tissue destruction at least to the depth of the muscularis mucosa (Figure 32.1). The word "peptic" reflects a belief (probably misplaced) that peptic activity is involved in pathogenesis. Peptic ulcers include ulcers in the stomach, pylorus, duodenum, or a Meckel's diverticulum, as well as ulcers at sites of gastrointestinal anastomosis (stomal ulcers) and at the gastroesophageal junction. The commonest symptom is pain. The most serious complications are bleeding and perforation.

Causes of peptic ulceration

It is only in the past 25 years that the causes of peptic ulcers have been identified and rational management defined.

Common causes

Most ulcers are directly caused by infection with *Helicobacter pylori* [1] or by nonsteroidal anti-inflammatory drugs (NSAIDs) [2,3], including aspirin [4] (Figure 32.2), which inhibit prostaglandin synthesis and abrogate mucosal defence mechanisms. In developed countries, duodenal ulcers are proportionally caused more commonly by *H. pylori* and gastric ulcers by NSAIDs, but either factor may produce an ulcer at either site. Absence of a history of NSAID use and a negative test for *H. pylori* should prompt a search for other causes, although in such patients *H. pylori* and NSAIDs are still the most likely causes. Tests for *H. pylori* have a low but measurable false negative rate and NSAIDs purchased directly and sometimes unknowingly in compound preparations, are easily ignored by doctors and patients.

Uncommon causes

Uncommon, but significant, causes of peptic ulcers include Crohn's disease, conditions causing acid hypersecretion (Zollinger-Ellison syndrome, multiple endocrine neoplasia, and mastocytosis [9]; see Chapter 112) severe physical stress such as being in intensive care, and mucosal ischemia due to

---

Textbook of Clinical Gastroenterology and Hepatology, Second Edition. Edited by C. J. Hawkey, Jaime Bosch, Joel E. Richter, Guadalupe Garcia-Tsao, Francis K. L. Chan.

critical celiac axis vascular disease and radiation. Gastric ulceration may also indicate gastric adenocarcinoma or gastric lymphoma

There is continuing debate about whether corticosteroids alone can cause ulcers [10,11], although the ability of corticosteroids to enhance NSAID-associated ulcers is well established (see below) [2,5]. Idiopathic ulcers are rare. Most are probably due to falsely negative *H. pylori* tests or sporadic or surreptitious NSAID use. If these causes are confidently excluded, rare conditions such as those described above should be sought. However, a small group of idiopathic peptic ulcers still exists

Epidemiology

The epidemiology of peptic ulceration reflects that of the main underlying causes (see Chapter 22 for *H. pylori* and Chapter 23 for NSAIDs). The early twentieth century saw a rapid rise in the incidence of duodenal ulceration in westernized societies [6]. *H. pylori* has been ubiquitous in the population for centuries, so a change in environment appears the most likely cause, and one possibility is the widespread adoption of smoking – an important co-factor for duodenal ulceration in *H. pylori*-colonized people. The prevalence of both *H. pylori* and peptic ulcer is falling in westernized societies [7], probably due to improvements in hygiene in the twentieth century(Figure 32.3). In other parts of the world such as Hong Kong where *H.*

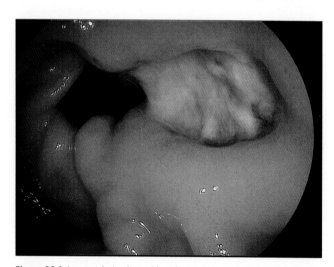

Figure 32.1 Large pyloric ulcer with red spot (minor bleeding stigma).

pylori remains common, the prevalence of peptic ulcer also remains high. As the prevalence of *H. pylori* infection has fallen, the importance of NSAIDs as a cause of peptic ulceration has increased, and low-dose aspirin is now the fastest growing cause of ulcer complications [8]. Recent studies [9–14] suggest that whilst uncomplicated ulcers continue to fall, this may not be so for ulcer complications.

Risk factors

The influence of risk factors depends largely but not entirely on whether the peptic ulcer is caused by *H. pylori* or NSAIDs [15–22] Peptic ulcer is an age-related disease for both *H. pylori* and NSAIDs (see Figure 32.3). In *H. pylori*-infected patients, smoking enhances the risk considerably [16]. Family history largely reflects "shared" *H. pylori* infection. A previous history of peptic ulcer increases risk for ulcers caused both by *H. pylori* infection and NSAID use. Risk may persist after NSAID cessation [8] which might explain some "idiopathic" ulceration. It is clear that different NSAIDs affect the risk of peptic ulcer to different extents, and that risk is highly dose dependent [19] (Figure 32.4). Risk factors in patients using *low-dose aspirin* are less well defined, but rates of ulcer bleeding are higher in patients with a past history and in elderly patients [22]. Risk factors for rare causes are unclear, and in some instances (e.g., Zollinger-Ellison syndrome) the underlying disease is a dominant influence.

Disease associations

Peptic ulcer is more common in patients with chronic obstructive lung disease, cirrhosis, coronary artery disease, and renal failure [7] and in coal miners, possibly because of shared risk factors, including *H. pylori* infection or hypergastrinemia.

Pathogenesis

It is a truism that mucosal integrity represents a balance between aggressive and protective factors. *H. pylori* infection and acid are the main aggressive factors. The main protective factors are mucus and bicarbonate secretion, hydrophobicity (waxiness) of epithelial cells, and mucosal blood flow. These are mediated by prostaglandins (and other mediators such as nitric oxide) and abrogated when their synthesis is inhibited by NSAIDs [2].

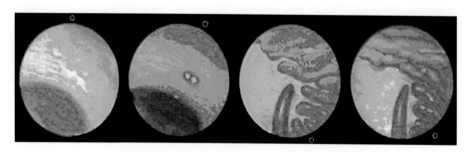

Figure 32.2 First demonstration of aspirin-induced gastric damage. (Reproduced with permission from Douthwaite AH, Lintott SAM. Gastropic observation of the effect of aspirin and certain other substances on the stomach. *Lancet.* 1938;ii:1222–1225.)

Upper GI Tract

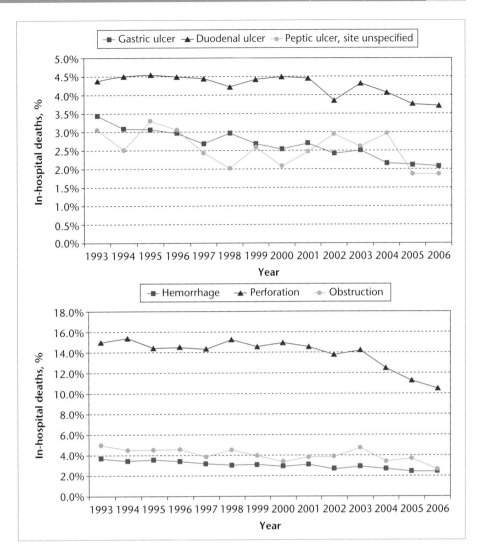

Figure 32.3 Recent trends in ulcer epidemiology. Top: Deaths from gastric ulcer and unspecified peptic ulcer. Bottom: Deaths from duodenal ulcer. (Reproduced with permission from Wang YR, Richter JE, Dempsey DT. Trends and outcomes of hospitalizations for peptic ulcer disease in the United States, 1993 to 2006. *Ann Surg.* 2010;251(1):51–58.)

H. pylori-associated ulcers

H. pylori colonization is lifelong in the absence of effective treatment [24] yet only about 15% of infected people develop peptic ulceration in their lifetime. The development of ulceration is due to a combination of bacterial virulence, host genetic susceptibility, and environmental co-factors.

Bacterial virulence

The best understood bacterial virulence factor is the *cag* pathogenicity island (*cag* PAI). *H. pylori* strains possessing this factor induce more inflammation and are more closely associated with peptic ulceration and gastric adenocarcinoma than *cag*-negative strains [23]. The *cag* PAI is a collection of genes encoding a bacterial type IV secretion system, a sort of molecular syringe through which at least one protein, CagA, is "injected" into epithelial cells [24]. Several signalling pathways are activated, resulting in epithelial cell changes and pro-inflammatory cytokine release, which induces inflammation [25]. A second virulence factor is the vacuolating cytotoxin, VacA. *H. pylori* strains producing more active forms are more closely

associated with disease [23,26]. Other factors that have been associated with increased strain pathogenicity include an adhesin, BabA, an outer membrane inflammatory protein, OipA [28], and a genetic marker of another type IV secretion system, *dupA* [27].

Host susceptibility

Genetic polymorphisms in some cytokine genes, such as interleukin-1β, increase the level of inflammation induced by *H. pylori* [27], induce the pan-gastritic pattern of inflammation, and increase the risk of *H. pylori*-associated gastric atrophy and adenocarcinoma. Peptic ulcer disease has been associated with inadequate regulatory T cell responses [28] and there is growing interest in the role of the innate immune responses [29].

Environmental factors

Smoking is an important risk factor for peptic ulceration in *H. pylori*-colonized people [16]. Its role in NSAID-associated ulcers is less clear.

Upper GI Tract

Localization of *H. pylori*-associated ulcers
Duodenal ulceration

Duodenal ulcers occur against a background of *H. pylori* colonization with a predominantly antral pattern of gastritis (Figure 32.5). Antral inflammation results in reduced somatostatin production by antral D cells and, as somatostatin normally has a negative feedback on gastrin, this results in

hypergastrinemia [30]. Gastrin stimulates the healthy gastric corpus to produce more acid. The increased acid load in the duodenum contributes to the formation of gastric metaplasia – a (possibly adaptive) change in the duodenal mucosa to resemble that in the stomach. *H. pylori*, which can colonize only gastric-type mucosa, can now colonize the duodenum and cause inflammation, damage, and ulceration (Figure 32.5).

Gastric ulceration

Gastric ulcers occur in *H. pylori*-colonized people with a corpus-predominant or pangastritis (Figure 32.5). Such persons also have hypergastrinemia, but acid production is unchanged or reduced because of the inflamed and damaged gastric corpus. This leads to a cycle of chronic damage with progressive atrophy of gastric glands and further hypochlorhydria. The pathogenesis of gastric ulceration in this environment is poorly understood, but ulcers usually occur in the transitional zone, between antrum and corpus mucosa, often on the lesser curve, where inflammation can be heavy. These people are also predisposed to develop distal gastric adenocarcinoma.

Nonsteroidal anti-inflammatory drugs (NSAIDs)
Mucosal defence

NSAIDs inhibit the synthesis of gastroduodenal prostaglandins, which are centrally important for mucosal protection via mucus and bicarbonate secretion and mucosal blood flow [2]. Abrogation of prostaglandin-dependent mechanisms is sufficient to cause local erosions, which deepen to form ulcers in the presence of acid and pepsin. A central role for pepsin is more likely in NSAID ulcers than in ulcers caused by *H. pylori*, as much greater changes in pH are needed to prevent damage [35] or heal ulcers [31,32].

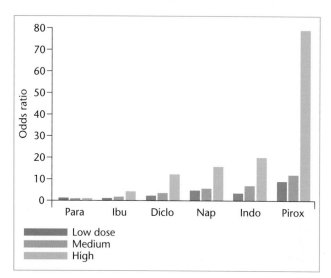

Figure 32.4 Differences in odds ratio for peptic ulcer bleeding with individual NSAIDs and doses. Paracetamol (acetaminophen) is also shown for comparison. Note: Confidence intervals were wide (not shown for groups). (Reproduced with permission from Lewis SC, Langman MJS, Laporte JR, *et al.* Dose-response relationships between individual nonaspirin nonsteroidal antiinflammatory drugs (NANSAIDs) and serious upper gastrointestinal bleeding: a meta-analysis based on individual patient data. *Br J Clin Pharmacol.* 2002;54(3):320–326.)

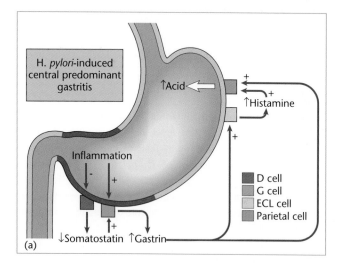

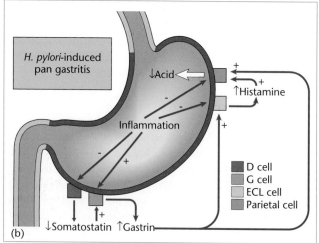

Figure 32.5 Hormonal changes in duodenal and gastric ulceration. **(a)** In *H. pylori*-induced antral predominant gastritis, the illustrated hormonal changes lead to hypergastrinemia and increased acid production from the uninflamed gastric corpus. The increased acid load on the duodenum may lead to ulceration (see text for full explanation). **(b)** In pangastritis, the same hormonal changes pertain, but the inflamed corpus produces reduced acid despite the hypergastrinemia. Such stomachs are at increased risk of gastric ulceration and adenocarcinoma.

Hemostasis

Aspirin inhibits thromboxane synthesis and platelet aggregation and reduced hemostasis likely contributes to ulcer bleeding in patients on low-dose aspirin.

Other ulcer types

Acid plays a dominant role in ulcers associated with gastrinomas, whether sporadic or occurring in the multiple endocrine neoplasia (MEN) 1 syndrome, and in systemic mastocytosis, where histamine stimulates acid secretion. Acid output is often increased in ulcers designated as idiopathic. Conversely, stress ulcers are associated with mucosal underperfusion and abrogation of defence mechanisms. Inflammatory pathogenic mechanisms in Crohn's disease and radiation are considered in Chapters 50 and 116 respectively.

Pathogenesis of symptoms

Pain is the hallmark symptom of peptic ulceration. The origin and pathogenesis of ulcer pain and ulcer-like pain are poorly understood. The mucosa is normally anesthetic, but contains fibers with the characteristics of acid-receptive nociceptors, which may be activated during mucosal injury and inflammation.

Pathology

Histologically, for a lesion to be an ulcer it must extend beneath the muscularis mucosa. More superficial lesions are classified as erosions (Figure 32.6). Endoscopically, a rough pragmatic equivalence is applied and erosions are commonly defined as lesions that are less than 3 mm in diameter and/or without discernible depth (Figure 32.6), whereas other lesions are classified as ulcers. Endoscopists are poor at discriminating NSAID-associated erosions and ulcers from those caused by *H. pylori* [39]. Histologically, erosions show localized superficial mucosal destruction with acute inflammation and local congestion. Acute ulcers are similar but with extension below the muscularis mucosa. Chronic peptic ulcers are additionally characterized by collagenous tissue in the base.

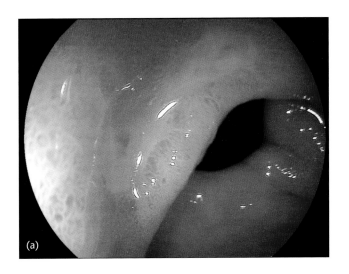

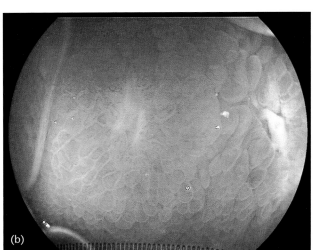

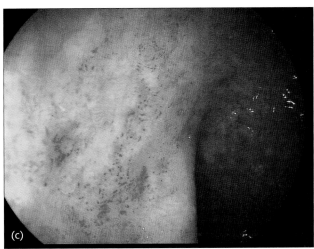

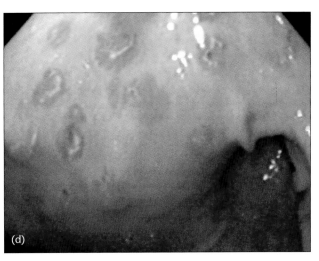

Figure 32.6 Differences between ulcers and erosions. (a) Ulcer with clear depth. (b–d) Superficial erosions. (b) Magnifying endoscopy shows erosions in villous duodenal mucosa.

Clinical presentation of uncomplicated ulcers
Duodenal ulceration
The classical symptom of duodenal ulceration caused by *H. pylori* is epigastric pain occurring before meals or overnight, relieved by antacids, milk, food, and acid-suppressing treatments [33,34]. The pain may radiate to the back, particularly in patients with posterior duodenal ulcers. If present, the pointing sign, in which a patient points to a discrete epigastric site of pain, is moderately predictive of duodenal ulceration. Because ulcers naturally form and heal, pain is classically episodic, typically with clusters of pain lasting for 1–3 months with asymptomatic spells in between. Duodenal ulcer pain is classically described as gnawing or a "hunger" pain, but the qualitative description of the pain is not very helpful in diagnosis. Moreover many presentations are atypical and uncomplicated duodenal ulcers may present with any combination of heartburn, anorexia, weight loss, or vomiting.

Gastric ulcer
Patients with gastric ulcer have a less stereotypical presentation. An epigastric location is common, but pointing is less so. Pain is more likely to occur soon after meals and somewhat less likely to be relieved by food. Anorexia, nausea, vomiting, and weight loss are more common than in duodenal ulcer and often lead to a suspicion of gastric cancer.

NSAID-associated ulcers
These are difficult to diagnose on the basis of symptoms. Drug-induced non-ulcer dyspepsia is common in NSAID users [35], whereas most peptic ulcers are silent, making dyspepsia a poor predictor. Nevertheless, the onset of epigastric pain in an NSAID user is associated with an increased likelihood of finding an endoscopic ulcer or the development of complications.

Differential diagnosis
Any cause of chronic recurrent upper abdominal pain (see Chapter 3) or "dyspepsia" (see Chapter 4) enters into the differential diagnosis of peptic ulcer disease.

Diagnostic approach
Several conditions (including functional dyspepsia, gastro-esophageal reflux disease, and gastric adenocarcinoma) commonly present with pain or discomfort centered predominantly in the upper abdomen and sometimes accompanied by the other symptoms detailed above. Examination is rarely helpful, and a definite diagnosis can be made only after investigation, usually upper gastrointestinal endoscopy. Because dyspeptic symptoms are so common, most healthcare systems reserve endoscopy for patients at higher risk of malignancy. This includes dyspeptic patients with "alarm" features such as overt GI bleeding, anemia due to GI blood loss, dysphagia, weight loss, persistent vomiting, or an upper GI mass. It also usually includes patients with new onset persistent dyspepsia above a specific age cut-off, typically 55 years.

Empiric management of dyspepsia
In patients with "simple dyspepsia", causes outside the gastrointestinal tract are excluded as far as possible by history and examination, and stopping any drugs that may be contributing to dyspepsia. In areas of high *H. pylori* prevalence, patients are then managed by testing for *H. pylori* using non-endoscopy-based tests such as the urea breath test, stool antigen test or (less accurately) serology, and treating those positive. This "test and treat" approach effectively treats ulcers (and those without ulcers) even when a firm diagnosis is never made [36–38]. Where the prevalence of *H. pylori* infection is low, empiric proton pump inhibitor (PPI) treatment is an alternative [37]. Management of dyspepsia is discussed further in Chapter 4.

Diagnostic tests
Where diagnosis is considered necessary, upper gastrointestinal endoscopy (see Chapter 123) is the investigation of choice. It is safe, accurate, and well tolerated by patients under light or no sedation. If possible, patients should avoid acid-suppressing agents for 4 weeks before endoscopy, as these drugs may heal ulcers and esophagitis, leading to a falsely negative endoscopy result. If possible, PPIs, antibiotics, and bismuth compounds should also be avoided for 4 weeks before endoscopy as these render biopsy-based tests for *H. pylori* unreliable. If a duodenal ulcer is found at endoscopy, biopsy samples should be taken from the gastric antrum and corpus to test for *H. pylori* (usually by biopsy urease test and/or histologic examination and from the duodenum if Crohn's disease is suspected. In patients with previous *H. pylori* treatment or multiple antibiotic courses for other conditions, biopsies should also be taken for microbiologic culture and antibiotic sensitivity testing, if this service is available. Where PPIs, bismuth compounds or antibiotics have recently been consumed, a positive biopsy urease test for *H. pylori* is still useful but a negative test is unreliable. The best approach is later to perform a reliable non-invasive test (urea breath test or stool antigen test) one month after stopping these agents. However, many practitioners use serology, which although less accurate can be done without waiting.

Similar tests are indicated for gastric ulceration, but additional biopsies should be taken from the ulcer rim to exclude carcinoma or lymphoma. The usual practice is also to check gastric ulcer healing 6–8 weeks after treatment is started and take further biopsies if healing is incomplete (although the pick-up rate for cancer if original biopsies are negative is very low). Barium radiology (see Chapter 132) is less accurate for picking up small ulcers and does not allow gastric biopsies to be taken to test for *H. pylori* or to exclude malignancy.

Diagnosis of the cause of an ulcer
H. pylori
This is most conveniently established at the time of endoscopy by urease testing and/or histology of antral and corpus

biopsies. Serology is less accurate. Other non-invasive testing (urea breath test or stool antigen test) is accurate but less convenient in situations where endoscopy is being performed anyway.

NSAIDs

Diagnosis depends on an accurate history, though this is not always forthcoming. There are no diagnostic tests for NSAID involvement, although measurement of serum thromboxane concentration has been considered.

Zollinger-Ellison syndrome

A random serum gastrin estimation is a useful screen but can be affected by food and PPIs. A fasting gastrin is more specific. The diagnosis is formally established by showing increased basal gastric acid output and a fasting gastrin level of less than 1000 pg/mL (10-fold increase) with an intragastric pH of 2.0, sometimes backed up by a secretin test (see Chapters 56 and 112).

Multiple endocrine neoplasia

This should be suspected where Zollinger-Ellison syndrome is associated with hyperparathyroidism (see Chapter 112).

Systemic mastocytosis

Systemic mastocytosis should be suspected in the presence of pruritus, urticaria or a characteristic rash (Figure 32.7). Diagnosis is based on the presence of infiltrates in bone marrow and/or extracutaneous organs, detection of c-*kit* mutations,

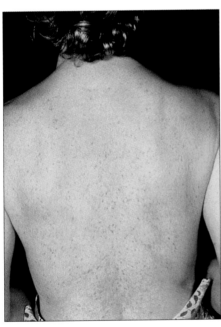

Figure 32.7 Cutaneous manifestations of systemic mastocytosis (urticaria pigmentosa). Patient presented with duodenal ulceration attributable to acid hypersecretion and diarrhea associated with intestinal involvement.

raised serum tryptase, and expression of CD2 and CD25 in c-*kit* positive mast cells [39].

Duodenal Crohn's disease

Duodenal involvement is reported in 0.5–13% of patients with Crohn's disease and recognized to cause duodenal ulcer with or without typical symptoms [40]. Thus, any patient not taking NSAIDs who is *H. pylori* negative should have duodenal biopsies and the possibility of Crohn's disease should be considered.

Stress ulcer

Ulcer bleeding occurring in the context of current or recent severe illness and/or intensive care should be assumed to be a stress ulcer (see below).

Celiac axis stenosis

The site may be atypical and pain-intense. Celiac axis angiography is necessary to establish this diagnosis.

Treatment and prevention
H. pylori-associated ulcers
Eradication of *H. pylori*

H. pylori eradication heals ulcers and prevents recurrence (Figure 32.8) [40]. Unfortunately, antibiotic resistance is increasing, and is a major problem in some countries [41,42,43]. Resistance to metronidazole is very common but is only partial and multi-drug regimens containing metronidazole retain near full efficacy. In contrast, resistance to clarithromycin (which is becoming common due to use of the drug for other infections, notably chest infections) leads to frequent treatment failure. In countries where clarithromycin resistance is less than 15%, triple therapy with a full dose PPI, clarithromycin 500 mg, metronidazole 400 mg, all twice daily is still commonly used. Two weeks treatment is slightly more effective than one, although it is unclear if this is cost-effective and side effects may be increased.

Where clarithromycin resistance is common, other regimens are becoming more widely used, for example quadruple therapy where amoxicillin 1 g twice a day is added to the above regimen (giving three effective drugs even if clarithromycin resistance is present) or alternatively the same drugs are used sequentially over 10 days with the PPI given over the whole period, amoxicillin 1 g twice a day, given for days 1–5, and clarithromycin 500 mg twice a day and metronidazole 400 mg three times a day given for days 6–10. Some physicians routinely check treatment success by urea breath test one month after the end of treatment, but others check only for large or complicated ulcers or if symptoms recur. When *H. pylori* status is not known, PPIs can be started and antibiotics added once *H. pylori* test results are available. If treatment fails, the most commonly-used second line regimen is full dose PPI twice a day, bismuth subcitrate or subsalicylate one tablet four times a day, tetracycline HCl 500 mg four times a day and

Upper GI Tract

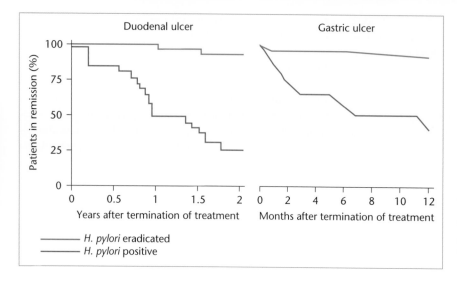

Figure 32.8 Ulcer relapse following *H. pylori* eradication. There is a marked reduction in relapse rates for duodenal and gastric ulcer following *H. pylori* eradication. (Reproduced with permission from Lind T, Megraud F, Unge P, *et al.* The MACH2 study: role of omeprazole in eradication of Helicobacter pylori with 1-week triple therapies. *Gastroenterology.* 1999;116:248–253.)

metronidazole 400 mg three times a day. This more complex regimen is now also used first-line by some practitioners. The further management of *H. pylori* treatment failures is discussed in Chapter 22.

Ancillary drug treatment

For duodenal ulcers, continuation of acid suppression after the antibiotic course is unnecessary, but some physicians give PPIs for a total of one month for very large or complicated ulcers. If this is done, checking for *H. pylori* eradication must be delayed for a further month. For gastric ulcers, which often heal more slowly, PPIs are usually continued until the repeat endoscopy.

Management of patients taking NSAIDs
Ulcer healing

PPIs accelerate healing compared with standard doses of H2 antagonists [32]. Misoprostol heals NSAID-associated ulcers but causes more side effects and is now seldom used.

Strategies to reduce risk of ulcer development

For NSAID users, removing the cause of the ulcer, by stopping the drug or switching to one that does not damage the stomach or duodenum, is the equivalent of *H. pylori* eradication. An alternative is to continue the NSAID where needed, at the lowest possible dose, and to give concurrent antiulcer prophylaxis, usually with a PPI.

Low-toxicity drugs

Ibuprofen at dosages of less than 1200 mg per day appears to confer less risk of bleeding peptic ulcer [23] than other NSAIDs (see Figure 32.4). Alternatively, and where higher doses are needed, selective COX-2 inhibitors have been shown to reduce the risk of ulcers that are detected endoscopically and clinically [44–53]. Clinical outcomes have been studied in large cohorts of patients (up to 18 500) for celecoxib, rofecoxib, and

lumiracoxib. The VIGOR and CLASS studies of rofecoxib and lumiracoxib showed a reduction in the risk of all ulcers of between 27% (celecoxib) and 57% (rofecoxib), and the TARGET study showed a 79% reduction in ulcer complications for lumiracoxib compared with ibuprofen or naproxen (Figure 32.9). Benefits are seen within a week [48] and across most risk factors [49]. While there has been some concern about the possibility that COX-2 inhibitors may enhance thrombotic complications of vascular disease, these properties may well be shared by non-selective NSAIDs and the balance of risks benefits clearly favours reduced gastrotoxicity [51]. The MEDAL study program showed etoricoxib to reduce the incidence of uncomplicated, but not complicated, ulcers, though this may be because PPI co-prescription was allowed [47].

Prophylactic co-prescription

Proton pump inhibitors have been shown to reduce development of endoscopic ulcers and relapse of endoscopic and clinically significant ulcers including those causing ulcer complications [52–58]. When combined with a COX-2 inhibitor the use of proton pump inhibitor has been associated with a zero rate of recurrent ulcer bleeding in patients who have already experienced one life threatening episode [58]. Generically available proton pump inhibitors have been sufficiently inexpensive that they offer highly cost effective ulcer prophylaxis in users of both NSAIDs and COX-2 inhibitors [54]. Standard doses of H_2 antagonists are not effective in preventing NSAID-associated gastric ulcer development [32]. The PGE-1 analogue misoprostol is effective against endoscopic and clinically complicated ulcers but seldom used because of the high level of drug related adverse effects [59].

H. pylori -positive NSAID or aspirin associated ulcers
NSAIDs

This is a controversial area. The evidence ranges from showing a benefit for *H. pylori* eradication in patients starting NSAIDs

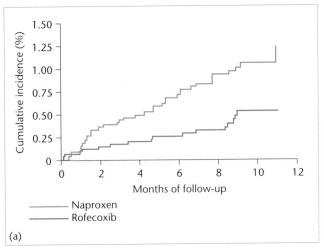
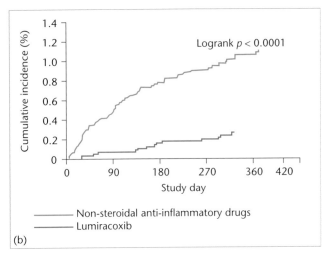

Figure 32.9 Results of VIGOR and TARGET outcome studies (primary outcomes). (a) VIGOR – perforations, ulcers, and bleeds. (b) TARGET – ulcer complications. Reproduced with data from [44] and [46].

[60,61] through to greater effectiveness of PPI prophylaxis in patients who remain infected [62]. Overall, *H. pylori* eradication alone is not sufficient protection against ulcer complications and such patients should receive a PPI and/or a COX-2 inhibitor.

Aspirin

It is possible that *H. pylori* eradication may be sufficiently effective to protect low-dose aspirin users [55], but until there are further data this cannot be recommended above PPI prophylaxis [55,57]. Reductions in the price of generic PPIs mean that it is probably cost effective to give all patients on low dose aspirin a PPI and certainly those with age over 65 or a past ulcer history. If funds allow, patients taking low-dose aspirin should receive PPI prophylaxis if they have any significant risk factor, such as age over 65 years or a past ulcer history.

Patients taking prophylactic aspirin and a non-aspirin NSAID

By competing at the level of the platelet, nonselective NSAIDs such as ibuprofen may substantially interfere with aspirin's ability to inhibit platelet aggregation and thereby prevent coronary heart disease [63–65]. These patients should use naproxen or diclofenac where there is either no evidence for such an inhibition (dicofenac) [63] or its consequences. Selective COX-2 inhibitors also avoid any pharmacodynamic interaction but in Europe their use in patients with established coronary heart disease is contraindicated. The USA FDA by contrast rules that non-selective NSAIDs and selective COX-2 inhibitors both increase the risk of myocardial infarction. Whether patients with cardiovascular risk factors who take aspirin as well as a COX-2 inhibitor have an increased risk of

myocardial infarction (as is the case for aspirin plus NSAID [64,65]) is not known. Therefore where local rules allow, prescribers should consider using a selective COX-2 inhibitor with aspirin to avoid an adverse pharmacodynamic interaction [63]. In patients taking aspirin and a coxib, a PPI should be used where the risk of aspirin alone would warrant it.

Complications and their management
Bleeding (Figure 32.10)
Epidemiology

Peptic ulcer is the commonest cause of acute upper gastrointestinal bleeding (see Chapters 20 and 146), accounting for nearly half of all instances and occurring in approximately 2–5 per 1000 of people aged over 60 years [5].

Clinical presentation

Hematemesis and/or melena are usually obvious, especially when accompanied by tachycardia or hypotension, usually leading to emergency hospital admission. Retrospective accounts of "melena" in well patients only occasionally indicate significant gastrointestinal bleeding.

Diagnosis and management

After resuscitation, patients with a significant bleed should undergo endoscopy, both to establish the diagnosis and to institute endoscopic management if stigmata of hemorrhage are present [66]. About 20–25% of patients, however, have no abnormality of pulse, blood pressure, hemoglobin, platelet count or urea, and in the absence of any suspicious past history such patients are at low risk of further bleeding, and can be discharged for subsequent out-patient endoscopic assessment [67].

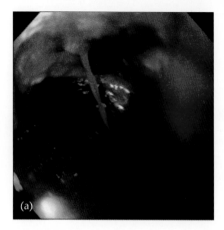
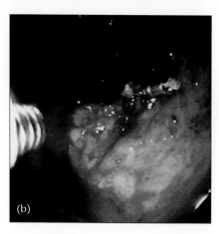

(a)   (b)

Figure 32.10 Bleeding ulcer. Arterial bleeding from a visible vessel in an ulcer **(a)** before and **(b)** after control by application of a hemoclip.

As detailed in Chapters 20 and 146, endoscopic therapy of bleeding peptic ulcers reduces rebleeding and the need for surgery, and may reduce mortality. The choices are injection therapy with epinephrine (adrenaline), light- or heat-based coagulation of the vessel, clipping **(Figure 32.10)** or a combination – using at least two modalities is better than using one alone. Patients with endoscopic stigmata suggesting high risk of rebleed are given a 72-hour infusion of intravenous proton pump inhibitor [66]. Conventionally, aspirin is stopped but this is ill-advised as patients are at particular risk of thrombosis, and mortality is much higher if aspirin is stopped in those who need it [68]. Pragmatically aspirin may be stopped for 48 hours and restarted once the patient is on PPI therapy.

Where *H. pylori* is the cause of the ulcer, eradication results in a substantial reduction in the subsequent risk of rebleeding [40]. Patients taking NSAIDs can resume these drugs if needed after healing if they take a PPI, as this has been shown substantially to reduce the readmission rate for ulcer complications over 6 months [54–58].

Mortality

In a large, comprehensive British survey the mortality rate was 8% in patients admitted because of bleeding peptic ulcer [69]. Patients die mainly as a result of pneumonia and the thrombotic complications of bleeding or surgery (deep vein thrombosis and pulmonary embolism, myocardial infarction), rather than exsanguination.

Perforation

(see also Chapters 22–24 and 156).

Epidemiology

The incidence of ulcer perforation is conventionally reported as about 7–10 per 100 000 population per annum [70]. A recent report suggests a higher incidence [71]. Perforation is more common in men than in women, in those with duodenal versus gastric ulcers, in cigarette smokers and in users of aspirin and NSAIDs [71] but presentation in the absence of risk factors is not uncommon. There is a diurnal and seasonal

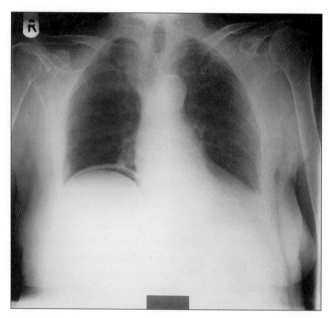

Figure 32.11 Chest radiograph showing air under the diaphragm in a patient with perforated peptic ulcer.

variation. Many perforated ulcers are *H. pylori* negative [72,73]. The reported incidence of *H. pylori* infection ranges from 0% to 100%.

Clinical presentation

This is usually stereotypical and obvious, with an abrupt onset of severe upper abdominal pain, rapidly spreading through the abdomen, and the development of symptoms and signs of peritonitis (see Chapter 156), hypotension, and shock.

Diagnosis

Diagnosis is largely based on history, examination, and plain radiography. Air within the abdominal cavity under the diaphragm is seen on plain abdominal and erect chest radiographs in most cases (Figure 32.11). Endoscopy is avoided because of theoretical risks of increased peritoneal soiling.

Management
Patients should be resuscitated with intravenous fluids and given broad-spectrum antibiotics (e.g., cefuroxime and metronidazole). Laparotomy to close the perforation should be carried out as soon as possible after resuscitation, although in patients with a high operative risk who are improving on conservative treatment, continued nonoperative management may be possible.

Prevention of recurrence
After successful recovery, management to prevent recurrence is standard (*H. pylori* eradication, NSAID avoidance). There are no direct data on the benefits of switching to a COX-2 inhibitor or taking PPI prophylaxis after perforation.

Mortality
The overall mortality rate is about 10%. Risk factors for death are age, co-morbid illness, delayed surgery, preoperative shock, heart rate, and a high serum creatinine level [70].

Penetration
Posterior perforation may result in digestive penetration into an adjacent organ rather than free perforation. Posterior duodenal ulcer penetration most commonly involves the pancreas, often resulting in different, more severe, pain than is typical. Other organs that may be involved include the left lobe of the liver, common bile duct (choledochoduodenal fistula), colon (gastrocolic fistula), lung, and pericardium. Except where fistulae have formed, treatment is by acid suppression with *H. pylori* eradication or NSAID cessation, as appropriate.

Gastric outlet obstruction
Epidemiology
Gastric outlet obstruction by peptic ulcers is relatively uncommon, probably affecting less than the quoted 2% of patients with ulceration. Obstruction occurs with (pre)pyloric or duodenal ulcers, especially in patients with a long history, and is thought particularly to be associated with NSAID use.

Clinical features
Obstruction should be suspected in patients with an ulcer who develop vomiting, particularly if projectile or occurring daily. Early satiety (60%), upper abdominal pain and distention (87%), and weight loss (65%) are common. A succussion splash is present in 25% or more of patients. Depending on severity, increases in serum urea concentration and electrolyte abnormalities (low K$^+$, metabolic alkalosis, low Na$^+$) are common.

Management
Nasogastric aspiration should be performed to empty the stomach prior to endoscopy. Aspiration of more than 200 mL after an overnight fast suggests delayed gastric emptying. At endoscopy, biopsy samples should be taken to exclude malignancy. Endoscopic balloon dilatation (see Chapter 150) and/

or treatment with acid suppression can restore gastric emptying. Some patients require surgery by antrectomy and Billroth 1 or 2 procedures (see Chapter 156).

Surgery for peptic ulcer
Nowadays, surgical intervention is rarely used for gastric or duodenal ulcers, except in the context of complications (see above).

Postoperative syndromes
Peptic ulcer surgery was an unphysiologic intervention that resulted in significant morbidity [78] including the following.

Dumping syndromes
These are characterized by flushing, palpitations, sweating, light-headedness, tachycardia, postural hypotension, and fatigue, likely due to rapid fluid shifts if symptoms occur within an hour or rebound hypoglycemia if they occurs 2–3 hours after a meal (see Chapter 37). The early dumping syndrome occurs 30–60 minutes after eating in patients who have had a gastrectomy. Dumping of food into the duodenum is thought to cause rapid fluid shifts, leading to faintness. Excessive release of vasoactive hormones may play a role. Octreotide may have therapeutic value. In the late dumping syndrome, dumping of food into the duodenum stimulates excessive insulin secretion resulting in rebound hypoglycemia 2–3 hours after a meal.

Postgastrectomy malnutrition
Most patients who have had a gastrectomy lose weight and/or become anemic or malnourished because of a combination of early satiety, impaired control of nutritional digestion and absorption, inadequate production of co-factors such as vitamin B12, and altered iron absorption. Problems develop over years and also include metabolic bone disease (vitamin D) and neuropathy (vitamin B12).

Stomal ulceration
After partial gastrectomy, ulcers may develop at the site of anastomosis and present with pain or sometimes complications. They can be managed with acid-suppressing drugs. The role of *H. pylori* in this situation is unclear, but eradication is wise.

Postgastrectomy neoplasia
Surgery for peptic ulcer is associated with an increased risk of later gastric cancer. This is discussed in Chapter 32.

Postvagotomy syndromes
Truncal vagotomy results in diarrhea in many patients [78]. Pathogenesis is multifactorial and management is symptomatic.

Meckel's diverticulum

This is an ileal diverticulum with acid-secreting heterotopic gastric mucosa that arises because of developmental abnormality in approximately 2% of the population. It can cause ulceration with pain or bleeding, as well as obstruction due to intussusception or volvulus. Diagnosis is often made incidentally during barium radiology. Technetium (99mTc) pertechnetate, which has an affinity for parietal cells, is the basis of the scan. Treatment is by surgical removal.

Stress ulcers

Severe medical stresses such as burns, head injuries, major trauma, sepsis, multisystem organ failure, or ventilation on an intensive care unit are associated with the development of stress ulcers in the stomach or duodenum that may bleed and are associated with a high mortality rate. Curling's ulcers are those associated with burns, and Cushing's ulcers with head injury. Stress ulcers are seen less commonly now than previously, possibly due to preventive measures in intensive care. In one large study, 31 of 2252 patients (1.4%) on an intensive care unit experienced clinically important bleeding [74].

Risk factors

A need for ventilation because of respiratory failure is the most important risk factor, increasing the chance of upper gastrointestinal bleeding by 15-fold [75,76]. The main ancillary risk factors are prolonged ventilation and coagulopathy. Sepsis, hepatic and renal failure, and glucocorticoids may enhance risk, although the evidence is less secure. Clinically important bleeding is extremely rare in patients with no risk factors [75–78].

Pathogenesis

The pathogenesis varies according to etiology. Reduced mucosal defence, largely because of poor blood flow that allows increased acid back diffusion, predisposes to stress ulcers in ventilated patients and after severe burns, despite an overall reduction in acid secretion. Cushing's ulcers differ in being associated with hypergastrinemia and hypersecretion of acid.

Clinical presentation

The most common presentation is with bleeding, manifesting as shock, hematemesis, or melena. This may occur at any time during a stressful illness, but is common at 10–14 days and may therefore present as the patient is improving in other respects. Perforation and penetration are much less common. Some patients may complain of antecedent pain.

Treatment and prevention

Once severe stress ulcer bleeding has occurred, the patient should be managed as for other ulcer bleeding; however, the mortality rate is high. Consequently, attention has focused on prophylaxis.

Prophylaxis

Treatment with H2 receptor antagonists, proton pump inhibitors and sucralfate have been shown to reduce endoscopic appearances of injury and/or blood in gastric aspirates but there is no clear evidence of an effect on survival or clinical outcome in either children or adults [76,77]. Where there is good general intensive care management, including with enteral nutrition, other specific measures are seldom needed.

Practical management

The following guidelines, updated from Tryba and Cook [78] are suggested:

- Stress ulcer prophylaxis should be restricted to patients with risk factors, particularly respiratory failure, coagulopathy, sepsis, shock, burns, head injury, or a history of peptic ulcer disease.
- Enteral nutrition, where given, probably reduces the incidence of ulcer bleeding.
- Where there is good general intensive care management, other specific measures are seldom needed.
- Alternatives are:
  1. Sucralfate 1 g six times daily by mouth.
  2. Enteral nutrition with sucralfate 1 g twice daily during a rest period when enteral nutrition is suspended.
  3. Ranitidine 50 mg by slow intravenous injection, then 125–250 mg/kg/h by infusion.

Cameron's ulcer

These ulcers typically occur in the neck of a big hiatus hernia, and are believed to arise on an ischemic basis [79]. They may be associated with iron deficiency anemia. They often respond to PPI therapy, but non-responsive ulcers can be cured by surgical intervention.

Prognosis and advice to patients with peptic ulcer

- Patients should be told the cause of their ulcer and be told to eat a normal diet.
- They should understand that the prognosis is very good in the absence of complications and particularly with definitive therapy.
- Patients given *H. pylori* treatment should be told of the importance of close compliance, warned of the common side effects with these multi-drug regimens, but told to continue despite these, unless they are very severe. The problem with failed treatment is that it very commonly results in antibiotic resistance making future treatment more difficult. After proven eradication of *H. pylori* in patients not taking NSAIDs, the relapse rate falls to less than 5%.
- Similarly, for patients using NSAIDs who stop these drugs, relapse is rare if they have no other risk factors such as *H. pylori* infection.

Upper GI Tract

- All patients on an NSAID should receive PPI prophylaxis with additionally a COX-2 inhibitor if they have significant risk. These patients should be told about the adverse effects of PPIs and COX-2 inhibitors, with an emphasis that the benefits of each therapy outweigh the risks.

SOURCES OF INFORMATION FOR PATIENTS AND DOCTORS

www.nlm.nih.gov/medlineplus/pepticulcer.html
www.kidshealth.org/parent/medical/digestive/peptic_ulcers.html
www.digestive.niddk.nih.gov/ddiseases/pubs/hpylori/
www.digestive.niddk.nih.gov/ddiseases/pubs/nsaids/
www.netdoctor.co.uk/diseases/facts/pepticulcertreatment. htm
  patients.uptodate.com/topic.asp?file=digestiv/9148

Current controversies

A number of recent findings may challenge conservative prescribers. These include fairly clear demonstrations suggesting that:

- All patients taking NSAIDs have reduced ulcer risk if they take a PPI. PPIs are not co-prescribed as commonly as they should be.
- The gastroduodenal benefits of selective COX-2 inhibitors outweigh any cardiac risks. However, vascular risks dominate current thinking.
- The risk of vascular thrombotic events may be similar for non-selective NSAIDs (except naproxen) and selective COX-2 inhibitors. However there is generally greater concern about COX-2 inhibitors.
- COX-2 inhibitors may be more suitable for patients needing aspirin for vascular protection because they lack the ability of non-selective NSAIDs to abrogate the effectiveness of aspirin. However the EMA contra-indicate COX-2 inhibitors in patients with vascular disease.
- Stopping aspirin in patients with bleeding peptic ulcers has been shown to increase mortality. Despite this, most doctors stop aspirin in these patients.
- Antibiotic resistance of *H. pylori* is increasing and varies between individuals and populations: the most effective treatment therefore also varies between individuals and populations.

There are also some wider controversies surrounding *H. pylori* management, which include:

- Should *H. pylori* (or at least pathogenic strains of *H. pylori*) be screened for and treated in some populations, with the aim of primary prevention of peptic ulcers and gastric cancer?
- *H. pylori* has co-evolved with humans over millennia. Does its absence from the human stomach of many individuals

for the first time in our evolutionary history have any disadvantages [15]?
- Can an effective vaccine for *H. pylori* be developed, and is it desirable?

References

1. Warren JR, Marshall B. Unidentified curved bacilli on gastric epithelium in active chronic gastritis. *Lancet*. 1983;i:1273–1275.
2. Hawkey CJ. Nonsteroidal anti-inflammatory drug gastropathy. *Gastroenterology*. 2000;119:521–535.
3. Hawkey CJ, Langman MJ. Non-steroidal anti-inflammatory drugs: overall risks and management. Complementary roles for COX- 2 inhibitors and proton pump inhibitors. *Gut*. 2003;52: 600–608.
4. Douthwaite AH, Lintott SAM. Gastropic observation of the effect of aspirin and certain other substances on the stomach. *Lancet*. 1938;ii:1222–1225.
5. Weil J, Langman MJ,Wainwright P *et al.* Peptic ulcer bleeding: accessory risk factors and interactions with non-steroidal antiinflammatory drugs. *Gut*. 2000;46:27–31.
6. Susser S. Civilisation and peptic ulcer. *Lancet*. 1962;i:115–118.
7. Higham J, Kang JY, Majeed A. Recent trends in admissions and mortality due to peptic ulcer in England: increasing frequency of hemorrhage among older subjects. *Gut*. 2002;50:460–464.
8. Taha AS, Angerson WJ, Prasad R, *et al.* Upper gastrointestinal bleeding and the changing use of COX-2 non-steroidal anti-inflammatory drugs and low-dose aspirin. *APT*. 2007;26 (8):1171–1178.
9. Post PN, Kuipers EJ, Meijer GA. Declining incidence of peptic ulcer but not of its complications: a nation-wide study in The Netherlands. *Aliment Pharmacol Ther*. 2006; 23(11):1587–1593.
10. Lassen Annmarie, Hallas Jesper, de Muckadell Ove, *et al.* Complicated and Uncomplicated Peptic Ulcers in a Danish County 1993–2002: a Population-Based Cohort Study. *Am J Gastroenterol*. 2006;101(5):945–953.
11. Cai S, Garcia Rodriguez LA, Masso-Gonzalez EL, Hernandez-Diaz S. Uncomplicated peptic ulcer in the UK: Trends from 1997 to 2005. *Aliment Pharmacol Ther*. 2009;30(10):1039–1048.
12. Sadic J, Borgstrom A, Manjer J, *et al.* Bleeding peptic ulcer – time trends in incidence, treatment and mortality in Sweden. *Aliment Pharmacol Ther*. 2009;30(4):392–398.
13. Ahsberg K, Hoglund P, Stael von Holstein C. Mortality from peptic ulcer bleeding: the impact of comorbidity and the use of drugs that promote bleeding. *Aliment Pharmacol Ther*. 2010;32 (6):801–810.
14. Wang YR, Richter JE, Dempsey DT. Trends and outcomes of hospitalizations for peptic ulcer disease in the United States, 1993 to 2006. *Ann Surg*. 2010;251(1):51–58.
15. Atherton JC, Blaser MJ. Co-adaptation of Helicobacter pylori and humans: ancient history and modern implications. *J Clin Invest*. 2009;119(9):2475–2487.
16. Borody TJ, George LL, Brandl S, *et al.* Smoking does not contribute to duodenal ulcer relapse after Helicobacter pylori eradication. *Am J Gastroenterol*. 1992;87:1390–1393.
17. Hawkey CJ, Laine L, Harper SE, *et al.* Rofecoxib Osteoarthritis Endoscopy Multinational Study Group. Influence of risk factors on endoscopic and clinical ulcers in patients taking rofecoxib or ibuprofen in two randomized controlled trials. *Aliment Pharmacol Ther*. 2001;15:1593–1601.

18. Hawkey CJ, Laine L, Harper SE, et al. Rofecoxib Osteoarthritis Endoscopy Multinational Study Group. Influence of risk factors on endoscopic and clinical ulcers in patients taking rofecoxib or ibuprofen in two randomized controlled trials. *Aliment Pharmacol Ther.* 2001; 15:1593–1601.

19. Blaser MJ, Atherton JC. Helicobacter pylori persistence: biology and disease. *J Clin Invest.* 2004;113:321–333.

20. Crabtree JE,Taylor JD,Wyatt JI, et al. Mucosal IgA recognition of Helicobacter pylori 120 kDa protein, peptic ulceration, and gastric pathology. *Lancet.* 1991;338:332–335.

21. Lewis SC, Langman MJS, Laporte JR, et al. Dose-response relationships between individual nonaspirin nonsteroidal anti-inflammatory drugs (NANSAIDs) and serious upper gastrointestinal bleeding: a meta-analysis based on individual patient data. *Br J Clin Pharmacol.* 2002;54(3):320–326.

22. Stack WA, Atherton JC, Hawkey GM, et al. Interactions between Helicobacter pylori and other risk factors for peptic ulcer bleeding. *Aliment Pharmacol Ther.* 2002;16:497–506.

23. Atherton JC. The pathogenesis of Helicobacter pylori-induced gastroduodenal disease. *Ann Rev Pathol Mech Dis.* 2006;1:63–96.

24. Odenbreit S, Puls J, Sedlmaier B, et al. Translocation of Helicobacter pylori CagA into gastric epithelial cells by type IV secretion. *Science.* 2000;287:1497–1500.

25. Argent RH, Kidd M, Owen RJ, et al. Determinants and consequences of different levels of CagA phosphorylation for clinical isolates of Helicobacter pylori. *Gastroenterology.* 2004;127: 514–523.

26. Atherton J, Cao P, Peek RM, et al. Mosaicism in vacuolating cytotoxin alleles of Helicobacter pylori: association of specific vacA types with cytotoxin production and peptic ulceration. *J Biol Chem.* 1995;270:17771–17777.

27. Macarthur M, Hold GL, El-Omar EM. Inflammation and cancer II. Role of chronic inflammation and cytokine gene polymorphisms in the pathogenesis of gastrointestinal malignancy. *Am J Physiol Gastrointest Liver Physiol.* 2004;286:G515–G520.

28. Robinson K, Kenefeck R, Pidgeon EL, et al. Helicobacter pylori-induced peptic ulcer disease is associated with inadequate regulatory T cell responses. *Gut.* 2008;57:1375–1385.

29. Peek RM, Fiske C, Wilson KT. The role of innate immunity in Helicobacter pylori-induced gastric malignancy. *Physiol Rev.* 2010;90:831–858.

30. Moss SF, Legon S, Bishop AE, et al. Effect of Helicobacter pylori on gastric somatostatin in duodenal ulcer disease. *Lancet.* 1992;340:930–932.

31. Elliott SL, Ferris RJ, Giraud AS, et al. Indomethacin damage to rat gastric mucosa is markedly dependent on luminal pH. *Clin Exp Pharmacol Physiol.* 1996;23:432–434.

32. Yeomans ND,Tulassay Z, Juhasz L, et al. A comparison of omeprazole with ranitidine for ulcers associated with nonsteroidal antiinflammatory drugs. Acid Suppression Trial: Ranitidine versus Omeprazole for NSAID-associated Ulcer Treatment (ASTRONAUT) Study Group. *N Engl J Med.* 1998;338:719–726.

33. Earlam R. Computerized questionnaire analysis of duodenal ulcer symptoms. *Gastroenterology.* 1976;71:314–317.

34. Horrocks JC, De Dombal FT. Clinical presentation of patients with "dyspepsia." Detailed symptomatic study of 360 patients. *Gut.* 1978;19:19–26.

35. Hawkey CJ, Talley NJ, Yeomans ND, et al. Improvements with esomeprazole in upper gastrointestinal symptoms in patients taking non-steroidal anti-inflammatory drugs including selective COX-2 inhibitors (NASA1 – SPACE1). *Am J Gastro.* 2005;100(5):1028–1036.

36. Malfertheiner P, Megraud F, O'Morain C, et al. Current concepts in the management of Helicobacter pylori infection: The Maastricht III Concensus Report. *Gut.* 2007;56:772–781.

37. Delaney BC, Qume M, Moayyedi P, et al. Helicobacter pylori test and treat versus proton pump inhibitor in initial management of dyspepsia in primary care: multicentre randomised controlled trial (MRC-CUBE trial). *BMJ.* 2008;336(7645): 651–654.

38. Duggan AE, Elliott CA, Miller P, et al. Clinical trial: a randomized trial of early endoscopy, Helicobacter pylori testing and empirical therapy for the management of dyspepsia in primary care. *APT.* 2009;29;1:55–68.

39. Castells MC. Mastocytosis: classification, diagnosis, and clinical presentation. *Allergy Asthma Proc.* 2004;25:33–36.

40. Lind T, Megraud F, Unge P, et al. The MACH2 study: role of omeprazole in eradication of Helicobacter pylori with 1-week triple therapies. *Gastroenterology.* 1999;116:248–253.

41. van Hogezand RA,Witte AM,Veenendaal RA, et al. Crohn's disease: review of the clinicopathologic features and therapy. *Inflamm Bowel Dis.* 2001;7:328–337.

42. Gerrits MM, van Vliet AH, Kuipers EJ, et al. Helicobacter pylori and antimicrobial resistance: molecular mechanisms and clinical implications. *Lancet Infect Dis.* 2006;6(11):699–709.

43. Raymond J, Lamarque D, Kalach N, et al. High level of antimicrobial resistance in French Helicobacter pylori isolates. *Helicobacter.* 2010;15(1):21–27

44. Bombardier C, Laine L, Reicin A et al. Comparison of upper gastrointestinal toxicity of rofecoxib and naproxen in patients with rheumatoid arthritis. VIGOR Study Group. *N Engl J Med.* 2000;343:1520–1528.

45. Silverstein F, Simon L, Faich G. Reporting of 6-month vs 12-month data in a clinical trial of celecoxib. *JAMA.* 2002;286:2399.

46. Schnitzer TJ, Burmester GR, Mysier E, et al. Comparison of lumiracoxib with naproxen and ibuprofen in the Therapeutic Arthritis Research and Gastrointestinal Event Trial (TARGET), reduction in ulcer complications: randomised controlled trial. *Lancet.* 2004;364;665–674.

47. Laine L, Curtis SP, Cryer B, et al. Assessment of upper gastrointestinal safety of etoricoxib and diclofenac in patients with osteoarthritis and rheumatoid arthritis in the Multinational Etoricoxib and Diclofenac Arthritis Long-term (MEDAL) programme: a randomised comparison. *Lancet.* 2007;369 (9560): 465–473.

48. Hawkey CJ, Weinstein WM, Stricker K, et al. Clinical trial: Comparison of the gastrointestinal safety of lumiracoxib with traditional nonselective nonsteroidal anti-inflammatory drugs early after the initiation of treatment – Findings from the Therapeutic Arthritis Research and Gastrointestinal Event Trial.

49. Hawkey CJ, Weinstein WM, Smalley W, et al. Effect of Risk Factors on Complicated and Uncomplicated Ulcers in the TARGET Lumiracoxib Outcomes Study. *Gastroenterology.* 2007;133 (1):57–64.

50. Rostom A, Muir K, Dube C, et al. Gastrointestinal Safety of Cyclooxygenase-2 Inhibitors: a Cochrane Collaboration Systematic Review. *Clin Gastroenterol Hepatol.* 2007;5(7):818–828.e5.

51. Van Der Linden MW, Van Der Bij S, Welsing P, et al. The balance between severe cardiovascular and gastrointestinal events among users of selective and non-selective non-steroidal anti-inflammatory drugs. *Ann Rheum Dis.* 2009;68(5):668–673.

52. Rostom A, Muir K, Dube C, *et al.* Prevention of NSAID-related upper gastrointestinal toxicity: A meta-analysis of traditional NSAIDs with gastroprotection and COX-2 inhibitors. *Drug Healthc Patient Saf.* 2009;1(1):47–71.

53. Hawkey CJ, Karrasch JA, Szczepanski L *et al.* Omeprazole compared with misoprostol for ulcers associated with nonsteroidal antiinflammatory drugs. Omeprazole versus Misoprostol for NSAID-induced Ulcer Management (OMNIUM) Study Group. *N Engl J Med.* 1998;338:727–734.

54. Latimer N, Lord J, Grant RL, *et al.* Cost effectiveness of COX 2 selective inhibitors and traditional NSAIDs alone or in combination with a proton pump inhibitor for people with osteoarthritis. *BMJ.* (Clinical research ed.) 2009;339:b2538.

55. Chan FK, Chung SC, Suen BY *et al.* Preventing recurrent upper gastrointestinal bleeding in patients with Helicobacter pylori infection who are taking low-dose aspirin or naproxen. *N Engl J Med.* 2001;344:967–973.

56. Chan FK, Hung LC, Suen BY *et al.* Celecoxib versus diclofenac and omeprazole in reducing the risk of recurrent ulcer bleeding in patients with arthritis. *N Engl J Med.* 2002;347:2104–2110.

57. Lai KC, Lam SK, Chu KM *et al.* Lansoprazole for the prevention of recurrences of ulcer complications from long-term low-dose aspirin use. *N Engl J Med.* 2002;346:2033–2038.

58. Chan FKL, Wong VWS, Suen BY, *et al.* Combination of a cyclo-oxygenase-2 inhibitor and a proton-pump inhibitor for prevention of recurrent ulcer bleeding in patients at very high risk: a double-blind, randomised trial. *Lancet.* 2007;369(9573):1621–1626.

59. Silverstein FE, Graham DY, Senior JR, *et al.* Misoprostol reduces serious gastrointestinal complications in patients with rheumatoid arthritis receiving nonsteroidal anti-inflammatory drugs. A randomized, double-blind, placebo-controlled trial. *Ann Intern Med.* 1995;123(4):241–249.

60. Chan FKL, Sung JJY, Chung SCS, *et al.* Randomised trial of eradication of Helicobacter pylori before nonsteroidal anti-inflammatory drug therapy to prevent peptic ulcers. *Lancet.* 1997;350(9083):975–979.

61. Huang JQ, Sridhar S, Hunt RH. Role of Helicobacter pylori infection and nonsteroidal anti-inflammatory drugs in peptic ulcer disease: a meta analysis. *Lancet.* 2002;359:14–22.

62. Hawkey CJ,Tulassay Z, Szczepanski L *et al.* Randomised controlled trial of Helicobacter pylori eradication in patients on nonsteroidal anti-inflammatory drugs: HELP NSAIDs study. Helicobacter Eradication for Lesion Prevention. *Lancet.* 1998;352:1016–1021 (Erratum, Lancet 1998;352:1634).

63. Catella-Lawson F, Reilly MP, Kapoor SC *et al.* Cyclooxygenase inhibitors and the antiplatelet effects of aspirin. *N Engl J Med.* 2001;345:1809–1817.

64. MacDonald TM,Wei L. Effect of ibuprofen on cardioprotective effect of aspirin. *Lancet.* 2003;361:573–574.

65. Patel TN, Goldberg KC. Use of aspirin and ibuprofen compared with aspirin alone and the risk of myocardial infarction. *Arch Intern Med.* 2004;164:852–856.

66. Barkun AN, Bardou M, Kuipers EJ, *et al.* International consensus recommendations on the management of patients with non-variceal upper gastrointestinal bleeding. *Ann Intern Med.* 2010;152(2):101–113.

67. Stanley AJ, Ashley D, Dalton HR, *et al.* Outpatient management of patients with low-risk upper-gastrointestinal haemorrhage: multicentre validation and prospective evaluation. *Lancet.* 2009;373(9657):42–47.

68. Sung JJY, Lau JYW, Ching JYL, *et al.* Continuation of low-dose aspirin therapy in peptic ulcer bleeding: a randomized trial. *Ann Intern Med.* 2010;152(1):1–9.

69. Hearnshaw SA, Logan RFA, Lowe D, *et al.* Use of endoscopy for management of acute upper gastrointestinal bleeding in the UK: results of a nationwide audit. *Gut.* 2010;59(8):1022–1029.

70. Svanes C. Trends in perforated peptic ulcer: incidence, etiology, treatment, and prognosis. *World J Surg.* 2000;24:277–283.

71. Taha AS, Angerson WJ, Prasad R, *et al.* Clinical trial: The incidence and early mortality after peptic ulcer perforation, and the use of low-dose aspirin and nonsteroidal anti-inflammatory drugs. *Aliment Pharmacol Ther.* 2008;28(7):878–885.

72. Reinbach DH, Cruickshank G, McColl KE. Acute perforated duodenal ulcer is not associated with Helicobacter pylori infection. *Gut.* 1993;34:1344–1347.

73. Gisbert JP, Pajares JM. Helicobacter pylori infection and perforated peptic ulcer: prevalence of the infection and role of antimicrobial treatment. *Helicobacter.* 2003;8:159–167.

74. Cook D, Heyland D, Griffith L, *et al.* Risk factors for clinically important upper gastrointestinal bleeding in patients requiring mechanical ventilation. Canadian Critical Care Trials Group. *Crit Care Med.* 1999;27:2812–2817.

75. Cook DJ, Fuller HD, Guyatt GH *et al.* Risk factors for gastrointestinal bleeding in critically ill patients. Canadian Critical Care Trials Group. *N Engl J Med.* 1994;339:377–381.

76. Janicki T, Stewart S. Stress-ulcer prophylaxis for general medical patients: a review of the evidence. *J Hosp Med.* 2007;2(2):86–92.

77. Quenot JP. When should stress ulcer prophylaxis be used in the ICU? *Curr Opin Crit Care.* 2009;15:139–143.

78. Tryba M, Cook D. Current guidelines on stress ulcer prophylaxis. *Drugs.* 1997;54:581–596.

79. Cameron AJ, Higgins JA. Linear gastric erosion: a lesion associated with large diaphragmatic hernia and chronic blood loss. *Gastroenterology.* 1986;91:338–342.

CHAPTER 33
Gastritis

Richard H. Lash and Robert M. Genta

Caris Diagnostics/Miraca; University of Texas Southwestern Medical Center, Irving, TX, USA

KEY POINTS

- Inflammation of the gastric mucosa *per se* does not usually produce symptoms
- **H. pylori gastrina**
  - Is the most common chronic infection in humans
  - Antrum-predominant *H. pylori* gastritis carries a 15–20% lifetime risk of peptic ulcer
  - Atrophic pangastritis is more common in less industrialized countries and populations with a high incidence of gastric adenocarcinoma
  - Carcinoma and lymphoma may present years after eradication of *H. pylori* infection
- **Autoimmune gastritis** can cause iron deficiency or pernicious anemia
- **Lymphocytic gastritis** may be associated with celiac disease, *H. pylori* infection, varioliform gastritis, and Ménétrier's disease
- **Chemical gastropathy**, caused by NSAIDs, alkaline reflux (bile or pancreatic secretion), or other chemical injury, is the most common pathologic finding in gastric biopsy specimens in the industrialized world

---

Introduction, including definition

The discovery of *Helicobacter pylori* catapulted gastritis onto centre stage [1]. Intensive research and voluminous literature followed. In this chapter the terms "body" or "gastric body" are used as synonymous with "corpus." The gastric mucosa is divided into four major regions, comprising different glandular components in differing proportions. From proximal to distal, they are: the **cardia, fundus, body** (corpus), and **antrum.** Histologically, the **gastric cardia** is a narrow band of mucosa juxtaposed to the squamous mucosa of the esophagus at the Z-line. Typical cardiac glands are of the mucous type, similar to those of the **gastric antrum**, but they often contain scattered acid-secreting gland elements. The **gastric fundus and body** contain a surface layer of mucus-producing glands with deeper layers of oxyntic glands. These oxyntic glands include parietal (acid-secreting) and chief (enzyme-secreting) cells as well as scattered endocrine cells. In the gastric antrum, the glands are of the mucous type, also with gastrin-producing endocrine cells. These histologic regions, however, do not necessarily correspond exactly to the gross anatomic landmarks.

Gastritis, simply defined as inflammation of the gastric mucosa, is a condition, **not a disease** [2]. With few exceptions, the inflammation of the gastric mucosa *per se* does not produce signs or symptoms. A subset of patients may have symptoms due to gastritis, but no independent tests are available to make that prediction in an individual patient. A second group of conditions characterized by gastric mucosal aberrations with little or no inflammation were historically included in classifications of gastritis, but are now categorized as **gastropathies** [2]. In some gastropathies there may be an inflammatory component, but the abnormal architectural changes are considered the dominant feature structurally and pathogenetically.

Classification

The classification of gastritis, outlined in Table 33.1, represents a modification of the **Updated Sydney System** and reflects current practice by most gastrointestinal pathologists and gastroenterologists [2]. Details of each type are provided in the following text.

Helicobacter pylori gastritis (see Chapter 22)
Definition

H. pylori infection is predicated on the identification of *H. pylori* organisms via a variety of diagnostic methods. Histologically, the typical findings are **chronic active gastritis.** "Chronic" refers to **mononuclear cell infiltrates**, especially lymphocytes and plasma cells, as well as eosinophils, with or without accompanying architectural distortion. "Active" refers to the presence of **neutrophils** infiltrating the epithelium and lamina propria. It is noteworthy that chronic active gastritis is neither specific for *H. pylori* infection nor is it present in all cases.

ESSENTIAL FACTS ABOUT *H. PYLORI* GASTRITIS

- It is the most common chronic infection in humans
- Mechanisms of transmission are unknown; prevalence is related to level of sanitation (15% to 80% in different populations)
- Two main types of pathology: antral-predominant non-atrophic (associated with risk for peptic ulcer) and atrophic pangastritis (associated with increased risk for gastric cancer)
- Treatment hinges on eradication of organism; therapies include combinations of antibiotics and proton pump inhibitors
- Eradication of *H. pylori* results in greatly decreased risk for peptic ulcer and decreased risk for intestinal-type gastric adenocarcinoma

---

Textbook of Clinical Gastroenterology and Hepatology, Second Edition. Edited by C. J. Hawkey, Jaime Bosch, Joel E. Richter, Guadalupe Garcia-Tsao, Francis K. L. Chan.

Table 33.1 Classification of gastritis with histologic correlations

Type of gastritis	Etiologic factors	Key Pathologic findings
Non-atrophic		
Helicobacter gastritis	*Helicobacter pylori* *Helicobacter heilmannii*	Multifocal chronic active gastritis with or without erosion/ulcer Lymphoid follicles characteristic Must exclude dysplasia and lymphoma
Other infectious gastritides	Bacteria (other than *H. pylori*) Viruses Fungi Parasites	Gastritis with or without ulcer/granuloma and identifiable organisms/viral cytopathic effect
Chemical gastropathy	Chemical irritation Bile NSAIDs ? Other agents	Foveolar hyperplasia Fibromuscular change of lamina propria Vascular dilatation
Lymphocytic	Idiopathic ? Immune mechanisms Gluten sensitivity Drug (*e.g.*, ticlopidine) ? *H. pylori*	Increased intraepithelial lymphocytes Must exclude *H. pylori* and lymphoma
Non-infectious granulomatous	Crohn's disease Sarcoidosis Wegener's granulomatosis and other vasculitides Foreign substances Idiopathic	Granulomas, typically non-caseating Occasionally identifiable organisms and foreign material
Eosinophilic	Food sensitivity ? Other allergies	Marked eosinophilia in mucosa and submucosa
Radiation Chemotherapy	Radiation injury (external and SIR spheres) Hepatic arterial infusion chemotherapy	Cytologically bizarre cells (both stromal and epithelial) with normal architecture Vascular changes Yttrium-90 spheres occasionally identifiable, often with ulceration
Atrophic		
Autoimmune	Autoimmunity Cross-reactivity with *H. pylori* antigens	Diffuse corporal atrophic gastritis with antral sparing IgG4-positive plasma cells in a minority
Multifocal atrophic	*Helicobacter pylori*, in association with dietary, environmental, and host factors	Patchy intestinal metaplasia/atrophy with involvement of corpus and antrum

Epidemiology

H. pylori gastritis is the most common chronic infection in humans [3]. It affects between three and four billion people, with a prevalence that varies from less than 20% in industrialized Western regions with ethnically homogeneous populations (*e.g.*, Scandinavia) to more than 80% in developing areas of the world (*e.g.*, parts of South America, equatorial Africa, Southeast Asia). Within countries, the most important predictor of high prevalence is **low socioeconomic status**. Improved socioeconomic conditions have resulted in a decreased prevalence of *H. pylori* in most Western countries and Japan.

Causes, risk factors, disease associations

Humans are the only important reservoir for *H. pylori*. **Helicobacter heilmannii**, a pathogen of dogs and cats, is responsible for approximately 1% of human *Helicobacter* infections; its histopathologic aspects and clinical associations are similar to those of *H. pylori* gastritis [4]. Transmission occurs primarily from human to human and is most efficient in **childhood,** as suggested by the finding that children and their parents are often infected by strains with identical genetic fingerprints [5–8]. *H. pylori* is a spiral, microaerophilic, urease-producing, Gram-negative bacterium. A number of proteins expressed by *H. pylori*, collectively known as **pathogenicity factors**, have been suspected of an association with particular manifestations of the infection (Table 33.2). However the virulence of *H. pylori* seems to be largely host-dependent, and none of these factors is unequivocally disease-specific [9,10]. *H. pylori* infection is associated with most duodenal and gastric ulcers that are not related to the use of nonsteroidal anti-inflammatory drugs (NSAIDs) and almost all primary **gastric lymphomas** of the mucosa-associated lymphoid tissue (MALT) [11]. In certain populations, a considerable proportion of infected subjects develop atrophic gastritis, a documented precursor of **gastric adenocarcinoma** [12,13].

Pathogenesis and pathology

Studies of the initial phases of *H. pylori* infection reveal acute mucosal inflammatory responses that usually involve all gastric regions and may be accompanied by antral erosions and subepithelial hemorrhages. The **chronic phase** is characterized by a mixed infiltrate in the lamina propria (usually most intense in its most superficial portions), consisting of lymphocytes, plasma cells, and variable amounts of eosinophils, with ongoing activity evidenced by neutrophilic infiltration (Figure 33.1).The intensity of inflammation is generally greater in the antrum and the cardia than in the gastric body, where it may be minimal despite visible bacterial colonization. This distribution of inflammation is described as **antrum-predominant gastritis**, the most common type of gastritis in Western populations.

In a proportion of infected subjects, the inflammation is equally intense in all gastric regions. This pattern, known as **pangastritis,** is associated with a progression toward glandular destruction with resulting atrophy and intestinal metaplasia. Atrophic pangastritis is the predominant phenotype in subjects from less industrialized areas of the world and particularly in populations with high incidence of gastric adenocarcinoma [2]. **Lymphoid follicles**, an expression of MALT (see Chapter 35), are virtually always found in infected stomachs, and their presence is a reliable indication of active or recently treated *H. pylori* gastritis. Their greatest density is in the region of the **incisura angularis** and the lowest in the proximal body greater curvature [14]. *H. pylori* pangastritis can usually be distinguished from classical autoimmune gastritis by the presence of disease in the antrum (not found in pure autoimmune gastritis) as well as less uniform atrophy/inflammation of the body and fundus (hence the former term "multifocal atrophic gastritis") [15]. Such an assessment requires adequate biopsy sampling (see "Diagnostic methods" below).

Clinical presentation

The relationship of chronic *H. pylori* gastritis with **dyspepsia** (see Chapter 4) remains unclear. *H. pylori* eradication in patients with nonulcer dyspepsia has not been shown conclusively to improve the dyspeptic symptoms. A subset may respond, but prediction of which patients belong to that subset is not possible at this time. Subjects with **antrum-predominant**

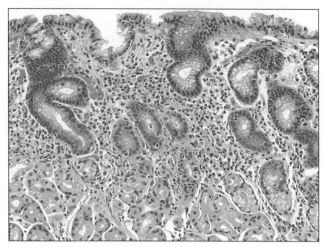

Figure 33.1 Biopsy of the gastric antrum showing moderate chronic active gastritis. The dark staining mixed inflammatory infiltrate is concentrated mostly in the upper portions of the mucosa. Various degrees of clear-staining edema and hemorrhage are seen in the subepithelial zone.

Table 33.2 Putative pathogenicity factors of *H. pylori* and their alleged associations

Putative pathogenicity factor	Characteristics	Associations
VacA (vacuolating cytotoxin)	Genotypes s1 (associated with CagA positivity and s2)	Not useful for predicting symptoms, presentation, degree of inflammation, or response to therapy
CagA(cytotoxin-associated gene product A)	Product of one of the genes in the *cag* pathogenicity island	Induction of cytokine expression in gastric epithelial cells, with raised mucosal levels of interleukin-8 and marked neutrophil infiltration. Increase risk of a symptomatic outcome (peptic ulcer and gastric cancer), but not in all populations. No predictive value in individual patients)
iceA (induced by contact with epithelium)	Bacterial restriction enzyme	No known biologic or epidemiologic evidence of a role for iceA as a virulence factor in *H. pylori*-related disease
babA (blood group antigen-binding adhesin)	Outer membrane protein, involved in adherence of *H. pylori* to Lewis-b (Leb) blood group antigens on gastric epithelial cells	No individual predictive value. Infection with *babA2* gene, *cagA*+ and *vocA* s1 ("triple-positive strains") may be related to duodenal ulcer risk

H. pylori **gastritis** have a lifetime risk for peptic ulcer disease of 15–20% (see Chapter 32). Most subjects who do not develop ulcer disease remain asymptomatic and are believed to have no increased risk for gastric adenocarcinoma (see Chapter 34); those with **pangastritis** also remain asymptomatic, but their gastric mucosa develops progressive destructive and reparative changes that result in expanding areas of glandular loss (atrophy) and replacement of the native gastric mucosa with an intestinal-type epithelium (intestinal metaplasia).

Atrophic gastritis is epidemiologically and biologically associated with **gastric adenocarcinoma** of the intestinal type, and patients with this phenotype account for much of the increased risk of cancer related to *H. pylori* infection [15]. Based on case-controlled and other retrospective epidemiologic studies, the overall gastric cancer risk for *H. pylori*-infected subjects has been estimated as **3- to 10-fold** that of the uninfected population [16]. *H. pylori* infection is also related to diffuse (**signet ring cell**) gastric cancer of the stomach, which accounts for 50% or more of all gastric cancers in some populations. Here there is no diffuse intestinal metaplasia or atrophy and no apparent dysplastic "soil." The risk for primary **gastric B-cell lymphoma**, a rare condition, is in the range of 5- to 7-fold that of noninfected subjects.

Both carcinoma and lymphoma may be diagnosed years or even decades after *H. pylori* infection has disappeared, possibly because of the combined effects of the hypochlorhydria related to atrophy, an inhospitable gastric environment brought upon by metaplasia and incipient epithelial and lymphoid neoplasia, and possibly incidental antibiotic treatments. Thus, it is likely that retrospective studies significantly underestimate the risk of neoplasia conferred by *H. pylori* infection. Studies taking into account the infecting strain of *H. pylori* (with regard to pathogenicity factors), the phenotype of gastritis, and the time elapsed between detection of the infection and the diagnosis of carcinoma, have raised the estimated risk to as much as **23-fold**.

Diagnostic methods (Table 33.3)

Testing for *H. pylori* should be performed only if treatment is intended. The diagnosis can be made by endoscopic biopsy of the gastric mucosa or by noninvasive methods, depending on the clinical setting. **Biopsy specimens** (ideally at least two from the antrum and two separately identified and submitted from the gastric body along the greater curve) are examined for the detection of *H. pylori* and for the diagnosis of gastritis (Figure 33.2). Special stains have been employed to identify the curved bacillary organisms with facility. A variety of histochemical stains have been employed, but the most sensitive and specific (both near 100%) is the immunohistochemical stain, which can also identify organisms after treatment with proton pump inhibitors and antibiotics (Figure 33.3). Organisms are typically found extracellularly in the lumen at the surface and in the superficial pit layer. After treatment, organisms can sometimes only be found in deep glands and intracellularly, often with atypical (coccoid) morphology. *H. heilmannii*

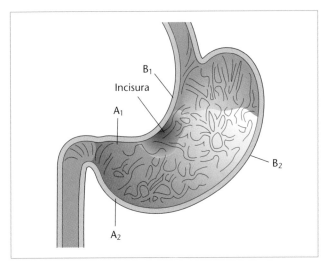

Figure 33.2 Biopsy protocol. Schematic representation of the biopsy protocol recommended by the Updated Sydney System when the objective is to map the severity and extent of gastritis. A minimum of two specimens is obtained from each of the antrum (A1 and A2 – lesser and greater curvature) and the corpus (B1 and B2 – lesser and greater curvature). In addition, one biopsy specimen from the incisura angularis (IA) is recommended to detect early atrophic and metaplastic changes, represented in blue. (This figure was published in *Clinical Gastroenterology and Hepatology*, Wilfred M. Weinstein, Christopher J. Hawkey, Jaime Bosch, Gastritis, Pages 223–232, Copyright Elsevier, 2005.)

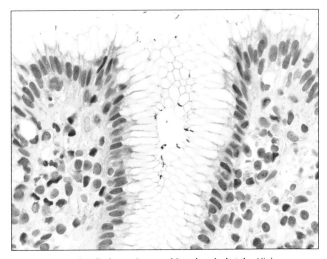

Figure 33.3 Anti-*Helicobacter* immunohistochemical stain. High-power photomicrograph of gastric mucosa with few *H. pylori* organisms, stained brown by an anti-*Helicobacter* immunohistochemical stain.

organisms have a characteristic tight spiral morphology and are two to three times longer (10 microns) than *H. pylori*.

A **urease test** on an antral biopsy specimen (Clotest®) permits the rapid detection of urease activity in the biopsy material, with a sensitivity of 80–100% and a specificity of 92–100%, although it is not known how well such tests work post-treatment. The urea breath test (UBT) is based on the detection of labelled carbon dioxide in a sample of the subject's breath after the ingestion of a meal containing ^{13}C and ^{14}C labeled urea. Although highly sensitive and specific, its use is largely limited by the need of administering the meal to the

Table 33.3 Invasive and non-invasive tests for the diagnosis of *H. pylori* infection

Test	Characteristics	Advantages	Disadvantages
Invasive methods			
Histopathologic examination of gastric mucosal biopsy	Detects current infection by direct observation with or without special staining techniques (immunohistochemistry is the most sensitive and specific)	Highly sensitive and specific Can discern *H. pylori* from *H. heilmannii* Allows the evaluation of associated conditions (intestinal metaplasia, dysplasia, carcinoma, lymphoma) Guarantees a permanent record	Invasive Sampling may affect yield
Smear, brush, and touch preparations (cytopathology)	Detects bacteria by direct observation of gastric exfoliated cells harvested by brushing	Inexpensive	Invasive Generally inaccurate, even with skilled operators Limited information on pathology of gastric mucosa
Bacterial culture	Detects bacterial growth in special media	100% specific Allows antibiotic sensitivity tests	Invasive Sensitivity is laboratory-dependent No information on pathology of gastric mucosa
Rapid urease tests	Detect current infection by bacteria-produced urease in fresh biopsy specimens	Highly sensitive Highly specific Rapid results (<2 hours)	Invasive No information on pathology of gastric mucosa
Non-invasive methods			
Urea breath tests	Detects current infection, relying on *H. pylori*-derived urease activity in the stomach	Sensitivity and specificity >90% Can be used in children Useful for initial diagnosis and to evaluate treatment	Requires ^{13}C or ^{14}C detection equipment Expensive in some settings No information on pathology of gastric mucosa
Laboratory-based serologic tests	Detect anti-*H. pylori* IgG in serum	Approved tests have high sensitivity and specificity (85%–90%) Inexpensive Useful for initial diagnosis	Specificity may be "population-specific" Detect evidence of past infection No information on pathology of gastric mucosa, except indirectly when combined with gastrin and pepsinogen ratio measurements ("serologic biopsy")
Simplified "in-office" immunoenzymatic tests	Detect anti-*H. pylori* IgG in serum or whole blood	Inexpensive Immediate results (<10 minutes) Moderate specificity and sensitivity (~85%)	Detect evidence of past infection No information on current infection Sensitivity and specificity <90% No information on pathology of gastric mucosa
Stool antigen assays	Detect *H. pylori* antigens in stools	Detects current infection Useful for determining eradication (8 weeks after therapy) Excellent specificity and sensitivity (>95%) Inexpensive	Specimen collection inconvenient No information on pathology of gastric mucosa
Urine tests	Detect anti-*H. pylori* IgG in urine	Inexpensive disposable kits Quick results (20 minutes) Recently developed tests (*e.g.*, RAPIRUN, URINELISA) have moderate specificity and sensitivity (~ 85%)	Not yet completely validated Sensitivity and specificity may be too low for clinical use Low specificity in children No information on pathology of gastric mucosa
Saliva tests	Detect anti-*H. pylori* IgA or IgG in saliva	Convenient collection of saliva	Low specificity and sensitivity (70% to 85% reported) Not approved, not readily available

patient and the relatively expensive analysers required for the evaluation of the breath sample. Culture of *H. pylori* with antibiotic sensitivity testing is not performed routinely for the initial diagnosis of *H. pylori* infection. Some laboratories have **high-quality culture** facilities for *H. pylori,* and culture may be used if a second course of therapy also fails to eradicate the organisms.

Indications for therapy

Primary indications for testing and treatment include:

- active peptic ulcer disease
- a history of documented peptic ulcer
- gastric MALT lymphoma.

Testing of asymptomatic subjects and patients with non-ulcer dyspepsia are not recommended, except when there is a documented history of gastric cancer in first-degree relatives. Despite the absence of data, many patients with life-dominating **non-ulcer dyspepsia** are treated if they have evidence of *H. pylori.* In children, testing for *H. pylori* is recommended when the symptoms are severe enough to justify therapy. In spite of, or perhaps because of, the many recommendations issued by gastroenterological associations and consensus groups, several issues regarding indications for therapy remain unresolved. In practice, treatment decisions are rarely based on evidence alone; frequently a number of patient- and doctor-driven considerations have the greatest weight in making these choices.

Therapy

The **Maastricht-III consensus** stated that for an eradication treatment regime to be considered effective, it should achieve an intention-to-treat eradication rate in excess of 80% [17]. However, eradication rates in practice for many of the most common regimens have fallen well below these levels in recent years, generally due to a combination of poor compliance and antibiotic resistance.

The recommended *first-line treatment* in published European and North American guidelines consists of a proton pump inhibitor (PPI) combined with amoxicillin and clarithromycin. However, while in 2000, eradication rates for standard triple therapy were in excess of 90%, recent studies have shown that this level has fallen below 70% and even as low as 60% in some areas. Therefore, Maastricht III guidelines [17] recommend substituting metronidazole for clarithromycin where resistance to that antibiotic, increasing in most countries, exceeds 15–20%. Although there has been debate on the optimal duration of therapy, the 2007 American College of Gastroenterology guidelines recommended 10-day treatment courses [18] and the most recent Maastricht consensus stated that 14 days of treatment had an advantage over 7 days in terms of eradication.

Since first-line therapy fails in approximately 20% of patients, several *second-line therapy* regimens have been developed. The most common are bismuth-based and levofloxacin-based therapies. Bismuth-based quadruple therapy consisting of a PPI, bismuth, tetracycline, and metronidazole for 10 days or

14 days has a reported efficacy between 75% and 95% in patients who failed first-line therapy. Levofloxacin-based therapy has grown in popularity in recent years; however, the rapidly increasing rate of quinolone resistance reported in several countries may soon limit its use [19].

Patients who fail both first and second-line therapy for *H. pylori* have been treated with empiric rescue regimens ("*third-line therapy*") that most commonly include rifabutin or furizoladone. These antibiotics have, however, serious side effects (including myelotoxicity) and their use may be limited to selected patients.

Recently, *sequential therapy* has been proposed to overcome clarithromycin resistance [20,21]. Hypothetically, during the first part of therapy, amoxicillin weakens the bacterial cell wall, which prevents the formation of the channels that block clarithromycin from binding to the bacterium and hence causes resistance to the antibiotic. A meta-analysis published in 2008 reported 93.4% eradication rates, compared with 76.9% for standard triple therapy [22]. Sequential therapy is not affected by bacterial factors (CagA status, bacterial load) and host factors (underlying disease, smoking), which until now have predicted the outcome of conventional eradication treatments. Even when strains were clarithromycin-resistant, the eradication rate with sequential therapy was 82.2% compared with 40.6% for triple therapy. Most studies on sequential therapy have been performed in Italy and this regimen is still untested in most countries. The American College of Gastroenterology "Guideline on the Management of *H. pylori* Infection" states that "sequential therapy may provide an alternative to clarithromycin-based triple therapy but requires validation within the United States before it can be recommended as a first-line therapy;" the European Maastricht III Consensus Report points out that "sequential treatment deserves further evaluation in different regions" [17,18].

Probiotics and vaccines may offer some alternatives in the future, but at the moment they are still in the early phases of evaluation.

A sensible approach for therapy in patients who fail a first- and second-line treatment involves *H. pylori* **culture and antibiotic testing**. However, susceptibility testing is limited by the fact that *in vivo* resistance may not accurately reflect *in vitro* resistance, notably with respect to metronidazole. Currently such an approach is carried out almost exclusively in specialized centres with research interest and expertise in the treatment of *H. pylori*; however, the development of newer technologies in the field of susceptibility testing may encourage this practice to become more widespread. This is likely to have substantial benefits and lead to more accurate prescribing and lower rates of resistance.

Autoimmune gastritis and pernicious anemia
Definition
Autoimmune gastritis is a chronic atrophic gastritis affecting the oxyntic gland mucosa (gastric body and fundus) and

commonly associated with circulating serum antiparietal cell and anti-intrinsic factor antibodies and intrinsic factor deficiency. In its endstage it is associated with vitamin B_{12} deficiency. Pernicious anemia is the vitamin B_{12} deficiency associated with chronic atrophic autoimmune gastritis.

> **ESSENTIAL FACTS ABOUT AUTOIMMUNE GASTRITIS**
>
> * Chronic corpus-restricted atrophic gastritis is associated with circulating serum anti-parietal cell and anti-intrinsic factor antibodies along with intrinsic factor deficiency
> * Affects predominantly older women. The prevalence is 1%–5% in persons over 60 years of age; higher in subjects with specific familial histocompatibility haplotypes (HLA-B8 and -DR3)
> * Pathology: dense mononuclear infiltrates in the corpus leading to progressive disappearance of oxyntic glands and intestinal metaplasia with resultant hypochlorhydria. Endocrine cell hyperplasia, carcinoid tumours, and inflammatory polyps are common
> * Vitamin B_{12} deficiency and macrocytic anemia ("pernicious anemia") characterize the advanced stage

Epidemiology

Autoimmune gastritis and pernicious anemia are diseases of older age, especially in women. The **prevalence** of pernicious anemia among Americans aged 60 years or older is 2.7% in women and 1.4% in men. There is a strong family association (see below) [23].

Pathogenesis

The high prevalence of specific familial **histocompatibility haplotypes** (HLA-B8 and -DR3) in patients with corpus-restricted atrophic gastritis and its association with other autoimmune conditions, strongly indicate an **autoimmune origin** [24]. **Autoantibodies** to parietal cells and to their secretory product, intrinsic factor, are present in the serum and gastric juice. The antigen recognized by parietal cell autoantibodies is gastric H^+/K^+-ATPase, the major protein of the membrane lining the secretory canaliculi of parietal cells, that secretes hydrogen ions in exchange for potassium ions [25]. During the course of the disease, both **parietal and chief cells disappear** progressively from the oxyntic glands. *H. pylori* infection may induce the formation of antibodies that cross react with parietal-cell antigens, and has been proposed as a possible etiologic factor in the pathogenesis of autoimmune gastritis. This correlation, however, remains unproven, and similarly, much stronger biologic, clinical, and epidemiologic evidence is needed before *H. pylori* can be viewed as the cause of autoimmune gastritis [26,27].

Pathology

Patients with autoimmune gastritis have a **corpus-restricted** chronic atrophic gastritis, and therefore the antral (and cardiac) mucosa is usually spared. **Mononuclear cell infiltrates** (plasma cells and lymphocytes) are found in the lamina propria between the gastric glands and may extend into the submucosa (Figure 33.4). Infiltrating plasma cells contain

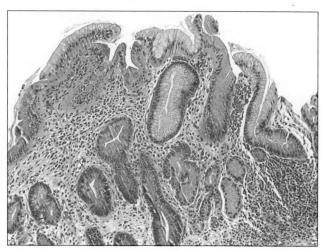

Figure 33.4 Autoimmune gastritis. Corpus mucosa with metaplastic atrophy, complete absence of oxyntic gland, and a dense mononuclear inflammatory infiltrate.

autoantibodies to the parietal cell antigen and to intrinsic factor. In the initial phases of the disease, individual parietal cells may be surrounded by lymphocytes or drop out from oxyntic glands.

As the disease progresses over a period of two to three decades, the oxyntic mucosa may be completely replaced by **pyloric/antral-type mucous glands, "pyloric metaplasia,"** and intestinal metaplasia. At this stage the inflammation becomes less intense. In patients with classic pernicious anemia, residual small nests of parietal and chief cells may persist, but their numbers are greatly reduced. The **hypochlorhydria** induces gastrin production from endocrine cells in the antrum, which in turn stimulates enterochromaffin-like (**ECL**) **cell hyperplasia**. This common finding is often subtle histologically but can be highlighted with the use of immunohistochemical stains for neuroendocrine differentiation. The range of ECL proliferation ranges from linear hyperplasia to microcarcinoid tumours. Such tumours are often multiple, are associated with various levels of background endocrine proliferation, and almost always are innocuous. In addition, benign gastric hyperplastic polyps are frequently seen in end-stage patients [28].

Clinical presentation

Most clinical manifestations of autoimmune gastritis become apparent when the parietal cell mass decreases beyond the critical point when the stomach becomes unable to produce sufficient amounts of acid, pepsinogens, and intrinsic factor. **Achlorhydria** occurs in the most advanced stages of the disease, but hypochlorhydria may also occur in patients with moderate numbers of surviving parietal cells, suggesting that anti-proton pump antibodies or inhibitory lymphokines released by subsets of inflammatory cells may participate in the inhibition of acid secretion. Patients with oxyntic gland atrophy and achlorhydria undergo **hyperplasia of gastrin-secreting endocrine cells** in the gastric antrum with resultant hypergastrinemia, typically correlating with the severity of the mucosal damage. Injury to chief cells leads to a reduction of pepsin activity in gastric juice and of pepsinogens in blood. Reduced **pepsinogen I** concentration (<20ng/mL) is a sensitive and specific indicator of atrophic gastritis. Patients with advanced autoimmune gastritis may develop:

- iron deficiency anemia
- pernicious anemia or
- combined anemia.

Hypochromic microcytic anemia (15% of patients) may be caused by achlorhydria, as **gastric acid** is important in the absorption of non-heme iron, which in Western diets supplies at least two-thirds of nutritional iron needs. Frank pernicious (macrocytic) anemia is usually preceded by chronic atrophic gastritis and reduced or absent acid secretion by approximately a decade, and is generally associated with a histologic pattern of end-stage atrophic gastritis. Thus a combined anemia may be present, and a considerable number of patients with severe atrophic oxyntic gland gastritis may still not fulfill the criteria for the diagnosis of pernicious anemia, but are clearly at risk for the development of vitamin B_{12} deficiency.

Disease associations
Autoimmune gastritis is a risk factor for:

- hyperplastic and adenomatous polyps
- carcinomas
- endocrine tumours

of the stomach. Polyps, found in 20–40% of patients with pernicious anemia, are mostly sessile, small, and multiple. Most are hyperplastic, but up to 10% may contain dysplastic foci [29]. The risk of gastric carcinoma is believed to be increased 3-fold, and that of gastric carcinoid tumours 13-fold, in patients with pernicious anemia [28]. The trophic action of gastrin may be responsible for the transformation of endocrine cells from hyperplastic to neoplastic.

Diagnostic methods
The diagnosis of autoimmune gastritis is frequently missed because patients (elderly people with anemia) are typically successfully treated by hematologists or general practitioners with iron and vitamin B_{12} supplements, and are not referred to gastroenterologists for the evaluation of atrophic gastritis, pepsinogen levels, or antiparietal cell antibodies. The diagnosis can be confirmed by a combination of histopathologic and serologic studies. A set of at least **four biopsy specimens** from the gastric mid-body on the greater curvature, along with two separately submitted from the antrum, should be obtained. The coexistence of severe and diffuse atrophic gastritis of the corpus with a normal antrum is virtually pathognomonic of autoimmune atrophic gastritis [2,30].

The atrophic gastritis is characterized histologically by **chronic inflammation** of the glandular mucosa with marked or complete **depletion of the parietal cell mass**, and intestinal and pyloric metaplasia. These findings can mimic antral gastritis and warrant the separate labeling of biopsies from these regions.

Serum antibodies to gastric parietal cells are found in 90% of patients with pernicious anemia and in about 30% of their non-anemic first-degree relatives. The demonstration of circulating intrinsic factor autoantibodies is almost diagnostic of autoimmune gastritis and is present in approximately 50%. Hypergastrinemia is the result of sparing of the antrum and stimulation of the gastrin-producing G cells by achlorhydria. A low serum pepsinogen concentration results from destruction of the chief cells.

Treatment
The standard treatment is regular monthly intramuscular injections of at least 100μg vitamin B_{12} to correct the vitamin deficiency. Hydroxycobalamin 1mg every 3 months is a common regimen. When indicated, iron supplements are given prior to B_{12} administration.

Other gastritides
Infectious gastritides due to agents other than *Helicobacter* spp
The acid environment of the normal stomach is inhospitable to most infectious agents. However, in subjects with atrophic gastritis and decreased acid secretion, in patients with impaired immune responses, or as part of systemic infections, a number of viruses, bacteria, and parasites can infect the stomach. These infectious gastritides (see Chapter 31, "Infections of the esophagus and stomach") are rare in otherwise healthy persons, but some (*e.g.*, cytomegalovirus) are not uncommon in immunocompromised patients. Their most important clinical and pathologic features are summarized in Table 33.4.

Lymphocytic gastritis
This is a distinctive type of pangastritis characterized by the presence of large numbers of mature lymphocytes infiltrating the surface and foveolar epithelium. The lamina propria is infiltrated by an often dense population of inflammatory cells in which lymphocytes and plasma cells predominate, although significant numbers of neutrophils and eosinophils are also present [31].

ESSENTIAL FACTS ABOUT LYMPHOCYTIC GASTRITIS

- Pangastritis characterized by large numbers of mature CD8+ lymphocytes infiltrating the surface and foveolar epithelium
- Prevalence: 0.1–1% of subjects undergoing gastric biopsies
- Etiology is unknown; it is not caused by *H. pylori* infection

Table 33.4 Infectious gastritides caused by agents other than *Helicobacter* spp.

Agent	Main characteristics	Pathology
Viral		
Rotaviruses, caliciviruses	Stomach may be infected during gastroenteritis	None known
Cytomegalovirus	Children Immunocompromised patients	Megaloblastic inclusions Mucosal erosions, ulcerations Rarely large-fold gastropathy
Bacteria		
Various	Overgrowth only in achlorhydric subjects	No detectable changes
Pyogenic bacteria (streptococci, staphylococci, *Escherichia coli*, *Proteus*, and *Haemophilus* spp.)	Phlegmonous gastritis Exceedingly rare	Large areas of purulent necrosis involving the full thickness of the gastric wall
Mycobacterium tuberculosis	Primary gastric tuberculosis rare Stomach may be involved in disseminated infections	Necrotizing granulomas may be found in the gastric mucosa
Treponema pallidum	Gastric involvement in secondary syphilis Rare, more common in HIV patients	Mixed inflammatory infiltrate, mostly plasma cells, and mucosal ulcerations. Swelling of gastric folds with erosions and ulcerations may mimic endoscopic appearance of lymphoma or carcinoma
Fungi		
Candida species **Histoplasma capsulatum** **Mucoraceae**	Only in immunocompromised patients	
Parasites		
Cryptosporidium spp. *Giardia intestinalis* *Strongyloides stercoralis*	Rarely found in the stomach, mostly immunocompromised patients	No inflammatory responses
Anisakidae	"Sushi worm" Many species of edible fishes have larvae of *Anisakidae* in their muscles. In a small proportion of individuals who eat infected fish, larvae penetrate the gastric wall causing a sudden onset of epigastric pain	Mostly eosinophilic response around penetrating larvae Dead larvae may elicit granulomas

Epidemiology

Lymphocytic gastritis is uncommon, found in 0.1–1% of subjects who undergo endoscopy with biopsy sampling.

Causes and pathogenesis

Because virtually all intraepithelial lymphocytes are CD8+ suppressor T cells (the same cells that form the intraepithelial infiltrate in celiac disease and lymphocytic colitis), an immune mechanism has been proposed. Lymphocytic gastritis is of interest primarily because of its clinical associations: approximately one-third of adults and up to half of children with **celiac disease** (see Chapter 40) have increased gastric intraepithelial lymphocytes, usually concentrated in the antrum. In most cases of lymphocytic gastritis *H. pylori* cannot be implicated, as the rate of infection in those with and without

lymphocytosis are similar. The first reports of lymphocytic gastritis featured endoscopic descriptions of large gastric folds with nodules and erosions, clinically accompanied by nausea, vomiting, and weight loss. These findings were presented as the signature lesions of a now rare disorder: diffuse **varioliform ("octopus-sucker") gastritis** [32].

Another unusual and **hypertrophic variant** of lymphocytic gastritis resembles Ménétrier's disease endoscopically, also in patients with protein loss. Case reports describe resolution of the intraepithelial lymphocytosis and symptomatology following a regimen of proton pump inhibitors. *H. pylori* has been found in some of these patients, and in a subset of these, eradication resulted in disappearance of the thick folds and lymphocytic gastritis. Although other putative disease associations include non-*Helicobacter* infections and Crohn's

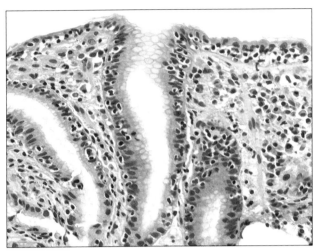

Figure 33.5 Lymphocytic gastritis. This is characterized by marked intraepithelial lymphocytosis and a variable plasma cell and lymphocyte infiltrate in the lamina propria.

disease, lymphocytic gastritis is most commonly seen in gastric biopsies where there is no known association.

Diagnostic methods

A substantial increase in **intraepithelial lymphocytes** (Figure 33.5) is accompanied by a spectrum of inflammation in the lamina propria ranging from a minor increase in chronic inflammatory cells with no activity to a marked chronic and active inflammation with erosions. In most cases the histologic picture can readily be distinguished from that of *H. pylori* chronic gastritis, in which (exclusive of focal lymphoepithelial lesions) few intraepithelial lymphocytes are present. The **diagnostic threshold** for lymphocytic gastritis is generally accepted as more than 25 intraepithelial lymphocytes per 100 epithelial cells, but in most cases the counts are greater than 50 [31].

Granulomatous gastritis

Granulomatous gastritis can be considered as a histopathologic placeholder to which gastric biopsies bearing granulomas are temporarily assigned while the condition responsible for their development is identified. In most cases the morphologic appearance of granulomas does not provide a useful clue to their etiology, except when

- foreign materials
- acid-fast bacilli or
- fungal forms

are found. Thus, a specific diagnosis can be made only by integrating histopathologic findings with clinical and laboratory information [33,34].

Etiology and pathogenesis

Granulomatous inflammation in the gastrointestinal mucosa can be found in patients with a variety of bacterial, fungal, and parasitic infections as well as certain immune disorders.

Primary **gastric tuberculosis** has been reported mostly from developing countries, typically manifesting as a large non-healing ulcer; disseminated tuberculosis also causes caseating granulomas (see Chapter 47). *Histoplasma capsulatum* rarely can cause gastric granulomatous inflammation. In gastric anisakiasis, fragments of helminthic cuticles may elicit the formation of foreign body granulomas.

The stomach may be involved in patients with Crohn's disease (see Chapter 50) and sarcoidosis. In **Crohn's disease**, the prevalence of gastric granulomas may be as high as 10%. However, more commonly, gastric biopsies appear largely normal but feature a focal chronic active inflammatory response, often limited to a few foveolae or oxyntic glands, termed "**focally enhanced gastritis**;" granulomas are not part of this response. While highly non-specific, this pattern of injury may be the first manifestation of Crohn's disease.

In **sarcoidosis**, involvement of the gastrointestinal tract rarely has any clinical importance, although outlet obstruction and bleeding have occasionally been reported. Endoscopic findings include nodularity, polypoid mucosal irregularity, erosions, ulcers, and segmental, usually distal, rigidity resembling linitis plastica. These gross changes reflect the presence of numerous small mucosal granulomas. Since the finding of gastric mucosal granulomas may precede the discovery of these diseases in other organs, the careful interpretation of gastric biopsy findings together with radiologic and serologic testing may lead to the diagnosis.

Other causes of granulomas include **foreign material**, such as suture material in patients who have undergone a partial gastrectomy, and food particles that may become engulfed in an ulcer crater. **Rare entities** causing gastric granuloma include immune-mediated vasculitis syndromes (see Chapter 111) and Wegener's granulomatosis.

The term "isolated (or idiopathic) granulomatous gastritis" should be applied only as a temporary diagnostic label to cases of granulomatous gastric inflammation for which no etiology has yet been determined. Even after careful evaluation, a large proportion of gastric granulomas will remain unexplained. These lesions are usually asymptomatic; as there is no information on their natural history or evolution, no treatment can be recommended [33,34].

Gastropathies

Reactive (or chemical) gastropathy

Reactive (or chemical) gastropathy is defined as the constellation of endoscopic and histologic changes caused by chemical injury to the gastric mucosa [35]. The term "chemical" is used broadly and refers to the gastric mucosa in some patients who take **NSAIDs** (see Chapter 23); it also includes patients with **alkaline reflux** after partial gastrectomy or those with poorly understood motility disorders resulting in **bile reflux**. No relationship has been established between the endoscopic or histologic appearance of the mucosa in patients who take NSAIDs and either dyspeptic symptoms or risk for gastric hemorrhage.

Interestingly, reactive gastropathy is only seen in 10–45% of those who take NSAIDs regularly. Biopsies at the edges of gastric erosions and ulcers often reveal the features of reactive or chemical gastropathy, even in settings other than those of NSAID ingestion.

ESSENTIAL FACTS ABOUT REACTIVE GASTROPATHY

- Also known as chemical gastropathy, it is the constellation of endoscopic and histologic changes caused by chemical injury to the gastric mucosa
- Most commonly associated with used of NSAIDs
- Highly prevalent (15% to 25%) in populations living in the industrialized world, particularly in the elderly
- Pathology: minimal or no inflammation, epithelial regeneration with foveolar hyperplasia, edema of the lamina propria, vascular congestion, and proliferation of the smooth muscle fibres

---

Histopathologic changes associated with reactive gastropathy include:

- Epithelial regeneration.
- Foveolar hyperplasia.
- Edema of the lamina propria.
- Proliferation of the smooth muscle fibres from the muscularis mucosae into the upper third of the mucosa (Figure 33.6).

However, both the specificity and predictive value of these features are low, and the diagnosis rests on the integration of clinical and histopathologic data [36]. When reactive gastropathy is found unexpectedly in a biopsy of normal-appearing gastric mucosa sampled to exclude *H. pylori*, the clinician should solicit a history that might reveal the etiology, usually chronic NSAID use or symptoms compatible with bile reflux.

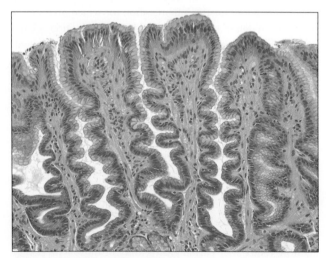

Figure 33.6 Reactive ("chemical") gastropathy. Hyperplastic "corkscrew" gastric foveolae and absence of inflammation: these features are seen in up to 45% of patients on chronic NSAIDs and in alkaline reflux gastropathy. They are virtually always present in the gastric mucosa adjacent to a Bilroth II anastomotic site.

Hemorrhagic gastropathies

This group of conditions, characterized by subepithelial hemorrhages and erosions, is related to:

- severe physical stress (see Chapter 32)
- the use of NSAIDs (see Chapter 23)
- the ingestion of large quantities of alcohol.

The most severe degrees of hemorrhagic gastropathy are those induced by stress in critically ill patients. Most patients admitted to an intensive care unit have mucosal lesions; approximately 20% of them have overt bleeding and 2–5% have life-threatening hemorrhage (see Chapter 32). The pathogenesis of stress-induced hemorrhagic gastropathy is incompletely understood, but when the mucosal defense mechanisms lose their integrity, luminal acid may exert a damaging effect. Vascular disturbances, in association with stasis, vasoconstriction, and increased vascular permeability, may contribute further to mucosal vulnerability [37].

Aspirin or other NSAIDs may induce acute mucosal injury, ranging from edema and hyperemia to multiple erosions and ulcerations. Such lesions may occur without warning symptoms in both first-time NSAID users and patients who have taken NSAIDs regularly for years. Except for generic risk factors (older age, female sex, and previous episodes), there is no way prospectively to identify NSAID users who are susceptible to severe gastric injury. Similar mucosal lesions, although usually less severe and only rarely eventuating to ulcer, can be caused by the ingestion of large quantities of alcohol. NSAIDs act by interfering with prostaglandin synthesis, while alcohol causes direct damage to the gastric mucosa, particularly at higher concentrations.

Acute hemorrhagic gastropathy is characterized by a hyperemic edematous mucosa with erosions and active bleeding. As the diagnosis is usually realized from the clinical context, gastric biopsies are rarely obtained. Nevertheless, in **immunocompromised patients**, it may be prudent to obtain biopsies to look for evidence of infection such as cytomegalovirus. Similarly, if hemorrhagic gastropathy is encountered outside of an expected clinical setting, biopsy to exclude a diffuse process like lymphoma or carcinoma should be performed.

Vascular gastropathies

This heterogeneous group of conditions is characterized by alterations in the gastric circulation and their effects on the gastric mucosa. From a morphologic and pathogenetic viewpoint, gastric antral vascular ectasia (GAVE) and portal hypertensive gastropathy are the best characterized.

Gastric antral vascular ectasia (GAVE)

GAVE, or "watermelon stomach," is a condition of unknown etiology frequently associated with atrophic gastritis, connective tissue disorders (particularly scleroderma), and sometimes portal hypertension. More than 70% of reported cases have occurred in women older than 65 years of age. Occult bleeding with iron deficiency anemia is present in almost 90% of patients, with melena or hematemesis in 60%. The picturesque name was inspired by the endoscopic appearance of "longitudinal antral folds seen converging on the pylorus, containing visible and ectatic vessels resembling the stripes on a watermelon." The prominent dilated vessels have also been compared to a large flat mushroom or honeycomb [38].

Histopathology

The lamina propria is expanded by **smooth muscle proliferation** and fibrosis, and contains **dilated mucosal capillaries** whose cross-sectional area is of the caliber of adjacent antral glands. Fibrin thrombi are characteristically found within at least some of the dilated capillaries. Other localized conditions (*e.g.*, gastric hyperplastic inflammatory polyps) may share some of these histopathologic characteristics; therefore, a diagnosis is possible only if there is appropriate endoscopic correlation. Sometimes the degree of histologic changes, particularly dilated capillaries, is minimal relative to the striking endoscopic appearance. This may be due to shrinkage of the vessels in biopsies with formalin fixation, and also reflects the fact that the primary and most striking leashes of abnormal vessels are in the submucosa.

Treatment

Endoscopic obliteration of the dilated vessels by **electrocoagulation** or **argon plasma coagulation** is effective and has greatly reduced the need for **antrectomy**. Recurrence (and the need for retreatment) is not uncommon. Because atrophic gastritis is a common accompaniment, patients with watermelon stomach should have biopsies taken from the mid-body greater curvature. If atrophic gastritis is present, the patient should be monitored for the development of **vitamin B$_{12}$** deficiency and dysplasia [39].

Portal hypertensive gastropathy

A proportion of patients with cirrhosis of the liver (see Chapter 97) have dilatation of the gastric mucosal vessels, more prominent in the proximal stomach; its prevalence parallels the severity of portal hypertension. Bleeding is relatively uncommon and rarely severe, except in patients with severe portal hypertension (see Chapter 97). The **endoscopic appearance** of portal hypertensive gastropathy (variously described as snake skin, mosaic, scarlatina rash, and cherry-red spots) is nonspecific and does not correlate well with the degree of portal hypertension. Because of the understandable reluctance to biopsy the stomach of a patient with apparent portal hypertensive gastropathy, the contribution of histopathology to the diagnosis of portal hypertensive gastropathy is of negligible importance.

Hypertrophic gastropathies

The classic description of hypertrophic gastropathies proposed by Ming is still useful because it serves as a scaffold that can be adapted to new and existing entities as they are recognized and better understood. The three classic types of hypertrophic gastropathy are:

1. Superficial foveolar (mucous neck region) hyperplasia with normal or atrophic deep oxyntic glands.
2. Hyperplasia of oxyntic glands with a largely unaffected mucous neck region.
3. A mixed type, in which both mucous neck and oxyntic glands show variable degrees of hyperplasia.

Type 1 corresponds to Ménétrier's disease, Type 2 to Zollinger-Ellison syndrome (see Chapter 112), and Type 3 incorporates a variety of conditions that may result from mixed glandular and foveolar hyperplasia, including:

- infections (*e.g.*, *H. pylori* infection, cytomegalovirus in children, syphilis)
- other diseases of uncertain etiology such as:
  - lymphocytic gastritis
  - eosinophilic gastroenteritis
  - sarcoidosis and
  - Cronkhite-Canada syndrome.

Ménétrier's disease

This rare condition is defined as an idiopathic diffuse enlargement of the gastric folds largely confined to the gastric body and fundus. When well established, the massive foveolar cell (mucous neck region) hyperplasia is associated with underlying **loss of parietal and chief cells**. The amount of **inflammation** is variable; some patients have multifocal superficial erosions whereas others have polypoid configurations of the hypertrophic mucosa. When accompanied by chronic active inflammation or intraepithelial lymphocytic infiltration, the large-fold variant of *H. pylori* gastritis or lymphocytic gastritis should be considered.

Clinical features

Most patients are men in their fifth or sixth decade who present with weight loss, epigastric and abdominal pain, nausea, and vomiting. The disease evolves over several years or decades, and eventually patients develop severe hypoalbuminemia as a consequence of the chronic protein loss. **Childhood Ménétrier's disease** is due to gastric cytomegalovirus infection, which may sometimes produce localized hypertrophic gastropathy in the gastric antrum or body of immunocompromised adults.

Pathology

Protein loss is caused by the large amounts of mucus and fluid secreted by hyperplastic foveolar cells. **Hypochlorhydria** is the rule in well-established cases. The pathogenesis is unknown, but it has been hypothesized that overproduction of **transforming growth factor (TGF)α** might explain several of the disturbances occurring in Ménétrier's disease. TGF, a mediator of gastric mucosal homeostasis produced by the gastric mucosa, inhibits acid secretion, stimulates mucosal repair after injury, and augments gastric mucin levels.

Treatment

A monoclonal antibody against the TGF receptor may hold some promise as a therapeutic agent. A variety of other treatments have been tried without uniform success. Occasionally, total gastrectomy is required because of the relentless hypoalbuminemia and the development of persistent anasarca. Ménétrier's disease appears to be associated with an increased risk of gastric adenocarcinoma; however, given the rarity of the disorder, it is unlikely that any cogent surveillance strategy will emerge.

Zollinger-Ellison syndrome (see Chapter 112)

The oxyntic mucosa in Zollinger-Ellison syndrome shows hyperplasia of the oxyntic compartment due to the trophic effect of circulating gastrin. As with atrophic gastritis, the hypergastrinemia can also stimulate proliferation of the ECL cells of the oxyntic mucosa, ranging from hyperplasia to the formation of gastric carcinoids.

Iatrogenic gastritis and gastropathies

Injury due to NSAIDs (hemorrhagic gastritis, erosion, ulcer, and reactive gastropathy) has been discussed above. However, a variety of therapeutic agents, including radioactive and chemical, administered orally, intravenously, and intra-arterially, can also cause damage to the gastric mucosa that is detectable endoscopically and histologically.

References

1. Marshall BJ. The 1995 Albert Lasker Medical Research Award. *Helicobacter pylori*. The etiologic agent for peptic ulcer. *JAMA*. 1995;274:1064–1066.
2. Dixon MF, Genta RM, Yardley JH, *et al*. Classification and grading of gastritis. The updated Sydney System. International workshop on the histopathology of gastritis, Houston 1994. *Am J Surg Pathol*. 1996;20:1161–1181.
3. Fennerty MB. *Helicobacter pylori*: why it still matters in 2005. *Cleve Clin J Med*. 2005;72 Suppl 2:S1–7; discussion S14–21.
4. Stolte M, Kroher G, Meining A, *et al*. A comparison of *Helicobacter pylori* and *H. heilmannii* gastritis. A matched control study involving 404 patients. *Scand J Gastroenterol*. 1997;32:28–33.
5. Elitsur Y, Adkins L, Saeed D, *et al*. *Helicobacter pylori* antibody profile in household members of children with *H. pylori* infection. *J Clin Gastroenterol*. 1999;29:178–182.
6. Luzza F, Mancuso M, Imeneo M, *et al*. Evidence favouring the gastro-oral route in the transmission of *Helicobacter pylori* infection in children. *Eur J Gastroenterol Hepatol*. 2000;12:623–627.
7. Malaty HM, Graham DY, Wattigney WA, *et al*. Natural history of *Helicobacter pylori* infection in childhood: 12-year follow-up cohort study in a biracial community. *Clin Infect Dis*. 1999;28:279–282.
8. Weyermann M, Adler G, Brenner H, *et al*. The mother as source of *Helicobacter pylori* infection. *Epidemiology*. 2006;17:332–334.
9. Yamaoka Y, Kato M, Asaka M. Geographic differences in gastric cancer incidence can be explained by differences between *Helicobacter pylori* strains. *Intern Med*. 2008;47:1077–1083.
10. Yamaoka Y, Ojo O, Fujimoto S, *et al*. *Helicobacter pylori* outer membrane proteins and gastroduodenal disease. *Gut*. 2006;55:775–781.
11. Isaacson PG, Du MQ. MALT lymphoma: from morphology to molecules. *Nat Rev Cancer*. 2004;4:644–653.
12. Correa P. A new paradigm for human carcinogenesis. *J Clin Gastroenterol*. 2000;30:341–342.
13. Cover TL, Blaser MJ. *Helicobacter pylori* in health and disease. *Gastroenterology*. 2009;136:1863–1873.
14. Genta RM, Hamner HW, Graham DY. Gastric lymphoid follicles in *Helicobacter pylori* infection: frequency, distribution, and response to triple therapy. *Hum Pathol*. 1993;24:577–583.
15. Correa P, Piazuelo MB. Natural history of *Helicobacter pylori* infection. *Dig Liver Dis*. 2008;40:490–496.
16. Sepulveda AR, Graham DY. Role of *Helicobacter pylori* in gastric carcinogenesis. *Gastroenterol Clin North Am*. 2002;31:517–35, x.
17. Malfertheiner P, Megraud F, O'Morain C, *et al*. Current concepts in the management of *Helicobacter pylori* infection: the Maastricht III Consensus Report. *Gut*. 2007;56:772–781.
18. Chey WD, Wong BC. American College of Gastroenterology guideline on the management of *Helicobacter pylori* infection. *Am J Gastroenterol*. 2007;102:1808–1825.
19. Graham DY, Yamaoka Y. One- or two-week triple therapy for *Helicobacter pylori*: questions of efficacy and inclusion of a dual therapy treatment arm. *Gut*. 2007;56:1021–1023.
20. Francavilla R, Lionetti E, Cavallo L. Sequential treatment for *Helicobacter pylori* eradication in children. *Gut*. 2008;57:1178.
21. Marshall B. Sequential therapy for *Helicobacter pylori*: a worthwhile effort for your patients. *Ann Intern Med*. 2008;148:962–963.
22. Jafri NS, Hornung CA, Howden CW. Meta-analysis: sequential therapy appears superior to standard therapy for *Helicobacter pylori* infection in patients naive to treatment. *Ann Intern Med*. 2008;148:923–931.
23. Toh BH, van D, I, Gleeson PA. Pernicious anemia. *N Engl J Med*. 1997;337:1441–1448.
24. Marshall AC, Alderuccio F, Murphy K, *et al*. Mechanisms of gastric mucosal cell loss in autoimmune gastritis. *Int Rev Immunol*. 2005;24:123–134.
25. Amedei A, Bergman MP, Appelmelk BJ, *et al*. Molecular mimicry between *Helicobacter pylori* antigens and H$^+$, K$^+$ -adenosine triphosphatase in human gastric autoimmunity. *J Exp Med*. 2003;198:1147–1156.
26. Appelmelk BJ, Faller G, Claeys D, *et al*. Bugs on trial: the case of *Helicobacter pylori* and autoimmunity. *Immunol Today*. 1998;19:296–299.
27. Negrini R. Is autoimmunity involved in the relationship between *Helicobacter pylori* infection, atrophic gastritis and gastric cancer? *Ital J Gastroenterol Hepatol*.1999;31:842–845.
28. Solcia E, Rindi G, Fiocca R, *et al*. Distinct patterns of chronic gastritis associated with carcinoid and cancer and their role in tumorigenesis. *Yale J Biol Med*. 1992;65:793–804.
29. Carmack SW, Genta RM, Graham DY, *et al*. Management of gastric polyps: a pathology-based guide for gastroenterologists. *Nat Rev Gastroenterol Hepatol*. 2009;6:331–341.
30. Rugge M, Correa P, Dixon MF, *et al*. Gastric mucosal atrophy: interobserver consistency using new criteria for classification and grading. *Aliment Pharmacol Ther*. 2002;16:1249–1259.

31. Carmack SW, Lash RH, Gulizia JM, *et al.* Lymphocytic disorders of the gastrointestinal tract: a review for the practicing pathologist. *Adv Anat Pathol.* 2009;16:290–306.

32. Haot J, Berger F, Andre C, *et al.* Lymphocytic gastritis versus varioliform gastritis. A historical series revisited. *J Pathol.* 1989; 158:19–22.

33. Ectors NL, Dixon MF, Geboes KJ, *et al.* Granulomatous gastritis: a morphological and diagnostic approach. *Histopathology.* 1993; 23:55–61.

34. Shapiro JL, Goldblum JR, Petras RE. A clinicopathologic study of 42 patients with granulomatous gastritis. Is there really an "idiopathic" granulomatous gastritis? *Am J Surg Pathol.* 1996; 20:462–470.

35. Genta RM. Differential diagnosis of reactive gastropathy. *Semin Diagn Pathol.* 2005;22:273–283.

33. El-Zimaity HM, Genta RM, Graham DY. Histological features do not define NSAID-induced gastritis. *Hum Pathol.* 1996;27: 1348–1354.

37. Laine L, Weinstein WM. Subepithelial hemorrhages and erosions of human stomach. *Dig Dis Sci.* 1988;33:490–503.

38. Gostout CJ, Viggiano TR, Ahlquist DA, *et al.* The clinical and endoscopic spectrum of the watermelon stomach. *J Clin Gastroenterol.* 1992;15:256–263.

39. Labenz J, Borsch G. Bleeding watermelon stomach treated by Nd-YAG laser photocoagulation. *Endoscopy.* 1993;25:240–242.

CHAPTER 34

Adenocarcinoma (gastric cancer and miscellaneous malignancy)

Dai-ming Fan and Kai-chun Wu

Fourth Military Medical University, Xi'an, China

ESSENTIAL FACTS ABOUT PATHOGENESIS

- Environmental factors:
  - Nitrates/nitrites
  - Excess salt
  - Lack of fresh fruits
  - Smoking
- Gene polymorphism
- *H.pylori* infection
- Chronic atrophic gastritis and intestinal metaplasia

ESSENTIALS OF DIAGNOSIS

- Symptoms: nospecific but epigastric pain, nausea and vomiting, dysphagia, weight loss are found in advanced stage
- Upper GI endoscopy: highly sensitive and specific for advanced cancer, chromoendoscopy and magnifying endoscopy useful for early cancer
- Reliable tumor markers not yet available

ESSENTIALS OF TREATMENT

- Eradication of *H.pylori* probably reduces the risk of gastric cancer
- Surgery: for resectable disease
- Early cancer: can be treated by EMR or ESD
- Chemotherapy (5-FU based) is the most common regime

Introduction and epidemiology

Gastric adenocarcinoma is the most frequently observed malignant gastric disease, and it accounts for nearly 90 to 95% of gastric neoplasms. It mostly occurs at the age of 55 to 70 years and is the second cause of all cancer deaths. Currently there is a worldwide decrease in prevalence and death rate, but there are still about 1 million new cases of gastric adenocarcinoma every year. There is a great gender and ethnic variation in the incidence of gastric cancer (Table 34.1), with the highest incidence in Japan, China, South America and Eastern Europe, and the lowest incidence in North America, Western Europe, Australia and New Zealand. At present, males are nearly 2 times more likely to have gastric adenocarcinoma than females.

Gastric adenocarcinoma can be subdivided into two subtypes: intestinal type and diffuse type. The intestinal type is better differentiated, characterized by cohesive neoplastic cells that form gland-like tubular structures. The diffuse type is less differentiated, characterized by individual cells which infiltrate and thicken the stomach wall. It results in a loss of distensibility of the gastric wall, and carries a poor prognosis. In high prevalence areas, the intestinal type is the predominant type, and is less likely to be found in areas where the frequency of gastric cancer is decreasing. In contrast, the incidence of diffuse type seems to be similar throughout the world.

Etiology and pathogenesis

Although many etiologic factors have been associated with gastric carcinoma, a definite etiology is still unknown. It is widely accepted that the development of gastric adenocarcinoma is a multifactorial and multi-step process [1] (Table 34.2).

The great geographic variation in the incidence of gastric cancer worldwide suggests that environmental factors contribute to the pathogenesis of gastric carcinogenesis. Immigrants from high- to low-incidence areas maintain their susceptibility to gastric cancer, while the risk for their offspring decreases to the level of the new areas. Epidemiologic studies find high nitrate concentrations in soil and drinking water in areas with high death rates from gastric cancer, and people in high-incidence areas prefer to ingest dried, smoked and salted foods which have a high concentration of nitrates and salt. These people also have a high prevalence of *Helicobacter pylori* infection. The nitrates are converted to carcinogenic nitrites by the bacteria. This process is enhanced by deficiency of fresh fruit, vegetables, and vitamins A and C.

Genetic factors also play an important role in gastric carcinogenesis. Epidemiologic studies have shown that gastric adenocarcinoma has familial clustering and higher prevalence rate (twice~three fold) in first degree relatives, especially in diffuse

---

Textbook of Clinical Gastroenterology and Hepatology, Second Edition. Edited by C. J. Hawkey, Jaime Bosch, Joel E. Richter, Guadalupe Garcia-Tsao, Francis K. L. Chan.
© 2012 Blackwell Publishing Ltd. Published 2012 by Blackwell Publishing Ltd.

Upper GI Tract

Table 34.1 Incidence rates of gastric cancer by race and gender in the United States

Race/ethnicity	Male (per 100,000 men)	Female (per 100,000 women)
All races	11.0	5.5
White	9.8	4.7
Black	16.8	9.0
Asian/Pacific Islander	18	10.0
American Indian/Alaska Native	15.5	7.9
Hispanic	14.9	9.3

Table 34.2 Risk factors for gastric adenocarcinoma

- Environmental:
  - nitrates/nitrites
  - excess salt
  - deficiency of fresh fruit, vegetables, vitamins A and C
  - smoking:
- Genetic:
  - familial gastric cancer
  - oncogene activation
  - tumor suppressor gene inactivation
  - DNA microsatellite instability
  - gene polymorphism:
- Infection:
  - *Helicobacter pylori* infection:
- Premalignant condition:
  - chronic atrophic gastritis and intestinal metaplasia
  - post-gastrectomy stumps

type. Several genetic mechanisms may account for the pathogenesis of gastric carcinogenesis: oncogene activation, tumor suppressor gene inactivation, DNA microsatellite instability and gene polymorphism. For example, loss of heterozygosity of the APC gene, mutation of p53 gene, and single nucleotide polymorphism of IL-1 have been observed in gastric adenocarcinoma. Patients carrying IL-1β genotype have a high rate of *H. pylori* infection and more severe mucosal inflammation, leading to increased risk of developing gastric cancer.

Retrospective and prospective studies have demonstrated a strong association between *H. pylori* infection and gastric cancer. *H. pylori* infection is significantly more common in patients with gastric cancer than in matched control groups, and more common in high cancer incidence than in low cancer incidence areas. *H. pylori* eradication can decrease the risk for gastric cancer in high-incidence areas. The mechanisms of *H. pylori*-induced gastric carcinogenesis remain unclear. Studies found that chronic atrophic gastritis and intestinal metaplasia are associated with an approximately 25-fold increase in gastric cancer. It is thought that these premalignant conditions represent intermediary steps to gastric adenocarcinoma.

Stem cell may also play an important role in the development and progression of gastric adenocarcinoma. Wang and his colleagues [2] found chronic infection with *Helicobacter* could induce the repopulation of the stomach with bone marrow-derived cells which subsequently progressed to intraepithelial cancer.

Clinical presentation

Early gastric cancer is a term which is applied to characterize early-stage of gastric adenocarcinoma. It is defined as gastric adenocarcinoma limited only to the mucosa and/or submucosa, no matter whether there is lymph node involvement and distant metastasis or not. In patients with early gastric cancer, they are often asymptomatic or have nonspecific symptoms. Physical examination may be unremarkable, so that it is difficult to diagnose gastric cancer in early-stage.

Advanced gastric adenocarcinoma is defined as gastric adenocarcinoma invaded beyond the submucosa. Epigastric pain is the most common symptom in advanced gastric adenocarcinoma, and it cannot be relieved by food or antacids. Nausea and vomiting are found in patients with gastric outlet obstruction; dysphagia and early satiety may be the major symptoms caused by diffuse lesions originating in the cardia. Weakness, fatigue, melena, hematemesis and anemia occur when the tumor bleeds. Some special signs may appear as a result of regional invasion or distant metastasis. Right upper quadrant pain, jaundice, and/or fever can occur when gastric cancer metastasizes to the liver. Lung metastases can cause cough, hiccups, and hemoptysis. Pain radiating to the back may indicate that the tumor has penetrated to the pancreas. Metastasis to the ovary is known as *Krukenberg's tumor*. In addition, intra-abdominal and supraclavicular lymph nodes are frequently involved. Left supraclavicular lymph node involvement is termed *Virchow's node*, and periumbilical nodal involvement is called *Sister Mary Joseph's node*. Physical examination may reveal an epigastric mass. Ascites, hepatomegaly, and *Virchow's node* may present when metastasis occurs.

Paraneoplastic syndromes may precede or occur concurrently. These include recurrent migratory thrombophlebitis, acanthosis nigricans, dermatomyositis and neuromyopathy.

Differential diagnosis
Benign gastric ulcer
Usually, there is no difficulty in distinguishing benign from malignant gastric ulcers by radiographic or endoscopic examination. A benign gastric ulcer is small and smooth with a regular base (Figure 34.1), whereas a malignant ulcer is large with an everted and irregular margin (Figure 34.2).

Gastric leiomyoma
Gastric leiomyoma arises from smooth muscle. It is usually located in the corpus or antrum. Radiographic examination usually reveals a smooth intramural filling defect, with or

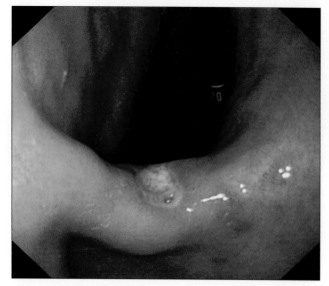

Figure 34.1 Benign gastric ulcer.

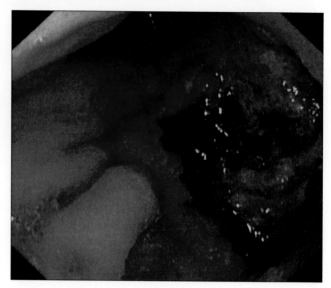

Figure 34.3 Gastric cancer in the antrum.

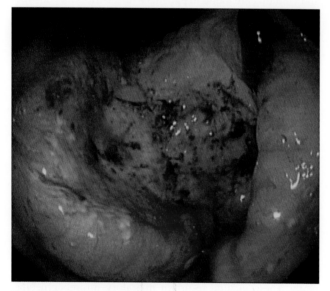

Figure 34.2 Malignant gastric ulcer.

without ulceration. Endoscopic ultrasonography is helpful in diagnosing gastric leiomyoma.

Primary gastric lymphoma

It is difficult to distinguish gastric adenocarcinoma from primary gastric lymphoma, because both of them present with similar clinical and radiographic appearance. The diagnosis of gastric lymphoma requires endoscopic biopsy or laparotomy. Microscopically, most gastric lymphoid tumors are non-Hodgkin's lymphomas that origin from B cells. Hodgkin's disease is extremely uncommon. Histologically, gastric lymphoma may range from well-differentiated, superficial disease to high-grade, large-cell lymphomas.

Diagnostic methods

Endoscopy and radiographic examination are the two main methods to diagnose gastric adenocarcinoma. Endoscopic ultrasonography, computed tomography and laboratory studies are also helpful in the diagnosis of gastric adenocarcinoma.

Upper gastrointestinal endoscopy is the first preferred diagnostic procedure. The advantages of endoscopy are that biopsies can be taken, small lesions evaluated more fully, and cancer can be localized and mapped. Gastric carcinoma of intestinal type occurs more often in the antrum (Figure 34.3), which is the area prone to *Helicobacter pylori* infection. Cancer may be detected as mucosal ulceration, polypoid mass, infiltrating lesion, or large gastric folds. When ulcers are observed, at least six biopsy specimens, from both the edge and the base of the ulcer, need to be obtained to enhance diagnostic yield. Early gastric cancer can only be found under careful examination by experienced endoscopists. Chromoendoscpy and magnifying endoscopy may improve the detection rate of early gastric cancer (Figure 34.4). Double-contrast radiographic examination is largely superseded by endoscopy. Decreased distensibility may be the only sign of a diffuse infiltrative carcinoma.

Endoscopic ultrasonography (EUS) utilizes high-frequency ultrasound transducers incorporated into the tip of a flexible endoscope. It can provide a good spatial resolution for using high-frequency sonic waves. It is often used to assess the extent and stage of tumor, including wall invasion and local lymph node involvement, and to help guide aspiration biopsies of lymph nodes to determine their features. EUS can also be used to provide accurate preoperative local staging of esophageal, pancreatic, and rectal malignancies, but distant metastases cannot be imaged satisfactorily.

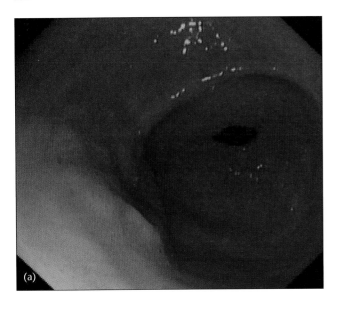
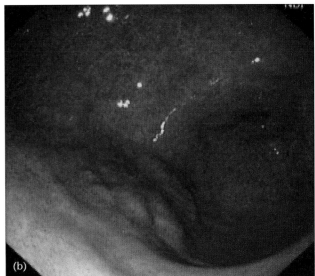
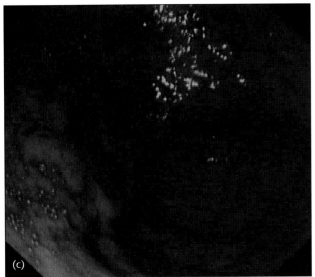

Figure 34.4 Endoscopic appearance of an early gastric cancer (a) in the antrum, (b) with narrow band imaging and (c) under chromoendoscopy.

High quality computed tomography (CT) scan is the most accurate, widely used, non-invasive performance for detecting distant metastases. Because CT scanning is excellent at detecting larger (>5 mm) or multiple metastases, abdominal and pulmonary CT scanning are performed to identify hepatic or pulmonary metastases. Usually, CT is combined with EUS to evaluate the staging of gastric tumor [3] (Table 34.3).

Laboratory studies may detect iron deficiency anemia. Abnormalities in liver tests generally may appear when distant metastases occur. Serologic markers, such as CEA and MG7, may be elevated in gastric adenocarcinoma, but there still is no sensitive and specific serologic marker available for gastric cancer.

Treatment and prevention

The only chance for cure of gastric cancer is surgical removal of the tumor and the adjacent lymph nodes. Even when the gastric cancer is not suitable for cure, palliative surgical resection is still an effective method to relieve symptoms [4]. Subtotal gastrectomy is often chosen for patients with distal cancers, but most proximal tumors need total gastrectomy. The prognosis after surgical resection depends on the staging of tumor, lymph node involvement, distant metastases and DNA aneuploidy.

Therapeutic endoscopy can also be applied to manage gastric adenocarcinoma. Early gastric cancer can be treated by endoscopic mucosal resection (EMR) or endoscopic

Table 34.3 Staging system for gastric adenocarcinoma

Stage	TNM	Characteristics
0	TisN0M0	node negative; limited to mucosa
IA	T1N0M0	node negative; invasion of lamina propria or submucosa
IB	T2N0M0	node negative; invasion of muscularis propria
II	T1N2M0 or T2N1M0	node positive; invasion beyond mucosa but within wall
	T3N0M0	node negative; extension through wall
IIIA	T2N2M0 or T3N1-2M0	node positive; invasion of muscularis propria or through wall
IIIB	T4N0-1M0	node negative; adherence to surrounding tissue
IV	T4N2M0	node positive; adherence to surrounding tissue
	T1-4N0-2M1	distant metastases

Table 34.4 Chemotherapy for gastric adenocarcinoma

Regimen	Dose	Response rate
FAM	5-FU 600 mg/m², ADM 30 mg/m², MMC 10 mg/m²	30%
EAP	VP16 120 mg/m², ADM 20 mg/m², DDP 40 mg/m²	40%
ELF	5-FU 500 mg/m², LV 200 mg/m², VP16 120 mg /m²	30%
FAMeC	5-FU 600 mg/m², ADM 30 mg/m², MeCCNU 125 mg/m²	30%
LV/FP	LV 20 mg/m², 5-FU 1000 mg/m², DDP 20 mg/m²	35–40%

 submucosal dissection (ESD) (Video 34.1). EMR is suitable for patients with intestinal type mucosal cancer less than 2 cm in diameter which has no lymph node metastasis. ESD is an innovative procedure that can remove larger lesions. For advanced gastric cancer, therapeutic endoscopy can provide palliative procedures such as stent placement and tumor ablation.

Gastric adenocarcinoma is resistant to radiotherapy. Meta-analysis shows that there is no survival benefit for radiotherapy. Radiotherapy may be applied for management of tumor bleeding, obstruction and pain as a palliative therapy.

Chemotherapy usually adopts postoperatively or preoperatively as an adjuvant therapy in patients with advanced gastric cancer, because gastric carcinoma has a low survival rate and high recurrence rates. The effect of chemotherapy with single-agent treatment is limited, with a low response rate of 20% to 30%, so combination regimens (Table 34.4) are often applied for gastric carcinoma which increases the response rate to 40% [5].

Epidemiologic studies suggest that eating more fresh fruit and vegetables, eating less salted foods and eradicating *Helicobacter pylori* can decrease the risk of gastric adenocarcinoma. The best way for prevention is to carry out an effective screening program in high-risk groups and in high-incidence areas, so that early discovery, early diagnosis and early treatment can be achieved.

Complications and their management
Bleeding
Gastric adenocarcinoma often produces chronic, occult bleeding which can result in anemia. However, acute and profuse bleeding may occur. Endoscopic therapy, angiographic therapy, or drug therapy are useful. Sometimes palliative surgery is necessary to stop bleeding.

Perforation
It is unusual to develop perforation in gastric cancer. When perforation occurs, abrupt and severe abdominal pain, abdominal muscular spasm, board-like rigidity of the abdomen, other manifestations of peritoneal irritation and shock may take place. The diagnosis can be confirmed by a plain abdominal radiograph with the patient standing. Management should start with correcting hemodynamic, fluid, and electrolyte imbalances, and emergency surgery is usually necessary.

Obstruction
This is often found in patients with tumors originating from the pylorus and cardia. Early satiety, nausea, vomiting, dysphagia, and weight loss are the main symptoms and signs for obstruction. Nasogastric suction, endoscopic stenting and palliative surgical resection are helpful.

Prognosis with or without treatment
About one third of patients who undergo a curative surgical resection are alive after 5 years. However, the survival of patients without any treatment is about 1 year. The overall 5-year survival rate in patients with gastric cancer is approximately 10%. The staging and TNM classification is the best prognostic indicator. Lymph node involvement, regional extension, distant metastases and tumor cell DNA aneuploidy often indicate poor prognosis.

> **SOURCES OF INFORMATION FOR PATIENTS AND DOCTORS**
>
> http://seer.cancer.gov/

References

1. Arend WP, Armitage JO, Clemmons DR, *et al. Cecil Medicine.* 23rd edition. 2007.

2. Houghton JM, Stoicov C, Nomura S, *et al.* Gastric cancer originating from bone marrow-derived cells. *Science.* 2004; 306(5701:1568.

3. Fauci AS, Kasper DL, Longo DL, *et al. Harrison's Principles of Internal Medicine.* 17th edition. 2008.

4. Feldman M, Scharschmidt BF, Sleisenger MH. *Sleisenger & Fordtran's Gastrointestinal and Liver Disease.* 6th edition. 2001. p. 733–748.

5. Allum WH, Griffin SM, Watson A, *et al.* Guidelines for the management of oesophageal and gastric cancer. *Gut.* 2002;Suppl5:v1–23.

CHAPTER 35

Gastric lymphoma

Andrea Grin[1] and Runjan Chetty[2]

[1]University of Toronto, Toronto, ON, Canada
[2]Oxford University Hospitals Trust, University of Oxford, Oxford, UK

ESSENTIALS FACTS ABOUT PATHOGENESIS

- Due to infection by *Helicobacter pylori* for most cases of MALT lymphoma and some cases of diffuse large B-cell lymphoma (DLBCL)
- Chronic infection leads to T-cell mediated B-cell proliferation and eventually results in deregulated monoclonal B-cell proliferation
- Recurrent chromosomal translocations, most commonly t(11;18), leads to *Helicobacter*-independent proliferation

ESSENTIALS OF DIAGNOSIS

- Signs and symptoms: non-specific; abdominal pain, anorexia, dyspepsia common
- Endoscopy: non-specific; may mimic gastritis or adenocarcinoma
- Pathology: endoscopic biopsy for histology and immunohistochemistry required
- Molecular diagnostics: the translocation t(11;18) predicts poor response to antibiotics. Difficult cases may require PCR for monoclonality

ESSENTIALS OF TREATMENT AND PROGNOSIS

Early-stage MALT
- *Helicobacter* eradication
- >80% 5-year survival

Helicobacter-negative, unresponsive Helicobacter-positive cases or cases with recurrent chromosomal translocation
- Single-agent chemotherapy, immunotherapy (rituximab) or radiotherapy

Advanced-stage MALT
- Chemotherapy or radiotherapy
- Not curative: treat symptoms and complications

Diffuse large B-cell lymphoma:
- Multi-agent chemotherapy and immunotherapy (R-CHOP)

Introduction and epidemiology

Primary gastric lymphoma is defined as a lymphoma that is predominantly located in the stomach. Lymph nodes, contiguous organs, other mucosal sites, and/or bone marrow may or may not be involved, but do not represent the major site of disease. Primary gastric lymphoma represents 1–5% of all gastric malignancies, but makes up 60–75% of all primary gastrointestinal non-Hodgkin lymphomas. While many histologic subtypes may occur in the stomach, **mucosa-associated lymphoid tissue (MALT) lymphoma** and **diffuse large B-cell lymphoma (DLBCL)** are the most common and account for >90% of cases (Table 35.1). The mean age at diagnosis is 57–64 years and men are affected slightly more often than women.

Causes and pathogenesis
Helicobacter pylori

Epidemiological studies have detected *H. pylori* in 60–90% of gastric MALT lymphoma cases [1,2] and the incidence of gastric MALT is higher in regions where *H. pylori* is endemic. Treatment of *H. pylori* infection results in complete regression of early-stage MALT and seropositive patients are more likely to develop gastric MALT lymphoma [3]. Primary DLBCL of the stomach may occur secondary to transformation from MALT lymphoma or may arise *de novo*. *H. pylori* is detected in approximately 35–55% of DLBCL cases.

Proposed mechanism of lymphomagenesis

H. pylori mediates lymphomagenesis through a mechanism of chronic antigen-dependent immune stimulation. Following infection with *H. pylori*, polyclonal B cells that are cross-reactive to auto-antigens proliferate with the help of *H. pylori*-specific T cells. Chronic infection leads to DNA damage, which inactivates cell cycle regulators and results in **monoclonal proliferation of B cells**. These cells remain dependent on *H. pylori* antigen stimulation and are susceptible to *H. pylori* eradication therapy until a chromosomal translocation occurs.

Cytogenetic and molecular alterations

The most common chromosomal translocation, occurring in approximately 30% of MALT lymphoma cases, is the **t(11;18) (q21;q21) translocation**, which results in fusion of the apoptosis inhibitor gene *API2* to the *MALT1* gene. Other translocations occur less frequently and include t(1;14)(p22;q32) and t(14;18)(q32;q21), which fuse the *BCL10* and *MALT1* genes,

Table 35.1 Frequency of histologic lymphoma types in the stomach

Histologic type	Percentage
DLBCL	56
With MALT	13
Without MALT	43
MALT	40
Peripheral T cell	1.5
Burkitt's/lymphoblastic	0.8
Mantle cell	0.7
Follicular	0.5

DLBCL, diffuse large B-cell lymphoma; MALT, mucosa-associated lymphoid tissue.

Table 35.2 Histological scoring of lymphoid infiltrate according to Wotherspoon *et al.* [4]

Score	Diagnosis	Histological features
0	Normal	Scattered plasma cells in lamina propria No lymphoid follicles
1	Chronic active gastritis	Small clusters of lymphocytes in lamina propria No lymphoid follicles No lymphoepithelial lesions
2	Chronic active gastritis with florid lymphoid follicle formation	Prominent lymphoid follicles with surrounding mantle zone and plasma cells No lymphoepithelial lesions
3	Suspicious lymphoid infiltrate, probably reactive	Lymphoid follicles surrounded by small lymphocytes that infiltrate diffusely in lamina propria and occasionally into epithelium
4	Suspicious lymphoid infiltrate, probably lymphoma	Lymphoid follicles surrounded by marginal zone cells that infiltrate diffusely in lamina propria and into epithelium in small groups
5	MALT lymphoma	Presence of dense infiltrate of marginal zone cells in lamina propria with prominent lymphoepithelial lesions

MALT, mucosa-associated lymphoid tissue.

respectively, to the IGH locus on chromosome 14. Primary gastric DLBCL may be t(11;18) positive; additional genetic alterations involve *BCL6*, *c-MYC*, and *p53*.

Clinical presentation

Abdominal pain is the most common symptom (75%), followed by anorexia and weight loss. **Weight loss** is related to disease location, as other B symptoms, such as fever and night sweats, are rare. Many patients also often complain of gastritis-like symptoms, such as **dyspepsia with nausea and vomiting**, which may contribute to delayed diagnosis. **Gastric bleeding** is present in approximately 20–30% of patients, but obstruction and perforation are uncommon. A palpable mass is only present in cases of advanced-stage or aggressive histology.

Differential diagnosis

Early MALT lymphoma may be difficult to distinguish from **chronic gastritis**. Widely infiltrative centrocyte-like cells and lymphoepithelial lesions favor MALT lymphoma, as outlined in the Wotherspoon histologic index (Table 35.2) [4]. B-cell monoclonality may be useful in some cases; however, monoclonal B cells may be detected in some cases of chronic gastritis.

MALT lymphoma typically shows a CD20+, CD5–, CD10–, Bcl-6, cyclin D1-immunophenotype. Aberrant expression of CD43 also supports the diagnosis of MALT lymphoma.

Cases of well-established gastric DLBCL may mimic adenocarcinoma and other aggressive lymphomas, such as Burkitt's lymphoma and the blastoid variant of mantle cell lymphoma. Immunohistochemistry and molecular diagnostics are useful diagnostic adjuncts in making this distinction.

Diagnostic investigation

Initial diagnosis relies on an adequate **biopsy** of sufficient size and depth to allow for initial histological interpretation with immunohistochemical stains (Figure 35.1). Superficial mucosal biopsies may be inconclusive. Sufficient material for additional molecular and cytogenetic investigations may also be required when the histological appearance is inconclusive, and are also important for prognosis and treatment. Polymerase chain reaction (PCR) and fluorescence *in situ* hybridization (FISH) may be performed on formalin-fixed, paraffin-embedded tissue.

Gastric MALT lymphoma may be multifocal; therefore, endoscopic biopsies at multiple sites are required to evaluate the extent of disease. Biopsies must be examined closely for *H. pylori*, using special stains if needed. If negative histologically, further tests for *H. pylori* (stool antigen test or urea breath test) should be done.

Multiple staging systems for primary gastric lymphoma exist (Table 35.3). An International Workshop in 1994 proposed the Lugano staging system, which is widely used. The Paris staging system is based on a TNM classification and is also in use.

Regardless of the system used, staging investigations are similar. Complete staging includes a physical examination

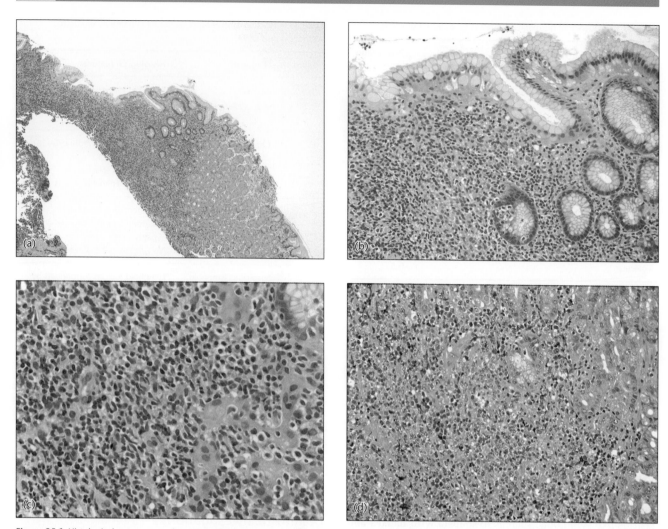

Figure 35.1 Histological appearance of gastric lymphoma. (a) Low power view of gastric mucosa-associated lymphoid tissue (MALT) lymphoma showing infiltration of the lamina propria. (b, c) The infiltrate is composed of small lymphocytes with a monocytoid appearance invading and destroying mucosal glands. (d) Diffuse large B-cell lymphoma of the stomach composed of sheets of large lymphoid cells.

Table 35.3 Comparison of the Lugano and Paris staging systems for primary gastrointestinal lymphomas

Lugano staging system		TNM Paris system	Tumor extension
Stage I	Confined to GI tract (single primary site or multiple, non-contiguous lesions)	T1N0M0	Mucosa, submucosa
		T2N0M0	Muscularis propria
		T3N0M0	Serosa
Stage II	Extending into abdomen		
	II₁ = local (para-gastric lymph nodes)	T1–3N1M0	Peri-gastric lymph nodes
	II₂ = distant (mesenteric, para-aortic, para-caval, pelvic, inguinal nodes)	T1–3N2M0	More distant regional lymph nodes
Stage IIE	Penetration of serosal to involve adjacent organs	T4N0M0	Invasion of adjacent organs
Stage IV	Disseminated extranodal involvement, or supra-diaphragmatic nodal involvement	T1–4N3M0	Spread to extra-abdominal lymph nodes
		T1–4,N0–3, M1	Distant metastases

with particular attention to peripheral lymphadenopathy and non-gastric MALT sites (Waldeyer's ring, eyes, skin). Laboratory investigations should include lactate dehydrogenase (LDH) and β₂-microglobulin. Bone marrow aspiration and biopsy is important as approximately 10% of cases are involved.

Accurate staging requires assessment of extent of disease, which may be evaluated using **computed tomography (CT)** scan with contrast. **Endoscopic ultrasound** has been shown to be more accurate in assessment of depth of invasion and locoregional lymph node involvement. Positron emission tomography (PET) scanning has been shown to be useful in DLBCL cases, but remains controversial in MALT lymphoma staging.

Treatment and prevention

While surgery was once considered the mainstay of treatment for gastric lymphoma, it is now reserved for the treatment of complications. Initial therapy for *H. pylori*-positive, gastric MALT lymphoma is **antibiotics** (oral omeprazole 20 mg b.i.d., clarithromycin 500 mg b.i.d., and either metronidazole 500 mg b.i.d. or amoxicillin 1000 mg b.i.d. for 1 week). Successful treatment of *H. pylori* may be verified with a **urea breath test** 1 month following antibiotic treatment. Close endoscopic follow-up of early-stage MALT lymphoma is recommended for evaluation of treatment response and to exclude large cell transformation. Endoscopy with biopsy every 3–6 months in the first year, followed by 6-month to 1-year intervals thereafter, is generally recommended.

Patients with successful eradication of *H. pylori* but residual lymphoma may be closely monitored or referred for further oncological treatment. A watch and wait strategy with regular endoscopies may be justified in patients with minimal histological residual disease as approximately one-third enter into late complete remission more than 12 months post-*H. pylori* eradication.

Patients with early-stage MALT resistant to antibiotics, who are negative for *H. pylori* or with recurrent translocations, are less likely to benefit from antibiotics. In these cases, locoregional radiotherapy or single-agent chemotherapy may be used. Radiotherapy is effective in achieving complete remission with 5-year disease-free and overall survival rates of 98% and 77%, respectively, in up to 90% of patients. Similarly, oral alkylating agents (chlorambucil or cyclophosphamide) or rituximab have shown similar results.

The treatment of DLBCL of the stomach is similar to its treatment at other anatomical sites. Chemo-immunotherapy using rituximab, cyclophosphamide, doxorubicin, vincristine, and prednisone (R-CHOP) is standard, with the possible addition of consolidation radiotherapy.

Treatment-related complications

Transient complications of gastric radiation include **anorexia, nausea, and vomiting**. Late toxicities are rarely severe and may include **ulceration, pancreatitis, and edema** [4,5]. Second malignancies may rarely occur in the radiation field. Perforation has been reported as a very rare late complication.

Patients receiving chemotherapy may become leukopenic. Bleeding may occur in 3–11% of patients with gastric DLBCL during chemotherapy, but rarely requires active surgical intervention such as angiography or gastrectomy. Gastric outlet obstruction secondary to scarring and fibrosis may occur as a late complication of chemotherapy, but perforation occurs very rarely.

Prognosis with and without treatment

MALT lymphoma is an indolent disease with a very good prognosis. The most important prognostic factor is disease stage: early-stage disease has a greater than 85% 5-year survival.

MALT lymphoma with the t(11;18) translocation often shows poor response to antibiotics and is locally aggressive, but has a low risk of large cell transformation.

Approximately 5–10% of patients with low-grade MALT who achieve complete remission status following *H. pylori* eradication relapse, due to re-infection with *H. pylori* [5].

MALT lymphoma with large cell transformation has a worse prognosis than MALT alone, but a better prognosis than primary DLBCL of the stomach. Five-year survival rates range from 73% to 84% for MALT with areas of DLBCL and 56–64% for DLBCL alone [6].

SOURCES OF INFORMATION FOR PATIENTS AND DOCTORS

http://www.nccn.org/professionals/physician_gls/PDF/nhl.pdf

References

1. Nakamura S, Yao T, Aoyagi K, Iida M, Fujishima M, Tsuneyoshi M. *Helicobacter pylori* and primary gastric lymphoma. A histopathologic and immunohistochemical analysis of 237 patients. *Cancer.* 1997;79:3–11.
2. Wotherspoon AC, Ortiz-Hidalgo C, Falzon MR, Isaacson PG. *Helicobacter pylori*-associated gastritis and primary B-cell gastric lymphoma. *Lancet.* 1991;338:1175–1176
3. Parsonnet J, Hansen S, Rodriguez L, *et al. Helicobacter pylori* infection and gastric lymphoma. *N Engl J Med.* 1994;330:1267–1271.
4. Wotherspoon AC, Doglioni C, Diss TC, Pan L, Moschini A, de Boni M, et al. Regression of primary low-grade B-cell gastric lymphoma of mucosa-associated lymphoid tissue type after eradication of *Helicobacter pylori. Lancet.* 1993;342:575–577.
5. Wundisch T, Thiede C, Morgner A, *et al.* Long-term follow-up of gastric MALT lymphoma after *Helicobacter pylori* eradication. *J Clin Oncol.* 2005;23:8018–8024.
6. Ferreri AJ, Freschi M, Dell'Oro S, Viale E, Villa E, Ponzoni M. Prognostic significance of the histopathologic recognition of low- and high-grade components in stage I-II B-cell gastric lymphomas. *Am J Surg Pathol.* 2001;25:95–102.

CHAPTER 36

Esophageal motility disorders

Peter J. Kahrilas

Feinberg School of Medicine, Northwestern University, Chicago, IL, USA

ESSENTIAL FACTS ABOUT PATHOGENESIS

- The best defined esophageal motility disorders are achalasia, reflux disease (Chapter 27), and diffuse esophageal spasm (DES)
- Achalasia is caused by autoimmune destruction of the esophageal myenteric plexus
- The neuromuscular pathology responsible for DES is unknown
- Esophageal dysmotility can occur as a secondary phenomenon in systemic diseases including scleroderma (Chapter 110), diabetes, malignancy, and Chagas disease
- Scleroderma and other collagen vascular diseases can be associated with connective tissue replacement of the esophageal muscularis propria

ESSENTIALS OF DIAGNOSIS

- Most common symptoms of motility disorders: dysphagia, chest pain, and heartburn
- Dysphagia for both solids and liquids is suggestive of a motility disorder like achalasia whereas uniquely solid food dysphagia suggests mechanical obstruction
- Severe regurgitation of retained esophageal contents, nocturnal aspiration and pulmonary complications can be the initial presentation of advanced achalasia
- Chest pain is frequent early in the course of achalasia
- DES is characterized by intermittent dysphagia and chest pain
- Differential diagnosis of achalasia includes Chagas disease and pseudoachalasia due to tumour infiltration (especially in older patients)
- Barium swallow and high resolution manometry can establish the diagnosis of achalasia

ESSENTIALS OF TREATMENT

- Achalasia: nitrates, calcium channel blockers, sildenafil, local injection of botulinum toxin, pneumatic dilatation and myotomy
- The laparoscopic Heller myotomy has become the preferred surgical procedure for achalasia
- DES: nitrates, calcium channel blockers, hydralazine, botulinum toxin and anxiolytics, although controlled data are limited

Introduction

A working, albeit restrictive, definition of an esophageal motility disorder is, "an esophageal disease attributable to symptomatic neuromuscular dysfunction in the smooth muscle, commonly associated with dysphagia, chest pain or heartburn." Employing this definition, there are relatively few primary esophageal motility disorders: achalasia, diffuse esophageal spasm (DES), absent peristalsis, and gastroesophageal reflux disease (see Chapter 28). Esophageal motility disorders can also be secondary phenomena in which case esophageal dysfunction is part of a more global disease as is the case with pseudoachalasia, Chagas disease, and scleroderma. Not included in this discussion are disease entities affecting the pharynx and proximal esophagus, impairment of which is almost always part of a more global neuromuscular disease process. Thus, the major focus of this chapter will be on the primary motility disorders, particularly achalasia and diffuse esophageal spasm. Mention will be made of the secondary motility disorders only to illustrate unique features.

A number of other manometric findings such as hypertensive or hypotensive peristalsis have been proposed as "esophageal motility disorders" during the last 30 years. However, the heterogeneity among these patients, combined with the absence of specific pathology or well-defined clinical implications, exclude them from the above definition of esophageal motility disorders [1], arguing to categorize them as "manometric variants" which is the nomenclature used hereafter.

Achalasia

Epidemiology

The incidence of achalasia is about 1/100,000 population, affecting both genders equally and usually presenting between age 25 and 60. Because achalasia is a chronic condition, its prevalence greatly exceeds its incidence; estimates range from 7.1–13.4/100,000. Achalasia has been reported in monozygotic twins, siblings, and children of affected parents. However, achalasia has also been reported in only one of a pair of monozygotic twins arguing against a strong genetic determinant. Emphasizing this point, a survey of 1012 first-degree relatives of 159 achalasics identified no affected relatives. A predisposing genotype has not been identified except in the rare triple A (alacrima, optic atrophy and achalasia) syndrome.

Textbook of Clinical Gastroenterology and Hepatology, Second Edition. Edited by C. J. Hawkey, Jaime Bosch, Joel E. Richter, Guadalupe Garcia-Tsao, Francis K. L. Chan.

Causes, risk factors, disease associations

The neuroanatomic change responsible for achalasia is loss of ganglion cells within the myenteric plexus. Excitatory (cholinergic) ganglionic neurons are potentially affected and inhibitory (nitric oxide) ganglionic neurons are necessarily impaired. Functionally, these neurons mediate deglutitive inhibition (including LES relaxation) and the propagation of peristalsis. Their absence explains the key physiologic abnormalities of achalasia: impaired LES relaxation and absent peristalsis. The degree of ganglion cell loss parallels disease duration with virtual aganglionosis being noted in long-standing cases. No risk factors for achalasia have been identified. Parkinson's disease and achalasia share many common features and may be related.

Pathogenesis

The ultimate cause of ganglion cell degeneration in achalasia is gradually being unraveled, with increasing evidence of an **autoimmune process** attributable to a latent infection with **human herpes virus 1 (HSV-1)** combined with genetical susceptibility [2]. Antibodies against myenteric neurons have been repeatedly shown in serum of achalasia patients especially in patients with HLA DQA1*0103 and DQB1*0603 alleles. Furthermore, anti-HSV-1 antibodies and HSV-1 DNA were isolated in 84% and 63% of achalasics, respectively, potentially implicating HSV-1 in the majority of achalasia cases.

Pathology

The destruction of ganglion cells in the esophageal wall of achalasics is associated with disintegration of the axoplasm and myelin sheaths within the vagus nerve supplying the esophagus and degenerative changes in the dorsal motor nucleus of the vagus. With respect to the esophagus itself, long-standing achalasia is characterized by progressive dilatation and sigmoidization of the esophageal body with hypertrophy of the LES. However the myosites themselves are microscopically normal. These changes are less pronounced early in the course of the disease.

Clinical presentation

Clinical manifestations of achalasia may include dysphagia, regurgitation, chest pain, weight loss, and aspiration pneumonia.

Most patients report **solid and liquid food dysphagia**. With a dilated esophagus and absent peristalsis, patients often compensate by eating slowly, drinking a lot while eating, and straightening the back, raising their arms, or standing while swallowing. Strangely, despite the severe dysphagia, significant weight loss is unusual.

Regurgitation occurs when food, fluid, and secretions are retained in the dilated esophagus. The regurgitant is often recognized as food that has been eaten hours, or even days, previously. It tends to be non-bilious, non-acid, and mixed with copious amounts of saliva that has mucoid characteristics, often described as slime by the patient. Some

patients induce vomiting to relieve the associated discomfort. Classically, patients will complain of regurgitant on their bed sheets and have often found it necessary to sleep with several pillows or upright in a chair. Patients with advanced achalasia are at risk for **bronchopulmonary complications** (bronchitis, pneumonia, or lung abscess) from chronic regurgitation and aspiration.

Chest pain is frequent early in the course of achalasia (**spastic achalasia**), and is usually thought to result from esophageal spasm. Patients describe a squeezing, pressure-like retrosternal pain, sometimes radiating to the neck, arms, jaw, and back. Paradoxically, many patients complain of heartburn. However, an unresolved issue is whether or not this "heartburn" is related to gastroesophageal reflux or simply the patient's way of perceiving and/or reporting esophageal pain. Treatment of achalasia is less effective in relieving chest pain than it is in relieving dysphagia or regurgitation. However, unlike dysphagia or regurgitation, chest pain may improve spontaneously.

An interesting, but fortunately rare, symptom of achalasia is airway compromise and stridor as a result of the dilated esophagus compressing the membranous trachea. In severe cases, this condition may require emergency treatment.

Differential diagnosis

The distinction between spastic achalasia and diffuse esophageal spasm can be subtle [3]. The differential diagnosis also includes Chagas disease and pseudoachalasia. These disorders may resemble achalasia so closely that conventional diagnostic tests are misleading. A rare genetic achalasia syndrome, **Familial adrenal insufficiency with alacrima**, has also been described. This is inherited as an autosomal recessive trait that manifests itself with the childhood onset of autonomic nervous system dysfunction including achalasia.

Chagas disease

Chagas disease is endemic in areas of central Brazil, Venezuela, and northern Argentina. Chagas disease is spread by the bite of reduvid (kissing) bug that transmits the culprit protozoan, *Trypanosoma cruzi*. After infection, an acute septicemia develops that varies in severity from being unnoticed to being fatal. The chronic phase of the disease develops years later and results from destruction of autonomic ganglion cells throughout the body, including the heart, gut, urinary tract, and respiratory tract. Chronic cardiomyopathy with conduction system disturbances and arrhythmias is the most common cause of death. The digestive tract organs most often affected are the esophagus, duodenum, and colon resulting in megaesophagus, megaduodenum, or megacolon. The **diagnosis** of Chagas disease is confirmed by a serologic test utilizing complement fixation or polymerase chain reaction.

Pseudoachalasia

Tumor infiltration (especially carcinoma in the gastric fundus) can completely mimic the functional impairment seen with idiopathic achalasia. The resultant pseudoachalasia accounts for up to 5% of suspected cases and is more likely with advanced age, abrupt onset of symptoms (<1yr), and weight loss in excess of 7 kg. Hence, endoscopy should be part of the initial evaluation of achalasia. A clue to the presence of pseudoachalasia is feeling more than slight resistance as the endoscope traverses the gastroesophageal junction. If suspicious of pseudoachalasia, endoscopic biopsy, computed tomography, magnetic resonance imaging, or endoscopic ultrasound should be considered for further evaluation.

Adenocarcinoma of the stomach accounts for more than half of pseudoachalasia cases with a myriad of tumors (pancreatic, oat cell, hepatoma, bronchogenic, esophageal squamous cell, prostate, lymphoma) accounting for the remainder. These tumors produce an achalasia syndrome by infiltrating the wall of the esophagus, in essence causing a malignant obstruction at the LES with proximal esophageal dilatation.

Similarly, pseudoachalasia can result from esophageal infiltration by **amyloid, sphingolipids, eosinophilic esophagitis, and sarcoidosis** or mechanical obstruction by **pancreatic pseudocysts, neurofibromatosis**, or most recently **lapband prostheses** used in bariatric surgery. Although often mentioned in the literature, it is exceedingly rare that an achalasic syndrome occurs as a paraneoplastic syndrome without direct tumor stenosis of the esophagogastric junction.

Diagnostic methods

A barium swallow X-ray or esophageal manometry can demonstrate the anatomic and physiologic abnormalities of achalasia.

Radiology

The characteristic X-ray is of a dilated intra-thoracic esophagus with impaired emptying, an air-fluid level, absence of a gastric air bubble, and an esophagogastric junction that tapers to a point giving the distal esophagus a beak-like appearance. Occasionally, an epiphrenic diverticulum is observed. With long-standing achalasia, the esophagus may assume a **sigmoid configuration**. In any event, the characteristic radiographic findings depend upon esophageal dilatation that is not present early in the course of the disease, thereby accounting for radiography's limited sensitivity.

Esophageal manometry

With esophageal manometry, intraluminal pressure sensors quantify the contractility of the esophagus and its sphincters. With high resolution manometry, sufficient pressure sensors are employed such that intraluminal pressure can be monitored as a continuum along the length of the esophagus, much as time is viewed as a continuum in line tracings of conventional manometry. When high resolution manometry is coupled with algorithms to display data as pressure topography plots, esophageal contractility is visualized with isobaric conditions among sensors indicated by isocoloric regions on the pressure topography plots. Figure 36.1a depicts a normal swallow in a high resolution esophageal pressure topography plot encompassing both sphincters and the intervening esophagus; the relative timing of sphincter relaxation and segmental peristaltic contractions are all readily demonstrated. Apart from improving the sensitivity of manometry in the detection of achalasia, high resolution esophageal pressure topography has also defined a clinically relevant subclassification of achalasia [4]. A diagnosis of achalasia requires both absent peristalsis and impaired deglutitive EGJ relaxation [5]. In its most obvious form, this occurs with negligible pressurization within the esophagus (Figure 36.1b). Alternatively, there can still be substantial esophageal pressurization. In fact, a very common pattern encountered is achalasia with esophageal compression and pan-esophageal pressurization (Figure 36.1c). The third, less common pattern is of spastic achalasia in which there is a spastic contraction within the distal esophageal segment (Figure 36.1d). In a series of 99 consecutive patients with newly diagnosed achalasia, 21 had the pattern in Figure 36.1b, 49 the pattern of Figure 36.1c, and 29 the pattern of Figure 36.1d [4].

Endoscopy

Endoscopy is relatively insensitive in the detection of achalasia except in advanced disease but is valuable to rule out pseudoachalasia. In advanced disease, the esophagus may be so full of food as to require lavage or even days of a liquid diet before endoscopy is feasible. With progressive dilatation and stasis, erythema, friability, and superficial ulcerations may be seen. Whitish plaque consistent with *Candida* can be seen; this is usually asymptomatic. The achalasic LES has a pinpoint appearance and does not open with air insufflation. Nonetheless, the instrument should pass with minimal pressure applied. Resistance, or a feeling of stiffness as the endoscope crosses the gastroesophageal junction, should raise the suspicion of pseudoachalasia and any visible abnormalities should be biopsied.

Treatment

Because there is no known way of preventing or reversing achalasia, treatments are aimed at reducing lower esophageal sphincter pressure. This can be done by pharmacologic therapy, forceful dilation, or surgical myotomy.

The optimal approach is debatable given the lack of high quality treatment trials and the failure of any existing trials to account for the variable response rates among the recently described achalasia subtypes; logistic regression analysis found achalasia with esophageal compression (Figure 36.1c) to be a predictor of positive treatment response while spastic achalasia (Figure 36.1d) and absent pressurization (Figure 36.1b) were predictive of negative treatment response.

Pharmacological therapy

Nitrates or calcium channel blockers, administered prior to eating, can relieve dysphagia in achalasics by reducing LES pressure. An uncontrolled trial of isosorbide dinitrate

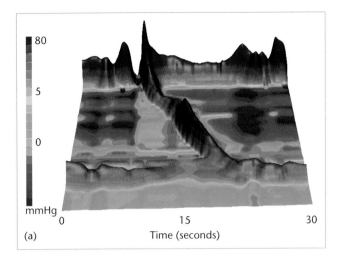

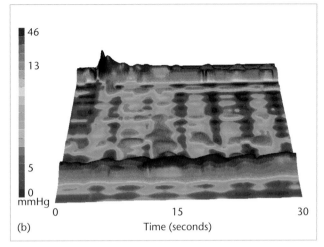

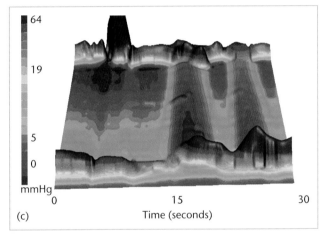

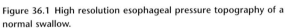

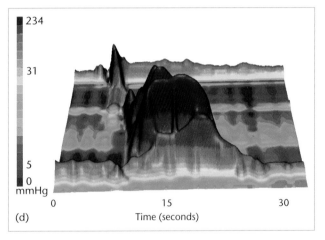

Figure 36.1 High resolution esophageal pressure topography of a normal swallow.

(a) and three subtypes of achalasia: classic (b), with esophageal compression (c) and spastic achalasia (d). All are characterized by impaired LES relaxation and absent peristalsis. However classic achalasia has minimal pressurization of the esophageal body while substantial fluid pressurization is observed in achalasia with esophageal compression and rapidly propagated spastic contractions are observed with spastic achalasia. The conventional term "vigorous" achalasia could be used to describe either Panel b or c which have extremely different treatment outcomes.

(Isordil™) reported marked relief of dysphagia but prominent side effects, particularly headache. Nifedipine™ (Procardia™) 10–30 mg was significantly better than placebo in a group of patients with early achalasia followed for 6–18 months. However, subsequent placebo-controlled crossover trials have found minimal benefit with nifedipine and limiting side effects, especially flushing, dizziness, headache, peripheral edema, and orthostasis.

Sildenafil™ decreases LES pressure by blocking the enzyme that destroys cyclic guanosine monophosphate induced by nitric oxide. In a double-blinded placebo controlled trial, 50 mg of sildenafil caused a significant decrease in LES pressure and relaxation pressure [6]. Therapeutic trials for achalasia have not yet been done.

Botulinum toxin injection

Botulinum toxin is a potent inhibitor of acetylcholine release from nerve endings. In achalasia, 80–100 units of botulinum toxin are injected into the LES with a sclerotherapy catheter.

The toxin binds to presynaptic, parasympathetic nerve endings reducing the non-myogenic component of LES pressure. Using this technique, Pasricha reported improved dysphagia in 66% of achalasics for 6 months [7]. However, the botulinum toxin effect is eventually reversed by axonal regeneration and subsequent studies report minimal continued efficacy after one year [8].

Pneumatic dilation

An achalasia dilator is a non-compliant, cylindrical balloon that can be positioned across the LES and inflated to a diameter of at least 3 cm. The only design currently available in the US, the **Rigiflex™ dilator**, is positioned fluoroscopically over a guidewire and is available in 3.0, 3.5, and 4.0 cm diameters. A European alternative is the **Witzel™ dilator**, a polyethylene balloon mounted onto an endoscope overtube so that the retroflexed endoscope can be used to monitor balloon position during inflation.

A cautious approach to dilation with the Rigiflex dilators is to initially use the 3 cm dilator and follow up with a 3.5 cm dilation 2–4 weeks later if the initial dilation was insufficient. The reported efficacy of dilation ranges from 32% to 98% [8]. Patients with a poor result or rapid recurrence of dysphagia are unlikely to respond to additional dilations but subsequent response to myotomy is not influenced.

The **major complication** of pneumatic dilation is esophageal perforation with a reported incidence ranging from 1 to 5%. Most perforations are clinically obvious but cautious practitioners routinely obtain a fluoroscopic examination following every pneumatic dilation. If a perforation appears confined, or intramural, conservative management is appropriate. If any substantial leak has occurred, or if worsening pain and fever occur during observation, **surgical repair** should be pursued quickly. Patients with perforation from pneumatic dilation that is surgically repaired within 6–8 hours have outcomes comparable to patients undergoing elective Heller myotomy.

Heller myotomy

The most common surgical procedure for achalasia is a myotomy, sometimes accompanied by an anti-reflux procedure (partial fundoplication). Myotomy can be carried out laparoscopically as well as through a thoracotomy. The appeal of myotomy is that it is more predictable than pneumatic dilation with surgical series reporting good to excellent results in 62–100% of patients [8] and 95% symptom resolution versus 51% in one controlled trial [9].

Laparoscopic myotomy is effective and much less invasive than an open procedure and is increasingly used at an early stage. In a recent report of 136 achalasics who underwent laparoscopic myotomy accompanied by a partial fundoplication there was one death and only 3 patients required conversion to an open procedure [10]. Relief of dysphagia was obtained in 93%, with failure usually attributable to extreme esophageal dilatation. Thus, laparoscopic Heller myotomy has become the preferred surgical procedure for achalasia.

Treatment failures

Occasionally, patients fail to respond to even a well done pneumatic dilation or myotomy. In such refractory cases of achalasia, esophageal resection with gastric pull-up or interposition of a segment of transverse colon may be the only option other than gastrostomy feeding. Indications for this intervention include irresolvable dysphagia, cancer, and perforation during dilation. Although excellent long term functional results can be achieved, the reported mortality of this surgery is about 4%, consistent with the mortality rate of esophagectomy done for other indications.

Complications and management

In achalasia, esophageal dilatation predisposes to **aspiration** and **stasis esophagitis**. Aspiration is best dealt with by effective treatment of achalasia, whether pneumatic dilation or surgery. Prolonged stasis esophagitis is the likely explanation for the association between achalasia and **esophageal squamous cell cancer**. Tumors develop after years of achalasia, usually in a greatly dilated esophagus. A population-based analysis in Sweden suggested that the overall squamous cell cancer risk for achalasics was increased 17-fold compared to controls.

Diffuse esophageal spasm

Epidemiology

No population-based studies exist on the prevalence of other esophageal motility disorders. Referencing their detection rate to that of achalasia, the prevalence of diffuse esophageal spasm is similar to that of achalasia (or lower if more restrictive diagnostic criteria are utilized) while the prevalence of the "manometric variants" is up to ten times greater.

Causes, risk factors and disease associations

The neuromuscular pathology responsible for diffuse esophageal spasm is unknown. As for risk factors and conditions associated with diffuse esophageal spasm, none are established. Certainly "manometric variants" and esophageal spasm occur more commonly in patients with gastroesophageal reflux disease, but in such cases it is probably best to think of the reflux disease as the parent entity.

Pathogenesis

Although there is no defined histopathology in spasm, physiologic evidence again implicates myenteric plexus neuronal dysfunction. Vagal impulses mediating peristalsis reach all levels of the smooth muscle esophagus simultaneously, activating myenteric plexus neurons which then act on the muscle. Inhibitory ganglionic neurons hyperpolarize the myocytes and inhibit contraction while excitatory ones depolarize the cells prompting contraction. At each locus, the net effect results from the balance between these controlling influences. Experimental evidence suggests that some **diffuse esophageal spasm** patients primarily exhibit a **defect of inhibitory interneuron function** leading to rapidly propagated, "simultaneous" contractions; while in others the defect is of excess excitation leading to high amplitude repetitive contractions.

Pathology

There are few histopathologic studies of DES. The most striking reported pathologic change is diffuse muscular hypertrophy or hyperplasia with thickening of up to 2 cm in the distal two thirds of the esophagus. However, this finding is neither sensitive nor specific for DES. Similarly, no consistent evidence of neuropathology has been reported.

Clinical presentation

The major symptoms of **diffuse esophageal spasm** are **dysphagia and chest pain**. Weight loss is rare. Dysphagia is usually intermittent, sometimes related to swallowing specific substances or **liquids at extreme temperature**. In some

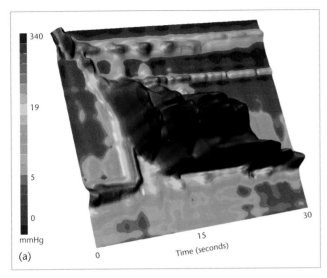

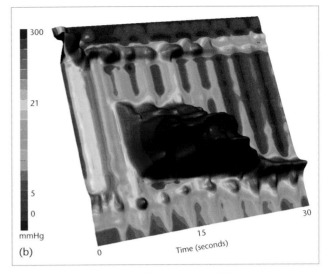

Figure 36.2 High resolution esophageal pressure topography of the two major variants of esophageal spasm: spastic nutcracker (a) and diffuse esophageal spasm (b).
Spastic nutcracker is defined by the extraordinarily high distal contractile integral (greater than 8000 mm (Hg/cm)/s with repetitive high amplitude contractions but normal contractile front velocity. Diffuse esophageal spasm is similar but primarily defined by a contractile front velocity greater than 10 cm/s.

Upper GI Tract

instances, patients experience episodes of esophageal obstruction while eating that persists until relieved by emesis. Esophageal chest pain is very similar to angina; described as crushing or squeezing in character, often radiating to the neck, jaw, arms, or midline of the back. Pain episodes may last from minutes to hours, but swallowing is usually not impaired. The mechanism producing pain is poorly understood.

Differential diagnosis

Unlike angina pectoris, which is a pain it can closely mimic, DES is not life threatening. Features suggesting esophageal as opposed to a cardiac pain include pain that is non-exertional, prolonged, interrupts sleep, is meal-related, is relieved with antacids, and is accompanied by heartburn, dysphagia, or regurgitation. However, each of these characteristics still exhibits some overlap with cardiac pain which should always be carefully considered first. Furthermore, even within the spectrum of esophageal diseases, both chest pain and dysphagia are also characteristic of peptic or infectious esophagitis. Only after these more common entities have been excluded by evaluation and/or treatment, should DES be pursued as the etiology of chest pain.

Diagnostic methods

Diffuse esophageal spasm is defined by **manometry or barium radiography** but the abnormal motor events are usually intermittent and there are no uniform definitions. Although DES has no pathognomonic endoscopic features, endoscopy is nonetheless useful to identify structural lesions and inflammation. Radiographically, a "**corkscrew esophagus**," "**rosary bead esophagus**," **pseudodiverticula,** or **curling** are indicative of DES. With conventional manometry, the hallmark features of DES are **simultaneous contractions** intermixed with some normal peristalsis, but with high-resolution esophageal pressure topography, it is becoming apparent that these criteria are not useful as neither of these features is essential [3,11]. Rather, the topographic criteria useful in identifying a spastic disorder accounting for symptoms of chest pain and/or dysphagia are of high amplitude, prolonged, repetitive distal esophageal contractions with or without rapid propagation velocity, as illustrated in Figure 36.2. The LES typically functions normally.

Treatment

Little controlled data exist regarding pharmacological therapy of DES. Long-term studies are not available, uniform definitions of DES have not been used, and the entire basis for this therapy is anecdotal. Uncontrolled trials of small numbers of DES patients report clinical response to **nitrates, calcium channel blockers, hydralazine, botulinum toxin,** and **anxiolytics**. The only controlled trial showing efficacy was with an anxiolytic. Consistent with this, success has also been reported using behavioral modification and biofeedback.

If dysphagia becomes so severe that weight loss is observed or if pain becomes unbearable, surgical therapy consisting of a **Heller myotomy** across the LES with **proximal extension** to include the involved area of spasm, or even esophagectomy should be considered. However, there are no controlled studies of these treatments and their indication is extremely rare.

Miscellaneous motility disorders (manometric variants)

Patients undergoing manometric evaluation for chest pain and/or dysphagia are found to have "manometric variants," most commonly hypertensive or hypotensive peristalsis, more frequently than either achalasia or DES. Among such individuals, there is a high prevalence of reflux and of psychiatric diagnoses, particularly anxiety and depression. Evidence also suggests a lower visceral pain threshold in this group and symptoms of irritable bowel syndrome may be seen in more than 50% of these patients [12]. Therapy of these conditions is as poorly defined as are the entities themselves. In view of the unproven value of detecting these conditions, current practice guidelines do not support pursuing them or rendering specific treatments. Rather, we should not overlook therapy aimed at the most common esophageal disorder, GERD, or more global conditions such as depression or somatization neurosis that are often coexistent in these patients.

Scleroderma esophagus (hypotensive LES and absent esophageal peristalsis) (see Chapter 110) was initially described as a manifestation of scleroderma or other collagen vascular diseases and thought to be specific for these disorders. However, this nomenclature subsequently proved unfortunate and has been discarded in the most current classification [11] because an estimated half of qualifying patients do not have an identifiable systemic disease and often reflux disease is the only identifiable association. When scleroderma esophagus occurs as a manifestation of a collagen vascular disease, the histopathological findings are of infiltration and destruction of the esophageal muscularis propria with collagen deposition and fibrosis. The pathogenesis of absent peristalsis and LES hypotension in the absence of a collagen vascular disease is unknown.

Prognosis with and without treatment

No mortality rate has been established for any of the esophageal motility disorders making their prognosis excellent, regardless of treatment. Nonetheless, it is indisputable that some people have died of complications of achalasia, whether aspiration pneumonia, lung abscesses or squamous cell cancer of the esophagus. Although no relevant corroborative data exist, the likelihood of incurring these complications is probably reduced by effective therapy.

Current controversies and their future resolution

Because achalasia is a rare condition, the relative merits of dilation, laparoscopic Heller myotomy, and botulinum toxin injection are still debated. Appropriate diagnostic criteria for DES remain controversial. It is increasingly recognized that reflux and visceral hyperalgesia are more relevant entities in

the genesis of chest pain. This controversy may be resolved in the future with careful clinical studies of chest pain patients. Whether "manometric variants" are of clinical relevance remains very controversial.

SOURCES OF INFORMATION FOR PATIENTS AND DOCTORS

www.nature.com/gimo/contents/p+1/full/gimo18.html
www.nidcd.nih.gov/health/voice/dysph.asp
www.cks.nhs.uk/patient_information_leaflet/dysphagia

References

1. Pandolfino JE, Kahrilas PJ. The second American Gastroenterological Association technical review on the clinical use of esophageal manometry. *Gastroenterology*. 2005;128:209–229.
2. Boeckxstaens GE. Achalasia: Virus-induced euthanasia of neurons? *Am J Gastroenterol*. 2008;103:1598–1612.
3. Pandolfino JE, Ghosh SK, Rice J, et al. Classifying esophageal motility by pressure topography characteristics: a study of 400 patients and 75 controls. *Am J Gastroenterol*. 2008;103:27–37.
4. Pandolfino JE, Kwiatek MA, Nealis T, et al. Achalasia: a new clinically relevant classification by high resolution manometry. *Gastroenterology*. 2008;135:1526–1533.
5. Ghosh SK, Pandolfino JE, Rice J, et al. Impaired deglutitive EGJ relaxation in clinical esophageal manometry: a quantitative analysis of 400 patients and 75 controls. *Am J Physiol*. 2007;293: G878–G885.
6. Bortolotti M, Mari C, Lopilato C, et al. Effects of sildenafil on esophageal motility of patients with idiopathic achalasia. *Gastroenterology*. 2000;118:253–7.
7. Spiess AE, Kahrilas PJ. Treating achalasia: from whalebone to laparoscope. *JAMA*. 1998;280:638–642.
8. Annese V, Bassotti G, Coccia G, et al. A multicentre randomised study of intrasphincteric botulinum toxin in patients with oesophageal achalasia. GISMAD Achalasia Study Group. *Gut*. 2000;46:597.
9. Csendes A, Braghetto I, Henriquez A, et al. Late results of a prospective randomised study comparing forceful dilatation and oesophagomyotomy in patients with achalasia. *Gut*. 1989; 30:299.
10. Chapman JR, Joehl RJ, Murayama KM, et al. Achalasia treatment: improved outcome of laparoscopic myotomy with operative manometry. *Arch Surg*. 2004;139;508–513.
11. Pandolfino JE, Fox MR, Bredenoord AJ, et al. High resolution manometry in clinical practice: utilizing pressure topography to classify oesophageal motility disorders. *Neurogastroenterol Mot*. 2009;21:796–806.
12. Rao SS, Gregersen H, Hayek B, et al. Unexplained chest pain: the hypersensitive, hyperreactive, and poorly compliant esophagus. *Ann Intern Med*. 1996;124:950.

CHAPTER 37
Gastric motility disorders

Jan Tack

University of Leuven; University Hospital Gasthuisberg, Leuven, Belgium

---

ESSENTIAL FACTS ABOUT PATHOPHYSIOLOGY

- Impaired gastric reservoir function (impaired accommodation): functional dyspepsia
- Visceral hypersensitivity: functional dyspepsia
- Delayed gastric emptying: functional dyspepsia and gastroparesis
- Absence of gastric or small bowel phase 3 activity: bezoar formation and bacterial overgrowth
- Too rapid delivery of nutrients into the small bowel: dumping syndrome

---

ESSENTIALS OF DIAGNOSIS

- Exclusion of organic disease is mandatory
- Measurement of gastric emptying rate is the most frequently used test, but its contribution to determining treatment is limited

---

ESSENTIALS OF TREATMENT

- Prokinetics are the drugs of choice for gastroparesis and functional dyspepsia with motility-like symptoms
- A subset of functional dyspepsia patients may respond to *Helicobacter pylori* eradication
- Refractory patients may benefit from centrally acting therapies (antidepressants, psychotherapy, hypnotherapy)
- Dumping syndrome may respond to dietary measures, acarbose or somatostain analogs

---

Introduction

A large number of patients present with symptoms that are related to meal ingestion or that refer to the gastroduodenal region. These **symptoms** include chronic or recurrent epigastric pain, epigastric burning, post-prandial fullness or early satiation (inability to finish a normal sized meal), upper abdominal bloating, belching, nausea, and vomiting. When conventional diagnostic means (endoscopy, histology, radiology, biochemistry) do not identify an underlying histological, biochemical, or structural abnormality that can consistently explain the patient's symptoms, abnormal gastric **sensorimotor function** is often thought to be the underlying mechanism.

Hence, a number of methods have been developed to study gastric motor and sensory function, and a number of conditions in which abnormal gastric motor or sensory function is present can be identified.

Normal gastric motor function
Functional anatomy

Functionally, the stomach can be divided into a proximal part and a distal part, each with different motor functions. The **proximal stomach** mainly serves to provide a reservoir to the meal. The main function of the **distal part** of the stomach is to grind and empty the meal from the stomach (Figure 37.1).

Structures involved in the **control of gastric motility** include smooth muscle cells, interstitial cells of Cajal, enteric nerves and the vagus nerve, and gastrointestinal peptides. The **muscle layers** of the stomach consist of an outer longitudinal layer, and an inner circular muscle layer. In the proximal stomach, near the lesser curvature, an intermediate oblique muscle layer is also present. The **myenteric plexus** is found between the circular and longitudinal muscle layers in the stomach and is built up of ganglia that contain the cell bodies of intrinsic neurons and glial cells. Although these neurons receive input from vagal and sympathetic extrinsic nerves, the gastric myenteric plexus has major **functional autonomy**. The **vagus nerve** has primarily a sensory role, as up to 90% of its fibers are afferents, with cell bodies in the nodose ganglion, which convey information to the nucleus of the solitary tract in the brain stem. After processing of incoming information, vagal motor neurons in the dorsal motor nucleus or in the **nucleus ambiguus** can become activated. These so-called **vago-vagal reflexes** provide the control of several physiological processes, including the regulation of gastric motility and secretion. The splanchnic or **sympathetic innervation** of the stomach originates from spinal segments 6–9. They mainly inhibit motility through presynaptic inhibition of acetylcholine release from the myenteric plexus.

Smooth muscle cells in the proximal stomach do not display electrical oscillatory activity and the motor response in this region is characterized by a tonic contractile activity. Smooth

---

Textbook of Clinical Gastroenterology and Hepatology, Second Edition. Edited by C. J. Hawkey, Jaime Bosch, Joel E. Richter, Guadalupe Garcia-Tsao, Francis K. L. Chan.

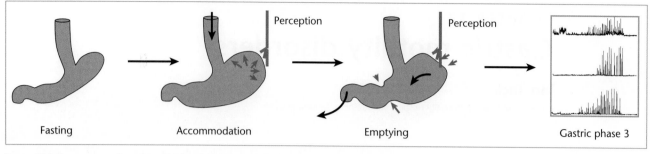

Figure 37.1 Components of gastric motor function during and after meal ingestion, and during the interdigestive state. (This figure was published in *Clinical Gastroenterology and Hepatology*, Wilfred M. Weinstein, Christopher J. Hawkey, Jaime Bosch, Gastric motility disorders, Pages 1–6, Copyright Elsevier, 2005.)

muscle cells in the distal part of the stomach display rhythmic electrical activity, the so-called slow waves, and phasic contractile activity. **Slow waves** are oscillations of the membrane potential at a frequency of three cycles/minute, which are triggered from a pacemaker area in the corpus near the greater curvature. Interstitial **cells of Cajal**, a specialized type of cell of mesodermal origin, located near the myenteric plexus, generate the slow waves, which determine the timing of **gastric contractions**. Action potential discharge, driven by neurotransmitter release from the myenteric plexus, occurs at the crest of a slow wave. Thus, the slow waves determine the maximal frequency of contractions, while enteric neuronal discharge determines the number of spikes and the strength of the contraction.

Interdigestive motility

In the fasting state, motility of the proximal gastrointestinal tract is dominated by the **migrating motor complex (MMC)**, a cyclical motor pattern of the stomach and small intestine. The MMC consists of three different phases, of which phase III, a few minutes of intense contractions at maximal frequency (three per minute in the stomach, 12 per minute in the duodenum), is the most characteristic one. **Phase I** is characterized by the absence of contractile activity, while **phase II** displays irregular contractile activity. The average MMC cycle lasts between 90 and 120 minutes, but with a large inter- and intra-individual variability. The MMC originates from the stomach or proximal small intestine and migrates distally at 1–4 cm/minute. The main role of **phase III** is thought to be the evacuation of indigestible particles from the stomach and the small bowel, and to maintain low counts of bacteria in the upper gastrointestinal tract [1].

Gastric reservoir function

When food is ingested, the MMC is suppressed and upper gastrointestinal motility switches to the fed or **post-prandial pattern**. During fasting, a high muscle tone in the proximal stomach is mediated by vagal tone. During and after ingestion of a meal, a vago-vagally–mediated relaxation of the proximal stomach occurs, which provides the meal with a reservoir and enables a gastric volume increase without a rise in pressure [2]. The gastric antrum probably also contributes to gastric storage capacity, through inhibition of phasic and tonic contractile activity.

Gastric emptying

After ingestion of a meal, **peristaltic waves** move from the mid-corpus to the pylorus. In the antrum, these contractions will grind the food and mix it with gastric juices through retropulsion, to finally lead to propulsion and evacuation to the duodenum. The **flow of chyme** from the stomach to the duodenum is pulsatile and is determined by a balance between antral contractions and duodenal resistance, and is titrated by the degree of pyloric relaxation. The **rate of emptying** depends on the caloric content and physical characteristics of the meal. Liquid meals empty from the stomach in a linear fashion. Emptying of a **solid meal** follows a biphasic pattern: during the lag phase, which can take up to 60 minutes, solids are redistributed in the stomach and broken down to smaller particles. Particles less than 1 mm in diameter can pass through the pylorus during the emptying phase.

Gastric motility disorders

Disordered gastric motility occurs when the processes of interdigestive motility, gastric reservoir function or gastric emptying are not properly controlled. **Conditions** associated with disordered gastric motility include functional dyspepsia, gastroparesis, dumping syndrome, and (other) postoperative conditions. The absence of gastric phase III activity promotes **gastric bezoar formation**, whereas the absence of ths small intestinal phase III promotes **bacterial overgrowth** [1] (see Chapter 42). Impaired **gastric accommodation** may lead to inability to ingest large meals and weight loss [3]. Severely delayed emptying leads to a **gastroparesis** syndrome with symptoms attributable to prolonged gastric stasis and fermentation of food [4]. Abnormally rapid gastric emptying may lead to duodenal caloric overload and **dumping syndrome** [5].

Symptoms

The symptoms that occur in patients with gastric motility disorders are non-specific, and include post-prandial fullness and bloating, early satiation (inability to finish a normal sized meal), nausea, vomiting, epigastric pain and burning, and loss

Upper GI Tract

of appetite. In more severe cases, this may lead to weight loss and in extreme cases, to inability to be fed orally. Depending on the underlying cause, these symptoms may be intermittent or continuous. The correlation between symptom pattern, symptom severity, and the presence or severity of disordered motility is often poor and variable. Nevertheless, a number of studies have reported associations between the symptom pattern and abnormalities of gastric motor function [6].

Small-scale studies in general have failed to find a correlation between delayed gastric emptying and symptom pattern [6]. A number of large-scale studies, mainly in single-center cohorts from Europe, found that patients with **delayed solid emptying** reported more frequent and more severe post-prandial fullness, nausea. and vomiting. This was not confirmed in large multicenter studies in the USA [6,7]. An association of gastric emptying and post-prandial dyspeptic symptoms has been reported, but **rapid gastric emptying** has most clearly been implicated in (postoperative) dumping syndrome [5,8]. Considering **impaired accommodation**, some studies have reported an association with early satiety and weight loss, while others have not reported such an association [6].

Diagnostic tests

Prior to considering the evaluation of gastric motor activity, **organic disease** needs to be excluded with confidence. Skillful evaluation and clear exposition can be valuable in the initial management of patients with relatively minor symptoms and absence of alarm symptoms. Often, however, exclusion of organic disease may require upper GI endoscopy and exclusion of abnormalities of electrolyte balance, glycemia, and thyroid function. **Tests of gastric motor function** can be considered, and may aid diagnostic labeling, but their contribution to determining the treatment approach is generally limited [9]. In the absence of alarm symptoms or risk factors, the optimal indication and timing of additional examinations in patients with symptoms suggestive of gastric motility disorders have not been established, but algorithms have been proposed [8–10].

Radionuclide gastric emptying measurement is considered the standard method to assess **gastric emptying** rate [11]. Solid and liquid emptying can be assessed separately or simultaneously. The solid and/or liquid meal is labeled with a (different) radioisotope, usually ^{99}Tc or ^{111}In. A gamma-camera measures the number of counts in an investigator-determined region of interest (total, proximal or distal stomach, small intestine) over a relevant time frame after ingestion of a meal. Mathematical processing involves corrections for distance to the camera and isotope decay, and curve fitting, allowing the calculation of the half emptying time, the lag phase, and the fraction of labeled meal that is present in the stomach at different time points (Figure 37.2). **Scintigraphy** also has the potential to provide information on distribution of the meal

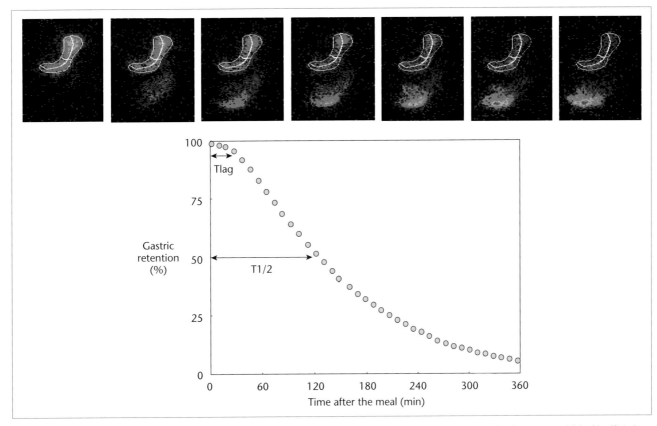

Figure 37.2 Scintigraphic images (upper panel) and example of a gastric emptying scintigraphy curve for solid food. (This figure was published in *Clinical Gastroenterology and Hepatology*, Wilfred M. Weinstein, Christopher J. Hawkey, Jaime Bosch, Gastric motility disorders, Pages 1–6, Copyright Elsevier, 2005.)

over the proximal and distal stomach, but this is not routinely applied [12]. **Disadvantages** include the use of radioactive labels, considerable cost, and poor level of standardization of meal composition and measuring times between different laboratories. To address the lack of standardization, a **standard protocol** has been proposed by the American Societies for Neurogastroenterology and Motility and for Nuclear Medicine, but the proposed test meal is limited by a lack of lipid content [13].

Breath tests can also be used to measure gastric emptying rates, by labeling the solid (or liquid) phase of the meal with a ^{13}C-containing substrate (octanoic acid, acetic acid, glycin or spirulina) [14]. With emptying of the substrate from the stomach, it is rapidly metabolized with generation of $^{13}CO_2$ which appears in the breath [14]. Breath sampling at regular intervals and mathematical processing of the $^{13}CO_2$ content over time allows the calculation of a gastric emptying curve. The **advantages** of this test are the use of non-radioactive materials and the ability to perform the test outside a hospital setting. **Disadvantages** are the absence of standardization of meal, substrate, and curve fitting models by different groups [14].

Ultrasound allows the diameter of the gastric antrum to be measured as a marker of the emptying rate of a liquid meal [15]. However, the ultrasound technique is time-consuming, likely to be observer-dependent, and not suitable for solid meals. Moreover, antral volume is not only influenced by the gastric emptying rate, but also by redistribution of the meal inside the stomach, e.g., in case of impaired accommodation. To account for some of these limitations, complex technologies have been described which allow assessment of proximal and distal gastric volumes [16], but this approach is mainly experimental.

Antro-pyloro-duodenal manometry quantifies contractility patterns of normal and abnormal interdigestive motility and gastric emptying. This is mainly a research tool, with clinical application in the investigation of generalized motility disorders, including chronic idiopathic intestinal pseudo-obstruction (CIIP) [17].

Assessment of **proximal stomach motor function** is still a research topic. The **gastric barostat** consists of a computer-driven pump connected to an oversized balloon, which can be positioned in the proximal or distal stomach. Measurement of volume changes in an isobaric mode allows changes in gastric tone to be measured after a meal. Due to its invasive nature, application of barostat measurements is restricted to research [18].

Imaging of stomach volumes using **single-photon emission computed tomography (SPECT)** or **magnetic resonance imaging (MRI)** also allows gastric volume responses to meal ingestion to be assessed, but these are also used only in research [19,20]. **Nutrient challenge tests** have been proposed as an alternative for the non-invasive estimation of gastric accommodation [21]. However, the test may be affected by other aspects such as taste or central effects [22].

Cutaneous electrodes allow measurement of electrical activity of the stomach. This so-called electrogastrography (EGG) provides information on the frequency and regularity of gastric pacemaker activity, as well as changes in power of the signal after meal ingestion. Although easy to use because of its non-invasive nature, EGG is still considered an experimental tool [23].

Therapeutic considerations
Not all patients with gastric motility disorders will require drug therapy. **Reassurance and explanation** of the nature of the disorder takes away the fear of a serious disease in the majority of patients. Although their efficacy is not proven, dietary and lifestyle adjustments are usually recommended.

Gastroparesis
Delayed gastric emptying in the absence of mechanical obstruction is often referred to as "gastroparesis." The most important **pathophysiological abnormalities** in gastroparesis include fundal hypomotility, antral hypomotility, gastric arrhythmia, and lack of antropyloroduodenal coordination. However, delayed gastric emptying is also present in up to 30% of functional dyspepsia patients [6]. Although there are some differences in symptom pattern associated with delayed emptying [6,7], the distinction between functional dyspepsia with delayed gastric emptying and idiopathic gastroparesis has not been clarified. Moreover, the presence of delayed gastric emptying is not stable over time in a large group of patients [24].

A number of **drugs**, such as anticholinergics, opioids, L-dopa, tricyclic antidepressants, and phenothiazines may contribute to a slowing of gastric emptying. When drug effects are ruled out, the **predominant causes** of gastroparesis are idiopathic (33%), diabetes mellitus (24%), and post-surgical (19%) [25]. Gastroparesis may occur in both type I and type II diabetes, with prevalences that vary largely depending on the study and on the definition of gastroparesis. **Diabetic gastroparesis** involves mainly solid meals and is often associated with the presence of autonomic neuropathy. Poor glycemic control may also contribute to delayed emptying, which in its turn may also impair glycemic control. **Vagotomy** causes rapid emptying of liquids and delayed emptying of solids. However, after partial gastrectomy, a complex situation exists that may lead to gastric stasis, or in contrast, to rapid emptying with dumping syndrome. Gastroparesis has also been associated with a number of less prevalent conditions such as **anorexia nervosa** and **renal failure**. When no underlying cause is apparent, the patient is referred to as having idiopathic gastroparesis. In some of these cases, an acute onset and the presence of viral antibodies suggest involvement of acute infections in the pathogenesis of gastroparesis [25,26].

Clinical suspicion of gastroparesis warrants ruling out of mechanical causes and serum electrolyte imbalances, usually followed by empirical treatment with a **gastroprokinetic drug** like domperidone or metoclopramide [8,27]. The former is the drug of choice as metoclopramide may be associated with extrapyramidal side effects. In the past, **cisapride** was frequently used in gastroparesis, but the drug's availability has been suspended because of an enhanced risk of QT prolongation with cardiac arrhythmias. Short-term studies in diabetic and post-surgical gastroparesis have reported beneficial effects of treatment with **erythromycin** (three doses of 250–500 mg), a macrolide antibiotic that has prokinetic properties by acting as a motilin receptor agonist [27,28]. Attempts to develop macrolide prokinetics devoid of antibiotic properties have been disappointing [29,30]. Overall, the evidence that classical gastroprokinetics like metoclopramide, domperidone, cisapride or erythromycin are effective in gastroparesis is far from overwhelming [27]. There are only anecdotal reports supporting the efficacy of **other prokinetic drugs** such as mosapride, renzapride, levosulpiride, and clonidine in diabetic gastroparesis [8,27].

Anecdotal evidence suggests the use of intrapyloric injection of **botulinum toxin** in idiopathic or diabetic gastroparesis, but in two controlled studies no benefit over saline injection was found [31,32]. In refractory cases with severe weight loss, hospitalization for parenteral nutrition may be required, and in case of rapidly recurring weight loss percutaneous endoscopic jejunostomy feeding tube insertion can be considered [8]. **Home parenteral nutrition** is another option, but it is not devoid of potentially life-threatening complications like septicemia or thromboembolism. **Gastric electrical stimulation** has been proposed as an alternative for the treatment of refractory gastroparesis patients, but there is a lack of evidence of major efficacy [33,34].

Functional dyspepsia

Functional dyspepsia is defined as the presence of early satiation, post-prandial fullness or epigastric pain or burning, in the absence of organic disease that readily explains the symptoms [35]. Dyspeptic symptoms are highly prevalent in the general population, and are often attributed to functional dyspepsia after additional investigations (mainly endoscopy). From a pathophysiological point of view, functional dyspepsia is most likely a **heterogeneous disorder** and an accurate diagnostic test is lacking. Pathophysiological studies have revealed the presence of delayed gastric emptying, impaired gastric accommodation, and hypersensitivity to gastric distension in subsets of functional dyspepsia patients [6,35].

In (functional) dyspepsia, empirical **proton pump inhibitor therapy** is most often the initial approach, but this is probably mainly helpful to identify patients with underlying gastro-esophageal reflux disease, rather than to treat true dyspepsia [6,36,37]. Motility-type dyspeptic symptoms are unlikely to respond to acid-suppressive therapy, and the same is probably true for *Helicobacter* eradication in those who are infected (a minority in most Western countries) [36,37]. **Prokinetic drugs** are widely used in the treatment of motility-like functional dyspepsia, but the evidence of efficacy is in fact limited [6,36,37]. In **refractory patients**, centrally acting therapeutic interventions can be used, such as low-dose antidepressants, hypnotherapy, and psychotherapy [6,36,37].

Dumping syndrome

Dumping syndrome is characterized by vasomotor and gastrointestinal symptoms that can be attributed to rapid gastric emptying [5]. Dumping syndrome occurs mainly after partial or complete gastrectomy, but may also be observed after vagotomy, both intentional or unintentional at the time of surgery at the gastroesophageal junction. **Symptoms** typically occur after meal ingestion and are subdivided into "early dumping" and "late dumping" symptoms (Table 37.1). Most patients suffer from early dumping, or a combination of early and late dumping, whereas isolated late dumping is rare. Severe dumping may lead to weight loss from fear of food ingestion and major impairment of quality of life.

Symptoms of early dumping are explained in part by the rapid passage of **hyperosmolar contents** into the small bowel, accompanied by a shift of fluids from the intravascular compartment to the lumen and the release of a number of **gastrointestinal peptides**, including enteroglucagon, vasoactive intestinal peptide, peptide YY, pancreatic polypeptide, and neurotensin. **Late dumping** occurs 1–3 hours postprandially and is characterized by symptoms of hypoglycemia (Figure 37.3). Rapid gastric emptying induces a high glucose concentration in the intestinal lumen. Glucose is rapidly absorbed, which brings about a peak insulin secretion. Because of the long half-life of insulin and the often very transient character of the initial rise in glycemia, reactive glycemia occurs when all sugars have been absorbed.

The diagnosis of dumping syndrome should be suspected in cases with suggestive symptoms in a predisposing setting (e.g., after gastric or esophageal surgery). Confirmation of the diagnosis can be obtained by the demonstration of hypoglycemia at the time of symptoms, or by a **modified oral glucose**

Table 37.1 Early and late symptoms of dumping syndrome

Early dumping		Late dumping
Gastrointestinal symptoms	Vasomotor symptoms	Hypoglycemia
Abdominal pain	Flushing	Transpiration
Diarrhoea	Palpitations	Palpitations
Borborygmi	Transpiration	Hunger
Bloating	Tachycardia	Weakness
Nausea	Hypotension	Confusion
	Syncope	Tremor
		Syncope

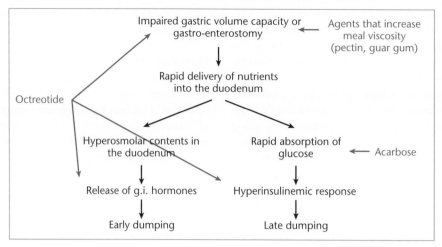

Figure 37.3 Pathophysiology and therapeutic approach in postoperative dumping syndrome.

challenge test: 50 g of glucose are ingested with water, and for 3 hours at 30-minute intervals glycemia, hematocrit, and pulse rate are noted. The test is considered positive if there is initial hyperglycemia and late hypoglycemia (<60 mg/dL) or an early rise in hematocrit of >3% or an early rise in pulse rate of >10 bpm [5].

Dietary measures are the first step in the treatment of dumping syndrome. Patients are instructed to divide their calorie intake over at least six meals, and to avoid drinking with meals and for the first 2 hours post-prandially. Rapidly absorbed carbohydrates are eliminated with accordingly increased intake of fat and proteins. Certain **food additives**, like pectin, guar gum, and glucomannan, form a gel with carbohydrates, and can theoretically be used to slow gastric emptying of the meal and to improve dumping symptoms, but their clinical efficacy is questionable. **Acarbose** is an inhibitor of intestinal alpha-glucosidase, which slows carbohydrate digestion and blunts post-prandial rises in glycemia, which is beneficial in late dumping [5].

If these first-line measures fail, **somatostatin analogs** can be considered, as they slow gastric emptying and inhibit the release of gastrointestinal peptides. They are administered either subcutaneously three times daily, or intramuscularly once every 2–4 weeks as a slow-release formulation. Patient preference seems to be for the slow-release formulations [5].

In exceptionally difficult-to-manage patients, **surgery** with the creation of a proximal short antiperistaltic intestinal loop can be considered [38].

SOURCES OF INFORMATION FOR PATIENTS AND DOCTORS

http://digestive.niddk.nih.gov/ddiseases/pubs/gastroparesis/
http://www.aci.gi.org/patients/gihealth/gastroparesis.asp
http://www.diabetes.org/living-with-diabetes/complications/
  gastroparesis.html

References

1. Vantrappen G, Janssens J, Hellemans J, Ghoos Y. The interdigestive motor complex of normal subjects and patients with bacterial overgrowth of the small intestine. *J Clin Invest*. 1977;59: 1158–1166.
2. Azpiroz F, Malagelada JR. Vagally mediated gastric relaxation induced by intestinal nutrients in the dog. *Am J Physiol*. 1986;251: G727–735.
3. Tack J, Piessevaux H, Coulie B, Caenepeel P, Janssens J. Role of impaired gastric accommodation to a meal in functional dyspepsia. *Gastroenterology*. 1998;115:1346–1352.
4. Parkman HP, Camilleri M, Farrugia G, *et al*. Gastroparesis and functional dyspepsia: excerpts from the AGA/ANMS meeting. *Neurogastroenterol Motil*. 2010;22:113–133.
5. Tack J, Arts J, Caenepeel P, De Wulf D, Bisschops R. Pathophysiology, diagnosis and management of postoperative dumping syndrome. *Nat Rev Gastroenterol Hepatol*. 2009;6:583–590.
6. Tack J, Bisschops R, Sarnelli G. Pathophysiology and treatment of functional dyspepsia. *Gastroenterology*. 2004;127:1239–1255.
7. Talley NJ, Locke GR 3rd, Lahr BD, *et al*. Functional dyspepsia, delayed gastric emptying, and impaired quality of life. *Gut*. 2006;55:933–939.
8. Tack J. The difficult patient with gastroparesis. *Best Pract Res Clin Gastroenterol*. 2007;21:379–391.
9. Tack J. Gastric motor disorders. *Best Pract Res Clin Gastroenterol*. 2007;21:633–644.
10. Tack J, Talley NJ. Gastroduodenal disorders. *Am J Gastroenterol*. 2010;105:757–763.
11. Parkman HP, Hasler WL, Fisher RS; American Gastroenterological Association. American Gastroenterological Association technical review on the diagnosis and treatment of gastroparesis. *Gastroenterology*. 2004;127:1592–1622.
12. Piessevaux H, Tack J, Walrand S, Pauwels S, Geubel A. Intragastric distribution of a standardized meal in health and functional dyspepsia: correlation with specific symptoms. *Neurogastroenterol Motil*. 2003;15:447–455.
13. Abell TL, Camilleri M, Donohoe K, *et al*.; American Neurogastroenterology and Motility Society and the Society of Nuclear Medicine. Consensus recommendations for gastric emptying scintigraphy: a joint report of the American Neurogastroen-

terology and Motility Society and the Society of Nuclear Medicine. *Am J Gastroenterol.* 2008;103:753–763.

14. Verbeke K. Will the 13C-octanoic acid breath test ever replace scintigraphy as the gold standard to assess gastric emptying? *Neurogastroenterol Motil.* 2009;21:1013–1016.

15. Ricci R, Bontempo I, Corazziari E, La Bella A, Torsoli A. Real time ultrasonography of the gastric antrum. *Gut.* 1993;34: 173–176.

16. Gilja OH, Detmer PR, Jong JM, *et al.* Intragastric distribution and gastric emptying assessed by three-dimensional ultrasonography. *Gastroenterology.* 1997;113:38–49.

17. Verhagen MA, Samsom M, Jebbink RJ, Smout AJ. Clinical relevance of antroduodenal manometry. *Eur J Gastroenterol Hepatol.* 1999;11:523–528.

18. Kindt S, Tack J. Impaired gastric accommodation and its role in dyspepsia. *Gut.* 2006;55:1685–1691.

19. Kim DY, Delgado-Aros S, Camilleri M, *et al.* Noninvasive measurement of gastric accommodation in patients with idiopathic nonulcer dyspepsia. *Am J Gastroenterol.* 2001;96:3099–3105.

20. Kunz P, Feinle C, Schwizer W, Fried M, Boesiger P. Assessment of gastric motor function during the emptying of solid and liquid meals in humans by MRI. *J Magn Reson Imaging* 1999; 9:75–80.

21. Tack J, Caenepeel P, Piessevaux H, Cuomo R, Janssens J. Assessment of meal induced gastric accommodation by a satiety drinking test in health and in severe functional dyspepsia. *Gut.* 2003; 52:1271–1277.

22. Tack J. Drink tests in functional dyspepsia *Gastroenterology.* 2002;122:2093–2094.

23. Parkman HP, Hasler WL, Barnett JL, Eaker EY; American Motility Society Clinical GI Motility Testing Task Force. Electrogastrography: a document prepared by the gastric section of the American Motility Society Clinical GI Motility Testing Task Force. *Neurogastroenterol Motil.* 2003;15:89–102.

24. Tougas G, Chen Y, Luo D, *et al.* Tegaserod improves gastric emptying in patients with gastroparesis and dyspeptic symptoms. *Gastroenterology.* 2003;124 (Suppl):A54–A54.

25. Horowitz M, Su YC, Rayner CK, Jones KL. Gastroparesis: prevalence, clinical significance and treatment. *Can J Gastroenterol.* 2001;15:805–813.

26. Tack J, Demedts I, Dehondt G, *et al.* Clinical and pathophysiological characteristics of acute-onset functional dyspepsia. *Gastroenterology.* 2002;122:1738–1747.

27. Sturm A, Holtmann G, Goebell H, Gerken G. Prokinetics in patients with gastroparesis: a systematic analysis. *Digestion.* 1999;60:422–427.

28. Janssens J, Peeters TL, Vantrappen G, *et al.* Improvement of gastric emptying in diabetic gastroparesis by erythromycin. Preliminary studies. *N Engl J Med.* 1990;322:1028–1031.

29. Talley NJ, Verlinden M, Geenen DJ, *et al.* Effects of a motilin receptor agonist (ABT-229) on upper gastrointestinal symptoms in type 1 diabetes mellitus: a randomised, double blind, placebo controlled trial. *Gut.* 2001;49:395–401.

30. Talley NJ, Verlinden M, Snape W, *et al.* Failure of a motilin receptor agonist (ABT-229) to relieve the symptoms of functional dyspepsia in patients with and without delayed gastric emptying: a randomized double-blind placebo-controlled trial. *Aliment Pharmacol Ther.* 2000;14:1653–1661.

31. Arts J, Holvoet L, Caenepeel P, *et al.* Clinical trial: a randomized-controlled crossover study of intrapyloric injection of botulinum toxin in gastroparesis. *Aliment Pharmacol Ther.* 2007;26:1251–1258.

32. Friedenberg FK, Palit A, Parkman HP, Hanlon A, Nelson DB. Botulinum toxin A for the treatment of delayed gastric emptying. *Am J Gastroenterol.* 2008;103:416–423.

33. Abell T, McCallum R, Hocking M, *et al.* Gastric electrical stimulation for medically refractory gastroparesis. *Gastroenterology.* 2003;125:421–428.

34. McCallum RW, Snape W, Brody F, Wo J, Parkman HP, Nowak T. Gastric electrical stimulation with Enterra therapy improves symptoms from diabetic gastroparesis in a prospective study. *Clin Gastroenterol Hepatol.* 2010;8:947–954.

35. Tack J, Talley NJ, Camilleri M, *et al.* Functional gastroduodenal disorders. *Gastroenterology.* 2006;130:1466–1479.

36. Moayyedi P, Delaney BC, Vakil N, Forman D, Talley NJ. The efficacy of proton pump inhibitors in nonulcer dyspepsia: a systematic review and economic analysis. *Gastroenterology.* 2004;127:1329–1337.

37. Moayyedi P, Soo S, Deeks J, Delaney B, Innes M, Forman D. Pharmacological interventions for non-ulcer dyspepsia. *Cochrane Database Syst Rev.* 2006;(4):CD001960.

38. Arts J, Caenepeel P, Bisschops R, *et al.* Efficacy of the long-acting repeatable formulation of the somatostatin analogue octreotide in postoperative dumping. *Clin Gastroenterol Hepatol.* 2009;7: 432–437.

Upper GI Tract

CHAPTER 38
Food allergy and intolerance

Stephan C. Bischoff and Katrin Feuser
University of Hohenheim, Stuttgart, Germany

ESSENTIAL FACTS ABOUT PATHOGENESIS

- The pathogenesis is multifactorial; genetic, environmental and nutritional factors play a role
- The hygiene hypothesis suggests that reduced microbial challenge is a major cause for the increase of allergic and autoimmune diseases

ESSENTIALS OF DIAGNOSIS

- Diagnosis is based on thorough clinical history with regard to the triggering food
- Elimination diet and subsequent open provocation test helps substantiate suspicion of food allergy or intolerance
- Gold standard: double-blind placebo-controlled food challenges (DBPCFC)
- Skin prick test, measurement of specific IgE in serum or organ-specific challenges (e.g., nasal, bronchial or intestinal provocations) confirm history and distinguishes between allergy and intolerance
- Hydrogen breath test following oral challenge are suitable tests to assess carbohydrate malabsorption; other food intolerance often requires DBPCFC

ESSENTIALS OF TREATMENT

- Individual diet counseling is required for adequate avoidance, education of the patients regarding to the proper reading of packaged food labels and ingredient lists, and prevention of diet-induced malnutrition
- Patients at risk for anaphylactic reactions need to wear and use epinephrine-containing syringe for emergency anaphylactic reactions
- In case of food allergy, elimination diet can be accompanied optionally by supplementary medical therapy with oral cromolyn and topical corticosteroids

Introduction

Abnormal reactions following food ingestion are commonly defined as adverse reactions to food [1]. The expression "adverse reactions to food" represent an umbrella term of immune-mediated food allergies and non-immune-mediated food intolerances (Figure 38.1) [2]. The underlying mechanisms of food allergy involving the immune system are distinct from other adverse reactions to food. Food allergy and food hypersensitivity are entities used interchangeably, but they are reserved for those reactions that are mediated by the immune system. Most food intolerances are caused by enzyme deficiencies as in case of lactose intolerance; however, the causes of intolerance reactions are often versatile and not completely understood. Intolerance can be subdivided into enzymatic, pharmacological and chemical as well as idiopathic intolerance [3].

Food Allergy
Epidemiology
Gastrointestinal discomfort from adverse reactions to food is common in the general population; however, only in a few cases are the symptoms due to immunologic reactions [4]. The incidence of immune-mediated food allergies among children is 4–6% and among adults 1–2% [1,5]. Geographic differences and eating habits as well as age all affect the development of food allergies. The common foods causing allergic reactions among infants and young children are cow's milk, eggs, wheat, and soy, whereas seafood, peanuts, and tree nuts are more common in adults (Table 38.1) [6].

Clinical presentation
The skin, gastrointestinal tract, and respiratory tract are the most common organ systems involved in food-induced allergic reactions. The gastrointestinal symptoms following food ingestion are variable and nonspecific. They depend on the target organ responses, the type of allergic reaction as well as characteristics of the triggering allergens, and range from swelling and itching around the lips, tongue, mouth, and laryngeal edema (oral allergy syndrome), reflux, nausea and vomiting (gastric reactions), abdominal pain, malassimilation, vitamin deficiency, and diarrhea or obstipation (colon reactions) [3,7]. Generally, symptoms occur shortly after food ingestion, thus facilitating the identification of the triggering foods.

Textbook of Clinical Gastroenterology and Hepatology, Second Edition. Edited by C. J. Hawkey, Jaime Bosch, Joel E. Richter, Guadalupe Garcia-Tsao, Francis K. L. Chan.
© 2012 Blackwell Publishing Ltd. Published 2012 by Blackwell Publishing Ltd.

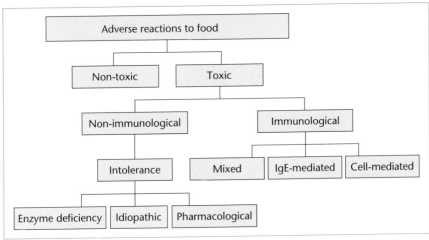

Figure 38.1 EAACI classification of adverse reaction to food based on the pathogenetic mechanism. (Modified from Bruijnzeel-Koomen C, Ortolani C, Aas K, *et al.* Adverse reactions to food. European Academy of Allergology and Clinical Immunology Subcommittee. *Allergy.* 1995;50:623–635.)

Table 38.1 Common antigens in gastrointestinal food allergy

Food	Non-food
cows milk	bacteria
peanut	virus
hazelnut	fungi
grain	worms
legumes	inhaled antigens (e.g., pollens)
eggs	chemicals
fish	drugs
meat	others
crustaceans	
others	

Allergic inflammation

The immune reactions following food ingestion can be divided into three general types (Figure 38.1): immunoglobulin (Ig) E-mediated type, also termed as type I or immediate type reaction, cell-mediated reactions (IgE-antibodies are not detectable), and mixed disorders (IgE and non-IgE mechanisms) [8]. The IgE-antibody dependent disease, which is also involved in bronchial asthma, urticaria, atomic eczema and seasonal rhinitis, is the best characterized immunologic reaction to food [9]. IgE-mediated allergies occur in 3 phases, first the sensitization phase, second the effector phase, consisting of an acute phase as well as a facultative late phase response, and third the chronic phase. The sensitization phase is characterized by the induction of allergen-specific IgE-antibodies in individuals with genetic predisposition. The acute phase is initiated by a re-exposure to the antigen and characterized by clinical manifestations [10,11]. The acute response can be followed by a late-phase reaction within 2 to 24 hours after allergen exposure. This phase is characterized by cellular infiltration of the tissue with inflammatory cells, such as eosinophils, basophils, and Th2 cells (Figure 38.2). The chronic phase is the result of repetitive late phases, which cause persistent infiltration of granulocytes and lymphocytes and subsequent chronic structural changes of the tissue [3,11].

Pathophysiology

Genetic and environmental factors are risk factors for the development of allergic reactions. In the meantime it is generally acknowledged that individual factors such as the psychological constitution, namely multiple neuronal factors, influence the generation of allergic reactions, too (Figure 38.3) [11].

Development of intestinal inflammation requires a sufficient quantity of allergen in the intestine as well as a hyper-reactive mucosal immune system. Bacteria, virus, and toxins might trigger the loss of an immunological tolerance and induce development of hypersensitivity of the mucosal immune system toward luminal antigens in selected individuals [9]. The gastrointestinal tract, the largest immune organ of the body, must simultaneously control the uptake of potentially harmful food proteins, microbes, toxins and chemicals, and allow colonization with commensal bacteria as well as uptake of nutrients. The complex functional entity that does this job is the gastrointestinal barrier serving as protector against invading pathogens or allergens, but also as sensor to the luminal environment from which nutrients and fluids come from [12].

Diagnosis (Table 38.2)

Guidelines and position papers for the evaluation and treatment of food allergies have been published by the American Academy of Allergy, Asthma and Immunology (AAAAI), the European Academy of Allergy and Clinical Immunology (EAACI) and the German Association for Allergology and Clinical Immunology (DGAKI) [13–15]. The basis of successful food allergy management is a clear medical history with regard to the specific foods triggering the symptoms. Open

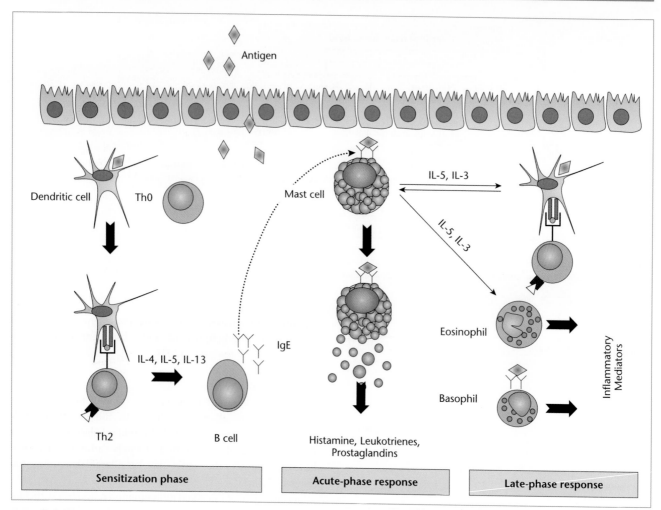

Figure 38.2 Phases of allergic response. (Modified from Bischoff SC. Food allergies. *Curr Treat Options Gastroenterol.* 2007;10:34–43.)

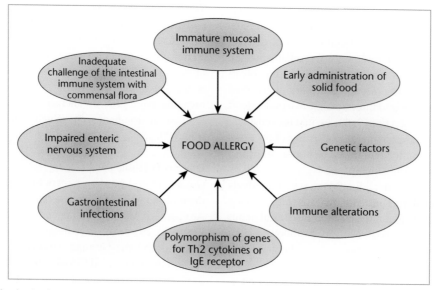

Figure 38.3 Risk factors for the development of gastrointestinal food allergies.

Table 38.2 Diagnosis of food allergies

Medical history
Symptoms
Atopy
Family history
Others

Laboratory studies
Routine laboratory parameters
Serum IgE/specific IgE (RAST, CAP)
EPX in serum and feces
Basophil histamine-release test (BHR)
Cellular allergen stimulation test (CAST)

Provocation test
Skin prick test
Elimination diet
Open provocation test
Double-blind placebo-controlled food challenge
Colonoscopic allergen provocation (COLAP) test

Gastroenterological examination
Endoscopy
X-ray
Sonograph of the abdomen
Histology of biopsy specimens

provocation tests may be helpful to substantiate suspicion, although they are subjective and require confirmation by objective testing [9]. Skin prick tests, measurement of specific IgE by using appropriate tests (formerly RAST, now CAP tests and others), and a few other laboratory measurements (e.g., measurements of eosinophils, eosinophil mediators, or mast cell mediators) are helpful to confirm the diagnosis or to make it more precise. Double-blind placebo-controlled food challenge (DBPCFC) is considered as the gold standard for diagnosing food allergies and should be performed in ambiguous cases. Food antigens are administered orally, by nasogastric tube, or via gelatine capsules. However, such procedures have several limitations with regard to food allergy manifesting in the gastrointestinal tract. The technique is widely not available and false negative results occur. Because of the lack of standardized readouts of reactions/symptoms the test is rather a subjective one even though it is performed in a DBPC fashion [4]. A new approach to overcome the limitations of double-blind placebo-controlled food challenges is local testing, e.g., by the colonoscopic allergen provocation (COLAP) test [3].

Treatment

The cornerstone of successful food allergy treatment is to avoid the exposure to the offending food. If trace amounts of allergen are sufficient to induce severe anaphylactic reactions the avoidance of the offending allergen is of particular importance. Patients need extensive education about how to avoid high-risk situations, the administration of epinephrine syringes in case of severe anaphylactic reactions and the proper reading of packaged food labels [8]. Such an education requires individual diet counseling by professional personnel. At present it is unclear if oral desensitization, injection immunotherapy, or prophylactic medications are beneficial in the prevention or therapy of food allergy. Some reports show that such therapies may be of benefit, but if the offending food cannot be identified or elimination is not feasible, antiallergenic medication is sometimes unavoidable [4].

Food intolerance

Food intolerance is an adverse reaction to food or a food group that occurs without direct involvement of the immune system. Food poisoning is caused by toxic substances in food and causes gastrointestinal symptoms in anyone who eats the food. It should not be mistaken for food intolerance, although similar symptoms can appear. Gas production, intermittent diarrhea, constipation, headache, and a nonproductive cough are typical symptoms of food intolerance [16]. Food intolerance is divided into three distinct forms (Figure 38.1). The diagnostic approach is often confusing, because of the uncertain etiology, the rather nonspecific symptomatology, the relative inaccessibility of the affected organ, and, most importantly, the lack of appropriate diagnostic means in many cases. Approximately 20–30% of the population of industrialized countries reports having at least some episodes of adverse reactions to food during their lifetime [4].

Enzyme deficiencies

Lactose intolerance is the most common food intolerance. It is provoked by enzyme deficiency and is common throughout the world. The disaccharide β-galactose-1,4-glucose, also named lactose, is present in the milk of mammals. Furthermore, dairy products and many processed foods contain lactose in different amounts. Lactase, a β-galactosidase, hydrolyses lactose to the monosaccharides, glucose and galactose. Lactase is mainly present on the apical surface of enterocytes in the jejunum [17].

Epidemiology

Lactose intolerance exists in three distinct types: primary, secondary, and congenital lactose intolerance. Primary lactase deficiency is inherited and most common. The incidence varies within different ethnic backgrounds [17]. In some Asian countries the prevalence is almost 100%. In the USA, 15% of the Whites, 50% of the Hispanics, and 80% of the Blacks exhibit lactose intolerance. Lactase activity is detected first by week 8 of gestation; it reaches its peak by birth [16]. However, lactase activity starts to decrease within the first months of life. Approximately 30% of the world population conserves the lactase activity beyond weaning and into adulthood, likely because of dairy farming in north Europe since approximately 10 000 BC [18].

Small and Large Bowel

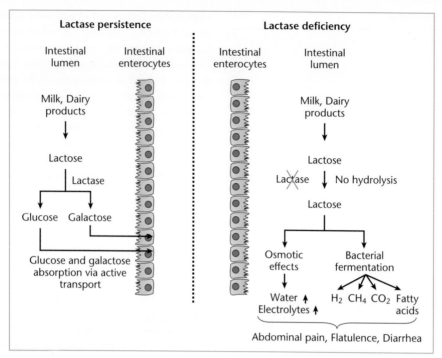

Figure 38.4 Pathophysiology of lactose malabsorption and intolerance.

Secondary lactase deficiency is caused by small intestine disease which damages the brush border, e.g., viral gastroenteritis, Crohn's disease and giardiasis. Usually the lactase activity returns to normal following healing of the underlying disease. Congenital lactase deficiency is inherited as an autosomal recessive disorder; the patients have no lactase activity from birth. Congenital lactase intolerance is very rare, with only few reported cases worldwide [16].

Pathophysiology and clinical presentation

Lactose intolerance typically presents with abdominal pain, flatus, diarrhea, and borborygmi. In some cases it causes constipation, nausea, and vomiting as well as systemic symptoms like headache or muscle pain. Symptom development is directly related to the pathophysiology of lactose intolerance. The inability to break down the lactose in the small intestine and to absorb disaccharides causes the fermentation of the lactose by the bacterial microbial flora (Figure 38.4). The high osmotic pressure of lactose results in an increased water and electrolyte secretion into the bowel lumen. In the colon, the disaccharide becomes hydrolyzed by the commensal microbiota to glucose and galactose; the monosaccharides becoming now available for bacterial fermentation which results in the production of short chain fatty acids, but also gases such as hydrogen, methane and carbon dioxide [18].

Diagnosis

The most reliable test confirming lactose intolerance (and other carbohydrate intolerances) is the hydrogen breath test. This test is non-invasive, inexpensive, and not labor-intensive. The breath hydrogen levels are determined, after fasting for 12 hours, before and after oral administration of 50 g lactose dissolved in water or tea. The principle of the test is that unabsorbed lactose becomes fermented by the intestinal microbiota in the colon whereby hydrogen is generated. Luminal hydrogen crosses the gastrointestinal barrier, enters the blood stream and is expired via the bronchi. An increase of breath hydrogen level above 20 ppm over the baseline within 3 hours of lactose ingestion indicates lactose intolerance. However, the occurrence of symptoms after ingestion of 50 g lactose does not exclude the likely possibility that patients can tolerate smaller amounts of lactose [17].

WORK UP FOR SUSPECTED FRUCTOSE/ LACTOSE INTOLERANCE

Clear clinical history
- Symptoms: abdominal distension, flatulence, abdominal cramping, diarrhea
- Symptoms are directly related to the quantity of ingested fructose/ lactose

Avoidance diet
- All sources of the suspected substance have to be eliminated, requiring the reading of food labels to identify hidden sources
- Generally a 2-week trial
- Resolutions of symptoms when suspected substance is removed from the diet, as well as recurrence of the symptoms when the substance is reintroduced, are very suggestive signs of intolerance
- Resolution of symptoms upon elimination of the suspected substance from the diet may not confirm intolerance. For instance, a patient can be sensitive to milk protein, so that symptoms of allergy resolve if milk is withdrawn from the diet

(Continued)

- Dieticians should advise the patients to make sure that the avoidance diet is nutritionally adequate

Hydrogen breath test
- In case of lactose/fructose intolerance
- Not invasive, inexpensive, not labour-intensive, more reliable than history
- Administration of 50 g fructose/lactose solved in still water or tea after a fasting phase of 12 hours
- Breath hydrogen levels are determined before and after oral administration
- Increase of breath hydrogen level above 20 ppm over baseline within 3 hours of ingestion indicate intolerance
- Factors that may produce false-negative or false-positive results are:
  - conditions affecting the intestinal flora (antibiotics)
  - lack of hydrogen-producing bacteria
  - ingestion of high-fibre diets before the test
  - small intestinal bacterial overgrowth
  - intestinal motility disorders

Blood testing
- Lactose intolerance is based on a single chain polymorphism
- Most commonly caused by the CC genotype of the C>T polymorphism located 13 910 base pairs upstream of the lactase-phlorizin hydrolase gene
- Genetic test results and breath test results are well correlated, hence gene tests are not common in lactose intolerance diagnosis

Stool analysis
- Measurement of reducing substances in the stool provides an indication of the absorption of carbohydrates
- The reducing substances have to be measured in the liquid portion and not in the solid portion
- Acid stool (pH level less than 5.5) indicates carbohydrate malassimilation

Therapy

Generally, people suffering from lactose intolerance do not have to remove lactose from their diet totally as small amounts of lactose are tolerated in most cases. Milk and dairy products are major sources of calcium and vitamins. Therefore, they should be consumed daily. For example hard cheeses are good sources of calcium. They contain little lactose and are tolerated by most of the people suffering from primary lactose deficiency [17]. Moreover, almost lactose-free dairy products are widely available. Alternatively, lactase preparations might be used to improve digestion of dairy products.

Pharmacological intolerance

In case of pharmacological intolerance, abnormal reactions occur due to the consumption of vasoactive amines and other food substances with pharmacological activity. The occurrence is dose-dependent and in most cases co-factors are necessary, thus not every exposure results in symptoms. Vasoactive amines are dopamine, histamine, norepinephrine, phenylethylamine, serotonin, tryptamine, and tyramine. But also methylxanthines (caffeine, theophylline, theobromine), capsaicin of red pepper, and alcohol can induce pharmacological intolerance [19].

Histamine, a diamine, is a chemical mediator which triggers allergic response. Histamine in foodstuffs arises from decarboxylation of histidine by microorganisms [20]. Cheese, alcoholic beverages, as well as fermented foods show high amounts of histamine. Furthermore, histamine is generated in the colon by intestinal bacteria which decay histidine to histamine. Normally, ingested histamine becomes rapidly inactivated by the diamine oxidase (Figure 38.5). People suffering from histamine intolerance show impaired diaminoxidase activity, which results in a decelerated histamine inactivation.

Idiopathic intolerance

Adverse reactions to food which cannot be classified in the above-mentioned categories are summarized as idiopathic intolerance. Mainly, reactions to food additives have to be considered in this category but also food aversions. The additives are employed in any stage of food production e.g., as

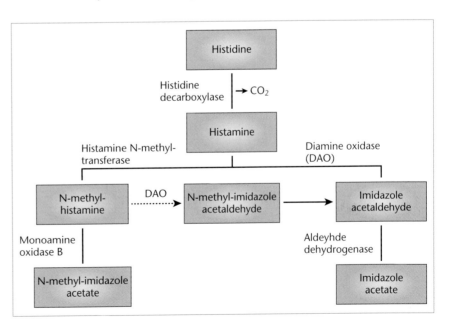

Figure 38.5 Histamine metabolism. (Modified from Maintz L, Novak N. Histamine and histamine intolerance. *Am J Clin Nutr.* 2007;85:1185–1196.)

food colorings, preservatives, or antioxidants. The maximum amount of food additives in foodstuffs is determined by law and considered as harmless [21]. The prevalence of hypersensitivity reactions to food additives seems to be rather low in contrast to the public perception. The investigation of the precise prevalence of food additive intolerance is difficult due to the large number of food additives under suspicion. European studies estimated the prevalence at 0.2–7% depending on the type of challenge [22–24]. Depending on the severity of the reactions, the identified additives have to be avoided in all their forms. Hence, commercially prepared foods should be restricted as much as possible [25].

References

1. Zuberbier T, Edenharter G, Worm M, *et al*. Prevalence of adverse reactions to food in Germany – a population study. *Allergy*. 2004;59:338–345.
2. Montalto M, Santoro L, D'Onofrio F, *et al*. Adverse reactions to food: allergies and intolerances. *Dig Dis*. 2008;26:96–103.
3. Bischoff SC. Gastrointestinal Allergy. In Holgate ST, Church MK, Lichtenstein LM, editors. *Allergy*. 3rd edition. Elsevier, London; 2006. p. 129–141.
4. Bischoff SC, Crowe SE. Gastrointestinal food allergy: new insights into pathophysiology and clinical perspectives. *Gastroenterology*. 2005;128:1089–1113.
5. Zuidmeer L, Goldhahn K, Rona RJ, *et al*. The prevalence of plant food allergies: a systematic review. *J Allergy Clin Immunol*. 2008;121:1210–1218.
6. Bischoff SC, Crowe SE. Food allergy and the gastrointestinal tract. *Curr Opin Gastroenterol* 2004;20:156–161.
7. Vighi G, Marcucci F, Sensi L, *et al*. Allergy and the gastrointestinal system. *Clin Exp Immunol*. 2008;153,Suppl 1:3–6.
8. Sicherer SH, Sampson HA. Food Allergy: Recent advances in pathophysiology and treatment. *Annu Rev Med*. 2009;60:261–277.
9. Bischoff SC. Food allergies. *Curr Treat Options Gastroenterol*. 2007;10:34–43.
10. Herz U. Immunological basis and management of food allergy. *J Pediatr Gastroenterol Nutr*. 2008;47,Suppl 2:S54–S57.
11. Sellge G, Bischoff SC. The Immunological basis of IgE-mediated reactions. In Metcalfe DD, Sampson HA, Simon RA, editors. *Food Allergy: Adverse reactions to foods and food additives*. 4th edition. Blackwell Publishing, Chichester; 2008. p. 15–28.
12. Chehade M, Mayer L. Oral tolerance and its relation to food hypersensitivities. *J Allergy Clin Immunol*. 2005;115:3–12.
13. Chapman JA, Bernstein IL, Lee RE, *et al*. Food allergy: a practical parameter. *Ann Allergy Asthma Immunol*. 2006;96,(3 suppl 2): S1–S96.
14. Niggemann B, Erdmann S., Fuchs T, *et al*. Standardization of oral food challenges in food allergies. *Allergo J*. 2006;4:262–270.
15. Bindslev-Jensen C, Ballmer-Weber BK, Bengtsson U, *et al*. Standardization of food challenges in patients with immediate reactions to foods – position paper from the European Academy of Allergology and Clinical Immunology. *Allergy*. 2004;59: 690–697.
16. Ozdemir O, Mete E, Catal F, *et al*. Food intolerances and eosinophilic esophagitis in childhood. *Dig Dis Sci*. 2009;54:8–14.
17. Harrington LK, Mayberry JF. A re-appraisal of lactose intolerance. *Int J Clin Pract*. 2008;62:1541–1546.
18. Lomer MC, Parkes GC, Sanderson JD. Review article: lactose intolerance in clinical practice – myths and realities. *Aliment Pharmacol Ther*. 2008;27:93–103.
19. Ortolani C, Pastorello EA. Food allergies and food intolerances. *Best Pract Res Clin Gastroenterol*. 2006;20:467–483.
20. Al Belushi I, Poole S, Deeth HC, *et al*. Biogenic amines in fish: roles in intoxication, spoilage, and nitrosamine formation – a review. *Crit Rev Food Sci Nutr*. 2009;49:369–377.
21. Randhawa S, Bahna SL. Hypersensitivity reactions to food additives. *Curr Opin Allergy Clin Immunol*. 2009;9:278–283.
22. Fuglsang G, Madsen G, Halken S, *et al*. Adverse reactions to food additives in children with atopic symptoms. *Allergy*. 1994;49: 31–37.
23. Wilson N, Scott A. A double-blind assessment of additive intolerance in children using a 12 day challenge period at home. *Clin Exp Allergy*. 1989;19:267–272.
24. Park HW, Park CH, Park SH, *et al*. Dermatologic adverse reactions to 7 common food additives in patients with allergic diseases: a double-blind, placebo-controlled study. *J Allergy Clin Immunol*. 2008;121:1059–1061.
25. Wilson BG, Bahna SL. Adverse reactions to food additives. *Ann Allergy Asthma Immunol*. 2005;95:499–507.
26. Bruijnzeel-Koomen C, Ortolani C, Aas K, *et al*. Adverse reactions to food. European Academy of Allergology and Clinical Immunology Subcommittee. *Allergy*. 1995;50:623–635.
27. Maintz L, Novak N. Histamine and histamine intolerance. *Am J Clin Nutr*. 2007;85:1185–1196.

CHAPTER 39
Maldigestion and malabsorption

Arvey I. Rogers[1] and Ryan D. Madanick[2]
[1]University of Miami Miller School of Medicine, Miami, FL, USA
[2]University of North Carolina School of Medicine, Chapel Hill, NC USA

ESSENTIAL FACTS ABOUT PATHOGENESIS

- Malabsorption results from impaired digestion and/or absorption of dietary macro- and micronutrients
- It can result in generalized malabsorption as in severe celiac disease or isolated malabsorption as for example in hypolactasia
- Steatorrhea results from impairment of lipid assimilation due to effects on lipolysis, micellarization, uptake and delivery

ESSENTIALS OF DIAGNOSIS

- A high index of suspicion in patients with chronic diarrhea, especially with loss of weight or nutrient deficiencies
- Certain etiologies, such as celiac disease, can be screened for during the evaluation with specific serologic tests
- Other cases require investigation for evidence of steatorrhea and determination of etiology through directed history and examination, laboratory studies, and rationally-selected diagnostic tests

ESSENTIALS OF TREATMENT AND PROGNOSIS

- Nutrient deficiencies should be corrected and pancreatic enzyme supplements given pragmatically whilst investigation is ongoing
- Fundamental treatment depends upon the cause

Introduction and definition

Malabsorption syndromes include disorders resulting from impaired digestion and/or impaired absorption. **Malabsorption** is the result of defective nutrient uptake or transport by the intestinal mucosa, whereas **maldigestion** denotes the impaired breakdown of macronutrients [1]. Etiologies are varied, but there are common presenting signs and symptoms. To accurately diagnose a malabsorption syndrome, it must be suspected on clinical grounds. Suspicion requires confirmation, and once confirmed, its etiology can usually be established [2]. Some understanding of the biochemical and physiologic aspects of the assimilation of dietary foodstuffs (macro and micronutrients) enhances an appreciation of the various manifestations of malabsorption. We will first present the essentials of carbohydrate, protein, and fat assimilation, and include key points regarding the assimilation of vitamin B$_{12}$. We will then focus on clinical strategies to evaluate a patient suspected of having a malabsorption syndrome. Many of the specific disease processes associated with malabsorption (e.g., celiac disease, bacterial overgrowth, exocrine pancreatic insufficiency) are discussed more completely in their respective chapters. Bile acid malabsorption will be discussed in detail in Chapter 43 and protein-losing enteropathies will be discussed in Chapter 44.

Physiology of assimilation: the essentials
Absorption sites

- Absorption of macro- and micronutrients occurs along a 3-meter length of small intestine (duodenum, jejunum, ileum).
- Carbohydrates, proteins, and lipids are absorbed in the duodenum-jejunum, a process completed at a point 100 cm distal to the duodenojejunal junction.
- Calcium, iron, zinc, folic acid, and the fat soluble vitamins A, D, E, and K are absorbed in the proximal intestine.
- The ileum can assume the absorptive function of macronutrients if the proximal intestinal structure or function is impaired.
- Vitamin B$_{12}$ and bile salts are absorbed in the ileum; the duodenum-jejunum cannot assume this function.

Carbohydrates

- Ingested as polysaccharides (starch), disaccharides (lactose, sucrose), and monosaccharides (glucose, fructose); absorbed only as monosaccharides.
- Polysaccharides digested primarily by salivary and pancreatic *amylases* to disaccharides, trisaccharides and branched oligosaccharides.
- Brush border enzymes hydrolyze the products of amylase digestion to monosaccharides.
- Glucose (and galactose) absorption occurs primarily through secondary active transport across the brush border membrane utilizing a sodium dependent co-transporter (*SGLT1*), which couples two sodium ions with one monosaccharide molecule [3].

Textbook of Clinical Gastroenterology and Hepatology, Second Edition. Edited by C. J. Hawkey, Jaime Bosch, Joel E. Richter, Guadalupe Garcia-Tsao, Francis K. L. Chan.

Small and Large Bowel

- Glucose (and galactose) accumulates intracellularly and enters the interstitial space by facilitated diffusion utilizing a basolateral transport protein (*GLUT2*).
- The sodium ions that enter the enterocyte (absorbing epithelial cell) are transported into the blood by a Na^+/K^+-pump in the basolateral membrane.
- Fructose is absorbed by facilitated diffusion utilizing an apical fructose-specific transport protein (*GLUT5*) as well as the basolateral transport protein (*GLUT2*). The human small intestine does not have an unlimited capacity to absorb fructose; its absorption is enhanced when ingested with glucose.
- Unabsorbed disaccharides are metabolized by colonic bacteria to short chain fatty acids that are absorbed by the colon (colonic salvage).

Proteins

- Sources include ingested food, intestinal juices, sloughed epithelial cells.
- The **chief cells** in the stomach produce **pepsin**, which plays a minor role in initiating digestion and yields amino acids and polypeptides.
- These products of hydrolysis stimulate release of **cholecystokinin** (CCK) from the duodenum and jejunum.
- CCK stimulates the pancreas to secrete both endopeptidases (**trypsin, chymotrypsin**, and **elastase**) and exopeptidases (**carboxypeptidase** A and B) as inactive precursors (e.g., **trypsinogen**).
- The brush border enzyme, **enterokinase**, activates trypsinogen to trypsin, which then autocatalyzes trypsinogen and all other peptidase precursors to their active forms.
- The active peptidases digest the polypeptides to amino acids (AA) and 4–6 AA residue peptides.
- Brush border peptidases digest the oligopeptides to tri- and dipeptides, some of which are absorbed intact and further digested to AA by intracellular peptidases.
- AA are neutral, basic, acidic, and L-isomers, which are absorbed by active, passive, and facilitated diffusion mechanisms.

Lipids

Long chain triglycerides

Four distinct and interrelated stages characterize the assimilation of dietary long-chain lipids: lipolytic, micellarization, cellular, and delivery.

Lipolytic stage

- **Lipases** (lingual, gastric, pancreas) incompletely digest long-chain triglycerides (TGs) to fatty acids (FAs), monoglycerides (MGs), diglycerides (DGs), and glycerol.
- Lipolysis is enhanced by both bicarbonate (yielding an intestinal pH of 6.8), and the detergent properties of conjugated bile salts.
- **Pancreatic co-lipase** facilitates binding of lipase to TG droplets, thus preventing the inhibition of lipase by bile salts.

Micellarization stage

- Defined as the solubilization of a complex mixture of the products of lipolysis into a **micelle**.
- Requires conjugated bile acids (CBAs), reaching a critical micellar concentration of $>2–3\,mol/m^3$.
- The resulting structure is a mixed micelle, consisting of CBAs, FAs, MGs, and some DGs, capable of solubilizing other fat-soluble substances and facilitating their absorption.
- The mixed micelle facilitates absorption of lipids through the epithelial cell plasma membrane (unstirred water layer).

Cellular stage

- Mixed micelles diffuse into the epithelial cell.
- Bile salts remain intraluminal, undergo absorption in the ileum via active transport sodium-dependent mechanisms, return to the liver via the **enterohepatic** (portal venous) circuit, and are recycled 4–6 times with each meal.
- Absorbed FAs bind to cellular proteins, are transported to the smooth endoplasmic reticulum where they undergo activation by acetyl CoA, and are esterified with alpha-glycerophosphate or 2-MGs to TG and phospholipid.
- **Chylomicrons** (TGs, phospholipids, cholesterol esters, apoprotein) undergo synthesis in the Golgi apparatus.

Delivery stage

- **Apoprotein B** synthesis is essential for the synthesis and transfer of synthesized chylomicrons into the lymphatics.
- Lymphatics are intraintestinal (lamina propria lacteals) and extraintestinal (cisterna chyli, thoracic duct).
- The process of transfer occurs via exocytosis.

Medium chain triglycerides (MCTs)

- Include FAs of 6–10 carbons in length.
- TGs are hydrolyzed readily by intraluminal pancreatic lipases, but MCTs do not require lipases for assimilation.
- Unhydrolyzed MCTs may be absorbed intact by the duodenojejunal epithelial cell.
- Intracellular MCT lipases can hydrolyze TGs to FAs.
- FAs do not undergo esterification; they are absorbed into the portal circulation bound to albumin.

Vitamin B_{12} (cobalamin)

- Cleaved from dietary sources by gastric hydrochloric acid secreted by the **oxyntic (parietal) cell**.
- At gastric pH < 3, gastric **intrinsic factor (IF)** secreted by the oxyntic cell has a poor binding affinity for the vitamin.
- Salivary **R-protein** is bound to the free vitamin in the stomach and is cleaved from the vitamin by pancreatic trypsin in the proximal small intestine.
- B_{12} then undergoes binding to IF in the duodenum.
- The stable B_{12}–IF complex attaches to specific receptor sites on epithelial cells of the terminal ileum.
- Once inside the epithelial cell, the complex is split, and the free vitamin is bound to **transcobalamin II** and circulated via the enterohepatic circulation.

Differential diagnosis

The differential diagnosis of malabsorption syndromes is impressive (Table 39.1). A detailed description of the individual conditions is beyond the scope of this chapter. Broadly, the categories may be recalled with a simple mnemonic, "LIMPS," as:

L Luminal disorders
I Infectious diseases
M Mucosal disorders
P Post-operative malabsorption
S Systemic disorders

Table 39.1 Causes of malabsorption ("LIMPS")

Luminal disorders
Exocrine pancreatic insufficiency
Bile acid deficiency
Zollinger-Ellison syndrome
Small bowel bacterial overgrowth

Infectious diseases
Tropical sprue
Whipple's disease
Parasitic diseases
    Protozoa (giardiasis)
    Tapeworms
Mycobacterium avium-intracellulare

Mucosal (*small intestinal*) disorders
Celiac disease (gluten-sensitive enteropathy)
Collagenous sprue
Lactase insufficiency
Crohn's disease
Lymphoma
Eosinophilic gastroenteritis
Systemic mastocytosis
Immunoproliferative small intestinal disease
Lymphangiectasia
Radiation enteritis
Chemotherapy-induced injury
Mesenteric vascular disease
Abetalipoproteinemia
Autoimmune enteropathy [22]

Postoperative malabsorption
After gastric surgery
After small bowel resection
After bariatric surgery

Systemic disorders
Endocrine disorders
    Diabetic enteropathy
    Hypothyroidism
    Hyperthyroidism
    Addison disease
Collagen vascular diseases
    Scleroderma
    Vasculitis
Amyloidosis
AIDS enteropathy
Graft-versus-host disease

After Farrell JJ. Overview and diagnosis of malabsorption syndrome. *Semin Gastrointest Dis.* 2002;13:182–190, with permission from Elsevier.

Approaching the patient with suspected malabsorption

The evaluation of a patient with possible malabsorption proceeds through three logical stages: (1) **suspicion** of malabsorption (based on signs, symptoms, and laboratory abnormalities); (2) **confirmation** of the presence of malabsorption; and (3) **defining the etiology** of the malabsorption. The separate stages are interdependent and proceed concurrently. The following section will focus on a rational approach to a patient whose presentation leads the clinician to **suspect** malabsorption. A thorough "bedside" evaluation and a limited number of laboratory tests should provide sufficient data to proceed from suspicion to confirmation.

Suspecting Malabsorption
"Bedside" Evaluation

The clinical manifestations of malabsorption range from covert, mild, subtle symptoms, to overt evidence of severe end-organ damage, depending upon the etiology and stage at presentation. **Clinical manifestations** may result from the **malabsorption** itself (e.g., diarrhea), the consequences of nutritional deficiency of the malabsorbed substance (e.g., iron-deficiency anemia with celiac disease), or the **underlying etiology** (e.g., abdominal pain with chronic pancreatitis). There is a plethora of **signs and symptoms** that should alert the clinician to the possibility of malabsorption, and it is incumbent upon the examiner to recognize and appreciate the possible significance of these features (Table 39.2). Many of the symptoms are nonspecific but should provide the initial evidence to the clinician that a malabsorption syndrome may be present. **Chronic diarrhea** is the most common symptom of malabsorption. However most chronic diarrheal disorders are not the result of a malabsorption syndrome (Chapter 6). When diarrhea is the presenting complaint, additional information should be sought to assess the likelihood that malabsorption exists. If **steatorrhea** is present, a patient may complain of visible oil in the toilet water; large, pale stools that float on the surface or are excessively foul-smelling point to steatorrhea (most floating stools do so because of gas, not fat). **Isolated carbohydrate malabsorption** may result in increased gas production, which leads to flatulence, bloating, and/or abdominal distension.

Malabsorption syndromes resulting from diffuse intestinal malabsorption may lead to **deficiencies of vitamins and other micronutrients**, and most of the clinical consequences are manifested in extraintestinal organ systems. As a consequence, the patient may not readily provide clinical clues without specific attention to the abnormality. Syndromes of **fat malabsorption** may result in deficiencies of the fat-soluble vitamins A, D, E, and K. **Musculoskeletal symptoms** such as tetany, muscle weakness, bone pain and osteomalacia occur as a consequence of vitamin D deficiency and hypocalcemia. **Ecchymoses** and easy bleeding can result from the coagulopathy associated with vitamin K deficiency. Vitamin A deficiency may lead to **night blindness**. Vitamin E deficiency, although rarely symptomatic, can lead to **neuropathy and retinopathy**.

Table 39.2 Clinical clues to the recognition of malabsorption

Signs and symptoms	Laboratory abnormalities
Gastrointestinal	**Hematologic**
Diarrhea	Anemia:
Constipation (rarely)	• Microcytic anemia
Steatorrhea	– Iron deficiency
Flatulence	• Macrocytic anemia
Bloating, distention	– Vitamin B$_{12}$ deficiency
Abdominal pain	– Folate deficiency
Glossitis	Hypersegmented PMNs
Cheilosis	Lymphopenia
Stomatitis	Eosinophilia
Ascites	Hypoprothrombinemia
Blood in stool (occult)	**Biochemical**
Musculoskeletal	Hypokalemia
Fractures	Hypocalcemia
Bone pain	Hypomagnesemia
Muscle weakness	Hypophosphatemia
Tetany	Hypoalbuminemia
Clubbing	Hypocholesterolemia
Rheumatologic	Hypotriglyceridemia
Arthralgias	Elevated alkaline phosphatase
Rheumatoid arthritis	Elevated serum bilirubin
Neurologic	Elevated serum folate levels
Paresthesias	
Peripheral neuropathy	
Night blindness	
Dementia	
Dermatologic	
Edema	
Acrodermatitis	
Hyperpigmented dermatitis	
Follicular dermatitis	
Koilonychia	
Dermatitis herpetiformis	
Hematologic	
Ecchymoses	
Easy bleeding	
Endocrinologic	
Amenorrhea	
Infertility	
Decreased libido	
Constitutional	
Weakness	
Fatigue	
Weight loss	
Cachexia	

PMNs: polymorphonucleocytes.

Diffuse intestinal malabsorption can also present with deficiencies of water-soluble vitamins and micronutrients. Cheilosis, glossitis, and stomatitis can result from deficiency of vitamin B complex, vitamin B$_{12}$, and iron. Iron deficiency also causes **microcytic anemia** and koilonychia (spoon-shaped nails). Both vitamin B$_{12}$ and folate deficiency can result in macrocytic anemia. However vitamin B$_{12}$ deficiency can be associated with **neurologic manifestations** such as peripheral neuropathy, whilst folate deficiency is not. Dermatologic manifestations can result from micronutrient deficiency, such as **perioral acrodermatitis (**zinc) or **hyperpigmented dermatitis** (niacin). **Amenorrhea** may complicate chronic illness, weight loss, and hypoproteinemia, all of which may be

associated with malabsorption. **Weight loss** in adults and **growth retardation** in children may indicate a malabsorption syndrome though other causes are common (Table 39.2) (see Chapter 12).

When evaluating a patient who presents with unusual, inexplicable, or disparate signs or symptoms, a **focused history and physical** should be performed to elicit additional information that could explain the consequences (clinical observations) and shed further light on the possible etiology of malabsorption. Much of this information can be elucidated with a thorough medical, social, and family history. Because of the exhaustive list of etiologic considerations, a complete listing of all pertinent inquiries is beyond the scope of this chapter. However, certain points should routinely be queried, as they may heighten the suspicion for malabsorption. Many of these are detailed in Table 39.3. Based on the initial assessment, the clinician should decide if lipid malabsorption (i.e., steatorrhea) is likely, as this judgment will help focus the remainder of the evaluation.

Initial evaluation

Although no laboratory finding is specific for malabsorption, **routine blood tests** can help to amplify the suspicion by identifying metabolic or hematologic consequences of malabsorption. First-line laboratory studies should include a **complete blood count** and differential, a complete **chemistry profile**, **coagulation studies**, and a **lipid profile**. Some additional specific (e.g., thyroid-stimulating hormone) and nonspecific (e.g., erythrocyte sedimentation rate (ESR) or C-reactive protein) tests can also be considered in the first-line evaluation as screening tests. However, most specialized laboratory tests (Table 39.4) should be ordered only if there is a strong likelihood of the disorder in question (e.g., **gastrin** in the Zollinger-Ellison syndrome (Chapter 112); cortisol or cortico-trophin levels in suspected Addison disease, etc.). A plain abdominal film may show calcification with chronic pancreatic insufficiency.

Confirmatory Tests without further evaluation

The reliability of screening tests for celiac disease and the ease of obtaining duodenal biopsy samples means that diagnosis is made and management instituted without formal confirmation of malabsorption. Similarly, a history implicating milk in the production of diarrhea should lead to rapid testing for hypolactasia. In more cryptic cases a formal process of confirming malabsorption and investigating its cause is required.

Confirming malabsorption
Fat

The initial step in evaluating a patient with suspected lipid malabsorption is confirming the presence of **steatorrhea**, defined as the excretion of at least 7g of fat in a 24-hour stool collection [2]. A simple screening test is the **qualitative Sudan III stain**. The test has limited value in patients with mild degrees of steatorrhea, i.e., 7–10g/24h. When the patient is ingesting an adequate amount of fat (75–100g/24h), the test is

Table 39.3 Questions to help identify possible etiology

Question	Potential etiology
History of present illness	
Do certain types of food products tend to provoke symptoms?	
• Dairy products	Lactase deficiency
• Dietetic candies and beverages; apples, pears, grapes, whole fruits and juices, honey	Fructose intolerance
Is abdominal (or back) pain a strong component in the presentation?	Chronic pancreatitis, pancreatic neoplasm, mesenteric vascular disease
Has there been a change in color of urine or stool?	Pancreatic neoplasm, cholestasis
Is pruritus present?	Cholestasis (intra- or extrahepatic)
Past medical history	
Is there a previous diagnosis of a malabsorptive disorder?	Crohn's disease, celiac disease, etc.
Is there a history of:	
• Prior gastrointestinal surgery (resection, bypass)?	• SBBO; pancreatitocibal asynchrony
• Liver disease?	• Cirrhosis
• Pancreatitis?	• Exocrine pancreatic insufficiency
• Immune deficiency or suppression?	• Infections, AIDS enteropathy, giardiasis
• Atherosclerosis or hypercoagulable state?	• Mesenteric vascular disease
• Diabetes?	• Exocrine pancreatic insufficiency, diabetic enteropathy, SBBO
• Radiation therapy?	• Strictures, fistulae, SBBO
• Dermatitis herpetiformis?	• Celiac sprue
• Chemotherapy?	• Small intestinal mucositis, mucosal atrophy
• Systemic sclerosis?	• SBBO
• Bone marrow transplantation?	• Graft-versus-host disease
Is there a previous diagnosis that may represent a consequence of a malabsorptive disorder, such as:	
• Peptic ulcer disease, erosive esophagitis?	• Zollinger-Ellison syndrome
• Nephrolithiasis? Gallstones?	• Crohn's disease
• Arthritis?	• Whipple's disease, Crohn's disease
• Cardiomyopathy?	• Amyloidosis
Is the patient ingesting a medication known to be associated with malabsorption?	Orlistat, acarbose, laxatives
Social history	
Is there a history of heavy alcohol use?	Cirrhosis, exocrine pancreatic insufficiency
Family history	
Is there a family history of a diarrheal disorder?	Crohn's disease, lactase deficiency, celiac disease

SBBO, small bowel bacterial overgrowth.

expected to be positive in approximately 80–90% of patients with true steatorrhea. False positive tests may occur in patients who are ingesting mineral oil, excessive nut oils, or using suppositories containing oils. In many laboratories an assay for fecal elastase is used to screen for malabsorption.

Carbohydrates

The most helpful screening test for isolated disaccharide malabsorption may simply be a well-documented history of dietary intolerance to the implicated disaccharide (i.e., lactose, sucrose). **Stool examination for pH and osmotic gap** are indirect tests that may indicate the presence of carbohydrate malabsorption. An acidic fecal pH (under 5.5) results from bacterial fermentation of malabsorbed carbohydrate. Although the sensitivity of the test is questionable at best, the specificity for carbohydrate malabsorption increases as the pH declines [4]. Stool osmotic gap is measured in the fecal supernatant and is calculated as follows based on the assumption that normal stool osmolarity is close to that of serum:

$$290\,mosm/L - 2\,([Na^+]_{stool} + [K^+]_{stool})$$

An osmotic gap greater than 50–100 mosm/L suggests the presence of an unmeasured solute, such as a malabsorbed carbohydrate. It is not however specific for carbohydrate malabsorption since the ingestion of a poorly absorbed ion (e.g., magnesium, sulfate, phosphate) or compound (e.g., sorbitol, lactulose), whether intentional or unintentional, also yields an elevated stool osmotic gap. Carbohydrate fermentation within the stool collection container may exaggerate the osmotic gap [1].

Hydrogen breath tests can also demonstrate carbohydrate malabsorption. In patients with carbohydrate malabsorption, an orally-administered disaccharide such as lactose remains undigested and passes into the colon. There it is fermented by the colonic bacteria, thus yielding a rise in breath hydrogen at 2–3 hours by 20 ppm from baseline [1,5]. In the case of small bowel bacterial overgrowth, the peak will occur within 1 hour and will be more prominent than the colonic peak. These tests

Table 39.4 Selected laboratory tests that may help define the etiology

Test	Potential etiology
Blood	
TSH[a]	Hypothyroidism, hyperthyroidism
ESR, C-reactive protein[a]	Crohn's disease, lymphoma, vasculitis
Glucose[a]	Diabetic enteropathy, chronic pancreatitis
Liver enzymes, bilirubin[a]	Cirrhosis
B$_{12}$, Folate	SBBO (elevated serum folate); tropical sprue (low levels of both)
HIV antibody, CD4$^+$ cell count	AIDS enteropathy
Anti-endomysial and tissue transglutaminase antibodies	Celiac disease
Antinuclear antibodies	Connective tissue disorders
Anti-mitochondrial antibody	Primary biliary cirrhosis
Intrinsic factor antibody	Pernicious anemia (rare cause of malabsorption)
Gastrin	Zollinger-Ellison syndrome
ACTH, cortisol	Addison disease
Leukocyte differential[a]	
Lymphocytes	Lymphangiectasia (lymphopenia)
Eosinophils	Eosinophilic gastroenteritis (eosinophilia), parasitism (strongyloidiasis)
Stool	
Ova and parasites	Parasitic disease
Giardia antigen	Giardiasis
Chymotrypsin, elastase	Chronic pancreatitis

[a]1st line tests

ACTH, adrenocorticotropic hormone; AIDS, acquired immune deficiency syndrome; ESR, erythrocyte sedimentation rate; HIV, human immunodeficiency virus; SBBO, small bowel bacterial overgrowth; TSH, thyroid-stimulating hormone.

may be falsely negative in the approximately 15% of patients who produce methane instead of hydrogen [5].

Inasmuch as dietary sources of fructose usually contain glucose, which enhances the absorption of fructose, there are no standards regarding the amount and concentration of fructose to be utilized in breath testing with fructose alone. When fructose malabsorption is suspected, a rational management approach to prove a cause and effect association would be to eliminate fructose ingestion [6].

Vitamin B$_{12}$ (Cobalamin)

Cobalamin deficiency is assessed initially by measurement of serum vitamin B$_{12}$. When this serum test is borderline or equivocal, an elevated **serum methylmalonic acid** confirms cobalamin deficiency [7]. Yet these tests do not differentiate between malabsorption of the vitamin and inadequate intake. The **Schilling test** provides both a confirmation of vitamin B$_{12}$ malabsorption as well as a differential assessment of the etiology of the malabsorption. In part I of the Schilling test, 1 µg of radiolabeled vitamin B$_{12}$ is administered orally, and its excretion is measured in a 24-hour urine collection. An injection of non-radiolabeled vitamin B$_{12}$ is administered as well in order to saturate the hepatic binding sites. At least 7% to 10% of the administered dose should be recovered in the urine to

be considered normal. When part I is abnormal, part II, which involves administration of vitamin B$_{12}$ along with oral intrinsic factor, is performed. In the presence of normal renal function and an adequate urine collection, normal excretion in part II of the test indicates intact ileal absorption of B$_{12}$ and a high likelihood that the patient has pernicious anemia. Persistent abnormalities during part II are the result of ileal dysfunction (e.g., Crohn's disease), small bowel bacterial overgrowth, or exocrine pancreatic insufficiency. The latter two etiologies may be teased out by repeating the test after the administration of antibiotics or pancreatic enzymes respectively.

Determining the etiology of malabsorption

Many cases of malabsorption (e.g., celiac disease or isolated carbohydrate malabsorption) seldom require sophisticated testing. If steatorrhea or other consequences of malabsorption (e.g., anemia, osteopenia, etc.) are confirmed, an etiology must be pursued. Isolated carbohydrate malabsorption rarely requires sophisticated testing. There is no single algorithm by which to approach each situation, and the sequence of testing is not hard and fast. Some of the tests that assess function (**Schilling test, D-xylose test, lactose hydrogen breath test**) both confirm malabsorption and help to pinpoint the etiology. A brief discussion about anatomic studies (radiologic, endoscopic, and histologic) and the D-xylose test follows, and a suggested course of evaluation concludes the chapter.

Endoscopic and histologic evaluation

If celiac disease is suspected, confirmation is a simple matter of taking 4–6 biopsies from the second part of duodenum. With modern endoscopes, lack of villi is obvious at the time of endoscopy. For more cryptic cases upper gastrointestinal endoscopy +/− enteroscopy with small bowel biopsy should be performed [8] with biopsy even if the mucosa is normal. Some diseases such as eosinophilic gastroenteritis, are patchy in nature, so biopsies should be obtained from different portions of the intestine (Table 39.5) [9,10].

Wireless capsule endoscopy (WCE, see Chapter 128) was introduced in 2001 as a method of directly imaging the small intestinal mucosa throughout the entire jejunum and ileum. WCE has been found to be useful in confirming mucosal pathology in patients with suspected non-stricturing small bowel Crohn's disease and celiac disease [11–14]. It may also prove to be beneficial in uncovering other mucosal diseases, such as Whipple's disease and lymphangiectasia, in patients with malabsorption syndrome and should be considered in selected cases, such as those with negative duodenal biopsies [14,15]. One limitation of the present versions of capsule endoscopes is the inability to obtain mucosal biopsies. Newer deep enteroscopic techniques (single-balloon, double-balloon, and spiral enteroscopy) show promise in their ability to evaluate the distal jejunum and ileum and obtain biopsies from areas with diseased mucosa (see Chapter 127). Similar to WCE, these advanced endoscopic techniques have been useful in diagnosing Crohn's disease and other small bowel diseases [16–18]. However since deep enteroscopy is newer,

Table 39.5 Diagnostic small bowel histology

Disease	Pathognomonic histologic findings
Generalized histologic abnormalities	
Abetalipoproteinemia	Lipid (triglyceride) accumulation in lamina propria; vacuolization of enterocytes
Collagenous sprue	Collagen band below atrophic mucosa
Mycobacterium avium-intracellulare	PAS-positive foamy macrophages with acid-fast bacilli
Whipple's disease	PAS-positive foamy macrophages (Gram-positive, acid fast-negative bacilli in lamina propria)
Patchy histologic abnormalities	
Amyloidosis	Congo red-positive deposits
Crohn's disease	Non-caseating granulomas
Eosinophilic gastroenteritis	Eosinophilic infiltration
Lymphangiectasia	Ectatic lymph vessels
Lymphoma	Clonal expansion of lymphocytes
Mastocytosis	Mast cell infiltration
Parasites	Parasites seen

After Högenauer C, Hammer HF. Maldigestion and malabsorption. In: Feldman M, Friedman LS, Sleisinger MH, editors, Sleisinger & Fordtran's *Gastrointestinal and Liver Disease*. 7th edn. Philadelphia: Saunders, 2002:1751–1782, with permission from Elsevier.
PAS, periodic acid-Schiff.

Table 39.6 Radiographic findings on small bowel series

Finding	Interpretation
Decreased small bowel length	Short bowel syndrome
Small bowel diverticula	SBBO
Fistula(e)	Crohn's disease, radiation enteropathy
Hypomotility	SBBO, diabetic enteropathy, scleroderma, amyloidosis
Dilatation	Celiac disease, systemic sclerosis
Stricture	Crohn's disease, radiation enteropathy
Tumor (with or without ulcers)	Lymphoma
Ulcers	Crohn's disease, NSAID enteropathy, vasculitis
Jejunization of ileum, barium flocculation	Celiac disease
Thickened folds	Eosinophilic gastroenteritis, giardiasis, Whipple's disease
Dilution of barium column	Zollinger-Ellison syndrome

NSAID, nonsteroidal anti-inflammatory drug; SBBO, small bowel bacterial overgrowth.

more invasive and less widely available than WCE, the body of literature to document the utility of these procedures in patients with small bowel diseases, especially malabsorption syndrome, is much smaller. Currently the role of these endoscopic procedures in the evaluation of patients with malabsorption syndrome remains to be defined.

Radiologic examinations

Advances in endoscopy mean that radiology (particularly barium studies) is less central to investigation than previously. Nevertheless, a small bowel series can be valuable in assessing the anatomy and mucosa of the small bowel. Although the negative predictive value of a small bowel series is low, an abnormal study is quite valuable and may guide further diagnostic testing (Table 39.6). **Enteroclysis**, or small bowel enema, is another radiographic technique for assessing small bowel disease; however, its use is limited by the need for small bowel intubation with a nasoenteric tube. **CT enterography**, a technique that improves visualization of the wall and lumen of the small bowel (see Chapter 133), is gaining popularity as a method of detecting small intestinal pathology. This technique has predominantly been studied for the diagnosis and staging of Crohn's disease [19]. To date, there are limited data on its use in detecting celiac disease or other mucosal disorders of the small bowel [20]. Cross-sectional imaging with CT enterography has the advantage of detecting mural and intramural pathology, as well as extraluminal pathology such as abdominal lymphadenopathy, which could occur in Crohn's disease or lymphoma. The gross and ductal anatomy of the

pancreas can also be assessed if chronic pancreatitis is a consideration.

D-Xylose Testing

As with radiology, testing **D-xylose** absorption is less routine than previously but may be valuable in cryptic cases. After ingesting a 25 g dose of D-xylose, the 1- or 2-hour serum value should be at least 25 mg/dL, and an adequate 5-hour urine collection should yield at least 4 g of the compound. Failure to achieve these levels suggests malabsorption as a result of proximal small bowel disease. The test may also be abnormal when there is proximal small intestinal bacterial overgrowth. False positive tests can occur with renal impairment, delayed gastric emptying, ascites (from third-spacing) and prokinetic or antimotility drug use [21].

Steatorrhea: Problem-Solving

There are a number of courses to take to arrive at an etiology for malabsorption. Most importantly, if a diagnosis is strongly considered, the appropriate specific diagnostic studies should be pursued prior to embarking on a potentially costly and exhaustive evaluation.

Once steatorrhea has been confirmed, defining its etiology requires only that the challenged clinician consider which of one or several stages of lipid assimilation has been compromised. Recalling which organ system (and its key factor) facilitates a particular stage sharpens the focus. A limited number of disorders may be the culprits that impair the function of a particular stage (Table 39.7). A focused inquiry into the

Table 39.7 Stages of lipid assimilation with key factors, disorders, and pathophysiology

Stage	Main organ system(s)	Key factor(s)	Representative disorders	Pathophysiology
Lipolytic	Pancreas	Lipase	Chronic pancreatitis Co-lipase deficiency Pancreatic cancer ZES Gastric surgery	Impaired lipase production or delivery Inhibition of lipase activity Impaired lipase delivery Inhibition of lipase activity Impaired mixing of fat and lipase (pancreaticocibal asynchrony)
Micellarization	Liver and biliary tract	Conjugated bile salts	Chronic liver disease Biliary obstruction SBBO	Impaired bile salt synthesis Impaired bile salt delivery Deconjugation of bile salts
	Terminal ileum	Enterohepatic circulation	Crohn's disease, ileal resection, bypass	Impaired enterohepatic circulation → reduced bile salt pool
Cellular	Duodenum and jejunum	Enterocyte (absorbing epithelial cell)	Celiac disease, tropical sprue Giardiasis Mesenteric vascular insufficiency	Enterocyte inflammation +/- atrophy Physical interference with absorbing unit Enterocyte atrophy
		Apolipoprotein B (ApoB), chylomicron	Abetalipoproteinemia	Defective or absent apoB → impaired chylomicron synthesis
Delivery	Lymphatic circulation	Lymphatic lacteals	Whipple's disease Lymphangiectasia	Lacteal obstruction Ectatic lymphatic channels
		Cisterna chyli, thoracic duct	Retroperitoneal fibrosis, tuberculosis, lymphoma	Extraintestinal lymphatic obstruction

SBBO, small bowel bacterial overgrowth; ZES, Zollinger-Ellison syndrome.

Table 39.8 Defining an etiology for steatorrhea

Suspected etiology	Confirmatory findings
Chronic pancreatitis	Pancreatic calcifications; pancreatic ductal abnormalities on CT; carbohydrate intolerance; improvement with enzyme replacement
Celiac disease	Family history; presence of anti-endomysial and/or tissue transglutaminase antibodies; abnormal small bowel biopsy; improvement with gluten restriction
Tropical sprue	Travel to or spending more than 30 days in Caribbean, southern India, or Southeast Asia; acute diarrhea→chronic diarrhea; megaloblastic anemia; abnormal small bowel biopsy; exclusion of celiac disease and parasitism; improvement on antibiotic therapy within 30 days.
Small bowel bacterial overgrowth (SBBO)	Gastro or enteroparesis; jejunal diverticula; surgical blind loops; enterocolonic fistulae; small bowel obstruction; chronic acid suppression; impaired B_{12} absorption; raised serum folate levels; improvement with antibiotic treatment
Crohn's disease	Ileal disease; prior ileal resection; extensive proximal small bowel disease; fistulae→bacterial overgrowth; obstruction→bacterial overgrowth
Giardiasis	Presence of parasite on small bowel biopsy, string test, or duodenal aspirate; identification of parasite or antigen in stool
Chronic liver and/or biliary tract disease	Evidence of liver or biliary tract disease on CT, US, MRCP/ERCP or hepatic biopsy
Lactase deficiency[a]	Acid pH on fresh stool; osmotic gap in stool supernatant; predisposing condition; positive H_2 breath test; improvement on lactose-free diet
Bile acid (cholerrheic) diarrhea[a]	Prior ileal resection or known ileal disease (<60–90 cm resected or diseased); improvement with bile acid sequestrant treatment (cholestyramine)
Surreptitious laxative use[a]	Fecal supernatant osmotic gap

[a]Non-steatorrheal malabsorptive syndromes.

Table 39.9 Application and interpretation of selected tests in steatorrhea

Stage of lipid assimilation	Diagnostic tests and expected findings		
	D-xylose absorption	Schilling (B$_{12}$ absorption)	Small bowel biopsy
Lipolytic	Normal	Normal[a]	Normal
Micellarization	Normal	Normal or abnormal[b]	Normal[c]
Cellular	Abnormal	Normal[d]	Abnormal
Delivery	Normal	Normal	Abnormal lymphatics

[a]May be abnormal if exocrine pancreatic insufficiency exists and will normalize with pancreatic enzyme supplementation.
[b]Normal with liver or biliary disease; abnormal with ileal dysfunction, resection, or bypass; or small bowel bacterial overgrowth (SBBO), which may normalize with antibiotics.
[c]Minimal inflammatory changes may be seen in some cases of SBBO.
[d]Unless cellular abnormalities extend to the ileum, e.g., tropical sprue.

patient's history will lead the astute clinician to consider possible etiologies. A careful review and interpretation of routine laboratory tests, selected specialized blood studies and stool examinations, as well as radiologic, endoscopic, and histologic studies will usually enable the identification of a specific etiology. A synthesis of findings that may be helpful in defining an etiology is presented in Table 39.8.

If the diagnosis still remains elusive, two of the previously discussed functional tests, the D-xylose and Schilling tests, can help determine the location of the pathophysiology. The decision about which to perform first depends on the previous evaluation and local availability. If vitamin B$_{12}$ deficiency is present, or if there is a concern for bacterial overgrowth or ileal dysfunction, a Schilling test should be performed first. If the diagnosis still is uncertain, the D-xylose test can then be used to document or disprove the small intestine as the site of malabsorption. If mucosal disease remains in the differential diagnosis, WCE should be performed. At the present time, deep enteroscopy cannot be routinely recommended when the prior testing is unrevealing. Should all of these tests be normal, then further evaluation of the liver and biliary tract is warranted (Table 39.9).

References

1. Farrell JJ. Overview and diagnosis of malabsorption syndrome. *Semin Gastrointest Dis.* 2002;13:182–190.
2. Hogenauer C, Hammer HF. Maldigestion and malabsorption. In: Feldman M, Friedman LS, Sleisinger MH, editors, Sleisinger & Fordtran's *Gastrointestinal and Liver Disease.* 7th edn. Philadelphia: Saunders, 2002:1751–1782.
3. Wright EM, Hirayama BA, Loo DF. Active sugar transport in health and disease. *J Intern Med.* 2007;261:32–43.
4. Eherer AJ, Fordtran JS. Fecal osmotic gap and pH in experimental diarrhea of various causes. *Gastroenterology.* 1992;103:545–551.
5. Romagnuolo J, Schiller D, Bailey RJ. Using breath tests wisely in a gastroenterology practice: an evidence-based review of indications and pitfalls in interpretation. *Am J Gastroenterol.* 2002;97:1113–1126.
6. Skoog SM, Bharucha AE. Dietary fructose and gastrointestinal symptoms: a review. *Am J Gastroenterol.* 2004;99:2046–2050.
7. Elin RJ, Winter WE. Methylmalonic acid: a test whose time has come? *Arch Pathol Lab Med.* 2001;125:824–827.
8. Babbin BA, Crawford K, Sitaraman SV. Malabsorption work-up: utility of small bowel biopsy. *Clin Gastroenterol Hepatol.* 2006;4:1193–1198.
9. Talley NJ, Shorter RG, Phillips SF, *et al.* Eosinophilic gastroenteritis: a clinicopathological study of patients with disease of the mucosa, muscle layer, and subserosal tissues. *Gut.* 1990;31:54–58.
10. Talley NJ. Eosinophilic gastroenteritis. In: Feldman M, Friedman LS, Sleisinger MH editors. *Sleisinger & Fordtran's Gastrointestinal and Liver Disease.* 7th edn. Philadelphia: Saunders; 2002:1972–1982.
11. Triester SL, Leighton JA, Leontiadis GI, *et al.* A meta-analysis of the yield of capsule endoscopy compared to other diagnostic modalities in patients with non-stricturing small bowel Crohn's disease. *Am J Gastroenterol.* 2006;101:954–964.
12. Spada C, Riccioni ME, Urgesi R, *et al.* Capsule endoscopy in celiac disease. *World J Gastroenterol.* 2008;14:4146–4151.
13. Ersoy O, Akin E, Ugras S, *et al.* Capsule endoscopy findings in celiac disease. *Dig Dis Sci.* 2009;54:825–829.
14. Sturniolo GC, Di Leo V, Vettorato MG, *et al.* Clinical relevance of small-bowel findings detected by wireless capsule endoscopy. *Scand J Gastroenterol.* 2005;40:725–733.
15. Delvaux M, Gay G. Capsule endoscopy: technique and indications. *Best Pract Res Clin Gastroenterol.* 2008;22:813–837.
16. Oshitani N, Yukawa T, Yamagami H, *et al.* Evaluation of deep small bowel involvement by double-balloon enteroscopy in Crohn's disease. *Am J Gastroenterol.* 2006;101:1484–1489.
17. Mensink PB, Groenen MJ, van Buuren HR, *et al.* Double-balloon enteroscopy in Crohn's disease patients suspected of small bowel activity: findings and clinical impact. *J Gastroenterol.* 2009;44:271–276.
18. Yano T, Yamamoto H. Current state of double balloon endoscopy: the latest approach to small intestinal diseases. *J Gastroenterol Hepatol.* 2009;24:185–192.
19. Tochetto S, Yaghmai V. CT enterography: concept, technique, and interpretation. *Radiol Clin North Am.* 2009;47:117–132.
20. Paulsen SR, Huprich JE, Fletcher JG, *et al.* CT enterography as a diagnostic tool in evaluating small bowel disorders: review of clinical experience with over 700 cases. *Radiographics.* 2006;26:641–657.
21. Craig RM, Ehrenpreis ED. D-xylose testing. *J Clin Gastroenterol.* 1999;29:143–150.
22. Akram S, Murray JA, Pardi DS, *et al.* Adult autoimmune enteropathy: Mayo Clinic Rochester experience. *Clin Gastroenterol Hepatol.* 2007;5:1282–1290.

CHAPTER 40
Celiac disease

Daniel A. Leffler,[1] Andrés Cárdenas[2] and Ciarán P. Kelly[1]

[1]Beth Israel Deaconess Medical Center, Harvard Medical School, Boston, MA, USA
[2]University of Barcelona, Barcelona, Spain

ESSENTIAL FACTS ABOUT PATHOGENESIS

- Incidence c. 1–2% in individuals of European, North African, Middle Eastern, and North Indian descent
- HLA DQ2 or DQ8 are necessary predisposing factors for the development of celiac disease. In a minority of these individuals, gluten derived from proteins in wheat, rye, barley and related grains triggers an immune reaction
- Active celiac disease causes damage to the small intestinal mucosa and produces auto-antibodies which may be involved in the systemic manifestations of celiac disease
- Untreated celiac disease is associated with numerous symptoms, diseases and complications

ESSENTIALS OF DIAGNOSIS

- Celiac disease can present at any age and prevalence is similar between men and women
- Initial assessment; tissue transglutaminase (TTG), endomysial antibody (EMA), or deamidated antigliadin peptide (DGP) serology are more accurate than antigliadin antibodies (AGA)
- **All patients at high risk for celiac disease or who are positive for TTG, EMA or DGP should have the diagnosis confirmed with duodenal biopsy**
- Intestinal and serologic tests normalize on a gluten-free diet

ESSENTIALS OF TREATMENT

- Strict gluten-free diet (GFD) is the only accepted treatment for celiac disease
- Less than 50 mg of gluten per day can cause persistent enteropathy
- Management should be multidisciplinary and always include a dietician knowledgeable about celiac disease and the GFD
- Persistent or recurrent symptoms, known as non-responsive celiac disease, are common and have a variety of causes
- Inadvertent gluten exposure is the most common cause
- Refractory celiac disease is a rare complication of celiac disease and is typically treated with corticosteroids or immunomodulators
- Type 2 refractory celiac disease (increased D3+/CD8– or [oligo] clonal intestinal T cells) predisposes to T-cell lymphoma, with a high mortality

Introduction

Celiac disease is characterized by malabsorption resulting from inflammatory injury to the small intestinal mucosa following **gluten ingestion**. In celiac disease there is clinical and histological improvement when a strict gluten-free diet is followed, and relapse when dietary gluten is reintroduced [1,2]. Celiac disease is a common disorder causing **clinical manifestations** in 0.3–1% of the population in the Western world, causing considerable morbidity and increased mortality, particularly from **lymphom**a [3–6].

The **pathogenesis** of celiac disease is related to inappropriate intestinal T-cell activation in HLA-DQ2 or DQ8 positive individuals triggered by antigenic cereal peptides from wheat, barley or rye. There is a wide variety of **presentations** that range from asymptomatic enteropathy to severe chronic diarrhea, weight loss, iron deficiency anemia and nutritional deficiencies.

Extraintestinal manifestations of celiac disease such as osteopenia or neurological disorders and associated conditions such as type I diabetes mellitus or hypothyroidism are commonly present. Although newer highly sensitive and specific serologic tests are available for the diagnosis of celiac disease, the demonstration of characteristic histological abnormalities in a **biopsy of the small intestine** remains the diagnostic gold standard.

Treatment consists of lifelong avoidance of dietary gluten to control symptoms and to prevent complications.

Epidemiology and the Spectrum of Disease

The true prevalence of celiac disease is not well documented because many patients are asymptomatic or have atypical symptoms. A multicenter Italian study identified seven new cases of childhood celiac disease for each known celiac patient, leading to the term the "**celiac iceberg**" [7–9]. Based on a recent Finnish study, the estimated prevalence of celiac disease among school children is at least 1 in 99. This estimate includes asymptomatic cases which were diagnosed based on serology and histology [10].

Textbook of Clinical Gastroenterology and Hepatology, Second Edition. Edited by C. J. Hawkey, Jaime Bosch, Joel E. Richter, Guadalupe Garcia-Tsao, Francis K. L. Chan.
© 2012 Blackwell Publishing Ltd. Published 2012 by Blackwell Publishing Ltd.

Contrary to past belief, celiac disease is common in many populations of European, Middle Eastern, North African, and North Indian descent [8,11]. Most series report a slight **female preponderance**, however in North America approximately 75% of diagnosed patients are female [12]. This is likely due to differences in healthcare utilization between men and woman rather than a major gender difference in the disease itself.

The **mortality rate** in patients not adhering to a strict gluten-free diet exceeds that of the general population mainly due to an increased risk for malignancy [13,14] although risk of death from cardiovascular and respiratory disease also appears to be elevated [6]. Treated patients adhering to a strict gluten-free diet appear to have no significant difference in mortality rates when compared to the general population [15,16], however on a population level, possibly due to imperfect gluten avoidance or to associated auto-immunity, mortality may not return to baseline [6].

Celiac disease classically presents with symptoms of **severe chronic diarrhea, nutritional deficiencies and anemia**. Although cases of classical celiac disease still occur, the majority of patients now present with atypical and more subtle manifestations such as iron deficiency anemia, short stature, dermatitis herpetiformis, or infertility. Cases of **silent celiac disease** in which the disease is identified by a serological test in an asymptomatic individual are increasingly common.

Latent celiac disease refers to individuals who are positive for serologic tests of celiac disease (tissue transglutaminase (TTG), endomysial antibody (EMA), or deamidated antigliadin peptide (DGP)) but have no evidence of enteropathy on intestinal biopsy. **Refractory celiac disease,** defined as symptomatic severe small intestinal villous atrophy mimicking celiac disease, but not responding to at least 6 months of a strict gluten-free diet, can be a life-threatening complication. This rare condition should only be diagnosed after carefully excluding concealed or inadvertent gluten ingestion, other causes of villous atrophy and overt intestinal lymphoma.

Pathogenesis

Celiac disease is perhaps the best understood autoimmune disorder. The identification of gluten as the trigger for celiac disease in the 1950s has allowed investigation into initial steps in pathogenesis in a fashion difficult or impossible in most other diseases [17,18]. Exposure of the intestinal mucosa to water-insoluble protein moieties of wheat gluten, or similar prolamins from the cereal grains barley and rye is necessary for celiac disease activation. Exactly how gluten passes though the mucosal lining is controversial and may occur via breaks in tight junctions [19,20] or by dendritic cell sampling [21–23]. In the submucosa of the small intestine, gluten peptides are selectively **deamidated** by the native enzyme tissue transglutaminase (TTG) [24]. The normal function of TTG is in collagen cross-linking and tissue remodeling; however, gluten peptides which have been deamidated by TTG have greatly increased **affinity for α/β heterodimer antigen binding** grooves of certain HLA binding sites on antigen presenting cells [25] (Figure 40.1).

It is also known that only the **HLA types DQ2 and DQ8** bind tightly enough to deamidated gluten peptides to stimulate an immune reaction. It is for this reason that celiac disease is limited to individuals with this genetic profile [26,27]. HLA class II molecules are glycosylated transmembrane heterodimers (α- and β- chains) organized in three related subregions: DQ, DR, and DP and encoded within the HLA class II region of the major histocompatibility complex on chromosome 6p. The HLA-DQ($\alpha1*501,\beta1*02$) heterodimer, known as HLA-DQ2 is present in over 95% of patients. The related DQ($\alpha1*0301,\beta1*0302$) heterodimer, known as HLA-DQ8 is found in almost all of the remainder. However, approximately 40% of individuals in Western populations carry either HLA DQ2 or DQ8 clearly indicating that these genes are necessary but not sufficient for development of celiac disease. Other genetic factors have proven elusive and aside from gluten exposure, environmental factors which may precipitate celiac disease in an at risk individual are largely speculative [28]. There is a high concordance in monozygotic twins, and an approximately 10 percent prevalence among first-degree relatives of individuals with celiac disease [29–31].

Binding of deamidated gluten to the HLA DQ2 or DQ8 molecules in patients with celiac disease activates T-lymphocytes expressing the **α/β T-cell receptor** [32]. The T-lymphocytes then activate **B lymphocytes** to production of immunoglobulins and other T-lymphocytes to secrete **cytokines** such as IFN-γ, IL-4, IL-5, IL-6, IL-10, TNFα, and TGFβ. These cytokines cause damage to enterocytes, stimulate migration of lymphocytes to the epithelium, and induce aberrant cell-surface expression of HLA-class II molecules on the luminal surface of enterocytes. This event may enable additional, more direct, antigen presentation by epithelial cells to sensitized T-lymphocytes. While T-cells mediate enteropathy, antibodies to TTG, gliadin and deamidated gliadin peptides (DGP) do not appear to be directly toxic to the intestine, although deposits of IgA anti-TTG can be found in the intestinal mucosa [33]. Beyond the great utility of antibodies to TTG and DGP for the diagnosis of celiac disease, there is growing evidence that autoantibodies to TTG may play a direct role in the **extraintestinal manifestations** of celiac disease, including dermatitis herpetiformis, neurological disorders and thyroid disease [34–36].

Histology

Celiac disease primarily affects the mucosa of the small intestine. The mucosal abnormalities are most evident proximally and decrease in severity with distal progression, but in severe disease even the ileum may be involved. Although enteropathy is often diffuse in a minority of patients, disease is patchy and may even affect only the jejunum or duodenal bulb [37,38]. For this reason, multiple biopsies are recommended for diagnosis of celiac disease.

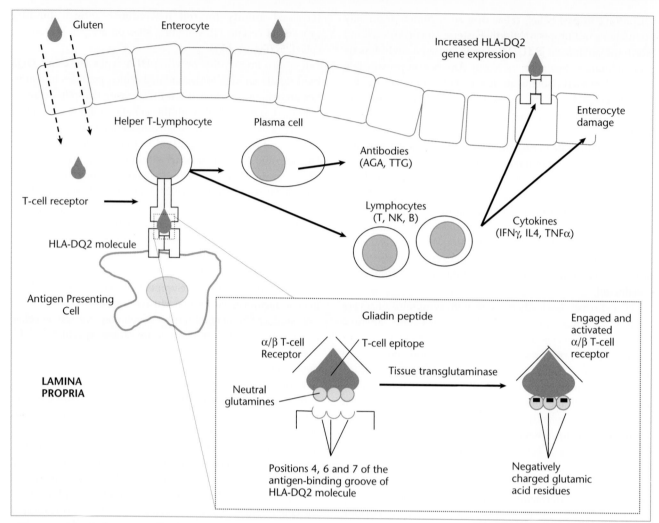

Figure 40.1 Pathogenesis of celiac disease.
Gluten is absorbed and presented in conjunction with HLA-DQ2 or DQ8 cell-surface antigens by antigen-presenting cells. Tissue transglutaminase (TTG) deamidates gliadin peptides, generating negatively charged residues of glutamic acid from neutral glutamines (inset). Because negatively charged residues are preferred in positions 4, 6, and 7 of the antigen-binding groove of HLA-DQ2, deamidated gliadin produces a stronger T-cell response. These lymphocytes then activate other lymphocytes to generate cytokines, such as interferon-γ, interleukin-4, and tumor necrosis factor α (TNF-α), which lead to villous damage and enteritis. Induction of aberrant HLA class II cell-surface antigens on the enterocytes may permit these cells to present additional antigens to the sensitized lymphocytes. AGA, antigliadin antibodies. (Modified with permission from Farrell RJ, and Kelly CP. Celiac sprue. *N Engl J Med.* 2002;346:180–188. Copyright Massachusetts Medical Society.)

The mucosal surface of biopsy specimens from untreated patients with severe lesions reveals a flat mucosa with absence of normal intestinal villi. Histological features include **loss of the normal villous structure** with a variable reduction in the villous height i.e., partial or subtotal villous atrophy, which may be grossly visible on endoscopy (Figure 40.2) [39]. The intestinal **crypts are hyperplastic**, markedly elongated and open onto a flattened absorptive surface. The total thickness of the mucosa is only slightly reduced in most instances, because crypt hyperplasia compensates for the absence or shortening of the villi. These architectural changes together with the reduction in mature, fully differentiated villous enterocytes decrease both the epithelial surface available and its capacity for digestion and absorption.

The **cellularity of the lamina propria** is increased, consisting largely of plasma cells and lymphocytes. The number of IgA, IgM, and IgG-producing plasma cells is increased two- to six-fold; but as in normal mucosa, IgA-producing cells predominate. Polymorphonuclear leukocytes, eosinophils, and mast cells may also contribute substantially to the increased cellularity of the lamina propria. Although the number of **intraepithelial lymphocytes** (IEL) observed per 100 enterocytes is increased in untreated celiac disease, the total number of IEL may not be increased, because the absorptive surface area is markedly reduced (Figure 40.3) [39,40]. In untreated celiac disease, as in the healthy small intestine, lamina propria T-cells are predominantly **CD4 positive** (helper) while the IELs are mainly CD8 positive (suppressor) cells. The density

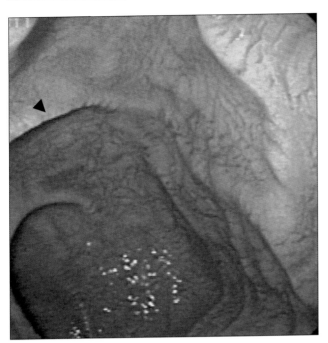

Figure 40.2 Endoscopic appearance of celiac disease with scalloping (arrowhead), flattening and atrophy of the duodenal mucosal folds, and a reticular, mosaic fissured pattern evident over the duodenal mucosa.

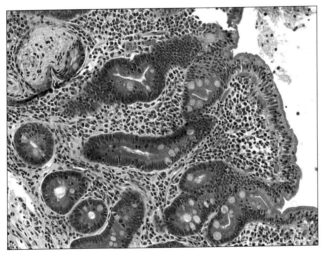

Figure 40.3 Histological appearance of the duodenal mucosa shown in Figure 40.2.
There is an increased number of intraepithelial lymphocytes and increased chronic inflammatory cells in the lamina propria. Note the architectural changes of focal epithelial injury and near complete absence of normal intestinal villi. The crypts are markedly elongated and open onto a flattened absorptive surface. (Courtesy of Maria L. Botero, MD, Beth Israel Deaconess Medical Center.)

of cells in both compartments returns to normal on a gluten-free diet [41].

Clinical Features

Celiac disease can present with a wide spectrum of gastro-intestinal and extraintestinal manifestations (Table 40.1). Hence

Table 40.1 Clinical presentations of celiac disease

Classical features	Other features
Chronic diarrhea	**General**
Iron deficiency anemia	Short stature
Abdominal pain	Delayed puberty
Irritability and depression	Clubbing
Abdominal distention	Edema
Failure to thrive	
Weight loss	**Gastrointestinal**
Malaise	Bloating
Anorexia	Recurrent aphthous stomatitis
	Steatorrhea
	Flatulence
	Vomiting
	Constipation
	Extraintestinal
	Folate deficiency
	Vitamin K and/or D deficiency
	Persistent hypertransaminasemia
	Thrombocytosis
	Osteomalacia, osteoporosis, fractures
	Dental enamel hypoplasia
	Arthralgia, arthropathy
	Peripheral neuropathy
	Ataxia
	Epilepsy (± cerebral calcification)
	Night blindness
	Female and male infertility
	Recurrent spontaneous abortions
	Poor academic performance
	Follicular keratosis, alopecia, easy bruising

(Modified with permission from Farrell RJ and Kelly CP. Diagnosis of celiac sprue. *Am J Gastroenterol.* 2001;96:3237–3246.)

celiac disease is easily missed unless it is included in the differential diagnosis of a multitude of symptoms, signs and laboratory abnormalities.

Children In children, celiac disease usually presents between 4 and 24 months of age with symptoms such as failure to thrive, impaired growth, vomiting, diarrhea, abdominal distention, wasting, hypotonia, anorexia, and irritability. Infants may have difficulty gaining weight, have pubertal delay and short stature. Other manifestations in childhood include constipation, recurrent abdominal pain, increased liver enzymes, recurrent or severe aphthous stomatitis, arthralgia, and dental enamel defects. Children may also have significant **behavioral problems**, such as depression, irritability and poor academic performance.

Adult patients Some adult patients are of short stature or give a history of undiagnosed diarrhea and abdominal pain in childhood. Nonetheless symptomatic celiac disease often develops de novo in adult life. Celiac disease can also be diagnosed in patients of **advanced age**; in fact approximately 30

Small and Large Bowel

percent of cases present after the age of 65 years [42]. Gastrointestinal symptoms can include large-volume or nocturnal diarrhea, flatulence, and weight loss. In many cases gluten sensitive enteropathy results in symptomatic lactose intolerance. Steatorrhea is less common and often indicates severe and extensive enteropathy. Dyspepsia and bloating are common and may lead to an erroneous diagnosis of irritable bowel syndrome. The diagnosis of celiac disease in adults is often delayed especially if patients present with multiple, mild and nonspecific symptoms consistent with irritable bowel syndrome.

Many patients initially present with **atypical symptoms** and as a result celiac disease is initially undiagnosed or misdiagnosed in over 50% of cases leading to an average 11 years of symptoms prior to diagnosis [12]. Adults with celiac disease are more likely to present with extraintestinal symptoms (Table 40.1). CR8 2NG due to malabsorption is the most common clinical presentation for adult celiac disease. Other **laboratory abnormalities** include macrocytic anemia secondary to folate deficiency, elevated prothrombin time resulting from vitamin K deficiency, and/or vitamin D deficiency leading to hypocalcemia [43].

Osteopenic bone disease develops as a result of impaired calcium absorption due to defective calcium transport, impaired Vitamin D absorption and binding of intraluminal calcium to unabsorbed fatty acids. Patients may present with bone pain and fractures, paresthesias, muscle cramps and even tetany. Osteoporosis is common in both adults and children with celiac disease [44,45]. Measurement of vitamin D status is recommended in patients with newly diagnosed celiac disease because osteopenia or osteoporosis are common and indicate a need for calcium and vitamin D supplementation in addition to treatment with a gluten-free diet [43,46]. In addition, bone mineral density measurement is recommended after one year on a gluten-free diet. Earlier bone densitometry is not generally recommended as there is significant improvement in bone density during the first year of celiac disease treatment [3,47]. Women may present with **infertility** or recurrent spontaneous abortions, and it is common for infertile women with celiac disease to become pregnant after commencing a gluten-free diet [48].

Ataxia is the most common severe **neurological disorder** associated with celiac disease and in some patients progressive gait and limb ataxia may be the only indication of celiac disease [49]. Patients presenting with nonhereditary progressive ataxia are frequently found to have evidence of gluten sensitivity and the disorder is believed to be auto-immune and possibly mediated by antibodies that cross-react between intestinal and neuronal tissue transglutaminase [35]. Peripheral neuropathy, muscle weakness and sensory loss may also develop in celiac disease. Although the association of epilepsy and celiac disease is well recognized, the underlying cause is again unknown [50].

Malignant diseases occur more frequently in patients with untreated celiac disease. Representative and reliable data are difficult to obtain but one recent large study found that the relative risk for malignancy in celiac disease was 30% higher than in the general population [51]. Although the risk of malignancy and mortality normalized in general with gluten withdrawal, data are conflicting as to whether these risks return fully to that of the baseline population [6,13]. Enteropathy associated intestinal T-cell lymphoma is the most commonly recognized fatal complication of celiac disease. Additional celiac disease-associated malignancies include other non-Hodgkin lymphomas, esophageal and oropharyngeal squamous carcinoma and small bowel adenocarcinoma.

Associated conditions

Many conditions that are associated with celiac disease are listed in Table 40.2. **Dermatitis herpetiformis** (DH); a skin disorder in which intensely pruritic papulovesicular lesions appear symmetrically over the extensor surfaces of the extremities, buttocks, trunk, neck and scalp, deserves special mention since it is invariably associated with gluten sensitive enteropathy. The diagnosis of DH is confirmed by performing immunoflouoresence which shows granular IgA deposits in an area of normal skin unaffected by blistering [34]. The treatment of choice for DH and the associated celiac disease is a lifelong strict gluten-free diet, however drug therapy with dapsone may be necessary as an adjunctive agent, especially early after diagnosis.

The most common **autoimmune disorders** associated with celiac disease are insulin-dependent diabetes mellitus (IDDM) and autoimmune thyroiditis with hypothyroidism [52]. The reported prevalence of celiac disease in patients with IDDM is approximately 4 percent and vice versa. Chronic diarrhea, other gastrointestinal symptoms, nutritional deficiencies, or unexplained episodes of hypoglycemia should alert the practitioner to the possibility of celiac disease in patients with IDDM. The relationship between celiac disease and other organ-specific autoimmune disorders may simply reflect shared HLA-haplotype associations. However, it has also been suggested that untreated celiac disease may increase the risk for autoimmunity through chronic uncontrolled lamina propria T-cell activation or decreased integrity of the intestinal mucosa. At this point it is unclear whether adoption of a gluten-free diet in celiac disease can lower the risk of subsequent autoimmune disorders [53,54].

Diagnosis
Serological tests

A diagnostic approach to celiac disease is described in Figure 40.4. The availability of a highly sensitive and specific serological test: the **IgA tissue transglutaminase** assay has greatly simplified the approach to making the diagnosis of celiac disease (see below). If the clinical suspicion of celiac disease is

Table 40.2 Associated diseases and complications of celiac disease

Associated conditions*	Complications*
Definite associations	Refractory celiac disease (circa 1%)
Hyposplenism	Enteropathy-associated T-cell lymphoma (2–10%)
Dermatitis herpetiformis	Carcinoma
IgA deficiency	(oropharyngeal, esophageal, small intestinal)
Autoimmune thyroid disease	Ulcerative jejunoileitis
Sjögren's syndrome	Collagenous sprue
Type 1 diabetes mellitus	
Microscopic colitis	
Rheumatoid arthritis	
Down syndrome	
IgA mesangial nephropathy	
Other reported associations	
Inflammatory bowel disease	
Sarcoidosis	
Congenital heart disease	
Addison disease	
Systemic lupus erythematosus	
Vasculitis	
Polymyositis	
Autoimmune hepatitis	
Primary biliary cirrhosis	
Recurrent pericarditis	
Cystic fibrosis	
Fibrosing alveolitis	
Lung cavities	
Pulmonary hemosiderosis	
Myasthenia gravis	
Schizophrenia	

(Modified with permission from Farrell RJ and Kelly CP. Diagnosis of celiac sprue. *Am J Gastroenterol.* 2001;96:3237–3246).

low (e.g., symptoms typical of irritable bowel syndrome), a negative serological test has a high negative predictive value; which would preclude the need for small bowel biopsy. Because the specificity of the IgA TTG test is high (>95%) the positive predictive values are also high even in low-risk populations [26].

Nonetheless, a positive serological test for celiac disease should be confirmed by **biopsy of the small intestine** before starting treatment with a gluten-free diet for the remainder of the patient's lifetime. When the index of suspicion is high, (e.g., chronic watery diarrhea, family history of celiac disease, iron deficiency anemia), both serology and a small bowel biopsy should be performed. The incidence of **IgA deficiency** is sixteen times greater among patients with celiac disease compared to the general population. This occasionally results in a falsely negative IgA TTG test. Thus measurement of total serum IgA levels are often performed together with IgA TTG (1,2,7,12). In cases of IgA deficiency, IgG deamidated gliadin peptide (DGP-IgG) is the preferred test.

Other serologic Tests

Serologic tests have revolutionized the diagnostic approach to celiac disease. These tests are useful for diagnosing individuals with suspected disease, evaluating those with atypical or extraintestinal manifestations and to monitor response to gluten-free diet. It is worth noting however, that serologic tests are of limited utility in monitoring gluten-free diet adherence [55]. Numerous serologic tests are available in addition to IgA TTG including **IgA-antiendomysial antibodies** (EMA), IgA and IgG anti-gliadin antibodies (AGA) and most recently IgA and IgG antibodies to **deamidated gliadin peptide** (DGP) (Table 40.3). IgA-antiendomysial antibodies are detected by indirect immunofluoresence using sections of human umbilical cord or monkey esophageal smooth muscle. The IgA-antiendomysial antibody tests have a sensitivity of 85–98 percent and specificity 97–100 percent [27]. Tissue transglutaminase is the autoantigen recognized by the antiendomysial antibody. An IgA-ELISA to detect human recombinant tissue transglutaminase is now widely available and is more sensitive, but marginally less specific than the antiendomysial antibody assay. The anti-endomysial antibody assay has been supplanted largely by TTG due to the lower cost and lower inter-observer variability of the latter assay. False-positive IgA TTG results are unusual and are usually low titer. False-negative IgA TTG are more common especially in mild enteropathy, in children under 2 years of age, and in patients with IgA deficiency as noted earlier.

Although **IgA- and IgG-antigliadin** antibody tests have been widely used for over 2 decades their clinical utility is in rapid decline since their diagnostic accuracy is substantially lower than any of the more recent serologic tests. In many normal individuals as well as patients with esophagitis, gastritis, gastroenteritis and inflammatory bowel disease, the antigliadin antibody tests, especially the IgG antigliadin assays, are falsely positive. Thus the positive predictive value

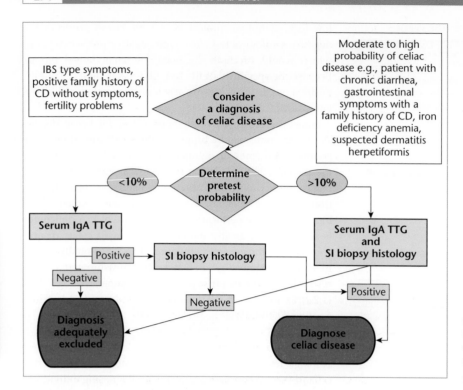

Figure 40.4 Diagnostic approach to celiac disease. TTG, tissue transglutaminase. (Modified with permission from Farrell RJ and Kelly CP. Diagnosis of celiac sprue. *Am J Gastroenterol.* 2001;96:3237–3246).

Table 40.3 Sensitivity and specificity of serological tests in patients with untreated celiac disease [70,71]

Serological test	Sensitivity*	Specificity*
IgA human tissue transglutaminase antibodies	93–95%	95–98%
IgA endomysial antibodies	85–98%	97–100%
IgA/IgG deamidated gliadin peptide	86–95%	93–96%
IgA guinea pig tissue transglutaminase antibodies	95–98%	94–95%
IgA antigliadin antibodies	75–90%	82–95%
IgG antigliadin antibodies	69–85%	73–90%

*Wide variations are reported between different laboratories and assays. (Modified with permission from Farrell RJ and Kelly CP. Diagnosis of celiac sprue. *Am J Gastroenterol.* 2001;96:3237–3246.)

of antigliadin antibody tests in both symptomatic and asymptomatic subjects is **unacceptably low**.

Monitoring

IgA-antigliadin antibody and IgA TTG appear to show similar sensitivities to changes in dietary gluten intake. Thus, serial IgA TTG testing is the standard test used to monitor immunologic response to treatment with a gluten-free diet. The levels of IgA TTG will typically reduce by 50% within 3 months of starting treatment with a strict gluten-free diet. IgG antibody

levels take substantially longer to normalize and are therefore less useful in monitoring treatment compliance and response. Deamidated gliadin peptide antibodies appear to be as accurate as TTG-IgA, and currently the composite DGP-IgG assay is the test of choice for individuals with IgA deficiency where it is more sensitive than TTG-IgG.

Other blood tests

Iron, folate, and/or vitamin D deficiency and secondary hyperparathyroidism are often present in patients with untreated celiac disease. Vitamin B_{12} deficiency is less common because celiac disease typically does not affect the ileum. Vitamin B_{12} deficiency may occur also as a complication of small intestinal bacterial overgrowth. For unclear reasons features of hyposplenism with **Howell-Jolly bodies** and thrombocytosis are seen in older untreated patients. Untreated celiac disease is often associated with mild elevation of serum transaminase levels, thus celiac disease should always be considered in patients with persistent and unexplained hypertransaminasemia. Liver enzyme levels revert to normal on a gluten-free diet unless there is co-existent liver disease.

Endoscopy and Small Intestine Biopsy

Histologic examination of a small intestinal biopsy, usually obtained during duodenoscopy, still retains its place as the gold standard for diagnosing celiac disease [56]. **Multiple (at least 6) biopsies** should be taken from the second and third portions of the duodenum in order to provide sufficient biopsy material to diagnose a sometimes mild and patchy enteropathy. In adults, the duodenal bulb has typically been avoided due to architectural distortion produced by Brunner's glands or peptic duodenitis, however there is increasing evidence that, in children at least, biopsies of the duodenal bulb may be warranted [37].

During **endoscopy** gross evidence of celiac enteropathy such as complete or partial loss of the normal duodenal folds, scalloped folds, mucosal nodularity or a fissured, mosaic pattern may be recognized (Figure 40.2). These endoscopic features, singly or in combination, have greater than 90% specificity for celiac disease but lack sensitivity in that over 40% of patients with biopsy-proven celiac disease have normal appearing duodenal mucosa at endoscopy [57]. Thus, biopsy is indicated whenever celiac disease is suspected regardless of the endoscopic appearance of the duodenal mucosa.

The characteristic histological appearance of the small bowel in patient with untreated celiac disease is described above (see also Figure 40.3). The severity and extent of the histological abnormalities of celiac disease vary greatly; surprisingly however, differences in degree and extent of villous atrophy do not seem to predict severity of symptoms [38,58].

Radiological tests

Small bowel barium X-rays, abdominal computed tomography, magnetic resonance enterography, or capsule endoscopy may be indicated in a small subset of celiac disease patients that do not respond to treatment with a strict gluten-free diet or in those with marked weight loss, abdominal pain, a palpable abdominal mass, profound hypoalbuminemia, gastrointestinal bleeding or obstruction in which complications such as lymphoma, or ulcerative jejunoileitis are suspected. Diffuse bone demineralization may be evident on plain films but **bone mineral density** testing is indicated in newly diagnosed celiac disease to provide a more sensitive and quantitative evaluation of bone mineral content. Osteoporosis or significant osteopenia in a patient with celiac disease indicates the need for oral calcium and/or vitamin D supplementation and monitoring of calcium, vitamin D, PTH concentrations and bone health.

Repeat Biopsy and Gluten Challenge

Even though an initial small bowel biopsy is required to establish the diagnosis, serologic testing for TTG auto-antibodies has dramatically reduced the need for repeat biopsies to confirm mucosal recovery on treatment and/or the recurrence of celiac enteropathy during subsequent gluten challenge. In short, a positive IgA TTG serology in combination with abnormal small bowel histology that is consistent with celiac disease, combine to provide an absolute diagnosis of celiac disease that does not require any routine re-evaluation. Nonetheless, a second biopsy may be needed for patients with a **poor clinical response** to gluten-free diet or in those where the initial diagnosis is less secure [1,3,59].

A **gluten challenge** is indicated when the diagnosis of celiac disease is in doubt during a period of gluten restriction (e.g., patients who began a gluten-free diet without histological confirmation of celiac disease). Gluten challenge should be started

with caution as some patients are exquisitely sensitive to gluten. If a small amount of gluten (a piece of a cracker or bread) is well tolerated, the portion can be doubled every 3 days until the equivalent of four slices of bread is ingested daily and continued for 6 to 8 weeks or until symptoms develop. At that point serological tests and biopsy are repeated. If serology and biopsy are both negative at 6 to 8 weeks, these individuals should be monitored for signs and symptoms of celiac disease on a normal diet for at least 6 months, after which serologic tests should again be checked and another small bowel biopsy considered.

Therapy

The mainstay of therapy for celiac disease is strict adherence to a **gluten-free diet**. Treatment represents a lifelong commitment, can be expensive and is socially inconvenient. These issues may limit compliance for all age groups but particularly for children and teenagers. Consequently it is very important that the diagnosis is made correctly and unambiguously before recommending treatment. Products that contain **wheat gluten**, or are produced from **barley or rye** must be avoided. Gluten is present in many dietary items because wheat flour is widely used in processed foods as a thickener and inexpensive filler. Furthermore, gluten-free grain can become **contaminated with wheat**, if producers use the same equipment to process both gluten-containing and gluten-free foods. As a result, complete elimination of gluten from the diet is a challenge to achieve and maintain. Patient education is of crucial importance and an effective gluten-free diet requires extensive, repeated counseling and instruction of the patient by the physician and a skilled dietician. It also requires a motivated patient that will read labels carefully and critically.

In recent years the CR8 2NG for individuals with celiac disease has been proven [60–62]. Although a tiny minority of patients may have an immunologic reaction to oat proteins, problems arise more commonly due to consumption of oats contaminated by wheat or barley. Thus, it is important that oats come from a **dedicated gluten-free source**. Currently, it is generally recommended that oats be avoided in all newly diagnosed patients until remission is achieved on a strict gluten-free diet. Afterwards, non-contaminated oats from a reliable source can be introduced and continued if well tolerated. Patients with untreated celiac disease often have secondary lactase deficiency and thus need to avoid dairy products initially. After 3–6 months of treatment and mucosal healing dairy products can be reintroduced if tolerated.

More than half of patients **improve within four weeks** of beginning a gluten-free diet [63]. In many, symptomatic improvement is noticed within 48 hours, although it can take months to achieve full clinical remission. **Serologic and histological improvement** usually lag behind symptom response and for this reason it is rarely helpful to repeat either serologic tests or biopsy after less than three months of treatment. Lack of clinical or histologic response, known as **non-responsive** celiac disease, has a number of etiologies, however the most common is ongoing gluten exposure [59,64]. Other common causes of non-responsive celiac disease include co-existing irritable bowel syndrome, lactose intolerance, microscopic colitis, small intestinal bacterial overgrowth and refractory celiac disease [59,64].

In addition to a gluten-free diet, all patients with clinical evidence of malabsorption should take a gluten-free **multivitamin tablet** daily along with a calcium and vitamin D supplement. Iron, folate vitamin B_{12} and zinc supplements may also be needed to replete body stores in those with deficiencies. In patients with **hyposplenism**, prophylactic antibiotics before invasive procedures and pneumococcus vaccination should be considered. In rare instances, intravenous corticosteroid therapy may be required for critically ill patients with acute celiac crisis manifested by severe diarrhea, dehydration, weight loss, acidosis, hypocalcemia, and hypoproteinemia, or the even more rare condition of gliadin shock complicating gluten challenge.

Refractory celiac disease

Refractory celiac disease is a diagnosis of exclusion defined as symptomatic severe celiac enteritis that does not respond to at least 6 months of a strict gluten-free diet and is not accounted for by other causes of villous atrophy or by intestinal lymphoma [65]. Although previously thought of as universally morbid, it is increasingly recognized that refractory celiac disease has a wide clinical spectrum [65,66].

Refractory celiac disease is divided pathologically into Type I and Type II disease. **Type I refractory celiac disease** is characterized by normal CD3/CD8 intraepithelial lymphocyte markers and no clonal T-cell population, while **type II disease** has either a high percentage of CD3+, CD8−, intraepithelial lymphocytes or a colonal/oligoclonal intestinal T-cell population. This designation is of great clinical importance as individuals with Type I disease have good long-term outcomes, while those with Type II disease have high mortality, largely due to the development of **enteropathy-associated T-cell lymphoma** [67,68].

In studies from Europe, approximately half of patients with refractory celiac disease are Type II; however this proportion appears to be much less in the United States. T-cell populations in Type II refractory celiac disease also appear to have destructive properties related to their cytotoxic phenotype, which lead to mucosal ulceration, lymph-node cavitation and progression to overt lymphoma. Therapy with **corticosteroids and other immunosuppressant drugs** such as azathioprine or cyclosporine may be beneficial in the short term but death from malnutrition, immunocompromise and lymphoma is frequent. Although the data are not conclusive, most published studies indicate that strict adherence to a gluten-free diet reduces the risk of all celiac disease-associated malignancies including enteropathy-associated T-cell lymphoma [13,69].

References

1. Farrell RJ, and Kelly CP. Celiac sprue. *N Engl J Med*. 2002;346: 180–188.

2. Green PH and Cellier C. Celiac disease. *N Engl J Med*. 2007;357: 1731–1743.

3. Rostom A, Murray JA, and Kagnoff MF. American Gastroenterological Association (AGA) Institute technical review on the diagnosis and management of celiac disease. *Gastroenterology*. 2006; 131:1981–2002.

4. Dube C, Rostom A, Sy R, *et al*. The prevalence of celiac disease in average-risk and at-risk Western European populations: a systematic review. *Gastroenterology*. 2005;128:S57–67.

5. Accomando S and Cataldo F. The global village of celiac disease. *Dig Liver Dis*. 2004;36:492–498.

6. Ludvigsson JF, *et al*. Small-intestinal histopathology and mortality risk in celiac disease. *JAMA*. 2009;302:1171–1178.

7. Kamin DS and Furuta GT. The iceberg cometh: establishing the prevalence of celiac disease in the United States and Finland. *Gastroenterology*. 2004;126:359–361, discussion 361.

8. Catassi C, Fabiani E, Rätsch IM, *et al*. The coeliac iceberg in Italy. A multicentre antigliadin antibodies screening for coeliac disease in school-age subjects. *Acta Paediatr Suppl*. 1996;412:29–35.

9. Catassi C, Rätsch IM, Fabiani E, *et al*. Coeliac disease in the year 2000: exploring the iceberg. *Lancet*. 1994;343:200–203.

10. Maki M, Mustalahti K, Kokkonen J, *et al*. Prevalence of Celiac disease among children in Finland. *N Engl J Med*. 2003;348: 2517–2524.

11. Catassi C. The global village of celiac disease. *Recent Prog Med*. 2001;92:446–450.

12. Green PHR, Stavropoulos SN, Panagi SG, *et al*. Characteristics of adult celiac disease in the USA: results of a national survey. *Am J Gastroenterol*. 2001;96:126–131.

13. West J, Logan RF, Smith CJ, *et al*. Malignancy and mortality in people with coeliac disease: population based cohort study. *BMJ*. 2004;329:716–719.

14. Rubio-Tapia A, Kyle RA, Kaplan EL, *et al*. Increased Prevalence and Mortality in Undiagnosed Celiac Disease. *Gastroenterology*. 2009;137:88–93.

15. Collin P, Pukkala E, and Reunala T. Malignancy and survival in dermatitis herpetiformis: a comparison with coeliac disease. *Gut*. 1996;38:528–530.

16. Collin P, Reunala T, Pukkala E *et al*. Coeliac disease–associated disorders and survival. *Gut*. 1994;35:1215–1218.

17. van Berge-Henegouwen GP and Mulder CJ. Pioneer in the gluten-free diet: Willem-Karel Dicke 1905–1962, over 50 years of gluten-free diet. *Gut*. 1993;34:1473–1475.

18. Dicke WK, Weijers HA, and van De Kamer JH. Coeliac disease. II. The presence in wheat of a factor having a deleterious effect in cases of coeliac disease. *Acta Paediatr*. 1953;42:34–42.

19. Tripathi A, Lammers KM, Goldblum S, *et al*. Identification of human zonulin, a physiological modulator of tight junctions, as prehaptoglobin-2. *Proc Natl Acad Sci USA*. 2009;106: 16799–16804.

20. Lammers KM, Lu R, Brownley J, *et al*. Gliadin induces an increase in intestinal permeability and zonulin release by binding to the chemokine receptor CXCR3. *Gastroenterology*. 2008;135:194–204,e3.

21. Agarwal S and Mayer L. Gastrointestinal manifestations in primary immune disorders. *Inflamm Bowel Dis*. 2010 Apr;16 (4):703–11.

22. Raki M, Schjetne KW, Stamnaes J *et al.* Surface expression of transglutaminase 2 by dendritic cells and its potential role for uptake and presentation of gluten peptides to T cells. *Scand J Immunol.* 2007;65:213–220.

23. Raki M, Tollefsen S, Molberg O, *et al.* A unique dendritic cell subset accumulates in the celiac lesion and efficiently activates gluten-reactive T cells. *Gastroenterology.* 2006;131:428–438.

24. Schuppan D. Current concepts of celiac disease pathogenesis. *Gastroenterology.* 2000;119:234–242.

25. Qiao SW, Bergseng E, Molberg O *et al.* Antigen presentation to celiac lesion-derived T cells of a 33-mer gliadin peptide naturally formed by gastrointestinal digestion. *J Immunol.* 2004;173: 1757–1762.

26. van de Wal Y, Kooy YM, Drijfhout JW, *et al.* Unique peptide binding characteristics of the disease-associated DQ(alpha 1*0501, beta 1*0201) vs the non-disease-associated DQ(alpha 1*0201, beta 1*0202) molecule. *Immunogenetics.* 1997;46:484–492.

27. Balas A, Vicario JL, Zambrano A *et al.* Absolute linkage of celiac disease and dermatitis herpetiformis to HLA-DQ. *Tissue Antigens.* 1997;50:52–56.

28. Sollid LM and Lie BA. Celiac disease genetics: current concepts and practical applications. *Clin Gastroenterol Hepatol.* 2005;3: 843–851.

29. Hogberg L, Fälth-Magnusson K, Grodzinsky E *et al.* Familial prevalence of coeliac disease: a twenty-year follow-up study. *Scand J Gastroenterol.* 2003;38:61–65.

30. Fasano A, Berti I, Gerarduzzi T *et al.* Prevalence of celiac disease in at-risk and not-at-risk groups in the United States: a large multicenter study. *Arch Intern Med.* 2003;163:286–292.

31. Greco L, Romino R, Coto I, *et al.* The first large population based twin study of coeliac disease. *Gut.* 2002;50:624–628.

32. Schuppan D Junker Y and Barisani D. Celiac Disease: From Pathogenesis to Novel Therapies. *Gastroenterology,* 2009.

33. Kaukinen K, Peräaho M, Collin P *et al.* Small-bowel mucosal transglutaminase 2-specific IgA deposits in coeliac disease without villous atrophy: a prospective and randomized clinical study. *Scand J Gastroenterol.* 2005;40:564–572.

34. Zone JJ. Skin manifestations of celiac disease. *Gastroenterology.* 2005;128:S87–S91.

35. Hadjivassiliou M, *et al.* Autoantibodies in gluten ataxia recognize a novel neuronal transglutaminase. *Ann Neurol.* 2008;64: 332–343.

36. Duntas LH, Does celiac disease trigger autoimmune thyroiditis? *Nat Rev Endocrinol.* 2009;5:190–191.

37. Weir DC, Glickman JN, Roiff T *et al.* Variability of histopathological changes in childhood celiac disease. *Am J Gastroenterol.* 2009.

38. Murray JA, Rubio-Tapia A, Van Dyke CT *et al.* Mucosal atrophy in celiac disease: extent of involvement, correlation with clinical presentation, and response to treatment. *Clin Gastroenterol Hepatol.* 2008;6:186–193, quiz 125.

39. Rubin CE, Brandborg LL, Phelps PC, Taylor HC Jr. Studies of celiac disease. I. The apparent identical and specific nature of the duodenal and proximal jejunal lesion in celiac disease and idiopathic sprue. *Gastroenterology.* 1960;38:28–49.

40. Niazi NM, Leigh R, Crowe P, Marsh MN Morphometric analysis of small intestinal mucosa. I. Methodology, epithelial volume compartments and enumeration of inter-epithelial space lymphocytes. *Virchows Arch A Pathol Anat Histopathol.* 1984;404: 49–60.

41. Jarvinen TT, Kaukinen K, Laurila K *et al.* Intraepithelial lymphocytes in celiac disease. *Am J Gastroenterol.* 2003;98:1332–1337.

42. Rashtak S and Murray JA. Celiac disease in the elderly. *Gastroenterol Clin North Am.* 2009;38:433–446.

43. Kupper C. Dietary guidelines and implementation for celiac disease. *Gastroenterology.* 2005;128:S121–S127.

44. Jatla M, Zemel BS, Bierly P, Verma R. Bone mineral content deficits of the spine and whole body in children at time of diagnosis with celiac disease. *J Pediatr Gastroenterol Nutr.* 2009;48: 175–180.

45. Bianchi ML and Bardella MT. Bone in celiac disease. *Osteoporos Int.* 2008;19:1705–1716.

46. Pazianas M, Butcher GP, Subhani JM *et al.* Calcium absorption and bone mineral density in celiac after long term treatment with gluten-free diet and adequate calcium intake. *Osteoporos Int.* 2005;16:56–63.

47. Barera G Beccio S, Proverbio MC, Mora S. Longitudinal changes in bone metabolism and bone mineral content in children with celiac disease during consumption of a gluten-free diet. *Am J Clin Nutr.* 2004;79:148–154.

48. Tata LJ, Card TR, Logan RF *et al.* Fertility and pregnancy-related events in women with celiac disease: a population-based cohort study. *Gastroenterology.* 2005;128:849–855.

49. Hadjivassiliou M, Sanders DS, Woodroofe N *et al.* Gluten ataxia. *Cerebellum.* 2008;7:494–498.

50. Bushara KO. Neurologic presentation of celiac disease. *Gastroenterology.* 2005;128:S92–S97.

51. Askling J, Linet M, Gridley G *et al.* Cancer incidence in a population-based cohort of individuals hospitalized with celiac disease or dermatitis herpetiformis. *Gastroenterology.* 2002;123: 1428–1435.

52. Barton SH and Murray JA. Celiac disease and autoimmunity in the gut and elsewhere. *Gastroenterol Clin North Am.* 2008;37: 411–428,vii.

53. Viljamaa M, Kaukinen K, Huhtala H *et al.* Coeliac disease, autoimmune diseases and gluten exposure. *Scand J Gastroenterol.* 2005;40:437–443.

54. Ventura A, Magazzu G, and Greco L, Duration of exposure to gluten and risk for autoimmune disorders in patients with celiac disease. SIGEP Study Group for Autoimmune Disorders in Celiac Disease. *Gastroenterology.* 1999;117:297–303.

55. Leffler DA, Edwards George JB, Dennis M *et al.* A prospective comparative study of five measures of gluten-free diet adherence in adults with coeliac disease. *Aliment Pharmacol Ther.* 2007;26:1227–1235.

56. Schuppan D and Kelly CP. Is duodenal biopsy required in all patients with suspected celiac disease? *Nat Clin Pract Gastroenterol Hepatol.* 2007.

57. Oxentenko AS, Grisolano SW, Murray JA *et al.* The insensitivity of endoscopic markers in celiac disease. *Am J Gastroenterol.* 2002;97:933–938.

58. Malamut G, Matysiak-Budnik T, Grosdider E *et al.* Adult celiac disease with severe or partial villous atrophy: a comparative study. *Gastroenterol Clin Biol.* 2008;32:236–242.

59. Leffler DA, Dennis M, Hyett B *et al.* Etiologies and predictors of diagnosis in nonresponsive celiac disease. *Clin Gastroenterol Hepatol.* 2007;5:445–450.

60. Koskinen O, Villanen M, Korponay-Szabo I, *et al.* Oats do not induce systemic or mucosal autoantibody response in children with coeliac disease. *J Pediatr Gastroenterol Nutr.* 2009;48: 559–565.

Small and Large Bowel

61. Garsed K and Scott BB. Can oats be taken in a gluten-free diet? A systematic review. *Scand J Gastroenterol*. 2007;42:171–178.

62. Kemppainen T, Janatuinen E, Holm K, *et al*. No observed local immunological response aT-cell level after five years of oats in adult coeliac disease. *Scand J Gastroenterol*. 2007;42:54–59.

63. Murray JA, Watson T, Clearman B, Mitros F. Effect of a gluten-free diet on gastrointestinal symptoms in celiac disease. *Am J Clin Nutr*. 2004;79:669–673.

64. Abdulkarim AS, Burgart LJ, See J, Murray JA. Etiology of non-responsive celiac disease: results of a systematic approach. *Am J Gastroenterol*. 2002;97:2016–2021.

65. Abdallah H, Leffler D, Dennis M, Kelly CP. Refractory celiac disease. *Curr Gastroenterol Rep*. 2007;9:401–405.

66. Kaukinen K, Peräaho M, Lindfors K *et al*. Persistent small bowel mucosal villous atrophy without symptoms in coeliac disease. *Aliment Pharmacol Ther*. 2007;25:1237–1245.

67. Rubio-Tapia A, Kelly DG, Lahr BD, *et al*. Clinical staging and survival in refractory celiac disease: a single center experience. *Gastroenterology*. 2009;136:99–107, quiz 352–353.

68. Cellier C Delabesse E, Helmer C *et al*. Refractory sprue, coeliac disease, and enteropathy-associated T-cell lymphoma. French Coeliac Disease Study Group. *Lancet*. 2000;356:203–208.

69. Holmes GK, Prior P, Lane MR *et al*. Malignancy in coeliac disease–effect of a gluten-free diet. *Gut*. 1989;30:333–338.

70. Farrell RJ and Kelly CP. Diagnosis of celiac sprue. *Am J Gastroenterol*. 2001;96:3237–3246.

71. Lewis, N.R. and Scott, B.B. Meta-analysis: deamidated gliadin peptide (DGP) antibody and tissue transglutaminase (TTG) antibody compared as screening tests for coeliac disease. *Aliment Pharmacol Ther*. 2010 Jan;31(1):73–81.

CHAPTER 41
Short bowel syndrome

Christian S. Jackson[1] and Alan L. Buchman[2]

[1]Loma Linda VA Healthcare System; Loma Linda University Medical Center, Loma Linda, CA, USA
[2]Feinberg School of Medicine, Northwestern University, Chicago, IL, USA

ETIOLOGY OF SHORT BOWEL SYNDROME

Children	Adults
Congenital jejunal or ileal atresia	
Resections for Crohn's disease, trauma, pseudo-obstruction, necrotizing enterocolitis, gastroschisis, omphalocele, midgut volvulus, intussusception	Resections for Crohn's disease, trauma, radiation enteritis, pseudo-obstruction, mesenteric vascular events (mesenteric venous thrombosis, mesenteric arterial thrombosis or embolism), midgut volvulus (now, post-bariatric surgery as well), intussusception, tumors (including desmoids)

DEFINITION AND DIAGNOSIS OF SHORT BOWEL SYNDROME (SBS)

- ≤200 cm of bowel remaining in an adult post-operatively
- Direct measurement of viable intestine left in situ after resection as measured on the anterior mesenteric border (preferred method)
- Opisometer to trace residual bowel length after barium small follow through radiographic (alternate method)

TREATMENT OF SHORT BOWEL SYNDROME

Medical management
Treatment of diarrhea
Diphenoxylate (2–4 mg qid)
Loperamide (2–4 mg qid)
Codeine (15–60 mg qid)
Tincture of opium (0.6–2.5 mL qid)
Clonidine (0.3 mg patch weekly)
Octreotide (100 µg SQ bid)
Proton Pump Inhibitors (first 6 months postoperatively)

Dietary management
Hyperphagia (1.5–2 times usual pre-operative food intake)
Increased starch, soluble fiber, and complex carbohydrate intake (patients with residual colon in continuity with small bowel only)
Oral Rehydration Fluid (1–3 L/day)
Calcium supplementation (1–2 g/day)
Micronutrient Supplementation if necessary (water and/or fat soluble vitamins, trace metals including Zn, Cu, and Se)
Growth Hormone

Surgical management
Re-anastomosis of Residual Small Intestine to Residual Colon
Intestinal Tapering (STEP, Bianchi in selected individuals)
Intestinal Transplantation

Introduction

Short bowel syndrome (SBS) is defined in adults as <200 cm of small intestine. The normal adult intestine ranges 300–800 cm in length depending on sex, age, and measuring technique [1–4]. SBS can be congenital (intestinal atresia), or can occur secondary to one or more enterectomies. The presence of SBS does not necessarily denote **intestinal failure,** which is defined as the inability to maintain nutrition or fluid/electrolyte autonomy. Therefore, not all individuals with SBS will require parenteral nutrition (PN), and 50% of those that due can be successfully weaned from PN within a year [5]. There are individuals with a full complement of intestine, but with malabsorptive syndrome such as refractory sprue, chronic intestinal pseudoobstruction, radiation enteritis) who have a **functional** short bowel, and therefore **intestinal failure** [9]. Patients at greatest nutritional risk are those with jejunocolic or ileocolonic anastomoses and <60 cm of residual small intestine or an end jejunostomy with <115 cm of residual small intestine [5–9].

Incidence and prevalence

The incidence of SBS is difficult to assess in the United States due to the absence of a national registry, and lack of an appropriate ICD-9 code. However, based on population data from Europe, there are likely at most 10 000 patients in the USA with SBS and intestinal failure [8]. Extrapolation of data gathered

Textbook of Clinical Gastroenterology and Hepatology, Second Edition. Edited by C. J. Hawkey, Jaime Bosch, Joel E. Richter, Guadalupe Garcia-Tsao, Francis K. L. Chan.
© 2012 Blackwell Publishing Ltd. Published 2012 by Blackwell Publishing Ltd.

from the Oley Foundation Home PN Registry (www.oley.org), which ended in 1992, suggested approximately 40 000 patients required home PN each year in the USA, of which approximately 26% had SBS [10].

Etiology of short bowel syndrome

SBS may be an acquired condition or a congenital condition. Infants may be born with ileal or jejunal atresia. SBS may result from surgical resection(s) such as multiple resections for recurrent Crohn's disease, massive enterectomy for a catastrophic vascular event such as mesenteric arterial embolism or thrombosis, venous thrombosis, midgut volvulus, trauma, tumor resection, or radiation enteritis. In children **gastroschisis**, necrotizing enterocolitis, midgut volvulus and extensive aganglionosis are the common causes for surgical resection resulting in SBS.

Diagnostic methods

Remaining viable intestine should be measured along the antimesenteric border at the time of resection, being careful not to overstretch the bowel. Bowel length can be estimated radiologically using an opisometer when there are no overlying loops [3,4,11]. Recently, citrulline has been used as a biomarker of small bowel mass; a post-absorptional serum concentration of <20 µmol/L is predictive of intestinal failure [12,13]. Citrulline is a protein not derived from food or proteolysis and is not incorporated in body proteins, but is synthesized in enterocytes from glutamine [14].

Oral intake and dietary management

"Hyperphagia" (the oral intake of 1.5–2.0 times usual food intake) should be encouraged [15]. Patients with <100 cm of residual jejunum have a net secretory response to dietary intake and fluid intake, which results in enhanced dehydration and electrolyte depletion [16]. Specific dietary management (e.g., high fat, low fat, high carbohydrate, low carbohydrate) has little role in these patients, and at times [17,21] oral intake may need to be restricted in order to reduce fluid losses. There is little data to support the use of peptide-based diets when compared to intact protein. Some patients may be lactase deficient, owing to diminished mucosal surface area, although the majority of patients with SBS do not exhibit lactose intolerance. It is to be noted that not only do patients with SBS have nutrient malabsorption, but medication malabsorption as well, greater than conventional doses may be necessary along with serum monitoring of drug or metabolite concentrations.

When >60 cm of terminal ileum has been resected, vitamin B$_{12}$ deficiency may develop. When >100 cm has been resected, fat maldigestion may occur secondary to bile salt malabsorption. Bile salt replacement using an ox bile extract has been described in a few case reports. In general, fat absorption was increased, but diarrhea was also increased [18,19].

When <100 cm, of terminal ileum has been resected, cholestyramine may be useful to treat bile salt-induced diarrhea, but may enhance malabsorption if used when >100 cm has been resected [20].

In those patients who have colon continuity, a high complex carbohydrate with starch and soluble fiber may result in enhanced fluid and energy absorption via carbohydrate salvage [21]. Malabsorbed carbohydrates (often 50% of oral consumption) pass into the colon where they undergo fermentation by indigenous bacterial flora to short chain fatty acids (SCFA) (butyrate, acetate, and proprionate), among other products. These can be absorbed by enterocytes as an energy source, and also serve to stimulate both colonic sodium and water absorption. Energy absorption in patients with an intact colon may be as great as 2 MJ (400–500 kcal) per day. Some medium chain triglycerides (MCT) and amino acids may also be absorbed by the colon.

Fluid and electrolyte management and control of diarrhea

Massive enterectomy is associated with gastric hypersecretion for approximately the first 6 months postoperatively [22,23]. These patients will benefit from the use of intravenous H2 antagonists or intravenous proton pump inhibitors to reduce the loss of fluid [24–26]. Massive enterectomy is also associated with rapid intestinal transit resulting in large amounts of fluid loss which require chronic control with anti-diarrheal agents, such as diphenoxylate and loperamide hydrochloride to increase intestinal transit time. The typical dose required is 4–16 mg/day in 4 divided doses. If these medications are ineffective, then additional medications such as codeine (15–60 mg 4 times daily) or tincture of opium (0.6–2.5 mL 4 times daily) should be used. Clonidine stimulates colonic chloride and fluid absorption and may be administered transcutaneously [27]. If all of these agents fail, octreotide may be used. Though the mechanism for the reduction of sodium and water loss is unclear, there is evidence that its use (100 µg subcutaneous 3 times daily) can reduce daily jejunostomy volume [28,29]. Octreotide should be used as a last resort because it may increase the risk for cholelithiasis and because of a reduction in splanchnic protein synthesis, may adversely impact on intestinal adaptation [30]. Growth hormone stimulates proximal renal tubular reabsorption of sodium, and results in fluid retention, and has led to a reduction in PN requirements in some patients with SBS [31]. Glucagon-like peptide II (GLP-II) administration has been associated with small bowel increased fluid absorption and decreased PN requirements in preliminary studies [32–34].

Several other growth factors may also be involved in intestinal adaptation following massive enterectomy, and also represent potential future therapeutic targets (Figure 41.1).

Isotonic glucose-based oral rehydration solutions (ORS) should be used to improve hydration and to decrease PN fluid requirements. Patients with <100 cm of residual jejunum are at

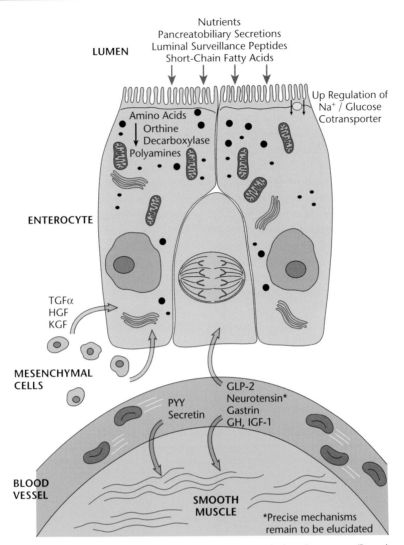

Figure 41.1 Gastrointestinal hormones and other factors involved in the post-resection intestinal adaptation process. (Reproduced with permission from Cisler JJ, Buchman AL. Intestinal Adaptation in Short Bowel Syndrome. *J Invest Med.* 2005:402–413.)

significant risk for the development of dehydration because they secrete more sodium (Na) and fluid than they orally consume. Glucose promotes salt and water via stimulation of sodium-linked transport [35]. Commercially available ORS, and especially the solution recommended by the World Health Organization (WHO) are effective [36]. In patients with colon incontinence, the sodium concentration may not be as critical, as the colon avidly absorbs sodium and water against a steep electrochemical gradient, as long as sufficient sodium and water is provided in the diet. In patients without jejunum, but who have an ileum, the presence of glucose is not as critical, because ileal water absorption is not affected by the presence of glucose [46].

Patient with SBS should routinely be provided with oral calcium supplementation (1000–1500 mg/day). This may also help reduce the risk for calcium oxalate nephrolithiasis in those patients with residual colon incontinence with their small bowel by finding dietary oxalate. In addition to Na and water

losses, significant quantities of magnesium (Mg) are lost in the jejunal or ileal effluent. Magnesium deficiency impairs parathyroid hormone release, which may result in impaired vitamin D-dependent calcium absorption. Since oral magnesium replacement is problematic, periodic parenteral magnesium replacement may be necessary [37].

Long-term PN is associated with complications including catheter-related infections, catheter-related occlusion (thrombotic and non-thrombotic), hepatobiliary complications, metabolic bone disease, renal dysfunction, memory deficits and neurologic problems [38–45]. In a cohort study of 124 adults with nonmalignant SBS enrolled in a 13-year period, survival and PN-dependence probabilities were reported as 86% and 49% at 2 years, and 75% and 45% at 5 years. Thirty-two of the 60 patients with permanent intestinal failure (53%), and 8 of the 64 (12.5%) with transient intestinal failure, died during follow-up. PN-related complications accounted for 22% of deaths in patients with permanent intestinal failure [46]. Those with the least residual intestine, and therefore who required the most PN, had the lowest survival. Patients that require long-term PN must be properly trained in its administration, use and care of their catheter, and infusion equipment.

Surgical management

The most important surgical procedure is re-anastomosis of the residual small bowel to the residual colon. This procedure carries relatively low mortality and morbidity rates and allows for enhanced energy absorption from short chain fatty acids (SCFA) produced from the bacterial fermentation of unabsorbed carbohydrate by colonic microflora. Longitudinal intestinal lengthening and tailoring (Bianchi procedure [47]) may be useful in patients with segmental intestinal dilation which has been rendered nonfunctional due to dysmotility and bacterial overgrowth. In this procedure, the surgeon divides the dilated bowel, creates two hemi-loops and anastomoses the hemi-loops in an end-to-end fashion, thereby doubling the bowel length [47]. Although the surface area is not truly increased, bowel function may improve, allowing reduction or elimination of PN. Nearly all of the approximately 100 operations reported have been undertaken in children. This procedure should be attempted only as a last resort before

intestinal transplantation, and it should be performed only in centers with significant experience.

A less complex procedure that has largely replaced the Bianchi, the serial transverse enteroplasty (STEP) developed by Kim, is a novel technique during which a linear surgical stapler is applied from alternating and opposite directions along the intestine's mesenteric border to incompletely staple and divide the dilated intestine [48]. This procedure leads to the tapering of the intestine in a zig-zag pattern, which results in nutrients being channeled along a narrower, but longer intestine. Rather than an intestinal lengthening procedure, this technique is better described as an intestinal tapering procedure. Results reported from an international registry (childrenshospital.org/cfapps/step/index.cfm) comprising 100 patients, mostly children, have indicated the procedure increases intestinal length by approximately 50%, and has resulted in close to a 100% increase in nutrient absorption [49,50]. These improvements in some individuals, however, may have been due in part to increased segmental absorption observed as part of the natural post-enterectomy adaption process. Nevertheless, the tapering of a dilated, essentially nonfunctional, loop of bowel may decrease bacterial overgrowth and improve nutrient absorption.

Table 41.1 Patient and graft survival rates at 1, 3, 5, and 10 years following isolated intestine, intestine/liver, and multivisceral transplants

Organ	Number of transplants	Month post-transplant	Survival rate patient/graft (%)	95% Conf. limits
Intestine alone	590	12	84.8/81.1	[81.7,88.0] [77.7,84.4]
		36	68.0/58.2	[63.6,72.4] [53.7,62.6]
		60	57.2/44.2	[52.0,62.4] [39.3,49.1]
		120	46.2/25.5	[38.8,53.6] [19.5,31.4]
Liver/intestine	430	12	63.3/60.8	[58.5,68.0] [56.1,65.5]
		36	52.0/49.1	[47.1,57.0] [44.2,53.9]
		60	48.1/44.8	[43.1,53.1] [39.9,49.7]
		120	40.0/36.7	[34.4,45.6] [31/3,42.1]
Multivisceral	649	12	71.8/68.7	[68.2,75.4] [65.0,72.4]
		36	58.7/54.7	[54.5,62.9] [50.6,58.9]
		60	51.4/45.9	[46.6,56.2] [41.2,50.6]
		120	36.1/31.5	[28.1,44.1] [24.3,38.7]

Based on OPTN data as of February 25 2010 for transplant performed from 1990 to October, 2008. Provided by the United Network for Organ Sharing (UNOS). This work was supported in part by Health Resources and Services Administration contract 234–2005–370011C. The content is the responsibility of the author alone and does not necessarily reflect the views or policies of the Department of Health and Human Services, nor does mention of trade names, commercial products, or organizations imply endorsement by the U.S. Government.

Intestinal transplantation

The first attempt at intestinal transplantation occurred in dogs in 1959 and since that time, the true success of intestinal transplantation occurred with the introduction of tacrolimus in 1990 [51]. As of May 31, 2007 (the most recent data from the International Small Bowel Transplant Registry www.intestinaltransplant.org), 1720 transplantation procedures had been performed worldwide in 1608 patients, 909 of whom were still alive. This experience included 746 isolated intestine, 594 intestine-liver, and 380 multi-visceral transplants. Patients who have undergone transplantation more recently, generally have better survival because of improved technique and optimized immunosuppressive regimens. Mean hospitalization was 56 days for isolated intestine, 76 days for intestine-liver, and 62 days for multi-visceral transplant recipients. Additional information can be found in the International Intestinal Transplant Registry website, (http://intestinaltransplant.org), which is updated every 2 years (last time in 2007). Additional survival data provided by the United Network for Organ Sharing (UNOS) Administration through 2008, organized by type of intestinal transplant can also be found in Table 41.1. Although outcomes have improved, currently long-term patient survival following intestine, intestine-liver, or multi-visceral transplantation is inferior to that of continued PN, in the absence of life-threatening complications of PN. These complications, namely the development of irreversible liver disease, loss of venous access, and chronic dehydration, serve as the backbone for Medicare-approved indications for intestinal transplantation.

References

1. Crenn P, Haniche M, Valleur P, et al. Surgical versus radiological evaluation of remaining small bowel length in short bowel syndrome (abstr). *Gastroenterology*. 1996;110:A321.
2. Bryant J. Observations upon the growth and length of the human intestine. *Am J Med Sci*. 1924;167:499–520.
3. Fanucci A, Cerro P, Fraracci L, et al. Small-bowel length measured by radiology. *Gastrointestinal Radiol*. 1984;9:349–351.
4. Nightingale JMD, Bartram CI, Lennard-Jones JE. Length of residual small bowel after partial resection: correlation between radiographic and surgical measurements. *Gastrointest Radiol*. 1991;16:305–306.
5. Messing B, Crenn P, Beau P, et al. Long term survival and parenteral nutrition dependence in adult patients with short bowel syndrome. *Gastroenterology*. 1999;117:1043–1050.
6. Carbonnel F, Cosnes J, Chevret S, et al. The role of anatomic factors in nutritional autonomy after extensive bowel resection. *JPEN J Parenter Enteral Nutr*. 1996;20:275–280.
7. Nightingale JMD, Lennard-Jones JE, Gertner DJ et al. Colonic preservation reduces need for parenteral therapy, increases incidence of renal stones, but does not change high prevalence of gallstones in patients with short bowel. *Gut*. 1992;33:1493–1497.
8. Buchman AL, Scolapio J, Fryer J: AGA technical review on SBS and intestinal transplantation. *Gastroenterology*. 2003;124:1111–1134.
9. O'Keefe SJ, Buchman AL, Fishbein TM, et al. Short bowel syndrome and intestinal failure: consensus definitions and overview. *Clin Gastroenterol Hepatol*. 2006;4:6–10.
10. Oley Foundaton. *North American home parenteral and enteral nutrition patient registry and annual report*. Albany, NY: Oley Foundaton; 1994
11. Shatani T, Clark MA, Lee JR, et al. Reliability of radiologic measurement of small intestinal length. *Colorectal Dis*. 2004;6: 327–329.
12. Sigalet DL, Lam V, Boctor D. The assessment, and glucagon-like peptide-2 modulation, of intestinal absorption and function. *Semin Pediatr Surg*. 2010;19:44–49.
13. Crenn P, Messing B, Cynober L, et al. Citrulline as biomarker of intestinal failure due to enterocyte mass reduction. *Clin Nutr*. 2008;27:328–339.
14. Curis E, Crenn P, Cynober L. Citrulline and the gut. *Curr Opin Clin Nutr Care*. 2007;10:620–626.
15. Crenn P, Morin MC, Joly F, et al. Net digestive absorption and adaptive hyperphagia in adult short bowel syndrome patients. *Gut*. 2004;53:1279–1286.
16. Nightingale JMD, Lennard-Jones JE, Walker ER, et al. Jejunal efflux in short bowel syndrome. *Lancet*. 1990;336:765–768.
17. Woolf GM, Jeejeebhoy KN. Dietary management of short bowel syndrome. *Gastroenterology*. 1983;85:218–219.
18. Little KH, Schiller LR, Bilhartz LE, et al. Treatment of severe steatorrhea with ox bile in an ileectomy patient with residual colon. *Dig Dis Sci*. 1992;37:929–933.
19. Fordtran JS, Bunch F, Davis GR. Ox bile treatment of severe steatorrhea in an ileectomy-ileostomy patient. *Gastroenterology*. 1982;82:564–568.
20. Hoffman AF, Poley R. Role of bile acid malabsorption in pathogenesis of diarrhea and steatorrhea in patients with ileal resection. *Gastroenterology*. 1972;62:918–934.
21. Norgaard I, Hansen Bs, Mortensen PB. Colon as a digestive organ in patient with short bowel. *Lancet*. 1994;343:373–376.
22. Windsor CWO, Fejfar J, Woodward DAK. Gastric secretion after massive small bowel resection. *Gut*. 1969;10:779–786.
23. Williams NS, Evans P, King RFGJ. Gastric acid secretion and gastrin production in the short bowel syndrome. *Gut*. 1985;26: 914–919.
24. Jacobsen K, Ladefoged K, Stage JG, et al. Effects of cimetidine on jejunostomy effluents in patients with severe short bowel syndrome. *Scand J Gastroenterol*. 1986;21:824–828.
25. Nightingale JMD, Walker ER, Farthing MJG, et al. Effect of omeprazole on intestinal output in the short bowel syndrome. *Aliment Pharmacol Ther*. 1991;5:405–412.
26. Jeppesen PB, Staun M, Tjellesen L, et al. Effect of intravenous ranitidine and omeprazole on intestinal absorption of water, sodium and macronutrients in patients with intestinal resection. *Gut*. 1998;43:763–769.
27. Buchman AL, Fryer J, Wallin A, et al. Clonidine reduces diarrhea and sodium loss in patients with proximal jejunostomy: a controlled study. *JPEN J Parenter Enteral Nutr*. 2006;30:487–491.
28. O'Keefe SJ, Peterson ME, Fleming CR. Octreotide as an adjunct to home parenteral nutrition in the management of permanent end-jejunostomy syndrome. *JPEN*. 1994;18:26–34.
29. Ladefoged K, Christensen KC, Hegnhoj J, et al. Effect of a long-acting somastattin analogue SMS 201–995 on jejunostomy effluents in patients with severe short bowel syndrome. *Gut*. 1989;30:943–949.

30. O'Keefe SJ, Haymond MW, Bennet WM, *et al.* Long-acting soma-tostatin analogue therapy an dprotein metabolism in patients with jejunostomies. *Gastroenterology.* 1994;107:379–378.

31. Byrne TA, Wilmore DW , Iyer K, *et al.* Growth hormone, glutamine, and an optimal diet reduces parenteral nutrition in patients with short bowel syndrome: a prospective, randomized, placebo-controlled, double-blind clinical trial. *Ann Surg.* 2005;242:655–661.

32. Jeppesen PB, Hartmann B, Thulesen J *et al.* Glucagon-like peptide 2 improves nutrient absorption in short bowel patients with no colon. *Gastroenterology.* 2001;120:806–815.

33. Jeppesen PB, Sanguinetti EL, Buchman AL, *et al.* Teduglutide (ALX-0600), a dipeptidyl peptidase IV resistant glucagon-like peptide 2 analogue, improves intestinal function in short bowel syndrome patients. *Gut.* 2005;54:1224–1231.

34. Okeefe SJD, Gilroy R, Jeppesen PN *et al.* Teduglutide, a novel GLP-2 analog in the management of short bowel syndrome (SBS) patients dependent on parenteral nutrition : a multicenter, multinational placebo controlled trial (abstr) *Gastroenterology.* 2008;134,A–37

35. Fortran JS. Stimulation of active and passive sodium absorption by sugars in the human jejunum. *J Clin Invest.* 1975;55:728–737.

36. World Health Organization. *Treatment and prevention of dehydration in diarrhea disease: a guide for use at the primary level.* WHO: Geneva; 1976.

37. Buchman AL. Etiology and Initial Management of Short Bowel Syndrome. *Gastroenterology.* 2006;130:S5–S15.

38. Buchman AL, Moukarzel A, Goodson B *et al.* Catheter related infections associated with home parenteral nutrition and predictive factors for the need of catheter removal in their treatment. *JPEN J Parenter Enteral Nutr.* 1994;18:297–302.

39. Buchman AL, Misra S, Moukarzel A, *et al.* Catheter thrombosis and superior/inferior vena cava syndrome are rare complications of long term parenteral nutrition. *Clin Nutr.* 1994;13:356–360.

40. Buchman AL, Iyer K, Fryer J. Parenteral nutrition-associated liver disease and the role for isolated intestine and intestine/liver transplantation. *Hepatology.* 2006;43:9–19.

41. Roslyn JJ, Pitt HA, Mann LL *et al.* Gallbladder disease in patients on long-term parenteral nutrition. *Gastroenterology.* 1993;84:148–154.

42. Buchman AL, Moukarzel A, Ament ME, *et al.* Serious renal impairment is associated with long-term parenteral nutrition. *J Parent Enteral Nutr.* 1993;17:438–444.

43. Buchman AL, Moukarzel A. Metabolic bone disease associated with total parenteral nutrition. *Clin Nutr.* 2000;19:217–231.

44. Buchman AL, Sohel M, Brown M, *et al.* Verbal and visual memory improve after choline supplementation in long-term total parenteral nutrition: a pilot study. *JPEN J Parenter Enteral Nutr.* 2001;25:30–35.

45. Idoate MA, Martinez AJ, Bueno J, *et al.* The neuropathology of intestinal failure and small bowel transplantation. *Acta Neuropathol.* 1999;97:502–508.

46. Messing B, Lemann M, Landais P, *et al.* Prognosis of patients with nonmalignant chronic intestinal failure receiving long term parenteral nutrition. *Gastroenterology.* 1995;108:1005–1010.

47. Bianchi A. Intestinal loop lengthening–a technique for increasing small intestinal length. *J Pediatr Surg.* 1980;15:145–151.

48. Kim HB, Fauza D, Garza J, *et al.* Serial transverse enteroplasty (STEP): a novel bowel lengthening procedure. *J Pediatr Surg.* 2003;38:425–429.

49. Modi BP, Javid PJ, Jaksic T, *et al.* First report of the international serial transverse enteroplasty data registry: indications, efficacy, and complications. *J Am Coll Surg.* 2007;204:365–371.

50. Sudan D, Thompson J, Botha J, *et al.* Comparison of intestinal lengthening procedures for patients with short bowel syndrome. *Ann Surg.* 2007;246:593–604.

51. Abu Elmugad K, Reyes J, Todo S, *et al.* Clinical intestinal transplantation: new perspectives and immunologic considerations. *J Am Coll Surg.* 1998;186:512–517.

Small and Large Bowel

CHAPTER 42

Small intestinal bacterial overgrowth

Ahmed Abu Shanab,[1] Rodrigo M. Quera[2] and Eamonn M. M. Quigley[1]

[1]University College Cork, Cork, Ireland
[2]Clinica Las Condes, Santiago, Chile

ESSENTIAL FACTS ABOUT PATHOGENESIS

- Disorders leading to alterations in one or more of the intrinsic defensive systems (gastric acid, motility) may be associated with SIBO
- The most common disorders associated with SIBO are intestinal dysmotility syndromes and chronic pancreatitis
- Systemic sclerosis, Crohn's disease and radiation enteropathy are commonly complicated by SIBO
- SIBO may be the presenting feature of jejunal diverticulosis and results from associated dysmotility
- IBS, *per se*, may not linked to SIBO but SIBO can lead to IBS-like symptoms

---

ESSENTIALS OF DIAGNOSIS

- The diagnosis of SIBO must be mindful of the clinical context and of the limitations of all available diagnostic tests
- Based on jejunal aspirates, SIBO is defined as the presence of $\geq 10^5$ colony forming units (CFU) per mL of bacteria in the proximal small bowel
- Jejunal aspirates are invasive, subject to contamination and fail to identify the >60% of the microbiota that is unculturable
- In hydrogen breath tests, the diagnosis of SIBO is established when the concentration of exhaled H_2 increases by more than 10 parts per million (ppm) over baseline on two consecutive samplings, or if the fasting breath hydrogen level exceeds 20 ppm

---

ESSENTIALS OF TREATMENT AND PROGNOSIS

- The primary goal should be the treatment or correction of any underlying disease or defect, when possible
- Several of the clinical conditions associated with SIBO, such as visceral myopathies and multiple jejunal diverticula, are not reversible; management is then based on antibiotic therapy
- Antibiotic treatment remains primarily empirical
- A single 7- to 10-day course of antibiotic may improve symptoms for up to several months in between 46 and 90% of cases
- For those who relapse, rotating antibiotic schedules are preferred
- The poorly absorbed antibiotic rifaximin offers considerable promise in SIBO

Introduction and epidemiology

In the healthy host, enteric bacteria colonize the alimentary tract at and soon after birth, and the composition of the intestinal microflora remains relatively constant throughout life [1]. Because of peristalsis and the antimicrobial effects of gastric acidity, the stomach and proximal small intestine contain relatively small numbers of bacteria; jejunal cultures may not detect any bacteria in up to 33% of healthy people. When bacterial species are present, they are usually lactobacilli, enterococci, oral streptococci, and other Gram-positive aerobic or facultative anaerobes reflecting the bacterial flora of the oropharynx. The bacterial counts of coliforms rarely exceed 10^3 colony forming units CFU/mL in jejunal juice. The microbiology of the terminal ileum represents a transition zone between the relatively sparse and predominantly aerobic flora of the jejunum and the dense population of anaerobes found in the colon. Bacterial colony counts may be as high as 10^9 CFU/mL in the terminal ileum immediately proximal to the ileocecal valve, with a predominance of Gram-negative organisms and anaerobes. On crossing into the colon, the concentration and variety of enteric flora change dramatically. Concentrations as high as 10^{12} CFU/mL may be found, comprised mainly of anaerobes such as bacteroides, porphyromonas, bifidobacteria, lactobacilli, and clostridia.

The normal enteric bacteria influence a variety of intestinal functions [1]. Unabsorbed dietary sugars are salvaged by bacterial dissacaridases, converted into short-chain fatty acids, and used as an energy source by the colonic mucosa. Vitamins and nutrients such as folate and vitamin K are produced by enteric bacteria. The relationship between the host's immune system and nonpathogenic flora is important in protecting the host from colonization by pathogenic species. Bacterial metabolism of some medications (such as sulfasalazine), within the intestinal lumen, is essential for the release of active moieties.

Although small intestinal bacterial overgrowth (SIBO) is usually defined in quantitative terms, as the number of colony forming units (CFU) per mL, the interpretation of such definitions must be mindful, firstly, of the location, in the intestine,

---

Textbook of Clinical Gastroenterology and Hepatology, Second Edition. Edited by C. J. Hawkey, Jaime Bosch, Joel E. Richter, Guadalupe Garcia-Tsao, Francis K. L. Chan.
© 2012 Blackwell Publishing Ltd. Published 2012 by Blackwell Publishing Ltd.

from where the sample was obtained and, secondly, of the fact that the majority of bacterial species in the gut remain unculturable. Thus, molecular techniques such as genomics and metabolomics suggest that as much as 60% of the normal flora has not been identified by culture-based methods. Alternatively, the diagnosis may be based on the presence of such consequences of SIBO as malabsorption, combined with a positive result from such noninvasive diagnostic methods as breath tests. These reservations notwithstanding, SIBO is usually, and pending the validation of a more accurate methodology based on molecular microbiology, defined as the presence of $\geq 10^5$ CFU per mL of bacteria in the proximal small bowel [2–4].

The prevalence of SIBO is directly dependent on the characteristics of the study population and the diagnostic method employed to detect or define bacterial overgrowth. If a breath test is employed as the diagnostic method, prevalence will vary further depending on the nature and dose of substrate used . While large-scale population studies of SIBO prevalence have yet to be performed, SIBO has been described in 0–12.5 % of apparently healthy individuals on the basis of the glucose breath test, 20–22% by the lactulose breath test and 0–35% by the ^{14}C D-xylose breath test. The elderly may be especially susceptible to SIBO due both to a lack of gastric acid and the consumption of a disproportionately large number of drugs that can cause hypomotility. Although SIBO has been diagnosed in up to 35% of apparently healthy elderly subjects with hypochlorhydria by the ^{14}C D-xylose breath test, others have described SIBO as an important cause of occult malabsorption in the elderly [5].

Causes and pathogenesis

The most important defensive factors against SIBO are gastric acid and small intestinal motility [4]. In the stomach, acid kills and suppresses the growth of most organisms that enter from the oropharynx. In the small bowel, the cleansing action of aborad propulsive forces and, especially, phase III of the interdigestive migrating motor complex, limits the ability of bacteria to colonize the small intestine. Other protective factors include the integrity of the intestinal mucosa and its protective mucus layer, the enzymatic activities of intestinal, pancreatic and biliary secretions, the protective effects of some of the commensal flora, such as lactobacilli, and the mechanical and physiological properties of the ileocecal valve. Small intestinal dysmotility, rather than fasting hypochlorhydria or immunodeficiency, is probably the major contributor to SIBO in elderly subjects.

Disorders leading to alterations in one of more of these defensive systems may be associated with SIBO (Table 42.1). The most common disorders associated with SIBO are intestinal dysmotility syndromes and chronic pancreatitis. The cause of SIBO in chronic pancreatitis is multi-factorial and includes a decrease in intestinal motility consequent upon the inflammatory process, the effects of narcotics on gut motility and

Table 42.1 Clinical conditions associated with SIBO

Small intestinal stasis
Anatomic abnormalities
- Small intestinal diverticulosis
- Surgical (Billroth II, end-to-side anastomosis)
- Strictures (Crohn's disease, radiation, surgery)

Abnormal small intestinal motility
- Diabetic autonomic neuropathy
- Scleroderma
- Amyloidosis
- Hypothyroidism
- Idiopathic intestinal pseudo-obstruction
- Radiation enteritis
- Crohn's disease

Abnormal communication between proximal and distal gastrointestinal tract
- Gastrocolic or jejunocolic fistula
- Ileo-cecal valve resection

Multifactorial
- Liver disease
- Irritable bowel syndrome
- Celiac disease
- Chronic pancreatitis
- Immune deficiency (e.g., AIDS, severe malnutrition)
- End-stage renal disease
- The elderly

intestinal obstruction. Stagnation and/or recirculation of intestinal contents resulting from fistulas, enterostomies and anastomoses also predispose to SIBO; thus explaining the frequent association of SIBO with Crohn's disease, radiation enteropathy and reconstructive surgery. Diverticula in the jejunum occur in 0.07% to 2% of the population and tend to be large and multiple, whereas those in the ileum are small and single; SIBO has been reported in between 10–40% and 6–40% of jejunal and ileal diverticula, respectively. Jejunal diverticula are twice as frequent in men and are observed predominantly among those over 60 years of age. Disorders of intestinal motility such as progressive systemic sclerosis, visceral myopathies and neuropathies play an important role in the formation of the small bowel diverticula.

Recently, SIBO has been associated with disorders such as irritable bowel syndrome, celiac disease, nonalcoholic fatty liver disease and spontaneous bacterial peritonitis; the true status of these associations remains uncertain. Most contentious has been the proposal that IBS is linked to SIBO. While initial reports, using the lactulose breath test, described SIBO in up to 84% of subjects with IBS, many subsequent studies using a variety of methodologies have failed to confirm this association [6]. We believe that IBS, per se, may not be linked to SIBO but that SIBO can lead to IBS-like symptoms, and that positive responses to antibiotic therapy in IBS most likely reflect effects on the colonic flora rather than SIBO. SIBO has been implicated as one of the causes of a failure to respond to a gluten-free diet among celiac patients; eradication of SIBO may lead to disappearance of persisting symptoms [7]. In both experimental and clinical studies, SIBO has been reported in association with portal hypertension and cirrhosis and linked to the development of both porto-systemic encephalopathy and spontaneous bacterial peritonitis [8].

Clinical presentation

The clinical consequences of SIBO relate to a number of factors including bacterial metabolism, direct injury to the mucosa, effects on postprandial motility, and the impact of altered food intake, secondary to the gastrointestinal symptoms induced by SIBO. The resultant symptoms vary greatly and depend on the severity of SIBO, as well as on the underlying cause. Although symptoms may be nonspecific, some, such as the combination of diarrhea, steatorrhea, postprandial bloating, and vitamin deficiency may be regarded as highly suggestive of SIBO (Table 42.2). Laboratory investigations may reveal anemia, which is usually macrocytic because of malabsorption of vitamin B_{12} as a result of the binding and incorporation of this vitamin into the bacteria. Levels of both folate and vitamin K are, however, usually normal or elevated in the context of SIBO due to bacterial synthesis of these vitamins. A microcytic anemia can result from bleeding from ulcers or erosions. In advanced cases, micronutrient deficiency and evidence of malnutrition may also be present.

Differential diagnosis

It is obvious from the above that the differential diagnosis of SIBO is potentially vast and, on the one hand, includes the many causes of the malabsorption syndrome and, on the other, any disorder that can lead to diarrhea [9], bloating or abdominal discomfort. In many instances, symptoms related to SIBO are non-specific and are readily confused with those related to irritable bowel syndrome, functional dyspepsia, celiac disease and Crohn's disease.

Diagnostic investigation

The diagnosis of SIBO should be entertained in any patient with a clinical condition known to be associated with SIBO and who has compatible gastrointestinal symptoms (Figure 42.1). The diagnosis of SIBO remains problematic [2,3]; several invasive and noninvasive diagnostic methods of differing sensitivity and specificity are available (Table 42.3).

Although aspiration and direct culture of jejunal contents is regarded by many as the gold standard for the diagnosis of SIBO, this method has several limitations, including the potential for contamination by oropharyngeal bacteria during the procedure itself, the observation that bacterial overgrowth may be patchy and thus missed by a single aspiration and the possibility that overgrowth may involve only the more distal portions of the small bowel out of reach to conventional intubation techniques. Furthermore, the culture of anaerobic organisms requires meticulous microbiologic technique and the majority of the gut flora is not readily cultured by usual laboratory methods. Overall, the reproducibility of jejunal aspiration and culture has been reported to be as low as 38%, in comparison to 92% for breath tests.

The principle behind the use of breath tests is that the administration of a dose of carbohydrate (D-xylose, lactulose, or glucose) when metabolized by the contaminating flora leads to the production of hydrogen which is absorbed and ultimately excreted in the breath [10]. Because hydrogen production is a normal phenomenon, patient preparation is vital for test accuracy. Therefore, the ingestion of certain foods, such as bread, fiber, and pasta; cigarette smoking, the actions of the oral bacteria and the presence of lung disease can affect diagnostic accuracy. In these tests, the diagnosis of SIBO is established when the concentration of H_2 exhaled increases by more than 10 parts per million (ppm) over baseline on two consecutive samplings, or if the fasting breath hydrogen level exceeds 20 ppm (Figure 42.2). Fermentation of residual carbohydrate by oropharyngeal bacteria may also contribute to elevated levels of hydrogen and, thus, to an overestimation of the fasting breath hydrogen level. Rinsing the mouth with a chlorhexidine-containing mouth wash prior to breath collection can solve this problem.

The interpretation of breath tests may be especially problematic in the context of disorders associated with impaired gastric emptying (false negative results) or rapid intestinal transit (false positive results) [10,11]. Furthermore, between 15 and 27% of the population will not produce hydrogen; breath tests reliant on the measurement of hydrogen alone may therefore provide a significant number of false negative results. The combination of measurements of both hydrogen and methane, end products of anaerobic bacterial metabolism in the intestine, may avoid this problem.

Table 42.2 Clinical characteristics of SIBO

Symptoms
- Abdominal discomfort
- Bloating
- Flatulence
- Diarrhea/steatorrhea
- Nausea
- Weight loss
- Neuropathy

Clinical Findings
- Fat and carbohydrate malabsorption
- Vitamin deficiencies: cobalamin (vitamin B_{12}) and fat-soluble vitamins (A, D, E, K)
- Hypoproteinemia and hypoalbuminemia
- Iron deficiency

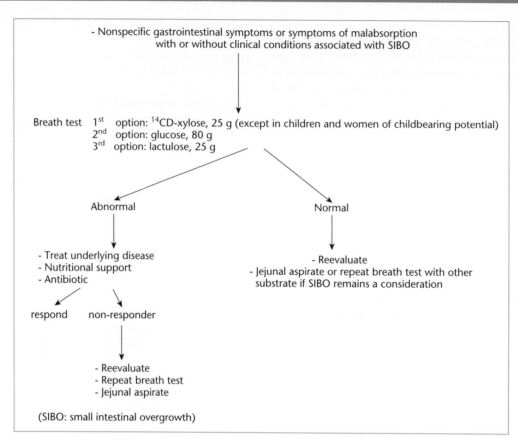

Figure 42.1 Algorithm for the evaluation and management of small intestinal bacterial overgrowth.

Table 42.3 Diagnostic methods for SIBO

Test	Sensitivity (%)	Specificity (%)	Ease of performance
Culture of jejunal aspirate	100	100	poor
Culture of small bowel biopsy	90.3	100	poor
^{14}C D-xylose BT	14.3–95	100	excellent
Glucose BT	6–93	78–100	excellent
Lactulose BT	6–68	44–70	excellent
Rice breath hydrogen	33–81	67–91	excellent
G-L chromatography jejunal fluid	56	100	poor
Bile acid BT	33–70	60–76	excellent

BT, breath test; G-L chromatography jejunal fluid, gas–liquid chromatography for volatile fatty acids in jejunal fluid.

Among the various substrates available, the sensitivity and specificity of the xylose breath test appears to be superior. As the administration of ^{14}C is associated with radiation exposure, the ^{13}C xylose breath test, using a stable isotope, has been used, as an alternative, in children and women of childbearing age. The lactulose breath test is safe, easy to perform and applicable to children and women of childbearing age. As lactulose is not absorbed in the normal small intestine, normal individuals should produce a peak at 2–3 hours, reflecting the arrival of the substrate into the colon, assuming that the colonic flora is intact. In SIBO, another peak occurs within 1 hour of ingestion and is less prominent than the colonic peak. As glucose is

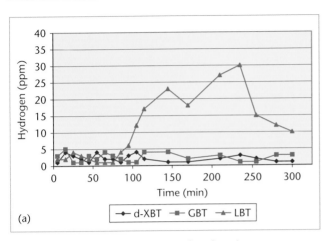 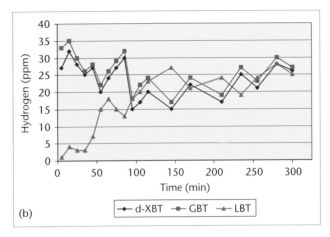

(a)

(b)

Figure 42.2 Non-invasive diagnostic test (breath test).
(a) Normal D-xylose breath test (d-XBT), glucose hydrogen breath test (GBT), and lactulose breath test (LBT). **(b)** Abnormal D-xylose breath test (d-XBT), glucose hydrogen breath test (GBT), and lactulose breath test (LBT); illustrating, in each instance, a breath hydrogen excretion pattern suggestive of bacterial overgrowth.

rapidly absorbed from the proximal small bowel, only proximal overgrowth can be detected by a glucose breath test. The fact that any peak is abnormal in this test is its main advantage over those using nonabsorbable substrates such as lactulose.

Treatment and prevention

There are three components to the treatment of SIBO; firstly, treating the underlying disease; secondly, eradicating overgrowth; and thirdly addressing any associated nutritional deficiencies. The primary goal should be the treatment or correction of any underlying disease or defect, when possible.

Unfortunately, several of the clinical conditions that are associated with SIBO, such as visceral myopathies and multiple jejunal diverticula, are not readily reversible. Management is then based on antibiotic therapy. Its objective should not be to eradicate the bacterial flora but to alter it in a way that leads to symptomatic improvement. Although ideally the choice of antimicrobial agents should reflect *in vitro* susceptibility testing, this is usually impractical as many different bacterial species, with different antibiotic sensitivities typically coexist. Antibiotic treatment remains, therefore, primarily empirical. Effective antibiotic therapy must cover both aerobic and anaerobic enteric bacteria; different schedules have been suggested (Table 42.4). In general, a single 7- to 10-day course of antibiotic may improve symptoms for up to several months in between 46 and 90% of patients with SIBO and render breath tests negative in 20–75%. Because of recurrent symptoms, some patients will need either repeated (e.g., the first 5 to 10 days out of every month) or continuous courses of antibiotic therapy [12]. For the latter, rotating antibiotic regimens are recommended to prevent the development of resistance (Table 42.4). Decisions on management should be individualized and consider such risks of long-term antibiotic therapy as diarrhea, *Clostridium difficile* infection, intolerance, bacterial resistance, and costs. We recommend the use of antibiotics with less toxicity and

Table 42.4 Antibiotic therapy for SIBO

- Ciprofloxacin (250 mg bid)
- Norfloxacin (800 mg/day)
- Metronidazole (250 mg tid)
- Trimethoprim-sulfamethoxazole (1 double strength bid)
- Doxycycline (100 mg bid)
- Amoxicillin-clavulanic acid (500 mg tid)
- Tetracycline (250 mg qid)
- Chloramphenicol (250 mg qid)
- Neomycin (500 mg bid)
- Rifaximin (1200 to 1600 mg/day in 2–4 divided doses)

lower systemic absorption; 7-day regimes incorporating ciprofloxacin, norfloxacin, amoxicillin-clavulanic acid, or metronidazole would, therefore, appear to be a good option. Where available, the minimally absorbed antibiotic rifaximin seems to offer an excellent option [13]. To date, there is not good evidence for efficacy of probiotics in the primary therapy of SIBO; the concept that probiotics might prevent relapse after successful antibiotic therapy is an attractive, though unproven, one.

The role of prokinetic agents among those with stasis and dysmotility is also unproven and the range of options is now limited. As octreotide stimulates propagative phase III activity in the small intestine, low doses (50 μg per day) have been advocated for patients who do not respond to antibiotics, cannot tolerate them, or develop antibiotic-related complications. Non-absorbable purgative solutions may improve gastrointestinal symptoms in children with short bowel syndrome and SIBO.

Nutritional support is an important component of the management of SIBO and may include dietary modifications such as lactose-free diet, replacement of vitamin deficiencies (especially fat soluble vitamins) and correction of deficiencies in nutrients such as calcium, magnesium and B_{12}. As mucosal damage, if present, may persist for some time even after complete eradication of bacterial overgrowth, nutritional support may be required over a prolonged period of time.

Complications and their management

Impaired absorption of nutrients can be attributed to the intraluminal effects of proliferating bacteria combined with mucosal injury. Carbohydrate malabsorption results from a combination of carbohydrate degradation by bacteria and a loss of the activity of brush border disaccharidases resulting from enterocyte damage. Protein malnutrition is also multifactorial and results from intraluminal utilization of dietary protein by bacteria, impaired absorption, and the development of a protein-losing enteropathy. In one third of patients, SIBO is severe enough to cause deficiencies of such vitamins such as vitamin B_{12} and fat-soluble vitamins (A, D, and E). Although the gross histological features of the small bowel are usually normal, bacterial overgrowth may be associated with a reduction in villus height, crypt depth and mucosal thickness, an increase in intraepithelial lymphocytes and focal areas of ulceration and erosion. These changes are reversible following successful antibiotic treatment.

Prognosis with and without treatment

Little is known of the natural history of SIBO other than its potential to lead to complications and protein-losing enteropathy, as described above. Given the metabolic potential of the microbiota, some have questioned the advisability of eradicating SIBO, in the context of the short bowel syndrome, for example, unless symptoms or complications directly referable to SIBO are present.

References

1. Guarner F, Malagelada JR. Gut flora in health and disease. *Lancet.* 2003;361:512–519.
2. Khoshini R, Dai SC, Lezcano S, *et al.* A systematic review of diagnostic tests for small intestinal bacterial overgrowth. *Dig Dis Sci.* 2008;53:1443–1454.
3. Abu-Shanab A, Quigley EM. Diagnosis of small intestinal bacterial overgrowth: the challenges persist! *Expert Rev Gastroenterol Hepatol.* 2009;3:77–87.
4. Rana SV, Bhardwaj SB. Small intestinal bacterial overgrowth. *Scand J Gastroenterol.* 2008:1–8.
5. McEvoy A, Dutton J, James OF. Bacterial contamination of the small intestine is an important cause of occult malabsorption in the elderly. *Br Med J.* 1983;287:789–793.
6. Ford AC, Spiegel BM, Talley NJ, *et al.* Small intestinal bacterial overgrowth in irritable bowel syndrome: systematic review and meta-analysis. *Clin Gastroenterol Hepatol.* 2009;7:1279–1286.
7. Rubio-Tapia A, Barton SH, Rosenblatt JE, *et al.* Prevalence of small intestine bacterial overgrowth diagnosed by quantitative culture of intestinal aspirate in celiac disease. *J Clin Gastroenterol.* 2009;43:157–161.
8. Pande C, Kumar A, Sarin SK. Small-intestinal bacterial overgrowth in cirrhosis is related to the severity of liver disease. *Aliment Pharmacol Ther.* 2009;29:1273–1281.
9. Fan X, Sellin JH. Review article: Small intestinal bacterial overgrowth, bile acid malabsorption and gluten intolerance as possible causes of chronic watery diarrhoea. *Aliment Pharmacol Ther.* 2009;29:1069–1077.
10. Simren M, Stotzer PO. Use and abuse of hydrogen breath tests. *Gut.* 2006;55:297–303.
11. Romagnuolo J, Schiller D, Bailey R. Using breath test wisely in a gastroenterology practice: an evidence-based review of indications and pitfalls in interpretation. *Am J Gastroenterol.* 2002;97:1113–1126.
12. Lauritano EC, Gabrielli M, Scarpellini E, *et al.* Small intestinal bacterial overgrowth recurrence after antibiotic therapy. *Am J Gastroenterol.* 2008;103:2031–2035.
13. Koo HL, Dupont HL. Rifaximin: a unique gastrointestinal-selective antibiotic for enteric diseases. *Curr Opin Gastroenterol.* 2010;26:17–25.

CHAPTER 43

Bile acid malabsorption

Linda Wedlake and Jervoise Andreyev

The Royal Marsden NHS Foundation Trust, London, UK

The rule of halves:
Half of the most common chronic disorders are undetected, half those detected are not treated and half those treated are not controlled.

From: Julian Tudor-Hart: Rule of halves: implications of increasing diagnosis and reducing dropout for future workload and prescribing costs in primary care. *Br J Gen Pract.* 1992;42:116–119, with permission.

ESSENTIAL FACTS ABOUT PATHOGENESIS

Three categories of bile acid malabsorption

Type 1 is caused by ileal disease:
- e.g., Crohn's disease, radiation, surgical resection

Type 2 is "ideopathic" has two main types
- congenital bile acid malabsorption, which is rare
- diarrhea-predominant IBS

Type 3 includes all other causes for example:
- vagotomy, post-cholecystectomy
- microscopic colitis

In type 1 and congenital type 2, absorption of bile acids fail because of defective ileal mechanisms. In types 2 and 3, terminal ileum function may be normal. Overproduction of bile acids by the liver, overwhelming normal absorptive mechanisms is usually the cause

ESSENTIALS OF DIAGNOSIS

- Bile acid malabsorption is a chronic disease and deserves diagnosis by a definitive test
- Main symptom is episodic loose stool, often explosive, and/or steatorrhea
- Patients may have normal stool or even be constipated between diarrhoeal episodes
- Diarrhea may be nocturnal, unpredictable and is often associated with urgency
- SeHCAT ([75]selenium homocholic acid taurine) scan is sensitive and specific but not universally available
- Serum 7 alpha-hydroxy-4-cholesten-3-one levels may be as sensitive but are less specific
- Serum FGF19 is a newly described diagnostic test
- Quantification of fecal bile acids is reliable but obsolete
- Therapeutic trials assessing response to bile acid sequestrants are of limited reliability

ESSENTIALS OF TREATMENT AND PROGNOSIS

- Bile acid sequestrants are the definitive treatment
- Colesevelam 1.25 g tds appears to be better tolerated and more potent than older agents (colestyramine and colestipol)
- For mild symptoms or sequestrant intolerance or incomplete response to sequestrants, dietary fat restriction and/or anti-diarrheal medication may help
- Trace element and fat soluble vitamin supplements may be required

The physiology of bile acid turnover, absorption, and malabsorption

The enterohepatic system: bile acid turnover and synthesis

Bile acids are detergents that are important for fat digestion. An efficient enterohepatic recirculation system maintains a pool for recirculation (Figure 43.1) [1,2] and prevents them reaching the colon where they have a profound irritant effect. Typically less than 5% of the total daily amount secreted by the liver (15–25 g) is lost in feces [3] with more than one third of the original pool remaining after a week [4].

As well as recirculation, the bile acid pool is maintained by *de novo* synthesis of primary bile acids (cholic and chenodeoxycholic acids) as a result of hydroxylation of cholesterol, through the rate-limiting enzyme CYP7A1. They are subsequently conjugated with glycine and taurine and secreted in response to dietary fats [5]. Bacterial deconjugation and dehydroxylation converts 20% to secondary bile acids (deoxycholic, lithocholic and ursodeoxycholic acids).

Reabsorption

The most important mechanism for the conservation of bile acids is the apical sodium-dependent bile acid transporter (ABST) expressed in the terminal ileum [6]. This transporter aggressively recaptures both conjugated and unconjugated bile acids with a preference for conjugated forms reducing luminal concentrations from 10 mmol/L to 0.6 mmol/L [4]. Intracellular transport is mediated via a cytosolic bile acid-binding protein, and an anion exchange mechanism allows basolateral efflux of bile acids from enterocytes into the portal blood for return to the liver [7].

Small and Large Bowel

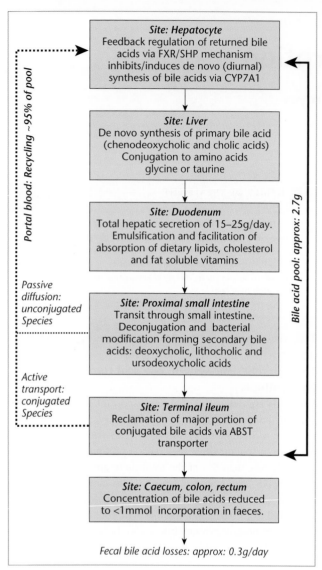

Portal blood: Recycling ~95% of pool

Site: Hepatocyte
Feedback regulation of returned bile acids via FXR/SHP mechanism inhibits/induces de novo (diurnal) synthesis of bile acids via CYP7A1

Site: Liver
De novo synthesis of primary bile acid (chenodeoxycholic and cholic acids) Conjugation to amino acids glycine or taurine

Site: Duodenum
Total hepatic secretion of 15–25 g/day. Emulsification and facilitation of absorption of dietary lipids, cholesterol and fat soluble vitamins

Passive diffusion: unconjugated Species

Site: Proximal small intestine
Transit through small intestine. Deconjugation and bacterial modification forming secondary bile acids: deoxycholic, lithocholic and ursodeoxycholic acids

Active transport: conjugated Species

Bile acid pool: approx: 2.7 g

Site: Terminal ileum
Reclamation of major portion of conjugated bile acids via ABST transporter

Site: Caecum, colon, rectum
Concentration of bile acids reduced to <1 mmol incorporation in faeces.

Fecal bile acid losses: approx: 0.3 g/day

Figure 43.1 Bile acid flux.

Passive absorption of deconjugated bile acids, which are uncharged, also contributes a small fraction of bile acid conservation. The balance between synthesis and loss changes little with age [8]. Bile acids returning to the hepatocyte exert feedback control on their own synthesis via the rate-limiting enzyme cholesterol 7α-hydroxylase (CYP7A1). Interruption of the enterohepatic circulation (i.e., loss of bile acids) induces CYP7A1 activity and thus increased synthesis [7]. A metabolite of the neutral pathway "C4" (7α-hydroxy-4-cholesten-3-one) mirrors bile acid synthesis [9–11].

Physiology of malabsorption

Damage, disease, surgical resection, blockade or mutation of the ABST transporter results in bile acid malabsorption. The length of segment over which ABST is expressed varies, but resection of as little as 10 cm may lead to significant malabsorption, which can be aggravated by dysregulation of feedback signalling and increased ileal motility or secretory activity.

Non-absorbed bile acids reaching the colon in concentrations >1–2 mmol increase permeability (mediated by enteric neurones), motility, water secretion and inhibition of water and electrolyte absorption, all potentially leading to diarrhea [12]. The secretory effect of bile acids can be modified by deconjugation, dehydroxylation and side chain modification by colonic microflora.

Factors contributing to diarrhea

In normal subjects, daily fecal bile acid output is 0.315 g/day compared to patients with diarrhea where losses may reach 1.4 g/day [13]. **Colonic water secretion** (which starts when concentrations of bile acids reach 1–2 mmol/L) is partly dependent on the bile acids present. Deoxycholic acid induces secretion at concentrations of 3 mmol/L and chenodeoxycholic at 5 mmol/L. The **solubility of bile acids** is increased when the pH of the stool is more alkaline. Increased levels of solubilized bile acids, increases permeability and motility, promoting diarrhea. On the other hand, if large amounts of **short chain fatty acids** are present (from fermentation of dietary starch and soluble non-starch polysaccharide) this may acidify stool and reduce solubility of bile acids. **Dietary fibre** has the potential to sequester bile acids directly, also reducing the risk of diarrhea.

Diarrhea and/or steatorrhea

Malabsorption of bile acids coupled with severe depletion of the bile acid pool impairs the ability to emulsify and absorb dietary lipids, resulting in both diarrhea and steatorrhea. The rare genetic ABST transporter defect causes diarrhea, steatorrhea (fecal fat >6 g/day) and failure to thrive from birth [14]. Adults with substantial ileal resections (>100 cm) may also present with more severe diarrhea, steatorrhea (fecal fat >20 g/day) and weight loss compared to patients with shorter resections [15]. However, severe bile acid malabsorption may occur with resections as short as 10 cm [16].

Malabsorption, ileal uptake and the size of the bile acid pool

It is now realized that not all idiopathic bile acid malabsorption is due to a defect in the transporter. Defective feedback regulation in the liver resulting in inappropriately high synthesis and a paradoxically expanded bile acid pool may be sufficient to overload uptake mechanisms despite up-regulation of the ABST protein [17,18].

Effects of malabsorption on intestinal transit

Faster transit in patients with idiopathic bile acid malabsorption may result in reduced absorption.

It has been shown that bile acids infused directly into the distal 40 cm of the ileum inhibit jejunal and ileal motility [19] although in idiopathic bile acid malabsorption this inhibition is lost [20]. Finally, secretion of chloride ions during phase III of the migrating motor complex in the small intestine is reportedly increased in patients with bile acid malabsorption [21] and may contribute to volume overload.

The epidemiology of bile acid malabsorption

Conventionally bile acid malabsorption is categorized as due to:

1. Disease or resection involving the terminal ileum
2. Idiopathic or congenital causes
3. Other causes (Table 43.1).

A more useful distinction lies between disease states characterized by defective absorption and those where bile acid production is also increased, overwhelming the absorptive capacity of the small bowel.

A review of 18 studies (15 prospective) totaling 1223 patients indicates that the true frequency of bile acid malabsorption in patients wrongly labeled as diarrhea-predominant irritable bowel syndrome is as high as 32%. When these patients were treated with colestyramine, 96% with severe, 80% with moderate and 70% with mild bile acid malabsorption responded well. Extrapolating these results suggests that there could be 10 million people in Europe and North America who are diagnosed as "diarrhea-predominant irritable bowel syndrome" who in fact have bile acid malabsorption [22].

In addition, bile acid malabsorption affects more than 100,000 of the 5 million survivors of pelvic cancer treated with radiotherapy [23], and several hundred thousand patients with Crohn's disease [24,25]. Other populations at increased risk of bile acid malabsorption are listed in Table 43.1. Well conducted prospective population studies suggest the frequency of bile acid malabsorption has not changed over 30 years [22,26].

Symptoms of bile acid malabsorption

Often described as **watery diarrhea** with or without an element of steatorrhea, this bland description does not do justice to the potential misery of bile acid malabsorption. While the stool can be watery, many patients say it is mostly soft rather than liquid. They usually describe extremely erratic, completely unpredictable, intermittently **severe and explosive symptoms** sometimes interspersed with days or weeks of completely normal stool. Defecation is often very **urgent**, may wake at night and be associated with foul smelling wind, abdominal pain and recurrent episodes of fecal incontinence. Stool volume may be normal or increased. When small bowel bacterial overgrowth (e.g., due to vagotomy or pelvic radiotherapy) is concomitant with bile acid malabsorption the degree of the **abdominal pain with associated vomiting** may be so severe that "subacute obstruction" is mistakenly diagnosed.

Steatorrhea is also more common than widely appreciated. Most patients and many clinicians fail to differentiate between diarrhea and steatorrhea although careful routine enquiry (presence of a film of oil in the lavatory pan) will alert the clinician without necessitating unpleasant 3-day fecal fat collections. Some patients describe steatorrhea predictably following a rich (e.g., high fat) meal, whilst in others symptoms occur more intermittently.

Diagnosis of bile acid malabsorption

A thorough clinical history should raise the possibility of bile acid malabsorption (Table 43.1) even in those patients with complex conditions and more than one cause for their symptoms. Since the condition is usually lifelong requiring ongoing medication, a definitive diagnostic test is indicated.

SeHCAT scanning

Under-diagnosis of bile acid malabsorption is widespread. The SeHCAT ([75]selenium homocholic acid taurine) test, which is the simplest and most reliable, is only available in nine European countries and in Australia and Canada. Even in the UK, more than half of gastroenterologists never or seldom use the test and 50% of all requests for SeHCAT tests come from only ten hospitals [27].

This reliable test became available in 1983 [28,29]. Selenium-75-homocholic acid taurine (the taurine conjugate of a synthetic bile acid) "SeHCAT" is administered orally. Gamma radiation emitted over the abdominal area at baseline (3 hours after SeHCAT capsule administration) and several days later is measured with an uncollimated gamma camera. Whilst various test protocols have been used, most centres now report 7-day retention of <5% of baseline value as being indicative of severe malabsorption, 5–10% moderate and 10–15% mild bile acid malabsorption. These cut-offs correlate well with response to treatment [22]. Levels greater than 15% are normal. The SeHCAT test has a reported sensitivity of between 89 and 97% and specificity of between 99 and 100% [28,30]. When repeated in the same patients, the results are highly reproducible [8]. The SeHCAT scan gives a dose of 0.26 mSV of radiation, equivalent to one month's background radiation, or similar to the dose from 2–3 chest X-rays. It should be used cautiously in women who could be pregnant.

24-hour fecal bile acid excretion

This test is unpleasant, expensive and requires considerable laboratory expertise. Collection of total (24-hour) fecal excretion and centrifugation of the stool homogenate allows measurement of the concentration of bile acids in the aqueous phase either enzymatically or by gas liquid chromatography.

Plasma C7α-hydroxy-4-cholestene-3-one ("C4") assay

In countries where the SeHCAT scan is not available, an alternative simple diagnostic test based on serum concentrations of 7α-hydroxy-4-cholestene-3-one ("C4") [9–11] can be undertaken. This test is more reliable than a therapeutic trial but is probably not as sensitive (90%) and definitely not as specific (79%) as a SeHCAT scan [11]. 7α-hydroxy-4-cholestene-3-one is a marker of the initial step in the synthesis of bile acids and is induced in patients with impaired enterohepatic recycling of bile acids.

Fibroblast growth factor 19 (FGF 19)

FGF19, produced in ileal enterocytes, has recently been shown to be a negative regulator of bile acid synthesis in the liver. Serum levels increase after meals, consistent with a feedback

Table 43.1 Frequency of bile acid malabsorption in symptomatic patients not responding to conventional treatment

Cause of bile acid malabsorption	Frequency of bile acid malabsorption in symptomatic patients not responding to conventional treatment	References	Comments
Type 1 bile acid malabsorption			
Right hemicolectomy	High	[38,39]	15–17% of all patients Diarrhea may improve with time
Crohn's (previous surgery)	97–100%	[24,25]	60% response rate to cholestyramine
Crohn's (no previous surgery)	32–54%	[24,25]	60% response rate to cholestyramine
HIV	8–84%	[40–42]	Especially associated with cryptosporidium infection 85% response rate to cholestyramine
Cystic fibrosis	33%	[43,44]	
Acutely during pelvic radiotherapy	44–57%	[45–47]	
Radiation enteropathy with diarrhea	1–83%	[48–52]	
Cancer chemotherapy	No published data		Anecdotal experience that this is the cause for symptoms in some patients
Untreated celiac disease	0–31%	[53,54]	
Type 2 bile acid malabsorption			
Diarrhea predominant IBS SeHCAT < 5% retention at 7 days (severe) SeHCAT < 10% retention at 5 days (moderate) SeHCAT < 15% retention at 5 days (mild)	4–13% (aggregate of all studies 10%) 12–65% (aggregate of all studies 32%) 18–53% (aggregate of all studies 26%)	Summarized in reference [21]	18 studies Response rates to colestyramine are 96% in severe, 80% in moderate and 70% in mild malabsorption
Congenital bile acid malabsorption	Rare		
Type 3 bile acid malabsorption			
Post infective diarrhea	N/A	[55]	
Diabetic diarrhea	4–47%	[51,55,56]	
Thyroid disease	N/A	[57]	Thyrotoxicosis, medullary carcinoma
Microscopic / lymphocytic / collagenous colitis	27–44% patients CC 9–60% patients LC	[58–60]	
Post cholecystectomy	12–96%	[51,61–63]	Increased risk in women?
Post vagotomy	8–100%	[51,64–66]	
Chronic pancreatitis	N/A	[67,68]	
Myotonic dystrophy	60%	[69]	
Scleroderma	High	[70]	A frequent problem
Drug related	N/A		Omeprazole, metformin

CC, collagenous colitis; LC, lymphocytic colitis; N/A, not available.

role on bile acid synthesis. Defective production of FGF19 seems to occur in bile acid diarrhea and serum FGF19 levels may be a useful new diagnostic marker [17,30].

Therapeutic trial using a bile acid sequestrant: an inadequate diagnostic method?

The commonest alternative to a formal diagnostic test is a therapeutic trial using a bile acid sequestrant. These drugs may take up to 10 days of adequate dosing to achieve a clinically evident response. However, one in four patients prescribed colestyramine or colestipol are unable to tolerate more than a single dose. An early side effect can be worsening diarrhea or steatorrhea. These drugs may also have non-specific effects, which lead to an apparent response when bile acid malabsorption is not present. So, except perhaps in patients who have undergone a right hemicolectomy and immediately develop severe diarrhea, it seems inappropriate to make a life-changing diagnosis or deny a lifetime of effective treatment on the basis of a potentially flawed therapeutic trial when alternative definitive tests are available.

^{14}C cholyglycine breath test, ^{14}C cholyglycine stool test

These tests are obsolete but important historically [12]. ^{14}C-glycine-labelled cholyglycine was ingested and non-absorbed radioactive cholyglycine reaching the colon was deconjugated by colonic bacteria, metabolized and absorbed to give $^{14}CO_2$ in the breath. Bacterial overgrowth could give false positive results, which can be excluded if the breath test was combined with fecal ^{14}C analysis. Concomitant assessment of intestinal transit was also required.

Other tests

Colonoscopy and terminal ileal biopsies may be normal in bile acid malabsorption unless there is associated collagenous colitis or terminal ileal disease. However, in the presence of raised inflammatory markers, anemia or in those with a sudden change in bowel habit, colonoscopy may be indicated to exclude macroscopic or microscopic inflammation, neoplasia or infection. Vitamin B_{12} levels are reduced in only one third of patients so are not a reliable marker of bile acid malabsorption [31].

Treatment of bile acid malabsorption

Medication

There is no licensed treatment for bile acid malabsorption. However, **bile acid sequestrants** which are licensed treatments for cholesterol lowering but have been used (off label) for bile acid malabsorption for many years. **Colestyramine** (initially 4–8 g daily) and **colestipol** (initially 5 g × 1–2/day) are effective in controlling diarrhea. However, up to 25% of people cannot tolerate the taste/consistency or develop unacceptable nausea, heartburn, wind, bloating or worsening diarrhea even when taken with meals (which is anecdotally thought to be better than consumption on an empty stomach

as recommended by the data sheet). Colestyramine is frequently reported to worsen steatorrhea.

The newer colesevelam hydrochloride 1.25 g tds appears to have advantages such as better affinity, specificity and sequestration ability for bile acids than colestyramine [33,34], effectiveness when colestyramine has failed or is not well tolerated [32,35] and improvement of steatorrhea when present. This reduces the risk of renal oxalate stone formation. It works by interrupting the recycling of bile acids, diverting endogenous cholesterol for synthesis of replacement bile acids. Colesevelam is more expensive than colestyramine and colestipol and not recommended by some agencies for this reason.

Aluminium hydroxide has bile-acid-binding properties *in-vitro* comparable with those of colestyramine. A single small study showed that large doses can reduce bowel frequency and daily stool weights [36].

Two other agents have in the past been suggested as well tolerated and effective but neither are available currently. One is **enteric-coated colestyramine**, the other is **cholylsarcosine**, a synthetic bile acid which may be particularly helpful in patients with massive small bowel resections as it seems to improve fat absorption but does not stimulate colonic secretion.

Anti-diarrheal agents **Anti-diarrheal** drugs such as **codeine phosphate** or **loperamide** (taken 30–60 minutes before main meals, up to four times a day) can be effective. In those with more severe symptoms, they are probably best used on a regular basis to try to pre-empt the development of diarrhea. However, many patients still report unpredictable episodes of diarrhea despite taking anti-diarrheal drugs regularly and the optimal dose is difficult to define. Anti-diarrheal drugs are least effective when patients with bile acid malabsorption have episodes of steatorrhea.

Dietary changes

Low fat diets (40 g of fat/day) may improve bowel function even in severe bile acid malabsorption but they are difficult to sustain especially when eating outside the home. Replacement of a large proportion of long chain triglycerides in the diet with **medium chain triglycerides** (MCTs) may help by reducing biliary secretions. However, there are few natural sources of MCTs and they are unpalatable. MCT-rich diets need long-term supervision by a qualified dietitian to ensure that the patient does not become deficient in essential nutrients. If all other treatments fail, long-term symptomatic improvement has been achieved by gastrostomy feeding using such diets [37].

Vitamins and lipids

Prolonged use of bile acid sequestrants may cause hypertriglyceridemia, fat soluble vitamin and trace element deficiency. Clinical experience suggests that approximately 20% of patients will have vitamin or trace element deficiency at presentation or will develop it with time. Baseline checks and annual monitoring of lipid and vitamin levels is therefore sensible. Vitamin B_{12} levels should be checked in patients in whom the diagnosis is suspected or confirmed. Fat soluble vitamin status (vitamin A, D, E and K) and trace elements should be checked periodically in all patients with chronic malabsorptive syndromes. Data are conflicting as to whether long-term usage increases the risk of gallstones.

Conclusions

Bile acid malabsorption is a real and often humiliating disease, which occurs considerably more frequently than generally recognized and is often misdiagnosed as irritable bowel syndrome. The disease is easier to understand if it is thought about not only in terms of terminal ileal dysfunction but also as a condition in which disordered regulation of bile acid production in the liver occurs, overwhelming absorptive mechanisms. Definitive diagnostic testing is recommended when the condition is suspected. This facilitates management. New therapeutic options to treat bile acid malabsorption are emerging.

References

1. Duane WC, Adler RD, Bennion LJ, *et al.* Determination of bile acid pool size in man: a simplified method with advantages of increased precision, shortened analysis time and decreased isotope exposure. *J Lipid Res.* 1975;16:155–158.
2. Chiang JY. Bile acids: regulation of synthesis. *J Lipid Res.* 2009;50:1955–1966.
3. Hofmann AF. The continuing importance of bile acids in liver and intestinal disease. *Arch Intern Med.* 1999;159:2647–2658.
4. Bajor A. *Bile acid induced diarrhea: Pathophysiological and clinical aspects.* University of Gothenburg Gothenburg, Sweden; 2008.
5. Galman C, Angelin B, Rudling M. Bile acid synthesis in humans has a rapid diurnal variation that is asynchronous with cholesterol synthesis. *Gastroenterology.* 2005;129:1445–1453.
6. Ung KA, Olofsson G, Fae A, *et al.* In vitro determination of active bile acid absorption in small biopsy specimens obtained endoscopically or surgically from the human intestine. *Eur J Clin Invest.* 2002;32:115–121.
7. Alrefai WA, Gill RK. Bile acid transporters: Structure, function regulation and pathophysiological implications. *Pharm Res.* 2007;10:1803–1823.
8. Bajor A, Kilander A, Sjövall H, *et al.* The bile acid turnover rate assessed with the (75)SeHCAT test is stable in chronic diarrhea but slightly decreased in healthy subjects after a long period of time. *Dig Dis Sci.* 2008;53:2935–2940.
9. Eusufzai S, Axelson M, Angelin B, *et al.* Serum 7alpha-hydroxy-4-cholesten-3-one concentrations in the evaluation of bile acid malabsorption in patients with diarrhea: correlation to SeHCAT test. *Gut.* 1993;34:698–701.
10. Brydon WG, Nyhlin H, Eastwood MA, *et al.* Serum 7alpha-hydroxy-4-cholesten-3-one and selenohomocholytaurine (SeHCAT) whole body retention in the assessment of bile acid induced diarrhea. *Eur J Gastroenterol Hepatol.* 1996;8:117–123.
11. Sauter GH, Munzing W, Von Ritter C, *et al.* Bile acid malabsorption as a cause of chronic diarrhea. Diagnostic value of 7alpha-hydroxy-4-cholesten-3-one in serum. *Dig Dis Sci.* 1999;44:14–19.
12. Fromm H, Malavolti M. Bile acid-induced diarrhea. *Clin Gastroenterol.* 1986;15:567–582.
13. Porter JL, Fordtran JS, Santa Ana CA, *et al.* Accurate enzymatic measurement of fecal bile acids in patients with malabsorption. *J Lab Clin Med.* 2003;141:411–418.
14. Oelkers P, Kirby LC, Heubi JE, *et al.* Primary bile acid malabsorption caused by mutations in the ileum sodium-dependent bile acid transporter gene (SLC10A2). *J Clin Invest.* 1997;99:1880–1887.
15. Hofmann AF, Poley JR. Role of bile acid malabsorption in pathogenesis of diarrhea and steatorrhea in patients with ileal resection. I. Response to cholestyramine or replacement of dietary long chain triglyceride by medium chain triglyceride. *Gastroenterology.* 1972;62:918–934.
16. Kurien M, Evans KE, Leeds JS, *et al.* Bile acid malabsorption: An under-investigated differential diagnosis in patients presenting with diarrhea predominant irritable bowel syndrome type symptoms. *Scandinavian Journal of Gastroenterology,* 2011; Early Online, 1–5.
17. Bajor A, Kilander A, Fae A, *et al.* Normal or increased bile acid uptake in isolated mucosa from patients with bile acid malabsorption. *Eur J Gastroenterol Hepatol.* 2006;18:397–403.
18. Hofmann AF, Mangelsdorf DJ, Kliewer SA. Chronic diarrhea due to excessive bile acid synthesis and not defective ileal transport: a new syndrome of defective fibroblast growth factor 19 release. *Clin Gastroenterol Hepatol.* 2009;7:1151–1154.
19. Penagini R, Spiller RC, Misiewicz JJ, *et al.* Effect of ileal infusion of glycochenodeoxycholic acid on segmental transit, motility, and flow in the human jejunum and ileum. *Gut.* 1989;30:609–617.
20. Sadik R, Abrahamsson H, Ung KA, *et al.* Accelerated regional bowel transit and overweight shown in idiopathic bile acid malabsorption. *Am J Gastroenterol.* 2004;99:711–718.
21. Bajor A, Ung KA, Ohman L, *et al.* Indirect evidence for increased mechanosensitivity of jejunal secretomotor neurones in patients with idiopathic bile acid malabsorption. *Acta Physiol (Oxf).* 2009;197:129–137.
22. Wedlake L, A'Hern R, Russell D, *et al.* Systematic review: the prevalence of idiopathic bile acid malabsorption as diagnosed by SeHCAT scanning in patients with diarrhea-predominant irritable bowel syndrome. *Aliment Pharmacol Ther.* 2009;30:707–717.
23. Andreyev HJN. Gastrointestinal symptoms following therapeutic pelvic radiotherapy: a new understanding to improve the management of symptomatic patients. *Lancet Oncol.* 2007;8:1007–1017.
24. Nyhlin H, Merrick MV, Eastwood MA. Bile acid malabsorption in Crohn's disease and indications for its assessment using SeHCAT. *Gut.* 1994;35:90–93.
25. Smith MJ, Cherian P, Raju GS, *et al.* Bile acid malabsorption in persistent diarrhea. *J R Coll Physicians Lond.* 2000;34:448–451.
26. Basumani P, Smith MJ, Srinivas M, *et al.* Bile acid malabsorption: two decades on. *Gut.* 2008;57(Suppl 1):A20.
27. Khalid U, Lalji A, Stafferton R, *et al.* Bile acid malabsoption: a forgotten diagnosis? *Clin Med.* 2010;10:1–3.
28. Merrick MV, Eastwood MA, Ford MJ. Is bile acid malabsorption underdiagnosed? An evaluation of accuracy of diagnosis by measurement of SeHCAT retention. *BMJ.* 1985;290:665–668.
29. Hofmann AF. Progress in idiopathic bile acid malabsorption. *Gut.* 1998;43:738–739.
30. Sciarretta G, Vicini G, Fagioli G, *et al.* Use of 23-selena-25-homocholoytaurine to detect bile acid malabsorption in patients

with ileal dysfunction or diarrhea. *Gastroenterology.* 1986;91: 1–9.

31. Walters JR, Tasleem AM, Omer OS, *et al.* A new mechanism for bile acid diarrhea: defective feedback inhibition of bile acid biosynthesis. *Clin Gastroenterol Hepatol.* 2009;7:1189–1194.

32. Wedlake L, Thomas K, Lalji A, *et al.* Effectiveness and tolerability of colesevelam hydrochloride for bile-acid malabsorption in patients with cancer: a retrospective chart review and patient questionnaire. *Clin Ther.* 2009;31:2549–2558.

33. Donovan JM, von Bergmann K, Setchell KD, *et al.* Effects of colesevelam HC1 on sterol and bile acid excretion in patients with type IIa hypercholesterolemia. *Dig Dis Sci.* 2005;50:1232–1238.

34. Insull WJ. Clinical utility of bile acid sequestrants in the treatment of dyslipidemia: a scientific review. *South Med J.* 2006;99: 257–273.

35. Puleston J, Morgan H, Andreyev HJN. New treatment for bile salt malabsorption. *Gut.* 2005;54:441–442.

36. Sali A, Murray WR, MacKay C. Aluminium hydroxide in bile-salt diarrhea. *Lancet.* 1977;2:1051–1053.

37. Nelson LM, Carmichael HA, Russell RI, *et al.* Use of an elemental diet (Vivonex) in the management of bile acid-induced diarrhea. *Gut.* 1977;18:792–794.

38. Jewkes AJ, Windsor CW, Ward RS, *et al.* Relationship between bile acid malabsorption using the 75Se homocholic acid taurine scanning method and diarrhoea following right hemicolectomy. *Br J Surg.* 1989;76(7):707–708.

39. Ho YH, Low D, Goh HS. Bowel function survey after segmental colorectal resections. *Dis Colon Rectum.* 1996;39(3):307–310.

40. Sciarretta G, Bonazzi L, Monti M, *et al.* Bile acid malabsorption in AIDS-associated chronic diarrhea: a prospective 1-year study. *Am J Gastroenterol.* 1994;89(3):379–381.

41. Cramp ME, Hing MC, Marriott DJ, *et al.* Bile acid malabsorption in HIV infected patients with chronic diarrhoea. *Aust N Z J Med.* 1996;26(3):368–371.

42. Bjarnason I, Sharpstone DR, Francis N, *et al.* Intestinal inflammation, ileal structure and function in HIV. *AIDS.* 1996;10(12): 1385–1391.

43. Weber AM, Roy CC, Morin CL, Lasalle R. Malabsorption of bile acids in children with cystic fibrosis. *N Engl J Med.* 1973;289(19): 1001–1005.

44. Stryker J, Hepner G, Mortel R. The effect of pelvic irradiation on ileal function. *Radiology.* 1977;124:213–216.

45. Fernández-Bañares F, Villá S, Esteve M, *et al.* Acute effects of abdominopelvic irradiation on the orocecal transit time: its relation to clinical symptoms, and bile salt and lactose malabsorption. *Am J Gastroenterol.* 1991;86(12):1771–1777.

46. Yeoh E, Lui D, Lee N. The mechanism of diarrhoea resulting from pelvic and abdominal radiotherapy; a prospective study using selenium-75 labelled conjugated bile acid and cobalt-58 labelled cyanocobalamin. *Br J Radiol.* 1984;57:1131–1136.

47. Ludgate S, Merrick M. The pathogenesis of post-irradiation chronic diarrhoea: measurement of SeHCAT and B12 absorption for differential diagnosis determines treatment. *Clinical Radiology.* 1985;36:275–278.

48. Arlow F, Dekovich A, Priest R, Beher W. Bile acids in radiation-induced diarrhea. *South Med J.* 1987;80(10):1259–1261.

49. Danielsson A, Nyhlin H, Persson H, *et al.* Chronic diarrhoea after radiotherapy for gynaecological cancer: occurrence and aetiology. *Gut.* 1991;32(10):1180–1187.

50. Ford GA, Preece JD, Davies IH, Wilkinson SP. Use of SeHCAT test in the investigation of diarrhoea. *Postgrad Med J.* 1992;68: 272–276.

51. Andreyev HJN, Vlavianos P, Blake P, *et al.* Gastrointestinal symptoms after pelvic radiotherapy: is there any role for the gastroenterologist? *Int J Radiol Biol Phys.* 2005;62(5):1464–1471.

52. Vuoristo M, Miettinen TA. The role of fat and bile acid malabsorption in diarrhoea of coeliac disease. *Scand J Gastroenterol Suppl.* 1987;22(3):289–294.

53. Gillberg R, Andersson H. Labelled bile salt excretion and diarrhoea in coeliac disease. *Scand J Gastroenterol Suppl.* 1980;15(8): 969–972.

54. Niaz SK, Sandrasegaran K, Renny FH, Jones BJ. Bile acid malabsorption and post-infective diarrhoea. *J R Coll Physicians Lond.* 1997;31(1):53–56.

55. Scarpello J, Sladen G. Malabsorption in relation to abdominal irradiation and quadruple chemotherapy for lymphosarcoma. *Postgrad Med J.* 1977;53(618):218–221.

56. Condon JR, Robinson V, Suleman MI, *et al.* The cause and treatment of postvagotomy diarrhoea. *Br J Surg.* 1975;62(4):309–312.

57. Raju GS, Dawson B, Bardhan KD. Bile acid malabsorption associated with Graves' disease. *J Clin Gastroenterol.* 1994;19(1):54–56.

58. Ung KA, Gillberg R, Kilander A, Abrahamsson H. Role of bile acids and bile acid binding agents in patients with collagenous colitis. *Gut.* 2000;46(2):170–175.

59. Fernandez-Bañares F, Esteve M, Salas A, *et al.* Bile acid malabsorption in microscopic colitis and in previously unexplained functional chronic diarrhea. *Dig Dis Sci.* 2001;46(10):2231–2238.

60. Ung KA, Kilander A, Willén R, Abrahamsson H. Role of bile acids in lymphocytic colitis. *Hepatogastroenterology.* 2002;49(44): 432–437.

61. Sciarretta G, Furno A, Mazzoni M, Malaguti P. Post-cholecystectomy diarrhea: evidence of bile acid malabsorption assessed by SeHCAT test. *Am J Gastroenterol.* 1992;87(12):1852–1854.

62. Eusufzai S. Bile acid malabsorption in patients with chronic diarrhea. *Scand J Gastroenterol Suppl.* 1993;28(10):865–868.

63. Fromm H, Tunuguntla AK, Malavolti M, *et al.* Absence of significant role of bile acids in diarrhea of a heterogeneous group of postcholecystectomy patients. *Dig Dis Sci.* 1987;32(1):33–44.

64. Smith MJ, Cherian P, Raju GS, *et al.* Bile acid malabsorption in persistent diarrhoea. *J R Coll Physicians Lond.* 2000;34(5): 448–451.

65. al-Hadrani A, Lavelle-Jones M, Kennedy N, *et al.* Bile acid malabsorption in patients with post-vagotomy diarrhoea. *Ann Chir Gynaecol.* 1992;81(4):351–353.

66. Thompson D, Wild R, Merrick MV, *et al.* Cholelithiasis and bile acid absorption after truncal vagotomy and gastroenterostomy. *Br J Surg.* 1994;81(7):1037–1039.

67. Dutta SK, Anand K, Gadacz TR. Bile salt malabsorption in pancreatic insufficiency secondary to alcoholic pancreatitis. *Gastroenterology.* 1986;91(5):1243–1249.

68. Madsen JL, Graff J, Philipsen EK, *et al.* Bile acid malabsorption or disturbed intestinal permeability in patients treated with enzyme substitution for exocrine pancreatic insufficiency is not caused by bacterial overgrowth. *Pancreas.* 2003;26(2):130–133.

69. Rönnblom A, Andersson S, Danielsson A. Mechanisms of diarrhoea in myotonic dystrophy. *Eur J Gastroenterol Hepatol.* 1998; 10(7):607–610.

70. Pazzi P, Putinati S, Bagni B, *et al.* Bile acid malabsorption in progressive systemic sclerosis. *Gut.* 1988;29(4):552–553.

Small and Large Bowel

CHAPTER 44
Protein-losing disorders of the gastrointestinal tract

Simon Murch

Warwick Medical School, Coventry, UK

CAUSES OF EXCESSIVE INTESTINAL PROTEIN LOSS

Lymphatic obstruction
Congenital – lymphangiectasia, Hennekam syndrome
Acquired – e.g., TB, retroperitoneal fibrosis, Whipple's disease, sarcoidosis, lymphoma, radiotherapy, endometriosis, thoracic duct obstruction

Excessive mesenteric venous pressure
Constrictive pericarditis, congestive cardiac failure, tricuspid incompetence
Malrotation
Congenital cardiac disease following Fontan surgery

Loss of the gut epithelial barrier
Ulcerating lesions
IBD
Pseudomembraneous colitis
Graft versus host disease
Amyloidosis
Malignancy
Ulcerative jejuno-ileitis
Non-ulcerating lesions
Congenital enterocyte heparan sulfate deficiency (very rare)
Congenital disorders of glycosylation (rare)
Cystic fibrosis
Kwashiorkor
Ménétrier's disease
Enteropathies – e.g., celiac disease, autoimmune enteropathy
Eosinophilic enterocolitis
Connective tissue disorders – notably SLE
Henoch-Schönlein purpura
AIDS
Bacterial overgrowth, parasites e.g., *strongloides, trichuris*

CLINICAL PRESENTATION

Nephrotic syndrome-like presentation of hypoalbuminia
 • Peripheral or facial edema, ascites, occasionally anasarca
 • Potential secondary peritonitis, venous thrombosis
Diarrhea – a variable feature, more common in acute onset PLE
Symptoms due to associated malabsorption
Immunodeficiency – if associated enteric lymphocyte loss (lymphangiectasia)
Symptoms of underlying condition – e.g., cardiac, inflammatory, metabolic

TREATMENT AND PREVENTION

1. Treatment of underlying cause
 • Enteropathy – appropriate dietary exclusion, immunosuppression etc.
 • Cardiac lesions – reduce right atrial pressure, relieve pericardial constriction
 • Lymphatic obstruction – surgical resection if localized lesion
2. Augment barrier to protein leakage
 • Heparin therapy may reduce protein loss
3. Treat hypoalbuminemia as necessary
 • Fluid intake restriction; avoid excess IV fluid therapy
 • 20% albumin infusion with diuretic cover
4. Minimize complications
 • Use medium chain triglycerides for main fat source if lymphatic obstruction
 • Give antibiotic cover if immunodeficient with ascites (e.g., splenectomy)
 • Check micronutrient and fat soluble vitamin status
5. Prevention. Avoid inappropriate malnutrition states. This is not restricted to the developing world, and occurs frequently in chronically hospitalized, post-surgical and elderly patients

Introduction

Many conditions can cause excess protein leakage from the gastrointestinal tract. This can be severe, exceeding 20 grams or more daily in IBD [1]. Protein-losing enteropathy (PLE) can occur as part of generalized impairment of intestinal function, accompanied by secretory diarrhea and malabsorption. In other conditions, protein losses may be predominant, and only fat absorption compromised.

Protein leakage may be restricted to the stomach, associated with giant hypertrophy of the gastric rugae (Ménétrier's disease) or may be due to either focal or diffuse pathology within the small intestine or colon. The causes of excess enteric protein loss can broadly be divided into two groups, due either to loss of barrier function of the epithelium, or to raised pressure within the lymphatics or mesenteric veins.

The prognosis of acute enteric protein-losing states is generally good, unless part of a broader pathological process. By contrast, chronic protein-losing conditions of more than moderate severity can have a poor prognosis.

Textbook of Clinical Gastroenterology and Hepatology, Second Edition. Edited by C. J. Hawkey, Jaime Bosch, Joel E. Richter, Guadalupe Garcia-Tsao, Francis K. L. Chan.
© 2012 Blackwell Publishing Ltd. Published 2012 by Blackwell Publishing Ltd.

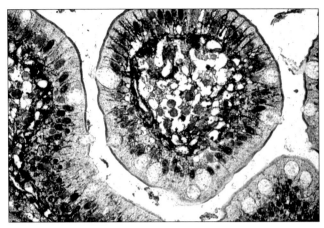

(a)

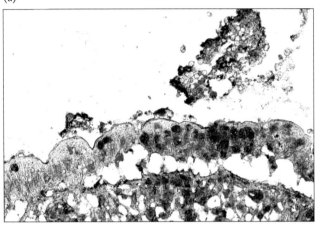

(b)

Figure 44.1 A common mechanism of enteric protein loss – reduction of epithelial heparan sulfate proteoglycan expression. These negatively charged GAGs provide an electrostatic barrier to albumin leakage. (a) Dense HSPG expression (black) on subepithelial basement membrane and between enterocytes in normal terminal ileum. Macrophages are stained red. Similar findings are seen throughout the gut. (b) Loss of basement membrane and epithelial HSPG in active Crohn's disease, associated with dense macrophage infiltration.

Epidemiology

There are a large number of potential causes of protein-losing enteropathy (Figure 44.1). Inflammatory bowel disease is one of the most common causes of persistent intestinal protein loss, although losses may be seen in a variety of mucosal and systemic inflammatory disorders. In developing countries, increased enteric protein loss may occur in kwashiorkor, a form of protein energy malnutrition in which edema occurs as a consequence of hypoalbuminemia. There is a very high incidence of complications, and death is common.

Pathogenesis and pathology

There has been recent advance from both clinical and basic scientific studies in the understanding of protein-losing enteropathy. The major factors are excess hydrostatic pressure within mesenteric veins or lymphatics and impaired epithelial

barrier function. Both factors may occur together, and may then synergise to amplify transepithelial protein leak.

Molecular basis of lymphangiectasia

A number of molecules play important roles in lymphatic development, including vascular-endothelial growth factors (VEGF)-C and D, their receptor VEGF-R3 and the transcription factors FOXC2 and Sox18 [2]. Mutations in these molecules have been shown to block lymphogenesis in mice and have been associated with congenital lymphatic disorders such as Milroy's disease. VEGF-C gene therapy has been successful in some mouse models of congenital lymphatic abnormality. This may offer a potential future therapeutic direction in intestinal lymphangiectasia, in which VEGF-C and Sox18 expression appears to be downregulated [2].

HSPG loss and albumin leak

The major regulator of albumin flux across many membranes is the negative charge provided by sulphated glycosaminoglycan (GAG) such as heparan sulphate, due to interaction with arginyl residues in the albumin molecule [3,4]. A critical component of the gut epithelial barrier is thus the expression of GAG chains by heparan sulfate proteoglycans (HSPG) on the basolateral epithelial surface [5] (Figures 44.1, 44.2).

The first indications of a role for intestinal HSPG in gut physiology came from findings of severe congenital PLE in infants born without epithelial HSPG [5]. Episodic life-threatening PLE occurred in an infant with a congenital disorder of n-glycosylation (CDG-1c) [6]. During PLE episodes, epithelial HSPG was trapped within the endoplasmic reticulum, preventing its appropriate localization on the basolateral epithelial surface. These findings prompted basic scientific studies, in which a critical role for HSPG in preventing PLE was identified first in epithelial cell lines and then in epithelial HSPG-deficient mice [7–10]. In both models, epithelial HSPG loss synergises with proinflammatory cytokines, notably TNF-α and interferon-γ. Losses are maximal when increased hydrostatic pressure occurs together with decreased epithelial HSPG in the presence of proinflammatory cytokines [8,9].

While inborn errors of HSPG expression are rare, recent findings in Zambian infants with kwashiorkor, demonstrate that there is significant reduction of HSPG expression throughout the intestinal mucosa [11] (Figure 44.3). This concords with previous evidence suggesting global impairment of HSPG synthesis in this form of malnutrition. It is possible, because of the multiple roles of HSPG in physiology, that HSPG loss may contribute to many specific features of kwashiorkor.

In inflammatory conditions such as IBD, there is widespread loss of epithelial and matrix HSPG's [12]. These are reduced through inflammatory degradation of their glycan chains by matrix degrading metalloproteases (MMP's), released from inflammatory cells. MMPs are inhibited by naturally occurring antagonists, the tissue inhibitors of metalloproteases (TIMP's). In active IBD, mucosal MMP expression overwhelms the TIMP response [13]. The cytokines TNF-α and IL-1 are pivotal

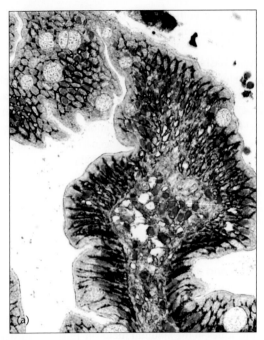
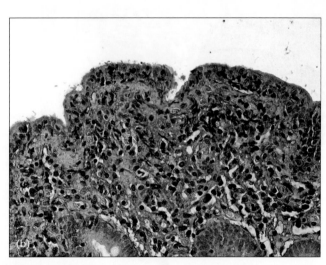

Figure 44.2 Pressure and the epithelial barrier – the two determinants of protein leakage. (a) Preserved duodenal epithelial HSPG expression in a child with lymphangiectasia. Dilated lymphatic spaces may be seen within the lamina propria. Here protein loss occurs because of raised pressure. (b) Grossly reduced duodenal epithelial HSPG expression in a Zambian child with kwashiorkor. Epithelial barrier function is thus compromised.

inducers of this enhanced MMP response [14]. Activated T cells produce MMPs, and thus other conditions associated with increased infiltration of activated intraepithelial lymphocytes may manifest albumin leakage.

Clinical implications of basic findings

Severe excess mesenteric lymphatic pressure alone may be sufficient to cause severe PLE, as seen in congenital or acquired lymphangiectasia. This pressure may be sufficient to induce small breakdowns in epithelial integrity, as evidenced by endoscopic findings of focal chylous leak and consequent circulating lymphopenia. The extent of protein loss in lymphangiectasia may be reduced by stratagems to reduce lymphatic pressure, such as reduction of long chain triglyceride intake. Substitution of medium chain triglycerides, which are absorbed directly into the portal vein without requiring lymphatic drainage, may reduce but not prevent protein loss.

By contrast to lymphatic obstruction, raised mesenteric venous pressure may predispose to enteric protein loss, but appears to require additional impairment of the epithelial barrier. In the severe PLE that occurs in up to 4–10% of patients after Fontan surgery for congenital cardiac defects, raised mesenteric vascular pressure is necessary but insufficient on its own to induce protein leakage. The PLE usually begins some time after surgery, but with no detectable change in right atrial pressure. However, once established, the PLE is relentless and often fatal, unless cardiac transplantation is possible. It is currently unknown why some cases develop PLE and

others do not, and the relationship to pressure is quite variable. It is likely that the epithelial barrier to protein leak may be impaired, for as yet unknown reasons, in those who go on to develop PLE. Therapy with full molecular weight heparin, to augment epithelial barrier function, has proven to be clinically useful.

Clinical presentation of protein-losing enteropathy

This will depend upon the underlying cause, and the primary initial manifestations of PLE may depend on the underlying disease. Syndromes associated with primary lymphangiectasia include yellow nail syndrome, in which nail dsystrophy is seen, and Hennekam, Turner and Noonan syndromes, in which there are characteristic facial, cardiac or neurological features.

Regardless of underlying cause, the effects of uncompensated intestinal protein loss will be those of hypoalbuminemia, and may therefore mimic nephrotic syndrome. Thus the first sign may be swelling of the legs or dependent areas with peripheral edema, which occurs due to loss of plasma oncotic pressure. In more severe cases, facial and periorbital edema may be seen, and anasarca may develop. Secondary complications include peritonitis or venous thrombosis.

Physical examination may simply show peripheral edema of variable severity, or may elicit signs of the underlying medical condition. Cardiac examination is important to exclude signs of tricuspid regurgitation or constrictive

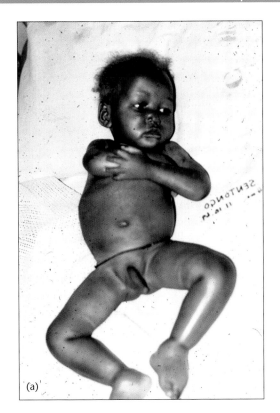

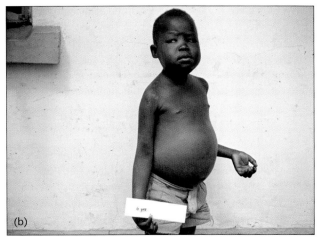

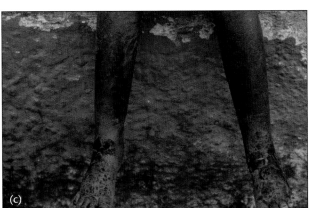

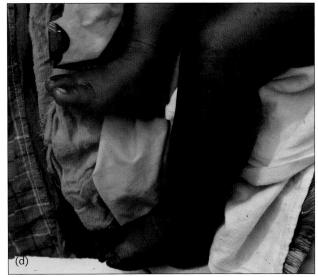

Figure 44.3 Clinical features of kwashiorkor in Ugandan children. (a) Characteristic peripheral edema and ascites in an infant. (b) 6-year-old with ascites and facial edema. (c) Leg ulceration in an adult with kwashiorkor. (d) Gangrene of left leg due to arterial thrombosis in an infant with kwashiorkor. (Photographs courtesy of Dr Jake McKinnon.)

pericarditis. In cases where the PLE is due to structural abnormalities within the lymphatic system (lymphangiectasia), there may be evidence of lymphedema in one or both of the lower limbs.

Differential diagnosis

In infants presenting with severe PLE, an inherited cause is more likely than in older children. Lymphedema of the lower limbs suggests lymphangiectasia, and this diagnosis is supported by findings of lymphopenia. Transferrin glycosylation should be checked to exclude a congenital disorder of glycosylation (CDG). Cystic fibrosis and intestinal malrotation can present as apparently isolated infantile PLE. Enterocyte heparan sulfate deficiency is very rare, but should be considered in cases where there is no evidence of lymphangiectasia and endoscopic biopsies are normal.

Excess protein leak can occur in celiac disease or food-sensitive enteropathy, and mucosal biopsy is an important part of the investigation of the hypoalbuminemic infant without proteinuria. Several rare infantile IBD syndromes may induce widespread ulceration, while older children may have classic IBD. Henoch-Schönlein purpura is an important cause of acute enteric protein loss in childhood, and may sometimes occur without the clasic accompanying skin rash. While Ménétrier's disease is rare in childhood, quite extensive gastric ulceration can occur after viral infections, particularly influenza. *Helicobacter pylori* infection is rarely associated with severe protein loss in childhood.

In adults there is a wide variety of medical conditions that can cause enteric protein loss (see box). Associated lymphopenia suggests localized or diffuse lymphangiectasis, as does macroscopic evidence of focal lymphatic leak at endoscopy. Cardiac disease, autoimmune disorders and malignancy are more common causes of PLE in adults than children.

Investigation

The major differential diagnosis in the initial establishment of a protein-losing enteropathy is protein loss from the renal tract, and thus it is important to perform urinalysis for protein in all cases. The objectives of investigation are to confirm and localize excess enteric protein loss, then identify any potentially treatable underlying cause. In particular, it is important to exclude cardiac abormalities and to consider the possibility of a multisystem disease such as SLE.

The detection of excess α1-antitrypsin in stools provides formal confirmation of excess protein loss, but this may be misleadingly negative in states of profound hypoproteinemia. A formal 24-hour stool collection can be performed to determine α1-antitrypsin clearance, which may provide greater specificity than single-sample testing. Technetium-labelled albumin scintigraphy may demonstrate enhancement within the bowel and may sometimes identify the site of albumin leakage. Ultrasonography may demonstrate less specific features of bowel wall thickening and mesenteric edema, while CT scanning may be helpful to identify focal bowel wall thickening in localized segmental lymphangiectasia. The results of lymphoscintigraphy have been poor in intestinal lymphangiectasia, but it is occasionally helpful in identifying a focal lesion.

The hallmark finding on initial blood investigation is a reduction in serum albumin and globulins. There may be apparent relative preservation of globulins if there is an underlying inflammatory cause. Inflammatory markers should always be checked, and evidence of lymphopenia sought.

As Ménétrier's syndrome is a relatively common cause of intestinal protein loss, endoscopy is an important component of investigation, and should be performed early. This should be combined with colonoscopy to exclude ulcerating colonic lesions. Multiple biopsies should be performed even if appearances are macroscopically normal. Video capsule endoscopy and push enteroscopy have both been used to identify focal (potentially resectable) lymphangiectasia, and should be considered if lymphopenia suggests this diagnosis. Barium follow-through should be considered to exclude malrotation, particularly in younger patients, while computed tomography or abdominal MRI may identify localized resectable lymphangiectatic segments.

In cases of ongoing PLE without clear underlying diagnosis, echocardiography should be performed to exclude disorders such as constrictive pericarditis. Hydrogen breath testing should also be considered, to exclude small bowel bacterial overgrowth.

The spectrum of ancillary investigations may be dictated by the age of the patient and the results of more general assessment. However milder variants of some conditions considered essentially pediatric, notably cystic fibrosis and congenital disorders of glycosylation, are increasingly being recognized in previously undiagnosed adults. By contrast, some conditions thought previously to be found almost exclusively in adults, such as Whipple's disease, amyloidosis and eosinophilic gastroenteropathy are being seen more commonly in childhood.

Treatment and prevention

In cases of secondary PLE, recognition and treatment of the underlying cause is essential. Such treatment may vary from as simple as a gluten-free diet in celiac disease to complex immunosuppressive therapy in IBD or other immunopathologies. Treatment has even included cardiac transplantation in individual cases of intractable PLE of cardiac origin.

Few medications have been shown to be specifically beneficial in protein-losing gastrointestinal states. There have been isolated reports of success with tranexamic acid administration. Heparin therapy, using full molecular weight heparin, can induce significant improvement in some cases, at doses lower than are required for systemic anticoagulation. A very promising development has been identification of a heparin analogue which has similar effects upon intestinal protein leak but without anticoagulant effects [9,10].

Octreotide is sometimes helpful in cases of severe PLE, particularly if associated with secretory diarrhea. Even in the absence of a defined mucosal inflammatory state, some cases do respond to empirical use of corticosteroids, at least in the short term, and the use of these and other immunosuppressants should clearly be considered in cases of intractable or life-threatening PLE.

Prognosis

The prognosis of enteric protein loss depends largely on the underlying condition, and the extent of PLE. In states of very high protein loss, the outcome can be very poor. Thus small bowel transplantation has now been carried out in cases of severe congenital lymphangiectasia. In other primary conditions such as SLE, or following Fontan operation, the development of significant enteric protein loss can be a complication of very adverse significance. In other cases, the loss of protein may be transient and easily dealt with. The current lack of effective therapies for intestinal protein loss contributes to the poor prognosis in many cases.

References

1. Beeken WL, Busch HJ, Sylwester DL. Intestinal protein loss in Crohn's disease. *Gastroenterology.* 1972;62:207–215.

2. Hokari R, Kitagawa N, Watanabe C, *et al.* Changes in regulatory molecules for lymphangiogenesis in intestinal lymphangiectasia with enteric protein loss. *J Gastroenterol Hepatol.* 2008;23: e88–e95.

3. Powers MR, Blumenstock FA, Cooper JA, *et al.* Role of albumin arginyl sites in albumin-induced reduction of endothelial hydraulic conductivity. *J Cell Physiol.* 1989;141:558–564.

4. Comper WD, Laurent TC. Physiological function of connective tissue polysaccharides. *Physiol Rev.* 1978;58:255–315.

5. Murch SH, Winyard PJD, Koletzko S, *et al.* Congenital enterocyte heparan sulfate deficiency is associated with massive albumin loss, secretory diarrhoea and malnutrition. *Lancet.* 1996;347: 1299–1301.

6. Westphal V, Murch S, Kim S, et al. A congenital disorder of glycosylation (CDG-Ic) impairs heparan sulfate proteoglycan accumulation in small intestine epithelial cells and contributes to protein-losing enteropathy. *Am J Pathol.* 2000;157:1917–1925.

7. Bode L, Eklund EA, Murch SH , Freeze HH. Heparan sulfate loss causes protein leakage and amplifies TNFα-response in an *in vitro* model of protein-losing enteropathy. *Am J Physiol Gastrointest Liver Physiol.* 2005;288:G1015–G1023.

8. Bode L, Murch S, Freeze HH. Heparan sulfate plays a central role in a dynamic in vitro model of protein-losing enteropathy. *J Biol Chem.* 2006;281:7809–7815.

9. Bode L, Salvestrini C, Park PW, *et al.* Heparan sulfate and syndecan-1 are essential in maintaining intestinal epithelial barrier function. *J Clin Invest.* 2008;118:229–238.

10. Lencer W. Patching a leaky intestine. *New Engl J Med.* 2008; 359:526–528.

11. Amadi B, Fagbemi AO, Kelly P, *et al.* Reduced production of sulfated glycosaminoglyans occurs in Zambian children with kwashiorkor but not marasmus. *Am J Clin Nutr.* 2009;89: 592–600.

12. Murch SH, MacDonald TT, Walker-Smith JA, *et al.* Disruption of sulphated glycosaminoglycans in intestinal inflammation. *Lancet.* 1993;341:711–714.

13. Heuschkel RB, MacDonald TT, Monteleone G, *et al.* Imbalance of stromelysin-1 and TIMP-1 in the mucosal lesions of children with inflammatory bowel disease. *Gut.* 2000;47:57–62.

14. Pender SLF, Fell JME, Chamow SM, *et al.* A p55 TNF receptor immunoadhesin prevents T cell-mediated intestinal injury by inhibiting matrix metalloproteinase production. *J Immunol.* 1998;160:4098–4103.

Small and Large Bowel

CHAPTER 45
Infective diarrhea

Michael J. G. Farthing[1] and Anna Casburn-Jones[2]

[1]University of Sussex, Brighton, UK
[2]St Mary's Hospital, London, UK

ESSENTIAL FACTS ABOUT CAUSATION

- Diarrhea occurs during intestinal infection as a result of increased secretion or decreased absorption, or a combination of each
- Increased secretion is usually activated by secretory enterotoxins (e.g., cholera, enterotoxigenic *E. coli*) resulting in watery diarrhea
- Decreased absorption occurs because of mucosal injury caused by microbial attachment or invasion, cytolethal cytotoxins and/or induction of chemoattractants
- Enteropathogens that are invasive or elaborate cytotoxins may cause an inflammatory colitis
- Invasive organisms cause systemic complications including hemolytic uremic syndrome (EHEC infections), non-septic arthritis and Reiter's syndrome, Guillain-Barré (*C. jejuni*), septic arthritis (*Salmonella*) and post-infective irritable bowel syndrome

---

ESSENTIALS OF DIAGNOSIS

- The context in which diarrhea occurs, the presence of blood in the stool and other clinical features should enable a restricted range of possibilities to be considered
- Most acute non-bloody diarrhea can be managed supportively without specific diagnosis
- Stool culture and toxin testing, and endoscopy and biopsy are most useful where specific diagnosis is needed

---

ESSENTIALS OF TREATMENT

- Fluid and electrolyte replacement, usually via the oral route with saline and potassium and carbohydrate, is the cornerstone of management
- A minority of patients require intravenous or formal oral rehydration treatment
- Specific antibiotic treatment is valuable in travellers diarrhea (quinolones or rifaximin), dysenteric illnesses, persistent diarrhea and immunosuppressed patients

---

Introduction and definition

Infections of the gastrointestinal tract are the most common intestinal disorders. They have their major impact in the developing world and are still responsible for the deaths of up to two million people each year. The seventh **cholera pandemic** continues to take lives in the Indian subcontinent, Africa, and Latin America. Despite industrialization, wealth, and public health interventions to ensure water quality and sewage disposal, intestinal infections still have a major impact in the Western world, including both food-borne and waterborne infections.

Food-borne disease accounts for about 70% of cases of acute diarrheal disease, which is related to many factors including the widespread contamination of poultry flocks with *Salmonella* and *Campylobacter* species and the use of raw or partially cooked foods such as eggs. However, in the UK there has been a significant decrease in the annual cases of *Salmonella enteritidis* phage type 4, the type commonly associated with food poisoning from chickens, suggesting that tighter controls are working.

Large outbreaks of **waterborne disease** have been reported in Europe and North America, commonly due to the protozoa *Cryptosporidium parvum* and *Giardia intestinalis*. The importance of an infective cause of colitis is now widely recognized following the steady increase in reports of *Campylobacter* infections in the UK (Figure 45.1) and a series of major outbreaks of enterohemorrhagic *Escherichia coli* (EHEC) infection with a reported mortality rate of 1–2% and a relatively high incidence of serious complications such as the hemolytic–uremic syndrome.

The increase in **foreign travel** has further contributed to the importance of infectious colitis in individuals living in the industrialized world as has the increasing use of broad-spectrum antibiotics and associated **antibiotic-related diarrhea** and pseudomembranous colitis due to infection with *Clostridium difficile*. A particularly virulent strain of the organism (NAP-1) has been increasingly isolated in nosocomial diarrhea with a high morbidity and mortality.

In the past 10–15 years development of diagnostic methods has led to **noroviruses** (previously known as Norwalk-like viruses) being recognized as major causes of gastroenteritis in adults and children. In the United States norovirus infection accounts for 90% of outbreaks previously considered iatrogenic for which no agent was previously identified. Other viral

---

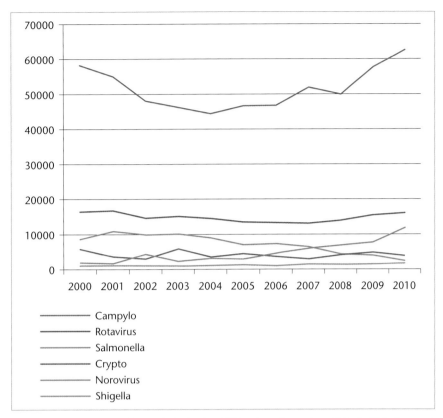

Figure 45.1 Laboratory reporting of gastrointestinal pathogens in England and Wales. Annual reporting of intestinal infective agents by the Health Protection Agency.

causes of diarrhea in children and adults include rotaviruses and adenoviruses.

Diarrhea is usually **defined** as an increase in stool frequency (more than three stools in 24 hours) almost invariably associated with an increase in stool liquidity. Acute infectious diarrhea usually resolves within 5–10 days; persistent diarrhea is defined as diarrhea that has continued for more than 14 days. **Dysentery** is diarrhea associated with blood and accompanied by fever. An increase in bowel frequency also occurs in some functional bowel disorders such as irritable bowel syndrome, although in this case stool weight does not exceed the generally accepted upper limit of 200 g per 24 hours.

Epidemiology

Reservoirs

The major reservoirs of human enteropathogens are **food, water, and other humans**. Certain infective agents are carried by animals that act as a reservoir for human infection; these conditions are known as **zoonoses** (Table 45.1). Almost any of the major bacterial, viral, and protozoal enteropathogens can enter the alimentary tract using food or drink as a vehicle. A recent example was a major outbreak of *Cyclospora cayetanensis* infection following ingestion of contaminated raspberries.

Table 45.1 Zoonotic infections of the alimentary tract

Bacteria	*Salmonella* spp.
	Campylobacter jejuni
	Enterohemorrhagic *E. coli*
	Yersinia enterocolitica
Protozoa	*Giardia intestinalis*
	Cryptosporidium parvum
	Balantidium coli

Domestic water supplies, swimming pools, sea water, and inland freshwater lakes and rivers also harbor enteropathogens; this may occur through contamination by animal and sometimes human feces, and by inadequate disposal of raw sewage. Despite adequate chlorination and acceptable coliform counts, the cysts of *Giardia* and *Cryptosporidium* can survive in municipal water supplies.

Transmission

Intestinal infections are generally transmitted by the **fecal–oral route**. In humans this occurs either through ingestion of contaminated food or fluids or by direct person-to-person

CAUSES AND RISK FACTORS

Microbial pathogens responsible for food-borne diarrheal disease

Organism	Source	Incubation period (h)	Symptoms	Recovery
Gut colonization				
Salmonella spp.	Eggs, poultry	12–48	Diarrhea, blood, pain, vomiting, fever	2–14 days
Campylobacter jejuni	Milk, poultry	48–168	As above	7–21 days
EHEC	Beef	24–168	As above	7–21 days
V. parahaemolyticus	Seafood	2–48	As above (blood less common)	2–30 days
Y. enterocolitica	Milk, pork	2–144	Diarrhea, fever, pain	1–3days
Clostridium perfringens	Spores in food especially meat	8–22	Diarrhea, pain	1–3 days
Pre-formed toxins				
Staphylococcus aureus	Transmitted to food by humans	2–6	Nausea, vomiting, pain (diarrhea)	few hours
Bacillus cereus	Spores in food, reheated rice	1–2	As above	few hours
Clostridium botulinum	Spores in home-bottled or home- canned food	18–36	Transient diarrhea, paralysis	10–14 days

EHEC, enterohemorrhagic *E. coli*.

contact. The latter is particularly important when only small infective doses are required to initiate infection such as in **shigellosis.**

Vibrio cholerae and other noncholera vibrios are transmitted by contaminated water, shellfish, and other seafood, and by person-to-person contact. Direct transmission of *Giardia* is common in day-care centers when young children are in close contact. Intimate sexual contact, notably oroanal sex, is commonly associated with transmission of **enteropathogens**, including bacterial and protozoal enteropathogens. Classic **sexually transmitted diseases** such as gonorrhea, syphilis and chlamydia may be introduced directly into the rectum during anal intercourse resulting in infective proctitis. **Viruses**, such as the norovirus, can be spread by direct person-to-person contact but also by aerosol, probably as a result of vomiting which is an important early symptom of the illness. This probably explains why this infection spreads so rapidly through cruise ships, hotels, and hospital wards [1].

Infective dose

The infective dose is an important determinant of whether clinical infection occurs following ingestion of an enteropathogen. For **V. cholerae** the standard infective dose is high at around 10^9 vibrios, but may fall to 10^3 in individuals with low gastric acidity. For **Shigella** the dose is low at 10^1–10^2 organisms, with a similar number of cysts being required to initiate infection with *Giardia*.

Seasonality

Seasonality is recognized to occur in a number of intestinal infections. In **cholera**, for example, infection is more common in the warmer, wetter months of the year, whereas **rotavirus diarrhea** in the northern hemisphere peaks in the winter months. Enteric adenovirus infections, however, occur at similar frequencies throughout the year.

Causes, risk factors, disease associations
Causes

Infective diarrhea presents as a variety of clinical patterns, recognition of which may assist clinical diagnosis and early management. The three major patterns are:

(1) Acute watery diarrhea.
(2) Bloody diarrhea (dysentery), usually due to an infective colitis.
(3) Persistent diarrhea, sometimes with steatorrhea and evidence of an enteropathy.

However, there is considerable overlap between these clinical patterns with some organisms such as *Shigella* sp. and *Campylobacter jejuni* presenting initially as acute watery diarrhea but then progressing to a dysenteric illness with fever and bloody diarrhea. Similarly, giardiasis may start as acute watery diarrhea but eventually become persistent with features of malabsorption.

Host and environmental risk factors

There are a number of important clinical settings in which the risk of intestinal infection is increased.

Age Individuals at the **extremes of age** are more susceptible to the acquisition of infection and are at greater risk of its consequences. This probably relates to increased exposure in infants and young children, although breastfed infants are

CAUSES AND RISK FACTORS

Causes of infectious diarrhea by clinical pattern

Enteropathogen	Acute watery diarrhea	Dysentery	Persistent diarrhea
Viruses			
Rotavirus	+	–	–
Enteric adenovirus (types 40, 41)	+	–	–
Norovirus	+	–	–
Astrovirus	+	–	–
Cytomegalovirus	+	+	+
Bacteria			
Vibrio cholerae and other vibrios	+	–	–
Enterotoxigenic E. coli (ETEC)	+	–	–
Enteropathogenic E. coli (EPEC)	+	–	+
Enteroaggregative E. coli (EAEC)	+	–	+
Enteroinavsive E. coli (EIEC)	+	+	–
Enterohemorraghic E. coli (EHEC)	+	+	–
Shigella spp.	+	+	+
Salmonella spp.	+	+	+
Campylobacter spp.	+	+	+
Yersinia spp.	+	+	+
Clostridium difficile	+	+	+
Mycobacterium tuberculosis	–	+	+
Protozoa			
Giardia intestinalis	+	–	+
Cryptosporidium parvum	+	–	+
Isospora belli	+	–	+
Cyclospora cayetanensis	+	–	+
Entamoeba histolytica	+	+	+
Balantidium coli	+	+	+
Fungi			
Microsporidia	+	–	+
Helminths			
Schistosoma spp.	–	+	+

Table 45.2 Prevalence of microbial enteropathogens in travelers' diarrhea

Enteropathogens	Reported isolation rates (%)
Bacteria	
ETEC	20–75
EAEC	13–16
Salmonella spp.	0–16
Shigella spp.	0–30
Campylobacter jejuni	1–11
Aeromonas and Plesiomonas spp.	1–57
Vibrio parahaemolyticus	1–16
EIEC	5–7
Protozoa	
Giardia lamblia	0–9
Entamoeba histolytica	0–9
Cryptosporidium parvum	1–10
Cyclospora cayetanensis	?
Viruses	
Rotavirus	0–36
Norovirus	4–15
Multiple pathogens	9–22
No pathogen isolated	15–55

ETEC, enterotoxigenic E. coli; EAEC, enteroaggregative E. coli; EIEC, enteroinvasive E. coli.

protected. Immune defence is suboptimal at both extremes of age.

Travel Gastrointestinal infection affects 30–50% of travelers from Western countries to the developing world and is commonly due to infection of the small intestine with **enterotoxigenic E. coli (ETEC)**, but can also be caused by a variety of other microorganisms (Table 45.2) [2,3]. The impact of travelers' diarrhea is usually viewed solely from the point

of view of the tourist. However, there are important implications for business travelers, the military (as was clearly identified during the first Gulf War), and for tourism-dependent economies of countries in the developing world. (See also Chapter 46.)

Food poisoning Food-borne infection is an important source of intestinal diarrheal disease. Although many episodes of food poisoning are due to true infection of the small intestine, others such as **staphylococcal food poisoning** relate to the ingestion of a preformed toxin.

Disease associations

Immunodeficiency and HIV/AIDS Immunocompromisation has long been recognized as an important risk factor for intestinal infection, but with the advent of **HIV infection** a unique spectrum of opportunistic infectious intestinal disease has become apparent. Many of these infections can be life-threatening when there is a background of profound immune deficiency (Table 45.3). The prevalence of these infections has, however, decreased dramatically in regions of the world that are able to afford highly active antiretroviral therapy. (See also Chapter 114.)

Protozoal infections such as *Giardia* are more common in **congenital forms of immune deficiency**, such as in defective immunoglobulin production. The use of **immunosuppressive drugs** for the treatment of cancer and to prevent organ

Table 45.3 Enteropathogens responsible for HIV-related diarrhea

Protozoa	Cryptosporidia
	Giardia intestinalis
	Isospora belli
	Cyclospora cayetanensis
	Shigella spp.
	Campylobacter spp.
	Clostridium difficile
	Mycobacterium avium complex
Fungi	*Microsporidium* spp.
Viruses	Cytomegalovirus

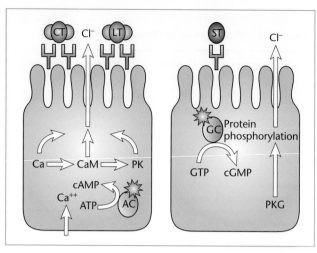

Figure 45.2 Intracellular mechanisms by which bacterial enterotoxins – cholera toxin (CT), *Escherichia coli* heat-labile toxin (LT), and heat stable toxin (ST) – activate adenylate cyclase (AC) and guanylate cyclase (GC), and through a series of second messengers such as calcium–calmodulin (CA, CaM) and protein kinases (PK) promote chloride ion secretion. cAMP, cyclic adenosine monophosphate; cGMP, cyclic guanosine monophosphate; PKG, protein kinase G.

rejection following transplantation renders these individuals at increased risk of intestinal infection. Of particular importance is the helminth *Strongyloides stercoralis*, which under such conditions can produce the hyperinfection syndrome that has a high mortality rate.

Impairment of nonimmune host defence mechanisms Gastric acidity has been recognized to be an important impediment to the acquisition of intestinal infection. **Cholera** and **giardiasis** are particular examples where gastric acid appears to be important in preventing infection. With the development of potent acid-suppressive agents such as the **H2-receptor antagonists** and the **proton pump inhibitors**, it is now clear that these drugs do increase the risk of intestinal infection, particularly in older age groups in which the overall increased risk may approach 10-fold [4].

Pathogenesis

Diarrhea occurs during intestinal infection as a result of two major disturbances of normal intestinal physiology:

Increased intestinal secretion of fluid and electrolytes, predominantly in the small intestine, generally activated by secretory enterotoxins such as cholera toxin, the related heat labile ETEC toxins, acting through adenylate cyclase (Figure 45.2), and heat stable toxins of ETEC (acting through guanylate cyclase), *Yersinia enterocolitica*, *V. cholerae* non-O1 and enteroaggregative *E. coli*. Enterotoxin-related secretory diarrhea may be partly mediated by a variety of endogenous secretagogues and via neuronal pathways [5,6,7].

Decreased absorption of fluid, electrolytes, and sometimes nutrients because of

- Osmotic effects of incompletely absorbed nutrients.
- Impaired fluid, electrolyte, and nutrient absorption in the small or large intestine, occurring as a result of mucosal injury caused by:

– Attachment processes (enteropathogenic *E. coli* and *Cryptosporidium parvum*).
– Enterocyte invasion (rotavirus).
– Inflammatory responses with viruses, parasites such as *Entamoeba histolytica*, and bacteria such as *Shigella* sp. and *Salmonella* sp., often involving cytolethal cytotoxins and/or induction chemoattractants causing an acute inflammatory response.

Such disturbances can involve both the small intestine and the colon and are described in detail in Chapter 6.

Pathology
Small intestine

In the **enterotoxin-mediated diarrheas** there is no gross injury to the intestine. However, there is a spectrum of subtle pathology ranging from the mildest microvillus disruption (*G. intestinalis*, *C. parvum*, and EPEC adherence with pedestal formation) to overt enteropathy. In the latter there can be mild to severe partial villus atrophy (*G. intestinalis*, *C. parvum*, and the intracellular protozoa, *Microsporidium*, *Cyclospora*, and *Isospora*) [8]. Villus atrophy is almost invariably associated with increased numbers of mucosal and intraepithelial lymphocytes. With norovirus infection there is broadening and blunting of the intestinal villi and crypt cell hyperplasia in the proximal jejunum.

The **invasive enteropathogens** such as *Salmonella* and *Yersinia* species commonly produce an ileitis that manifests as a nonspecific inflammatory response in the mucosa and sub-mucosa. *Yersinia* can produce classic aphthoid ulcers in the terminal ileum.

Colon

Invasive colonic enteropathogens such as *Salmonella* spp., *Shigella* spp., *and Campylobacter jejuni* commonly produce a **macroscopic colitis**. In addition to a loss of vascular pattern and erythema there may be discrete ulceration. The histologic appearances of colonic mucosa in the later stages of infection with invasive enteropathogens are often indistinguishable from those of nonspecific inflammatory bowel disease. However, if biopsies are taken within the first 24–72 hours, features that might suggest infectious colitis include:

- Mucosal edema.
- Straightening of the glands.
- An acute inflammatory infiltrate including polymorphonuclear leukocytes, which can sometimes be seen penetrating the epithelium [9].

In *C. difficile* infection (see Chapter 54), there may be the typical appearances of pseudomembranous colitis; histologically there is an acute inflammatory infiltrate combined with the typical "erupting volcano" lesion, which is the histologic counterpart of pseudomembrane. Some organisms can be identified in mucosal biopsies, including:

- The trophozoites of *E. histolytica*
- Ova of *Schistosoma* sp.
- *C. parvum*
- The "owl's eye" inclusion bodies indicative of cytomegalovirus infection.

Clinical presentation

Acute watery diarrhea: viruses

Rotavirus infection, the most common cause of acute diarrhea in infants and young children, is often preceded by a brief prodromal illness with fever and mild respiratory symptoms, followed by vomiting and diarrhea. If fluid and electrolyte losses are not replaced promptly, dehydration and metabolic acidosis soon follow. The degree of dehydration can be assessed clinically by noting skin tone and tissue turgor, intraocular tension, and, in young infants, depression of the anterior fontanelle. In addition, there may be dryness of mucous membranes. As the degree of dehydration increases, there is impairment of consciousness ultimately leading to stupor and coma. Typically the illness lasts about 7 days. **Adenovirus infection** results in a more prolonged illness with pronounced respiratory symptoms. **Norovirus infection** causes watery diarrhea and/or vomiting, often associated with abdominal cramps and constitutional features.

Bacterial causes Acute watery diarrhea in adults is usually bacterial in origin, most commonly due to **ETEC in travelers** or one of the **food-borne pathogens** in the indigenous population of industrialized countries. ETEC usually begins after a short incubation period and on average lasts 3–5 days. Watery diarrhea is often accompanied by anorexia, nausea, vomiting, abdominal cramps, bloating, and low-grade fever. In adults, severe dehydration is uncommon, although this may become clinically important in infants and young children and in the elderly [10].

Mild **cholera** may be indistinguishable from other agents that produce acute watery diarrhea. However, when severe, diarrhea begins abruptly, with stool volume rates of up to 1 L/h. Fecal output is highest in the first 24–48 hours but, provided stool losses are matched by either oral or intravenous fluid and electrolyte replacement, stool volumes decline progressively over a 5-day period. Fever is usually absent, but vomiting is common in the early stages of the illness.

Bloody diarrhea, dysentery, and colitis

The organisms responsible for acute bloody diarrhea are:

- The invasive **bacterial enteropathogens** (*Shigella* spp., *Salmonella* spp., *Campylobacter jejuni*, and EHEC).
- The **protozoan** *E. histolytica*.

There is often a **prodromal illness** of low-grade fever, headache, anorexia, and lassitude. The incubation period is variable, and can range from 1 to 7 days. After an initial period of watery diarrhea, stool volume may actually decrease with the appearance of **blood and mucus** in the stools. Moderate or severe, cramping, lower **abdominal pain** is an important feature of a dysenteric illness, as is **tenesmus** and rectal **prolapse,** particularly in children with shigellosis. There may be fever and mild abdominal distention with some tenderness over the colon. Clinically it is difficult to distinguish acute infectious colitis from nonspecific inflammatory bowel disease. Any form of severe colitis can give rise to abdominal tenderness, **distention**, and in some cases reduced bowel sounds due to ileus.

Proctosigmoidoscopy should form part of the initial clinical assessment and may confirm the presence of colitis. Although some forms of **infective proctitis** do have specific features that might favour a diagnosis of infection (Table 45.4), ulceration in the rectum can occur in infection and in nonspecific inflammatory bowel disease; **pseudomembrane** may be a feature of ischemic colitis as well as *C. difficile* infection. In addition, the endoscopic appearances in the rectum may be normal in many forms of infective colitis that may be limited to the right colon.

Persistent diarrhea

In adults, *G. intestinalis* is the most common cause of persistent diarrhea, often associated with anorexia, abdominal bloating, substantial weight loss, and overt steatorrhea. The other intracellular protozoa are also relatively common causes of

Table 45.4 Endoscopic appearances of the rectum in infective proctitis

Endoscopic appearances	Clinical diagnosis
"Colitis" but may be normal	Salmonellosis Shigellosis Yersiniosis Tuberculosis *Clostridium difficile* infection Amebiasis
Deep ulcers	Amebiasis Tuberculosis Syphilis
Pseudomembrane	*Clostridium difficile* infection
Vesicles	Herpes simplex virus
Beads of pus	Gonorrhea

persistent diarrhea, particularly in the immunocompromised (see Table 45.3). **In children**, EPEC is an important organism to consider. Any cause of persistent diarrhea in infants and young children can result in failure to thrive and growth retardation. *Strongyloides stercoralis* infection may also cause chronic diarrhea and malabsorption, although this is more common in the hyperinfection syndrome. Amebic colitis can persist in a relatively indolent manner without there being overt blood loss.

Differential diagnosis

Acute watery diarrhea

Noninfectious causes of watery diarrhea include:

- Drugs, bile salt malabsorption.
- Neuroendocrine diarrheas, Poma, carcinoid syndrome, medullary carcinoma of the thyroid).
- Laxative abuse and sorbitol ingestion should also be considered.

Bloody diarrhea and colitis

Diarrhea with blood presents a major diagnostic challenge for the clinician because of the importance of distinguishing infection from nonspecific **inflammatory bowel disease** and other inflammatory conditions of the colon. The clinical differentiation of infection from these other conditions is usually not easy, although infective colitis generally has a relatively abrupt onset and cramping lower abdominal pain often emerges as the most disruptive symptom, which is usually not the case in ulcerative colitis.

Physical examination rarely distinguishes between infection and nonspecific inflammatory bowel disease unless there are obvious **perianal stigmata** of Crohn's disease, or other

typical **extraintestinal manifestations** of inflammatory bowel disease such as erythema nodosum, aphthous ulceration, pyoderma gangrenosum, and arthralgia. However, **joint symptoms** may accompany infection due to certain invasive enteropathogens and may form part of a Reiter's syndrome. The presence of physical signs suggestive of **HIV infection** include cutaneous Kaposi sarcoma, choroidoretinitis, hairy leukoplakia, and oral candidiasis.

Persistent diarrhea

There is a long list of conditions that cause persistent diarrhea, including:

- Small bowel disorders such as celiac disease and other enteropathies.
- Bacterial overgrowth.
- Lactose intolerance.
- Inflammatory bowel disease.
- Pancreatic insufficiency in all its many forms will also result in chronic diarrhea and malabsorption.
- Many drugs.
- Neuroendocrine diarrheas.

Occasionally patients may fabricate diarrhea by adding water or urine, so-called factitious diarrhea.

Diagnostic methods

Although the majority of episodes of acute infective diarrhea resolve without the need to identify a specific etiologic agent, persistent diarrhea and bloody diarrhea usually always require further investigation. This is particularly important in severely ill patients when delay in starting appropriate treatment might significantly alter the outcome. Confident exclusion of an infective etiology is rarely achieved in less than 24–48 hours and, although imprecise, clinical assessment is important for guiding management during this early phase of the illness.

Routine laboratory investigations are of limited diagnostic value because anemia, a raised neutrophil count, and evidence of an inflammatory process with a raised erythrocyte sedimentation rate, C-reactive protein, and platelet count occur in infective colitis and nonspecific inflammatory bowel disease. The cornerstone of evidence-based management is microbiological identification of the etiologic agent.

Microbiology

Light microscopic examination of three sequential fecal specimens continues to be important for the identification of all **enteropathogenic protozoa**.

- It is essential to examine fresh specimens if there is a requirement to identify the free-living forms (trophozoites) in giardiasis and amebiasis as these organisms lose their motility at room temperature and rapidly disintegrate.

- Protozoal cysts, oocysts, and sporocysts are more robust and survive storage. *Balantidium coli* is a large motile ciliate and can sometimes be seen with a hand lens.
- Fecal microscopy is also of potential value in identifying the ova of *Schistosoma* spp., and a skilled parasitologist can identify the various subspecies by ova morphology.

Stool culture will usually isolate the classic invasive enteropathogens provided appropriate culture conditions are employed. However, it is unusual for a bacterial enteropathogen to be identified in less than 24–48 hours, and for the slower growing organism such as *Yersinia enterocolitica* and *Campylobacter jejuni* information may not be forthcoming for 3–5 days.

Multiplex genetic assays

Identification of specific toxins is clinically relevant for *C. difficile* toxins A and B and for **Shiga toxin** producing isolates of EHEC.

Blood culture should be performed in ill patients with fever and other systemic symptoms. Invasive organisms that produce an enteric fever-like illness, including *Salmonella* spp., *C. jejuni*, and *Y. entercolitica*, can be detected by this approach.

Serology is of limited value in the diagnosis of intestinal infection. However, in amebic colitis, serology is positive in 80–90% of patients and is an important screening test alongside fecal microscopy if amebiasis is an important diagnostic possibility. Serology can detect *Y. enterocolitica* infection, although results are not usually positive for at least 10–14 days after the onset of the illness, and therefore the results may become available only as the diarrhea resolves.

Enzyme-linked immunosorbent assays are now available for the diagnosis of **strongyloidiasis** and **schistosomiasis**, and should be regarded as first-line screening tests for travelers returning from endemic areas. They are of little value in the indigenous population once an infection has been diagnosed and treated, because antibodies may persist for months or even years after the initial infection.

Endoscopy

If rigid sigmoidoscopy reveals the presence of colitis in the rectum, it is usually unnecessary to pursue this further with a more extensive examination of the colon and distal ileum. A **rectal biopsy** should, however, be taken for histologic examination. If the rectum is normal, it is usually appropriate to examine the proximal colon endoscopically. However, the endoscopic differentiation between acute infectious colitis and other forms of colitis is difficult. Appearances of *Shigella*, *Salmonella*, and *Campylobacter* infections are macroscopically indistinguishable from nonspecific inflammatory bowel dis-

eases. These infections may produce a predominantly right-sided colitis that macroscopically resembles ulcerative colitis.

An experienced endoscopist may be able to identify the typical **amebic ulcers**, which are shallow lesions with undermined edges often covered with a yellow exudate. The intervening mucosa appears normal, and this distinguishes it from ulcerative colitis and other invasive bacterial infections of the colon. However, the diagnosis must be confirmed by microscopic examination of ulcer slough for trophozoites.

The presence of **pseudomembranes** in the colon – appearing as pale, white-yellow excrescences on the epithelium that, when removed, leave an area of spontaneous bleeding separated by areas of normal mucosa – is generally indicative of *C. difficile* infection, although pseudomembrane is not specific for this condition and may occur in ischemia.

Multiple colonic biopsies should always be taken, as in some instances it may be possible to detect the presence of an enteropathogen directly in tissue (*E. histolytica*, *Schistosoma* spp., and **cytomegalovirus**).

Radiology and ultrasonography

A supine **plain abdominal radiograph** can be invaluable in assessing the severity and extent of infectious colitis. A gas-filled colon devoid of feces is consistent with total colitis; loss of haustration and colonic dilatation is indicative of severe inflammation. The examination is also useful for detecting free air in the abdominal cavity, a sign of colonic perforation.

Ultrasonography may reveal bowel wall thickening in invasive ileocolitis and enlarged lymph nodes in yersiniosis and abdominal tuberculosis. The examination may also be invaluable in detecting complications of intestinal infections such as amebic liver abscess.

Treatment and prevention

Fluid and electrolyte replacement via the oral route is usually sufficient except when losses are very severe or there is associated profound vomiting. Dehydration occurs more quickly in infants and young children, and therefore early administration of an oral rehydration solution is advised to prevent dehydration and acidosis [15]. In severe dehydration in infants and young children, intravenous fluids are advisable. Food should be commenced as soon as the individual wishes to eat and drink normally. Breastfeeding should be continued in infants.

In adults formal oral rehydration is usually not required, but it is recommended that they should increase oral fluids such as salty soups (sodium) and fruit juices (potassium), and take carbohydrates (salty crackers, rice, bread, pasta, potatoes), to provide glucose for glucose–sodium co-transport.

Antidiarrheal therapy

Antimotility agents act by increasing intestinal transit time and enhancing the potential for reabsorption of fluid and electrolytes. The most commonly used is loperamide which may have some antisecretory activity. Not all clinical trials have shown it to be superior to placebo. It is probably most effective when combined with an antibiotic [11].

Antimotility agents are not recommended for infants and very young children owing to concerns about respiratory depression or in dysentery because of the risk of colonic dilatation [19]. Antimotility agents have also been thought in the past to increase the fecal carriage of gut enteropathogens, but there is little evidence that this is the case.

Antisecretory agents

There is an ongoing search for the agents that will directly inhibit secretory processes [12]. An important approach has been the development of an enkephalinase inhibitor, **racecadotril**, which has pro-absorptive activity via its ability to potentiate endogenous enkephalins in the intestine [13]. This is an effective agent for reducing stool weight and bowel frequency; it can be used safely in children and does not cause rebound constipation, which can be a problem with antimotility agents [14].

The **thiazolidinone moieties** that inhibit the cystic fibrosis transmembrane regulator (CFTR) protein may also hold promise for the future as the basis for drug development [15]. This protein is integral to the chloride channel on the apical membrane of the intestinal epithelial cell that is an essential component of the secretory process. Further clinical evaluation is required to determine whether this is or will be a valuable addition to the management of secretory diarrhea.

Crofelemer, initially known as SP303, is a naturally occurring proanthocyanidin with chloride channel blocking activity. It has been shown to have antisecretory action mediated through the CFTR. A double-blind randomized controlled trial reduced the duration of travelers' diarrhea (see Chapter 46) by 29% [16]. Further phase 2 and 3 studies are underway and already suggest that this agent will find a place in the treatment regimens for a variety of acute and possibly chronic infective diarrheas.

It is now well established that the **enteric nervous system** (ENS) is involved in the promotion of intestinal secretion. A number of neurotransmitters have been identified in the ENS; many are thought to be involved in intestinal secretion and are therefore potential pharmacologic targets for the treatment of watery diarrhea [17].

Antimicrobial therapy

Antibiotic therapy for infectious diarrhea is controversial. Mild illnesses probably do not need antibiotic treatment, although there are some infections in which **treatment is recommended**: dysenteric shigellosis, cholera, pseudomembranous enterocolitis, and some protozoal infections.

There are several diseases for which the indications are less clear but **treatment is usually recommended**: infection with the noncholera vibrios, prolonged or protracted infection with *Yersinia*, early in the course of campylobacteriosis, *Aeromonas*,

and *Plesiomonas* infections, and outbreaks of EPEC diarrhea in nurseries.

Patients should be treated if they are debilitated, particularly with malignancy, if immunosuppressed, have an abnormal cardiovascular system, have valvular, vascular, or orthopedic prostheses, have hemolytic anemia (especially if salmonellosis is involved), or are extremely young or old. Treatment is also advised for those with prolonged symptoms and those who relapse.

Acute watery diarrhea

Antibiotic therapy is controversial unless the illness is severe or due to cholera. Indiscriminate use of antibiotics may contribute to the emergence of antibiotic resistance and exposes the individual to severe unwanted side effects such as the Stevens-Johnson syndrome or pseudomembranous colitis.

However, in **travelers' diarrhea** (see Chapter 46) antimicrobial therapy is unequivocally effective and is recommended for severe infections or when the individual is unable to tolerate a diarrheal illness because of work or other commitments. **Quinolone antibiotics** are now the treatment of choice; standard doses for 3–5 days can reduce the severity and duration of illness by at least 50% [18], but single dose regimens have similar efficacy [19]. Recently there has been renewed interest in a nonabsorbed locally active antibiotic, **rifaximin**, for the treatment of traveler's diarrhea. This drug has been shown to be as effective as ciprofloxacin but with the potential advantage of only minimal systemic absorption [20].

Dysentery

Antibiotics are recommended for the treatment of dysentery due to most organisms [21]. However, antibiotic therapy for *Campylobacter* and EHEC infection remains controversial. In *Campylobacter* **infection** there is good evidence that antibiotics do not alter the natural course of the illness if they are started more than 4 days after the onset of symptoms.

Antimicrobial therapy in **EHEC infection** remains controversial for two reasons: (1) antibiotics do not significantly improve outcome, especially if started well after infection was established [22]; and (2) there is anecdotal evidence that antibiotics can promote the development of hemolytic–uremic syndrome. Antibiotics are thought to increase the lysis of organisms and the release of shiga-like toxin (verotoxin) and endotoxin.

Persistent diarrhea

Most of the enteropathogens that cause persistent diarrhea are amenable to antimicrobial therapy [21]. *Cryptosporidium parvum* is, however, difficult to treat and is resistant to most antimicrobial agents. Paromomycin has been shown to have some efficacy in one open study [23], but a more recent randomized controlled trial has indicated that this drug is no better than placebo [24]. Recent studies have shown that high-dose albendazole or nitazoxanide may be the most efficacious agents in cryptosporidiosis [25,26].

TREATMENT AND PREVENTION

Antimicrobial therapy for acute infectious diarrhea

Organism	Efficacy of Antimicrobial Therapy	Drug of choice	Alternative choice
Bacteria			
Vibrio cholerae	Proven	Tetracycline 500 mg qds 3 days Ciprofloxacin 1000 mg single dose	TMP-SMX, doxycycline, norfloxacin, ciprofloxacin: 3 days
ETEC	Proven	Ciprofloxacin 500 mg bd 3–5 days Norfloxacin 400 mg bd, 3–5 days	Ciprofloxacin 500 mg single dose
EPEC	Possible		
EIEC	Possible	? same as Shigella spp.	
EHEC	Controversial	See text	

Shigella spp.	Proven efficacy in dysenteric
	    shigellosis
		TMP-SMX 2 tabs bd 5 days[a]
		Ciprofloxacin 500 mg bd 5 days
		Other quinolones –norfloxacin,
		    fleroxacin, cinoxacin
			Short-term quinolone
			Cefixime 400 mg daily
			5–7 days OR
			other third generation
			    cephalosporins
			Nalidixic acid 1 g qds 5–7 days

Salmonella spp.	Doubtful efficacy in enterocolitis Proven efficacy in severe salmonellosis (dysentery, fever)	Ciprofloxacin 500 mg bd 10–14 days 3rd gen cephalosporins 10–14 days Carrier state: Norfloxacin 400 mg bd 28 days	TMP-SMX ampicillin, amoxicillin

Campylobacter spp.	Possible efficacy in campylobacter
	    enteritis
	Proven efficacy in campylobacter
	    dysentery/sepsis
		Ciprofloxacin 500 mg bd 7–14 days	Azithromycin 500 mg od 7–14 days

Yersinia spp.	Doubtful efficacy in Yersinia
	    enteritis
	Proven efficacy in Yersinia
	    septicemia
		Ciprofloxacin 500 mg bd 7–10 days	Tetracycline 250 mg qds 7–10 days

Clostridium difficile	Proven	Metronidazole 400 mg tds 7–10 days	Vancomycin 125 mg qds 7–10 days Rifaximin 400–800 mg bd 14 days
Protozoa			
Cryptosporidium parvum	Possible	Nitazoxanide 500 mg bd 14 days	Paromomycin 25–35 mg/kg 14 days
Isospora belli	Proven	TMP-SMX 2 tabs qds 10 days	Ciprofloxacin, nitazoxanide
Cyclospora cayetanensis	Proven	TMP-SMX 2 tabs bd 7 days	Ciprofloxacin, nitazoxanide
Entamoeba histolytica	Proven	Metronidazole 750 mg tds 5 days Diloxanide furoate 500 mg tds 10 days	Paromomycin 25–35 mg/kg tds 7–10 days

Antimicrobial therapy is not indicated for acute viral diarrhea such as that due to rotavirus, enteric adenoviruses and norovirus.
[a]TMP/SMX (trimethoprim-sulfamethoxazole) is of limited value because of resistance patterns.
(Modified and updated from Casburn-Jones AC, Farthing MJG. Management of infectious diarrhea. *Gut.* 2004;53:296–305, with permission.)

Small and Large Bowel

Microsporidia are also difficult to treat and have variable sensitivity to many agents. Albendazole is effective in treating *Encephalitozoon intestinalis* but not very effective in treating *Enterocytozoon bieneusi*. *C. cayetanensis* infection can be treated effectively with trimethoprim–sulfamethoxazole.

Probiotics

There is increasing evidence that a variety of probiotics, notably *Lactobacillus sp.* and *Bifidobacteria sp* are effective in treating acute infective gastroenteritis in adults and children. In an early multicenter trial *Lactobacillus* GG was shown to reduce the duration of rotavirus episodes but had no effect on bacterial diarrheas [27]. A recent meta-analysis supports the view that probiotics can shorten the duration of acute diarrheal illness in children by 1 day [28]. There is also growing evidence that probiotics can be effective in both the treatment and prevention of *C. difficile* infections [29].

Prevention

Primary prevention of gastrointestinal infection can be achieved by interruption of the fecal–oral transmission route. This involves ensuring the availability of high quality drinking water, adequate sanitation to ensure the safe disposal of feces, and clear guidelines on personal hygiene to minimize person-to-person transmission. In addition, guidelines and legislation are required to ensure the highest standards in animal

TREATMENT AND PREVENTION

Antimicrobial therapy of persistent infectious diarrhea

Enteropathogen	Antimicrobial therapy	Alternatives
Protozoa		
Giardia intestinalis	Metronidazole 400 mg tds 7–10 days	Tinidazole 2 g single dose
Cryptosporidium parvum	Nitazoxanide 500 mg bd 14 days	Paromomycin 25–35 mg/ kg 14 days
Cyclospora cayetanensis	TMP-SMX 2 tabs bd 7 days	Ciprofloxacin, nitazoxanide
Isospora belli	TMP-SMX 2 tabs qds 10 days	Ciprofloxacin, nitazoxanide
Fungi		
Microsporidia	Albendazole 400 mg bd 14–28 days	
Encephalitozoon intestinalis	Fumagillin 60 mg od 14 days	
Enterocytozoon bieneusi		
Helminths		
Strongyloides stercoralis	Albendazole 400 mg od 3 days	Thiabendazole 25 mg/kg bd 2–3 days
Schistosoma spp	Praziquantel 2–3 doses on day 1	Ivermectin 100–200 μg/ kg od 2 days
S. mansoni, S. haematobium	Praziquantel 40 mg/kg/d	
S. japonicum	Praziquantel 60 mg/kg/d	
Virus		
Cytomegalovirus	Ganciclovir 5 mg/kg bd iv 3–6 weeks	Foscarnet 90 mg/kg bd iv 3–6 weeks Maintenance therapy required

Modified from Casburn-Jones AC, Farthing MJG. Management of infectious diarrhea. *Gut.* 2004; 53:296–305, with permission.

husbandry, food production, and subsequent food handling, with regular surveillance procedures to ensure that these standards are maintained. In the UK this is now the responsibility of the Foods Standards Agency.

Chemoprophylaxis

Broad-spectrum antibiotics taken at approximately half the therapeutic dose can prevent certain intestinal infections, particularly **cholera** (tetracycline) and **travelers' diarrhea** (fluoroquinolones). Their use in travelers' diarrhea, however, is not generally recommended because of concerns about adverse effects and emerging drug resistance. The nonantibiotic preparation bismuth subsalicylate is an alternative, but is less effective than antibiotics.

Probiotics

The concept that the gut can be colonized with harmless bacteria that will protect against the harmful effects of enteropathogens has been around for more than a century, since the time of Louis Pasteur. The evidence for their efficacy as a prophylactic remains controversial but some studies have clearly

demonstrated a protective effect against rotavirus infection in children. This is a rapidly developing field and it is likely that genetically modified organisms with improved efficacy will be available in the future.

Immunoprophylaxis

Although parenteral vaccines for cholera and typhoid have been available for many years, their efficacy is low. The major thrust of vaccine development in recent years has focused on oral vaccines to ensure that there is the capacity for a local protective immune response in the gut. A whole cell–B subunit oral **cholera vaccine** has been subjected to extensive field trials and shown to be moderately effective. More recently, a genetically engineered live oral cholera vaccine has been developed which appears to be as effective after a single dose.

These cholera vaccines also have some protective effects against **travelers' diarrhea** caused by other organisms, and the whole cell–B subunit vaccine is currently marketed in some countries for travelers' diarrhea. Although there have been successful attempts to develop vaccines against **rotavirus infection**, particularly a tetravalent rhesus assortant vaccine,

Small and Large Bowel

the program has been seriously curtailed by the occurrence of an important adverse effect, namely intussusception. Vaccines for *Shigella* and *Salmonella* are also under development.

Complications and their management
Dehydration and acidosis
Although the majority of deaths worldwide from intestinal infection are still due to dehydration and acidosis, this aspect of the illness should always be possible to manage by oral or intravenous rehydration. In recent years it has become increasingly clear that death also occurs as a result of the complications of infection, particularly those due to the invasive enteropathogens.

Hemolytic–uremic syndrome
Shigella dysenteriae type 1 infection has been known for several decades to cause hemolytic–uremic syndrome, and it is now well established that this is also responsible for a substantial proportion of the mortality associated with **EHEC infection.** Hemolytic–uremic syndrome, which consists of a triad of features – acute renal failure, thrombocytopenia, and microangiopathic hemolytic anemia – is also described with *Salmonella typhi, Campylobacter jejuni,* and *Yersinia pseudotuberculosis* infections. It occurs in about 6% of patients with EHEC infection and carries a mortality rate of 3–5% [30].

Nonseptic arthritis and Reiter's syndrome
These symptoms are commonly associated with several invasive organisms including *Salmonella* spp., *Shigella* spp., *Y. enterocolitica*, and. More than 70% of patients who develop nonseptic arthritis are **HLA-B27 positive**. Nonseptic arthritis may be associated with iritis and conjunctivitis, which may occur in up to 90% of patients with arthritis following shigellosis and in up to 25% of those with *Salmonella, Campylobacter, Yersinia* infections.

The term **Reiter's syndrome** is reserved for the classic triad of symptoms consisting of arthritis, urethritis, and conjunctivitis. Again, HLA-B27 positivity strongly predicts the likelihood of developing Reiter's syndrome and is indicative of its severity.

Guillain-Barré syndrome
There is now a clear link between *C. jejuni* **infection** and the Guillain-Barré syndrome. If the syndrome follows *Campylobacter* infection, it appears to be predominantly a motor disorder and has a particularly poor outcome with an increased risk of requiring ventilatory support and of having severe disability at 1 year.

Septic arthritis
Purulent synovitis during enteric infection is relatively rare, occurring in 0.2–2.5% of individuals with *Salmonella* infection. Infection is usually monoarticular, involving the large joints.

Symptoms begin within 2 weeks of the gastrointestinal symptoms, but may occur as late as 7 weeks. There is no association with HLA-B27.

Chronic carrier state
Prolonged carriage is well recognized in *Salmonella* infection, particularly in the presence of renal stones or gallstones. Eradication can be achieved in more than 80% of cases by administration of amoxicillin or a quinolone for 4–6 weeks at standard doses.

Hypolactasia
Temporary or persistent depression in brush border enzyme activity is common following infections that affect the small bowel. Clinically the most common consequence is **milk intolerance**, due to hypolactasia.

Irritable bowel syndrome
There is now good evidence that acute intestinal infection can lead on to irritable bowel syndrome (IBS, see Chapter 62) following clearance of the enteropathogen, now known as post-infectious IBS [31]. It has been proposed that this may be related to subclinical "inflammation" and an increase in 5-HT containing enterochromaffin cells. Management is the same as for other causes of irritable bowel syndrome.

Prognosis with and without treatment
Many acute intestinal infections are self-limiting and will resolve without specific treatment. Even infections such as cholera and intestinal amebiasis that benefit from antibiotic therapy will resolve without treatment, provided supportive therapy is given. Antibiotic therapy, however, is vital when there is evidence of bacteremia and systemic complications. Similarly, patients with impaired immunity are also less likely to clear infections naturally and thus it is wise to give antibiotic therapy early in the course of the illness. It is this group that is most likely to succumb to an intestinal infection. Death is also more likely in infants and young children, but is generally avoidable provided that fluid and electrolyte losses are replaced promptly. The hemolytic–uremic syndrome has a significant mortality when associated with *Shigella dysenteriae* and EHEC infection.

What to tell patients
Avoidance
Travelers should be made aware of the risk factors associated with intestinal infection and given advice about an avoidance strategy "Boil it, cook it, peel it, or forget it" [32]. This is clearly described on a number of travel health websites. Immunocompromised patients should be aware of their susceptibility and take avoidance measures at all times, whether or not they are traveling.

Self-therapy

Individuals should be made aware of the importance of early oral rehydration during an attack of acute infectious diarrhea. Some travelers may want advice on the use of an antibiotic should they develop diarrhea during a trip abroad in which they could not afford to be unwell for 2–3 days [33].

The time to seek medical advice

When diarrhea persists for more than 2–3 weeks it is entirely reasonable for a patient to seek medical advice. The same would apply to patients experiencing bloody diarrhea, especially when associated with high fever. Patients with immune deficiency should have a particularly low threshold for seeking self-referral.

Current controversies and their future resolution

- The role of antibiotic therapy in a number of infective diarrheas – more high quality randomized controlled trials are needed.
- The role of probiotics and prebiotics in the prevention and treatment of infective diarrhea – more high-quality clinical trials with established probiotic preparations and the development of new agents with enhanced capacity to colonize the human intestine are necessary.
- The role of antisecretory drugs in the management of watery diarrhea – further clinical trials of established agents and a search for agents that will target novel sites in the enterocyte and the enteric nervous system are required.

SOURCES OF INFORMATION FOR PATIENTS AND DOCTORS

Adults: http://www.patient.co.uk/showdoc/23069066/
Children: http://www.patient.co.uk/showdoc/23069067/

References

1. Lopman B, Vennema H, Kohli E, et al. Increase in viral gastroenteritis outbreaks in Europe and epidemic spread of new norovirus variant. *Lancet*. 2004;363:682–688.
2. Farthing MJG, DuPont HL, Guandalini S, et al. Treatment and prevention of travellers' diarrhea. *Gastroenterol Internat*. 1992;5:162–175.
3. DuPont HL. Systematic review: the epidemiology and clinical features of traveller' diarrhea. *Aliment Pharmacol Ther*. 2009;30:187–196
4. Neal KR, Scott HM, Slack RCB. Omeprazole as a risk factor for *Campylobacter* gastroenteritis: case control study. *BMJ*. 1996;312:414–415.
5. Field M, Fao M, Chang EB. Intestinal electrolyte transport and diarrheal disease. *N Engl J Med*. 1989;321:879–883.
6. Turvill JL, Mourad FH, Farthing MJG. Crucial role for 5-HT in cholera toxin but not *Escherichia coli* heat-labile enterotoxinintestinal secretion in rats. *Gastroenterology*. 1998;115:883–890.
7. Salim AFM, Phillips AD, Walker-Smith JA, et al. Sequential changes in small intestinal structure and function during rotavirus infection in neonatal rats. *Gut*. 1995;36:231–238.
8. Farthing MJG, Kelly MP, Veitch AM. Recently recognised microbial enteropathies and HIV infection. *J Antimicrob Chemother*. 1996;37:61–70.
9. Nostrant TT, Kumar NB, Appelman HD. Histopathology differentiates acute selflimited colitis from ulcerative colitis. *Gastroenterology*. 1987;92:318–328.
10. Farthing MJG. Dehydration and rehydration in children. In: Arnaud MJ, editor. *Hydration throughout life*. Paris: John Libbey Eurotext; 1998. p.159–173.
11. Murphy GS, Bodhidatta L, Echeverria P, et al. Ciprofloxacin and loperamide in the treatment of bacillary dysentery. *Ann Intern Med*. 1993;118:582–586.
12. Farthing MJG, Casburn-Jones A, Banks MR. Getting control of intestinal secretion: thoughts for 2003. *Dig Liv Dis*. 2003;35:378–385.
13. Farthing MJG. Enkephalinase inhibition: a rational approach to anti-secretory therapy for acute diarrhea. *Aliment Pharmacol Ther*. 1999;13(Suppl 6):1–2.
14. Salazar-Lindo E, Santisteban-Ponce J, Chea-Woo E, et al. Racecadotril in the treatment of acute watery diarrhea in children. *N Eng J Med*. 2000;343:463–467.
15. Ma T, Thiagarajah JR, Yang H, et al. Thiazilinone CFTR inhibitor identified by high throughput screening blocks cholera toxin-induced intestinal fluid secretion. *J Clin Invest*. 2002;110:1651–1658.
16. DiCesare D, DuPont HL, Mathewson JJ, et al. A double-blind, randomized, placebocontrolled study of SP 303 (Provir) in the symptomatic treatment of acute diarrhea among travelers to Jamaica and Mexico. *Am J Gastroenterol*. 2002;97:2585–2588.
17. Farthing MJ. Novel targets for the control of secretory diarrhea. *Gut*. 2002;50(Suppl 3):iii15–iii18.
18. Mattila L, Peltola H, Siitonen A, et al. Short-term treatment of traveler's diarrhea with norfloxacin: a double-blind, placebo controlled study during two sessions. *Clin Infect Dis*. 1993;17:779–782.
19. Salam I, Katelaris P, Leigh-Smith S, et al. A randomised placebo-controlled trial of single dose ciprofloxacin in treatment of travellers' diarrhea. *Lancet*. 1994;344:1537–1539.
20. DuPont HL, Jiang Z-D, Ericsson CD, et al. Rifaximin versus ciprofloxacin for the treatment of traveler's diarrhea: a randomised, double-blind clinical trial. *Clin Infect Dis*. 2001;33:1807–1815.
21. Casburn-Jones AC, Farthing MJG. Management of infectious diarrhea. *Gut*. 2004;53:296–305.
22. Prouix F, Turgeon JPJ, Delage G, et al. Randomized, controlled trial of antibiotic therapy for *Escherichia coli* O157-H7 enteritis. *J Pediatr*. 1992;121:299–303.
23. Bissuel F, Cotte L, Rabodonirina M, et al. Paromomycin: an effective treatment for cryptosporidial diarrhea in patients with AIDS. *Clin Infect Dis*. 1994;18:447–449.
24. Hewitt RG, Tiannoutsos CT, Higgs ES et al. Paromomycin: no more effective than placebo for treatment of cryptosporidiosis in patients with advanced immunodeficiency virus infection. AIDS Clinical Trial Group. *Clin Infect Dis*. 2000;31:1084–1092.
25. Bailey JM, Erramouspe J. Nitazoxanide treatment for giardiasis and cryptosporidiosis in children. *Ann Pharmacother*. 2004;38:634–640.

26. Farthing MJG. Clinical aspects of human cryptosporidiosis. *Contrib Microbiol*. 2000;6:50–74.

27. Guandalini S, Kirjavainen PV, Zikri MA, *et al*. *Lactobacillus* GG administered in oral rehydration solution to children with acute diarrhea: a multicenter European trial. *J Pediatr Gastroenterol Nutr*. 2000;30:54–60.

28. Huang JS, Bousvaros A, Lee JW, *et al*. Efficacy of probiotic use in acute diarrhea in children: a meta-analysis. *Dig Dis Sci*. 2002;47:2625–2634.

29. Leffler DA, LaMont JT. Treatment of *Clostridium difficile*-associated disease *Gastroenterology*. 2009;136:1899–1912.

30. Boyce TG, Swerdlow DL, Griffin PM. *Escherichia coli* O157:H7 and the hemolytic–uremic syndrome. *N Engl J Med*. 1995;333:364–368.

31. Spiller RC, Garsed K. Postinfectious irritable bowel syndrome. *Gastroenterology*. 2009;136:1979–1988.

32. Kozicki M, Steffen R, Schar M. "Boil it, cook it, peel it, or forget it": does this rule prevent travelers' diarrhea? *Int J Epidemiol*. 1985;14:169–172.

33. Casburn-Jones AC, Farthing MJ. Traveler's diarrhea. *J Gastroenterol Hepatol*. 2004;19:610–618.

Small and Large Bowel

CHAPTER 46

Travelers' diarrhea

Andrew W. DuPont[1] and Herbert L. DuPont

[1]The University of Texas Health Science Center at Houston, Houston, TX, USA
[2]The University of Texas-Houston School of Public Health, Houston, TX, USA

ESSENTIALS FACTS ABOUT PATHOGENESIS

- Traveler's diarrhea is a food-borne infective illness occurring in travelers, particularly those who live close to the local population
- Enterotoxigenic *Escherichia coli* is the commonest pathogen, followed by enteroaggregative and enteroinvasive *E. coli*

ESSENTIALS OF DIAGNOSIS

- More than 80% of travelers with diarrhea have uncomplicated traveler's diarrhea
- Fever or bloody stools suggest a dysenteric illness
- Most traveler's diarrhea can be managed presumptively without recourse to investigation

---

ESSENTIALS OF TREATMENT AND PREVENTION

- Bismuth subsalicylate (antisecretory) and loperamide (antimotility) reduce the number of stools, but loperamide may cause abdominal pain
- Specific treatment is with a fluoroquinolone, azithromycin or rifaximin A single dose is effective in most cases
- Irritable bowel syndrome is a common consequence of traveler's diarrhea that may require more prolonged treatment (see Chapter 62)
- Because of the risk of selection for drug resistance, careful hygiene ± bismuth subsalicylate is preferred to antibiotics for prophylaxis
- Vaccines against enterotoxigenic *E. coli* are under development

---

Introduction

Traveler's diarrhea is typically defined as a clinically important illness with at least three unformed stools over a 24-hour period and one or more additional signs or symptoms of enteric infection, such as abdominal discomfort and cramps, nausea, and vomiting, in a person traveling from an industrialized region to a less hygienic tropical or semi-tropical region.

Epidemiology

Annually more than 600 million people travel outside their country, with more than 100 million visiting tropical and subtropical regions hyperendemic for diarrhea. The world can be divided broadly into three levels of diarrhea risk to the international traveler [1]. The **low-risk areas** include northern Europe, the United States, Canada, Japan, Australia, and New Zealand, with diarrhea occurring in 2–4% of those visiting these regions. Those traveling from the low-risk areas to the **high-risk regions** of Latin America, South Asia (Indian subcontinent), and much of Africa have an approximately 40% chance of developing illness. Countries of the northern Mediterranean, the Caribbean, Russia, China, and South-East Asia (e.g., Thailand) comprise a third category of **intermediate risk** where travelers experience rates of illness varying from 10% to 20%.

Protective immunity develops within months of living in endemic areas, presumably through repeated exposure to enteric pathogens found in food, with the most striking immunity developing against the major cause of illness in many settings – enterotoxigenic *Escherichia coli* (ETEC). The finding of short-term immunity in international travelers has given hope for control of disease through immunoprophylactic approaches.

Causes, risk factors, and disease associations

Illness rates are increased in adventure travelers, missionaries, Peace Corps volunteers, and others working or living close to the local population and staying in inexpensive hotels or camps. The **age of the traveler** influences the rate of acquisition of diarrhea with two peaks of increased rate: travelers aged 0–2 years and those younger than 30 years of age (see Chapters 6 and 45). It has been well established that **food** is the major source of enteric infection among international travelers [2]. There is clearly an association with illness rates and the location of food consumption, with lowest rates when food is self-prepared in apartments and higher rates when it is eaten in the homes of local people or in public restaurants.

Foods and beverages can be categorized as **high or low risk** based on several principles. Contamination of food and beverages may be diminished or eliminated by heating to at least 59°C (food that is steaming hot). Recontamination becomes a

---

Textbook of Clinical Gastroenterology and Hepatology, Second Edition. Edited by C. J. Hawkey, Jaime Bosch, Joel E. Richter, Guadalupe Garcia-Tsao, Francis K. L. Chan.
© 2012 Blackwell Publishing Ltd. Published 2012 by Blackwell Publishing Ltd.

problem when food is cooked too early before consumption, as is commonly the case for hamburgers obtained from non-fast food chains. **Other generally safe foods** include those that are dry (bread), those that have been peeled (fruit), and those with a high sugar content (jellies, honey, and syrup) or low pH if refrigerated between use.

Host factors

Some international travelers are able to remain well during periods of risk, whereas others with a similar travel experience and risk factors may be affected repeatedly.

Genetic factors

These appear to explain a proportion of illness susceptibility variation among travelers to high-risk areas. Possession of certain **blood groups** predisposes persons to **norovirus** gastro-enteritis or to **cholera**, which constitutes an unexplained genetic association with enteric infectious diseases. The occurrence of diarrhea due to the **two major pathogens** in this setting, ETEC and enteroaggregative *E. coli* (EAEC), appears to also show **genetic associations**. It is likely in humans that **ETEC receptors** are present or absent on a genetic basis, explaining relative susceptibility to this pathogen. In EAEC diarrhea, the major mediator of the inflammatory diarrhea appears to be release of **intestinal interleukin-8 (IL-8)**. It has been shown that among US travelers to Mexico, where EAEC diarrhea commonly occurs, susceptibility to this form of diarrhea is determined by **genetic polymorphism** in the **promoter region of the *IL-8* gene** [3].

Gastric acid

For more than a century investigators have supported the idea that decreased gastric acidity predisposes to enteric infection by bacterial pathogens, although the association remains largely unstudied for travelers. It appears intuitive that travelers with hypochlorhydria or achlorhydria would be at increased risk for diarrhea when traveling to the tropics, although the association may not be as strong as once thought.

Pathogenesis and pathology

The major causes of diarrhea among international travelers to high-risk tropical and subtropical areas are a variety of bacterial pathogens (approximately 80% of cases) (Table 46.1). The **diarrheagenic *E. coli*** (ETEC, EAEC, and enteroinvasive *E. coli*) explain over **50% of illness** in most areas [4]. ETEC strains contain up to **three important virulence characteristics**, including an attachment ligand called colonization factor antigens as well as two toxins – cholera-like heat-labile toxin (LT) and a low molecular weight and inflammatory heat-stable toxin (ST). All ETEC strains produce one of the following: LT only; ST only; and ST plus LT (see Chapter 45).

Other important bacterial agents include *Shigella*, *Salmonella*, *Campylobacter*, *Aeromonas*, and *Plesiomonas* species. Parasitic pathogens explain fewer than 5% of cases and viruses

Table 46.1 Geographic considerations in the microbial etiology of travelers' diarrhea

Geographic area	Characteristic etiology
All regions of the tropical and semi-tropical developing world	Bacterial enteropathogens, especially ETEC and EAEC
Thailand	Ciprofloxacin-resistant *Campylobacter*
Russia (St Petersburg)	*Giardia* and *Cryptosporidium*
Nepal (springtime, early summer)	Cyclospora

EAEC, enteroaggregative *E. coli*; ETEC, enterotoxigenic *E. coli*.

(particularly noroviruses) about 10%. ***Cyclospora*** has been shown to be an important cause of spring or early summertime diarrhea in travelers to Nepal, and *Giardia* and *Cyclospora* have been commonly identified in travelers to Russia, particularly St Petersburg. In Thailand, ciprofloxacin-resistant ***Campylobacter*** may cause diarrhea in international visitors [5]. Resistant *Campylobacter* is an important cause of diarrhea with worldwide occurrence, and should be considered as the major cause of fluoroquinolone-unresponsive travelers' diarrhea regardless of region.

Clinical presentation

More than 80% of travelers with diarrhea will experience **watery diarrhea without significant fever** that, left untreated, typically consists of passage of 13 unformed stools over a 5-day interval. Those affected characteristically experience **abdominal cramps** and pain that is temporarily debilitating (see also Chapters 6 and 45).

In fewer than 10% of travelers with diarrhea, **febrile dysentery** (bloody stools) may occur and is most often due to strains of *Shigella*, *Campylobacter*, *Salmonella*, non-cholera vibrios, and *Aeromonas*. In approximately 10% of cases, **vomiting** is the predominant symptom, likely due to infection with viruses (mostly noroviruses) or ingestion of the preformed toxin of *Staphylococcus* or *Bacillus cereus*.

Travelers' diarrhea regularly forces a change in itinerary, confining 20–46% to bed for 1 day or more. Between 4% and 17% will seek care from a local physician and nearly 0.2% require local hospitalization. In 10% of patients, diarrhea lasts for more than a week, and in 2–10% it persists for more than 1 month [6].

In an important subset of those with travelers' diarrhea, a chronic illness develops that is compatible with **post-infectious irritable bowel syndrome** [7], and in a small number **inflammatory bowel disease** may be precipitated or unmasked. Other potential causes of protracted illness include **disaccharidase deficiency** and **small bowel overgrowth**, as well as **Brainerd diarrhea**, a chronic diarrheal illness of unknown etiology that may last for years and can often be traced to the consumption of raw (unpasteurized) milk or untreated surface water.

Differential diagnosis

In most cases of travelers' diarrhea a bacterial pathogen should be suspected. When vomiting is the primary symptom of the illness, viral gastroenteritis or food-borne intoxication is the most likely explanation of illness. For those with persistent illness, parasitic agents and post-infectious irritable bowel syndrome should be considered as possible causes of illness.

Diagnostic methods

Most traveler's diarrhea can be managed presumptively without recourse to investigations. Laboratory testing should be done for a limited number of indications, including persistent diarrhea (see Chapter 45), fluoroquinolone-resistant illness, or when the traveler has a serious underlying medical condition, such as acquired immune deficiency syndrome (AIDS). In cases of prolonged symptoms in which stool studies have been unrevealing (e.g., negative tests for parasites including *Giardia* and *Cryptosporidium* antigens) and a dietary association has not been found (e.g., lactose intolerance), endoscopic and/or radiographic studies may be indicated. **Endoscopic evaluation** of the small bowel with aspiration or biopsy can help to diagnose parasitic infections; proctosigmoidoscopy or colonoscopy can be used to evaluate for persistent colonic infection and to rule out inflammatory bowel disease in the appropriate setting.

Treatment and prevention

Symptomatic treatment will help to control the passage of unformed stools and allow travelers to function when they develop illness. **Bismuth subsalicylate** works through its salicylate-mediated antisecretory properties and will decrease the number of stools passed by 40%. The antimotility drug **loperamide** is more effective, reducing the number of stools passed by 60%, but it may produce objectionable post-treatment constipation or abdominal pain. Novel antisecretory drugs may safely offer more physiological relief of symptoms and may in the future become standard treatment for the symptoms of travelers' diarrhea.

Antibacterial drugs represent the mainstay of therapy for traveler's diarrhea (Table 46.2). A single dose is effective in treating most cases [8] and will shorten illness by 1–2 days [9].

Choice of drug

When **trimethoprim** resistance became widespread, the **fluoroquinolones** became standard therapy. **Azithromycin** is as effective as the fluoroquinolones in shortening the duration of diarrhea after the initiation of therapy and has the advantages of being effective against ciprofloxacin-resistant *Campylobacter*; it can be given safely to children and, potentially,

Table 46.2 Antibacterial therapy of acute travelers' diarrhea*

Antibacterial agent	Dose and duration	Comments
Ciprofloxacin	750 mg once; can repeat next morning if not well and repeat again on third day if needed	Not to be used in pregnant women or children *Campylobacter* resistance is a growing problem *Clostridium difficile* colitis is a rare complication
Levofloxacin	500 mg once; can repeat next morning if not well and repeat again on third day if needed	**Not** to be used in pregnant women or children *Campylobacter* resistance is a growing problem *Clostridium difficile* colitis is a rare complication
Azithromycin	1000 mg once	Safe in all patients and can be used in children and pregnant women
Rifaximin	200 mg t.i.d. or 400 mg b.i.d. for 3 days	Safe in all patients and can be used in children

*All drugs shorten illness by more than 1 day compared with placebo.

pregnant women with illness. These absorbable drugs, including fluoroquinolones and azithromycin, are effective in treating most cases of travelers' diarrhea with a single dose [8]. Where available, **rifaximin may be the drug of choice** for nonfebrile, non-dysenteric illness. Rifaximin is as effective as ciprofloxacin in treating afebrile, non-dysenteric travelers' diarrhea [10].

Prevention

The key to **prevention** of travelers' diarrhea is careful **food and beverage selection**. This approach, while potentially successful, is often not followed. Drugs can be used to prevent the illness. **Bismuth subsalicylate** will prevent 65% of the disease that would occur without daily use. A **fluoroquinolone** is more effective, preventing approximately 80% of the disease that would otherwise occur. Use of prophylaxis with systemically absorbed antimicrobials is currently **not recommended** for all travelers in view of potential side effects of the drugs and concern about the development of general resistance. The **poorly absorbed drug rifaximin** has been shown to be efficacious in the prevention of diarrhea among travelers to Mexico with minimal effect on normal fecal flora, and can be recommended in a subset of travelers [11]. Vaccines are under development against ETEC, the principal cause of travelers' diarrhea [12].

Complications and prognosis

Travelers' diarrhea is a non-fatal condition. Although the diarrhea may be severe, the major concern other than short-term disability is the production of post-infectious chronic illness, most importantly post-infectious irritable bowel syndrome. These patients should be worked up and treated.

Future considerations

Rates of diarrhea during international travel have not changed since studies were initiated 50 years ago. Local governments should be encouraged to work with restaurants, hotels, and tour operators to improve the hygiene for international travelers [13]. If this is not possible, the restaurants and hotels should work independently to create safe havens where persons can remain disease-free while in the area of risk. Preventive medications and vaccines are likely to have important future roles in reducing rates of illness among international travelers.

SOURCES OF INFORMATION FOR PATIENTS AND DOCTORS

http://www.traveldoctor.co.uk/diarrhoea.htm
http://www.masta-travel-health.com/
http://www.who.int/ith/en/
http://wwwn.cdc.gov/travel/

References

1. DuPont HL. Systematic review: the epidemiology and clinical features of travellers' diarrhoea. *Aliment Pharmacol Ther.* 2009;30:187–196
2. Adachi JA, Mathewson JJ, Jiang Z-D, *et al.* Enteric pathogens in Mexican sauces of popular restaurants in Guadalajara, Mexico and in Houston, Texas. *Ann Intern Med.* 2002;136:884–887.
3. Jiang ZD, Okhuysen PC, Guo DC, *et al.* Genetic susceptibility to enteroaggregative *Escherichia coli* diarrhea – polymorphism in interleukin-8 promoter region. *J Infect Dis.* 2003;188:506–511.
4. Shah N, DuPont HL, Ramsey DJ. Global etiology of travelers' diarrhea: Systematic review from 1973 to the present. *Am J Trop Med Hyg.* 2009;80:609–614.
5. Tribble DR, Sanders JW, Pang LW, *et al.* Traveler's diarrhea in Thailand: randomized, double-blind trial comparing single-dose and 3-day azithromycin-based regimens with 3-day levofloxacin regimen. *Clin Infect Dis.* 2007;44:338–346.
6. DuPont HL, Capsuto EG. Persistent diarrhea in travelers. *Clin Infect Dis.* 1996;22:124–128.
7. Okhuysen PC, Jiang Z-D, Carlin L, *et al.* Post-diarrhea chronic intestinal symptoms and irritable bowel syndrome in North American travelers to Mexico. *Am J Gastroenterol.* 2004;99:1774–1778.
8. Salam I, Katelaris P, Leigh-Smith S, Farthing MJG. Randomized trial of single-dose ciprofloxacin for travelers' diarrhea. *Lancet.* 1994;344:1537–1539.
9. DuPont HL, Ziang ZD, Belkind-Gerson J, *et al.* Treatment of travelers' diarrhea: randomized trial comparing rifaximin, rifaximin plus loperamide, and loperamide alone. *Clin Gastroenterol Hepatol.* 2007;5:451–456.
10. Taylor DN, Bourgeois AL, Ericsson CD, *et al.* A randomized, double-blind, multicenter study of rifaximin compared with placebo and with ciprofloxacin in the treatment of travelers' diarrhea. *Am J Trop Med Hyg.* 2006;74:1060–1066.
11. DuPont HL, Jiang Z-D, Okhuysen PC, *et al.* A randomized, double-blind, placebo-controlled trial of rifaximin to prevent travelers' diarrhea. *Ann Intern Med.* 2005;142:805–812.
12. Frech SA, DuPont HL, Bourgeois AL, *et al.* Use of a patch containing heat-labile toxin from *Escherichia coli*: against travellers' diarrhoea: a phase II, randomized, double-blind, placebo-controlled field trial. *Lancet.* 2008;371:2019–2025.
13. Ashley DV, Walters C, Dockery-Brown C, *et al.* Interventions to prevent and control food-borne diseases associated with a reduction in traveler's diarrhea in tourists to Jamaica. *J Travel Med* 2004;11:364–367.

Small and Large Bowel

CHAPTER 47
Abdominal tuberculosis

Bhupinder Anand

Baylor College of Medicine; Michael E. DeBakey VA Medical Center, Houston, TX, USA

ESSENTIAL FACTS ABOUT PATHOGENESIS

- Abdominal tuberculosis is due to *Mycobacterium tuberculosis* infection
- Infection is from swallowed sputum, lymphatic and blood spread, and by local extension
- Incidences are increasing, in part because of HIV, in developing countries but now falling in the USA
- Ileo-cecal involvement is commonest

ESSENTIALS OF DIAGNOSIS

- Low grade/spiking fever malaise, anorexia and weight loss
- Most patients get abdominal pain, most commonly right iliac fossa with subacute obstruction
- Differential diagnosis includes Crohn's disease
- Plain and barium radiology may show obstruction and ileo-cecal contraction/scarring
- Endoscopy, biopsy, acid fast bacilli staining, culture and PCR (for rapid 48-hour diagnosis) are usually needed.
- Ultrasound and CT may be of value
- The interferon gamma release assay is cheaper and more specific than tuberculin skin testing in diagnosing TB
- Tubercular ascites characterized by high protein, lymphocytic response and raised adenosine deaminase

---

ESSENTIALS OF TREATMENT

- Quadruple therapy (rifampin, isoniazid, pyrazinamide, and ethambutol) for 2 months followed by rifampin and isoniazid for 4 more months

---

Introduction

The term abdominal tuberculosis encompasses disease of the gastrointestinal tract, peritoneum, lymph nodes, and intra-abdominal organs such as liver and spleen (Table 47.1). The majority of patients have associated pulmonary tuberculosis. The infection spreads to the abdomen more frequently in cavitory lung disease compared to predominantly fibrotic lesions. The risk of acquiring tuberculosis is increased greatly in the presence of HIV infection.

Epidemiology

Nearly one-third of the world's population (2 billion people), are infected with the organism *Mycobacterium tuberculosis*. In 2007, a total of 9.3 million new TB cases were diagnosed worldwide; roughly 15% (1.4 million) occurred in people with HIV. Most of the newly diagnosed cases as well as the deaths (1.8 million a year) occurred in developing countries. In the US, after the resurgence of tuberculosis in the 1980s due to the **AIDS epidemic**, new infections have declined to 4.2 cases per 100000, the lowest level in 50 years [1].

Pathogenesis

Infection with **M. tuberculosis** is responsible for nearly all cases of abdominal tuberculosis; other mycobacterium (see below) are encountered infrequently. From the point of entry (usually the lungs), the tubercle bacillus reaches the gastrointestinal tract by several routes: swallowed sputum, lymphatic spread, bloodstream and from the adjacent tissues and pelvic organs. In immunocompetent individuals, the influx of specific lymphocytes and monocytes localizes the infection to a specific area. If the immune response is inadequate, the infection can spread locally, and systemically by lympho-hematogenous dissemination.

Pathology
Intestinal tuberculosis

The **sites of involvement** in order of decreasing frequency are: ileo-cecum, colon, jejunum, rectum and anal canal, duodenum, stomach, and esophagus. Three pathological forms are described; these are not mutually exclusive and can be seen in the same patient (Table 47.1).

Ulcerative variety

Mucosal ulcers are seen which may be localized to one area or may involve a variable length of the bowel, with normal intervening mucosa [2]. The ulcers are located **transversely**; when the entire circumference is involved, the diseased bowel develops in a "napkin-ring-like" contraction. The ulcers are

---

Textbook of Clinical Gastroenterology and Hepatology, Second Edition. Edited by C. J. Hawkey, Jaime Bosch, Joel E. Richter, Guadalupe Garcia-Tsao, Francis K. L. Chan.
© 2012 Blackwell Publishing Ltd. Published 2012 by Blackwell Publishing Ltd.

Table 47.1 Classification of abdominal tuberculosis

Gastrointestinal
- Ulcerative (presence of ulcers, which may be single, multiple or diffuse)
- Hypertrophic (mass lesion)
- Fibrotic (stricture formation)

Peritoneal
- Ascites (localized, generalized)
- Fibrotic or dry form (peritoneal adhesions, rolled up omentum)
- Mixed form

Nodal
- Mesenteric adenitis
- Mesenteric abscess

Visceral disease
- Liver, spleen, urinary tract, genital organs

Table 47.2 Characteristic symptoms and signs of abdominal tuberculosis

Symptoms
- Systemic: fever, night sweats, weight loss, menstrual abnormalities
- Abdominal:
  Pain: right iliac fossa, diffuse
  Change in bowel habit
  Subacute intestinal obstruction: episodic colicky pain, distention, borborygmi
  Malabsorption: diarrhea, bulky stools
- Organ-specific:
  Esophagus: dysphagia
  Stomach and duodenum: ulcer-like pain, gastric outlet obstruction
  Colon: ulcerative colitis-like picture – diarrhea with blood and mucus

Signs
- General: sick appearing, febrile, emaciated patient
- Peripheral lymphadenopathy
  Cervical, inguinal, axillary
  Nodes are often fused ("matted"), fixed to tissues, sinus tracks
- Abdomen:
  Distention
  - localized (mass, loculated ascites)
  - generalized (intestinal obstruction, ascites)
  Intestinal obstruction: visible peristalsis, borborygmi
  Mass lesions: ileocecal mass, rolled up omentum, hepatosplenomegaly, nodal mass
  Doughy feel: diffuse peritoneal involvement
  Fistulae: cutaneous, perianal, internal

Small and Large Bowel

generally superficial and do not penetrate the muscularis mucosa. The corresponding mesenteric surface shows increase in fat content and enlarged lymph nodes. Histology reveals granulation tissue, with neutrophils and microabscesses. The characteristic **tuberculous granulomas**, comprising of lymphocytes, plasma cells and Langhans giant cells are seen in the ulcer bed. Rarely, colonic tuberculosis may present as a diffuse disease, resembling ulcerative colitis.

Hyperplastic lesion

There is marked thickening of the bowel wall, measuring up to 3 cm in width. The mucosal surface may develop a **cobble-stone pattern**. The bowel assumes a tubular form with narrowing of the lumen. The hypertrophic variety is typically seen in the **ileo-cecal region**. The intestinal lesion together with the enlarged lymph nodes may present as an abdominal mass. Histology shows exuberant granulomatous tissue extending from the mucosa to the serosa, accompanied with hypertrophy of the muscularis layer.

Sclerotic form

This abnormality is characterized by areas of marked narrowing of the bowel. Patients may develop a single stricture or multiple strictures. The **proximal bowel is dilated** and enteroliths are noted at the stricture site. Histology shows diffuse fibrosis extending from the submucosa to the serosa. Granulation tissue is limited to the bowel segment adjacent to the strictured areas.

Peritoneal tuberculosis

The classic appearance is of **grayish white "miliary" nodules** scattered over the peritoneum. In addition, fibrous bands or adhesions are common. The adhesions are mostly thin, but when thick and dense they divide the peritoneal cavity into compartments, with the formation of loculated ascites. In some cases, the fibrotic response is so exuberant that the peritoneal cavity is completely obliterated, encasing the intestines like a cocoon. The **omentum** may become thickened, presenting as a transversely placed mass ("rolled-up" omentum). Histology of the miliary nodules usually shows caseating necrosis and tuberculous granulomas. Clinically, the most frequent presentation of peritoneal disease is with **ascites.**

Nodal tuberculosis

Isolated involvement of mesenteric nodes is uncommon. Enlarged lymph nodes may cause extrinsic compression and narrowing of the bowel lumen. Inflamed nodes can produce **traction diverticula**, seen mostly in the esophagus and colon.

Clinical presentation

The peak age at presentation is between 30 and 50 years. There is no gender difference in the West but women outnumber men 2:1 in developing countries. Although most patients have an **indolent illness,** between 10% and 30% patients experience an **acute presentation**, with an average duration of symptoms of **1–2 weeks**. The acute illness, which may arise as a primary disease or as reactivation of latent infection, manifests with features of **peritonitis, bowel obstruction and perforation** (see Table 47.2).

Systemic symptoms

Patients commonly present with **fever, malaise, anorexia and weight loss**. Fever is usually low grade, with an evening spike. Sweating can be profuse, often drenching clothes and bed sheets. Patients with lung disease develop productive cough. Menstrual abnormalities including amenorrhea are seen in 20% patients. Women may become sterile because of pelvic disease.

Abdominal symptoms

Most patients present with **abdominal pain**. The pain is localized to the site of the disease, usually the right iliac fossa but can be diffuse and nonspecific. Typically, patients experience episodes of subacute **intestinal obstruction** with colicky pain, distention, and borborygmi, relieved to some extent by vomiting. The bowel habit is erratic, with episodes of diarrhea and constipation. Additional symptoms are related to involvement of a specific site: **dysphagia** with esophageal disease, **ulcer-like pain** and gastric **outlet obstruction** in duodenal involvement, and **diarrhea** with blood in diffuse colonic disease.

Physical examination

Patients appear **sick and emaciated**. A low grade temperature is noted. Peripheral **lymphadenopathy** should be carefully sought as it provides an easy source of diagnosis. Diseased nodes frequently fuse together ("matted") and form adhesions with the surrounding tissues. On examination, the nodes appear "fixed" and **sinus tracks** may form through the overlying skin. A palpable mass in the right iliac fossa is typical, but masses may be felt at other sites including the epigastrium (rolled-up omentum). **Visible peristalsis** is noted in subacute bowel obstruction. Tenderness is localized to the site of disease. Diffuse tenderness with a **"doughy" feel** is suggestive of peritoneal involvement. Presence of an uneven abdominal distention indicates loculated ascites. Fecal **fistulae,** and perianal fistulae and fissures may be noted. Enlargement of **liver and spleen** indicates involvement of these organs.

Differential diagnosis

Lymphoma, carcinoma and **amoeboma** can mimic abdominal tuberculosis. However, the condition most difficult to differentiate from tuberculosis is **Crohn's disease** (Table 47.3). Both can involve any part of the gastrointestinal tract, produce skip lesions, have a predilection for the ileo-cecal area, and histology shows inflammatory cells with granulomas.

Diagnostic methods

Confirmation of the diagnosis requires the **identification of M. tuberculosis**. However, the organism is usually difficult to detect and a definitive diagnosis is possible only in a minority of individuals. Therefore, a **therapeutic trial** is justified in endemic countries (see Table 47.4).

Indirect tests

A high sedimentation rate is a common but nonspecific finding. An abnormal **chest X-ray** (seen in 30% patients) is helpful. A positive tuberculin skin test (TST) is useful in nonendemic

Table 47.3 Characteristics of intestinal tuberculosis and Crohn's disease

Characteristic	Tuberculosis	Crohn's disease
Epidemiology	developing countries	developed countries
Clinical findings		
Intestinal obstruction	50%	<10%
Diarrhea	30%	>80%
Fistulae	<10%	30%
Anal lesions	<5%	30%
Extra-intestinal lesions	<5%	30%
Pathology		
Ulcers	superficial, transverse	deep, longitudinal
Granulomas	confluent	discrete
Caseation, AFB	present	absent
Investigations		
Positive tuberculin test	90%	never
Abnormal chest X-ray	30%	never
Treatment		
Steroid use	worsening of disease	beneficial response
Clinical course	cured with treatment	relapses despite treatment

countries, but not in endemic areas because of high positive rates in healthy individuals and after BCG inoculation. Moreover, false-negative results are common in immunosuppressed conditions like AIDS. An alternative technique is the **interferon gamma release assay (IGRA)**. The test involves incubating the patient's blood with synthetic proteins which represent *M. tuberculosis* proteins; interferon gamma released by sensitized leucocytes is measured. The IGRA test provides greater specificity at lower cost, requires a single patient visit and is not affected by prior BCG vaccination [3].

Imaging studies

Plain X-rays may show **dilated bowel loops**, with air-fluid levels. Calcified nodes may be noted.

Barium study, best performed by the enteroclysis technique, is useful in establishing the location and extent of the disease, and identification of fistulae. The classic radiological features

Table 47.4 Diagnostic tests in abdominal tuberculosis

Laboratory tests
- Elevated sedimentation rate (nonspecific finding)
- Positive tuberculin test (low specificity in endemic countries)
- Serological tests (not reliable)
- Interferon gamma release assay (more specific)

Imaging studies
- Chest X-ray: very helpful if abnormal, and sputum is AFB +ve
- Flat films: dilated bowel loops, air-fluid levels, calcified nodes
- Barium study: location and extent of bowel disease; fistulae and sinus tracts
- Ultrasound/CT scan: assessment of free fluid, nodal disease, bowel wall thickness, mass lesions, disease of pelvic organs.

Endoscopy and biopsy
- Evaluation of diseased area
- Histopathology: granulomas, caseation necrosis, staining for AFB
- Culture for *M. tuberculosis*
- PCR for *M. tuberculosis*

Ascitic fluid analysis
- Exudate, high lymphocyte count
- AFB and culture (low yield)
- Elevated adenosine deaminase (high yield)

Laparoscopy
- Peritoneum: thickened, irregular, dull appearance
- Adhesions
- Miliary nodules: high positive yield at histology

AFB, acid fast bacilli.

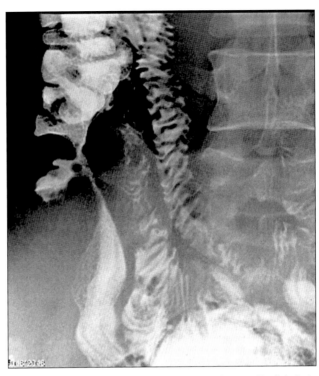

Figure 47.1 Narrow ileum opening into a contracted cecum (Sterlin's sign) (Courtesy of Drs. Nirmal Kumar and Veena Chaudhary, Maulana Azad Medical College, New Delhi, India).

are: contracted terminal ileum with a wide open ileo-cecal valve (**Fleischner sign**) and a narrow ileum opening into a contracted cecum (Figure 47.1). Overlapping bowel loops may interfere with an accurate assessment, especially in the presence of bowel adhesions.

Ultrasonography is very useful in detecting small quantities of fluid. Other abnormalities identified are: fibrous strands; enlarged nodes with hypoechoic centers (secondary to caseation necrosis); alternating pattern of echogenic and echo-free layers (club sandwich appearance) produced by diseased bowel loops with intervening fluid collection [4].

Computed tomography (Figure 47.2) provides a better assessment of bowel wall thickness and mass lesions. Disease nodes are enlarged in size, with low density centers and peripheral enhancement after contrast injection. There may be diffuse or localized fluid collection, and abnormality of pelvic organs may be present [5].

Endoscopy and biopsy

Diseased areas should be examined if located within the reach of an endoscope. **Biopsy specimens** should be used for histopathology, acid fast bacilli (AFB) staining, and culture. **PCR** can be performed on the tissue specimens and provides a rapid diagnosis (within 48 hours), with higher sensitivity and

specificity [6]. Overall, a definitive diagnosis by endoscopy is made in one-third of patients. An important advantage of endoscopy however, is that conditions such as lymphoma and carcinoma can be excluded.

Tuberculous ascites

The ascitic fluid has high **protein content** (>2.5g%), with a predominant lymphocytic response. A positive culture is obtained in <20% and AFB are detected infrequently (<5%). Ascitic fluid **adenosine deaminase**, an enzyme released by stimulated T-cells, has a high sensitivity (100%) and specificity (97%) [7]. **Laparoscopy** is very useful in patients with peritoneal disease [8]. The usual findings are thickening of the peritoneum and presence of nodules. Biopsy of nodules confirms the diagnosis in most patients. In view of the presence of adhesions, care should be taken to avoid inadvertent bowel perforation.

Treatment and prevention

Medical therapy comprises an "**induction phase**" of four drugs: isoniazid, rifampin, pyrazinamide and ethambutol or streptomycin administered daily for 2 month (Table 47.5). The patient is then switched to the "**continuation phase**" with two drugs: isoniazid and rifampin daily for 4 months. Twice weekly directly observed therapy (DOT), has been found to be equally effective. While a 6-month course is acceptable in drug-sensitive infection, a 3-drug continuation phase (containing ethambutol) over a longer duration (9–12 months) should

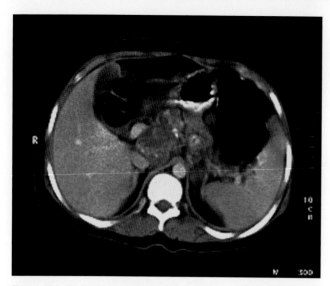

Figure 47.2 CT scan showing enlarged retroperitoneal lymph nodes (Courtesy of Drs. Nirmal Kumar and Veena Chaudhary, Maulana Azad Medical College, New Delhi, India).

be used in countries with high prevalence of drug-resistant tuberculosis.

Emergence of **resistant forms** of *M. tuberculosis* is an area of much concern. Recently extensively drug-resistant TB (XDR-TB) has been identified in several countries including Europe and the USA [9]. In addition to isoniazid and rifampin (termed multidrug-resistant organisms), these organisms are resistant to fluoroquinolone, and aminoglycosides. The treatment of XRD-TB is a major challenge and requires the use of multiple second-line drugs such as pyrazinamide, streptomycin, amikacin, kanamycin, and para-aminosalicylic acid.

Adverse reactions

The most dreaded adverse reaction is hepatitis, since **fulminant hepatitis** can occur in susceptible individuals, often within 2 weeks of starting treatment. Hepatitis is seen more frequently (four times) with combined isoniazid and rifampin than isoniazid alone. Both drugs should be discontinued until transaminases become normal. Isoniazid is restarted in increasing doses under close monitoring of transaminase levels. Treatment should continue with a second drug other than rifampin (see Table 47.5).

Table 47.5 Medical treatment of tuberculosis

Drug	Daily dose	Adverse effects	Action
Isoniazid	5 mg/kg	Hepatitis	Stop if liver enzymes elevated (x3 ULN)
		Peripheral neuropathy	Prophylactic vitamin B6
		Interaction with phenytoin and carbamazepine	
Rifampin	10 mg/kg	Hepatitis	Same as for isoniazid
		Thrombocytopenia	Monitor blood counts
		Skin rash	
		Several drug interactions	
Pyrazinamide	15–30 mg/kg	Hepatitis	Same as for isoniazid
		Gout	Monitor uric acid
		Skin rash	
		Avoid in pregnancy	
Ethambutol	15–25 mg/kg	Optic neuritis, color blindness	Baseline visual check; F/U as needed
Streptomycin	15 mg/kg	Ototoxicity	Baseline audiography; F/U as needed
		Nephrotoxicity	Baseline renal tests; F/U as needed

F/U, follow up; ULN, upper limit of normal.

Complications and their management

The most common complication is acute **intestinal obstruction**. Less frequent complications include: perforation, malabsorption, fistulae, and bleeding from a penetrating ulcer. Emergent **surgery** is required for complications such as free perforation, complete intestinal obstruction and acute bleeding. The most common indication for elective surgery is failure of medical therapy, usually for intestinal strictures. Other indications are: bowel adhesions, abdominal abscess secondary to localized perforation, and fistulae. The current surgical approach to intestinal strictures is stricturoplasty. Peritoneal adhesions are treated by adhesiolysis and placement of reabsorbable cellulose membranes over the peritoneal surface.

Prognosis

Most patients respond well to treatment. Systemic symptoms subside within weeks, while the mucosal abnormalities take longer to disappear. Eventually, 70% patients have **resolution** of the radiologic abnormality [10]. **Non compliance** and emergence of **resistant bacteria** are the primary reasons for treatment failure. Effort should be made to obtain culture and drug sensitivity before initiating therapy. Patients with resistant bacteria should receive at least 3 drugs and treatment should be given for **12–24 months.** Lack of clinical response should prompt repeat susceptibility testing. DOT is encouraged when compliance is an issue. Moreover, all patients should be tested for HIV.

What to tell patients

Tuberculosis can involve any part of the intestinal tract. The main defect is narrowing of the intestines resulting in abdominal pain, distention and vomiting. Other symptoms are: fever, sweating, decrease in appetite and weight. Treatment consists of multiple drugs which should be taken for several months. Tuberculosis is a curable disease, if treatment is started early. Poor compliance results in emergence of resistant bacteria which are difficult to eradicate.

Current controversies and their future resolution

Mycobacterium tuberculosis is a difficult organism to culture. The traditional method (Lowenstein-Jensen media) takes 6 weeks to confirm the diagnosis. The use of liquid broth (Bactec™ system) has reduced the culture time to 2 weeks. Current research is directed at producing more rapid diagnostic tests utilizing nucleic acid amplification techniques [11,12]. One test uses DNA probe (GenProbe™) to target mycobacterial RNA. Another employs the polymerase chain reaction to amplify bacterial DNA.

Other mycobacterial infections

The family Mycobacteriaceae is divided into two groups: tuberculous and nontuberculous mycobacteria (Table 47.6).

Table 47.6 Classification and clinical syndromes of mycobacterial species

Organism	Clinical syndromes
Tuberculous species	
Mycobacterium complex	
• *M. tuberculosis*	localized or disseminated
• *M. bovis*	lung, genitourinary, disseminated
• *M. africanum*	rare, exclusive to Africa
Mycobacterium lepra	leprosy
Nontuberculous species	
Rapidly growing	
• *M. fortuitum* group	lung, skin, soft tissues, catheter-related infections
• *M. chelonei/abscessus* group	lung, bone, nodes, skin, soft tissues
Slowly growing	
• *M. avium* complex	lung, disseminated (mostly HIV +ve)
• *M. kansasii*	lung, bone, disseminated (mostly HIV +ve)
• *M. xenopi*	lung
• *M. scrofulaceum*	lung, nodes, bones
• *M. haemophilum*	skin, soft tissues, bone
Intermediately growing	
• *M. marinum*	skin (swimming pool), bone

Tuberculous forms include **Mycobacterium tuberculosis complex** which contains *M. tuberculosis*, *M. bovis* and *M. africanum*. **Mycobacterium bovis** was once a common cause of infection but has been largely eradicated because of pasteurization of milk, and stringent control measures in dairy herds. However, *M. bovis* infection is still reported from developed and undeveloped countries. Active disease is mostly seen in immunesuppressed individuals. The main sites of involvement are lungs and the genitourinary tract [13]. Treatment is similar to *M. tuberculosis*, except for pyrazinamide which is ineffective. *M. africanum* is a rare cause of disease, seen exclusively in Africa.

Nontuberculous mycobacteria ("atypical mycobacteria") are ubiquitous in the environment. There are nearly 50 species that cause disease. The most important is **Mycobacterium avium complex (MAC)** which includes *M. avium* and *M. intracellulare*. Pulmonary infection can occur in healthy individuals resulting in productive cough, hemoptysis, fever and weight loss. Children often present with lymphadenitis. The enlarged nodes are nontender and usually localized to one area. Disseminated MAC infection, seen in AIDS patients with CD4 usually <100/mm^3, is associated with fever, sweating, weight loss, diarrhea and hepatosplenomegaly. The gastrointestinal tract is frequently involved and shows **blunted villi** containing histiocytes loaded with AFB. **Treatment** consists of three drugs: clarithormycin (500 mg b.i.d) or azithromycin (500 mg/day), ethambutol (15 mg/kg per day), and rifabutin (300 mg/day). Patients with CD4 ≤50/mm^3 should receive prophylaxis with clarithormycin or azithromycin.

References

1. Trends in tuberculosis – United States, 2008. *MMWR Morb Mortal Wkly Rep.* 2009;58:249–253.
2. Tandon HD, Prakash A. Pathology of intestinal tuberculosis and its distinction from Crohn's disease. *Gut.* 1972;13:260–269.
3. de Perio MA, Tsevat J, Roselle GA, *et al.* Cost-effectiveness of interferon gamma release assays vs. tuberculin skin tests in health care workers. *Arch Intern Med.* 2009;169:179–187.
4. Kedar RP, Shah PP, Shivde RS, *et al.* Sonographic findings in gastrointestinal and peritoneal tuberculosis. *Clin Radiol.* 1994;49:24–29.
5. Suri, S, Gupta, S, Suri, R. Computed tomography in abdominal tuberculosis. *Br J Radiol.* 1999;72:92–98.
6. Anand BS, Schneider FE, El-Zaatari FAK, *et al.* Diagnosis of intestinal tuberculosis by polymerase chain reaction on endoscopic biopsy specimens. *Am J Gastroenterol.* 1994;89:2248–2249.
7. Riquelme, A, Calvo, M, Salech, F, *et al.* Value of adenosine deaminase (ADA) in ascitic fluid for the diagnosis of tuberculous peritonitis: a meta-analysis. *J Clin Gastroenterol.* 2006;40:705–710.
8. Krishnan P, Vayoth SO, Dhar P, *et al.* Laparoscopy in suspected abdominal tuberculosis is useful as an early diagnostic method. *ANZ J Surg.* 2008;78:987–989.
9. Madariaga MG, Lalloo UG, Swindells S. Extensively drug-resistant tuberculosis. *Am J Med.* 2008;121:835–844.
10. Anand BS, Nanda R. Sachdev GK. Response of tuberculous stricture to antituberculous treatment. *Gut.* 1988;29:62–69.
11. Nucleic acid amplification tests for tuberculosis. *MMWR Morb Mortal Wkly Rep.* 1996;45:950–951.
12. Lye, WC. Rapid diagnosis of Mycobacterium tuberculous peritonitis in two continuous ambulatory peritoneal dialysis patients, using DNA amplification by polymerase chain reaction. *Adv Perit Dial.* 2002;18:154–157.
13. Hlavsa, MC, Moonan, PK, Cowan, LS, *et al.* Human tuberculosis due to Mycobacterium bovis in the United States, 1995–2005. *Clin Infect Dis.* 2008;47:168–175.

Small and Large Bowel

CHAPTER 48

Parasites

John Croese

The Townsville Hospital, Townsville, QLD, Australia

Introduction

The parasite–host relationship reflects an antagonistic coevolution governed by frequency-dependent selection [1]. Polymorphic alleles that are present in both protagonists flux over time (sympatric) and space (allopatric) [2]. Least virulent clones tend to be the most infectious, a selection advantage. Resistant hosts are naturally favoured creating a dynamic "arms race." As a consequence and also due to adaptive immunity, coexistent infections, general health and many other variables, a parasite behaves differently depending on the strain, its evolutionary relationship to and the circumstances of the host. Geographical context is important. Also important is the evolutionary stresses these durable parasites have had on the genetic traits of the host [3,4]. Adapted parasites regulate the host immunity to avoid expulsion, and in so doing, have shaped a predisposition to autoimmune diseases [3,4,5].

In endemic locales, typically poor without sanitation, indigenous populations harbor several parasites which individually and collectively limit virulence, but causes growth retardation, reduced cognitive development and accrue significant mortality [6,7]. Most infections are asymptomatic. For the traveller, a more pronounced virulence results in overt disease. The benefits arising from the disappearance of parasites are profound. Recently though, observational studies and clinical trials that identified a benefit from *Trichuris suis* in inflammatory bowel disease suggest that an evolutionary adaptation to helminths is contributing to the growth in autoimmune diseases [8,9,10]. Clinical trials testing the health benefits of helminths are underway. The immunobiology of once exotic helminths has a new relevance.

Protozoa and microsporidia

Protozoa and microsporidia are unicellular eukaryotes. They are classified according to shape as flagellate (*Giardia intestinalis*), amoeboid (*Entamoeba histolytica*), ciliate (*Balantidium coli*) and sporozoan, which includes coccidia (*Cryptosporidium parvum* and *Isospora belli*) and microsporidia. Giardiasis, cryptosporidiosis, amebiasis are familiar diseases. Globally, over 50 million infections with *E. histolytica* causing 100 000 deaths occur annually [7]. *Cryptosporidia* spp. and *G. intestinalis* are common in the USA, the latter with an estimated prevalence of 0.7 per cent [11]. Many infections including those

Small and Large Bowel

Textbook of Clinical Gastroenterology and Hepatology, Second Edition. Edited by C. J. Hawkey, Jaime Bosch, Joel E. Richter, Guadalupe Garcia-Tsao, Francis K. L. Chan.
© 2012 Blackwell Publishing Ltd. Published 2012 by Blackwell Publishing Ltd.

with traditional pathogens are asymptomatic, particularly in endemic populations.

Cause and pathogenesis

Fecal-oral spread and contamination of food and water by hardy cysts and spores account for most infections. In young children, virulence may be attenuated which obscures the role of day-care facilities as the source of community outbreaks. Epidemics imply either contamination of food, often imported from an endemic area, or water sourced from a catchment compromised by human or animal habitation (*Cryptosporidium* spp.). Endemic infections in domestic pets and farm animals are common and may account for sporadic and recurrent infections.

The pathogenesis of most protozoa is not known. They inhabit the surface of enterocytes (*E. histolytica* and *G. intestinalis*) or invade the cell membrane (*C. parvum* and microsporidia). The secretory diarrhea which is common to most is associated with the loss of microvilli, villous blunting and chronic inflammatory infiltrates. Both virulence and resistance are linked to the intensity of interferon-γ and T cell responses. With the exception of *I. belli*, eosinophilia does not accompany protozoan infections. Pathogenicity is often strain-specific. *Entamoeba histolytica* that bind to the cell wall, invade and induce an ulcerating colitis are distinct from clones that cause liver abscesses.

Clinical presentation

Amebic infections including 90 percent with *E. histolytica* are asymptomatic but are linked to malnutrition and growth retardation. Amebic dysentery has a sub-acute onset sometimes accompanied by fever and can progress to a fulminant colitis.

Acute infections with protozoa cause secretory diarrhea, flatulence, nausea and mild upper abdominal pain which resolve after 3 weeks. Chronic infection with *G. intestinalis* causing malabsorption is common, and most protozoa can induce a post-enteritis irritable bowel syndrome. In immuno-compromised populations, *Cryptosporidia* spp., *I. belli* and microspora cause debilitating diarrhea and are difficult to eradicate.

Diagnosis

Infections are diagnosed by fecal microscopy, although poor sensitivity is a problem. Simple precautions will improve detection:

- Inform the laboratory of the clinical circumstance and provide a differential diagnosis as special stains are available but not routinely applied.
- Provide 3 wet stools freshly submitted as excretion may be intermittent.

When suspected infections are chronic and standard methods fail:

- Collect tissue samples for histology.
- Negotiate with reference laboratories to test feces, serum and tissue using antibody (ELISA) and molecular (PCR) assays, and electron microscopy as appropriate.

Treatment and prevention

Mainstream therapies and dosages for acute infections are listed in Table 48.1. Asymptomatic infections do not warrant treatment except in food handlers. Hygiene will limit cross-infection in families and institutions. Isolation of carriers with diarrhea is recommended for childcare settings.

Helminths

Roundworms (nematodes), tapeworms (cestodes) and flukes (trematodes) remain endemic in many developing nations. Anthropophilic species are generally of low virulence. Zoonoses are uncommon but produce acute illnesses characterized by eosinophilia.

Cause and pathogenesis

Helminths have complex lifecycles. Uniquely, *E. vermicularis* (pinworm) is spread person-to-person and remains universally endemic. Ova from *A. lumbricoides*, *Trichuris* spp., *Ancylostoma duodenale* and *Necator americanus* are shed in feces and require moist soil conditions to develop into infective larvae. They have disappeared from urban populations. Infection with *S. stercoralis* is similar, but it is capable of autoinfection and may remain cryptic long after the initial contact is forgotten. *Schistosoma* spp. (bilharziasis) are endemic in African, Asian and South American populations that share habitats with snails, an essential vector. Depending on the species, adult flukes reside in the portal system and deposit ova that are excreted in feces and urine. Ova also circulate to reach the liver and lungs causing granulomatous inflammation and fibrosis.

Adapted helminths are "masters of regulation." They modify the generic Th2 inflammation provoked by excreted and secreted derivates to minimize the damage caused by invasion and attachment.

Infection with a zoophilic species is largely determined by local culture. *Ancylostoma ceylanicum* (a hookworm of civet cats acquired through contact with contaminated soil) and *Trichostrongylus* spp. (common in herbivores acquired from vegetables fertilized with manure) can achieve patency in humans. Only a single Anisakidae (parasites of cetaceous mammals acquired from consuming uncooked fish) or *Ancylostoma caninum* (ubiquitous in domesticated dogs acquired from contaminated soil) is ever found, and then only at endoscopy or after a small bowel resection. Characteristically, these exotic parasites are virulent, but occasionally are found serendipitously (Figure 48.1).

Clinical presentation

Portal hypertension (Symmers' fibrosis) is an end-stage development in schistosomiasis although many infections are

Table 48.1 Therapeutic options for intestinal protozoa infections in adults

Organism	Classification	Drug and dose	Duration	Pregnancy
Bloody diarrhea *Entamoeba histolytica*	Amoeba	Metronidazole 800 mg t.i.d.	5–10 days	B
Balantidium coli	Ciliate	Tetracycline 500 mg t.i.d. Metronidazole 800 mg t.i.d.	10 days 10 days	D B
Secretory diarrhea *Giardia intestinalis*	Flagellate	Tinidazole 2 g (single dose)		C
Cryptosporidium parvum	Coccidian	Nitazoxanide 500 mg b.d.	3 days	B
Isospora belli	Coccidian	Co-trimoxazole 960 mg q.i.d.	10 days	C
Cyclospora cayatenensis	Coccidian	Co-trimoxazole 960 mg q.i.d.	10 days	C
Enterocytozoon bieneusi	Microsporidian	Albendazole 400 mg b.d.	28 days	C
Encephalitozoon intestinalis	Microsporidian	Albendazole 400 mg b.d.	28 days	C
Disputed pathogen *Dientamoeba fragilis*	Flagellate	Metronidazole 800 mg t.i.d.	10 days	B
Blastocystis hominis	Unclassified	Metronidazole 800 mg t.i.d.	10 days	B
Sarcocystis hominis	Coccidian	Co-trimoxazole 960 mg q.i.d.	10 days	C

(Adapted from Pierce KK, Kirkpatrick BD. Update on human infections caused by intestinal protozoa. *Curr Opin Gastroenterol.* 2009;25:12–17.)

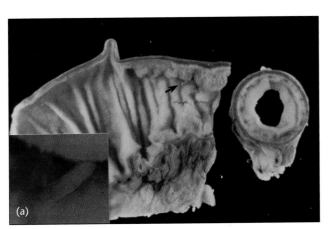 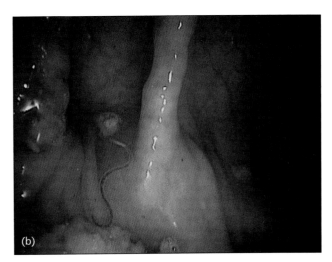

Figure 48.1 **(a)** Idiopathic acute eosinophilic small bowel obstruction correctly diagnosed several years after presentation by an astute medical student as caused by *Ancylostoma caninum* [12]. **(b)** A small adult *Ancylostoma caninum* feeding in the transverse colon found serendipitously during a surveillance colonoscopy.

Small and Large Bowel

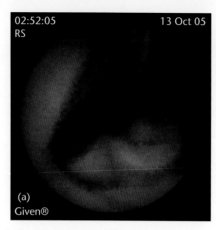

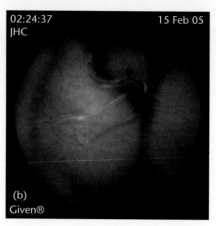

Figure 48.2 (a) Likely a single adult *Ascaris lumbricoides* (Video 48.2) found unexpectedly in a researcher undergoing capsule endoscopy as part of a series to evaluate experimental *Necator americanus* infection. This large worm was not present in prior or subsequent examinations and relevant ova were not detected in serial fecal examinations. Infection was probably acquired during trekking in one of several endemic regions. The wave of asymptomatic eosinophilic enteritis that accompanied the expulsion of immature hookworms is thought to have dislodged the ascarid [13]. (b) Feeding, paired *Necator americanus* in a Crohn's disease patient experimentally infected (Video 48.1) [14]. Experimental light infection with *N. americanus* is safe and in modern sanitary environments infected individuals pose no risk to others [15].

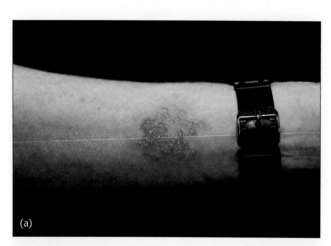

Figure 48.3 (a) An unusually intense pustular rash caused by experimental inoculation with *Necator americanus* (author). The entry points of the 50 larvae are easily counted. (b) The responses to 10 *Necator americanus* larvae or fewer have been typically pruritic with identifiable entry points, but without blistering.

unrecognized. Unwary travellers may experience swimmer's itch (cercarial dermatitis), a febrile illness characterized by lymphadenopathy, hepato-splenomegaly and eosinophilia (acute schistosomiasis or Katayama fever) and granulomatous colitis.

Generally, most helminth infections are asymptomatic. Capsule endoscopy highlights how elusive infection can be (Figure 48.2a). Experimental *N. americanus* infection may cause a pruritic rash and mild enteritis in naïve hosts when the inoculum exceeds 10 larvae (Figure 48.2b, Figure 48.3), but once established does not cause symptoms or anemia.

Infection with a zoophilic helminth typically provokes a severe gastritis or enteritis characterized by pain, diarrhea or obstruction and eosinophilia, although the blood changes may take days to develop.

Diagnosis

Infections are detected by fecal microscopy, although most commercial laboratories screen only if alerted. Scant infections usually require concentration or culture techniques (Harada-Mori). Screening serial fecal cultures and serology for *S. stercoralis* are prudent when considering migrants and veterans from endemic areas for an immune suppressive therapy.

Treatment and prevention

Mainstream therapies and dosages for helminth infections are listed in Table 48.2.

Future directions

In endemic areas, reinfection and drug resistance are undermining eradication programs. Vaccination is an alternative

Table 48.2 Therapeutic options for helminth infections in adults

Organism	Common name	Drug and dose	Duration	Pregnancy
Nematodes (roundworms)				
Ascaris lumbricoides	Roundworm	Mebendazole 100 mg b.i.d.	3 days	C
Necator americanus	Hookworm	Albendazole 400 mg (single dose)		C
Ancylostoma duodenale	Hookworm	Albendazole 400 mg (single dose)		C
Strongyloides stercoralis		Thiabendazole 1500 mg t.i.d.	2 days	C
Trichuris trichiura	Whipworm	Mebendazole 100 mg b.i.d.	3 days	C
Enterobius vermicularis	Threadworm	Mebendazole 100 mg (single dose)	2 weeks apart	C
Trematodes (flukes)				
Schistosoma mansoni	Schistosome	Praziquantel 1.2 g t.i.d.	1 day	B
Schistosoma japonicum	Schistosome	Praziquantel 1.2 g t.i.d.	1 day	B
Fasciola hepatica	Sheep liver fluke	Praziquantel 1.8 g t.i.d.	2 days	B
Clonorchis sinensis	Liver fluke	Praziquantel 1.8 g t.i.d.	2 days	B
Cestodes (tapeworms)				
Taenia saginata	Beef tapeworm	Praziquantel 1.2 g (single dose)		B
Taenia solium	Pork tapeworm	Praziquantel 1.2 g (single dose)		B
Echinococcus granulosus	Hydatid	Albendazole 400 mg b.i.d.	28 days × 3 14 days apart	C
Hymenolepis nana	Dwarf tapeworm	Praziquantel 1.8 g (single dose)		B
Diphyllobothrium latum	Fish tapeworm	Praziquantel 1.2 g (single dose)		B

Small and Large Bowel

strategy, but effective vaccines are proving elusive. In similar vein, research into the mitigating effects of helminths on vaccination targeting other infectious diseases (HBV and influenza) and helminth-enhanced virulence of other diseases (HIV and tuberculosis) is largely unaddressed. Unexpectedly, the diseases associated with modernity are providing a new impetus for helminth research.

Parasites are linked to autoimmunity in observational studies and clinical trials. A better prognosis for multiple sclerosis tied to unspecified parasites which correlated with altered myelin-specific B and T cell responses has been reported. Similarly, *S. stercoralis* appears protective against autoimmune liver disease. *Trichuris suis* (pig whipworm) reduced the activity of Crohn's disease and ulcerative colitis in separate clinical trials. In one well researched case, self-infection with *T. trichiura* was reported effective in ulcerative colitis unresponsive to conventional treatment. In celiac disease, experimental infection with *N. americanus* inhibited gluten-specific Th1 and Th17 immunological responses, but not pathology following a robust gluten challenge.

Clinical trials using helminths in complex diseases will increase over the next decade. Currently in progress are trials using pig whipworms and human hookworms in autoimmune and atopic diseases as diverse as autism, multiple sclerosis, hay fever and peanut hypersensitivity. Eventually this list will likely include irritable bowel syndrome and coronary artery disease. The pharmacological potential of parasite derivatives is commanding new interest. As these helminths reside in the intestine, old enemies will have a new relevance to gastroenterologists.

References

1. Ebert D. Host-parasite coevolution: Insights from the Daphnia-parasite model system. *Curr Opin Microbiol.* 2008;11:290–301.
2. Decaestecker E, Gaba S, Raeymaekers JA, *et al.* Host-parasite 'Red Queen' dynamics archived in pond sediment. *Nature.* 2007;450:870–873.

3. Fumagalli M, Pozzoli U, Cagliani R, *et al.* Parasites represent a major selective force for interleukin genes and shape the genetic predisposition to autoimmune conditions. *J Exp Med.* 2009;206: 1395–1408.

4. Rook GAW. The broader implications of the hygiene hypothesis. *Immunology.* 2009;126:3–11.

5. Maizels RM, Balic A, Gomez-Escobar N, *et al.* Helminth parasites – masters of regulation. *Immunol Rev.* 2004;201:89–116.

6. Jackson JA, Friberg IM, Little S, *et al.* Immunity against helminths and immunological phenomena in modern human populations: coevolutionary legacies? *Immunology.* 2009;126:18–27.

7. Pierce KK, Kirkpatrick BD. Update on human infections caused by intestinal protozoa. *Curr Opin Gastroenterol.* 2009;25:12–17.

8. Weinstock JV, Elliott DE. Helminths and the IBD hygiene hypothesis. *Inflamm Bowel Dis.* 2009;15:128–133.

9. Correale J, Farez M, Razzitte G. Helminth infections associated with multiple sclerosis induce regulatory B cells. *Ann Neurol.* 2008;64:187–199.

10. Aoyama H, Hirata T, Sakugawa H, *et al.* An inverse relationship between autoimmune liver diseases and Strongyloides stercoralis infection. *Am J Trop Med Hyg.* 2007;76:972–976.

11. Pawlowski SW, Warren, CA, Guerrant R. Diagnosis and treatment of acute or persistent diarrhea. *Gastroenterology.* 2009;136: 1874–1886.

12. Walker NI, Croese J, Clouston AD, *et al.* Eosinophilic enteritis in north-eastern Australia. *Am J Surg Path.* 1995;19:328–337.

13. Croese J, Wood, MJ, Melrose W, *et al.* Allergy controls the population density of Necator americanus in the small intestine. *Gastroenterology.* 2006;131:402–409.

14. Croese J, O'Neil J, Masson J, *et al.* A proof of concept study establishing Necator americanus in Crohn's patients and reservoir donors. *Gut.* 2006;55:136–137.

15. Mortimer K, Brown A, Feary J, *et al.* Dose-ranging study for trials of therapeutic infection with Necator americanus in humans. *Am J Trop Med Hyg.* 2006;75:914–920.

Small and Large Bowel

CHAPTER 49
Ulcerative colitis

Fergus Shanahan

University College Cork, Cork, Ireland

ESSENTIAL FACTS ABOUT PATHOGENESIS

Etiology

A convergence of genetic susceptibility, environmental modifers and immune-mediated tissue injury

Pathogenesis – major theories

1. An organ-specific autoimmune disease with immune reactivity against the colonic mucosa; the bacterial flora are required but play a permissive role priming the development of the mucosal immune response
2. An abnormal immune reactivity against components of the colonic flora in which the mucosa is subject to innocent bystander injury
3. A heterogeneous syndrome or group of conditions with different causes but with a final common pathway of tissue damage

Disease modifiers

Industrialized society	A complex array of lifestyle and environmental factors
Smoking	Impact differs from that in Crohn's disease
	Smoking is less common in colitis than in general population.
	A history of recent cessation of smoking is common prior to onset or relapse
Enteric infections	Occasionally precipitate relapse
Appendectomy	Apparently protective against risk of developing colitis
Stress	Unproven adverse effect in humans but persuasive evidence in animal models
Drugs	Relapses have been linked with usage of antibiotics and NSAIDs and other barrier breakers

ESSENTIALS OF DIAGNOSIS

Clinical presentation

Colitis

Bloody diarrhea

Peri-defecatory abdominal cramping

Proctitis

Urgency of defecation

Tenesmus

Mucous discharge, pruritus ani

Proximal constipation and fecal loading in some patients

Systemic features

Fatigue, malaise, arthralgia, fever and weight loss (mild, depending on severity)

Extraintestinal manifestations

Rarely, may occur before the onset of colonic symptoms

Colonoscopy/sigmoidoscopy

Diffuse continuous involvement with non-granulomatous inflammation

Exclusion of other disorders (mainly infectious colitides)

Evidence of chronicity (relapses and remissions)

Differential diagnosis – causes of bloody diarrhea that mimic ulcerative colitis

Inflammatory

Crohn's disease

Behçet disease

Infectious colitides (examples)

Campylobacter

Salmonella

Shigella

C. difficile

Enterohaemorrhagic *E. coli*

Sexually transmitted proctitides

Cytomegalovirus

Herpes simplex

Chlamydia

Neoplastic

Colorectal cancer

Vascular

Ischemic colitis

Iatrogenic

Irradiation

Non-steroidal anti-inflammatory drugs

Textbook of Clinical Gastroenterology and Hepatology, Second Edition. Edited by C. J. Hawkey, Jaime Bosch, Joel E. Richter, Guadalupe Garcia-Tsao, Francis K. L. Chan.
© 2012 Blackwell Publishing Ltd. Published 2012 by Blackwell Publishing Ltd.

ESSENTIALS OF TREATMENT – INDUCTIVE AND MAINTENANCE

General and supportive
- Patient education and psychosocial support
- Specialist multidisciplinary hospital care
- Diet and nutrition (particularly in childhood and adolescence)
- Osteopenia prophylaxis
- Thromboembolism prophylaxis for immobilized patients
- Drugs to avoid (e.g., anticholinergics in acute colitis; antibiotics and NSAIDs unless specifically indicated)
- Vigilance and precautions against opportunistic infections
- Long term follow-up including dysplasia surveillance

Anti-inflammatory or immunomodulatory drug therapy
- Aminosalicylates (topical or oral)
- Corticosteroids (topical or systemic) for induction only
- Purine analogues (6-mercaptopurine, azathioprine) for maintenance only
- Cyclosporine for induction only
- Infliximab (anti-TNF) – an alternative to cyclosporine for induction, suitable for maintenance also

Surgery
- Total colectomy with end ileostomy
- Colectomy with ileal pouch-anal anastomosis (IPAA)

Table 49.1 The changing face of ulcerative colitis

Historically accepted feature	Changing patterns
Incidence higher than Crohn's disease	The opposite has emerged in some recent studies from Europe
Incidence follows a north-south gradient	This has become less evident
Male to female ratio	The male/female ratio has changed over several decades with slight male predominance now
Ethnicity e.g., Jewish background is a good predictor of risk for colitis	This is no longer true and is subject to numerous confounding variables

Introduction

Ulcerative colitis is a chronic relapsing and remitting inflammatory disease of the colorectal mucosa. Along with Crohn's disease, these two major forms of inflammatory bowel disease represent distinct syndromes with overlapping features. Unlike Crohn's disease, where the inflammatory process is transmural and may affect any part of the alimentary tract, uncomplicated ulcerative colitis is confined to the mucosa and restricted to the large bowel. Together, these differences in disease distribution account for much of the differences in disease progression and risk of complications between the two disorders. Both forms of inflammatory bowel disease are responsible for much personal suffering that is occasionally disabling; they impose a significant burden on healthcare resources and have important economic implications including work absenteeism.

Ulcerative colitis was one of the first areas in clinical medicine to enter the arena of what is now popularly referred to as evidence-based medicine. A half century ago, Sidney Truelove and colleagues conducted one of the first double-blind controlled clinical trials in gastroenterology in showing the efficacy of corticosteroids in ulcerative colitis [1]. Although corticosteroids remain a cornerstone treatment for moderate-severe ulcerative colitis, improved understanding of the pathogenesis of the disorder and continued application of evidence-based approaches have expanded medical and surgical therapeutic options. In addition to the influence of scientific advances on diagnostics and therapy, few disorders have changed face over time to such a degree as with ulcerative colitis. Once considered rare, ulcerative colitis has become a major gastroenterologic problem in the developed world. Traditionally accepted

risk factors such as Jewish ethnicity and high socio-economic status are either less evident today or are being challenged along with several other earlier epidemiologic observations (Table 49.1). Changes include an apparent shift in disease distribution with proportionately more patients presenting with proctitis rather than pancolitis than in the past.

As discussed later, much of the changing face of ulcerative colitis probably reflects environmental and lifestyle changes associated with modern industrialized societies [2,3]. However, the most important change may relate to doctor-patient relationships. For example, comparisons of current with earlier editions of classic textbooks of internal medicine reflect the changing attitudes of clinicians toward patients with ulcerative colitis. Unsubstantiated linkages of patients' personality or behavioral traits with susceptibility to colitis have been replaced with objectivity and compassion.

Epidemiology

Ulcerative colitis has become a worldwide problem. While improvements in diagnostic techniques have contributed to increased detection rates, there appears to have been a real increase in incidence in many countries over the past fifty years; in some areas this has reached a plateau. Although more common in the Western world than in Africa, Asia or South America, the incidence seems to increase as countries become developed and industrialized. In developing countries, the appearance and rising incidence of ulcerative colitis tends to precede that of Crohn's disease. After an interval of one to two decades, the latter then follows a similar trend [2,3]. A north-south geographic gradient has appeared in many reports, but this appears to be becoming less distinct. More important than geographic latitude, may be variations in socio-economic development and urban/rural differences; there is about a two-fold higher incidence for ulcerative colitis in urban areas. Features of a modern lifestyle associated with developed or industrialized nation status are summarized in Table 49.2.

Table 49.2 Changing lifestyle and environment linked with socio-economic development that may confer increased risk of ulcerative colitis

Improved sanitation and hygiene
Refrigeration
Reduced consumption of fermented food products
Decline in prevalence of *H. pylori* infection
Decline in endemic parasitism
Life on concrete – reduced exposure to soil microbes
Increased antibiotic usage
Vaccinations
Smaller family size
Delayed or altered pattern of exposure to childhood mucosal infections

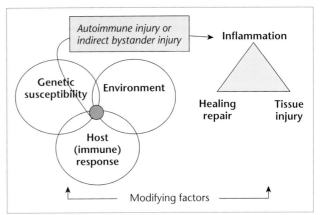

Figure 49.1 Contributory elements in the pathogenesis of ulcerative colitis. The immunoinflammatory response mediates tissue damage either by indirect innocent bystander injury or by direct autoimmune reactivity. Genetic susceptibility and environmental modifiers may act either at the level of the immune response or at the end organ. More than one gene is involved and several environmental modifiers have been implicated including the colonic flora, cigarette smoking, and non-steroidal anti-inflammatory drugs. (This figure was published in *Clinical Gastroenterology and Hepatology*, Wilfred M. Weinstein, Christopher J. Hawkey, Jaime Bosch, Ulcerative colitis, Pages 1–15, Copyright Elsevier, 2005.)

Ethnic variations in the epidemiology of ulcerative colitis were once thought to represent good predictors of risk, but this is no longer the case. Although ulcerative colitis appears to be more common in Jews, this appears to apply to a subset i.e., those of Ashkenazi descent. Confounding variables such as socio-economic status and migration between geographic areas of high and low prevalence, have diminished the apparent impact of ethnicity.

Reported incidences for ulcerative colitis from North America and northern Europe have been in the range of 10–20 new cases per 100 000 population (associated prevalence rates are about 150–250/100 000). Age-specific incidence rates for ulcerative colitis are usually described as bimodal with a major peak age of onset at 20–40 years and a later minor peak occurring after the age of 60 years. The male/female ratio for ulcerative colitis appears to have shifted from a female toward a marginal male predominance, particularly in patients with proctitis. The opposite trend appears to apply to Crohn's disease and might be influenced by smoking patterns.

Smoking is the most consistent polarising influence on inflammatory bowel disease, conferring protection against ulcerative colitis, in contrast to an increased risk for Crohn's disease. Indeed, patients with ulcerative colitis often relate the onset to recent cessation of cigarette smoking. The mechanism of these intriguing effects is unclear although smoking has been shown to influence mucosal immunity, colonic mucus production and motility [4].

Another consistent observation has been the apparent protective effect of appendectomy against development of ulcerative colitis. Patients with ulcerative colitis are significantly less likely to have had appendectomy compared with controls, particularly if the procedure has been performed before the age of 20 [5]. One interpretation of this might be that appendectomy has a direct protective effect in reducing the

risk of ulcerative colitis. This has been supported by evidence from an animal model of colitis (T cell receptor-α knockout mice) where resection of the cecal patch at one month of age attenuates subsequent development of colitis [6]. This interpretation has also prompted some investigators to perform appendectomy as a form of treatment. Alternatively, appendicitis rather than appendectomy *per se* might be inversely associated with ulcerative colitis. This is suggested by large population-based and national cohort studies where the risk of colitis was not reduced in cases where a non-diseased appendix was resected [7,8]. A third interpretation might be that the factors which predispose to development of ulcerative colitis also protect against appendicitis.

Causes, risk factors and disease associations

A simple explanation for the cause of ulcerative colitis has not emerged; a single cause and effect relation seems unlikely. As with most chronic inflammatory disorders, ulcerative colitis probably represents an interaction amongst genetic predisposing factors, environmental influences and endogenous modifiers. The outcome is activation of the intestinal immune system and a continual cycle of inflammation and healing (Figure 49.1). In common with chronic inflammatory disorders in other organs, ulcerative colitis may be a heterogeneous syndrome, comprised of different conditions with different causes but with a similar final common pathway of tissue injury.

Genetic factors

Advances in the genetics of inflammatory bowel disease have continued apace over the past decade, generating insights into pathogenesis, particularly in Crohn's disease but more recently in ulcerative colitis also. However, it is noteworthy that known genetic associations are thought to account for only about 20% of susceptibility, with both ulcerative colitis and Crohn's disease being polygenic, many genetic loci remaining to be identified. In addition, there is emerging interest in epigenetic factors, which are heritable changes in gene expression that occur without alterations in DNA sequences. Furthermore, concordance rates for monozygotic twins confirm the importance of non-genetic factors and suggest that a genetic influence is not as strong in ulcerative colitis (6–14%) as it is in Crohn's disease (44–50%).

While genome-wide association scans (GWAS) have been particularly successful in Crohn's disease, there has been progress in ulcerative colitis. As with many immune-mediated disorders, several genes in the human leukocyte antigen (HLA) region or major histocompatibility complex (MHC) on chromosome 6 have been linked with ulcerative colitis and confirmed by GWAS. It has also emerged that while some genetic predisposing factors are shared between ulcerative colitis and Crohn's disease, others are specific for either condition [9]. In addition to linkage with the MHC locus, associations between ulcerative colitis and the IL23R, IL10 loci and loci on chromosomes 1p36 and 12q15 have been reported. More recently, reported associations focus attention on candidate genes involved in the maintenance of epithelial barrier function and a first genetic link between ulcerative colitis and colon cancer has been described [10,11]. Future fine mapping and functional studies are likely to clarify these associations and should inform rational design and targeting of novel drug therapy.

Environmental factors

The importance of non-genetic or environmental factors in ulcerative colitis is indicated by the relatively low concordance rate in monozygotic twins (6–14%). Similar epidemiologic patterns and temporal trends in disease frequency suggest that some environmental risk factors for inflammatory bowel disease are probably common to Crohn's disease and ulcerative colitis. In contrast, as discussed earlier, other environmental influences such as appendectomy in early life and smoking are either specific to colitis or have opposing effects on the two forms of inflammatory bowel disease. There is some evidence that non-steroidal anti-inflammatory drugs (NSAIDs) may trigger exacerbation or the onset of ulcerative colitis. Reduced mucosal cytoprotective eicosanoids seems a likely mechanism.

The pattern of exposure to environmental microbes, particularly in early life, may be the most important exogenous factor influencing risk of developing inflammatory bowel disease. Elements of a modern lifestyle in developed societies (Table 49.2) have altered the pattern of microbial exposure. This has important implications for the development and education of the immune system. Development of the mucosal immune system is incomplete at birth and continual fine-tuning of cytokine responses and T cell repertoires occurs throughout childhood and adolescence. Since the function of the immune system is to sense microbial danger within the environment, immune education requires appropriate exposure to indigenous colonising flora in early life and to episodic infections, both of which prime and condition the intestinal immune response [2,12]. As with any sensory organ, inappropriate or inadequate stimulatory input may lead to dysfunction and errors of immune perception.

The most persuasive evidence implicating the indigenous flora, or components thereof, in the pathogenesis of ulcerative colitis is from animal models of colitis. A diversity of defects, either at the level of mucosal barrier function or at the level of immunoregulation, has been associated with the development of colitis in experimental animals. Irrespective of the underlying genetic defect in these models, the colitis does not occur in a germ-free environment and only develops after colonization with commensal bacterial flora. This suggests the flora either has a permissive role by priming the development of the immunoinflammatory response or in some instances may have a more direct pro-inflammatory effect [13,14]. In humans, there is some evidence for a loss of immunologic tolerance to the flora with the development of autoreactive antibodies that are cross-reactive with components of the flora and epithelial and non-epithelial antigens. None of these autoimmune phenomena has been shown to mediate tissue damage but have been explored for diagnostic purposes (see below).

While many clinical and experimental observations support the concept that ulcerative colitis is causally related to direct exposure to alimentary bacterial and other antigens, some observations are difficult to reconcile in this context. Firstly, the striking demarcation of disease distribution in subtotal colitis does not conform to the limits of bacterial exposure. Secondly, ulcerative colitis has been reported to occur in an autotransplanted colonic neovagina where there is no exposure to alimentary antigens [15]. This might be explained by inter-mucosal traffic of immune cells, cross-reactivity with vaginal microbes or may represent a subset of disease that is not due to direct microbial exposure.

Endogenous modifiers

Endogenous outcome modifiers include the brain-gut axis, placebo response, coping skills, and positive and negative emotional factors including psychologic stress [4,16]. Although logistically difficult to quantify and study in humans, the role of stress has been demonstrated well in animals with experimental colitis. Stress-induced reactivation of colitis has been adoptively transferred and is dependent on T cells. It appears that stress may adversely affect mucosal barrier function and promote uptake of bacterial antigens which activate previously sensitized mucosal T cells.

Disease associations

Extraintestinal disease associations and manifestations may occur in up to 5–10% of patients [17]. Some are true disease associations, whereas other conditions are complications or

Table 49.3 Extraintestinal disease associations and manifestations/complications

Organ or system	Manifestation or complication	Disease association
General/constitutional[a]	Weight loss, anemia, malaise Growth retardation Hypercoagulation syndromes Amyloidosis	
Skin and buccal mucosa		Erythema nodosum[a] Pyoderma gangrenosum Oral aphthous ulcers
Musculoskeletal	Osteopenia[a] Avascular necrosis[a,b]	Spondyloarthropathy Peripheral arthritis[a]
Liver and biliary tract		Sclerosing cholangitis
Ocular		Uveitis/iritis[a] Episcleritis[a] Conjunctivitis[a]
Pulmonary		Varied and non-specific including drug-induced

[a]tends to be related to activity of the colitis.
[b]This has traditionally been linked with steroid therapy but there are several reports of avascular necrosis occurring without steroid exposure and may be related to hypercoagulability.

manifestations secondary to the inflammatory activity or are side effects of its treatment (Table 49.3). Those involving the joints (peripheral arthritis and spondyloarthropathy), skin (erythema nodosum, pyoderma gangrenosum), eye (uveitis, episcleritis) and liver (sclerosing cholangitis) are the most common.

Articular disease is the most common extracolonic manifestation/disease association of ulcerative colitis. This includes axial arthropathies (ankylosing spondylitis and isolated sacroiliitis) and peripheral arthropathies. The former are unrelated to the inflammatory activity in the colon, whereas the latter consist of two patterns: **pauciarticular**, which affects large joints (<5 joints) and is usually self-limiting and associated with colitis activity (type 1); **polyarticular** (>5 joints), affects a wide range of joints but particularly the metacarpophalangeal joints and is independent of colitis activity (type 2). Both forms of peripheral arthropathy are non-erosive. Recently, distinct HLA gene associations have been differentially linked with each pattern of arthropathy associated with ulcerative colitis.

The most common skin manifestation is erythema nodosum, which is related to the activity of the colitis. In most cases it

occurs at the time of diagnosis or prior to presentation. In up to one third of cases it may be recurrent. Pyoderma gangrenosum is a more serious, albeit less common, problem. Unlike erythema nodosum, its clinical course is frequently independent of the activity of the colitis. The lesions are characteristically painful, beginning as one or more lumps usually on the lower limbs, which develop into pustules that breakdown and leave a necrotic centre with undermined violaceous edges. Because the lesions exhibit pathergy (i.e., may be extended by trauma), surgical debridement should be avoided. In contrast, to erythema nodosum, pyoderma gangrenosum tends to be indolent if not aggressively treated with immunosuppression.

Ocular involvement presents with an acute painful red eye and is usually linked with active colitis and involves the anterior chamber (iritis, episcleritis, scleritis, and uveitis). HLA genes such as B27 appear to have an important role in predisposing to these conditions in patients with ulcerative colitis.

Abnormalities in liver tests are common in patients with ulcerative colitis and may be due to various factors such as sepsis, malnutrition, treatment with parenteral nutrition, adverse drug effects, and transfusion-associated viral infections. However, clinically significant liver disease is far less common and present in about 5%. In contrast to most other extra intestinal manifestations/associations, liver disease is more common in ulcerative colitis than in Crohn's disease. Primary sclerosing cholangitis is by far the most common clinically significant liver disease associated with ulcerative colitis. In some patients it may precede the onset of colitis. It is unrelated to colitis activity, is unaffected by colectomy and may even occur years after colectomy. There is an increased risk not only of cholangiocarcinoma but also of colorectal cancer in patients with ulcerative colitis who have sclerosing cholangitis. Although a miscellany of other non-specific liver disorders have been associated with inflammatory bowel disease, including autoimmune hepatitis, such diagnoses should be made with caution and only if sclerosing cholangitis has been excluded and if cholangiography is normal.

Pathogenesis

The colonic mucosa is a functional barrier between the internal milieu and a living mass of antigenic bacteria within the lumen. Antigenic presence maintains the mucosal immune system in a state of controlled physiologic inflammation. This requires precise regulation to avoid excessive reactivity to the indigenous flora, whilst remaining on ready-alert for responsiveness against episodic challenge with pathogens. Tissue injury and colitis are an expected outcome if breakdown of mucosal immunoregulation occurs with excessive inflammatory responses to innocuous bacterial antigens or if there is failure to turn off appropriate immune responses after resolution of infection with a pathogen.

The balance of mucosal cytokines is influenced by genetic and environmental factors, including the composition of the

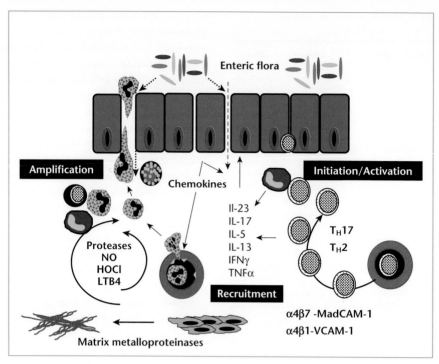

Figure 49.2 Immune-mediated tissue injury in ulcerative colitis. (This figure was published in *Clinical Gastroenterology and Hepatology*, Wilfred M. Weinstein, Christopher J. Hawkey, Jaime Bosch, Ulcerative colitis, Pages 1–15, Copyright Elsevier, 2005.)

luminal flora. It is important to appreciate the plasticity and dynamic nature of the immune response, depending on the nature of the stimulus and the response over time. A diversity of cytokines with overlapping functions may be produced at different phases of the mucosal inflammatory response, a feature that may account, in part, for disappointing results when certain cytokines have been targeted therapeutically. While the mucosal cytokine profiles of Crohn's disease and ulcerative colitis overlap, the former has traditionally been considered to be an IL-12-dependent T_H1 response (associated mainly with IL-1, IL-6, TNF-α, and interferon-γ, IFN-γ), the latter has been considered to be a non-T_H1 or modified T_H2 response (with increased mucosal interleukin IL-5 and IL-10, IL-13). This overly simplistic view has been challenged with the discovery of an additional subset of T helper, T_H17 cells which produce the proinflammatory cytokines, IL17 and IL22. T_H17 cells are activated by IL6 and transforming growth factor-beta (TGFβ) and their survival and differentiation is promoted by by IL23. The IL23/T_H17 pathway is activated in both Crohn's disease and ulcerative colitis [9,18,19].

The control of cytokine production and immune activation involves transcription factors that bind to the gene promoter regions. Of these, nuclear factor-kappa B (NF-κB) is a pivotal regulator of pro-inflammatory cytokines within the mucosal epithelium and immune system. Mucosal expression of NF-κB is enhanced in patients with ulcerative colitis, and its activation is influenced by cytokines such as TNF-α thereby creating the basis of a positive feedback or amplification loop. NF-κB is also activated by bacterial signals from the lumen via Toll-like receptors (TLRs) which are pattern recognition receptors

on the surface of enterocytes and on antigen presenting cells of the immune system. Increased epithelial expression of TLR4 which recognizes bacterial lipopolysaccharide has been described in ulcerative colitis. The molecular basis of host-flora interactions including a search for polymorphisms of TLRs that might predispose to inappropriate responses to lumenal bacteria in ulcerative colitis is now a focal area of research.

Enhanced humoral immunity is more evident in ulcerative colitis than Crohn's disease. Mucosal plasma cells from patients with ulcerative colitis produce high levels of immunoglobulins and, in contrast with those from controls or patients with Crohn's disease, preferentially produce IgG1 subclass antibodies which can activate complement. In addition, a variety of autoantibodies, including anti-colon and anti-neutrophil cytoplasmic antibodies (ANCA), are detectable in the sera of most patients. Deposits of complement and IgG1 anti-epithelial antibodies directed against epithelial tropomyosins are detectable within the epithelium in ulcerative colitis but the autoantibodies do not otherwise have pathogenic potential. They probably reflect disturbed immunoregulation and appear to be cross-reactive between self- and bacterial antigens.

In both forms of inflammatory bowel disease, the downstream effects of unrestrained T cell activation and cytokine release are similar. Upregulation of vascular adhesion molecules facilitate recruitment of additional effector cells causing amplification of the inflammatory response and the generation of activated matrix metalloproteinases, such as stromolysin-1, which mediate tissue destruction (Figure 49.2). Thus, irrespective of whether the initiating mechanism of immune activation is autosensitization or microbial stimulation or both, the final common pathway of tissue damage involves transmigration of neutrophils and other acute inflammatory cells from the vasculature through the mucosa and into the lumen.

The molecular basis of both the transendothelial and transepithelial migration are multi-step processes requiring cell-cell contacts using a series of adhesion molecules that are upregulated under the influence of cytokines. Further amplification of the inflammatory process occurs due to disruption of mucosal barrier function by the transepithelial migration of neutrophils, enhancing ingress of bacterial-derived chemotactic peptides and antigens. Tissue injury is mediated in a non-specific fashion by release of inflammatory mediators released by the transmigrating cells. These include reactive oxygen metabolites and matrix metalloproteinases. Some neutrophil-derived mediators such as leukotriene B4 (LTB4) which is the most potent chemotactic factor within the inflamed mucosa cause additional amplification of the inflammatory response by increasing inflammatory cell recruitment and activation.

Pathophysiology of symptoms

Diarrhea in ulcerative colitis is multifactorial. Inflammation may inhibit fluid absorption and/or increase secretion. Mechanisms of reduced absorption include: (i) decreased colonic surface area with epithelial denudation in severe cases, (ii) neural and hormonal inhibition of salt absorption, (iii) increased motor activity and transit in some cases, and (iv) increased osmolar load from nutrient malabsorption such as impaired colonic salvage of carbohydrate. In contrast, increased secretion is due to inflammation-derived secretagogues including arachidonic acid metabolites, leakage of plasma from denuded mucosa and loss of barrier function. Bowel frequency and urgency in colitis are due not only to increased stool volume (diarrhea) but may also arise because of irritability and reduced compliance of the inflamed rectum. It is noteworthy that despite increased stool frequency, proximal colonic transit may be reduced (proximal constipation) particularly in patients with proctitis or left-sided colitis. Bleeding is secondary to the adverse effects of inflammation on the mucosal microvasculature. Mucosal capillaries become engorged, leaky and occasionally thrombosed. Bleeding is almost always present when ulcerative colitis is severe enough to cause diarrhea, and if absent, another diagnosis should be suspected. Similarly, resolution of inflammation should lead to control of bleeding; if it doesn't, an alternative source of blood loss should be suspected.

Pathology

Despite its name, inflammation rather than ulceration is the cardinal feature of ulcerative colitis. Indeed, mucosal ulceration is usually evident only in severe advanced disease, whereas it is a defining feature of early lesions in Crohn's disease. Ulcerative colitis is a disease of the colorectal mucosa;

it begins in the rectum at the anal verge and characteristically extends to a variable degree proximally in a diffuse continuous manner without skip areas. Progression or regression of the upper limit of the extent of the colitis is variable and unpredictable over time. When the disease is limited to the rectum or left side of the colon, its upper limit is often remarkably well demarcated from the proximal non-inflamed mucosa. It is noteworthy, however, that in some patients, particularly those with long standing disease that has been treated, the degree of inflammation may appear variable and give a false impression of patchiness or skip lesions [20]. A mistaken diagnosis of Crohn's disease in this situation can be avoided if biopsies are taken which confirm the histologic continuity of the inflammatory process. It is also important to be aware that a "cecal patch" of inflammation has been described in patients with ulcerative colitis; this appears as an area of erythema around the appendiceal orifice. In patients with distal colitis, it does not imply Crohn's disease.

Macroscopically or endoscopically, the mucosa in acutely active ulcerative colitis appears hyperaemic, granular and friable – bleeding easily when touched. As the condition becomes more severe, punctate ulceration appears and may become confluent and leave islands of inflammatory tissue. When the clinical course is one of frequent severe recurrences with extensive ulceration, *"pseudopolyps"* (more correctly termed *inflammatory polyps*) and mucosal bridging may develop due to undermining of the mucosa by confluency of ulceration. When the colitis is inactive or "burnt out," inflammatory polyps persist and the intervening mucosa is smooth and atrophic. While these inflammatory polyps do not have the neoplastic implications of true adenomatous polyps, they make accurate dysplasia surveillance more difficult. Unlike Crohn's disease, fibrosis is not a prominent feature of the healing phase of ulcerative colitis. Over time, shortening of the colon and a reduction in diameter are due to thickening and contracture of its muscle layer. This is usually best illustrated by barium enema which confirms the colonic foreshortening along with loss of haustral folds, an increase in retrorectal space, and, rarely, the appearance of benign non-fibrotic strictures.

Because ulcerative colitis is primarily a mucosal disease, its histologic features can be fully assessed using endoscopic biopsies. Cardinal features of acute disease include vascular congestion, edema, goblet cell mucin depletion, crypt abscess formation and inflammatory cell infiltration of the lamina propria. Crypt abscesses are collections of neutrophils that have migrated across the crypt epithelium into the lumen. They also occur in infectious colitides and in Crohn's disease. The inflammatory infiltrate in the lamina propria consists mainly of plasma cells and lymphocytes with a moderate increase in eosinophils and mast cells. Ulceration, if it occurs, is superficial and only becomes penetrating to the propria muscularis when the disease is fulminant or if toxic megacolon occurs. As disease activity subsides, crypt abscesses and mucin depletion resolves. Inflammatory cell infiltrates diminish more slowly. Regenerative changes within the epithelium become prominent. However, evidence of disease chronicity persists and is useful for distinguishing the disease from acute infectious colitis. This includes distortion of gland architecture such as shortening, branching and loss of parallelism. In addition, Paneth cells metaplasia in the base of the crypts is a feature of long-standing ulcerative colitis.

Clinical presentation

The onset of symptoms in patients with ulcerative colitis, although more abrupt than with Crohn's disease, is frequently gradual and intermittent, becoming progressively more severe and persistent over a period of weeks or months. Bloody diarrhea or the passage of blood and mucus are the cardinal symptoms of ulcerative colitis and are present in over 90% of patients at presentation. Nocturnal diarrhea is common and should always prompt suspicion of organic disease. Depending on the severity of inflammation, there may be urgency and tenesmus (best described as "dry heaves in the rectum"). Cramping and abdominal pain are usually mild or absent. If pain is particularly severe or persistent, an alternative diagnosis or a complication such as microperforation should be considered. Weight loss is usually not a feature at presentation or is minimal, except in childhood and adolescence where weight gain and growth may be delayed. When inflammation is confined to the rectum (proctitis), patients often complain of passing fresh blood and mucus and may have constipation. It is common for such patients to have an empty distal colon and rectum combined with fecal loading of the proximal colon.

Physical examination is usually unremarkable when the disease is mild or moderate. Systemic signs are absent and general health is usually maintained, particularly in patients with proctitis. Even patients with severe disease or pancolitis may appear deceptively healthy. Abdominal examination may be normal or exhibit mild tenderness over the sigmoid colon. Rectal examination is usually normal except for the presence of blood. Unlike Crohn's disease, perianal lesions are not a characteristic feature of ulcerative colitis. If they arise, they are nonspecific and secondary to diarrhea, and include excoriation, superficial abscess formation, hemorrhoids, mucosal prolapse, and superficial fissures. Fistula formation is rare and should raise suspicion of Crohn's disease.

With increasing severity of disease, anemia, fever, tachycardia and fluid depletion become apparent (Table 49.4). Further deterioration with the development of severe persistent abdominal pain or distension may signal the development of a complication such as toxic megacolon or perforation.

Laboratory markers of the presence of severe inflammation include a raised erythrocyte sedimentation rate (ESR) or C-reactive protein, leukocytosis and thrombocytosis and anemia. Hypokalemia, hypoalbuminemia and elevated urea suggest severe pancolitis with fluid and electrolyte depletion.

Table 49.4 Truelove and Witts' classification of clinical severity of ulcerative colitis

Variable	Mild[a]	Severe	Fulminant
Bowel frequency	<4/day	>6	>10
Blood in stool	Intermittent	Frequent	Continuous
Temperature (C)	Normal	>37.5	>37.5
Pulse	Normal	>90	>90
Hemoglobin	Normal	<75% baseline	Transfusion required
ESR (mm/hr)	≤30	>30	>30
Plain film X-ray		Colonic air, edema, thumbprinting	Colonic dilatation
Physical signs		Abdominal tenderness	Distention and tenderness

[a]Moderate disease severity includes features of both mild and severe disease.

Various activity indices have been devised to quantify disease severity. It is important to appreciate that these relate only to the degree of clinical activity at a given time and do not take into account the disease distribution or the clinical course of disease over time or the responsiveness to therapy. The Truelove and Witts classification (Table 49.4) is a classic and still used in reporting clinical trials. However, few clinicians routinely use this or any formal activity index in daily practice. An example of a simple activity index that is convenient because it does not require any laboratory values and includes key questions that are used routinely by clinicians in assessing disease severity, is shown in Table 49.5 [21].

Extracolonic disease associations Occasionally, patients with ulcerative colitis may present with one of the extracolonic disease associations and in some cases, one or more of these manifestations may precede the onset of colitis by several years. However, it is noteworthy that some patients may not complain of colonic symptoms but have endoscopic and histologic evidence of inflammatory activity.

Differential diagnosis

No single clinical, endoscopic, histologic or other marker is diagnostic of ulcerative colitis. The diagnosis requires consideration of the composite clinical picture over time. In effect, the diagnosis rests upon: (a) a clinical picture compatible with colitis, usually bloody diarrhea or blood and mucus; (b) exclusion of other disorders which are mainly infectious colitides that mimic acute ulcerative colitis; (c) demonstration of

Table 49.5 Simple clinical assessment of activity of ulcerative colitis based on history and not requiring detailed physical examination or laboratory tests

Symptom	Variable	Score[b]
Stool frequency	1–3	0
	4–6	1
	7–9	2
	>9	3
Nocturnal frequency	1–3	1
	4–6	2
Urgency of defecation	Hurry	1
	Immediately	2
	Incontinence	3
Blood in stool	Trace	1
	Occasionally frank	2
	Usually frank	3
General well being	Very well	0
	Slightly below par	1
	Poor	2
	Very poor	3
	Terrible	4
Extracolonic manifestations[a]		1 per manifestation

[a]Includes arthritis, pyoderma gangrenosum, erythema nodosum, uveitis.
[b]A score of ≥3–5 is consistent with active disease
(Walmsley RS, *et al.* A simple clinical colitis activity index. *Gut.* 1998;43:29–32).

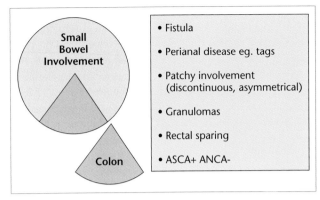

Figure 49.3 Endoscopic, histologic and serologic features of colitis suggesting Crohn's versus ulcerative colitis in patients with indeterminate colitis. However, it is noteworthy that the endoscopic appearances may become patchy after treatment and granulomas are present in only a minority of endoscopic series of Crohn's colitis. In addition, the sensitivity and accuracy of serology (ANCA and ASCA) is insufficient to be recommended for routine use. (This figure was published in *Clinical Gastroenterology and Hepatology*, Wilfred M. Weinstein, Christopher J. Hawkey, Jaime Bosch, Ulcerative colitis, Pages 1–15, Copyright Elsevier, 2005.)

chronicity. While a wide range of conditions might present with blood per rectum or with diarrhea, these symptoms seldom occur alone in ulcerative colitis; in practice, the differential diagnosis can be resolved, firstly, into the distinction between ulcerative colitis and acute infectious colitis; and secondly, the distinction between ulcerative colitis and colonic Crohn's disease.

Ulcerative colitis versus acute infectious colitis

At first presentation, the most important differential diagnosis to be excluded is acute infectious colitis. This is particularly true when the inflammation is confined to the rectosigmoid. When the duration of symptoms exceeds three weeks, a first presentation of ulcerative colitis is more likely than an infectious etiology. However, a specific infectious pathogen cannot be detected in all cases of acute self-limited colitides and a negative stool examination for pathogens or parasites does not necessarily imply a diagnosis of ulcerative colitis. In such circumstances, the histopathologic features of rectal biopsy may be helpful. Distorted crypt architecture favors a diagnosis of chronic ulcerative colitis over acute infectious colitis. Plasmacytosis in the lamina propria extending to the mucosal base (basilar plasmacytosis) is another marker of the chronic condition over a self-limited colitis. Regardless of the findings in the acute phase of the illness, the best differential approach is

patient follow-up and observation of the clinical course of colitis over time.

Ulcerative colitis versus colonic Crohn's disease

Differentiating Crohn's disease from ulcerative colitis is usually not difficult; the presence of small bowel disease immediately rules out ulcerative colitis. Difficulty arises only when Crohn's disease is confined to the colon, which occurs in up to 25% of patients with Crohn's disease (**Figure 49.3**).

In most of these cases, the combined endoscopic, histopathologic and radiologic features are sufficiently characteristic to permit a differential diagnosis, but in 5–10% of cases the colitis is indeterminate. Patchy, asymmetrical involvement and rectal sparing, with or without histopathologic evidence of granulomas, is consistent with Crohn's disease. Although granulomas may be found in 60% of resected specimens, they are found in only about 20% of patients with Crohn's disease in endoscopic series. Furthermore, while diffuse continuous involvement is characteristic of ulcerative colitis, some degree of patchiness is expected when the condition becomes chronic and after treatment [19]. Therefore, the colonoscopic examination performed at the time of first presentation is the most helpful in distinguishing ulcerative colitis from Crohn's colitis. However, in some patients the differential diagnosis is impossible and even examination of the surgically resected colon may not be definitive because the inflammatory process frequently becomes transmural if the condition becomes fulminant or progresses to toxic megacolon.

Diagnostic methods

Diagnosis is based on the composite clinical picture and not on the basis of endoscopy, histology or any other single disease marker. Colonoscopy is the critical diagnostic test. Plain abdominal radiology of the abdomen provides useful information regarding the extent of colonic involvement and the presence of right-sided fecal loading in patients with proctitis. It is particularly useful in monitoring patients for the development of toxic megacolon. While a barium enema may show characteristic appearances, barium studies are no longer necessary for the diagnosis of ulcerative colitis and should be avoided in acute severe disease to avoid increasing the risk of toxic megacolon.

The immunologic disturbances in patients with inflammatory bowel disease include various serum antibody markers such as perinuclear antineutrophil cytoplasmic antibodies (pANCA) and anti-*Saccharomyces cerevisiae* antibodies (ASCA) [22]. Since these two antibody markers are differentially and oppositely expressed in ulcerative colitis and Crohn's disease, their role in differential diagnosis has been investigated. Detection of pANCA in ulcerative colitis and ASCA in Crohn's disease has a high degree of specificity for these conditions respectively, but sensitivity is modest in both cases (55–65%). When combined testing for both markers is performed, diagnostic accuracy in terms of specificity and positive predictive value increases to greater than 95% but sensitivity decreases by about 10%. However, in patients with Crohn's disease confined to the colon, the prevalence of ASCA is relatively low and the sensitivity of ASCA positivity alone or in combination with ANCA negativity was only 45% and 32% respectively in one study [23]. Thus, serologic testing for ANCA and ASCA is least helpful in the subset of patients where the differential diagnosis is most problematic (i.e., Crohn's confined to colon vs ulcerative colitis) [22]. Furthermore, up to 15% of patients with Crohn's disease of the colon have been reported to be ANCA positive. Finally, a prospective study of ANCA and ASCA in patients with indeterminate colitis showed that serology was unhelpful in over half of the patients and its accuracy otherwise was insufficient to justify routine use of serology [24].

Treatment and prevention

There is no specific, curative treatment for ulcerative colitis – the emphasis is on supportive measures and judicious use of potentially toxic anti-inflammatory and immunosuppressive drugs on an individualized basis. The objectives of therapy are to improve quality of life, to reduce the risk of disease-related complications, and to avoid the need for surgery. The single most important aspect of disease management is access for the patient to a physician who is interested in the disease, compassionate and committed to long-term care.

General measures

As with every chronic illness, patient education is a pivotal component of successful long-term management. This includes guidance on the nature of the disease and reasonable expectations for therapy. In some cases, stress may exacerbate colitis

and perhaps trigger relapse. Advice from a counsellor, particularly for patients without strong family support, may improve ability to cope with the uncertainties of the disease.

A well balanced diet with minimal restrictions is encouraged. This is particularly important in children and adolescents with colitis. Emphasis is placed on maintaining adequate caloric intake and avoidance of excessive weight loss or malnutrition. A requirement for specific dietary supplements should be anticipated. These include iron for patients at risk of developing depleted iron stores and anemia due to chronic blood loss. Calcium is indicated to offset risk of metabolic bone disease in patients receiving corticosteroid therapy. A pragmatic exercise programme such as a regular walking routine has also been shown to help prevent bone thinning in those taking corticosteroids. Consensus guidelines on management of inflammatory bowel disease-related osteoporosis have been published [25,26]. In addition, the health benefit of dietary supplementation with folic acid is increasingly recognized and recommended by several clinicians.

For hospitalized patients with active severe disease, consideration should be given to use of preventive measures against thromboembolic disease. This may include wearing support stockings or the use of low molecular weight heparin. Active inflammatory bowel disease is associated with a procoagulant state and thromboembolism is an important cause of mortality in this young age group. Baseline investigations at first presentation or when patients are first seen should anticipate immunosuppression and plan for preventive strategies against opportunistic infections (**Table 49.6**).

Induction of remission

The current status of commonly used drugs for both the induction and maintenance of remission in ulcerative colitis is summarized in Table 49.7 and is contrasted with their roles in Crohn's disease. The characteristics of these drugs are covered in Chapter 50 and elsewhere [27]; considerations regarding their usage will be summarized here. While treatment should be individualized, a general strategy for drug usage is shown in Figure 49.4.

For patients with mild-to-moderate ulcerative colitis, aminosalicylates remain the cornerstone treatment of active disease and for maintenance of remission [27]. Efficacy is dose-dependent; consequently, patients should receive maximum tolerated doses before resorting to the use of systemic steroids (Figure 49.5). For patients with distal or left-sided disease, topical aminosalicylate enemas alone or in combination with oral aminosalicylates are at least as good, or in most studies better, than steroid enemas. Budesonide retention enemas have some advantage over prednisolone enemas because of low systemic activity due to high first-pass hepatic metabolism. Therefore, prolonged usage is less likely to impair endogenous cortisol responsiveness. In practice, foam enema preparations are easier for patients to retain in the bowel and are associated with better adherence than liquid formulations (Table 49.8).

Table 49.6 Diagnostic baseline data used in planning treatment of ulcerative colitis

Blood tests (for markers of systemic impact and severity of inflammation)
- Raised ESR and C-reactive protein
- Thrombocytosis and leukocytosis
- Presence or absence of anemia
- Hypoalbuminemia (marker of chronicity and severity)
- Liver enzymes (to screen for co-morbidity)

Stool examination (to rule out infectious colitides)
- Microscopy for ova/parasites
- Culture
- *C. difficile* toxin

Serology (selected patients)
- Serum pANCA, ASCA (optional - not for routine use)
- HIV, amebiasis, (selected patients)

Conventional radiology
- Plain film of abdomen (to monitor for colonic dilatation)
- Chest X-ray (if TB suspected or immunosuppressive contemplated)
- Barium enema (neither necessary nor desirable in most patients)
- Barium small bowel study (only if Crohn's suspected)

Endoscopy
- This is the mainstay of diagnosis, particularly the initial examination of the untreated patient; diffuse continuous pattern of erythema, granularity and friability with exudate – followed by ulceration in advanced severe cases
- After treatment, the appearances may become patchy
- Biopsy can help exclude co-incidental CMV infection

Plan
- Anticipate use of purine analogues (TPMT status)
- Anticipate risk of opportunistic infections
- Establish vaccination, infection and travel history
- Serology for varicella, hepatitis B and C, γ–IFN release assay (selected cases)

Table 49.7 Current status and contrasting roles of drugs used for induction and maintenance of remission in ulcerative colitis and Crohn's disease

	Ulcerative colitis		Crohn's disease	
	Acute	Maintenance	Acute	Maintenance
Aminosalicylates	+	+	+	−
Corticosteroids	+	−	+	−
Purine analogues	−	+	−	+
Methotrexate	−	−	+	+
Cyclosporine	+	−	−	−
Anti-TNF-α (infliximab)	+	+	+	+

(+) established role; (−) no conclusive role.

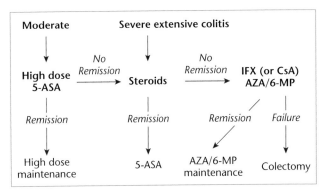

Figure 49.4 Algorithm for drug therapy of ulcerative colitis. 5-ASA, 5-aminosalicylate; IFX, infliximab; CsA, cyclosporine; AZA, azathioprine; 6-MP, 6-mercaptopurine. (This figure was published in *Clinical Gastroenterology and Hepatology*, Wilfred M. Weinstein, Christopher J. Hawkey, Jaime Bosch, Ulcerative colitis, Pages 1–15, Copyright Elsevier, 2005.)

Once the clinical assessment indicates that the colitis is moderately severe, there is nothing to be gained from postponing corticosteroid medication. The goal of treatment is to prevent progression to severe or fulminant disease and to achieve reduced inflammatory activity and remission. Corticosteroids should be prescribed at high dosage (e.g., 40 mg/d prednisolone) to bring the condition under control and tapered as the clinical course permits. The tapering regimen should be individualized but typically is not linear and will be by weekly decrements of 5 mg/d while tapering from 40 mg/d to 20 mg/d, and thereafter by 2.5 mg/d decrements weekly. It should be noted that the most troublesome symptoms of patients with pancolitis may be due to proctitis (tenesmus, urgency and bleeding). For such patients, the addition of a topical corticosteroid foam enema may hasten relief and enable the systemic steroids to be tapered more rapidly.

Patients presenting with acute severe or fulminant ulcerative colitis require admission to hospital for treatment and

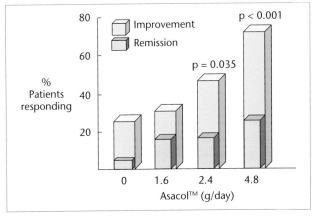

Figure 49.5 Dose-dependent influence of aminosalicylates on ulcerative colitis. (This figure was published in *Clinical Gastroenterology and Hepatology*, Wilfred M. Weinstein, Christopher J. Hawkey, Jaime Bosch, Ulcerative colitis, Pages 1–15, Copyright Elsevier, 2005.)

Table 49.8 A selection of pitfalls and useful tips

Pitfalls and tips

- Despite its name, ulcerative colitis is seldom an ulcerating disease; ulcers arise in advanced severe/fulminant disease
- The appearance of relative rectal sparing or patchy disease distribution in patients with longstanding treated ulcerative colitis is not a reason to change the diagnosis to Crohn's disease
- Common causes of treatment failure include inadequate dosing with aminosalicylates or corticosteroids and/or insufficient duration of steroid treatment
- Remember to prescribe calcium supplements with steroids
- Patient satisfaction and compliance with topical enema therapy is far superior if foam rather than liquid preparations are prescribed
- The forgotten order – stop all antispasmodics and antidiarrheals in patients with acute colitis to reduce risk of toxic megacolon
- Treatment with purine analogues requires at least three months before clinical efficacy is manifest – continuation with steroid therapy in the interim is required
- Record and document advice and warnings given to patients, express level of risk in simple terms and in perspective

observation. The emphasis is on careful clinical assessment and vigilance for emergence of toxic megacolon. There is no place for full colonoscopy or barium enema at this stage of the disease; these procedures are not necessary, can be deferred and may precipitate toxic megacolon. Surgical consultation should be obtained at the outset and a joint physician-surgeon team approach is important. The four components of management are intravenous fluid and electrolyte replacement, broad spectrum antibiotic coverage, intravenous corticosteroids and discontinuation of all opiate or anticholinergic, antispasmodic or anti-diarrheal drugs because they are risk factors for toxic megacolon. Aminosalicylates are not likely to have a significant therapeutic effect at this advanced stage of the disease. Nutrition should continue to be given by the enteral route; parenteral nutrition should be avoided, if possible, because it is usually unnecessary and because of the risk of complications including central vein thrombosis and sepsis. Prophylaxis against thromboembolism should be instituted.

Irrespective of the extent of colitis, an important subset of patients is resistant to aminosalicylates and corticosteroids (up to 16% in one study) [28]. For severe disease, intravenous cyclosporine is an effective option either alone or in conjunction with steroids. Although initial reports used a relatively high dose (4 mg/kg per day) of cyclosporine, it is clear that lower doses (2 mg/kg per day) are safer and equally effective [27]. Cyclosporine should only be used by experienced clinicians in referral centres where blood levels can be monitored. Prophylaxis against *Pneumocystis carinii* with co-trimoxazole should be considered [4]. The advantage of cyclosporine is its rapid action. However, because of its potential toxicity, the drug cannot be recommended as a routine oral therapy over the long term. It is noteworthy that of the patients with severe disease treated with cyclosporine and in whom a colectomy is

initially avoided, at least half will require colectomy within the following year. In the transition to long-term therapy, consideration should be given to switching to azathioprine/6-mercaptopurine in those patients who respond to steroids and/or cyclosporine in the acute phase.

For many clinicians, infliximab (anti-TNF; 5 mg/kg ivi) will be a preferable option to cyclosporine; it has been shown to be an effective rescue therapy for induction of remission [27, 29], appears to be safer and less complicated than cyclosporine but more expensive. Other biologic agents including adalimumab (anti-TNF given subcutaneously), visilizumab (anti-CD3) and selective anti-adhesion molecule strategies have been tested in ulcerative colitis and appear promising but data are limited as outlined in American and European consensus documents [27,30]. As with all immunomodulatory and immunosuppressive drugs including corticosteroids, vigilance against opportunistic infections is important, particularly in malnourished patients. Precautionary planning against opportunistic infections has been assisted by the publication of European guidelines [31].

Surgical intervention should not be delayed if there is failure of medical therapy or clinical deterioration despite aggressive medical therapy. Persistent pain (other than cramping associated with defecation) is a particularly worrisome development as is any evidence for colonic dilatation on abdominal X-ray films. In addition, a requirement for blood transfusion is a sinister development. Indeed, for acutely ill patients, surgery is often the conservative approach and may be safer than prolonged immunosuppressive therapy.

Maintenance therapy

The long-term goal is to keep patients in remission and to minimize frequency of relapses. The efficacy of medical therapy is judged in terms of quality of life and ability to work and function socially. Assessment of disease activity at regular follow-up visits is primarily on a symptomatic basis and not on endoscopic or biopsy findings. Patients should not be subjected to repeated radiologic or endoscopic procedures just "to see how things are."

Most patients with ulcerative colitis can be successfully maintained with aminosalicylates and intermittent brief courses of corticosteroids. Controlled clinical trials have confirmed the efficacy of sulfasalazine and the aminosalicylates in prevention of relapses. Adherence to aminosalicylates can be improved by once daily dosing rather than divided dosing without loss of efficacy, and this appears to hold for older formulations as well as extended release formulations such as MMX mesalazine. Corticosteroids are indicated only for breakthrough symptoms and have no role as a maintenance therapy.

Evidence from controlled studies of the prophylactic efficacy of azathioprine or 6-mercaptopurine in ulcerative colitis is sparse, but these drugs remain the treatment of choice for patients who fail to respond to aminosalicylates and corticosteroids [32]. The starting dose for 6-mercaptopurine is 50 mg/day and may be adjusted to 1.5 mg/kg per day in 25 mg/day increments depending on clinical response after 3–6 months. The dose for azathioprine is about twice that for 6-mercaptopurine. The rate-limiting enzyme for catabolism of these purine analogue drugs is thiopurine methyltransferase (TPMT), which is variably expressed due to genetic polymorphism. Therefore, assessment of TPMT genotype in advance of prescribing purine analogues is recommended, where available, so that rare (<1%) homozygotes with low or absent levels of the enzyme can be identified and for whom the drug should be contraindicated. In addition, heterozygotes (10%) with intermediate levels of enzyme activity may require dosage adjustment. The use of enzyme and metabolite levels to monitor drug therapy has also been proposed but studies have been conflicting. Irrespective of whether these assays are used, they do not preclude the need for regular blood counts to monitor for delayed bone marrow suppression. Patients should be advised to have a monthly full blood count.

There is insufficient supporting evidence for methotrexate as a maintenance therapy in ulcerative colitis, although this requires further study [27,32]. Cyclosporine, although an effective inductive agent for severe colitis, cannot be recommended as a maintenance therapy because of its toxicity, whereas infliximab (anti-TNF) is effective and relatively safe in selected patients, such as those who cannot tolerate purine analogues.

Alternative or emerging therapeutic strategies

A wide range of immunosuppressive drugs including mycophenolate mofetil and other agents have been studied in ulcerative colitis with encouraging results [27]. Results with other agents including heparin, nicotine, fish oils, leukopheresis, epidermal growth factor, antibiotics and leukotriene inhibitors have been disappointing in most instances despite early promise [4]. It seems likely that the next biologic therapy to move from the research bench to the bedside will be based on antagonising alpha-4 integrins [33] (Figure 49.2). Some new strategies are particularly intriguing and include the use of helminths, most notably the ova of the pig whipworm *Trichuris suis* which transiently colonizes the gut but is non-pathogenic in humans. A randomized trial in mild-moderate active colitis showed significant efficacy over placebo [34].

An alternative therapeutic strategy is to target the microbial environment within the colon [35]. The rationale for using probiotics is based on the notion that inflammatory bowel disease is due to an abnormal host immune response to some but not all components of the indigenous colonic bacteria. Accordingly, bacteria such as lactobacilli and bifidobacteria that lack proinflammatory potential have been successfully used as probiotics in experimental rodent models of enterocolitis. Other bacteria including *E. coli* strain Nissle 1917, a nonpathogenic coliform, have also been reported to have efficacy equivalent to that of mesalazine as a maintenance therapy in human ulcerative colitis [27]. Additional controlled trials of probiotic strategies are underway.

Surgical management

There are three main groups of indications for colectomy in ulcerative colitis. First, emergency colectomy is indicated for acute fulminating course or toxic megacolon. Second, elective colectomy becomes a serious consideration for patients in whom medical therapy has either failed to restore an acceptable quality of life or in whom there is unacceptable drug toxicity, such as a requirement for continual steroids despite optimal aminosalicylate and immunosuppressive drug therapy. Third, detection of either low grade or high grade dysplasia, particularly if confirmed by a second pathologist, is an indication for colectomy.

In emergency situations, a subtotal colectomy with ileostomy is often the procedure of choice. This can be converted to a total colectomy with permanent ileostomy by resecting the rectal stump at a later time, once the patient has recovered physically and emotionally. Alternatively, the option to proceed at a later stage to surgical creation of an ileal pouch and subsequent pouch-anal anastomosis may be exercised. The choice of procedure will depend on several individual variables including the age of the patient, co-morbidity, coping skills and ability to psychosocially adjust to stoma care. Where possible, in elective situations, patients should be counselled well in advance and given realistic expectations. Stoma care should be outlined by an experienced stoma therapist. It is important that patients understand there can be no guarantee regarding the distinction between ulcerative colitis and Crohn's disease in advance of surgery. They should also appreciate that any continent pouch procedure may fail and require repeat surgery; complications may necessitate complete surgical revision, possibly ending with a standard ileostomy. Pregnant women with a pouch should be offered Caesarian section instead of vaginal delivery to reduce risk of incontinence due to sphincter injury.

Pouchitis

The cumulative frequency of developing pouchitis after colectomy with ileal pouch-anal anastomosis (IPAA) increases with duration of follow-up and may be up to 50% after ten years. The condition is tantamount to a human experimental model of ulcerative colitis in a colonized pouch, and should be considered as a recurrence of ulcerative colitis [36]. It is largely confined to patients who have IPAA performed for ulcerative colitis and is much less common in those having it performed for familial adenomatous polyposis. The mainstay of treatment for pouchitis is antibiotics. Many patients will respond to metronidazole 200–400 mg three times daily for one to two weeks or longer. Alternatives to metronidazole include ciprofloxacin or similar broad spectrum agents. Some patients may require the addition of aminosalicylates, topical steroids or even immunosuppressive drugs. Probiotics have been explored as a preventive strategy following induction of remission with antibiotics, and controlled trials have been positive [37, 38] but clinical experience has been disappointingly variable.

Complications and their management
Toxic megacolon

Toxic megacolon is a medical emergency. It may occur as a complication of any form of severe colitis. Occasionally, it is the presenting feature. Risk factors for development of this complication include the use of anticholinergics, opiates, hypokalemia , hypomagnesemia, and barium enema or colonoscopic procedures in the setting of fulminant disease. Dilatation may involve the entire colon but appears maximal in the transverse colon radiographically. This is because air tends to rise in the upright position. In affected areas, the inflammatory process which is usually confined to the mucosa, extends into the muscle layer, perhaps due to bacterial overgrowth. There is bowel wall thinning and paralysis of motor function. The texture of the bowel wall has been likened to wet tissue paper; perforation with systemic sepsis poses a major threat with a mortality rate up to 30%. The cardinal symptoms of toxic dilatation are abdominal tenderness, guarding, tympany, and reduced or absent bowel sounds. Diagnosis is confirmed by plain abdominal radiograph; a continuous column of colonic air usually precedes onset of dilatation. Loss of haustral markings and an irregular luminal border may be visible with nodular defects indicating islands of inflammatory necrotic mucosa alternating with areas of ulceration. Gas shadows within the wall of the colon are a particularly ominous sign. It is important to recognize that the patient's clinical status may change over a period of hours from toxic dilatation to perforation and shock. Immediate treatment includes discontinuation of any precipitating drug, correction of fluid and electrolyte imbalances, and broad spectrum antibiotics. Colonic decompression may be achieved with a soft rectal tube and a long nasoenteral tube. Colonic gas can also be redistributed by intermittent repositioning of the patient from supine to prone position. However, unless prompt resolution occurs with these strategies, emergency colectomy should be performed.

Colitis-associated cancer

The risk of developing colorectal cancer in ulcerative colitis increases with disease duration, severity, and extent of disease [39,40], and also appears to be adversely influenced by the presence of sclerosing cholangitis [41], a positive family history of sporadic colorectal cancer [42], and backwash ileitis [43].

The pathogenesis of colitis-associated carcinogenesis differs from that of sporadic colorectal cancer [44,45]. While the two forms of cancer share many molecular abnormalities, the timing or sequence of molecular events distinguishes the two neoplastic pathways. For example, abnormalities of the p53 tumor suppressor gene are a relatively early event in chronic colitis, occasionally preceding dysplasia, but are observed late in the pathogenic sequence of sporadic colorectal carcinoma. In addition, mutation or deletion of the APC tumor suppressor gene tends to be late and uncommon in colitis-associated cancer, but an early event in sporadic colon cancer. The two neoplastic processes also differ in relation to expression of cell cycle regulatory proteins. Multiple mechanisms appear to predispose to colitis-associated cancer. Inflammatory signals increase oxidative stress, which promotes DNA mutagenesis and also activate pro-survival or anti-apoptotic pathways in epithelial cells, which contribute to tumor promotion. Inflammation also creates an environment conducive to tumor growth, angiogenesis, migration, and invasion of tumor cells [44].

While prophylactic colectomy is the only certain method of avoiding progression to colorectal cancer, this is seldom an attractive option. Therefore the management of cancer risk in patients with colitis depends on surveillance colonoscopy. Surveillance colonoscopy has not been shown to reduce mortality from colitis-associated cancer and a randomized controlled trial has not yet been performed.

Several problems associated with surveillance endoscopy as currently practised have been highlighted [46,47]. These include a poor understanding on the part of most gastroenterologists of the true meaning of the term dysplasia. Many gastroenterologists do not appreciate that dysplasia means neoplasia confined to the epithelium and is not pre-neoplasia. Secondly, there is a lack of consistency and consensus on the optimal number of biopsies taken at endoscopy. This influences sampling error. For example, it has been estimated that 65 biopsies are required to have a 95% confidence of finding the highest grade of neoplasm (dysplasia or cancer), and 33 biopsies are required to find the highest degree of dysplasia [48]. However, many now feel that careful attention to detail and targeted biopsies may be more important than a multiplicity of random biopsies. Thirdly, even if pathologists receive adequate biopsy material, their inter-observer agreement for diagnosing low-grade dysplasia is only about 60% for experienced, specialized pathologists. It is, therefore, not surprising that gastroenterologists have inconsistent approaches to the management of low-grade dysplasia. This is disturbing because a confirmed finding of low-grade dysplasia is a strong predictor of progression to invasive cancer, and early colectomy should be a serious consideration [49]. Fourthly, if clinicians wait for the development of high grade dysplasia before recommending colectomy, it may be too late to prevent invasive cancer. The progression of low-grade to high-grade dysplasia is not evident in all cases and once high-grade dysplasia is detected, an invasive cancer will already be present in up to 30% of cases, in many of which it will be advanced (Dukes C) [46,47].

Developments that promise to improve the accuracy of surveillance colonoscopy in identifying those patients at particular risk of colitis-associated cancer include the introduction of magnifying or high-resolution endoscopy coupled with mucosal dye staining (chromoendoscopy) [47]. In addition, a more fundamental understanding of the molecular events underlying the inflammation-dysplasia-cancer sequence promises to facilitate the development of a molecular profile of the genetic alterations in the colonic epithelia conferring increased risk of cancer [45].

Since colitis-associated cancer appears to be a result of chronic inflammation, it is plausible to conclude that effective therapy can reduce the risk of cancer. Perhaps because of this, recent reports indicate that the risk of colitis-associated cancer may be much lower today than originally reported from earlier times [50,51]. A chemoprophylactic effect of aminosalicylates against colitis-associated cancer has been proposed based on retrospective data but this remains unproven [52]. In the absence of definitive data, aminosalicylates are appropriate and could reasonably be combined with other preventive strategies, such as the use of folic acid and calcium supplements with putative chemopreventive effects.

Prognosis

The clinical course of ulcerative colitis in individual patients is impossible to predict but its relapsing nature is revealed by population-based studies showing a one year risk of relapse in the range of 50%, even in patients receiving maintenance aminosalicylates. Follow-up studies of patients with ulcerative colitis have shown that only half the patients are in remission at any time. In untreated patients, the relapse rate is 50–70% over one year, as estimated from the placebo-treated groups in clinical trials of aminosalicylate therapy [32]. The likelihood of surgery becoming a necessity for any patient is much more difficult to estimate because of so many individual variables and because it is almost certainly changing with the increasing use of more effective drugs including immunosuppressive agents.

The clinical course of patients in the placebo-controlled limb of clinical therapeutic trials may reveal lessons regarding the clinical course of ulcerative colitis. In one analysis, the mean placebo response for clinical symptoms was similar to that for more objective measures such as endoscopy and histology (25–30%). More importantly, the only factor that appeared to influence the placebo response was the number of doctor-patient contacts [53]. This is circumstantial support for regular follow-up but is not necessarily at variance with the concept of guiding patients to help themselves [54]. Thus, guided self-management of ulcerative colitis has some advantages for patients but should not be a substitute for regular contact with a committed experienced clinician.

While early studies indicated a reduced life expectancy in patients with ulcerative colitis creating difficulties for patients seeking life insurance, recent studies have been less pessimistic. Some, but not all population-based studies have since shown either improved or equivalent survival for ulcerative colitis relative to the general population. Interpretation of the data may be confounded by subtle variables in methods and design [55]. It appears that while survival has improved, some clinical subsets of ulcerative colitis such as pancolitis and older age may still have reduced life expectancy. Indeed, it has been speculated that a higher mortality rate from cancers or infections might be the price paid for avoiding colectomy [55].

What to tell patients

Perhaps the most important thing to tell patients is that they should take some responsibility for their own management. A minimal expectation should be that patients know precisely the names and dosages of their medications and have a reasonable understanding and perspective on the risks, benefits and alternatives of the different drug strategies. As with any chronic disease, patients who are well informed at the outset are likely to comply with medical advice and not seek cures by doctor-hopping. Removing fear of the unknown by frank discussion of prognosis and worst case scenarios is important for some patients. It may also be helpful to let patients observe the colonoscopic appearance of themselves while in relapse and remission so that they have a tangible rather than abstract understanding of the disease process. With regard to the risk of developing colon cancer, patients and physicians need to know that the risk increases with time but the ability of the clinician to detect it by colonoscopic surveillance is limited and may not change over time. Patients need to be aware of the difficulty distinguishing Crohn's disease from ulcerative colitis and that an absolute guarantee cannot be given in advance of surgery. It is increasingly important to document that patients have been advised of drug side-effects. In explaining the risk of side effects, simple language that places risk in perspective is essential. For example, if the risk of developing a lymphoma while on immunosuppressive or immunomodulatory drugs is thought to be about 6/10 000, it is helpful to place this in context by informing the patient that the lifetime risk of developing colon cancer in the general population is about 6/100.

For patients who wish to join or make contact with support groups and sources of patient-oriented information, the following sources are recommended: in the United States, the Crohn's and Colitis Foundation of America (http://www.ccfa.org); in Europe the European Federation of Crohn's and Ulcerative colitis associations (EFCCA, http://www.efcca.org) and similar national organizations are easy to access by the internet in other continents.

Current controversies and their future resolution

The biotech and genotech boom has made it possible to develop drug strategies that mimic or antagonize any mediator or receptor involved in the inflammatory cascade. Thus, drug development is no longer a problem, but prediction of individual responsiveness and the development of biomarkers including pharmacogenomics to facilitate individualized treatment are now required and are being pursued.

Most drug strategies are directed toward suppression of the host inflammatory or immune response. In this respect, it is likely that the next group of immunomodulators to be introduced to the clinic will be antagonism of mucosal homing of lymphocytes by monoclonal inhibition of α-4 integrins. However, the role of the bacterial flora in relation to the pathogenesis of colitis, which may be permissive or stimulatory, will drive research into the therapeutic manipulation of the enteric microbial microenvironment with prebiotics and probiotics.

For patients who avoid colectomy with improved medical therapy, there is an acute need to resolve the deficiencies of current dysplasia practices. New molecular markers for identifying those at increased risk of neoplasia are likely to emerge, and targeting of endoscopic biopsy material may be improved by techniques such as chromoendoscopy.

Irrespective of advances in molecular medicine and diagnostics, the traditional principles of good patient care are unlikely to be replaced. The science of the art of the doctor-patient relationship can still be a fruitful area of research. For example, if the mechanisms underlying the placebo response were understood, and if the conditions favoring enhancement of the response could be harnessed, the outcome for most patients could be improved substantially.

SOURCES OF INFORMATION FOR PATIENTS AND DOCTORS

patients.uptodate.com/topic.asp?file=digestiv/10728
www.clevelandclinic.org/gastro/ibd/patient/colitis.htm
www.patient.co.uk/showdoc/23068968
www.patient.co.uk/showdoc/611/
www.gastro.org
www.nacc.org.uk/content/home.asp

References

1. Truelove SC, Witts LT. Cortisone in ulcerative colitis: a final report on a therapeutic trial. *Br Med J.* 1955;2:1041–1048.
2. Bernstein CN, Shanahan F. Disorders of a modern lifestyle-reconciling the epidemiology of inflammatory bowel diseases. *Gut.* 2008;57:1185–1191.
3. Shanahan F, Bernstein CN. The evolving epidemiology of inflammatory bowel disease. *Curr Opin Gastroenterol.* 2009;25: 301–305.
4. Farrell RJ, Peppercorn MA. Ulcerative colitis. *Lancet.* 2002;359: 331–340.
5. Koutroubakis IE, Vlachonikolis IG, Kouroumalis EA. Role of appendicitis and appendectomy in the pathogenesis of ulcerative colitis: a critical review. *Inflamm Bowel Dis.* 2002;8:277–286.
6. Mizoguch A. Misoguchi E, Chiba C, *et al.* Role of the appendix in the development of inflammatory bowel disease in TCR-alpha mutant mice. *J Exp Med.* 1996;184:707–715.
7. Andersson RE, Olaison G, Tysk C, *et al.* Appendectomy and protection against ulcerative colitis. *N Engl J Med.* 2001;15;344: 808–814.
8. Frisch M, Pedeersen BV, Andersson RE. Appendicitis, mesenteric lymphadenitis, and subsequent risk of ulcerative colitis: cohort studies in Sweden and Denmark. *BMJ.* 2009;338:b716.
9. Abraham C, Cho JH. Inflammatory bowel disease. *N Engl J Med.* 2009;361:2066–2078.
10. UK IBD Genetics Consortium, Barrett JC, Lee JC, *et al.* Genome-wide association study of ulcerative colitis identifies three new susceptibility loci, including the HNF4A region. *Nat Genet.* 2009;41:1330–1334.
11. Asano K, Matsushita T, Umeno J, *et al.* A genome-wide association study identifies three new susceptibility loci for ulcerative colitis in the Japanese population. *Nat Genet.* 2009;41:1325–1329.
12. Shanahan F. Gut Microbes: from bugs to drugs. *Am J Gastroenterol.* 2010;105:275–279.
13. Strober W, Fuss IJ, Blumberg RS. The immunology of mucosal models of inflammation. *Annu Rev Immunol.* 2002;20:495–549.
14. Garrett WS, Lord GM, Punit S, *et al.* Communicable ulcerative colitis induced by T-bet deficiency in the innate immune system. *Cell.* 2007;131:33–45.
15. Froese DP, Haggitt RC, Friend WG. Ulcerative colitis in the autotransplanted neovagina. *Gastroenterology.* 1991;100:1749–1752.
16. Mawdsley JE, Rampton DS. The role of psychological stress in inflammatory bowel disease. *Neuroimmunomodulation.* 2006;13: 327–336.
17. Orchard T. Extraintestinal complications of inflammatory bowel disease. *Curr Gastroenterol Rep.* 2003;5:512–517.
18. Shanahan F. Host-flora interactions in inflammatory bowel disease. *Inflamm Bowel Dis.* 2004; 10 Suppl 1: S16–S24.
19. Mayer L. Evolving paradigms in the pathogenesis of IBD. *J Gastroenterol.* 2010;45:9–16.
20. Bernstein CN, Shanahan F, Weinstein WM. Patchiness of mucosal inflammation in treated ulcerative colitis. A prospective study. *Gastrointest Endosc.* 1995;42:232–237.
21. Walmsley RS, Ayres RCS, Pounder RE, Allen RN. A simple clinical colitis activity index. *Gut.* 1998;43:29–32.
22. Shanahan F. Inflammatory bowel disease: immunodiagnostics, immunotherapeutics and ecotherapeutics. *Gastroenterology.* 2001;120:622–635.
23. Quinton J-F, Sendid B, Reumaux D, *et al.* Anti-Saccharomyces cerevisiae mannan antibodies combined with antineutrophil cytoplasmic autoantibodies in inflammatory bowel disease: prevalence and diagnostic role. *Gut.* 1998;42:788–791.
24. Joossens S, Reinisch W, Vermeire S, *et al.* The value of serologic markers in indeterminate colitis: a prospective follow-up study. *Gastroenterology.* 2002;122:1242–1247.
25. American Gastroenterological Association: medical position statement: guidelines on osteoporosis in gastrointestinal diseases. *Gastroenterology.* 2003;124:791–794.
26. Bernstein CN, Leslie WD, Leboff MS. AGA technical review on osteoporosis in gastrointestinal diseases. *Gastroenterology.* 2003;124:795–841.
27. Travis SPK, Stange EF, Lemann M, *et al.* European evidence-based consensus on the management of ulcerative colitis: current management. *J Crohns Colitis.* 2008;2:24–62.
28. Faubion WA Jr, Loftus EV Jr, Harmsen WS, *et al.* The natural history of corticosteroid therapy for inflammatory bowel disease: a population-based study. *Gastroenterology.* 2001;121: 255–260.
29. Rutgeerts P, Sandborn WJ, Feagan BG, *et al.* Infliximab for induction and maintenance therapy for ulcerative colitis. *N Engl J Med.* 2005;353:2462–2476.
30. Hanauer SB, Rutgeerts P, Clark M, *et al.* AGA institute consensus development conference on the use of biologics in the treatment of inflammatory bowel disease. *Gastroenterology.* 2007;133:312–339.

Small and Large Bowel

31. Rahier JF, Ben-Horin S, Chowers Y, *et al.* European evidence-based consensus on the prevention, diagnosis and management of opportunistic infections in inflammatory bowel disease. *J Crohns Colitis.* 2009; dol:10.1016/j.crohns.2009.02.010.

32. Feagan BG. Maintenance therapy for inflammatory bowel disease. *Am J Gastroenterol.* 2003;98:Suppl. S6–S17.

33. Sandborn WJ, Yednock TA. Novel approaches to treating inflammatory bowel disease: targeting alpha-4 integrin. *Am J Gastroenterol.* 2003;98:2372–2382.

34. Summers RW, Elliott DE, Urban Jr JF, *et al.* Trichuris suis therapy for active ulcerative colitis: a randomised controlled trial. *Gastroenterology.* 2005;128:825–832.

35. Shanahan F. Physiological basis for novel drug therapies used to treat the inflammatory bowel diseases I. Pathophysiological basis and prospects for probiotic therapy in inflammatory bowel disease. *Am J Physiol Gastrointest Liver Physiol.* 2005;288: G417–G421.

36. Sandborn WJ. Pouchitis following ileal pouch-anal anastomosis: definition, pathogenesis, and treatment. *Gastroenterology.* 1994;107:1856–1860.

37. Gionchietti P, Rizzello F, Venturi A, *et al.* Oral bacteriotherapy as maintenance treatment in patients with chronic pouchitis: a double blind, placebo-controlled trial. *Gastroenterology.* 2000;119: 305–309.

38. Mimura T, Rizzello F, Helwig U, *et al.* Once daily high dose probiotic therapy (VSL#3) for maintaining remission in recurrent or refractory pouchitis. *Gut.* 2004;53:108–114.

39. Rutter M, Saunders B, Wilkinson K, *et al.* Severity of inflammation is a risk factor for colorectal neoplasia in ulcerative colitis. *Gastroenterology.* 2004;126:451–459.

40. Eaden JA, Abrams KR, Mayberry JF. The risk of colorectal cancer in ulcerative colitis: a meta-analysis. *Gut.* 2001;48:526–535.

41. Shetty K, Rybicki L, Brzezinski A, *et al.* The risk for cancer or dysplasia in ulcerative colitis patients with primary sclerosing cholangitis. *Am J Gastroenterol.* 1999; 94: 1643–1649.

42. Nuako KW, Ahlquist DA, Mahoney DW, *et al.* Familial predisposition for colorectal cancer in chronic ulcerative colitis: a case control study. *Gastroenterology.* 1998;115:1079–1083.

43. Heuschen UA, Hinz U, Allemeyer EH, *et al.* Backwash ileitis is strongly associated with colorectal carcinoma in ulcerative colitis. *Gastroenterology.* 2001;120:841–847.

44. Shanahan F. Relation between colitis and colon cancer. *Lancet.* 2001;357:246–247.

45. Brentnall TA. Molecular underpinnings of cancer in ulcerative colitis. *Curr Opin Gastroenterol.* 2003;19:64–68.

46. Shanahan F. Colitis-associated cancer – time for new strategies. *Aliment Pharmacol Ther.* 2003;18 Suppl 2:6–9.

47. Bernstein CN. The color of dysplasia in UC. *Gastroenterology.* 2003;124:1135–1138.

48. Rubin CE, Haggitt RC, Burmer GC, *et al.* DNA aneuploidy in colonic biopsies predicts future development of dysplasia in ulcerative colitis. *Gastroenterology.* 1992; 103: 1611–1620.

49. Ullman T, Croog V, Harpaz N, *et al.* Progression of flat low-grade dysplasia to advanced neoplasia in patients with ulcerative colitis. *Gastroenterology.* 2003;125:1311–1319.

50. Lakatos PL, Lakatos L. Risk for colorectal cancer in ulcerative colitis: changes, causes and management strategies. *World J Gastroenterol.* 2008;14:3937–3947.

51. Rutter MD, Saunders BP, Wilkinson KH, *et al.* Thirty-year analysis of a colonoscopic surveillance program for neoplasia in ulcerative colitis. *Gastroenterology.* 2006;130:1030–1038.

52. Bernstein CN, Blanchard JF, Metge C, *et al.* Does the use of 5-aminosalicylates in inflammatory bowel disease prevent the development of colorectal cancer? *Am J Gastroenterol.* 2003;98: 2784–2788.

53. Ilnychyj A, Shanahan F, Anton PA, *et al.* The placebo response in ulcerative colitis. *Gastroenterology.* 1997;112:1854–1858.

54. Robinson A, Thompson DG, Wilkin D, *et al.* Guided self-management and patient-directed follow-up of ulcerative colitis: a randomised trial. *Lancet.* 2001;358:976–981.

55. Loftus Jr. E.V. Mortality in inflammatory bowel disease. *Gastroenterology.* 2003;125:1881–1895.

CHAPTER 50
Crohn's disease

Séverine Vermeire,[1] Gert Van Assche[2] and Paul Rutgeerts[2]
[1]University Hospital Gasthuisberg, Leuven, Belgium
[2]University of Leuven, Leuven, Belgium

Small and Large Bowel

ESSENTIAL FACTS ABOUT PATHOGENESIS

- Crohn's disease has a multifactorial etiology
- Mucosal inflammation originates from an abnormal activation of the mucosal immune system in the gut, due to loss of tolerance against bacterial antigens in a genetically predisposed individual
- Crohn's disease is characterized by a T-helper 1 and 17 cytokine response
- Advances in inflammatory bowel disease genetics have identified more than 50 Crohn's disease genes, of which the *NOD2/CARD15* gene has been most studied
- The best recognized environmental factor that predisposes to Crohn's disease is cigarette smoking
- A general dysbiosis has been described in Crohn's disease and the most replicated findings have been the association of adherent-invasive *Escherichia coli* and a reduction in the number of *Faecalibacterium prausnitzii*

ESSENTIALS OF DIAGNOSIS

- Referral from primary to secondary care is often delayed by a failure to distinguish Crohn's disease from irritable bowel syndrome
- Laboratory findings that raise the suspicion of Crohn's disease include a raised platelet count, sedimentation rate or C-reactive protein, anemia or hypoalbuminemia
- Colonoscopy is used to obtain histological confirmation of terminal ileum or large bowel involvement
- Discontinuous inflammation and non-caseating granulomata are highly suggestive of Crohn's disease
- Increasingly, magnetic resonance imaging is preferred to barium studies for small bowel imaging because of the hazards of cumulative eradication
- Capsule endoscopy allows visualization of a small bowel mucosa

---

ESSENTIALS OF TREATMENT

- Salicylates are of limited efficacy
- Corticosteroids, including budesonide, methotrexate, and anti-TNF agents, are all superior to placebo and aminosalicylates for induction of remission
- Immunosuppressive drugs (azathioprine, 6-mercaptapurine or methotrexate) and anti-TNF agents are effective for consolidation and maintenance of remission
- Combining an anti-TNF and immunosuppressive agent is superior to either treatment alone
- Choice of traditional treatment escalation (bottom up) versus initial intensive (top down) treatment varies from country to country
- Metronidazole and ciprofloxacin are valuable, particularly as adjunctive treatment in perianal disease

---

Introduction and definition

Crohn's disease is a chronic inflammatory disease of the gastrointestinal tract that develops mostly in young people between the ages of 15 and 25 years. Common symptoms include diarrhea, abdominal cramps, and weight loss. The exact cause of the disease is still unknown, but current data suggest that the gut flora triggers sustained inflammation in a genetically susceptible host [1]. In this chapter, an overview on the different aspects of Crohn's disease is given, including the epidemiology, pathogenesis, clinical presentation, (differential) diagnosis, complications, and treatment.

Although clinical descriptions of diarrhea and blood loss go back thousands of years, clear descriptions of ulceration and enteritis date only from the 19th century. Doctors at Mount Sinai Hospital in New York had shown interest in tuberculosis-like ileocecal enteritis without the presence of tubercle bacilli. On December 11th 1931, Dr Burril Crohn wrote to the American Gastroenterological Association: "I have an important scientific contribution I would like to present before the American Gastroenterological Association. I have discovered, I believe, a new intestinal disease, which we have named Terminal Ileitis. I would like to present the facts before the Association in connection with the general subject of Benign Granulomata of the Intestinal Tract . . .". Burril Crohn, together with his colleagues Ginzburg and Oppenheimer, presented their findings in May 1932 to the American Gastroenterological Association. The report was followed later that year by the landmark article entitled "Regional ileitis: a pathologic and clinical entity," by the same authors [2].

Epidemiology

Almost eight decades later, the exact cause of Crohn's disease remains unknown, although the **incidence** is higher, having risen between the 1950s and 1970s [3]. In Copenhagen, Denmark, the incidence rose from 1 to 4.1 per 100 000 per year between 1962 and 1987 [4]. With a prevalence of 1–2 per 1000, the disease has become an important entity in North America and Western Europe [3,5,6]. The incidence of Crohn's disease now averages 5–6 per 100 000 population and has been increasing worldwide, although the increase has been slowing in

---

highly affected countries [3]. The onset of the disease occurs most often in the second or third decade of life, but a second and smaller peak is seen between 50 and 60 years.

Geographic variations

Geographically, there is a **north–south gradient** in many countries of the northern hemisphere [7]. In Europe, age-adjusted incidence rates of 10 cases per 100000 have been reported for Norway [8] versus 0.9 per 100000 for Spain [9] and 3.4 per 100000 in Italy [10]. There is also something of an West–East gradient, with low incidence rates in Japan. This West–East gradient may reflect differences in lifestyle, although important ethnic differences are observed. The highest risk occurs in **Ashkenazi Jews**, who are reported to have a 2–8-fold greater risk, followed by North American and northern European Caucasian people. African-Americans and Asians carry the lowest risk. Other ethnic groups, such as the Roma gypsies in Hungary, have a considerably lower prevalence than the average surrounding population.

Inheritance

Family studies have further underscored the genetic etiology of the disease. They have shown the risk for a patient with inflammatory bowel disease (IBD) of having a first-degree relative who suffers from the same disease to be around 10% [11–13]. Hence first-degree relatives of patients with Crohn's disease are 10 times more likely also to develop the disease. Familial aggregation data further suggest the λs (relative risk of disease for a sibling of an affected individual) to be around 15–30 for Crohn's disease [5–7] (Table 50.1). Important direct evidence for genetic factors comes from twin studies (Table 50.2). The published twin studies have shown that concordance rates in monozygotic twins are much higher than those in dizygotic twins (33% versus 4%) [14–16]. There has also been significant phenotypic concordance described in monozygotic concordant pairs with Crohn's disease in contrast to ulcerative colitis, both at diagnosis and longitudinally, supporting a genetic influence not only on disease occurrence but also on disease course [17]. However, as the concordance is not 100%, non-genetic, environmental factors must also be involved.

Table 50.1 Family studies in inflammatory bowel disease, implicating the relative risk to a sibling

Reference	Relative risk of Crohn's disease
Orholm et al. [12]	10
Satsangi et al. [13]	15–35
Peeters et al. [11]	13

Table 50.2 Concordance for Crohn's disease in twin studies

Reference	Concordance	
	Monozygotic twins	Dizygotic twins
Tysk et al. [14]	8/18 (44%)	1/26 (4%)
Thompson et al. [15]	5/25 (20%)	3/46 (7%)
Orholm et al. [16]	5/10 (50%)	0/27

Causes, risk factors, and disease associations

Crohn's disease is a chronic inflammatory disease with a complex and multifactorial etiology. The current hypothesis is that a normal luminal flora drives an inappropriate activation of the mucosal immune system in a genetically susceptible host and that this activation is triggered by yet unknown environmental factors. To date, very few risk factors have been identified; **smoking** is probably the best known [3,18]. Smokers have not only an increased risk for the development of Crohn's disease (Table 50.3), but also present with more severe disease in comparison with non-smoking patients and have a higher relapse rate for the disease after surgery [18,19]. Despite these well described associations, the mechanism by which cigarette smoking affects Crohn's disease is not known.

Several studies have shown that high levels of **hygiene** in childhood predispose to Crohn's disease [3], an observation that could plausibly explain the rise in incidence during the 20th century. Most studies have found breastfeeding to be protective, an observation that might imply importance for early immune programming.

Diet has been proposed to be an important etiologic factor. Patients with Crohn's disease are more likely to eat a diet high in unrefined carbohydrates, but whether this is causal or consequential is unclear.

Infectious agents have been put forward as risk factors, and one of the most discussed putative agents has been *Mycobacterium avium* subspecies *paratuberculosis*. *M. avium* is an acid-fast bacillus that causes Johne's disease (enteritis) in cattle. Whether it can cause Crohn's disease is controversial and any mode of transmission is unclear, but some evidence suggests that humans may become infected via contaminated milk [20].

Crohn's disease has been associated with **other immune-mediated disorders** such as psoriasis, ankylosing spondylitis, multiple sclerosis, and arthritis. In addition, associations with rare genetic diseases such as the Hermansky–Pudlak syndrome and Turner syndrome have been described.

Pathogenesis

The current idea about the pathophysiology of IBD is that the intestinal flora, in conjunction with yet unidentified environmental factors, triggers and drives an aberrant immune

Table 50.3 Effect of smoking on risk of Crohn's disease

Small and Large Bowel

Reference	Year	Study period	Site of disease	Data collection	Length of follow-up	Outcome Non smokers	Smokers	Ex-smokers	Statistical analysis
Sutherland et al. [110]	1990	1966–1983	SB + IC + LB	Questionnaire	Mean 10–8 years	Reoperation rate (n = 85) 5 years 29% 10 years 41%	(n = 89) 5 years 36% 10 years 70%		p = 0.007 RR 2.1
Lindberg et al. [111]	1992	No record	SB + IC + LB	Questionnaire	10 years	Reoperation rate 10 years postop. (n = 81) 26%	(n = 54) 42% (heavy smokers: >10/day)		p = 0.015 RR 1.79
Cottone et al. [112]	1994	1973–1991	SB + IC + LB	Questionnaire	Mean 8–2 years	(n = 53) Clinical recurrence[a] rate 6 years postop. 40% Reoperation rate 6 years postop. 8% Endoscopic recurrence rate 1 year postop. 35%	(n = 110) 73% 24% 70%	(n = 19) 59% 21% 27%	p = 0.006[c] RR 1.4 p = 0.005[c] RR 2.0 p = 0.002[c] RR 4.3
Breuer-Katschinski et al. [113]	1996	1989–1992	SB + IC + LB	Questionnaire	No record	Reoperation rate (n = 143) 5 years 26% 10 years 33%	(n = 144) 5 years 43% 10 years 64%		p < 0.00 RR 3.1
Cosnes et al. [114]	1996	1974–1995	SB + IC + LB	Personal interview	No record	Crude reoperation rate (n = 89) 22%	(n = 115) 30%		n.s.
Timmer et al. [115]	1998	1990–1993	SB + IC + LB	Personal interview	48 weeks	Relapse[b] rate 48 weeks postop. (n = 53) 30%	(n = 59) 53%	(n = 40) 35%	p = 0.02[c] RR 2.1
Medina et al. [116]	1998	No record	SB + IC + LB	No record	No record	Crude symptomatic recurrence rate (n = 14) 86%	(n = 26) 50%		n.s.
Yamamoto & Keighley [117]	1999	1975–1990	IC alone	Personal interview and questionnaire	Median 8–1 years	Reoperation rate (n = 79) 5 years 19% 10 years 36%	(n = 62) 5 years 35% 10 years 55%		p = 0.007 RR 2.3
Yamamoto et al. [118]	1999	1960–1996	LB alone	Personal interview and questionnaire	Median 18–6 years	Reoperation rate (n = 36) 5 years 11% 10 years 15% 15 years 18%	(n = 33) 5 years 25% 10 years 46% 15 years 52%		p = 0.005 RR 3.0

CDAI, Crohn's Disease Activity Index; IC, ileocecal; LB, large bowel; n.s. not significant; RR, relative risk; SB, small bowel. [a]CDAI > 150; [b]CDAI > 150 or increase of CDAI > 60; [c]smokers *versus* non-smokers.

response in a genetically susceptible host, resulting in chronic inflammation of the gut (Figure 50.1).

Genetics

The genetic predisposition is based on several lines of evidence, including wide variations in the incidence and prevalence of Crohn's disease among different populations, co-segregation of the disease with a variety of uncommon Mendelian and more common polygenic disorders (Figure 50.2), and familial aggregation of the disease [11–13]. As previously explained, first-degree relatives of an affected patient have a risk of IBD that is **4–20 times** as high as that among the background population; the absolute risk of IBD is approximately **7%** among first-degree family members. In multicase families (three or more cases of IBD), both genetic and environmental factors cluster and we recently described a 57-fold increase in incidence of IBD among first-degree relatives in such families [21].

In the past decade and since the start of genetic research in other complex disorders, great advances have been made and more than 50 susceptibility genes or loci have so far been identified through genome-wide linkage and association studies (Figure 50.3). The first gene for Crohn's disease, *NOD2/CARD15*, was identified in 2001 [22,23]. This gene encodes a cytoplasmic protein designated Nod2 and is expressed in monocytes/macrophages, epithelial cells, and Paneth cells, where it serves as an intracellular cytosolic pattern-recognition receptor (PRR) for peptidoglycan-derived muramyldipeptide. It therefore represents a key player in the innate immune system and is involved in the regulation of nuclear factor-kappa B activation and controlled cell death (apoptosis) [24]. Around 40% of Crohn's disease patients of West European or North American origin carry at least one of the three major disease-associated variants (R702W, G908R, L1007fsinsC) in Nod2, compared with only 0.5–20% of healthy controls [25,26]. Individuals carrying these variants have an increased and dose-dependent risk of developing Crohn's disease. Whereas the relative risk is two to four times higher in subjects heterozygous for any one of the variants, it increases to over **20-fold** in homozygous or compound heterozygous subjects.

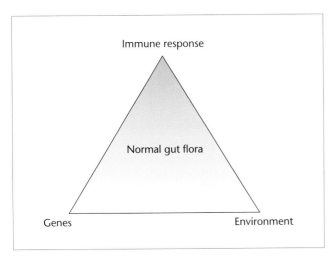

Figure 50.1 Current pathogenic model of Crohn's disease. (This figure was published in *Clinical Gastroenterology and Hepatology*, Wilfred M. Weinstein, Christopher J. Hawkey, Jaime Bosch, Crohn's disease, Pages 359–376, Copyright Elsevier, 2005.)

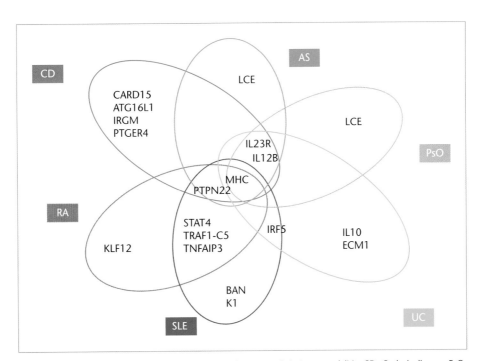

Figure 50.2 Genetic flower: genetic classification of immune-mediated disorders. AS, ankylosing spondylitis; CD, Crohn's disease; PsO, psoriasis; RA, rheumatoid arthritis; SLE, systemic lupus erythematosus; UC, ulcerative colitis.

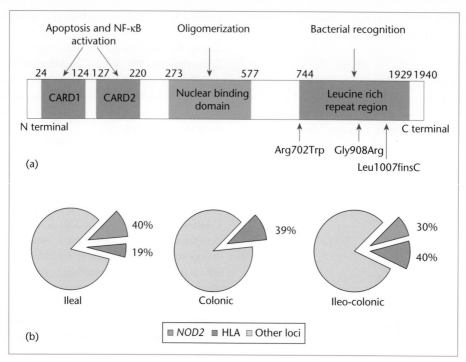

Figure 50.3 Genetic influences on inflammatory bowel disease. (a) Structure of the *NOD2* gene and sites of polymorphism. (b) Proportional contribution of *NOD2* polymorphisms to Crohn's disease at different sites. (Adapted with permission from Hugot JP, Chamaillard M, Zouali H, *et al.* Association of CARD15 leucine-rich repeat variants with susceptibility to Crohn's disease. *Nature.* 2001;411:599–603.)

The variants are predominantly associated with a phenotype of **ileal inflammation**. This has been explained by the preferential expression of Nod2 in the **Paneth** cells at the base of the crypts of Lieberkühn, where the protein protects the multipotent stem cells and the epithelial barrier against bacteria by secretion of antimicrobial peptides (lysozyme and defensins). Both in animal models of colitis as well as in humans with Crohn's disease, a lack of human **alpha-defensins** (HD-5 and HD-6) has been demonstrated, regardless of the *NOD2* genetic status [27,28]. However, the expression of defensins is even further reduced in *NOD2* mutant carriers. Whether the three *NOD2* variants really lead to a loss or gain of function of the Nod2 receptor is still subject to controversy, and by which mechanisms this change in function increases the susceptibility to Crohn's disease is still under investigation.

A recent pathway that has been identified through the results of the genome-wide association studies (GWAS) is the **autophagy pathway**. A non-synonymous SNP in *ATG16L1* (rs2241880 or Thr300Ala), and several non-coding polymorphisms within and around the *IRGM* gene were found to be highly associated with Crohn's disease [29–31]. Autophagy (derived from the Greek for "self-eating") is a fundamental biological process, originally described as an adaptation of the yeast cell to starvation, and is highly conserved amongst eukaryotes. Through the formation of **autophagosomes**, damaged or excess cell organelles are degraded and recycled, in support of cellular anabolic needs. Relatively recently, it has become clear that autophagy has other important roles, namely

in **cell death** and in the **defense against micro-organisms**. The process not only plays a role in the sequestration and direct elimination of intracellular pathogens (viruses, parasites, and bacteria), but it is also implicated in antigen presentation to the innate and adaptive immune system. Especially in the gut mucosa, exposed to a dense microbial load, the contribution of autophagy to host defense may be important. It is clear that, although some of the effects on immune regulation and bacterial clearance may explain the link between *ATG16L1*, *IRGM*, and Crohn disease, more research is needed in order to determine if defective or excessive autophagy determines this risk.

Immunology

Acute inflammation in the gut of patients with Crohn's disease is characterized by infiltration of granulocytes and mononuclear cells, and by epithelial cell necrosis [32]. The chronic phase of the transmural inflammation is frequently accompanied by fibrosis and bowel strictures. The mucosal inflammation in established Crohn's disease is dominated by CD4+ lymphocytes with a type 1 helper T cell (Th1) and Th17 phenotype (see Figure 50.1), characterized by the production of interferon-γ and interleukin (IL)-2 and IL-17.

These cytokines activate macrophages, which in turn produce IL-12, IL-18, and macrophage migration inhibitory factor, which further stimulate Th1 cells in a self-sustaining cycle. Just as importantly, activated macrophages produce a potent mix of cytokines, which amplify the inflammatory reaction. These cytokines include tumor necrosis factor (TNF)-α, IL-1, IL-6, chemokines, and growth factors, as well as metabolites of arachidonic acid (e.g., prostaglandins and leukotrienes) and reactive oxygen metabolites such as nitric oxide.

A central signaling molecule in macrophages is the transcription factor **NF-κB**. Inflammation in Crohn's disease is characterized by increased expression of **adhesion molecules** on endothelial cells and leukocytes. This is responsible for further recruitment of additional leukocytes from the vascular space to sites of disease activity, and is important in maintaining inflammation. There is increasing evidence that these inflammatory events are due to loss of tolerance against bacterial antigens. An important mechanism of tolerance induction is **cell apoptosis**, the physiological process of programmed cell death. This balance between T-cell death and survival is essential to maintain immune homeostasis. In Crohn's disease, there appears to be a resistance to apoptotic stimuli and this is further underscored by an increased Bcl-2/Bax ratio in the inflamed mucosa, and decreased Bax expression with a high Bclx1/Bax ratio in isolated mucosal T cells [33]. Monocytes/macrophages are also important in providing the first line of intestinal defense, and abnormal apoptosis of monocytes/macrophages may be relevant to the pathogenesis of IBD.

Bacteria

Observations derived from patients suffering from Crohn's disease or ulcerative colitis, and from experimental animal models of colitis, show that the **gut microflora** is involved in the etiopathogenesis of IBD. Crohn's disease lesions are located mainly in regions of the gut colonized by large numbers of bacteria (ileum, colon), and diversion of the fecal stream from inflamed sites often results in clinical improvement in the patient and prevents postoperative recurrence of Crohn disease [34]. Moreover, infusion of intestinal contents into excluded ileum of patients with Crohn's disease re-induced inflammation [35]. An increased association of luminal bacteria with the mucous layer of patients with IBD compared with controls has been reported. Antibiotic therapy results in transient clinical improvement of Crohn disease, and treatment with metronidazole/ornidazole prevents recurrence of Crohn disease after surgery to some extent [36,37]. Results from experiments on germ-free rodents with a dysfunctional immune system (gene knockout or transgenic animals), in which intestinal inflammation is absent, have indicated that bacteria are indispensable contributors to the pathogenesis of the chronic intestinal inflammation.

Despite many attempts, **specific pathogens** have not been identified as the cause of IBD. *M. paratuberculosis*, *Listeria monocytogenes*, and measles virus have been candidate pathogens, but data have been inconclusive so far. The hypothesis that a gut microbiota of "abnormal composition" might be present has also not been proven, but this is extremely difficult to study. With conventional methods, up to 90% of the total microscopic count cannot be cultured.

More recently, culture-independent techniques have shown that the microbiota in patients with IBD is characterized by high concentrations of bacteria in contact with the mucosa, instability, presence of high numbers of unusual bacteria, and reduction in the biodiversity. This complex phenomenon is also called **dysbiosis** and is believed to be crucial in the pathogenesis of the disease [38]. Swidsinski *et al.* performed cultures of washed colonoscopic biopsies of Crohn's disease patients and validated microbial cultures by quantitative polymerase chain reaction (PCR) with subsequent cloning and sequencing, fluorescence *in situ* hybridization, and electron microscopy. The authors found high concentrations of mucosal bacteria in patients with bowel inflammation and a correlation was seen with the severity of the disease [39].

The group of Colombel in Lille have isolated *Escherichia coli* strains from ileal biopsy specimen of patients with Crohn's disease that are able to adhere to and invade cultured epithelial cells. These adherent invasive *E. coli* (AIEC) are able to survive and replicate in macrophages without inducing cell death of the infected cells [40–42]. The cells, however, release high levels of TNF-α. Several groups have confirmed these findings and further shown that the number of *E. coli* seems restricted to inflamed mucosa and correlates with the severity of ileal disease. Besides the AIEC which are associated with Crohn disease, the group of Joel Dore in Paris showed that *Faecalibacterium prausnitzii* is underrepresented in Crohn disease patients in mucosal samples [43]. *F. prausnitzii* is a butyrate-producing bacteria of which the anti-inflammatory properties are being studied at present.

Bacterial antigens

There is evidence that patients with IBD have a **loss of tolerance** to specific bacterial and possibly also auto-antigens [44]. They display antibodies against oligomannan epitope [anti-*Saccharomyces cerevisiae* antibody (ASCA)], outer membrane protein C of *E. coli* (anti-OmpC), an epitope of *Pseudomonas fluorescens* (anti-I2), and pancreas proteins [pancreatic antibodies (PAB)] [45,46]. The epitopes for the different antibodies have either not been identified or it is not clear what the significance of the antibodies is, although higher antibody responses are observed in patients with more complicated disease, including strictures and fistulae [46].

Pathology

Inflammation in Crohn's disease is patchy and focal, at both the histological and the macroscopic level. Discontinuous bowel involvement with interspersed uninvolved segments (skip lesions) is typical of Crohn's disease . The earliest lesion of Crohn's disease is the aphthous ulceration (Figure 50.4a). Macroscopically, tiny ulcers are surrounded by a halo of erythema. Histologically, inflammation is focal. Microfistulization from aphthous ulcers is then associated with deeper inflammation that may be associated with cobblestoning (Figure 50.4c). Inflammation typically extends beyond the mucosa and through to the serosa (Figure 50.5). Increasing fistulization may result in macroscopic tracks between loops of bowel to

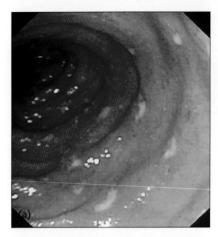
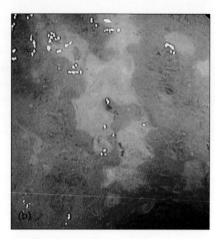
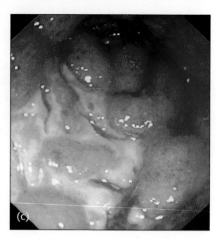

Figure 50.4 Mucosal ulceration in Crohn's disease. (a) Aphthous ulcers as the first manifestation of Crohn's disease. (b) Longitudinal ulcers in the colon, typical of Crohn's disease. (c) Serpiginous ulcers interspersed by nodular thickening – the typical cobblestone pattern.

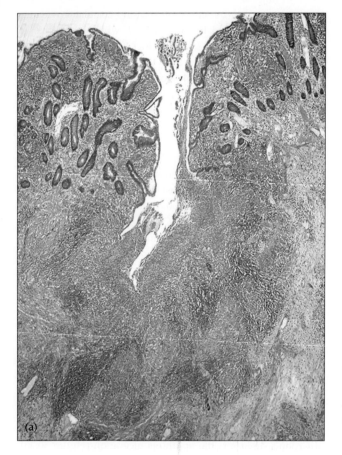
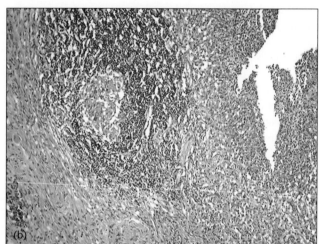
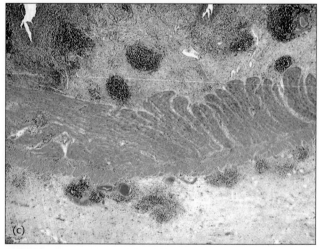

Figure 50.5 Histologic features in Crohn's disease. (a) Mucosal ulceration with microfissuring, and transmural inflammation with numerous lymphoid aggregates. (b) Microfissure with adjacent granuloma. (c) String of lymphoid aggregates on either side of muscularis propria in both mucosa and serosa. (Courtesy of Dr Philip Kaye, University Hospital, Nottingham, UK.)

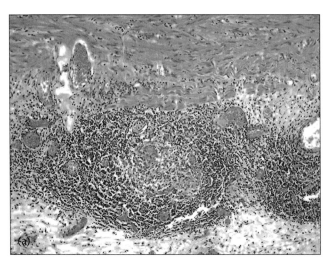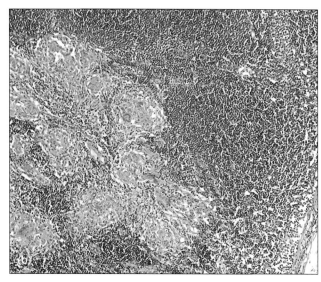

Figure 50.6 Granuloma in Crohn's disease. (a) In serosa. (b) In draining lymph node. (Courtesy of Dr Philip Kaye, University Hospital, Nottingham, UK.)

adjacent organs, or to the skin. Non-caseating granulomas, which are highly suggestive but not absolutely diagnostic of Crohn's disease, have been reported in 15–70% of patients (Figure 50.6).

Clinical presentation

Crohn's disease may typically affect the entire gastrointestinal tract from the mouth to the anus in a discontinuous and transmural way, with a preference for the terminal ileum and right colon. Clinical symptoms of Crohn's disease vary, but classically the most common symptoms have been:

- **Diarrhea**: this may arise by a number of mechanisms, including colonic involvement, bile acid malabsorption (especially after terminal ileal resection), and small bowel malabsorption
- **Weight loss**: may variously be due to inflammatory cachexia, malabsorption, and anorexia (Figure 50.7)
- **Abdominal pain**: most often located in the right lower quadrant (implying terminal ileal involvement).

Crohn's disease may present with more general symptoms, such as fatigue, anemia, or pyrexia of unknown origin.

Symptoms by site

The clinical features of Crohn's disease can thus be very variable, but in most cases are predictable from the site of disease:

- **Mouth:** oral Crohn disease is characterized by aphthous ulceration, often on a background of mucosal edema greater than that seen with simple mouth ulcers
- **Esophagus**: this is rare but may cause dysphagia or pain

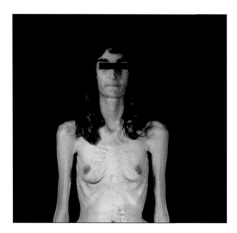

Figure 50.7 Patient with extensive small bowel Crohn's disease and extreme weight loss.

- **Stomach and duodenum**: asymptomatic gastric involvement is not uncommon. Duodenal involvement may result in typical ulcer symptoms. Stricturing may result in symptoms of gastric outlet obstruction
- **Small bowel**: diffuse extensive mucosa involvement can lead to malabsorption (see Chapter 39), protein-losing enteropathy (see Chapter 44), diarrhea (see Chapter 6), and sometimes steatorrhea. Segmental thickening or stricturing results in painful obstructive symptoms and may lead to bacterial overgrowth
- **Ileocecal involvement**: symptoms of obstruction due to inflammatory swelling or stricturing are common, with post-prandial bloating, pain, and borborygmi, particularly after consumption of fibrous vegetables or fruit. Transmural inflammation and local sepsis result in matting of local loops of bowel and a palpable inflammatory mass

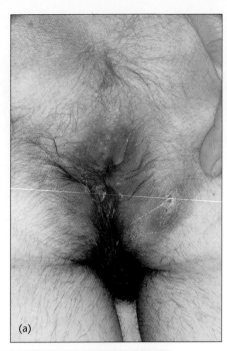 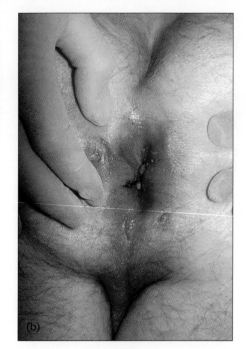

Figure 50.8 (a, b) Two examples of perianal Crohn's disease.

- **Colon**: typically, colonic involvement results in diarrhea that, in contrast to that seen in ulcerative colitis, is seldom bloody and more often associated with abdominal pain
- **Perianal disease**: nowadays, one of the first symptoms may also relate to perianal disease, and 20–80% of patients with Crohn's disease show anal involvement with abscesses, fistulae, or fissures (Figure 50.8). These account for considerable morbidity [47] (Figure 50.8).

The disease may behave in different ways in different individuals. Symptoms of post-prandial abdominal pain, abdominal distension, or nausea should raise the suspicion of a stricture. **Strictures** are characterized by narrowing of the lumen and thickening of the bowel wall, with or without prestenotic dilatation (Figure 50.9). Other symptoms, such as fecal loss per vagina or pneumaturia, imply the presence of fistulae to the vagina or bladder, respectively. Fistulae to the abdominal wall may result in a purulent or feculent discharge (Figure 50.10). Fistulae between loops of bowel may present with early passage of undigested food and otherwise unexplained weight loss.

Extraintestinal manifestations

Up to 40% of patients with Crohn's disease suffer from extraintestinal symptoms (Table 50.4, Figure 50.11). Some, such as erythema nodosum, iritis, or peripheral arthritis, occur intermittently at times of disease activity. Typically, the activity-related arthritis involves two or three medium-sized joints. Other extraintestinal symptoms, such as ankylosing spondylitis or sclerosing cholangitis, represent disease associations

unaffected by changes in Crohn's disease activity. Others, such as gallstones or renal stones, are a metabolic consequence of Crohn's disease or its treatment. Bile acid loss from malabsorption due to terminal ileal involvement or resection predisposes to gallstone formation. The consequently increased absorption of oxalate predisposes to renal stones. Extraintestinal manifestations of IBD are of importance because they may represent the only symptom index of disease activity. Moreover, they do not only follow intestinal symptoms, but sometimes precede them by years. Where extraintestinal manifestations reflect overall disease activity, treatment of the intestinal inflammation – either medical or surgical – usually helps in the resolution of these complications.

Special situations
Pediatric disease

Crohn's disease commonly presents in children and adolescents. Active disease impairs physical growth, and this may be the first symptom to come to light. Otherwise, children and adolescents suffer symptoms similar to those in adults, although the consequences of Crohn's disease for personal and sexual development may dominate the effect that Crohn's disease has in this age group.

Pregnancy

Overall, there appears to be little pregnancy-related variation in Crohn's disease activity, but women may display an individually stereotyped pattern of remission or relapse with successive pregnancies. Crohn's disease reduces fertility, implying that many women need to continue full treatment during

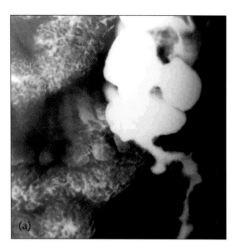
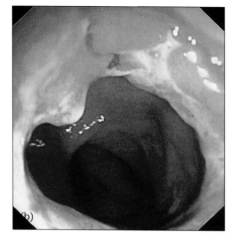
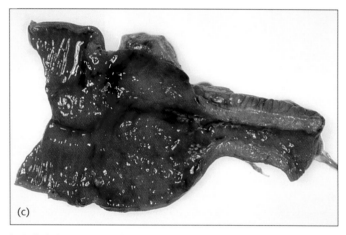

Figure 50.9 Fibrostenotic Crohn's disease. (a) Small-bowel follow-through of a Crohn's disease patient showing extensive involvement of the ileum with stenosis. (b) Crohn's disease colonic stricture. (c) Resected specimen showing fibrostenosis with proximal dilatation.

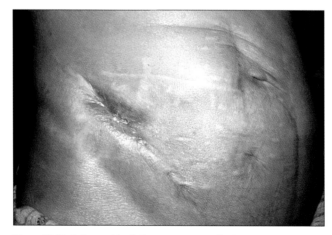

Figure 50.10 Active and healed enterocutaneous fistulae.

Table 50.4 Extraintestinal manifestations of IBD

Organ or system	Condition
Skin	Erythema nodosum[a]
	Pyoderma gangrenosum[a,b]
Joint	Peripheral arthritis[a]
	Sacroiliitis
	Ankylosing spondylitis
Eye	Iritis, uveitis, and episcleritis[a]
Biliary	Gallstones
	Sclerosing cholangitis[b]
	Cholangiocarcinoma[b]
Renal	Stones
	Amyloid

[a]Varies with bowel activity.
[b]More common in ulcerative colitis.

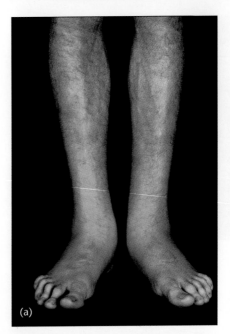
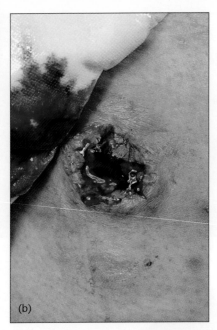
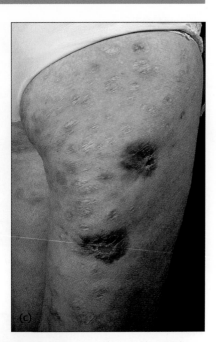

Figure 50.11 Some skin manifestations of Crohn's disease. (a) Erythema nodosum. (b) Active pyoderma gangrenosum. (c) Active pyoderma with multiple healed lesions. Activity of pyoderma gangrenosum generally follows bowel activity, but not always.

conception. (Male patients should cease sulfasalazine as this drug produces sperm abnormalities.) Active disease probably increases the rate of spontaneous abortion, premature labor, and stillbirth. Limited evidence suggests that most drugs are not harmful to the baby (with the exception of methotrexate), and certainly appear to pose less threat than active disease.

Proposed classifications

Given the heterogeneous presentation of Crohn disease, several classification systems have been proposed over the years. The most recent classification, also known as the Montreal classification, resulted from an international working party of the World Congress of Gastroenterology in 2005 [48] and includes:

- Age at diagnosis: younger than 16 years (A1), between 17 and 40 years (A2), and older than 40 years (A3).
- Location: terminal ileum (L1), colon (L2), ileocolon (L3), isolated upper gastrointestinal (L4) (L4 is a modifier that can be added to L1–L3 when concomitant upper gastrointestinal disease is present).
- Behavior: non-stricturing, non-penetrating (B1), stricturing (B2), penetrating (B3); p is perianal disease modifier and is added to B1–B3 when concomitant perianal disease is present.

Differential diagnosis

Initial diagnosis

Although Crohn's disease causes many symptoms, the diagnosis should not be difficult to make. Nevertheless, patients may take several years before the diagnosis is established, usually as a result of failure to distinguish it from irritable bowel syndrome. Gastrointestinal symptoms normally call attention to the part of the gastrointestinal tract involved, and endoscopy or radiology will show changes compatible with Crohn's disease. Under these circumstances, the challenge is often to establish that it is Crohn's disease rather than another pathology that is responsible for inflammation.

Systemic manifestations

Differential diagnosis is more difficult when the presentation is with predominantly **non-gastrointestinal symptoms**. Crohn's disease should enter into consideration in patients with pyrexia of unknown origin, failure to thrive or loss of weight (see Chapter 12), abdominal pain (see Chapter 19), intra-abdominal abscess (see Chapter 121), anemia [49] or extraintestinal manifestations such as erythema nodosum. Penetrating Crohn's disease in the ileocecal region may mimic appendicitis and/or cause iliopsoas irritation, infection, or abscess characterized clinically by pain on hip extension.

Acute infection

The clinical picture of Crohn's disease, certainly in the presence of an acute onset, is very similar to an acute infectious episode. *Yersinia* **infection** may resemble Crohn's disease, given its preferential location in the terminal ileum. Differential diagnosis also includes other colitides (vascular, drug induced, or toxic), and a check should always be made for a history of foreign travel, drug and medication intake, and sexual habits. Differential diagnosis with other disorders, such as lymphocytic or collagenous colitis, is another possibility. In its chronic phase, Crohn's disease is characterized by histological lesions very similar to those seen in **intestinal tuberculosis**. Mycobacteria (especially *M. paratuberculosis*) remain one of the putative causal agents of Crohn's disease, and antimycobacterial therapies have been tried [50].

Distinction from other colitides

Differential diagnosis between Crohn's disease and ulcerative colitis (see Chapter 49) can usually be made based on clinical, radiological, endoscopic, and histological determinations. Crohn's disease may affect any part of the gastrointestinal tract (most commonly the terminal ileum) and is characterized by the presence of discontinuous transmural inflammation, whereas ulcerative colitis affects only the large bowel in a continuous way and is restricted to the mucosa. Both diseases may be complicated by extraintestinal manifestations (skin, eyes, joint) or colorectal malignancy. Microscopic colitis (see Chapter 52) and infectious colitides can sometimes be difficult to distinguish, especially where inflammation is patchy. A precise classification for about 10–15% of patients presenting with colonic inflammation remains difficult in practice. These patients are categorized as having "indeterminate colitis" (see Chapter 51).

Diagnostic methods

The diagnosis of Crohn's disease is based on a combination of symptoms, radiological examination, endoscopy, and histological criteria. **Laboratory findings** consistent with Crohn's disease include a raised platelet count [51] or erythrocyte sedimentation rate, and increased levels of acute-phase proteins (particularly C-reactive protein), anemia due to iron, vitamin B_{12}, or folate deficiency, or chronic disease [49]. Hypoalbuminemia associated with protein-losing enteropathy, and deficiencies of vitamins and minerals, are fairly common. The inflammation in Crohn's disease typically affects the entire gastrointestinal tract. **Colonoscopy** is a frequent diagnostic maneuver [52]. Intestinal Crohn's disease is most frequently located in the terminal ileum, and in patients with colonic involvement, the rectum is often spared, making colonoscopy more appropriate than limited sigmoidoscopy. Discontinuous inflammation and aphthous or longitudinal ulcers are often seen as the first manifestation (see Figure 50.4a, b). At a later stage, serpiginous ulcers interspersed by nodular thickening (the so-called cobblestone pattern) occur (see Figure 50.4c). A **Crohn's Disease Endoscopic Index of Severity (CDEIS)** and simple endoscopic score for Crohn's disease (SES-CD) have been devised that have prognostic significance and are used principally in research [53,54]. **Histological changes** include an abnormal mucosal architecture and increased cellularity of the lamina propria with infiltration of neutrophils (see Figure 50.5). However, the histological hallmark of Crohn's disease is the **granuloma**, which is seldom found in ulcerative colitis [55]. A granuloma is defined as a collection of monocytes/macrophages and other inflammatory cells with or without giant cells, and is reported in 15–70% of patients. In contrast to tuberculosis, central necrosis and caseation are very rare, and should raise the suspicion of tuberculosis. Small-bowel follow-through (SBFT) remains an important radiological examination for assessing the extent of small bowel involvement and for detecting fistulous tracks or strictures (see Figure 50.9). SBFT should be performed at least once, usually at the time of diagnosis, in every patient.

Treatment and prevention

Medical treatment and treatment goals

Patients with Crohn's disease require extensive treatment because of the chronic relapsing nature of the disease. The medical advances in Crohn's disease over the past years have altered our treatment goals. Improvement of symptoms is no longer satisfactory and modification of the clinical course has become a major goal. With the therapeutic options available, the goals are to bring patients into remission, taper steroids and avoid their further use, maintain patients in remission, induce mucosal healing, and reduce hospitalizations and surgeries. In children, promotion of growth is an additional goal. Given that the clinical symptoms of Crohn's disease patients in part reflect transmural and/or superficial mucosal inflammation, treatments that induce healing of the intestinal mucosa may therefore provide particular clinical benefits. If a treatment induces profound and long-lasting mucosal healing, it may reduce complications, including the need for surgical interventions, and therefore it is hypothesized that such a drug could potentially slow down or even stop the progression of the disease. Medical management includes a combination of systemic corticosteroids, budesonide, immunosuppressive agents, antibiotic treatment, and biological therapies such as anti-TNF-α antibodies (infliximab, adalimumab, certolizumb pegol). Therapy can be divided into agents that are effective for induction of and for maintenance of remission.

Induction of remission

Drugs that have been shown to be effective in randomized controlled trials include sulfasalazine, antibiotics, budesonide, oral corticosteroids, infliximab, adalimumab, and certolizumab pegol.

Maintenance of remission

Patients who relapse within 6–12 months after discontinuation of induction therapy should be given induction therapy again, but should also receive maintenance therapy with an immunosuppressive agent (azathioprine, 6-mercaptopurine, or methotrexate) or anti-TNF (Figure 50.12). The degree of disease activity also plays a role: sulfasalazine and antibiotics are effective in mild-to-moderate (colonic) disease, whereas steroids and infliximab are reserved for more severe active disease.

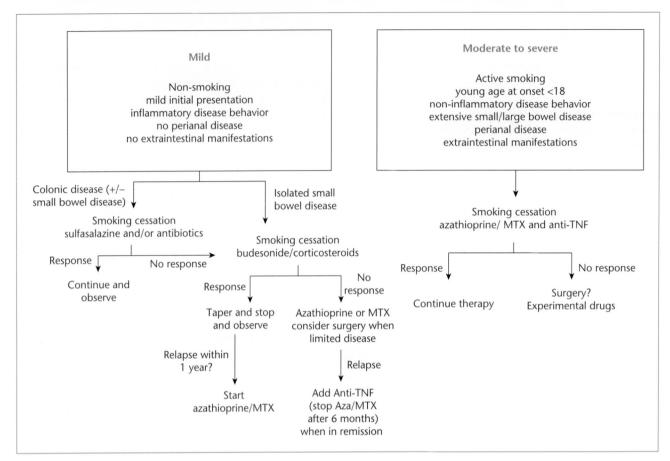

Figure 50.12 Treatment algorithm of Crohn's disease. Anti-TNF, antitumor necrosis factor; Aza, azathioprine; MTX, methotrexate.

5-aminosalicylates

Although aminosalicylates are widely used in the treatment of Crohn's disease, the scientific evidence supporting this practice is poor [56]. High doses of mesalazine (4 g/day) are effective in mild-to-moderate Crohn's disease, although not all studies have shown consistent results. A meta-analysis of 15 randomized controlled trials of mesalazine maintenance therapy involving a total of 2097 patients showed that it significantly reduced the risk of symptomatic relapse in 13%, but only in the post-surgical setting and in patients with ileitis and prolonged disease duration [57]. In the medical setting, the benefit was not significant. However, in practice, mesalazine compounds are often started as initial therapy in newly diagnosed mild-to-moderate Crohn's disease.

Corticosteroids

Prednisone and prednisolone have an efficacy in active disease that is superior to placebo, antibiotics, and mesalazine. Corticosteroids inhibit T-cell activation and proinflammatory cytokine production. However, in a prospective trial by Munkholm et al. [58], 36% of patients with Crohn's disease were steroid dependent and 20% steroid resistant after 1 year. Corticosteroids are further associated with a multitude of side effects, both short term (gastrointestinal intolerance and

dyspepsia, moon facies, acne, hypertension, hyperglycemia, depression, and psychosis) and long term (osteoporosis, cataract, growth failure). **Budesonide**, a synthetic glucocorticosteroid, provides the efficacy of a corticosteroid without the corticosteroid toxicity. It has a high ratio of topical to systemic activity owing to its extensive first-pass metabolism in the liver. In a study by Rutgeerts et al. [59], budesonide 9 mg/day was as effective as prednisone 40 mg/day in inducing remission. These findings have been confirmed in at least two subsequent studies [60,61].

Azathioprine and 6-mercaptopurine

Azathioprine and its metabolite 6-mercaptopurine (6-MP) offer a therapeutic advantage over placebo in the maintenance of remission in Crohn's disease. In the Candy and Wright study of 1995, 63 patients with active Crohn's disease treated with prednisolone were randomized to either azathioprine (2.5 mg/kg) or placebo [62]. At 15 months, 42% of patients receiving azathioprine were in remission, compared with 7% of those receiving placebo ($p = 0.001$).

Azathioprine is, however, associated with a number of **side effects**, including bone marrow toxicity, pancreatitis, and hepatotoxicity (see Chapter 143). A number of these adverse events are related to the metabolism of azathioprine by the enzyme **thiopurine methyltransferase** (TPMT). The activity of TPMT is genetically regulated and several polymorphisms have been described within the gene [63]. Approximately 11% of the population is heterozygous for the common TPMT polymorphisms and around 1 in 300 is a homozygous mutant. Heterozygotes show decreased activity of TPMT, and homozygotes have almost absent TPMT activity [64]. A deficiency of TPMT is associated with an increased risk of bone marrow suppression and neutropenia [65].

Dosage recommendations for azathioprine and 6-MP vary with the patient's genotype. In patients with the wild-type genotype (normal enzyme activity), a standard dose (2–2.5 mg/kg daily for azathioprine and 1–1.25 mg/kg daily for 6-MP) may be started. Patients who are **homozygous mutants** (absent enzyme activity), however, are known to develop early pancytopenia following the introduction of azathioprine. Azathioprine is not recommended in these patients. Heterozygous patients (intermediate enzyme activity) should be started at 50–60% of the dose. **Close monitoring** of the blood count and liver function tests are important – and mandatory if the genotype is not known. **Other side effects** of azathioprine, such as pancreatitis, fever, myalgia, and arthralgia, are type I hypersensitivity reactions. In the unlikely event of such an adverse event, azathioprine should be stopped; rechallenge is not recommended.

Methotrexate

The folate antagonist methotrexate is used as an immunomodulator in Crohn's disease and other inflammatory conditions such as rheumatoid arthritis. A double-blind placebo-controlled multicenter study of weekly injections of methotrexate in patients who had chronically active Crohn's disease despite receiving prednisone for a minimum of 3 months showed that methotrexate, administered at a dose of 25 mg once weekly, was more effective than placebo in improving symptoms and reducing the need for prednisone [66].

A follow-up trial showed that maintenance therapy with methotrexate (15 mg intramuscularly, once weekly) in patients with chronically active Crohn's disease who entered remission after 4–6 months of treatment with 25 mg methotrexate was beneficial compared with placebo [67]. Methotrexate is typically used as a second-line immunosuppressive drug for patients unresponsive to or intolerant of azathioprine (see Chapter 143).

Antibiotics

Antibiotics have been used empirically by many physicians for many years in the treatment of Crohn's disease, although no causative microorganism has been identified for Crohn's disease and there is a lack of controlled trials to validate this approach [68]. This includes antimycobacterial strategies [69] based on the possibility of mycobacterial infection. In addition, as well as their antibacterial action, some antibiotics, such as metronidazole and quinolones, have potential immunosuppressive properties. Enteric bacteria play a role in the pathogenesis of certain complications of Crohn's disease, including abscesses and fistulae, and antibiotics are used successfully for these complications. The most commonly used antibiotics are metronidazole and ciprofloxacin.

Metronidazole

This is an imidazole compound with activity against protozoa and most Gram-negative and Gram-positive anaerobic bacteria. Several uncontrolled trials, as well as clinical experience, suggest the drug is efficacious for **perianal complications** of Crohn's disease, but no controlled trials have been published to support this [70–72]. Metronidazole is sometimes also used where a secondary infective component is suspected elsewhere in the gastrointestinal tract (e.g., with complex matted distal ileum or suspected enteroenteric fistulization), started at a dose of 20 mg/kg (typically 400 mg three times daily) (see Chapter 143). The dose can be halved once improvement or remission has been achieved.

Side effects occur in 1–20% of patients and most often include nausea, gastrointestinal intolerance, neurotoxicity, and metallic taste. Metronidazole is usually given in courses lasting up to 3 months to patients with active perianal disease. Long-term treatment can give rise to peripheral neuropathy, characterized by paresthesias in the extremities. The adverse effects are reversible with discontinuation of the drug, although the neuropathy may sometimes continue after metronidazole is stopped. The antibiotic seems to be safe, although some mutations and teratogenicity have been reported in animal studies. Available evidence suggests that metronidazole does not affect fetal outcome adversely. However, caution is warranted and, until more data are available, the drug should be discontinued in women who wish to conceive.

Ciprofloxacin

This is a quinolone with a selective action against *E. coli* and aerobic Enterobacteria; it is therefore a selective suppressive agent for intestinal microflora. Ciprofloxacin has been used for both perianal disease and ileitis, as well as ulcerative colitis and pouchitis (see Chapter 49). In a number of open studies, ciprofloxacin either alone or in combination with metronidazole was effective in controlling symptoms and active disease, and in the treatment of fistulae and abscesses [73,74].

A combination of metronidazole and ciprofloxacin, which is effective against many enteric bacteria, has been reported to be effective in the treatment of acute Crohn's disease as an alternative to steroids. Prantera *et al.* randomized 41 patients with refractory or steroid-dependent Crohn's disease to a combination of 1000 mg ciprofloxacin and either 1000 mg metronidazole or methylprednisolone 0.70–1 mg/kg for 12 weeks [74]. Some 45% of patients (10 of 22) achieved remission with metronidazole versus 63% (12 of 19) with methylprednisolone. The most common side effects are gastrointestinal complaints.

Small and Large Bowel

Antimycobacterial agents

M. paratuberculosis has been identified in tissues from a higher proportion of patients with Crohn's disease than controls, suggesting that this organism may be one of the causes of Crohn's disease, although this is controversial. The possible involvement of *M. paratuberculosis* in Crohn's disease has led several investigators to use antimycobacterial therapy. A recent meta-analysis of the effect of antimycobacterial therapy in Crohn's disease concluded that this therapy is effective in maintaining remission in some patients following a course of corticosteroids combined with antimycobacterial therapy to induce remission [69]. Treatment of Crohn's disease with antimycobacterial therapy does not seem to be effective without a course of corticosteroids to induce remission.

Probiotics

There are many different preparations of probiotic lactobacilli, and some evidence showing that they are of value in Crohn's disease, although this is not conclusive [68].

Biological therapy
Anti-TNF-α antibodies

The management of IBD entered a new era at the beginning of the 1990s with the development of biological therapies that selectively block the inflammatory cascade [75]. Biological therapies have been developed thanks to an increasing knowledge regarding disease pathogenesis, and their production has been precipitated by the techniques of molecular biology. One of the first biological treatments involves chimeric antibodies to TNF-α: **infliximab** (Remicade®). TNF-α plays a central role in the inflammatory reaction observed in IBD. Infliximab is a mouse–human chimeric monoclonal IgG1 antibody against TNF-α. It is prescribed in the USA and Europe for the treatment of active therapy-resistant Crohn's disease [76,77] and for active fistulizing Crohn's disease [78,79]. Response rates of 75–80% are reached after a single infusion of infliximab 5 mg/kg, with up to 50% of patients entering clinical remission. The underlying reasons for the lack of response seen in 25% of patients are not known, and efforts are being made to identify factors predictive of response or failure [80–82].

Most patients relapse 8–12 weeks after initial infusion. **Retreatment** with infliximab every 8 weeks maintains clinical benefit, as shown in the ACCENT I study but also in real-life clinical practice [79,83]. In the ACCENT II study of infliximab maintenance treatment for fistulizing Crohn's disease, about two-thirds responded initially (>50% reduction in the number of draining fistulae), and of these, 62% who received placebo maintenance experienced a loss of response after a median of 14 weeks compared with 42% of those given maintenance treatment (median time to loss of response >40 weeks) [77]. Infliximab is also capable of inducing colonic **mucosal healing** assessed on the CDEIS. Also in children, infliximab has shown good efficacy, as demonstrated by the REACH study [84]. This study furthermore showed the superiority of q8 weekly infusions over q12 weekly infusions.

The comparative efficacy of infliximab and azathioprine therapy alone or in combination for Crohn's disease was evaluated in the recent double-blind randomized SONIC trial, which compared infliximab monotherapy, azathioprine monotherapy, and the two drugs combined in 508 adults with moderate-to-severe Crohn's disease who had not undergone previous immunosuppressive or biological therapy [85]. The corticosteroid-free clinical remission at week 26 (the primary end-point) was 56.8% in the combination group, as compared with 44.4% in the infliximab monotherapy arm and 30.0% in the azathioprine arm ($p < 0.001$ for the comparison with combination therapy and $p = 0.006$ for the comparison with infliximab). Also, the mucosal healing rates at this time point were highest in patients receiving combination therapy (43.9%), as compared with 30.1% in patients receiving infliximab and 16.5% in patients receiving azathioprine ($p < 0.001$ for the comparison with combination therapy and $p = 0.02$ for the comparison with infliximab). This study advocates the use of combination therapy in patients who are immunomodulator naïve.

Because the cost of anti-TNF agents is high and their long-term safety is uncertain, the UK National Institute for Health and Clinical Excellence (NICE) has recommended that these agents be limited to approximately the most severe 10% of patients and that a trial of withdrawal should be considered after 1 year. There is evidence that colonoscopic assessment is useful with approximately 60% of those without ulcers not relapsing rapidly on withdrawal. By contrast, Van Assche *et al.*, who showed that in patients failing immunomodulators, the introduction of infliximab is efficacious, advocate stopping the immunomodulators and continuing with infliximab monotherapy after 6 months [86]. This is an area where practice differs significantly from one country to another.

More humanized anti-TNF antibodies have been tested in more recent years. **Adalimumab** (Humira®) is a fully human antihuman TNF-α monoclonal antibody and certolizumab pegol is a pegylated anti-TNF Fab fragment. Results of the CLASSIC, CHARM, and PRECISE trials on efficacy and safety of adalimumab and certolizumab pegol respectively have shown also good efficacy for induction and maintenance of remission [87–91]. In a subanalysis of CHARM, adalimumab therapy was also more effective than placebo for inducing fistula healing [91]. Adalimumab has been approved for treatment of Crohn's disease. So far, certolizumab has only been approved in the USA and Switzerland.

Antibodies to anti-TNF agents

The presence of murine elements is associated with a risk of immunogenicity. In a prospective study of 125 infliximab-treated patients, 61% developed antibodies to infliximab (ATI), previously known as human antichimeric antibodies (HACA), after the fifth infusion [92]. ATI are more likely to develop when infliximab is given episodically and without concomitant immunomodulators. ATI are clearly associated with infusion reactions and loss of response to the drug. **Acute infusion** reactions are anaphylactoid and accompanied by dyspnea, chest tightness, urticaria, and headache. They should be treated with antihistamines, steroids, or epinephrine (adrenaline), and can be reduced in patients known to suffer them or to be at risk by prior use of immunosuppressives, including steroids.

Delayed hypersensitivity usually occurs several days after the infusion in a patient who typically has not had infliximab for at least a year. Symptoms are of myalgia and atrophy, fever, rash, pruritus and urticaria, edema, sore throat, and dysphagia. These can be reduced with immunosuppression and intravenous steroids [92,93]. Infliximab-treated patients should therefore receive concomitant immunosuppression with azathioprine, 6-MP, or methotrexate.

To avoid the problem of immunogenicity, more humanized anti-TNF antibodies have been developed. The incidence of antibodies to **adalimumab** and **certolizumab** pegol is lower than that of infliximab, although 2.6% of patients developed antibodies in the CLASSIC II study. In our own experience, 9% of patients (15 of 168) developed antibodies to adalimumab and all had undetectable serum concentrations of adalimumab [94].

Safety of anti-TNF agents
TNF-α is a key molecule in the inflammatory cascade, so it is not surprising that blocking it leads to an increase in the number of infectious events. The most frequently reported side effect is upper respiratory tract infection. In our single-center experience of the first 734 patients with IBD treated with infliximab and a control group of 666 patients not treated with infliximab [median follow-up of 58 months (IQR 33–88) and 144 months (IQR 83–163), respectively], 112 severe adverse events occurred in 93 patients (13%) treated with infliximab and 157 in 126 (19%) control patients (OR 1.33; 95% CI 0.56–3.00, $p = 0.45$) [95]. There was no difference between the two groups in mortality, malignancies, and infection rate, although concomitant treatment with steroids was the only independent risk factor for infections in patients treated with infliximab (OR 2.69; 95% CI 1.18–6.12; $p = 0.018$).

In addition, a reactivation of latent tuberculosis has been seen. American and European guidelines for the use of anti-TNF now recommend that all patients undergo chest radiography and/or skin purified protein derivative (PPD) test before therapy is administered [96].

Anti-TNF treatment is further contraindicated for moderate-to-severe heart failure, and caution should be exercised when administering it to patients with mild **heart failure** [97]. Although infliximab may induce antinuclear antibodies in almost 50% of patients, and this seems a class effect of all anti-TNFs, these autoantibodies are not associated with clinical manifestations of drug-induced lupus [98]. Finally, around 20% of patients under long-term anti-TNF therapy may develop **psoriasiform-like cutaneous lesions**. Topical therapy is effective in most and needs to be stopped only in very few patients.

Adhesion molecules
Adhesion molecules play a role in the trafficking of leukocytes in normal and inflamed gut. They are also involved in local lymphocyte stimulation and antigen presentation within the intestinal mucosa. In IBD, most of the adhesion factors are upregulated. Therapeutic compounds directed against trafficking of lymphocytes toward the gut mucosa have been developed as a novel class of drugs in the treatment of Crohn's disease. α4 Integrins are important mediators of leukocyte migration across the vascular endothelium. They form heterodimers with subunits β7 and β1, and interact with vascular cell adhesion molecule 1 (VCAM-1) and mucosal addressin cell adhesion molecule 1 (MadCAM-1), respectively. In this way they are involved in the recruitment of leukocytes to the place of inflammation.

The **anti-α4 integrin antibody** natalizumab (Antegren®) is a humanized mouse monoclonal antibody containing approximately 5% mouse-derived protein. The ENACT study randomized 905 patients to natalizumab 300 mg at weeks 0, 4, and 8, or to placebo. At 12 weeks, 42% of patients with severe luminal Crohn's disease characterized by a raised C-reactive protein level entered into remission, compared with 29% of placebo-treated patients [99]. Vedolizumab is a humanized monoclonal antibody to anti-α4β7 integrin. A double-blind placebo-controlled dose-finding trial in 185 patients with active Crohn's disease showed its biological activity [100].

Autologous stem cell transplantation
A number of case reports and case series of lymphoablation and autologous hematopoietic stem cell transplantation (HCT) have shown that this therapy may induce long-lasting remission in patients with severe Crohn's disease refractory to all conventional drugs [101]. This therapy is believed to reset the immunological system to "zero." At present, more than 1000 patients have been transplanted for autoimmune disease in Europe, along with the three major multinational randomized trials for Crohn's disease (the ASTIC study) [102], systemic sclerosis (the ASTIS study), and multiple sclerosis (the ASTIMS study).

Surgical treatment
Surgery should be reserved for patients in whom medical treatment fails to control the inflammation, or for complications such as strictures, abscesses, or fistulae. Sands *et al.* showed that 20% of patients with Crohn's disease required surgery within 3 years of their diagnosis, and almost 5% had already had major surgery at the time of diagnosis [103]. The most common risk factor for surgery is **smoking**, whereas isolated colonic involvement is seen as a negative risk factor for early surgery. The most common operations used in Crohn's disease (see Chapter 156) are listed in Table 50.5. Temporary or permanent defunctioning may be used for downstream disease, and as an adjunct to surgery for fistulae, where standard surgical procedures are accompanied

Table 50.5 Most common operations used for patients with Crohn's disease

Site	Indication	Operation
Gastroduodenal	Outlet obstruction	Gastrojejunostomy Duodenal strictureplasty
Small intestine	Obstruction	Strictureplasty Segmental resection
Ileocecal	Obstruction or pain	Ileal resection or right hemicolectomy Resection and ileostomy
Colonic	Obstruction	Colonic resection and ileostomy
	Pain	Colonic resection and ileorectal anastomosis
	Other symptoms not controlled medically	Segmental resection
Anorectal	Uncontrolled by medical treatment	Temporary defunctioning colostomy Colonic resection and ileostomy Colonic resection and ileorectal anastomosis
	Recurrent abscess formation	Seton stitch

by challenging individual dissections. **Perianal abscesses** may require drainage, but the surgical approach to perianal disease should be conservative because of poor healing. Postoperative recurrence at sites of anastomosis, often fibrostenotic, is common and in some patients appears to occur with accelerated rapidity. There is some evidence that prophylactic immunosuppression with azathioprine or 6-MP after surgery reduces the relapse rate. Given that the disease may recur after surgery, bowel-saving operations should be performed to prevent short bowel syndrome (SBS). Operative techniques have changed significantly over the past few years, and techniques such as **strictureplasty** are much less invasive and may prevent SBS. Therapy for recurrent anorectal Crohn's disease follows the same rules, and proctectomy remains the last option. In addition, emergency surgery in recurrent Crohn's disease follows the same rules as in elective surgery.

Nutritional therapy

Ensuring adequate nutrition and replacement, or prevention of specific deficiencies, is of central importance in the management of Crohn's disease. In addition, there is some evidence that nutritional therapy reduces disease activity, although not as effectively as with glucocorticoids [104]. Enteral diet therapy is used, particularly for children. There is some limited evidence that specific dietary exclusions might be of value (see Chapter 38).

Helminths

The possibility that nematode infection could result in improvements in IBD by inducing a global Th1 to Th2 immunological response has been investigated. These studies have been triggered by the observation that Crohn's disease is characterized by a Th1 response and that IBD is rare in countries where nematode infection is prevalent. As yet, the data are uncontrolled, requiring evaluation in randomized clinical trials and also demonstrating an effect on mucosal healing [105].

Complications and their management
Fibrostenosis

Inflammation of the bowel of patients with Crohn's disease does not only result in ulceration but may also lead to fibrostenosis after healing. Intestinal fibrostenosis is a frequent and debilitating complication of Crohn's disease, resulting in small bowel obstruction that requires surgery (strictureplasty or resection). Repeated bowel resection may potentially result in SBS. Colonic strictures can be managed by endoscopic dilatation, with some success [106]. More than one-third of Crohn's disease patients have a clear stenosing disease phenotype, often in the absence of luminal inflammatory symptoms.

Short bowel syndrome

Patients with Crohn's disease are at high risk for postoperative recurrence (60% after 15 years) and often undergo multiple operations. SBS is defined as a remaining bowel length of less than 180 cm with associated malabsorption. Several factors, including aggressive resectional therapy, but also surgical complications and errors in initial diagnosis, may contribute to the development of SBS. Therefore, bowel-saving operations should be performed whenever possible (see also Chapters 41 and 144).

Colorectal cancer (see Chapters 58 and 59)

Colorectal cancer (CRC) remains a feared complication of colitis. Although the risk is probably highest for total ulcerative colitis, it has become clear that less extensive colitis and Crohn's colitis also increase the risk. IBD cancers are preceded by dysplasia, and the relative risk increases by 0.5–1.0% per annum, and starts typically about 10 years after diagnosis. Currently, the main preventive strategy is a secondary one: surveillance colonoscopy after 8 years of disease duration. CRC tends to occur at the site of overt disease and develops at an earlier age (mean 50 years) than in sporadic non –IBD-associated CRC (70 years). Cancer should also be suspected in a *de novo* stricture of the colon, as this is associated with a 5–10-fold increased risk of colonic cancer. The increased risk of colonic cancer exists in patients with Crohn's disease even when disease is confined to the small bowel, and patients also have an increased risk of developing extraintestinal and reticuloendothelial tumors, as well as anovulval and malignant melanoma.

The **treatment of CRC** includes segmental resection, total proctocolectomy, subtotal colectomy, and palliative procedures. The prognosis is no worse after operation than that of sporadic non–IBD-associated colonic cancer. There have been recent reports that mesalazine given in a dose of 1.2 g/day may reduce the risk of colonic carcinoma. Other studies have suggested a role for folate and ursochol as chemopreventive agents.

Adenocarcinoma of the small bowel is extremely rare, compared with adenocarcinoma of the large bowel. Although only few small bowel cancers have been reported in patients with Crohn's disease, the number is significantly increased in relation to the expected number [107]. Most small bowel cancers in Crohn's disease are adenocarcinomas. They present at a younger age, more diffusely, and more distally than *de novo* cancers, usually making them undiagnosable at a curable early stage; indeed, two-thirds present with intestinal obstruction.

Fistulae

Fistulae consist of an abnormal communication between the lumen of the gut and the mesentery and/or another organ or the abdominal wall or skin. Symptoms such as fecal loss per vagina or pneumaturia (bladder fistula) imply the presence of a fistula. Fistulae also occur between bowel and skin (enterocutaneous), and between any two segments of bowel, sometimes resulting in malnutrition and eating-induced diarrhea (e.g., duodenocolic or ileosigmoid fistula). Before the introduction of infliximab, antibiotics were the only non-surgical treatment for fistulae, and often needed to be given over a very long period of time, leading to adverse effects and non-adherence.

The introduction of infliximab has dramatically improved the management of fistulizing Crohn's disease [76,77] However, despite closure of draining external orifices after infliximab therapy, fistulous tracks with varying degrees of residual inflammation may persist, and may cause recurrent fistulae and pelvic abscesses [108] (Figure 50.13). Whether complete fistula fibrosis occurs over time with repeated infliximab infusions is not known, and is the subject of current studies.

Abscess formation

In some patients, penetrating transmural disease and fistulization may result in local abscess formation (see Chapter 121). Frank perforation is unusual. If an abscess is suspected, the patient should be started on broad-spectrum antibiotics and the abscess identified by computed tomography (CT), usually accompanied by attempts at CT-guided percutaneous drainage. If this is not possible or the patient is ill with signs of local inflammation (e.g., iliopsoas irritation), surgical exploration and drainage should be carried out.

Bleeding

Although the diarrhea of Crohn's disease is characteristically non-bloody, rapid bleeding is recognized as an uncommon but occasionally life-threatening complication.

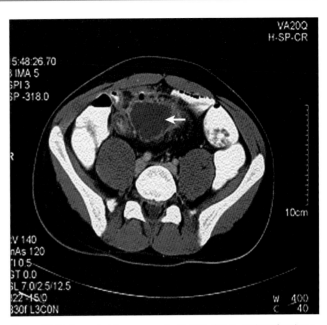

Figure 50.13 Computed tomogram of a Crohn's disease patient showing a large abscess (arrow).

Malnutrition

Patients with Crohn's disease become malnourished (see Figure 50.7) for many reasons, including anorexia (see Chapter 14), vomiting, malabsorption (see Chapter 39), protein-losing enteropathy (see Chapter 44), small bowel bacterial overgrowth (see Chapter 42), and intestinal bypass because of fistula formation. Vitamin supplementation and caloric support are of central importance in Crohn's disease. Enteral nutrition is preferred to parenteral where possible, because of both its enterotropic and therapeutic effects.

Bone disease

Patients with Crohn's disease are prone to osteopenic bone disease and osteoporosis [109] Persistent inflammation, malnutrition, and use of corticosteroids are all contributory. Many would give calcium and vitamin D with steroids prophylactically (although there is no firm evidence of benefit). Patients with established osteoporosis, diagnosed by dual X-ray absorptiometry (DEXA) scanning, can be treated with bisphosphonates.

Prognosis and what to tell patients

Crohn's disease typically involves relapse and remission between relatively good and relatively poor health. Most patients are likely to require surgery at some time. Typical estimates are that up to 57% of patients require at least one surgical resection and that on average approximately 15 years elapse between resections, although the disease is very variable. When planning a family, patients need to know that there is a strong genetic component and that their children have a 10-fold increased risk of developing IBD. They should also know that smoking cessation substantially reduces activity and symptom burden. Patients with Crohn's disease have been shown to have a somewhat reduced life-expectancy throughout the course of the disease. Some of this may, however, be attributable to the cardiovascular consequences of smoking [110].

SOURCES OF INFORMATION FOR PATIENTS AND DOCTORS

http://www.angelfire.com/ga/crohns/
http://www.patient.co.uk/showdoc/23068969/
http://www.patient.co.uk/showdoc/222/
http://www.gastro.org/generalPublic.html
http://www.nacc.org.uk/content/home.asp

References

1. Podolsky DK. Inflammatory bowel disease. *N Engl J Med.* 2002; 347:417–429.

2. Crohn BB, Ginzburg L, Oppenheimer GD. Regional ileitis: a pathologic and clinical entity. *JAMA.* 1932;99:1323–1328.

3. Loftus EV Jr, Sandborn WJ. Epidemiology of inflammatory bowel disease. *Gastroenterol Clin North Am.* 2002;31:1–20.

4. Munkholm P, Langholz E, Nielsen OH, Kreiner S, Binder V. Incidence and prevalence of Crohn's disease in the county of Copenhagen, 1962–87: a sixfold increase in incidence. *Scand J Gastroenterol.* 1992;27:609–614.

5. Loftus EV Jr, Silverstein MD, Sandborn WJ, Tremaine WJ, Harmsen WS, Zinsmeister AR. Crohn's disease in Olmsted County, Minnesota, 1940–1993: incidence, prevalence, and survival. *Gastroenterology.* 1998;114:1161–1168.

6. Loftus EV Jr, Schoenfeld P, Sandborn WJ. The epidemiology and natural history of Crohn's disease in population-based patient cohorts from North America: a systematic review. *Aliment Pharmacol Ther.* 2002;16:51–60.

7. Shivananda S, Lennard-Jones J, Logan R, *et al.* Incidence of inflammatory bowel disease across Europe: is there a difference between north and south? Results of the European Collaborative Study on Inflammatory Bowel Disease (EC-IBD). *Gut.* 1996;39:690–697.

8. Moum B, Ekbom A, Vatn MH, *et al.* Inflammatory bowel disease: re-evaluation of the diagnosis in a prospective population based study in south eastern Norway. *Gut.* 1997;40:328–332.

9. Martinez-Salmeron JF, Rodrigo M, de Teresa J, *et al.* Epidemiology of inflammatory bowel disease in the Province of Granada, Spain: a retrospective study from 1979 to 1988. *Gut.* 1993;34:1207–1209.

10. Ranzi T, Bodini P, Zambelli A, *et al.* Epidemiological aspects of inflammatory bowel disease in a north Italian population: a 4-year prospective study. *Eur J Gastroenterol Hepatol.* 1996;8:657–661.

11. Peeters M, Nevens H, Baert F, *et al.* Familial aggregation in Crohn's disease: increased age adjusted risk and concordance in clinical characteristics. *Gastroenterology.* 1996;111:597–603.

12. Orholm M, Munkholm P, Langholz E, *et al.* Familial occurrence of inflammatory bowel disease. *N Engl J Med.* 1991;324:84–88.

13. Satsangi J, Grootscholten C, Holt H, Jewell DP. Clinical patterns of familial inflammatory bowel disease. *Gut.* 1996;38:738–741.

14. Tysk C, Lindberg E, Jarnerot G, *et al.* Ulcerative colitis and Crohn's disease in an unselected population of monozygotic and dizygotic twins. A study of heritability and the influence of smoking. *Gut.* 1988;29:990–996.

15. Thompson NP, Driscoll R, Pounder RE, *et al.* Genetic versus environment in inflammatory bowel disease: results of a British twin study. *BMJ.* 1996;312:95–96.

16. Orholm M, Binder V, Sorensen TI, *et al.* Concordance of inflammatory bowel disease among Danish twins. Results of a nationwide study. *Scand J Gastroenterol.* 2000;35:1075–1081.

17. Halfvarson J, Jess T, Bodin L, Järnerot G, Munkholm P, Binder V, Tysk C. Longitudinal concordance for clinical characteristics in a Swedish-Danish twin population with inflammatory bowel disease. *Inflamm Bowel Dis.* 2007;13:1536–1544.

18. Thomas GA, Rhodes J, Green JT, Richardson C. Role of smoking in inflammatory bowel disease: implications for therapy. *Postgrad Med J.* 2000;76:273–279.

19. Cosnes J, Beaugerie L, Carbonnel F, Gendre JP. Smoking cessation and the course of Crohn's disease: an intervention study. *Gastroenterology.* 2001;120:1093–1099.

20. Greenstein RJ. Is Crohn's disease caused by a mycobacterium? Comparisons with leprosy, tuberculosis, and Johne's disease. *Lancet Infect Dis.* 2003;3:507–514.

21. Joossens M, Van Steen K, Branche J, *et al.* Familial aggregation and antimicrobial response dose-dependently affect the risk for Crohn's disease. *Inflamm Bowel Dis.* 2010;16:58–67.

22. Hugot JP, Chamaillard M, Zouali H, *et al.* Association of CARD15 leucine-rich repeat variants with susceptibility to Crohn's disease. *Nature.* 2001;411:599–603.

23. Ogura Y, Bonen DK, Inohara N, *et al.* A frameshift mutation in *CARD15* associated with susceptibility to Crohn's disease. *Nature.* 2001;411:603–606.

24. Hisamatsu T, Suzuki M, Reinecker HC, Nadeau WJ, McCormick BA, Podolsky DK. CARD15/NOD2 functions as an antibacterial factor in human intestinal epithelial cells. *Gastroenterology.* 2003;124:993–1000.

25. Esters N, Pierik M, Claessens G, *et al.* Mutations in NOD2/CARD15 in Crohn's Disease patients and their unaffected siblings. *Gastroenterology.* 2002;122:A-295, M1406.

26. The first convincing linkage replication for a non-Mendelian disease: Crohn's disease and chromosome 16, by the IBD International Genetics Consortium. *Am J Hum Genet.* 2000;68:1165–1171.

27. Kobayashi KS, Chamaillard M, Ogura Y, *et al.* Nod2-dependent regulation of innate and adaptive immunity in the intestinal tract. *Science.* 2005;307:731–734.

28. Wehkamp J, Salzman NH, Porter E, *et al*; Reduced Paneth cell alpha-defensins in ileal Crohn's disease *Proc Natl Acad Sci U S A.* 2005;102:18129–18134.

29. Rioux JD, Xavier RJ, Taylor KD, *et al.* Genome-wide association study identifies new susceptibility loci for Crohn disease and implicates autophagy in disease pathogenesis. *Nat Genet.* 2007;39:596–604.

30. Hampe J, Franke A, Rosenstiel P, *et al.* A genome-wide association scan of nonsynonymous SNPs identifies a susceptibility variant for Crohn disease in ATG16L1. *Nat Genet.* 2007;39:207–211.

31. Parkes M, Barrett JC, Prescott NJ, *et al.* Wellcome Trust Case Control Consortium, Cardon L, Mathew CG. Sequence variants in the autophagy gene IRGM and multiple other replicating loci

Small and Large Bowel

contribute to Crohn's disease susceptibility. *Nat Genet.* 2007; 39:830–832.

32. Neurath MF. Mucosal immunity in Crohn's disease. *Inflamm Bowel Dis.* 2004;10 (Suppl 1):S29–S31.

33. Ina K, Itoh J, Fukushima K, Kusugami K, *et al.* Resistance of Crohn's disease T cells to multiple apoptotic signals is associated with a Bcl-2/Bax mucosal imbalance. *J Immunol.* 1999;163:1081–1090.

34. Rutgeerts P, Geboes K, Peeters M, *et al.* Effect of faecal stream diversion on recurrence of Crohn's disease in the neoterminal ileum. *Lancet.* 1991;338:771–774.

35. D'Haens GR, Geboes K, Peeters M, Baert F, Penninckx F, Rutgeerts P. Early lesions of recurrent Crohn's disease caused by infusion of intestinal contents in excluded ileum. *Gastroenterology.* 1998;114:262–267.

36. Rutgeerts P, Hiele M, Geboes K, *et al.* Controlled trial of metronidazole treatment for prevention of Crohn's recurrence after ileal resection. *Gastroenterology.* 1995;108:1617–1621.

37. Rutgeerts P, Van Assche G, Vermeire S, *et al.* Ornidazole for prophylaxis of postoperative Crohn's disease recurrence: a randomized, double-blind, placebo-controlled trial. *Gastroenterology.* 2005;128:856–861.

38. Tamboli CP, Neut C, Desreumaux P, Colombel JF. Dysbiosis in inflammatory bowel disease. *Gut.* 2004;53:1–4.

39. Swidsinski A, Ladhoff A, Pernthaler A, *et al.* Mucosal flora in inflammatory bowel disease. *Gastroenterology.* 2002;122: 44–54.

40. Masseret E, Boudeau J, Colombel JF, *et al.* Genetically related *Escherichia coli* strains associated with Crohn's disease. *Gut.* 2001;48:320–325.

41. Boudeau J, Glasser AL, Masseret E, Joly B, Darfeuille-Michaud A. Invasive ability of an *Escherichia coli* strain isolated from the ileal mucosa of a patient with Crohn's disease. *Infect Immun.* 1999;67:4499–4509.

42. Glasser AL, Boudeau J, Barnich N, Perruchot MH, Colombel JF, Darfeuille-Michaud A. Adherent invasive Escherichia coli strains from patients disease survive and replicate within macrophages without inducing host cell death. *Infect Immun.* 2001;69:5529–5537.

43. Sokol H, Pigneur B, Watterlot L, *et al.* Faecalibacterium prausnitzii is an anti-inflammatory commensal bacterium identified by gut microbiota analysis of Crohn disease patients. *Proc Natl Acad Sci U S A.* 2008;105:16731–16736.

44. Landers CJ, Cohavy O, Misra R, *et al.* Selected loss of tolerance evidenced by Crohn's disease-associated immune responses to auto- and microbial antigens. *Gastroenterology.* 2002;123: 689–699.

45. Sendid B, Colombel JF, Jacquinot PM, *et al.* Specific antibody response to oligomannosidic epitopes in Crohn's disease. *Clin Diagn Lab Immunol.* 1996;3:219–226.

46. Ferrante M, Henckaerts L, Joossens M, *et al.* New serological markers in inflammatory bowel disease are associated with complicated disease behaviour. *Gut.* 2007;56:1394–1403.

47. Singh B, Mortensen NJMcC, Jewell DP, George B. Perianal Crohn's disease. *Br J Surg.* 2004;91:801–814.

48. Silverberg MS, Satsangi J, Ahmad T, *et al.* Toward an integrated clinical, molecular and serological classification of inflammatory bowel disease: Report of a Working Party of the 2005 Montreal World Congress of Gastroenterology. *Can J Gastroenterol.* 2005;19 (Suppl A):5–36.

49. Wilson A, Reyes E, Ofman J. Prevalence and outcomes of anemia in inflammatory bowel disease: a systematic review of the literature. *Am J Med.* 2004;116 (Suppl 7A):44S–49S.

50. Afdhal NH, Long A, Lennon J, *et al.* Controlled trial of antimycobacterial therapy in Crohn's disease. Clofazimine versus placebo. *Dig Dis Sci.* 1991;36:449–453.

51. Danese S, Motte Cd Cde L, Fiocchi C. Platelets in inflammatory bowel disease: clinical, pathogenic, and therapeutic implications. *Am J Gastroenterol.* 2004;99:938–945.

52. Hommes DW, van Deventer SJ. Endoscopy in inflammatory bowel diseases. *Gastroenterology.* 2004;126:1561–1573.

53. Mary JY, Modigliani R. Development and validation of an endoscopic index of the severity for Crohn's disease: a prospective multicentre study. Groupe d'Etudes Thérapeutiques des Affections Inflammatoires du Tube Digestif (GETAID). *Gut.* 1989;30:983–989.

54. Daperno M, D'Haens G, Van Assche G, *et al.* Development and validation of a new, simplified endoscopic activity score for Crohn's disease: the SES-CD. *Gastrointest Endosc.* 2004;60: 505–512.

55. Kleer CG, Appelman HD. Surgical pathology of Crohn's disease. *Am J Surg Pathol.* 1998;22:983–989.

56. Travis SP, Stange EF, Lémann M, *et al.*; European Crohn's and Colitis Organisation. European evidence based consensus on the diagnosis and management of Crohn's disease: current management. *Gut.* 2006;55 (Suppl 1):i16–i35.

57. Camma C, Giunta M, Rosselli M, Cottone M. Mesalamine in the maintenance treatment of Crohn's disease: a meta-analysis adjusted for confounding variables. *Gastroenterology.* 1997;115: 1465–1473.

58. Munkholm P, Langholz E, Davidsen M, Binder V. Frequency of glucocorticoid resistance and dependency in Crohn's disease. *Gut.* 1994;35:360–362.

59. Rutgeerts P, Lofberg R, Malchow H, *et al.* A comparison of budesonide with prednisolone for active Crohn's disease. *N Engl J Med.* 1994;331:842–845.

60. Campieri M, Ferguson A, Doe W, Persson T, Nilsson LG. Oral budesonide is as effective as oral prednisolone in active Crohn's disease. The Global Budesonide Study Group. *Gut.* 1997;41:209–214.

61. Bar-Meir S, Chowers Y, Lavy A, *et al.* Budesonide versus prednisone in the treatment of active Crohn's disease.The Israeli Budesonide Study Group. *Gastroenterology.* 1998;115:835–840.

62. Candy S, Wright J, Gerber M, Adams G, Gerig M, Goodman R. A controlled double blind study of azathioprine in the management of Crohn's disease. *Gut.* 1995;37:674–678.

63. Weinshilboum RM, Sladek SL. Mercaptopurine pharmacogenetics: monogenic inheritance of erythrocyte thiopurine methyltransferase activity. *Am J Hum Genet.* 1980;32:651–662.

64. Yates CR, Krynetski EY, Loennechen T, *et al.* Molecular diagnosis of thiopurine *S*-methyltransferase deficiency: genetic basis for azathioprine and mercaptopurine intolerance. *Ann Intern Med.* 1997;126:608–614.

65. Colombel JF, Ferrari N, Debuysere H, *et al.* Genotypic analysis of thiopurine *S*-methyltransferase in patients with Crohn's disease and severe myelosuppression during azathioprine therapy. *Gastroenterology.* 2000;118:1025–1030.

66. Feagan BG, Rochon J, Fedorak RN, *et al.* Methotrexate for the treatment of Crohn's disease.The North American Crohn's Study Group Investigators. *N Engl J Med.* 1995;332:292–297.

67. Feagan BG, Fedorak RN, Irvine EJ, *et al.* A comparison of methotrexate with placebo for the maintenance of remission in Crohn's disease. North American Crohn's Study Group Investigators. *N Engl J Med.* 2000;342:1627–1632.

68. Sartor RB. Therapeutic manipulation of the enteric microflora in inflammatory bowel diseases: antibiotics, probiotics, and prebiotics. *Gastroenterology.* 2004;126:1620–1633.

69. Borgaonkar MR, MacIntosh GD, Fardy JM. A meta-analysis of antimycobacterial therapy for Crohn's disease. *Am J Gastroenterol.* 2000;95:725–729.

70. Bernstein LH, Frank MS, Brandt LJ, *et al.* Healing of perineal Crohn's disease with metronidazole. *Gastroenterology.* 1980;79:357–365.

71. Rosen A, Ursing B, Alm T, *et al.* A comparative study of metronidazole and sulfasalazine for active Crohn's disease: the Cooperative Crohn's Disease Study in Sweden. I. Design and methodological considerations. *Gastroenterology.* 1982;83:541–549.

72. Sutherland L, Singleton J, Sessions J, *et al.* Double blind, placebo controlled trial of metronidazole in Crohn's disease. *Gut.* 1991;32:1071–1075.

73. Turunen U, Färkkilä V, Valtonen V, *et al.* Long-term outcome of ciprofloxacin treatment in severe perianal or fistulous Crohn's disease. *Gastroenterology.* 1993;104:A793.

74. Prantera C, Zannoni F, Scribano ML, *et al.* An antibiotic regimen for the treatment of active Crohn's disease: a randomized, controlled trial of metronidazole plus ciprofloxacin. *Am J Gastroenterol.* 1996;91:328–332.

75. Rutgeerts P, Van Assche G, Vermeire S. Optimizing anti-TNF treatment in inflammatory bowel disease. *Gastroenterology.* 2004;126:1593–1610.

76. Present DH, Rutgeerts P, Targan S, *et al.* Infliximab for the treatment of fistulas in patients with Crohn's disease. *N Engl J Med.* 1999;340:1398–1405.

77. Sands BE, Anderson FH, Bernstein CN, *et al.* Infliximab maintenance therapy for fistulizing Crohn's disease. *N Engl J Med.* 2004;350:876–885.

78. Targan SR, Hanauer SB, van Deventer SJ, *et al.* A short-term study of chimeric monoclonal antibody cA2 to tumor necrosis factor alpha for Crohn's disease. Crohn's Disease cA2 Study Group. *N Engl J Med.* 1997;337:1029–1035.

79. Hanauer SB, Feagan BG, Lichtenstein GR, *et al.* Maintenance infliximab for Crohn's disease: the ACCENT I randomised trial. *Lancet.* 2002;359:1541–1549.

80. Parsi MA, Achkar JP, Richardson S, *et al.* Predictors of response to infliximab in patients with Crohn's disease. *Gastroenterology.* 2002;123:707–713.

81. Vermeire S, Louis E, Carbonez A, *et al.* Logistic regression of clinical parameters influencing response to infliximab. *Am J Gastroenterol.* 2002;97:2357–2363.

82. Arnott ID, McNeill G, Satsangi J. An analysis of factors influencing short-term and sustained response to infliximab treatment for Crohn's disease. *Aliment Pharmacol Ther.* 2003;17:1451–1457.

83. Schnitzler F, Fidder H, Ferrante M, *et al.* Long-term outcome of treatment with infliximab in 614 patients with Crohn's disease: results from a single-centre cohort. *Gut.* 2009;58:492–500.

84. Hyams J, Crandell W, Kugathasan S, *et al.*; REACH Study Group. Induction and maintenance infliximab therapy for the treatment of moderate-to-severe Crohn's disease in children. *Gastroenterology.* 2007;132:863–873.

85. Colombel JF, Sandborn WJ, Reinisch W, *et al.* SONIC Study Group. Infliximab, azathioprine, or combination therapy for Crohn's disease. *N Engl J Med.* 2010;362:1383–1395.

86. Van Assche G, Magdelaine-Beuzelin C, D'Haens G, *et al.* Withdrawal of immunosuppression in Crohn's disease treated with scheduled infliximab maintenance: a randomized trial. *Gastroenterology.* 2008;134:1861–1868.

87. Hanauer SB, Sandborn WJ, Rutgeerts P, *et al.* Human anti-tumor necrosis factor monoclonal antibody (adalimumab) in Crohn's disease: the CLASSIC-I trial. *Gastroenterology.* 2006;130:323–333; quiz 591.

88. Colombel JF, Sandborn WJ, Rutgeerts P, *et al.* Adalimumab for maintenance of clinical response and remission in patients with Crohn's disease: the CHARM trial. *Gastroenterology.* 2007;132:52–65.

89. Sandborn WJ, Feagan BG, Stoinov S, *et al.* Certolizumab pegol for the treatment of Crohn's disease. *N Engl J Med.* 2007;357:228–238.

90. Schreiber S, Khaliq-Kareemi M, Lawrance IC, *et al.* PRECISE 2 Study Investigators. Maintenance therapy with certolizumab pegol for Crohn's disease. *N Engl J Med.* 2007;357:239–250. Erratum in: *N Engl J Med.* 2007;357:1357.

91. Colombel JF, Schwartz DA, Sandborn WJ, *et al.* Adalimumab for the treatment of fistulas in patients with Crohn's disease. *Gut.* 2009;58:940–948.

92. Baert F, Noman M, Vermeire S, *et al.* Influence of immunogenicity on the longterm efficacy of infliximab in Crohn's disease. *N Engl J Med.* 2003;348:601–608.

93. Vermeire S, Noman M, Van Assche G, Baert F, D'Haens G, Rutgeerts P. Effectiveness of concomitant immunosuppressive therapy in suppressing the formation of antibodies to infliximab in Crohn's disease. *Gut.* 2007;56:1226–1231.

94. Karmiris K, Paintaud G, Noman M, *et al.* Influence of trough serum levels and immunogenicity on long-term outcome of adalimumab therapy in Crohn's disease. *Gastroenterology.* 2009;137:1628–1640.

95. Fidder H, Schnitzler F, Ferrante M, *et al.* Long-term safety of infliximab for the treatment of inflammatory bowel disease: a single-centre cohort study. *Gut.* 2009;58:501–508.

96. Keane J, Gershon S, Wise RP, *et al.* Tuberculosis associated with infliximab, a tumor necrosis factor alpha-neutralizing agent. *N Engl J Med.* 2001;345:1098–1104.

97. Chung ES, Packer M, Lo KH, *et al.* Randomized, double-blind, placebocontrolled, pilot trial of infliximab, a chimeric monoclonal antibody to tumor necrosis factor-alpha, in patients with moderate-to-severe heart failure: results of the Anti-TNF Therapy Against Congestive Heart Failure (ATTACH) trial. *Circulation.* 2003;107:3133–3140.

98. Vermeire S, Noman M, Van Assche G, *et al.* Autoimmunity associated with anti-tumor necrosis factor alpha treatment in Crohn's disease: a prospective cohort study. *Gastroenterology.* 2003;125:32–39.

99. Sandborn WJ, Colombel JF, Enns R, *et al.* International Efficacy of Natalizumab as Active Crohn's Therapy (ENACT-1) Trial Group; Evaluation of Natalizumab as Continuous Therapy (ENACT-2) Trial Group. Natalizumab induction and maintenance therapy for Crohn's disease. *N Engl J Med.* 2005;353:1912–1925.

100. Ghosh S, Goldin E, Gordon FH, *et al*. Natalizumab for active Crohn's disease. *N Engl J Med*. 2003;348:24–32.

101. Oyama Y, Craig RM, Traynor AE, *et al*. Autologous hematopoietic stem cell transplantation in patients with refractory Crohn's disease. *Gastroenterology*. 2005;128:552–563.

102. Sullivan KM, Muraro P, Tyndall A. Hematopoietic cell transplantation for autoimmune disease: updates from Europe and the United States. *Blood Marrow Transplant*. 2010;16:S48–S56.

103. Sands BE, Arsenault JE, Rosen MJ, *et al*. Risk of early surgery for Crohn's disease: implications for early treatment strategies. *Am J Gastroenterol*. 2003;98:2712–2718.

104. Griffiths AM, Ohlsson A, Sherman PM, *et al*. Meta-analysis of enteral nutrition as a primary treatment of active Crohn's disease. *Gastroenterology*. 1995;108:1056–1067.

105. Hunter MM, McKay DM. Helminths as therapeutic agents for inflammatory bowel disease. *Aliment Pharmacol Ther*. 2004; 19:167–177.

106. Thienpont C, D'Hoore A, Vermeire S, *et al*. Long-term outcome of endoscopic dilatation in patients with Crohn's disease is not affected by disease activity or medical therapy. *Gut*. 2010;59:320–324.

107. Munkholm P. The incidence and prevalence of colorectal cancer in inflammatory bowel disease. *Aliment Pharmacol Ther*. 2003;18 (Suppl 2):1–5.

108. Van Assche G, Vanbeckevoort D, Bielen D, *et al*. Magnetic resonance imaging of the effects of infliximab on perianal fistulizing Crohn's disease. *Am J Gastroenterol*, 2003;98:332–339.

109. Harpavat M, Keljo DJ, Regueiro MD. Metabolic bone disease in inflammatory bowel disease. *J Clin Gastroenterol*. 2004;38: 218–224.

110. Card T, Hubbard R, Logan RF. Mortality in inflammatory bowel disease: a population based cohort study. *Gastroenterology*. 2003; 125:1583–1590.

111. Sutherland LR, Ramcharan S, Bryant H, Fick G. Effect of cigarette smoking on recurrence of Crohn's disease. *Gastroenterology*. 1990;98:1123–1128.

112. Lindberg E, Jarnerot G, Huitfeldt B. Smoking in Crohn's disease: effect on localization and clinical course. *Gut*. 1992;33: 779–782.

113. Cottone M, Rosselli M, Orlando A, *et al*. Smoking habits and recurrence in Crohn's disease. *Gastroenterology*. 1994;106: 643–648.

114. Cosnes J, Carbonnel F, Beaugerie L, Le Quintrec Y, Gendre JP. Effects of cigarette smoking on the long-term course of Crohn's disease. *Gastroenterology*. 1996;110:424–431.

115. Timmer A, Sutherland LR, Martin F. Oral contraceptive use and smoking are risk factors for relapse in Crohn's disease. The Canadian Mesalamine for Remission in Crohn's Disease Study Group. *Gastroenterology*. 1998;114:1143–1150.

116. Medina C, Vergera M, Casellas F, Lara F, Naval J, Malagelada JR. Influence of the smoking habit in the surgery of inflammatory bowel disease. *Rev Enferm Dig*. 1998;90:771–778.

117. Yamamoto T, Keighley MR. The association of cigarette smoking with a high risk of recurrence after ileocolonic resection for ileocecal Crohn's disease. *Surg Today* 1999;29:579–580.

118. Yamamoto T, Allan RN, Keighley MR. Smoking is a predictive factor for outcome after colectomy and ileorectal anastomosis in patients with Crohn's colitis. *Br J Surg* 1999;86: 1069–1070.

Small and Large Bowel

CHAPTER 51
Indeterminate colitis

Stephan R. Targan[1] and C. J. Hawkey[2]

[1]Cedars-Sinai IBD Center, Los Angeles, CA, USA
[2]Nottingham Digestive Diseases Centre, University of Nottingham and Nottingham University Hospitals, Nottingham, UK

ESSENTIAL FACTS ABOUT PATHOGENESIS

Indeterminate colitis shares features of ulcerative colitis or Crohn's disease and may develop into one or other of them. Indeterminate colitis is more common in younger than older patients

---

ESSENTIALS OF DIAGNOSIS

- Typical symptoms include abdominal pain, bleeding, diarrhea and weight loss
- Colonoscopic features include colonic erosions and ulcers, pancolitis with rectal sparing and early onset in childhood
- Histological features include diffuse transmucosal lamina propria cellular increase and patchy inflammation
- Increase in patchy inflammation histologically
- The incidence of colorectal cancer appears to be high

ESSENTIALS OF TREATMENT

- There are few specific clinical trials but reasons to believe aminosalicylates, corticosteroids, immunosuppressive drugs, anti-TNF agents and cyclosporine may be valuable
- Surgery may be needed but the optimal choice of operation is debated
- There is a higher rate of pouch failure with emergence of features of Crohn's disease than in patients with ulcerative colitis

---

Introduction and definition

The term "indeterminate colitis" was originally introduced to describe the colitis observed in surgical specimens that could not accurately be classified as ulcerative colitis (UC) or Crohn's disease (CD) [1–3]. Subsequently the term indeterminate colitis has been extended and applied to patients who have not yet undergone colectomy. Some authorities argue that indeterminate colitis represents a distinct clinical entity, whereas others believe it is simply a problem of classification at the time of evaluation [1–4]. There has been an increasing tendency, particularly in the pediatric world, to extend the purely pathological definition into one considered to have characteristic clinical features. These include abdominal pain, bleeding, diarrhea and weight loss with macroscopic features of erosions and

ulcers in the colon, pancolitis with rectal sparing, early onset in childhood and diffuse transmucosal lamina propria cellular increase and patchy inflammation histologically [5]. A recent meta analysis suggests that indeterminate colitis is more common in children accounting for 12.7% of all cases of IBD versus 6% in adults [6].

An alternative view has been taken by the Montreal group on the classification of inflammatory bowel disease, who suggested that the term indeterminate colitis still be reserved for colectomy specimens and that a new term colonic Inflammatory Bowel Disease Unclassified (IBDU) be introduced [7].

Advances in our understanding of the pathogenesis of mucosal inflammation in animal models and humans suggest that IBD represents a heterogeneous group of diseases based on clinical, subclinical, and genetic characteristics (Figure 51.1). For example, **CARD15 (NOD2)** variants have been shown to be associated not only with CD but also with younger age of disease onset, ileal involvement, and a tendency to develop strictures [8–10]. This notion of disease heterogeneity has been further supported by the development of several animal models of IBD with distinct phenotypes and immunologic features following selective manipulation of a variety of genes, including those of proinflammatory or immunoregulatory cytokines [11]. Given this premise and its extrapolation to human disease, indeterminate colitis may in fact be a distinct manifestation within the IBD spectrum.

Between 5% and 23% of the initial diagnoses of IBD are classified as indeterminate colitis with an incidence of approximately 2.4 per 100000 [6,12–14], with indeterminate colitis accounting for a higher proportion of childhood than adult cases of inflammatory bowel disease [6] (Figure 51.2). Indeterminate colitis has been associated with a higher risk of colorectal cancer development and increased mortality compared with UC [15,16]. The cumulative incidence of colectomy in patients with indeterminate colitis in a population-based study was four times higher than in patients with definite UC [16]. Although many patients with indeterminate colitis will be reclassified as having CD or UC on long-term follow-up evaluation, a significant proportion of them will still carry the diagnosis of indeterminate colitis [12].

Textbook of Clinical Gastroenterology and Hepatology, Second Edition. Edited by C. J. Hawkey, Jaime Bosch, Joel E. Richter, Guadalupe Garcia-Tsao, Francis K. L. Chan.
© 2012 Blackwell Publishing Ltd. Published 2012 by Blackwell Publishing Ltd.

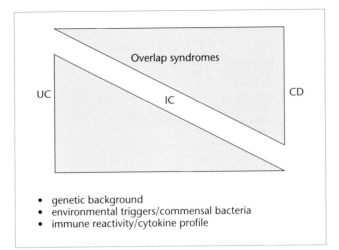

- genetic background
- environmental triggers/commensal bacteria
- immune reactivity/cytokine profile

Figure 51.1 IBD represents heterogeneous syndromes of mucosal inflammation. At the extreme ends of the spectrum, classic cases of ulcerative colitis (UC) and Crohn's disease (CD) are seen. The phenotypic expression of these diseases is influenced by the genetic background of the individual, the environmental triggers of the disease, the mucosal cytokine profile, and specific immune reactivity to luminal bacterial flora, which could be interrelated. IC, indeterminate colitis. (This figure was published in *Clinical Gastroenterology and Hepatology*, Wilfred M. Weinstein, Christopher J. Hawkey, Jaime Bosch, Indeterminate colitis, Pages 1–3, Copyright Elsevier, 2005.)

Pathogenesis and pathology

The pathogenesis of indeterminate colitis is similar to that of UC or CD. Inappropriate activation of the mucosal immune system in response to commensal bacterial antigens of the colon initiates a cascade of events leading to mucosal inflammation and epithelial cell dysfunction [11]. The pathology of indeterminate colitis has been described in surgical specimens and includes macroscopic features such as total severe colitis, segmental disease with rectal sparing, and variation in disease severity in different parts of the colon. The microscopic features may include fissuring ulcers, mucosal islands with a regular epithelium, preserved goblet cells, and mild inflammation and transmural inflammation associated with severe ulceration [1–5]. Granulomas and transmural lymphoid aggregates are not present. However, given the limitations of the precolectomy evaluation of mucosal biopsies in patients with indeterminate colitis (inability to evaluate for transmural lymphoid aggregates and granulomas in the deeper layers of the bowel and the potential effect of prior treatment), the physician should often rely on the evaluation of multiple biopsy specimens from the ileum and colon in combination with endoscopy to establish a definitive diagnosis [2]. The absence of diagnostic features of CD (such as granulomas) in the biopsy specimens in repeated histopathologic evaluations of the ileum and colon would indicate that the patient has indeterminate colitis. One study classified patients as having indeterminate colitis if they had isolated colitis, endoscopy was inconclusive, and microscopy indicated 'active and patchy transmucosal chronic inflammation with minimal or moderate architectural distortion and an absence of diagnostic features for either CD or UC.

Clinical presentation

The typical clinical presentation of indeterminate colitis includes symptoms related to colitis such as abdominal pain, diarrhea, rectal bleeding, and tenesmus. Systemic manifestations are frequently observed, such as fever, weight loss, and anemia. The diagnosis of indeterminate colitis is made more frequently in children than in adults and is associated with early onset of disease. Data are limited but colon cancer, with a relatively poor prognosis, has been associated with indeterminate colitis.

Paediatric patients with Crohn's disease have a higher incidence of colitis associated with polymorphisms in the TNF-alpha promoter gene [17] and an absence of NOD-2 [9,10].

Differential diagnosis

By definition, indeterminate colitis refers to chronic idiopathic colitis that cannot be differentiated from UC and CD at the initial presentation. Distinction from UC or CD becomes clinically important in medically refractory cases when surgery is contemplated, particularly because patients with indeterminate colitis have a higher frequency of pouch failure than those with UC and this may unmask an underlying diagnosis of Crohn's disease [3].

In patients with indeterminate colitis the probability of having a diagnosis of CD on follow-up evaluation was increased in patients with fever at their initial presentation, segmental endoscopic lesions, or extraintestinal complications, and in current smokers, whereas the probability of having a diagnosis of UC was increased in patients who had not undergone appendectomy before diagnosis [3]. The development of new endoscopic modalities such as the wireless capsule has assisted in the diagnostic evaluation of patients with indeterminate colitis. A subset of such patients, despite normal radiographic studies of the small bowel, will be found to have small bowel lesions characteristic of CD.

Children with immune deficiency disorders including chronic granulomatous disease, Wiskott-Aldrich syndrome, common variable immune deficiency disease, immune disregulation polyendocrinopathy, enteropathy X-linked syndrome or glycogenosis type 1B [6,17] may present as inflammatory bowel disease.

Investigation

An important component of investigation is to differentiate from ulcerative colitis, particularly for those patients who may require surgery, in view of the high rate of pouch failure when done for indeterminant colitis. Upper GI endoscopy, by detecting extra colonic lesions has a role in this process [18]. Preliminary results from the use of wireless capsule endoscopy suggests this may confer less benefit than once hoped for [19]. Much emphasis has been placed on the development of serological testing.

Serologic testing in patients with an initial diagnosis of indeterminate colitis may be helpful in categorizing the disease

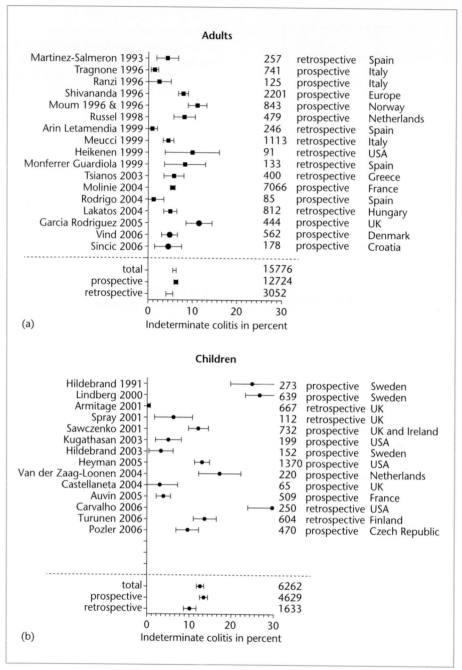

Figure 51.2 Proportion of patients with inflammatory bowel disease where the condition is indeterminate colitis in adults and in children.

and predicting the follow-up diagnosis [11,20]. The most extensively studied serologic markers in IBD include perinuclear antineutrophil cytoplasmic antibody (pANCA) and anti-*Saccharomyces cerevisiae* antibody (ASCA). As subclinical indicators of immune dysregulation, these markers can be used in IBD to stratify patients based on clinical, immunologic, and genetic characteristics. pANCA is detected in the serum of 60–70% of patients with UC and in 10–20% of patients with CD. ASCA is present in 50–70% of patients with CD and in 6–14% of patients with UC. ASCA is rarely expressed in individuals who do not have IBD and thus is highly specific for

CD [11]. In a prospective study, pANCA and ASCA were studied in 97 patients with indeterminate colitis. ASCA-positive pANCA-negative indeterminate colitis predicted evolution to CD in 80% of the patients [20]. ASCA-negative pANCA-positive indeterminate colitis predicted UC in 64% of patients, whereas this combination was 100% predictive of UC or "UC-like CD." The latter represents cases of CD with left-sided colonic involvement, which resemble UC both clinically and endoscopically. Interestingly, almost half of patients with indeterminate colitis were negative for both of these serologic markers, and most of these patients (85%) continued to carry the diagnosis of indeterminate colitis on follow-up evaluation (mean follow-up 10 years). The immune reactivity to other bacterial antigens such as OmpC, I2, and CBir (flagellin) are likely to improve further the classification of patients with indeterminate colitis, although this has yet to be achieved [21].

Treatment and prevention

Randomized controlled trials of medical therapies in IBD have included only well documented cases of UC or CD. As many patients with indeterminate colitis will eventually be found to have either UC or CD, any therapy that is effective in both diseases may prove useful in the treatment of indeterminate colitis [3,5]. The goals of medical treatment in indeterminate colitis are the same as those for other forms of IBD, namely induction and maintenance of remission.

Aminosalicylates

The mainstay of medical treatment for mild to moderately active indeterminate colitis includes the use of 5-aminosalicylates (5-ASAs). There are three delivery systems for oral aminosalicylates and several topical (rectal) formulations. The oral formulations include azo-bond conjugates (sulfasalazine, olsalazine, and balsalazide), pH-dependent mesalazine with varied Eudragit (USP) coatings (Asacol®, Salofalk®, and Claversal®), and time/pH-release formulations of mesalazine encapsulated into ethylcellulose beads (Pentasa®) [3]. As indeterminate colitis usually involves the entire colon, combined administration of oral and topical 5-ASA may have an additive therapeutic effect.

Corticosteroids

In patients with indeterminate colitis who fail to respond to 5-ASA treatment, or those with severe disease, corticosteroids are often required to induce remission. However, corticosteroids have no maintenance benefit in patients with CD or UC, and should not be used long-term in patients with indeterminate colitis either [3].

Immunosuppressive drugs

In cases where indeterminate colitis becomes steroid-dependent, immunomodulatory treatment with 6-mercaptopurine (6-MP) or azathioprine (AZA) should be initiated [3]. In patients who are intolerant to 6-MP or AZA, or fail to respond adequately, methotrexate can be tried. This drug has been shown to be effective for the induction and maintenance of remission in steroid-dependent chronic active CD, but is less effective in UC. However, its efficacy in indeterminate colitis is unknown.

Anti-TNF agents

These drugs are highly effective in the treatment of inflammatory and fistulising Crohn's disease but less so for the treatment of ulcerative colitis. In one retrospective study of 20 patients with severely active and refractory indeterminate colitis, treatment with infliximab led to a response in 16 out of 20 patients. Eight of these were eventually reclassified as having Crohn's disease [22]. In another series of patients with medically refractory indeterminate colitis, infliximab was effective in 67% of patients, several of whom avoided colectomy [23].

Ciclosporin

May also be effective in patients with indeterminate colitis who have failed to respond to corticosteroid treatment, similar to patients with UC. The use of 6-MP or AZA is required for maintenance of remission in these patients.

Surgery

As discussed above, the risk of major surgery is increased several-fold in patients with indeterminate colitis compared with those with UC. Ileal anal-pouch anastomosis (IPAA) has been considered the gold standard surgical treatment for UC and is generally contraindicated in patients with CD owing to the high incidence of complications, including pelvic abscess, fistula, and pouch failure, which may require pouch excision [24]. The major decision regarding surgical treatment of indeterminate colitis is whether to perform restorative proctocolectomy (IPAA) or total colectomy with ileostomy or, in patients with rectal sparing, subtotal colectomy with ileorectal anastomosis [25]. The outcome of patients operated on for indeterminate colitis with IPAA who did not develop CD in long-term follow-up is reportedly as good as in those operated on for UC, although other studies have reported a higher incidence of complications in patients operated on for indeterminate colitis. This discrepancy may be related to differences in the definition of indeterminate colitis used in different studies. Nevertheless, the development of CD following IPAA for either UC or indeterminate colitis is associated with a poor long-term outcome [3]. Extensive evaluation of patients with an upper gastrointestinal series/small bowel follow-through or even wireless capsule endoscopy should be performed to rule out CD of the small bowel before performing an IPAA. Patients with indeterminate colitis should be offered IPAA if there is no strong reason to suspect CD, provided they are informed of the increased risks of pouch failure in indeterminate colitis.

Conclusion

Indeterminate colitis was originally reported in colectomy specimens to describe inflammatory processes that could not be classified definitively as either UC or CD. Recently, the term has been extended to include cases of chronic IBD without small bowel inflammation, and inconclusive diagnostic features of either UC or CD. Although long-term follow-up may change the diagnosis to either UC or CD, a significant number of patients will still have indeterminate colitis. The heterogeneity of IBD supports the idea that, although indeterminate colitis may represent a problem of classification at the time of initial evaluation in some patients, others may truly represent a distinct disease entity. Medical therapies are similar to those used for the treatment of UC, and sometimes CD. Surgical treatment may be needed in those patients with severe treatment-resistant disease.

References

1. Price AB. Overlap in the spectrum of nonspecific inflammatory bowel disease – colitis indeterminate. *J Clin Pathol.* 1978;31:567–577.
2. Geboes K, Colombel JF, Greenstein A, *et al.* Indeterminate colitis: a review of the concept – what's in a name? *Inflamm Bowel Dis.* 2008;14:850–857.
3. Tremaine WJ. Indeterminate colitis – definition, diagnosis and management. *Aliment Pharmacol Ther.* 2007;25:13–17.
4. Odze R. Diagnostic problems and advances in inflammatory bowel disease. *Mod Pathol.* 2003;16:347–358.
5. Romano C, Famiani A, Gallizzi R, *et al.* Indeterminate colitis: a distinctive clinical pattern of inflammatory bowel disease in children. *Pediatrics.* 2008;122:e1278–e1281.
6. Prenzel, F, Uhlig, HH. Frequency of indeterminate colitis in children and adults with IBD – a meta-analysis *J Crohn's Colitis.* 2009;3:277–281.
7. Telakis E, Tsironi E. Indeterminate colitis – definition, diagnosis, characteristics and management. *Ann Gastroenterol.* 2008;21:173–179.
8. Cho JH. The genetics and immunopathogenesis of inflammatory bowel disease. *Nat Rev Immunol.* 2008;8:458–466.
9. Meinzer U, Idestrom M, Alberti C, *et al.* Ileal involvement is age dependent in pediatric Crohn's disease. *Inflamm Bowel Dis.* 2005;11:639–644.
10. Levine A, Kugathasan S, Annese V, *et al.* Pediatric onset Crohn's colitis is characterized by genotype-dependent age-related susceptibility. *Inflamm Bowel Dis.* 2007;13:1509–1515.
11. Papadakis KA, Targan SR. Serologic testing in inflammatory bowel disease: its value in indeterminate colitis. *Curr Gastroenterol Rep.* 1999;1:482–485.
12. Wells AD, McMillan I, Price AB, *et al.* Natural history of indeterminate colitis. *Br J Surg.* 1991;78:179–181.
13. Stewenius J, Adnerhill I, Ekelund G *et al.* Ulcerative colitis and indeterminate colitis in the city of Malmö, Sweden. A 25-year incidence study. *Scand J Gastroenterol.* 1995;30:38–43.
14. Meucci G, Bortoli A, Riccioli FA *et al.* Frequency and clinical evolution of indeterminate colitis: a retrospective multicentre study in northern Italy. GSMII (Gruppo di Studio per le Malattie Inflammatorie Intestinali). *Eur J Gastroenterol Hepatol.* 1999;11:909–913.
15. Stewenius J, Adnerhill I, Anderson H *et al.* Incidence of colorectal cancer and all cause mortality in non-selected patients with ulcerative colitis and indeterminate colitis in Malmö, Sweden. *Int J Colorectal Dis.* 1995;10:117–122.
16. Branco BC, Harpaz N, Sachar DB, *et al.* Colorectal carcinoma in indeterminate colitis. *Inflamm Bowel Dis.* 2009;15:1076–1081.
17. Ruemmele FM, Moes N, de Serre NP, *et al.* Clinical and molecular aspects of autoimmune enteropathy and immune dysregulation, polyendocrinopathy autoimmune enteropathy X-linked syndrome. *Curr Opin Gastroenterol.* 2008;24:742–748.
18. Castellaneta SP, Afzal NA, Greenberg M, *et al.* Diagnostic role of upper gastrointestinal endoscopy in pediatric inflammatory bowel disease. *J Pediatr Gastroenterol Nutr.* 2004;39:257–261.
19. Murrell Z, Vasiliauskas E, Melmed G, *et al.* Preoperative wireless capsule endoscopy does not predict outcome after ileal pouch-anal anastomosis. *Dis Colon Rectum.* 2010;53:293–300.
20. Joossens S, Reinisch W, Vermeire S *et al.* The value of serologic markers in indeterminate colitis: a prospective follow-up study. *Gastroenterology.* 2002;122:1242–1247.
21. Benor S, Russell GH, Silver M, *et al.* Shortcomings of the inflammatory bowel disease serology 7 panel. *Pediatrics.* 2010;125:1230–1236.
22. Gornet JM, Couve S, Hassani Z, *et al.* Infliximab for refractory ulcerative colitis or indeterminate colitis: an open-label multicentre study. *Alim Pharmacol Ther.* 2003;18:175–181.
23. Papadakis KA, Treyzon L, Abreu MT, *et al.* Infliximab for the treatment of medically refractory indeterminate colitis. *Aliment Pharmacol Ther.* 2003;18:741–747.
24. Wolff BG. Is ileoanal the proper operation for indeterminate colitis: the case for. *Inflamm Bowel Dis.* 2002;8:362–365;discussion 368–369.
25. Lindsey I, Warren BF, Mortensen NJM. Indeterminate colitis; surgical approaches. In: Bayless T, Hanauer S, editors. *Advanced therapy of inflammatory bowel disease.* Lewiston NY: BC Decker; 2001. pp. 241–244.

CHAPTER 52
Microscopic colitis

Frank Hoentjen,[1] Chris Mulder[2] and Gerd Bouma[2]

[1]Radboud University Medical Center, Nijmegen, The Netherlands
[2]Vrije Universiteit Medical Center, Amsterdam, The Netherlands

---

ESSENTIAL FACTS ABOUT PATHOGENESIS

- Microscopic colitis encompasses the closely related conditions of lymphocytic colitis and collagenous colitis
- A female preponderance and strong associations with celiac disease (>20%), thyroid disease (~20%) and diabetes (~10%) and other autoimmune conditions suggest an autoimmune pathology
- Case reports suggest a causal role for NSAIDs, PPIs and other drugs in collagenous colitis
- Incidence rates vary between 7.1 and 12.6 per 100 000 person-years
- The female to male ratio is between 2:1 and 7:1

ESSENTIALS OF DIAGNOSIS

- Classically: older female patients with watery non-bloody diarrhea
- No abnormalities in laboratory, radiology and endoscopic findings
- Histopathology: intraepithelial lymphocytosis with (collagenous colitis) or without (lymphocytic colitis) a thickened subepithelial collagenous band
- Proximal and distal colonic biopsies are required due to the patchy nature of the disease

---

ESSENTIALS OF TREATMENT

- Stop all NSAIDs and other colitis-inducing medication
- Budesonide is the mainstay for induction of remission and maintenance therapy
- Thiopurines, mesalamine, and cholestyramine, are other treatment options
- Microscopic colitis can be self-limiting
- No increased risk of malignancy
- High recurrence rates are reported without maintenance therapy

---

Introduction

Chronic diarrhea is a frequently reported symptom and a common reason for referral to a gastroenterologist. Microscopic colitis is now recognized as a relatively frequent cause of diarrhea, especially in elderly women. The term microscopic colitis refers to both **lymphocytic and collagenous colitis** [1–3]. The first case of collagenous colitis was published in 1976 by Lindström, who described a new entity in a patient in which **chronic watery diarrhea** was associated with a thick, **subepithelial collagen deposition** in biopsy samples of endoscopically normal colonic mucosa [1]. The term **lymphocytic colitis** was proposed in 1989 to describe patients with pronounced lymphocytic inflammation in the absence of a thickened collagen band on histological evaluation [3]. These entities are now well-accepted gastrointestinal diseases and microscopic colitis is recognized as an inflammatory condition of unknown cause affecting especially the large bowel. This chapter will provide an overview of recent advances in the epidemiology, pathogenesis, diagnostics, and management of microscopic colitis.

Epidemiology

In the past, microscopic colitis was considered a rare disorder. More recently, the epidemiology of microscopic colitis was investigated in several studies and it has become apparent that microscopic colitis is a common cause of diarrhea, especially in middle-aged or elderly patients. Collagenous colitis is a disease predominantly affecting elderly women, with a **female to male ratio** around 7:1 [4,5]. The peak incidence is **around 65 years** with an age range between 10 and 90 years [4,6,7]. The **incidence of collagenous colitis** varies widely across studies, between 0.6 and 7.1 per 100 000 inhabitants [8,9]. Reported **incidence rates for lymphocytic colitis** vary between 4.4 and 12.6 per 100 000 person-years, and the female preponderance is less pronounced than in collagenous colitis (2:1) [6,8]. The peak onset for lymphocytic colitis is comparable to that of collagenous colitis, with similar age ranges [6,7].

The incidence of microscopic colitis is **rising**. For example, in Olmsted County, USA, the annual incidence for collagenous and lymphocytic colitis increased between 1985 and 2001 from 0.3 and 0.5 to 7.1 and 12.6, respectively [8]. In fact, by the end of this study period, the incidence of microscopic colitis exceeded that of Crohn's disease and ulcerative colitis in that area [8]. This increase can, at least in part, be explained by an increased awareness of the condition but at this point it cannot be excluded that the true incidence is rising as well.

Textbook of Clinical Gastroenterology and Hepatology, Second Edition. Edited by C. J. Hawkey, Jaime Bosch, Joel E. Richter, Guadalupe Garcia-Tsao, Francis K. L. Chan.

Causes and pathogenesis
Genetics

Despite a well-defined description of the pathology, the **etiology of microscopic colitis is unknown**. Many potential pathophysiologic mechanisms have been investigated in patients with microscopic colitis. However, these studies are typically small, and the results are often inconsistent. It is likely that microscopic colitis is a histological phenotype resulting from various underlying pathophysiological mechanisms. The current working hypothesis is that disease occurs as the consequence of a specific **immune reaction** in the intestine to various noxious agents in **predisposed individuals**. Whether or not this relates to a genetic predisposition is so far unknown. **Familial occurrence** has been reported occasionally [10–13]. In addition, associations with alleles of the **HLA-DR3-DQ2-TNFA-380*2** ancestral haplotype have been described irrespective of the co-occurrence of celiac disease, although these findings need to be interpreted with great care because of the small sample size [14,15].

So far there is no compelling evidence that the microscopic colitis and collagenous colitis are manifestations of the same disease in different stages of development. There are however some arguments that support this thesis. Both increased numbers of **intraepithelial lymphocytes** and a **thickened collagenous band** are frequently observed in one patient. In addition, **co-occurrence** of lymphocytic colitis and collagenous colitis within one family has been described, as well as **conversion** from lymphocytic colitis to collagenous colitis [11–13].

Autoimmune factors

There are multiple features that suggest that microscopic colitis might be an **autoimmune** disease. Microscopic colitis is associated with various **autoimmune diseases. Celiac disease** was detected in over 20% of patients with collagenous colitis [16], and vice-versa, patients with celiac disease have a relative risk of 7.9 for the development of microscopic colitis [9]. It must be noted however that the association with celiac disease is highly variable across different studies. For example, in one study the prevalence of celiac disease occurring in lymphocytic colitis was found to be 27%, but no cases of celiac disease in association with collagenous colitis were found in that study [17]. In another study involving 59 patients with microscopic colitis, no celiac disease was identified [18].

In addition to celiac disease, **thyroid diseases** are found in up to 20% of patients, **diabetes** in 10% and **rheumatoid arthritis** in 2.5% of microscopic colitis patients [6,19]. **Other autoimmune diseases** have been reported such as CREST syndrome, Sjögren's syndrome, psoriasis, Raynaud phenomenon, dermatomyositis, polymyalgia rheumatica, Wegener's granulomatosis, Behçet disease and SLE (Table 52.1) [6,20–22].

In addition to the correlation with other autoimmune diseases, the described HLA class II association, the **response to steroids** and the **female predominance lend** further support to the possibility that microscopic colitis is an autoimmune disease. Increased prevalence of **auto antibodies**, including

Table 52.1 Reported associations of microscopic colitis and other autoimmune diseases

Disease	Association (%)	Reference
Celiac disease	6–10 %	[6]
Thyroid disease	Up to 20 %	[6,19]
Diabetes mellitus	Up to 10 %	[6]
Rheumatoid arthritis	Up to 2.5 %	[6]

antinuclear antibodies (ANA), perinuclear anti-neutrophil cytoplasmic antibodies (pANCA), and anti-Saccharomyces cerevisiae antibodies have been reported in small data sets [4,6,22].

The **cytokine response** associated with microscopic colitis has so far been studied in one study. In this study, upregulated mucosal mRNA levels of interferon-gamma, TNF alpha and IL-15 were found. This Th1 cytokine profile is reminiscent of that in celiac disease [23]. Whether or not the patients in this small study had concomitant celiac disease is unknown.

Luminal agents

It has been suggested that a luminal agent or an immunological reaction against an endogenous antigen produced by enterocytes might trigger microscopic colitis [7]. The observation that diversion of the fecal stream can normalize or reduce the histopathological changes in collagenous colitis supports this thesis [24]. These fecal agents presumably cause **epithelial leakage** and **vacuolization of the enterocytes**. This weakens the epithelial barrier resulting in **thickening of the subepithelial collagen layer**, constructing a new barrier. The predominant abnormalities of microscopic colitis in the **proximal colon** support the luminal agent hypothesis. The luminal agent might be phagocytosed by macrophages and then presented to immunocompetent cells stimulating the immune system and initiate a cascade of inflammatory reactions involving fibroblast proliferation, possibly responsible for the excessive collagen deposits [25].

The possibility of an **infectious etiology** for microscopic colitis is supported by the finding of acute inflammation in a biopsy specimen and/or a history suggesting an acute gastrointestinal infection in many patients with microscopic colitis. Microbiological studies in microscopic colitis however have so far not provided a clear explanation. *Yersinia enterocolitica* and *Clostridium difficile* have been suggested but formal evidence is lacking [26]. Resolution of collagenous colitis after **antibiotic treatment** for *Helicobacter pylori* and the observed improvement after treatment with bismuth support this possibility [27,28].

Drugs

Adverse drug effects have been suggested to be associated with the development of microscopic colitis. Best known are

65. Pardi DS, Loftus EV, Jr., Tremaine WJ, *et al.* Treatment of refractory microscopic colitis with azathioprine and 6-mercaptopurine. *Gastroenterology.* 2001;120:1483–1484.

66. Vennamaneni SR, Bonner GF. Use of azathioprine or 6-mercaptopurine for treatment of steroid-dependent lymphocytic and collagenous colitis. *Am J Gastroenterol.* 2001;96:2798–2799.

67. Riddell J, Hillman L, Chiragakis L, *et al.* Collagenous colitis: oral low-dose methotrexate for patients with difficult symptoms: long-term outcomes. *J Gastroenterol Hepatol.* 2007;22:1589–1593.

68. Wildt S, Munck LK, Vinter-Jensen L, *et al.* Probiotic treatment of collagenous colitis: a randomized, double-blind, placebo-controlled trial with Lactobacillus acidophilus and *Bifidobacterium animalis subsp. Lactis. Inflamm Bowel Dis.* 2006;12:395–401.

69. Jarnerot G, Tysk C, Bohr J, Eriksson S. Collagenous colitis and fecal stream diversion. *Gastroenterology.* 1995;109:449–455.

70. Fuss IJ, Marth T, Neurath MF, *et al.* Anti-interleukin 12 treatment regulates apoptosis of Th1 T cells in experimental colitis in mice. *Gastroenterology.* 1999;117:1078–1088.

71. Cruz-Correa M, Milligan F, Giardiello FM, *et al.* Collagenous colitis with mucosal tears on endoscopic insufflation: a unique presentation. *Gut.* 2002;51:600.

72. Koulaouzidis A, Henry JA, Saeed AA. Mucosal tears can occur spontaneously in collagenous colitis. *Endoscopy.* 2006;38:549.

73. Wickbom A, Lindqvist M, Bohr J, *et al.* Colonic mucosal tears in collagenous colitis. *Scand J Gastroenterol.* 2006;41:726–729.

74. Smith RR, Ragput A. Mucosal tears on endoscopic insufflation resulting in perforation: an interesting presentation of collagenous colitis. *J Am Coll Surg.* 2007;205:725.

75. Allende DS, Taylor SL, Bronner MP. Colonic perforation as a complication of collagenous colitis in a series of 12 patients. *Am J Gastroenterol.* 2008;103:2598–2604.

Small and Large Bowel

CHAPTER 53

Eosinophilic disorders of the gastrointestinal tract

Jon A. Vanderhoof[1] and Rosemary J. Young[2]

[1]Children's Hospital; Harvard Medical School, Boston, MA, USA
[2]Boys Town National Research Hospital, Boys Town, NE, USA

ESSENTIAL FACTS ABOUT PATHOGENESIS

- Eosinophilic disorders of the GI tract are thought to arise on an allergic basis
- A personal or family history of immune hypersensitivity is common but not universally present
- Mechanisms are not well understood but appear to involve eosinophil recruitment by activated Th2 cells producing IL-4, IL-5 and IL-13

ESSENTIALS OF DIAGNOSIS

- Eosinophilic esophagitis: any age but children and males predominate. Main symptom is dysphagia +/− abdominal pain or symptoms of reflux
- Eosinophilic gastroenteritis: diarrhea, and malabsorption +/− peripheral eosinophilia
- Eosinophilic colitis: diarrhea , malabsorption, bloody diarrhea with mucus in infants. Severe constipation with rectal bleeding in older children and adults
- Diagnostic approach: histologic evidence of eosinophil infiltration and exclusion of parasite infection
- Eosinophils in submucosal, muscular, or serosal layers are considered abnormal
- Peripheral eosinophilia, hypoalbuminemia, and elevated IgE, ESR and fecal α-1 antitrypsin are additional diagnostic clues
- There may be a spectrum between eosinophilic esophagitis and part treated reflux with eosinophilic esophageal infiltrate

ESSENTIALS OF TREATMENT

- Eosinophilic esophagitis: dietary exclusion of six most common allergens, topically (budesonide, montelukast, aerosolized or systemic steroids)
- Strictures may require dilatation
- Eosinophilic gastroenteritis: allergen avoidance, corticosteroids, cromolyn sodium, montelukast, ketotifen or suplatast tosilate (Th2 inhibitor)
- Enterocolitis: dietary change, probiotics and laxatives if constipation
- Novel/investigational treatments: omalizumab (anti-IgE), treatments targeting IL-5, eosinophil selective adhesion molecules, eotaxin or eosinophil apoptosis

Introduction

The true extent of eosinophilic disease in the gastrointestinal tract is largely unknown but the incidence is increasing and it appears to affect all age groups. The clearly defined syndrome of classic eosinophilic gastroenteritis has been recognized for a number of years. More recently, it has been appreciated that eosinophilic diseases may also affect localized areas in isolation such as the esophagus and large intestine. Therapies range from dietary avoidance to the use of anti-inflammatory medications and agents which modulate the immune system.

Pathogenic processes

Eosinophils are thought to be recruited in excess numbers by eotaxin, a chemoattractant produced by irritation in the epithelial cells from allergens, infection or other non-specific modes of tissue injury [1]. The mechanism that stimulates eosinophil formation is not well understood but interleukin (IL)-5, IL-4, IL-13 and tumor necrosis factor produced by **activated Th2 and mast cells** appear to recruit and activate eosinophils in response to tissue injury [2–4]. The activated eosinophils degranulate and generate other cytotoxic inflammatory cytokines causing tissue damage and subsequent development of symptoms.

Allergic esophagitis and eosinophilic esophagitis

Clinico-pathological features

Although some have suggested merely an increased awareness, as with many atopic diseases, allergic or eosinophilic esophagitis (EoE) appears to be increasing in prevalence [5]. These patients may present at any age from **early childhood to adulthood** although at both ages there appears to be a **male predominance** with some seasonality noted with presentation suggesting a role for aeroallergens [6,7]. While symptoms of gastroesophageal reflux including vomiting and heartburn may be present, the more typical presentation is one of **dysphagia with abdominal pain [8]** being a predominant symptom in children [9,10]. Frequently, **recurrent food impaction** in the esophagus occurs. The disorder should be suspected in the presence of poor response to aggressive treatment of gastroesophageal reflux with proton pump inhibitors. Testing for allergens via skin prick tests or patch testing should be considered if there is any personal or family history of atopy [11].

Diagnosis

Endoscopy with biopsy, intraesophageal pH testing, and radiography may be useful in the evaluation of EE. **Endoscopy** often reveals concentric rings or trachealization typical of esophageal spasm (Figure 53.1). Small white patches of exudate (clusters of eosinophils) have been noted in eosinophilic infiltration of the esophagus [12]. Regardless of visual appearance and because EE is patchy in distribution, general recommendations are for biopsies of the distal, mid and proximal esophagus whenever EE is suspected [13,14]. **Biopsies** reveal dense eosinophilic infiltrate within the esophageal epithelium with greater than 15 eosinophils per high power field suggested as being diagnostic [12] (Figure 53.2). **Radiography** to evaluate for malrotation in children and esophageal caliber in all ages may also be helpful. Intraesophageal pH testing is often normal in EE and beneficial to distinguish symptoms from gastroesophageal reflux disease. The concurrent existence of both eosinophilic and reflux esophagitis is not uncommon.

Treatment, prevention and complications

Treatment of EE may involve **dietary restrictions**, medication therapy and/or esophageal dilatation. Clinicopathologic remission, primarily studied in children, has been shown by delivering all the caloric needs via a hypoallergenic amino acid formula [15]. Although targeted food elimination based on

allergy testing may be useful it has also been shown the **removal of the 6 most common allergens** also results in significant improvement [16]. If symptoms are severe, systemic steroid therapy may be required. In many cases **topical steroids such as fluticasone**, an inhalable corticosteroid that is swallowed, has been shown to be of particular benefit in both children and adults [17,18]. A comparative study of systemic versus topical steroids demonstrated greater histologic improvement with the systemic therapy; however similar degrees of symptom abatement and time to relapse when therapy was discontinued was seen in both groups [19]. **Budesonide** mixed in a slurry solution has also been suggested [20]. Monitoring of therapy is problematic because it has been shown that significant esophageal inflammation may be present despite few apparent symptoms [21].

The primary complication with EE is the development of strictures. **Esophageal dilatation** may be used to treat fixed strictures but is associated with increased complications [22]. Preventive measures have not been clearly identified.

Eosinophilic gastroenteritis

Clinico-pathological features

Eosinophilic gastroenteritis (EG) is present when eosinophilic inflammatory changes occur distal to the esophagus and are accompanied by gastrointestinal symptoms [23]. Although quite rare it typically appears in adulthood around the third to fifth decade of life. There are **3 identified subtypes** including mucosal (most common), muscularis and serosal which produce varying symptoms. It is suspected that in many cases an allergic component is involved; however other conditions such as inflammatory bowel disease, parasitic infections, connective tissue diseases and drug-induced hypersensitivy have also been associated with EG [22] (see Chapters 50–52).

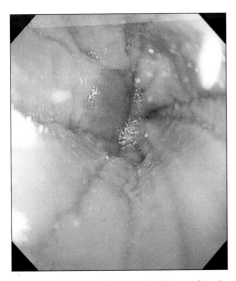

Figure 53.1 Endoscopy. Concentric rings and white exudates in a 29-year-old male with dysphagia. Histology confirmed eosinophilic esophagitis. (Image courtesy of Dr Paul Fortun.)

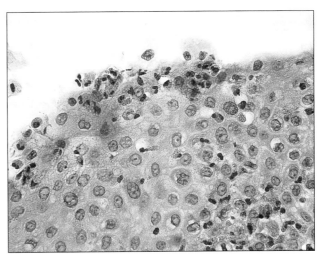

Figure 53.2 Esophageal squamous epithelium. Esophageal squamous epithelium infiltrated by abundant eosinophils with bright orange granules (H&E ×200). This biopsy is from a 16-year-old boy who presented with food impaction. (Image courtesy of Dr Philip Kaye.)

Classic eosinophilic gastroenteritis often begins with mild and variable symptoms making the diagnosis difficult. Mucosal disease often presents with symptoms similar to inflammatory bowel disease[23], and abdominal pain and obstructive symptoms occur with muscularis eosinophlia. Serosal inflammation may result in bloating and ascites [25]. In many cases, there is a family history of allergic disorders but the true cause is somewhat obscure.

Diagnosis

The diagnosis of eosinophilic gastroenteritis is based on the presence of gastrointestinal symptoms, the demonstration of eosinophilic infiltration in gastrointestinal biopsies, and the exclusion of other causes. Generally, visual endoscopic findings of the upper and lower gastrointestinal tract are normal. In severe cases endoscopic visualization may reveal lymphoid hyperplasia, thickened folds, erythema and mucosal irritation [22].

Histology In children it has been found that up to 30 eosinophils per high power field are normally present in the ileum with progressively decreasing numbers throughout the colon. In these areas they are presumed to be present to protect against parasitic and allergic irritants [26]. Although there is no general agreement on what increased level constitutes a pathological condition in mucosal disease, when combined with other features such as eosinophils infiltrating the epithelium and crypts, esoinophil degranulation or eosinophils in the gastric antrum or fundus (typically not present in these locations), the diagnosis becomes clearer [24,27].

Laparoscopy is required to evaluate for muscularis or serosal disease with the presence of any eosinophils in these layers being considered abnormal. Eosinophilic infiltrates can be patchy in nature and necessitate multiple biopsy specimens for appropriate identification.

Peripheral eosinophilia, an elevated immunoglobulin E (IgE) and sedimentation rate, hypoalbuminemia, increased **fecal α–1 antitrypsin** or the presence of fecal eosinophils may assist in the diagnosis of eosinophilic gastroenteritis.

Radiologic findings are uncommon but in severe cases, thickened intestinal folds, esophageal narrowing and antral stenosis may be identified on barium studies.

Ultrasonography may also demonstrate gastrointestinal wall thickening and/or ascites [28].

Treatment, prevention and complications

Since the etiology of eosinophilic gastroenteritis is not known, treatment of the condition primarily relies on management of symptoms. **Avoidance of certain allergens** is rarely helpful in widespread eosinophilic disease. Anti-inflammatory medications are therefore generally utilized. If symptoms are severe, initiation of high-dose systemic **corticosteroid therapy** may

often be required; subsequent maintenance with less potent anti-inflammatory agents and diet therapy may be useful. Other medications specifically targeting control of eosinophils have been explored. Case reports of **cromolyn sodium** and more recently **montelukast** have demonstrated success [29,30]. **Ketotifen**, which inhibits secretion of mast cell mediators such as histamine, and **suplatast tosilate**, a selective T-helper-2 cytokine IL-4 and IL-5 inhibitor, have been used in some cases of eosinophilic gastroenteritis with success [31,32]. **Acid suppression** may be used for patients with upper gastrointestinal symptoms. Treatment of other symptoms such as nausea may include medications such as **ondansetron** or prokinetic agents such as **metaclopramide**. Recently in a small series, **Omalizumab**, a humanized ant-IgE antibody proved to be of benefit in an open label trial of EG [33]. **Therapies under** investigation include anti-interleukin 5, eosinophil selective adhesion molecules, a monoclonal eotaxin antibody and substances which enhance eosinophil apoptosis [34,35].

Eosinophilic colitis
Infantile
Clinico-pathological features

It is estimated that 2% and 7% of infants experience allergic enterocolitis. In most cases the reaction is to **cows' milk protein** through a non-IgE-mediated mechanism characterized by inflammatory changes in the small bowel or colon [20]. About half of the babies who are allergic to milk also turn out to be allergic to **soy** [36]. Some have been shown to be allergic to fragments of cows' milk protein in extensively hydrolyzed infant formulas and even to the cows' milk protein fragments present in breast milk [37–38]. Allergic infants seem to be more common in families with a strong history of food allergy [39]. **Atopic dermatitis** may accompany the inflammatory changes in the gut.

Infants with inflammatory changes predominantly in the small bowel disease will present with **diarrhea, malabsorption, and poor intake**. Chronic irritability is common and, because of delayed gastric emptying, gastroesophageal reflux is also common. In infants with predominantly large bowel inflammatory changes, bloody stools containing large quantities of mucus are more typical [40,41].

Some infants who react to cows' milk protein do so through an **IgE-mediated mechanism**. In this situation, symptoms are often quite abrupt in onset and, likewise, resolve quickly if the antigen is removed [42]. Cutaneous and systemic manifestations are common, including **anaphylaxis, wheezing, or atopic eczema**.

Diagnosis

The true incidence of non-IgE mediated enterocolitis in babies is often difficult to determine because the presentation may be subtle and few, if any, laboratory parameters can reliably diagnose the condition. Generally the condition is suspected based on presenting symptoms however confirmation **via small** bowel and rectal biopsies is confirmatory. In infants with non-IgE-mediated allergic enterocolitis, IgE testing to a specific antigen either by skin test or RAST test is not of significant benefit [41].

Treatment, prevention and complications
Response to **dietary intervention** with removal of the offending protein is often delayed for a period of days to weeks, often taking up to 2–3 weeks for the inflammatory changes to clear and symptoms to totally resolve. Although soy protein formulas are often used as the initial therapeutic modality in such infants, many of these infants will relapse after a few days or weeks on soy with recurrence of symptoms and reappearance of histologic inflammatory changes [42]. Allergic enterocolitis in infants commonly resolves on **protein hydrolysate formulas** provided the proteins in the formulas are extensively hydrolyzed [43]. Partially hydrolyzed infant formulas are frequently not beneficial and should be avoided in such infants [37]. Occasionally, the use of an **amino acid-based infant formula** is required for a small number of such infants [44]. Breast-fed infants are typically treated by **eliminating cows' milk** and occasionally certain other common dietary antigens from the mother's diet [45].

Investigation into the prevention of allergic enterocolitis has included the use of **probiotics** by the mother prior to delivery as well as given to the infant immediately after birth but have not yielded consistent benefits [46]. Avoidance of cow's milk protein by the mother prior to delivery does not appear to be beneficial and may result in inadequate nutrition [47,48].

Older children and adults
Clinico-pathological features
The association of ongoing allergic, non-IgE mediated, colitis in older children and adults has also been identified [49–51]. The clinical characteristics of this syndrome include **severe constipation** with extreme difficulty in expelling stool, **rectal bleeding** as well as unresponsiveness to traditional medical management. A prior history of multiple food intolerance as an infant may precede the clinical syndrome [52–54]. Abdominal pain accompanies the constipation and is frequently periumbilical and poorly described [52].

Diagnosis
Diagnosis is suggested by the presence of colonic lymphoid nodular hyperplasia and intra-epithelial and lamina propria eosinophilia may be present in both **rectal and duodenal biopsies** [55,56].

Treatment, prevention and complications
Following a short course of laxative therapy, prolonged **dietary restriction** of suspected food protein allergens is required. Resolution of symptoms is commonly seen with restriction of cow's milk protein and wheat protein-free diets [53,55]. Adults may respond better to anti-inflammatory therapy [57]. Prevention would most likely be obtained with restriction of allergic

dietary proteins in those with a family history of atopy; however this has not been proven. As this is a newly recognized condition, long-term complications have not been identified.

Conclusion
Eosinophilic disorders of the gastrointestinal tract are rarely known to be fatal and, although previously considered to be rare, seem to be on the increase. This is probably due to greater awareness of the condition and better diagnostic modalities. Although treatment traditionally responds to immunosuppression with corticosteroids, current knowledge of the pathophysiological mechanisms has led to the use of alternative therapies including restrictive diet and other pharmacologic agents targeted at decreasing the eosinophilic response. Placebo-controlled trials are often lacking.

> **SOURCES OF INFORMATION FOR DOCTORS AND PATIENTS**
>
> http://www.emedicine.com/med/topic688.htm
> http://www.naspghan.org

References
1. Garcia-Zepeda EA, Rothenberg ME, Ownbey RT, et al. Human eotaxin is a specific chemoattractant for eosinophil cells and provides a new mechanism to explain tissue eosinophilia. Nat Med. 1996;2:449–456.
2. Rankin SM, Conroy DM, Williams TJ. Eotaxin and eosinophil recruitment: implications for human disease. Mol Med Today. 2000;6:20–27.
3. Mishra A, Hogan S, Lee J, et al. Fundamental signals that regulated eosinophil homing into the gastrointestinal tract, J Clin Invest. 1999;103:1719–1727.
4. Kato M, Kephart GM, Talley NJ, et al. Eosinophil infiltration and degranulation in normal human tissue. Anat Rec. 1998;252:418–425.
5. Chehade, Mirna; Sampson, Hugh A. Epidemiology and etiology of eosinophilic esophagitis. Gastrointest Endosc Clin N Am. 2008;18:33–44.
6. Prasad GA, Smyrk TC, Schleck C, et al. Seasonal variation in the incidence of eosinophilic esophagitis over 30 years: a population based study (abstract). Gastroenterology. 2008;134:A–619.
7. Franciosi JP, Tam V, Liacouras CA, et al. A case-control study of sociodemographic and geographic characteristics of 335 children with eosinophilic esophagitis. Clin Gastroenterol Hepatol. 2009;7:415–419.
8. Müller S, Pühl S, Vieth M, Stolte M. Analysis of symptoms and endoscopic findings in 117 patients with histological diagnoses of eosinophilic esophagitis. Endoscopy. 2007;39:339–344.
9. Pentiuk S, Putnam PE, Collins MH, et al. Dissociation between symptoms and histological severity in pediatric eosinophilic esophagitis. J Pediatr Gastroenterol Nutr. 2009;48:152–160.
10. Flood EM, Beusterien KM, Amonkar MM, et al. Patient and caregiver perspective on pediatric eosinophilic esophagitis and

newly developed symptom questionnaires. *Curr Med Res Opin.* 2008;24:3369–3381.

11. Ferre-Ybarz L, Nevot Falco S, Plaza-Martin AM. Eosinophilic oesophagitis: Clinical manifestations and treatment options. The role of the allergologist. *Allergol Immunopathol.* 2008;36:358–365.

12. Khan S, Orenstein SR. Eosinophilic gastroenteritis: epidemiology, diagnosis and management. *Paediatr Drugs.* 2002;4:563–570.

13. Furuta GT, Forbes D, Boey C, et al. Eosinophilic Gastrointestinal Diseases Working Group. Eosinophilic gastrointestinal diseases (EGIDs). *J Pediatr Gastroenterol Nutr.* 2008;47:234–238.

14. Yantiss RK, Odze RD. Optimal approach to obtaining mucosal biopsies for assessment of inflammatory disorders of the gastrointestinal tract. *Am J Gastroenterol.* 2009;104:774–783.

15. Kelly KJ, Lazenby AJ, Rowe PC, et al. Eosinophilic esophagitis attributed to gastroesophageal reflux: improvement with an amino acid-based formula. *Gastroenterology.* 1995;109:1503–1512.

16. Kagalwalla AF, Sentongo TA, Ritz S, et al. Effect of six-food elimination diet on clinical and histologic outcomes in eosinophilic esophagitis. *Clin Gastroenterol Hepatol.* 2006;4:1097–1102. Epub 2006 Jul 21.

17. Faubion WA Jr, Perrault J, Burgart LJ, et al. Treatment of eosinophilic esophagitis with inhaled corticosteroids. *J Pediatr Gastroenterol Nutr.* 1998;27:90–93.

18. Teitelbaum JE, Fox VL, Twarog FJ, et al. Eosinophilic esophagitis in children: immunopathological analysis and response to fluticasone propionate. *Gastroenterology.* 2002;122:1216–1225.

19. Schaefer ET, Fitzgerald JF, Molleston JP, et al. Comparison of oral prednisone and topical fluticasone in the treatment of eosinophilic esophagitis: a randomized trial in children. *Clin Gastroenterol Hepatol.* 2008;6:165–173.

20. Host A. Frequency of cow's milk allergy in childhood. *Ann Allergy Asthma Immunol.* 2002;89(Suppl 1):33–37.

21. Pentiuk S, Putnam PE, Collins MH, et al. Dissociation between symptoms and histological severity in pediatric eosinophilic esophagitis. *J Pediatr Gastroenterol Nutr.* 2009;48:152–160.

22. Yan BM, Shaffer EA. Primary eosinophlic disorders of the gastrointestinal tract. *Gut.* 2009;58:721–732.

23. Katsanos KH, Zinovieva E, Lambri E, et al. Eosinophilic-Crohn overlap colitis and review of the literature. *Journal of Crohn's and Colitis* 2011;5:256–261.

24. Khan S, Orenstein SR. Eosinophilic gastroenteritis: epidemiology, diagnosis and management. *Paediatr Drugs.* 2002;4:563–570.

25. Pratt CA, Demain JG, Rathkopf MM. Food allergy and eosinophilic gastrointestinal disorders: guiding our diagnosis and treatment. *Curr Probl Pediatr Adolesc Health Care.* 2008;38:170–88.

26. Lowichik A, Weinberg AG. A quantitative evaluation of mucosal eosinophils in the pediatric gastrointestinal tract. *Mod Pathol.* 1996;9:110–114.

27. Talley NJ, Shorter RG, Phillips SF, et al. Eosinophilic gastroenteritis: a clinicopathological study of patients with disease of the mucosa, muscle layer, and subserosal tissues. *Gut.* 1990;31:54–58.

28. Buljevac M, Urek MC, Stoos-Veic T. Sonography in diagnosis and follow-up of serosal eosinophilic gastroenteritis treated with corticosteroid. *J Clin Ultrasound.* 2005;33:43–46.

29. Perez-Millan A, Martin-Lorente JL, Lopez- Morante A, et al. Subserosal eosinophilic gastroenteritis treated efficaciously with sodium cromoglycate. *Dig Dis Sci.* 1997;42:342–344.

30. Vanderhoof JA, Young RJ, Hanner TL, et al. Montelukast: use in pediatric patients with eosinophilic gastrointestinal disease. *J Pediatr Gastroenterol Nutr.* 2003;36:293–294.

31. Melamed I, Feanny SJ, Sherman PM, Roifman CM. Benefit of ketotifen in patients with eosinophilic gastroenteritis. *Am J Med.* 1991;90:310–314.

32. Shirai T, Hashimoto D, Suzuki K, et al. Successful treatment of eosinophilic gastroenteritis with suplatast tosilate. *J Allergy Clin Immunol.* 2001;107:924–925.

33. Foroughi S, Foster B, Kim N, et al. Anti-IgE treatment of eosinophil-associated gastrointestinal disorders. *J Allergy Clin Immunol.* 2007;120:594–601.

34. Nutku-Bilir E, Hudson SA, Bochner BS. Interleukin-5 priming of human eosinophils alters siglec-8 mediated apoptosis pathways. *Am J Respir Cell Mol Biol.* 2008;38:121–124.

35. Bochner BS. Verdict in the case of therapies versus eosinophils: the jury is still out. *J Allergy Clin Immunol.* 2004;113:3–9.

36. Rozenfeld P, Docena GH, Añón MC, et al. Detection and identification of a soy protein component that cross-reacts with caseins from cow's milk. *Clin Exp Immunol.* 2002;130:49–58.

37. Vanderhoof JA, Murray ND, Kaufman SS, et al. Intolerance to protein hydrolysate infant formulas: an underrecognized cause of gastrointestinal symptoms in infants. *J Pediatr.* 1997;131:741–744.

38. Pumberger W, Pomberger G, Geissler W. Proctocolitis in breast fed infants: a contribution to differential diagnosis of haematochezia in early childhood. *Postgrad Med J.* 2001;77:252–254.

39. Chandra RK. Five-year follow-up of high-risk infants with family history of allergy who were exclusively breast-fed or fed partial whey hydrolysate, soy, and conventional cow's milk formulas. *J Pediatr Gastroenterol Nutr.* 1997;24:380–388.

40. Fox VL. Gastrointestinal bleeding in infancy and childhood. *Gastroenterol Clin North Am.* 2000;29:37–66.

41. Sicherer SH. Clinical aspects of gastrointestinal food allergy in childhood. *Pediatrics.* 2003;111:1609–1616.

42. Kaplan MS. Complications in children with a severe allergy to cow milk. *Ann Allergy.* 1993;71:529–532.

43. Rozenfeld P, Docena GH, Añón MC, et al. Detection and identification of a soy protein component that cross-reacts with caseins from cow's milk. *Clin Exp Immunol.* 2002;130:49–58.

44. de Boissieu D, Dupont C. Allergy to extensively hydrolyzed cow's milk proteins in infants: safety and duration of amino acid-based formula. *J Pediatr.* 2002;141:271–273.

45. Pumberger W, Pomberger G, Geissler W. Proctocolitis in breast fed infants: a contribution to differential diagnosis of haematochezia in early childhood. *Postgrad Med J.* 2001;77:252–254.

46. Kopp MV, Salfeld P. Probiotics and prevention of allergic disease. *Curr Opin Clin Nutr Metab Care.* 2009;12:298–303.

47. Arshad SH. Food allergen avoidance in primary prevention of food allergy. *Allergy.* 2001;56(Suppl 67):113–116.

48. Arvola T, Holmberg-Marttila D. Benefits and risks of elimination diets. *Ann Med.* 1999;31:293–298.

49. Iacono G, Cavataio F, Montalto G, et al. Intolerance of cow's milk and chronic constipation in children. *N Engl J Med.* 1998;339:1100–1104.

50. Carroccio A, Di Prima L, Iacono G, et al. Multiple food hypersensitivity as a cause of refractory chronic constipation in adults. *Scand J Gastroenterol.* 2006;41:498–504.

51. Shah N, Lindley K, Milla P. Cow's milk and chronic constipation in children. *N Engl J Med.* 1999;340:891–892.

52. Vanderhoof JA, Perry D, Hanner TL, et al. Allergic constipation: association with infantile milk allergy. *Clin Pediatr (Phila).* 2001;40:399–402.

53. Daher S, Tahan S, Solé D, *et al.* Cow's milk protein intolerance and chronic constipation in children. *Pediatr Allergy Immunol.* 2001;12:339–342.

54. Ravelli A, Villanacci V, Chiappa S, *et al.* Dietary protein-induced proctocolitis in childhood. *America Journal of Gastroenterology.* 2008;103:2605–2612.

55. Carroccio A, Iacono G, Di Prima L, *et al.* Food hypersensitivity as a cause of rectal bleeding in adults. *Clin Gastroenterol Hepatol.* 2009;7:120–122.

56. Iacono G, Ravelli A, Di Prima L, *et al.* Colonic lymphoid nodular hyperplasia in children: relationship to food hypersensitivity. *Clin Gastroenterol Hepatol.* 2007;5:361–366.

57. Gaertner WB, MacDonald JE, Kwaan MR, *et al.* Eosinophilic Colitis: University of Minnesota Experience and Literature Review. *Gastroenterology Review and Practice.* 2011;1–6.

Small and Large Bowel

CHAPTER 54

Pseudomembranous colitis

Tanya M. Monaghan and Yashwant R. Mahida

Nottingham University Hospitals, Nottingham, UK

ESSENTIAL FACTS ABOUT PATHOGENESIS

- *Clostridium difficile* is a Gram positive, anerobic, spore forming, toxin-producing bacillus which is responsible for most cases of pseudomembranous colitis
- Intestinal disease is largely mediated by two exotoxins secreted by the bacterium, designated toxin A and toxin B
- The predominant risk factor associated with acquisition of *Clostridium difficile* is disruption of the protective colonic microflora by broad spectrum antibiotics, especially in the elderly

ESSENTIALS OF DIAGNOSIS

- Usually based on detection of *C. difficile* toxins in stool sample, either by enzyme-linked immunosorbent assays (ELISAs) or bioassay
- Flexible sigmoidoscopy (with biopsies) is helpful in facilitating a rapid diagnosis of pseudomembranous colitis and is particularly beneficial for patients for whom there is a high index of suspicion of *Clostridium difficile* infection

ESSENTIALS OF TREATMENT

- Mild disease may resolve following discontinuation of offending antibiotics
- Oral metronidazole is the standard first line therapy for treating mild disease
- Vancomycin is recommended for treatment of severe *C. difficile* infection
- Patients with very severe disease may benefit from early surgery and there is currently a need for robust criteria that will enable such patients to be identified
- The management of recurrent infection remains a substantial therapeutic challenge. Various strategies have been proposed

Introduction

Pseudomembramous colitis is a severe, acute, exudative colitis which is usually due to infection by toxigenic strains of **Clostridium difficile**. *C. difficile* is a Gram-positive, anerobic, spore-forming and toxin-producing bacillus that was first identified as the causative agent of antibiotic-associated pseudomembranous colitis in 1978 [1]. Since then, this pathogen

has become the leading cause of hospital-acquired infectious diarrhea worldwide.

Epidemiology

Over the last 20 years, there has been a progressive increase in the number of reported cases of *C. difficile* infection. In England, more than 50 000 cases of *C. difficile* infection were reported in 2007 – a **50-fold increase since 1990.**

Since 2001–2002, there have been a number of reports of **epidemics of *C. difficile* infection in hospitalised patients** in several countries, together with reports of more severe disease in those over the age of 65 years [1]. Molecular studies in isolates from different countries have reported that a **hypervirulent strain** of *C. difficile*, designated NAP1/027, has been responsible for outbreaks and more severe and refractory disease [1,2]. However, other strains (including PCR ribotypes 001, 053, 078 and 106) have also been implicated. Moreover, there have been reports of more severe disease in non-traditional hosts such as young seemingly healthy adults, children in the community and some individuals without anti-microbial exposure [1].

Risk factors for the development of *C. difficile*-associated disease include advancing age and the use of broad-spectrum antibiotics and chemotherapeutic or immunosuppressant agents. Although a causal relationship has not been established, a number of epidemiological studies have reported an association between proton pump inhibitors and *C. difficile* infection [3]. A 2- to 3-fold increase in frequency of *C. difficile* infection has also been reported in patients with inflammatory bowel disease [1].

Causes and pathogenesis

C. difficile is **transmitted** via highly resistant spores which contaminate surfaces in the vicinity of an affected patient and are capable of surviving for months or even years. After ingestion, the spores convert to metabolically active vegetative forms and *C. difficile* multiplies to colonise the large intestine, especially when the resident microbial flora has been disrupted by broad-spectrum antibiotics.

The intestinal disease in *C. difficile* infection is mediated by two high molecular weight exotoxins (designated **toxins A and B**) that are secreted by the bacterium [4]. Following internalization by host cells, both toxins inactivate small regulatory proteins of the **Ras superfamily of GTPases** [5]. In the intestinal epithelial cells, initial changes include:

- loss of barrier function
- secretion of pro-inflammatory cytokines
- disruption of the cell cytoskeleton, followed by programmed cell death [6,7].

In contrast to lymphocytes, epithelial cells and monocytes/macrophages are highly susceptible to *C. difficile* toxin-induced cell death [8,9]. It is believed that the responses to *C. difficile* toxins by mucosal epithelial cells and underlying cells in the lamina propria lead to recruitment of polymorphonuclear cells, monocytes and lymphocytes to the intestinal mucosa as part of a prominent inflammatory response. In those colonised with toxigenic *C. difficile*, the host **humoral immune response** to the secreted toxins may determine the development of disease, its severity and risk of recurrence [1].

Clinical presentation

Following colonization with toxigenic *C. difficile*, individuals may become asymptomatic carriers or develop colonic disease. The clinical presentation of *C. difficile*-associated disease can range from mild diarrhea to life-threatening pseudomembranous colitis, toxic megacolon and sepsis.

Diarrhea: Diarrhea is the usual presenting symptom. Most affected individuals tend to experience fairly mild to moderate (2–6 stools/day) non-bloody, watery diarrhea with some **abdominal cramping** and tenderness. Evidence of peritoneal signs should immediately raise suspicion for fulminant colitis. Other indicators of severe disease include the presence of profuse diarrhea and systemic symptoms such as **fever, anorexia, nausea, vomiting and malaise**. It is important to recognise that some patients with severe pseudomembranous colitis may have little or no diarrhea as a result of **toxic megacolon** and **paralytic ileus**. In these patients, abdominal distension, marked leukocytosis and dilated and inflamed colon on abdominal radiography and computed tomography (CT) may provide important clues regarding the diagnosis [1].

Differential diagnosis

The majority of cases of antibiotic-associated diarrhea may not be due to *C. difficile* infection [1]. A wide range of microorganisms can also cause diarrhea and include protozoa (e.g., *Giardia*, *Cryptosporidium*), pathogenic bacteria (e.g., *Shigella*, *E. coli* 0157:H7, *Campylobacter*, *Salmonella*) and viruses (e.g., rotavirus, enteric adenoviruses) [10]. Other diagnoses to consider include inflammatory bowel disease, ischemic colitis

(appearances similar to pseudomembranous colitis can sometimes be seen, but there is often a sharp demarcation between diseased and normal parts of the left colon) and drug-induced diarrhea. Pseudomembranous colitis is often seen in patients with the more severe form of *C. difficile* infection and is very uncommon in other infections that cause colonic inflammation. However, rarely, enteric pathogens such as enterotoxigenic *C. perfringens* and *Shigella* may also cause pseudomembranous colitis.

Diagnostic investigation
Laboratory studies

The diagnosis of *C. difficile* infection typically involves demonstration of the presence of toxigenic *C. difficile* or (more commonly) its **toxins A and/or B** in a stool sample. The majority of clinical laboratories now use enzyme-linked **immunosorbent assays** (ELISAs) for toxin A or toxins A and B. Assays that test for the presence of both toxins are preferable as toxin A-negative, toxin-B positive strains can also cause disease. These assays have the advantages of being relatively quick and easy to perform, with results available the same day. However, if the prevalence of *C. difficile* toxin positive stool samples is low, their positive predictive value may be unacceptably low and in this case, a two-stage testing strategy may be required [11].

Prior to the availability of specific ELISAs, *C. difficile* toxins in stool samples were detected using a **culture cytotoxicity assay**, which is still considered by many to be the "gold standard." Although it may have greater sensitivity than ELISAs for toxin detection, the main disadvantages of this assay are that it takes 24–48 hours to obtain a result, requires greater laboratory resources and expertise and is much more expensive.

To avoid false negative test results due to potential problems with toxin degradation, stool samples should be **refrigerated** prior to testing. In some patients with pseudomembranous colitis due to *C. difficile* infection, repeat stool tests may be negative [12]. **Flexible sigmoidoscopy** (see below) and/or culture for toxigenic *C. difficile* may be required. For the latter, the stool sample is cultured in selective medium, with requirement for further tests to confirm that the cultured *C. difficile* is toxigenic. Since it would take 3–4 days to obtain a result (and is more expensive), this test is not routinely used for diagnostic purposes in most hospitals. However, direct culture of *C. difficile* has demonstrated utility in investigating outbreaks as isolates can be **genotyped**, and for assessing the antimicrobial susceptibility of *C. difficile* strains [1]. Sensitive molecular techniques involving PCR technology to detect the presence of *C. difficile* toxin genes *tcdA* (toxin A) and *tcdB* (toxin B) in stool samples are currently being adapted and simplified for consideration of routine laboratory use.

Imaging

Abdominal radiography and CT of the abdomen are useful in the context of severe disease and help in detecting complications such as toxic dilatation and perforation. Since intestinal inflammation shows up as mucosal enhancement, CT of the abdomen can also be helpful in the assessment of the extent and severity of pseudomembranous colitis.

Endoscopy

In the relevant clinical context, the characteristic appearance of pseudomembranes at sigmoidoscopy is highly suggestive of *C. difficile* infection, even in the presence of negative stool tests for *C. difficile* toxin [12]. Macroscopically, pseudomembranes are appreciated as multiple raised discrete **plaques of yellow-white exudate** up to 2 cms in diameter separated by normal or mildly hyperemic mucosa (Figure 54.1). These lesions can easily be removed during endoscopy, revealing an **erythematous inflamed mucosa**. In more advanced cases, the pseudomembranes may coalesce to form a confluent exudative membrane covering most of the surface of the colon. Rarely, severe untreated cases may progress to **broad ulceration** of the mucosal surface. Pseudomembranous colitis or the characteristic histological changes may not be seen in inflammatory bowel disease patients with *C. difficile* infection.

Unprepped **bedside flexible sigmoidoscopy** (with biopsies) can facilitate rapid diagnosis of pseudomembranous colitis, before the results of stool *C. difficile* toxin test are available, or if the results are negative [12]. This bedside approach may also facilitate the identification of other causes of diarrhea and minimizes the risks of contaminating other sites with *C. difficile* spores.

Histology

Three types of histopathological lesion of *C. difficile*-associated pseudomembranous colitis have been described in biopsy material, colectomy specimens and those obtained at postmortem [13].

- **Type 1 "summit lesions"** manifest as a focal area of epithelial necrosis and an exudate consisting of polymorphonuclear cells, fibrin and "nuclear dust" (Figure 54.2).
- **In type 2 lesions**, the major feature comprises a well-defined group of disrupted glands, distended by mucin and polymorphonuclear cells. There is usually loss of the superficial half of their epithelial lining and they are surmounted by a **cloud of epithelial debris**, fibrin, mucus, and polymorphonuclear cells ("the pseudomembrane").
- **Type 3 lesions** have been described as showing complete structural **necrosis of the mucosa**, with a thick covering of fibrin, mucus, and inflammatory debris [13].

In mild disease, biopsy specimens may demonstrate only nonspecific changes such as intraepithelial infiltration by polymorphonuclear cells.

Treatment and prevention
Infection prevention and control

As this infection is often acquired by hospital patients receiving broad-spectrum antibiotics (which lead to disruption of the protective resident microbial flora, thereby allowing colonization by *C. difficile*), **prevention strategies** are of major importance [1]. In addition to prevention of cross-infection (such as patient isolation, cohorting of infected individuals, enhanced environmental and equipment cleaning), there is also a need for the prudent use of antimicrobial agents (for example, limiting duration of antibiotic exposure, using automatic stop dates, avoiding broad-spectrum antibiotics where possible and restricting intravenous antibiotics). Participation in local, regional and national surveillance programs is also encouraged.

Treatment of an acute episode

In an acute episode, treatment is best guided by the severity of the disease as assessed by bowel frequency (with the caveat that some patients with severe pseudomembranous colitis may have little or no diarrhea due to toxic megacolon and

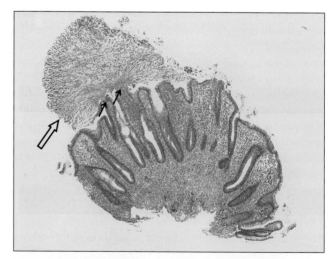

Figure 54.2 Type 1 summit lesion. Photomicrograph of histological section of colonic mucosal biopsy from a patient with pseudomembranous colitis, showing areas of focal epithelial necrosis (thin arrows) associated with an eruption of inflammatory exudate (summit lesion; outline arrow), which is composed of neutrophils, fibrin, mucus and necrotic epithelial cells (hematoxylin and eosin).

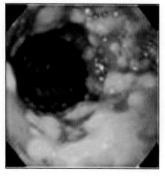

Figure 54.1 Endoscopic image of pseudomembranous colitis.

paralytic ileus), abdominal pain, nausea (and vomiting in those with paralytic ileus), pyrexia and abdominal tenderness. Leukocytosis, raised CRP level and low albumin level are also often seen in severe disease.

In those with mild diarrhea, cessation of the offending antibiotics may be all that is necessary. This approach can be considered in circumstances in which the patient can be monitored such that antibiotic treatment can be commenced if there is lack of response or deterioration within the first 2–3 days [1,12].

Although a number of new antibiotic and non-antibiotic based therapeutic agents are presently being investigated [1], oral **metronidazole** or **vancomycin** remains the mainstay of treatment. A recent clinical trial has confirmed clinical experience over many years that vancomycin is superior to metronidazole in the treatment of severe (but not mild) *C. difficile*-associated disease [14]. As it is more cost-effective and reduces selection pressure for the emergence of vancomycin-resistant *enteroccoci*, metronidazole is often recommended as initial treatment for **mild disease**, with the option of changing to oral vancomycin if there is inadequate or lack of response. Patients with pseudomembranous colitis at endoscopy or appearances consistent with colitis on abdominal CT should be treated with **vancomycin**. In the presence of vomiting and/ or ileus, adequate levels of antibiotic may not be achieved in the colonic lumen following oral administration. **Intravenous metronidazole** which is secreted into the lumen of the inflamed colon may, therefore, need to be added to high dose (e.g., 500 mg qds) oral (or via nasogastric tube) **vancomycin**. Clinical trial evidence for combination treatment in this subgroup of patients with severe *C. difficile* infection is awaited.

Intravenous **immunoglobulin treatment** is often considered in patients with severe disease and it is anticipated that controlled clinical trial evidence for its use will be available in the near future. Retrospective case studies suggest that in those with severe *C. difficile*-associated colitis (such as those requiring admission to the intensive care unit because of cardiorespiratory compromise), **emergency colectomy** may be more beneficial than medical treatment. However, postoperative mortality if often high and prospective studies are required. Currently, an early combined medical and surgical cooperative approach is recommended in patients with severe disease [1].

Treatment of recurrent disease

Recurrent *C. difficile*-associated disease is a common management problem occurring in **15–35% of patients**, despite successful treatment of the initial episode [1]. The disease typically recurs within 1 to 3 weeks following completion of treatment of the initial episode. However, late recurrences up to 2 months later also occur and some patients may suffer multiple recurrences.

Disease recurrence may reflect germination of persistent spores of the original strain or re-infection with a new strain of *Clostridium difficile* [1].

The risk of recurrent disease is **higher** in those that have previously had more than one episode of infection and has been shown to be related to the host's humoral immune response to *C. difficile* toxins [1]. **Management** of recurrent *C. difficile*-associated disease is predominantly based on published clinical experience and case series. Treatment for a first recurrence of *C. difficile* infection is usually identical to that for the primary episode. For subsequent recurrences, a prolonged tapering or pulse-dosing regimen of vancomycin is often used. In a controlled clinical trial, addition of the **probiotic yeast *S. boulardii*** to standard antibiotics has been reported to significantly reduce the recurrence rate [15].

Several **other therapeutic interventions** have been reported for treating multiple recurrences, illustrating the need for a single effective approach [16]. The interventions include:

- probiotics
- prebiotics (oligofructose)
- antibiotics (rifaximin)
- toxin-binders (tolevamer)
- fecal bacteriotherapy
- immune-based treatments such as normal pooled intravenous immunoglobulin.

New therapeutic strategies are also being tested. These include vaccination against *C. difficile* and its toxins, monoclonal antibodies and antimicrobial agents that are active against *C. difficile*, but cause minimal disruption to the resident microbial flora [1].

Complications and their management

Toxic dilatation of the colon that does not respond to aggressive medical treatment requires **surgery**; as does colonic perforation.

Prognosis with and without treatments

In those with mild *C. difficile* infection, the disease may resolve by stopping the offending antibiotics. In the majority of treated cases of *C. difficile*-induced pseudomembranous colitis, recovery occurs within 7 days. Mortality is often high in elderly frail patients with multiple co-existing illnesses who develop severe pseudomembranous colitis due to *C. difficile* infection. There is a need for robust criteria to enable not only the identification of patients that will benefit from surgery, but also the timing of colectomy.

SOURCES OF INFORMATION FOR DOCTORS AND PATIEENTS

http://www.statistics.gov.uk/hub/search/index.html?newquery=clostridium+difficile

www.cdc.gov/hai/organisms/cdiff/cdiff_infect.html

www.hpa.org.uk/Topics/InfectiousDiseases/InfectionsAZ/ClostridiumDifficile/

References

1. Monaghan T, Boswell T, Mahida YR. Recent advances in *Clostridium difficile*-associated disease. *Gut*. 2008;57:850–860.

2. Gerding DN, Muto CA, Owens RC Jr. Treatment of *Clostridium difficile* infection. *Clin Infect Dis*. 2008;46(Suppl 1):S32–S42.

3. Leonard J, Marshall JK, Moayyedi P. Systematic review of the risk of enteric infection in patients taking acid suppression. *Am J Gastroenterol*. 2007;102:2047–2056; quiz 2057.

4. Voth DE, Ballard JD. Clostridium difficile toxins: mechanism of action and role in disease. *Clin Microbiol Rev*. 2005;18:247–263.

5. Aktories K, Just I. Clostridial Rho-inhibiting protein toxins. *Curr Top Microbiol Immunol*. 2005;291:113–145.

6. Mahida YR, Makh S, Hyde S, *et al*. Effect of *Clostridium difficile* toxin A on human intestinal epithelial cells: induction of interleukin 8 production and apoptosis after cell detachment. *Gut*. 1996;38:337–347.

7. Johal SS, Solomon K, Dodson S, *et al*. Differential effects of varying concentrations of clostridium difficile toxin A on epithelial barrier function and expression of cytokines. *J Infect Dis*. 2004;189:2110–2119.

8. Mahida YR, Galvin A, Makh S, *et al*. Effect of *Clostridium difficile* toxin A on human colonic lamina propria cells: early loss of macrophages followed by T-cell apoptosis. *Infect Immun*. 1998; 66:5462–5469.

9. Solomon K, Webb J, Ali N, *et al*. Monocytes are highly sensitive to *Clostridium difficile* toxin A-induced apoptotic and nonapoptotic cell death. *Infect Immun*. 2005;73:1625–1634.

10. Samuel S, Mahida YR. Intestinal Infections: mimics and precipitants of relapse. In: Irving P, Rampton DS, Shanahan F, editors. *Clinical Dilemmas in Inflammatory Bowel Disease*. Oxford: Blackwell Publishing; 2006. pp. 217–221.

11. Planche T, Aghaizu A, Holliman R, *et al*. Diagnosis of *Clostridium difficile* infection by toxin detection kits: a systematic review. *Lancet Infect Dis*. 2008;8:777–784.

12. Johal SS, Hammond J, Solomon K, *et al*. Clostridium difficile associated diarrhea in hospitalised patients: onset in the community and hospital and role of flexible sigmoidoscopy. *Gut*. 2004;53:673–677.

13. Price AB, Davies DR. Pseudomembranous colitis. *J Clin Pathol*. 1977;30:1–12.

14. Zar FA, Bakkanagari SR, Moorthi KM, *et al*. A comparison of vancomycin and metronidazole for the treatment of *Clostridium difficile*-associated diarrhea, stratified by disease severity. *Clin Infect Dis*. 2007;45:302–307.

15. McFarland LV, Surawicz CM, Greenberg RN, *et al*. A randomized placebo-controlled trial of *Saccharomyces boulardii* in combination with standard antibiotics for *Clostridium difficile* disease. *JAMA*. 1994;271:1913–1918.

16. Surawicz C. Reining in recurrent *Clostridium difficile* infection – who's at risk? *Gastroenterology*. 2009;136:1152–1154.

CHAPTER 55

Ischemia/ischemic colitis

Aliya G. Hasan and Joel S. Levine

University of Colorado Denver, Aurora, CO, USA

ESSENTIAL FACTS ABOUT PATHOGENESIS

- Nonocclusive mesenteric ischemia caused by congestive heart failure or hypotension cause the majority of cases. Vascular occlusion due to embolus and thrombosis are less commonly seen
- More than 90% of patients are >60 years of age. Most are women
- Preventable or treatable causes such as cocaine, exogenous estrogens, vasculitis, and coagulopathy should be considered

ESSENTIALS OF DIAGNOSIS

- Classically: a transient colitis with crampy lower abdominal pain, hematochezia, and urgent desire to defecate, usually improving in 48–72 hours. Uncommonly progresses to gangrene and infarction
- Commonly: sepsis in obtunded patient after acute myocardial infarction, hypotension, or aortic surgery
- Importantly: exclude infarction, enteric infections (*C. difficile*, *Salmonella*), mesenteric ischemia, and diverticulitis with stool cultures; imaging (CT scan, ultrasound with/without Doppler)
- Segmental inflammation on colonoscopy with edema and hemorrhage on histology are the gold standards for diagnosis

ESSENTIALS OF TREATMENT

- Intravenous fluids, oxygen, stop potentially causal drugs, bowel rest, and antibiotics if the symptoms are moderate to severe; with nasogastric decompression for ileus
- Optimize cardiopulmonary function
- Exploratory laparoscopy or laparotomy with any suggestion of infarction during careful monitoring

Introduction and epidemiology

Colonic ischemia is different in many respects from the less common small bowel mesenteric ischemia or infarction. Ischemic colitis is most frequently found in the elderly; a clear precipitating factor may not be defined; and most cases are nonocclusive without embolism or thrombosis [1]. Angiography is rarely helpful in either diagnosis or management. In a majority, the condition resolves with conservative management, but a poor outcome is common when colonic infarction occurs in the setting of medical co-morbidities.

More than 90% of reported patients are over the age of 60. Women account for approximately two-thirds of the cases, perhaps because of the use of estrogens. Colonic ischemia can account for up to 20% of acute lower gastrointestinal bleeding. Fatal ischemia has been estimated as 1.7/100000 person years, with higher rates in patients over 80 [2].

Causes and pathogenesis

The majority of patients with ischemic colitis have nonocclusive mesenteric ischemia. Although most are elderly, a specific inciting cardiovascular event may not be identified. At presentation, some patients may have previously unsuspected arrhythmias, atherosclerosis, or heart failure [3]. In most elderly with ischemic colitis, congestive heart failure, any event associated with hypotension, myocardial infarction, cardiac surgery, aortic aneurysm repair, some medications (digitalis, estrogens, pseudoephedrine, vasopressin, sumatriptan, alosteron, interferon), and obstructing lesions of the colon such as diverticulitis or colonic cancer is apparent. Elective endovascular aneurysm repair has a decreased risk of ischemic colitis compared to elective open repair (0.5% vs. 1.9%) and emergent open (up to 60%) procedures [4]. Ischemic colitis due to mesenteric vein thrombosis may be associated with an underlying coagulopathy. In younger patients with ischemic colitis, related conditions include connective tissue disorders (e.g., polyarteritis nodosa, systemic lupus erythematosus), cocaine and methamphetamine use, oral contraceptives and pregnancy, strenuous physical exertion (marathon runners), sickle cell disease, and coagulopathies [5].

Most of the colon's blood supply comes from branches of the superior mesenteric artery (SMA) and the inferior mesenteric artery (IMA). Branches of the internal iliac artery supply the rectum, with abundant collaterals between the three vascular systems. Two watershed regions that have fewer collaterals, and thus are more susceptible to decreased blood flow and ischemia then the rest of the colon, are the splenic flexure (SMA and IMA) and the rectosigmoid (IMA and internal iliac).

The right colon is affected in 8% of cases, transverse in 15%, splenic flexure in 23%, descending colon in 23%, sigmoid in 23%, and rectum in 24% [6]. Nonocclusive injuries involve longer discontinuous segments, whereas atheromatous embolism (uncommon) involves smaller isolated segments. Grossly there may be mucosal erythema and edema that may evolve into reddish-purple lobular mucosal swellings, difficult to distinguish from a colonic neoplasm. Ultimately the mucosa may slough and leave large linear ulcerations and a cobblestone appearance. Gangrenous bowel may appear green to black. Sometimes the picture is indistinguishable from a diffuse or patchily distributed colitis. Reversible colopathy involves the superficial half of the mucosa with submucosal hemorrhage and superficial crypt loss. Ischemic colitis is one of the recognized causes of pseudomembranous colitis. Transient colitis may involve full-thickness mucosal ulceration with evidence of mucosal regeneration. Fulminant colitis shows complete mucosal loss with complete crypt destruction, and chronic ulcerating ischemic colitis may mimic inflammatory bowel disease. Fibrosis may eventually lead to stricture formation. Gangrene is associated with transmural destruction of the mucosa and muscularis propria, with eventual perforation through the serosa. Many endoscopic changes, especially those at the milder end of the spectrum, may resemble other disorders, such as inflammatory bowel disease, solitary rectal ulcer, antibiotic-associated pseudomembranous colitis, and infectious colitis. Histology remains the gold standard for diagnosis [7].

Clinical presentation

Most patients present with acute onset, variably severe, crampy lower abdominal pain, rectal bleeding, or urgent bloody diarrhea. Infarction should be suspected with severe constant pain and disproportionately little abdominal tenderness to palpation. Blood loss is usually mild, but significant bleeding can occur. However, it is essential to consider colonic ischemia in <u>any</u> patient with recent hypotension (myocardial infarction, aneurism repair, surgery) and unexplained hematochezia, fever, or sepsis, as such patients may be intubated, obtunded, or sedated and unable to relate pain.

The clinical spectrum of ischemic colitis includes reversible transient colitis, gangrene, chronic ulcerating ischemic colitis, stricture formation, and fulminant colitis. Most patients have a benign, self-limiting ischemic colitis. The symptoms subside in 24–48 hours, and endoscopic lesions heal by 1–2 months. Peritoneal signs, if present, are usually transient; but if they persist for more than a few hours, colonic infarction is suspect. Patients with isolated right sided ischemia may be more likely to have gangrene and an unfavorable outcome [8]. Colonic infarction presents with persisting peritonitis, acidosis, and hypotension. Emergent laparotomy is required. Uncommonly patients have a chronic ulcerating ischemic colitis characterized by recurrent fevers, bloody diarrhea, and sepsis. Rarely ischemia causes a protein-losing colopathy, but colonic strictures do not usually manifest with obstructive symptoms.

Differential diagnosis

In patients with the common acute colopathy, differential diagnoses include acute infectious colitis (*Clostridium difficile,*

Campylobacter, Shigella, E.coli O157:H7, *Salmonella*), small bowel mesenteric ischemia, diverticulitis, and colonic obstruction (cancer, fecal impaction, solitary rectal ulcer). In the obtunded post-operative patient other causes of sepsis, fever, or hypotension should be considered. Diverticular disease, Crohn's disease, and cancer are more common causes of the chronic ischemic symptoms of altered bowel function and lower abdominal pain. Pain from acute small bowel mesenteric ischemia is mainly periumbilical and constant, with infrequent bloody diarrhea. Ischemic symptoms have been rarely reported secondary to hydrogen peroxide enemas or from retained glutaraldehyde on an inadequately rinsed endoscope.

Diagnostic investigation

Careful drug and medication history with screens for illegal drugs, when appropriate, is important. In all patients, stool studies should be sent to rule out infectious colitis. Clinical presentation and follow-up with complete resolution helps to differentiate ischemic colitis from Crohn's disease or ulcerative colitis. However, ischemic colitis uncommonly presents as a chronic ulcerating or inflammatory disease that can be quite difficult to differentiate from inflammatory bowel disease.

Ischemic colitis should be considered in all patients with acute onset, crampy abdominal pain with blood in the stool. As soon as ischemia is considered in the differential, imaging of the abdomen is crucial. Plain radiography is often nondiagnostic early on, but severe changes of thumbprinting and pneumatosis may be identified in 30% [9]; colonic dilatation is a more ominous potential finding. Computed tomograms (CT) early in the course of the disease may be normal or show nonspecific segmental bowel thickening, but will help to exclude diverticulitis and small bowel ischemia, and localize the area of inflamed colon. Gas in the mesenteric veins and pneumatosis are seen in more advanced disease (Figure 55.1). Ultrasound can be a useful adjunct to CT when the diagnosis is in doubt, showing greater wall thickness, loss of wall stratification, and absence of color flow on Doppler [10]. Magnetic

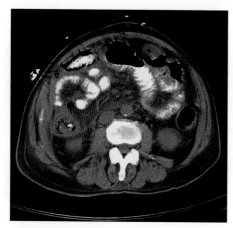

Figure 55.1 Computed tomogram of the abdomen. Scan illustrates *Pneumatosis coli* at the hepatic flexure.

resonance angiography and duplex ultrasonography may detect a high-grade arterial stenosis [11], yet such a stenosis may have nothing to do with the clinical presentation. If the patient is very ill, with infarction possible, exploratory surgery should be strongly considered.

Careful colonoscopy with biopsy is the preferred diagnostic test (Video 55.1). Insufflation with air is minimized as overdistention of the colon may further reduce colonic blood flow. If an apparent ischemic segment is encountered, biopsies are taken and the procedure is aborted. Biopsies should include the edge of the ulceration and 1 cm of noninvolved tissue. Sometimes the ulcerated mucosa does not reveal its source of injury, but the adjacent mucosa may reveal histologic "footprints" of ischemia. Usually, pale or cyanotic and edematous mucosa with ulcerations (Figure 55.2), petechial bleeding, and bluish hemorrhagic nodules are seen on endoscopy (Figure 55.3). The distribution of these lesions is segmental and there is an abrupt transition from injured to normal mucosa. Although black mucosa should suggest gangrene, colonoscopy is not helpful in distinguishing ischemic from infarcted bowel [12]. Angiography is rarely useful in this primarily nonocclusive disease with circulation affected at the arteriolar level. In most patients, blood flow has returned to normal by the time of clinical presentation. Delayed diagnosis of ischemia and development of sepsis, acidosis, or peritonitis increase the morbidity and mortality associated with surgical resection. This has led some vascular surgeons to recommend routine endoscopy after aneurism repair. Laparoscopy may be better tolerated than laparotomy for the diagnosis of ischemic colitis in an elderly population. Laparoscopy is also helpful after surgical resection for a second look, to assess viability of the bowel. Intraperitoneal pressures should not exceed 10–15 mm Hg with laparoscopy, as the pneumoperitoneum may further reduce blood flow to the colon [13].

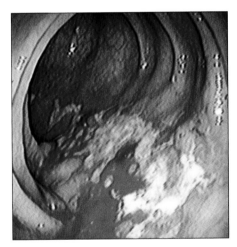

Figure 55.2 Localized ischemic ulcer. Localized ischemic ulcer of the splenic flexure in a patient with nonocclusive mesenteric ischemia; resolution was complete without therapy.

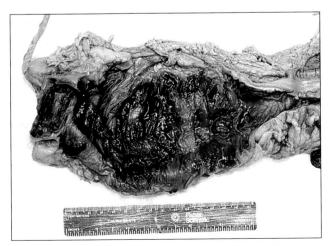

Figure 55.3 Ischemia and infarction. Ischemia and infarction of the cecum at autopsy in a patient with embolism to the superior mesenteric artery.

Treatment and prevention

Supportive measures are directed at reducing the progression to infarction. Oxygen is started, potentially causal drugs are withdrawn, and intravenous fluids are given to ensure adequate colonic perfusion. Correction of anemia, arrhythmia, hypovolemia, or congestive heart failure is undertaken. Avoidance of oral intake is desirable until the course is defined, and nasogastric tube suction may be required if ileus is present. Empiric antibiotic coverage is given in moderate to severe cases, theoretically to reduce bacterial translocation across the damaged colon. Patients need to be monitored for persistent fever, bleeding or diarrhea, leukocytosis, acidosis, and peritoneal signs. Regular plain films of the abdomen and periodic CT imaging should be used to follow slowly resolving cases. In selected cases colonoscopy is repeated in 1–2 months to assure the process has healed and to exclude cancer. Ischemic colitis from *mesenteric vein thrombosis* should be assessed for underlying hypercoagulable states. Anticoagulation therapy is started and continued for at least 6 months if there is an underlying coagulopathy or a cardiac source [14]. In those unusual patients with a clearly defined cause (e.g., vasculitis, polycythemia, embolism), therapy is directed at the primary disease.

Complications and their management

Patients need to be monitored for clinical worsening and signs of peritonitis. The team management approach should include early surgical consultation. Emergent surgery is indicated if the patient's condition deteriorates, infarction becomes evident, or there is massive hemorrhage, recurrent fevers, or sepsis. Toxic megacolon is associated with significant (50–70%) rates of operative mortality and morbidity in this setting [15]. A second-look operation in 12–24 hours may be needed to see whether there is ischemic change beyond the original resection margins. In patients undergoing aortoiliac surgery, recognition of postoperative ischemic colitis is important, because prompt intervention may be required [16]. Routine sigmoidoscopy has not been shown to improve survival [12].

A minority develop chronic ischemic colitis associated with features that may include recurrent abdominal pain, bacteremia, bloody diarrhea, sepsis, strictures, weight loss, and protein-losing enteropathy. Such patients may need segmental resection. Strictures may be symptomatically improved with endoscopic balloon dilatation. Idiopathic inflammatory bowel disease must be excluded because corticosteroid therapy in ischemic colitis may lead to perforation.

Prognosis with and without treatment

Most patients resolve completely with supportive care. Many patients never have another episode of ischemia. Anticoagulation has no role in the common patient with nonocclusive disease. With colonic infarction and gangrene, the mortality rate in the elderly with multiple co-morbid conditions may approach 50–75% with surgery, and is universally fatal with nonsurgical management.

SOURCES OF INFORMATION FOR PATIENTS AND DOCTORS

www.mayoclinic.com/health/ischemic-colitis/DS00794
www.nlm.nih.gov/MEDLINEPLUS/ency/article/000258.htm

References

1. Higgins PDR, Davis KJ, Laine L. Systematic review: the epidemiology of ischaemic colitis. *Aliment Pharmacol Ther*. 2004;19:729–738.
2. Acosta S, Ögren M, Sternby N, *et al*. Fatal colonic ischaemia: a population-based study. *Scand J Gastroenterol*. 2006;41:1312–1319.
3. Collett, Even C, Bouin M, *et al*. Prevalence of electrocardiographic and echocardiographic abnormalities in ambulatory ischemic colitis. *Dig Dis Sci*. 2000;45:23–25.
4. Perry RJT, Martin MJ, Eckert MJ, *et al*. Colonic ischemia complicating open vs endovascular abdominal aortic aneurysm repair. *J Vasc Surg*. 2008;48:272–277.
5. Preventza OA, Lazarides K, Sawyer MD. Ischemic colitis in young adults; a single institution experience. *J Gastrointest Surg*. 2001;5:388–392.
6. Price AB. Ischemic colitis. In: Williams GT, editor. *Current topics in pathology: gastrointestinal pathology*. New York: Springer; 1990; 81:229–246.
7. Zou X, Cao J, Yao Y. Endoscopic findings and clinicopathologic characteristics of ischemic colitis: a report of 85 cases. *Dig Dis Sci*. 2009; 54:2009-2015.
8. Sotiriadis J, Brandt LJ, Behin DS, *et al*. Ischemic colitis has a worse prognosis when isolated to the right side of the colon. *Am J Gastroenterology*. 2007;102:2247–2252.
9. Smerud MJ, Johnson CD, Stephens DH. Diagnosis of bowel infarction: comparision of plain films and CT scans in 23 cases. *AJR Am J Roentgenol*. 1990;154:99–103.
10. Taorel P, Aufort S, Merigeaud S, *et al*. Imaging of ischemic colitis. *Radiol Clin North Am*. 2008;46:909–924.
11. Ernst O, Asnar V, Sergent G, *et al*. Comparing contrast-enhanced breath-hold MR angiography and conventional angiography in the evaluation of mesenteric circulation. *AJR Am J Roentgenol*. 2000;174:433–439.
12. Houe T,Thorboll JE, Sigild U, *et al*. Can colonoscopy diagnose transmural ischaemic colitis after abdominal aortic surgery? An evidence-based approach. *Eur J Vasc Endovasc Surg*. 2000;19:304.
13. Kleinhaus S, Sammartano R, Boley SJ. Effects of laparoscopy on mesenteric blood flow. *Arch Surg*. 1978;113:867–869.
14. American Gastroenterological Association. Medical position statement: guidelines on intestinal ischemia. *Gastroenterology*. 2000;118:951–953.
15. Longo WE,Ward D,Vernava AM *et al*. Outcome of patients with total colonic ischemia. *Dis Colon Rectum*. 1997;40:1448–1454.
16. Van Damme H, Creemers E, Limet R. Ischaemic colitis following aortoiliac surgery. *Acta Chir Belg*. 2000;100:21–27.

CHAPTER 56
Small bowel tumors

Matthew P. Spinn[1] and Sushovan Guha[2]

[1]University of Texas Health Science Center Houston – Medical School, Houston, TX, USA
[2]The University of Texas MD Anderson Cancer Center, Houston, TX, USA

ESSENTIALS FACTS ABOUT PATHOGENESIS

- Small bowel tumors are uncommon and elusive; they account for <3% of all gastrointestinal neoplasms and <0.4% of all cancers in the USA
- Adenocarcinomas, carcinoid tumors, and adenomas are more common than benign or malignant mesenchymal tumors, or lymphomas
- Incidence of adenocarcinoma and malignant carcinoids is greater in African-Americans
- There is a slight male predominance
- Up to 25% are associated with hereditary conditions (familial adenomatous polyposis, hereditary non-polyposis colon cancer, Peutz–Jeghers syndrome), and/or synchronous tumors (up to 25%) in colon, breast, endometrium, and prostate
- Small bowel malignancy may complicate celiac disease and Crohn's disease
- Pathogenesis is unclear but the molecular changes in adenocarcinomas mimic colonic adenocarcinomas

ESSENTIALS OF DIAGNOSIS

Presentation
- Two-thirds of small bowel tumors detected at surgery are malignant
- Most benign tumors do not present in life, but are found at autopsy
- Suspect small bowel tumors in elderly males of African-American ethnicity and with predisposing conditions, including FAP, HNPCC, and Peutz–Jeghers syndrome
- Suspect small bowel tumors in patients with refractory celiac disease (on a gluten-free diet) or development of treatment-resistant symptomatic Crohn's disease strictures
- Negative initial work-up (EGD, colonoscopy, and CT) for abdominal pain, weight loss, anemia, small bowel obstruction, and gastrointestinal bleeding should trigger high suspicion of small bowel neoplasms
- Non-specific symptoms cause delay in diagnosis
- Malignant neoplasms more often have gastrointestinal symptoms
- Adenocarcinoma presents in the sixth to seventh decades with lymphomas usually diagnosed a decade earlier

Imaging
- Endoscopy for proximal polyps
- For more distal disease, barium studies, CT enteroclysis, capsule, balloon or spiral enteroscopy
- Upper gastrointestinal series with small bowel follow-through (UGI-SBFT) and enteroclysis are common methods to evaluate intraluminal pathology distal to the ligament of Trietz

- CT enteroclysis is a more sensitive and specific imaging modality for small bowel disease
- In pediatric patients with suspected intussusception, perform ultrasound and look for "target" sign

Endoscopic techniques
- Diagnostic and therapeutic
- Esophagogastroduodenoscopy (EGD) with enteroscopy
- Single- and double-balloon enteroscopy
- Spiral enteroscopy

Surgery
- Diagnosis mainly intraoperative, but this may change with new techniques

ESSENTIALS OF TREATMENT

Adenocarcinoma
- Relatively resistant to radiotherapy
- Chemotherapy cannot be recommended outside of clinical trials
- Surgical resection is the mainstay of treatment

Small bowel lymphoma
- Rarely diagnosed before surgery
- Complete resection of the primary tumor and a wedge resection of the mesentery should be performed along with extensive lymph node resection
- Adjuvant chemotherapy, radiotherapy or both may improve survival
- 5-year survival 20–38% across all unselected pathologies

Introduction

Small bowel tumors are extremely elusive and pose a unique challenge to clinicians across medical specialties. Table 56.1 depicts the classification of small intestinal neoplasms into primary benign and malignant epithelial, neuroendocrine, mesenchymal, lymphoproliferative, and metastatic lesions. Primary tumors of the small bowel are rare, and their clinical presentation is non-specific. Consequently, preoperative diagnosis remains the exception rather than the rule.

Primary neoplasms of the small intestine are notorious for their insidious presentation and vague symptoms. These non-specific symptoms, coupled with the lack of physical findings,

Table 56.1 Classification of SB neoplasms

Primary

Benign
- Adenoma – non-ampullary small bowel, ampullary/periampullary
- Neuroendocrine – carcinoid, G-cell, D-cell, EC-cell, gangliocytic paraganglioma
- Mesenchymal – stromal (GIST), neurogenic (neurofibroma), smooth muscle (leiomyomas), lipoctye (lipoma), desmoid, vascular (hemangioma)
- Lymphoproliferative – nodular lymphoid hyperplasia

Malignant
- Adenocarcinoma – non-ampullary small bowel and ampullary
- Neuroendocrine – carcinoid
- Mesenchymal – stromal (GIST), autonomic nerve (plexosarcoma), smooth muscle (leiomyosarcoma), lipocyte (liposarcoma), malignant fibrous histiocytoma, Kaposi's sarcoma, angiosarcoma
- Lymphoproliferative:
  ○ B-cell lymphoma:
    – Mucosa-associated lymphoid tissue (MALT) type – marginal zone, immunoproliferative small intestinal disease (IPSID)
    – Mantle cell lymphoma
    – Other types (large B-cell, lymphocytic, follicular center)
    – Immunodeficiency related – acquired immune deficiency syndrome (AIDS), common variable immunodeficiency (CVID) with hypogammaglobulinemia, selective IgA deficiency, post-transplant
  ○ T-cell lymphoma:
    – Enteropathy-associated T-cell lymphoma (EATL)
    – Adult T-cell leukemia/lymphoma
    – Human T-lymphotropic virus 1 (HTLV-1)

Metastatic
- Malignant melanoma
- Bronchogenic carcinoma – large cell carcinoma
- Breast carcinoma
- Gastric signet-ring cell carcinoma

often cause a significant delay in reaching a diagnosis. Since the small bowel has been a relatively inaccessible area to standard endoscopic techniques, **contrast radiography** has been regarded historically as the gold standard diagnostic modality. The management of primary malignant small bowel tumors is invariably **surgical**. However, adjuvant **chemotherapy** and **radiotherapy** may be warranted, depending on the type of tumor. The most common primary malignant small bowel neoplasms in Western countries are **adenocarcinomas**, followed by **carcinoid tumors**, small bowel lymphomas, and gastrointestinal stromal tumors (GISTs) [1].

Epidemiology

The small intestine represents 75% of the length and 90% of the surface area of the alimentary tract; yet it accounts for **<3% of all gastrointestinal (GI) neoplasms** and <0.4% of all cancers in the USA [2]. An estimated 5260 new cases of small intestinal cancer were diagnosed in the USA in 2003, with an estimated **1130 deaths** reported in the same year [3]. In 2008, the expected

number of new cases of small intestinal cancer and deaths due to this cancer was estimated to be 6110 and 1110, respectively [4]. The average annual age-adjusted incidence per 100 000 persons for cancer of the small intestine, when age-standardized to the US 2000 population, is 1.9 in men and 1.4 in women.

From 1975 to 2000, the **rates increased** by almost 50%. This trend reflected increases for adenocarcinomas, malignant carcinoid tumors, and lymphomas in women [5]. A preponderance of benign tumors are **seen at autopsies**, the most frequent being adenomas and mesenchymal tumors. Malignant small bowel tumors represent the majority of those **detected during surgery** [3]. Approximately two-thirds of small bowel tumors detected at surgery are malignant; >95% of these are adenocarcinomas, carcinoids, lymphomas or sarcomas [2]. Adenocarcinomas and carcinoid tumors are the most common small bowel malignancies, with an annual incidence of 3.9 and 3.7 cases, respectively, per million people in the USA, followed by GIST (1.3/million) and lymphomas (1.1/million) [3]. There is a slight **male** predominance, and the mean age at presentation is 60 years.

Patients with small bowel lymphomas are usually diagnosed a decade earlier. Small bowel malignancies are associated with several **heritable conditions** that affect the GI tract (Table 56.2). **Geographically**, small bowel malignancies are high among the Maori of New Zealand and ethnic Hawaiians, and low in India, Romania, and other parts of Eastern Europe. The incidence of small bowel adenocarcinoma and malignant carcinoids is greater in **African-Americans** than in Caucasians [2]. In addition, up to 25% of affected patients have **synchronous cancers** involving the colon, endometrium, breast, and prostate.

Causes and pathogenesis

The reason for the low incidence of small intestinal carcinogenesis, in comparison with the colon, remains obscure [6,7]. There is no single hypothesis or set of experimental data to explain the paucity of small bowel adenocarcinomas compared with colonic, gastric, pancreatic, and esophageal adenocarcinomas, which is rather remarkable given the overlapping geographic- and age-related distribution of small bowel and colon cancers. The unique microenvironment has been proposed in a global sense to explain the **decreased susceptibility**, but no specific factors have been identified.

Experimental evidence supports the notion that the small intestine affords a **protective milieu** against malignant transformation [2,7]. The pathogenesis of specific types of small bowel tumors is discussed elsewhere. Little is known regarding the pathogenesis of primary small intestinal lymphoma. While the majority appears to have no overt predisposing cause, analogous to *Helicobacter pylori* in the stomach, nevertheless, there are well-defined clinicopathological associations, including **chronic antigenic stimulation** from chronic infections, which may shed some light on the pathogenesis of small intestinal lymphoma.

Table 56.2 Clinical conditions predisposing to small bowel neoplasms

Clinical condition	Type of small bowel lesion
Familial adenomatous polyposis (FAP)	Adenoma, adenocarcinomas
Gardner's syndrome	Adenoma, adenocarcinomas
Peutz–Jeghers syndrome	Adenocarcinoma
Hereditary non-polyposis colorectal cancer (HNPCC)	Adenocarcinoma
Crohn's disease	Adenocarcinoma, lymphoma (B-cell)
Ileostomy and ileal conduits	Adenocarcinoma
Ileo-pouch anal anastomosis (IPAA)	Adenoma, adenocarcinoma
Celiac disease	Lymphoma (T-cell), adenocarcinomas
Chronic infection/antigenic stimulation	Immunoproliferative small intestinal disease (IPSID)
Immunodeficiency diseases:	Lymphoma (B-cell and rarely T-cell)
Common variable immunodeficiency . . . (CVID) with hypogammaglobulinemia	
Selective IgA deficiency	
X-linked	
AIDS	
Von Recklinghausen's disease	Paraganglioma
Multiple endocrine neoplasia 2b (MEN 2b)	Ganglioneuroma

Other risk factors
- Male gender
- Increasing age
- African-American ethnicity
- High-fat diet

Table 56.3 Clinical presentations and common locations of primary small bowel neoplasms

Symptom/sign	Location	Type
Jaundice + GI bleeding	Ampulla	Adenoma, adenocarcinoma
Occult GI bleeding, anemia	Duodenum	Adenoma, adenocarcinomas
Flushing + diarrhea	Ileum, jejunum	Carcinoid-mid gut (metastatic)
Intestinal obstruction	Jejunum, ileum	Lipoma
Intussusception + melanin pigmentation	Jejunum, ileum	Peutz–Jeghers syndrome
GI bleeding, perforation	Jejunum, ileum	Gastrointestinal stromal tumor (GIST)
Fever + diarrhea + weight loss	Ileum, jejunum	Lymphoma

Rarely, patients with **hereditary non-polyposis colon cancer (HNPCC)** (see Chapter 59) present with small bowel adenocarcinoma. Patients with **Peutz–Jeghers syndrome** develop hamartomas of the small bowel (see Chapter 59), with symptoms including bleeding, obstruction or intussusception. Although these hamartomas are presumably non-neoplastic, there is a risk of adenocarcinoma after the development of focal dysplastic (adenomatous) changes. Patients with **celiac disease** (see Chapter 42) have an increased risk for enteropathy-associated T-cell lymphomas (EATL) as well as adenocarcinoma. Because the risk for both of these malignancies appears to be very small (<1%), there is no established role for surveillance with any imaging modality; neither is there in **Crohn's disease**-associated adenocarcinoma or lymphoma. Small bowel cancer cases have been found to resemble controls across socioeconomic status. In regard to **tobacco** and **alcohol use** as risk factors for small bowel cancer, there are conflicting results. However, more recent studies suggest that there is an association. Consumption of alcohol has been associated with small bowel adenocarcinomas independently of smoking history [2,5].

Predisposing conditions

The primary role of the gastroenterologist with respect to small bowel neoplasms is to identify patients who are at an increased risk. A number of **disease states are associated** with an increased incidence of small bowel neoplasms, as illustrated in Table 56.2 [1,7]. At least 70% of patients with familial adenomatous polyposis (FAP) will develop adenomas in the region of the ampulla of Vater. However, only about 5–8% will develop duodenal adenocarcinoma.

Predictors of cancer risk include number, size, histology, and degree of dysplasia (modified Spigelman's score) [8].

Clinical presentation

Mostly, patients present with **non-specific symptoms and signs**.

Perforation and **gross bleeding** are rare. In Table 56.3, clinical presentations and common locations of some selected small bowel neoplasms are presented. Patients with malignant small bowel neoplasms more often have GI symptoms, compared to those with benign tumors, which are usually discovered at autopsy. However, the clinical presentation alone does not distinguish between benign and malignant lesions [1].

Table 56.4 Overall frequency of symptoms

Symptom/sign	Frequency (%)
Abdominal pain	42–83
Weight loss	23–87
Anemia	18–75
GI bleeding	13–68
Intestinal obstruction	16–65
Abdominal mass	19–29
Jaundice	18–30
Anorexia	18–25

When the different subtypes of small bowel malignancy are considered together (Table 56.4), 65% present with **intermittent abdominal pain** that is typically dull, crampy, and radiates to the back, 50% present with **anorexia** and **weight loss**, while only 25% present with signs and symptoms of bowel obstruction. Bowel **perforation**, which occurs in fewer than 10% of patients, is most common among those with lymphoma or sarcoma. Of the most common specific types of small bowel tumors, GIST, gut/pancreatic endocrine tumors, and carcinoid syndrome are discussed in Chapters 34, 112, and 113 respectively.

Adenocarcinoma

Adenocarcinoma (non-ampullary) is the most common primary malignant tumor of the small intestine in Western countries, accounting for approximately 30–50% of all primary malignant small bowel tumors. The annual **incidence** in the US is approximately 3.9 cases per million persons. These tumors are mainly **located** in decreasing order of frequency in the duodenum, jejunum, and ileum, except in the setting of **Crohn's disease** where they occur in the ileum. The proximal location of most small bowel adenocarcinomas may reflect the presence of higher concentrations of bile (and/or pancreatic juice), previously linked to increased risk for adenocarcinoma [9,10]. **Peak incidence** is in the sixth to seventh decades of life, with a male preponderance. Unlike ampullary and periampullary carcinomas, which are usually circumscribed and polypoid, small bowel adenocarcinomas are usually large, **annular**, **constricting**, and **centrally ulcerated** masses with circumferential involvement of the bowel wall.

Microscopically, these tumors are very similar to their colonic counterparts, but with a higher proportion of poorly differentiated tumors. These tumors are also similar in their development to adenomatous polyps and share genetic susceptibility [1,8]. Most of the duodenal adenocarcinomas become symptomatic much earlier than other small bowel tumors. Yet, most small bowel carcinomas are already metastatic at the time of diagnosis. Unlike the large bowel, small bowel mucosa contain lymphatics that course through the villi extending near the luminal surface, and invasion of mucosal tumor into these lymphatics may account for this tendency of early metastasis [11].

Lymphoma

Primary small bowel lymphoma is the **third most common primary** malignant neoplasm of the small intestine and accounts for 15–20% of all malignant small bowel tumors. Although the GI tract is the most common extranodal site for lymphomas, it accounts for only approximately 5–20% of all lymphomas and is quite uncommon in Western countries. The small bowel is the **second most common site** of primary GI lymphoma after the stomach [11]. Several types of small bowel lymphoma exist, and the particular type is largely dependent upon the geographical location. The majority are **B-cell non-Hodgkin's lymphomas (NHL)**. The B-cell NHL can be divided into two major categories; immunoproliferative and non-immunoproliferative small bowel disease [11]. **Immunoproliferative** small intestinal disease (IPSID) is extremely rare in the USA. IPSID is found primarily in the Middle East, **Mediterranean countries**, and North Africa, where it is endemic and affects young adults of lower socioeconomic status.

Non-immunoproliferative small bowel disease encompasses several subtypes. One subtype is the **intestinal mucosa-associated lymphoid tissue (MALT)** lymphoma, also called **extranodal marginal zone B-cell lymphoma**, which is most commonly seen in middle-aged men. Most patients with intestinal MALT lymphoma present with a single **exophytic mass**, commonly located in the distal ileum and causing symptoms of intestinal obstruction, perforation, or GI bleeding. In contrast to the stomach, where MALT lymphomas are usually of low grade, those of the intestine are **frequently of high grade** [11]. Unlike gastric MALT lymphoma (see Chapter 35), no association between *Helicobacter pylori* infection and intestinal MALT lymphoma has been established. Those rare cases of **T-cell NHL are usually EATL** associated with underlying **celiac disease** [11].

Differential diagnosis

The differential diagnosis depends on the predominant clinical symptoms/signs at the initial presentation. These consist of:

- Common causes of small bowel obstruction – adhesions or strictures, endometriosis, congenital pancreatic rest, splenosis, and enteric duplication cysts
- Causes of abdominal pain (see Chapter 3) – peptic ulcer disease, cholelithiasis, pancreatitis, functional bowel disorder to diverticular disease, appendicitis, and endometriosis
- Anemia and obscure causes of bleeding (see Chapter 13) – peptic, non-steroidal anti-inflammatory drugs (NSAIDs)/ medication-induced erosions and ulcers, and vascular lesions (e.g., vascular ectasia and Dieulafoy's lesion) [7].

Table 56.5 Diagnostic modalities of suspected small bowel neoplasms

Diagnostic tests	Utility
Radiology	
Abdominal X-rays	±
Small bowel follow-through (SBFT)	+
Enteroclysis	++
Ultrasound	+
CT scan	++
CT + enteroclysis	+++
MRI	++
Angiography	+
MRI + enteroclysis	+++
Endoscopy	
Esophagogastroduodenoscopy (EGD)	+
Push enteroscopy	+++
Sonde enteroscopy	++
Intraoperative enteroscopy	++++
Colonoscopy with ileoscopy	++
Endoscopic ultrasound (EUS)	Ampullary lesions
Wireless capsule endoscopy	++
Double- or single-balloon enteroscopy	+++
Spiral enteroscopy	+++
Nuclear medicine	
Octreotide scintigraphy	Neuroendocrine tumors
Gallium-67 scan	±
Surgery	
Explorative laparotomy	++++
Laparoscopy	+++

Diagnostic investigations

Most patients with small bowel tumors present with non-specific symptoms/signs and the diagnosis is significantly delayed by 7–12 months [1]. The clinical presentation usually dictates the order of imaging, and endoscopic and surgical modalities used for diagnosis as shown in Table 56.5 (see Chapters 34 and 113 for the specific diagnosis of GISTs and carcinoid syndrome, respectively).

Plain abdominal X-rays may show small bowel obstruction or free air, prompting an exploratory laparotomy. Patients with chronic symptoms of abdominal pain, nausea, vomiting, and weight loss, and signs of gastrointestinal bleeding usually have undergone an unrevealing work-up [colonoscopy, upper endoscopy, and computed tomography (CT) of the abdomen].

An **upper gastrointestinal series with small bowel follow-through (UGI-SBFT)** and enteroclysis remains the most common method to evaluate small bowel intraluminal pathology distal to the ligament of Trietz. The sensitivity of UGI-SBFT is usually <50–60% [12]. Small bowel enteroclysis, which requires duodenal intubation and injection of barium and methylcellulose directly into the small bowel, reveals a sensitivity of >90% in the majority of studies [12]. It is the most

useful preoperative diagnostic modality in patients suspected of having proximal small bowel tumors. **Abdominal CT** may provide information on the local invasiveness as well as the metastatic spread of the disease [13]. Multidetector row helical **CT enteroclysis** allows depiction of small bowel disease in patients suspected of having small bowel conditions, as well as allowing detection of extraluminal disease [14]. There is no role for transcutaneous abdominal ultrasonography (see Chapter 125) in the evaluation of patients with suspected small bowel tumors except in pediatric patients with suspected intussusception, where the classic "target sign" can be seen [12].

Upper endoscopy with a side-viewing duodenoscope is well suited for the identification of duodenal tumors, and may have a therapeutic role in selected instances [7]. **"Push" enteroscopy** without an overtube (using a pediatric colonoscope or specialized enteroscope) may allow visualization of the proximal 50–100 cm of jejunum. In contrast, extended small bowel enteroscopy using a 120-degree, forward-viewing, 2560-mm, balloon-tipped endoscope (**Sonde enteroscopy**) can allow visualization of up to 70% of the small bowel mucosa. The Sonde technique, while not widely available, relies upon small bowel peristalsis to advance the endoscope; in one report, it permitted successful intubation of the terminal ileum in 77% of cases within 8 hours [1]. The invention of capsule endoscopy created a major breakthrough in the evaluation of the small intestine. However, this tool has several limitations, such as inability to take a tissue sample and difficulty in handling the device.

Wireless capsule endoscopy (see Chapter 128) may visualize small bowel mucosa for sources of obscure GI bleeding/anemia, and recurrent abdominal pain. However, it is contraindicated in the presence of strictures identified in prior imaging studies [15]. Until 2001, direct endoscopic visualization of whole small bowel without surgery was virtually impossible. **Double-balloon enteroscopy** (DBE) (see Chapter 127), introduced in 2001, completely changed the approach to small bowel diseases, since capsule endoscopy has diagnostic yields similar to intraoperative enteroscopy and DBE has full diagnostic and therapeutic capabilities. The agreement between DBE and other diagnostic procedures, either endoscopic (CE) or radiological (SBFT/enteroclysis, abdominal CT) was high [16]. **A single-balloon enteroscopy** (SBE) system for the examination of the small intestine has recently been introduced. This SBE system consists of a dedicated endoscope without an attached balloon, an overtube with a balloon, and an air controller to inflate or deflate the balloon of the overtube. The two techniques have never been compared head to head [17]. **Spiral enteroscopy** is a new technique for deep small-bowel intubation that uses a special overtube [Discovery Small Bowel (DSB)] to pleat the small bowel. Preliminary studies reveal this to be a means of rapid, safe, and effective deep small-bowel intubation. Depth of insertion into the small bowel and total procedure time compare favorably with other deep enteroscopy techniques [18].

Table 56.6 Management of small bowel neoplasms

Key points
- Location
- Histological grading (Grade 1–4 and Grade X)
- Clinical classification (cT0–4, XN0–1, XM0–1, X) and staging (Stage 0–IV)

Benign neoplasms
- Endoscopy (see Chapter 149): cautery and polypectomy, endoscopic mucosal resection (EMR), endoscopic ampullectomy, intraoperative enteroscopy with polypectomy
- Surgery: laparoscopy and laparotomy

Malignant neoplasms
- Surgery: Whipple, segmental/wedge resections, right hemicolectomy, and lymph node dissection
- Adjuvant chemotherapy: 5-fluorouracil/folinic acid (5-FU/FA), mitomycin C, adriamycin, and irinotecan
- Adjuvant chemotherapy (lymphoma): CHOP or BACOP hybrid regimens
- Adjuvant chemotherapy + radiotherapy: CHOP-based regimens + whole abdomen (WAR), involved-field (IF), or intensity-modulated radiotherapy (IMRT) – sequentially, alternately, or concomitantly

---

Explorative laparotomy and laparoscopy are often required to evaluate patients suspected of having small bowel tumors when most of the imaging work-up is inconclusive and also to obtain adequate tissue samples in case of suspected small bowel lymphoma [1].

Treatment/management and prevention

The management of small bowel tumors, outlined in Table 56.6, depends on several variables: the histological subtype, whether it is malignant or benign, the stage of the tumor if it is malignant, and its location within the small bowel. The management of benign lesions of the small bowel largely depends on their size, location, and malignant potential. Tubular adenomas may be cured with simple **endoscopic polypectomy or local resection**. Adenomas with villous features can be managed in a similar fashion as long as the resected specimen does not contain invasive carcinoma. The management of **duodenal adenomas in FAP** (see Chapter 34) is more complex. The majority of patients can be managed **expectantly**. This involves surveillance by upper endoscopy with a side-viewing duodenoscope for optimal assessment of the ampulla. **Endoscopic treatment** of duodenal adenomas has a role in FAP, including cautery, bipolar probe, argon plasma coagulation (APC) or Nd-YAG laser, endoscopic mucosal resection (EMR), and endoscopic ampullectomy, all of which may be used for non-familial adenomas as well (see Chapters 147–149) [1,7]. Patients with **Peutz–Jeghers syndrome** should undergo upper endoscopy and biopsy of hamartomas to look for adenomatous foci in the polyps, UGI-SBFT, and enteroclysis, or possibly wireless capsule endoscopy to evaluate the entire small bowel [19]. Polyps >5 mm should

be endoscopically resected if they are accessible. Those >15 mm or symptomatic should be considered for **laparotomy with intraoperative enteroscopy and polypectomy** because bleeding and intussusception are common [19]. Patients with celiac disease who become symptomatic after years of quiescent disease while strictly adhering to a gluten-free diet should be thoroughly investigated for a small bowel cancer. In patients with **Crohn's disease**, development of a symptomatic small bowel stricture that does not respond to steroids and immunosuppressive drugs should be considered for enteroscopy (double- or single-balloon, or spiral) to obtain biopsies to rule out malignancy [16–18]. Surgical resection may be needed to rule out any malignancy and resection [1].

Surgery is the mainstay of therapy for all small bowel tumors, although the type of operation and the histological subtype, stage, and location of the tumor dictate the need for adjuvant therapy. Overall, the prognosis is poor with the 5-year survival rate between 20% and 38% [20].

Adenocarcinoma

Duodenal tumors involving the first and second portions usually lead to a **Whipple resection**. Tumors in the third and fourth portions of the duodenum usually require a wider segmental resection, although a Whipple procedure may be done additionally. **Jejunal and proximal ileal adenocarcinomas** are treated with segmental resection, including mesentery and associated lymph nodes. Tumors involving the **terminal ileum** are treated like right-sided colonic tumors, with right hemicolectomy and lymph node dissection [1]. The role of **adjuvant chemotherapy** in this subgroup of patients is clearly undefined. There are no proven benefits of 5-fluorouracil/folinic acid (5-FU/FA), mitomycin C, and adriamycin in metastatic disease. A novel camptothecin analog, **irinotecan**, is being evaluated in clinical trials for adjuvant chemotherapy and metastatic disease. Thus, chemotherapy cannot be recommended in these patients outside of clinical trials. Small bowel adenocarcinoma is relatively resistant to radiotherapy [7].

Lymphoma

Small bowel lymphoma is rarely diagnosed before surgery. Complete resection of the primary tumor and a wedge resection of mesentery should be performed along with extensive lymph node resection. Adjuvant chemotherapy, radiotherapy, or both may improve survival.

Metastatic cancer

The small bowel frequently is involved in metastatic disease. Clinical presentation may include symptoms of abdominal pain, intestinal obstruction, and bleeding. Any extra-abdominal or intra-abdominal malignancy can metastasize to the small bowel with melanoma being the most common malignancy to metastasize to the small bowel. Systemic chemotherapy may be offered for the primary malignancy. Palliative resection may be considered in advanced cases. Overall, survival rates are poor for these patients.

References

1. Abu-Hamda EM, Hattab EM, Lynch PM. Small bowel tumors. *Curr Gastroenterol Rep.* 2003;5:386–393.

2. Neugut AI, Jacobson JS, Suh S, Mukherjee R, Arber N. The epidemiology of cancer of the small bowel. *Cancer Epidemiol Biomarkers Prev.* 1998;7:243–251.

3. Jemal A, Clegg LX, Ward E, *et al.* Annual report to the nation on the status of cancer, 1975–2001, with a special feature regarding survival. *Cancer.* 2004; 101:3–27.

4. Jemal A, Siegel R, Ward E, *et al.* Cancer statistics, 2008. *CA Cancer J Clin.* 2008;58:71–96.

5. Schottenfeld D, Beebe-Dimmer J, Vigneau F. The epidemiology and pathogenesis of neoplasia in the small intestine. *Ann Epidemiol.* 2009;19:58–69.

6. Lowenfels AB. Why are small-bowel tumours so rare? *Lancet.* 1973;1:24–26.

7. Gill SS, Heuman DM, Mihas AA. Small intestinal neoplasms. *J Clin Gastroenterol.* 2001;33:267–282.

8. Spigelman AD, Talbot IC, Penna C, *et al.* Evidence for adenoma-carcinoma sequence in the duodenum of patients with familial adenomatous polyposis. The Leeds Castle Polyposis Group (Upper Gastrointestinal Committee). *J Clin Pathol.* 1994;47: 709–710.

9. Delaunoit T, Neczyporenko F, Limburg P, *et al.* Pathogenesis and risk factors of small bowel adenocarcinoma: a colorectal cancer sibling? *Am J Gastroenterol.* 2005;100:703–710.

10. Lowenfels AB. Does bile promote extra-colonic cancer? *Lancet.* 1978;2:239–241.

11. Riddell RH, Petras RE, Williams GT, Sobin LH. *Tumors of the Intestines.* Washington, DC: Armed Forces Institute of Pathology, 2003.

12. Nolan DJ. Imaging of the small intestine. *Schweiz Med Wochenschr.* 1998;128:109–114.

13. Horton KM, Fishman EK. Multidetector-row computed tomography and 3-dimensional computed tomography imaging of small bowel neoplasms: current concept in diagnosis. *J Comput Assist Tomogr.* 2004;28:106–116.

14. Boudiaf M, Jaff A, Soyer P, *et al.* Small-bowel diseases: prospective evaluation of multi-detector row helical CT enteroclysis in 107 consecutive patients. *Radiology.* 2004;233:338–344.

15. Eliakim R. Wireless capsule video endoscopy: Three years of experience. *World J Gastroenterol.* 2004;10:1238–1239.

16. Almeida N, Figueiredo P, Lopes S, Gouveia H, Leitão MC. Double-balloon enteroscopy and small bowel tumors: a South-European single-center experience. *Dig Dis Sci.* 2009;54:1520–1524.

17. Tsujikawa T, Saitoh Y, Andoh A, *et al.* Novel single-balloon enteroscopy for diagnosis and treatment of the small intestine: preliminary experiences. *Endoscopy.* 2008;40:11–15.

18. Akerman PA, Agrawal D, Cantero D, Pangtay J. Spiral enteroscopy with the new DSB overtube: a novel technique for deep peroral small-bowel intubation. *Endoscopy.* 2008;40:974–978.

19. McGarrity TJ, Kulin HE, Zaino RJ. Peutz–Jeghers syndrome. *Am J Gastroenterol.* 2000;95:596–604.

20. Howe JR, Karnell LH, Menck HR, Scott-Conner C. The American College of Surgeons Commission on Cancer and the American Cancer Society. Adenocarcinoma of the small bowel: review of the National Cancer Data Base, 1985–1995. *Cancer.* 1999;86: 2693–2706.

Small and Large Bowel

Small and Large Bowel

CHAPTER 57

Biology and genetics of colorectal cancer and polyps and polyposis

Ajay Goel[1] and Christian Arnold[2]

[1]Baylor University Medical Center, Dallas, TX, USA
[2]Klinikum Friedrichshafen, Friedrichshafen, Germany

ESSENTIAL FACTS ABOUT PATHOGENESIS

- 25% of colon cancer patients have some degree of familial background
- Multistep carcinogenesis is caused by mutations in oncogenes and tumor suppressor genes
- Colorectal neoplasia is the result of a heterogeneous collection of genetic abnormalities
- Three different genetic signatures are characteristically seen in colorectal cancer: chromosomal instability, microsatellite instability, and CpG island methylator phenotype
- Familial adenomatous polyposis (FAP) is caused by a germline mutation in the *APC* gene, which predisposes the carrier to develop a large number of adenomas
- *MYH*-associated polyposis is an hereditary colorectal cancer condition that is caused by germline mutations in the base excision repair *MYH* gene
- Lynch syndrome or hereditary non-polyposis colorectal cancer is caused by germline mutations in one of the DNA MMR genes
- Sporadic adenomatous polyps are commonly initiated by loss of the *APC* gene, followed by the sequential mutation of oncogenes and inactivating mutations at tumor suppressor genes
- Polyps evolving through the "serrated pathway" may account for 8–18% of all colon cancers

ESSENTIALS OF DIAGNOSIS

- Screening methods for colorectal cancer can be used to search for molecular abnormalities in the feces or blood
- Cancer prevention and cancer detection tests have to be routinely used to prevent/detect adenoma formation as early as possible

ESSENTIALS OF TREATMENT

- The genetic characteristics of a colorectal tumor are of prognostic value in terms of growth characteristics and therapeutic response
- The use of non-steroidal anti-inflammatory drugs (NSAIDs) such as sulindac and celecoxib can induce regression of adenomas in FAP

Introduction

Colorectal neoplasia is one of the most common malignancies in the Western world. The lifetime risk of colorectal cancer in the Western population is 5–6%. Over 50% of the population will develop an adenomatous polyp by the age of 70, but only one-tenth of these will proceed to cancer [1]. This chapter reviews the genetics, molecular biology, and familial aspects of adenomatous polyp and cancer development in the colon. Readers are directed to other chapters for reviews of the epidemiology, pathology, prevalence, and incidence rates, and growth characteristics of colonic polyps.

The term "polyp" always refers to the adenoma, as this is clinically the most important lesion. Non-neoplastic polyps, including juvenile polyps, inflammatory polyps, and hamartomas, do not confer an increased risk for cancer unless adenomatous (neoplastic) tissue evolves within these lesions. Moreover, many of the paradigms developed for tumor development in general have been understood in the context of colorectal neoplasia, making this a cornerstone for understanding tumor biology.

Inherited susceptibility to colorectal cancer

It appears that some individuals are more prone to colorectal cancer than others are. About 25% of colon cancer patients have some degree of familial background, and 15% have a strong family history involving a first- or second-degree relative [1]. Those individuals with one affected first-degree relative have a two- to three-fold increased risk of developing colon cancer compared to the general population. The relative risk for colorectal cancer increases further with the number of affected individuals, early age of onset, and the level of relatedness (Table 57.1).

Genetic principles of colorectal carcinogenesis
Adenoma–carcinoma sequence

Several lines of evidence suggest that most colorectal cancers begin as colorectal adenomas, giving rise to a colorectal cancer that evolves in a normal–adenoma–cancer sequence (Figure

Textbook of Clinical Gastroenterology and Hepatology, Second Edition. Edited by C. J. Hawkey, Jaime Bosch, Joel E. Richter, Guadalupe Garcia-Tsao, Francis K. L. Chan.
© 2012 Blackwell Publishing Ltd. Published 2012 by Blackwell Publishing Ltd.

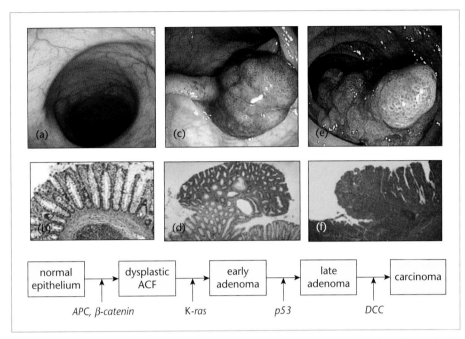

Figure 57.1 Adenoma to carcinoma sequence in colorectal cancer. Endoscopic and histological appearance, together with associated molecular alterations (based on Fearon and Vogelstein [2]) in lesions in the adenoma to carcinoma sequence. (a, b) Normal colonic epithelium. (c, d) Adenomatous polyp. (e, f) Colonic adenocarcinoma. ACF, aberrant crypt foci; *APC*, adenomatous polyposis coli gene; *DCC*, deleted in colon cancer gene.

57.1; see Video 57.1). This sequence was initially proposed by Bert Vogelstein's group and is also referred to as "classical vogelgram" [2] (see later). If one compares the mutational spectrum of tiny adenomas against larger adenomas, adenomas that contain foci of cancer, and invasive cancers, the number of mutations or genetic alterations increases with the pathological severity of the lesion.

Additional evidence suggests that most colorectal cancers evolve from benign neoplasms that antedate them. First, individuals with familial adenomatous polyposis (FAP) are predisposed to developing hundreds – even thousands – of adenomatous polyps, and because so many polyps occur, these patients inevitably develop colorectal cancer over time, typically two to three decades after the adenomas are first found. Second, those populations with higher incidences of colorectal cancer also have higher incidences of colorectal adenomas, usually occurring one or more decades earlier in life. Third, it is not unusual to find remnant adenomatous tissue immediately adjacent to or surrounding an emerging colorectal cancer, suggesting that the cancer arose from an antecedent colorectal adenoma.

Multistep carcinogenesis: role of oncogenes and tumor suppressor genes

Our understanding of colorectal carcinogenesis has evolved into a concept of sequential accumulation of mutations in multiple genes involved in complex pathways that regulate colonic epithelial growth. Multistep carcinogenesis is best considered in the context of **genomic instability**, which encompasses processes that generate many random alterations in the genome through several diverse mechanisms. Whereas most of these alterations would be expected to be neutral at best and deleterious at worst, some serendipitously produce a growth or survival advantage for the mutated cell. This permits clonal expansion, and the unstable milieu facilitates additional rounds of mutation and selection. Mutated genes that are critical for tumor development can be grouped into two broad conceptual classes: tumor suppressor genes and oncogenes.

Oncogenes are altered versions of normal genes (proto-oncogenes) that encode proteins that participate in the regulation of cell growth. Specific mutations in proto-oncogenes typically lead to the overexpression of the protein and a resultant acceleration of cell growth. The best example of an oncogene in the context of colorectal neoplasia is the **K-*ras* proto-oncogene**. This gene ordinarily serves in a signal transduction pathway required for ordinary cell proliferation. Mutations in K-*ras* can be found in approximately half of all colorectal cancers [3,4].

Tumor suppressor genes are genes whose normal expression leads to inhibition of cell proliferation; their inactivation permits colonic epithelial cells to grow as signals to stop are ignored. The best example in the context of the colorectal adenoma is the **adenomatous polyposis coli (*APC*) gene**.

Thus, mutations in oncogenes are "activating" point mutations or other rearrangements that lead to their overexpression, while mutations in tumor suppressor genes participate in colorectal carcinogenesis by bi-allelic "inactivation" of a growth regulatory gene. For many colorectal cancer syndromes, disease-defining genes have been identified (Table 57.2).

Small and Large Bowel

Table 57.1 Inherited risks of colorectal cancer

Risk group	Proportion of all CRC	Lifetime risk of CRC
Sporadic cancer, general population	60–80%	5%
Familial cancers	20–30%	
One first-degree relative with CRC		2–3-fold increase
Two first-degree relatives with CRC		3–4-fold increase
One second- or third-degree relative with CRC		1.5-fold increase
Two second- or third-degree relatives with CRC		2–3-fold increase
One first-degree relative with adenoma		2-fold increase
One first-degree relative with adenoma, age <60 years		2–3-fold increase
Hereditary syndromes	2–8%	
Hereditary non-polyposis colonic cancer	1–6%	80%
Familial adenomatous polyposis	1%	100%
Hamartomatous polyposis syndromes	<1%	2–50%

CRC, colorectal cancer.

Adapted and reprinted with permission from Burt RW, Ahnen DJ. Genetics of colon cancer. In: Yamada T, editor. *Gastroenterology Updates*, vol. 3. Philadelphia: JB Lippincott, 1998:1–16

Genomic instability in colorectal cancer

No single mechanism for carcinogenesis is common to all colorectal cancers. Colorectal neoplasia is the result of a heterogeneous collection of genetic abnormalities that leads to abnormal cell growth. One can characterize neoplasms based upon the predominant form of mutation found in the tumor and define the type of "genomic" or "epigenomic" instability in a particular colorectal neoplasm. The three main general patterns are:

- Chromosomal instability (genomic)
- Silencing by promoter methylation (epigenetic)
- Microsatellite instability (genomic).

There is a complex interaction amongst these with one type of genetic signature possibly a consequence of one or another of the other two. Nevertheless, characterization of neoplasms is often based on the predominate form of mutation found in the tumor.

Chromosomal instability

One of the most common aberrations in colorectal cancers is **aneuploidy**, in which the integrity of chromosomal replication is altered. This can result in chromosomal duplications, deletions, and rearrangements This type of global nuclear aberration is referred to as chromosomal instability (CIN). Chromosomal deletions and rearrangements often lead to loss of tumor suppressor genes, referred to as loss of heterozygosity [5].

Silencing by promoter methylation

Another mechanism for loss of tumor suppressor genes is their **silencing by promoter methylation.** About half of human genes have clusters of cytosine–guanine (CpG) sequences in their promoters. A group of enzymes called **DNA methyltransferases** can covalently transfer methyl groups to the cytosine residues. When a critical number of cytosines in the "CpG island" of a promoter are methylated, the gene is permanently silenced (Figure 57.2). The methylation of cytosines is stably passed on to subsequent generations of that cell. In certain tumors, there is excessive and widespread methylation of gene promoters. Such tumors are said to have the **CpG island methylator phenotype** [6]. The exact mechanism of the CpG island methylator phenotype is still unknown; however, it is believed that methylation of multiple CpG sequences causes cellular chromatin to adopt a "closed" configuration state, which causes transcriptional inactivation of the tumor suppressor gene. If the small proportion of hereditary colon cancers is excluded (3–5%), it is believed that most sporadic colonic tumors develop either through chromosomal instability or CpG island methylator phenotype pathways [7].

It is not yet clear what proportion of tumors develop via the CpG island methylator phenotype pathway, but this mechanism is considered to be very common, and as many as 50% of all colon cancers may demonstrate signatures for this type of epigenetic instability [7,8]. CpG island methylator phenotype tumors evolve as a result of the inactivation of multiple tumor suppressor genes [9,10]. Genes that are targets of the CpG island methylator phenotype include *MLH1, APC, p16, MGMT, RUNX3, SFRP2,* **and** *PTEN.* Although the majority of these genes are primarily silenced by aberrant methylation of their promoter regions, some may also be inactivated as a result of mutations or deletions. However, the current concept is that there are many different ways to disrupt the normal restraints on cell growth, movement, and invasion. Each cancer does this with a unique combination of mutations, deletions, amplifications, or promoter methylation.

While CpG island methylator phenotype involves *de novo* **hypermethylation** of cytosine residues within "CpG-rich" sequences (CpG islands within gene promoters) in cancer cells, hypomethylation of CpG-poor sequences (intronic CpG sites) is believed to be another possible mechanism leading to increased chromosomal instability. Intronic CpG sites are a common mechanism for keeping various retroviruses and proto-oncogenes silenced in healthy cells by methylation: however, demethylation of these sites may lead to reactivation of various proto-oncogenes and an increased chromosomal instability in cancer cells.

Microsatellite instability

A third type of genetic signature is microsatellite instability (MSI), which is a "mutator phenotype." While a proportion of colorectal neoplasias develops via MSI (~12–15%) or CpG island methylator phenotype (~35–50%), these pathways overlap as MSI in sporadic colon cancers occurs as a result of

Table 57.2 Genes implicated in colorectal carcinogenesis

Gene	Chromosome location	Presumed function	Associated inherited syndrome	Comment
Tumor suppressor				
APC	5q21	Regulation of β-catenin/Wnt signaling; cell migration; cell–cell adhesion; chromosome segregation	Familial adenomatous polyposis	Somatic mutations in 60–80% of sporadic colonic cancers; thought to be the rate-limiting step in tumor initiation
p53	17p13	Transcription factor; regulates cell cycle and apoptosis	Li-Fraumeni syndrome	Mutations occur late in colorectal carcinogenesis
DCC	18q21	Cell adhesion molecule; regulates cell migration; apoptosis		Mutations occur late in carcinogenesis, and may indicate a poor prognosis
TGFβIIR		TGF-β receptor component; inhibition of cell proliferation	HNPCC-like syndrome with late-onset tumors	Mutations occur late at carcinoma stage; found in most MSI-high tumors
SMAD2	18q21	Transcription factor in TGF-β pathway		Mutations found in 10% of colorectal cancers
SMAD4	18q21	Transcription factor in TGF-β pathway	Juvenile polyposis	Mutations found in 25% of colorectal cancers
STK11/LKB1	19p	Serine/threonine protein kinase	Peutz–Jeghers syndrome	
PTEN	10q23	Phosphoinositide 3-phosphatase; tyrosine phosphatase	Cowden's disease, sporadic cases of juvenile polyposis	Possible target of MMR dysfunction
Oncogenes				
K-ras	12p	Guanosine triphosphate hydrolase (GTPase); activation of growth pathways		Participates in an intermediate stage of carcinogenesis
CTNNB1 (β-catenin)	3p22	Signal transduction protein; upregulates growth- related genes; cell–cell adhesion	50% of colonic cancers lacking APC mutations, but no inherited syndrome identified	Found in 50% of tumors lacking APC mutations (a small fraction of all sporadic tumors)
c-src	20q11	Tyrosine kinase		Mutations found only in metastatic tumors
DNA mismatch repair				
hMSH2	2p16	Recognizes mismatches	30% of HNPCC cases	
hMLH1	3p21	Excises mismatches	30% of HNPCC cases	
hPMS1	2q32		Rare	
hPMS2	7p22	Excises mismatches	Rare	
hMSH6	2p16	Binds to hMSH2 and single base-pair mismatches	Variant form of HNPCC	
hMSH3	5q11	Binds to hMSH2 and longer base-pair mismatches		
Base excision repair				
MYH	1p	DNA glycosylase, helps repair oxidative DNA damage	Recessive inheritance and multiple adenomas cases lacking	May account for 30% of multiple adenoma dominant inheritance

HNPCC, hereditary non-polyposis colorectal cancer; MMR, mismatch repair; MSI, microsatellite instability; TGF, tumor growth factor.

Small and Large Bowel

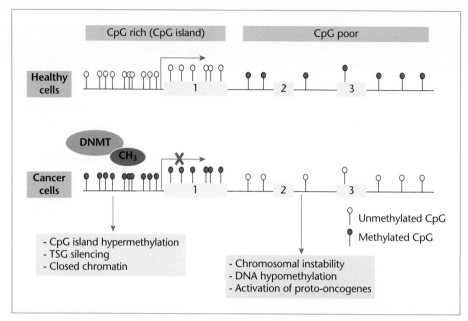

Figure 57.2 CpG island hypermethylation (left panel).and hypomethylation of CpG poor regions (right panel). CpG island methylation: more than half of tumor suppressor genes in humans have a preponderance of CpG dinucleotide (cytosine–guanine) sequences within their gene promoters. In cancer cells methyl (CH₃) groups are transferred onto CpG dinucleotides by DNA methyltransferases (DNMTs). Adherent methylation of the promoter region results in chromatin compaction and silencing of transcription. In addition to hypermethylation of CpG islands within gene promoters, cancer cells also undergo a simultaneous hypomethylation of their CpG-poor regions (intronic CpG sites), which leads to increased chromosomal instability as a consequence of demethylation and a resultant reactivation of the proto-oncogenes. TSG, tumor suppressor gene.

methylation-induced silencing of the *MLH1* gene. In many of these tumors, alterations in the *APC*, K-*ras*, or *p53* genes are not found. It is not certain how these tumors develop; however, in the presence of MSI, one frequently finds **stabilizing mutations in the β-catenin gene** that render it resistant to inactivation in the presence of wild-type *APC* [11]. Most colorectal cancers with MSI are apparently diploid or near diploid. MSI is primarily a consequence of **inactivation of the DNA mismatch repair (MMR) system**, and is characterized by very **frequent mutations at simple repeat sequences (microsatellites)** (Figure 57.3). In this case, the predominant outcome is inactivation of tumor suppressor genes that have "microsatellite" repeat sequences (typically a stretch of mononucleotides that is repeated 7–10 times) that are strategically located in the gene. The characteristic signature of MSI is the deletion of one element in the repetitive sequence, which creates a frameshift in the coding sequence, inactivating gene expression.

Such critically-located microsatellite sequences are **relatively uncommon** in human genes, but a few human genes encoding microsatellites are critical in the control of epithelial cell growth [12]. Examples of these genes are the transforming growth factor beta-1 receptor II **gene**, which encodes a sensitive A_{10} sequence in exon 3 [13], and the **BAX gene**, which encodes a G8 sequence [14]. This phenotype is always caused by loss of the DNA mismatch repair system, and is seen either in association with germline mutations in the DNA *MMR* genes (**Lynch syndrome**) or the acquired methylation-induced silencing of the *MLH1* gene [7,15,16].

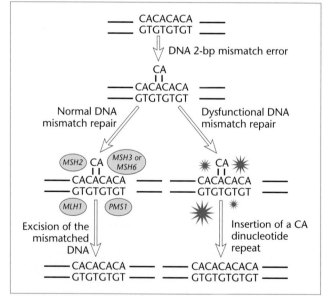

Figure 57.3 DNA mismatch repair. In normal cells insertion of a CA dinucleotide as a result of slippage error is excised by the mismatched repair genes *MSH2*, *MSH3* or *MSH6*, *MLH1*, and *PMS1* (left-hand sequence). Similar mechanisms can repair single base-pair mismatches. If mismatch repair genes are inactivated, in cancer the error is not corrected and the resulting strand contains an additional CA repeat (or single base pair). (This figure was published in *Clinical Gastroenterology and Hepatology*, Wilfred M. Weinstein, Christopher J. Hawkey, Jaime Bosch, Biology and genetics of colorectal cancer, Pages 397–406, Copyright Elsevier, 2005.)

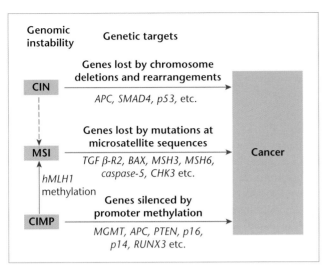

Figure 57.4 Genomic instability in colorectal cancers. Most tumors evolve predominately through one of three mechanisms – chromosomal instability (CIN), microsatellite instability (MSI), and hypermethylation in the CpG island methylator phenotype (CIMP). Genetic targets of these processes are shown. In addition, there is interaction between the three mechanisms. For instance, almost all sporadic MSI tumors arise as a consequence of methylation of the *MLH1* gene, suggesting a strong overlap between MSI and CpG island methylator phenotype mechanisms. Similarly, a weaker overlap exists between a smaller proportion of MSI and chromosomal instability neoplasms.

Table 57.3 Hereditary syndromes predisposing to colorectal cancer

	Gene responsible
Strongly predispose to cancer	
Familial adenomatous polyposis (FAP)	*APC* (dominant) and *MYH* (recessive)
Lynch syndrome (HNPCC)	*hMLH1, hMSH2, hMSH6, PMS1, PMS2,*
	hMLH3, EXO1
Weaker cancer risk	
Peutz–Jeghers syndrome	*STK11 (or LKB1)*
Juvenile polyposis	*SMAD4/MADH4 or BMPR1A*
Cowden's disease	*PTEN/MMAC1*
Bannayan–Ruvalcaba syndrome	*PTEN*
Li-Fraumeni syndrome	*p53*
Bloom syndrome	*Blm*

All of the above concepts highlight the fact that a significant degree of overlap exists between various forms of genetic and epigenetic mechanisms of genomic instability in the colon (Figure 57.4).

Familial colon cancer

Although familial colon cancer accounts for <5% of all colorectal neoplasms, it plays an important role in identifying elevated risks for cancer, and these diseases have been particularly helpful in gaining an understanding of polyp biology [17]. Various hereditary syndromes and their disease-associated genes are listed in Table 57.3.

Familial adenomatous polyposis

Familial adenomatous polyposis (FAP), accounting for <1% of all colorectal cancers, is caused by **a germline mutation in the *APC* gene**, which predisposes the carrier to develop a very large number of adenomas (>100 in number) at a young age. The *APC* gene has been termed a "gatekeeper gene" [18]. Inactivation of *APC* appears to be sufficient to permit the colonic epithelial cell to ignore signals from its environment to stop proliferating, which leads to **clonal expansion**. Ongoing proliferation of colonic epithelial cells at the top of the colonic crypt leads to the formation of the adenomatous polyp. A very large number of adenomatous polyps develop in FAP, and because additional mutations may accrue in this expanding clone, these patients eventually develop cancer. The gatekeeper concept implies that loss of the *APC* gene opens the gate for ongoing proliferation. Of interest, **spontaneous regression** of (small) colorectal adenomas has been observed in FAP, and the use of **non-steroidal anti-inflammatory drugs (NSAIDs)**, such as sulindac and celecoxib, can induce regression of adenomas in this disease [19].

Attenuated familial adenomatous polyposis

Attenuated familial adenomatous polyposis (AFAP) is a variant form of FAP, in which the inherited predisposition to colorectal cancer is characterized by fewer than 100 adenomatous polyps in the colon. The polyps tend to occur 10–20 years later than in classic FAP. AFAP is transmitted in an autosomal dominant manner.

MYH-associated polyposis

MYH-associated polyposis (MAP) is a hereditary colorectal cancer caused by **germline mutations in the base excision repair *MYH* gene**. MAP patients often appear clinically to have mild and late-onset FAP, but this disease is inherited in an autosomal recessive manner. Approximately 1–2% of Caucasians are asymptomatic carriers of *MYH* mutations. As a result, the disease often looks like a *de novo* mutation, since neither parent will have polyposis. Bi-allelic mutations in *MYH* were first associated with polyposis in siblings with multiple adenomatous polyps but without other history suggesting FAP [20,21]. When the polyps were evaluated, the mutational pattern suggested a defect in the base excision repair system, in which *MYH* plays a part.

Lynch syndrome

Lynch syndrome or **hereditary non-polyposis colorectal cancer (HNPCC)** is caused by a **germline mutation in one of the DNA *MMR* genes**, usually *hMSH2*, *hMLH1*, *hMSH6 or hPMS2* [22,23]. The DNA MMR system plays a "caretaker" function [18]. The presence of the one intact (wild-type) MMR allele permits normal MMR activity in the cell [24,25]. Loss of the remaining wild-type allele from a colonic epithelial cell in Lynch syndrome causes loss of DNA MMR activity and permits accelerated accumulation of point or insertion/ deletion mutations in simple repetitive sequences (see Figure 57.3). Therefore, Lynch syndrome is mechanistically different from FAP, since FAP involves germline inactivation of a structural gene that restrains cell proliferation, whereas Lynch syndrome is caused by mutational inactivation of a gene required to maintain genomic integrity, which then **permits mutations** at "target genes" that actually regulate cell growth [26,27].

Multistep carcinogenesis in sporadic polyps

Sporadic adenomatous polyps are not homogeneous lesions. Some are initiated by **loss of the *APC* gene** [28], followed by the sequential mutation of oncogenes and inactivating mutations at tumor suppressor genes (Figure 57.1). Vogelstein *et al.* outlined the sequence of events by which this takes place [2,29]. They found allelic losses of the *APC* gene in a similar proportion of adenomatous polyps regardless of whether these were small, large, or malignant. Thus, it was concluded that inactivation of the *APC* gene was sufficient to permit formation of the adenoma but *APC* loss did not directly participate in progression to a more advanced lesion. Mutations in the **K-*ras* oncogene** were almost never found in tiny adenomas, but were present in half of larger adenomas and in about 90% of very large villous adenomas [3,4,29]. It was concluded that K-*ras* mutations mediated accelerated growth of the adenomas but were not sufficient to initiate the adenoma. It was subsequently found that bi-allelic inactivation of the *p53* gene mediated the **adenoma-to-carcinoma transition** [30]. Thus, two genes were given specific temporal locations in the tumor development scheme, in which *APC* inactivation marked the initiation of the adenoma and *p53* inactivation marked the conversion to carcinoma [31].

APC

Some adenomatous polyps have one or two mutated copies of the *APC* gene. The *APC* gene regulates a signal transduction pathway in which the WNT ligand stimulates cell proliferation. WNT signaling leads to the expression of the *β-catenin* gene, which then activates a cascade of genes involved in cell proliferation. This leads to an increased rate of proliferation and an enhanced ability of adenoma cells to adhere to one another. When signaled to do so, the APC protein is produced in the developing colonic cell, which leads to degradation of β-catenin, which inhibits cell proliferation and allows the cell to die and detach from the crypt [11].

Some colorectal adenomas have wild-type copies of *APC*. These polyps often have **mutations in the *β-catenin* gene** that prevent this protein from being degraded on interaction with the APC protein. Additionally, inactivating mutations have been found in other genes that are downstream in the WNT signaling cascade, such as *WISP-3* [32].

K-ras

Similarly, not every adenomatous polyp or colorectal cancer has a mutated copy of the K-*ras* gene. Some tumors progress through the adenoma stage, develop *p53* mutations, and convert to cancers without incurring K-*ras* mutations. Colorectal neoplasms with K-*ras* mutations tend to be **exophytic or pedunculated**, while those without this mutation tend to be the **flat adenomas and cancers** [33–35]. The oncogenic potential of K-*ras* is manifested through its interaction with several effector proteins, of which the **raf kinases** are among the best characterized. Raf is a major proliferative and antiapoptotic effector, and it was shown that B-raf, one of the raf kinases, is mutationally activated in ~15% of colorectal cancers [36]. K-*ras* and B-*raf* mutations are mutually exclusive in colorectal neoplasia, and activating mutations in either of these genes may have similar consequences in tumorigenesis

p53

This gene can be inactivated by multiple different pathways. The most common form of genetic inactivation of *p53* is a point mutation of one allele followed by a loss of heterozygosity event in the other. In certain other experimental systems, *p53* can be inactivated by the overexpression of a normal cellular protein that binds and inactivates it (MDM-2), or by the presence of a viral oncoprotein such as T antigen or other transforming genes.

DCC

The *DCC* (deleted in colon cancer) gene is a candidate **tumor suppressor gene** located on chromosome 18q that encodes a molecule homologous to several other cell adhesion molecules that appear to regulate growth pathways and apoptosis. **Increased loss of heterozygosity events** at chromosome 18q were believed previously to be a key molecular event in colorectal pathogenesis. Recent data indicate that *DCC* may act as a conditional tumor suppressor gene. In this scenario, *DCC* may prevent cell growth in the absence of one of its ligands, **netrin-1**, which is a frequent target of epigenetic silencing [37].

Alternative pathways for neoplastic evolution
Serrated pathway

A proposed alternative pathway of multistep carcinogenesis for colorectal cancer involves serrated polyps as precursors for colorectal cancer [38,39] (Figure 57.5). This pathway is referred to as the **serrated pathway** because of the pathological appearance of the early lesions. This pathway may explain 8–18% of all colon cancers, and it has been suggested that it accounts

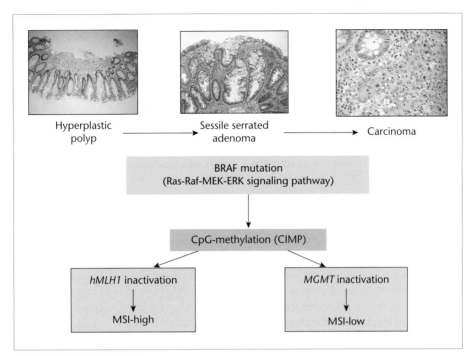

Figure 57.5 Alternate serrated pathway to colon cancer. This phenotype may account for ~18% of all non-familial colon cancers. Serrated polyps have a peculiar histopathological appearance, and are often associated with mutations in the B-*raf* gene, and an overall abrogation of Ras–Raf–Mek–Erk signaling pathway. Serrated adenomas with hypermethylation of the *MLH1* gene acquire a MSI-high phenotype, while the ones with methylation of *MGMT* promoter are characterized as MSI-low.

for the **non-familial MSI tumors**. Serrated lesions include hyperplastic-type aberrant crypt foci (ACF), hyperplastic polyps, sessile serrated adenomas, admixed polyps, and serrated adenomas [40]. The histopathological characteristics predicting the severity of cancer risk of these polyps are unknown. Serrated adenomas and carcinomas typically evolve through the activation of the "Ras–Raf–MEK–ERK signaling pathway" by an **activating mutation in** *BRAF*, display excessive CpG island methylator phenotype though **inactivation of** *hMLH1* **or** *MGMT*, and, consequently, are MSI [41].

Hamartomatous polyposis

Germline mutations in the *PTEN*, *SMAD4*, **and** *BMPR1* genes can lead to the development of hamartomatous polyps (typically juvenile polyps). Germline mutations in these three genes account for 30–40% of patients with **juvenile polyposis syndrome (JPS)**. The histological features of these polyps suggest that an alteration in the lamina propria or other supportive tissues is the underlying lesion that leads to polyp growth. Thus, one can think of the development of these lesions as a result of a defect in the environment in which the epithelial cells grow, and these genes have been tentatively termed "landscaper genes."

Inflammatory bowel disease-associated colorectal cancer

Colorectal cancer is a serious complication in patients with **ulcerative colitis or Crohn's disease**. Interestingly, **MSI** is frequently found in ulcerative colitis-associated dysplasia or

cancer, and also in up to 50% of non-dysplastic chronically inflamed mucosal biopsies [42–44]. Studies have failed to identify germline mutations in the *MMR* genes of these patients, but have identified *hMLH1* **promoter methylation** as a possible cause of MSI. The largest fraction of ulcerative colitis-associated dysplastic lesions or cancers, however, demonstrates a specific subtype of MSI, called MSI-low [42]. The prevailing hypothesis is that excess amounts of **free radicals overwhelm DNA repair pathways**, leading to the accumulation of damaged DNA. It has been shown that oxidative stress may temporarily relax the MMR system, and thereby allow insertion/deletion mutations [45–47].

Clinical implications

Knowledge of the molecular pathogenesis of polyp biology, colorectal cancer, and colorectal cancer syndromes has made it possible to use screening methods to search for molecular abnormalities in the feces or blood that indicate the occurrence of a polyp or cancer [48–50]. Several commercially available **diagnostic tests** are in clinical practice to search for the molecular abnormalities characteristic for the genetic defects. All of these tests rely on the integrity and relative stability of the DNA in the stool shed by the adenomatous polyp or cancer. Another approach is to search for **germline mutations** in familial cancer syndromes like FAP or Lynch syndrome [51]. Once an individual is identified, peripheral blood is used to identify the genetic defect, which is beneficial for the siblings of the patient in terms of early screening and tumor

Small and Large Bowel

prevention. However, even though the knowledge of colorectal carcinogenesis has broadened in recent years, guidelines for polyp surveillance have still to be followed strictly, as inconsistencies have implications for large-scale follow-up studies on natural history of colonic polyps and reoccurrence after endoscopic polypectomy.

The genetic characteristics of a colorectal tumor have also been shown to be of prognostic value in terms of growth characteristics and therapeutic response. For instance, MSI cancers have a better prognosis than microsatellite stable sporadic colorectal cancers. On the other hand, MSI cancers seem to have a poorer response once treated with 5-fluorouracil compared to sporadic cancers [52,53]. Other molecular markers like *p53*, *DCC* or *TGFβRII* have been shown to be predictive for outcome, but are still far from being used by clinicians in therapeutic decisions [54]. Only knowledge of the K-*ras* status implicates the response to the inhibition of the epithelial growth factor receptor (EGFR) by the tyrosine kinase inhibitors cetuximab and bevacizumab, which are commonly used as combination first-, second- or third-line chemotherapeutic agents in colorectal cancers with the wild-type K-*ras* allele.

Conclusions

The molecular characterization of colorectal tumorigenesis has opened a wide spectrum of screening tools for early diagnosis and prevention of colorectal cancer. A number of molecular markers have been defined and are currently under investigation for use in the choice adequate treatment regimens and to predict survival and response to therapies. In general, molecular screening tests have to be compared with conventional screening methods and validated in prospective trials in the immediate future.

References

1. Johns LE, Houlston RS. A systematic review and meta-analysis of familial colorectal cancer risk. *Am J Gastroenterol*. 2001;96: 2992–3003.
2. Fearon ER, Vogelstein B. A genetic model for colorectal tumorigenesis. *Cell*. 1990;61:759–767.
3. Bos JL, Fearon ER, Hamilton SR, *et al*. Prevalence of ras gene mutations in human colorectal cancers. *Nature*. 1987;327: 293–297.
4. Forrester K, Almoguera C, Han K, Grizzle WE, Perucho M. Detection of high incidence of K-ras oncogenes during human colon tumorigenesis. *Nature*. 1987;327:298–303.
5. Kern SE, Fearon ER, Tersmette KW, *et al*. Clinical and pathological associations with allelic loss in colorectal carcinoma [corrected]. *JAMA*. 1989;261:3099–3103.
6. Toyota M, Ohe-Toyota M, Ahuja N, Issa JP. Distinct genetic profiles in colorectal tumors with or without the CpG island methylator phenotype. *Proc Natl Acad Sci U S A*. 2000;97:710–715.
7. Goel A, Nagasaka T, Arnold CN, *et al*. The CpG island methylator phenotype and chromosomal instability are inversely correlated in sporadic colorectal cancer. *Gastroenterology* 2007;132:127–138.
8. Shen L, Toyota M, Kondo Y, *et al*. Integrated genetic and epigenetic analysis identifies three different subclasses of colon cancer. *Proc Natl Acad Sci U S A*. 2007;104:18654–18659.
9. Toyota M, Issa JP. CpG island methylator phenotypes in aging and cancer. *Semin Cancer Biol*. 1999;9:349–357.
10. Goel A, Arnold CN, Niedzwiecki D, *et al*. Characterization of sporadic colon cancer by patterns of genomic instability. *Cancer Res*. 2003;63:1608–1614.
11. Morin PJ, Sparks AB, Korinek V, *et al*. Activation of beta-catenin-Tcf signaling in colon cancer by mutations in beta-catenin or APC. *Science*. 1997;275:1787–1790.
12. Duval A, Reperant M, Compoint A, *et al*. Target gene mutation profile differs between gastrointestinal and endometrial tumors with mismatch repair deficiency. *Cancer Res*. 2002;62:1609–1612.
13. Markowitz S, Wang J, Myeroff L, *et al*. Inactivation of the type II TGF-beta receptor in colon cancer cells with microsatellite instability. *Science*. 1995;268:1336–1338.
14. Rampino N, Yamamoto H, Ionov Y, *et al*. Somatic frameshift mutations in the BAX gene in colon cancers of the microsatellite mutator phenotype. *Science*. 1997;275:967–969.
15. Kane MF, Loda M, Gaida GM, *et al*. Methylation of the hMLH1 promoter correlates with lack of expression of hMLH1 in sporadic colon tumors and mismatch repair-defective human tumor cell lines. *Cancer Res*. 1997;57:808–811.
16. Herman JG, Umar A, Polyak K, *et al*. Incidence and functional consequences of hMLH1 promoter hypermethylation in colorectal carcinoma. *Proc Natl Acad Sci U S A*. 1998;95:6870–6875.
17. Kinzler KW, Vogelstein B. Lessons from hereditary colorectal cancer. *Cell*. 1996;87:159–170.
18. Kinzler KW, Vogelstein B. Cancer-susceptibility genes. Gatekeepers and caretakers. *Nature*. 1997;386:761–763.
19. Giardiello FM, Hamilton SR, Krush AJ, *et al*. Treatment of colonic and rectal adenomas with sulindac in familial adenomatous polyposis. *N Engl J Med*. 1993;328:1313–1316.
20. Al-Tassan N, Chmiel NH, Maynard J, *et al*. Inherited variants of MYH associated with somatic G:C-->T:A mutations in colorectal tumors. *Nat Genet*. 2002;30:227–232.
21. Wang L, Baudhuin LM, Boardman LA, *et al*. MYH mutations in patients with attenuated and classic polyposis and with young-onset colorectal cancer without polyps. *Gastroenterology*. 2004;127:9–16.
22. Peltomaki P, Vasen HF. Mutations predisposing to hereditary nonpolyposis colorectal cancer: database and results of a collaborative study. The International Collaborative Group on Hereditary Nonpolyposis Colorectal Cancer. *Gastroenterology*. 1997;113:1146–1158.
23. Clendenning M, Senter L, Hampel H, *et al*. A frame-shift mutation of PMS2 is a widespread cause of Lynch syndrome. *J Med Genet*. 2008;48:340–345.
24. Koi M, Umar A, Chauhan DP, *et al*. Human chromosome 3 corrects mismatch repair deficiency and microsatellite instability and reduces N-methyl-N'-nitro-N-nitrosoguanidine tolerance in colon tumor cells with homozygous hMLH1 mutation. *Cancer Res*. 1994;54:4308–4312.
25. Hawn MT, Umar A, Carethers JM, *et al*. Evidence for a connection between the mismatch repair system and the G2 cell cycle checkpoint. *Cancer Res*. 1995;55:3721–3725.
26. Kim H, Jen J, Vogelstein B, Hamilton SR. Clinical and pathological characteristics of sporadic colorectal carcinomas with DNA replication errors in microsatellite sequences. *Am J Pathol*. 1994;145:148–156.
27. Konishi M, Kikuchi-Yanoshita R, *et al*. Molecular nature of colon tumors in hereditary nonpolyposis colon cancer,

familial polyposis, and sporadic colon cancer. *Gastroenterology.* 1996;111:307–317.

28. Powell SM, Zilz N, Beazer-Barclay Y, *et al.* APC mutations occur early during colorectal tumorigenesis. *Nature* 1992;359:235–237.

29. Vogelstein B, Fearon ER, Hamilton SR, *et al.* Genetic alterations during colorectal-tumor development. *N Engl J Med.* 1988;319:525–532.

30. Baker SJ, Fearon ER, Nigro JM, *et al.* Chromosome 17 deletions and p53 gene mutations in colorectal carcinomas. *Science* 1989;244:217–221.

31. Boland CR, Sato J, Appelman HD, Bresalier RS, Feinberg AP. Microallelotyping defines the sequence and tempo of allelic losses at tumour suppressor gene loci during colorectal cancer progression. *Nat Med* 1995;1:902–909.

32. Thorstensen L, Diep CB, Meling GI, *et al.* WNT1 inducible signaling pathway protein 3, WISP-3, a novel target gene in colorectal carcinomas with microsatellite instability. *Gastroenterology.* 2001;121:1275–1280.

33. Chiang JM, Chou YH, Chou TB. K-ras codon 12 mutation determines the polypoid growth of colorectral cancer. *Cancer Res.* 1998;58:3289–3293.

34. Yashiro M, Carethers JM, Laghi L, *et al.* Genetic pathways in the evolution of morphologically distinct colorectal neoplasms. *Cancer Res.* 2001;61:2676–2683.

35. Yashiro M, Laghi L, Saito K, *et al.* Serrated adenomas have a pattern of genetic alterations that distinguishes them from other colorectal polyps. *Cancer Epidemiol Biomarkers Prev.* 2005;14:2253–2256.

36. Davies H, Bignell GR, Cox C, *et al.* Mutations of the *BRAF* gene in human cancer. *Nature.* 2002;417:949–954.

37. Shin SK, Nagasaka T, Jung BH, *et al.* Epigenetic and genetic alterations in Netrin-1 receptors UNC5C and DCC in human colon cancer. *Gastroenterology.* 2007;133:1849–1857.

38. Jass JR. Serrated route to colorectal cancer: back street or super highway? *J Pathol.* 2001;193:283–285.

39. Jass JR. Hyperplastic polyps of the colorectum-innocent or guilty? *Dis Colon Rectum.* 2001;44:163–166.

40. Young J, Jass JR. The case for a genetic predisposition to serrated neoplasia in the colorectum: hypothesis and review of the literature. *Cancer Epidemiol Biomarkers Prev.* 2006;15:1778–1784.

41. Kambara T, Simms LA, Whitehall VL, *et al.* BRAF mutation is associated with DNA methylation in serrated polyps and cancers of the colorectum. *Gut.* 2004;53:1137–1144.

42. Brentnall TA, Crispin DA, Bronner MP, *et al.* Microsatellite instability in nonneoplastic mucosa from patients with chronic ulcerative colitis. *Cancer Res.* 1996;56:1237–1240.

43. Laghi L, Randolph AE, Chauhan DP, *et al.* JC virus DNA is present in the mucosa of the human colon and in colorectal cancers. *Proc Natl Acad Sci U S A.* 1999;96:7484–7489.

44. Ricciardiello L, Baglioni M, Giovannini C, *et al.* Induction of chromosomal instability in colonic cells by the human polyomavirus JC virus. *Cancer Res.* 2003;63:7256–7262.

45. Campregher C, Luciani MG, Gasche C. Activated neutrophils induce an hMSH2-dependent G2/M checkpoint arrest and replication errors at a (CA)13-repeat in colon epithelial cells. *Gut.* 2008;57:780–787.

46. Chang CL, Marra G, Chauhan DP, *et al.* Oxidative stress inactivates the human DNA mismatch repair system. *Am J Physiol Cell Physiol.* 2002;283:C148–C154.

47. Gasche C, Chang CL, Rhees J, Goel A, Boland CR. Oxidative stress increases frameshift mutations in human colorectal cancer cells. *Cancer Res.* 2001;61:7444–7448.

48. Ahlquist DA, Skoletsky JE, Boynton KA, *et al.* Colorectal cancer screening by detection of altered human DNA in stool: feasibility of a multitarget assay panel. *Gastroenterology.* 2000;119:1219–1227.

49. Dong SM, Traverso G, Johnson C, *et al.* Detecting colorectal cancer in stool with the use of multiple genetic targets. *J Natl Cancer Inst.* 2001;93:858–865.

50. Sidransky D, Tokino T, Hamilton SR, *et al.* Identification of ras oncogene mutations in the stool of patients with curable colorectal tumors. *Science.* 1992;256:102–105.

51. Grady WM. Genetic testing for high-risk colon cancer patients. *Gastroenterology.* 2003;124:1574–1594.

52. Carethers JM, Smith EJ, Behling CA, *et al.* Use of 5-fluorouracil and survival in patients with microsatellite-unstable colorectal cancer. *Gastroenterology.* 2004;126:394–401.

53. Ribic CM, Sargent DJ, Moore MJ, *et al.* Tumor microsatellite-instability status as a predictor of benefit from fluorouracil-based adjuvant chemotherapy for colon cancer. *N Engl J Med.* 2003;349:247–257.

54. Arnold CN, Goel A, Blum HE, Boland CR. Molecular pathogenesis of colorectal cancer: implications for molecular diagnosis. *Cancer.* 2005;104:2035–2047.

CHAPTER 58

Colorectal cancer: screening and surveillance

Austin G. Acheson and John H. Scholefield

Nottingham University Hospitals, Nottingham, UK

ESSENTIAL FACTS ABOUT PATHOGENESIS

- Many colorectal cancers arise from adenomatous polyps
- Identification of the genes responsible for hereditary cancers has led to improvement in care (see Chapter 57)

ESSENTIALS OF DIAGNOSIS

- The goals of screening are to detect early cancers before they metastasize, and resect advanced adenomas to prevent cancer
- Colorectal cancer has a long preclinical phase during which curable asymptomatic neoplasia can be detected
- Advanced adenomas (greater than 1 cm, with villous tissue or high- grade dysplasia) are the target of screening
- Annual fecal occult blood tests achieve a 15–30% reduction in the colorectal cancer mortality rate
- Screening with flexible sigmoidoscopy reduces mortality for colorectal cancer by 30%
- Virtual colonoscopy and testing of stool DNA may be future screening options

ESSENTIALS OF TREATMENT

- Treatment should be tailored to the natural history and molecular biology of the specific cancer being assessed (see Chapter 59)

Introduction

Screening for colorectal cancer uses a simple test to identify those individuals in an average-risk population who are most likely to have colorectal neoplasia. Once identified a more definitive diagnostic evaluation is then justified. The term surveillance describes the periodic performance of colonoscopy or other investigations in high-risk individuals such as those who have previously had adenomatous polyps or cancer, inflammatory bowel disease, or those with a genetic predisposition to colon cancer.

In 1968 Wilson and Junger published World Health Organization (WHO) guidelines regarding suitability of conditions for screening. Colorectal cancer fulfils these WHO criteria in a number of ways. First, it is a major public health problem worldwide and is the second most common cause of cancer mortality in the USA and UK. Second, precancerous adenomas can be readily detected and removed at colonoscopy thus preventing these adenomas transforming into malignant lesions [1]. The progression from adenoma to carcinomas takes place over a prolonged period of time (10–20 years) [2]. Third, surgical treatment for colorectal cancer can be curative with localized or early-stage disease having a better prognosis than more advanced disease. Finally, there are a number of highly sensitive, specific, safe, and cost effective screening tests currently available for colorectal cancer such as fecal occult blood testing and flexible sigmoidoscopy. These factors all contribute towards diagnosing this common cancer at an earlier stage with the aim of improving overall survival.

National guidelines in the USA recommend that physicians screen those at average risk of colorectal cancer over the age of 50 years [3]. These guidelines also suggest that prior to screening patients should be assessed for any other risks of colorectal cancer that may then indicate the need for a more intensive screening programme. If the screening test is positive then an appropriate diagnostic evaluation test is performed. If the screening test is negative then repeat screening should be performed at an appropriate interval for the method used. In the UK, a National Bowel Cancer Screening Programme has recently started but this is presently only offered to those over the age of 60 years.

This chapter presents the current screening guideline recommendations and discusses the pros and cons of each screening approach. It also outlines the surveillance guidelines for those who have had colonoscopic polypectomy or curative surgery for cancer.

Options for population screening

Unlike breast cancer and some other malignancies in which a single screening test is recommended, several tests have been evaluated within colorectal cancer screening programs. Each

---

Textbook of Clinical Gastroenterology and Hepatology, Second Edition. Edited by C. J. Hawkey, Jaime Bosch, Joel E. Richter, Guadalupe Garcia-Tsao, Francis K. L. Chan.
© 2012 Blackwell Publishing Ltd. Published 2012 by Blackwell Publishing Ltd.

of these options has some advantages and disadvantages and will be discussed in turn.

Fecal occult blood test

The fecal occult blood test (FOBT) is the one that has received most attention as a screening tool, with several large prospective randomized controlled trials published. The principle behind this test is that blood from cancers or polyps can be detected from stool samples. There are three types of FOBT available: guaiac impregnated paper method, immunochemical assays, and heme-porphyrin assays. Guaiac tests are by far the most frequently used. The guaiac paper turns blue when the heme molecule reacts with hydrogen peroxide. It is not specific for human hemoglobin and ingested red meat can give rise to false positives as can the ingestion of foodstuffs containing naturally occurring peroxidises such as parsnips, broccoli, and cauliflower. False negatives can also occur following the ingestion of vitamin C.

Many studies have concentrated on improving the sensitivity and specificity of the FOBT. Desiccation of the slides can decrease the sensitivity, and rehydrating the samples can significantly improve this, but also often increases the positivity rate resulting in large numbers of patients proceeding to colonoscopy, and therefore increasing the cost of the screening programme. Immunochemical tests are more sensitive and maintain good specificity compared with guaiac tests but they are more expensive and have not been subject to large prospective trials. Heme-porphyrin requires fluorescent spectrometry to interpret the results, and this complexity means it is rarely used in population screening.

Testing of feces for cellular abnormalities such as fecal mutant DNA or protein products can be performed. One such stool test (SDT-1, "PreGen-Plus test" Exact Sciences, Marlborough, Massachusetts, USA) has been compared with standard hemoccult test in the only reported multicentre study. Sensitivity of the DNA test and the FOBT for cancer was 52% and 13% respectively, with specificity for both tests of 95% [4]. Further large controlled trials are needed before these techniques can be considered cost effective for population screening.

An FOBT is the only screening option that has been shown to be effective in randomized controlled trials. Many of these trials have used different designs and methodologies but, despite the variability, some comparisons can be made and the larger trials each deserve further discussion. The three largest published randomized trials in the literature (Minnesota, Denmark, and Nottingham) have all used the guaiac impregnated paper test – hemoccult. Each of these trials has shown a reduction in mortality from colorectal cancer of at least 15% at 8–10 year median follow up, which is comparable with breast-cancer screening.

The Minnesota trial was not a true population study but rather a volunteer-based screening program comparing annual and biennial FOB testing with a control group. Compliance in this study was good (80%). Rehydration of the samples did occur resulting in a high positivity rate that resulted in 38% of the annual screened subjects having a colonoscopy. After 13 years of follow up, this study reported a 33% statistically significant reduction in mortality in the annual screened group versus controls. However, the Minnesota trial has received criticism because of the high colonoscopy rate in those screened, and this should be taken into account when noting mortality rates from other studies [5].

The Danish study was a true population study of 60 000 individuals between 45 and 74 years old and used hemoccult testing but no rehydration. The positive rate in the screened group was low (1.1%) and the overall reduction in mortality from colorectal cancer was 18% but this did not achieve statistical significance [6].

The Nottingham study is the largest of the three and is a true population-based study. Over 150 000 individuals were recruited with 50% offered biennial hemoccult testing but again no rehydration. Initial compliance was just over 50% and the positivity rate was 2.1%. At 8 years follow up a 15% reduction in mortality from colorectal cancer was reported and this was of a similar magnitude to that obtained from the Danish study [7].

Symptom questionnaires

Several studies including the Nottingham FOB screening trial have investigated the value of simple questionnaires looking at the common symptoms of bowel cancer. Compliance in these studies was poor and the conclusions reached suggest that, although symptoms are common within the community, they are poor predictors of cancer and therefore this approach has little value as a population screening tool [8].

Flexible sigmoidoscopy

Flexible sigmoidoscopy is an accurate and inexpensive test, but it is not without its complications. In particular it is associated with a small risk of perforation (<0.1%). A single flexible sigmoidoscopy around the age of 60 years has been argued as a cost-effective way of reducing the incidence and mortality of colorectal cancer. Approximately 70% of colorectal cancers or advanced adenomas should be detected by a 60 cm flexible sigmoidoscopy [9]. Despite being potentially a good screening tool, one of the drawbacks of this procedure is the associated high colonoscopy rate triggered by the detection of polyps. In the UK flexible sigmoidoscopy trial, there was a 5% colonoscopy rate. Other studies suggested that this rate may be even higher, and this increased workload clearly may have a rate-limiting effect on introducing this as a population screening process [10].

Initial data from the UK flexible sigmoidoscopy trial showed that compliance rates are approximately 40% [11]. Over 11 years, a single flexible sigmoidoscopy results in a reduction in the incidence of colorectal cancer by 23% and mortality by 33% [12]. These impressive data are under consideration by public health bodies around the world but flexible sigmoidoscopy may ultimately be regarded as the most effective and cost effective method of population screening.

Fecal occult blood test and flexible sigmoidoscopy

Combining these two tests has some attraction as a screening tool as it largely corrects the limitations of performing either option alone. However, despite potentially improving cancer detection rates there is evidence that compliance rates are significantly reduced [13].

Barium enema

Although included in the guideline options, a double contrast barium enema is rarely used due to its poor sensitivity at detecting neoplasia. Some studies have shown that up to 15% of colorectal cancers can be missed by barium enema examinations. It has more of a role in the surveillance of high-risk groups when colonoscopy has failed, is contraindicated, or is unavailable, rather than a screening tool for average-risk individuals [14]. It is also becoming less widely used due to the advantages of computed tomography (CT) colonography.

Colonoscopy

Limitations for the use of colonoscopy as a screening tool includes issues of risk, cost, patient acceptability, and capacity. It goes against the guidelines set out by WHO for a screening test as previously discussed as it is an expensive, complex, invasive, definitive diagnostic, and therapeutic investigation. For this reason most colonoscopies should be reserved for high-risk individuals rather than population screening. No large controlled trials of its use in population screening exist.

Virtual colonoscopy (CT colonography)

Virtual colonoscopy (CT colonography) presently requires full bowel preparation along with insufflation of air per rectum during the procedure. The investigation is less invasive than colonoscopy and generally takes only 5 minutes to perform. However, not only does the test involve a substantial radiation dose, the interpretation of the images requires extensive training and may take approximately 20–30 minutes by an experienced radiologist.

Although this technique is expensive to set up it is a sensitive test reported at detecting 90% of adenomas >1 cm with a false positive rate of 17%. Sensitivity and specificity for small polyps is unfortunately low [15].

The role of virtual colonoscopy in population screening is uncertain. The technique is still evolving and improvements in stool subtraction techniques, reducing the radiation dose, and the development of automated polyp detection using computer algorithms to reduce reporting times may make this test a more feasible and effective screening tool in the future.

Surveillance of high-risk individuals

There are several groups in which there is an above-average risk of developing colorectal cancer (Table 58.1) and colonoscopy is generally advised as part of a surveillance programme in each group.

There is substantial evidence that the lifetime risk of developing colorectal cancer is related to a strong family history, particularly when first-degree relatives are affected at a young age (Table 58.2) [16]. Although the frequency of colonoscopy is not agreed it is generally perceived that it should be tailored to the perceived risk to result in effective surveillance [17].

For patients at risk of hereditary nonpolyposis colorectal cancer, colonoscopy should be carried out every 2 years beginning at the age of 20–25 years, or 10 years earlier than the youngest familial case. Genetic testing should be offered to

Table 58.1 Risk factors for colorectal cancer

No inherited disposition
Age
Colorectal adenomas/carcinomas
Inflammatory bowel disease
Previous cholecystectomy
Previous uterosigmoid diversion
Previous gastric surgery

Inherited predisposition
Familial adenomatous polyposis (FAP)
Hereditary nonpolyposis colorectal cancer (HNPCC) or Lynch syndromes
Turcot syndrome
Muir–Torre syndrome
Peutz–Jeghers syndrome
Gorlin syndrome
Cowden disease

Table 58.2 Causes and risk factors: familial risk of colonic cancer

Familial setting	Approximate lifetime risk of colonic cancer
General population risk in the USA	6%
One first-degree relative with colonic cancer[a]	Increased 2–3-fold
Two first-degree relatives with colonic cancer[a]	Increased 3–4-fold
First-degree relative with colonic cancer diagnosed at ≤50 years	Increased 3–4-fold
One second- or third-degree relative with colonic cancer[b,c]	Increased about 1.5-fold
Two second-degree relatives with colonic cancer[b]	Increased about 2–3-fold
One first-degree relative with adenomatous polyp[a]	Increased about 2-fold

[a]First-degree relatives include parents, siblings, and children.
[b]Second-degree relatives include grandparents, aunts, and uncles.
[c]Third-degree relatives include great-grandparents and cousins.
(Reprinted with permission from Burt RW. Colon cancer screening. *Gastroenterology* 2000;119:837–853. © American Gastroenterological Association.)

relatives of those known to have an inherited mismatch repair gene mutation.

Patients with longstanding total colitis (>8–10 years) are at increased risk of developing colorectal cancer and are often entered into a 1–2 yearly colonoscopic surveillance program with multiple biopsies taken. Patients are at more risk if the colitis affects the whole colon and therefore surveillance in those with less extensive disease or Crohn's colitis is more controversial and varies throughout the world [18].

Surveillance after polypectomy

It is accepted that patients with adenomatous polyps may have an increased risk of developing further more advanced polyps or carcinomas in the future. Guidelines regarding the frequency of follow-up post polypectomy have largely been based on the results of the National Polyp study from the USA. This multicenter prospective trial excluded high-risk patients with previous colorectal cancer, inflammatory bowel disease, familial adenomatous polyposis, malignant polyps, and sessile adenomas with a base larger than 3 cm. Between 1980 and

1990, 1418 post-polypectomy patients were randomized into two groups: one had a follow-up colonoscopy at 1 year and then every 3 years, the second had colonoscopy every 3 years only. The results of this study showed that in the former group more adenomas were detected (42% v 32%) but the majority of these were small tubular adenomas of little clinical significance. However, 3.3% of patients in each group were found to have advanced adenomas (defined as an adenoma >1 cm, or with high-grade dysplasia or invasive carcinoma) suggesting that these can be detected as well by one examination at 3 years as by two examinations in 3 years. This study concluded that 1-year follow-up colonoscopy was no longer necessary in the majority of cases. The chances of having advanced adenomas is increased if the index adenoma is large (>1 cm), multiple (>3 cm), or if there is a strong family history of colorectal cancer [19].

Post-polypectomy recommendations are based primarily on the evidence from the above study, and the current trend in the UK is to pursue the guidelines developed by Atkin and Saunders in 2002 [20] by stratifying patients into low-, intermediate-, and high-risk groups (Figure 58.1). Others still

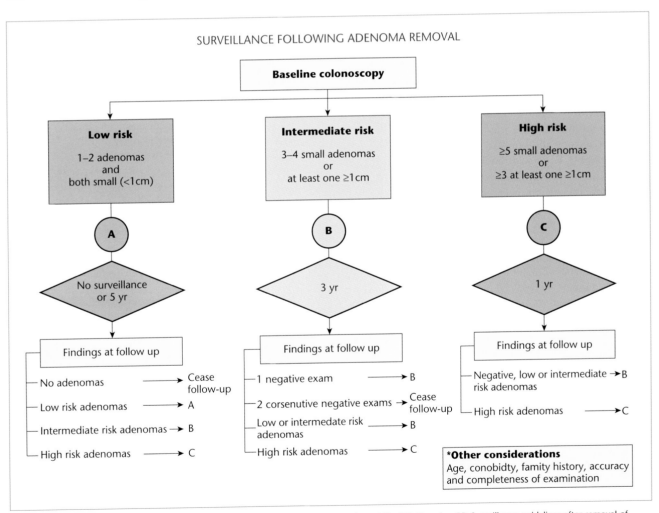

Figure 58.1 Surveillance following adenoma removal. (Reproduced with permission from Atkin WS, Saunders BP, Surveillance guidelines after removal of colorectal adenomatous polyps., *Gut*. 2002 Oct;51(Suppl 5):V6–V9.)

continue to follow a more intensive protocol for adenoma sur-veillance, but many of these lack a clear evidence base.

Surveillance following surgery for colorectal cancer

The follow up of patients following surgery for colorectal cancer remains controversial with no consensus among physicians as to the frequency, techniques used, or benefits of surveillance. The aims of follow up are to detect early surgical complications, identify synchronous or metachronous lesions, and detect treatable recurrent disease, as well as facilitating audit and providing psychological support for patients and their families.

In the past, many have argued that following up patients after surgery did not alter outcome. However, with the development of multidisciplinary team meetings along with improvements in survival following chemotherapy and liver surgery, this is no longer considered acceptable. There are now ongoing large prospective randomized trials in the United Kingdom (FACS) and Europe (GILDA) that are attempting to address some of the uncertainties regarding the intensity and benefits of surveillance. However until the results of these studies are available, patients who are not part of a trial are followed up in a varied program that usually includes outpatient visits, clinical examination, as well as hematological, endoscopic and radiological evaluation.

Approximately 80% of local and distant recurrences occur within 2 years of surgery and this has lead to a more intensive follow up during this time interval. These recurrences generally occur outside the bowel with anastomotic recurrences being very rare. Even with intensive surveillance regimens, symptomatic recurrences frequently occur between investigations, asymptomatic recurrences often go undetected, and curative treatment of locally recurrent colorectal cancer is only rarely possible. Several meta-analyses have been performed over recent years and the majority of these do suggest a survival benefit for patients followed more intensively. However, many of the studies included are underpowered and it is therefore difficult to draw firm conclusions. Nevertheless, one point on which most studies agree is that liver imaging is essential in those with minimal co-morbidities [21,22]. Approximately 30% of colorectal cancer patients will develop post-operative liver metastases of which approx 30% will be considered resectable. Specialist hepatobiliary units report 5-year disease-free survival from such surgery in up to 35% of cases [23]. Similarly, pulmonary metastasectomy has reported 5-year survival rates of 24–64% [24]. Therefore it is acceptable to offer patients who are considered fit for a liver or lung resection a yearly chest and abdominal CT in the first 2 years after surgery.

The role of serum carcinoembryonic antigen (CEA) measurements is unclear. There is evidence that a rising CEA helps to detect asymptomatic recurrences earlier but there is still no evidence that this lead time has any survival advantages [25].

Despite the uncertainty of the benefit, many surgeons still perform regular 3- to 6-monthly CEA measurements as part of their surveillance program and again the FACS trial may help to clarify this.

Colonoscopy is important in the identification of both synchronous and metachronous lesions but again there is no evidence that it has an impact on survival. If the whole colon was not visualized before surgery it should be performed 3–6 months post-operatively to produce a clean colon. Occasionally interval cancers are found within 2 years of surgery and some surgical guidelines therefore recommend a further colonoscopy 1 year after surgery to clear all polyps/cancers. Repeat colonoscopic surveillance should then be performed at 5-yearly intervals to detect metachronous lesions in fit patients [19,26].

In conclusion, until the results of ongoing larger prospective randomized controlled trials are available there is no uniform opinion for the follow up of colorectal cancer, but evidence would suggest that it is reasonable to offer CT imaging within the first 2 years after surgery along with 5-yearly colonoscopy. Follow up should cease in elderly or frail patients.

References

1. Kune GA, Kune S, Watson LF. History of colorectal polypectomy and risk of subsequent colorectal cancer. *Br J Surg.* 1987;74: 1064–1065.
2. Stryker SJ, Wolff BG, Culp CE, *et al.* Natural history of untreated colonic polyps. *Gastroenterology.* 1987;93:1009–1013.
3. Winawer S, Fletcher R, Rex D, *et al.* Colorectal cancer screening and surveillance: clinical guidelines and rationale – Update based on new evidence. *Gastroenterology.* 2003;124:544–560.
4. Imperiale TF, Ransohoff DF, Itzkowitz SH, *et al.* Fecal DNA versus fecal occult blood for colorectal-cancer screening in an average-risk population. *N Engl J Med.* 2004;351:2704–2714.
5. Mandel JS, Bond JH, Church TR, *et al.* Reducing mortality from colorectal cancer by screening for fecal occult blood. Minnesota Colon Cancer Control Study. *N Engl J Med.* 1993;328: 1365–1371.
6. Kronborg O, Fenger C, Olsen J, *et al.* Randomised study of screening for colorectal cancer with faecal-occult-blood test. *Lancet.* 1996;348:1467–1471.
7. Hardcastle JD, Chamberlain JO, Robinson MH, *et al.* Randomised controlled trial of faecal-occult-blood screening for colorectal cancer. *Lancet.* 1996;348:1472–1477.
8. Farrands PA, Hardcastle JD. Colorectal screening by a self-completion questionnaire. *Gut.* 1984;25:445–447.
9. Austoker J. Cancer prevention: setting the scene. *BMJ.* 1994;308: 1415–1420.
10. Atkin WS, Edwards R, Wardle J, *et al.* Design of a multicentre randomised trial to evaluate flexible sigmoidoscopy in colorectal cancer screening. *J Med Screen.* 2001;8:137–144.
11. Selby JV, Friedman GD, Quesenberry CP, Jr., *et al.* A case-control study of screening sigmoidoscopy and mortality from colorectal cancer. *N Engl J Med.* 1992;326:653–657.
12. Atkin WS, Edwards R, Kralj-Hans I *et al.* Once-only flexible sigmoidoscopy screening in prevention of colorectal cancer: a multicentre randomised controlled trial. *Lancet.* 2010 May 8;375(9726):1624–1633.

13. Berry DP, Clarke P, Hardcastle JD, *et al.* Randomized trial of the addition of flexible sigmoidoscopy to faecal occult blood testing for colorectal neoplasia population screening. *Br J Surg.* 1997;84:1274–1276.

14. Rex DK, Rahmani EY, Haseman JH, *et al.* Relative sensitivity of colonoscopy and barium enema for detection of colorectal cancer in clinical practice. *Gastroenterology.* 1997;112:17–23.

15. Fenlon HM. Virtual colonoscopy. *Br J Surg.* 2002;89:1–3.

16. Lovett E. Family studies in cancer of the colon and rectum. *Br J Surg.* 1976;63:13–18.

17. Stephenson BM, Murday VA, Finan PJ, *et al.* Feasibility of family based screening for colorectal neoplasia: experience in one general surgical practice. *Gut.* 1993;34:96–100.

18. Lennard-Jones JE, Melville DM, Morson BC, *et al.* Precancer and cancer in extensive ulcerative colitis: findings among 401 patients over 22 years. *Gut.* 1990;31:800–806.

19. Winawer SJ, Zauber AG, O'Brien MJ, *et al.* Randomized comparison of surveillance intervals after colonoscopic removal of newly diagnosed adenomatous polyps. The National Polyp Study Workgroup. *N Engl J Med.* 1993;328:901–906.

20. Atkin WS, Saunders BP. Surveillance guidelines after removal of colorectal adenomatous polyps. *Gut.* 2002;51 Suppl 5:V6–V9.

21. Schoemaker D, Black R, Giles L, *et al.* Yearly colonoscopy, liver CT, and chest radiography do not influence 5-year survival of colorectal cancer patients. *Gastroenterology.* 1998;114:7–14.

22. Tjandra JJ, Chan MK. Follow-up after curative resection of colorectal cancer: a meta-analysis. *Dis Colon Rectum.* 2007;50: 1783–1799.

23. Mayo SC, Pawlik TM. Current management of colorectal hepatic metastasis. Expert Rev *Gastroenterol Hepatol.* 2009;3:131–144.

24. Watanabe K, Nagai K, Kobayashi A, *et al.* Factors influencing survival after complete resection of pulmonary metastases from colorectal cancer. *Br J Surg.* 2009;96:1058–1065.

25. Northover J. Carcinoembryonic antigen and recurrent colorectal cancer. *Gut.* 1986;27:117–122.

26. Barlow AP, Thompson MH. Colonoscopic follow-up after resection for colorectal cancer: a selective policy. *Br J Surg.* 1993;80:781–784.

Small and Large Bowel

CHAPTER 59

Colorectal cancer: a multidisciplinary approach

Rachel S. Midgley,[1] Haitham M. Al-Salama,[2] A. Merrie,[3] N. Mortensen,[1] and David J. Kerr[1,4]

[1]University of Oxford, Oxford, UK
[2]Qatar Foundation, Doha, Qatar
[3]University of Auckland, Auckland, New Zealand
[4]Weill-Cornell College of Medicine, New York, NY, USA

ESSENTIAL FACTS ABOUT PATHOGENESIS

- Most colorectal cancers arise from adenomatous polyps
- Identification of the genes responsible for hereditary cancers has led to improvement in care (see Chapter 57)

ESSENTIALS OF DIAGNOSIS

- Fecal occult blood tests – blood from cancers or polyps can be detected from stool samples
- Flexible sigmoidoscopy – accurate and inexpensive but associated with a small risk of perforation
- Colonoscopy – expensive, complex, invasive, definitive diagnostic method
- Virtual colonoscopy and testing of stool DNA may be future options

(see Chapter 58)

ESSENTIALS OF TREATMENT

- The proportion of patients with colorectal cancer diagnosed at an earlier, treatable stage is increasing
- The treatment algorithm needs to be tailored to the natural history and molecular biology of the specific cancer being assessed
- Most chemotherapy regimens have a narrow therapeutic window
- 5-Fluorouracil (5-FU) has been the mainstay of colorectal cancer chemotherapy for 4 decades; combination of novel cytotoxic agents has led to improved effectiveness
- Biological agents such as cetuximab and bevacizumab are now being integrated into the therapeutic repertoire
- 5-FU is only active in the S phase of the cell cycle, therefore continuous infusion may be more effective against cycling cells than bolus regimens
- Both preoperative radiotherapy and total mesorectal incision have reduced local recurrence rates in rectal cancer
- Immunotherapy and gene therapy offer hope for future advances in management

Introduction

Colorectal cancer (CRC) is a significant cause of morbidity and mortality in the Western World. In North America, western Europe, Australasia, and Japan the **incidence** exceeds 40 per 100 000 of the population in males and 25–30 per 100 000 in females. Significantly, in Africa and in Central and South America the incidence is typically less than 5 per 100 000. Some of this discrepancy in incidence may be explained by genetic variability, as described in Chapter 57, but it is likely to be due largely to differences in diet (low in fiber, high in fat) and the increasingly sedentary lifestyles observed in the West. Many patients presenting with CRC are symptomatic, although the number of patients who are asymptomatic and whose cancers are detected by screening is increasing with the gradual introduction of formal screening programs (see Chapter 58).

The most **common symptoms** that patients describe are rectal bleeding, a change in bowel habit, pain, and occasionally a palpable mass or fatigue secondary to anemia; the latter two symptoms are more common in patients with right-sided tumors. There has been a clear-cut shift towards **earlier diagnosis** of colorectal cancer. In France, one cancer registry showed that, in 1976, 40% of patients had stage I or stage II disease at diagnosis, whereas this figure had risen to 57% by 1991. Over the same period, the percentage of patients with stage IV (advanced) disease decreased from 34% to 22% [1].

This stage migration has probably contributed to the increase in **overall survival** observed for this disease since 1980. For most countries in Europe, the 5-year survival rate from colorectal cancer has increased from 40% to approximately 55% in the past 20 years. However, a number of other factors that will be described in this chapter have contributed significantly to the observed improvement in prognosis for CRC. **Surgical advances** and the evolution of **effective postoperative care** have reduced perioperative mortality and the likelihood of

---

Textbook of Clinical Gastroenterology and Hepatology, Second Edition. Edited by C. J. Hawkey, Jaime Bosch, Joel E. Richter, Guadalupe Garcia-Tsao, Francis K. L. Chan.

local recurrence. Preoperative **radiotherapy** for rectal cancer has also diminished local recurrence rates. **Chemotherapy** administered after surgery appears to have an impact on the risk of metastatic disease and also on overall survival of patients with colonic tumors.

Overview: what happens when a patient is diagnosed with colorectal cancer?

When a patient is diagnosed with colorectal cancer, they should be **staged** to assess local and distant disease (Table 59.1). For **colonic tumors** this usually means **colonoscopy** with biopsy and **computed tomography** (CT) of the chest, abdomen, and pelvis. **Rectal tumors**, particularly those in the lower two-thirds of the rectum, should also be assessed by pelvic **magnetic resonance imaging (MRI)** or **endoscopic ultrasonography (EUS),** as precise local staging is necessary to determine the appropriate first-line treatment.

Ideally, the results of staging investigations should then be discussed at a **multidisciplinary meeting**. Meetings of such teams allow face-to-face contact between surgeons, radiation oncologists, radiologists, pathologists, and specialist nurses, streamlining the patient's care and standardizing protocols for each clinical situation based on best available evidence. Figure 59.1 (a) and (b) show how the pertinent factors are considered for each patient and how the decision about the treatment pathway is made. For example, if the patient were fit and well with a tumor in the colon, surgery to remove the primary tumor would be the first line of treatment followed by assessment of operative histology and consideration of adjuvant chemotherapy. Conversely, for a patient who has a tumor in

the mid third of the rectum that extends into the mesorectum, and an associated large lymph node, downstaging chemoradiotherapy prior to surgery would be sensible in order to increase the chances of a clear (R_0) resection margin.

Colonic and rectal tumors: the anatomic, therapeutic, and molecular distinction

Rectal tumors, probably because of their anatomic location and difficulty in achieving clear planes of resection at surgery, tend to recur locally within the pelvis. Conversely, **colonic tumors** tend to seed early to distant sites, leading to liver and lung metastases. These differences have determined the pattern of therapy for the two sites of disease. Whereas patients with colonic tumors tend to undergo excision followed by chemotherapy to prevent distant recurrence, those with rectal tumors often have preoperative radiotherapy or chemoradiotherapy, followed by resection to prevent local recurrence.

Colonic and rectal tumors may also differ at the **molecular level**. Colorectal carcinogenesis is a multistep pathway (see Chapter 57). [2] Two proteins that are central to this tumorigenic pathway are p53 and APC (the adenomatous polyposis coli protein). One study has suggested that tumors of colonic and rectal origin differ in terms of the relative importance of these proteins [3]. The *APC* **mutations** may be less important in rectal cancer. Furthermore, the **p53 pathway** appeared more important in the rectal tumors. Expression of mutated *p53* was more consistent in rectal tumors (64% versus 29% for colonic tumors) and there was a correlation between positive mutated *p53* expression and worse disease-free survival ($p=0.008$). No such expression or outcome correlation existed for the colonic

Table 59.1 Staging and survival of patients with colorectal cancer

TNM system				Approx. 5-year survival rate (%)	Dukes' classification
Stage	Tumor	Lymph nodes	Metastasis		
0	T0	N0	M0		
I	T1	N0	M0	97	A
I	T2	N0	M0	90	
II	T3	N0	M0	78	B
II	T4	N0	M0	63	
III	Any T	N1	M0	56–66	C
III	Any T	N2	M0	26–37	
IV	Any T	Any N	M1	1	D

T1, tumor invades submucosa; T2, tumor invades muscularis propria; T3, tumor invades through muscularis propria into subserosa, or into nonperitonealized pericolis or perirectal tissues; T4, tumor directly invades other organs or structures, and/or perforates visceral peritoneum; N0, no regional lymph node metastasis; N1, metastasis in one to three regional lymph nodes; N2, metastasis in four or more regional lymph nodes; M0, no distant mestastasis; M1, distant metastasis.

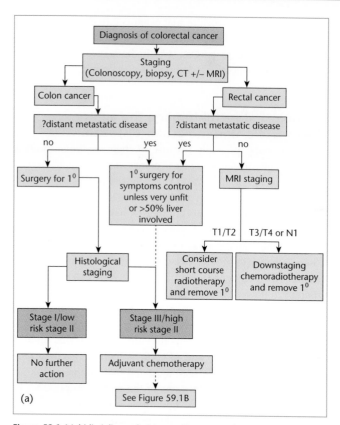

(a)

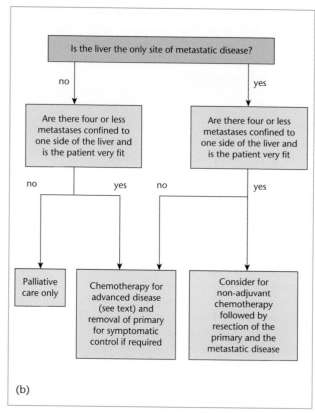

(b)

Figure 59.1 Multidisciplinary decision-making approach to patients with colorectal cancer. (a) Treatment pathway for primary colorectal cancer (CRC). (b) Treatment pathway when distant metastatic disease is present at diagnosis. (This figure was published in *Clinical Gastroenterology and Hepatology*, Wilfred M. Weinstein, Christopher J. Hawkey, Jaime Bosch, Colorectal cancer: a multidisciplinary approach, Pages 421–430, Copyright Elsevier, 2005.)

tumors [3]. It could be that this difference in disease-free survival for patients with rectal tumors that were *p53* mutation positive or negative reflected the relative radiation resistance or sensitivity of the two groups. It is clear then that there is evidence to suggest that treating colonic and rectal tumors as distinct entities in terms of therapy is appropriate. For the data on the role of *p53* malignancy associated with ulcerative colitis see Chapter 49.

Surgery for colorectal cancer

Assessment

Surgery with curative intent is aimed at removing the tumor and the corresponding lymphatic drainage to allow accurate staging, and is the primary form of treatment for CRC. All patients being considered for surgery should have a histologic diagnosis, imaging of the colon, and staging for metastatic disease prior to discussion at a multidisciplinary meeting. **Imaging of the colon** can be accomplished using a variety of techniques, discussed elsewhere in this book (see Chapters 124, 132 and 136). Staging for metastatic disease involves imaging the liver and lungs, and can also be accomplished by a variety of techniques: ultrasonography, CT, MRI, and positron emission tomography (PET). Accuracy of detection of liver metastases is optimal with MRI or intraoperative

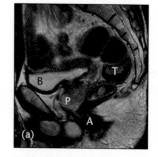

(a)

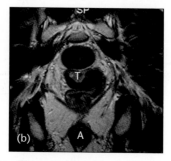

(b)

Figure 59.2 Pelvic MRI demonstrating a T2 tumor of the mid rectum. (a) Sagittal section. (b) Coronal section. This is a T2 tumor as it can be seen involving, but not invading through, the full thickness of the bowel wall. A, anus; B, bladder; P, prostate; T, tumor; S, sacrum.

ultrasonography, but CT remains an accurate and readily available imaging technique.

Local staging of rectal cancer has undergone revolutionary changes. Current best practice is for all rectal cancers to be assessed with MRI with a body coil, or with EUS to assess the extent of tumor spread, clearance of surgical margins, and, more recently, lymph node involvement (Figure 59.2). This determines the need for and type of preoperative adjuvant treatment. Formal assessment also includes careful physical examination including rigid sigmoidoscopy to determine the position of the tumor in relation to the anal sphincters, and assessment of function of the anal sphincters. This may need to be done under anesthesia to enable an accurate assessment; if there is concern about anal sphincter function, preoperative assessment of anal physiology may be useful.

Surgery for colonic cancer

Segmental resection of the colon is based on lymphovascular drainage. The principles of anatomic dissection apply to both colonic and rectal surgery, with sharp dissection in the planes of embryologic fusion. This is usually done in an open surgical fashion; however, the **laparoscopic approach** is gaining acceptance for some patients, and a discussion of the technique and comparison with the open technique is given in Chapter 157. Surgery for obstructing CRC carries a high mortality rate. The development of self-expanding **colorectal stents** shows promise in relieving acute obstruction to allow surgery to be performed in an elective setting after appropriate staging and assessment [4].

Surgery for rectal cancer

A high local recurrence rate in patients with rectal cancer (25%) was traditionally the driving force behind the use of preoperative and postoperative radiotherapy, as discussed below. However, the adoption of anatomic rectal excision, best known as **total mesorectal excision (TME)**, has seen these recurrence rates drop to under 10%. [5,6] Rarely has a change in surgical practice produced such a significant improvement in outcome. Total mesorectal excision is a careful extrafascial excision of the rectum and mesorectum down to the pelvic floor, thereby excising the tumor and surrounding lymphatic drainage *en bloc*. Although there has been much debate about semantics and terminology, essentially TME is used for **low and middle rectal cancers**. For **high rectal cancers**, 5 cm of mesorectum distal to the tumor is taken to ensure adequate clearance within the mesorectum.

Low anterior resection is the preferred treatment of choice for low rectal cancers, except for tumors with inadequate distal clearance (<2 cm) and in cases where the sphincter mechanism is not adequate for continence. In these instances **abdominoperineal excision** remains the treatment of choice. Increasingly adjuvant chemoradiotherapy is utilized in the treatment of these patients.

For reconstruction of low anterior resections the **use of a short-term colonic J pouch** has been shown to improve short term postoperative neorectal function with a decreased anastomotic leak rate due to theoretically better perfusion at the anastomosis. The pouch should be no bigger than 5 cm at the level of the pelvic floor; if it is longer or more cephalad, impaired evacuation can occur. **Local excision** of rectal cancer is generally restricted to early rectal cancers that are mobile on clinical examination, stage T1 on endoanal ultrasonography (Figure 59.3), and well differentiated on biopsy, or in less fit patients. The major problem is that prediction of lymph node involvement is difficult. Local excision can be done via **transanal endoscopic microsurgery** or by per anal disc

excision. The principles in both are the same: to excise the lesion in a full-thickness manner with a cuff of normal surrounding tissue (Figure 59.4).

Impotence and retrograde ejaculation in men are recognized complications of pelvic surgery. The adoption of the TME approach and a better understanding of the anatomy and physiology of the pelvic autonomic nervous system (Figure 59.5) have been accompanied by a parallel decline in the rates of sexual dysfunction. Spontaneous resolution of these problems can occur up to 1 year after surgery; in addition, treatment with sildenafil and drugs with similar actions are generally successful [7].

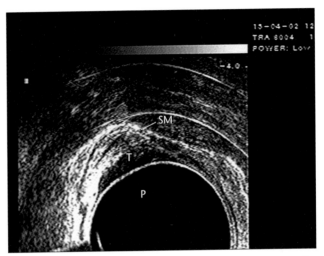

Figure 59.3 Endoanal ultrasound scan demonstrating a T1 rectal cancer. P, endorectal ultrasound probe; T, tumor; SM, submucosa.

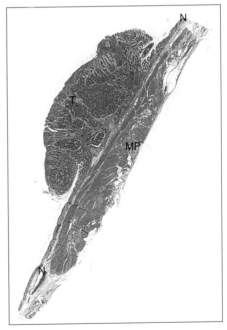

Figure 59.4 T1 rectal cancer. Histologic section of a T1 rectal cancer following full-thickness complete local excision. N, normal mucosa; T, T1 tumor; MP, muscularis propria.

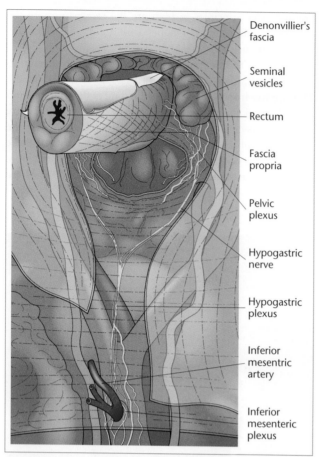

Denonvillier's fascia

Seminal vesicles

Rectum

Fascia propria

Pelvic plexus

Hypogastric nerve

Hypogastric plexus

Inferior mesentric artery

Inferior mesenteric plexus

Figure 59.5 Pelvic anatomy. Dissection in the extrafascial (total mesorectal excision) plane, with autonomic nerves and seminal vesicles exposed. (Reproduced with permission of and acknowledgment to Mr Ian Bissett, University of Auckland, New Zealand.)

Chemotherapy for colorectal cancer

Basic concepts of cancer chemotherapy

Advanced versus adjuvant setting and traditional trial paradigms

Chemotherapy can be given in either the advanced disease setting or the adjuvant setting. In advanced disease, where there is distant metastasis or inoperable local recurrence, chemotherapy is administered to palliate symptoms or to prolong life with no expectation of cure. In the **adjuvant setting**, chemotherapy is administered to patients after potentially curative surgery in an attempt to decrease the risk of recurrence and death from the disease. Therefore the goal is cure for a proportion of the patients treated. The different objectives in these two scenarios determine the balance between toxicity and quality of life that clinicians and patients are prepared to accept from such therapy. When novel chemotherapeutic agents are being assessed, they are first tested in the advanced disease setting where a rough assessment of their efficacy in terms of tumor response rates, as well as their toxicity, can be made. The agents go through phase I, phase II, and then randomized phase III trials (comparison with the "gold standard" treatment) in patients with advanced disease, and finally they are tested in

Table 59.2 Traditional trial paradigm for novel anticancer agents

Phase I
Dose finding and toxicity assessment
Number of arms: 1
Setting: advance disease
Numbers: 10 to 20

Phase II
First efficacy testing
Number of arms: 1 or 2
Setting: advance disease
Numbers: 10 to 50 (more if two arms)

Phase III
Efficacy testing against gold standard
Measured by response rate
Number of arms: 2 or more
Setting: advance disease first
Numbers: 100s

Phase III adjuvant
Efficacy testing against gold standard
Measured by disease-free and overall survival differences
Number of arms: 2 or more
Setting: adjuvant after removal of primary
Numbers: many 100s or 1000s

(This table was published in *Clinical Gastroenterology and Hepatology*, Wilfred M. Weinstein, Christopher J. Hawkey, Jaime Bosch, Colorectal cancer: a multidisciplinary approach, Pages 421–430, Copyright Elsevier, 2005.)

the adjuvant arena (Table 59.2). The process from first clinical trial to being accepted for use in the adjuvant setting to prevent recurrence of disease takes somewhere between 12 and 15 years.

Important pharmacologic concepts in chemotherapy

Cytotoxic drugs tend to have **steep dose–response curves**: the higher the plasma level that can be achieved, the greater the chance of response. Furthermore, the drugs generally have a **narrow therapeutic window**, which means there is little difference in the plasma concentration required to bring about tumor cytotoxicity and that which induces significant toxicity to normal tissues. In general, chemotherapy doses are calculated according to the patient's individual **body surface area** (determined by their height and weight), although there are a number of genetic polymorphisms and differences in renal or hepatic physiology that can cause deficiencies in the metabolism of cytotoxic drugs, leading to greatly enhanced toxicity. Oncologists grade patients' toxicity on a scale from 1 to 4. Generally toxicity equal to or greater than grade 3 or repeated episodes of grade 2 toxicity necessitates dose reduction for future cycles of chemotherapy (Table 59.3).

Routes of administration

Although historically chemotherapy has always been given intravenously, attempts are constantly being made to formulate drugs that are predictably absorbed through the bowel mucosa. This has huge implications on patient acceptability and cost of administration.

Table 59.3 National cancer institute common toxicity criteria for some common chemotherapy toxicities

	Grade 1	Grade 2	Grade 3	Grade 4
Mucositis	Soreness or erythema	Erythema, ulcers – can eat solids	Erythema, ulcers – liquid diet only	Alimentation not possible
Nausea	Able to eat reasonable intake	Can eat but decreased intake	No significant intake	
Vomiting	1 episode in 24 h	2–5 episodes in 24 h	6–10 episodes in 24 h	>10 episodes or requiring parenteral nutrition
Diarrhea	Increase of 2–3 stools per day compared to pre-treatment	Increase of 4–6 stools or nocturnal stools	Increase of 7–9 stools per day or malabsorption	Increase of 10 or more stools per day or grossly bloody stools, dehydration
Fatigue	Increased fatigue – able to conduct normal activities	Moderate difficulty performing some activities	Severe loss of ability to perform some activities	Bedridden or disabling
Neutropenia ($\times 10^9$/L)	1.5–1.9	1.0–1.4	0.5–0.9	<0.5

Regional delivery of chemotherapy via the hepatic artery

The majority of metastatic CRC is confined to the liver. Also, it has been known for many years that micrometastases within the liver derive their blood supply from the hepatic artery, whereas normal hepatocytes derive their supply predominantly from the portal vein. Furthermore, a number of chemotherapy drugs are largely metabolized during their first pass through the liver. Hence relatively high doses of drug can be administered directly to the liver, while still keeping systemic exposure low. Randomized trials comparing hepatic arterial infusion with systemic therapy have given conflicting results, but many have suffered from poor trial design. Most have confirmed a higher response rate, but evidence of improved survival has been lacking [8].

Chemotherapy for advanced colorectal cancer: the evidence

When considering chemotherapy for advanced CRC the risks and benefits must be weighed carefully. A randomized trial more than 10 years ago established that chemotherapy with **5-fluorouracil (5-FU)**-based regimens improved median survival from 5 to 10 months when compared with best supportive care for patients with metastatic CRC. There was also evidence of an improvement in **quality of life** in responding patients. The major dose-limiting **toxicities** of the common CRC chemotherapy regimens are mucositis with soreness of the mouth, diarrhea (usually controlled by drugs such as loperamide or diphenoxylate), plantar–palmar erythema, and mild myelosuppression (usually manifesting as a fall in neutrophil count).

5-Fluorouracil

5-Fluorouracil has been the mainstay of CRC chemotherapy for over 40 years. It is an antimetabolite and a pro-drug. It is converted into its active form, fluorodeoxyuridine monophosphate (FdUMP), within the cell. This metabolite binds to the enzyme **thymidylate synthase**, blocking its action and preventing pyrimidine, and therefore DNA, synthesis (Figure 59.6). 5-Fluorouracil can also be falsely incorporated into RNA, interfering with protein synthesis. An interesting feature of 5-FU metabolism is the presence of a degree of genetic polymorphism governing the enzyme that inactivates FdUMP: dihydropyrimidine dehydrogenase (DPD). Approximately 1 to 2% of the Caucasian population exhibits severely depressed levels of DPD, and these individuals demonstrate exaggerated and prolonged plasma levels of FdUMP, leading to augmented toxicity such as prolonged neutropenia and complete alopecia.

As one of the major effects of 5-FU is disruption of DNA replication, the drug is largely active in the **S phase of the cell cycle.** Given the small fraction of cells in S phase at any one time, it was suggested that infusional regimens might have a greater "hit" against cycling cells than bolus regimens. Indeed, a meta-analysis in advanced CRC, comparing infusional 5-FU against bolus 5-FU treatment (given on five consecutive days every 4 weeks – Mayo regimen), found that infusional therapy delivered a higher response rate and prolonged progression-free survival but only a negligible improvement in median survival. **Infusional 5-FU** regimens are now the standard of care in Europe and in many parts of the United States. However, with infusional regimens it must be remembered that, unless patients want to be confined to hospital for the duration of their chemotherapy, central line insertion, with all the incumbent risks of infection and thrombophlebitis, is a prerequisite for such therapy. **Leucovorin (folinic acid; FA)** is given with 5-FU as it provides a further mechanism to augment the efficacy of 5-FU. The addition of FA increases the pool of reduced folate in the cell and stabilizes the FdUMP–thymidylate synthase complex. Studies have shown that the addition of leucovorin (FA) to 5-FU in bolus regimens doubles the response rate.

Small and Large Bowel

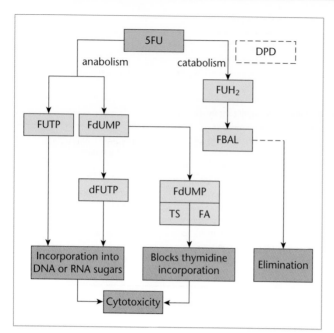

Figure 59.6 Metabolism of 5-fluorouracil (5FU). dFUTP, fluorodeoxyuridine triphosphate; DPD, dihydropyridine dehydrogenase; FA, leucovorin (folinic acid); FBAL, fluoro-β-alanine; FdUMP, fluorodeoxyuridine monophosphate; FUH2, dihydrofluorouracil; FUTP, fluorouridine triphosphate; TS, thymidine synthase. (This figure was published in *Clinical Gastroenterology and Hepatology*, Wilfred M. Weinstein, Christopher J. Hawkey, Jaime Bosch, Colorectal cancer: a multidisciplinary approach, Pages 421–430, Copyright Elsevier, 2005.)

Novel cytotoxics

Irinotecan

Irinotecan, also known as CPT-11, is a potent inhibitor of **topoisomerase I**, an enzyme essential for DNA supercoiling. Randomized studies have shown that in patients whose advanced CRC has become resistant to treatment with 5-FU response rates of up to 15% are achievable with single-agent irinotecan, resulting in a statistically significant overall survival benefit when compared with best supportive care alone. The use of irinotecan in the first-line setting was initially avoided because of concerns about its toxicity. Irinotecan can be a difficult drug for patients to tolerate, with approximately one-quarter to one-third of patients suffering grade 3 or 4 diarrhea. Neutropenia, nausea, and alopecia are also reported frequently. However, with greater experience of the drug and an evolving ability to deal with the toxicities, there has been increasing interest in the use of irinotecan in combination with 5-FU as first-line palliative CRC therapy. Randomized phase III studies have now shown that **triple therapy** with infusional 5-FU–leucovorin–irinotecan gives better response rates, increased median time to progression, and increased median survival compared with single- or double-agent combinations.

Oxaliplatin

Oxaliplatin is a third-generation platinum compound that induces **DNA cross-linkages and apoptotic cell death**. Unlike the related agents cisplatin and carboplatin, it does have

activity against human CRC. There is evidence that oxaliplatin acts in a synergistic way with 5-FU, the combination achieving response rates of up to 50% when used in first-line therapy. Infusional 5-FU plus oxaliplatin as first-line treatment for advanced CRC resulted in a doubled response rate compared with 5-FU alone [9]. Oxaliplatin has no renal and minimal hematologic toxicity. It does, however, cause a particular dysesthesia precipitated by cold, as well as a cumulative sensory neuropathy.

Oral 5-fluorouracil analogs

Tablet equivalents of 5-FU, such as uracil–ftorafur (UFT) or capecitabine, have been the subject of four multicenter trials in patients with advanced CRC comparing oral UFT plus FA or capecitabine with intravenous 5-FU. These studies demonstrated approximately equal efficacy and similar median survival times. There was less mucositis, neutropenia, and alopecia but more hand–foot syndrome (erythema desquamation of the palms and soles) and diarrhea with oral agent administration. The capecitabine / oxaliplatin has now become commonplace in the therapeutic armoury, but capecitabine / irinotecan is still only given cautiously and infrequently, because of the overlapping toxicity of sever diarrhea between the two drugs.

Novel biological agents

Bevacizumab

Bevacizumab (Avastin), a monoclonal antibody that targets the **vascular endothelial growth factor (VEGF)** receptor. It works by preventing the formation of tumor blood vessels, diminishing the delivery of blood, oxygen, and nutrients necessary for the tumor cell growth. Combined with chemotherapy, bevacizumab is used as first-line treatment for patients suffering advanced or metastatic CRC. A phase III clinical trial has shown that the combination addition of **bevacizuamb** to the **irinotecan/5-FU/leucovorin chemotherapy** regimen increased median survival by 5 months and increased progression-free survival by approximately 4 months [10]. Another randomized phase III trial concluded that adding bevacizumab to the FOLFOX4 (oxaliplatin, leucovorin, and 5-FU) chemotherapy regimen in previously-treated metastatic CRC patients increased the overall survival as well as progression-free survival period [11]. Uncommon, though serious, **side effects** include gastrointestinal and non-gastrointestinal perforation, increased risk of thromboembolic events and impaired wound healing.

Cetuximab

Epidermal growth factor receptor (EGFR) is overexpressed in many CRC cells. Cetuximab, **an EGFR antagonist**, is a monoclonal antibody that halts cell growth and promotes apoptosis. Cetuximab has been used with and without irinotecan, and has mainly been utilized to date in advanced or metastatic CRC that is chemo-resistant or in patients who cannot tolerate irinotecan. There is evidence from phase II and phase III clinical trials to suggest that it can increase response rates compared with irinotecan alone and improve progression-free survival [12]. However it is only recommended in CRC patients with normal (non-mutated) KRAS gene status in their tumours, as no benefit is gained in patients whose tumour is KRAS mutant [13,14]. Cetuximab **side effects** include severe nausea, vomiting, hypersensitivity, paronychial infections and, more commonly, an acne-like dermatologic rash.

Chemotherapy for advanced colorectal cancer: what is the standard of care?

There is general consensus in Europe and the United States that combination chemotherapy should become the standard of care in the therapy of **advanced CRC**. However, the specific sequencing with respect to oxaliplatin and irinotecan is still a point of contention. One large study compared the delivery of 5-FU–FA–oxaliplatin in combination for first-line therapy, followed by 5-FU–FA–irinotecan on progression, with the reverse sequence. There was no difference in overall survival; however, in both arms median survival was in excess of 20 months, which compares very favourably to historic controls [15]. The present United Kingdom **National Institute for Clinical Excellence** guidelines allow for infusional 5-FU–FA only as the first-line treatment, with single-agent irinotecan on progression. Capecitabine can be substituted for infusional 5-FU if it is considered that the oral drug would be better tolerated by the patient. Although capecitabine is a more expensive drug than 5-FU, there are many cost savings with respect to line complications and chemotherapy nurse administration time. For patients with potentially resectable metastases confined to the liver, a first-line combination of 5-FU–FA–oxaliplatin is recommended. This is based on a large French series in which patients initially deemed to have borderline irresectable liver disease were given this combination and one in eight patients was converted to resectability.

Adjuvant chemotherapy for colorectal cancer: the evidence

Despite the best efforts of the surgeon in the 80% of colorectal tumors that are deemed operatively curable, 50% of these patients will subsequently relapse and die from their disease. This is as a result of occult tumor cells that are present at the time of the operation, either locally, in the lymph nodes, or at distant sites (spread by hematogenous routes), but are too small to detect by available radiologic techniques. Adjuvant chemotherapy is administered in an attempt to eradicate the cells before they become large functional tumor masses.

The role of **adjuvant chemotherapy** in increasing the chance of cure from CRC is now well established, but it has taken many years to prove the extent of the benefit. In 1990, results showed a 33% reduced odds of death and 41% reduced risk of recurrence amongst patients with Dukes' C colonic cancer who received adjuvant 5-FU–levamisole after surgery compared with surgery alone [16]. **Levamisole** has been superseded by

FA, as in the setting of advanced CRC. Subsequent large prospective randomized trials showed convincing evidence of improved 3-year disease-free survival and overall survival in patients treated with 5-FU–FA, with a 25–30% decrease in the odds of dying from colonic cancer (or an absolute improvement in survival rate of 5–6%) compared with surgery-alone controls. Subsequently, a large phase III trial suggested that oral **capecitabine** administered for 6 months may be superior to bolus 5-FU–FA in the adjuvant treatment of stage III CRC with respect to recurrence-free survival and was as good with respect to disease-free survival [17]. More recently a large randomized trial has indicated that adding **oxaliplatin** to 5-FU-based treatment in the adjuvant setting of stage III colon cancer can improve disease-free survival and overall survival, although the overall survival benefits are small and the extra neurotoxicity is significant. Based upon these trials clinicians tend to decide whether their individual patient's tumour characteristics warrant the additional toxic costs of oxaliplatin. If so the patient receives 6 months of 5-FU or capecitabine plus oxaliplatin; if not, most commonly they receive 6 months of capectabine alone. **Bevacizumab** and **cetuximab** are now being assessed in the adjuvant setting.

The role of **chemotherapy in stage II (Dukes' B) colonic cancer** is less certain. Adjuvant therapy in this setting is not at present recommended as standard practice for all patients in Europe. However, data from the **QUASAR trial** in patients with stage II colonic cancer randomized to chemotherapy or surgery alone suggest a small but statistically significant improvement in the overall survival in the chemotherapy-treated patients. It is possible that there will be a subset of stage II patients who have specific poor prognostic factors (perforation, obstruction, T4 tumors) that will derive most benefit from adjuvant therapy. This will be a question addressed in future trials. In the United States the consensus is a little different, and many patients with stage II disease are receiving adjuvant chemotherapy.

Adjuvant chemotherapy for rectal tumors is another contentious issue. Because of the anatomic constraints within the pelvis, local recurrence rather than distant metastasis has historically been the main problem and the major determinant of outcome. Based on this, the role of the oncologist has been largely restricted to radiotherapy. However the **QUASAR1 study** also demonstrated benefits from adjuvant chemotherapy for rectal cancer patients, and therefore this is appropriate for selected individuals.

Radiotherapy and chemoradiotherapy for rectal cancer

Radiotherapy as an adjuvant treatment to surgery in the treatment of rectal cancer has been assessed in a series of trials and proven benefit has been established. The postoperative radiotherapy approach has been largely superseded by preoperative radiotherapy, either with a short (1 week) course of radiotherapy or the more traditional longer course [18]. Both

Small and Large Bowel

regimens allow for a decrease in dose requirements, decreased small bowel irradiation, significantly decreased local recurrence rates by up to 50%, and, in some studies, an increase in overall survival has been suggested.

Chemoradiation: The integration of chemotherapy with the preoperative regimen appears to prime the tissue for radiotherapy effect, allowing increased tumor downstaging, with complete pathologic response in some tumors (Figure 59.7). With continual improvement in preoperative imaging, nodal status can now be accurately predicted on MRI [19], enabling early identification of patients who may benefit from combined neo-adjuvant chemoradiotherapy. There is no rigid consensus about which patients should receive preoperative radiotherapy. The initial dramatic results shown with preoperative radiotherapy probably reflect the historic unacceptably high local recurrence rates that were prevalent prior to the widespread adoption of anatomic rectal surgical techniques (discussed below). Despite improvements in surgery to a general high standard, however, studies still demonstrate that the administration of preoperative radiotherapy does further decrease local recurrence rates. However, this is a proportional effect, so the benefit to patients with early tumors that have a low rate of local recurrence is quite moderate [20]. It is accepted that patients with T4 tumors and tumors with invasion within 2 mm of the enveloping fascia of the mesorectum (fascia propria) on imaging benefit from long-course preoperative (chemo)radiotherapy, and it is generally accepted that patients with T3 tumors, tumors with MRI evidence of lymph node metastases, tumors in the most distal 5 cm of the rectum, and anterior tumors in men also benefit from radiotherapy.

Pathology and prognosis of colorectal cancer

Many factors impact on the prognosis of patients with CRC. Accurate clinicopathologic staging remains the mainstay for decision-making with regard to further adjuvant treatment. The **histologic staging** is of paramount importance; detailed assessment of the resected specimen enables precise staging to be done (Figure 59.8). Particular to rectal cancer is assessment of the circumferential margin; this is the **TME resection margin**. Involvement or encroachment of this by tumor is highly predictive of the development of local recurrence [21]. Several staging systems for CRC exist of which the **tumor node metastasis (TNM) system**, summarized in Table 59.1, is

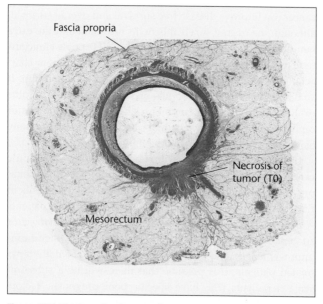

Figure 59.7 Histology showing complete response. Full-mount histologic section of rectal cancer showing complete regression following chemoradiotherapy – histologic stage T0.

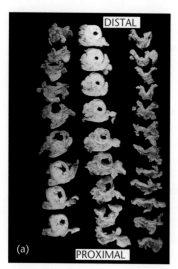
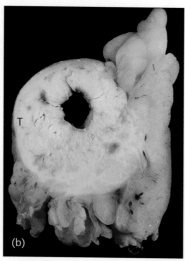
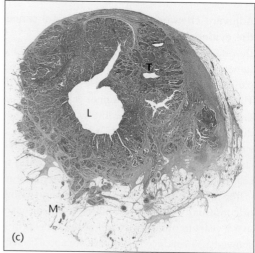

Figure 59.8 Histologic staging. (a) Multiple gross transverse sections taken from a formalin-fixed specimen of an extended right hemicolectomy for a transverse colonic cancer. (b) Appearance of a gross transverse section of the tumor; this is circumferential and obstructing, and stage T3 as it has invaded beyond the bowel wall. (c) Full-mount histologic appearance of the cancer – histologic grade pT3 N0 M1 (stage III). L, lumen; M, mesocolon; T, tumor.

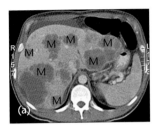 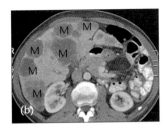

Figure 59.9 Computed tomogram showing bilobar hepatic metastases from colorectal cancer. Axial sections from oral (a) and intravenous (b) contrast-enhanced scans (portal venous phase). M, metastases.

Table 59.4 Recurrence of rectal cancer related to technique and adjuvant Treatment

Technique	Recurrence (%)
Conventional surgery	25
Postop. radiotherapy	15–20
Preop. radiotherapy	10–15
Total mesorectal excision	10
Preop. radiotherapy	2–5

the most comprehensive. This is reviewed regularly and takes into account factors such as the circumferential resection margin. Also, systematic reviews have consistently demonstrated that higher patient volumes and increased specialization of individual surgeons are associated with improved survival and decreased morbidity [22].

Follow-up of patients with colorectal cancer

There is some evidence is accumulating to suggest that intensive follow-up, including liver imaging, is associated with a decrease in mortality rate, perhaps because a greater proportion of patients are picked up with operable metastatic disease [23]. However the issue of follow-up for CRC remains a contentious issue and there is little clarity or uniformity on this matter.

Recurrence of colorectal cancer

Most episodes of recurrence present within 2 years; the most common site is in the **liver** (33%) (Figure 59.9), followed by **lung** (20%), and then **local recurrence** (20%), which is mainly in the pelvis. Rectal cancer is more likely than colonic cancer to present with local recurrence. The chance of local recurrence is influenced by several factors including tumor stage, surgical technique, and the use of adjuvant (chemo)radiotherapy. Treatment of local recurrence is difficult. After thorough imaging with MRI and/or PET, radiotherapy followed by excision, which may include sacrectomy and pelvic exenteration, can yield acceptable long-term results in patients who have complete excision of the disease. However, careful patient selection is required.

Surgery for metastatic disease

Colorectal cancer liver metastases are present in 18% of patients at diagnosis (Table 59.4). The natural history without any intervention is poor, with an average life expectancy of 5 to 10 months. The short-term outlook is better in unilobular and solitary metastases, with a **1-year survival** rate of up to 77% and a **3-year survival** rate of 23%. Imaging for hepatic metastases is best performed using **triphasic helical CT**, with scans performed before the administration of arterial contrast

and during arterial and portal venous phases, and repeated after a delay. **Chemotherapy** can be offered to many patients with hepatic metastatic disease to palliate symptoms and prolong life (see above). However, **hepatic resection** is the only potentially curative modality for isolated hepatic disease. Outcome is influenced largely by patient selection. Median survival of the order of 25–45% at 5 years can be achieved and is determined by a variety of factors: deferred presentation after primary resection, no extrahepatic disease, resectable pattern of metastases (not necessarily solitary), sufficient hepatic reserve, and a fit patient. Imaging (including MRI of the liver and CT of the chest and abdomen) is usually performed prior to consideration of resection, and liver function tumor markers are assessed. All patients should be discussed at a multidisciplinary meeting.

Liver failure can be a major complication following resection and is related to age, extent of resection, remnant size and quality, presence of chronic liver disease, and steatosis. For those patients who survive the operation without undue complications, consideration is now being made of "adjuvant" systemic or hepatic arterial chemotherapy. Although this is not advocated in Europe because of a perceived lack of adequate randomized evidence, it is practised by a number of centers in North America.

Other modalities have been assessed in the therapy of isolated liver metastases; both radiofrequency ablation and cryotherapy can be useful in conjunction with resection; preoperative embolization stimulates growth of the hepatic remnant; and hepatic artery chemotherapy can be administered.

Surgery for pulmonary metastases is also worth considering. Development of lung lesions in a resectable pattern is less common than with liver metastases. However, for patients with limited disease, a 5-year survival rate of up to 25% can be obtained.

Novel strategies to treat colorectal cancer

There are other new exciting therapies predicated upon basic science advances that are now entering the clinical arena. These are "translational approaches" that really do bridge the gap between basic medical science and clinical treatment, such as immunotherapy and gene therapy. These treatments are likely to have greatest impact in the curable adjuvant setting, where tumor burden is low. Clearly larger-scale treatment trials for any new therapies are required before they can be used in clinical practice.

Immunotherapy

Immunotherapy in CRC can involve rather **non-specific stimulation** of the host immune system through administration of BCG (Bacillus Calmette–Guerin) or cytokines, or more directed strategies such as **anti-idiotypic monoclonal antibodies**, or the use of **virus vaccines**. Early trials of vaccines constructed with vaccinia virus or fowlpox virus backbones flanking inserted tumor-associated antigen genes such as *CEA* and *MUC1* have been completed. Disease stabilization and minimal toxicity have been documented. Furthermore, in-vitro post-vaccination testing of peripheral blood lymphocytes found specific lytic activity against carcinoembryonic antigen (CEA)-expressing tumor cells.

Gene therapy

Cancer gene therapy encompasses a myriad of genetic manipulation strategies including the insertion of genes encoding cytokines, expression of tumor suppressor genes to abort excessive proliferation, and insertion of drug resistance genes into healthy cells to allow aggressive cytotoxic therapy. However, phase I trials are now under way using an innovative technique termed virus-directed enzyme pro-drug therapy (VDEPT). This involves insertion of genes into cells that are capable of metabolizing pro-drugs. Retroviral vectors linking the *CEA* promoter to the structural gene for the bacterial enzyme cytosine deaminase have been formulated. The cytosine deaminase metabolizes the pro-drug 5-fluorocytosine to 5-FU, but transduction should occur only in CEA-expressing cells (i.e., CRC cells). The objective is to confer selectivity of the cytotoxic agent, allowing a 10000-fold higher concentration of the 5-FU in the tumor and in neighboring bystander cells than in the systemic circulation.

References

1. Faivre-Finn C, Bouvier AM, Mitry E, *et al*. Chemotherapy for colon cancer in a well defined French population: Is it under- or over-prescribed? *Aliment Pharmacol Ther*. 2002;16:353–359.
2. Fearon ER, Hamilton SR, Vogelstein B. Clonal analysis of human colorectal tumors. *Science*. 1987;238:193–197.
3. Kapiteijn E, Liefers GJ, Los LC, *et al*. Mechanisms of oncogenesis in colon versus rectal cancer. *J Pathol*. 2001;195:171–178.
4. Khot UP, Lang AW, Murali K, *et al*. Systematic review of the efficacy and safety of colorectal stents. *Br J Surg*. 2002;89:1096–1102.
5. Heald RJ, Husband EM, Ryall RDH. The mesorectum in rectal cancer surgery – the clue to pelvic recurrence? *Br J Surg*. 1982;69:613–616.
6. McCall JL, Cox MA, Wattchow DA. Analysis of local recurrence rates after surgery alone for rectal cancer. *Int J Colorectal Dis*. 1995;10:126–132.
7. Keating JP. Sexual function after rectal excision. *Aust N Z J Surg*. 2004;74:248–259.
8. Kerr DJ, McArdle CS, Ledermann J, *et al*. Intrahepatic arterial versus intravenous fluorouracil and folinic acid for colorectal cancer liver metastases: a multicentre randomised trial. *Lancet*. 2003;361:368–373.
9. de Gramont A, Figer A, Seymour M, *et al*. Leucovorin and fluorouracil with or without oxaliplatin as first-line treatment in advanced colorectal cancer. *J Clin Oncol*. 2000;18:2938–2947.
10. Hurwitz H, Fehrenbacher L, Novotny W, *et al*. Bevacizumab plus irinotecan, fluorouracil, and leucovorin for metastatic colorectal cancer. *N Engl J Med*. 2004;350:2335–2342.
11. Giantonio BJ, Catalano PJ, Meropol NJ *et al*. Bevacizumab in combination with oxaliplatin, fluorouracil, and leucovorin (FOLFOX4) for previously treated metastatic colorectal cancer: results from the Eastern Cooperative Oncology Group Study E3200. *J Clin Oncol*. 2007;25:1539–1544.
12. Cunningham D, Humblet Y, Siena S, *et al*. Cetuximab monotherapy and cetuximab plus irinotecan in irinotecan-refractory metastatic colorectal cancer. *N Engl J Med*. 2004;351:337–345.
13. Allegra CJ, Jessup JM, Somerfield MR, *et al*. American Society of Clinical Oncology provisional clinical opinion: testing for KRAS gene mutations in patients with metastatic colorectal carcinoma to predict response to anti-epidermal growth factor receptor monoclonal antibody therapy. *J Clin Oncol*. 2009;27:2091–2096.
14. Heinemann V, Stintzing S, Kirchner T, *et al*. Clinical relevance of EGFR- and KRAS-status in colorectal cancer patients treated with monoclonal antibodies directed against the EGFR. *Cancer Treat Rev*. 2009;35:262–271.
15. Douillard JY, Sobrero A, Carnaghi C, *et al*. Metastatic colorectal cancer: integrating irinotecan into combination and sequential chemotherapy. *Ann Oncol*. 2003;14:7–12.
16. Moertel CG, Fleming TR, Macdonald JS, *et al*. Levamisole and fluorouracil for adjuvant therapy of resected colon carcinoma. *N Engl J Med*. 1990;322:352–358.
17. McKendrick JJ, Cassidy J, Chakrapee-Sirisuk G, *et al*. Capecitabine is resource-saving compared with IV bolus 5FU/LV in adjuvant chemotherapy for Dukes' C colon cancer patients: Medical resource utilization data from a large phase III trial (X-ACT). *Proc ASCO*. 2004;23:265 (Abstract).
18. Colorectal Cancer Collaborative Group. Adjuvant radiotherapy for rectal cancer: a systematic overview of 8507 patients from 22 randomised trials. *Lancet*. 2001;358:1291–1304.
19. Brown G, Radcliffe AG, Newcombe RG, *et al*. Preoperative assessment of prognostic factors in rectal cancer using high-resolution magnetic resonance imaging. *Br J Surg*. 2003;90:355–364.
20. Kapiteijn E, Marijnen CA, Nagtegaal ID, *et al*. Dutch Colorectal Cancer Group. Preoperative radiotherapy combined with total mesorectal excision for resectable rectal cancer. *N Engl J Med*. 2001;345:638–646.
21. Quirke P, Durdey P, Dixon MF, Williams NS. Local recurrence of rectal adenocarcinoma due to inadequate surgical resection. *Lancet*. 1986;ii: 996–999.
22. Hodgson DC, Fuchs CS, Ayanian JZ. Impact of patient and provider characteristics on the treatment and outcomes of colorectal cancer. *J Natl Cancer Inst*. 2001;93:501–515.
23. Jeffery GM, Hickey BE, Hider P. Follow-up strategies for patients treated for nonmetastatic colorectal cancer (Cochrane Review). In: *The Cochrane Library*, 2004, Issue 3. Chichester, UK: John Wiley.

CHAPTER 60
Obstruction and volvulus

Rakesh Bhardwaj[1] and Michael C. Parker[2]

[1]Darent Valley Hospital, Dartford, UK
[2]Fawkham Manor Hospital, Fawkham, UK

ESSENTIAL FACTS ABOUT PATHOGENESIS

- Causes of mechanical obstruction include adhesions and hernias (small bowel), malignant diverticular disease or volvulus (large bowel), and malignancy or Crohn's disease (both sites)
- Mechanical obstruction needs to be distinguished from functional/pseudo-obstruction of neurogenic, pharmacological, and other etiologies

ESSENTIALS OF DIAGNOSIS

- In patients with acute abdominal distension and pain, the goal is to distinguish functional and mechanical obstruction and determine the site and cause of the latter
- Plain radiographs still play an important role in early assessment
- Sigmoid volvulus gives an omega loop sign and cecal volvulus a coffee bean sign on plain abdominal film
- Computed tomography is the most sensitive and specific diagnostic tool
- Contrast enemas may also be needed

ESSENTIALS OF TREATMENT

- In fit patients, significant persistent obstruction due to malignancy, hernia, diverticular disease, and volvulus should be managed by definitive or palliative surgery
- Colonic decompression is sufficient for many cases of sigmoid volvulus, especially in frail patients
- Recurrence is common following surgery for adhesion-related obstruction
- Prophylactic measures versus adhesions (careful handling, diligent hemostasis, keeping the bowel moist, starch-free gloves, laparoscopic approach, etc.) are important
- Management of pseudo-obstruction involves correction of underlying causes, colonoscopic decompression, and neostigmine/pirolostigmine.

Introduction

The management of intra-abdominal bowel obstruction involves differentiation between functional or mechanical obstruction, and in the latter case an accurate determination of the precise level of obstruction in order to facilitate efficient clinical resolution. This chapter focuses on established concepts in the management of pseudo-obstruction, malignant and benign colonic obstruction, small bowel obstruction, and volvulus, with particular reference to surgery. We have deemed it appropriate to include in this second edition some of the recent advances in each of the above categories. This includes:

- **Diagnostic improvements**
- Role of **medical therapies** for functional obstruction
- Recent minimally invasive advances, which include:
  - **Colonic stent use**
  - Increasing role of **laparoscopic strategies**.

We have assumed the reader understands the common etiological factors which induce obstruction and volvulus and some of the material included in this chapter does refocus on established concepts.

Radiological determination of bowel obstruction

Though **plain radiographs** still play a vital role in the early assessment of a patient, the role of **computed tomography** (CT) is well established. This is in part due to protocol optimization, faster scan times, the use of remote technologies, and a general acceptance of the value of this tool in the emergency setting. CT is of particular use to the laparoscopic surgeon as it allows appropriate planning of surgery.

Comparison of CT with plain radiography in the evaluation of small bowel obstruction shows comparable sensitivity, though CT is more specific in determining closed-loop obstruction and may identify a malignant or inflammatory process (Figure 60.1). CT is particularly useful to identify a transition point between proximally dilated and distally collapsed bowel, though this identification can be quite challenging.

The **viability of the small bowel** can be difficult to interpret clinically; **plain radiological signs** include:

- Edematous bowel walls
- Pneumatosis and gas in the portal vein.

Small and Large Bowel

Textbook of Clinical Gastroenterology and Hepatology, Second Edition. Edited by C. J. Hawkey, Jaime Bosch, Joel E. Richter, Guadalupe Garcia-Tsao, Francis K. L. Chan.
© 2012 Blackwell Publishing Ltd. Published 2012 by Blackwell Publishing Ltd.

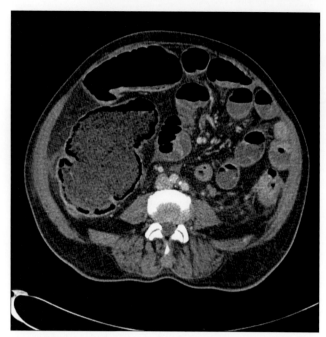

Figure 60.1 CT scan showing an obstructing descending colonic lesion with a proximally dilated cecum. (Courtesy of Mr P. Hanek, Consultant Surgeon, Darent Valley Hospital, Dartford, UK.)

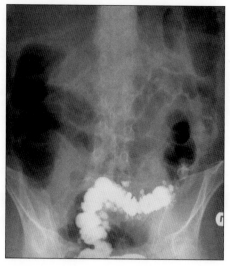

Figure 60.2 "Cut-off" of water-soluble contrast medium with an obstructing sigmoid lesion.

CT signs of ischemia may include:

- Ascites
- Asymmetric enhancement of bowel loops
- Circumferential thickening of the bowel wall
- Pneumatosis intestinalis and hemorrhage into the mesentery.

Colonic obstruction may reveal itself with dilated, gas-filled colonic loops proximal to the obstruction, with diminished or absent gas patterns distally on a plain X-ray. In the presence of a competent ileocecal valve, colonic distension ensues rapidly. However, if the ileocecal valve is incompetent, gas may flow into the small bowel. Cecal diameters of 9–12 cm are traditional measures of impending colonic ischemia and perforation. The site of the point of obstruction may not correlate with the plain radiographic appearance. A **contrast-enhancing enema** is recommended in order to differentiate mechanical from colonic pseudo-obstruction (Ogilvie's syndrome) (Figure 60.2). However in most instances this can be used in conjunction with a CT. In cases where contrast enemas are contraindicated, such as toxic megacolon, CT is of particular benefit. Focal points of mid- and hind-gut **volvulus** can be misinterpreted on a plain radiograph. The "**whirl sign**" (also known as the whirlpool sign) is essential to recognize in cases where midgut volvulus is suspected and plain radiography is unhelpful. It is seen when the bowel rotates around the mesentery, with the mesenteric vessels creating the whirls. It is seen in midgut and cecal volvulus. It represents the swirling appearance of the mesentery and superior mesenteric vein around the superior mesenteric artery.

Though **magnetic resonance imaging (MRI)** has the advantage of providing no radiation exposure to the patient, its role is not widespread in the acute setting. There is no doubt of its sensitivity and specificity, but once again technological advances are awaited. Beall *et al.* reported a correct diagnosis of small and large bowel obstruction with CT in 71% and with MRI in 95% of 44 patients [1]. Causes included fibrous adhesions, malignancy, Crohn's disease, intra-abdominal abscesses, hernias, lymphoma, intussusception, and an anastomotic stricture.

Pseudo-obstruction

Acute colonic pseudo-obstruction, **Ogilvie's syndrome**, refers to marked dilatation of the colon without an identifiable obstructing lesion. The etiology is uncertain; whilst Ogilvie in 1948 proposed that the sympathetic activity of the colon |was interrupted, allowing unopposed sacral parasympathetic innervation, recent work has supported the theory that the condition is due to sympathetic overactivity and/or parasympathetic suppression.

The condition is related to recent surgery, trauma, severe illness or medication. Evaluation in the critically ill patient includes excluding mechanical obstruction and other causes of toxic megacolon, and observing the patient's clinical state for signs of colonic ischemia and perforation. The precise **cecal diameter**, as measured on a plain X-ray or CT, that indicates impending colonic perforation varies amongst patients. Though work by Lowman and Davis in 1956 showed that in 19 surgically treated patients who had cecal perforation or "impending" perforation, cecal diameters were above 9 cm. Vanek and Al-Salti reviewed 400 cases and highlighted that perforation or ischemia was not seen unless the cecum was at least 12 cm [2].

Initial treatment includes correction of underlying causes, metabolic irregularities, and cessation of drugs that decrease colonic motility (narcotics, anticholinergics, and calcium channel antagonists). **Supportive therapy** with nasogastric suction and rectal tubes may be beneficial. **Colonoscopic decompression** is technically challenging, risks perforation, but may be effective; however, recurrence is common, often necessitating repeat endoscopy. Recurrences can be decreased by insertion of a drainage tube into the right colon with endoscopic assistance.

Neostigmine is effective in providing rapid relief of acute colonic pseudo-obstruction. Ponec *et al.* studied 21 patients with a cecal diameter of at least 10 cm and observed rapid colonic decompression in 10 of 11 patients randomly assigned to receive intravenous neostigmine (2.0 mg) and in none of 10 patients who received saline [3].

Chronic intestinal pseudo-obstruction, characterized by long-standing intestinal dilatation and dysmotility without mechanical obstruction, can be diffuse or specific to an isolated segment of gut. It can result from interference at any level of the brain–gut axis; its origins can be classified broadly into neuropathic or myogenic and may be associated with evidence of autonomic neuropathy and generalized smooth muscle dysfunction. A clue to diagnosis may be evidence of multiple laparotomies. **Symptoms** include recurrent abdominal pain, distension, diarrhea, and constipation. Useful modalities that aid diagnosis include **histology and intestinal manometry**. **Treatment** is aimed at limiting symptoms, restoring normal intestinal propulsion, and maintaining adequate nutrition. Though exciting developments are being explored with modulating enteric transmission, small bowel transplantation may be indicated in those dependent on parenteral nutrition and who are refractory to treatment. O'Dea *et al.* examined the role of a cholinesterase inhibitor, **pyridostigmine**, in patients with slow-transit constipation and pseudo-obstruction. Whilst only one of the former showed improvement, all seven of the latter patients included in the study had some improvement with few side effects [4].

Malignant obstruction

Colorectal carcinomas account for the majority of cases of large bowel obstruction with one-third of colonic cancers presenting with obstruction. Approximately half of **splenic flexure tumors** obstruct, as compared with approximately a quarter of left colonic tumors and up to a third of right-sided lesions. However, few **rectosigmoid cancers** present with obstruction. The rapidity of onset of symptoms may reflect the level of obstruction. **Cecal or ascending colonic obstruction** may present with colicky abdominal pain, abdominal distension, and vomiting indicative of small bowel dilatation. In the presence of a competent ileocecal valve, cecal distension may occur rapidly.

With left-sided colonic obstruction, **absolute constipation** may be a predominant feature; pain, colonic distension, and vomiting may be late presenting features. Clinical examination may identify a palpable **abdominal or rectal mass** indicative

of a malignant lesion, and hepatomegaly, which may reflect metastases. An assessment of the patient's co-morbidities is essential to plan intervention. The patient may be too frail initially to undergo operative intervention without adequate resuscitation and physiological optimization. Although a single contrast **water-soluble enema** can demonstrate complete obstruction, **CT** can do this and also demonstrates metastatic spread, which may influence management.

When **surgery** is undertaken the presence of local and distant disease will influence whether the procedure is regarded as curative or palliative, though in some instances resection of the obstructing lesion is an entirely justifiable palliative procedure. For right-sided and transverse colon lesions, a single-stage procedure such as a right or an extended right hemicolectomy is recommended. Usually a **primary anastomosis** is feasible, but analyses of leak rates in anastomoses constructed in the emergency situation (10%) have prompted some authors to suggest in cases where anastomotic healing may be in doubt, that exteriorization of the divided bowel may be suitable. Carcinomas of the **transverse colon** often necessitate resection of part of the greater omentum and those near or at the splenic flexure may prove difficult to remove as mobilization of the splenic flexure is required. If the disease does not permit resection, a palliative bypass may suffice.

The management of **left-sided colonic neoplasms** has evolved. One now aims to provide a tailored solution for each case; this includes the role of established technologies that include colonic stents, the appreciation of staged resectional procedures, and the role of laparoscopic approaches both in the emergency setting and after stabilization of the patient with endoluminal stents (as a bridge to surgery). The formation of a **transverse colostomy** as a primary definitive procedure for a distal localized obstruction can be regarded by the colorectal purist to be suboptimal, though in some instances it is appropriate. A **two-stage procedure**, which is resection and formation of a proximal end colostomy, as described by Hartmann, with closure of the rectal stump or creation of a mucous fistula and subsequent reversal, allows a simple solution. Some patients do not advance to reversal but when this is offered, leak rates seem to be lower if this is left for at least 6 months. The problem with a formal Hartmann's procedure is that the reversal often requires a laparotomy (although laparoscopic proponents are increasingly suggesting a laparoscopic approach should be attempted where feasible). A **side-to-end anastomosis** next to a protecting end colostomy (STEC procedure), proposed by Santulli and Blanc in 1961, has been revisited in the literature with Meijer *et al.*'s report in 10 patients [5] and Fukami *et al.*'s case report [6]. The advantage of this technique is that stomal closure can be performed under local anesthetic.

There are two surgical options if a **single-stage procedure** is undertaken. The first involves an oncological **resection of the tumor**, often with on-table colonic irrigation and primary anastomosis. The second option involves **resection of the entire colon** proximal to the obstructing tumor and creation

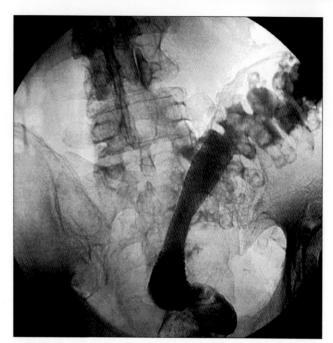

Figure 60.3 Insertion of a self-expanding metal stent to relieve an obstructing sigmoid carcinoma.

of an ileosigmoid or ileorectal anastomosis; this of course has the advantage of removing synchronous tumors. The SCOTIA Study Group conducted a randomized prospective evaluation of single-stage treatment for malignant left-sided colonic obstruction in 91 patients, comparing subtotal colectomy in 47 patients with segmental resection following intraoperative resection in 44 patients [7]. They showed no significant difference in operative mortality, hospital stay, anastomotic leakage or wound sepsis.

Endoluminal stents provide a safe option in those who are initially medically unfit to tolerate an operative procedure as it allows immediate relief of an acute obstructive lesion prior to planned curative resection (bridge to surgery); they are also effective for palliation of advanced colorectal cancer, avoiding a stoma. An ideal colonic stent is one that can be inserted easily transrectally, can negotiate the colonic folds, be comfortably deployed, allow a sufficient channel for fecal material to pass, and remain in position (Figure 60.3).

Khot *et al.* conducted a detailed systematic review of the literature on the use of self-expanding metal stents from 1990 to January 2001 and revealed 58 publications, with analysis of outcomes possible for 29 of these papers [8]. For the 598 subjects selected in this review, the intended treatment for 336 (56%) was palliative and 262 (44%) were treated with the intention of surgical intervention at a later date. In the whole group clinical success was reported in 525 (88%) of cases. Importantly, of those 233 patients selected for surgery and successfully stented, 212 (91%) went on to have a successful **one-stage surgical resection** of the colonic segment. Saida *et al.*, comparing long-term prognosis of emergency surgery in 40 cases against stents as a preoperative "bridge to surgery" in 44 cases,

showed leak rates of 11% versus 3%, and a 5-year survival rate of 44 versus 40% [9]. In the UK, recent **cost analyses** demonstrated that stents save £685 per stented patient.

Two recent reviews have revisited the literature with respect to **stenting in the acute setting.** Trompetas used the PubMed and Cochrane databases and concluded that colonic stenting was the best option either for palliation or a bridge to surgery, with reduced morbidity and mortality rates [10]. Tilney *et al.* focused on a comparison of colonic stenting and open surgery, with 10 studies included and outcomes reported for 451 patients [11]. In their analysis stents proved successful in 226 (92.6%) patients; the hospital stay was shorter for the stent group by approximately 8 days, with lower mortality and fewer complications. Significantly, the "bridge to surgery" did not influence survival.

Improvements in stent and endoscopic technology and assessment of lesion size has also influenced **optimal stent usage.** Cennamo *et al.* suggest the use of a side viewing endoscope to negotiate sharply angulated and very stenotic lesions at the distal sigmoid [12]. Jung *et al.* examined factors associated with successful long-term outcomes and concluded that those with short segment obstruction and more distally located lesions have better long-term results [13]. Lee *et al.* in their non-randomized series of 80 patients compared covered and uncovered stents and concluded that **covered stents** resulted in more late stent migration and loss of function in the long term [14]. Small and Baron compared the **Enteral Wallstent** and the **Precision Colonic Ultraflex** stent in the palliative setting [15]. They suggested that though both relieved obstruction adequately with similar rates of early occlusion and migration, the former stent resulted in a higher rate of delayed complications (perforation, occlusion, migration, and erosion) and re-intervention.

Kim *et al.* compared dual-design stents and concluded that stents with flared ends and bent ends were equally safe and effective, having similar perforation and migration rates [16]. Park *et al.* compared **stent with laparoscopic resection** versus one-stage resection with colonic lavage [17]. They concluded that the operative time was shorter, anastomotic failure lower, return of gut function more rapid, and postoperative hospital stay shorter in the former group. Recent trials have sought to answer some of the questions posed by many of the retrospective non-randomized trials reported over the last two decades. With this in mind, it shall be interesting to await the results of the **Dutch Stent-in-2 study** and the **UK-based CReST trial.**

Lesser invasive strategies can sometimes be of use in rectal tumors but are employed in few centers. These include cryotherapy, electrocoagulation, photodynamic therapy, and ablation with a neodymium-yttrium aluminum garnet (Nd-YAG) laser.

Obstruction from diverticular disease
Obstruction from diverticular disease often occurs as a result of the complications of severe inflammation.

McConnell *et al.* found that women were more likely to present with obstruction; in their series of 934 patients requiring surgical resection for diverticular disease, 61 had obstructive symptoms [18]. Assessment may be made on clinical grounds alone, but usually involves hematological analysis, urinalysis, and plain radiography. A **water-soluble enema** permits identification of complete obstruction, with extravasation of the contrast in cases of perforation, though a CT scan with oral, rectal or intravenous contrast is often required to accurately identify the local inflammatory complications, such as abscesses or fistula formation. **Resection and diversion** is a safe surgical option with obstruction due to diverticulitis, though primary anastomosis with on-table lavage is an alternative where there is minimal contamination of the peritoneal cavity. Laparoscopic approaches with drainage of intra-abdominal abscesses for the inflammatory complications can settle the patient prior to an elective resection.

Small bowel obstruction: adhesions

Fevang *et al.* studied factors that influenced complications and deaths after operations for small bowel obstruction in 877 patients undergoing 975 operations over a 30-year period [19]. **Adhesions** accounted for 526 (54%) procedures; **incarcerated hernias** 293 (30%), and **small bowel volvulus** 30 (3%). **Other causes** included Crohn disease, radiation injury, gallstone, and foreign body obstruction.

Logistic regression analysis showed that **death rate** was increased by:

- Advanced age
- Co-morbidity
- Non-viable strangulation
- Treatment delay of >24 hours.

Parker *et al.* conducted a 10-year follow-up of 12 584 patients who underwent lower abdominal surgery in 1986 [20]. In the study period, 430 abdominal interventions for direct adhesion-related disease were identified, 200 of which were for small bowel obstruction. The authors raised concerns over the cost and manpower-related effort expended on the treatment of adhesions and advocated the use of new **adhesion prevention strategies.**

Volvulus

Volvulus is the torsion of a segment of bowel and mesentry. The reported **incidence** in Western societies ranges from 1.4 to 1.7 per 100 000 persons. Patients may present with **recurrent abdominal pain** and in the emergency situation **severe abdominal pain** with **distension**. The **sigmoid colon** is commonly affected (Figure 60.4), followed in descending order of frequency by the **cecum**, splenic flexure, and transverse colon. Once the colonic segment torts, distension occurs in the obstructed loop with subsequent ischemia, gangrene, and

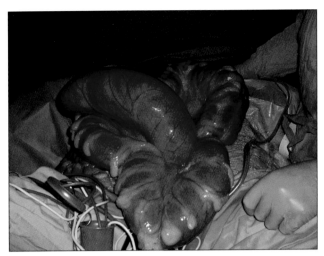

Figure 60.4 Grossly distended sigmoid colon resulting from acute volvulus. (Courtesy of Mr P. J. Webb, Consultant Surgeon, Medway Maritime Hospital, Gillingham, UK.)

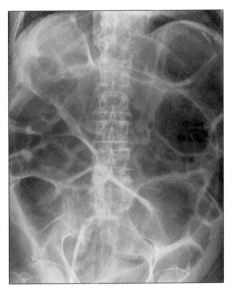

Figure 60.5 Coffee bean sign.

perforation. The diagnosis is often made on clinical grounds with plain radiography, although water-soluble enemas and CT are useful ("**whirl sign**"). With sigmoid volvulus, a loop arising from the left iliac fossa, the "**omega loop**" sign, may be identified on plain abdominal X-ray, and the "**coffee bean**" (Figure 60.5) sign is demonstrable in the right iliac fossa with cecal volvulus. Fluid levels within the obstructed loop and thickened bowel loops may also be noted.

In the case of a non-viable sigmoid colon either a **Hartmann's procedure**, a **Paul Mikulicz** or **primary anastomosis** with on-table colonic lavage is appropriate. Conservative management strategies for sigmoid volvulus with a viable sigmoid colon, such as a drainage tube or colonoscopic decompression, are more suited to elderly patients and those with severe concurrent disease as recurrence rates are high. Even when a delayed surgical procedure is advocated after **initial decompression**, Chung *et al.* reported that of 14 (48%) of 29 patients who refused surgery after endoscopic decompression, 12 (86%) developed **recurrent volvulus** in a median time of 2.8 months [21]. For recurrent sigmoid volvulus in patients unfit for major surgery, percutaneous **endoscopic fixation** of the sigmoid colon has been advocated with good outcomes [22]. Operative detorsion and sigmoid fixation, though simple, has recurrence rates of up to 50%; in order to reduce this, extra-peritonealization of the sigmoid colon is practiced by some; this may also be performed laparoscopically.

Due to the paucity of randomized trials to demonstrate the superiority of a particular operative technique in treating sigmoid volvulus, Kuzu *et al.* reported on **primary resection**, with or without anastomosis in 106 consecutive patients, 57 of whom had primary colonic anastomosis [23]. Of the 57 who had primary anastomoses constructed, dehiscence was observed in four (7%); the mortality in the total group was seven of 106 (6.6%). These results compared favorably with a review of 880 cases from 1952 to 2000 identified by the authors.

Liang *et al.* reported the effective **laparoscopic treatment of a sigmoid volvulus** with a primary anastomosis in 14 patients over a 4-year period with an average operative time of 196 minutes [24]. Cartwright-Terry *et al.* showed similar encouraging results in nine patients over a 6-year period. The median operative time in this series was 115 minutes [25]. Alternatives to sigmoid resection in cases of a non-gangrenous sigmoid colon include **mesosigmoidoplasty**, which aims to reduce the ability of the long and narrow sigmoid mesocolon to rotate around its axis. Bach *et al.* proposed a **modification of the technique** in which instead of just the peritoneal cover being adjusted, all layers of the sigmoid colon were shortened and widened [26]. Ten of 12 patients who underwent this procedure required no further intervention and during a short follow-up of 4–8 months there were no complaints of abdominal pain. Mehendale *et al.* showed in two patients the feasibility of this technique laparoscopically [27].

Colonoscopic treatment of cecal volvulus is not recommended as recurrence rates are high. Cecopexy and cecostomy should be reserved for elderly and frail patients. Cecal resection and anastomosis is the preferred option.

The "**ileosigmoid knot**," first described by Parker in 1845, is a form of sigmoid volvulus in which the ileum wraps itself around the base of the sigmoid and causes a closed loop obstruction of both the ileum and colon. Operative intervention is mandatory as endoscopic attempts to correct the abnormality are usually unsuccessful. Whilst resection of both involved bowel segments is often required, there is some merit in unwrapping of the torted segments if there is viable bowel present. If a segment of small bowel necessitates resection, anastomosis of the ileal ends is safe and the recent trend is to resect the sigmoid colon and to construct a primary anastomosis. Raveenthiran described the successful surgical management of an ileosigmoid knot in seven cases treated over a 6-year period from 1994 [28]. In all cases the sigmoid colon

was gangrenous. After initial deflation of the distended bowel loops, the knot was unraveled in five patients. In all patients a primary ileoileal and/or colocolic anastomosis was constructed, though in one patient an ileocolic anastomosis was necessary as the resected small bowel was close to the ileocecal valve.

Conclusions

Advances in imaging, critical care, endoscopic and laparoscopic strategies continue to enable clinicians to target specific treatments for the treatment of both small and large bowel obstruction. Rapid differentiation between mechanical and functional obstruction is crucial. Operative intervention is not always indicated, but when surgery is necessary a balance between resolution of the underlying disease process and further therapy is required. Stents continue to be used widely and the confidence in laparoscopic approaches ensures optimal therapeutic strategies continue to be employed.

References

1. Beall DP, Fortman BJ, Lawler BC, *et al.* Imaging bowel obstruction: a comparison between fast magnetic resonance imaging and helical computed tomography. *Clin Radiol.* 2002;57:719–724.
2. Vanek VW, Al-Salti M. Acute pseudo-obstruction of the colon (Ogilvie's syndrome). An analysis of 400 cases. *Dis Colon Rectum.* 1986;29:203–210.
3. Ponec RJ, Saunders MD, Kimmey MB. Neostigmine for the treatment of acute colonic pseudo-obstruction. *N Engl J Med.* 1999;15:137–141.
4. O'Dea CJ, Brookes JH, Wattchow DA. The efficacy of treatment of patients with severe constipation or recurrent pseudo-obstruction with pyridostigmine. *Colorectal Dis.* 2010;12:540–548.
5. Meijer WS, Vermeulen J, Gosselink MP. Primary resection and side-to-end anastomosis next to an end-colostomy in the management of acute malignant obstruction of the left bowel: an alternative in selected patients. *Tech Coloproctol.* 2009;13:123–126.
6. Fukami Y, Terasaki M, Sakaguchi K, Murata T, Ohkubo M, Nishi-mae K. Side-to-end anastomosis in a colostomy for acute malignant large-bowel obstruction: side-to-end anastomosis with a colostomy (STEC procedure). *Surg Today.* 2009;39:265–268.
7. The SCOTIA Study Group. Single stage treatment for malignant left sided colonic obstruction: a prospective randomised clinical trial comparing subtotal colectomy with segmental resection following intra-operative irrigation. *Br J Surg.* 1995;82:1622–1627.
8. Khot UP, Lang AW, Murali K, Parker MC. Systematic review of the efficacy and safety of colorectal stents. *Br J Surg.* 2002; 89:1096–1102.
9. Saida Y, Sumiyama Y, Nagao J, *et al.* Long-term prognosis of preoperative "bridge to surgery" expandable metallic stent insertion for obstructive colorectal cancer: comparison with emergency operation. *Dis Colon Rectum.* 2003;46(10Suppl):S44–49.
10. Trompetas V. Emergency management of malignant acute left-sided colonic obstruction. *Ann R Coll Surg Engl.* 2008;90: 181–186.

11. Tilney HS, Lovegrove RE, Purkayastha S, *et al.* Comparison of colonic stenting and open surgery for malignant large bowel obstruction. *Surg Endosc.* 2007;21:225–233.

12. Cennamo V, Fuccio L, Laterza L, *et al.* Side-viewing endoscope for colonic self-expandable metal stenting in patients with malignant colonic obstruction. *Eur J Gastroenterol Hepatol.* 2009;21:585–586.

13. Jung MK, Park SY, Jeon SW, *et al.* Factors associated with the long-term outcome of a self-expandable colon stent used for palliation of malignant colorectal obstruction. *Surg Endosc.* 2009;3:356–359.

14. Lee KM, Shin SJ, Hwang JC, *et al.* Comparison of uncovered stent with covered stent for treatment of malignant colorectal obstruction. *Gastrointest Endosc.* 2007;66:931–936.

15. Small AJ, Baron TH. Comparison of Wallstent and Ultraflex stents for palliation of malignant left-sided colon obstruction: a retrospective, case-matched analysis. *Gastrointest Endosc.* 2008;67:478–488.

16. Kim JH, Song HY, Li YD, *et al.* Dual-design expandable colorectal stent for malignant colorectal obstruction: comparison of flared ends and bent ends. *AJR Am J Roentgenol.* 2009;193:248–254.

17. Park IJ, Choi GS, Kang BM, *et al.* Comparison of one-stage managements of obstructing left-sided colon and rectal cancer: stent-laparoscopic approach vs. intraoperative colonic lavage. *J Gastrointest Surg.* 2009;13:960–965.

18. McConnell EJ, Tessier DJ, Wolff BG. Population-based incidence of complicated diverticular disease of the sigmoid colon based on gender and age. *Dis Colon Rectum.* 2003;46:1110–1114.

19. Fevang BT, Fevang J, Stangeland L, Soreide O, Svanes K, Viste A. Complications and death after surgical treatment of small bowel obstruction: A 35-year institutional experience. *Ann Surg.* 2000;231:529–537.

20. Parker MC, Ellis H, Moran BJ, *et al.* Postoperative adhesions: ten-year follow-up of 12,584 patients undergoing lower abdominal surgery. *Dis Colon Rectum.* 2001;44:822–829.

21. Chung YF, Eu KW, Nyam DC, *et al.* Minimizing recurrence after sigmoid volvulus. *Br J Surg.* 1999;86:231–233.

22. Daniels IR, Lamparelli MJ, Chave H, Simson JN. Recurrent sigmoid volvulus treated by percutaneous endoscopic colostomy. *Br J Surg.* 2000;87:1419.

23. Kuzu MA, Aslar AK, Soran A, *et al.* Emergent resection for acute sigmoid volvulus: results of 106 consecutive cases. *Dis Colon Rectum.* 2002;45:1085–-1090.

24. Liang JT, Lai HS, Lee PH. Elective laparoscopically assisted sigmoidectomy for the sigmoid volvulus. *Surg Endosc.* 2006;20:1772–-1773.

25. Cartwright-Terry T, Phillips S, Greenslade GL, Dixon AR. Laparoscopy in the management of closed loop sigmoid volvulus. *Colorectal Dis.* 2008;10:370–372.

26. Bach O, Rudloff U, Post S. Modification of mesosigmoidoplasty for nongangrenous sigmoid volvulus. *World J Surg.* 2003;27:1329–1332.

27. Mehendale VG, Chaudhari NC, Mulchandani MH. Laparoscopic sigmoidopexy by extraperitonealization of sigmoid colon for sigmoid volvulus: two cases. *Surg Laparosc Endosc Percutan Tech.* 2003;13:283–285.

28. Raveenthiran V. The ileosigmoid knot: new observations and changing trends. *Dis Colon Rectum.* 2001;44:1196–2000.

Small and Large Bowel

CHAPTER 61

Constipation and constipation syndromes

Adil E. Bharucha and Madhusudan Grover

Mayo Clinic, Rochester, MN, USA

ESSENTIAL FACTS ABOUT PATHOGENESIS

- Metabolic disorders (e.g., hypothyroidism), neurological diseases, colonic tumors, and medications are the most common organic causes of chronic constipation
- Maladaptive patterns (e.g., excessive straining during defecation) may predispose to defecatory disorders, which result from inadequate relaxation of pelvic floor muscles (i.e., dyssynergia) or failure to generate adequate propulsive forces during defecation
- There is a marked depletion of colonic nerves and interstitial cells of Cajal in a subset of patients with slow-transit constipation

ESSENTIALS OF DIAGNOSIS

- Exclude secondary causes by clinical assessment, selected blood tests, and lower gastrointestinal endoscopy when indicated
- Defecatory disorders are common and should be considered in every patient with chronic constipation. Anorectal functions and colonic transit should be assessed in patients who do not respond to dietary fiber supplementation and laxatives, and perhaps sooner in patients with clinical features suggestive of pelvic floor dysfunction
- Anorectal manometry and rectal balloon expulsion tests generally suffice for identifying or excluding defecatory disorders. Defecography may be necessary when these test results contradict each other, differ from the clinical impression, or if a rectocele is suspected
- Assessment of colonic motor activity by intraluminal techniques, i.e., manometry and/or a barostat, is available in selected centers and useful in selected patients with chronic constipation, particularly prior to subtotal colectomy

ESSENTIALS OF TREATMENT

- First-line approaches include dietary fiber supplementation, osmotic, and, if necessary, stimulant laxatives
- When increasing dietary fiber content, start with a low amount and increase gradually. Consider an alternative fiber preparation if necessary
- Magnesium salts and polyethylene glycol may be better tolerated in severe constipation than are lactulose and sorbitol. This is because gas production is not an issue
- Stimulant laxatives (e.g., bisacodyl suppositories) should be used as "rescue" agents if there are no bowel movements for 2–3 days. Stimulant laxatives should be synergized with the gastrocolonic response by administering them 30 minutes after meals
- Newer agents should be considered in patients who do not respond to or tolerate first-line approaches
- Pelvic floor retraining by biofeedback therapy is superior to laxatives for defecatory disorders

- After excluding defecatory disorders, a subtotal colectomy should be considered for patients with medically-refractory slow-transit constipation who do not have pelvic floor dysfunction or severe abdominal pain
- In patients with fecal impaction, treatment will fail unless the colon is completely evacuated; monitor with abdominal X-ray if necessary
- If fecal impaction is suspected and digital rectal examination is negative, obtain a simple abdominal X-ray to look for high impaction
- Use gastrografin to assess general colon structure and to assist in colon evacuation; barium is not necessary and could harden with retention in severe constipation
- Recommend a rectocele repair cautiously in constipated women and only when digital compression of the bulge into the vagina greatly improves defecation
- Do not recommend segmental resection of the colon to shorten the bowel or remove loops of colon in constipated patients

FALLACIES AND MISCONCEPTIONS

- Normal bowel frequency is one bowel movement daily
- Chronic constipation with excessive residence time of stools in the colon leads to autointoxication
- A colon that is "too long" (dolichocolon) may cause constipation and should be shortened
- Colonic function normally deteriorates with ageing
- The most common cause of chronic constipation is decreased dietary fiber and fluid intake
- Chronic use of laxatives may lead to dependency, tolerance, and less responsive constipation

Table 61.1 Salient features of normal colonic motor activity

- Colonic motor activity is intermittent, variable and unpredictable, increasing during the day and more so after meals [78]
- Motor activity is comprised of tone (i.e., sustained motor activity) and phasic activity, which includes propagated and nonpropagated contractions [79]. Phasic pressure activity and tone are measured by manometry and a barostat, respectively
- The relationship between colonic motor activity and transit is incompletely understood since only one third of propulsive colonic contents were associated with propagated contractions [80]. High-amplitude propagated contractions (HAPC), which are ≥75 mmHg, occur an average of 5 times per day, especially upon awakening and after meals, and often induce mass migration of colonic contents

Introduction

Chronic constipation is a common symptom, which can impair quality of life [1]. This chapter will deal with "functional" disorders causing chronic constipation, which can be classified in two ways. Specialists generally use an algorithm that relies on assessments of colonic transit and anorectal function to subcharacterize constipated patients into one of the three groups: normal transit constipation, slow transit constipation, and pelvic floor dysfunction [2]. In contrast to this system, the Rome II criteria, which are extensively used in epidemiological studies and therapeutic trials, consider symptoms and anorectal assessments to classify constipated patients as follows: irritable bowel syndrome (IBS), functional constipation (FC), and pelvic floor dysfunction [3,4]. Thus, both classification systems recognize that pelvic floor dysfunction can cause constipation.

Epidemiology

In North America, the prevalence of chronic constipation in the community ranges from 12% to 19% [5], is higher in women (median female to male ratio of 2.2:1), and increases with age in studies that define constipation by self-report [5] but not when defined by symptom criteria [6–8]. Several studies, which have been reviewed elsewhere [5], have consistently identified lower socioeconomic status as a risk factor for chronic constipation. Most individuals with self-reported constipation do not seek healthcare for this symptom. The distribution of constipation subtypes among people with constipation in the community or presenting for primary care is unknown. However, defecatory disorders are common at tertiary centers; in a study of 70 consecutive patients with chronic constipation, 50% had anorectal dysfunctions [9]. Constipated individuals, especially those who also have abdominal pain, have a poorer quality of life [8,10] and work-related productivity [11]. The economic burden associated with constipation is considerable, with an average healthcare cost of approximately $235 million in the United States in 2001 [11].

Pathophysiology
Colonic motor dysfunctions

Table 61.1 highlights the salient features of normal colonic motor activity in humans. Most studies evaluating colonic motor activity in humans have measured phasic pressure activity by manometry but not colonic tone. These studies revealed colonic motor dysfunction – i.e., fewer high amplitude propagated contractions (HAPCs), reduced phasic contractile responses to a meal and pharmacological stimuli (e.g., bisacodyl) – in some patients with slow transit constipation [12–17]. Together, these studies suggest that colonic motor dysfunction causes slow transit constipation. However, this concept is not supported by assessments of colonic tone and phasic pressure activity, which reveal that fasting and/or postprandial colonic tone and/or compliance are reduced not only in 40–50% of patients with slow transit constipation but in a similar proportion of patients normal transit constipation and defecatory disorders [18]. Moreover, these motor assessments reveal patterns of colonic motor disturbances (e.g., increased sigmoid phasic pressure activity with normal fasting and postprandial tone), which may correspond to specific phenotypes in chronic constipation [18] (Figure 61.1). These patterns may provide an alternative approach for classifying chronic constipation.

Some patients with slow transit constipation have impaired contractile responses to bisacodyl or to cholinesterase inhibitors (neostigmine or edrophonium), reflecting more severe colonic motor dysfunction. Colonic inertia is defined by impaired contractile responses to physiological (i.e., a meal) and pharmacological stimuli [19].

While routine colonic histopathological assessments (i.e., hematoxylin/eosin and Masson's trichrome) stains are unremarkable, special stains reveal a marked reduction in the number of nerve fibers and interstitial cells of Cajal (ICCs) in the sigmoid colon in slow transit constipation, and more so in chronic megacolon [20–22]. This loss of ICCs may be of pathophysiological significance since ICCs are required for generating electrical slow waves in smooth muscle and for transducing/amplifying signals between nerves and smooth

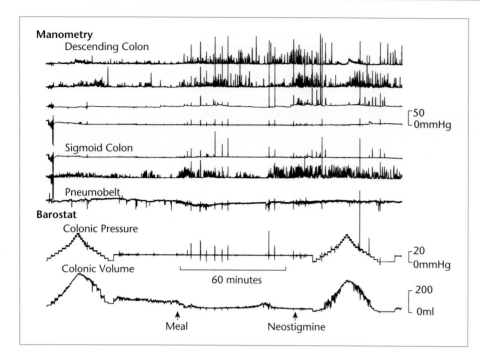

Figure 61.1 Normal fasting, post-prandial and post-neostigmine tonic and phasic colonic motor activity in a patient with slow-transit constipation. Observe reduced balloon volume, reflecting increased colonic tone, after a meal and after neostigmine. Manometry showed increased phasic pressure activity in the sigmoid colon after a meal and also in the descending colon after neostigmine. The principal component analysis revealed a high score for factor 2. (Reproduced with permission from Ravi K, Bharucha AE, Camilleri M, Rhoten D, Bakken T, Zinsmeister AR. Phenotypic variation of colonic motor functions in chronic constipation. *Gastroenterology.* 2010; 138:89–97.)

muscle [23]. The relative importance of loss of nerves versus ICCs needs to be clarified, as does the etiology of nerve/ICC loss. For example, it is unclear to what extent, if any, these findings are attributable to chronic laxative use.

Other studies observed downregulation of progesterone dependent contractile G-proteins and upregulation of inhibitory G-proteins in resected colonic specimens of slow transit constipation, which is intriguing since slow transit constipation is more common in women [24]. However, colonic water absorption is not abnormal in patients with constipation [25].

Defecatory disorders

Normal defecation requires propulsive forces coordinated with relaxation of the puborectalis and the external anal sphincter (Figure 61.2). Defecatory disorders result from inappropriate contraction or inadequate relaxation of pelvic floor muscles (dyssynergia) or failure to generate adequate propulsive forces during defecation [4]. While defecatory disorders have been attributed to maladaptive learning of defecation, perhaps secondary to excessive straining, patients often have other disturbances, including rectal hyposensitivity, rectoceles, perineal laxity (manifested as excessive perineal descent), delayed colonic transit, and colonic motor dysfunctions [18,26,27]. Up to 50% of patients with defecatory disorders have delayed colonic transit [18], which may result from physical obstruction by retained stool, rectocolonic inhibitory reflexes initiated by retained stool, or coexistent colonic motor dysfunction unrelated to pelvic floor dysfunction [28]. Rectal hyposensitivity and delayed transit can improve after biofeedback treatment (Figure 61.3), suggesting that, in some patients, these features are consequences of defecatory disorders [29].

Clinical assessment

The clinical assessment should, in particular, characterize bowel habits to ascertain if constipation is real or perceived, evaluate risk factors for constipation, (e.g., medications, inadequate dietary calorie and fiber intake, and a history of abuse), and identify clinical features of a defecatory disorder. Bowel habits should be documented by bowel diaries and by pictorial representations of stool form, particularly since self-reported stool frequency is unreliable [30]. In contrast to stool frequency, stool form is reasonably correlated with colonic transit [31].

Two or more of the following six symptoms are necessary to diagnose functional constipation by Rome III criteria: infrequent bowel habits, excessive straining, anal digitation, or a sense of anorectal blockage during defecation, a sense of incomplete evacuation after defecation, and hard stools [3]. Some of these symptoms (e.g., anal digitation and the sense of anorectal blockage during defecation) suggest pelvic floor dysfunction, particularly if patients report difficult evacuation not only with hard but also with soft stools.

Symptoms of constipation may begin in childhood. A long-term follow-up study of childhood constipation observed that one third of children followed beyond puberty continued to have severe constipation [32]. Other patients report that symptoms began after an event, e.g., hysterectomy or a fall with sacral injury. However, a case-control study observed a higher incidence of abdominal pain but not constipation after a hysterectomy [33].

In addition to bowel symptoms, patients may have abdominal pain, upper gastrointestinal symptoms, and urogynecological symptoms. The Rome III criteria for IBS require that abdominal pain be associated with two of three features: pain

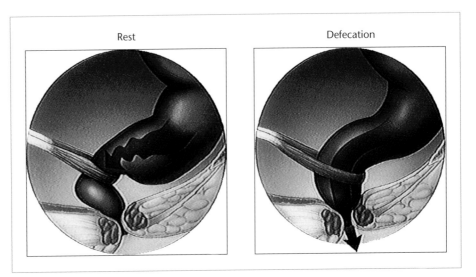

Figure 61.2 Anorectum and puborectalis muscle at rest (left panel) and during defecation (right panel). The puborectalis and anal sphincters relax allowing opening of the anal canal and perineal descent during defecation. (Reproduced from Bharucha AE, Wald A. Anorectal Diseases. In: Yamada *et al.*, editors. *Atlas of Gastroenterology, 4th edn.* Oxford; Hoboken: Wiley-Blackwell; 2009, pp. 491–507, with permission.)

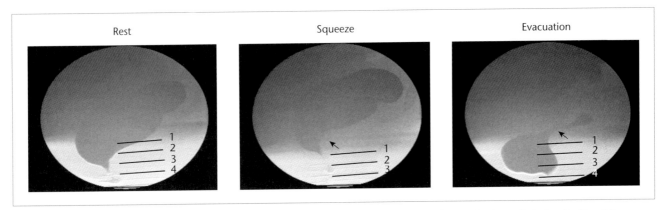

Figure 61.3 Anorectal images at rest, squeeze, and evacuation acquired by barium defecography in a patient with difficult defecation. During squeeze, the puborectalis indentation (black arrow) was more prominent and the anorectal junction was elevated by 2 cm. Perineal motion was measured by markings on the commode at 1 cm intervals. Evacuation was associated with reduced perineal descent (1 cm), paradoxical contraction of the puborectalis, and a rectocele, which retained barium paste. (Reproduced with permission from Bharucha AE. Update of tests of colon and rectal structure and function. *Journal of Clinical Gastroenterology.* 2007; 40:96–103.)

relieved by defecation and/or associated with a change in stool form (e.g., hard stools) and/or associated with a change in stool frequency [3]. In contrast, patients with functional constipation who also have abdominal pain (i.e., painful constipation), lack these associated symptoms [8]. In a community-based study, women with constipation-predominant IBS and painful constipation reported poorer general health, more somatic symptoms, and a greater impact of bowel symptoms on quality of life than women with constipation alone (i.e., painless constipation) [8]. Urogynecological symptoms (irregular menses, nocturia, and hesitancy), and systemic features (malaise) may coexist [34]. Psychosocial disturbances are also common. Patients with transit delays in two or three regions (e.g., stomach, small intestine and colon) were more likely to have low levels of hypochondriasis, and high levels of depression and anger control [35].

Abdominal examination may reveal tenderness to palpation or palpable stool. A careful digital rectal examination is extremely useful for identifying anorectal dysfunction. Patients with defecatory disorders may have anismus (i.e., high anal resting pressure), inadequate perineal descent, or, conversely, excessive perineal descent (i.e., ballooning of the perineum), with or without rectal prolapse. Anal inspection may also reveal fissures.

Chronic megacolon, not due to Hirschsprung disease, generally represents the end stage of slow transit constipation, characterized by persistent colonic dilatation [36]. Patients present with abdominal distention, constipation, or paradoxically even with normal bowel habits.

Differential diagnosis

With the exception of certain metabolic disorders (hypothyroidism, hypo- or hypercalcaemia, diabetes mellitus), most secondary causes (e.g., Parkinson's disease) of constipation will be associated with other clinical features of the underlying condition (Table 61.2). Medications, particularly

Table 61.2 Secondary causes of chronic constipation

Metabolic and endocrine disorders:
- Diabetes mellitus
- Hypothyroidism
- Hypercalcemia, hypokalemia
- Pregnancy
- Porphyria
- Panhypopituitarism
- Pheochromocytoma

Neurogenic disorders
Peripheral
- Hirschsprung disease
- Chagas disease
- Neurofibromatosis
- Ganglioneuromatosis
- Autonomic neuropathy
- Hypoganglionosis
- Intestinal pseudo-obstruction
Central
- Multiple sclerosis
- Spinal cord lesions
- Parkinson's disease
- Shy–Drager syndrome
- Trauma to nervi erigentes
- Cerebrovascular accidents

Collagen vascular and muscle disorders
- Systemic sclerosis
- Amyloidosis
- Dermatomyositis
- Myotonic dystrophy

Table 61.3 Some commonly-used drugs associated with chronic constipation

Analgesics
- Nonsteroidal anti-inflammatory agents

Anticholinergics
- Antispasmodics
- Antidepressants
- Antipsychotics
- Antiparkinsonian drugs (some)

Cation-containing agents
- Iron supplements
- Aluminum (antacids, sucralfate)
- Metallic intoxication (arsenic, lead, mercury)

Other agents
- Opiates
- Antihypertensives
- Vinca alkaloids
- Anticonvulsants
- Calcium channel blockers
- 5-HT$_3$ antagonists

anticholinergic agents and opiates, are common and often overlooked causes of chronic constipation (Table 61.3). Colonic tumors should be considered in patients over 50 years, or those who have relatively acute symptoms, and/or alarm features (e.g., anemia, weight loss, or a history of gastrointestinal bleeding). After excluding these secondary causes, anorectal functions and colonic transit should be evaluated as detailed below.

Diagnostic tests

As a minimum, a complete blood count and, to be complete, serum calcium, fasting glucose, and thyroid stimulating hormone should be assessed. Depending on the patient's age and clinical features, endoscopy, either a flexible sigmoidoscopy or colonoscopy, should be performed. Plain abdominal radiographs may reveal excessive colonic stool and/or dilatation. Then anorectal functions and colonic transit should be evaluated in patients who have not responded to simple measures (e.g., laxatives) as detailed below.

Assessment of colonic transit

Radio-opaque markers, scintigraphy, and the wireless pH-pressure capsule technique provide comparable measurements of colonic transit. With the radio-opaque marker technique, the numbers of markers remaining in the colon are counted on plain X-rays of the abdomen a few days after patients ingest commercially available radiopaque markers (Sitz capsule). One approach is to administer a capsule containing 20 markers on day 1; delayed colonic transit is manifest by 8 or more markers on day 3 or 5 or more markers on day 5 on plain X-rays [37]. Alternatively a capsule containing 24 radio-opaque markers is given on days 1, 2, and 3 and remaining markers seen on a plain abdominal X-ray on days 4 and 7 are counted [38]. With this technique, a total of 68 or fewer markers remaining in the colon is normal while more than 68 markers indicates slow transit. During scintigraphy, a capsule containing radioisotope, typically ^{111}In, is administered orally. Its pH-sensitive delayed-release coating disintegrates at an alkaline pH within the distal ileum, releasing the radioisotope in the ascending colon. Scans taken 24 and 48 hours after administration of the capsule detect the distribution of radioactivity in the colon [39]. While radiopaque markers and scintigraphy entail similar total body radiation exposure [40], colonic transit can be assessed in 48 hours by scintigraphy and in 5–7 days by radiopaque markers. Moreover, scintigraphy can simultaneously assess gastric, small intestinal, and colonic transit.

The wireless pH-pressure capsule technique relies on changes in pH to identify when it is emptied from the stomach to the small intestine and subsequently to the colon and eventually expelled. Colonic transit measured by the capsule and radio-opaque markers is correlated [41]. The capsule can also measure colonic pressure activity [42].

Intraluminal assessments of colonic motility

Perhaps the commonest indication for intraluminal testing is to evaluate colonic motor activity in patients with medically-refractory chronic constipation, usually when surgery (i.e., subtotal colectomy) is being considered [18]. Phasic and tonic activity are recorded by manometric sensors and a barostat respectively. Compared with manometry, a barostat is more sensitive for recording contractions that do not occlude the lumen. A barostat can also record colonic relaxation, sensation, and pressure–volume relationships. These devices are generally positioned in the colon by flexible endoscopy, after cleansing the rectosigmoid and occasionally the entire colon. Findings are discussed in the section on Pathophysiology.

Anorectal functions

Rectal balloon expulsion test: Patients are asked to expel a 4-cm rectal balloon filled with 50 ml of warm water while seated on a commode; usually, this requires less than 1 minute [43]. Alternatively, patients are asked to expel a rectal balloon, connected over a pulley to weights, in the left lateral decubitus position. Patients with pelvic floor dysfunction require more external traction (>200 gm) to expel the balloon. Because the test is simple and highly (>85%) sensitive and specific for diagnosing defecatory disorders, it is an invaluable screening assessment.

Anorectal manometry: Patients with defecatory disorders may have a high anal resting pressure or anismus (i.e., ≥90 mmHg) [44]. The recto-anal pressure gradient (i.e., rectal–anal pressure) during simulated evacuation is also used to identify defecatory disorders [4]. Current concepts suggest that asymptomatic people have a positive gradient. However, the precise techniques to measure and analyze this gradient need to be refined, particularly since our clinical experience and studies suggest that a considerable proportion of asymptomatic people have an abnormal gradient [45]. Consequently, the utility of an abnormal gradient alone to diagnose defecatory disorders is unclear. Except for Hirschprung disease, the recto-anal inhibitory reflex is preserved in chronic constipation. Rectal sensation may also be reduced in chronic constipation and in defecatory disorders [27].

Defecography: Barium or magnetic resonance (MR) defecography is useful in patients with suspected structural abnormalities or to confirm the diagnosis when only one test (either anorectal manometry or rectal balloon expulsion) is abnormal [44]. Defecography can detect structural abnormalities (rectocele, enterocele, rectal prolapse) and assess functional parameters (anorectal angle at rest and during straining, perineal descent, anal diameter, indentation of the puborectalis, amount of rectal and rectocele emptying). The diagnostic value of defecography has been questioned, primarily because normal ranges for quantified measures are inadequately defined, and because some parameters such as the anorectal angle cannot be measured reliably because of variations in rectal contour. Moreover, similar to anorectal manometry, a small fraction of asymptomatic healthy people have features of disordered defecation during proctography. While there is no true gold standard diagnostic test for defecation disorders, an integrated consideration of findings with the clinical features generally suffices to confirm or exclude defecation disorders. Magnetic resonance defecography provides an alternative approach for imaging anorectal motion and rectal evacuation in real time without radiation exposure (Figure 61.4). In a controlled study, MR defecography identified disturbances of evacuation and/or squeeze in 94% of patients with suspected defecation disorders [26].

Management

Simple and inexpensive approaches – including fiber supplementation, osmotic laxatives (e.g., polyethylene glycol, milk of magnesia), timed evacuation with stimulant suppositories – should be tried initially, particularly in primary care [46–48] (Table 61.4). Thereafter, newer agents should be considered. However, this "step-care" approach for managing chronic

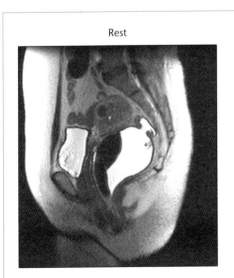
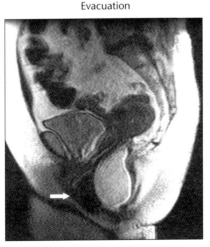

Rest   Evacuation

Figure 61.4 Excessive perineal descent during evacuation associated with a rectocele (white arrow). (Reproduced with permission from Bharucha AE, Fletcher JG, Seide B, Riederer SJ, Zinsmeister AR. Phenotypic variation in functional disorders of defecation. *Gastroenterology*, 2005; 128:1199–1210.)

Small and Large Bowel

Table 61.4 Preferred laxatives for managing constipation

Laxative	Usual adult dose[a]
Bulk-forming laxatives	
Natural (e.g., psyllium)	7–10 g/day
Synthetic (e.g., methylcellulose, polycarbophil)	4–6 g/day
Osmotic laxatives	
Polyethylene glycol	8–25 g/day
Lactulose	15–60 mL/day
Sorbitol (70%)	15–60 mL/day
Saline laxatives:	
magnesium hydroxide	2400 mg (30 mL)
Stimulant laxatives	
Diphenylmethanes	
Bisacodyl	10 mg up to 3 times/week
	10-mg suppository
Secretory agents	
Lubiprostone	8 or 24 µg b.i.d.

[a]Oral except where indicated otherwise.

constipation has not been evaluated in clinical trials since the inclusion criteria for these trials were primarily anchored by symptoms alone, rather than by lack of responsiveness to previous therapy.

Dietary and lifestyle modifications

Many patients with constipation benefit from simple measures, such as eating regular meals including breakfast and not deferring the call to defecate. Patients should be counseled to avoid straining during defecation. Though widely recommended and probably beneficial to overall health, there is little evidence to suggest that increasing fluid intake or exercise improves constipation [49,50]. Gradually increasing dietary fiber supplementation over several weeks is a useful first step, particularly in primary care; many patients will benefit considerably. Alternative agents should be considered for patients who don't tolerate a particular preparation (e.g., psyllium). Patients should be informed that the benefits of a fiber supplement are less pronounced than laxatives. An uncontrolled study of 149 constipated patients treated with plantago for 6 weeks reported a better response in normal transit (85%) than slow transit constipation (20%) or defecatory disorders (37%) [51].

Laxatives

Over-the-counter laxative preparations are generally safe, often effective, and widely used. Among laxatives, the use of polyethylene glycol 3350 (PEG) is backed by considerable evidence, including a 6-month controlled trial; milk of magnesia, sorbitol, and lactulose are other osmotic agents, which are also widely used and probably safe, even for long-term use [52]. Isosmotic PEG-based solutions and sorbitol also accelerate

colonic transit in chronic constipation and health, respectively [53,54]. Among elderly constipated men, a 4-week trial suggested that sorbitol (70% syrup, 15–60 mL daily) was cheaper, better tolerated, and equivalent to lactulose for improving symptoms [55].

Glycerol and bisacodyl suppositories induce colonic HAPCs, generally within 15–30 minutes after administration [56]. Oral bisacodyl takes longer (6–8 hours) to work. Both agents are effective "rescue" agents when patients miss a bowel movement for 2–3 days. To synergize pharmacological therapy with the gastrocolonic response, these suppositories should preferably be administered 15 minutes after a meal. Surface-active agents such as docusates are relatively expensive and of little use as stool softeners in slow-transit constipation. Of the diphenylmethane derivatives, phenolphthalein was withdrawn from the US market after animal studies suggested the compound may be carcinogenic; there is no evidence in humans to support this claim. The **anthraquinones** senna, cascara, sagrada, aloe, and rhubarb are common constituents of herbal and over-the-counter laxatives. These agents are metabolized to active forms by colonic bacteria, may undergo enterohepatic cycling, and can cause melanosis coli, which refers to brownish colonic mucosal pigmentation associated with apoptotic cell death. The incidence of cathartic colon associated with chronic laxative use has declined [57]. The available evidence does not implicate an association between anthraquinones and colorectal carcinoma [58].

Newer agents

Controlled trials demonstrate that three newer agents (**lubiprostone**, **prucalopride**, and **linaclotide**) are effective for treating chronic constipation. While the serotoninergic 5-HT$_4$ partial agonist tegaserod was withdrawn from the market, another 5-HT$_4$-receptor agonist, prucalopride has been approved by the European Medicines Evaluation Agency (EMEA). Lubiprostone, which is an oral bicyclic fatty acid (i.e., a prostone), and linaclotide, which is a first-in-class, 14-aminoacid peptide, stimulate intestinal secretion by activating epithelial type 2 chloride channels (ClC-2) and activating guanylate cyclase-C (GC-C), respectively. Trials of these newer agents were anchored by similar eligibility criteria and endpoints, which were based on complete spontaneous bowel movements (CSBMs). These are defined as bowel movements that were not preceded, within a 24-hour period, by suppositories, enemas, or laxatives (i.e., were spontaneous) and also provided satisfactory relief (i.e., were complete). Patients enrolled in these trials had fewer than three CSBMs weekly at baseline. The primary endpoint was more than three CSBMs per week, except for lubiprostone, where the primary endpoint was spontaneous bowel movements (SBMs) rather than CSBMs. Since there are no head-to-head comparisons of the three newer agents, relative efficacy can only be gauged by comparisons across studies, since inclusion criteria and study design were similar. For the endpoint of CSBMs, the number needed to treat (NNT), based on published articles only, is 3.5

for linaclotide (4 week trial) [59], and 5.3, 7.1, and 8.4 in three trials, all of 12-weeks duration, for prucalopride [60–62]. The lubiprostone studies did not provide data for CSBMs. For SBM reported weekly rather than across all 4 weeks, the NNT was 3.3 for the fourth week of therapy [63]. For polyethylene glycol, the NNT for CSBM responders, defined by improvement for 50% or more of weeks in a 6-month study, was 2.4 [47]. In addition to increasing stool frequency and reducing stool consistency and straining, these agents also improved abdominal discomfort. However, patients enrolled in these trials had relatively mild abdominal discomfort.

Lubiprostone delayed gastric emptying but accelerated small bowel and colonic transit in healthy subjects [64]. There are no published data on its effects on colonic transit in chronic constipation. The FDA-approved dose for chronic constipation is 24 μg orally b.i.d. and for constipation-predominant IBS is 8 μg orally bid [65]. Similar results were observed in subpopulation analyses for gender, race, and elderly patients (≥65 years of age) [66,67]. Nausea, which affects 30% of patients and necessitates stopping treatment in 8.7%, can be reduced by taking lubiprostone with food or by decreasing the dose to 24 μg once daily.

Prucalopride was approved by the EMEA based on three large multicenter studies, which were published recently after issues pertaining to potential carcinogenicity were resolved. Prucalopride also accelerated intestinal and colonic transit in healthy subjects and in constipation-predominant IBS [68].

Linaclotide activates guanylate cyclase-C and increases cyclic guanosine monophosphate (cGMP), thereby inducing signaling pathways that stimulate chloride and bicarbonate secretion through CFTR channel-dependent and, to a lesser extent, channel-independent mechanisms [69]. Linaclotide also inhibits sodium absorption from the lumen via a sodium proton exchanger [70]. Linaclotide accelerated colonic transit in chronic constipation [71].

Biofeedback therapy

Defecatory disorders are managed by pelvic floor retraining using biofeedback therapy. Using feedback provided by activity recorded by instrumentation, either surface electromyography (EMG) or anal manometric sensors, patients are taught to synchronize abdominal wall motion with anal relaxation during defecation. While precise regimens vary across centers, typically 5 or 6 weekly sessions are necessary. An alternative approach is to provide more intensive therapy with two or three sessions daily over 2 weeks. Controlled studies show that pelvic floor retraining was superior to laxatives alone for improving symptoms and anorectal functions in defecatory disorders [72,73]. This improvement was sustained at 12 and 24 months. An abnormal rectal balloon expulsion test predicted the response to biofeedback therapy [29]. Other than an ileostomy or colostomy, therapeutic options for patients who have not responded to laxatives or pelvic floor retraining are limited; the role of sacral nerve stimulation and pelvic floor injection of botulinum toxin, which have been evaluated in small, uncontrolled studies with limited follow-up, is unclear [74,75].

Surgery

Laparoscopic or open colectomy is reserved for patients with medically refractory severe slow transit constipation without a defecatory disorder. Questionnaire-based studies suggest that approximately 80–90% of patients are satisfied after a subtotal colectomy for constipation, provided defecatory disorders are excluded by careful assessment and managed by biofeedback therapy before surgery [76]. Patients who have pelvic floor dysfunction may continue to experience abdominal discomfort, bloating, and difficult evacuation after surgery [76,77]. A subtotal colectomy with an ileorectal anastomosis is preferred; the rectum is also removed when indicated (megarectum). Some patients with refractory pelvic floor disorders may require a colostomy. In patients with upper gastrointestinal symptoms, gastric and small intestinal transit should be assessed before a colostomy.

Acknowledgements

This work was supported in part by USPHS NIH Grant R01 DK78924.

References

1. Talley NJ, Lasch KL, Baum CL. A gap in our understanding: chronic constipation and its comorbid conditions. *Clin Gastroenterol Hepatol* 2009;7:9–19.
2. Lembo A, Camilleri M. Current concepts: Chronic constipation. *N Engl J Med*. 2003;349:1360–1368.
3. Longstreth GF, Thompson WG, Chey WD, Houghton LA, Mearin F, Spiller RC. Functional bowel disorders. *Gastroenterology*. 2006;130:1480–1491.
4. Bharucha AE, Wald A, Enck P, *et al*. Functional anorectal disorders. *Gastroenterology*. 2006;130:1510–1518.
5. Higgins PD, Johanson JF. Epidemiology of constipation in North America: a systematic review. *Am J Gastroenterol*. 2004;99:750–759.
6. Drossman DA, Li Z, Andruzzi E, *et al*. U.S. householder survey of functional gastrointestinal disorders. Prevalence, sociodemography, and health impact. *Digest Dis Sci*. 1993;38:1569–1580.
7. Talley NJ, Fleming KC, Evans JM, *et al*. Constipation in an elderly community: a study of prevalence and potential risk factors. *Am J Gastroenterol*. 1996;91:19–25.
8. Bharucha AE, Locke GR, Zinsmeister AR, *et al*. Differences between painless and painful constipation among community women. *Am J Gastroenterol*. 2006;101:604–612.
9. Surrenti E, Rath DM, Pemberton JH, *et al*. Audit of constipation in a tertiary referral gastroenterology practice. *Am J Gastroenterol*. 1995;90:1471–1475.
10. Chang L, Toner BB, Fukudo S, *et al*. Gender, age, society, culture, and the patient's perspective in the functional gastrointestinal disorders. *Gastroenterology*. 2006;130:1435–1446.
11. Martin BC, Barghout V, Cerulli A. Direct medical costs of constipation in the United States. *Manag Care Interface*. 2006;19:43–49.
12. Bassotti G, Gaburri M. Manometric investigation of high-amplitude propagated contractile activity of the human colon. *Am J Physiol*. 1988;255:G660–G664.

13. Bazzocchi G, Ellis J, Villanueva-Meyer J, et al. Postprandial colonic transit and motor activity in chronic constipation. Gastroenterology. 1990;98:686–693.

14. De Schryver AM, Samsom M, Smout AI. Effects of a meal and bisacodyl on colonic motility in healthy volunteers and patients with slow-transit constipation. Digest Dis Sci. 2003;48:1206–1212.

15. Hagger R, Kumar D, Benson M, et al. Colonic motor activity in slow-transit idiopathic constipation as identified by 24-h pancolonic ambulatory manometry. Neurogastroenterol Motil. 2003;15:515–522.

16. Herve S, Savoye G, Behbahani A, et al. Results of 24-h manometric recording of colonic motor activity with endoluminal instillation of bisacodyl in patients with severe chronic slow transit constipation. [see comment]. Neurogastroenterol Motil. 2004;16:397–402.

17. Rao SS, Sadeghi P, Batterson K, et al. Altered periodic rectal motor activity: a mechanism for slow transit constipation. Neurogastroenterol Motil. 2001;13:591–598.

18. Ravi K, Bharucha AE, Camilleri M, et al. Phenotypic Variation Of Colonic Motor Functions In Chronic Constipation. Gastroenterology. 2010;138:89–97.

19. Bassotti G. If it is inert, why does it move? Neurogastroenterol Motil. 2004;16:395–396.

20. He CL, Burgart L, Wang L, et al. Decreased interstitial cell of cajal volume in patients with slow-transit constipation. Gastroenterology. 2000;118:14–21.

21. Lyford GL, He CL, Soffer E, et al. Pan-colonic decrease in interstitial cells of Cajal in patients with slow transit constipation. [see comment]. Gut. 2002;51:496–501.

22. Wedel T, Spiegler J, Soellner S, et al. Enteric nerves and interstitial cells of Cajal are altered in patients with slow-transit constipation and megacolon. Gastroenterology. 2002;123:1459–1467.

23. Huizinga JD, Zarate N, Farrugia G. Physiology, injury, and recovery of interstitial cells of Cajal: basic and clinical science. Gastroenterology. 2009;137:1548–1556.

24. Xiao ZL, Pricolo V, Biancani P, et al. Role of progesterone signaling in the regulation of G-protein levels in female chronic constipation. Gastroenterology. 2005;128:667–675.

25. Devroede G, Soffie M. Colonic absorption in idiopathic constipation. Gastroenterology. 1973;64:552–561.

26. Bharucha AE, Fletcher JG, Seide B, et al. Phenotypic Variation in Functional Disorders of Defecation. Gastroenterology. 2005;128:1199–1210.

27. Gladman MA, Lunniss PJ, Scott SM, et al. Rectal hyposensitivity. Am J Gastroenterol. 2006;101:1140–1151.

28. Law NM, Bharucha AE, Zinsmeister AR. Rectal and colonic distension elicit viscerovisceral reflexes in humans. Am J Physiol Gastrointest Liver Physiol. 2002;283:G384–G389.

29. Chiarioni G, Salandini L, Whitehead WE. Biofeedback benefits only patients with outlet dysfunction, not patients with isolated slow transit constipation. Gastroenterology. 2005;129:86–97.

30. Ashraf W, Park F, Lof J, et al. An examination of the reliability of reported stool frequency in the diagnosis of idiopathic constipation. Am J Gastroenterol. 1996;91:26–32.

31. Degen LP, Phillips SF. How well does stool form reflect colonic transit? Gut. 1996;39:109–113.

32. van Ginkel R, Reitsma JB, Buller HA, et al. Childhood constipation: longitudinal follow-up beyond puberty. Gastroenterology. 2003;125:357–363.

33. Sperber AD, Morris CB, Greemberg L, et al. Constipation does not develop following elective hysterectomy: a prospective, controlled study. Neurogastroenterol Motil. 2009;21:18–22.

34. Preston DM, Lennard-Jones JE. Severe chronic constipation of young women: 'idiopathic slow transit constipation'. Gut. 1986;27:41–48.

35. Bennett EJ, Evans P, Scott AM, et al. Psychological and sex features of delayed gut transit in functional gastrointestinal disorders. Gut. 2000;46:83–87.

36. Bharucha A, Phillips S. Megacolon: acute, toxic, and chronic. Curr Treat Opt Gastroenterol. 1999;2:517–523.

37. Bouchoucha M, Devroede G, Arhan P, et al. What is the meaning of colorectal transit time measurement? Dis Colon Rectum. 1992;35:773–782.

38. Metcalf AM, Phillips SF, Zinsmeister AR, et al. Simplified assessment of segmental colonic transit. Gastroenterology. 1987;92:40–47.

39. Camilleri M, Zinsmeister AR. Towards a relatively inexpensive, noninvasive, accurate test for colonic motility disorders. Gastroenterology. 1992;103:36–42.

40. Stivland T, Camilleri M, Vassallo M, et al. Scintigraphic measurement of regional gut transit in idiopathic constipation. Gastroenterology. 1991;101:107–115.

41. Rao SS, Kuo B, McCallum RW, et al. Investigation of Colonic and Whole Gut Transit with Wireless Motility Capsule and Radioopaque Markers in Constipation. Clin Gastroenterol Hepatol. 2009;7:537–544.

42. Hasler WL, Saad RJ, Rao SS, et al. Heightened colon motor activity measured by a wireless capsule in patients with constipation: relation to colon transit and IBS. Am J Physiol Gastrointest Liver Physiol. 2009;297:G1107–G1114.

43. Rao SS, Hatfield R, Soffer E, et al. Manometric tests of anorectal function in healthy adults. Am J Gastroenterol. 1999;94:773–783.

44. Bharucha AE. Update of tests of colon and rectal structure and function. J Clin Gastroenterol. 2006;40:96–103.

45. Ravi K, Zinsmeister AR, Bharucha AE. Do Rectoanal Pressures Predict Rectal Balloon Expulsion in Chronic Constipation? Gastroenterology. 2009;136:A–101.

46. Kienzle-Horn S, Vix JM, Schuijt C, et al. Efficacy and safety of bisacodyl in the acute treatment of constipation: a double-blind, randomized, placebo-controlled study. Aliment Pharmacol Ther. 2006;23:1479–1488.

47. Dipalma JA, Cleveland MV, McGowan J, et al. A randomized, multicenter, placebo-controlled trial of polyethylene glycol laxative for chronic treatment of chronic constipation. Am J Gastroenterol. 2007;102:1436–1441.

48. Bijkerk CJ, de Wit NJ, Muris JW, et al. Soluble or insoluble fibre in irritable bowel syndrome in primary care? Randomised placebo controlled trial. BMJ 2009;339:b3154.

49. Meshkinpour H, Selod S, Movahedi H, et al. Effects of regular exercise in management of chronic idiopathic constipation. Dig Dis Sci. 1998;43:2379–2383.

50. Chung BD, Parekh U, Sellin JH. Effect of increased fluid intake on stool output in normal healthy volunteers. J Clin Gastroenterol. 1999;28:29–32.

51. Voderholzer WA, Schatke W, Muhldorfer BE, et al. Clinical response to dietary fiber treatment of chronic constipation. Am J Gastroenterol. 1997;92:95–98.

52. Ramkumar D, Rao SS. Efficacy and safety of traditional medical therapies for chronic constipation: systematic review. [see comment]. Am J Gastroenterol. 2005;100:936–971.

53. Corazziari E, Badiali D, Habib FI, *et al*. Small volume isosmotic polyethylene glycol electrolyte balanced solution (PMF-100) in treatment of chronic nonorganic constipation. *Dig Dis Sci*. 1996; 41:1636–1642.

54. Skoog SM, Bharucha AE, Camilleri M, *et al*. Effects of an osmotically active agent on colonic transit. *Neurogastroenterol Motil*. 2006;18:300–306.

55. Lederle FA, Busch DL, Mattox KM, *et al*. Cost-effective treatment of constipation in the elderly: a randomized double-blind comparison of sorbitol and lactulose. *Am J Med*. 1990;89:597–601.

56. Louvel D, Delvaux M, Staumont G, *et al*. Intracolonic injection of glycerol: a model for abdominal pain in irritable bowel syndrome? *Gastroenterology*. 1996;110:351–361.

57. Joo JS, Ehrenpreis ED, Gonzalez L, *et al*. Alterations in colonic anatomy induced by chronic stimulant laxatives: the cathartic colon revisited. *J Clin Gastroenterol*. 1998;26:283–286.

58. Nusko G, Schneider B, Schneider I, *et al*. Anthranoid laxative use is not a risk factor for colorectal neoplasia: results of a prospective case control study. *Gut*. 2000;46:651–655.

59. Lembo AJ, Kurtz CR, MacDougall JE, *et al*. Efficacy of linaclotide for patients with chronic constipation. *Gastroenterology*. 2010; 138:886–895.

60. Tack J, van Outryve M, Beyens G, *et al*. Prucalopride (Resolor) in the treatment of severe chronic constipation in patients dissatisfied with laxatives. *Gut*. 2009;58:357–365.

61. Quigley EM, Vandeplassche L, Kerstens R, *et al*. Clinical trial: the efficacy, impact on quality of life, and safety and tolerability of prucalopride in severe chronic constipation–a 12-week, randomized, double-blind, placebo-controlled study. *Aliment Pharmacol Ther*. 2009;29:315–328.

62. Camilleri M, Beyens G, Kerstens R, *et al*. Safety assessment of prucalopride in elderly patients with constipation: a double-blind, placebo-controlled study. *Neurogastroenterol Motil*. 2009; 21:1256–e117.

63. Johanson JF, Morton D, Geenen J, *et al*. Multicenter, 4-week, double-blind, randomized, placebo-controlled trial of lubiprostone, a locally-acting type-2 chloride channel activator, in patients with chronic constipation. *Am J Gastroenterol*. 2008;103: 170–177.

64. Camilleri M, Bharucha AE, Ueno R, Burton D, *et al*. Effect of a selective chloride channel activator, lubiprostone, on gastrointestinal transit, gastric sensory, and motor functions in healthy volunteers. *Am J Physiol Gastrointestinal Liver Physiol*. 2006;290: G942–G947.

65. Drossman DA, Chey WD, Johanson JF, *et al*. Clinical trial: lubiprostone in patients with constipation-associated irritable bowel syndrome–results of two randomized, placebo-controlled studies. *Aliment Pharmacol Ther*. 2009;29:329–341.

66. Schey R, Rao S. Lubiprostone for the treatment of adults with constipation and irritable bowel syndrome. *Digestive Dis Sci*. 2011;56:1619–1625.

67. Camilleri M, Beyens G, Kerstens R, *et al*. Safety assessment of prucalopride in elderly patients with constipation: a doublblind, placebo-controlled study. *Neurogastroenterol Motil*. 2009: 21:1256–e117.

68. Camilleri M, Kerstens R, Rykx A, *et al*. A placebo-controlled trial of prucalopride for severe chronic constipation. *N Engl J Med*. 2008;358:2344–2354.

69. Joo NS, London RM, Kim HD, *et al*. Regulation of intestinal Cl- and HCO3-secretion by uroguanylin. *Am J Physiol*. 1998;274: G633–G644.

70. Donowitz M, Cha B, Zachos NC, *et al*. NHERF family and NHE3 regulation. *J Physiol*. 2005;567:3–11.

71. Andresen V, Camilleri M, Busciglio IA, *et al*. Effect of 5 days linaclotide on transit and bowel function in females with constipation-predominant irritable bowel syndrome. *Gastroenterology*. 2007;133:761–768.

72. Chiarioni G, Whitehead WE, Pezza V, *et al*. Biofeedback is superior to laxatives for normal transit constipation due to pelvic floor dyssynergia. *Gastroenterology*. 2006;130:657–664.

73. Rao SS, Seaton K, Miller M, *et al*. Randomized controlled trial of biofeedback, sham feedback, and standard therapy for dyssynergic defecation. *Clin Gastroenterol Hepatol*. 2007;5:331–338.

74. Vitton V, Roman S, Damon H, *et al*. Sacral nerve stimulation and constipation: still a long way to go. *Dis Colon Rectum*. 2009;52:752–753; author reply 753–754.

75. Maria G, Cadeddu F, Brandara F, *et al*. Experience with type A botulinum toxin for treatment of outlet-type constipation. *Am J Gastroenterol*. 2006;101:2570–2575.

76. Nyam DC, Pemberton JH, Ilstrup DM, *et al*. Long-term results of surgery for chronic constipation. *Dis Colon Rectum*. 1997; 40:273–279.

77. Kamm MA, Hawley PR, Lennard-Jones JE. Outcome of colectomy for severe idiopathic constipation. *Gut*. 1988;29:969–973.

78. Hagger R, Kumar D, Benson M, *et al*. Periodic colonic motor activity identified by 24-h pancolonic ambulatory manometry in humans. *Neurogastroenterol Motil*. 2002;14:271–278.

79. Rao SS. Constipation: evaluation and treatment of colonic and anorectal motility disorders. *Gastrointest Endosc Clin N Am*. 2009;19:117–139, vii.

80. Cook IJ, Furukawa Y, Panagopoulos V, *et al*. Relationships between spatial patterns of colonic pressure and individual movements of content. *Am J Physiol Gastrointest Liver Physiol*. 2000;278:G329–G341.

Small and Large Bowel

CHAPTER 62
Irritable bowel syndrome

Robin Spiller
Nottingham Digestive Diseases Centre and NIHR Biomedical Research Unit, University of Nottingham and Nottingham University Hospitals, Nottingham, UK

ESSENTIAL FACTS ABOUT PATHOGENESIS

- Age: peak incidence in 20s and 30s
- Risk factors: female predominance, around half of patients have preceding anxiety or depression, severe adverse life events in the preceding 9 months, or an episode of gastroenteritis
- Early learning environment is as important as genetic influences

---

ESSENTIALS OF DIAGNOSIS

- Symptoms of recurrent abdominal pain and/or discomfort associated with a disturbed bowel habit. Rome III criteria provide more restrictive diagnosis
- Alarm features warrant further investigation, as shown in the alarm features Text Box.

ESSENTIALS OF TREATMENT

- Confident diagnosis and explanation
- Exploration of patient's beliefs and concerns
- Cognitive behavioural therapy
- Hypnosis
- Treatment of anxiety with low-dose tricyclic antidepressants
- Ispaghula husk for constipation
- Loperamide for diarrhea
- Mebeverine and/or low-dose tricyclic antidepressants for pain with mixed bowel pattern
- 5-HT$_4$ receptor agonists may be effective with constipation while 5-HT$_3$ receptor antagonists are effective for IBS patients with diarrhea predominance

---

ROME III DIAGNOSTIC CRITERIA FOR IRRITABLE BOWEL SYNDROME*

Recurrent abdominal pain or discomfort for *3 or more days per month in the last 3 months* associated with two or more of the following:

- Improvement with defecation
- Onset associated with a change in frequency of stool
- Onset associated with a change in form (appearance) of stool

*Criteria fulfilled for the last 3 months with symptom onset 6 months or more prior to diagnosis.

Though not life threatening, these symptoms cause considerable anxiety resulting in frequent healthcare consultations. Recent studies suggest that around 4% of all consultations in primary care are for functional diseases and of these more than half are for IBS [2], whilst IBS patients account for around 40% of the workload in gastroenterology specialist practice. Experienced primary care physicians are quite good at diagnosing IBS without using the Rome Criteria, but by using nongastrointestinal (non-GI) features instead. Factors that predict a diagnosis of IBS in primary care include multiple previous consultations for non-GI symptoms, previous medically unexplained symptoms, and fear of cancer, which was found in 46% of such patients. The other important predictor was a history of symptoms for more than 2 years [2].

Introduction

Irritable bowel syndrome (IBS) is one of the commonest conditions seen in gastroenterological practice. It is characterized by recurrent chronic abdominal pain and discomfort associated with disordered bowel habit. The bowel habit can vary between constipation and diarrhea, often with disordered defecation and associated bloating. This plethora of sometimes contradictory symptoms led to confusion and inconsistency in the literature until an international coordinating committee produced the Rome Criteria. These criteria have been revised and the current version, known as the Rome III criteria [1] has been widely adopted in both surveys and scientific studies.

FACTORS FAVORING A DIAGNOSIS OF IBS VERSUS OTHER DIAGNOSES IN PRIMARY CARE [2]

Doctor's observations
- Polysymptomatic
- Multiple previous consultations for non-GI symptoms
- Previous medically unexplained symptoms
- Symptoms >6 months

Patient's observations
- Fear of cancer
- Stress aggravates
- Dissatisfied with consultation

Textbook of Clinical Gastroenterology and Hepatology, Second Edition. Edited by C. J. Hawkey, Jaime Bosch, Joel E. Richter, Guadalupe Garcia-Tsao, Francis K. L. Chan.

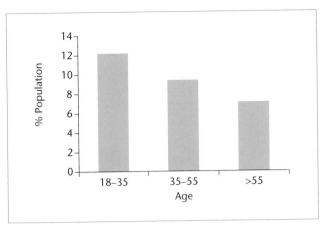

Figure 62.1 Age-related incidence of irritable bowel syndrome (IBS). The proportion of the population reporting IBS symptoms in this telephone survey of over 40 000 Europeans shows a progressive fall from age 18–55 years. (Reproduced with permission from Hungin AP, Whorwell PJ, Tack J, *et al*. The prevalence, patterns and impact of irritable bowel syndrome: an international survey of 40 000 subjects. *Aliment Pharmacol Ther.* 2003;17: 643–650.)

Epidemiology

Both in outpatients and in the general population IBS is one of the commonest disorders. Incidence varies, depending on the precise criteria used. Using the Rome I, II, or III criteria gives an incidence of between 5% and 10%, with a female predominance [3]. Recent large surveys suggest a peak in incidence in the second and third decade of life with a decline thereafter (Figure 62.1) [4]. The condition is found throughout the world in both urban and rural environments and in the tropics as well as in the temperate zones. In the UK, consultation rates are around 14 per thousand person years for females and 4 per thousand for males. This equates to more than 850 000 consultations per annum, an average of 1.6 contacts per year. The total number of visits by IBS patients to primary care clinics was around double this when non-GI consultations were included. Indeed, it is characteristic of IBS patients that they consult more for non-GI symptoms than non-IBS patients. Recent studies in the USA suggest IBS patients visit their primary care physician more often than non-IBS sufferers, 4.2 versus 1.3 times per year, and take more days off work, 6.4 versus 3.0 days per annum [5].

Healthcare burden

The estimated direct and indirect costs of IBS to the US employer in 1998 was $4527 compared with $3276 for a non-IBS employee. Although IBS management is relatively cheap owing to a lack of effective drugs, the ensuing time off work ensures that the indirect costs are high and absenteeism costs were $901 versus $528 for non -IBS employees [6]. Quality of life assessments such as the SF36 indicate that IBS sufferers have considerable impairment in quality of life, both in physical and emotional zones. Indeed, the impairment in social and emotional functioning was comparable with depression (not surprising considering the frequent overlap between the two syndromes), while the impairment in physical function was on average worse than in both diabetes and hypertension.

Predictors of healthcare utilization

The determinants of consultation for IBS have been extensively studied. Health anxiety, female sex, and physical and sexual abuse in childhood increase the risks of consultation. Increasing age also increases the probability of consultation for IBS, as it does for other symptoms. Ethnicity also plays a role and, in the United States, whites are more likely than blacks to seek care. Cultural factors are important: in the Asian subcontinent, in some communities, men are more likely to seek care than women. The factors listed above are, however, less important than the perceived severity of symptoms which is, in most studies, the strongest predictor of healthcare seeking. Studies in tropical countries have shown a prevalence of IBS similar to that in the West, though the relative frequency of diarrhea and constipation varies from country to country.

Causes and risk factors

Since the condition is quite heterogeneous, it is no surprise to learn that there is no single cause. The condition appears to be determined by both central brain and peripheral gut factors. Central factors include personality, early-life environment, and anxiety while peripheral factors include both visceral hypersensitivity and abnormal motility. Incidence studies show annual incidence of around 2% to 4 % [7,8] with females outnumbering males 3:2. Onset of symptoms can be gradual or may be precipitated by an adverse life event such as divorce, bereavement, or being made redundant [9]. It can also follow an acute infectious gastroenteritis [10] and war trauma. Anxiety, depression, and somatization are commoner in patients attending outpatient clinics with IBS compared with normal controls, but the difference is much less when IBS sufferers who are not patients are studied in the community. There are several prospective studies looking at risk factors for developing IBS in the general population. One estimate comes from the General Practice Research Database (GPRD) in the UK, which is a prospective survey of over 580 000 British primary care records. The annual incidence of new diagnoses of IBS in this unselected population is around 0.4%, with female sex and a history of bacterial food poisoning being the strongest predictors of developing IBS during the next year [8]. The Leeds *Helicobacter pylori* eradication trial followed individuals for 10 years and showed that factors predicting the development of IBS were, in order of importance, lower quality of life at baseline, odds ratio (OR) 4.41; 2.92–6.65, female gender (OR 2.14; 1.56–2.94), and dyspepsia at baseline (OR 1.77; 1.28–2.46 [11]. A study over a shorter period suggested that high levels of medial consultation, anxiety, sleep problems, and somatic symptoms also increased the risk of developing IBS between 2- and 5-fold [12].

Non-GI symptoms that are commonly associated with IBS are helpful in making the diagnosis. These include headache, neck pain, palpitations, sleep disturbance, backache, and lethargy [13]. A substantial proportion of people with fibromyalgia also suffer from IBS as do those with functional dyspepsia,

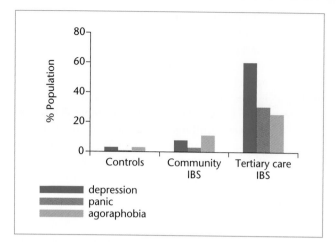

Figure 62.2 Incidence of lifetime psychiatric diagnosis in irritable bowel syndrome (IBS). Percentage of patients with a lifetime diagnosis of depression, panic, and agoraphobia, showing that while IBS patients in the community have a modest increase in psychiatric diagnosis, those in tertiary care have a much more substantial increase with nearly 60% experiencing a lifetime diagnosis of depression. (Reproduced with permission from Walker EA *et al*. The relationship of current psychiatric disorder to functional disability and distress in patients with inflammatory bowel disease. *Gen Hosp Psychiat*. 1996;18:220–229.)

those with coexisting IBS having more severe dyspeptic symptoms [14].

Pathogenesis

The three key factors are psychological abnormalities (including anxiety, depression and somatization), abnormal gut motility, and visceral hypersensitivity, which are each abnormal in about one third of cases [15]. As already discussed, psychosocial stressors associated with poor quality of life, severe adverse life events, or infectious gastroenteritis are known risk factors that may be followed by abnormalities of sensation and motor function.

Anxiety, depression, and somatization

There is an increasing excess of anxious and hypochondriacal individuals in the IBS populations as one moves up the referral pyramid, from the community setting through primary care to secondary and even tertiary care. The proportion of patients with an overt psychiatric diagnosis peaks in tertiary care, with a lifetime incidence of a psychiatric diagnosis as high as 60% compared with 2% in community samples of IBS and 1% of normal controls (Figure 62.2) [16]. An enrichment of anxious patients in secondary care is guaranteed by the referral process. Those that are not reassured in primary care are likely to insist on referral to secondary care, thereby increasing the proportion of anxious individuals.

Many psychological characteristics are heavily influenced by childhood experiences. Abuse of either a sexual or physical nature is commoner in a range of painful conditions like IBS or fibromyalgia, and animal experiments suggest that emotional trauma in early life can induce long-lasting visceral hypersensitivity [17].

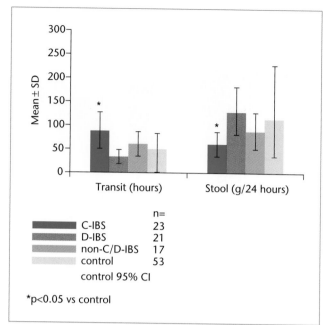

Figure 62.3 Whole gut transit and stool weight in subtypes of IBS. Graph shows that patients with constipation-predominant IBS (C-IBS) have longer transit and smaller stool weights than those with diarrhea-predominant IBS (D-IBS); even in normal subjects there is considerable variability drawn. (Reproduced from Cann PA *et al*. Irritable bowel syndrome: relationship of disorders in the transit of a single solid meal to symptom patterns. *Gut*. 1983;24:405–411, with permission from BMJ Publishing Group Ltd.)

Disordered motility

Bowel habits in the normal population vary widely, with gender, diet, and exercise all playing a part. Patients with IBS who have predominant diarrhea have transit times that are at the lower limit of normal, while those complaining of constipation tend to have transit time at the upper limit of normal (Figure 62.3) The stool weights tend to be inversely proportional to transit time but in both cases the IBS values lie within the normal range. Variability in bowel habit, both frequency and consistency, is however greater in IBS and around 50% of patients describe both hard and soft stools, which may occur on the same day. Though not part of the definition, many subjects experience exacerbation of pain and urgent bowel movements after eating. This gastrocolonic response to feeding is part of normal physiology but can be exaggerated in IBS. Some studies have shown enhanced response to a range of stimulants including cholecystokinin (CCK) as well as the stress hormone corticotrophin releasing factor (CRF), with excessive propulsive activity.

Previous studies of intestinal motility in IBS using ambulatory manometry have shown small differences with increased frequency of contractions but such techniques are highly invasive and poorly tolerated by patients. More recently, using noninvasive magnetic resonance imaging (MRI) we have been able to show decreased volume of small bowel contents with accelerated transit, a feature which correlates well with anxiety levels (Figure 62.4) [18].

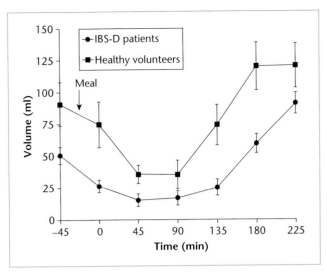

Figure 62.4 Decreased small bowel water content in irritable bowel syndrome (IBS). Small bowel water content as measured by magnetic resonance imaging (MRI) shows reduced fasting and postprandial levels in diarrhea-predominant IBS (IBS-D) patients compared with healthy controls. This was associated with reduced small bowel transit time, which correlated negatively with anxiety score on the Hospital Anxiety and Depression Scale. (Reproduced with permission from Marciani L, Cox EF, Hoad CL, *et al.* Postprandial changes in small bowel water content in health and irritable bowel syndrome. *Phys Med Biol.* 2007;52:6909–6922.)

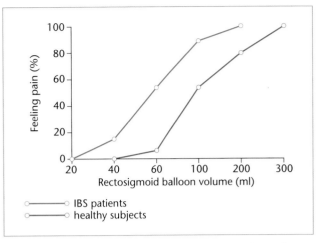

Figure 62.5 Increased sensitivity to rectal distention in irritable bowel syndrome (IBS) versus controls. The volume of the rectal sigmoid balloon needed to induce a sensation of pain was decreased in IBS patients compared with controls. (Reproduced from Ritchie J. Pain from distension of the pelvic colon by inflating a balloon in the irritable colon syndrome. *Gut.* 1973;14:125–132, with permission from BMJ Publishing Group Ltd.)

One of the normal functions of GI motor patterns is to rapidly expel swallowed air and gas derived from colonic fermentation of food residues. While the normal gut can deal with an infusion of gas of up to 30 mL/min without excessive distention, IBS patients retain more gas and experience more distention, even when an infusion rate of just 12 mL/min is used [12].

Patients with IBS often complain of bloating. This means different things to different patients. It is important to distinguish visible distension with the need to loosen clothing, which is much commoner in patients with underlying constipation, from a sensation of bloating without actual distension, which is more a reflection of visceral hypersensitivity [19]. The fact that bloating can come on so rapidly after a trigger such as eating was mysterious until imaging studies showed abdominal protuberance is induced by lowering the diaphragm and relaxing the abdominal walls [20]. This acute response may be a reflex that reduces pain but appears to be involuntary.

Visceral hypersensitivity

It is a common experience that performing a colonoscopy with air insufflation often causes excessive pain and discomfort in a patient with IBS compared with other patients. This has been formalized using a balloon placed in the rectum and distended to fixed pressures. With such a technique, IBS patients demonstrate greater pain at lower pressures and volumes (Figure 62.5). They also report an abnormally extensive somatic referral, with pain felt not only in the anal region where normal

subjects experience it, but also in the abdomen [21]. Thus, normal cutaneous stimuli induced by contact of clothes are interpreted as painful and patients often feel the need to wear lose clothing. This phenomenon, allodynia, is typical of hypersensitivity induced by inflammation or chronic stimulation of spinal pain pathways and reflects neural plasticity whereby chronic stimulation of visceral nociceptive C fibers facilitates neurotransmission in adjoining nerves from somatic tissue. More recent studies have suggested that this feature is not universal and only perhaps one third are truly hypersensitive [15].

Cerebral influences are also important. Visceral hypersensitivity in some patients is due to anticipation of discomfort and even sham distentions can induce the perception of pain. Even those IBS patients who do not initially show hypersensitivity can be induced to show it by repetitive painful distention of the sigmoid colon. Whereas under these circumstances normal volunteers show a degree of habituation, IBS patients show a fall in threshold or "wind up." Brain imaging using functional MRI and positron emission tomography (PET) scanning has shown increased activation of the anterior cingulate and impaired activation of brainstem nuclei in IBS (Figure 62.6). These changes are noted both during actual and sham distentions and represent an anticipation of discomfort [22]. Much of the change seen in the arousal network, including the amygdala and anterior cingulated cortex habituate and the visceral hypersensitivity, is less apparent if the tests are repeated four times over a 12-month period even though symptoms remain unaltered. This suggests that IBS patients cope less well with the stress of the experimental procedure than healthy controls [23]. Recent evidence shows that IBS patients show fewer preparatory deactivations particularly in the brain stem, which normal subjects show when anticipating a painful stimulus

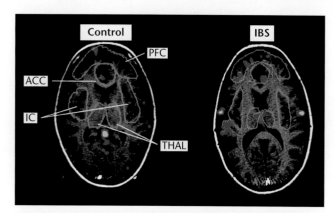

Figure 62.6 Abnormal central processing of visceral stimuli in irritable bowel syndrome (IBS). These functional magnetic resonance (fMRI) images show increased cerebral blood flow in IBS patients during rectal distention compared with controls. This increase was particularly noted in the anterior cingulate cortex (ACC), thalamus (THAL), prefrontal cortex (PFC), and insular cortex (IC). The anterior cingulate is the area of the brain activated by anticipation of pain and some activation can be seen equally during true or sham distentions. (Reproduced from *Gastroenterology*, Prather CM *et al.* Tegaserod accelerates orocecal transit in patients with constipation-predominant irritable bowel syndrome, 2000;118:463–468, with permission from the American Gastroenterological Association.)

[24]. This supports the idea that IBS patients have defective diffuse noxious inhibitory control (DNIC). This describes the inhibitory descending neural activity originating in the mid brain, which inhibits transmission of ascending afferent activity in response to painful peripheral stimuli. These descending anti-nociceptive pathways include both serotonergic and noradrenergic nerves whose activities are decreased in depression. This may partially explain why antidepressants are among the most effective treatments for IBS even in the absence of overt depression. Some of their benefit may be by enhancing these anti-nociceptive pathways.

Pathology

Conventional radiology and microscopy in IBS is normal. However, several studies have indicated subtle abnormalities in motor patterns, transit, and mucosal histology. Those in whom IBS develops after infection have been shown to have increased numbers of lymphocytes and enteroendocrine cells. Others have similarly shown increases not only in lymphocyte numbers but also in cytokine mRNA indicating ongoing low-grade inflammation (for review see Garsed 2009 [10]). Recent surveys indicate that between 6% and 17% of cases arise in such a way [25]. The importance of low-grade inflammation in other types of IBS is as yet unclear but visceral sensitization can be readily induced in laboratory animals by inflammation of both biological and chemical nature. More recently the importance of the mast cell is being recognized. Animal studies indicate that chronic stress increases mast cell numbers [26], while human studies suggest increased mast cell numbers close to afferent enteric nerves correlate with pain severity in

IBS [27]. The same group also showed an increased release of histamine and other mediators from colonic mucosal biopsies of IBS patients, which activate afferent nerves and could cause pain [28]. Several small studies have suggested that agents which reduce mast cell numbers – mesalmine (mesalazine) – or which stabilize them – cromolyn (cromoglycic acid) can improve symptoms but these findings need repeating in larger randomized placebo controlled trials (RCTs).

Food intolerance

Some patients experience symptoms only when they eat certain foods, and they can avoid these by elimination diets. The best example is lactose intolerance found in 1 in 10 of the Caucasian population but as many as 90% of Orientals. Most patients learn to associate milk ingestion with symptoms; hence, they avoid milk and do not present with IBS. However, there is a small subgroup that does not recognize their lactose intolerance and may benefit from being put on a restricted lactose intake. Another common dietary intolerance is that for wheat, which is a substantial part of the western diet. Around 15% of wheat starch is malabsorbed and therefore enters the colon where it is fermented to various products depending on the precise bacterial flora. Random controlled trials of bran have shown this increases flatulence and in clinical practice restricting wheat may alleviate bloating and flatulence. While food intolerances causing urticaria or asthma are clearly due to mast-cell activation, in the absence of such manifestation an allergic basis for food intolerances seems unlikely in most case of IBS.

Clinical presentation

The commonest reason for consultation is abdominal pain, which is typically described as severe, often colicky, exacerbated by eating, and relieved by defecation. The release by defecation is variable and not always consistent. The pain is typically central or lower abdominal and bilateral. It is generally indicated by a circular movement of the outstretched hand and not precisely localized. Radiation to the back and perianal region is not uncommon. The pain is typically episodic with bouts lasting between 2 and 5 days followed by some days with freedom before symptoms return. The bowel habit varies and in most series around half alternate between diarrhea and constipation, often on the same day. The remainder are either predominantly constipated or have predominantly diarrhea. During a constipated phase patients pass small hard stools, often straining with some difficulty. They may also notice mucus with the stool. Loose stools are often associated with urgency and even incontinence. Patients with a mixed habit may pass solid stool first thing in the morning and then pass increasingly liquid stool over the next few hours. This pattern is probably an exaggeration of the normal reflex emptying of the colon after overnight quiescence with sequential emptying of rectal, sigmoid, descending, transverse, and finally ascending colon contents causing the progression from formed to loose stool. Other patients may describe days of diarrhea followed by days of constipation.

Non-gastrointestinal symptoms

Patients with IBS typically suffer from many other medically unexplained conditions including chronic backache, headache, and fibromyalgia and, in some, irritable bladder. Common features include sleep disturbance, health anxiety, somatization, and often lack of a close personal contact with whom to share anxieties and concerns. The presence of multiple somatic complaints, medically unexplained is typical and should make the diagnosis more secure.

Differential diagnosis

The differential diagnosis of abdominal pain and constipation is limited once intestinal obstruction is excluded. By contrast abdominal pain and diarrhea has many causes.

DIFFERENTIAL DIAGNOSIS OF ABDOMINAL PAIN AND DIARRHEA

- Crohn's disease
- Microscopic colitis
- Hypolactasia
- Celiac disease
- Tropical sprue
- Small bowel contamination
- Giardiasis
- Bile salt malabsorption
- Radiation enteritis
- Colonic cancer
- Diverticular disease

Apart from Crohn's disease, most of the conditions that present with abdominal pain and diarrhea are for the most part associated with only mild discomfort often relieved by defecation. However, they can all be mistaken for IBS. Since the incidence of colonic cancer and diverticular disease rises steeply after age 50 years, most guidelines suggest that when new symptoms develop after this age the colon should be imaged.

A diagnosis can be made with some security providing the Rome criteria are satisfied in the absence of alarm symptoms (see Text Box), a set of criteria with high specificity but only modest sensitivity so that around one third of patients ultimately diagnosed as IBS fail to meet these criteria (Figure 62.7) [14]. The diagnosis is made more secure by a history of more than 2 years. A normal blood count also increases the reliability of the diagnosis. Associated features that support the diagnosis include bloating, sense of incomplete evacuation, passage of mucous per rectum, and/or straining at stool. Other factors that may be helpful include previous multiple presentations with medically unexplained conditions, somatization, and failure of reassurance by primary care practitioners.

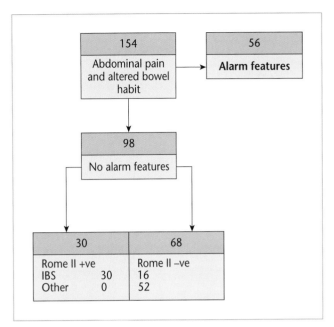

Figure 62.7 Diagnostic value of Rome II criteria. 154 patients with possible irritable bowel syndrome (IBS) were studied, of whom 56 were excluded because of alarm features. Of the 98 with no alarm features who met the Rome II criteria, all 30 were finally diagnosed with IBS after full evaluation. A further 16 out of the remaining 68 patients were diagnosed as IBS after full evaluation, giving the Rome II criteria in the absence of alarm features, a modest sensitivity of just 65% but high specificity of 100%. (Reprinted by permission from Macmillan Publishers Ltd: Vanner *et al.* Predictive value of the rome criteria for diagnosing the irritable bowel syndrome. *Am J Gastroenterol.* 1999;94:2912–2917.)

ALARM FEATURES [3,29]

Symptoms warranting further investigation:
- Documented weight loss
- Nocturnal symptoms
- Family history of colon cancer
- Blood mixed with the stool
- Recent antibiotic use
- Relevant abnormalities on physical examination
- Age >50 years
- Short history of symptoms
- Male sex

Diagnostic methods

In primary care, provided the Rome criteria are met in the absence of alarm features, the diagnosis is reasonably secure on clinical grounds since the *a priori* probabilities strongly favor IBS. However, in secondary care, patients will have been referred because of some diagnostic uncertainty, which may alter the probabilities, particularly in those with diarrhea. For these patients, some useful screening tests are indicated.

Positive results in these screening tests are in practice rare (usually <5%) but are probably cost effective, since for some (e.g., celiac patients) this will lead to a lifelong cure. In subjects over the age of 50 years with a short history, imaging of the

---

SCREENING TESTS FOR PATIENTS WITH DIARRHEA-PREDOMINANT IBS

1. Hematology
   Hemoglobin
   Mean red cell volume (MCV)
   Erythrocyte sedimentation rate (ESR)
   Serum vitamin B$_{12}$, red cell folate
   Ferritin
2. Biochemistry
   Calcium & albumin
   Liver function tests
   Thyroid function
3. Immunology
   Endomysial antibodies
   C reactive protein (CRP)
4. Stool examination
   Microscopy – ova cysts, parasites and fat globules
   Calprotectin

---

colon should be carried out to avoid mistaking colon cancer for IBS though this is actually extremely uncommon. This age cut-off may be altered if there is a family history of colon cancer, particularly at an early age, in which case, screening colonoscopy is probably warranted even without symptoms. Anxiety and depression can be assessed by means of the Hospital Anxiety and Depression Scale [15], while multiple somatic symptoms are easily assessed using the Personal Health Questionnaire (PHQ15) [30]. High scores should lead to consideration of psychological treatments.

Treatment and prevention

Treatments can be considered under the following headings: dietary, psychological, and pharmacological.

Dietary treatment

Identification of lactose intolerance and adoption of a low-lactose diet can be effective treatment, although this has been somewhat disappointing in the UK, probably because most patients in whom lactose intolerance is the cause of their symptoms will have recognized this and will not consult a doctor. Furthermore, many IBS patients do not take enough lactose to induce symptoms and hence restricting lactose intake produces no benefit. A variety of other exclusion diets have been described. The principle is to exclude common dietary offenders such as wheat, dairy products, citrus fruits, chocolate, nuts, and onions. If symptoms resolve then each food item can be added back to the diet and over a number of months the culprit responsible for symptoms can be identified and excluded. This can be successful in some leading to sustained (>12 months) improvements in over half the patients who agree to take part in such studies [30]. Unfortunately, unless adequately supervised this can lead to nutritionally inadequate diets, as some patients exclude progressively more and more items in a vain attempt to limit symptoms. Other

diets have been described which specifically exclude sources of poorly absorbed fermentable polysaccharide. These diets have been shown to not only reduce 24-hour H$_2$ and CH$_4$ production, but also to alter the fermentation profile of colonic organisms [32]. More recently diets reducing fermentable oligosaccharides (such as fructans, raffinose, inulin), disaccharides (lactose), monosaccharides (fructose), and polyhydric alcohols (sorbitol; FODMAPs) have been reported to be of benefit, mainly by reducing osmotically active poorly absorbed sugars from fruit and wheat such as fructose and sorbitol whose intake has recently increased in the western diet [33].

Psychological treatment

Since anxiety and depression are common associated features, treatment of these may be warranted on their own merits. Where excessive anxiety exists, treatment of this may result in resolution of bowel symptoms.

A range of psychological treatments has been shown to be of benefit including psychotherapy, cognitive behavioral therapy, hypnotherapy, and relaxation therapy but many of the trials are methodologically suspect [18]. Controlled trials are difficult since the placebo effect of any therapy in IBS is high, and adequate controls for psychological therapy are difficult to devise. Controlled trials of both behavioral and relaxation therapy showed symptoms improved after both but this was equal in both treatment and placebo groups [19]. By contrast both psychotherapy [20] and hypnotherapy [21] have been shown in large placebo-controlled trials to produce long lasting benefit in otherwise resistant patients. Hypnotherapy has a particular advantage in that patients can be taught to self administer treatment, which can be used indefinitely at no additional cost.

Pharmacological treatment
Anxiolytics and antidepressants

Patients with IBS are typically rather intolerant of drugs and may require very small doses of antidepressants. Therefore, while the full therapeutic dose of amitriptyline is 150 mg at night, IBS patients may typically manage on as little as 10–25 mg. Amitriptyline has a number of advantages over more selective serotonin reuptake inhibitors (SSRIs) in that it also has antihistaminic effects, which give it a mild sedative effect. This is particularly helpful for agitation and insomnia, which is common in IBS of all types and undoubtedly contributes to the lethargy and fatigue frequently associated with IBS. A recent meta-analysis of a range of different tricyclics [22] suggested that the number needed to treat (NNT) to achieve one responder over and above that achieved by placebo was 3.2. This is comparable to the NNT for common treatments for allergic rhinitis, migraine, or hypertension.

Antispasmodics

Although many trials of antispasmodics have been of inadequate power and design meta-analysis and clinical experience suggest there may be a small benefit, the NNT being 4.5. The

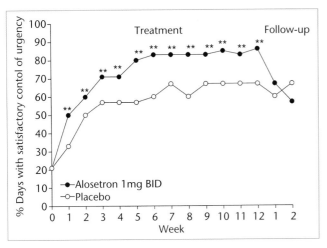

Figure 62.8 Alosetron reduced urgency in 801 female IBS patients with diarrhea. Note rapid onset and relapse on discontinuation. (Reproduced from Lembo *et al. Am J Gastroenterol.* 2001;96:2662–2670 by kind permission of the editors.)

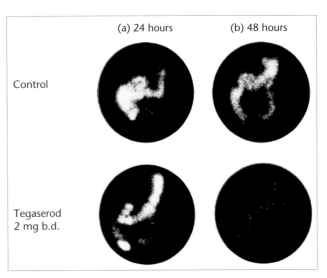

Figure 62.9 The effect of a 5-HT$_4$ agonist on colonic transit. At 24 hours, isotope in the tegaserod-treated patient is filling the transverse colon (a), while at 48 hours it has virtually all been expelled (b). In contrast, in the control conditions at 48 hours, the isotope is seen outlining the entire colon, thus showing the accelerating effect of tegaserod on colonic transit. (Reproduced from *Gastroenterology*, Prather CM *et al.* Tegaserod accelerates orocecal transit in patients with constipation-predominant irritable bowel syndrome, 2000;118:463–468, with permission from the American Gastroenterological Association.)

commonest one prescribed in the United Kingdom is mebeverine, which has the merit of being extremely safe and cheap. It is a smooth muscle relaxant that can reduce the muscular contractions [23] that may underlie symptoms in some IBS patients.

Opiates

Opiates act as analgesics by stimulating central descending anti-nociceptive pathways and also inhibiting pain pathways at the level of the spinal cord. They also inhibit intestinal secretions and propulsive motor patterns and improve diarrheal symptoms. Codeine is a highly effective antidiarrheal agent but poorly tolerated because of central effects such as nausea and sedation. Loperamide is a μ-opioid receptor agonist that does not cross the blood-brain barrier and is hence largely free of CNS side effects. It improves diarrhea but has less effect on pain, and some patients complain that it actually aggravates the sensation of bloating [24].

Serotonin antagonists

5-HT$_3$ antagonists were developed initially for the treatment of chemotherapy-induced nausea and vomiting caused by massive 5-hydroxytryptamine (5-HT) release, and for this condition these drugs (ondansetron and granisetron) are dramatically effective and safe. They also slow intestinal transit and cause constipation as a side effect. A second-generation 5-HT$_3$ receptor antagonist, alosetron, designed to be gut selective with minimal central nervous system effects was highly successful in treating diarrhea-predominant IBS. It slows colonic transit, increases stool consistency, and reduces IBS symptoms (Figure 62.8), the NNT being 7 [34]. Unfortunately, after more than 450 000 prescriptions it was abruptly withdrawn owing to adverse effects. These included severe constipation in a substantial proportion of patients, in some cases inducing ileus and intestinal obstruction. While this side effect can be seen as

merely an extension of its desired therapeutic effect, which could have been controlled by more careful prescribing, the other rare (1 in 700) side effect of ischemic colitis was unexplained. This was transient, self-limiting, and benign in nearly all cases with only a small proportion of patients requiring hospitalization. Nevertheless, these two adverse effects led to the drug's withdrawal, though it is now available under special license in the United States. In spite of this, alosetron did demonstrate the effectiveness of 5-HT$_3$ antagonists in the treatment of diarrhea IBS. Ramosetron is a related 5-HT$_3$ antagonists recently shown in large RCT to be effective in the treatment of diarrhea IBS at a dose of 5 μg, with an NNT of 5 [35].

5-HT$_4$ agonists: Pharmacological studies show that 5-HT$_4$ agonists stimulate peristalsis and intestinal secretions. Constipated patients have reduced frequency of propulsive motor patterns and serotonin agonists acting on the 5-HT$_4$ receptor have been shown to accelerate colonic transit, increase stool frequency (Figure 62.9), and improve symptoms in IBS patients where constipation is the predominant symptom. Although tegaserod, a 5-HT$_4$ agonist has been withdrawn owing to a rare association with thrombotic events, a more specific 5-HT$_4$ agonist (prucalopride), shown to be effective in the treatment of resistant constipation (NNT: 7–8) and constipated IBS, has recently been launched.

Complications

Irritable bowel syndrome does not develop into other diseases and as such there are no true complications. However, IBS patients are often not diagnosed as such and their symptoms may be misinterpreted as chronic cholecystitis, pelvic inflammatory disease, and a range of other conditions, which can all result in unnecessary abdominal surgery [26]. The same study also showed that patients with unrecognized IBS who attended gynecological clinics fared worse and were more likely to still be symptomatic at the end of 1-year follow-up. Therefore, it is important that the condition is recognized and that the patient sees a single physician who can prevent them being repeatedly referred to different surgeons with the attendant risk of further unnecessary surgery.

Prognosis

Irritable bowel syndrome is a diagnosis that can be made with some confidence and in which the diagnosis is rarely revised. The prognosis for survival is therefore excellent; however, IBS remains a chronic cause of substantial impairment of quality of life, which may last for many decades. Regrettably, there are no large prospective studies, so data on long-term prognosis is weak and largely based on cross-sectional studies. One small prospective survey of postinfective IBS found that over a 6-year period around 40% of patients had recovered [27]. Other small studies have suggested that chronic ongoing life stressors or the presence of psychiatric disorders reduce the chances of resolution of symptoms, which certainly fits with clinical experience.

What to tell the patient
Reassurance

Patients need reassurance that the physician understands and appreciates their symptoms. The physician should also make it clear that he or she is confident of the diagnosis from the symptoms and normal physical examination in the absence of alarm features. They also need to know that if any investigations are ordered, they are expected to be normal. This is important to avoid an endless series of negative tests, which leads the patient to believe that their condition is not understood. They should be told that the condition is chronic but benign.

Explanation of symptoms

Some attempt should be made to explain the symptoms in a way the patient can understand. That the pain can arise from distention of the gut or forceful contractions is readily acceptable, as is the concept that their guts may be hypersensitive. Introducing the idea that hypersensitivity may be due to abnormal processing of visceral stimuli by the brain allows one to then explain how antidepressants might help by enhancing descending pain-inhibiting pathways. The idea that abnormal contractions might be due to dietary intolerances allows one to explore the possible precipitation of symptoms by certain foods.

Self-help groups and sources of information

There are many self-help groups, which produce material of variable usefulness. Other reputable sites are provided by national health services. Good examples are given in the Sources Box. However, many sites on the web are of lesser value, either being hospital advertisements or attempts to sell unproven therapies.

SOURCES

http://www.theibsnetwork.org/
http://www.iffgd.org/
http://www.patient.co.uk/health/Irritable-Bowel-Syndrome.htm

Current controversies and their future resolution

While all agree that IBS has both central and peripheral components the precise balance is a matter of much debate, with some groups arguing that the peripheral elements are epiphenomena secondary to a primarily psychologically driven illness. Substantial efforts have been made to understand the pharmacology of visceral pain particularly focused on receptors that are upregulated by inflammation such as purinergic (P2X3), vanilloid (VR-1), and acid-sensitive ion channels (ASIC3). However translation of animal studies to human therapies has proved difficult, and there is doubt as to whether the animal models of visceral hypersensitivity can be used to predict clinical efficacy. Abnormalities in 5-HT metabolism in the mucosa of the various subtypes of IBS have been described, with decreased release in constipated IBS patients and increased release in those with diarrhea-predominant IBS. Increased 5-HT could be due to impaired activity of the serotonin transporter (SERT) but initial reports of reduced SERT in the colonic mucosa have not been reproduced. 5-HT_3 receptor antagonists are undoubtedly effective but whether the side effect of ischemic colitis is a general phenomenon affecting all such drugs is unclear. Anti-inflammatory agents such as mesalamine have shown some promise but as yet the trials are either anecdotal or poorly designed or else too small to be confident that there is a real benefit. All current IBS trials have comparatively large NNTs suggesting that there is considerable need for objective markers to identify subtypes who will respond to specific therapies in the future.

References

1. Longstreth GF, Thompson WG, Chey WD, *et al.* Functional bowel disorders. *Gastroenterology.* 2006;130:1480–1491.
2. Thompson WG, Heaton KW, Smyth GT, *et al.* Irritable bowel syndrome in general practice: prevalence, characteristics, and referral. *Gut.* 2000;46:78–82.
3. Spiller R, Aziz Q, Creed F, *et al.* Guidelines on the irritable bowel syndrome: mechanisms and practical management. *Gut.* 2007; 56:1770–1798.

4. Hungin AP, Whorwell PJ, Tack J, *et al.* The prevalence, patterns and impact of irritable bowel syndrome: an international survey of 40,000 subjects. *Aliment Pharmacol Ther.* 2003;17:643–650.

5. Hungin AP, Chang L, Locke GR, *et al.* Irritable bowel syndrome in the United States: prevalence, symptom patterns and impact. *Aliment Pharmacol Ther.* 2005;21:1365–1375.

6. Leong SA, Barghout V, Birnbaum HG, *et al.* The Economic Consequences of Irritable Bowel Syndrome: A US Employer Perspective. *Arch Intern Med.* 2003;163:929.

7. Locke GR, III, Yawn BP, Wollan PC, *et al.* Incidence of a clinical diagnosis of the irritable bowel syndrome in a United States population. *Aliment Pharmacol Ther.* 2004;19:1025–1031.

8. Rodriguez LA, Ruigomez A. Increased risk of irritable bowel syndrome after bacterial gastroenteritis: cohort study. *Br Med J.* 1999;318:565–566.

9. Creed F, Craig T, Farmer R. Functional abdominal pain, psychiatric illness, and life events. *Gut.* 1988;29:235–242.

10. Garsed K, Spiller R. Postinfectious Irritable Bowel Syndrome. *Gastroenterology.* 2009;136:1979–1988.

11. Ford AC, Forman D, Bailey AG, *et al.* Irritable bowel syndrome: a 10-yr natural history of symptoms and factors that influence consultation behavior. *Am J Gastroenterol.* 2008;103:1229–1239.

12. Nicholl BI, Halder SL, Macfarlane GJ, *et al.* Psychosocial risk markers for new onset irritable bowel syndrome–results of a large prospective population-based study. *Pain.* 2008;137: 147–155.

13. Vandvik PO, Wilhelmsen I, Ihlebaek C, *et al.* Comorbidity of irritable bowel syndrome in general practice: a striking feature with clinical implications. *Aliment Pharmacol Ther.* 2004;20:1195–1203.

14. Corsetti M, Caenepeel P, Fischler B, *et al.* Impact of coexisting irritable bowel syndrome on symptoms and pathophysiological mechanisms in functional dyspepsia. *Am J Gastroenterol.* 2004;99:1152–1159.

15. Camilleri M, McKinzie S, Busciglio I, *et al.* Prospective study of motor, sensory, psychologic, and autonomic functions in patients with irritable bowel syndrome. *Clin Gastroenterol Hepatol.* 2008;6:772–781.

16. Walker EA, Katon WJ, Jemelka RP, *et al.* Comorbidity of gastrointestinal complaints, depression, and anxiety in the Epidemiologic Catchment Area (ECA) Study. *Am J Med.* 1992;92:26S–30S.

17. Mayer EA, Collins SM. Evolving pathophysiologic models of functional gastrointestinal disorders. *Gastroenterology.* 2002;122: 2032–2048.

18. Marciani L, Cox EF, Hoad CL, *et al.* Postprandial changes in small bowel water content in health and irritable bowel syndrome. *Phys Med Biol.* 2007;52:6909–6922.

19. Agrawal A, Houghton LA, Lea R, *et al.* Bloating and distention in irritable bowel syndrome: the role of visceral sensation. *Gastroenterology.* 2008;134:1882–1889.

20. Accarino A, Perez F, Azpiroz F, *et al.* Abdominal distention results from caudo-ventral redistribution of contents. *Gastroenterology.* 2009;136:1544–1551.

21. Mertz H, Naliboff B, Munakata J, *et al.* Altered rectal perception is a biological marker of patients with irritable bowel syndrome. *Gastroenterology.* 1995;109:40–52.

22. Mertz H, Morgan V, Tanner G, *et al.* Regional cerebral activation in irritable bowel syndrome and control subjects with painful and nonpainful rectal distention. *Gastroenterology.* 2000;118: 842–848.

23. Naliboff BD, Berman S, Suyenobu B, *et al.* Longitudinal change in perceptual and brain activation response to visceral stimuli in irritable bowel syndrome patients. *Gastroenterology.* 2006;131: 352–365.

24. Berman SM, Naliboff BD, Suyenobu B, *et al.* Reduced brainstem inhibition during anticipated pelvic visceral pain correlates with enhanced brain response to the visceral stimulus in women with irritable bowel syndrome. *J Neurosci.* 2008;28:349–359.

25. Longstreth GF, Hawkey CJ, Mayer EA, *et al.* Characteristics of patients with irritable bowel syndrome recruited from three sources: implications for clinical trials. *Aliment Pharmacol Ther.* 2001;15:959–964.

26. Santos J, Benjamin M, Yang PC, *et al.* Chronic stress impairs rat growth and jejunal epithelial barrier function: role of mast cells. *Am J Physiol Gastrointest Liver Physiol.* 2000;278:G847–G854.

27. Barbara G, Stanghellini V, De Giorgio R, *et al.* Activated mast cells in proximity to colonic nerves correlate with abdominal pain in irritable bowel syndrome. *Gastroenterology.* 2004;126: 693–702.

28. Barbara G, Wang B, Stanghellini V, *et al.* Mast cell-dependent excitation of visceral-nociceptive sensory neurons in irritable bowel syndrome. *Gastroenterology.* 2007;132:26–37.

29. Brandt LJ, Chey WD, Foxx-Orenstein AE, *et al.* An evidence-based position statement on the management of irritable bowel syndrome. *Am J Gastroenterol.* 2009;104(Suppl 1):S1–S35.

30. Kroenke K, Spitzer RL, Williams JB. The PHQ-15: validity of a new measure for evaluating the severity of somatic symptoms. *Psychosom Med.* 2002;64:258–266.

31. Atkinson W, Sheldon TA, Shaath N, *et al.* Food elimination based on IgG antibodies in irritable bowel syndrome: a randomised controlled trial. *Gut.* 2004;53:1459–1464.

32. King TS, Elia M, Hunter JO. Abnormal colonic fermentation in irritable bowel syndrome. *Lancet.* 1998;352:1187–1189.

33. Shepherd SJ, Gibson PR. Fructose malabsorption and symptoms of irritable bowel syndrome: guidelines for effective dietary management. *J Am Diet Assoc.* 2006;106:1631–1639.

34. Cremonini F, Delgado-Aros S, Camilleri M. Efficacy of alosetron in irritable bowel syndrome: a meta-analysis of randomized controlled trials. *Neurogastroenterol Motil.* 2003;15:79–86.

35. Matsueda K, Harasawa S, Hongo M, *et al.* A randomized, double-blind, placebo-controlled clinical trial of the effectiveness of the novel serotonin type 3 receptor antagonist ramosetron in both male and female Japanese patients with diarrhea-predominant irritable bowel syndrome. *Scand J Gastroenterol.* 2008;43:1202–1211.

Small and Large Bowel

CHAPTER 63
Diverticular disease of the colon

Anish A. Sheth and Martin H. Floch
Yale University School of Medicine, New Haven, CT, USA

ESSENTIAL FACTS ABOUT PATHOGENESIS

Risk factors:
- Low fiber-diet
- Increasing age
- Obesity
- Decreased physical activity
- Connective tissue disease (i.e., Ehlers–Danlos syndrome)

ESSENTIALS OF DIAGNOSIS

Acute diverticulitis
- Clinical presentation
  - Left-lower quadrant abdominal pain
  - Fever
  - Abdominal tenderness +/− rebound
- Investigation
  - Complete blood count
  - Abdominal X-ray (free air indicates perforation)
  - CT scan abdomen/pelvis

Diverticular bleeding
- Clinical presentation
  - Painless hematochezia
- Investigation
  - 99mTc scintigraphy
  - Angiography
  - Colonoscopy

TREATMENT

Acute diverticulitis
- Uncomplicated
  - Broad-spectrum antibiotics
  - Bowel rest
- Complicated
  - CT-guided abscess drainage
  - Surgical resection
  - Colonoscopic stenting (stricture)

Diverticular bleeding
- Angiography
  - Vasopressin injection
  - Arterial embolization
- Colonoscopy
  - Epinephrine injection
  - Bipolar cautery
  - Endoclip placement

Introduction

Left-sided diverticular disease of the colon is one of the most common medical conditions affecting industrialized nations. Its incidence has increased over the past several decades from less than 10% to figures as high as 50% in those over age 60 years [1,2]. The largest post-mortem study revealed a diverticulosis rate of 35–50% [3]. The incidence of perforated diverticulitis has also increased over the past two decades [4].

Inflammatory and bleeding complications occur in 25% of patients and can range in severity from mild, self-limited bouts of abdominal pain to severe episodes of diverticulitis and diverticular bleeding requiring surgery.

A less common form of diverticular disease occurring in Asian populations affecting the right colon differs in several ways from left-sided disease.

Causes and pathogenesis

Left-sided diverticula are **pseudodiverticula** because herniation is limited to the mucosal and submucosal layers (Figure 63.1). In contrast, diverticula seen in Asian-predominant right-colon disease are **true diverticula**, with herniation involving all bowel wall layers. Diverticula form at weak points in the bowel wall, typically where the vasa recta penetrate colonic circular smooth muscle.

Epidemiologic studies have linked fiber-poor diets with development of left-sided diverticulosis [1]. Industrialized regions (North America, Europe) have significant higher rates of diverticular disease than less developed regions (Africa, Asia).

Fiber-deficient diets result in smaller volume stools and increased intracolonic pressures [5]. Excessive intraluminal pressures are generated when the sigmoid colon undergoes forceful contractions, a process known as "segmentation" [5] (Figure 63.2).

The pathogenesis of diverticular inflammation is unclear. Altered peri-diverticular bacterial flora may play a role in triggering inflammation [7]. Peri-diverticular inflammation, regardless of cause, leads to increased intradiverticular pressure and eventual microperforation. Chronic manifestations of diverticular disease, including chronic pain and irritable bowel syndrome (IBS)-like presentations, are caused by low-level mucosal inflammation and enhanced visceral sensitivity [7].

Textbook of Clinical Gastroenterology and Hepatology, Second Edition. Edited by C. J. Hawkey, Jaime Bosch, Joel E. Richter, Guadalupe Garcia-Tsao, Francis K. L. Chan.
© 2012 Blackwell Publishing Ltd. Published 2012 by Blackwell Publishing Ltd.

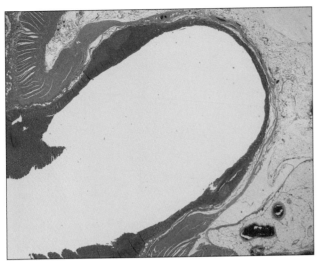

Figure 63.1 Diverticulosis Histology: Histology shows herniation of mucosal and submucosal layers. (Slide courtesy of Dhanpat Jain, MD.)

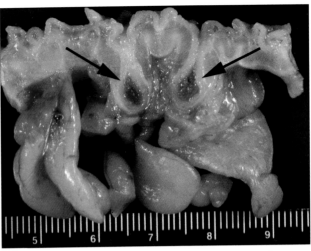

Figure 63.3 Diverticulosis gross pathology: sigmoid resection specimen shows gross appearance of colonic diverticula. (Slide courtesy of Dhanpat Jain, MD.)

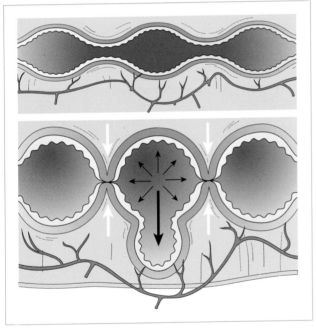

Figure 63.2 Colonic segmentation results in diverticula formation. Lumen obliterating contractions in patients with low volume stools causes elevated intracolonic pressures. High pressures promote mucosal herniation through weak points in the colonic wall. (This figure was published in *Clinical Gastroenterology and Hepatology*, Wilfred M. Weinstein, Christopher J. Hawkey, Jaime Bosch, Diverticular disease of the colon, Pages 1–9, Copyright Elsevier, 2005.)

Pathology

Surgical and postmortem specimens reveal structural changes in areas of the colon affected by diverticulosis (Figure 63.3). Grossly, the colon appears thickened and contracted, a morphological change termed **mychosis**. This corrugated appearance is due to bowel shortening and increased elastin deposition [6].

Segmental colitis associated with diverticula (SCAD) is a unique form of chronic colitis limited to the areas of the colon with diverticula [8]. Colonoscopic findings mimic those of inflammatory bowel disease (IBD) with friable peri-diverticular mucosa but the notable absence of aphthous ulcerations typically seen in Crohn's disease.

Clinical presentation
Diverticulitis
Diverticular inflammation typically presents acutely with the triad of **left-lower quadrant abdominal pain** (70%), **fever** (60%), and **elevated white blood cell count** (55%). The diagnosis is often made on clinical grounds in patients who have had prior episodes of diverticulitis but may be difficult in first-time presenters or those who are immunocompromised.

Physical examination in patients with contained microperforation classically reveals left lower quadrant tenderness and focal rebound tenderness. Patients with abscess or phlegmon may also have a palpable mass (20%) [9]. Free diverticular perforation leads to diffuse abdominal tenderness, rebound, and signs of systemic toxicity.

The severity of acute diverticulitis can vary from mild, uncomplicated disease caused by contained microperforation to complicated disease characterized by generalized peritonitis. Perforated diverticulitis confers a six-fold increase in mortality compared with healthy controls [10].

Other complications of acute diverticulitis include abscess, phlegmon, and fistula formation (Table 63.1), the latter most commonly occurring between the sigmoid diverticula and bladder. Diverticular inflammation can also lead to stricture formation and colonic obstruction.

Chronic diverticular disease can present with IBS-type symptoms. Patients with SCAD present similarly to patients with IBD with abdominal pain, bleeding, and diarrhea.

Table 63.1 Complications of diverticulitis

- Abscess
- Bleeding (rare)
- Fistula
- Phelgmon
- Obstruction
- Sepsis
- Stricture

Diverticular bleeding

Diverticular bleeding occurs in approximately 5% of patients with diverticulosis and presents with painless hematochezia. The cardinal manifestations of diverticulitis (i.e., pain, fever) are notably absent. Bleeding can be mild and self-limited in nature or life threatening in patients with significant underlying comorbidities.

Differential diagnosis
Diverticulitis

Conditions mimicking diverticulitis include appendicitis (especially in cases of right-sided diverticular disease), perforated colon cancer, inflammatory, ischemic and infectious colitis, as well as gynecologic processes such as endometriosis, ruptured ovarian cyst, and tubo-ovarian abscess. Patients with acute diverticulitis typically present with constipation, helping to differentiate this process from other colonic inflammatory conditions.

Diagnostic investigation

Diverticulosis is most commonly detected in asymptomatic patients who undergo abdominal imaging or screening colonoscopy (Figure 63.4). Diagnostic investigation for patients with symptomatic disease is based on clinical presentation.

Diverticulitis

Computed tomography (CT) of the abdomen/pelvis with oral and intravenous contrast is the current gold standard (accuracy 98–100%) for diagnosis of acute diverticular disease [10,11] (Figure 63.5). The most specific finding on CT scan is increased soft tissue density in pericolonic fat.

Buckley and Hinchey classifications are commonly used to stage acute diverticulitis based on criteria such as degree of bowel thickening, abscess size, and degree of perforation (see Tables 63.2 and 63.3) [11].

Symptoms of chronic diverticular disease (i.e., low-level pain, diarrhea) are best assessed with colonoscopy. Peridiverticular mucosa should be biopsied if endoscopic evidence of inflammation is visualized. Exclusion of colorectal carcinoma is another important aspect of endoscopic evaluation.

Diverticular bleeding

Two main strategies are currently employed in the evaluation of lower gastrointestinal (GI) bleeding: nuclear scanning

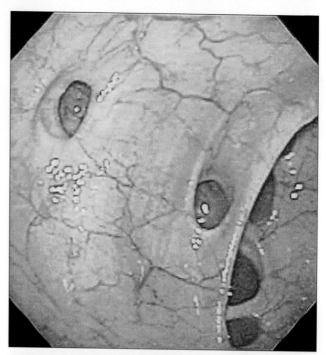

Figure 63.4 Colonoscopic appearance of sigmoid diverticulosis.

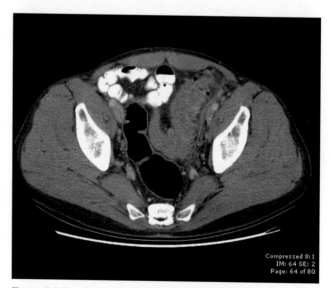

Figure 63.5 Sigmoid diverticulitis: Computed tomography (CT) scan in patient with uncomplicated sigmoid diverticulitis showing pericolonic fat stranding. (Image courtesy of Gary Israel, MD.)

Table 63.2 Hinchey classification (perforated diverticulitis)

Stage	CT findings
I	Pericolonic abscess or phlegmon
II	Pelvic, intra-abdominal or retroperitoneal abscess
III	Generalized purulent peritonitis
IV	Generalized fecal peritonitis

Table 63.3 Buckley classification

Stage	CT findings
Mild	Bowel wall thickening, fat stranding
Moderate	Bowel wall thickening >3 mm, phlegmon, or small abscess
Severe	Bowel wall thickening >5 mm, frank perforation with subdiaphragmatic air, abscess >5 cm

followed by angiography, and rapid-preparation colonoscopy. Choice of strategy depends largely on locally available technology and expertise.

Treatment and prevention

Diverticulitis

Acute, uncomplicated diverticulitis can be managed with broad-spectrum antibiotic therapy. Outpatient treatment with ciprofloxacin 500 mg p.o. twice daily and metronidazole 500 mg p.o. three times daily for 7 to 10 days is feasible for patients with minimal symptoms and ability to maintain oral intake.

Hospitalized patients should receive intravenous antibiotics. Effective regimens include: ampicillin (2 g IV every 6 hours), gentamicin (1.5–2 mg/kg IV every 8 hours), and metronidazole (500 mg IV every 8 hours), or piperacillin-tazobactam (3.375 g IV every 6 hours).

Routine surgical intervention after a single episode of acute diverticulitis is not recommended as only 25% will have recurrent attacks [12]. Patients should be advised to maintain a high-fiber diet (25–35 g daily). Ongoing studies are evaluating the efficacy of probiotics and 5-aminosalicylates in the prevention of recurrent disease.

The timing of surgical resection in patients with recurrent disease is evolving. The belief that patients with recurrent disease are at high risk for developing severe, complicated disease with subsequent attacks led to guidelines calling for surgical resection after the second episode of diverticulitis. A recent study shows that patients with recurrent attacks who have had more than two episodes have similar morbidity and mortality rates to patients who have had two or fewer attacks.

The optimal timing of surgical intervention in patients with diverticulitis who are less than 40 years old is unclear. Initial reports describing more virulent disease among young patients with diverticulitis have been challenged.

Treatment of patients with chronic, low-level symptoms is an active area of investigation. Uncontrolled studies have shown benefit with 5-aminosalicylate compounds, rifaximin, and probiotics [13].

Diverticular bleeding

Treatment mainstays include angiographic injection and embolization and endoscopic therapy. Angiographic injection of vasopressin is effective in temporary cessation of bleeding

in 91% of patients, thereby allowing for semi-elective endoscopic or surgical intervention. Angiographic embolization of a bleeding vessel can offer definitive therapy but can cause intestinal infarction in 20% of cases.

If an actively bleeding diverticulum is visualized during colonoscopy, therapy can be delivered (Video 63.1). Endoscopic treatment options include four-quadrant epinephrine injection, bipolar cautery, and endoclip placement..

Surgical resection is advocated for recalcitrant or recurrent diverticular bleeding and is required in up to 25% of cases. Laparoscopic segmental resection with primary anastomosis is the treatment of choice. Surgical intervention can be performed as salvage therapy following angiographic or colonoscopy localization when bleeding persists or recurs.

Complications and their management

The majority of patients with acute diverticulitis will present with uncomplicated disease, but 25% of patients will experience complicated diverticulitis characterized by generalized peritonitis, abscess, fistulae, or stricture.

Peritonitis

Diagnosis is made based on clinical examination and CT scan findings. Hinchey classification of CT findings in perforated diverticulitis includes Stage III and IV disease, corresponding to purulent and fecal peritonitis, respectively. Mortality increases with peritonitis severity: 6% in purulent peritonitis and 35% in fecal peritonitis.

Treatment of acute diverticulitis complicated by peritonitis is resection of the affected colon segment with end colostomy and Hartmann's pouch. Anastomosis is typically undertaken 3–6 months after recovery. There is emerging data to support the safety of single-stage laparoscopic sigmoid resection with primary anastomosis in patients with peritonitis [14].

Abscess

Abscess formation is common during acute diverticulitis, occurring in 16% of cases (Figures 63.6 and 63.7). Small abscesses can be treated simply with intravenous antibiotics and bowel rest. Abscesses larger than 4 cm should undergo CT-guided drainage. Drains are left in place until drain output falls to less than 10 mL per 24 hours and clinical improvement is seen. Drainage allows for semi-elective colon surgery and increases the chance of single stage operation (resection with primary anastomosis).

Fistula

Fistula formation can occur after a single bout of acute diverticulitis and is an indication for surgical intervention. Colovesicular and colovaginal fistulas are the most common sites of disease (Figure 63.8). Fistula diagnosis is most commonly made with CT scanning. Laparoscopic resection of the affected colon segment is the mainstay of treatment. Several options

Small and Large Bowel

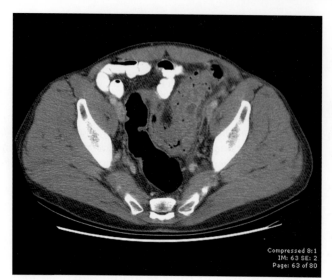

Figure 63.6 Sigmoid diverticulitis with abscess: Computed tomography (CT) scan showing complicated sigmoid diverticulitis with intramural abscess. Small abscesses (<4 cm) may respond to antibiotic therapy alone and typically do not require drainage. (Image courtesy of Gary Israel, MD.)

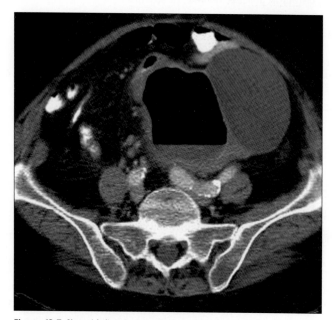

Figure 63.7 Sigmoid diverticulitis with large abscess: Computed tomography (CT) scan showing complicated sigmoid diverticulitis with large pericolonic abscess. Large diverticular abscesses should be managed with CT-guided catheter drainage in addition to intravenous antibiotics. (Image courtesy of Gary Israel, MD.)

for bladder closure exist in the setting of a colovesicular fistula depending on the location and size of the communication.

Stricture

Colonic strictures are a rare complication of diverticular disease. Patients present with symptoms of large-bowel obstruction and treatment options include endoscopic dilation and stenting as well as surgical resection with primary anastomosis.

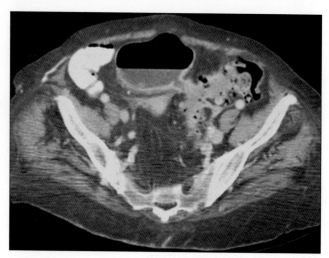

Figure 63.8 Colovesicular fistula: Computed tomography (CT) scan showing colovesicular fistula. This is the most common site of fistula formation in diverticular disease. (Image courtesy of Gary Israel, MD.)

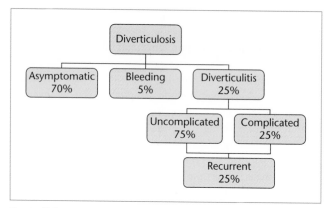

Figure 63.9 Natural history of diverticular disease.

Prognosis with and without treatment (Figure 63.9)

Of patients with diverticulosis, 70% will remain asymptomatic, 5% will suffer bleeding complications, and 25% will experience one or more episodes of diverticulitis. There is some evidence that maintenance of a high-fiber diet (>25 g/day) and physical activity may help prevent diverticular disease complications.

Patients who have experienced one episode of diverticulitis have a 25% chance of recurrent disease [12]. Recent studies have shown that subsequent episodes of diverticulitis are not necessarily more severe, and they do not confer an increased mortality.

SOURCES OF INFORMATION FOR PATIENTS AND DOCTORS

http://www.utdol.com/online/content/
    topic.do?topicKey=digestiv/6237
http://digestive.niddk.nih.gov/ddiseases/pubs/diverticulosis/
http://www.mayoclinic.com/health/diverticulitis/DS00070

References

1. Painter NS, Burkitt DP. Diverticular disease of the colon: a deficiency disease of Western civilization. *Br Med J.* 1971;2:450–454.

2. Parra-Blanco A. Colonic diverticular disease: pathophysiology and clinical picture. *Digestion.* 2006;73(Suppl 1):47–57.

3. Hughes LE. Postmortem survey of diverticular disease of the colon. II. The muscular abnormality of the sigmoid colon. *Gut.* 1969;10:344–351.

4. Humes DJ, Solaymani-Dodaran M, Fleming KM, Simpson J, Spiller RC, West J. A population-based study of perforated diverticular disease incidence and associated mortality. *Gastroenterology.* 2009;136:1198–1205.

5. Painter NS, Burkitt DP. Diverticular disease of the colon, a 20th century problem. *Clin Gastroenterol.* 1975;4:3–21.

6. West AB, Losada M. The pathology of diverticulosis coli. *J Clin Gastroenterol.* 2004;38(Suppl):S11–16.

7. Floch CL. Diagnosis and management of acute diverticulitis. *J Clin Gastroenterol.* 2006;40(Suppl 3):S136–144.

8. Peppercorn MA. Drug-responsive chronic segmental colitis associated with diverticula: a clinical syndrome in the elderly. *Am J Gastroenterol.* 1992;87:609–612.

9. Parks TG. Natural history of diverticular disease of the colon. *Clin Gastroenterol.* 1975;4:53–69.

10. Buckley O, Geoghegan T, O'Riordain DS, Lyburn ID, Torreggiani WC. Computed tomography in the imaging of colonic diverticulitis. *Clin Radiol.* 2004;59:977–983.

11. Hinchey EJ, Schaal PG, Richards GK. Treatment of perforated diverticular disease of the colon. *Adv Surg.* 1978;12:85–109.

12. Janes S, Meagher A, Frizelle FA. Elective surgery after acute diverticulitis. *Br J Surg.* 2005;92:133–142.

13. Di Mario F, Comparato G, Fanigliulo L, *et al.* Use of mesalazine in diverticular disease. *J Clin Gastroenterol.* 2006;40(Suppl 3): S155–159.

14. Constantinides VA, Tekkis PP, Athanasiou T, *et al.* Primary resection with anastomosis vs. Hartmann's procedure in nonelective surgery for acute colonic diverticulitis: a systematic review. *Dis Colon Rectum.* 2006;49:966–981.

Small and Large Bowel

CHAPTER 64

Megacolon and pseudo-obstruction

Eamonn M. M. Quigley

University College Cork, Cork, Ireland

ESSENTIAL FACTS ABOUT PATHOGENESIS

- Acute megacolon, or Ogilvie syndrome, is associated with an underlying medical condition or the postoperative state in over 90% of cases
- Risk factors for the development of Ogilvie syndrome following surgery include: advanced age, obesity, immobility, and use of patient-controlled analgesia
- Colonic motor dysfunction and megacolon are common in neurological disorders
- Secondary causes of chronic intestinal pseudo-obstruction (CIP) include: connective tissue disorders and scleroderma, in particular, neurological disorders, skeletal muscle diseases, metabolic disorders, and drugs and toxins

ESSENTIALS OF DIAGNOSIS

- Progressive abdominal distention is the clinical hallmark of acute megacolon
- Abdominal distension, often asymptomatic, is the usual presenting feature of chronic megacolon, typically, in the context of chronic and severe slow-transit constipation
- The typical history of chronic intestinal pseudo-obstruction (CIP) is of repeated admissions with symptoms, signs, and radiological evidence of "obstruction" with no convincing cause for obstruction being found
- In the diagnosis of acute megacolon, a plain abdominal X-ray may be the only essential investigation
- The definitive diagnoses of CIP can only be provided by pathological examination of full-thickness biopsies by an expert pathologist

ESSENTIALS OF TREATMENT

- Find and, where possible, treat any underlying disorder
- In resistant cases, therapy should begin with cholinergic agonists e.g., neostigmine
- Surgical intervention and the placement of a tube cecostomy where there is a high risk of perforation and pharmacological approaches and colonoscopic attempts at decompression have failed
- Surgery will also be necessary in those who progress to ischemia or perforation
- The management of Hirschsprung's disease and of megacolon related to Chagas disease is primarily surgical

Introduction and epidemiology

Because of the relative inaccessibility of the small intestine and colon and the additional difficulties posed, in the colon, by the presence of solid or semisolid fecal material, our understanding of small intestinal and colonic motility lags behind that of other organs of the gastrointestinal tract.

Motility in the small intestine is arranged into two basic patterns: fasting and post-prandial. During fasting, small intestinal motility is organized into three distinct patterns of motility, which occur in sequence, slowly migrate along the length of the bowel, and synchronize with motor events in contiguous organs; these are the three phases of the migrating motor complex (MMC), which is most readily identified by the third of these patterns, phase III (or the activity front), an uninterrupted burst of phasic contractions. Once a meal is ingested, the MMC is abolished and replaced by apparently irregular contractile activity whose duration and intensity are related to the size and composition of the ingested meal; this fed response promotes mixing of the meal with digestive enzymes and bile to optimize digestion and assimilation of the meal.

Our understanding of colonic motility is less complete; at first sight colonic motility appears complex and almost uninterpretable [1]. As a generalization, it can be stated that colonic motility, in humans, presents alternating periods of activity and quiescence. Some recognizable patterns have been identified in the active periods: individual phasic contractions, propagating contractions, propagating bursts or clusters of contractions, and, most recognizable of all, high-amplitude propagating contractions (HAPCs). The latter are more prevalent in children than in adults, are associated with the mass movement of fecal material over segments of the colon, and may be accompanied by the passage of flatus or the urge to defecate. Colonic motility is influenced by food intake (the gastrocolonic reflex), diurnal variation, exercise, and stress. In comparison with the small intestine, the colon is more susceptible to the influences of the autonomic and central nervous

Small and Large Bowel

systems, a fitting arrangement given our necessity to regulate the time and place of voluntary defecation.

In clinical terms, the most useful classification of colonic dysmotility identifies two principal disorders: acute colonic pseudo-obstruction (including Ogilvie syndrome) and chronic motor disorders (including chronic megacolon); both may be manifestations of a more generalized motility disorder, chronic intestinal pseudo-obstruction (CIP).

The precise prevalence rates of megacolon and pseudo-obstruction, in strict epidemiological terms, are unknown. Of these disorders, acute megacolon, or Ogilvie syndrome, may well be the most common, with inherited disorders of enteric muscle and nerve being distinctly rare. Consequently, rates for the occurrence of Ogilvie syndrome in relation to certain surgical procedures, or in the context of certain clinical scenarios, have been reported, but, with the exception of congenital disorders such as aganglionosis [2], age-specific rates for any of these conditions in the population at large are not available.

Causes and pathogenesis

Acute megacolon may be a manifestation of a variety of disorders. Toxic megacolon, for example, is a dreaded complication of ulcerative colitis and, indeed, virtually any cause of colitis, be it inflammatory, infectious, or ischemic. Acute colonic pseudo-obstruction, or Ogilvie syndrome, is defined as an acute dilatation of the colon without evidence of mechanical obstruction distal to the dilated segment (Figure 64.1) [3].

Oglivie syndrome is associated with an underlying medical condition or the postoperative state in over 90% of cases. Risk factors for the development of Ogilvie syndrome in an individual patient following surgery include: advanced age, obesity, immobility, and use of patient-controlled analgesia.

There are many potential causes of chronic megacolon. Though, typically, a disease of childhood, Hirschsprung's disease may occasionally present in adult life. In Chagas disease, chronic infection with the protazoan *Trypanosoma cruzi* leads to a similar loss of inhibitory neurons in various parts of the gastrointestinal tract, including the anorectum and colon, and to the development of megacolon (Figure 64.2). Colonic motor dysfunction is common in neurological disorders, and chronic megacolon has been described in Parkinson disease, multiple sclerosis (Figure 64.3), motor neuron disease, Alzheimer's disease, autonomic neuropathies and in relation to spinal cord injury, among others. The description of enteric neural changes in the myenteric plexus of the colon among patients who had chronically used anthroquinone-type laxatives led to the assumption that these agents were neurotoxic; more recent studies among patients with chronic idiopathic, slow-transit constipation suggest that such changes may be

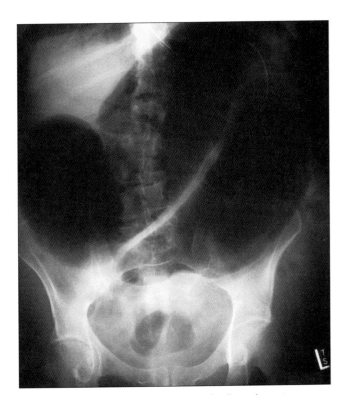

Figure 64.1 Ogilvie syndrome. Plain abdominal radiograph – note prominent dilatation of right and transverse colon with preservation of haustrae.

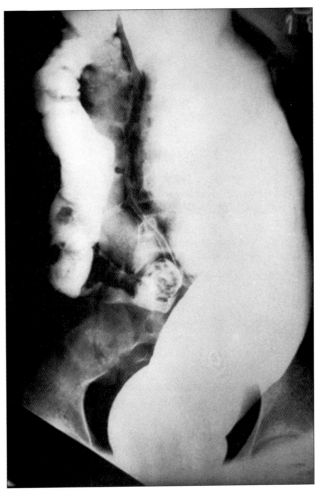

Figure 64.2 Megacolon and megarectum in Chagas disease.

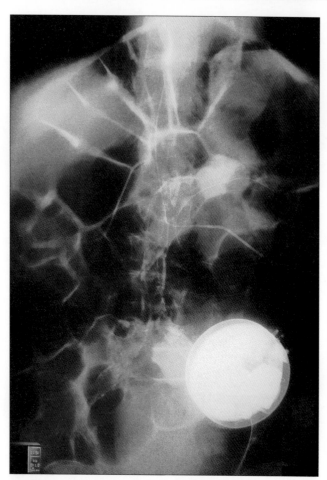

Figure 64.3 Megacolon in multiple sclerosis and paraplegia. Note the presence of an implanted system for the delivery of baclofen.

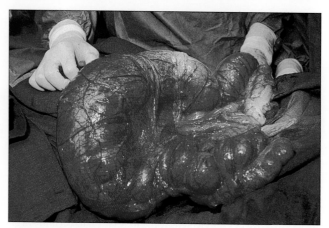

Figure 64.4 Idiopathic chronic megacolon. Appearances of the colon at the time of colectomy for chronic intractable megacolon.

linked to constipation *per se* and not to the use of laxatives. In some instances, chronic megacolon may occur in the absence of any discernable cause: idiopathic megacolon (Figure 64.4). In such instances, megacolon usually occurs in a background of chronic constipation and is assumed to represent the expression of a degenerative disorder of intestinal nerve and/or muscle, though the exact nature of the basic defect remains to be defined.

Several of the disorders listed above may be accompanied by a more generalized disorder of intestinal motility, CIP [4], which may be idiopathic or secondary; idiopathic examples may, in turn, be hereditary or acquired. Hirschsprung's disease provides a good, albeit rare, example of an inherited idiopathic enteric neuropathy that predominantly (though not exclusively) affects the colon. Neuronal intestinal dysplasia (a disorder sometimes associated with Hirschsprung's disease), which features neural hyperplasia, has been described in up to 30% of children with pseudo-obstruction; the criteria for the diagnosis of this entity have, however, been questioned. In contrast to Hirschsprung's disease, most other causes of chronic intestinal pseudo-obstruction tend to diffusely affect the entire gastrointestinal tract. While a variety of inherited syndromes involving intestinal myopathy or neuropathy, as well as other extra-intestinal features, have been described, these disorders, even taken collectively, are rare with secondary forms of pseudo-obstruction being far more common. Secondary causes of CIP include: connective tissue disorders and scleroderma, in particular, neurological disorders, skeletal muscle diseases, metabolic disorders, and drugs and toxins [4]. Chronic intestinal pseudo-obstruction has also been described as a non-metastatic manifestation of a number of malignancies.

Clinical presentation

Progressive abdominal distention is the clinical hallmark of acute megacolon; in the postoperative state distention is, typically, evident by the fourth postoperative day. Lower abdominal pain and nausea and vomiting are present in 60–80% and 50%, respectively. It is important to realize that, while the vast majority of patients with Ogilvie syndrome are completely constipated, megacolon can develop in individuals who continue to pass both stool and flatus. Only 40% of patients will have hypoactive or absent bowel sounds. Abdominal distension, often asymptomatic, is the usual presenting feature of chronic megacolon and usually occurs in the context of chronic and severe slow-transit constipation.

Though CIP may involve any part of the gastrointestinal tract and result in symptoms related to that organ (e.g. GERD, dysphagia, achalasia, gastroparesis, constipation, megacolon), symptoms referable to small-intestinal obstruction classically dominate the clinical picture. Indeed, the typical history of the patient with CIP is that of repeated admissions with symptoms, signs and radiological evidence of "obstruction" with no convincing cause for obstruction being found. Unfortunately, these patients have usually been subjected to a number of fruitless laparotomies before the diagnosis is even entertained. Attention to the clinical context should prompt suspicion of

CIP. The concept of CIP has recently been extended to include a sub-occlusive syndrome among those patients with chronic or recurrent gastrointestinal symptoms (abdominal pain, nausea, vomiting, altered bowel habit) who have manometric or other evidence of dysmotility [5,6]; recently, a neuropathological basis has been provided to support this concept [7]. The term enteric dysmotility (ED) has been proposed as a new diagnostic label for patients with disturbed intestinal motility and severe symptoms but no radiological signs of pseudo-obstruction [5].

Differential diagnosis

In the patient with acute megacolon, the main differential diagnoses to be considered are, firstly, toxic megacolon and, secondly, acute colonic obstruction due to carcinoma, stricture, volvulus, or intussusception.

Toxic megacolon should be obvious from the patient's history and clinical presentation and obstruction may be suspected by the prominence of pain in the symptomatology, as well as by clinical and radiographic findings. It is important to note that, on X-ray, haustral markings are preserved in Ogilvie syndrome, in contrast to both toxic megacolon and obstruction.

With regard to chronic megacolon, subacute or chronic obstruction related to carcinoma and stricture again looms large in the differential diagnosis. In the patient with chronic small-intestinal or colonic motor dysfunction without megacolon, symptom overlap is to be expected with Crohn's disease, other causes of acute or chronic low-grade intestinal obstruction and even with the more severe cases of irritable bowel syndrome (IBS). With regard to the latter, the presence of symptoms, signs, or radiographic or manometric evidence of a generalized motor abnormality should suggest CIP rather than IBS. Most challenging is the differentiation of sub-occlusive CIP, or ED, from severe IBS; here one needs recourse to highly specialized testing [6,8].

Diagnostic investigation

In the diagnosis of acute megacolon, a plain abdominal X-ray may be the only essential investigation. Typically, there is dilatation of the cecum and ascending and transverse colon with less gaseous distention in the left colon (see Figure 64.1). If obstruction needs to be ruled out abdominal computed tomography (CT) is undoubtedly the best option. If colonoscopy is contemplated, the endoscopist needs to be mindful of the risk of a cecal perforation due to the closed loop phenomenon if obstruction is complete.

As with acute megacolon, plain abdominal radiography is very useful in the assessment of chronic megacolon. The role of manometric studies in the evaluation of patients with suspected disorders of colonic motor function continues to evolve but its diagnostic value remains to be established, especially in adults.

The diagnosis of CIP is not easy and the key is to suspect it, ever mindful of the fact that obstruction is much more common than pseudo-obstruction. Conventional imaging techniques, CT, small bowel contrast studies, CT or magnetic resonance enterography or enterosocopy (fiberscopic or capsule) serve primarily to exclude other causes for the patient's symptoms. Definitive diagnoses can only be provided by pathological examination of full-thickness biopsies by an expert pathologist [9]. Pathologically, chronic pseudo-obstruction is usually separated into those disorders that predominately involve intestinal muscle (the myopathies) and those that predominately affect the enteric nervous system or the autonomic nerves that supply the gut (the neuropathies). Small intestinal manometry, a highly specialized technique, has been advanced as a diagnostic test for CIP. Accordingly, myopathic disorders are identified by the presence of a marked reduction in the amplitude of individual contractions while patterns of organization are retained; in contrast, neuropathies feature the retention of the amplitude of individual contractions (as the enteric muscle is intact) but motor activity is disorganized to a greater or lesser extent. There have, however, been few direct assessments of the predictive accuracy of these manometric findings and not all have supported the ability of manometry to reliably differentiate myopathy from neuropathy [10]. Manometry assumes special importance in the differentiation of ED from IBS; here a normal manometric study may assume considerable importance. In the assessment of the patient with suspected CIP or ED the diffuse nature of these disorders, in many instances, must also be borne in mind, and more accessible tests such as esophageal manometry and gastric emptying scintigraphy may provide important corroborative evidence.

Treatment and prevention

The first step in the management of acute megacolon is to search for and, where possible, treat any underlying disorder [4]. Many cases will resolve spontaneously as the associated primary disorder improves; patient positioning may also promote resolution. In resistant cases, therapy should begin with a pharmacological approach.

Cholinergic agonists are effective: in their placebo controlled trial, Ponec and colleagues reported that 10 of their 11 patients who received neostigmine in a dose of 2 mg intravenously had prompt colonic decompression compared with none of the 10 patients who received placebo [11]. The median time for response was 4 minutes.

Given the risk of spontaneous perforation with its associated high mortality, colonoscopy has, for some time, played an important role in the management of patients with megacolon and significant cecal distention. By definition, the colon will not be prepared in these patients and the procedure may, therefore, be technically difficult. An overall success rate in achieving a reduction in cecal diameter of approximately 70% has been reported but the recurrence rate has been as high as

40%. Colonoscopy should be reserved for those who fail conservative therapy in view of its risks in Ogilvie syndrome.

Surgical intervention and the placement of a tube cecostomy, in particular, may become necessary in the patient with megacolon who appears at high risk of perforation and has failed pharmacological and colonoscopic attempts at decompression. Clearly, surgery will also be necessary in those who unfortunately progress to ischemia or perforation. In all of these situations, surgery has been associated with high morbidity and mortality rates.

The management of Hirschsprung's disease and of megacolon related to Chagas disease (see Figure 64.2) is primarily surgical and the approach will depend on the extent of the aganglionic segment. There are few prospective studies of any intervention in the management of other varieties of chronic megacolon; again, the main option is colectomy (see Figure 64.4), which may be indicated on the basis of intractable symptoms and risk of perforation.

Complications and their management

The overall risk of perforation, the main complication of acute megacolon, is low, in the region of 3%, but mortality following perforation, in this context, may be as high as 50%. Cecal diameter is valuable in predicting risk of perforation; a diameter in excess of 9 cm is abnormal and when greater than 12 cm indicates a significant risk of perforation.

Perforation rates in chronic megacolon seem especially low, perhaps reflecting the adaptation of the colon to slow distension; the dilated sigmoid may be prone to volvulus, however.

Small-intestinal bacterial overgrowth (SIBO) is a common complication of CIP, and its assessment and management are dealt with in detail in Chapter 42 of this volume. SIBO together with the patient's inability or reluctance to eat due to the precipitation of symptoms may result in malnutrition and even intestinal failure, a topic dealt with in Chapter 41 of this volume. Home parenteral nutrition may be required [12], and some of these patients may proceed to intestinal transplantation [13]. Considerable excitement surrounds the possibility that enteric nervous system stem cells may provide a curative approach for those with neuropathies [14]. Pharmacological options for the management of CIP have declined with the withdrawal of both cisapride and tegaserod and the application of a "black box" to metoclopramide. Symptomatic therapy remains the order of the day and, typically, will include anti-nausea or anti-emetic preparations (as detailed in Chapters 5 and 37); prokinetic options are confined to cholinomimetics, domperidone and the aforementioned metoclopramide.

References

1. Quigley EM. What we have learned about colonic motility: normal and disturbed. *Curr Opin Gastroenterol.* 2010;26:53–60
2. Ieiri S, Suita S, Nakatsuji T, Akiyoshi J, et al. Total colonic aganglionosis with or without small bowel involvement: a 30-year retrospective nationwide survey in Japan. *J Pediatr Surg.* 2008;43:2226–2230.
3. Quigley EM. Acute intestinal pseudo-obstruction. *Curr Treat Options Gastroenterol.* 2000;3:273–285.
4. Stanghellini V, Cogliandro RF, de Giorgio R, et al. Chronic intestinal pseudo-obstruction: manifestations, natural history and management. *Neurogastroenterol Motil.* 2007;19:440–452.
5. Wingate DL, Hongo M, Kellow JE, et al. Disorders of gastrointestinal motility: towards a new classification. *J Gastroenterol Hepatol.* 2002;17:S1–S14.
6. Lindberg G, Iwarzon M, Tornblom H. Clinical features and long-term survival in chronic intestinal pseudo-obstruction and enteric dysmotility. *Scand J Gastroenterol.* 2009;44:692–699.
7. Lindberg G, Törnblom H, Iwarzon M, et al. Full-thickness biopsy findings in chronic intestinal pseudo-obstruction and enteric dysmotility. *Gut.* 2009;58:1084–1090.
8. Iwarzon M, Gardulf A, Lindberg G. Functional status, health-related quality of life and symptom severity in patients with chronic intestinal pseudo-obstruction and enteric dysmotility. *Scand J Gastroenterol.* 2009;44:700–707.
9. Knowles CH, De Giorgio R, Kapur RP, et al. Gastrointestinal neuromuscular pathology: guidelines for histological techniques and reporting on behalf of the Gastro 2009 International Working Group. *Acta Neuropathol.* 2009;118:271–301.
10. van den Berg MM, Di Lorenzo C, et al. Morphological changes of the enteric nervous system, interstitial cells of cajal, and smooth muscle in children with colonic motility disorders. *J Pediatr Gastroenterol Nutr.* 2009;48:22–29.
11. Ponec RJ, Saunders MD, Kimmey MB. Neostigmine for the treatment of acute colonic pseudo-obstruction. *N Engl J Med.* 1999;341:137–141.
12. Amiot A, Joly F, Alves A, Panis Y, et al. Long-term outcome of chronic intestinal pseudo-obstruction adult patients requiring home parenteral nutrition. *Am J Gastroenterol.* 2009;104:1262–1270.
13. Sauvat F, Grimaldi C, Lacaille F, et al. Intestinal transplantation for total intestinal aganglionosis: a series of 12 consecutive children. *J Pediatr Surg.* 2008;43:1833–1838.
14. Metzger M, Caldwell C, Barlow AJ, et al. Enteric nervous system stem cells derived from human gut mucosa for the treatment of aganglionic gut disorders. *Gastroenterology.* 2009;136:2214–2225.

CHAPTER 65

Splanchnic vascular disorders

J. Hajo van Bockel,[1] Robert H. Geelkerken[2] and Jeroen J. Kolkman[2]

[1]Leiden University Medical Center, Leiden, The Netherlands
[2]Medisch Spectrum Twente, Enschede, The Netherlands

ESSENTIAL FACTS ABOUT PATHOGENESIS

- The intestine receives between 10 and 20% of resting and up to 35% of postprandial cardiac output
- Obstruction of the celiac artery and/or superior mesenteric artery may lead to postprandial splanchnic ischemia
- The gut can compensate by its abundant collateral circulation if obstruction occurs gradually
- Heavy physical exercise can induce symptomatic splanchnic ischemia

ESSENTIALS OF DIAGNOSIS

- The classic triad of postprandial pain, epigastric bruit, and weight loss is present in only a minority of patients with chronic splanchnic ischemia
- A high index of suspicion is required for diagnosis
- Duplex ultrasound, magnetic resonance imaging (MRI), computed tomography (CT) angiography, and gastrointestinal tonometry are useful for assessment of the splanchnic vasculature

ESSENTIALS OF TREATMENT

- Treatment plan should incorporate surgical risk, vascular status, and life expectancy
- The "gold standard" is vascular surgical reconstruction of both the obstructed celiac artery and superior mesenteric artery
- Percutaneous transluminal angioplasty or retrograde endovascular recanalization is preferred in patients with cachexia, comorbidity, or limited life expectancy

Introduction

Splanchnic vascular disorders encompass a spectrum of acute and chronic occlusive and aneurysmal disorders affecting the vessels of the abdominal viscera. Of these relatively uncommon disorders, splanchnic ischemia occurs most frequently. Vascular disorders of the splanchnic circulation are mostly asymptomatic but occasionally catastrophic. Prospective randomized studies on the diagnosis and treatment are not available. Therefore, current opinions on assessing chronic occlusive splanchnic disorders are at best based on prospective cohort studies and personal experience.

Epidemiology

Chronic splanchnic disease is characterized by asymptomatic significant stenosis in the celiac artery (CA), the superior mesenteric artery (SMA), and/or the inferior mesenteric artery (IMA). Atherosclerosis is responsible for most cases. The natural history of chronic splanchnic disease has not been well documented. Most patients will remain asymptomatic but in some the stenosis will progress to occlusion causing chronic or acute splanchnic syndrome with symptoms of intestinal angina.

Anatomy and pathophysiology

An abundant and variable collateral circulation exists between the celiac, superior mesenteric and inferior mesenteric artery. The intestinal villous microvasculature system permits arteriovenous shunting of oxygen, resulting in lower oxygen tension at the tip of the villi than at the base. Consequently, ischemic damage to the intestinal mucosa begins at the tip of the villi and extends toward the base if ischemia is prolonged.

Clinical presentation

Chronic splanchnic syndrome or chronic mesenteric ischemia

Classically, chronic splanchnic syndrome (CSS) results from occlusive disease of splanchnic arteries, which fail to meet the increased metabolic demand after meals. The intestine receives 10–20% of resting and up to 35% of postprandial cardiac output, and 70% of this volume supplies the mucosa. During reduced circulatory volume states, the splanchnic arteries show early and profound vasoconstriction to maintain perfusion of vital organs. This effect is mediated by the adrenergic system, and underlies the non-occlusive mesenteric ischemia (NOMI) that is common in the ICU and peri-operative period. [1] Stimulation of the sympathetic nervous system, and specific medication such as digoxin may have similar effects.

The typical symptoms of CSS involve upper abdominal pain provoked by eating, weight loss due to fear of eating, and pain

---

Textbook of Clinical Gastroenterology and Hepatology, Second Edition. Edited by C. J. Hawkey, Jaime Bosch, Joel E. Richter, Guadalupe Garcia-Tsao, Francis K. L. Chan.
© 2012 Blackwell Publishing Ltd. Published 2012 by Blackwell Publishing Ltd.

on exercise or even mental stress. The typical postprandial pain occurs within the first hour after eating and diminishes within 2 hours. Weight loss is invariably caused by reduction of caloric intake due to fear of eating. Exercise-induced pain is caused by decreased splanchnic blood flow. The classic triad of postprandial pain, epigastric bruit, and weight loss is present in only a minority of patients. Chronic splanchnic syndrome may also appear as unexplained gastroduodenal ulcer disease and (right-sided) ischemic colitis.

A distinction should be made between patients with single-vessel (i.e., occlusive disease of the celiac or superior mesenteric artery) and those with multivessel involvement. The single-vessel disease group is characterized by a relatively low incidence of ischemic symptoms and, after interventions, a very low complication rate and a high success rate. The multivessel disease group is characterized by more pronounced ischemic symptoms. After intervention, there is a significant complication and morbidity rate but also a high success rate, but when left untreated, mortality by bowel infarction as well [2]. Patients with advanced multivessel CSS seem to develop more atypical symptoms including pain not associated with meals, diarrhea, or dyspepsia-like complaints.

Celiac axis compression syndrome
Isolated occlusive disease of the CA is due to compression by the arcuate ligament of the diaphragm, the so-called "celiac axis compression syndrome" or "median arcuate ligament syndrome" (Figure 65.1). The existence of this syndrome was controversial [3]. After open celiac axis revascularization, 83% of the patients were free of symptoms.

Differential diagnosis
Chronic splanchnic syndrome should be considered in patients with unexplained chronic abdominal pain, especially if it occurs postprandially and/or in smokers. Absence of weight loss or a bruit does not exclude this possibility.

Diagnostic methods
Duplex ultrasound
Duplex ultrasound (US) is the most widely used screening tool for detection of splanchnic arterial stenosis. The physiological differences between patients and inherent technical difficulties make splanchnic duplex US results difficult to interpret. The influence of respiration, meal, exercise, anatomic variations, and collateral circulation on commonly used duplex US parameters has not been clarified. There is poor correlation of anatomical information and abdominal symptoms. Consequently, if duplex US clearly demonstrates significant stenosis in the CA and SMA origins, this may not be sufficient evidence for the existence of chronic splanchnic syndrome.

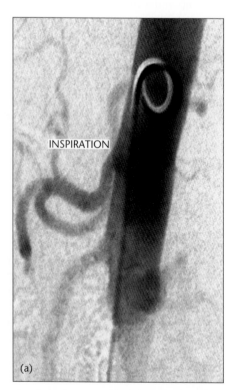
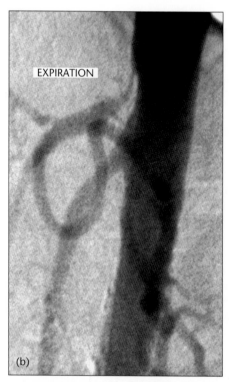

Figure 65.1 Lateral aortal angiography in celiac artery compression syndrome. Normal celiac artery in inspiration (a) and 95% celiac artery stenoses in expiration (b), when the celiac artery is pulled up towards the median arcuate ligament.

Magnetic resonance angiography

Contrast-enhanced magnetic resonance angiography (MRA) can visualize the celiac, superior mesenteric artery, and inferior mesenteric artery in a single breath-hold of 20–25 seconds. The data can be reconstructed in any desired plane. The orifices of the splanchnic vessels can therefore always be visualized with MRA.

Functional magnetic resonance imaging

With functional magnetic resonance imaging (fMRI), functional information on splanchnic blood flow can also be obtained. Flow velocities and total flow volumes can be measured in the mesenteric vessels using two-dimensional cine phase contrast velocity mapping.

Computed tomography angiography

Computed tomography (CT) angiography is increasingly used for visualization of the splanchnic arteries. When using multislice technology with a slice thickness of 1–2 mm, it combines excellent spatial resolution, assessment of collaterals with low invasiveness, and the detection of alternative diagnoses. In most cases it can be used for revascularization planning and be an alternative for visceral angiography. The main drawback of CT angiography is the high radiation burden [4,5].

Tonometry

Tonometry is based on a general characteristic of ischemic tissues in which lack of oxygen results in increased production of acids, which are buffered locally leading to increased PCO_2 (Figure 65.2). CO_2 rapidly diffuses over different membrane layers, therefore a luminal PCO_2 will equal mucosal PCO_2. Interestingly, mucosal ischemia is invariably associated with increased gastrointestinal PCO_2. The latter can be measured using a balloon-tipped catheter, the tonometer, attached to a modified capnograph, the Tonocap. An increased PCO_2 gradient between the systemic circulation and the gastrointestinal mucosa indicates mucosal CO_2 production and therefore ischemia [6]. Ischemia can be provoked by meal ingestion or submaximal exercise.

Angiography

Digital subtraction angiography (DSA) of the splanchnic circulation is still considered the gold standard for assessment of vascular anatomy and relevant stenoses in the splanchnic vessels (Figure 65.3). For diagnostic purposes DSA has been replaced by CT angiography in many centers. Now, angiography is currently almost exclusively used during intervention.

Multidisciplinary approach

A reliable diagnosis of chronic splanchnic syndrome, based on a proven causal relationship between the occlusive disease and the symptoms, can be very difficult. Apart from precise anatomic information on the vasculature, functional proof of ischemia is required. Currently, only tonometry has proven diagnostic accuracy for that purpose. A multidisciplinary

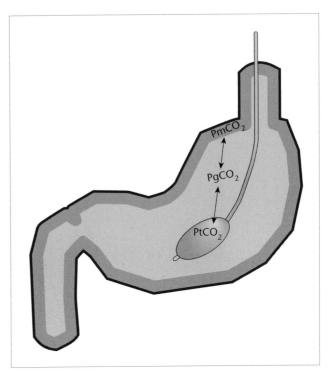

Figure 65.2 Scheme of gastric tonometry. CO_2 diffuses rapidly over different membranes, therefore the tonometer PCO_2 ($PtCO_2$) will be in equilibrium with gastric luminal PCO_2 ($PgCO_2$) and mucosal PCO_2 ($PmCO_2$). The PCO_2 can be measured from the catheter either from injected saline using blood gas analyzers or by gas analysis using modified capnopgraphs. The underlying physiological principle is that ischemia is always associated with increased mucosal PCO_2.

approach including the gastroenterologist, vascular surgeon, and interventional radiologist can be of value in interpretation of symptoms and tests, and agreeing a management plan.

Treatment and prevention
Chronic splanchnic syndrome or chronic mesenteric ischemia

Conservative medical treatment such as eating more and smaller meals, using proton pump inhibitors to diminish the oxygen demand of the gastric mucosa, refraining from smoking, and using vasodilative drugs to diminish vasospasm are often used. The effect of these therapies is unknown.

A variety of surgical and endovascular techniques, such as re-implantation, transarterial and transaortic endarterectomy, antegrade and retrograde aortovisceral bypass using vein or arterial autograft bypasses and prosthetic bypasses, have been advocated for repairing the splanchnic vessels (Figure 65.4). However, the efficacy for the various techniques is usually based on local experience rather than evidence. The best long-term results are reported from surgical repair of more than one artery [7,8]. Percutaneous transluminal angioplasty is gaining favor, with reports of similar secondary patency achieved compared to open repair but with lower morbidity (Figure 65.5). The current approach is "best breed:" endovascular

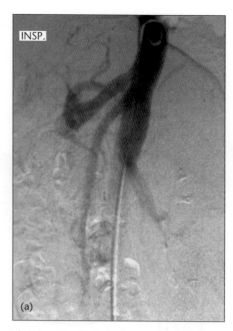
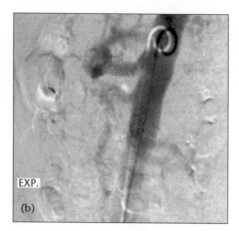

Figure 65.3 Lateral aortal angiography. Normal celiac artery and superior mesenteric artery in inspiration (a) and 70% stenoses in expiration (b).

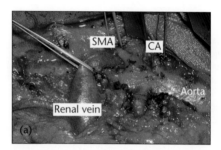
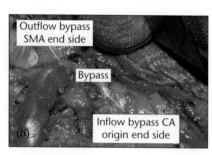
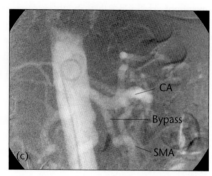

Figure 65.4 In-vivo view of the celiac and proximal part of superior mesenteric artery after left retroperitoneal visceral rotation (a), and in-vivo autologous bypass to celiac and superior mesenteric artery (b). Post-reconstruction lateral aortal angiography (c).

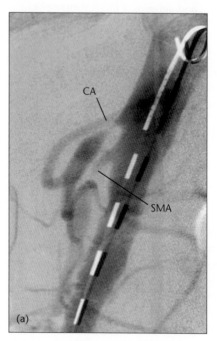
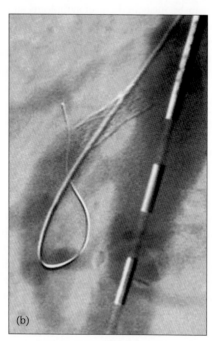
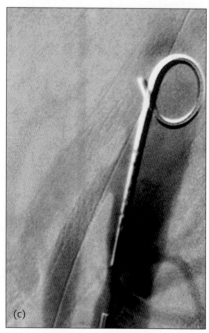

Figure 65.5 Lateral aortal angiography. Two-vessel chronic splanchnic syndrome. (a) Severe stenoses in celiac and superior mesenteric artery. Bridge® stents in the celiac (b) and the superior mesenteric artery (c).

treatment with minor morbidity, albeit a lower patency on long term follow-up in case of high cardiopulmonary risk, elderly age, cachexia, or hostile abdomen [7,9]. Operative repair, more demanding for patients but with a proven excellent long-term patency is clearly the superior option for relatively young and vital patients.

Celiac axis compression syndrome

The surgical treatment of celiac artery compression syndrome consists of decompression of the celiac artery at the diaphragm. Intraoperative duplex evaluation is essential to detect irreversible stenosis. The latter can only be treated by vascular reconstruction. Recently, release of the arcuate ligament can be performed laparoscopically or endoscopically. Stent placement should not be performed since repeated pressure from the arcuate ligament with each respiratory cycle damages metal stents.

References

1. Kolkman JJ, Mensink PB. Non-occlusive mesenteric ischaemia: a common disorder in gastroenterology and intensive care. *Best Pract Res Clin Gastroenterol.* 2003;17:457–473.

2. Mensink PB, van Petersen AS, Geelkerken RH, Otte JA, Huisman AB, Kolkman JJ. Clinical significance of splanchnic artery stenosis. *Br J Surg.* 2006;93:1377–1382.

3. Holland AJ, Ibach EG. Long-term review of coeliac axis compression syndrome. *Ann R Coll Surg Engl.* 1996;78:470–472.

4. Horton KM, Fishman EK. Multidetector CT angiography in the diagnosis of mesenteric ischemia. *Radiol Clin North Am.* 2007;45:275–288.

5. Iannaccone R, Laghi A, Passariello R. Multislice CT angiography of mesenteric vessels. *Abdom Imaging.* 2004;29:146–152.

6. Kolkman JJ, Otte JA, Groeneveld AB. Gastrointestinal luminal PCO2 tonometry: an update on physiology, methodology and clinical applications. *Br J Anaesth.* 2000;84:74–86.

7. van Petersen AS, Kolkman JJ, Beuk RJ, Huisman AB, Doelman CJ, Geelkerken RH. Open or percutaneous revascularization for chronic splanchnic syndrome. *J Vasc Surg.* 2010;51:1309–1316.

8. Geelkerken RH, Van Bockel JH, De Roos WK, Hermans J, Terpstra JL. Chronic mesenteric vascular syndrome. Results of reconstructive surgery. *Arch Surg.* 1991;126:1101–1106.

9. Davies RS, Wall ML, Silverman SH, *et al.* Surgical versus endovascular reconstruction for chronic mesenteric ischemia: a contemporary UK series. *Vasc Endovascular Surg.* 2009;43:157–164.

Small and Large Bowel

CHAPTER 66

Drug-induced damage to the small and large intestine

Ingvar Bjarnason, Zeino Zeino and Guy Sisson

King's College Hospital, London, UK

ESSENTIAL FACTS ABOUT PATHOGENESIS

- Drug use is second only to infectious diseases as a cause of diarrhea
- NSAID enteropathy is the most common of the drug-induced small bowel diseases
- The combined effect of inhibition of COX-1 and COX-2 and a topical effect increase intestinal permeability leading to intestinal inflammation and ulcers
- NSAIDs are a risk factor for clinical relapse in patients with inflammatory bowel disease (IBD) and diverticular complications and may cause a drug-related colitis *de novo*

ESSENTIALS OF DIAGNOSIS

- Drug causes of intestinal disease are often missed: a high index of suspicion is important
- This should include:
  - **Diarrhea:** proton pump inhibitors, aminosalicylates, beta blockers, other cardiac drugs, and statins
  - **Constipation:** tricyclic anti-depressants, anti-cholinergics, anti-parkinsonian drugs and opiates
  - **Colitis:** antibiotics, chemotherapeutic agents, NSAIDs, penicillamine, oral gold, micophenolate
- Presentation with NSAIDs:
  - Classically: asymptomatic +/− iron deficiency anemia and/or hypoalbuminemia
  - Rarely: gastrointestinal bleeding, intestinal perforation, or small-bowel obstruction
- Diagnosis of NSAID enteropathy is best made by capsule or other enteroscopy

ESSENTIALS OF TREATMENT

- Most symptoms resolve on drug withdrawal
- For NSAIDs a COX-2 selective agent avoids most of the associated intestinal toxicity
- Surgery may be required for the serious complications of NSAID-enteropathy

Introduction and epidemiology

The gastrointestinal tract is a frequent site for adverse drug reactions and may account for 20–40% of all drug-induced side effects [1]. This may be by virtue of the fact that most drugs are ingested, exposing both the stomach and small bowel to high concentrations of drugs. However, other routes of administration are not without intestinal complications, for example, peptic ulceration from topical non-steroidal anti-inflammatory gels or debilitating diarrhea following intravenous systemic chemotherapy.

Small- and large-bowel side effects of drugs may manifest in a variety of ways and can even mimic symptoms suggestive of malignancy. The most important issue in diagnosis is awareness. There may be a strong temporal association between ingestion of the drug and symptoms (e.g., acute constipation with codeine-containing analgesics) in which case a detailed knowledge of the pharmacologic action of the drug will alert to this possibility. In other cases, when drugs cause structural damage – e.g., non-steroidal anti inflammatory drug (NSAID) enteropathy – the temporal relationship between ingestion and symptoms is delayed and knowledge of the anticipated side effects is essential. Some drugs are notorious for aggravating underlying pathology (e.g., tricyclic anti-depressants increase the severity of constipation in Parkinson's disease) and some side effects may be idiosyncratic.

Small intestinal disease

The approach to the diagnosis of drug induces symptoms depends on the cause. It is particularly important to note that if the side effects are pharmacological it is sufficient to discontinue the drug or counteract its action; endoscopy, in one form or another, or intestinal functional tests are useful when structural disease is suspected. However the precise mechanism of damage is almost always complex involving numerous biochemical and physiological pathways.

The most common types of drug-induced problems are due to their propensity to cause **mucosal damage**. This damage is

Textbook of Clinical Gastroenterology and Hepatology, Second Edition. Edited by C. J. Hawkey, Jaime Bosch, Joel E. Richter, Guadalupe Garcia-Tsao, Francis K. L. Chan.
© 2012 Blackwell Publishing Ltd. Published 2012 by Blackwell Publishing Ltd.

Table 66.1 Drugs causing small (and sometimes large) intestinal mucosal ulceration and hemorrhage

- NSAIDs
- Potassium
- Cocaine
- Chemotherapeutic agents (to name a few):
  - Actinomycin D
  - Bleomycin
  - Cytosine
  - Arabinoside
  - Doxorubicin
  - 5-Fluorouracil
  - Methotrexate
  - Vincristine
  - Docetaxel and paclitaxel
  - Irinotecan
- Oral contraceptive pills
- Gold
- Arsenic

characterized by inflammation sometimes associated with malabsorption, bleeding, and protein loss, which may progress to ulceration, which is in turn associated with serious complications such as perforation, overt bleeding, and strictures. Table 66.1 shows the drugs that are most commonly associated with de-novo small-bowel mucosal damage.

Potassium salts are now formulated in such a way as to minimize the risk of mucosal damage (e.g., a controlled-release wax matrix system). **Oral contraceptive pills** may rarely cause mesenteric venous and arterial thrombosis, which lead to ischemia and necrosis of the small bowel. **Chemotherapeutic agents** affect cells with a rapid turnover, including those of the gastrointestinal tract, and can cause erosive enteritis, features of which include pain, bleeding, ileus, diarrhea, and vomiting. Apart from NSAIDs, serious outcomes are unusual with these drugs.

NSAID enteropathy (see Chapter 25)

NSAID-enteropathy is a prototype for drug-induced mucosal damage.

Conventional NSAIDs that inhibit **cyclo-oxygenase** (COX) 1 and 2 frequently cause damage through the gastrointestinal tract [2,3]. The stomach is often adversely affected (NSAID gastropathy) [4], but NSAID enteropathy is equally prevalent [4] and is associated with almost identical serious outcomes [5].

Pathogenesis

Almost all the information on the pathogenesis of NSAID enteropathy comes from studies in rodents. We can take the prevailing and **simplistic view** [6] that NSAID-induced COX-1 inhibition causes damage because this leads to very low levels of mucosal prostaglandins that are essential for the maintenance of intestinal integrity. Alternatively, we can explore the pathogenesis further in and the situation is rather more

complex. The single most important point is that selective COX-1 inhibition or absence (COX-1 knockout animals) appears to have no pathophysiological consequences, and does not lead to gastrointestinal damage [3]. Rather, NSAIDs initiate small-bowel damage by a **combination of different biochemical actions**, namely various combinations of the topical effect, COX-1 inhibition, and COX-2 inhibition [2,3].

How the damage develops is a matter of controversy. One suggestion is that the biochemical effects of these drugs lead to cellular damage, which is then relayed over to tissue damage. Hence the topical effect damages with the epithelial cells occur via an interaction with surface membrane lipid [7] or an effect to uncouple mitochondrial **oxidative phosphorylation** (leading to depletion of cellular ATP) [5]. At the same time the primary pathophysiologic consequence of COX-1 inhibition (and decreased prostaglandins) is a compromise in the microcirculation to the mucosa with impaired oxygenation, which causes or exacerbates reductions in cellular ATP. Given the cellular damage this leads to tissue damage, relayed through increased intestinal permeability. This shifts the balance between the luminal aggressors and mucosal defense in favor of the former, which allows **commensal luminal bacteria** access to the mucosa. This elicits an inflammatory neutrophil response. The neutrophils are activated on contact with the bacteria and undergo a **respiratory burst** and degranulation, both of which damage the surrounding tissue. COX-2 inhibition may then play a significant role by compromising inflammatory responses and resolution.

Prevalence and diagnosis

Fifty to sixty per cent of patients receiving conventional NSAIDs develop NSAID enteropathy within a few weeks of ingestion. The prevalence and severity of the inflammation is similar with all the acidic NSAIDs. NSAID enteropathy is characterized by **low-grade inflammation** and it is predominantly mid small intestine in location. This inflammation can be documented with the use of intestinal **permeability tests** or with stool markers such as **fecal calprotectin** concentrations [8], but these markers of damage are not specific for NSAIDs.

Video capsule endoscopy (see Chapter 128) is now the preferred method for the non-invasive diagnosis of NSAID enteropathy [9]. The appearances of damage vary. Firstly, there may be scattered **petechiae** with or without evidence of intraluminal blood. Secondly, there are distinct mucosal lesions comprising ulcers and erosions collectively known as "**mucosal breaks**." These mucosal breaks (Figure 66.1) are sometimes seen to bleed. In some patients on conventional NSAIDs there is evidence of semilunar diaphragms (Figure 66.2). These represent the early developmental phase of "**diaphragm disease**," one of the serious outcomes of NSAID enteropathy (Figure 66.3) [10]. Even when strictures and ulcers are present there is usually insufficient distortion for these to be detected by barium studies. Double balloon or Sonde enteroscopy play a very limited role in the diagnosis.

Small and Large Bowel

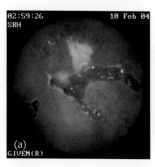 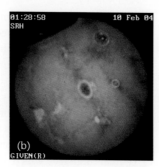

Figure 66.1 Video capsule endoscopic image in a patient on non-steroidal anti-inflammatory drugs (NSAIDs) who presented with abdominal pain and a mild anemia. (a) There is a clear-cut small bowel ulcer with a white base. (b) There is an erosion at 7 o'clock with a linear ulcer. These appearances are not easily distinguishable from that seen in Crohn's disease.

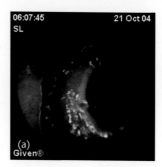 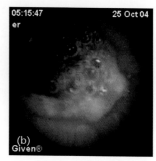

Figure 66.2 Video capsule endoscopic images of "diaphragm" strictures that are pathognomonic for NSAID-induced damage. (a) A semilunar diaphragm with a leading edge of inflammation (circular ulcer) which represents an early stage of fully developed NSAID-induced "diaphragm" disease. (b) A fully developed "diaphragm" stricture of the small bowel whereby the capsule image shows the circular ulcer and proximal fluid accumulation (which bubbles). The capsule may not pass and, in these cases, patients have presented with symptoms of intermittent subacute small bowel obstruction.

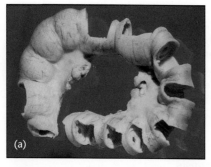 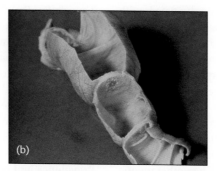 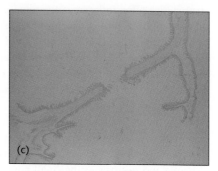

Figure 66.3 "Diaphragm" disease of the small bowel. The surgical resection specimens in parts (a) and (b) were inflated with formalin under pressure. (a) Patient on long-term NSAIDs presented with symptoms of subacute small bowel obstruction and underwent laparotomy. A segment of small bowel was resected. The exterior shows regular and multiple dimples and when opened up these represent the "diaphragms" with marked luminal compromise. (b) Surgical resection specimen from a patient on NSAIDs who presented with complete obstruction. There is prestenotic dilation of the bowel to a concentric "diaphragm" that has closed the lumen to a pinhole. (c) Characteristic histopathology of NSAID-induced "diaphragm" disease of the small bowel. The diaphragm is composed of mucosal fibrosis with minimal acute inflammation at the lesion tip. The muscularis propria is not seen within the diaphragm (which would be pathognomonic of congenital developmental abnormalities).

Complications

NSAID enteropathy, despite being associated with erosions and ulcers, is probably asymptomatic, although many patients on NSAIDs have symptoms reminiscent of **irritable bowel syndrome** (Chapter 62). Many clinicians do not therefore perceive it as a clinical problem. However, the consequences of this pathology can lead to management problems and the serious events of perforation, overt bleeding, and strictures mandate case-specific treatment.

Bleeding

Figure 66.4 shows that virtually all patients with NSAID enteropathy bleed and there is a significant correlation between the inflammation and bleeding. This bleeding is mild, ranging from 1 to 8 mL/day, which by itself is usually insufficient to lead to an **iron deficiency anemia** [11]. However, in patients with active rheumatoid arthritis who may have an impaired appetite, hypochlorhydria (due to co-treatment with proton pump inhibitors, etc.), or malabsorption of iron the low-grade bleeding may be an important contributory factor for the development of iron deficiency anemia. The iron deficiency is difficult to diagnose (may require bone marrow examination) as the normal blood film appearances (hypochromic microcytosis) are overshadowed by the features seen in the **anemia of chronic disease** (normochromic macrocytosis). Many rheumatologists have a rule of thumb to **initiate iron supplementation** in their rheumatoid patients when the hemoglobin level falls below 10 g/L. However oral iron supplementation is often tolerated badly (abdominal pain and constipation) and intravenous iron must be administered with great caution in patients with inflammatory arthropathies. **Video capsule endoscopy** is the preferred technique to provide a positive diagnosis.

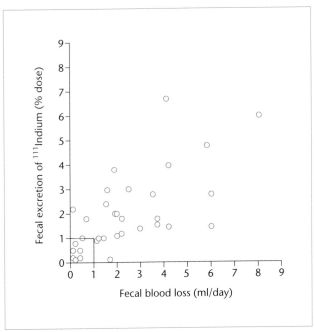

Figure 66.4 Intestinal inflammation and blood loss. Patients with rheumatoid and osteoarthritis on long-term NSAIDs underwent simultaneous study to assess intestinal inflammation (indium-111-labeled white cell fecal excretion) and blood loss (chromium-51-labeling of red cells). There is a significant correlation between the intestinal inflammatory activity and the intestinal bleeding. Patients with no inflammation (white cell excretion of less than 1%) do not bleed excessively (normal blood loss of less than 1 mL/day). (Reproduced with permission from Hayllar J, et al. Nonsteroidal antiinflammatory drug-induced small intestinal inflammation and blood loss. Effects of sulfasalazine and other disease-modifying antirheumatic drugs. *Arthr Rheum.* 1994;37:1146–1150.)

Protein loss

Most of the patients with NSAID enteropathy have a mild **protein-losing enteropathy** of little clinical significance as the liver has a substantial reserve capacity to produce albumin. However, about 10% of hospitalized patients with rheumatoid arthritis have symptomatic (peripheral edema, congestive heart failure, and even ascites) **hypoalbuminemia** as a complication of NSAID enteropathy, in which case targeted treatment for the enteropathy is called for.

Serious outcomes

Serious outcomes are defined as overt bleeding, perforation, and strictures usually originating from ulcers. The prevalence of these complications in NSAID-induced gastropathy and enteropathy are very similar with absolute annual prevalence rates of about 1%. Clinically, overt rectal bleeding may occur from discrete small-bowel ulcers and these are diagnosed by angiography and usually require surgery. **Small-bowel perforation**, presenting as an acute abdomen, is also perceived as a rare complication of NSAID enteropathy, and also requires immediate surgery. It is also worrying that a large autopsy study showed that some patients on NSAIDs had an unexpected (undiagnosed) perforated small-bowel ulcer that had contributed to their death [12].

"**Diaphragm**" **disease** of the small bowel is found in 1–2% of long term users of NSAIDs. These are multiple (ranging from 3 to over 100), concentric, thin (2–3 mm), fibrous septa that may narrow the lumen to a pinhole (see Figure 66.3). An increasing number is being described at colonoscopy (cecum and right colon) in patients on sustained release formulations of NSAIDs. Most patients with "diaphragm" strictures have had recurrent iron deficiency **anemia** and at times **hypoalbuminemia**, suggestive of a severe NSAID enteropathy. They present with symptoms of intermittent **sub-acute small-bowel obstruction**, i.e., postprandial pain, nausea, and vomiting. Conventional small-bowel barium studies do not show these strictures with any consistency. **Capsule enteroscopy**, however, shows the early lesions of semilunar diaphragms (see Figure 66.3) or the classical fully developed stricture (Figure 66.2b)

Treatment

When NSAID enteropathy leads to problematic **iron deficiency** or **hypoalbuminemia** this should be treated according to conventional lines, such as iron supplementation, but consideration should also be given to treating the **intestinal inflammation** itself. As yet there are only uncontrolled comparative efficacy trials for NSAID enteropathy [5].

The following **algorithm** is largely based on personal experience. The first line approach is to **discontinue** NSAIDs if possible. Treatment with **metronidazole** (any anaerobic antimicrobial is likely to be effective) 400 mg twice a day for 4 to 6 weeks reduces the inflammation, bleeding, and protein loss, even if patients continue their NSAID intake. The effectiveness of the treatment can be monitored with serial **fecal calprotectin** measurements. Serum albumin levels, if low, usually start improving after 2 to 3 weeks of treatment, but the benefit for

Table 66.2 Drugs causing mucosal hemorrhage

- Anticoagulants
- Antiplatelet drugs
- Thrombolytic drugs
- Glycogen IIb/IIIa inhibitors
- Levodopa

Table 66.3 Drugs causing malabsorption

Mucosal damage
- Allopurinol
- Colchicine
- Methotrexate
- Methyldopa
- Metformin
- Neomycin
- NSAIDs
- Chemotherapeutic agents

Interaction
- Tetracycline chelates calcium
- Cholestyramine binds iron and vitamin B$_{12}$
- Thiazides impair Na$^+$ transport
- Aluminum and magnesium hydroxides precipitate calcium and phosphate ions
- Lipase inhibitors (used for weight control) interfere with ingested lipid digestion
- α-glucosidase inhibitors (used in diabetics) interferes with carbohydrate digestion

hemoglobin levels is not immediately evident unless iron supplements are also given. Where patients wish to continue their NSAIDs, we consider treatment with **sulfasalazine** 1 g three times a day for the long term. Alternatively, misoprostol (200 µg 3 to 4 times a day) can be given to heal or prevent the enteropathy. Consideration of prescribing COX-2 selective agents should be made at an early stage. These drugs are free of small-intestinal side effects when taken short term and safer than NSAIDs when taken long term.

The serious consequences of NSAID enteropathy (overt bleeding, perforation, and strictures) need to be dealt with as a matter of urgency and by surgery.

Summary

Conventional acidic NSAIDs frequently cause small-bowel inflammation. Investigation of NSAID enteropathy provides a blueprint for the investigation of the other drug-induced small bowel damage.

Other (non-NSAID) drug-induced injury of the small and large intestine

The clinical impact of adverse effects on the small and large intestine should not be underestimated and although we have placed certain drugs under a specific heading there is a significant variability in how patients may present.

Hemorrhage

A variety of drugs can give rise to intestinal bleeding (Table 66.2) usually by virtue of interfering with hemostatic mechanisms and without discrete mucosal lesions. The risk of bleeding is dependent on a number of factors that include drug dose, clotting parameters, concomitant medications, and comorbid disorders. **Warfarin**, in particular, is notorious for causing overt gastrointestinal bleeding. In half of such cases, the bleeding site will be in the small bowel. Diagnosis is by capsule enteroscopy, but a specific lesion may not be seen. Rarely, these drugs cause intramucosal hematomas that can present with obstructive symptoms.

Malabsorption (and maldigestion)

Drugs may have a direct effect on intestinal mucosa causing a generalized impairment of absorption or they may interact with particular absorption pathways leading to selective malabsorption (both concepts may involve maldigestion). Table 66.3 lists the drugs more commonly associated with this pathology. Some of the drugs that cause mucosal damage and

malabsorption interfere with **cell mitoses** and may cause subtotal or partial **villous atrophy**. This may manifest as an iron deficiency anemia, low serum folates, or even hypocalcemia. Fat malabsorption presenting as mild steatorrhea may also be a presenting feature.

Motility

Small-bowel motility may be influenced by drugs but to a lesser extent than the colon (see Chapter 139). Table 66.4 shows drugs that are commonly associated with motility problems of both the small and large intestine. Increased motility of the small bowel may result in **diarrhea** (see Chapter 6), although clinically it may be difficult to tell whether such symptoms are, in fact, attributable to small- or large-intestinal pathology. Increased motility may be the result of interference with the normal fluid and electrolyte balance of the gut. **Magnesium salts** predictably cause an osmotic diarrhea as do the laxatives lactulose and polyethylene glycol. **Digoxin** inhibits the sodium–potassium pump involved in the active transport of water and electrolytes across the cell membrane and occasionally leads to problematic diarrhea. A drug-induced neuropathy may produce profuse diarrhea similar to that seen in diabetic autonomic neuropathy; **vincristine** has been associated with such a phenomenon. Beta blockers are an often missed cause of diarrhoea.

Drugs may also reduce motility. Occasionally, this may be so severe as to cause a paralytic ileus. **Tricyclic antidepressants** and **loperamide** are good examples of such a drug reaction. The antimuscarinic, **antiparkinsonian drugs** such as benzhexol, benzatropine, and orphenadrine frequently inhibit motility contributing to severe constipation (see Chapter 61) whereas the **dopaminergic, antiparkinsonian drugs** selegiline and entacapone may cause either diarrhea or constipation. Interestingly, levodopa appears to have no adverse effect on

Table 66.4 Drugs affecting intestinal motility

Increased motility (diarrhea)	Decreased motility (constipation)
Gastrointestinal drugs	**Anticholinergic pharmacology**
Laxatives	Anticholinergic drugs
Magnesium antacids	Tricyclic antidepressants
Misoprostol	Antiparkinsonian drugs
Proton pump inhibitors	Atropine
5-amino salicylates	Hyoscine
Cardiac drugs	**Other drugs**
Beta blockers	Opiate drugs
Digitalis	Vincristine
Quinidine	Sucralfate
Procainamide	Aluminum/calcium antacids
Diuretics	Calcium channel blockers
ACE inhibitors	Cholestyramine
Hydralazine	
Lipid-lowering drugs	
Clofibrate	
Gemfibrozil	
Statins N	
Europsychiatric drugs	
Lithium	
Fluoxetine	
Sodium valproate	
Ethosuximide	
Miscellaneous	
NSAIDs	
Thyroxine	
Colchicine	
Theophylline	
Chemotherapeutic agents	

Table 66.5 Drugs that cause colitis

Antibiotics
- Amoxicillin
- Ampicillin
- Clindamycin
- Erythromycin
- Cephalosporins

Drugs causing ischemic colitis
- Oral contraceptive pill
- Chemotherapeutic agents – 5-fluorouracil, cisplatin
- Danazol
- Vasopressin
- Clindamycin

Miscellaneous
- NSAIDs
- Methyldopa
- Penicillamine
- Gold (oral)

gut motility. Usually, cessation of the drug results in resolution of the dysmotility and symptoms. However, this may not be practicable, in particular with the constipation seen in Parkinson's disease, and patients are frequently prescribed drugs to combat constipation.

Large intestinal disease

Drug-induced colonic disease is not as common as that of the small bowel, presumably as most drugs are completely absorbed before reaching the colon. There are isolated case reports of drugs causing colitis but motility problems may be more common.

Colitis

Antibiotics commonly cause diarrhea but a more serious adverse effect is **pseudomembranous colitis** (see Chapter 54). Originally attributed to clindamycin, although virtually any antibiotic can cause it, pseudomembranous colitis is the result of *Clostridium difficile* overgrowth of the colon when such broad-spectrum antibiotics have killed the normal flora. *Clostridium difficile* produces a toxin that causes diarrhea; the most severe form of the disease is colitis. The antibiotics more

commonly associated with pseudomembranous colitis are listed in Table 66.5. Apart from NSAIDs, which have already been discussed and frequently cause proctitis when give as a suppository (and may cause strictures), drug-induced colitis is rarely seen in clinical practice. Drug-induced colitis can usually be distinguished from classical inflammatory bowel disease (ulcerative colitis and Crohn's disease) by endoscopic and histologic features and by elimination of suspect drugs.

Dysmotility

Many of the agents shown in Table 66.4 that affect the small bowel, giving rise to diarrhea or constipation, also affect the colon. Of note, however, is the excessive use of laxatives. Apart from the diarrhea that may be provoked by their use (or misuse), anthraquinones such as senna can damage the myenteric plexus of the colon when used chronically, although whether the association is causal is now questioned (see Chapter 64). This atonic (cathartic) colon can result in constipation often resulting in the use of further purgatives. Long-term anthraquinone use can also lead to melanosis coli.

Conclusion

A number of commonly used drugs are associated with gastrointestinal side effects that may cause symptoms suggestive of serious underlying disease. In many cases it is sufficient to discontinue the drug and switch to another drug with a similar action. When the drugs have caused structural damage it may also be necessary to treat the inflammation or ulcers.

With the increased use of drugs in the aging population and increasing tendency for prescribing multiple drugs in the long term, it is likely that the side effects discussed in this chapter will become more frequent. Furthermore, there are a number of considerations when the above drugs are used in patients with pre-existing disease. For instance, in patients with ulcerative colitis and Crohn's disease, it may be prudent to avoid NSAIDs (may cause clinical relapse of disease) and the choice of chemotherapeutic agents in those that develop extraintestinal malignancy requires special consideration. Patients with a history of diverticulitis should avoid NSAIDs as these drugs predispose to diverticular complications.

References

1. Geboes K, De Hertogh G, Ectors N. Drug-induced pathology in the large intestine. *Curr Diagn Pathol.* 2006;12:239–247.
2. Wallace JL, McKnight W, Reuter BK, Vergnolle N. Dual inhibition of both cyclooxygenase (COX)-1 and COX-2 is required for NSAID induced erosion formation. *Gastroenterology.* 2000;119: 704–714.
3. Sigthorsson G, Simpson RJ, Walley M, *et al.* COX-1 and 2, intestinal integrity and pathogenesis of NSAID enteropathy in mice. *Gastroenterology.* 2002;122:1913–1923.
4. Hawkey CJ. Nonsteroidal anti-inflammatory drug gastropathy. *Gastroenterology.* 2000;119:521–535.
5. Bjarnason I, Hayllar J, Macpherson AJ, Russell AS. Side effects of nonsteroidal anti-inflammatory drugs on the small and large intestine. *Gastroenterology.* 1993;104:1832–1847.
6. Hawkey CJ. COX-2 inhibitors. *Lancet.* 1999;353:301–314.
7. Lichtenberger LM, Zhou Y, Dial EJ, Raphael RM. NSAID injury to the gastrointestinal tract: evidence that NSAIDs interact with phospholipids to weaken the hydrophobic surface barrier and induce the formation of unstable pores in membranes. *J Pharm Pharmacol.* 2006;58:1421–1428.
8. Tibble J, Sigthorsson G, Foster R, *et al.* Faecal calprotectin: A simple method for the diagnosis of NSAID-induced enteropathy. *Gut.* 1999;45:362–366.
9. Maiden L, Thjodleifsson B, Seigal A, *et al.* Long-term effects of nonsteroidal anti-inflammatory drugs and cyclooxygenase-2 selective agents on the small bowel: a cross-sectional capsule enteroscopy study. *Clin Gastroenterol Hepatol.* 2007;5:1040–1045.
10. Bjarnason I, Zanelli G, Smethurst P, *et al.* Clinico-pathological features of nonsteroidal antiinflammatory drug-induced small intestinal strictures. *Gastroenterology.* 1988;94:1070–1074.
11. Hayllar J, Price AB, Smith T, *et al.* Nonsteroidal antiinflammatory drug-induced small intestinal inflammation and blood loss: effect of sulphasalazine and other disease modifying drugs. *Arthr Rheum.* 1994;37:1146–1150.
12. Allison MC, Howatson AG, Torrance CJ, Lee FD, Russell RI. Gastrointestinal damage associated with the use of nonsteroidal antiinflammatory drugs. *N Engl J Med.* 1992;327:749–754.

Small and Large Bowel

CHAPTER 67

Acute appendicitis

John Simpson and David J. Humes

Nottingham University Hospitals, Nottingham, UK

ESSENTIAL FACTS OF PATHOGENESIS

- The etiology of appendicitis is unknown
- The condition most often occurs in the first and second decade of life but no age is exempt
- The condition is more common in males than females (1.4:1)
- The incidence of appendicitis and appendicectomy rates have fallen over the last two decades

ESSENTIALS OF DIAGNOSIS

- The diagnosis of appendicitis is essentially clinical and rarely requires specialist investigation
- Simple bedside and laboratory tests should be used to exclude other pathologies and provide additional evidence to support the clinical diagnosis
- In cases of diagnostic uncertainty computed tomography has a higher sensitivity and specificity than ultrasound scanning
- Magnetic resonance imaging is used in those patients where radiation exposure would not be acceptable, for example, pregnancy

ESSENTIALS OF TREATMENT

- Antibiotics should be commenced once a diagnosis is made
- Surgery should be undertaken without delay once a diagnosis is made
- The choice of laparoscopic or open surgery depends on the facilities available and the surgeon's experience

TERMINOLOGY

- Simple appendicitis – inflamed appendix, in the absence of gangrene, perforation, or abscess around the appendix
- Complicated appendicitis – perforated or gangrenous appendicitis or the presence of periappendicular abscess
- Negative appendicectomy – term used for an operation performed for suspected appendicitis, in which the appendix is found to be normal on histological evaluation

Introduction

Acute appendicitis is the most common surgical condition requiring emergency surgery. It results from inflammation of the vermiform appendix, which is a tubular structure attached to the base of the cecum at the confluence of the taeniae coli.

Many patients present with a typical history and examination findings and the diagnosis is predominantly a clinical one. Appendicectomy is the treatment of choice and is increasingly performed as a laparoscopic procedure. This chapter reviews the presentation, investigation, treatment, and complications of acute appendicitis and appendicectomy.

Epidemiology

Appendicitis is the most common abdominal emergency and accounts for more than 280 000 surgical operations in the United States per annum [1]. Despite over a century of research, the exact etiology of the condition is unknown but is probably multifactorial with luminal obstruction and dietary and familial factors having all been suggested [2]. Appendicitis most commonly occurs between the ages of 10 and 20 years but no age is exempt [3]. There is a male preponderance with a male to female ratio of 1.4:1 and the overall lifetime risk is 8.6% for males and 6.7% for females in the United States [3]. Over recent decades, there has been a declining trend in the appendicitis and appendicectomy rates but the reasons behind this are unknown [4,5].

Diagnosis

The diagnosis of acute appendicitis necessitates a thorough history and examination [6].

History

Patients with acute appendicitis present primarily with abdominal pain. Murphy initially described the diagnostic sequence of colicky central abdominal pain, followed by vomiting with migration of the pain to the right iliac fossa, but this sequence may only be present in 50% of patients [7]. Typically, patients describe a peri-umbilical colicky pain, which during the first 24 hours intensifies becoming constant and sharp and migrating to the right iliac fossa. This initial pain represents referral phenomena due to the visceral innervation of the midgut and the localization is due to involvement of the parietal peritoneum following progression of the inflammatory process. Loss of appetite is frequently a predominant feature,

---

DIFFERENTIAL DIAGNOSIS OF ACUTE APPENDICITIS

Surgical
- Intestinal obstruction
- Intussusception
- Acute cholecystitis
- Perforated peptic ulcer
- Mesenteric adenitis
- Meckel's diverticulitis
- Colonic/appendicular diverticulitis
- Pancreatitis
- Rectus sheath hematoma

Urological
- Right ureteric colic
- Right pyelonephritis
- Urinary tract infection

Gynecological
- Ectopic pregnancy
- Ruptured ovarian follicle
- Torted ovarian cyst
- Salpingitis / pelvic inflammatory disease

Medical
- Gastroenteritis
- Pneumonia
- Terminal ileitis
- Diabetic ketoacidosis
- Preherpetic pain on the right 10th and 11th dorsal nerves
- Porphyria

Table 67.1 Anatomical considerations in the presentation of acute appendicis

Retrocecal/retrocolic (75%)
- Right loin pain is often present with tenderness on examination
- Muscular rigidity and tenderness to deep palpation are often absent due to protection form the overlying cecum
- The psoas muscle may be irritated in this position leading to hip flexion and exacerbation of the pain on hip extension (psoas stretch sign)

Subcaecal and pelvic appendix (20%)
- Suprapubic pain and urinary frequency may predominate
- Diarrhea may be present due to irritation of the rectum
- Abdominal tenderness may be lacking but rectal or vaginal tenderness may be present on the right
- Microscopic hematuria and leucocytes may be present on urinalysis

Pre- and post-ileal (5%)
- Signs and symptoms may be lacking
- Vomiting may be more prominent
- Diarrhea due to irritation of the distal ileum

with constipation and nausea also often seen. Profuse vomiting may be indicative of developing generalized peritonitis following perforation but is rarely a major feature in simple appendicitis. A meta-analysis of the symptoms and signs associated with a presentation of acute appendicitis was unable to identify any one diagnostic finding but stressed the importance of a history of migratory pain in the diagnosis of appendicitis [8].

This classical presentation can be influenced by the anatomical position of the appendix and the age of the patient (Table 67.1) [9]. Patients at the extremes of age, or those who are immunocompromised can present diagnostic difficulty due to a non-specific presentation often with subtle clinical signs. Young children can appear withdrawn and the elderly may present with confusion – there must be a high index of suspicion for acute appendicitis in these groups of patients.

Examination

The patient is often flushed, pyrexic (up to 38°C) and tachycardic. There may be dry tongue and an associated fetor oris. Abdominal palpation reveals localized tenderness and muscular rigidity following localization of the pain to the right iliac fossa. Patients often find movement and coughing exacerbates the pain and reveals localization in the right iliac fossa. Rebound tenderness is present, but eliciting this sign can often distress the patient and is best avoided. The site of maximal tenderness is typically said to be over McBurney's point which

lies two-thirds of the way along a line drawn from the umbilicus to the anterior superior iliac spine [10]. Per rectal and vaginal examination may be normal although there may be tenderness on the right side particularly in patients with a pelvic appendix. In complicated appendicitis, a pelvic abscess or inflammatory phlegmon can sometimes be felt. The most reliable clinical findings indicating a diagnosis of acute appendicitis are percussion tenderness, guarding, and rebound tenderness[8].

Further specific examination techniques that may aid in the diagnosis of appendicitis are the psoas stretch sign, the obturator sign [11] and Rovsig's sign (palpation of the left iliac fossa causes pain in the right iliac fossa).

Investigations

Specialist investigations are seldom required to confirm a diagnosis of acute appendicitis as the diagnosis is predominantly a clinical one. There is no specific diagnostic test for appendicitis but the judicious use of simple urine and blood tests, particularly inflammatory indices, should allow the exclusion of other pathologies and provide additional evidence to support or refute a clinical diagnosis of appendicitis (Table 67.2) [8]. Scoring systems and algorithms have been proposed to aid the diagnosis of acute appendicitis but have not been widely used [12–14].

In straightforward cases of appendicitis radiological imaging is not necessary. However, specialist radiological investigations can be valuable in supplementing clinical suspicion in equivocal cases or high-risk cases, and the choice of investigation lies predominantly between ultrasound (US) and computed tomography (CT). From a diagnostic perspective, in both children and adults, CT had a significantly higher sensitivity and specificity than the more operator-dependant technique of US (0.91–0.95 and 0.93–0.96 vs 0.83–0.88, 0.78–0.84)

Table 67.2 Investigation of acute appendicitis

Investigation	Significance
Urinalysis	40% have leucocytes and microscopic hematuria
Pregnancy test	To exclude pregnancy
Full blood count	Neutrophil (>75%) predominant leucocytosis is present in 80–90%.
C-reactive protein (CRP)	A raised CRP level may be present but its absence should not exclude a diagnosis of appendicitis

[15]. However, from a safely perspective, exposure to radiation should be considered, especially in children.

Whether the increased use of imaging modalities has reduced the negative appendicectomy rate is unclear. A longitudinal study reported that the introduction of US and CT scanning had not influenced the negative appendicectomy rate suggesting that this was related to the inconsistent performance characteristics of the tests [16]. However, these findings are not supported by earlier studies on the use of CT scanning alone, which demonstrated a decrease in the number of unnecessary admissions and appendicectomies [17,18] and also a decrease in the use of hospital resources. Magnetic resonance imaging (MRI) can also be used the for the diagnosis of appendicitis, although its use tends to be restricted to cases where exposure to radiation and diagnostic difficulties preclude the use of other modalities, for example, pregnancy [19,20].

Treatment

Herbert Fitz was the first author to publish on the need for early diagnosis and surgery in the management of acute appendicitis [21]. Appropriate resuscitation, analgesia, and expedient appendicectomy with perioperative antibiotics is the treatment of choice. Withholding analgesia on the grounds that it may affect the clinical picture and patient assessment is not justified. The use of broad spectrum perioperative (1–3 doses) antibiotics has been shown to decrease the incidence of postoperative wound infection and intra-abdominal abscess formation [22].

Timing of surgery

In a study by Abou-Nukta *et al.* [23], it was demonstrated that there were no significant differences in complications between early (<12 hours post-presentation) or later (12–24 hours post-presentation) appendicectomy. However, this did not take into account the actual time from the onset of symptoms to presentation, which can have a bearing on the rate of perforation [24]. The average rate of perforation at presentation is between 16% and 30% following 36 hours from the onset of symptoms, and the risk of perforation is 5% for every 12 hour period

[25,26]. Other studies have also suggested that the risk of developing advanced pathology and postoperative complications increases with time [27]. Therefore, once a diagnosis of acute appendicitis is made, appendicectomy should be performed without any unnecessary delays.

Operative procedure

Classically, open appendicectomy has been carried out through a muscle-splitting gridiron incision over McBurney's point, made perpendicular to a line joining the umbilicus and anterior superior iliac spine. However, it may also be undertaken through a more horizontally placed and cosmetically acceptable Lanz's incision. The proportion of open procedures performed has fallen with the increased use of laparoscopic techniques. Compared with open surgery, a systematic review found that laparoscopic appendicectomy in adults reduces wound infections, postoperative pain, duration of hospital stay, and time taken to return to work, although it was found that the number of intra-abdominal abscesses was increased following the laparoscopic approach [28]. However, these findings were not shared by a recent study, which found no significant differences between the two procedures although the laparoscopic procedure took longer to perform [29]. The laparoscopic group, however, had better quality-of-life scores at 2 weeks postoperatively.

In children, laparoscopic appendicectomy reduced the number of wound infections and the length of hospital stay compared with open surgery, but found no significant differences in postoperative pain, time to mobilization, or proportion of intra-abdominal abscesses [28].

Although in the light of some of these findings laparoscopic appendicectomy (Figure 67.1) is becoming increasingly common, it is often technically more demanding and requires specialist equipment. As a result, the method of approach for performing an appendicectomy is dictated by the level of experience of the operating surgeon and facilities available.

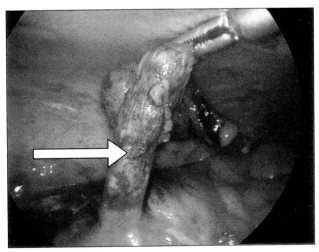

Figure 67.1 Laparoscopic appendicectomy. Arrow shows the inflamed appendix.

Laparoscopic techniques also afford the ability to perform diagnostic laparoscopy initially, which may demonstrate alternate pathology as the cause of the presentation.

Non-operative resolution of early appendicitis can occur and antibiotics alone can be used to treat appendicitis if there are no facilities for appendicectomy [30,31]. However, trials have shown 14–35% readmission rate associated with antibiotic treatment and, because of the high recurrence rate and relatively low morbidity and mortality associated with appendicectomy, early operative intervention remains the treatment of choice. These data nevertheless do provide support for the immediate commencement of intravenous antibiotics once a diagnosis of appendicitis is made and the patient is waiting for surgery.

Complications

Appendicectomy is regarded as a relatively safe procedure with a mortality rate for non-perforated appendicitis of 0.8 per 1000 [32]. The mortality and morbidity rates are related to the stage of disease and an increased mortality of 5.1 per 1000 [32] is seen in cases of perforation. The average rate of perforation at presentation is between 16% and 30% [25,26,32]. This is significantly increased in the elderly and young children where figures can be up to 97% usually due to a delay in diagnosis [11,33].

The increased mortality and morbidity associated with perforation has been used as justification for high rates of negative appendicectomy quoted as between 20% and 25% [32]. Despite this, complications can also occur following removal of a normal appendix, and there is a continued drive by the surgical community to reduce the numbers of negative procedures [34–36].

Wound infection

The rate of postoperative wound infection is determined by the intraoperative contamination and the use of perioperative antibiotics has been shown to decrease the rates of wound infections [22]. Rates of infection vary from <5% in simple appendicitis to 20% in cases with perforation and gangrene.

Intra-abdominal abscess

Postoperative intra-abdominal or pelvic abscesses may form following gross contamination of the peritoneal cavity. Patient presents with a swinging pyrexia and the diagnosis can be confirmed by ultrasound or CT. Abscesses can be treated radiologically with a percutaneous drain, although open or per rectal drainage may be required for a pelvic abscess. The use of perioperative antibiotics has been shown to decrease rates of abscess formation [22].

Special considerations
Pregnancy

Appendicitis has an incidence of 0.15 to 2.10 per 1000 pregnancies [37] and is the most common non-obstetric emergency requiring surgery in pregnancy. It was previously thought that there was an equal incidence in pregnant and non-pregnant women but a recent large scale case control study has suggested a reduction in the incidence of appendicitis during pregnancy, particularly during the third trimester [38].

Due to anatomical displacement of the appendix by the gravid uterus, clinical presentation is frequently atypical or may be mistaken for the onset of labor. Nausea and vomiting are often present, and tenderness may be located anywhere on the right hand side of the abdomen although it may be minimal if the inflamed appendix is displaced posteriolaterally.

In cases of simple appendicitis maternal mortality is negligible but this rises to 4% with advanced gestation and perforation. Fetal mortality ranges from between 0% and 1.5% in cases of simple appendicitis to between 20% and 35% in cases of perforation [37]. In a recent systematic review of laparoscopic appendicectomy versus open appendicectomy in pregnancy it was highlighted that although the laparoscopic approach was possibly associated with similar or slightly better rates of preterm delivery, this procedure was associated with a higher rate of fetal loss compared with the open technique [39]. The rates of negative appendicectomy have always been higher due to concern regarding perforation but as a negative appendicectomy is not complication free in pregnant women, the risk of misdiagnosis versus perforation from a delayed diagnosis must be carefully considered [39,40].

According to a large historical cohort study, a perforated appendix during childhood does not appear to have a long-term detrimental effect on subsequent fertility [41].

Appendix mass

In patients with a delayed presentation, a tender mass with overlying muscle rigidity may be felt in the right iliac fossa and the presence of the inflammatory phlegmon may be confirmed by US or CT (Figure 67.2). In an otherwise well patient, the initial management is conservative with appropriate resuscitation and intravenous broad-spectrum antibiotics. In the majority of cases the mass will decrease in size over the

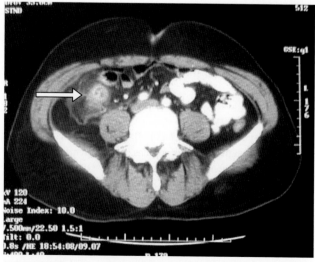

Figure 67.2 Computed tomogram showing an inflammatory mass (arrow) in the right iliac fossa secondary to acute appendicitis.

Small and Large Bowel

subsequent days as the inflammation resolves, although the patient requires careful observation to detect early signs of progression of the inflammatory process. The classical management following resolution of the mass is an interval appendicectomy, although a conservative approach with outpatient follow up has been suggested but no definitive evidence exists to support this [42]. It is imperative, however, that the presence of underlying neoplasia is excluded.

Appendix abscess

Patients present with a tender mass and swinging pyrexia, and tachycardia blood tests reveal raised inflammatory markers. The abscess is most frequently located in the lateral aspect of the right iliac fossa but may be pelvic; a rectal examination is useful to identify a pelvic collection. The abscess can be demonstrated by US or CT, and percutaneous radiological guided drainage may be performed. Open drainage has the added advantage of allowing a simultaneous appendicectomy to be performed [42].

Chronic (recurrent) appendicitis

It is known that minor episodes of appendiceal inflammation can settle spontaneously, although the natural history of these episodes remains unclear. Many studies however, have now clearly demonstrated that inflammation through many areas of the gastrointestinal tract can result in long-standing alterations in enteric nerve neurotransmitters, which can alter gut perception. Whether episodes of appendiceal inflammation result in "neuroimmune appendicitis" and right iliac fossa symptoms requires further work, but it represents an interesting concept [43].

Inflammatory bowel disease

A recent large Scandinavian epidemiological study showed an observed lower risk of ulcerative colitis following appendicectomy [44]. However, the association was restricted to appendectomies performed for appendicitis or mesenteric lymphadenitis before the age of 20 years. Without these conditions, appendicectomy had no impact on subsequent risk on development of the condition.

The influence of appendicectomy in Crohn's disease is less clear, with some evidence suggesting a delayed onset of disease in patients following appendicectomy, although contradictory evidence also exists to suggest an increased risk of developing the condition dependant on the patient's age, sex, and diagnosis at the time of operation. Some authors have also suggested diagnostic bias as a explanation for the increased risk of developing Crohn's disease following appendicectomy [45].

SOURCES OF INFORMATION FOR PATIENTS AND DOCTORS

http://www.nhs.uk/conditions/appendicitis/Pages/Introduction.aspx

---

Acknowledgments

This chapter is an updated version of a review by the authors in the *BMJ* 2006;333:530–534.

References

1. National Center for Health Statistics. Ambulatory and Inpatient Procedures in the United States, 1996. *National Center for Health Statistics Series 13. [No. 139]* 2004.
2. Larner AJ. The aetiology of appendicitis. *Br J Hosp Med.* 1988;39: 540–542.
3. Addiss DG, Shaffer N, Fowler BS, Tauxe RV. The epidemiology of appendicitis and appendectomy in the United States. *Am J Epidemiol.* 1990;132:910–925.
4. Kang JY, Hoare J, Majeed A, Williamson RCN, Maxwell JD. Decline in admission rates for acute appendicitis in England. *Br J Surg.* 2003;90:1586–1592.
5. Andersson R, Hugander A, Thulin A, Nystrom PO, Olaison G. Indications for operation in suspected appendicitis and incidence of perforation. *BMJ.* 1994;308:107–110.
6. Beasley SW. Can we improve diagnosis of acute appendicitis? *BMJ.* 2000;321:907–908.
7. Murphy J. Two thousand operations for appendicitis, with deductions from his personal experience. *Am J Med Sci.* 1904;128: 187–211.
8. Andersson R. Meta-analysis of the clinical and laboratory diagnosis of appendicitis. *Br J Surg.* 2004;91:28–37.
9. Buschard K, Kjaeldgaard A. Investigation and analysis of the position, fixation, length and embryology of the vermiform appendix. *Acta Chir Scand.* 1973;139:293–298.
10. McBurney C. Experiences with early operative interference in cases of diseases of the vermiform appendix. *NY Med J.* 1889; 50:676–684.
11. Wagner JM, McKinney WP, Carpenter JL. Does this patient have appendicitis? *JAMA.* 1996;276:1589–1594.
12. Alvarado A. A practical score for the early diagnosis of acute appendicitis. *Ann Emerg Med.* 1986;15:557–564.
13. Paulson EK, Kalady MF, Pappas TN. Suspected Appendicitis. *N Engl J Med.* 2003;348:236–242.
14. Tzanakis N, Efstathiou S, Danulidis K, *et al.* A New Approach to Accurate Diagnosis of Acute Appendicitis. *World J Surg.* 2005; 29:1151–1156.
15. Terasawa T, Blackmore CC, Bent S, Kohlwes RJ. Systematic Review: Computed Tomography and Ultrasonography To Detect Acute Appendicitis in Adults and Adolescents. *Ann Intern Med.* 2004;141:537–546.
16. Flum DR, McClure TD, Morris A, Koepsell T. Misdiagnosis of Appendicitis and the Use of Diagnostic Imaging. *J Am Coll Surg.* 2005;201:933.
17. Rao PM, Rhea JT, Novelline RA, Mostafavi AA, McCabe CJ. Effect of Computed Tomography of the Appendix on Treatment of Patients and Use of Hospital Resources. *N Engl J Med.* 1998;338:141–146.
18. Rao PM, Rhea JT, Rattner DW, Venus LG, Novelline RA. Introduction of appendiceal CT: impact on negative appendectomy and appendiceal perforation rates. *Ann Surg.* 1999;229:344–349.
19. Nitta N, Takahashi M, Furukawa A, Murata K, Mori M, Fukushima M. MR imaging of the normal appendix and acute appendicitis. *J Mag Res Imaging.* 2005;21:156–165.
20. Cobben LP, Groot I, Haans L, Blickman JG, Puylaert J. MRI for Clinically Suspected Appendicitis During Pregnancy. *Am J Roentgenol.* 2004;183:671–675.

21. Fitz R. Perforating inflammation of the vermiform appendix, with special refrence to its early diagnosis and treatment. *Trans Assoc Am Physicians.* 1886;1:107–144.

22. Andersen BR, Kallehave FL, Andersen HK. Antibiotics versus placebo for prevention of postoperative infection after appendicectomy. *Cochrane Database Syst Rev* 2005(3):CD001439.

23. Abou-Nukta F, Bakhos C, Arroyo K, *et al.* Effects of Delaying Appendectomy for Acute Appendicitis for 12 to 24 Hours. *Arch Surg.* 2006;141:504–507.

24. Temple CL, Huchcroft SA, Temple WJ. The natural history of appendicitis in adults. A prospective study. *Ann Surg.* 1995;221: 278–281.

25. Bickell NA, Aufses JAH, Rojas M, Bodian C. How Time Affects the Risk of Rupture in Appendicitis. *J Am Coll Surg.* 2006;202: 401–406.

26. Braveman P, Schaaf VM, Egerter S, Bennett T, Schecter W. Insurance-Related Differences in the Risk of Ruptured Appendix. *N Engl J Med.* 1994;331:444–449.

27. Ditillo MF, Dziura JD, Rabinovici R. Is it safe to delay appendectomy in adults with acute appendicitis? *Ann Surg.* 2006;244: 656–660.

28. Sauerland S, Lefering R, Neugebauer EA. Laparoscopic versus open surgery for suspected appendicitis. *Cochrane Database Syst Rev* 2004(4):CD001546.

29. Katkhouda N, Mason RJ, Towfigh S, Gevorgyan A, Essani R. Laparoscopic versus open appendectomy: a prospective randomized double-blind study. *Ann Surg.* 2005;242:439–448; discussion 48–50.

30. Eriksson S, Granstrom L. Randomized controlled trial of appendicectomy versus antibiotic therapy for acute appendicitis. *Br J Surg.* 1995;82:166–169.

31. Styrud J, Eriksson S, Nilsson I, *et al.* Appendectomy versus Antibiotic Treatment in Acute Appendicitis. A Prospective Multicenter Randomized Controlled Trial. *World J Surg.* 2006;30:1033.

32. Blomqvist PG, Andersson RE, Granath F, Lambe MP, Ekbom AR. Mortality after appendectomy in Sweden, 1987–1996. *Ann Surg.* 2001;233:455–460.

33. Grosfeld JL, Weinberger M, Clatworthy HW, Jr. Acute appendicitis in the first two years of life. *J Pediatr Surg.* 1973;8:285–293.

34. Flum DR, Koepsell T. The Clinical and Economic Correlates of Misdiagnosed Appendicitis: Nationwide Analysis. *Arch Surg.* 2002;137:799–804.

35. Benjamin IS, Patel AG. Managing acute appendicitis. *BMJ.* 2002;325:505–506.

36. Jones PF. Suspected acute appendicitis: trends in management over 30 years. *Br J Surg.* 2001;88:1570–1577.

37. Guttman R, Goldman RD, Koren G. Appendicitis during pregnancy. *Can Fam Physician.* 2004;50:355–357.

38. Andersson REB, Lambe M. Incidence of appendicitis during pregnancy. *Int J Epidemiol.* 2001;30:1281–1285.

39. Walsh CA, Tang T, Walsh SR. Laparoscopic versus open appendicectomy in pregnancy: a systematic review. *Int J Surg.* 2008;6: 339–344.

40. McGory ML, Zingmond DS, Tillou A, Hiatt JR, Ko CY, Cryer HM. Negative appendectomy in pregnant women is associated with a substantial risk of fetal loss. *J Am Coll Surg.* 2007;205: 534–540.

41. Andersson R, Lambe M, Bergstrom R. Fertility patterns after appendicectomy: historical cohort study. *BMJ.* 1999;318:963–967.

42. Ahmed I, Deakin D, Parsons SL. Appendix mass: do we know how to treat it? *Ann R Coll Surg Engl.* 2005;87:191–195.

43. Di Sebastiano P, Fink T, di Mola FF, *et al.* Neuroimmune appendicitis. *The Lancet* 1999;354:461.

44. Frisch M, Pedersen BV, Andersson RE. Appendicitis, mesenteric lymphadenitis, and subsequent risk of ulcerative colitis: cohort studies in Sweden and Denmark. *BMJ.* 2009;338:b716.

45. Kaplan GG, Pedersen BV, Andersson RE, Sands BE, Korzenik J, Frisch M. The risk of developing Crohn's disease after an appendectomy: a population-based cohort study in Sweden and Denmark. *Gut.* 2007;56:1387–1392.

Small and Large Bowel

CHAPTER 68
Anorectal diseases

Steven D. Wexner and Giovanna M. da Silva
Cleveland Clinic Florida, Weston, FL, USA

Hemorrhoidal disease

ESSENTIALS FACTS ABOUT PATHOGENESIS

- Prevalence: 4.4% in the United States, similar in both genders, peak 45–65 years of age
- Risk factors: chronic straining, constipation
- Pathogenesis: weakening of the supporting tissues with slippage of cushions

ESSENTIALS OF DIAGNOSIS

- Internal hemorrhoids: painless bleeding, prolapse
- Patients >40 years old or with atypical symptoms: colonoscopy to exclude cancer
- External hemorrhoids: painful perianal mass when thrombosed

ESSENTIALS OF TREATMENT

- All grades: high-fiber diet, increased water intake
- Grades I–III: rubber band ligation, sclerotherapy, and infrared coagulation
- Grades II–IV: stapled hemorrhoidopexy or hemorrhoidectomy

Hemorrhoids are cushions of submucosal tissue composed of blood vessels, smooth muscle fibers, and supporting connective tissue, normally present in the anal canal. The term "hemorrhoids" is also applied to situations when these cushions become symptomatic. The prevalence rate is 4.4% in the United States, similar in both genders, with a peak from 45 to 65 years of age.

Causes and pathogenesis
Hemorrhoids are the result of slippage of the anal cushions due to weakening of the supporting tissues. The prolapse hinders the venous flow leading to dilatation and engorgement of the anal cushions, exposing them to complications such as edema, thrombosis, and bleeding. Predisposing factors include conditions associated with chronic straining, constipation, diarrhea, and increased intra-abdominal pressure such as with pregnancy.

Hemorrhoids are classified as internal, external, or combined. Internal hemorrhoids are located proximal to the dentate line and are covered by insensate columnar mucosa or transitional epithelium. External hemorrhoids are located below the dentate line, covered with squamous epithelium rich in nerve endings.

Clinical presentation
The most common symptoms of internal hemorrhoids are **bleeding per rectum** and **prolapsing tissue.** The bleeding is bright red and painless, and it usually follows evacuation; blood may drip into the commode or stain the toilet paper. Prolapse occurs during straining or heavy lifting causing discomfort, feeling of incomplete evacuation, mucus discharge, and pruritus. Prolapsing hemorrhoids can be complicated by incarceration and strangulation secondary to thrombosis, causing severe pain and requiring urgent surgery (Figure 68.1). Internal hemorrhoids are classified according to the degree of prolapse: Grade I – bleeding without prolapse; Grade II – prolapse on straining that spontaneously reduces; Grade III – prolapse that requires manual reduction; and Grade IV – irreducible prolapse (Figure 68.2).

External hemorrhoids are usually asymptomatic unless thrombosis develops, which is frequently due to trauma and straining. They present as a painful blue lump at the anal verge.

Differential diagnosis
Hemorrhoidal bleeding needs to be differentiated from neoplasia, polyps, inflammatory bowel disease, anal fissure, abscess, fistula, and prolapse. It is rarely dark, melenic, or mixed with stool. Patients older than 40 years or with atypical symptoms should undergo complete colonic investigation to exclude cancer. Inflammatory bowel disease is marked by bloody diarrhea. If pain is present, anal fissure and abscess must be considered. Prolapsing hemorrhoids may be confused with rectal prolapse, polyps, hypertrophied papillae, or skin tags.

Diagnostic methods
A careful history characterizing bleeding, protrusion, pain, and bowel habits will often lead to the correct diagnosis. The

Textbook of Clinical Gastroenterology and Hepatology, Second Edition. Edited by C. J. Hawkey, Jaime Bosch, Joel E. Richter, Guadalupe Garcia-Tsao, Francis K. L. Chan.
© 2012 Blackwell Publishing Ltd. Published 2012 by Blackwell Publishing Ltd.

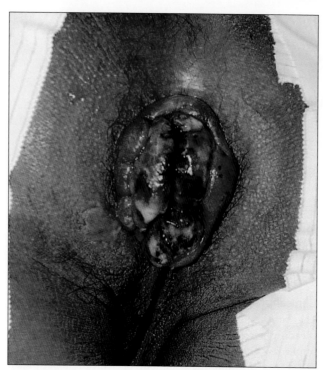

Figure 68.1 Strangulated hemorrhoids. (Courtesy of Dr Laurence Sands, University of Miami, Miami, FL, USA.)

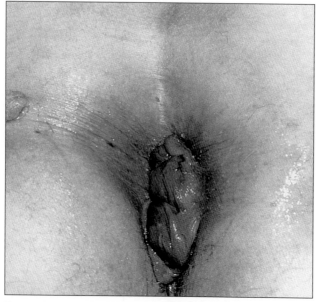

Figure 68.2 Prolapsing internal hemorrhoids. Radial folds of prolapsing internal hemorrhoids with an internal component.

perianal area is inspected to exclude other diseases. Anoscopy permits visualization of the internal hemorrhoids as they bulge into the lumen.

Treatment and prevention

Medical treatment aims to promote soft, formed, regular bowel movements with a high-fiber diet (20–30 g/day),

bulking agents (psyllium husk: e.g., Metamucil™, 1 packet 1–3 times/day) and generous water intake (six 8-ounce glasses of water/day). Warm sitz baths are helpful to relax the anal sphincter.

The minority of patients who do not respond to conservative treatment and those with second- or third-degree hemorrhoids are good candidates for office procedures, such as rubber band ligation (RBL), infrared coagulation, or sclerotherapy. The most common method used in the United States is RBL (Figure 68.3). Randomized trials demonstrated RBL to be superior to sclerotherapy [1] and similarly effective to infrared coagulation with a success rate of 96.8%, although associated with more post-procedural pain [2].

Surgery is the definitive treatment and can be done by standard hemorrhoidectomy or by stapled hemorrhoidopexy (procedure for prolapse and hemorrhoids; PPH). A meta-analysis of 29 trials including 2056 patients showed PPH to be significantly less painful than hemorrhoidectomy, with similar complication rates, although with higher recurrence rates [3]. Both techniques can be used for second- and third-degree hemorrhoids. Hemorrhoidectomy is a better option for grade IV hemorrhoids, when there is an external component or other condition that requires surgery such as fissure or fistula.

More recently, the Doppler-guided hemorrhoidal artery ligation technique has been introduced as an option for patients who are candidates for hemorrhoidectomy [4]. The technique uses a proctoscope containing a Doppler transducer to identify and selectively ligate the hemorrhoidal vessels. The procedure appears to be effective and associated with minimal morbidity and pain. Treatment of thrombosed external hemorrhoids requires excision if symptoms are of less than 48–72 hours. If symptoms are present for more than 72 hours and if the pain is improving the patient can be conservatively managed.

Complications and their management

Hemorrhoidectomy, RBL, and PPH can be complicated by pain, bleeding, urinary retention, and, rarely, sepsis. Pain can be managed with sitz baths, high-fiber diet, and analgesics. When accompanied by fever and dysuria, sepsis should be suspected and the patient examined under anesthesia with possible abscess drainage. Bleeding may occur 7 to 10 days after the procedure when the band falls off, and this is usually managed by cauterization or suture ligation. Urinary retention is managed by catheterization. Fecal incontinence and stenosis are complications of the surgical procedures, which may require surgical repair.

Prognosis with and without treatment

The majority of the hemorrhoidal symptoms permanently abate after adequate therapy with or without surgery. Untreated hemorrhoids may rarely lead to anemia, thrombosis, or incarceration.

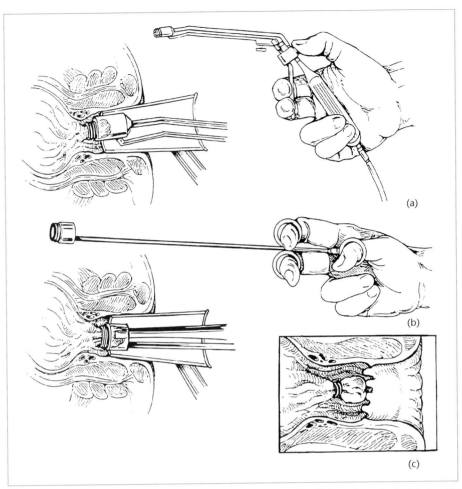

Small and Large Bowel

Figure 68.3 Rubber band ligation. Using an anoscope, a rubber band is placed on the hemorrhoidal tissue above the dentate line. (Adapted from Beck DE, Wexner SD, eds. Fundamentals of anorectal surgery, 2nd edn. London: W.B. Saunders; 1998, with permission from Elsevier.)

Anal fissure

ESSENTIALS FACTS ABOUT PATHOGENESIS

- Epidemiology: common problem, especially in teenagers and young adults
- Causes: constipation, diarrhea, trauma to the anal canal
- Pathogenesis: lack of tissue support, poor perfusion and increased anal pressure impair fissure healing in the posterior anal area

ESSENTIALS OF DIAGNOSIS

- Symptoms: pain with defecation, scant bleeding
- Examination: tear in the midline, sphincter spasm
- Fissures that are non-midline, multiple, painless, and non-healing should be evaluated for specific diseases

ESSENTIALS OF TREATMENT

- Conservative: increased fluid intake, fiber supplements, warm sitz baths
- Medical: nitrates, calcium channel blockers and botulinum toxin type A (Botox®)
- Surgical: sphincterotomy for prior treatment failure. Risk of incontinence

Anal fissure is a painful linear tear in the anoderm. It is a very common problem, the precise incidence of which is unknown. It affects all age groups from both genders, particularly teenagers and young adults.

Causes and pathogenesis

Anal fissure usually results from the traumatic passage of large and hard stool or prolonged diarrhea. Approximately 90% of fissures are located in the posterior midline, which may be explained by the elliptical configuration of the sphincter mechanism, resulting in weakness of the posterior midline. Anal fissure has also been hypothesized as an ischemic ulcer as the associated internal sphincter spasm causes reduced blood flow, impairing fissure healing, especially in the posterior region where there is a paucity of arterioles.

Clinical presentation

Anal fissure typically presents with **severe pain** initiated by the passage of stool, lasting minutes to hours after bowel movement. The pain is knifelike, cutting, or tearing. It is often associated with streaks of **bright red blood** in the stool and/

or on the toilet paper. Other symptoms include pruritus, swelling, prolapse, and discharge.

Differential diagnosis

Specific pathologies causing anal fissures should be investigated whenever fissures are non-midline, non-healing, multiple, broad, deep, irregular, painless, or extend above the dentate line. Alternative etiologies include inflammatory bowel disease, tuberculosis, HIV infection, leukemia, syphilis, and anal carcinoma. A careful medical history, physical examination, cultures, and biopsy of the fissure help to differentiate most of these conditions.

Diagnostic methods

Diagnosis is made by history and physical examination. In acute anal fissures, gentle spread of the buttocks will reveal a tear with a flat edge extending from the anal verge to the dentate line. Chronic fissures have raised edges and a deeper base with exposure of the internal sphincter (Figure 68.4). There is often an associated "sentinel" skin tag at the distal portion of the fissure, and a proximal hypertrophied papilla; sphincter tone is usually increased.

Treatment and prevention

Initial treatment consists of increased fluid and fiber supplements, warm sitz baths for 10–15 minutes 2 or 3 times per day, topical anesthetics (2% lidocaine before defecation) and steroid ointment. Up to 50% of acute fissures (less than 4–6 weeks) respond to these conservative measures.

Pharmacological agents are offered to patients who do not respond to conservative therapy, and to patients with chronic anal fissure. Theses agents work by chemically reducing internal sphincter pressure and increasing blood flow. **Topical glyceryl trinitrate (GTN; 0.2%)** has a 33% to 68% success rate

with a relapse rate of 50%. The ointment is applied in the anal canal 2 or 3 times daily for 6–8 weeks. Headache is the major side effect (20–30% of cases) and is dose related. Recent meta-analysis of calcium channel blocker treatment showed 2% diltiazem to be as effective as GTN, with similar recurrence rates but fewer side effects, including headache and hypotension [5]. The medication is applied 3 times/day for 6-8 weeks. **Botulinum toxin A** (BTX-A; Botox®) has a success rate of 60% to 80%. Usually 20–30 U of BTX-A is injected in the internal sphincter. Up to 12% of patients may experience temporary incontinence. Lateral internal sphincterotomy is usually reserved for patients who relapse or fail nonsurgical methods. It is associated with a healing rate of 90–100%.

A Cochrane review demonstrated that pharmacological therapy for chronic anal fissure, acute fissure, and fissure in children is marginally better than is placebo, and for chronic fissures in adults is far inferior than surgery [6]. However, due to low morbidity, drugs are used as an adjunct in the first-line therapy before considering surgical therapy, which has a very high cure rate, but with a risk of incontinence.

Complications and management

Side effects of pharmacological treatments are transient and resolve with conservative management and cessation of the medication. Sphincterotomy may be complicated by hematoma, abscess, and fecal incontinence in up to 30% of patients, and may be permanent. Abscess is managed by surgical drainage and incontinence with injection of bulking agents or sphincter repair.

Prognosis with or without treatment

Most anal fissures heal in 10–14 days with conservative treatment. Fissures that fail to heal in 6 weeks become chronic, requiring further treatment. Patients should be aware of the possibility of recurrence, especially with non-surgical therapy.

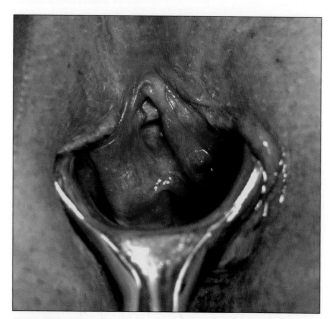

Figure 68.4 Anal fissure. (Courtesy of Dr Badma Bashankaev, Cleveland Clinic, Weston, FL, USA.)

Anorectal abscess

ESSENTIAL FACTS ABOUT PATHOGENESIS

- Epidemiology: more common in males, third decade
- Pathogenesis: acute infection of the perirectal spaces secondary to infection of the anal glands
- Classification: intersphincteric, perianal, ischiorectal, supralevator, submucosal, and postanal

ESSENTIALS OF DIAGNOSIS

- Symptoms: pain, swelling, warmth and fever
- Physical findings: erythema, warmth, induration, fluctuance
- Supralevator and intersphincteric abscesses may lack external manifestation

ESSENTIALS OF TREATMENT

- Surgery: incision and drainage
- Complications: necrotizing fasciitis, septic shock, death
- Prognosis: 40% result in fistula, 10–37% recurrence rate

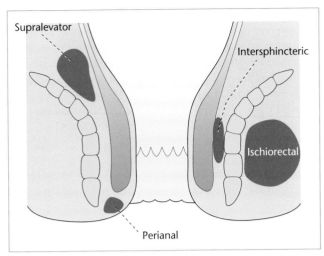

Figure 68.5 Classification of anorectal abscess. (Adapted from Beck DE, Wexner SD, eds. Fundamentals of anorectal surgery, 2nd edn. London: W.B. Saunders; 1998, with permission from Elsevier.)

Anorectal abscess is an acute infection of the perirectal tissues. The estimated annual incidence ranges between 68 000 and 96 000 in the United States. It is more common in males, in the third decade, and in warm climates.

Causes and pathogenesis

The majority of the anorectal abscesses result from non-specific infection of the anal glands (cryptoglandular origin). The abscesses may extend to the perirectal spaces and are classified as: intersphincteric, perianal, ischiorectal, and supralevator (Figure 68.5).

Clinical presentation

Anal abscess presents with pain, swelling, warmth, and fever. The pain is constant and is worsened by defecation. Occasionally the patient will describe spontaneous foul-smelling drainage with subsequent improvement of the pain. Patients with intersphincteric and supralevator abscesses may complain of severe rectal pain accompanied by dysuria, or urinary retention without an external manifestation. Immunocompromised, diabetic, and older patients may lack or have diminished symptoms of infection.

Differential diagnosis

Differential diagnosis includes anal fissure, thrombosed external hemorrhoid, hidradenitis suppurativa, pilonidal abscess, infected epidermoid cyst, and sexually transmitted disorders. Pain secondary to anal fissure occurs after bowel movement and disappears minutes to hours later. Thrombosed hemorrhoids are marked by acute onset of pain without fever. Hidradenitis abscesses are usually multiple accompanied by several draining sinus tracts. Infected epidermoid cysts and pilonidal abscesses are usually located remote from the anal canal, the latter in the intergluteal area.

While 90% of the abscesses result from non-specific cryptoglandular infection, 10% may result from diseases such as inflammatory bowel disease (Crohn's), trauma, malignancy (carcinoma, leukemia, lymphoma), and infection (tuberculosis, actinomycosis, lymphogranuloma venereum). In these situations, an appropriate investigation is warranted. Treatment and surgical outcomes differ for each of these conditions.

Diagnostic methods

Diagnosis is usually established by history and physical examination. Inspection reveals erythema, warmth, induration, and fluctuance. Intersphincteric or supralevator abscesses may lack external manifestation, and a delay in diagnosis can be disastrous. Digital examination reveals a tender mass. If tenderness precludes adequate assessment, patients should be examined under anesthesia; computed tomography (CT) and magnetic resonance imaging (MRI) are helpful in complex cases.

Treatment and prevention

Treatment is incision and drainage. Care must be taken not to drain a supralevator abscess originating in the pelvis through the levator plate, because a complex suprasphincteric fistula may develop. If a fistula is identified at the time of drainage, most surgeons opt to repair it in a separate visit to lessen the risk of incontinence.

Complications and management

Persistent drainage or recurrence can complicate the treatment course. In these cases, the presence of a fistula or an underlying pathology like Crohn's disease and malignancy should be investigated.

Prognosis with and without treatment

If left untreated or inadequately drained, anorectal abscess may result in necrotizing infection and even death, especially in diabetic or immunosuppressed patients. Approximately 40% of the abscesses will result in fistulas. Recurrence rates range from 10% to 37% of the cases. Close follow up until the wounds are completely healed is essential to prevent premature wound closure and recurrence.

Fistula-in-ano

ESSENTIAL FACTS ABOUT PATHOGENESIS

- Epidemiology: common disease, 2:1 male : female ratio, third and fourth decade
- Pathogenesis: cryptoglandular infection, incomplete healing of drained abscess
- Classification: intersphincteric, trans-sphincteric, extrasphincteric, and suprasphincteric

ESSENTIALS OF DIAGNOSIS

- Symptoms: pain, swelling and fever
- Exam: identification of the external and internal openings and fistula tract
- Differential diagnosis: inflammatory bowel disease, infections, trauma, and malignancy

Small and Large Bowel

ESSENTIALS OF TREATMENT

- Correct identification of all tracts and openings is essential for success
- Surgery: fistulotomy, sphincter-sparing techniques in cases of large portion of sphincter involved or in Crohn's disease

---

Anorectal abscess and fistula represent different points on the spectrum of the same disease. Abscess represents the acute stage and fistula the chronic phase. Anal fistula is a common disease with a male: female ratio of 2:1. It occurs predominantly in the third and fourth decade of life.

Causes and pathogenesis

Similar to anorectal abscesses, the majority of anal fistulas result from cryptoglandular infection and incomplete healing of the abscess. Consequently, the primary opening is the cryptoglandular area at the dentate line and the secondary opening is the skin where the abscess was drained. Fistulas are classified according to the relationship of the tract formed to the sphincter musculature and levator ani: intersphincteric, transsphincteric, extrasphincteric, and suprasphincteric, (Figure 68.6).

Clinical presentation

Anal fistula usually manifests as a small dimple area with chronic drainage of pus, bleeding, swelling, and discomfort often after abscess drainage.

Differential diagnosis

Similar to anal abscesses, differential diagnosis includes inflammatory bowel disease, infections, trauma, and malignancy.

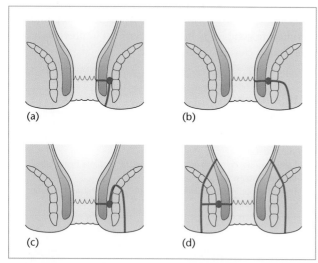

Figure 68.6 Classification of fistula in ano. (a) Intersphincteric; (b) trans-sphincteric; (c) suprasphincteric; (d) extrasphincteric. (Adapted from Vasilevski CA. Fistula in ano and abscess. In: Beck DE, Wexner SD, eds. Fundamentals of anorectal surgery, 2nd edn. London: W.B. Saunders; 1998, with permission from Elsevier.)

Diagnostic methods

The external opening can be identified discharging pus upon pressure or digital rectal examination. A tract can be subcutaneously palpated as a fibrous cord between the external opening and the anal orifice. The internal opening may be felt as an indurated nodule or pit or may be visualized by anoscopy. In cases of complex fistulas or unclear anatomy, anal ultrasound and MRI can be helpful, while sigmoidoscopy is useful to exclude underlying pathology.

Treatment and prevention

Treatment of fistula is surgical, with the goal to cure the fistula, avoid recurrence, and preserve continence. Identification of the primary opening and all side tracts with division of the least amount of muscle is the key factor for surgical success. Fistulas that involve significant portions of sphincters such as high transphincteric fistulas or those associated with Crohn's disease are treated with sphincter-sparing techniques such as loose-seton placement, endorectal advancement flap, fibrin glue, or collagen plug. These methods can be used in isolation or combined with variable results.

Complications and management

Recurrence is often due to failure to recognize the internal opening or inadequate management. Occasionally a secondary fistula may develop, raising suspicion for Crohn's disease. Partial fecal incontinence occurs in 5% to 30% of patients.

Prognosis with and without treatment

Fistulas rarely spontaneously heal. There is a very small risk of subsequent cancer development. The external opening may temporarily close leading to recurrent abscess or a more complex fistula, with the need of surgical intervention. The most common morbidity associated with surgery is fecal incontinence, especially if fistulotomy is performed. Recurrence is more likely to occur with complex fistula, and with failure to recognize the internal opening.

SOURCES FOR PATIENTS AND DOCTORS

http://www.fascrs.org/patients/
http://my.clevelandclinic.org/health/default.aspx

References

1. MacRae HM, McLeod RS. Comparison of hemorrhoidal treatments: a meta-analysis. *Can J Surg.* 1997;40:14–17.
2. Marques CF, Nahas SC, Nahas CS, *et al.* Early results of the treatment of internal hemorrhoid disease by infrared coagulation and elastic banding: a prospective randomized cross-over trial. *Tech Coloproctol.* 2006;10:312–317.
3. Shao WJ, Li GC, Zhang ZH, *et al.* Systematic review and meta-analysis of randomized controlled trials comparing stapled

haemorrhoidopexy with conventional haemorrhoidectomy. *Br J Surg.* 2008;95:147–160.

4. Walega P, Scheyer M, Kenig J, *et al.* Two-center experience in the treatment of hemorrhoidal disease using Doppler-guided hemorrhoidal artery ligation: functional results after 1-year follow-up. *Surg Endosc.* 2008;22:2379–2383.

5. Sajid MS, Rimple J, Cheek E, *et al.* The efficacy of diltiazem and glyceryltrinitrate for the medical management of chronic anal fissure: a meta-analysis. *Intl J Colorectal Dis.* 2008;23:1–6.

6. Nelson R. Non surgical therapy for anal fissure. *Cochrane Database of Systematic Reviews* 2006, Issue 4: CD003431.

CHAPTER 69

Acute pancreatitis

Georgios Papachristou, Vijay Singh, and David C. Whitcomb

University of Pittsburgh, Pittsburgh, PA, USA

ESSENTIAL FACTS ABOUT PATHOGENESIS

- Incidence: 35–60 per 100 000 per year and rising
- Risk: increased in alcoholics, the obese, and patients with gallstones
- Pathogenesis: any injury that leads to trypsinogen activation or activation of the immune system
- Genetic predisposition: mutations in cationic trypsinogen (PRSS1), cystic fibrosis transmembrane conductance regulator (CFTR), and serine protease inhibitor Kazal type 1 (SPINK1) for recurrent acute pancreatitis are most common genetic factors
- The magnitude of the acute inflammatory response determines the severity of the disease and related complications

ESSENTIALS OF DIAGNOSIS

- Acute pancreatitis requires 2 of 3 diagnostic signs
  - Amylase or lipase 3× upper limit of normal values
  - Characteristic sudden onset abdominal pain
  - Characteristic changes on abdominal images
- Early diagnosis of complications is critical for proper management
- The evidence of systemic inflammation and vascular leak, when persistent, is the best predictor of early organ failure and can be diagnosed at the bedside
- Hypovolemia is caused by a vascular leak syndrome and diagnosed by hypotension, tachycardia, and hemoconcentration

ESSENTIALS OF TREATMENT

- Aggressive fluid resuscitation should be initiated upon the diagnosis of acute pancreatitis and continued until signs of resuscitation are met, whether or not the clinical course is predicted to be severe
- Early endoscopic retrograde cholangiopancreatography (ERCP) with biliary sphincterotomy should be considered in selected patients to prevent bacterial cholangitis
- Enteral nutrition is the preferred route of nutrition in severe acute pancreatitis and should be started within 48 hours of admission
- Prophylactic antibiotics are not recommended, but may be considered in the presence of >30% pancreatic necrosis
- The etiology of an episode of acute pancreatitis should be systematically investigated, and the source of pancreatic injury treated before discharge, if possible

Introduction and epidemiology

Acute pancreatitis (AP) is an inflammatory syndrome initiated by pancreatic injury and activation of pancreatic digestive enzymes, leading to direct and indirect activation of the immune system. Population studies of patients with AP indicate a steadily increasing incidence, which ranges from 35 to 60 per 100 000 population. Acute pancreatitis currently accounts for 333 000 hospitalizations and 911 000 physician office visits with a hospitalization cost that exceeds $2 billion annually in the United States [1]. While most patients have a benign course, approximately 15% either present with or develop single or multiple organ involvement and/or pancreatic necrosis within the first 72 hours, resulting in prolonged hospitalization and significant morbidity and mortality [2]. The mortality rate from AP in large referral centers is fairly consistent at around 5–15% [3], with a slight but significant, reduction in case mortality in recent decades.

Causes and pathogenesis

The etiology of AP should be determined as early as possible to guide treatment and for planning to prevent recurrence. The most common etiologies are biliary (gallstones or sludge), alcohol, post-endoscopic retrograde cholangiopancreatography (ERCP), metabolic (hypertriglyceridemia, hypercalcemia), structural (pancreas divisum, pancreatic mass), and medication use (e.g., hydrochlorothiazide, azathioprine) [4,5], and others (Table 69.1). The initial work-up to determine the etiology of AP should include a detailed clinical history, blood chemistry (liver function tests, corrected serum calcium and triglyceride levels), and right upper quadrant ultrasonography to assess for gallstones or dilation of common bile duct. Approximately 20% of cases will be idiopathic.

Studies of AP in animal models and in humans following ERCP suggest that the first sign of injury is usually pain followed by a rise in serum amylase and lipase levels within the first hour of injury, peaking between 4 and 12 hours in mild cases [6]. Inflammatory cytokines (e.g., interleukin-6) then begin to increase at 8–12 hours, with maximal concentrations reached after 24–48 hours. Serum C-reactive protein (CRP) concentrations increase later, peaking at 72 hours.

Textbook of Clinical Gastroenterology and Hepatology, Second Edition. Edited by C. J. Hawkey, Jaime Bosch, Joel E. Richter, Guadalupe Garcia-Tsao, Francis K. L. Chan.
© 2012 Blackwell Publishing Ltd. Published 2012 by Blackwell Publishing Ltd.

Table 69.1 Risk factors and etiologies for acute pancreatitis

Susceptibility factors
- Duct obstruction
  - Gallstones
  - ERCP
  - Tumors
  - Anatomical abnormalities
  - Parasites
- Metabolic
  - Hyperlipidemia
  - Hypercalcemia
  - Acidosis (e.g. diabetic ketoacidosis)
- Toxins
  - Ethyl alcohol (high doses)
  - Organophosphorus insecticides (acetylcholinesterase inhibitors)
  - Scorpion toxin (Caribbean and South America varieties)
- Medications* (partial list)
  - Acetaminophen (paracetamol)
  - Azathioprine
  - Erythromycin
  - Estrogen
  - Exenatide (Byetta)
  - Furosemide
  - 6-Mercaptopurine
  - Metronidazole
  - NSAIDs
  - Pentamidine
  - Stavudine
  - Sulindac
  - Tetracycline
  - Valproic acid
- Genetic
  - Cystic fibrosis gene (*CFTR*)
  - Trypsinogen gene (*PRSS1*)
  - Pancreatic secretory trypsin inhibitor gene (*SPINK1*, recurrent only)
- Infectious
  - Viruses
  - Bacteria
- Trauma
  - Blunt or penetrating
  - Surgical
- Ischemia
- Idiopathic

Modifying factors
- Alcoholism (i.e., >2 drinks per day)
- Obesity (i.e., BMI >30)
- Genetic factors

*Multiple mechanisms, usually idiosyncratic reactions or linked to hypertriglyceridemia.
ERCP, endoscopic retrograde cholangiopancreatography; NSAIDs, non-steroidal anti-inflammatory drugs.

The acute inflammatory response to pancreatic injury can extend beyond the pancreas and trigger a systemic inflammatory response, which in turn may lead to multi-organ dysfunction, failure, and death. Systemic inflammation, previously known as the inflammatory response syndrome (SIRS) usually takes 12–36 hours to develop, leaving only a short window of opportunity for supportive intervention. The likelihood of systemic inflammation and/or organ dysfunction/failure is strongly influenced by pre-existing factors. The most important factors include obesity (especially visceral adipose tissue) [7], and chronic alcohol use (e.g., >2 drinks per day) [8]. Other factors (e.g., older age, female sex, genetic polymorphisms, metabolic state, and environmental variables) may also be important.

Clinical presentation

The pain associated with gallstone AP is typically sudden, epigastric, knife-like, and may radiate to the back. In some patients with alcoholic pancreatitis, hereditary pancreatitis, drug-induced pancreatitis, or some metabolic causes, the onset may be less abrupt, and the pain poorly localized. The pain is often unbearable and associated with severe nausea and vomiting but with minimal post-emetic improvement in nausea. For unknown reasons, some patients experience minimal pain.

The clinical diagnosis of AP is based on presence of at least two of the following three criteria: 1) abdominal pain characteristic of AP; 2) serum amylase and/or lipase three or more times the upper limit of normal; and/or 3) findings characteristic of AP on abdominal imaging studies. This definition includes patients with AP who have minimally elevated serum enzymes or with minimal or poorly described pain (e.g., infants and younger children or patients with altered mental status). It also excludes most patients with elevated serum digestive enzymes from other causes [9].

Differential diagnosis

Sudden onset of severe abdominal pain that may be similar to AP include myocardial infarction, dissecting aortic aneurism, mesenteric thrombosis, ischemia or infarction, vovlulus, intussusception, penetrating gastric or duodenal ulcers, biliary colic, and acute cholecystitis. Careful evaluation, including serial amylase levels, abdominal imaging, surgical consultation, and observation may be required to make the correct diagnosis in some cases.

Mild elevation of amylase and lipase (<3× upper limits of norm) occur in patients *without* AP in associated with other acute and chronic conditions [9]. However, mild elevations are also occasionally seen in patients *with* AP and significant pancreatic necrosis, or with pseudo-normalization in patients with diminished acinar cell mass from chronic pancreatitis or pancreatic resection (i.e., inappropriately normal when they should be low). Elevated trypsinogen activation peptide (TAP) levels or trypsinogen-2 levels are more specific than amylase or lipase, but are not widely available for clinical use.

Diagnostic investigation
Imaging
Abdominal imaging frequently performed in patients with AP includes computed tomography (CT) with or without contrast, magnetic resonance imaging (MRI) with or without

contrast, or transcutaneous ultrasound. Transcutaneous ultrasound is used to diagnose stones in the gallbladder or bile duct to help evaluate a possible biliary etiology and biliary complications. Contrast-enhanced CT has low sensitivity early in the course of AP until significant edema, fat stranding, and/or fluid collections develop; it is usually not needed to make a diagnosis and intravenous contrast has the potential of worsening pancreatic ischemia and necrosis, especially if performed before fluid resuscitation [10]. CT and MRI remain the most accurate methods for assessing later complications of acute pancreatitis (e.g., more than 48 hours after the onset of pain) including pancreatic necrosis, fluid collections, and other complications.

Scoring systems

Once the diagnosis of acute pancreatitis is established, the physician must determine the required level of care, including home, hospitalization, or intensive care unit (ICU). Multiple scoring systems have been used assess the severity of inflammation and predict the need for ICU care [11]. The most widely used scoring systems reflect the intensity of systemic inflammation, extra-pancreatic organ dysfunction (Marshall score, SOFA), or a combination (Ranson's, APACHE II, BISAP) [12,13]. The Atlanta criteria [14] include definitions of organ failure and/or local pancreatic complications, complemented by the presence of unfavorable multifactorial prognostic scores (Ranson ≥3 or APACHE II ≥8). Pancreas-specific scoring systems do not perform better than general ICU outcome prediction schemes. The predictive accuracy of most scores is generally approximately 80% [5], but they may be useful in focusing the physicians' attentions on early organ dysfunction.

The primary cause of early morbidity and mortality in AP is the development of systemic inflammation followed by organ dysfunction. Systemic inflammation is only seen with significant infections, including sepsis and septic shock, and in a few other non-infectious conditions including multiple trauma, severe burns, ischemia-reperfusion injury after cardiac arrest, and AP [15]. Systemic inflammation is identified clinically by the physiologic response to inflammatory cytokines (e.g., TNFα, IL-1). Systemic inflammation is diagnosed by two or more features of 1) temperature >38°C or <36°C; 2) heart rate >90 beats per minute; 3) resting rate of respiration (RR) >20/min; 4) white blood cell (WBC) count >12 000 or 5) PCO_2 <32 mmHg. Patients without systemic inflammation are at very low risk of severe complications or death. The development of systemic inflammation markedly increases the risk of complications, but in about half of cases it resolves within a day. If systemic inflammation persists for more than 48 hours, then the likelihood of a long and complicated course or death is markedly increased [12,16].

Other well-studied and reliable biomarkers used to diagnose a significant systemic inflammation include elevated serum levels of the cytokine IL-6 (>400 pg/mL), the leukocyte enzyme PMN elastase (>300 μg/L) and the acute phase protein CRP (>150 mg/L). CRP represents an acute phase response to pro-inflammatory cytokines, becomes an accurate marker of severe systemic inflammation 48 hours or more after admission, but has no correlation with severe organ dysfunction early in the course of AP.

Treatment and prevention

The most important role of the physician is to anticipate and, to the greatest degree possible, prevent serious complications of AP by assessing fluid status, providing rapid fluid resuscitation if needed, and controlling pain. Careful monitoring of vital signs, oxygen saturation, and urine output should be performed every 4 hours for the first 24 to 48 hours in hospitalized patients. Triage decisions to ICU transfer are based on the presence of hypotension, hypoxia, or tachypnea, all of which suggest high likelihood of severe disease [27].

Fluid resuscitation

Currently, it is often difficult to predict who will develop systemic inflammation, vascular leak syndrome, or multiple organ failure. Therefore, early and aggressive fluid resuscitation in the emergency department and close follow up is recommended to prevent or treat significant hypovolemia. One approach is to give one liter of lactated Ringer's solution followed by 250 to 300 milliliters per hour of intravenous fluids when cardiac status permits [5]. Another is to use guidelines for fluid resuscitation in septic shock [17]. Fluid resuscitation should be accomplished within 6 hours of admission with goals of maintaining a mean arterial blood pressure of >65 mmHg, urine output of at least 0.5 mL/kg/h, or central venous pressure of 8–12 mmHg [17]. Patients with persistent hypotension despite adequate fluid resuscitation should be started on vasopressors (e.g., dobutamine infusion up to 20 μg/kg/min [17]), while avoiding vasopressin because of a potential risk of mesenteric ischemia [18]. Special attention is needed for elderly patients, and those with cardiovascular disorders or renal insufficiency.

Patients with vascular leak syndrome who are fluid resuscitated will likely develop pulmonary edema. Anticipation of this complication and close monitoring of blood oxygenation is essential. Treatment escalation from supplemental oxygen to mechanical ventilation is determined by clinical conditions.

Pain control

Relief of abdominal pain is essential for patient comfort, but the amount and frequency of parenteral narcotic administration should be monitored closely. Parenteral narcotics, such as meperidine, morphine, fentanyl, and hydromorphone, are usually administered to relieve the pain. Oxygen saturation should be part of the vital signs measured in patients receiving narcotic agents due to respiratory drive suppression from narcotic agents [3].

Metabolic monitoring

Electrolyte and metabolic abnormalities, such as hypocalcemia (corrected for hypoalbuminemia), hypoalbuminemia, and hyperglycemia, can be seen in the setting of AP. Hyperglycemia is considered a marker of poor prognosis [13]. Serum glucose monitoring and use of sliding-scale insulin coverage is recommended. Case reports have suggested that patients with severe AP due to hypertriglyceridemia may benefit from plasma exchange [19].

Nutritional support

Acute pancreatitis represents a high catabolic state. In the majority of patients, oral intake is usually restored within 3 to 5 days of hospitalization, so nutritional support is not required. Clear liquids or low-fat [20] are initiated when abdominal pain and nausea subside and bowel sounds are present. In mild AP, nutritional support is only recommended when the clinician foresees that the patient will not be able to tolerate oral intake. In contrast, patients with severe AP have multiple nutrition needs and feeding should be started on nutritional support early in the course of the disease (e.g., within 48 hours [21]). When possible, enteral nutrition (EN) is preferred over total parenteral nutrition (TPN) because it reduces infections, systemic inflammation, ICU length-of-stay, possibly mortality, and costs less than TPN [21–23]. Enteral nutrition has been given by nasogastric (NG) and nasojejunal (NJ) approaches; the latter has a theoretic advantage of providing pancreatic rest and is superior to TPN in preserving intestinal function and splanchnic metabolism. Formulas with low fat content, fat in the form of medium-chain triglycerides, and proteins in the form of small peptides are better tolerated and show less stimulation of the pancreas [24], but probiotics should be avoided [25]. Enteral nutrition can be accomplished with ileus. Vigilant monitoring and quick changes in the feeding strategy may promote improved tolerance in those patients experiencing difficulty with initiation of EN.

Early endoscopic retrograde cholangiopancreatography

Most patients with gallstone pancreatitis have already passed the stone into the duodenum at the time of presentation and do not need early intervention with ERCP. An alanine transaminase (ALT) level three times the upper limit of normal has a positive predictive value of 95% for gallstone pancreatitis [26] with endoscopic ultrasound (EUS) or magnetic resonance cholangiopancreatography (MRCP) being the best test for excluding the diagnosis. Biliary obstruction from a gallstone impacted in the ampulla of Vater predisposes to bacterial cholangitis and worsens the outcome and severity of AP.

Therapeutic ERCP is indicated in patients with biliary AP and concomitant cholangitis (serum bilirubin level >1.2 mg/dL or dilated common bile duct on imaging and temperature >38.5°C) or cholestasis (serum bilirubin level >2.3 mg/dL or dilated common bile duct and temperature: ≤38.5°C) [27]. Early consultation with an experienced endoscopist or transfer to a tertiary facility may be needed, and the decision should be made as early as possible.

Preventing recurrence

Whenever possible, the etiology of pancreatitis should be determined and plans to prevent recurrence should be developed prior to hospital discharge. Medications associated with AP [4] should be discontinued. In AP due to gallstones, a cholecystectomy or sphincterotomy should be considered before discharge in mild cases or within a few months in more severe or complicated cases. If the etiology is hypertriglyceridemia, dietary measures, cessation of alcohol consumption, weight reduction, and pharmacologic management should be initiated with outpatient follow up. Identification of hypercalcemia requires attention to the underlying cause.

Complications and their management

Early complications of AP are related to extrapancreatic organ dysfunction while late complications are usually related to severe pancreatic damage. The most common complications are listed in Table 69.2.

Cardiovascular complications

The primary cardiovascular complications of AP are hypotension and shock. The etiology is primarily hypovolemia as a consequence of a vascular leak syndrome (VLS). The VLS occurs with endothelial cell activation leading to increased permeability to plasma proteins and solute, with extravasation of intravascular fluid into the tissues. Extravasation of fluid into the lungs results in pulmonary edema, while continued loss of intravascular fluid volume results in hemoconcentration, pre-renal azotemia, and eventually hypotension and hypovolemic shock [3,5]. Hypovolemia may also be worsened by patient vomiting and inability to hold ingested fluids, as well as the physician's orders to take nothing by mouth.

Early detection of the vascular leak syndrome and prevention of signification loss of intravascular fluid with appropriate therapy as outlined above may prevent many of the severe complications. Arterial or venous lactate >4 mmol/L suggests that shock has already resulted in tissue injury [17]. Patients with signs of hypovolemia require accurate and continuous monitoring of fluid status; in difficult cases the placement of a central line for measurement of central venous pressure should be considered.

Organ dysfunction and failure

Early **pulmonary dysfunction** is usually linked with pulmonary vascular leak and pulmonary edema and must be carefully assessed and treated with supplemental oxygen and, if necessary, mechanical ventilation. Pulmonary edema should *not* be treated with diuresis, as in congestive heart failure, because in the case of the vascular leak syndrome the diuresis will worsen hypovolemia and hypotension. Acute lung injury (ALI) can also occur as a consequence of inflammatory

Table 69.2 Common complications in acute pancreatitis

Pancreatic

Ductal
- Duct disruption
  - With fluid collections
    - Unorganized (previously called phlegmon)
    - Organized (pseudocysts)
  - With fistula
    - Pancreatic ascites
    - Pleural effusion
    - Cutaneous
- Duct obstruction
  - Pancreatic
    - Stone, stricture, or other with upstream ductal dilation
    - Stone, stricture, or other with upstream fluid leak
  - Biliary
    - Stone, stricture, or other with abnormal liver injury tests
    - Stone, stricture, or other with bacterial cholangitis

Vascular
- Pancreatic necrosis
- Portal vein thrombosis
- Splenic vein thrombosis
- Hemorrhage from pseudoaneurysms
  - Hemosuccus pancreaticus
  - Pseudocysts
  - Retroperitoneal

Inflammatory
- Pancreatic abscess
- Pseudocysts
- Post-necrotic fluid collections
  - Sterile pancreatic necrosis
  - Infected pancreatic necrosis
- Inflammatory mass

Peripancreatic
- Peripancreatic fat necrosis
- Duodenal stenosis – obstruction
- Colonic stenosis – obstruction

Extrapancreatic
- Abdominal compartment syndrome – (intra-abdominal pressure of 20–25 mmHg or higher)
- Systemic inflammatory complications
  - Systemic inflammatory response syndrome (SIRS)
  - Compensatory anti-inflammatory response syndrome (CARS)
  - Infections
- Distant organ dysfunction/failure
  - Vascular leak syndrome
  - Cardiovascular
    - Hypotension
    - Shock
  - Pulmonary
    - Pulmonary edema (capillary leak rather than heart failure)
    - Adult respiratory distress syndrome
  - Intestine
    - Ileus
    - Leaky gut syndrome
  - Renal
    - Pre-renal azotemia
    - Acute tubular necrosis

processes, and in severe cases acute respiratory distress syndrome (ARDS), defined as ALI with hypoxia ($PaO_2/FiO_2 \leq 200$ mmHg), may develop and require mechanical ventilation. After the first week, patients with severe AP may are also susceptible to bacterial pneumonia..

Renal dysfunction is a common complication of AP and is a poor prognostic sign. The etiology may be multifactorial, including pre-renal azotemia from hypovolemia or acute tubular necrosis from transient ischemia, toxic effects of CT contrast, or other factors. Elevated blood urea nitrogen (BUN) or creatinine on admission may be very useful in assessing fluid status, but time is required for either BUN or creatinine levels to rise. A rise in creatinine may reflect more widespread acute visceral organ hypotension and ischemic injury affecting other organs such as the pancreas [28].

Intestinal dysfunction is a central pathologic problem in AP. Gut mucosal injury from hypoperfusion and ischemia is a critically important early event because it strongly contributes to persistent systemic inflammation. The gut is the source of enteric bacteria that cause all types of infection during the later phase of immune paralysis. The primary sign of intestinal injury is ileus. Treatment includes correcting hypotension and hypoperfusion plus enteral nutrition.

Late complications

Late complications of AP are the result of damage caused during the early stages of local and systemic injury, plus susceptibility to infections related to the counter anti-inflammatory response syndrome (CARS). The most common problems are fluid collections and pseudocysts, pancreatic necrosis, infections, and nutritional deficits, but life-threatening compartment syndromes and hemorrhage must also be considered.

Pancreatic fluid collections are poorly organized and ill-defined collections within or near the pancreas that occur early in AP. Approximately half of these pancreatic fluid collections will be absorbed spontaneously within 4 to 6 weeks. Approximately 10–20% persist and progress to **pseudocysts**, which are well circumscribed and surrounded by a well-defined wall. Fluid collections are diagnosed by abdominal imaging studies. Persistence of the collections and the presence of high amylase concentrations suggest pancreatic duct disruption. Current practice is to manage fluid collections and pseudocysts conservatively unless they persist or grow due to duct disruption or compress other organs.

Pancreatic necrosis (PNec) is an infarction of the pancreas associated with hypovolemia, hemoconcentration, and increased creatinine. It is usually diagnosed by contrast-enhanced CT or MRI 48 hours or more after admission. Sterile PNec is best managed conservatively for the first 4-6 weeks to allow for clear demarcation between dead and viable tissue. Over this period, necrotic tissue progressively liquefies and eventually is encapsulated by granulation tissue.

Approximately one-third of patients with PNec develop infected necrosis [29], which is a major determinant of late morbidity and mortality. CT-guided percutaneous fine-needle aspiration with Gram stain and culture is often required for confirmation of the infected necrosis but has a false-negative rate of about 10% and should be repeated if clinically indicated in 5–7 days [30]. The utility of prophylactic antibiotics is marginal, and may be further diminished by the growing use of EN [22,23] or gut decontamination [31]. When antibiotics are used they should penetrate the necrotic material (e.g., imipenem–cilastin [32] or a fluoroquinolone with metronidazole) and are usually given for 14 days in patients with more than 30% pancreatic necrosis and then discontinued [3].

Treatment of PNec is evolving. Delayed open surgical intervention for 2 weeks or longer has been associated with reduced morbidity [33]. Minimally invasive approaches are becoming standardized and may reduce morbidity [30]. Endoscopic approaches are showing promise [34], and recent reports of medical treatment alone [35] has intensified debate on optimal management.

An **abdominal compartment syndrome**, defined as intra-abdominal pressure greater than 20–25 mmHg, is a life-threatening emergency that requires prompt surgical intervention. Abdominal compartment syndrome is caused by accumulation of fluid and intestinal gas resulting in impaired venous return, hemodynamic compromise, acute renal failure, reduced diaphragmatic excursion, and increased ventilator requirements [30]. Intra-abdominal pressure can be monitored with an indwelling urinary bladder catheter. Abdominal compartment syndrome is treated by decompression laparotomy, which results in a rapid, remarkable improvement in the patient's hemodynamic status, respiratory and renal function.

Splenic vein thrombosis is seen in up to 20% of patients with AP. Anticoagulation is currently not recommended during the acute stage of thrombosis, unless there is extension of the thrombus into the portal or superior mesenteric vein [36]. Late complications include gastric varacies and gastrointestinal bleeding. Whether or not early anticoagulation can prevent this long-term complication is unknown.

Arterial pseudoaneurysms are rare, late complications of AP. The most common reported site of pseudoaneurysms is the splenic artery, followed by the gastroduodenal and the pancreaticoduodenal artery. Pseudoaneurysms may bleed into a pseudocyst, resulting in sudden-onset abdominal pain: intra-abdominally, resulting in acute abdomen; or into the pancreatic duct, presenting as massive gastrointestinal bleeding (hemosuccus pancreaticus). Prompt and timely diagnosis can be challenging. Emergent angiography with embolization is considered the therapy of choice.

Discharge planning

Patients can be discharged when their pain is controlled with oral analgesics and they are able to eat and drink. Oral feeding can be started when abdominal tenderness is diminishing and the patient is hungry. Patients should be instructed to eat small, low-fat, carbohydrate–protein diets that can be increased in size over 3 to 6 days as tolerated. Pancreatic

exocrine insufficiency occurs in the majority of patients with severe acute pancreatitis and a subset of patients with milder disease [37] and may require pancreatic enzyme replacement therapy. In many cases pancreatic function returns over 12 to 18 months [37].

Prognosis with and without treatment

Treatment of mild acute pancreatitis can be managed at home with pancreatic rest and analgesics. Patients with more severe acute pancreatitis are at high risk of sudden death. The primary early challenge is that severe complications evolve over time, and early misclassification can be disastrous, and a prolonged observation period is warranted for patients at high risk (e.g., obese, alcohol users, the elderly) or if there is concern of complications. Aggressive hydration should be initiated during this observation period to minimize the chance of occult ischemic injury to visceral organs.

> ### SOURCES OF INFORMATION FOR PATIENTS AND DOCTORS
>
> MedlinePlus (patients and physicians): http://www.nlm.nih.gov/medlineplus/pancreaticdiseases.html
> National Institute of Diabetes and Digestive and Kidney Diseases (patients): http://digestive.niddk.nih.gov/ddiseases/pubs/pancreatitis/index.htm
> National Institute of Diabetes and Digestive and Kidney Diseases (physicians): http://www2.niddk.nih.gov/Research/ScientificAreas/Pancreas/
> National Pancreas Foundation (patients and physicians): http://www.pancreasfoundation.org/
> Pancreas.org (patients and physicians): http://www.pancreas.org/

References

1. NIDDK. Actue Pancreatitis. 2009; Available from: www2.niddk.nih.gov.
2. Isenmann R, Beger HG. Natural history of acute pancreatitis and the role of infection. *Best Pract Res Clin Gastroenterol.* 1999;13: 291–301.
3. Forsmark CE, Baillie J. AGA Institute technical review on acute pancreatitis. *Gastroenterology.* 2007;132:2022–2044.
4. Badalov N, Baradarian R, Iswara K, Li J, Steinberg W, Tenner S. Drug-induced acute pancreatitis: an evidence-based review. *Clin Gastroenterol Hepatol.* 2007;5:648–561 e3.
5. Whitcomb DC. Acute pancreatitis. *N Engl J Med.* 2006;354: 2142–2150.
6. Chen CC, Wang SS, Lu RH, Lu CC, Chang FY, Lee SD. Early changes of serum proinflammatory and anti-inflammatory cytokines after endoscopic retrograde cholangiopancreatography. *Pancreas.* 2003;26:375–380.
7. Martinez J, Sanchez-Paya J, Palazon JM, Suazo-Barahona J, Robles-Diaz G, Perez-Mateo M. Is obesity a risk factor in acute pancreatitis? A meta-analysis. *Pancreatology.* 2004;4:42–48.
8. Papachristou GI, Papachristou DJ, Morinville VD, Slivka A, Whitcomb DC. Chronic alcohol consumption is a major risk factor for pancreatic necrosis in acute pancreatitis. *Am J Gastroenterol.* 2006;101:2605–2610.

9. Neoptolemos JP, Kemppainen EA, Mayer JM, *et al.* Early prediction of severity in acute pancreatitis by urinary trypsinogen activation peptide: a multicentre study. *Lancet.* 2000;355:1955–1960.

10. Hotz HG, Schmidt J, Ryschich EW, *et al.* Isovolemic hemodilution with dextran prevents contrast medium induced impairment of pancreatic microcirculation in necrotizing pancreatitis of the rat. *Am J Surg.* 1995;169:161–166.

11. Arvanitakis M, Delhaye M, De Maertelaere V, *et al.* Computed tomography and magnetic resonance imaging in the assessment of acute pancreatitis. *Gastroenterology.* 2004;126:715–723.

12. Mofidi R, Duff MD, Wigmore SJ, Madhavan KK, Garden OJ, Parks RW. Association between early systemic inflammatory response, severity of multiorgan dysfunction and death in acute pancreatitis. *Br J Surg.* 2006;93:738–744.

13. Papachristou GI, Muddana V, Yadav D, *et al.* Comparison of BISAP, Ranson's, APACHE-II, and CTSI Scores in Predicting Organ Failure, Complications, and Mortality in Acute Pancreatitis. *Am J Gastroenterol.* 2010;105:435–441.

14. Bradley EL, 3rd. A clinically based classification system for acute pancreatitis. Summary of the International Symposium on Acute Pancreatitis, Atlanta, Ga, September 11 through 13, 1992. *Arch Surg.* 1993;128:586–590.

15. Castellheim A, Brekke OL, Espevik T, Harboe M, Mollnes TE. Innate immune responses to danger signals in systemic inflammatory response syndrome and sepsis. *Scand J Immunol.* 2009; 69:479–491.

16. Buter A, Imrie CW, Carter CR, Evans S, McKay CJ. Dynamic nature of early organ dysfunction determines outcome in acute pancreatitis. *Br J Surg.* 2002;89:298–302.

17. Dellinger RP, Levy MM, Carlet JM, *et al.* Surviving Sepsis Campaign: international guidelines for management of severe sepsis and septic shock: 2008. *Crit Care Med.* 2008;36:296–327.

18. Malay MB, Ashton JL, Dahl K, *et al.* Heterogeneity of the vasoconstrictor effect of vasopressin in septic shock. *Crit Care Med.* 2004;32:1327–1331.

19. Furuya T, Komatsu M, Takahashi K, *et al.* Plasma exchange for hypertriglyceridemic acute necrotizing pancreatitis: report of two cases. *Ther Apher.* 2002;6:454–458.

20. Jacobson BC, Vander Vliet MB, Hughes MD, Maurer R, McManus K, Banks PA. A prospective, randomized trial of clear liquids versus low-fat solid diet as the initial meal in mild acute pancreatitis. *Clin Gastroenterol Hepatol.* 2007;5:946–951; quiz 886.

21. McClave SA, Martindale RG, Vanek VW, *et al.* Guidelines for the Provision and Assessment of Nutrition Support Therapy in the Adult Critically Ill Patient: Society of Critical Care Medicine (SCCM) and American Society for Parenteral and Enteral Nutrition (A.S.P.E.N.). *J Parenter Enteral Nutr.* 2009;33:277–316.

22. Marik PE, Zaloga GP. Meta-analysis of parenteral nutrition versus enteral nutrition in patients with acute pancreatitis. *BMJ.* 2004;328:1407.

23. Mayerle J, Hlouschek V, Lerch MM. Current management of acute pancreatitis. *Nat Clin Pract Gastroenterol Hepatol.* 2005;2: 473–483.

24. McClave SA. Nutrition support in acute pancreatitis. *Gastroenterol Clin N Am.* 2007;36:65–74, vi.

25. Besselink MG, van Santvoort HC, Buskens E, *et al.* Probiotic prophylaxis in predicted severe acute pancreatitis: a randomised, double-blind, placebo-controlled trial. *Lancet.* 2008;371:651–659.

26. Tenner S, Dubner H, Steinberg W. Predicting gallstone pancreatitis with laboratory parameters: a meta-analysis. *Am J Gastroenterol.* 1994;89:1863–1866.

27. van Santvoort HC, Besselink MG, de Vries AC, *et al.* Early endoscopic retrograde cholangiopancreatography in predicted severe acute biliary pancreatitis: a prospective multicenter study. *Ann Surg.* 2009;250:68–75.

28. Mudanna V, Whitcomb DC, Khalid A, Slivak A, Papachristou GI. Elevated serum creatinine as a marker of pancreatic necrosis in acute pancreatitis. *Am J Gastroenterol.* 2009;104:164–170.

29. Banks PA, Freeman ML. Practice guidelines in acute pancreatitis. *Am J Gastroenterol.* 2006;101:2379–2400.

30. Hughes SJ, Papachristou GI, Federle MP, Lee KK. Necrotizing pancreatitis. *Gastroenterol Clin North Am.* 2007;36:313–323, viii.

31. Luiten EJ, Hop WC, Lange JF, Bruining HA. Controlled clinical trial of selective decontamination for the treatment of severe acute pancreatitis. *Ann Surg.* 1995;222:57–65.

32. Bassi C, Falconi M, Talamini G, *et al.* Controlled clinical trial of pefloxacin versus imipenem in severe acute pancreatitis. *Gastroenterology.* 1998;115:1513–1517.

33. Mier J, Leon EL, Castillo A, Robledo F, Blanco R. Early versus late necrosectomy in severe necrotizing pancreatitis. *Am J Surg.* 1997;173:71–75.

34. Papachristou GI, Takahashi N, Chahal P, Sarr MG, Baron TH. Peroral endoscopic drainage/debridement of walled-off pancreatic necrosis. *Ann Surg.* 2007;245:943–951.

35. Runzi M, Niebel W, Goebell H, Gerken G, Layer P. Severe acute pancreatitis: nonsurgical treatment of infected necroses. *Pancreas.* 2005;30:195–199.

36. Heider TR, Azeem S, Galanko JA, Behrns KE. The natural history of pancreatitis-induced splenic vein thrombosis. *Ann Surg.* 2004;239:876–880; discussion 80–82.

37. Keller J, Layer P. Human pancreatic exocrine response to nutrients in health and disease. *Gut.* 2005;54 Suppl 6:vi1–28.

CHAPTER 70
Chronic pancreatitis

Pascal O. Berberat,[1] Güralp O. Ceyhan,[1] Zilvinas Dambrauskas,[2] Markus W. Büchler,[3] and Helmut Friess[1]

[1]Technische Universität München, Munich, Germany
[2]Kaunas University of Medicine Hospital, Kaunas, Lithuania
[3]University of Heidelberg, Heidelberg, Germany

Pancreas and Biliary Tract

ESSENTIALS FACTS ABOUT PATHOGENESIS

- Incidence is approximately 6 per 100 000 population per year
- Alcohol is the main cause in the Western world (70%)
- The association between alcohol and pancreatitis complex is only partly dose dependent
- Other risk factors are genetic predisposition, smoking, and nutrition

ESSENTIALS OF DIAGNOSIS

- Mean age at onset is 40–60 years
- Endosonography detects earliest parenchymal changes
- Ductal changes can be detected early through endoscopic retrograde cholangiopancreatography (ERCP)
- CT scanning is widely available and shows complications
- Magnetic resonance cholangiopancreatography (MRCP) has the potential to be the "all-in-one" diagnostic investigation (including standard scan, MRCP, angiography) for the future

ESSENTIALS OF TREATMENT

Conservative treatment
- Pain control
- Avoidance of exacerbating factors (abstinence from alcohol and nicotine consumption and avoidance of fatty foods)
- Pancreatic enzymes to treat maldigestion, management of diabetes mellitus
- Stenting of the bile and pancreatic duct once only – then consider surgery

Surgical therapy:
- Indications should be considered when complications occur or conservative treatment fails
- Operations are longitudinal pancreaticojejunostomy (Pusteow and Partington–Rochelle procedures); pancreaticoduodenectomy (Whipple operation, classic and pylorus preserving); duodenum-preserving pancreatic head resection (Beger operation); longitudinal pancreaticojejunostomy and local pancreatic head excision (Frey operation); and central pancreatic head resection (Büchler–Farkas operation)

Introduction

Chronic pancreatitis is an inflammatory disease of the pancreas characterized by dysplastic ducts, foci of proliferating ductal cells, acinar cell degeneration, marked fibrosis, and unbearable abdominal pain. Consequently, patients with chronic pancreatitis exhibit variable degrees of pancreatic exocrine and endocrine dysfunction. Chronic pancreatitis is a complex disease, afflicting heavy drinkers in the majority of cases, but it is also associated with several other causes. Although much is known about the etiological background of the disease, there is still a large group of patients, perhaps 20–25% of the total, in whom the exact cause of the disease is unknown [1].

Epidemiology

There are only a few population-based estimates of frequency. Furthermore, the use of different classifications makes the comparison of different epidemiological studies difficult. However, five studies from the Czech Republic, Denmark, France, Germany, and the USA show similar frequency rates; approximately six cases per 100 000 inhabitants per year. Over time, the incidence of chronic pancreatitis has been increasing, as a result of the higher consumption of **alcohol**. More males than females are affected (ratio 5:1). Only idiopathic and hyperlipidemia-induced pancreatitis are more prevalent in females. Moreover, there are significant differences between races, as the frequency of chronic pancreatitis is greater amongst people of Asian and African descent and in populations native to India and Africa. The mean age of onset, in all subsets, is between the fourth and sixth decade of life. Only in idiopathic chronic pancreatitis has a bimodal age distribution been reported, designated as an early-onset form (median age 19.2 years) and late-onset form (median age 56.2 years), whereas hereditary pancreatitis begins in adolescence [2].

Table 70.1 Causes and risk factors

Common (90%)
- Excessive alcohol consumption (70%)
- Idiopathic (20%)

Rare (10%)
- Hyperparathyroidism
- Hypertriglyceridemia and other nutritional factors (tropical pancreatitis)
- Hereditary/genetic diseases and syndromes
- Pancreas divisum, anulare, stenosis of the papilla of Vater, and other anatomic abnormalities
- Autoimmune diseases
- Trauma

Causes, risk factors, and disease associations

Excessive alcohol consumption accounts for more than 70–80% of all cases. However, the association seems to be complex and only partly dose-dependent. Only a minority of heavy drinkers actually develop chronic pancreatitis, and those who drink moderately have also presented with the disease. Other factors, such as genetic predisposition or nutrition, may influence the development of alcoholic pancreatitis. In addition to alcohol consumption, smoking has been identified as an independent risk factor.

In approximately 20% of patients the disease has to be classified as **idiopathic chronic pancreatitis**. However, the discovery of the gain-of-function mutations in the cationic trypsinogen gene (*PRSS1*), the two loss of function mutations in the chymotrypsin C gene (*CTRC*), and the pancreatic secretory trypsin inhibitor gene (*SPINK1*) demonstrated that genetic alterations in the cytoprotective mechanism of the pancreas lead to chronic pancreatitis. This and the recognition of other gene mutations, such as the cystic fibrosis transmembrane conductance regulator (*CFTR*) mutation in patients with idiopathic chronic pancreatitis, has heightened the awareness and importance of hereditary factors in this disease. Rare causes of chronic pancreatitis include hyperparathyroidism, hypertriglyceridemia and other nutritional factors, anatomical abnormalities such as pancreas divisum, anulare or stenosis of the duct, and trauma. Tropical pancreatitis, found in Asia and Africa, is influenced by nutritional factors, leading to early endocrine insufficiency. Some infectious agents have been established as a cause of chronic pancreatitis with reasonable certainty, i.e., echinococcus, coxsackie virus, cytomegalovirus, mumps, human immunodeficiency virus (HIV), and microsporidia. Many autoimmune diseases may also be associated with chronic pancreatitis, but only Sjögren's syndrome is clearly related to this disease [3,4] (Table 70.1).

Pathogenesis

The pathogenesis of chronic pancreatitis remains controversial. Alcohol and other insults trigger multifactorial cascades in the pancreas, which lead to chronic inflammation, progressive fibrosis, pain, and loss of exocrine and endocrine function. Three main concepts have been proposed:

- **Increased viscosity of pancreatic juice** and formation of protein plugs, subsequently obstructing pancreatic ducts
- **Direct toxic effect of alcohol** and its metabolites on pancreatic acinar and ductal cells
- **Free radical injury** of the pancreatic parenchyma as a result of reduced hepatic detoxification.

However, none of these classic pathophysiological concepts can explain the morphological, functional, and clinical picture of chronic pancreatitis conclusively. Recent advances in modern cell and molecular biology have revealed new distinct mechanisms (Figure 70.1):

- **Growth factors** – many growth factors are overexpressed in human chronic pancreatitis. Transgenic mice that overexpress important growth factors, such as transforming growth factor (TGF)-β and TGF-α, develop severe pancreatic fibrosis and histological features also seen in humans with chronic pancreatitis.
- **Stellate cells** – evidence suggests that pancreatic fibrosis requires the differentiation and stimulation of specific cells called pancreatic stellate cells. It is thought that recurrent acinar cell injury, caused by oxidative stress (e.g., alcohol, ischemia), and other factors (Figure 70.1) result in cytokine and chemokine release from acinar cells and the activation of resident macrophages. These macrophages, in turn, suppress acute inflammation by releasing TGF-β and other cytokines, which stimulate stellate cells to produce collagen, and thereby promote fibrosis.
- **Other inflammatory mediators** – potent proteolytic enzyme systems, such as urokinase-dependent plasminogen activation, and inflammatory mediators, such as phospholipase A_2, also seem to be involved in the pathobiology of chronic pancreatitis.
- **Immune functions** – data suggest that decreased regulatory CD4 T cells and uncontrolled activation of CD8 T lymphocytes result in T-cell–mediated cytotoxicity [5,6].

Pathogenesis of symptoms
- **Pain** – the pathogenesis of pain is probably multifactorial, perhaps explaining why patients do not respond similarly to the same treatment modality [7];
- **Malabsorption** is due to deficiency of pancreatic enzymes
- **Diabetes mellitus.**

Pathology

In chronic pancreatitis the pancreas usually has a firm appearance with signs of calcification; duct obstruction by protein plugs or small calculi are occasionally seen. Histological evaluation of the tissue reveals dense fibrosis, destruction of acinar tissue and enlarged intrapancreatic nerves with dense fomation of neural networks. Only islets remain relatively unchanged. Signs of chronic inflammation with targeted immune cell infiltration of pancreatic nerves (pancreatic neuritis), vast infiltration by mononuclear cells, and marked

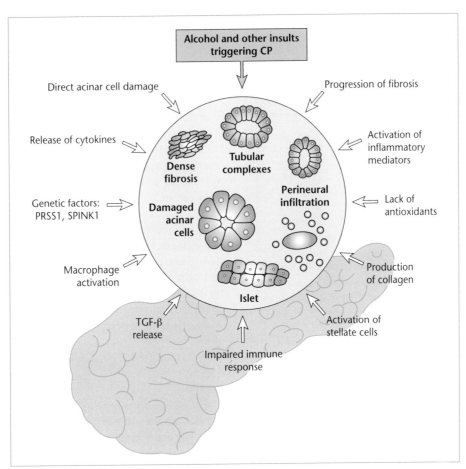

Figure 70.1 Pathogenesis of chronic pancreatitis. (This figure was published in *Clinical Gastroenterology and Hepatology*, Wilfred M. Weinstein, Christopher J. Hawkey, Jaime Bosch, Chronic pancreatitis, Pages 1–8, Copyright Elsevier, 2005.)

atrophy of the exocrine pancreas are characteristic of chronic pancreatitis (Figure 70.2).

Clinical presentation

Most patients with chronic pancreatitis have **pain in the upper abdomen**, which may radiate to the back. Exceptions include a minority of older patients with senile chronic pancreatitis, and a subset of patients with tropical pancreatitis who present at first with diabetes mellitus and may be pain free. Today the generation of pain is beleived to be directly associated with evident intrapancreatic neuropathic changes, as pancreatic neuritis and increased neural hypertrophy and density. Two types of pancreatic pain have been described:

- Type A pain refers to **recurrent episodic pain**, suggestive of acute exacerbation of chronic pancreatitis
- Type B pain refers to **continuous pain**.

Only a few patients with chronic pancreatitis are pain free.

Enzyme deficiency (**exocrine insufficiency**) due to pancreatic damage results in maldigestion and impaired absorption of food, especially of fats. Weight loss is characteristic of chronic pancreatitis. Patients may notice bulky, smelly stools due to too much fat (steatorrhea). Loss of insulin production may result in diabetes (**endocrine insufficiency**). Symptoms related to complications of pseudocyst include jaundice due to extrahepatic bile duct obstruction and signs of duodenal obstruction [8–10] (Table 70.2).

Differential diagnosis

The diagnosis of chronic pancreatitis in an advanced case is obvious, with typical symptoms such as upper abdominal pain, weight loss, steatorrhea, diabetes mellitus, history of alcohol use, and age approximately 45 years. In the initial stage of the disease, however, symptoms are often very non-specific. Similar pain can be caused by cancer of the pancreas, stones in the gallbladder and bile duct (biliary colic), or severe types of gastric or duodenal ulcer. All of these conditions have to be considered and appropriate diagnostic tests applied.

The most critical differential diagnosis is pancreatic cancer in patients with suspected chronic pancreatitis. The problem is many overlapping clinical symptoms and signs, such as jaundice, pain, and weight loss. However, there are some hints that are suggestive of possible pancreatic cancer, such as no history of alcohol abuse, older age (60–70 years), and significant constitutional symptoms (Table 70.3).

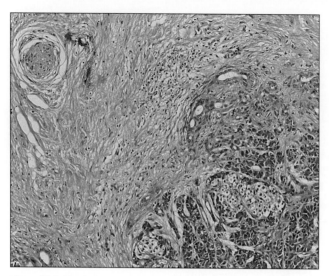

Figure 70.2 Histologic appearance of chronic pancreatitis. Section shows dense fibrosis, enlarged nerves with disruption of the perineurium tubular complexes, infiltration of mononuclear cells, and destruction of acinar tissue.

Table 70.2 Clinical presentation

(In order of frequency)
- Abdominal pain (>75%):
  – In upper abdomen, may radiate to the back
  – Lasts from hours to days, eventually continuous
  – Exacerbated by eating, drinking, alcohol
- Pancreatic insufficiency (late):
  – Maldigestion, steatorrhea and weight loss (exocrine insufficiency)
  – Signs of diabetes mellitus (endocrine insufficiency)
- Complications (rare):
  – Pseudocysts (10%, often asymptomatic)
  – Splenic vein thrombosis (10%)
  – Nausea and vomiting (duodenal obstruction, 10%)
  – Jaundice and pale or clay-colored stools (bile duct obstruction, 10%)
  – Pancreatic cancer (cumulative risk after 10 years: 2%, after 20 years: 4%)
  – Narcotic addiction (secondary to chronic pain)

Table 70.3 Differential diagnosis

- Pancreatic carcinoma
- Stones in gallbladder and bile duct
- Gastric or duodenal ulcer
- Irritable bowel syndrome
- Acute pancreatitis

Diagnostic methods
Function tests

The utility of pancreatic function testing to diagnose chronic pancreatitis is still debated. The majority believes that this is unnecessary and plays only a role in diagnosing early chronic pancreatitis without structural changes. Furthermore, these tests have limitations:

- Most tests for pancreatic exocrine function have good sensitivity and specificity only when severe pancreatic insufficiency is present (after loss of 90% of the secretory capacity of the pancreas)
- The secretin–cerulein stimulation test may diagnose mild disease. However, this procedure is invasive, very unpleasant, and expensive
- There is a lack of a widely accepted "gold standard" procedure.

The preferred exocrine function test today is the measurement of pancreatic enzymes in the stool, such as elastase-1 and chymotrypsin. Further indirect tests, which verify maldigestion and help to optimize enzyme treatment, are the quantitative fecal fat test, the pancreolauryl test, and various breath tests. However, non-invasive tests tend to perform poorly in patients with early chronic pancreatitis [11]. Poor endocrine function of the pancreas can be revealed by glucose tolerance tests, blood insulin, and C-peptide level measurements.

Imaging

The first-line non-invasive diagnostic investigations are transabdominal ultrasonography and computed tomography (CT). The main findings on **transabdominal ultrasonography (tUS)** are changes in the size, shape, contour, or echotexture of the gland, calcifications, and ductal dilatation. Dilatation of the main pancreatic duct above a diameter of 2 mm can be revealed by tUS.

CT is a highly accurate method (sensitivity 75–80%, specificity around 90%). **Magnetic resonance cholangiopancreatography (MRCP)** detects and better characterizes biliary and pancreatic strictures. However, tUS, CT, and MRCP cannot detect subtle early minor alterations and small branch chronic pancreatitis [12,13].

A sensitivity and specificity of >90% can be attained by **endoscopic retrograde cholangiopancreatography (ERCP)**. Even in early chronic pancreatitis with minimal changes, sensitivity of >65% may be achieved. Pancreatic juices can be collected within the pancreas for laboratory analysis, and tissue specimens can be taken when there is any suspicion of cancer. Moreover, therapeutic procedures such as dilatation and stenting are effective in relieving symptoms. The main disadvantage of ERCP is the risk of complications (such as bleeding, perforation and post-ERCP pancreatitis). If papillotomy is performed, the complication rate increases up to 5–10% (without papillotomy, 1.5%), and the risk of death is around 0.5%. (Figure 70.3).

Endoscopic ultrasonography (EUS) can detect more subtle and earlier minimal changes of chronic pancreatitis (sensitivity 80%, specificity 86%). This procedure also offers therapeutic options, such as EUS-guided fine-needle aspiration, pancreatic pseudocyst drainage, and celiac plexus neurolysis [13,14].

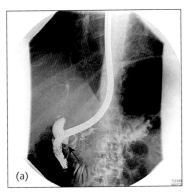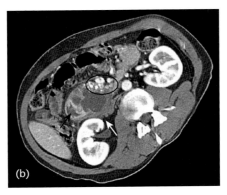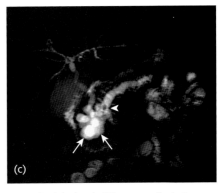

Figure 70.3 Imaging in chronic pancreatitis. (a) Endoscopic retrograde cholangiopancreatography (ERCP) – stenosis of the head of the pancreatic duct (arrow). (b) CT – cystic lesion (arrows) in the head of the pancreas with multiple calcification (circle) in the head and body. (c) Magnetic resonance cholangiopancreatography (MRCP) – cystic lesion (arrows) in the head, and duct dilatation (arrowhead).

However, EUS still has some drawbacks, e.g., the endosonographic definition of chronic pancreatitis is not universally agreed, the procedure requires sedation, and the accuracy is highly operator dependent [15].

Treatment and prevention

The treatment of patients with chronic pancreatitis is primarily conservative and revolves around:

- Management of malabsorption
- Management of diabetes mellitus
- Pain control.

Management of malabsorption

About 80% of patients with chronic pancreatitis can be managed by **dietary recommendations** and **pancreatic enzyme supplementation**. Reduction of steatorrhea and supplementation of calories are the main goals of nutritional therapy. Total abstinence from alcohol and frequent low-fat meals are the basis of dietary recommendations. The diet should be rich in carbohydrates (if diabetes mellitus is not present) and proteins (up to 1.0–1.5 g/day). Weight loss and/or steatorrhea (15 g/day) are indications for supplementation of pancreatic enzymes. Furthermore, malabsorption of proteins and carbohydrates, dyspepsia, meteorism, and diarrhea have also been taken as indications for the substitution of exocrine pancreatic function. Although evidence for the efficacy of pancreatic enzyme replacement is restricted to two randomized trials, their wide use, ease of administration, and lack of any significant side effects make them a first choice in the medical treatment of pain [16].

Pain control
Medical measures

Pain is the most common and most difficult problem. Pain may be treated interventionally or surgically, but medical treatment is generally the first-line therapy. For initial pain relief, non-narcotic analgesics and non-steroidal anti-inflammatory drugs

(NSAIDs) are recommended. Opioid analgesics should be prescribed for severe pain on an "as and when" required basis, but attention should be given to avoid addiction. Some patients with chronic pancreatitis suffer from depression, which lowers the visceral pain threshold. Therefore, antidepressants may have a positive additive effect in pain control. Overall, medical treatment seems to have potential benefit in 40–70% of patients with chronic pancreatitis and pain [17].

Endoscopic therapy

The next line of treatment for pain and the relief of other associated symptoms should be endoscopic therapy, when feasible. However, the prerequisite is a dilated main pancreatic duct and/or ductal obstruction by stones or stricture. The modalities include pancreatic sphincterotomy, stenting, and possibly lithotripsy to break large calculi. If endoscopic treatment fails in the first intent, surgical therapy should be considered. A recent randomized trial showed that surgical drainage is significantly more effective and efficient in pain reduction in comparison to endoscopic stent therapy [18].

Surgical intervention

There are a number of indications for surgical interventions in chronic pancreatitis, but the most common is **intractable pain** (Table 70.4). Two main types of surgical treatment are applied today: procedures that involve drainage and those that involve resection (Figure 70.4) [19].

- **Drainage procedures** – pancreaticojejunostomy (Pusteow and Partington–Rochelle procedures). These have the goals of reducing intrapancreatic pressure by draining the main pancreatic duct and preserving pancreatic tissue to avoid loss of pancreatic function
- **Procedures involving resection** – pancreaticoduodenectomy (Whipple operation or left resection). These are indicated in cases of a contracted duct, when an inflamed mass is present in the pancreatic head or tail, or when a pancreatic carcinoma is suspected

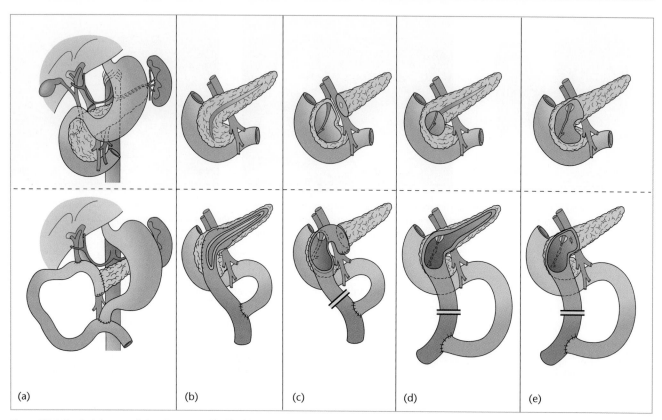

(a) (b) (c) (d) (e)

Figure 70.4 Surgical therapy of chronic pancreatitis. The five main procedures performed: (a) pylorus-preserving Whipple procedure; (b) pancreaticojejunostomy (Pusteow); (c) duodenum-preserving pancreatic head resection (Beger operation); (d) Frey operation; (e) Bern operation (new modification of the Beger operation). (This figure was published in *Clinical Gastroenterology and Hepatology*, Wilfred M. Weinstein, Christopher J. Hawkey, Jaime Bosch, Chronic pancreatitis, Pages 1–8, Copyright Elsevier, 2005.)

Table 70.4 Indications for surgical therapy in chronic pancreatitis

- Chronic pain: inadequate response to medical and/or endoscopic treatment
- Complications of neighboring structures: duodenal obstruction, common bile and/or pancreatic duct obstruction, portal and/or splenic vein obstruction
- Mass lesion in pancreatic head and suspected pancreatic cancer
- Effects of ductal rupture
- Persistent or symptomatic pseudocyst
- Pancreatic fistula unresponsive to other therapy
- Pancreatic ascites unresponsive to medical therapy

- **Procedures that combine resection and duct drainage** – (duodenum-preserving pancreatic head resection: Beger operation, Frey operation, Büchler–Farkas operation). These are generally very effective in pain relief, with long-term success rates in the range of 90%, along with good preservation of pancreatic function.

Randomized studies show that, at least in the early follow-up, organ-preserving procedures, such as the duodenum-preserving pancreatic head resection, the Frey operation, and Büchler-Farkas operation, show better results than the Whipple procedures. There seems not to be a significant difference between the three organ-preserving procedures in the outcome. However, the Frey operation and the Büchler–Farkas operation are technically less demanding than the duodenum-preserving pancreatic head resection. In the long-term (>10 years), duodenum-preserving pancreatic head resection provides similar outcome to the Whipple procedure.

Prevention
Avoidance of heavy alcohol consumption dramatically reduces the risk of developing chronic pancreatitis.

Complications and their management
The most important complications are pseudocysts, biliary strictures, splenic vein thrombosis, and ascites.

Pseudocysts (see also Chapter 72)
The pseudocyst is the most common local complication of chronic pancreatitis. Pseudocysts are either retention cysts or cysts that develop following acute exacerbation of chronic pancreatitis. Pseudocysts develop in approximately 10–25% of all patients with chronic pancreatitis and often may be asymptomatic, but they can also be the cause of persistent pain, obstruction symptoms or even abscess formation. Most pseudocysts regress spontaneously over time. If they become

Table 70.5 Prognosis with and without treatment

Treatment	Pain release	Exocrine insufficiency	Endocrine insufficiency	Complications
Natural course	Pain course of 10– 0 years	100%	80–90 %	50%
Medical treatment	Symptomatic	Reduction maldigestion (enzymes)	Control diabetes (insulin)	No effect
Endoscopic treatment	Selected patients	No effect	No effect	Removing stricture, drainage pseudocysts
Surgical treatment	85–95%	No effect	No effect or impairment	Removed

symptomatic or infected, treatment is needed. Primarily, pancreatic cysts and pseudocysts are usually managed by transcutaneous puncture or endoscopic drainage of the collections. Today, three different endoscopic procedures are used to drain pseudocysts:

- Transgastric drainage
- Transduodenal approaches
- The newer procedure of placement of a pigtail endoprosthesis through the papilla into the cyst.

If the endoscopic treatment fails or recurrence following successful endoscopic drainage occurs, surgical drainage procedures should be considered. Classically via cystgastrostomy or cystenterostomy, an open surgical drainage is performed. In specialized centers, this procedure may also be done laparoscopically. In some cases a resection may be indicated [20].

Biliary strictures

Stenosis of the common bile duct is usually treated by a single attempt at endoscopic stenting, especially in patients with acute cholestasis (before carrying out biliodigestive surgery). Plastic stents or Wallstents show good short- and medium to long-term results. Ascending cholangitis is the main complication with all stents, and long-term follow-up data are lacking. If jaundice recurs, definitive surgical therapy should be performed, especially in young patients. In patients with calcifying chronic pancreatitis, stenting has a failure rate of >90%.

Other complications

Splenic vein thrombosis is another important complication, and is seen in approximately 10% of patients with chronic pancreatitis. It may lead to the development of gastric fundal varices, which may cause bleeding.

Pancreatic ascites may develop following rupture of the main pancreatic duct, but this is an uncommon complication of chronic pancreatitis. The chronic inflammatory and **fibrosing process** may extend to adjacent organs, causing lumen narrowing of the duodenum, distal stomach, or transverse colon.

Prognosis with and without treatment

Chronic pancreatitis is a serious disease that may lead to disability and death. Although it is an incurable, progressive condition, the severity, frequency, and nature of symptoms can vary. Some people, especially those who cease alcohol consumption entirely, have very mild or occasional symptoms that are easily managed with medication. Other people, especially those who continue to consume alcohol, can experience disabling, daily pain that may require frequent hospitalization. Chronic pancreatitis is a risk factor in the development of pancreatic cancer (Table 70.5) [21].

SOURCES OF INFORMATION FOR PATIENTS AND DOCTORS

www.chirurgieinfo.com
www.pancreasfoundation.org
www.pancreas.org
www.pankreasinfo.com
http://patients.uptodate.com/topic.asp?file=digestiv/5269
http://www.patient.co.uk/showdoc/23069114/
http://www.patient.co.uk/showdoc/23364026/
http://www.chir.med.tu-muenchen.de/mric/content/e239/e588/index_ger.html
http://cchs-dl.slis.ua.edu/patientinfo/gastroenterology/pancreas/pancreatitis/chronic.htm
http://www.gastro.org/clinicalRes/brochures/pancreatitis.html

---

References

1. Tandon RK, Sato N, Garg PK. Chronic pancreatitis: Asia–Pacific consensus report. *J Gastroenterol Hepatol*. 2002;17:508–518.
2. Banks PA. Epidemiology, natural history, and predictors of disease outcome in acute and chronic pancreatitis. *Gastrointest Endosc*. 2002;56 (Suppl):S226–S230.
3. Whitcomb DC. Genetic predisposition to alcoholic chronic pancreatitis. *Pancreas*. 2003;27:321–326.
4. Treiber M, Schlag C, Schmid RM. Genetics of pancreatitis: a guide for clinicians. *Curr Gastroenterol Rep*. 2008;2:122–127.
5. Friess H, Kleeff J, Buchler MW. Molecular pathophysiology of chronic pancreatitis – an update. *J Gastrointest Surg*. 2003;7:943–945.

6. Charnley RM. Hereditary pancreatitis. *World J Gastroenterol.* 2003;9:1–4.

7. Hayakawa T, Naruse S, Kitagawa M, Ishiguro H, Jin CX, Kondo T. Clinical evidence of pathogenesis in chronic pancreatitis. *J Hepatobiliary Pancreat Surg.* 2002;9:669–674.

8. Mitchell RM, Byrne MF, Baillie J. Pancreatitis. *Lancet.* 2003; 361:1447–1455.

9. Petersen JM, Forsmark CE. Chronic pancreatitis and maldigestion. *Semin Gastrointest Dis.* 2002;13:191–199.

10. Farrell JJ. Overview and diagnosis of malabsorption syndrome. *Semin Gastrointest Dis.* 2002;13:182–190.

11. Lieb JG 2nd, Draganov PV. Pancreatic function testing: here to stay for the 21st century. *World J Gastroenterol.* 2008;14: 3149–3158.

12. Robinson PJ, Sheridan MB. Pancreatitis: computed tomography and magnetic resonance imaging. *Eur Radiol.* 2000;10:401–408.

13. Sugiyama M, Haradome H, Atomi Y. Magnetic resonance imaging for diagnosing chronic pancreatitis. *J Gastroenterol.* 2007;42 (Suppl 17):108–112

14. Chong AK, Hawes RH, Hoffman BJ, Adams DB, Lewin DN, Romagnuolo J. Diagnostic performance of EUS for chronic pancreatitis: a comparison with histopathology. *Gastrointest Endosc.* 2007;65:808–814.

15. Raimondo M, Wallace MB. Diagnosis of early chronic pancreatitis by endoscopic ultrasound. Are we there yet? *JOP.* 2004;5:1–7.

16. Khalid A, Whitcomb DC. Conservative treatment of chronic pancreatitis. *Eur J Gastroenterol Hepatol.* 2002;14:943–949.

17. Singh VV, Toskes PP. Medical therapy for chronic pancreatitis pain. *Curr Gastroenterol Rep.* 2003;5:110–116.

18. Cahen DL, Gouma DJ, Nio Y, *et al.* Endoscopic versus surgical drainage of the pancreatic duct in chronic pancreatitis. *N Engl J Med.* 2007;356:676–684.

19. Schafer M, Mullhaupt B, Clavien PA. Evidence-based pancreatic head resection for pancreatic cancer and chronic pancreatitis. *Ann Surg.* 2002;236:137–148.

20. Bhattacharya D, Ammori BJ. Minimally invasive approaches to the management of pancreatic pseudocysts: review of the literature. *Surg Laparosc Endosc Percutan Tech.* 2003;13:141–148.

21. Whitcomb DC, Pogue-Geile K. Pancreatitis as a risk for pancreatic cancer. *Gastroenterol Clin North Am.* 2002;31:663–678.

CHAPTER 71

Pancreatic exocrine tumors

Paula Ghaneh and John P. Neoptolemos

University of Liverpool, Liverpool, UK

Pancreas and Biliary Tract

ESSENTIAL FACTS ABOUT PATHOGENESIS

- Incidence: varies from 10 to 12 per 100 000 population
- Major risk factors: age, smoking, chronic pancreatitis, late-onset diabetes mellitus
- Inherited risk: hereditary pancreatitis, cancer family syndromes, familial pancreatic cancer
- Pathogenesis: precursor lesions – intraductal papillary mucinous neoplasms (IPMNs) and pancreatic intraepithelial neoplasms (PanINs)
- Molecular pathogenesis: mutations in *KRAS* oncogene, tumor suppressor genes, growth factors, angiogenic factors, apoptosis, developmental genes

ESSENTIALS OF DIAGNOSIS

- Early symptoms vague: e.g., dyspepsia, abdominal bloating
- Classical presentation of painless obstructive jaundice, weight loss, back pain
- Differential diagnosis chronic pancreatitis, other periampullary tumors, autoimmune pancreatitis
- Majority of patients present with advanced disease (85%)
- Multidetector computed tomography (CT) gold standard for diagnosis and staging
- Endoscopic retrograde cholangiopancreatography (ERCP)/percutaneous transhepatic cholangiography (PTC) and brushings for jaundiced patients
- Percutaneous biopsy only for patients not undergoing resection

ESSENTIALS OF TREATMENT

Unresectable
- Endoscopic biliary stent
- Endoscopic duodenal stent
- Percutaneous biliary stent
- Palliative bypass surgery
- Pancreatic enzyme supplements
- Analgesia
- Celiac plexus block
- Thoracoscopic splanchnicectomy
- Pancreas enzyme supplements
- Systemic chemotherapy: gemcitabine plus capectabine

Resectable
- Preoperative short covered metal stent preferred
- Kausch–Whipple pancreatoduodenectomy (KW-PPD)
- Pylorus-preserving pancreatoduodenectomy (PP-PPD)
- Total pancreatectomy
- Left pancreatectomy
- Adjuvant chemotherapy – avoid chemoradiation

Introduction

Pancreatic ductal adenocarcinoma is the commonest cancer affecting the exocrine pancreas and is the fourth or fifth leading cause of cancer-related death in the Western world [1]. Pancreatic cancer has a median survival of 3–6 months without treatment, which increases to around 24 months with surgical resection and adjuvant treatment [2]. Unfortunately, the late presentation and aggressive tumor biology of this disease mean that only a minority of patients can undergo potentially curative surgery. There have been major improvements in operative mortality and morbidity in the past decades through the development of specialist regional centers. Recent progress has been made in understanding the key molecular events in pancreatic cancer [3]. It is hoped that this knowledge will provide the basis for novel and effective diagnostic and therapeutic approaches in the near future.

Epidemiology

The incidence of pancreatic cancer increases with each decade resulting in four-fifths of cases occurring between the ages of 60 and 80 years. The peak incidence is in the 65–75 year age group with 60% of patients being older than 65 years of age [4]. The highest rates for pancreatic cancer are seen in Sweden, Denmark, Austria, the UK, New Zealand, and the USA and range from 12 to 20 per 100 000. The lowest rates are reported in Nigeria, Kuwait, Singapore, and regions of India with rates of 0.7 to 2.1 per 100 000 population. In 2002, there were 232 306 new cases of pancreatic cancer and 227 023 deaths worldwide [5]. In the USA in 2006 there were 33 730 new cases and 32 300 deaths.

The lifetime risk of developing pancreatic cancer in developed countries is 1%. From these figures pancreatic cancer represents 3% of all cancers, and 5% of all cancer deaths.

Causes

- Tobacco smoking is associated with a two-fold risk of developing pancreatic cancer and accounts for approximately 30% of all cases.
- Patients with diabetes mellitus of at least 5-years duration have a two-fold increased risk, and pancreatic cancer may

follow 2–3 years after a diagnosis of diabetes mellitus in elderly patients with no family history of diabetes mellitus.

- Chronic pancreatitis has an associated 5–15-fold risk and patients may have chronic pancreatitis for at least 20 years before the development of pancreatic cancer.
- The risk of developing cancer is even higher with hereditary pancreatitis (HP) with estimates of a 70- to 100-fold increase in risk. This is a rare disorder inherited as an autosomal dominant condition with an estimated 80% penetrance and an equal gender incidence [6].
- Other factors including previous surgery, *Helicobacter pylori* infection, pernicious anemia, virus infections, coffee drinking, and a western diet have weak or unclear roles in the causation of pancreatic cancer.
- The development of pancreatic cancer may be associated with inherited mutations and these account for 5–10% of all cases of pancreatic cancer. There are several inherited conditions that are associated with pancreatic cancer (Table 71.1).
- Familial pancreatic cancer itself is a rare disease and the mode of inheritance is unclear [7]. It is an autosomal dominant condition with an as yet unidentified causative mutation. Diagnostic criteria are: two or more first-degree relatives with pancreatic ductal adenocarcinoma (PDAC); one first-degree relative with early onset pancreatic cancer (age less than 50 years at diagnosis); or two or more second-degree relatives with pancreatic cancer, one of whom has early onset pancreatic cancer. In families with at least two first-degree relatives affected by pancreatic cancer, the

relative risk may be increased 18- to 57-fold depending on the number of pre-existing affected relatives.

Pathogenesis
Histological pathogenesis
The ductal phenotype gives rise to three distinct cancer precursor lesions with distinct, although overlapping, gene alterations: mucinous cystic neoplasms, intraductal papillary mucinous neoplasms (IPMNs), and pancreatic intraepithelial neoplasms (PanINs) [8] (Figure 71.1). Pancreatic intraepithelial neoplasms are classified into early and late lesions, starting with PanIN-1A, 1B (hyperplasia) and progressing to PanIN-2 and then to PanIN-3 or carcinoma in situ. It is important to note that the malignant potential of the early 1A lesion is unknown. It is only when the basement membrane is breached or satellites of tumor deposits are seen that the diagnosis of malignancy can be made. Associated with the development of the invasive phenotype is a dense collagenous reaction termed "desmoplasia."

Molecular pathogenesis
The molecular pathogenesis of pancreatic cancer involves an accumulation of genetic and molecular changes that results in a malignant phenotype with invasive potential [3]. Somatic mutations include activation of key oncogenes such as *KRAS* and inactivation of important tumor suppressor genes such as *TP53*, *CDKN2A*, and *SMAD4* in a large proportion of cases. Abnormalities in growth factors and growth factor receptors also contribute to the malignant phenotype. Disruption of the normal regulation of the extracellular matrix involving the matrix metalloproteinases (MMPs) and tissue inhibitors of matrix metalloproteinases (TIMPs) and increase in the expression of angiogenic factors such as vascular endothelial growth factor (VEGF) and platelet-derived endothelial cell growth factor (PDECGF) also contribute to the invasive potential of tumor cells. Reactivation of developmental signaling pathways in pancreatic cancer such as Notch and Hedgehog are also important factors in carcinogenesis. The role of polymorphisms in metabolic and DNA repair genes still has to be established.

Pathology
Ductal adenocarcinoma is the most common malignant tumor of the pancreas (Figure 71.2). Sixty-five per cent are located within the head, 15% in the body, 10% in the tail, and 10% are multifocal. Tumors of the head tend to present earlier with obstructive jaundice. Tumors of the body and tail tend to present later and are associated with a worse prognosis. There is often an intense desmoplastic reaction in the stroma surrounding these tumors. Pancreatic ductal adenocarcinoma must be distinguished from carcinomas of the intrapancreatic bile duct, ampulla of Vater, or duodenal mucosa as these tumors have a much better prognosis. In approximately 20% of cases it is not possible to distinguish the tissue of origin of

Table 71.1 Hereditary cancer syndromes affecting the pancreas

Syndrome	Gene mutation
Peutz-Jeghers syndrome	STK11/LKB1
Familial breast and ovarian cancer syndromes	BRCA1 and BRCA2
Familial atypical multiple mole melanoma (FAMMM)	TP16
Familial pancreatic cancer	BRCA2 in up to 20%; 4q32–34 ?
Hereditary pancreatitis	PRSS1 in up to 80%
von Hippel-Lindau disease	VHL
Ataxia telangiectasia	ATM
Li-Fraumeni syndrome	TP53
Cystic fibrosis	CFTR
Familial adenomatous polyposis (FAP)	APC
Hereditary nonpolyposis colon cancer (HNPCC)	MLH1, MSH2, MSH6, PMS1, PMS2

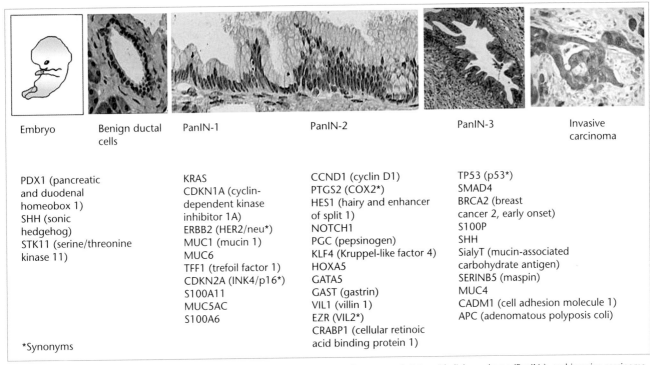

Embryo	Benign ductal cells	PanIN-1	PanIN-2	PanIN-3	Invasive carcinoma
PDX1 (pancreatic and duodenal homeobox 1) SHH (sonic hedgehog) STK11 (serine/threonine kinase 11)		KRAS CDKN1A (cyclin-dependent kinase inhibitor 1A) ERBB2 (HER2/neu*) MUC1 (mucin 1) MUC6 TFF1 (trefoil factor 1) CDKN2A (INK4/p16*) S100A11 MUC5AC S100A6	CCND1 (cyclin D1) PTGS2 (COX2*) HES1 (hairy and enhancer of split 1) NOTCH1 PGC (pepsinogen) KLF4 (Kruppel-like factor 4) HOXA5 GATA5 GAST (gastrin) VIL1 (villin 1) EZR (VIL2*) CRABP1 (cellular retinoic acid binding protein 1)	TP53 (p53*) SMAD4 BRCA2 (breast cancer 2, early onset) S100P SHH SialyT (mucin-associated carbohydrate antigen) SERINB5 (maspin) MUC4 CADM1 (cell adhesion molecule 1) APC (adenomatous polyposis coli)	

*Synonyms

Figure 71.1 Histological images of benign pancreatic ductal epithelial cells, progressive pancreatic intraepithelial neoplasms (PanINs), and invasive carcinoma, with associated genetic alterations. (Images kindly provided by Ali Shekouh and Jutta Luettges.)

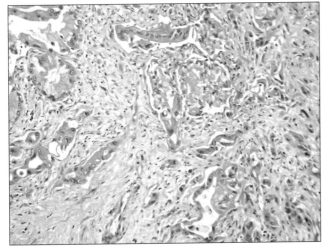

Figure 71.2 Pancreatic ductal adenocarcinoma. (Figure kindly supplied by Dr Fiona Campbell, Consultant Histopathologist, Department of Pathology, Royal Liverpool University Hospital Trust, Liverpool, UK.)

Table 71.2 Histological variants of malignant tumors of the exocrine pancreas

Histological type	Frequency	Features
Ductal adenocarcinoma	82%	Long term survival rare
Anaplastic	5%	Worse prognosis than ductal
Mucinous cystadenocarcinoma	3%	Variable
Acinar cell	2%	Variable prognosis
Mucinous non-cystic	2%	—
Adenosquamous	2%	Poor prognosis
Small cell	1%	Extremely poor prognosis
Squamous cell carcinoma	<1%	More aggressive than ductal
Intraductal papillary-mucinous	<1%	More favourable prognosis then ductal
Serous cystadenocarcinoma	rare	Prognosis similar to ductal
Pancreatoblastoma	rare	Childhood tumor; relatively good prognosis

cancers arising in the head of the pancreas, and the term "peri-ampullary cancer" is often applied. There are some uncommon types of tumor that are considered to be variants of pancreatic ductal adenocarcinoma. These account for a small percentage of the total number of malignant tumors of the pancreas (Table 71.2). Histological grading is outlined in Table 71.3. In addition

Pancreas and Biliary Tract

Table 71.3 Histological grading of ductal adenocarcinoma of the pancreas

Tumor grade	Glandular differentiation	Mucin production	Mitoses (per 10 high power fields)	Nuclear anaplasia
1	Well differentiated duct-like glands	Intensive	1–5	Little polymorphism, some polar arrangement
2	Moderately differentiated duct-like and tubular	Irregular	6–10	Some polymorphism
3	Poorly differentiated glands, mucoepidermoid and pleomorphic structures	Abortive	>10	Marked polymorphism, increased nuclear size

Table 71.4 UICC TNM clinical classification of pancreatic ductal adenocarcinoma

T – Primary tTumor

TX	Primary tumor cannot be assessed
T0	No evidence of primary tumor
Tis	Carcinoma in situ
T1	Tumor limited to the pancreas, 2 cm or less in greatest diameter
T2	Tumor limited to the pancreas, more than 2 cm in greatest diameter
T3	Tumor extends directly into any of the following duodenum, bile duct, peripancreatic tissues
T4	Tumor extends directly into any of the following stomach, spleen, colon, adjacent large vessels

N – Regional lymph nodes

NX	Regional lymph nodes cannot be assessed
N0	No regional lymph node metastasis
N1	Regional lymph node metastasis
N1a	Metastasis in a single regional lymph node
N1b	Metastasis in multiple regional lymph nodes

M – Distant Metastasis

MX	Distant metastasis cannot be assessed
M0	No distant metastasis
M1	Distant metastasis

Table 71.5 Stage grouping for pancreatic ductal adenocarcinoma

Stage	T	N	M
Stage 0	Tis	N0	M0
Stage I	T1 T2	N0	M0
Stage II	T3	N0	M0
Stage III	T1 T2 T3	N1	M0
Stage IVA	T4	Any N	M0
Stage IVB	Any T	Any N	M1

pancreas and also extrapancreatic cancers such as colorectal cancer. Mainstays of diagnosis are Computed tomography (CT), magnetic resonance cholangiopancreatography (Figure 71.4) and endoluminal ultrasonography with fine-needle aspiration and cyst fluid analysis (cytology, mucin, CEA, and CA19-9). Serous cystadenomas are nearly always benign and may be managed conservatively and kept under radiological surveillance. Side-branch IPMNs (Figure 71.5) that lack malignant features may also be managed conservatively with radiological monitoring: diameter less than 3 cm, absence of nodules and thick walls, CA19-9 25 kU/L, absence of recent-onset or worsened diabetes, absence of jaundice or of any other symptom. Resection is needed for all mucinous cystic neoplasms and main-duct IPMN.

to histological confirmation of the disease, the International Union Against Cancer (UICC) classification enables a standard staging exercise for tumors. For pancreatic tumors the TNM categories are shown in Table 71.4. The pathological classification (i.e., pT, pN, and pM) should correspond to the clinical T, N, and M categories. The stage grouping based on the UICC TNM classification (Table 71.5) has been shown to be a factor in predicting patient survival. Stages I and II are associated with better long-term survival.

Pancreatic cystic neoplasms

Pancreatic cystic neoplasms are being increasingly identified and comprise at least 15% of all pancreatic cystic masses. Most non-inflammatory pancreatic cysts are malignant or premalignant: main differential diagnosis is a pancreatic pseudocyst. The three main types are serous cystic neoplasms, mucinous cystic neoplasms and intraductal papillary mucinous neoplasms (IPMN) (Figure 71.3). Patients with pancreatic cysts have an increased risk of developing other cancers of the

Clinical presentation

Pancreatic cancer is relatively asymptomatic during its early course. With vague presenting symptomatology such as back and epigastric pain, until the systemic symptoms of weight loss, anorexia, and obstructive jaundice appear; it can be a difficult diagnosis to achieve requiring careful investigation. Pancreatic cancer classically presents with painless obstructive jaundice, weight loss, and back pain (70–90% of patients). Any one of these symptoms should be investigated in the older patient [9].

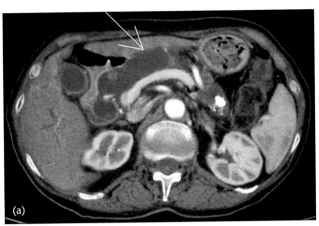

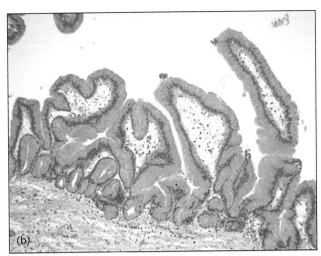

Figure 71.3 (a) Contrast enhanced multi-slice computed tomograph of a main-duct intraductal papillary mucinous neoplasm, demonstrating dilatation of the main pancreatic duct (arrow) (Figure kindly supplied by Dr Jonathan Evans, Consultant Radiologist, Department of Radiology, Royal Liverpool University Hospital Trust, Liverpool, UK.); (b) High power of

intraductal papillary mucinous neoplasm showing minimal atypia within the lining mucinous epithelium. (Figure kindly supplied by Dr Fiona Campbell, Consultant Histopathologist, Department of Pathology, Royal Liverpool University Hospital Trust, Liverpool, UK.)

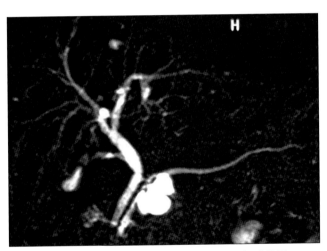

Figure 71.4 Magnetic resonance cholangiopancreatography (MRCP) demonstrating a side-branch intraductal papillary mucinous neoplasm.

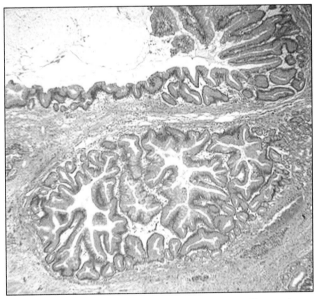

Figure 71.5 Low-power view of branch type intraductal papillary mucinous neoplasm showing papillary infoldings of lining epithelium. (Figure kindly supplied by Dr Fiona Campbell, Consultant Histopathologist, Department of Pathology, Royal Liverpool University Hospital Trust, Liverpool, UK.)

Early symptoms for pancreatic cancer have been reported. A combination of anorexia, and/or early satiety, and/or asthenia were reported in 22.3% of pancreatic cancer patients compared with 0.7% of controls. The symptoms appeared less than 6 months before the onset of pain and jaundice in 17% of patients. However, these symptoms are non-specific, and are unlikely to be acted on by patient or general practitioner alike.

More commonly the patient presents with abdominal pain. It is usually insidious pain originating in the epigastric region and radiating to the sides and/or back. The pain may be worse at night and in the postprandial period. Pain is the presenting symptom in between 31% and 79% of pancreatic cancer patients.

Jaundice arises from compression of the biliary tract. It can be the first manifestation of pancreatic cancer depending on the site of the tumor in 24–85%.

Weight loss is another common presenting symptom of pancreatic cancer. This can be due to anorexia, catabolic metabolism induced by the tumor, and malabsorption . However, weight loss is a common symptom in the elderly population, and not always as a result of malignancy.

Other presentations include diabetes mellitus and acute pancreatitis. Around 70% of patients with pancreatic cancer have impaired glucose tolerance (IGT) or diabetes. Newly diagnosed diabetes mellitus in the over 60s may herald pancreatic cancer when there is no family history of diabetes.

Pancreatic cancer can also present as acute pancreatitis in approximately 3% of cases. Acute pancreatitis of unknown aetiology in the over 50s should induce a suspicion of pancreatic cancer.

Patients may also present with acute cholangitis, duodenal obstruction, deep venous thrombosis, pruritus, steatorrhea, and thrombophlebitis migrans (as described by Trousseau based on his own pancreatic cancer). Signs may include jaundice, hepatomegaly, palpable gallbladder (Courvoisier's sign – 40%), cachexia, Troisier's sign (involved Virchow's node), an abdominal mass, and ascites. Persistent back pain and/or partial relief of pain by sitting upright usually indicates unresectable disease.

Differential diagnosis

The differential diagnosis depends on the clinical presentation of the patient:

- In the presence of jaundice, intrahepatic causes, cholangiocarcinoma, and benign causes such as gallstone disease or Mirizzi syndrome may be considered. Ultrasound scan and CT will differentiate these causes.
- Epigastric pain will need to be differentiated from benign gastric disease such as peptic ulcer disease, gastritis, or malignant gastric tumors. Endoscopic examination may be required.
- Back pain will need to be differentiated from musculoskeletal causes of back pain.
- An abdominal mass in the epigastrium needs to be differentiated from a hepatic, gastric, colonic or omental mass.
- Other causes of steatorrhea including malabsorption (e.g., celiac disease). Endoscopic examination may be carried out to differentiate these disease entities.
- The main diagnostic dilemma is that between pancreatic cancer and chronic pancreatitis both of which may present with very similar symptoms and may coexist. The diagnosis relies on improved imaging modalities as well as clinical acumen. omputed tomography is mandatory for the diagnosis of pancreatic cancer.

Diagnostic methods

Initial investigations will include blood tests for anemia, clotting profile, liver function tests, and serum CA19-9 in jaundiced patients.

- Transabdominal ultrasound is usually the initial investigation because most patients will present with jaundice. Tumors larger than 2 cm in size, dilatation of the biliary and main pancreatic ducts, and possible extrapancreatic spread, notably liver metastases may be detected, but a normal ultrasound scan does not rule out pancreatic cancer.
- If pancreatic cancer is suspected, multidetector computed tomography (MDCT) should always be performed. This

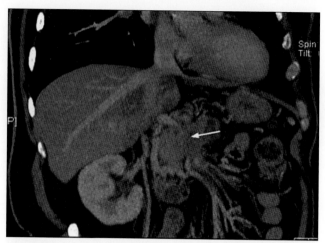

Figure 71.6 Coronal section of multislice computed tomograph demonstrating pancreatic tumor encasing the portal vein (arrow). This patient has unresectable disease. (Figure kindly supplied by Dr Jonathan Evans, Consultant Radiologist, Department of Radiology, Royal Liverpool University Hospital Trust, Liverpool, UK.)

can achieve diagnostic rates of 97% for pancreatic cancer (Figure 71.6). The accuracy for predicting unresectable lesions is 90%, but the accuracy of predicting resectable lesions is much less (80–85%). False negatives are mainly due to small hepatic metastases (<1 cm) and small peritoneal deposits.

- Magnetic resonance imaging (MRI) is an alternative to MDCT and is useful for patients who cannot receive intravenous contrast; and magnetic resonance cholangiopancreatography (MRCP) can also provide images of the biliary and pancreatic duct systems similar to endoscopic retrograde cholangiopancreatography (ERCP).
- The role of positron emission tomography (PET) remains to be proven.
- Endoscopic cholangiopancreatography (ERCP) visualizes the biliary tree and pancreatic duct and is used therapeutically to place stents to relieve jaundice. At the same time brush cytology is carried out. ERCP should be carried out after MDCT.
- Percutaneous transhepatic cholangiography (PTC) is used to visualize the biliary tree and relieve jaundice in patients who cannot undergo ERCP due to difficult anatomy or previous surgery.
- Endoscopic ultrasound (EUS) is increasingly being used (Figure 71.7) and demonstrates a sensitivity of 95% and specificity of 80% with a positive predictive value of 95% and negative predictive value of 80% for malignant masses. EUS can be combined with fine-needle aspiration (FNA) to obtain biopsy with a sensitivity of 86–96%. EUS is used for diagnosis particularly in patients who are not jaundiced and when there is a doubt about the diagnosis.
- Percutaneous FNA biopsy may be used to obtain a diagnosis in patients who are deemed inoperable on imaging or are unfit for resection.

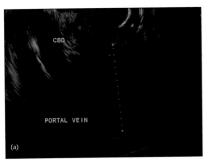
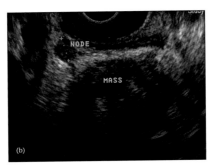
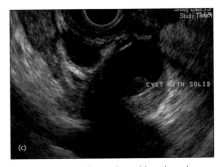

Figure 71.7 Endoluminal ultrasound demonstrating (a) a pancreatic tumor abutting the portal vein; (b) a pancreatic tumor and an enlarged lymph node; (c) a pancreatic tumor abutting the portal vein. (Figures kindly supplied by Dr Jonathan Evans, Consultant Radiologist, Department of Radiology, Royal Liverpool University Hospital Trust, Liverpool, UK.)

Treatment and prevention

Once the pancreatic cancer has been identified, the patient needs to be carefully assessed for fitness for major surgery and the tumor staged preoperatively for resectability (Table 71.6) using MDCT as the mainstay for this. Laparoscopy with laparoscopic ultrasound enables intraoperative scanning of the liver and pancreas to be performed and is highly predictive of resectability, altering the management of 15% of patients already assessed as resectable by MDCT. Selective laparoscopy based on the serum level of CA19-9 is a more efficient strategy, reducing the proportion of patients undergoing laparoscopic ultrasound from 100% to around 45% while increasing the yield from 15% to 25% [10]. Malignant cells can be identified in 7% to 30% of peritoneal washing samples from patients with pancreatic cancer. The relationship between positive cytology and survival is not entirely clear and requires further study [11].

Resectable disease
Principles of management
(Please refer to the accompanying management protocol on the website)

These are, broadly:

- To treat patients in a center of expertise with a high case load
- To consider preoperative biliary drainage in jaundiced patients
- To resect all tumor to achieve R0 resection
- To reduce/manage postoperative complications
- To consider adjuvant chemotherapy for all patients

Pre-operative biliary drainage

There is some evidence from a randomized controlled trial that preoperative plastic biliary stents increase complications [12]. In routine practice, however, stents are used to facilitate logistical planning of staging and treatment.

Short covered metal stents should be used and placed endoscopically if possible.

Table 71.6 Indicators of resectability in pancreatic cancer

Factors contraindicating resection	Factors that do not contraindicate resection
Liver, peritoneal, or other metastasis	Continuous invasion of duodenum, stomach, or colon
Uncertain whether distant lymph node metastasis influence prognosis	Lymph node metastasis within the operative field
Major venous encasement (>2 cm in length, >50% circumference involvement)	Venous impingement or minimal invasion of superior mesenteric and hepatic portal veins
Superior mesenteric, celiac, or hepatic artery encasement	Gastroduodenal artery encasement
Severe co-morbid illness	Age of patient
Cirrhosis with portal hypertension	

Surgical management

- The aim of surgery is to achieve an R0 resection (clear microscopic resection margins).
- Nevertheless, 30–60% of resections are R1 positive: complete clearance of macroscopic tumor with positive microscopic resection margins.
- Patients who have R2 resections (incomplete clearance of macroscopic tumor) should be treated as for locally advanced disease.

Tumors of the head of pancreas

The standard operation for tumors of the head of pancreas (Figure 71.8) is the Kausch–Whipple partial pancreatoduodenectomy (Figure 71.9). The most commonly used approach at the present time is the pylorus-preserving partial pancreatoduodenectomy (Figure 71.10). There is no difference in long-term outcome between these two approaches [13]. Pancreatojejunostomy, hepaticojejunostomy, and duodenojejunostomy are performed for the reconstruction. There is no significant difference between pancreatojejunostomy and pancreatogastrostomy [14].

Pancreas and Biliary Tract

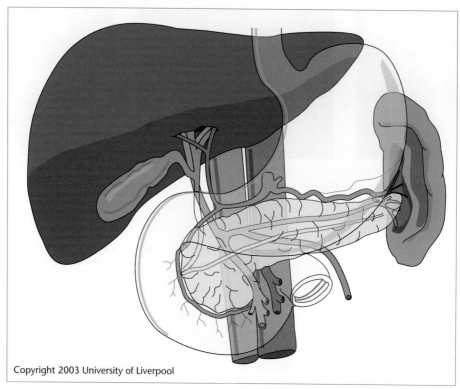

Figure 71.8 Normal preoperative anatomy of the pancreas.

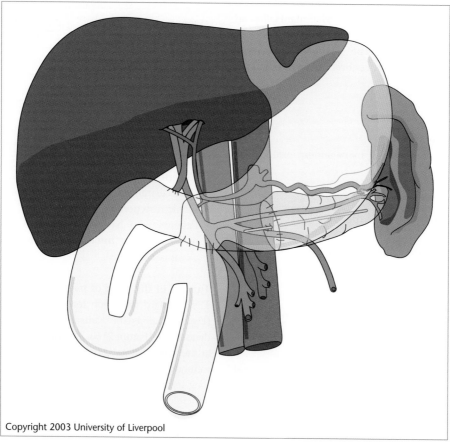

Figure 71.9 Pylorus-preserving Kausch–Whipple pancreatoduodenectomy.

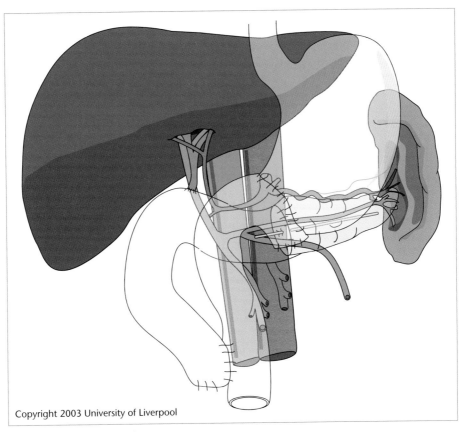

Copyright 2003 University of Liverpool

Figure 71.10 Classical Kausch–Whipple pancreatoduodenectomy.

- There is no survival advantage for extended radical lymphadenectomy in pancreatic cancer [15].
- There is no survival advantage to be gained by performing a total pancreatectomy for a tumor of the pancreatic head, unless it is to achieve R0 resection.
- Resection of the portal or superior mesenteric vein may be necessary to achieve an R0 resection and can be done with an acceptable morbidity.

Tumors of the body and tail of pancreas

A left pancreatectomy is performed, which includes splenectomy and en-bloc removal of the hilar lymph nodes.

Morbidity and mortality

- The overall mortality for major pancreatic resections is less than 5% in major centers.
- Postoperative morbidity is around 40%, so patients require high-dependency care for at least the first 24 hours after surgery.

Neo-adjuvant therapy

Indications are:
- To convert patients to resectability from being locally unresectable
- To be used with adjuvant therapy to improve overall survival

Results from small trials are useful to identify particular regimens and toxicity. A comparison of adjuvant and neo-adjuvant therapy did not demonstrate a significant difference in survival between the two groups. There is a suggestion that the proportion of R0 resections may be increased by neo-adjuvant therapy but this does not appear to translate into improved overall survival.

- To date there are no completed phase III studies of neo-adjuvant studies using either chemotherapy or chemoradiation.
- Neo-adjuvant therapy should only be assessed as part of a clinical trial [16].

Adjuvant chemotherapy

The results from two large randomized trials (ESPAC-1 and CONKO-1) show that adjuvant systemic chemotherapy will increase the 5-year survival from 9–12% with resection alone to 21–29% and 23% with either 5-fluourouracil (5FU) and folinic acid (FA) or gemcitabine (GEM), respectively [2,17].

The survival benefit is maintained irrespective of the type of operation used and whether or not patients develop postoperative complications.

The international ESPAC-3(v2) trial comparing adjuvant gemcitabine and 5FU randomized 1088 patients following surgery for pancreatic cancer. Median survival from resection of patients treated with 5FU/FA was 23.0 (95% CI: 21.1, 25.0) months and for patients treated with GEM this was 23.6 (95% CI: 21.4, 26.4) months. There was no statistically significant difference in survival estimates between the treatment groups (c^2_{LR}=0.7, p=0.39, HR_{GEM}=0.94 (95%CI: 0.81, 1.08) [18]. There was less toxicity in the gemcitabine group compared with 5FU and this is now the standard of care following surgery.

Adjuvant chemoradiotherapy
Improved survival seen in small randomized and non-randomized series of patients. This has not been confirmed in large randomised trials [19,20].

Chemoradiotherapy and follow-on chemotherapy
The RTOG 9704 trial [21] used background 5FU-based chemoradiotherapy together with pre- and post-chemoradiation systemic chemotherapy comprising either 5FU or gemcitabine. The results showed no difference between the two groups in of terms of median survival or 3-year survival in all patients.

Meta-analysis
The results of meta-analysis using individual patient data reject the use of chemoradiation and provide powerful evidence for systemic chemotherapy [22,23].

Unresectable disease
Approximately 70% of patients will present with unresectable disease. The treatment of patients who have unresectable pancreatic cancer due to localized advanced disease, and/or metastases consists of symptom control and palliative therapy

Pain relief
Intractable pain is a major problem, which necessitates the use of high-dose opiates.

Additional approaches include intraoperative, percutaneous CT-guided or EUS neurolytic celiac plexus block and bilateral or unilateral thoracoscopic splanchnicectomy.

Jaundice and duodenal obstruction
- Jaundice is best relieved using ERCP and biliary stent.
- A PTHC-endoscopy approach is employed only if ERCP is not technically possible.
- Main complications are acute cholangitis, bleeding, and peritonitis.
- Self-expanding metal (and covered) stents should be used for patients with a good performance status and favourable prognosis (locally advanced primary tumor <3 cm).
- Plastic stents should be used for those patients with metastases and tumors >3 cm in diameter.
- Endoscopically placed expandable metal stents are deployed for duodenal obstruction (occurs in approximately 15% of patients).

- Success rate is approximately 85%. Complications include perforation, fistula, bleeding, and recurrent obstruction due to stent migration or fracture.
- Surgical bypass (open and laparoscopic) can be used to relieve jaundice using a Roux-en-Y loop hepatojejunostomy, and duodenal obstruction by gastrojejunostomy, especially in younger patients and both can be achieved laparoscopically.

Weight loss
Weight loss is initially due to pancreatic exocrine insufficiency owing to obstruction of the main pancreatic duct as well as exclusion of bile acids from obstruction of the main bile duct. Fat maldigestion may also contribute to abdominal pain and bloating. Relief of biliary obstruction and pancreatic enzyme supplementation will alleviate these symptoms [24]

Cachexia can be a marked feature of the later stages of pancreatic cancer, with no good treatment.

Role of chemo-radiotherapy
External beam radiotherapy is used with 5FU or gemcitabine as a radiosensitizing agent (chemoradiotherapy). The main drawback is the limit on the dosage owing to the close proximity of adjacent radiosensitive organs. Newer techniques such as conformal radiotherapy are now being used, but these studies almost invariably employ follow-on chemotherapy once the chemoradiotherapy has been completed. Meta-analysis has demonstrated that chemoradiotherapy is better than radiotherapy alone but there is no survival difference between chemoradiotherapy plus follow-on chemotherapy and chemotherapy alone [25]. It should only be evaluated as part of a clinical trial.

Systemic chemotherapy
Pancreatic ductal adenocarcinoma is highly resistant to conventional methods of cytotoxic treatment and radiotherapy. Few chemotherapeutic agents have been shown to have reproducible response rates of more than 10%.

5FU is an inhibitor of thymidylate synthetase (essential for synthesis of DNA nucleotides) and has been the most widely used in advanced pancreatic cancer, with a median survival of around 5–6 months, and is better than the best supportive care.

The nucleoside analog, gemcitabine, has replaced 5FU as the preferred drug. Median survival increase in favor of gemcitabine compared with 5FU is 5.7 vs 4.4 months), the 1-year survival rate increase is 18% vs 2%, toxicity is relatively mild and there is a better clinical response (24% vs 5%, respectively).

A recent meta-analysis has confirmed that combination chemotherapy may improve the survival observed with gemcitabine alone [26]. Two agents in combination with gemcitabine have improved survival compared to gemcitabine alone. Capecitabine (Xeloda) is a new oral, fluoropyrimidine carbamate that is sequentially converted to 5FU by three enzymes located in the liver and in tumors, including pancreatic cancer, and demonstrated a trend towards improved survival compared with gemcitabine alone, which was significant in a meta-analysis [27]. Platinum based agents have also demonstrated improved survival. FOLFIRINOX combination has demonstrated high response rates and survival [28].

Novel therapy
There are many novel agents in early phase clinical trials that target specific molecular pathways and may ultimately improve outcome in these patients. [29]

Prevention
Avoiding alcohol and smoking are obvious preventative measures to reduce the risk of pancreatic cancer [30]. There are no clinical trials as yet for chemoprevention in pancreatic cancer. The majority of data has been generated in preclinical studies *in vitro* and *in vivo*. Dietary isoprenoids, somatostatin analogs, selective estrogen modulators and anti-androgen agents have shown some effects in preclinical studies. Aspirin, nonsteroidal anti-inflammatory drugs (NSAIDs) and selective COX-2 inhibitors have also been proposed. The anti-oxidants associated with green and black tea are also possible agents for chemoprevention. Vitamins C and E and selenium are also potential chemopreventative agents. The majority of the evidence for these compounds is based on in-vitro studies and therefore much work is still needed [31].

Complications of surgery
Surgery-related postoperative morbidity has also decreased in recent years, but it still ranges from 20% to 54% [32]. Many of the postoperative complications respond to medical treatment and radiological and endoscopic intervention.

Medical complications
Medical complications include those arising from the respiratory system (atelectasis, pneumonia, respiratory insufficiency), cardiovascular system (angina, myocardial infarction, arrhythmias, stroke, deep venous thrombosis, and pulmonary embolism), renal system (acute renal failure), as well as hepatic and metabolic disturbances, urinary tract infection, and central line infection.

Intra-abdominal abscess
Intra-abdominal abscess occurs in between 1% and 12% of patients. The usual cause is anastomotic leak at the pancreatojejunostomy, hepatojejunostomy, duodenojejunostomy, gastrojejunostomy, or the jejunojejunostomy. Contrast-enhanced CT is indicated. Preferred management is CT-guided percutaneous drainage.

Hemorrhage
Postoperative hemorrhage occurs in between 2% and 5% of patients. Bleeding within 24 hours is due to insufficient intraoperative hemostasis or bleeding from an anastomosis. Free intraperitoneal hemorrhage requires immediate reoperation. Management of anastomotic bleeding is initially conservative. Stress ulceration can be managed medically and/or endoscopically. Secondary haemorrhage (1–3 weeks after surgery) is commonly related to an anastomotic leak and secondary erosion of the retroperitoneal vasculature, or a pseudoaneurysm with a mortality rate of 15–58%. Investigations: contrast enhanced CT, endoscopy, selective angiography with embolization. Bleeding from a pancreatojejunostomy may require completion total pancreatectomy or refashioning of the anastomosis.

Fistula after pancreatoduodenectomy
Incidence of fistula after pancreatoduodenectomy ranges between 2% and 24%. The mortality risk from a major pancreatic fistula may be as high as 28%; the cause of death is retroperitoneal sepsis and hemorrhage. Most leaks, however, can be managed conservatively with little upset to the patient.

Delayed gastric emptying
Delayed gastric emptying is reported to be present in between 4% and 37% of patients after resection of the head of the pancreas. The etiology of delayed gastric emptying is not entirely clear but includes anastomotic edema and damage to the fragile vascular supply of the gastroduodenal neuroendocrine axis. Supportive measures include the use of erythromycin, metoclopramide, and cyclizine. Gastric function normalizes at 2–4 weeks following pancreatoduodenectomy. Although delayed gastric emptying almost invariably resolves with conservative treatment, operative correction is occasionally required.

Other uncommon major complications
Acute cholangitis indicates partial obstruction due to edema of the anastamosis or is associated with a local complication. Acute pancreatitis is rare and usually resolves with conservative management, but bleeding or infection may ensue, which may require surgical intervention. Small bowel obstruction is also managed conservatively but ischemia and necrosis may occur so that vigilance is required. Hepatic portal vein thrombosis is rare but, if detected early, percutaneous transhepatic thrombectomy should be performed. Chylous ascites is probably commoner than suggested by reports from series and can be troublesome – infection may ensue causing an abscess. External drainage of the ascites is necessary and may need to be supplemented with nil by mouth, total parenteral nutrition, and octreotide.

Prognosis with and without treatment

The most important determinants of survival in pancreatic cancer are:

- Surgical resectability
- Performance status

Overall survival is 0.4%. Median survival following surgical resection ranges between 11 and 20 months. Five-year survival ranges from between 7% and 25%. This can be improved to 29% with adjuvant chemotherapy. Median survival for advanced disease is between 3 and 6 months. This can be improved using systemic chemotherapy to over 7 months.

The other prognostic factors can be categorized into tumor-related, patient-related, and treatment-related groups.

Tumor-related factors

- Stage of tumor – patients with locally advanced disease have a better prognosis than those with metastatic disease
- Histological type – undifferentiated (anaplastic) carcinoma has a worse prognosis than ductal adenocarcinoma
- Grade of tumor differentiation – well-differentiated tumors have a better prognosis
- Lymph node involvement – and lymph node 8a involvement indicates poor prognosis
- A high lymph node ratio indicates a poor prognosis [33]
- Location – head lesions have better prognosis than those of body and tail
- Presence of perineural invasion is associated with decreased survival
- Resection margins involvement is associated with decreased survival (positive resection margin is defined as at least one cancer cell within 1 mm of any surface)
- Raised CA19.9 is a marker for poor prognosis [33]
- Molecular markers, e.g., KRAS mutation, TGF beta, VEGF, BAX, PD-ECGF, DPC4, S100A6, MUC4, MMPs

Patient-related factors

- Leukocytosis – elevated white cell count is associated with poor survival
- Elevated gamma glutamine transferase is a biomarker of cholestasis and has a poor prognosis
- Elevated C-reactive protein level is an independent prognostic marker in advanced disease
- Presence of severe pain is a poor prognostic factor in advanced disease
- High platelet/lymphocyte ratio indicates poor outcome [34]

Treatment-related factors

- Treatment center with expertise and high case load
- Resection
- Relief of jaundice and gastric outlet obstruction in advanced disease
- Systemic chemotherapy

SOURCES OF INFORMATION FOR PATIENTS AND DOCTORS

There are major sources of information for patients and clinicians on the internet, the following being the most useful:
http://www.cancerbacup.org.uk/Home
http://pancreas.org/
http://www.liv.ac.uk/surgery/europac.html
http://pathology.jhu.edu/pancreas/
http://www.pancreaticcancer.org.uk/
http://www.lctu.org.uk/
http://www.cancerhelp.org.uk/help/default.asp?page=2795

Patient information booklets concerning pancreatic cancer and its diagnosis and treatment are available from Solvay Healthcare Limited, Southampton, UK and there are a number of textbooks on the subject [35].

References

1. Parkin DM, Bray FI, Devesa SS. Cancer burden in the year 2000. The global picture. *Eur J Cancer*. 2001;37 Suppl 8:4–66.
2. Neoptolemos J, Stocken D, Freiss H, *et al*. A randomised trial of chemoradiotherapy and chemotherapy after resection of pancreatic cancer. *N Engl J Med*. 2004;350:1200–1210.
3. Ghaneh P, Costello E, Neoptolemos JP. Biology and management of pancreatic cancer. *Gut*. 2007;56:1134–1152.
4. Raimondi S, Maisonneuve P, Lowenfels AB. epidemiology of pancreatic cancer: an overview. *Nat Rev Gastroenterol Hepatol*. 2009;6:699–708.
5. http://www-dep.iarc.fr/
6. Howes N, Lerch MM, Greenhalf W, *et al*. Clinical and genetic characteristics of hereditary pancreatitis in Europe. *Clin Gastroenterol Hepatol*. 2004;2:252–261.
7. McFaul CD, Greenhalf W, Earl J, *et al*. Anticipation in familial pancreatic cancer. *Gut*. 2006;55:252–258.
8. Hruban RH, Takaori K, Klimstra DS, *et al*. An illustrated consensus on the classification of pancreatic intraepithelial neoplasia and intraductal papillary mucinous neoplasms. *Am J Surg Pathol*. 2004;28:977–987.
9. Shore S, Vimalachandran D, Raraty MG, Ghaneh P. Cancer in the elderly: pancreatic cancer *Surg Oncol*. 2004;13:201–210.
10. Halloran CM, Ghaneh P, Connor S, Sutton R, Neoptolemos JP, Raraty MG. Carbohydrate antigen 19.9 accurately selects patients for laparoscopic assessment to determine resectability of pancreatic malignancy. *Br J Surg*. 2008;95:453–459.
11. Kelly KJ, Wong J, Gladdy R, *et al*. Prognostic impact of RT-PCR-based detection of peritoneal micrometastases in patients with pancreatic cancer undergoing curative resection. *Ann Surg Oncol*. 2009;16:3333–3339.
12. van der Gaag NA, Rauws EA, van Eijck CH, *et al*. Preoperative biliary drainage for cancer of the head of the pancreas. *N Engl J Med*. 2010;362:129–137.
13. Diener MK, Heukaufer C, Schwarzer G, *et al*. Pancreaticoduodenectomy (classic Whipple) versus pylorus-preserving pancreaticoduodenectomy (pp Whipple) for surgical treatment of periampullary and pancreatic carcinoma. *Cochrane Database Syst Rev*. 2008;(2):CD006053.
14. Wente MN, Shrikhande SV, Müller MW, *et al*. Pancreaticojejunostomy versus pancreaticogastrostomy: systematic review and meta-analysis. *Am J Surg*. 2007;193:171–183.

Pancreas and Biliary Tract

15. Michalski CW, Kleeff J, Wente MN, Diener MK, Büchler MW, Friess H. Systematic review and meta-analysis of standard and extended lymphadenectomy in pancreaticoduodenectomy for pancreatic cancer. *Br J Surg.* 2007;94:265–273.

16. Ghaneh P, Smith R, Tudor-Smith C, Raraty M, Neoptolemos JP. Neoadjuvant and adjuvant strategies for pancreatic cancer. *Eur J Surg Oncol.* 2008;34:297–305.

17. Oettle H, Post S, Neuhaus P, *et al.* Adjuvant chemotherapy with gemcitabine vs observation in patients undergoing curative-intent resection of pancreatic cancer: a randomized controlled trial *JAMA.* 2007;297:267–277.

18. Neoptolemos JP, Stocken DD, Bassi C, *et al.*; European Study Group for Pancreatic Cancer. Adjuvant chemotherapy with fluorouracil plus folinic acid vs gemcitabine following pancreatic cancer resection: a randomized controlled trial. *JAMA.* 2010;304:1073–1081.

19. Klinkenbijl JH, Jeekel J, Sahmoud T, *et al.* Adjuvant radiotherapy and 5-fluorouracil after curative resection of cancer of the pancreas and periampullary region: phase III trial of the EORTC gastrointestinal tract cancer cooperative group. *Ann Surg.* 1999; 230:776–784.

20. Smeenk HG, van Eijck CH, Hop WC, *et al.* Long-term survival and metastatic pattern of pancreatic and periampullary cancer after adjuvant chemoradiation or observation: long-term results of EORTC trial 40891. *Ann Surg.* 2007;246:734–740.

21. Regine WF, Winter KA, Abrams RA, *et al.* Fluorouracil vs gemcitabine chemotherapy before and after fluorouracil-based chemoradiation following resection of pancreatic adenocarcinoma: a randomized controlled trial. *JAMA.* 2008;299:1019–1026.

22. Stocken DD, Büchler MW, Dervenis C, *et al.* Meta-analysis of randomised adjuvant therapy trials for pancreatic cancer. *Br J Cancer.* 2005;92:1372–1381.

23. Neoptolemos JP, Stocken DD, Tudor Smith C, *et al.* Adjuvant 5-fluorouracil and folinic acid vs observation for pancreatic cancer: composite data from the ESPAC-1 and -3(v1) trials. *Br J Cancer.* 2009;100:246–250.

24. Bruno MJ, Haverkort EB, Tijssen GP, Tytgat GN, van Leeuwen DJ. Placebo controlled trial of enteric coated pancreatin microsphere treatment in patients with unresectable cancer of the pancreatic head region. *Gut.* 1998;42:92–96.

25. Sultana A, Tudur Smith C, Cunningham D, *et al.* Systematic review, including meta-analyses, on the management of locally advanced pancreatic cancer using radiation/combined modality therapy. *Br J Cancer.* 2007;96:1183–1190.

26. Sultana A, Smith CT, Cunningham D, Starling N, Neoptolemos JP, Ghaneh P. Meta-analyses of chemotherapy for locally advanced and metastatic pancreatic cancer. *J Clin Oncol.* 2007;25:2607–2615.

27. Cunningham D, Chau I, Stocken DD, *et al.* Phase III randomized comparison of gemcitabine versus gemcitabine plus capecitabine in patients with advanced pancreatic cancer. *J Clin Oncol.* 2009;27:5513–5518.

28. Conroy T, Desseigne F, Ychou M, *et al.* FOLFIRINOX versus gemcitabine for metastatic pancreatic cancer. *N Engl J Med.* 2011;364:1817–1825.

29. Middleton G, Ghaneh P, Costello E, Greenhalf W, Neoptolemos JP. New treatment options for advanced pancreatic cancer. *Expert Rev Gastroenterol Hepatol.* 2008;2:673–696.

30. Vimalachandran D, Ghaneh P, Costello E, Neoptolemos JP. Genetics and prevention of pancreatic cancer. *Cancer Control.* 2004;11:6–14.

31. Ghaneh P, Greenhalf W, Neoptolemos JP. Factors involved in carcinogenesis and prevention in hepatobiliary cancer. In: *Structure of GI Oncology: A Critical MDT Approach.* Eds Jankowski, Sampliner, Kerr and Fong. Blackwell Publishing (Oxford) 2007.

32. Halloran CM, Ghaneh P, Bosonnet L, Hartley MN, Sutton R, Neoptolemos JP. Complications of pancreatic cancer resection. *Dig Surg.* 2002;19:138–146.

33. Smith RA, Bosonnet L, Ghaneh P, *et al.* Preoperative CA19-9 levels and lymph node ratio are independent predictors of survival in patients with resected pancreatic ductal adenocarcinoma. *Dig Surg.* 2008;25:226–232.

34. Smith RA, Bosonnet L, Raraty M, *et al.* Preoperative platelet-lymphocyte ratio is an independent significant prognostic marker in resected pancreatic ductal adenocarcinoma. *Am J Surg.* 2009 ;197:466–472.

35. Beger HG, Warshaw A, Buchler M, *et al. The Pancreas: An Integrated Textbook of Basic Science, Medicine, and Surgery.* Blackwell Publishing (Oxford) 2008.

Pancreas and Biliary Tract

CHAPTER 72

Cysts and pseudocysts of the pancreas

Brian G. Turner[1] and William R. Brugge[1,2]

[1]Massachusetts General Hospital, Boston, MA, USA
[2]Harvard Medical School, Boston, MA, USA

Pancreas and Biliary Tract

ESSENTIAL FACTS ABOUT PATHOGENESIS

- Prevalence: varies between 0.21% and 24.3%
- Risk: advanced age and genetic alterations are associated with cystic lesions
- Pathogenesis: serous cyst adenomas are associated with mutations in the VHL gene, mucinous with *KRAS* oncogene and *p53* mutations
- Serous cystadenomas occur more commonly in men, while mucinous cystic neoplasms are far more common in women

---

ESSENTIALS OF DIAGNOSIS

- Pancreatic cysts are often asymptomatic and incidentally found on imaging studies
- Differentiating between a pseudocyst and cystic neoplasm
- Calcifications in the pancreas or history of pancreatitis is suggestive of a pseudocyst
- Computed tomography (CT), magnetic resonance imaging (MRI), and endoscopic ultrasound (EUS) with fine needle aspiration (FNA) are useful in evaluating cysts
- Cyst fluid analysis (CEA and molecular markers) and cytology can be helpful in distinguishing benign and malignant lesions

---

ESSENTIALS OF TREATMENT

- Surgery for premalignant lesions is determined by symptoms, risk of malignancy, and surgical risk to patient
- Pseudocysts can be managed by surgery or drainage (endoscopic or radiologic)
- New potential therapies for premalignant lesions include introducing ethanol and chemotherapeutic agents into cystic lesions

---

Introduction

Cystic lesions of the pancreas are composed of a broad range of neoplastic cysts and inflammatory pseudocysts. The neoplastic cysts span the spectrum of malignancy, from benign cystadenomas to premalignant and frankly malignant lesions. With the widespread use of abdominal imaging, the lesions are increasingly identified in early stages of asymptomatic patients. There are three basic types of pancreatic cystic lesions: serous, mucinous, and inflammatory [1,2] (Table 72.1).

Epidemiology

Prevalence

The reported prevalence of lesions ranges from 0.21% on ultrasound imaging [3] to 24.3% in an autopsy study [4]. Screening magnetic resonance imaging (MRI) studies in 1444 patients in a general hospital population in the United States have demonstrated a prevalence rate of 19.6% [5]. This study included patients with known pancreatitis, jaundice, and biliary obstruction. A more recent study utilizing multidetector computed tomography (CT) reported a prevalence of 2.6% in a series of 2832 consecutive patients [6].

Clinical epidemiology

Surgical pathology studies estimate that serous cystadenomas (SCAs) account for approximately 1–2% of all exocrine pancreatic neoplasms [7]. Serous cystadenomas occur only in adults and are more commonly found in men. Patients have ranged in age from 18 to 91 years, with a median age in the seventh decade. Mucinous cystic neoplasms (MCNs) account for approximately 2–5% of all exocrine pancreatic tumors. Women are affected far more commonly than men (9:1 female:male ratio), with a mean age at diagnosis in the fifth decade. Intraductal papillary mucinous neoplasms (IPMNs) are closely associated with MCNs. Their true incidence is uncertain, but estimates range from 1% to 8% of all pancreatic tumors. Intraductal papillary mucinous neoplasms affect men and women equally or men predominantly, depending on the reported series, and they tend to occur in an older age group than MCNs. Finally, pancreatic pseudocysts have an incidence of 1.6–4.5% or 0.5–1 per 100 000 adults per year [8,9], and can complicate the clinical course in up to 30–40% of patients with chronic pancreatitis [10].

Causes, risk factors, and disease associations

Von Hippel–Lindau (VHL) disease is the best described genetic, inherited disorder associated with cystic lesions [11]. In a series of 158 prospectively evaluated patients with VHL, pancreatic involvement was observed in 122 patients (77.2%) and included true cysts (91.1%), serous cystadenomas (12.3%),

---

Table 72.1 Types of cystic lesion

- Serous (benign without malignant potential)
- Mucinous (pre-malignant or malignant)
- Inflammatory (fluid collections, pseudocysts)

Table 72.2 Pathogenesis of cystic lesions

Type of cystic lesion	Genetic alterations
Serous	Mutations of VHL gene (3p25)
Mucinous cystic neoplasms	Mutations of *KRAS*, *p53*
Intraductal papillary mucinous neoplasms	Mutations of *PIK3CA*, Expression of CDX2, MUC1, MUC2, and MUC5
Inflammatory	None

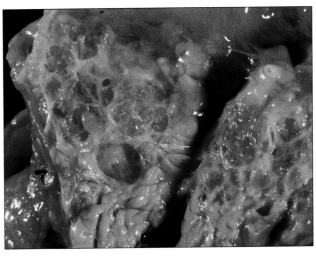

Figure 72.1 Serous cystadenoma. Gross pathology of a serous cystadenoma.

neuroendocrine tumors (12.3%), or combined lesions (11.5%). Pancreatic pseudocysts are peripancreatic fluid collections that arise in association with inflammatory conditions of the pancreas or disruption of the pancreatic duct due to surgery or trauma.

Pathogenesis (see Table 72.2)

Serous cystadenomas are strongly associated with mutations of the VHL gene, located on chromosome 3p25, and may play a sentinel role in sporadic cases [12]. In one study, 70% of the sporadic SCAs studied demonstrated loss of heterozygosity at 3p25 with a VHL gene mutation in the remaining allele [13]. The mutations in the VHL gene probably result in hamartomatous proliferation of the centro-acinar cells. Mucinous cystic neoplasms and intraductal papillary mucinous neoplasms are thought to have a different pathogenesis compared to SCAs. Mucinous cystic neoplasms frequently contain mutations of the *KRAS* oncogene and *p53* tumor suppressor gene; the frequency increases with increasing degrees of dysplasia in the tumor. The frequency of *KRAS* mutation in MCNs is linearly related to the grades of atypia [14]. However, the degree of atypia in IPMNs does not seem to correlate with the presence of *KRAS* mutations. Loss of heterozygosity (LOH) of the *p16* gene was observed with increasing degrees of histological atypia in IPMNs, whereas LOH of the *p53* gene was seen only in invasive carcinomas. Other genetic alterations include strong expression of MUC1, MUC2, and MUC5 in IPMN's [15].

Pancreatic pseudocysts have no epithelial lining. Two basic mechanisms describe pancreatic pseudocyst formation [16]. In the "ductal-leakage" mechanism, localized necrosis of a pancreatic duct may allow the leakage of fluid out of the pancreas and into spaces formed by organs adjacent to the pancreas. In a minority of pseudocysts the origin of the fluid is not leakage, but liquefactive necrosis of pancreatic tissue in severe acute pancreatitis.

Pathology

Serous cystadenomas (Figure 72.1)

Serous tumors have three variants based on gross morphology: microcystic, macrocystic, and solid. Microcystic SCAs are the most common and are composed of innumerable small cysts with a honeycomb-like appearance on cross-section. Large-diameter microcystic SCAs often have a fibrotic or calcified central scar. Macrocystic SCAs are composed of far fewer cysts with large cystic cavities mimicking the appearance of mucinous lesions. The cyst fluid from SCAs is thin, clear, and contains no mucin. The epithelial cells of all types of SCAs are similar in appearance with a cuboidal shape, glycogen-rich, clear cytoplasm, and small, regular centrally located nuclei [17].

Mucinous cystic neoplasms (Figure 72.2)

Grossly, MCNs are characteristically macrocystic with discrete cavities. In the absence of an associated mass, malignant transformation may be suspected with focal thickening, irregularity, or ulceration of the cyst lining. They are lined by mucin-secreting cells, and are categorized based on the degree of epithelial dysplasia: benign, borderline, and malignant. Mucinous cystic neoplasms of the pancreas often contain a highly cellular (so-called "ovarian") stroma. It occurs almost exclusively in female patients, although rare cases of MCNs with ovarian stroma in male patients have been encountered.

Intraductal papillary mucinous neoplasms

Intraductal papillary mucinous neoplasms originate in the pancreatic ductal system. The presence of a papillary tumor causes dilatation of the ducts as a result of tumor growth. The degree of ductal ectasia varies with the degree of mucin production, but duct dilatation evident on imaging studies or gross pathologic examination is a *sine qua non* of the diagnosis.

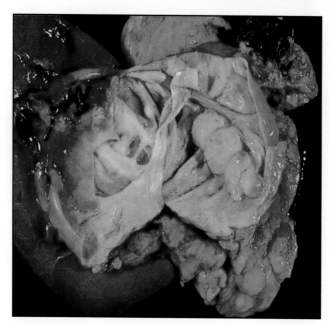

Figure 72.2 Mucinous cystic lesion. Gross pathology of a mucinous cystic lesion.

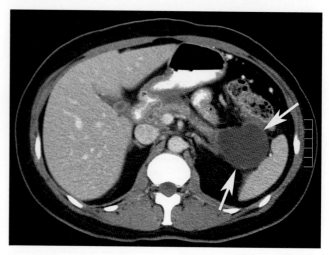

Figure 72.3 Pseudocyst. Abdominal computed tomograph of a simple, thin-walled pseudocyst indicated by white arrows.

The degree of dysplasia exhibited by the epithelium may range from mild to moderate to severe (carcinoma *in situ*). Intraductal papillary mucinous neoplasms originating from the main duct are much more likely to be malignant.

Pancreatic pseudocysts

Pathologic examination of pancreatic pseudocysts can reveal a fluid collection of necrotic fat, as well as a mixture of necrotic cells with surrounding granulation tissue. Persistence of the inflammatory collection results in the formation of a fibrotic pseudocapsule around the fluid. In a recent study of 42 patients with pseudocysts, 75% of cysts had histiocytes, neutrophils, or both. In addition, 31% contained yellow, pigmented material, and 24% showed fat necrosis [18].

Clinical presentation

Most patients with a pancreatic cystic lesion have no signs or symptoms related to the pancreatic lesion. Often the lesion is incidentally found on imaging studies performed for a variety of indications. Symptomatic patients commonly present with recurrent abdominal pain, nausea, and vomiting from mild pancreatitis. These symptoms often reflect the presence of a lesion connected to the main ductal system or duct obstruction. Chronic abdominal pain is a rare presentation of a benign cystic lesion and suggests a malignancy or pseudocyst. Pseudocysts may arise after an episode of acute pancreatitis or insidiously in the setting of chronic pancreatitis and are associated with chronic abdominal pain. Large pseudocysts can compress the stomach, duodenum, or bile duct, causing early satiety, vomiting, or jaundice.

Differential diagnosis

The most important differentiation is between a cystic neoplasm and a pseudocyst. Although pancreatic pseudocysts usually arise in association with pancreatitis, the acute episode of pancreatitis may not have been clinically apparent or the patient may have mild chronic pancreatitis. Evidence of inflammatory changes or calcifications in the pancreas suggests an associated cystic lesion is a pseudocyst. However, in the acute setting of mild pancreatitis, it may be difficult to differentiate between a cystic neoplasm that has caused pancreatitis and a pseudocyst that has formed as a result of pancreatitis. If a pancreatic pseudocyst can be excluded on the basis of a clinical history or imaging findings, attention should be focused on the differential between the types of cystic neoplasms. The principal differentiation is between mucinous and serous lesions because the fundamental difference in management is based on the neoplastic potential of mucinous lesions.

Diagnostic methods

Computed tomography (CT) is an excellent test for cystic lesions of the pancreas [19] (Figure 72.3) Magnetic resonance imaging (MRI) is used increasingly because of the lack of radiation exposure and the ability to image the pancreatic duct with MR cholangiopancreatography (MRCP). Although seen in less than 20% of lesions, demonstration of a central scar by CT or MRI is a highly diagnostic feature of an SCA. The honeycombed or microcystic appearance of the lesion is commonly used to provide a diagnosis. However, macrocystic SCAs are difficult to diagnose with cross-sectional imaging because of the morphologic similarities with mucinous lesions. Mucinous cystic neoplasms, in contrast, are commonly diagnosed with CT based on their unilocular or macrocystic characteristics (Figure 72.4). Though infrequent, the finding of peripheral calcification by CT is specific for an MCN.

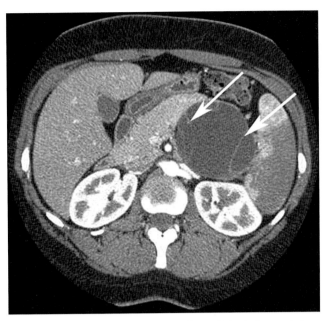

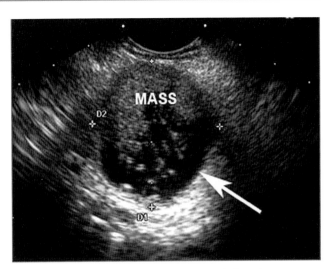

Figure 72.5 Mucinous lesion. Endoscopic ultrasound of a malignant mucinous lesion with a mass filling the cystic space. The white arrow indicates the outer wall of the cyst.

Figure 72.4 Septated, mucinous cystic neoplasm. Abdominal computed tomograph of a septated mucinous cystic neoplasm. White arrows indicate septations within the cyst.

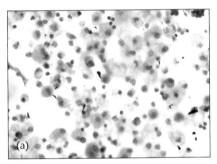

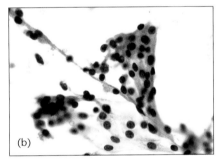

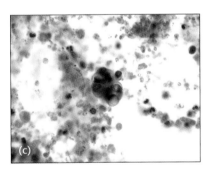

Figure 72.6 Cytology slides of aspirates from endoscopic ultrasound guided fine needle aspiration (EUS-FNA). (a) Pseudocyst aspirate – pseudocyst fluid contains epithelioid histiocytes, hematoidin pigment and proteinaceous debris but, by definition, no cyst lining epithelial cells. (b) Serous cystadenoma. benign cuboidal, non-mucinous epithelial cells line the delicate septa of serous cystadenomas and are difficult to aspirate intact

contributing to the high non-diagnostic rate. (c) Intraductal papillary mucinous neoplasms – in the background of blood and necrosis is a single intact cluster of moderately atypical epithelial cells with only a single residual mucin vacuole. Even a small number of such atypical cells is sufficient to warrant a suspicion of carcinoma.

Intraductal papillary mucinous neoplasms may involve the main pancreatic duct exclusively, a side branch, or both. Magnetic resonance cholangiopancreatography can demonstrate the diagnostic findings of pancreatic duct dilation, mural nodules, and ductal connection. The diagnosis of a pancreatic pseudocyst is more dependent upon the clinical history and the associated findings of chronic pancreatitis. Pseudocysts appear as unilocular fluid-filled cavities associated with parenchymal changes such as calcifications and atrophy.

Intraductal papillary mucinous neoplasms can be imaged with endoscopic retrograde cholangiopancreatography (ERCP) or endoscopic ultrasound (EUS). Contrast retrograde pancreatography will demonstrate the characteristic findings of mucinous filling defects within the duct, diffuse ductal dilation, and

cystic dilation of side branches. Endoscopic ultrasound has been increasingly used to diagnose cystic lesions of the pancreas and guide fine needle aspiration (FNA). The imaging features of cystic neoplasms by EUS are not always sufficient to accurately differentiate benign from malignant cystadenomas; however, the presence of an intramural nodule, mass lesion, or invasive tumor accurately predict malignancy (Figure 72.5). Cyst material, aspirated using EUS guidance, can be analyzed through the use of cytology and a variety of tumor markers (Figure 72.6). However, the low cellular content of cyst fluid has resulted in poor sensitivity in cytologic distinction between mucinous and non-mucinous lesions [20].

Cyst fluid CA 72-4 and carcinoembryonic antigen (CEA) concentrations are high (>192 ng/mL) in mucinous lesions and quite low (<5 ng/mL) in serous cystadenomas [20,21]. Cyst fluid DNA analysis can help to identify mucinous lesions [22]. The use of cyst fluid KRAS to identify mucinous lesions is highly specific (greater than 95%) and moderately sensitive (45%).

Treatment and prevention
Cystic neoplasms
The decision to resect a lesion is based on the presence or absence of symptoms, the risk of malignancy, and the surgical risk to the patient. High-risk patients with low-grade cystic neoplasms may be monitored with periodic CT/MRI or EUS-FNA. In 2006, the Sendai Consensus Guidelines for the management of IPMNs and MCNs of the pancreas was established. For an outline of management of side branch IPMNs [23] please refer to the accompanying management protocol on the website.

Mucinous cystic neoplasms are typically located in the tail of the pancreas and a distal pancreatectomy is highly effective treatment. Serous cystadenomas are resected by removing the involved portion of the pancreas: head (Whipple), body (middle pancreatectomy), or tail (tail resection). Since IPMNs invade the pancreas along ductal structures, frozen section histology is used during surgery to ensure negative margins. High-risk IPMNs involving the entire pancreas may require total pancreatectomy.

Pancreatic pseudocysts
Only 40% of pseudocysts less than 6 cm in diameter will require drainage due to complications or persistence. Small pseudocysts located in the tail of the pancreas and arising from acute biliary pancreatitis have a very high rate of spontaneous drainage. Prior to drainage, it is critical to confirm the diagnosis of a pseudocyst using fluid analysis and cytology.

Drainage of pseudocysts
Pancreatic pseudocysts may be drained using a variety of approaches. External drainage using CT/US guidance is a common approach and involves the percutaneous placement of a small drainage catheter.

Surgical drainage of pseudocysts is performed by providing a large anastomosis between the pseudocyst wall and the stomach or small bowel. Maturation of a pseudocyst wall over 4–6 weeks will allow the formation of a thick wall that will provide a more secure anastomosis. Surgical drainage is the best approach when the pseudocyst is complicated by areas of necrosis, infection, or involves adjacent organs such as the spleen. Cyst-gastrostomy is the easiest approach and requires less operating time than cyst-jejunostomy. Studies report overall success rates for surgical drainage of 90% with major complication rates of 9% and recurrence rates of 3%.

Endoscopic drainage of pseudocysts is an alternative to surgical or radiologic drainage [24]. This approach is used most commonly for uncomplicated, unilocular pseudocysts. Pseudocyst drainage is accomplished with either a transpapillary approach with ERCP or direct endoscopic stent placement across the stomach or duodenal wall (see Video 72.1) [25]. A transpapillary approach is used when the pseudocyst communicates with the main pancreatic duct, usually in the head of the pancreas. A transgastric or duodenal approach is used when the pseudocyst is directly adjacent to the gastroduodenal wall. Endoscopic US is used to determine the size, location, and thickness of the pseudocyst wall [26]. A wall thickness of more than 1 cm or the presence of large intervening vessels or varices precludes endoscopic drainage. Elective EUS-directed drainage can be performed with complication rates of 13%, success rates up to 90%, and recurrence rates of 10–20%. A recent study of laparoscopic, endoscopic, and open pancreatic cystgastrostomy for pancreatic pseudocyst demonstrated no significant difference in the overall success rates between groups [27] .

Complications and their management
Complications of cystic neoplasms are rare and consist of malignant invasion of local structures, such as the bile duct. Endoscopic stenting is the treatment of choice unless the lesion is surgically resectable. Bleeding and infection are the most common complications of pancreatic pseudocysts. Arterial pseudoaneurysms are the most common cause of intracystic and intraductal bleeding and should be managed with angiography.

Prognosis with and without treatment
The prognosis for resected cystic tumors of the pancreas is excellent [28]. There have been only rare reports of tumor recurrence in cases where the lesion was completely resected and no malignant tissue was in the resected specimen. Even for IPMNs containing carcinoma the 5-year survival is over 50% [29]. The worst prognosis is for advanced, transmural adenocarcinomas arising from mucinous lesions; the 5-year survival is only 30% for resected lesions.

Current controversies
With the widespread use of CT/MRI and EUS-FNA, cystic lesions continue to be identified at an early stage. Without a firm understanding of the natural history of IPMNs, it is difficult to know when and if surgical resection should be performed. Non-invasive therapies such as chemical ablation of pancreatic cysts would offer alternatives to surgical therapy. Groups have used ethanol injection, in the Ethanol Pancreatic Injection of Cysts (EPIC) trial [30], as well as combination ethanol/paclitaxel injection [31]. The EUS 2008 Working Group has offered comments on the current state of these promising therapies [32].

References

1. Brugge WR, Lauwers GY, Sahani D, Fernandez-del Castillo C, Warshaw AL. Cystic neoplasms of the pancreas. *N Engl J Med.* 2004;351:1218–1226.

2. Hamilton SaA, LA., ed *Pathology and Genetics. Tumors of the Digestive System.* 3rd ed. Lyon: IARC Press; 2000. World Health Organization Classification of Tumours; No. 2.

3. Ikeda M, Sato T, Morozumi A, *et al.* Morphologic changes in the pancreas detected by screening ultrasonography in a mass survey, with special reference to main duct dilatation, cyst formation, and calcification. *Pancreas.* 1994;9:508–512.

4. Kimura W, Nagai H, Kuroda A, Muto T, Esaki Y. Analysis of small cystic lesions of the pancreas. *Int J Pancreatol.* 1995;18: 197–206.

5. Zhang XM, Mitchell DG, Dohke M, Holland GA, Parker L. Pancreatic cysts: depiction on single-shot fast spin-echo MR images. *Radiology.* 2002;223:547–553.

6. Laffan TA, Horton KM, Klein AP, *et al.* Prevalence of unsuspected pancreatic cysts on MDCT. *AJR Am J Roentgenol.* 2008;191:802–807.

7. Compton CC. Serous cystic tumors of the pancreas. *Semin Diagn Pathol.* 2000;17:43–55.

8. Sandy JT, Taylor RH, Christensen RM, Scudamore C, Leckie P. Pancreatic pseudocyst. Changing concepts in management. *Am J Surg.* 1981;141:574–576.

9. Wade JW. Twenty-five year experience with pancreatic pseudocysts. Are we making progress? *Am J Surg.* 1985;149:705–708.

10. Boerma D, Obertop H, Gouma DJ. Pancreatic pseudocysts in chronic pancreatitis. Surgical or interventional drainage? *Ann Ital Chir.* 2000;71:43–50.

11. Hammel PR, Vilgrain V, Terris B, *et al.* Pancreatic involvement in von Hippel-Lindau disease. The Groupe Francophone d'Etude de la Maladie de von Hippel-Lindau. *Gastroenterology.* 2000;119: 1087–1095.

12. Moore PS, Zamboni G, Brighenti A, *et al.* Molecular characterization of pancreatic serous microcystic adenomas: evidence for a tumor suppressor gene on chromosome 10q. *Am J Pathol.* 2001;158:317–321.

13. Vortmeyer AO, Lubensky IA, Fogt F, Linehan WM, Khettry U, Zhuang Z. Allelic deletion and mutation of the von Hippel-Lindau (VHL) tumor suppressor gene in pancreatic microcystic adenomas. *Am J Pathol.* 1997;151:951–956.

14. Yoshizawa K, Nagai H, Sakurai S, *et al.* Clonality and K-ras mutation analyses of epithelia in intraductal papillary mucinous tumor and mucinous cystic tumor of the pancreas. *Virchows Arch.* 2002;441:437–443.

15. Hruban RH, Adsay NV. Molecular classification of neoplasms of the pancreas. *Hum Pathol.* 2009;40:612–623.

16. Byrne MF, Mitchell RM, Baillie J. Pancreatic Pseudocysts. *Curr Treat Options Gastroenterol.* 2002;5:331–338.

17. Pyke CM, van Heerden JA, Colby TV, Sarr MG, Weaver AL. The spectrum of serous cystadenoma of the pancreas. Clinical, pathologic, and surgical aspects. *Ann Surg.* 1992;215:132–139.

18. Gonzalez Obeso E, Murphy E, Brugge W, Deshpande V. Pseudocyst of the pancreas: the role of cytology and special stains for mucin. *Cancer Cytopathol.* 20 2009;117:101–107.

19. Curry CA, Eng J, Horton KM, *et al.* CT of primary cystic pancreatic neoplasms: can CT be used for patient triage and treatment? *AJR Am J Roentgenol.* 2000;175:99–103.

20. Brugge WR, Lewandrowski K, Lee-Lewandrowski E, *et al.* Diagnosis of pancreatic cystic neoplasms: a report of the cooperative pancreatic cyst study. *Gastroenterology.* 2004;126:1330–1336.

21. Frossard JL, Amouyal P, Amouyal G, *et al.* Performance of endosonography-guided fine needle aspiration and biopsy in the diagnosis of pancreatic cystic lesions. *Am J Gastroenterol.* 2003;98:1516–1524.

22. Khalid A, Zahid M, Finkelstein SD, *et al.* Pancreatic cyst fluid DNA analysis in evaluating pancreatic cysts: a report of the PANDA study. *Gastrointest Endosc.* 2009;69:1095–1102.

23. Tanaka M, Chari S, Adsay V, *et al.* International consensus guidelines for management of intraductal papillary mucinous neoplasms and mucinous cystic neoplasms of the pancreas. *Pancreatology.* 2006;6:17–32.

24. De Palma GD, Galloro G, Puzziello A, Masone S, Persico G. Endoscopic drainage of pancreatic pseudocysts: a long-term follow-up study of 49 patients. *Hepatogastroenterology.* 2002;49: 1113–1115.

25. Varadarajulu S. EUS followed by endoscopic pancreatic pseudocyst drainage or all-in-one procedure: a review of basic techniques (with video). *Gastrointest Endosc.* 2009;69(2 Suppl): S176–181.

26. Sanchez Cortes E, Maalak A, Le Moine O, *et al.* Endoscopic cystenterostomy of nonbulging pancreatic fluid collections. *Gastrointest Endosc.* 2002;56:380–386.

27. Melman L, Azar R, Beddow K, *et al.* Primary and overall success rates for clinical outcomes after laparoscopic, endoscopic, and open pancreatic cystgastrostomy for pancreatic pseudocysts. *Surg Endosc.* 2009;23:267–271.

28. Harper AE, Eckhauser FE, Mulholland MW. Resectional therapy for cystic neoplasms of the pancreas. *Am Surg.* 2002;68:353–357; discussion 357–358.

29. Kanazumi N, Nakao A, Kaneko T, *et al.* Surgical treatment of intraductal papillary-mucinous tumors of the pancreas. *Hepatogastroenterology.* 2001;48:967–971.

30. DeWitt J, McGreevy K, Schmidt CM, Brugge WR. EUS-guided ethanol versus saline solution lavage for pancreatic cysts: a randomized, double-blind study. *Gastrointest Endosc.* 2009;70: 710–723.

31. Oh HC, Seo DW, Lee TY, *et al.* New treatment for cystic tumors of the pancreas: EUS-guided ethanol lavage with paclitaxel injection. *Gastrointest Endosc.* 2008;67:636–642.

32. Ho KY, Brugge WR. EUS 2008 Working Group document: evaluation of EUS-guided pancreatic-cyst ablation. *Gastrointest Endosc.* 2009;69(2 Suppl):S22–27.

Pancreas and Biliary Tract

CHAPTER 73

Development and miscellaneous abnormalities

Erica Makin and Mark Davenport

King's College Hospital, London, UK

Development

The pancreas develops from the foregut between the fifth and eighth weeks of intrauterine life from multiple sources. The acinar exocrine cells, the epithelium of its duct system, and the endocrine islet cells are derived from endodermal precursors. Blood and lymphatic vessels together with stromal connective tissue develop from mesoderm, and its innervation arises from neural crest ectoderm. Pancreatic endocrine cells are initially located in the walls of the ducts. Proliferation and later migration into mesenchyme occurs to form the **Islets of Langerhans**.

Islet maturation occurs with polyhormonal cells evolving into monohormonal ones arranged to form a core of insulin-producing cells surrounded by the other cell types. Pancreatic endoderm originates as ventral and dorsal buds from the caudal part of the foregut (Figure 73.1A). The dorsal bud appears initially and grows between the leaves of the dorsal mesentery. The smaller ventral bud arises adjacent to the origin of the hepatic diverticulum and slightly caudal to the dorsal bud. The caudal foregut representing the developing duodenum elongates and bows ventrally to form a loop. It then rotates to the right and comes to lie against the dorsal body wall creating its characteristic C-shape (Figure 73.1B). The dorsal bud element now lies to the left of the duodenum and the ventral one to the right. Differential growth of the duodenal wall causes the growing ventral bud and developing bile duct to migrate dorsally with fusion of the two primordial elements. Thus, in the developed pancreas the entire body, tail, and the anterior part of the head, are derived from the dorsal bud leaving the posterior part derived from the ventral bud. The uncinate process is derived from both pancreatic elements. Initially, there are two independent duct systems, one for each of the primordia. A variable amount of fusion then occurs such that the original dorsal duct territory (tail and body) drains via the proximal ventral duct (of Wirsung). The original smaller proximal dorsal duct opening persists as the accessory duct (of Santorini) and in most adults drains a small portion of the head. Duct fusion is believed to occur in the seventh week of gestation. Failure or incomplete duct fusion is termed "pancreas divisum." Functional maturation of the pancreas is first evident in the third month of intrauterine life with the appearance of secretory acini at the end of ducts. Formation of trypsin occurs around 22 weeks' gestation but full exocrine function is only achieved by the second year of life [1].

Agenesis and hypoplasia

Agenesis of the entire pancreas is a very rare abnormality characterized by intrauterine growth retardation, severe metabolic acidosis, hyperglycemia, and meconium ileus and is

Pancreas and Biliary Tract

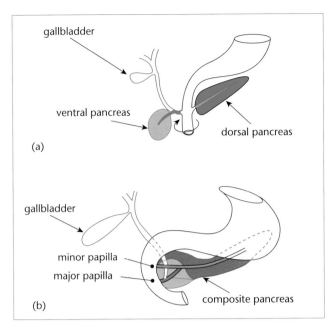

Figure 73.1 Development of the pancreas. (a) Schematic view of developing foregut (30–35 days) with opposing dorsal and ventral pancreatic anlagen. The latter having an intimate relationship with the liver bud and primitive bile duct. (b) Differential growth brings ventral anlage behind dorsal anlage where coalescence of ducts occurs (sixth week).

usually fatal. It is associated with point mutations in the *IPF1* (insulin promoter factor) gene, which encodes a transcription factor believed to be important in early pancreas development. **Partial agenesis** may involve either the dorsal or ventral anlage. Dorsal agenesis is the more common and may be hereditary. In **partial agenesis of the dorsal pancreas**, the accessory papilla, the terminal end of the main dorsal duct of Santorini, or the pancreatic body is present. Diabetes mellitus and polysplenia may be associated but presentation is most often with recurrent acute pancreatitis in the ventral moiety and subsequent exocrine pancreatic insufficiency. Imaging shows absence of the body and tail of the pancreas. Partial agenesis must be distinguished from atrophy or degeneration secondary to disease.

Pancreatic hypoplasia refers to paucity or underdevelopment of the pancreas. Typically, this affects the acini with preservation of ducts and may be part of the autosomal recessive Shwachman–Diamond syndrome characterized by exocrine pancreatic insufficiency and bone marrow dysfunction.

Congenital absence of the pancreatic islets is very rare and associated with intrauterine growth retardation and neonatal death. It may be inherited in an X-linked manner.

Ectopic (syn. heterotopic) pancreatic tissue

Pancreatic tissue may be present outside the confines of the gland itself. Most reported examples have been foregut-related (i.e., stomach, duodenum, and biliary tree), although other reported sites include small bowel, Meckel's diverticulum, and colon. Ectopic pancreatic tissue may contain both exocrine and endocrine elements. Although most cases are asymptomatic incidental findings, symptoms may result from extrinsic compression (e.g., causing obstructive jaundice or gastric outlet obstruction), peptic ulceration (causing bleeding), intussusception, or, rarely, malignant change. Symptomatic ectopic pancreas is treated by surgical resection.

Annular pancreas

The second part of the duodenum may be encircled by a band of pancreatic tissue and is termed an annular pancreas. This may be due to fixation of the ventral pancreatic bud prior to its rotation or, alternatively, splitting of the ventral bud with failure of involution of the left ventral element. The relationship of the annulus to the duodenum varies from juxtaposition to intramural "invasion." A large duct has been reported to run dorsally within the annulus, draining into the duct of Wirsung in about two-thirds of cases. Other anomalies such as duodenal atresia/stenosis, intestinal malrotation, esophageal atresia, distal small-bowel atresia, anorectal malformations, cardiac anomalies, and caudal regression syndrome have all been reported, and usually present during the neonatal period, while those presenting later are typically isolated. Down syndrome is not uncommon because of its relationship with duodenal atresia and a few familial cases have been described.

Clinical presentation

Although most cases of annular pancreas are probably clinically silent, a proportion will present with the underlying duodenal obstruction, typically within the first week of life with non-bilious vomiting; this is in contrast to duodenal obstruction secondary to duodenal atresia, which usually presents with bilious vomiting [2]. A minority will present much later in life and many cases are reported with the first symptoms only occurring in adulthood. There is usually vomiting and abdominal pain due to intermittent duodenal obstruction. Acute pancreatitis, peptic ulcer disease, and, rarely, biliary tract obstruction have all been associated with annular pancreas.

Diagnosis

The radiological feature of duodenal obstruction in infants is that of a "double bubble" appearance on a plain abdominal X-ray. Diagnosis can also be made on antenatal ultrasound by the presence of a constricting ring (hyperechogenic band) distal to the "double bubble" [3]. In older children and adults, further investigations may include an upper gastrointestinal contrast series to define the nature of the duodenal obstruction and endoscopic retrograde cholangiopancreatography (ERCP) or magnetic resonance cholangiopancreatography (MRCP) to visualize pancreatic ductal arrangement. Computed

Pancreas and Biliary Tract

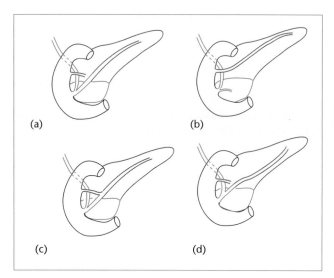

Figure 73.2 Variations and abnormalities of pancreatic ductal anatomy. (a) Normal arrangement; (b) pancreas divisum; (c) incomplete (functional) pancreas divisum; (d) common pancreatobiliary channel.

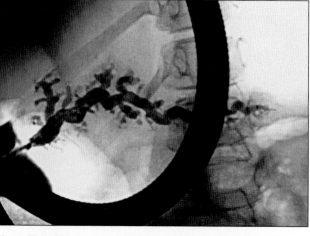

Figure 73.3 ERCP in a 6-year-old child with recurrent pancreatitis. The main pancreatic duct is filled by cannulating the minor papilla (i.e., pancreas divisum) and is dilated consistent with chronic obstruction. Symptoms relieved by longitudinal pancreaticojejunostomy.

tomography (CT) and, most recently, endoscopic ultrasound may allow visualization of the annulus itself.

Treatment

Duodenal obstruction is relieved by duodenoduodenostomy performed anterior to the annulus. No attempt should be made to divide the annulus itself as this carries a high risk of fistula formation. In the older child or adult presenting with pancreatitis, pancreatic duct arrangement needs to be investigated endoscopically and, in some cases, duct drainage procedures may be useful.

Pancreas divisum

Originally, the term pancreas divisum was confined to complete failure of fusion of the ventral and dorsal duct systems; however, this has been expanded to encompass variants due to abnormal fusion of the two duct systems. Figure 73.2 illustrates the concept of pancreas divisum. In most, the key observation is that the dorsal duct drains most of the gland via the minor accessory papilla (of Santorini) rather than the major ampulla of Vater. Pancreas divisum is a relatively common anatomical observation although there is discrepancy between the reported incidence at endoscopy (~5%) and that observed at autopsy (~10%). For this reason its relationship to pancreatic pathology has been questioned, at least in adults [4]. It is probable that it is not simply that the accessory duct drains most pancreatic exocrine secretions, but that there is also a relative accessory duct stenosis causing a raised ductal pressure. The term **"dominant dorsal duct syndrome"** has been coined to reflect this [5].

> **PANCREAS DIVISUM**
>
> - Failure of fusion of embryonic dorsal and ventral duct systems
> - Incidence: 5–10% (ERCP, autopsies)
> - Presentation: may be clinically silent, recurrent pancreatitis, recurrent abdominal pain
> - Diagnosis: ERCP, MRCP ± secretin
> - Treatment (when symptomatic)
>   - endoscopic – dorsal duct stenting/sphincterotomy,
>   - open surgery – dorsal duct sphincteroplasty, Puestow procedure
>
> ERCP, endoscopic retrograde cholangiopancreatography; MRCP, magnetic resonance cholangiopancreatography.

Clinical presentation

Clinical presentation has included recurrent abdominal pain, recurrent acute pancreatitis, and chronic pancreatitis, and in this setting usually affects the dorsal pancreas. Rarely, the ventral element drains exclusively by fine ducts into the dorsal duct, resulting in so-called ventral-segment pancreatitis.

Diagnosis

Pancreas divisum can only be definitively diagnosed by ERCP (Figure 75.3), as standard cannulation of the major papilla causes only ventral duct opacification. Similarly, MRCP may show non-communicating dorsal and ventral ducts, independent drainage sites, and a dominant dorsal pancreatic duct. However, there is still a significant false-negative rate and a range of supportive investigations has been advocated in adult practice. Therefore, intravenous secretin stimulation with detection of consequent dorsal duct dilatation by ultrasonography or MR pancreatography have been described [5].

Treatment

A suitable initial approach would be endoscopic dorsal duct stenting and/or sphincterotomy. Adult series suggest that most benefit is seen if the presenting symptoms have been recurrent pancreatitis rather than chronic pancreatic pain [6]. In children, if there has been symptomatic relief in terms of reduction in episode frequency then open surgical pancreatic duct drainage should be seriously considered. This can be achieved either by transduodenal accessory ductoplasty or by a retrograde duct drainage procedure (e.g., longitudinal pancreaticojejunostomy – Puestow procedure) [7].

Common pancreaticobiliary channel

The terminal parts of the common bile duct and the ventral pancreatic duct often unite outside of the medial wall of the duodenum to form a short common channel (see Figure 73.2D). The length of this varies from approximately 3 mm in infants to approximately 5 mm in children and adolescents. It is clearly pathological if it is long (>10 mm) and lies outside the sphincter of Oddi. It should be remembered that a common channel is a normal stage in pancreatic duct development and absorption of this into the wall of the duodenum occurs only towards the end of gestation.

Common channel is a frequent observation in choledochal malformations (~80%) and biliary atresia (~20%), and has a higher than expected incidence in gallbladder carcinoma (associated with activation of the *KRAS* oncogene and inactivation of the tumor suppressor gene *p53)*. There is some evidence that because the common channel allows free intermixing of bile and pancreatic juices it may actually cause some choledochal malformations by exposing biliary epithelium to activated proteolytic enzyme attack [8–10]. Conversely, acute pancreatitis may also occur, which is due to the abnormal presence of bile within the pancreatic duct triggering premature activation of secreted pancreatic enzymes.

Diagnosis

The gold standard is ERCP, but with advances in MRCP, particularly three-dimensional MRCP, diagnostic accuracy is reported to be 75% in adults. Percutaneous transhepatic cholangiography (PTC) has also been used in this respect and again can be used to clear the common channel of debris or calculi (Figure 73.4).

Treatment

The aim of surgical therapy is to separate pancreatic and biliary secretions and this is achieved by excision of the choledochal malformation, cholecystectomy, and Roux-en-Y hepaticojejunostomy. In addition, an ampullary drainage procedure either open or endoscopic needs to be considered if there is obvious stone/protein plug formation within the channel [11].

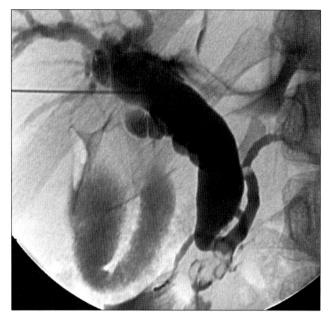

Figure 73.4 Percutaneous transheptic cholangiogram (PTC) in a 12-year-old girl with recurrent pancreatitis and intermittent jaundice. There is a fusiform choledochal dilatation, a dilated common channel containing radiolucent debris, and a dilated main pancreatic duct. Symptoms relieved by excision of choledochal malformation, hepaticojejunostomy-en-Roux, and a transduodenal sphincteroplasty.

COMMON PANCREATOBILIARY CHANNEL

- Abnormal early fusion of pancreas and common bile ducts, allowing pathological intermixing of biliary and pancreatic secretions
- Incidence: unknown
- Associations: choledochal malformations, biliary atresia, gallbladder dysplasia and malignancy
- Presentation: recurrent pancreatitis
- Diagnosis: ERCP, PTC, MRCP
- Management: surgical biliary diversion ± common channel clearance

ERCP, endoscopic retrograde cholangiopancreatography; MRCP, magnetic resonance cholangiopancreatography; PTC, percutaneous transhepatic cholangiography.

Congenital pancreatic duct strictures

This has been reported in about 3% of autopsies and usually involves the junction of the ventral and dorsal duct systems with consequent distal dorsal duct dilatation. Presentation is usually with recurrent acute pancreatitis and should be investigated with ERCP. Retrograde duct drainage will decompress the distal ducts satisfactorily [7].

Anomalous insertion of the common bile duct

This may occur into the third or fourth part of the duodenum and is often associated with a long common channel and

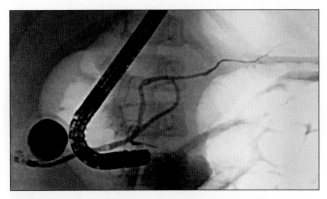

Figure 73.5 Endoscopic retrograde cholangiopancreatography (ERCP) in a 7-year-old girl with recurrent pancreatitis. There is a cyst anatomically adjacent to the gastric antrum that communicates by an accessory duct with the main pancreatic duct. Resection of the cyst showed this to be a foregut duplication cyst containing predominantly gastric mucosa.

choledochal malformation. In itself, it is usually asymptomatic; however, a few cases of recurrent pancreatitis have been reported. Symptomatic relief was achieved by hepaticojejunostomy and complete biliary diversion.

Enteric duplication cysts

These are, strictly speaking, not true pancreatic malformations. However, their close proximity to the gland and possible presentation with pancreatitis merits consideration here. Such duplications may be entirely within the pancreatic head and may present with pancreatitis due to duct obstruction and occasionally gastritis due to hypergastrinemia. A variety of imaging modalities have been suggested including ultrasonography, ERCP, CT, and intraoperative ultrasound. Gastric duplications abutting on the head of the pancreas may present with pancreatitis secondary to erosion or perforation of a

posterior peptic ulcer into the gland. Such cysts may also directly communicate with the pancreatic duct system causing pancreatitis by blockage of the ducts with mucus and debris (Figure 73.5).

References

1. Gittes GK. Developmental biology of the pancreas: A comprehensive review. *Develop Biol.* 2009;326:4–35.
2. Jimenez JC, Emil S, Podnos Y, Nguyen N. Annular pancreas in children: A Recent Decade's Experience. *J Pediatr Surg.* 2004;39: 1654–1657.
3. Dankovcik R, Jirasek JE, Kucera E, *et al.* Prenatal diagnosis of annular pancreas: reliability of the double bubble sign with periduodenal hyperechogenic band. *Fetal Diagn Ther.* 2008;24: 483–490.
4. Quest L, Lombard M. Pancreas divisum: opinio divisa. *Gut.* 2000;47:317–319.
5. Warshaw AL, Simeone JF, Schapiro RH, Flavin-Warshaw B. Evaluation and treatment of the dominant dorsal duct syndrome (pancreas divisum redefined). *Am J Surg.* 1990;159:59–64.
6. Heyries L, Barthet M, Delvasto C. *et al.* Long-term results of endoscopic management of pancreas divisum with recurrent acute pancreatitis. *Gastrointest Endosc.* 2002;55:376–381.
7. Tagge EP, Smith SD, Raschbaum GR, *et al.* Pancreatic ductal abnormalities in children. *Surgery.* 1991;110:709–717.
8. Stringer MD, Dhawan A, Davenport M, *et al.* Choledochal cysts: lessons from a 20 year experience. *Arch Dis Child.* 1995;73: 528–531.
9. Dabbas N, Davenport M. Congenital choledochal malformation: not just a problem for children. *Ann R Coll Surg Eng.* 2009;91: 100–105.
10. Chiu B, Lopoo J, Superina RA. Longitudinal pancreaticojejunostomy and selective biliary diversion for chronic pancreatitis in children. *J Pediatr Surg.* 2006;41:946–949.
11. Terui K, Yoshida H, Kouchi K, *et al.* Endoscopic sphicterotomy is a useful preoperative management for refractory pancreatitis associated with pancreaticobiliary maljunction. *J Pediatr Surg.* 2008;43:595–599.

CHAPTER 74

Cholelithiasis, choledocholithiasis, and cholecystitis

Franz Ludwig Dumoulin[1,2] and Tilman Sauerbruch[2]

[1]Gemeinschaftskrankenhaus Bonn, Bonn, Germany
[2]University of Bonn, Bonn, Germany

ESSENTIAL FACTS ABOUT PATHOGENESIS

- Prevalence: 10–15% in Western societies
- 80% cholesterol stones; <20% pigment stones
- Gallbladder stones: ~30% become symptomatic (mostly biliary pain, less often from complications)
- Bile duct stones: at least 50% become symptomatic
- Risk factors: genetic predisposition, older age, female gender, obesity, weight loss, pregnancy, terminal ileal disease, parenteral nutrition, drugs; lower than average incidence observed with increased physical activity, caffeine, statin use, alcohol consumption
- Prevention of gallstone formation to be considered during weight reduction using ursodeoxycholic acid 600 mg/day or during prolonged parenteral nutrition using cholecystokinin (CCK-8) 50 ng/kg body weight/day

ESSENTIALS OF DIAGNOSIS

Clinical presentation
- Asymptomatic cholecystolithiasis may be detected at routine abdominal ultrasound
- Symptomatic cholecystolithiasis is mostly due to biliary pain
- Bile duct stones may also present with complications (common complications: bile duct obstruction with jaundice, ascending cholangitis, acute biliary pancreatitis
- Rare complications: perforation with cholecystoenteric fistula and gallstone ileus, Mirizzi syndrome, gallbladder or bile-duct carcinoma)

Differential diagnosis
- Common: symptomatic cholecystolithiasis, cholecystitis, cholangiolithiasis, cholangitis, acute appendicitis, peptic ulcer disease, acute (biliary) pancreatitis, right kidney disease (e.g., pyelonephritis, stone), mesenteric infarction, aortic aneurysm, ileus, peritonitis
- Less common: liver disease (e.g., alcohol hepatitis, hepatic abscess), basal pneumonia with pleurisy or pulmonary embolism

Diagnostic methods
- Routine blood tests
- Blood cultures (in cases of suspected cholecystitis/cholangitis)
- Ultrasound (high sensitivity for gallbladder stones, cholecystitis, cholestasis; lower sensitivity for bile duct stones)
- Endoscopic ultrasound or magnetic resonance cholangiopancreatography (MRCP): high sensitivity and specificity for the detection of bile duct stones; preferred methods in patients with intermediate probability of bile duct stones or inaccessibility of bile ducts.

- Endoscopic retrograde cholangiopancreatography (ERCP) (percutaneous transhepatic cholangiography, PTC) with the potential for subsequent lithotripsy and stone extraction in patients with high suspicion of bile duct stones (e.g., jaundiced patients with dilated duct on ultrasound)
- Axial computed tomography (mandatory in cases of unclear diagnosis)

ESSENTIALS OF TREATMENT

Symptomatic cholecystolithiasis
- NSAIDs, spasmolytics (opioids) for treatment of acute biliary pain
- (Laparoscopic) cholecystectomy

Cholecystolithiasis associated with common bile duct stones
- NSAIDs, spasmolytics (opioids) for treatment of acute pain
- Preferably endoscopic stone extraction followed by (laparoscopic) cholecystectomy; palliative transpapillary stenting to be considered in patients unfit for surgery

Cholangitis
- Urgent endoscopic (nasobiliary) drainage, followed by treatment of choledocholithiasis/cholecystolithiasis

Cholecystitis
- Emergency medical therapy with fasting, fluid resuscitation, analgesics, antibiotics
- Early (preferably laparoscopic) cholecystectomy within 48 hours; alternatively, percutaneous or transpapillary drainage of the gallbladder to be considered in critically ill patients

Introduction and epidemiology

Gallstones (concretions mainly formed from cholesterol crystals) are common in Western societies. They are mostly formed from cholesterol crystals in cholesterol-supersaturated gallbladder bile. Crystals are then trapped in mucin, which overlays a dysfunctional gallbladder wall, and finally become stones. The most frequent symptom caused by sludge or gallstones is biliary colic, characterized by pain in the right upper quadrant and epigastrium. Most patients with gallbladder

Pancreas and Biliary Tract

stones (cholecystolithiasis), however, are asymptomatic. In contrast, bile duct stones (choledocholithiasis) more often induce biliary pain, jaundice, acute biliary pancreatitis, and/or ascending cholangitis. An inflammatory reaction of the gallbladder wall (cholecystitis) is usually initiated when a stone or sludge becomes impacted in the gallbladder neck or the cystic duct. Acalculous cholecystitis may occur as a consequence of an impaired microcirculation and/or infection of the gallbladder wall in the absence of gallstones.

Gallstone prevalence ranges from 10% to 15% in the Western world with considerable variation between different ethnic groups. Gallstones are more frequent in young women and prevalence increases with age. The highest prevalence (>70%) has been described in female Pima Indians at age 25 years [1]. A higher than average prevalence has also been reported in Chile, Alaska, Canada, and Bolivia. In contrast, African Americans, Asians, and sub-Saharan Africans have a lower than average risk [2]. The importance of genetic factors is further emphasized by the fact that first-degree relatives of index persons are 4.5 times more likely to develop gallstones, and that several single-gene defects associated with cholelithiasis have been identified (Table 74.1) [3–6]. In the majority of patients, however, a complex genetic predisposition, rather than single genes, promotes gallstone formation. A variety of

Table 74.1 Genes involved in cholesterol gallstone formation. (Modified from references 6 and 11.)

Gene symbols	Protein function	Potential mechanisms
ABCB4 (GBD1)	ATP binding cassette transporter B4	Biliary phospholipid secretion ↓
ABCB11	ATP binding cassette transporter B11	Biliary bile salt secretion ↓
ABCG5/G8 (GBD4)	ATP binding cassette transporters G5/G8	Biliary cholesterol secretion ↑
ARDB3	β₃ Adrenergic receptor	Gallbladder hypomotility
APOA1	Apolipoprotein A1	Biliary cholesterol secretion ↑ Secondary to reverse cholesterol transport ↑
APOB	Apolipoprotein B	Biliary cholesterol secretion ↑ Secondary to hepatic VLDL synthesis ↓ and intestinal cholesterol absorption ↑
CCK1R	Cholecystokinin 1 receptor	Gallbladder and small intestinal hypomotility
CYP7A1	Cytochrome P450 7A1	Bile salt synthesis ↓
ESR2	Oestrogen receptor 2	Cholesterol synthesis ↑

ATP, adenosine triphosphate; VLDL, very low density lipoprotein.

susceptibility loci have been mapped in the mouse and will help the future characterization of candidate genes in man [7,8].

Causes and pathogenesis
Causes and risk factors
Pregnancy and childbirth are important risk factors. Thus, sludge and/or gallstones develop in up to one third and 1–3% of all pregnancies, respectively. After pregnancy, sludge resolves in 60–70% and gallstones disappear in 20–30% [9]. Other risk factors are age, obesity, rapid weight loss, or weight fluctuations, while physical activity is associated with a lower risk for gallstone formation [1]. Consequently, up to 25% of patients with rapid weight loss and up to 50% of patients following gastric bypass develop sludge or gallstones. Moreover, the risk for gallstones increases with serum triglyceride levels, and there is an inverse correlation to high-density lipoprotein (HDL) cholesterol in serum. Clinical conditions associated with gallstone formation are parenteral nutrition, diseases of the terminal ileum, in particular Crohn's disease (see Chapter 50), pancreatic insufficiency including cystic fibrosis, and spinal cord injury. Black pigment stones, resulting from an increase in bilirubin output, are more frequently observed in chronic hemolysis and in up to 30% of patients with liver cirrhosis. A variety of drugs are known to increase the risk of gallstone or sludge formation including ceftriaxone, octreotide, estrogens, and lipid-lowering drugs such as clofibrate. Finally, bacterial cholangitis, which promotes bilirubin deconjugation, can contribute to the formation of brown pigment stones.

Gallstone formation
Gallstones are classified as cholesterol and pigment stones (Figure 74.1). Cholesterol stones consist of >50% cholesterol monohydrate crystals, bound in a matrix of glycoproteins often with a core of calcium bilirubinate. They account for up to 80% of the stones in the Western world. Three principal mechanisms contribute to their formation: secretion of bile supersaturated with cholesterol, accelerated nucleation of cholesterol crystals, and gallbladder hypomotility [11]. In bile, cholesterol is kept in aqueous solution by the detergent action of bile acids and phospholipids. An increase in cholesterol saturation results in the formation of unilamellar and finally unstable multilamellar vesicles. Accelerated nucleation time may be due to an excess of pronucleating factors (e.g., mucin glycoproteins) or a deficiency of antinucleating factors. Finally, gallbladder hypomotility has been found in many patients with gallstones [8]. Black pigment stones are predominantly found in patients with chronic hemolysis, liver cirrhosis, cystic fibrosis, or diseases of the terminal ileum [12]. They are composed of calcium bilirubinate and develop as a consequence of bilirubin supersaturation of bile along with biliary proteins and mucins serving as a nidus for crystallization. Brown pigment stones are mostly formed within the bile ducts as a

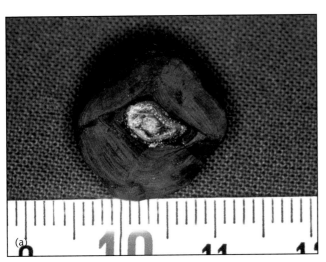
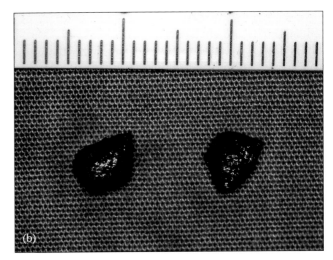

Figure 74.1 Gallbladder stones. (a) Endoscopically extracted mixed bile duct stone with a typical cholesterol core that had moved from the gallbladder and served as a nidus for the formation of a brown pigment shell in the common bile duct. (b) Black pigment gallbladder stones (scale bar = 1 cm).

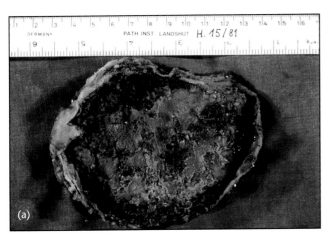
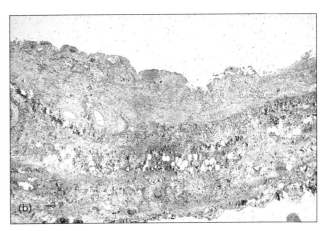

Figure 74.2 Acute cholecystitis. (a) Macroscopic appearance with typically thickened gallbladder wall and mucosal ulceration (scale bar = 1 cm). (b) Dense inflammatory infiltrate on histopathology.

consequence of bacterial infection and hydrolysis of glucuronic acid from bilirubin by bacterial beta-glucuronidase. This results in a decreased solubility of deconjugated bilirubin ultimately leading to the formation of stones consisting of calcium salts of unconjugated bilirubin, deconjugated bile acids, and varying amounts of cholesterol and saturated long chain fatty acids. There is growing evidence that subtle local inflammatory responses and their sequelae support stone formation [13].

Cholecystitis

More than 90% of patients with calculous cholecystitis have an obstruction of the cystic duct by the impaction of sludge or a gallstone in the gallbladder neck. Increased intraluminal pressure and bile trigger an inflammatory reaction within the gallbladder wall. In about 20–50% of cases, a secondary bacterial infection (most commonly by *Escherichia coli*, *Klebsiella*, and

enterococci) is observed [10]. In contrast, acalculous cholecystitis develops in the absence of gallstones as a result of ischemia and gallbladder stasis [14]. Acalculous cholecystitis is seen with an incidence of 0.2–3% in critically ill patients and/or in patients with vascular disorders (atherosclerosis, vasculitis) and may also result from primary microbial infection of the gallbladder. In acute cholecystitis, the gallbladder is usually distended and, besides bile, contains stones, sludge, and an inflammatory exudate (Figure 74.2a). Histological changes comprise an inflammatory infiltrate of polymorphous nuclear granulocytes with edema or, in advanced stages, necrosis (Figure 74.2b). In chronic cholecystitis, the inflammatory infiltrate is replaced by lymphocytes and plasma cells eventually resulting in mucosal atrophy and fibrous thickening of the gallbladder wall. Signs of vasculitis with ischemia and endothelial damage may dominate the histological picture in acute acalculous cholecystitis.

Clinical presentation
Cholelithiasis and choledocholithiasis

Biliary sludge results in stone formation in 12–80% of the patients, with an incidence of cholelithiasis ranging from 3% to 13% [9]. Cholelithiasis is asymptomatic in 60–80% of the patients. In two prospective studies on asymptomatic patients, biliary pain developed at a rate of 2% per year during the first 5 years; the overall incidence was 15–26% at 10 years. By that time, complications (cholecystitis, biliary obstruction, ascending cholangitis, pancreatitis) had developed in 3% of the patients and gallbladder carcinoma had been diagnosed in 1 of 161 patients [2]. Biliary pain due to intermittent obstruction of the cystic duct by a gallstone localizes to the mid-epigastrium or the right upper abdomen and may radiate to the back or to the right shoulder. It is colicky but waves of pain are of long duration, typically lasting from 15 minutes to several hours. They may be accompanied by nausea and/or vomiting. Once an episode of biliary pain has occurred, the risk of repeated attacks or complications ranges from 60% to 70%; in other words: approximately one third of the patients will remain free of further symptoms after a first episode of biliary pain. On the other hand, the majority of complications are preceded by episodes of biliary pain [2,15]. Abdominal discomfort following fatty meals may have a similar predictive value [16]. The natural history of choledocholithiasis is less well defined, but symptoms are more likely and complications are more severe than in cholelithiasis [2]. Consequently, biliary pancreatitis (possibly accompanied by pain from biliary obstruction) may be the first symptom of choledocholithiasis (see Chapter 69) [17].

Cholecystitis

Cholecystitis typically causes worsening pain lasting longer than 5 hours. It is located in the right upper quadrant and accompanied by signs of inflammation such as fever, chills, and, in severe cases, signs of sepsis. Jaundice may be present in patients with sepsis or as a consequence of Mirizzi syndrome (see below). On examination, there is tenderness in the right hypochondrium with or without a palpable mass. Pain and an arrest in inspiration upon deep palpation underneath the right costal margin (Murphy's sign) may be present and has a sensitivity and specificity of 65% and 87%, respectively [16].

Cholangitis

Ascending cholangitis is usually due to bile duct obstruction with subsequent infection by Gram-negative enteric bacteria or enterococci. It is a potentially life-threatening complication presenting with fever, chills, and, often, posthepatic jaundice; it necessitates emergency treatment. Concomitant cholecystitis or biliary pancreatitis should be ruled out. Long-term complications can be stricture formation, recurrent cholangitis with intrahepatic stone formation, and secondary biliary cirrhosis.

Other presentations

There are other well-recognized but rare presentations. Thus some patients may present with acute biliary pancreatitis (see Chapter 69). A stone impacted in the cystic duct may produce intermittent obstruction of the common bile duct (Mirizzi syndrome). Gallstones can erode the gallbladder wall resulting in cholecystoenteric fistula with or without subsequent duodenal obstruction (Bouveret syndrome) or gallstone ileus [18].

Differential diagnosis

The differential diagnosis of recurrent abdominal pain is large. In addition to the biliary tract, abdominal pain may originate from the chest, stomach, small intestine, colon, pancreas, kidneys, uterus, and ovaries. Moreover, ischemic, neurogenic (e.g., from herpes zoster), or musculosketetal pain, as well as pain of metabolic or toxic origin, should be considered [19]. Jaundice and pain suggest choledocholithiasis, while painless jaundice favors liver disease or malignant biliary obstruction. In patients with additional signs of inflammation, cholangitis and cholecystitis (see below) must be included in the list of possible differential diagnoses.

Fever, chills, and/or persistent pain localized in the right upper quadrant lasting longer than 12 hours are suggestive of cholecystitis and/or cholangitis. Differential diagnoses include acute appendicitis, acute pancreatitis, pyelonephritis or right kidney stones, peptic ulcer disease, alcohol hepatitis, hepatic abscess or tumor, and basal pneumonia with pleurisy. The differential diagnosis may be particularly challenging, since patients may indeed have more than one diagnosis (e.g., cholangitis and pancreatitis). Diagnosis of acalculous cholecystitis in mechanically ventilated, critically ill patients is notoriously difficult. A high grade of suspicion of cholecystitis as a possible focus in critically ill patients, with sepsis of unknown cause, is required [20].

Diagnostic methods
Cholelithiasis and choledocholithiasis

Physical examination during an episode of biliary colic may reveal right upper quadrant tenderness, but usually there is no tenderness between the attacks. Blood chemistry will be normal in the majority of patients but may show increases in serum bilirubin, alkaline phosphatase, gamma-glutamyl transpeptidase, and transaminases, particularly with cholangitis, or amylase in the case of biliary obstruction or pancreatitis. In cholangitis, signs of inflammation (fever, leukocytosis with left-shift, elevated C-reactive protein) may be seen and blood cultures may become positive. Transabdominal ultrasound is the best single test for the diagnosis of gallstones (Figure 74.3). Common bile duct stones may be visualized by ultrasound but in the majority of patients only indirect evidence, such as the presence of dilated bile ducts together with gallstones, can be obtained [21]. Endoscopic retrograde cholangiopancreatography (ERCP) and, in case of inaccessibility of the papilla or technical failure, percutaneous transhepatic cholangiography (PTC) remain the most important diagnostic tools for the imaging of bile duct stones (Figure 74.4a). The preferred diagnostic method in patients with a high suspicion for choledocholithiasis is ERCP since it allows subsequent therapeutic intervention [22] (please refer to the accompanying management protocol on the website). Endoscopic ultrasound has a similar diagnostic accuracy (Figure 74.4b), but its

precise role remains to be defined [21,23]. Magnetic resonance cholangiopancreatography (MRCP) has sensitivity and specificity of 90–95% for the detection of common bile duct stones (Figure 74.4c) and is well suited to rule out bile-duct stones in patients with low or intermediate clinical suspicion. In addition, it is the imaging method of choice if the biliary tract is inaccessible to endoscopy [24]. Axial computed tomography (CT) has its role in the work-up of abdominal pain or acute abdomen and is useful in ruling out calcified stones in patients who are evaluated for oral litholysis. Finally, intraoperative cholangiography can be performed in patients with an intermediate probability of cholangiolithiasis who undergo cholecystectomy.

Cholecystitis

Blood chemistry will show signs of inflammation and possibly of cholestasis; aerobe and anaerobe blood cultures may become positive [14]. Transabdominal ultrasound is the single most useful diagnostic tool with a sensitivity and specificity of >90% and >80%, respectively. Typical findings are thickening of the gallbladder wall, which, however, may also be present in patients with ascites or hypoalbuminemia, a positive sonographic Murphy's sign, emphysematous cholecystitis with gas bubbles in the gallbladder wall (so-called champagne sign), or signs of perforation or abscess formation (Figure 74.5a) [20,21]. Abdominal CT is useful, particularly if the initial diagnosis of abdominal pain is obscure (Figure 74.5b/c). Ultrasound is a less reliable diagnostic tool in critically ill patients but the presence of sludge together with the above signs is a useful hint. Murphy's sign, however, is rarely observed and CT should be performed in the critically ill with a high suspicion of cholecystitis [20].

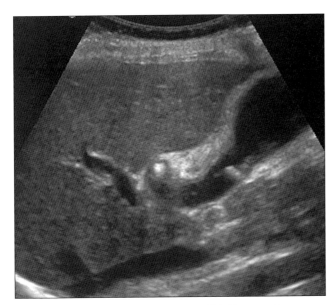

Figure 74.3 Transabdominal ultrasound of a gallbladder stone. A gallbladder stone is easily recognized by its hyperechoic signal with dorsal acoustic shadowing. In this young female patient small stones can be seen in the infundibulum and in the fundus of the gallbladder.

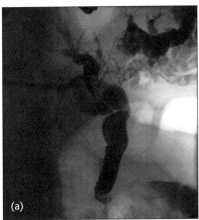 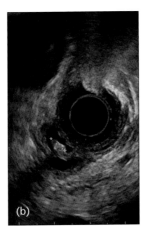 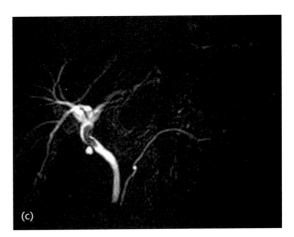

Figure 74.4 Detection of common bile duct stones. (a) Endoscopic retrograde cholangiopancreatography (ERCP) showing multiple intrahepatic stones. The 80-year-old patient had been cholecystectomized 20 years earlier. Note the dilated left-sided bile duct system with multiple filling defects. In such a patient the possibility for a genetic predisposition (e.g., *ABCB4* polymorphism) should be kept in mind. (b) Endoscopic ultrasound has a high sensitivity and specificity even for the detection of stones <5 mm.

(c) Magnetic resonance cholangiopancreatography (MRCP) has a similar sensitivity and specificity for the detection of common bile duct stones, although small stones in the distal part of the common bile duct are better visualized by endoscopic ultrasound (MRCP courtesy of PD Dr. W. Willinek and Prof. Dr. H.H. Schild, Department of Radiology, University of Bonn, Germany).

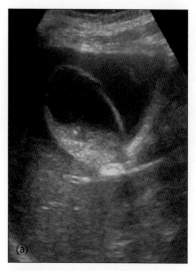
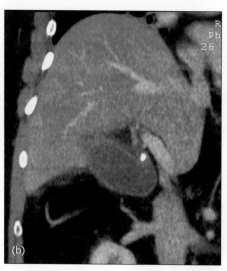
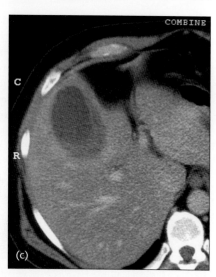

Figure 74.5 Diagnosis of cholecystitis. (a) Abdominal ultrasound showing a large pericholecystic fluid collection suggestive of perforated cholecystitis and gallbladder sludge. The diagnosis was confirmed at laparoscopic cholecystectomy. (b) Detection of a small stone obstructing the infundibulum of the gallbladder. (c) Computed tomography (CT) appearance of pericholecystitis as hypointense fluid collection in the same patient. (CT courtesy of Prof. Dr. H.H. Schild, Department of Radiology, University of Bonn, Germany).

Treatment and prevention
Cholecystolithiasis and choledocholithiasis
Preventive measures
Prevention of stone formation is possible in high-risk situations with ursodeoxycholic acid (UDCA), 600 mg/day p.o., as adjunctive therapy to weight reduction or with cholecystokinin octapeptide (CCK-8), 50 ng/kg body weight i.v., in patients receiving long-term total parenteral nutrition [9,25] although this approach may not effective pediatric patients [26]. In addition, statin use was found to be associated with a lower rate of cholecystectomy in women [27].

Asymptomatic cholelithiasis
Asymptomatic cholelithiasis is not an indication for cholecystectomy since the risk of complications from surgery outweighs the advantage of preventing possible complications from asymptomatic gallbladder stones including gallbladder cancer. However, cholecystectomy can be justified in some instances. These include patients undergoing bariatric surgery for morbid obesity [28] or receiving solid-organ transplantation other than cardiac transplant surgery [29]. Similarly, the prevention of gallbladder cancer may be an indication for cholecystectomy in male patients with gallbladder stones >3 cm (up to 10-fold increased risk for gallbladder cancer), in those with polyps >10 mm, or in those with a calcified gallbladder (cancer risk of 3–6% or up to 20%, respectively). Finally, there is a debate whether asymptomatic patients with multiple small gallbladder stones could profit from cholecystectomy to prevent biliary pancreatitis [25].

Symptomatic cholelithiasis
Emergency treatment of biliary colic is accomplished by spasmolytics (e.g., butylscopolamine [hyoscinebutyl bromide]

40 mg i.v.) and nonsteroidal anti-inflammatory drugs (NSAIDs; e.g., metamizol 1 g i.v., diclofenac 75 mg i.m.). Cholecystectomy, preferably by laparoscopic approach, should be performed to avoid the 50–70% rate of recurrence as well as the 1–2% risk of complications from gallstone disease. In selected patients who do not wish to undergo an operation and have solitary, non-calcified stones with a diameter of less than 20 mm and a well-contracting gallbladder, an attempt of extracorporeal shock wave lithotripsy (ESWL) and oral litholysis with UDCA (10–15 mg/kg body weight/day) for 6–12 months is justified [30] but has been abandoned in most centres because the stone recurrence rate is high [31,32]. Patients with tiny floating stones may profit from prolonged UDCA treatment alone.

Choledocholithiasis
Choledocholithiasis is an indication for treatment, probably also in asymptomatic patients, since complications occur more often and are more severe than in cholecystolithiasis. In the majority of patients, there is coexistent cholecystolithiasis and three options are available: surgical treatment with (laparoscopic) cholecystectomy and bile duct exploration [33]; endoscopic removal of bile duct stones followed by (laparoscopic) cholecystectomy; or flexible splitting [34]. While a surgical approach has the advantage of subjecting the patient to just one procedure, laparoscopic duct exploration is technically demanding and time consuming. On the other hand, endoscopic methods for bile-duct clearance with standard equipment (Dormia basket and balloon) are successful in over 90% of the patients (Figure 74.6; Videos 74.1 and 74.2). Treatment options for difficult stones include mechanical lithotripsy, extracorporeal shock wave lithotripsy [35] (Figure 74.7), and electrohydraulic or laser lithotripsy [36]. Alternatively, surgical bile-duct exploration remains a valuable option, in

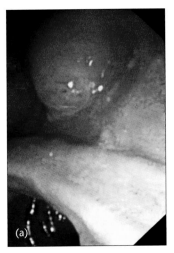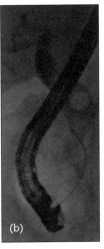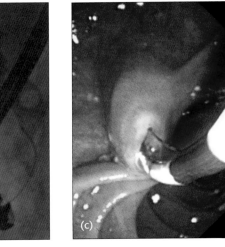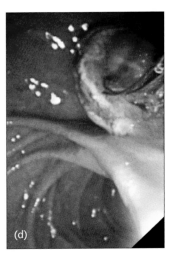

Figure 74.6 Endoscopic removal of common bile duct stones. In this jaundiced patient the bile duct was dilated on transabdominal ultrasound and we therefore proceeded directly to endoscopic retrograde cholangiopancreatography (ERCP). (a) Aspect of a swollen papilla during duodenoscopy. (b) ERCP image showing a filling defect in the distal part of the bile duct. (c) Endoscopic sphincterotomy is performed using a wire-guided sphincterotome. (d) The stone is extracted using a Dormia basket.

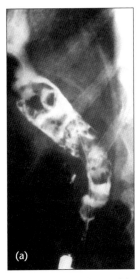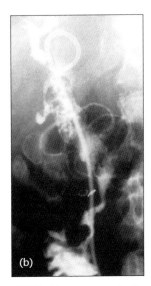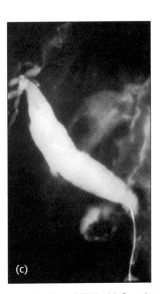

Figure 74.7 Efficacy of extracorporeal shock-wave lithotripsy (ESWL). (a) Multiple filling defects due to multiple common bile duct stones. (b) During endoscopic retrograde cholangiopancreatography (ERCP) a nasobiliary catheter is inserted for temporary biliary drainage and to facilitate visualization of stones for planned ESWL. (c) Complete duct clearance after two ESWL treatments and subsequent ERCP with extraction of stone fragments by Dormia basket and balloon.

particular for large impacted stones and in patients with an indication of cholecystectomy. Under certain circumstances (e.g., elderly patients unfit for surgery with difficult-to-treat bile-duct stones) endoscopic sphincterotomy and stenting are accepted alternatives. If ascending cholangitis complicates choledocholithiasis, emergency endoscopic placement of naso-biliary drainage along with antibiotic therapy and supportive measures are warranted.

Cholecystitis

Emergency treatment consists of fasting, fluid resuscitation, spasmolytics, and analgesia, preferably with NSAIDs.

In addition, intravenous antibiotic therapy covering Gram-negative enteric microorganisms (e.g., broad spectrum acyl-ureidopenicillins/third-generation cephalosporins/chinolones) should be started. Most patients respond to initial conservative medical treatment. However, up to 20% develop signs of advanced cholecystitis (fever >38°C, serum bilirubin >10 mg/dL or 170 μmol/L) and need emergency surgery to avoid complications such as gangrene, perforation, peritonitis, or sepsis [10]. The timing of surgery in the remaining 80% of patients is still under debate. Early laparoscopic surgery (within 48 hours of the onset of symptoms) is preferred, since these patients have lower conversion and complication rates and shorter hospital stays than those undergoing delayed (>5 days after the onset of symptoms) or interval (>6 weeks after the acute episode) laparoscopic surgery. The overall complication rates of the laparoscopic approach range from 9.0% to 15.0%, with bile duct injuries between 0.7% and 1.3%, which is comparable to complications for open cholecystectomy in these patients [37–40]. Percutaneous (ultrasound or CT-guided) drainage of the gallbladder is an alternative temporary treatment in patients unfit for surgery. The possibility of a bedside procedure renders this technique a valuable treatment option in critically ill patients. Cholecystostomy without subsequent cholecystectomy can be a definite treatment for acalculous cholecystitis.

Treatment pitfalls

Complications of gallstone disease may occur in combination, for example, pancreatitis and cholangitis, or ascending cholangitis with cholecystis. In these patients, concomitant complications must not be overlooked and should be treated promptly. Moreover, the acuity of cholecystitis, particularly acalculous cholecystitis, may be underestimated. Particularly in critically ill patients, a frequent interdisciplinary re-evaluation is warranted to proceed to emergency cholecystectomy (or cholecystotomy) if necessary.

Complications and their management

Cholecystolithiasis and choledocholithiasis

The single most frequent complication of gallstone disease is cholecystitis, which has been discussed above. Other complications are mostly due to migrating or impacted stones, which may result in a variety of complications such as ascending cholangitis, acute biliary pancreatitis (discussed in Chapter 69), Mirrizi syndrome, gallstones ileus (including Bouveret syndrome), choledocho- or cholecysto-enteric fistulae, and gallbladder cancer. Cholecystitis may become gangrenous (2–30%) or lead to gallbladder perforation (10%) with a mortality of 30%, as well as cholecysto-enteric fistulae and gallstone ileus (see above) and/or sepsis [10]. Early diagnosis of local complications by ultrasound and/or contrast-enhanced CT is important. Treatment consists of supportive measures and emergency cholecystectomy.

Rare complications

Mirizzi syndrome (Figure 74.8) and cholecystocholedochal fistula are two manifestations of the same process beginning with impaction of gallstone(s) in the gallbladder neck and subsequent obstruction of the hepatocholedochal duct and/or erosion with fistula formation. Presenting symptoms are pain, jaundice, and fever. It is important to make an accurate diagnosis (usually by ERCP). Surgical treatment is usually required, with laparoscopic procedures carrying a higher risk of complications. Endoscopic retrograde cholangiography with sphincterotomy, lithotripsy, and stone extraction may be helpful, in particular for poor surgical candidates. Fistula formation is

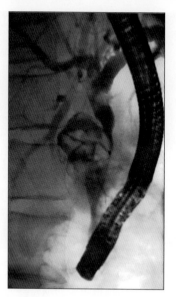

Figure 74.8 Mirizzi syndrome is a rare complication of cholelithiasis. On the endoscopic retrograde cholangiopancreatograph note the eccentric stenosis of the common hepatic duct in close vicinity to the cystic duct and the presence of multiple stones both in the gallbladder and the bile ducts. The patient underwent open cholecystectomy and a large defect in the wall of the common hepatic duct was diagnosed intraoperatively. Cystic stump insufficiency after open cholecystectomy occurred and this patient was treated by spincterotomy and temporary transpapillary stenting.

usually identified at cholangiography. Management may be expectant (e.g., for an asymptomatic choledochoduodenal fistula) or surgical (e.g., at the time of cholecystectomy). Treatment of gallstone ileus comprises supportive measures and emergency surgery [18].

Prognosis with and without treatment

Prognosis with treatment

The prognosis of cholelithiasis is good. Likewise, calculous cholecystitis usually follows a benign course. The overall mortality rate after surgical treatment is less than 0.1%. However, after cholecystectomy up to 10% of the patients complain of recurrent or persistent pain, which is referred to as "post cholecystectomy syndrome" [41]. In some cases, this may represent continuation of preoperative non-gallstone pain that was misattributed to coincidental gallstones. Acalculous cholecystitis in critically ill patients carries a poor prognosis, which depends on coexisting medical conditions and the mortality may be higher than 50% [14].

Prognosis without treatment

The natural history of asymptomatic gallstones has been described. Acute cholecystitis resolves spontaneously in half of the patients within 7–10 days; however, the rate of gangrenous cholecystitis with gallbladder perforation may be as high as 10%. If cholecystitis is treated without cholecystectomy, the recurrence rate is about 60% within 6 years. Ascending bacterial cholangitis has a high mortality rate if left untreated (e.g., when unrecognized). Acalculous cholecystitis carries a high mortality rate, even with appropriate treatment.

Harmful consequences of treatment

The risk of interventional endoscopy depends on patient characteristics and comorbidity as well as the techniques used and the skills of the endoscopist. Endoscopic sphincterotomy probably carries the highest risk, with pancreatitis as the most important complication (4.2–9.8%); mortality rates range between 0% and 0.4% [36,42]. The major complications of laparoscopic cholecystectomy are bile-duct injuries; these occur at a rate of 0.2–0.4%, which is similar to the rate reported for open cholecystectomy [43]. Bile-duct injuries comprise biliary strictures, which may be managed by endoscopic stent insertion or dilatation. Similarly, biliary leaks can be treated by endoscopic sphincterotomy and temporary stent insertion. However, large biliary leaks or a complete bile-duct obstruction usually require surgical repair. Other complications, such as injury to vessels, are less frequent. The risk of surgery also depends on patient selection and the experience of the laparoscopic surgeon. Patients with cholecystitis have a higher than average rate of bile-duct injury, and conversion to open surgery should be performed liberally [40,44].

SOURCES OF INFORMATION FOR PATIENTS AND DOCTORS

American Gastroenterological Association (AGA) patient center:
   http://www.gastro.org/patient-center
American College of Gastroenterology (ACG) patient information:
   http://patients.gi.org
Patient UK: www.patient.co.uk/
UpToDate for patients: (http://www.uptodate.com/patients/index.html

---

References

1. Carey MC, Paigen B. Epidemiology of the American Indians' burden and its likely genetic origins. *Hepatology*. 2002;36: 781–791.
2. Ko CW, Lee SP. Epidemiology and natural history of common bile duct stones and prediction of disease. *Gastrointest Endosc*. 2002;56:S165–169.
3. Lammert F, Miquel JF. Gallstone disease: from genes to evidence-based therapy. *J Hepatol*. 2008;48 Suppl 1:S124–135.
4. Hoblinger A, Lammert F. Genetics of biliary tract diseases: new insights into gallstone disease and biliary tract cancers. *Curr Opin Gastroenterol*. 2008;24:363–371.
5. Lammert F, Sauerbruch T. Mechanisms of disease: the genetic epidemiology of gallbladder stones. *Nat Clin Pract Gastroenterol Hepatol*. 2005;2:423–433.
6. Lammert F, Sauerbruch T. Pathogenesis of gallstones formation: updated inventory of human lithogenic genes. In: Carey MC, Dité P, Gabryelewicz A, Keim V, Mössner J, editors. *Future Perspectives in Gastroenterology (Falk Symposium 161)*. Dordrecht: Springer; 2008. p. 99–107.
7. Lammert F, Carey MC, Paigen B. Chromosomal organization of candidate genes involved in cholesterol gallstone formation: a murine gallstone map. *Gastroenterology*. 2001;120:221–238.
8. Kosters A, Jirsa M, Groen AK. Genetic background of cholesterol gallstone disease. *Biochim Biophys Acta*. 2003;1637:1–19.
9. Ko CW, Sekijima JH, Lee SP. Biliary sludge. *Ann Intern Med*. 1999;130:301–311.
10. Indar AA, Beckingham IJ. Acute cholecystitis. *BMJ*. 2002; 325:639–643.
11. Wang DQ, Cohen DE, Carey MC. Biliary lipids and cholesterol gallstone disease. *J Lipid Res*. 2009;50:S406–411.
12. Vitek L, Carey MC. Enterohepatic cycling of bilirubin as a cause of 'black' pigment gallstones in adult life. *Eur J Clin Invest*. 2003;33:799–810.
13. Maurer KJ, Carey MC, Fox JG. Roles of infection, inflammation, and the immune system in cholesterol gallstone formation. *Gastroenterology*. 2009;136:425–440.
14. Barie PS, Eachempati SR. Acute acalculous cholecystitis. *Curr Gastroenterol Rep*. 2003;5:302–309.
15. Besselink MG, Venneman NG, Go PM, *et al*. Is complicated gallstone disease preceded by biliary colic? *J Gastrointest Surg*. 2009;13:312–317.
16. Trowbridge RL, Rutkowski NK, Shojania KG. Does this patient have acute cholecystitis? *JAMA*. 2003;289:80–86.
17. van Erpecum KJ. Gallstone disease. Complications of bile-duct stones: Acute cholangitis and pancreatitis. *Best Pract Res Clin Gastroenterol*. 2006;20:1139–1152.
18. Abou-Saif A, Al-Kawas FH. Complications of gallstone disease: Mirizzi syndrome, cholecystocholedochal fistula, and gallstone ileus. *Am J Gastroenterol*. 2002;97:249–254.
19. Kalloo AN. Overview of differential diagnoses of abdominal pain. *Gastrointest Endosc*. 2002;56:S255–257.
20. Ko CW, Lee SP. Gastrointestinal disorders of the critically ill. Biliary sludge and cholecystitis. *Best Pract Res Clin Gastroenterol*. 2003;17:383–396.
21. Gandolfi L, Torresan F, Solmi L, Puccetti A. The role of ultrasound in biliary and pancreatic diseases. *Eur J Ultrasound*. 2003;16:141–159.
22. Lammert F, Neubrand MW, Bittner R, *et al*. [Short version of the updated S3 (level 3) guidelines for diagnosis and treatment of gallstones of the German Society for Digestive and Metabolic Diseases and the German Society for the Surgery of the Alimentary Tract]. *Dtsch Med Wochenschr*. 2008;133:311–316.
23. Sivak MV, Jr. EUS for bile duct stones: how does it compare with ERCP? *Gastrointest Endosc*. 2002;56:S175–177.
24. Fulcher AS. MRCP and ERCP in the diagnosis of common bile duct stones. *Gastrointest Endosc*. 2002;56:S178–182.
25. Venneman NG, van Erpecum KJ. Gallstone disease: Primary and secondary prevention. *Best Pract Res Clin Gastroenterol*. 2006;20: 1063–1073.
26. Tsai S, Strouse PJ, Drongowski RA, Islam S, Teitelbaum DH. Failure of cholecystokinin-octapeptide to prevent TPN-associated gallstone disease. *J Pediatr Surg*. 2005;40:263–267.
27. Tsai CJ, Leitzmann MF, Willett WC, Giovannucci EL. Statin use and the risk of cholecystectomy in women. *Gastroenterology*. 2009;136:1593–1600.
28. Uy MC, Talingdan-Te MC, Espinosa WZ, Daez ML, Ong JP. Ursodeoxycholic acid in the prevention of gallstone formation after bariatric surgery: a meta-analysis. *Obes Surg*. 2008;18: 1532–1538.

Pancreas and Biliary Tract

29. Kao LS, Kuhr CS, Flum DR. Should cholecystectomy be performed for asymptomatic cholelithiasis in transplant patients? *J Am Coll Surg*. 2003;197:302–312.

30. Howard DE, Fromm H. Nonsurgical management of gallstone disease. *Gastroenterol Clin North Am*. 1999;28:133–144.

31. Berr F, Mayer M, Sackmann MF, Sauerbruch T, Holl J, Paumgartner G. Pathogenic factors in early recurrence of cholesterol gallstones. *Gastroenterology*. 1994;106:215–224.

32. Sackmann M, Niller H, Klueppelberg U, *et al*. Gallstone recurrence after shock-wave therapy. *Gastroenterology*. 1994;106:225–230.

33. Fielding GA. The case for laparoscopic common bile duct exploration. *J Hepatobiliary Pancreat Surg*. 2002;9:723–728.

34. Binmoeller KF, Schafer TW. Endoscopic management of bile duct stones. *J Clin Gastroenterol*. 2001;32:106–118.

35. Sauerbruch T, Holl J, Sackmann M, Paumgartner G. Fragmentation of bile duct stones by extracorporeal shock-wave lithotripsy: a five-year experience. *Hepatology*. 1992;15:208–214.

36. Carr-Locke DL. Therapeutic role of ERCP in the management of suspected common bile duct stones. *Gastrointest Endosc*. 2002;56:S170–174.

37. Madan AK, Aliabadi-Wahle S, Tesi D, Flint LM, Steinberg SM. How early is early laparoscopic treatment of acute cholecystitis? *Am J Surg*. 2002;183:232–236.

38. Liu TH, Consorti ET, Mercer DW. Laparoscopic cholecystectomy for acute cholecystitis: technical considerations and outcome. *Semin Laparosc Surg*. 2002;9:24–31.

39. Kitano S, Matsumoto T, Aramaki M, Kawano K. Laparoscopic cholecystectomy for acute cholecystitis. *J Hepatobiliary Pancreat Surg*. 2002;9:534–537.

40. Gurusamy KS, Samraj K, Fusai G, Davidson BR. Early versus delayed laparoscopic cholecystectomy for biliary colic. *Cochrane Database Syst Rev*. 2008:CD007196.

41. Peterli R, Schuppisser JP, Herzog U, Ackermann C, Tondelli PE. Prevalence of postcholecystectomy symptoms: long-term outcome after open versus laparoscopic cholecystectomy. *World J Surg*. 2000;24:1232–1235.

42. Cotton PB, Geenen JE, Sherman S, *et al*. Endoscopic sphincterotomy for stones by experts is safe, even in younger patients with normal ducts. *Ann Surg*. 1998;227:201–204.

43. Lammert F, Neubrand MW, Bittner R, *et al*. [S3-guidelines for diagnosis and treatment of gallstones. German Society for Digestive and Metabolic Diseases and German Society for Surgery of the Alimentary Tract]. *Z Gastroenterol*. 2007;45:971–1001.

44. Hashizume M, Sugimachi K, MacFadyen BV. The clinical management and results of surgery for acute cholecystitis. *Semin Laparosc Surg*. 1998;5:69–80.

CHAPTER 75

Sphincter of Oddi dysfunction

Dana C. Moffatt, Stuart Sherman, and Evan L. Fogel

Indiana University Health, Indianapolis, IN, USA

ESSENTIAL FACTS ABOUT PATHOGENESIS

- In Sphincter of Oddi dysfunction (SOD) deranged contractility obstructs the flow of bile or pancreatic juice
- This results in biliary and/or pancreatic type pain
- Sphincter of Oddi dysfunction is a benign, non-calculous obstruction to flow of bile or pancreatic juice through the pancreaticobilary junction, with resultant intraductal hypertension leading to symptomatology
- The underlying cause is not known

ESSENTIALS OF DIAGNOSIS

- Severe episodic pain not relieved by bowel movements, postural change, or antacids, with exclusion of other structural cause
- Biliary and pancreatic subtypes are classified as type I (typical pain with both abnormal chemistry and ductal dilatation), type II (abnormal chemistry or ductal dilatation), or type III (pain without objective of abnormalities)
- Sphincter of Oddi dysfunction can cause unexplained acute pancreatitis
- The morphine-prostigmine provocative (Nardi) test is not recommended due to high false-positive rates.
- Diagnosis is made by sphincter manometry of both pancreatic and common bile duct during endoscopic retrograde cholangiopancreatography (ERCP)

ESSENTIALS OF TREATMENT

- A trial of medical therapy (muscle relaxants, amitriptyline, gabapentin) is justified in type II and III SOD despite limited evidence of efficacy
- Sphincterotomy is the endoscopic therapy of choice in appropriate patients
- Pancreatic sphincterotomy may improve outcome in patients with pancreatic sphincter dysfunction
- Placement of a prophylactic pancreatic stent during ERCP to prevent post-ERCP pancreatitis is now considered standard of care in patients with suspected SOD
- Surgical sphincteroplasty is an option in patients with recurrent sphincter stenosis or if ERCP is technically not feasible

Introduction

Sphincter of Oddi dysfunction (SOD) refers to an abnormal contractility of the sphincter of Oddi. It is a benign, noncalculus, obstruction to flow of bile or pancreatic juice through the pancreaticobilary junction. It may manifest clinically with typical biliary (right upper quadrant, radiating to the back/shoulder blade) or pancreatic pain (epigastric, radiating to mid-back), recurrent pancreatitis, abnormal liver enzymes, or abnormal pancreatic enzymes. Sphincter of Oddi dysfunction most commonly is recognized in patients post-cholecystectomy who develop pain similar to their preoperative biliary colic. Once common bile duct stones and other potential etiologies are ruled out, this residual group of patients has a high frequency of SOD [1].

Epidemiology

Sphincter of Oddi dysfunction most commonly occurs in middle-aged women, although patients of any age or sex may be affected. Although SOD typically is seen in the post-cholecystectomy state, it may occur with the gallbladder *in situ*. The epidemiology of SOD is unclear due to a paucity of population-based data and the considerable variation that exists in currently published literature, including variable patient-selection criteria, definition of SOD used, and whether or not one or both sphincter segments are studied by manometry. Eversman *et al.* performed sphincter of Oddi manometry (SOM) of both the biliary and pancreatic sphincter segments in 360 patients with intact sphincters [2]. In this series, 19% had abnormal pancreatic basal sphincter pressure alone, 11% had abnormal biliary basal sphincter pressure, and 31% had abnormal basal sphincter pressure in both segments for a total of 61% with abnormal sphincter manometry. Similar findings were reported by Americh and colleagues in a series of 73 patients [3]. These two studies highlight the need to evaluate both the bile duct and pancreatic duct during SOM. Furthermore, sphincter dysfunction may also cause recurrent pancreatitis, and manometrically documented SOD has been reported in 15–72% of patients previously labeled as having idiopathic pancreatitis.

Textbook of Clinical Gastroenterology and Hepatology, Second Edition. Edited by C. J. Hawkey, Jaime Bosch, Joel E. Richter, Guadalupe Garcia-Tsao, Francis K. L. Chan.

Pathogenesis and pathology

The sphincter of Oddi (SO) is a complex of smooth muscles that surrounds the terminal common bile duct, ventral pancreatic duct, and the common channel (ampulla of Vater) if present (Figure 75.1). Its primary role is to regulate bile and pancreatic juice flow and to prevent reflux of duodenal contents into the sterile biliary and pancreatic systems. The SO has both a variable basal pressure and phasic contractile activity, which are under both neural and hormonal control. The basal pressure appears to be the predominant mechanism regulating outflow of pancreaticobiliary secretion into the duodenum, while phasic contractions maintain the high-pressure zone responsible for inhibition of ductal reflux. Phasic wave contractions are linked to the migrating motor complex of the duodenum but are also affected by cholecystokinin (CCK), secretin, vasoactive intestinal peptide (VIP), and nitric oxide, while basal pressure is more clearly subject to relaxation when exposed to CCK, secretin, and VIP. Interestingly, sphincter function is not dependent on bile-duct innervation as the SO is still functional post liver transplant. Patients with type I SOD (Tables 75.1 and 75.2) may have disregulation of the above mentioned sphincter regulatory mechanisms. However, these type I patients are thought to have a stenotic sphincter rather than a sphincter in spasm, as pathological series of sphincteroplasty resection specimens have shown significant inflammation, reactive muscular hypertrophy, and fibrosis within the papillary zone in 60% of patients [4]. These pathophysiologic changes at the sphincter papillary orifice are likely responsible for ductal hypertension with resultant duct dilation, elevated liver enzymes, and biliary-type pain in patients with type I SOD. In patients with type II and III SOD (see Tables 75.1 and 75.2), the mechanism of dysfunction is not related to sphincter inflammation and scarring but is thought to be related to disregulation of stimulatory and/or inhibitory factors.

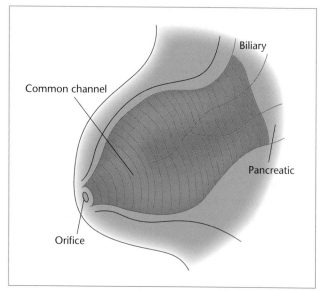

Figure 75.1 The sphincter of Oddi.

Table 75.1 Modified Milwaukee classification for biliary sphincter of Oddi dysfunction, post-cholecystectomy

Biliary type 1	Patients with biliary-type pain, abnormal ALT or alkaline phosphatase >2 times normal, and dilated CBD >12 mm diameter
Biliary type II	Patients with biliary-type pain and one of either: abnormal ALT or alkaline phosphatase >2 times normal OR dilated CBD >12 mm
Biliary type III	Patients with only biliary type-pain and no other abnormalities

ALT, alanine transaminase; CBD, common bile duct.
(Adapted with permission from Behar J, Corazziari E, Guelrud M, Hogan W, Sherman S, Toouli J. Functional gallbladder and sphincter of oddi disorders. *Gastroenterology.* 2006;130:1498–1509.)

Table 75.2 Modified pancreatic classification system for sphincter of Oddi dysfunction

Pancreatic type 1	Patients with pancreatic-type pain, abnormal amylase or lipase >1.5 times normal on any occasion, and dilated PD >6 mm diameter in the head or 5 mm in the body
Pancreatic type II	Patients with pancreatic-type pain and only one of: abnormal amylase or lipase >1.5 times normal on any occasion, OR dilated PD >6 mm diameter in the head or 5 mm in the body
Pancreatic type III	Patients with only pancreatic-type pain and no other abnormalities

PD, pancreatic duct.
(Adapted with permission from Behar J, Corazziari E, Guelrud M, Hogan W, Sherman S, Toouli J. Functional gallbladder and sphincter of oddi disorders. *Gastroenterology.* 2006;130:1498–1509.)

How does SOD cause pain?

From a theoretical point of view, this may be related to: (1) impedance of flow of bile and pancreatic juice resulting in ductal hypertension; (2) muscular ischemia of the sphincter arising from spastic contractions; and (3) hypersensitivity of the papilla and/or duodenum [5]. These mechanisms may potentially act alone or in concert to explain the genesis of pain.

Clinical presentation

Recently, the Rome III classification system provided diagnostic criteria for SOD, as illustrated in Table 75.3 [6]. Abdominal pain is the most common presenting symptom, thought to be due to predominant obstruction of biliary or pancreatic flow (see Tables 75.1 and 75.2) [1]. In biliary-type SOD, the pain is usually localized to the epigastric area or right upper quadrant and lasts anywhere from 30 minutes to several hours. Other features of SOD pain include radiation to the back or shoulder as well as nausea and vomiting, precipitated by food or narcotics. The pain may begin several years after cholecystectomy and is usually similar in character to the pain that initially

Table 75.3 Rome III criteria for functional biliary, gallbladder, and sphincter of Oddi disorders

Diagnostic criteria for functional gallbladder and sphincter of Oddi disorders

Must include episodes of pain located in the epigastrium and/or right upper quadrant and ALL of the following:
- Episodes lasting 30 minutes or longer
- Recurrent symptoms occurring at different intervals (not daily)
- The pain builds up to a steady level
- The pain is moderate to severe enough to interrupt the patient's daily activities or lead to hospital visit
- The pain is not relieved by bowel movements
- The pain is not relieved by postural change
- The pain is not relieved by antacids
- Exclusions of other structural disease that would explain the symptoms

Supportive criteria
The pain may present with one or more of the following:
- Pain is associated with nausea and vomiting
- Pain radiates to the back and/or right infrascapular region
- Pain awakens from sleep in the middle of the night

Diagnostic criteria for functional biliary sphincter of Oddi disorder:
Must include BOTH of the following:
- Criteria for functional gallbladder or sphincter of Oddi disorder met
- Normal amylase/lipase

Supportive criteria
Elevated serum transaminases, alkaline phosphatase or conjugated bilirubin temporally related to at least two pain episodes.

Diagnostic criteria for functional pancreatic sphincter of Oddi disorder
Must include BOTH of the following:
- Criteria for functional gallbladder or sphincter of Oddi disorder met
- Elevated amylase and/or lipase

(Adapted with permission from Behar J, Corazziari E, Guelrud M, Hogan W, Sherman S, Toouli J. Functional gallbladder and sphincter of oddi disorders. *Gastroenterology.* 2006;130:1498–1509.)

prompted gallbladder evaluation. Alternatively, patients may have continued pain that was not relieved by cholecystectomy. Jaundice, fever, or chills are rarely observed. Physical examination typically is negative or shows only mild abdominal tenderness. The pain is not relieved by trial medications for acid peptic disease or irritable bowel syndrome. Laboratory abnormalities, consisting of transient elevations of liver enzyme tests during episodes of pain that normalize during pain-free periods, may be observed.

Patients with pancreatic SOD may present with typical pancreatic pain (epigastric or left upper quadrant pain radiating to the back) with or without pancreatic enzyme elevation, or recurrent pancreatitis.

The association between SOD and chronic pancreatitis is poorly understood. It is not known whether the sphincter at times becomes dysfunctional as part of the overall scarring process, or whether it has a role in the pathogenesis of chronic pancreatitis. However, a high frequency of basal sphincter pressure abnormalities in the pancreatic sphincter has been identified. Tarnasky and colleagues [7] demonstrated that 20

of 23 patients (87%) with chronic pancreatitis had SOD. Sphincterotomy has been demonstrated to improve pain in a subset of patients with chronic pancreatitis in uncontrolled studies.

While the diagnosis of SOD is commonly made after cholecystectomy, SOD may also exist in the presence of an intact gallbladder. However, the symptoms due to SOD may be indistinguishable from gallbladder-type pain, resulting in the diagnosis of SOD being made after cholecystectomy or, less frequently, after gallbladder abnormalities have been excluded. Given the potential complications of ERCP in patients with suspected SOD (see below), empiric cholecystectomy may be considered as initial therapy prior to endoscopic retrograde cholangiopancreatography (ERCP) even in the setting of normal gallbladder evaluation.

Differential diagnosis

The clinical presentation of SOD may be mimicked by many organic pathologies including common bile duct stones, chronic pancreatitis, ampullary tumors, peptic ulcer disease, mesenteric ischemia, renal colic, as well as other functional disorders including irritable bowel syndrome, referred musculoskeletal pain, and functional dyspepsia. Given the 10–20% complication rate seen in the evaluation and therapy of patients with suspected SOD, the diagnosis should be treated as one of exclusion, with other diagnostic possibilities initially pursued with appropriate testing. As well, therapeutic trials with low-risk empirical medical therapies such as proton pump inhibitors, anti-spasmodics, and/or pain modulators should be made before proceeding with ERCP and SOM.

Diagnostic methods and classification

Initial investigations for patients with suspected SOD should include laboratory tests (liver enzymes, serum amylase, and/or lipase), and abdominal imaging (ultrasound or computed tomography [CT]). If at all possible, the sample for enzyme studies should be drawn during an acute attack of pain, although liver test abnormalities lack both sensitivity and specificity [8]. Mild elevations (<2× upper limit of normal) are common in SOD, whereas greater abnormalities are more suggestive of stones, tumors, and intrinsic liver disease. Imaging of the abdomen is usually normal but occasionally dilated bile ducts or pancreatic ducts may be found. Sphincter of Oddi dysfunction is subtyped according to whether the pain is biliary or pancreatic in nature and accompanied by abnormalities of biochemistry or imaging (see Tables 75.1 and 75.2) [1].

More detailed structural evaluation may be obtained with endoscopic ultrasound (EUS) and magnetic resonance imaging/magnetic resonance cholangiopancreatography (MRI/MRCP) in select patients. Several non-invasive tests have been designed in an attempt to identify those individuals with SOD. The morphine-prostigmine provocative test (Nardi test) has been shown to have an unacceptable rate of false-positive studies (>40% in patients with irritable bowel syndrome) and as such is no longer recommended. Quantitative hepatobiliary scintigraphy (HBS), with or without morphine provocation, may predict an abnormal SOM and response to biliary sphincterotomy [9]. However, abnormal results may be found in asymptomatic controls and HBS does not address the pancreatic sphincter, which may be the cause of the patient's symptoms. Measurement of the common bile duct (CBD) by US after either lipid-rich meal or secretin stimulation has been also been shown to have variable sensitivity (21–88%) and specificity (82–97%) [10,11]. More recently, our group has prospectively compared secretin-stimulated MRCP (sMRCP) with SOM [12]. Prediction of SOD based on sMRCP results was poor, with positive and negative predictive values of 67% and 33%, respectively. Considering the limitations of non-invasive testing, SOM demonstrating an elevated basal sphincter pressure over 40mmHg (either biliary or pancreatic) is still considered the gold standard for diagnosing SOD.

Performance of sphincter of Oddi manometry
See Video Clip 75.1.

Treatment
The therapeutic approach in patients with SOD is aimed at decreasing the resistance to flow of bile and pancreatic juice across the sphincter of Oddi. Although the emphasis of therapy is generally placed on definitive intervention such as surgical sphincteroplasty or endoscopic sphincterotomy, a trial of medical therapy is appropriate in patients with type III SOD, and in minimally symptomatic type II patients given the risks associated with ERCP and manometry. A therapeutic trial of nifedipine has been shown to reduce the total number of days with pain by 40%, and may also decrease total analgesic requirement [13]. Although limited data exist, non-specific muscle relaxants (hyoscyamine, dicyclomine) and pain modulators (amitriptyline, gabapentin) are also often used in clinical practice with variable success rates. Once the decision has been made to evaluate the highly symptomatic patient, endoscopic sphincterotomy remains the standard therapy for patients with manometrically confirmed SOD. Most data on endoscopic therapy relate to biliary sphincter ablation alone, and have reported highly variable outcomes (Table 75.4) This variability likely reflects the different criteria used to diagnose SOD, patient type (i.e., type I, II, or III), the method of data collection (retrospective versus prospective), and the definitions used for "improved outcome." In type I biliary SOD patients evaluated in five studies, biliary sphincterotomy led to clinical improvement in 57/67 (85%) patients with a 2-year follow-up [14]. A total of 177 type II biliary SOD patients were evaluated in 10 small studies, and 122 (69%) improved following biliary sphincterotomy alone with a mean of 3-year follow-up [14]. Of 169 type III patients culled from seven studies, only 62 (37%) improved following biliary sphincterotomy, with nearly 3-year follow-up [14]. These data suggest that the majority of biliary type I patients respond to biliary

Table 75.4 Response to biliary sphincterotomy alone in biliary sphincter of Oddi (SOD) patients

SOD type	n studies	n patients (total)	n improved (%)	Mean follow-up (months)
I	5	67	57 (85)	25.2
II	10	177	122 (69)	36.8
III	7	169	62 (37)	34.7

(Adapted with permission from Sgouros SN, Pereira SP. Systematic review: sphincter of Oddi dysfunction – non-invasive diagnostic methods and long-term outcome after endoscopic sphincterotomy. *Aliment Pharmacol Ther.* 2006 Jul 15;24(2):237–246.)

Table 75.5 Symptomatic improvement in pancreatic sphincter of Oddi (SOD) patients after pancreatic sphincterotomy

Author/year [ref.]	n	n improved (%)	Mean follow-up (months)
Pereira, 2006 [15]	13	7 (54)	30.2
Okolo, 2000 [16]	15	11 (73)	16
Elton, 1998 [17]	43	31 (72)	36.4
Soffer, 1994 [18]	25	16 (64)	13.7
Guelrud, 1995 [19]	27	22 (81)	14.7
Total	123	87 (71)	23.9

(Adapted with permission from Sgouros SN, Pereira SP. Systematic review: sphincter of Oddi dysfunction – non-invasive diagnostic methods and long-term outcome after endoscopic sphincterotomy. *Aliment Pharmacol Ther.* 2006 Jul 15;24(2):237–246.)

sphincterotomy alone, and performance of SOM is not necessary. Biliary type II patients may be more likely to respond to sphincter ablation than type III patients. Manometry is highly recommended in type II patients, and mandatory in type III patients. Recent data, however, suggest that the addition of pancreatic sphincterotomy to biliary sphincterotomy may offer additional benefit in patients with pancreatic sphincter hypertension, regardless of the presence of biliary SOD, as shown in Table 75.5. Furthermore, performance of an initial dual pancreatobiliary sphincterotomy was associated with a lower reintervention rate (70/285, 24.6%) than biliary sphincterotomy alone (31/95, 33%, $p < 0.05$) in one large study [20]. The additional benefit of pancreatic sphincter ablation may also be associated with a better long-term outcome than biliary sphincterotomy alone in patients with idiopathic recurrent pancreatitis and pancreatic SOD [20]. A randomized trial comparing biliary ES with combined pancreatobiliary ES in patients with idiopathic pancreatitis and SOD is currently underway at our institution.

Freeman and colleagues recently demonstrated that young patient age (< 40 years), normal pancreatic manometry, daily narcotic use, and presence of gastroparesis were all negative predictors of a favorable outcome, regardless of SOD type [21]. The authors proposed that SOD type may be less important as a predictor of outcome than previous studies have suggested. Confirmatory prospective studies are awaited.

Results from small series with botulinum toxin injected into the SO are intriguing, suggesting that response to injection may predict subsequent response to sphincterotomy. However, this technique requires two procedures to potentially achieve the same therapeutic outcome. Confirmatory data from larger trials are awaited. Balloon dilation of the papilla and trials of biliary stenting have been suggested as alternative methods to improve flow across the biliary sphincter. However, pancreatitis rates are unacceptably high with these techniques and cannot be recommended. Furthermore, pancreatic stent trials are strongly discouraged due to the potential for stent-induced pancreatic ductal injury. In patients with recurrent symptoms after initial response to sphincterotomy, repeat ERCP with SOM may be indicated to assess for sphincter stenosis. Surgical intervention with transduodenal biliary sphincteroplasty and transampullary septoplasty is another option [22]. Early surgical series demonstrated a 60–70% benefit with 1- to 10-year follow-up, but this approach has generally fallen out of favor as endoscopic intervention is associated with lower morbidity, better patient tolerance, lower cost, and improved cosmetic result. Today, surgical intervention in SOD tends to be reserved for recurrent sphincter stenosis following repeated endoscopic therapy, or in patients where ERCP is not technically feasible.

Complications

Patients with suspected SOD are at increased risk of post-ERCP complications, with most studies quoting complication rates 2–5 times higher than patients undergoing ERCP for common bile duct stones or pancreatobiliary malignancy. Pancreatitis is the most common complication, and historically has occurred in up to 30% of patients in some series. Several large multicenter studies and meta-analyses have identified suspected SOD as an independent risk factor for post-ERCP pancreatitis [23–26]. This increased risk of pancreatitis does not appear to be related to SOM itself [27], particularly when the aspirating catheter is used. Several important measures may be undertaken to decrease the incidence of post-ERCP pancreatitis in patients with suspected SOD, including use of the aspirating catheter for SOM, limiting perfusion rates to 0.2–1.0 mL/lumen/min, and utilizing prophylactic pancreatic stents in all patients with suspected SOD, whether or not sphincterotomy is performed [28,29]. As in all patients undergoing ERCP, limiting the number of pancreatic-duct injections [30] and the extent of pancreatic duct opacification [31] may further decrease pancreatitis rates. It has been suggested that use of a solid-state non-perfusion manometry catheter system

may also decrease pancreatitis rates, but additional studies are necessary.

While pharmacologic intervention remains an attractive alternative to decrease post-ERCP pancreatitis rates, available to all endoscopists, no agent is currently recommended for routine use. However, a recent meta-analysis evaluating the role of rectally-administered non-steroidal anti-inflammatory drugs (NSAIDs) suggested that these agents may be effective [32]. Further study in high-risk patients is necessary and a multicenter randomized trial is currently underway.

Despite these advances, complication rates remain significant in patients with suspected SOD. These patients should be counseled thoroughly on the risk–benefit ratio of undergoing ERCP with SOM, prior to proceeding with endoscopic intervention.

Prognosis with and without therapy

The natural history and long-term prognosis of patients with SOD is not well defined, with no population-based data nor data beyond 5–10 years of follow-up available. As described above, limited prospective data suggest that types I and II biliary SOD patients frequently respond to biliary sphincterotomy, but a pancreatic sphincterotomy may be required for those patients with pancreatic sphincter hypertension. There are no prospective controlled data available regarding type III patients. Currently a prospective randomized multicenter study is being undertaken to evaluate predictors and the long-term benefit of intervention with sphincterotomy in suspected type III SOD patients. It is anticipated that this much-needed study will further help to delineate the most appropriate interventions for this controversial, difficult-to-treat group of patients [33].

While progress is being made in both patient outcomes and prevention of complications (i.e., pancreatitis) in patients with suspected SOD, a thorough review of the risk–benefit ratio with individual patients remains mandatory prior to performance of ERCP and SOM.

References

1. Venu RP, Geenen JE, Hogan WJ. Sphincter of Oddi stenosis and dysfunction. In: Sivak MV, Jr., editor. *Gastroenterologic Endoscopy*, 2nd edition. Philadelphia: WB Saunders; 2000. p. 1023.
2. Eversman D, Fogel EL, Rusche M, Sherman S, Lehman GA. Frequency of abnormal pancreatic and biliary sphincter manometry compared with clinical suspicion of sphincter of Oddi dysfunction. *Gastrointest Endosc.* 1999;50:637–641.
3. Aymerich RR, Prakash C, Aliperti G. Sphincter of oddi manometry: is it necessary to measure both biliary and pancreatic sphincter pressures? *Gastrointest Endosc.* 2000;52:183–186.
4. Anderson TM, Pitt HA, Longmire WP, Jr. Experience with sphincteroplasty and sphincterotomy in pancreatobiliary surgery. *Ann Surg.* 1985;201:399–406.
5. Desautels SG, Slivka A, Hutson WR, *et al.* Postcholecystectomy pain syndrome: pathophysiology of abdominal pain in sphincter of Oddi type III. *Gastroenterology.* 1999;116:900–905.
6. Behar J, Corazziari E, Guelrud M, Hogan W, Sherman S, Toouli J. Functional gallbladder and sphincter of oddi disorders. *Gastroenterology.* 2006;130:1498–1509.

Pancreas and Biliary Tract

7. Tarnasky PR, Hoffman B, Aabakken L, *et al.* Sphincter of Oddi dysfunction is associated with chronic pancreatitis. *Am J Gastroenterol.* 1997;92:1125–1129.

8. Steinberg WM. Sphincter of Oddi dysfunction: a clinical controversy. *Gastroenterology.* 1988;95:1409–1415.

9. Thomas PD, Turner JG, Dobbs BR, Burt MJ, Chapman BA. Use of (99m)Tc-DISIDA biliary scanning with morphine provocation for the detection of elevated sphincter of Oddi basal pressure. *Gut.* 2000;46:838–841.

10. Rosenblatt ML, Catalano MF, Alcocer E, Geenen JE. Comparison of sphincter of Oddi manometry, fatty meal sonography, and hepatobiliary scintigraphy in the diagnosis of sphincter of Oddi dysfunction. *Gastrointest Endosc.* 2001;54:697–704.

11. Di Francesco V, Brunori MP, Rigo L, *et al.* Comparison of ultrasound-secretin test and sphincter of Oddi manometry in patients with recurrent acute pancreatitis. *Dig Dis Sci.* 1999; 44:336–340.

12. Aisen AM, Sherman S, Jennings SG, *et al.* Comparison of secretin-stimulated magnetic resonance pancreatography and manometry results in patients with suspected sphincter of oddi dysfunction. *Acad Radiol.* 2008;15:601–609.

13. Khuroo MS, Zargar SA, Yattoo GN. Efficacy of nifedipine therapy in patients with sphincter of Oddi dysfunction: a prospective, double-blind, randomized, placebo-controlled, cross over trial. *Br J Clin Pharmacol.* 1992;33:477–485.

14. Sgouros SN, Pereira SP. Systematic review: sphincter of Oddi dysfunction–non-invasive diagnostic methods and long-term outcome after endoscopic sphincterotomy. *Aliment Pharmacol Ther.* 2006 ;24:237–246.

15. Pereira SP, Gillams A, Sgouros SN, Webster GJ, Hatfield AR. Prospective comparison of secretin-stimulated magnetic resonance cholangiopancreatography with manometry in the diagnosis of sphincter of Oddi dysfunction types II and III. *Gut.* 2007;56:809–813.

16. Okolo PI, 3rd, Pasricha PJ, Kalloo AN. What are the long-term results of endoscopic pancreatic sphincterotomy? *Gastrointest Endosc.* 2000;52:15–19.

17. Elton E, Howell DA, Parsons WG, Qaseem T, Hanson BL. Endoscopic pancreatic sphincterotomy: indications, outcome, and a safe stentless technique. *Gastrointest Endosc.* 1998;47:240–249.

18. Soffer EE, Johlin FC. Intestinal dysmotility in patients with sphincter of Oddi dysfunction. A reason for failed response to sphincterotomy. *Dig Dis Sci.* 1994;39:1942–1946.

19. Guelrud M, Plaz J, Mendoza S, Beker R, Rojas O, Rossiter J. Endoscopic treatment in type II pancreatic sphincter dysfunction. . *Gastrointest Endosc.* 2005;41:398A.

20. Park SH, Watkins JL, Fogel EL, *et al.* Long-term outcome of endoscopic dual pancreatobiliary sphincterotomy in patients with manometry-documented sphincter of Oddi dysfunction and normal pancreatogram. *Gastrointest Endosc.* 2003;57:483–491.

21. Freeman ML, Gill M, Overby C, Cen YY. Predictors of outcomes after biliary and pancreatic sphincterotomy for sphincter of oddi dysfunction. *J Clin Gastroenterol.* 2007;41:94–102.

22. Sherman S, Lehman GA, Jamidar P, *et al.* Efficacy of endoscopic sphincterotomy and surgical sphincteroplasty for patients with sphincter of Oddi dysfunction (SOD): randomized, controlled study. *Gastrointest Endosc.* 1994;40:A125.

23. Cheng CL, Sherman S, Watkins JL, *et al.* Risk factors for post-ERCP pancreatitis: a prospective multicenter study. *Am J Gastroenterol.* 2006;101:139–147.

24. Freeman ML, DiSario JA, Nelson DB, *et al.* Risk factors for post-ERCP pancreatitis: a prospective, multicenter study. *Gastrointest Endosc.* 2001;54:425–434.

25. Freeman ML, Nelson DB, Sherman S, *et al.* Complications of endoscopic biliary sphincterotomy. *N Engl J Med.* 1996;335:909–918.

26. Masci E, Mariani A, Curioni S, Testoni PA. Risk factors for pancreatitis following endoscopic retrograde cholangiopancreatography: a meta-analysis. *Endoscopy.* 2003;35:830–834.

27. Singh P, Gurudu SR, Davidoff S, *et al.* Sphincter of Oddi manometry does not predispose to post-ERCP acute pancreatitis. *Gastrointest Endosc.* 2004;59:499–505.

28. Saad AM, Fogel EL, McHenry L, *et al.* Pancreatic duct stent placement prevents post-ERCP pancreatitis in patients with suspected sphincter of Oddi dysfunction but normal manometry results. *Gastrointest Endosc.* 2008;67:255–261.

29. Tarnasky PR, Palesch YY, Cunningham JT, Mauldin PD, Cotton PB, Hawes RH. Pancreatic stenting prevents pancreatitis after biliary sphincterotomy in patients with sphincter of Oddi dysfunction. *Gastroenterology.* 1998;115:1518–1524.

30. Freeman ML, Guda NM. Prevention of post-ERCP pancreatitis: a comprehensive review. *Gastrointest Endosc.* 2004;59:845–864.

31. Cheon YK, Cho KB, Watkins JL, *et al.* Frequency and severity of post-ERCP pancreatitis correlated with extent of pancreatic ductal opacification. *Gastrointest Endosc.* 2007;65:385–393.

32. Elmunzer BJ, Waljee AK, Elta GH, Taylor JR, Fehmi SM, Higgins PD. A meta-analysis of rectal NSAIDs in the prevention of post-ERCP pancreatitis. *Gut.* 2008;57:1262–1267.

33. Cotton PB. Sphincter of Oddi Dysfunction Type III: A Clinical Minefield. *AGA Perspectives.* 2009;5:9–10.

CHAPTER 76
Primary sclerosing cholangitis

Sombat Treeprasertsuk[1] and Keith D. Lindor[2]

[1]Chulalongkorn University, Bangkok, Thailand
[2]Arizona State University, Tempe, AZ, USA

ESSENTIAL FACTS ABOUT PATHOGENESIS

- Incidence: varies between 4 and 13 per million per year
- Risk: decreased among current and former smokers
- Pathogenesis: multifactorial and further studies are still required
- Genetic predisposition resulting in dysregulation of the immune system
- Toxic and infectious injuries related to intestinal transmigration of bacteria in patients with primary sclerosing cholangitis (PSC) and inflammatory bowel disease (IBD)

ESSENTIALS OF DIAGNOSIS

- Classically: male patients with mean age at onset during the fourth decade with pruritus and fatigue
- Commonly: cholestatic liver pattern with compatible liver enzyme abnormalities cholestasis with elevations in serum alkaline phosphatase (ALP) level of 3–5 times
- Commonly: IBD involving the colon, usually chronic ulcerative colitis
- Exclusion of secondary causes of biliary stricture, e.g., ischemia, cryptosporidiosis, trauma
- Cholangiographic finding: endoscopic retrograde cholangiopancreatography (ERCP) or magnetic resonance cholangiopancreatography (MRCP) of diffuse multifocal biliary strictures or beading pattern of intra- or extrahepatic bile ducts
- Liver biopsy is not necessary

ESSENTIALS OF TREATMENT AND PROGNOSIS

- No effective medical therapy is available
- Endoscopic management: currently used for patients with high-grade focal strictures of the bile ducts
- Liver transplantation: the best treatment in end stage PSC; it improves survival
- Manage complications: metabolic bone disease, chronic cholestasis, and cirrhosis complications
- Surveillance for the increased risk of hepatobiliary and colon cancer
- Prognosis: using Mayo PSC risk score for assessing the risk of patients and making treatment decisions

Introduction

Primary sclerosing cholangitis (PSC) is a chronic cholestatic liver disease with a male predominance that usually presents during the fourth decade of life. It is characterized by slowly progressive inflammation and fibrosis of the intra- and extrahepatic biliary trees, culminating with the development of biliary cirrhosis. The pathogenesis of PSC is multifactorial. It has a strong association with inflammatory bowel disease (IBD), especially ulcerative colitis. Currently, no effective medical therapy is available. Liver transplantation is the only treatment to improve the survival of patients with PSC.

Epidemiology

The incidence of PSC varies between 4 and 13 per million per year with a prevalence of 100 to 150 per million. Most of the data originates from Europe, Canada, and the United States (Table 76.1). The mean age at onset is during the fourth decade with a male predominance of 3:1 [1]. In children, PSC is less common than in adults and, when it presents in children, the mean age at initial presentation is 13 years.

Risk factors

Odds of having PSC are significantly decreased among current and former smokers regardless of their IBD status. Risk is increased in those with a family history of PSC, suggesting a genetic predisposition. The prevalence of PSC among first-degree relatives is 0.7% and the prevalence in siblings is 1.5% [2]. Other conditions reportedly associated with PSC include several autoimmune disorders, such as systemic lupus erythematosus, Sjögren's syndrome, celiac sprue, and rheumatoid arthritis.

Pathogenesis

The pathogenesis of PSC is multifactorial. A genetic predisposition resulting in dysregulation of the immune system is evident. Bergquist et al. reported a high prevalence of PSC in first-degree relatives of PSC patients, nearly 100 times higher than the general population [2]. The role of an immune-related process and other mechanisms such as toxic and infectious injuries related to intestinal transmigration of bacteria in patients with IBD has been considered. Further studies are still required in order to better understand the etiology of PSC.

Textbook of Clinical Gastroenterology and Hepatology, Second Edition. Edited by C. J. Hawkey, Jaime Bosch, Joel E. Richter, Guadalupe Garcia-Tsao, Francis K. L. Chan.
© 2012 Blackwell Publishing Ltd. Published 2012 by Blackwell Publishing Ltd.

Pancreas and Biliary Tract

Table 76.1 The incidence and prevalence of primary sclerosing cholangitis (PSC)

Authors, Country	Study period	PSC cases; Control	Mortality rate (Hazard ratio; HR)	Incidence (per million per year)	Prevalence (per million)
Bambha K, et al. [1], United States	1976–2000	22 PSC; 20000 age-adjusted US whites	—	Men: 12.5 (95% CI, 7–21) Women: 5.4 (95% CI, 2.2–11)	Men: 209 (95% CI, 95–324) Women: 63 (95% CI, 10–125)
Boberg KM, et al. [3], Norway	1986–1995	17 PSC; population of 130000 inhabitants	—	13	85
Card TR, et al. [4], United Kingdom	1991–2001	223 PSC; 2217 controls from the General Practice Research Database	HR 2.92 (95% CI 2.16–3.94)	4.1 (95% CI, 3.4–4.8)	—
Kaplan GG, et al. [5], Canada	2000–2005	49 PSC; population of the Calgary Health Region, 2001	—	Total: 9 Adults: 11.1 Children: 2.3 Small duct PSC: 1.5	—

Liver pathology

Common liver histological findings include periductal fibrosis and inflammation, portal edema and fibrosis, focal proliferation of bile ducts and ductules, focal bile duct obliteration, loss of bile ducts, and cholestasis. For histological staging, the commonly used criteria of Ludwig et al. [6] are as follows: stage I, cholangitis or portal hepatitis; stage II, periportal fibrosis or periportal hepatitis; stage III, septal fibrosis, bridging necrosis, or both; and stage IV, biliary cirrhosis (Figure 76.1). However, the sampling variability of liver biopsy is a major problem. It varies from 18% to 71%, and advanced liver disease (stages 3 or 4) was missed in 40% of the liver biopsy specimens [7]. In a previous study regarding of the role of liver biopsy in providing new information after PSC diagnosis by cholangiography, 98.7% of liver biopsies revealed no atypical findings and did not affect clinical management [8]. The role of liver biopsy in providing new information after PSC diagnosis by cholangiography is low and seldom affects clinical management.

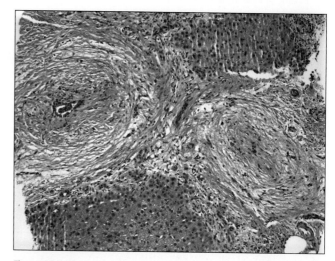

Figure 76.1 Histological staging showing stage IV, biliary cirrhosis.

Clinical presentation

Typical symptoms are pruritus and fatigue, although some patients (21%) are asymptomatic when investigated for liver test abnormalities in IBD. The course is a slowly progressive liver disease with inflammatory destruction of both intrahepatic and extrahepatic bile ducts [1] Three-quarters of patients with PSC in the US have IBD involving the colon, usually chronic ulcerative colitis (UC) [1]. Only 1% to 14% of PSC patients have colonic Crohn's disease. Concurrent PSC and IBD are common and the diagnosis of IBD precedes the diagnosis of PSC in 64%. The average time from onset of IBD to PSC is 9 years (range: 1.3– 23 years) [1]. However, both diseases have courses independent of the initial disease activity. The characteristics of UC in PSC patients are those of widespread quiescent colitis and rectal sparing. Some patients

(6–10%) may present with cholestasis for several years with normal endoscopic retrograde cholangiopancreatography (ERCP). Overt PSC may eventually develop in some [9]. These patients have been classified as having small-duct PSC, which may progress to large-duct PSC [10]. It may represent an earlier stage of PSC and is associated with a significantly better long-term prognosis. Small-duct PSC may recur after orthotopic liver transplantation (OLT) and it is not influenced by IBD. None of the patients with small-duct PSC develop cholangiocarcinoma (CCA) compared with the 11% of those with large-duct PSC who develop CCA [10].

Differential diagnosis

Several cholestatic liver diseases may mimic the clinical syndrome or the cholangiographic findings of PSC. Chronic

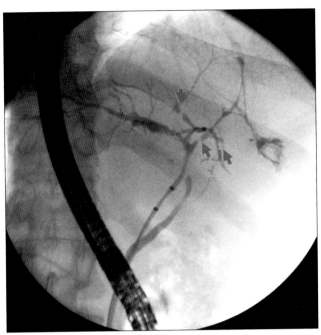

Figure 76.2 Endoscopic retrograde cholangiopancreatography (ERCP); the gold standard for primary sclerosing cholangitis (PSC) diagnosis showing typical changes of PSC, biliary strictures involving the bile duct in both hepatic lobes (red arrows).

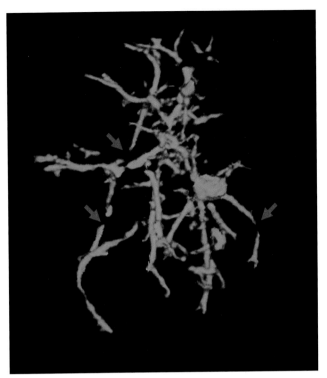

Figure 76.3 Magnetic resonance cholangiopancreatography (MRCP); a noninvasive and shows a good diagnostic accuracy for detection of biliary strictures in a patient with primary sclerosing cholangitis (PSC) in both hepatic lobes (red arrows).

cholestasis from any cause can lead to liver histological changes of bile duct stasis and Mallory–Denk bodies. The differential diagnosis includes primary biliary cirrhosis, autoimmune hepatitis, overlap syndrome with autoimmune hepatitis, cryptosporidiosis, and graft-versus-host disease. Clinical evaluation, the pattern of liver tests, and the lack of typical cholangiographic findings help excluded these diagnoses. Causes of secondary sclerosing cholangitis (SSC) including surgical trauma from cholecystectomy, intraductal stones, recurrent pancreatitis, ischemic injury, or abdominal injury should be considered in the differential diagnosis. Patients with SSC have a shorter survival free of transplant than PSC patients. Differentiating CCA from benign biliary strictures in PSC patients may be the most difficult problem.

Diagnostic methods

Patients with PSC commonly have a high serum alkaline phosphatase (ALP) level of 3–5 times the upper limit of normal and serum transaminase levels elevated to a mild degree. If hyperbilirubinemia develops, prompt investigation should be performed for identification of complicating stricture. Endoscopic retrograde cholangiopancreatography is still considered the gold standard for PSC diagnosis and to detect complications including biliary strictures, biliary stones, or CCA (Figure 76.2). The key diagnostic features for PSC are composed of the following: 1) cholangiographic findings by ERCP or magnetic resonance cholangiography (MRCP) showing diffuse multifocal biliary strictures or a beading pattern of intra- or

extrahepatic bile ducts with 2) compatible cholestatic liver enzyme abnormalities with elevations in serum ALP, with or without positive results of nonspecific autoantibodies such as, the perinuclear anti-neutrophil cytoplasmic antibodies (p-ANCAs) which are nonspecific, and 3) exclusion of secondary causes, which can cause biliary stricture (e.g., ischemia, cryptosporidiosis, trauma). Liver biopsies are not necessarily used for diagnosis [8]. Recently, MRCP has been increasingly used because it is noninvasive, shows good diagnostic accuracy for detection of strictures (Figure 76.3), and has no risk of pancreatitis, unlike ERCP.

Treatment and prevention

The evaluation of therapy in chronic liver diseases such as PSC is challenging because of the very slow progression of liver fibrosis and the difficulties related to the quantification of disease progression. Currently, no effective medical therapy is available. Orthotopic liver transplantation is the only treatment that improves survival. The goals of any treatment should be to emphasize symptom relief, manage complications, and provide surveillance for the increased risk of hepatobiliary and colon cancer.

Pharmacological approaches

Ursodeoxycholic acid (UDCA), a hydrophilic bile acid, is the most widely evaluated treatment of PSC. Several controlled

Table 76.2 Pharmacological therapies for primary sclerosing cholangitis with varied results

Pharmacological therapies	Dose	Results
Ursodeoxycholic acid (UDCA)	8–30 mg/kg/day	Improves liver tests, but high dose (28–30 mg/kg/day) UDCA therapy shows no improvement in survival and has a 2.2 times higher rate of liver decompensation than placebo
Silymarin (silibinin)	140 mg orally 3 times daily, for 1 year	Improves liver tests in approx. one-third of patients but not survival
Antibiotic prophylaxis for bacterial cholangitis		No benefit
Minocycline	100 mg orally twice daily, for 1 year	Significantly improves serum alkaline phosphatase (ALP) and Mayo risk score
Several immunosuppressive and antifibrotic agents, including corticosteroids, methotrexate, tacrolimus, pentoxifylline, colchicine, and penicillamine		No significant benefit or altered disease progression

and uncontrolled studies have consistently demonstrated that UDCA in a dose range from 8 to 30 mg/kg/day improves liver biochemistries [11]. However, high-dose UDCA therapy (28–30 mg/kg/day) does not improve survival and has a 2.2-fold higher rate of liver decompensation or CCA than placebo [12]. Other pharmacological therapies have shown varied results (Table 76.2).

Endoscopic therapy

Endoscopic management for PSC is currently used for patients with high-grade focal strictures of the bile ducts, which are associated with poor outcome. Dominant biliary strictures are managed by repeated angioplasty-type balloon dilation or biliary stent placement, which may lead to a better survival [13]. Complications occur in 9% of patients, mostly related to ERCP complications such as pancreatitis and post-sphincterotomy bleeding. The role of bile duct brushing with additional newer techniques such as fluorescence in-situ hybridization (FISH) showed promising results in improving the cytological diagnosis of biliary cancer. Biliary decompression with stent for endoscopic delivery of photodynamic therapy (PDT) shows improved CCA patient survival.

Surgical treatment

In the past, choledochoenteric anastomoses were used for major extrahepatic blockage or involvement of the extrahepatic bile ducts in patients with PSC [14]. However, previous biliary surgery is associated with poor outcome post OLT. Currently, dominant bile duct strictures are better managed by endoscopic treatment, and consequently there is no role for the surgical management of strictures.

Liver transplantation

In 2005, PSC accounted for 5% of candidates on the waiting list for OLT. Survival from OLT in PSC patients is excellent with 5-year survival rates of 83% to 88%, which are better than rates for other causes of liver diseases [13]. However, retransplantation rates are high and occur in 9% to 20% of PSC patients followed up for 2–5 years [15]. Most patients with recurrence have elevated ALP levels and biliary stricture by cholangiography at 90 days post OLT. For PSC patients with CCA, OLT has shown poor survival, with overall 5-year survival rates ranging from 9% to 28%. A recent study shows excellent survival as a result of neoadjuvant chemoradiotherapy followed by OLT for PSC patients with localized, node-negative hilar CCA [16].

Complications and management

The complications of PSC include metabolic bone disease, chronic cholestasis, and malignancy, especially CCA, which is the most lethal complication of PSC.

Chronic cholestasis and osteoporosis

Steatorrhea and vitamin deficiency (mainly vitamin A, D, or E), secondary to fat malabsorption, may occur during the late stages of the disease. Therefore, patients should be screened for fat-soluble vitamin deficiency such as 25-hydroxy vitamin D and 1,25-dihydroxy vitamin D and treated accordingly.

Therapies for cholestatic pruritus are often unsatisfactory. Currently, there is no FDA-approved therapy for cholestatic pruritus. UDCA does not improve pruritus. Cholestyramine, a bile-acid binding resin is a good choice and is partially effective in up to 85% of patients. Rifampicin may adversely affect liver enzymes but can be effective in controlling pruritus. Antihistamines, naltrexone, phenobarbital, and sertraline may have some beneficial effects.

Osteopenia occurs in approximately 9% of patients with PSC. Older patients with longer duration of IBD and more advanced liver disease are a high-risk group. Bone mineral density (BMD) is used for detection of osteoporosis and is measured by dual-energy X-ray absorptiometry (DEXA), which is currently the best predictor of fracture risk. BMD should be preformed in all newly diagnosed patients with PSC and thereafter at 2- to 3-year intervals. UDCA treatment does not affect the rate of bone loss. Aggressive supportive therapy including calcium and vitamin D supplements is reasonable. Further study of treatment for osteoporosis in PSC is needed.

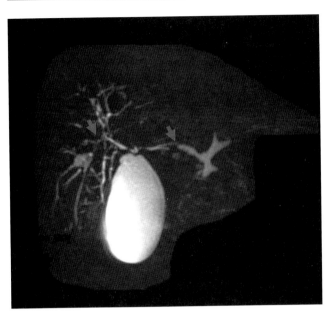

Figure 76.4 Cross-sectional magnetic resonance imaging (MRI) showing biliary strictures in PSC patient with moderate dilatation of both hepatic lobes with periductal enhancement (red arrows).

Hepatobiliary carcinoma
Cholangiocarcinoma
The lifetime risk of CCA is up to 14–20% in PSC patients evaluated for OLT, and the annual risk varies from 0.6% to 1.5% per year [17]. Cholangiocarcinoma is often detected at the same time or within 1 year of the diagnosis of PSC. Patients with concomitant PSC and CCA have a short median survival time of 5 months. Recently, a screening strategy was reported with high accuracy for detecting CCA using complementary studies, including serum carbohydrate antigen CA19-9 combined with liver imaging (ultrasonography, CT, or MRI) (Figure 76.4). Cholangiography (ERCP or MRCP) and cytologic examination are useful for confirming the diagnosis of CCA in patients with PSC [17]. Evaluation using FISH increases the sensitivity of bile duct cytology. In a recent study, 51% of PSC patients tested by FISH had positive results; only one-third of these patients had CCA [18]. FISH had 46% sensitivity and 88% specificity for the diagnosis of CCA in PSC patients [18]. Patients with PSC who have an early diagnosis of CCA may have a better outcome with 5-year survival of 82% for perihilar CCA treated with a combination of neoadjuvant chemoradiotherapy and OLT [19]. Arterial and portal venous complications are reported in 40% of patients receiving neoadjuvant chemoradiotherapy. For unresectable CCA, treatment with decompressing plastic biliary stents combined with PDT every 3 months may be an optional therapy with a 1-year survival rate of 30% [20].

Gallbladder carcinoma
The prevalence of a gallbladder mass in PSC patients undergoing cholecystectomy is 13.7% and 57% of them have adenocar-

cinoma of the gallbladder [21]. The histological findings from 72 gallbladders of PSC patients with liver explants and cholecystectomies include gallbladder dysplasia (37%) and gallbladder adenocarcinoma (14%) [22]. Gallbladder adenocarcinoma is associated with intrahepatic bile-duct dysplasia, CCA, IBD and older age [23]. Gallbladder polyps in PSC patients have a risk of malignancy and should be considered for cholecystectomy.

Hepatocellular carcinoma
The prevalence of hepatocellular carcinoma (HCC) in patients undergoing OLT for PSC is 2% compared to 6% in patients without PSC. Median duration of PSC before HCC detection is 8 years [23]. Concomitant presence of HCC and PSC has been reported sporadically.

Colorectal cancer
The risk of developing colorectal dysplasia or cancer in PSC patients is 9%, 31%, and 50% after 10, 20, and 25 years of disease duration, which are higher rates than those reported in comparable age- and IBD-severity matched patients without PSC (2%, 5%, and 10%, respectively) [24]. The 10-year and 20-year risk for colon cancer in PSC patients is 14% and 31%, respectively, which is significantly higher than rates in PSC patients without IBD (2% and 2%, respectively) [25]. Therefore, PSC patients with UC should receive colonoscopic surveillance at 1- to 2-year intervals from the time of the diagnosis of PSC [5,26].

Chronic liver disease complications
Approximately 17% to 36% of patients with PSC have esophageal varices at initial esophagogastroscopy while 20.2% developed new varices during the follow up and 20% of new varices were moderate or large . Non-invasive markers including a higher Mayo risk score and higher aspartate aminotransferase to alanine aminotransferase (AST/ALT) ratio were significantly associated with the presence of varices at initial endoscopy while lower platelet count and higher total bilirubin at 2 years were significantly associated with an increased risk of developing new varices [27,28].

Prognosis
Several models have been developed to predict disease progression and survival in PSC. However, the limitation of some models is the requirement of liver histology in the model and the lack of symptom variables [29]. A revised natural history model for PSC from the Mayo Clinic that does not include liver histology parameters and is based on patient age, bilirubin levels, albumin, AST levels, and history of variceal bleeding, can be used for assessing the risk of death in patients with PSC and making treatment decisions. This model is calculated as follows:

PSC risk score (R)

$$= 0.03\,(\text{age}\,[\text{year}]) + 0.54\,\log_e(\text{bilirubin}\,[\text{mg/dL}])$$
$$+ 0.54\,\log_e(\text{aspartate aminotransferase}\,[\text{U/L}])$$
$$+ 1.24\,(\text{variceal bleeding}\,[0/1]) - 0.84\,(\text{albumin}\,[\text{g/dL}])$$

A web-based calculator for this model is available at http://www.mayoclinic.org/gi-rst/mayomodel3.html or at http://www.psc-literature.org/mrscalc.htm

For post-OLT patients with PSC, the Child–Pugh score was better in predicting survival rate compared with the Mayo PSC risk score model.

A recent study shows that PSC patients with elevated IgG4 had more aggressive liver disease and had shorter time to OLT than PSC patients with normal IgG4 [30]. The mortality of PSC patients has remained unchanged during the last two decades and highlights the need for effective therapeutic strategies.

Natural history

Most patients may be anxious and need to know the natural history of PSC. We should emphasize that PSC is an uncommon disease and slowly damages the bile ducts. Many people with PSC have no symptoms, especially in the early stages of the disease. Common symptoms are fatigue and pruritus. The cause of disease is unknown. The bile ducts become damaged and bile accumulates in the liver. Liver cells are damaged gradually and cause scarring of the liver and, eventually, cirrhosis. Patients with PSC may develop liver failure 10 to 17 years after diagnosis, and some patients may finally need a liver transplant. Approximately three-quarters of patients with PSC also have IBD, especially UC. Patients with PSC and UC should be screened by colonoscopic surveillance due to the high risk of colon cancer. One of the serious complications of PSC is bile-duct cancer. Currently, there are no specific medications, herbs, or vitamin supplements to slow the disease progression. No specific lifestyle changes need to be implemented. Close monitoring is recommended. Orthotopic liver transplantation is the best modality of treatment to improve survival in end-stage PSC with excellent results. Referral to specialized centers should be considered, especially if the patients are interested in participating in clinical trials.

SOURCES OF INFORMATION FOR DOCTORS AND PATIENTS

http://www.liverfoundation.org/abouttheliver/info/psc/
http://www.gi.org/patients/gihealth/sclerosing.asp

Current controversies and future resolution

Understanding the role of cytokines, bacterial infection, cholangiocyte biology, genetic factors, and innate immunity may be required to develop innovative treatments. Results from small clinical trials of new pharmacological therapies,

including immunosuppressive agents, anticytokines, antibiotics, antifibrotic agents, and anti-tumor necrosis factor therapies, need confirmation with larger trials. Surveillance strategies for cancers related to PSC such as CCA and colon cancer are needed to establish guidelines for clinical practice. Distinguishing CCA from benign biliary strictures has important therapeutic and prognostic implications. Tumor serological markers, especially CA19-9, combined with cross-sectional liver imaging studies and additional molecular tests of bile-duct brushings may be helpful in the early diagnosis of CCA. Finally, new strategies to control disease activity of PSC post OLT are needed to prevent recurrent PSC.

References

1. Bambha K, Kim WR, Talwalkar J, *et al.* Incidence, clinical spectrum, and outcomes of primary sclerosing cholangitis in a United States community. *Gastroenterology.* 2003;125:1364–1369.
2. Bergquist A, Lindberg G, Saarinen S, *et al.* Increased prevalence of primary sclerosing cholangitis among first-degree relatives. *J Hepatol.* 2005;42:252–256.
3. Boberg KM, Aadlund E, Jahnsen J. Incidence and prevalence of primary biliary cirrhosis, primary sclerosing cholangitis and autoimmune hepatitis in a Norwegian population. *Scand J Gastroenterol.* 1998;33:99–103.
4. Card TR, Sulaymani-Dodoran M, West J. Incidence and mortality of primary sclerosing cholangitis in the United Kingdom: A population-based cohort study. *J Hepatology.* 2008;48:939–944.
5. Kaplan GG, Heitman SJ, Hilsden RJ, *et al.* Population-based analysis of practices and costs of surveillance for colonic dysplasia in patients with primary sclerosing cholangitis and colitis. *Inflamm Bowel Dis.* 2007;13:1401–1407.
6. Ludwig J, Barham SS, LaRusso NF, *et al.* Morphologic features of chronic sclerosing cholangitis and chronic ulcerative colitis. *Hepatology.* 1981;1:632–640.
7. Olsson R, Hagerstrand I, Broome U, *et al.* Sampling variability of percutaneous liver biopsy in primary sclerosing cholangitis. *J Clin Pathol.* 1995;48:933–935.
8. Burak KW, Angulo P, Lindor KD. Is there a role for liver biopsy in primary sclerosing cholangitis? *Am J Gastroenterol.* 2003;98:1155–1158.
9. Kaplan GG, Laupland KB, Butzner D, *et al.* The burden of large and small duct primary sclerosing cholangitis in adults and children: a population-based analysis. *Am J Gastroenterol.* 2007;102:1042–1049.
10. Angulo P, Maor-Kendler Y, Lindor KD. Small-duct primary sclerosing cholangitis: a long-term follow-up study. *Hepatology.* 2002;35:1494–1500.
11. Cullen SN, Rust C, Fleming K, *et al.* High dose ursodeoxycholic acid for the treatment of primary sclerosing cholangitis is safe and effective. *J Hepatol.* 2008;48:792–800.
12. Lindor KD, Kowdley KV, Luketic VA, *et al.* High-dose ursodeoxycholic acid for the treatment of primary sclerosing cholangitis. *Hepatology.* 2009;50:808–814.
13. Baluyut AR, Sherman S, Lehman GA, *et al.* Impact of endoscopic therapy on the survival of patients with primary sclerosing cholangitis. *Gastrointest Endosc.* 2001;53:308–312.
14. Campsen J, Zimmerman MA, Trotter JF, *et al.* Clinically recurrent primary sclerosing cholangitis following liver transplantation: a time course. *Liver Transpl.* 2008;14:181–185.

15. Roberts MS, Angus DC, Bryce CL, *et al.* Survival after liver transplantation in the United States: a disease-specific analysis of the UNOS database. *Liver Transpl.* 2004;10:886–897.

16. Heimbach JK. Successful liver transplantation for hilar cholangiocarcinoma. *Curr Opin Gastroenterol.* 2008;24:384–388.

17. Charatcharoenwitthaya P, Enders FB, Halling KC, *et al.* Utility of serum tumor markers, imaging, and biliary cytology for detecting cholangiocarcinoma in primary sclerosing cholangitis. *Hepatology.* 2008;48:1106–1117.

18. Bangarulingam SY, Bjornsson E, Enders F, *et al.* Long-term outcomes of positive fluorescence in situ hybridization tests in primary sclerosing cholangitis. *Hepatology.* 2010;51:174–180.

19. Rea DJ, Heimbach JK, Rosen CB, *et al.* Liver transplantation with neoadjuvant chemoradiation is more effective than resection for hilar cholangiocarcinoma. *Ann Surg.* 2005;242:451–458; discussion 458–461.

20. Prasad GA, Wang KK, Baron TH, *et al.* Factors associated with increased survival after photodynamic therapy for cholangiocarcinoma. *Clin Gastroenterol Hepatol.* 2007;5:743–748.

21. Buckles DC, Lindor KD, Larusso NF, *et al.* In primary sclerosing cholangitis, gallbladder polyps are frequently malignant. *Am J Gastroenterol.* 2002;97:1138–1142.

22. Lewis JT, Talwalkar JA, Rosen CB, *et al.* Prevalence and risk factors for gallbladder neoplasia in patients with primary sclerosing cholangitis: evidence for a metaplasia-dysplasia-carcinoma sequence. *Am J Surg Pathol.* 2007;31:907–913.

23. Leidenius M, Hockersted K, Broome U, *et al.* Hepatobiliary carcinoma in primary sclerosing cholangitis: a case control study. *J Hepatol.* 2001;34:792–798.

24. Broome U, Lofberg R, Veress B, *et al.* Primary sclerosing cholangitis and ulcerative colitis: evidence for increased neoplastic potential. *Hepatology.* 1995;22:1404–1408.

25. Claessen MM, Vleggaar FP, Tytgat KM, *et al.* High lifetime risk of cancer in primary sclerosing cholangitis. *J Hepatol.* 2009;50:158–164.

26. Vleggaar FP, Lutgens MW, Claessen MM. Review article: The relevance of surveillance endoscopy in long-lasting inflammatory bowel disease. *Aliment Pharmacol Ther.* 2007;26(Suppl 2):47–52.

27. Zein CO, Lindor KD, Angulo P. Prevalence and predictors of esophageal varices in patients with primary sclerosing cholangitis. *Hepatology.* 2004;39:204–210.

28. Treeprasertsuk S, Kowdley KV, Luketic VA, *et al.* The predictors of the presence of varices in patients with primary sclerosing cholangitis. *Hepatology.* 2010;51:1302–1310.

29. Kim WR, Therneau TM, Wiesner RH, *et al.* A revised natural history model for primary sclerosing cholangitis. *Mayo Clin Proc.* 2000;75:688–694.

30. Mendes FD, Jorgensen R, Keach J, *et al.* Elevated serum IgG4 concentration in patients with primary sclerosing cholangitis. *Am J Gastroenterol.* 2006;101:2070–2075.

Pancreas and Biliary Tract

CHAPTER 77
Cholangiocarcinoma

Konstantinos N. Lazaridis and Gregory J. Gores
Mayo Clinic, Rochester, MN, USA

ESSENTIAL FACTS ABOUT PATHOGENESIS

- The pathogenesis of cholangiocarcinoma is indeterminate
- Among established risk factors, primary sclerosing cholangitis is the most common, although the majority of cholangiocarcinoma cases remains idiopathic

ESSENTIALS OF DIAGNOSIS

- The diagnosis of cholangiocarcinoma is based on clinical, biochemical, and histopathological criteria
- Diagnosis of cholangiocarcinoma can be challenging in patients who have primary sclerosing cholangitis because the former mimics the latter
- Standard cytology has low sensitivity and specificity; recently fluorescent in-situ hybridization (FISH) of biliary scrapings has become the standard method of diagnosis

ESSENTIALS OF TREATMENT

- Surgical resection is the best approach to treat cholangiocarcinoma
- In selected cases, liver transplantation provides excellent survival to affected patients
- Biliary decompression in the form of biliary stenting or percutaneous drainage offers palliation
- Photodynamic therapy is a promising approach to alleviate the obstructive complications of cholangiocarcinoma and may improve survival

---

Introduction

Cholangiocarcinoma is a malignant tumor of the bile ducts that accounts for 10–15% of hepatobiliary malignancies [1]. Cholangiocarcinoma is an adenocarcinoma arising from the bile ducts with markers of cholangiocyte differentiation [2]. Despite progress in better understanding the biology of cholangiocarcinoma, this malignancy has a grave prognosis [3] and therapies are limited.

Epidemiology

Epidemiological studies from around the world have shown an increasing incidence of intrahepatic cholangiocarcinoma

[4,5]. The etiology of this finding remains unclear. The incidence of cholangiocarcinoma in the United States is approximately 7 cases per million [6]. Cholangiocarcinoma affects slightly more males than females. The peak age is the seventh decade in Western societies.

Risk factors and disease associations

Several established risk factors have been associated with the development of cholangiocarcinoma including primary sclerosing cholangitis (PSC), Caroli disease, congenital choledochal cyst, chronic hepatolithiasis, liver flukes such as *Clonorchis sinensis* and *Opisthorchis viverrini*, exposure to Thorotrast, chronic viral hepatitis, cirrhosis, and obesity. Nevertheless most patients diagnosed with cholangiocarcinoma do not have history of a known predisposing factor associated with the disease. The risk for developing cholangiocarcinoma in a patient with PSC is approximately 1.5% per year after diagnosis of the biliary disease [7]. An association between biliary–enteric drainage surgical procedures and development of cholangiocarcinoma has been reported [8]. A common feature of the many triggers that operate in cholangiocarcinogenesis is the presence of chronic inflammation in the biliary tree and/or persistent cholestasis.

Pathogenesis

Chronic inflammation of the bile ducts is likely a predisposing factor of malignant transformation of cholangiocytes, which leads to the development of cholangiocarcinoma. In fact, a number of genetic and somatic alterations could lead to cholangiocarcinoma. These mechanisms include pathways to: (1) develop apoptosis resistance and divert immune surveillance of cholangiocytes; (2) acquire telomerase activity resulting in immortalization and malignant propagation of bile ducts; (3) alter the expression of oncogenes and tumor suppressor genes leading to lack of cholangiocyte-cycle control. We now know that the inflammatory milieu within the bile ducts could cause cholangiocarcinogenesis via dysregulation or constitutive expression of growth factors,

---

Textbook of Clinical Gastroenterology and Hepatology, Second Edition. Edited by C. J. Hawkey, Jaime Bosch, Joel E. Richter, Guadalupe Garcia-Tsao, Francis K. L. Chan.

proinflammatory cytokines and their receptors. Moreover, proinflammatory cytokines can advance expression of inducible nitric oxide (NO) synthetase and thus produce NO locally that consequently causes DNA damage, inhibits DNA repair and apoptosis, promotes angiogenesis for tumor growth, and induces the expression of cyclooxygenase (COX)-2 that in turn restrains apoptosis and aids cell-growth and angiogenesis.

Pathology

Cholangiocarcinoma is a relatively slow growing, locally destructive tumor that could involve any port of the biliary tree (i.e., intra- and extrahepatic). Histologically, cholangiocarcinoma is a well- to poorly-differentiated tubular adenocarcinoma. The tumor forms glands with a prominent, dense, desmoplastic stroma. Other variants of cholangiocarcinoma include papillary adenocarcinoma, signet-ring carcinoma, squamous cell or mucoepidermoid carcinoma, and a lymphoepithelioma-like form.

Macroscopically, cholangiocarcinoma is classified into the extra- and intrahepatic types. Extrahepatic cholangiocarcinoma represents two-thirds of cholangiocarcinomas and is subdivided into: (1) hilar or upper-third; (2) middle third; and (3) distal third tumors. Hilar cholangiocarcinoma or Klatskin tumor accounts for approximately 60% of all extrahepatic biliary carcinomas. Based on gross appearance, extrahepatic cholangiocarcinoma is grouped into sclerosing, nodular, and papillary. Sclerosing cholangiocarcinoma is the most common and develops annular thickening of the bile ducts with infiltration and fibrosis of the periductal tissues. Intrahepatic cholangiocarcinoma represents about one-third of bile duct carcinomas and can be misdiagnosed as hepatocellular carcinoma. Intrahepatic cholangiocarcinoma may be solitary or multinodular; it may also be well-demarcated as a mass lesion or a diffuse, infiltrating neoplasm growing along the intrahepatic bile ducts.

Clinical presentation

Extrahepatic cholangiocarcinoma is characterized by symptoms, signs, and biochemical profile of cholestasis. Patients often present with jaundice, dark urine, pale stools, pruritus, malaise, and weight loss. The laboratory tests reveal an increased alkaline phosphatase and bilirubin. Serum CA19-9 is often elevated. Imaging studies demonstrate dilatation of the biliary tree and often localize the level of obstruction. Unilobular bile-duct obstruction is usually associated with atrophy of the affected lobe coupled with hypertrophy of the non-affected liver lobe (i.e., the atrophy–hypertrophy complex) [9]. An atrophied lobe usually signifies vasculature encasement by the tumor in the affected lobe.

Endoscopic retrograde cholangiopancreatography (ERCP) is used often to define the topography of cholangiocarcinoma

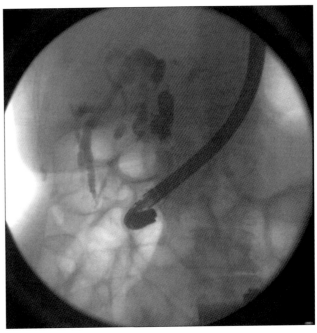

Figure 77.1 Hilar cholangiocarcinoma:. this endoscopic retrograde cholangiopancreatography illustrates the presence of a stricture at the hilum of the biliary system.

along the bile ducts. In addition, endoscopic biopsies and brush cytology of the bile ducts can be obtained during ERCP for pathological diagnosis of the obstructive lesion. An ERCP of a patient with a hilar cholangiocarcinoma is shown in Figure 77.1. Nevertheless, the pathological diagnosis could be challenging, because cholangiocarcinoma is a highly desmoplastic tumor consisting mainly of fibrous tissue with few aggregations of malignant cells. This desmoplastic reaction, which surrounds the bile ducts and extends into the submucosal space, causes only 30% of cholangiocarcinomas to be diagnosed by brush cytology Combined brush cytology and endoscopic biopsy increase the yield of positive finding to 40–50% of cholangiocarcinomas [3]. However, novel approaches including single-cell techniques such as fluorescent in-situ hybridization (FISH) offer promising tools to evaluate cellular aneuploidy and to assess the chromosomal duplication of cholangiocarcinoma [10]. In a recent study, FISH analysis doubled the diagnostic yield of cholangiocarcinoma compared with the standard brush cytology [10]. In clinical practice, however, it is not uncommon to make the diagnosis of cholangiocarcinoma based on clinical, laboratory, and imaging findings in the absence of tissue diagnosis. To this end, the diagnosis of cholangiocarcinoma in patients with PSC is challenging as the patient may have a dominant benign biliary stricture, which may be difficult to differentiate from cholangiocarcinoma. In this situation, sudden and unexpected clinical deterioration associated with progressive elevation of alkaline phosphatase, and serum CA19-9 values greater than 100U/L, in the absence of bacterial cholangitis, strongly

Table 77.1 Tumor node metastasis (TNM) pathological classification of extrahepatic cholangiocarcinoma

Stage	Tumor	Node	Metastasis
0	T_{is}	N_0	M_0
IA	T_1	N_0	M_0
IB	T_2	N_0	M_0
IIA	T_3	N_0	M_0
IIB	T_1–T_3	N_1	M_0
III	T_4	Any N	M_0
IV	Any T	Any N	M_1

T_{is}, carcinoma *in situ*; T_1, tumor invades subepithelial connective tissue (T_{1a}) or fibromuscular layer (T_{1b}); T_2, tumor invades perifibromuscular connective tissue; T_3, tumor invades adjacent structures, i.e., liver, pancreas, duodenum, stomach, gallbladder, colon; N_1, cystic duct, pericholedochal, hilar lymph node metastases; N_2: peripancreatic (head only), paraduodenal, periportal, celiac, superior mesenteric, posterior pancreaticoduodenal lymph node metastases; M_1, distant metastases.

Table 77.2 Tumor node metastasis (TNM) pathological classification of intrahepatic cholangiocarcinoma

Stage	Tumor	Node	Metastasis
I	T_1	N_0	M_0
II	T_2	N_0	M_0
III	T_3	N_0	M_0
IVA	T_4	N_0	M_0
	Any T	N_1	M_0
IVB	Any T	Any N	M_1

T_1, solitary tumor without vascular invasion; T_{2a}, solitary tumor with vascular invasion; T_{2b}, multiple tumors, with and without vascular invasion; T_3, tumor perforating the visceral peritoneum or involving the local extrahepatic structures by direct invasion; T_4, tumor with periductal invasion (periductal growth pattern); N_1, regional lymph node metastases; M_1, distant metastases.

Table 77.3 Proposed, preoperative T-stage criteria for hilar cholangiocarcinoma

Stage	Criteria
T1	Tumor involving biliary confluence +/– unilateral extension to second-order biliary radicles
T2	Tumor involving biliary confluence +/– unilateral extension to second-order biliary radicles, and ipsilateral portal vein involvement +/– ipsilateral hepatic lobar atrophy
T3	Tumor involving biliary confluence + bilateral extension to second-order biliary radicles; **or** unilateral extension to second-order biliary radicles with contralateral portal vein involvement; **or** unilateral extension to second-order biliary radicles with contralateral hepatic lobar atrophy; **or** main or bilateral portal vein involvement

suggest the development of cholangiocarcinoma complicating PSC.

The intrahepatic cholangiocarcinoma presents with non-specific symptoms of a liver mass. An abdominal mass on examination or imaging study may be the only presentation in asymptomatic patients. Usually, the alkaline phosphatase is elevated with a normal bilirubin. Serum tumor markers, such as CA19-9 and CEA are increased. The diagnosis of intrahepatic cholangiocarcinoma is made by the exclusion of other primary or metastatic liver masses that could mimic its clinical and imaging features. At times biopsy of the liver lesion is the only approach to make the correct diagnosis.

Staging

The aim of staging is to identify potential candidates for surgical resection (Tables 77.1 and 77.2). The value of TNM classification for extrahepatic cholangiocarcinoma is limited. During the clinical staging of extrahepatic cholangiocarcinoma, it is important to first define the proximal and distal boundaries of the tumor. This goal can be achieved by ERCP or percutaneous transhepatic cholangiography (PTC) or by magnetic resonance cholangiopancreatography (MRCP). Second, it is important to exclude vascular encasement by the tumor of the contralateral lobe prior to partial hepatectomy as well as vascular patency of the portal vein and hepatic artery (Table 77.3). Third, regional metastases should be excluded. Endoscopic ultrasound (EUS) is better than conventional abdominal imaging (i.e., computed tomography [CT], magnetic resonance imaging [MRI]) to assess for metastatic disease, particularly for regional lymph nodes, which can also be biopsied during EUS. Approximately 15–20% of patients with normal conventional abdominal imaging were found to have metastatic lymph-node involvement by EUS [11,12].

Therapy

The best treatment for intra- and extrahepatic cholangiocarcinoma is surgical excision [13]. To date, chemotherapy and/or radiation therapy for cholangiocarcinoma have not been evaluated in randomized, controlled trials. Consequently, there is no standard-of-care recommendation regarding chemotherapy for patients with unresectable disease [14]. Overall, palliative therapies provide symptom relief without affecting survival. (Please refer to the overview algorithm for the treatment of cholangiocarcinoma on the website.)

Surgical therapy

For extrahepatic cholangiocarcinoma, surgery should only be carried out with the intent to cure. Nevertheless, to achieve tumor-free margins, partial hepatic resection(s) are required. In fact, patients with positive surgical margins have survival comparable to patients receiving palliative care [15]. In patients with tumor-free margins, the 5-year survival is only 20–40% with an operative mortality of approximately 10% [15]. Following surgical resection, the main morbidity is infection. For intrahepatic cholangiocarcinoma, surgical resection provides the best outcome with 3-year survival between 40% and 60% [15]. Prognostic factors of unfavorable outcome following surgical resection of intrahepatic cholangiocarcinoma are shown on Table 77.4.

For patients who develop extrahepatic cholangiocarcinoma on the background of PSC the diagnostic dilemma is challenging – i.e., benign or malignant biliary stricture(s) (Figure 77.2). Such patients usually have end-stage liver disease and therefore cannot tolerate surgery. Also, cholangiocarcinoma in PSC is also associated with bile-duct dysplasia [16] posing a risk for recurrent de-novo cholangiocarcinoma development even following successful initial surgical

Table 77.4 Prognostic factors associated with unfavorable outcome after surgical treatment of intrahepatic cholangiocarcinoma

- Preoperative CA19-9 levels >1000 U/mL
- Multifocal disease
- Liver capsule invasion
- Lack of cancer-free surgical margins
- Lymph node involvement
- Mass-forming or periductal-infiltrating type cholangiocarcinoma growth
- Expression of MUC1 by cholangiocarcinoma cells

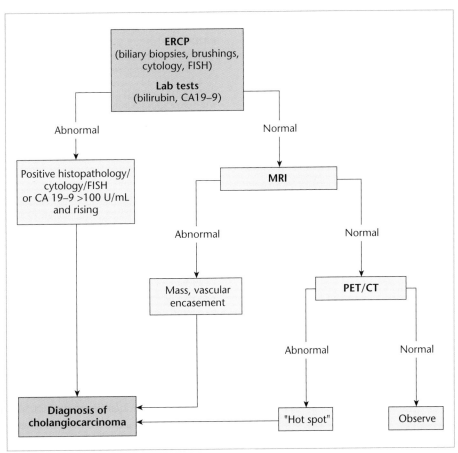

Figure 77.2 Primary sclerosing cholangitis (PSC) patient with suspicious bile duct stricture and/or rapid bilirubin increase. (CT, computed tomography; ERCP, endoscopic retrograde cholangiopancreatography; FISH, fluorescent in-situ hybridization; MRI, magnetic resonance imaging; PET, positron emission tomography.) (This figure was published in *Clinical Gastroenterology and Hepatology*, Wilfred M. Weinstein, Christopher J. Hawkey, Jaime Bosch, Cholangiocarcinoma, Pages 1–5, Copyright Elsevier, 2005.)

Table 77.5 Prognostic factors associated with unfavorable outcome after surgical treatment of extra-hepatic cholangiocarcinoma

- Late stage disease (TNM)
- Lymph node metastasis
- Vascular and perineural invasion
- Poor differentiation grade

resection (Table 77.5). In fact, the 5-year survival following diagnosis of cholangiocarcinoma complicating PSC is less than 10% [17]. In PSC patients with early stage cholangiocarcinoma, orthotopic liver transplantation is the best therapeutic approach.

Cholangiocarcinoma in the absence of PSC can be an indication for orthotopic liver transplantation in selected centers that have established protocols. In such cholangiocarcinoma transplant protocols, patients undergo preoperative chemo- and radiation therapy as well as preoperative exploratory laparotomy before receiving a liver transplant. At the Mayo Clinic, the 5-year post-liver transplantation survival for patients with TNM stage I and II cholangiocarcinoma is approximately 75% [18].

Palliative therapeutic approaches
Biliary stents
Endoscopic or percutaneous placement of biliary stents prevents obstructions of the biliary tree and restores near-normal bile flow [3]. Biliary stents improve symptoms of fatigue, anorexia, and pruritus but not survival [3]. A preplacement MRCP may be helpful to define the biliary anatomy in complex hilar tumors. The choice between a plastic or metallic stent depends on many aspects including expected survival and availability of stent exchange. A course of antibiotics, usually ciprofloxacin, is recommended after stent placement to prevent the development of cholangitis.

Photodynamic therapy (PDT)
This therapy involves the systemic pre-administration of a non-toxic, photosensitizer such as hematoporphyrin that accumulates mainly within the malignant cholangiocarcinoma cells [19]. Subsequently, the patient undergoes ERCP or PTC, during which a red laser light is used and energy is transferred from the photosensitizer to molecular oxygen causing cholangiocarcinoma cell death. A randomized, prospective controlled trial shows PDT to improve patient survival and quality of life when used in conjunction with biliary stenting [20]. Patients who may benefit from PDT are those with no improvement of cholestasis following stent placement alone.

Future therapeutic directions
Randomized, controlled clinical trials are needed to address and test the usefulness of novel chemotherapeutic agents and/or radiation therapy.

As we better understand the biology of cholangiocarcinoma, pharmacological inhibitors of highly expressed receptors in these tumors (i.e., cyclooxygenase-2, epidermal growth factor) should be used in future trials with or without chemotherapeutic drugs.

References
1. Blechacz B, Gores GJ. Cholangiocarcinoma: advances in pathogenesis, diagnosis, and treatment. *Hepatology.* 2008;48:308–321.
2. Gores GJ. Cholangiocarcinoma: current concepts and insights. *Hepatology.* 2003;37:961–969.
3. Khan SA, Davidson BR, Goldin R, *et al.* Guidelines for the diagnosis and treatment of cholangiocarcinoma: consensus document. *Gut.* 2002;51 Suppl 6:VI1–9.
4. Patel T. Worldwide trends in mortality from biliary tract malignancies. *BMC cancer.* 2002;2:10.
5. Khan SA, Toledano MB, Taylor-Robinson SD. Epidemiology, risk factors, and pathogenesis of cholangiocarcinoma. *HPB (Oxford).* 2008;10:77–82.
6. Patel T. Increasing incidence and mortality of primary intrahepatic cholangiocarcinoma in the United States. *Hepatology.* 2001;33:1353–1357.
7. Bergquist A, Broome U. Hepatobiliary and extra-hepatic malignancies in primary sclerosing cholangitis. *Best Practice Res.* 2001;15:643–656.
8. Tocchi A, Mazzoni G, Liotta G, Lepre L, Cassini D, Miccini M. Late development of bile duct cancer in patients who had biliary-enteric drainage for benign disease: a follow-up study of more than 1,000 patients. *Ann surg.* 2001;234:210–214.
9. Hadjis NS, Adam A, Gibson R, Blenkharn JI, Benjamin IS, Blumgart LH. Nonoperative approach to hilar cancer determined by the atrophy-hypertrophy complex. *Am J Surg.* 1989;157:395–39.
10. Moreno Luna LE, Kipp B, Halling KC, *et al.* Advanced cytologic techniques for the detection of malignant pancreatobiliary strictures. *Gastroenterology.* 2006;131:1064–1072.
11. Gores GJ. Early detection and treatment of cholangiocarcinoma. *Liver Transpl.* 2000;6:S30–34.
12. Gleeson FC, Rajan E, Levy MJ, *et al.* EUS-guided FNA of regional lymph nodes in patients with unresectable hilar cholangiocarcinoma. *Gastroint Endosc.* 2008;67:438–443.
13. Kloek JJ, Ten Kate FJ, Busch OR, Gouma DJ, Van Gulik TM. Surgery for extrahepatic cholangiocarcinoma: predictors of survival. *HPB (Oxford).* 2008;10:190–195.
14. Verslype C, Prenen H, Van Cutsem E. The role of chemotherapy in biliary tract carcinoma. *HPB (Oxford).* 2008;10:164–167.
15. Jarnagin WR, Fong Y, DeMatteo RP, *et al.* Staging, resectability, and outcome in 225 patients with hilar cholangiocarcinoma. *Ann Surg.* 2001;234:507–517; discussion 17–19.

16. Fleming KA, Boberg KM, Glaumann H, Bergquist A, Smith D, Clausen OP. Biliary dysplasia as a marker of cholangiocarcinoma in primary sclerosing cholangitis. *J Hepatol*. 2001;34:360–365.

17. Boberg KM, Bergquist A, Mitchell S, *et al*. Cholangiocarcinoma in primary sclerosing cholangitis: risk factors and clinical presentation. *Scand J Gastroenterol*. 2002;37:1205–1211.

18. Rosen CB, Heimbach JK, Gores GJ. Surgery for cholangiocarcinoma: the role of liver transplantation. *HPB (Oxford)*. 2008;10: 186–189.

19. Zoepf T. Photodynamic therapy of cholangiocarcinoma. *HPB (Oxford)*. 2008;10:161–163.

20. Ortner ME, Caca K, Berr F, *et al*. Successful photodynamic therapy for nonresectable cholangiocarcinoma: a randomized prospective study. *Gastroenterology*. 2003;125:1355–1363.

Pancreas and Biliary Tract

CHAPTER 78

Congenital abnormalities of the biliary tract

Daniel Dhumeaux,[1] Elie Serge Zafrani,[1] Daniel Cherqui,[2] and Alain Luciani[1]

[1]Henri Mondor Hospital, Créteil, France
[2]New York Presbyterian/Weill Cornell Medical College, New York, NY, USA

Pancreas and Biliary Tract

ESSENTIAL FACTS ABOUT PATHOGENESIS

Congenital cystic diseases of the intrahepatic biliary tract
- Family of bile duct malformations that are mostly related to abnormal remodeling of the embryonic ductal plate ("ductal plate malformation")
- The basic lesion consists of cysts that are either macroscopic or microscopic
- Since ductal plate malformation can occur simultaneously at different levels of the intrahepatic biliary tree, co-existence of several cystic disorders is common
- The liver disease is frequently associated with a variety of renal disorders that are related to congenital malformations of renal tubular segments

Congenital hepatic fibrosis
- Characterized by enlargement of portal spaces by abundant fibrous tissue containing numerous ectatic bile ducts
- Inherited and transmitted as an autosomal recessive trait with a prevalence of about 1 in 100 000
- The main consequence of the disease is portal hypertension, due to fibrous compression and/or hypoplasia of portal vein branches
- Variceal hemorrhage first occurs between the ages of 5 and 20 years
- It is occasionally complicated by recurrent bacterial cholangitis, even in the absence of Caroli's syndrome
- Hepatocellular and cholangiocellular carcinomas may be a complication

Von Meyenburg complexes
- Consist of groups of variably dilated bile ducts containing bile and embedded in fibrous tissue, mostly at the periphery of the portal tracts

Simple cyst of the liver
- Prevalence is about 3% in the adult population; the lesion predominates in females

Choledochal cysts
- Congenital dilatation of the common bile duct following four patterns, the most common being a diffuse fusiform dilatation of the common bile duct
- It occurs in 1 per 100 000 to 1 per 150 000 births, being more prevalent in Far Eastern countries, especially Japan

Paucity of interlobular bile ducts
- In children, there are two forms: syndromic paucity (Alagille's syndrome) and non-syndromic paucity
- In adults, paucity of interlobular bile ducts can have several causes; the idiopathic form may be a late-onset form of the non-syndromic paucity observed in children

ESSENTIALS OF DIAGNOSIS

Von Meyenburgh complexes
- Asymptomatic
- Commonly diagnosed incidentally at histological examination
- May be visualized at magnetic resonance cholangiography

Caroli's syndrome
- Characterized by cystic dilatations of large, segmental intrahepatic bile ducts that may be diffuse or confined to a lobe or a segment of the liver
- Usually associated with congenital hepatic fibrosis
- Usually asymptomatic for the first 5–20 years of life until it presents with recurrent cholangitis; unlike other types of cholangitis, the main and often the only symptom is fever (in the absence of abdominal pain)
- Invasive investigations of the biliary tree must be avoided

Simple cyst of the liver
- Aberrant dilated bile duct without communication with the biliary tree; the cyst is not septated and its fluid is clear
- Its diameter increases with age, ranging from a few millimeters to >20 cm
- The cyst is solitary in about 50% of cases
- Generally asymptomatic

Choledochal cysts
- Mainly diagnosed in children, but can also be diagnosed in adults; 80% of patients are female
- In children, the main symptom is an abdominal mass, whereas cholangitis, with or without jaundice, is the most frequent sign in adults
- Associated with adenocarcinoma, the prevalence of which markedly increases with age, reaching 15% in adults

ESSENTIALS OF TREATMENT

Congenital hepatic fibrosis
- Prevention and treatment of variceal bleeding
- Liver transplantation

Von Meyenburg complexes
- No therapy necessary

Caroli's syndrome
- Treatment consists of antibiotic therapy for cholangitis and ursodeoxycholic acid to prevent or treat intracystic stones
- In the localized form, partial hepatectomy is indicated
- Liver transplantation may be considered for patients with the diffuse form complicated by severe recurrent cholangitis

Textbook of Clinical Gastroenterology and Hepatology, Second Edition. Edited by C. J. Hawkey, Jaime Bosch, Joel E. Richter, Guadalupe Garcia-Tsao, Francis K. L. Chan.

Pancreas and Biliary Tract

Simple cyst of the liver
• When large cysts produce abdominal pain or are complicated, cyst resection or, more often, cyst fenestration, is the therapy of choice

Choledochal cysts
• Treatment of choice is (as far as possible) excision of the cyst, followed by choledochojejunostomy

Paucity of interlobular bile ducts
• Ursodeoxycholic acid
• Transplantation may be required in severe cases

Introduction

Congenital abnormalities of the biliary tract can affect both the intra- and extra-hepatic bile ducts. They are either inherited or not inherited, and can be divided into two main groups: cystic and non-cystic. It is now widely agreed that congenital cystic diseases of bile ducts belong to a family of bile duct malformations that are mostly related to abnormal remodeling of the embryonic ductal plate ("ductal plate malformation"). Although they are congenital, all of them can be diagnosed at any age of life. Contrary to congenital cystic diseases of bile ducts, congenital non-cystic diseases of bile ducts are probably not linked to a malformation process, but are rather the result of gradual destruction of bile ducts during fetal life. They are mainly diagnosed in children. Only those congenital abnormalities of the biliary tract that present in adults will be reviewed in this chapter.

Congenital cystic diseases of intrahepatic bile ducts

This category includes entities that differ in their prevalence, manifestations, and severity, but share at least three characteristics: (1) the basic lesion of the liver consists of **cysts** that are either macroscopic, and therefore easily recognized by imaging techniques, or microscopic, i.e., only found at histological examination of the liver; (2) a **ductal plate malformation** can account for these disorders; and (3) the liver disease is frequently associated with a variety of **renal disorders** that are related to congenital malformations of renal tubular segments.

Pathogenesis

Embryonic anomalies lead to congenital cystic diseases of the intrahepatic bile ducts. In normal embryos, at around the eighth week of gestation, a layer of cells originating from liver precursor cells, with the characteristics of biliary cells, surrounds each mesenchymal area containing the largest branches of the portal vein. This layer of cells, which is later partially duplicated by a second layer of the same cells, is referred to as the **ductal plate**. In the following weeks, ductal plates also appear more distally around smaller portal vein branches. After 12 weeks of gestation, the ductal plates are progressively remodeled along a gradient from the hilum to the periphery of the liver. This remodeling leads to: (1) dilatation of short

segments of the double-layered ductal plate to form tubular structures; (2) subsequent incorporation of these structures as individualized bile ducts into the mesenchyme surrounding portal vein branches; and (3) disappearance of most non-tubular portions of the ductal plate (Figure 78.1) [1].

Remodeling defects, which likely cause congenital cystic diseases of intrahepatic bile ducts, result in the persistence of an excess of embryonic bile duct structures, a phenomenon referred to as "ductal plate malformation." When the remodeling defect is complete, ductal plate malformation appears as a circular lumen containing a fibrovascular axis (Figure 78.2a).When it is incomplete, it may give rise either to a nearly circular lumen with an apparent polypoid projection of mesenchymal tissue (Figure 78.2b) or to an interrupted circle of dilated bile ducts around the fibrovascular axis (Figure 78.2c) [1,2].

When discussing ductal plate malformation as the basic component of congenital cystic diseases of the intrahepatic bile ducts, it is important to bear in mind that: (1) the different segments of the intrahepatic biliary tree develop during successive periods of fetal life; (2) ductal plate malformation can

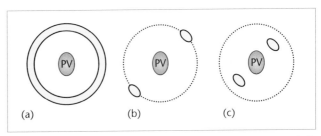

Figure 78.1 Schematic representation of the embryonic ductal plate and of its remodeling. (a). Initial ductal plate with the typical double layer of biliary cells. (b) Remodeling of the ductal plate, with tubular dilatation in some segments and disappearance of most of the ductal plate. (c) Incorporation of the tubular segments within the portal mesenchyme. Note the presence of a portal vein (PV) branch at the center of the embryonic portal space. (This figure was published in *Clinical Gastroenterology and Hepatology*, Wilfred M. Weinstein, Christopher J. Hawkey, Jaime Bosch, Congenital abnormalities of the biliary tract, Pages 575–582, Copyright Elsevier, 2005.)

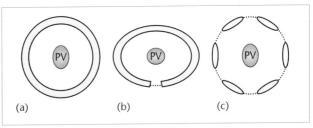

Figure 78.2 Schematic representation of the ductal plate malformation. (a) Complete lack of remodeling of the ductal plate, which appears as a continuous circular dilated duct. (b, c) Incomplete remodeling of the ductal plate, which appears as a dilated bile duct with a polypoid projection of mesenchymal tissue (b) or as an interrupted circle of dilated bile ducts (c). Note the presence of a portal vein (PV) branch at the center of the ductal plate malformation. (This figure was published in *Clinical Gastroenterology and Hepatology*, Wilfred M. Weinstein, Christopher J. Hawkey, Jaime Bosch, Congenital abnormalities of the biliary tract, Pages 575–582, Copyright Elsevier, 2005.)

be observed in segmental (Caroli's syndrome), interlobular (congenital hepatic fibrosis), or more peripheral bile ducts (von Meyenburg complexes, polycystic liver disease); and (3) ductal plate malformation occurring simultaneously at different levels of the intrahepatic biliary tree may explain the observed co-existence of these disorders.

Von Meyenburg complexes [1–4]

These are usually asymptomatic and are diagnosed incidentally at histological examination. They are often multiple and may occur in an otherwise normal liver or can be associated with congenital hepatic fibrosis, Caroli's syndrome, or polycystic liver disease. Von Meyenburg complexes consist of groups of more or less dilated bile ducts containing bile and embedded in fibrous tissue (Figure 78.3).They are located within or at the periphery of the portal tracts. Von Meyenburg complexes may be secondary to a ductal plate remodeling defect in the later phases of bile duct development, thus affecting the smallest branches of the intrahepatic biliary tree.

Congenital hepatic fibrosis [1–6]

Histologically, congenital hepatic fibrosis consists of enlargement of portal spaces by an abundant fibrous tissue containing

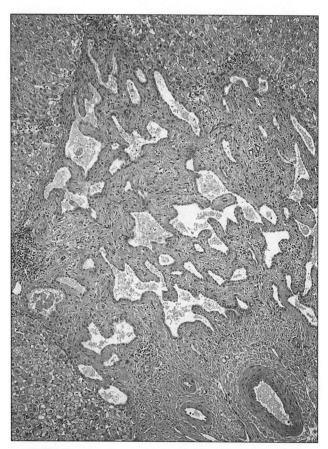

Figure 78.3 Von Meyenburg complexes. Multiple biliary channels are lined by a cuboidal epithelium and are embedded in dense fibrous tissue. Note the irregular outline of the ducts, with polypoid projections into dilated lumens, as seen in ductal plate malformation. Dilated bile ducts contain bile, indicating that they communicate with the rest of the biliary tree.

numerous, more or less ectatic bile ducts. Some bile ducts contain bile, indicating communication with the rest of the biliary tree. Bile ducts can be so dilated that they form cysts that are nonetheless not macroscopically visible, at least in congenital hepatic fibrosis not associated with Caroli's syndrome. Portal veins appear to be hypoplastic. The disease can be sporadic or familial. It is inherited and transmitted as an autosomal recessive trait. The mutant gene is not clearly identified. Due to a possible association between congenital hepatic fibrosis and recessive polycystic kidney disease, the gene *PKHD1*, which is involved in the renal disease, could be a candidate. This gene encodes bilbrocystin, a protein localized in the primary cilium of biliary epithelcal cells. Its mutation may be the cause of congenital hepatic fibrosis. However, several cases of congenital hepatic fibrosis associated with protein-losing enteropathy have been linked to a congenital phosphomannose isomerase deficiency [7]. In this disorder, protein hypoglycosylation secondary to the enzyme deficiency has been suggested to play a role in the defective embryonic development of intrahepatic bile ducts, but the mechanism by which protein hypoglycosylation leads to ductal plate malformation remains to be elucidated.

The prevalence of congenital hepatic fibrosis is about 1 in 100 000. The main consequence of the disease is **portal hypertension**, due to fibrous compression or, more probably, hypoplasia of portal vein branches. The first bleeding episode secondary to ruptured gastroesophageal varices usually occurs between the ages of 5 and 20 years, sometimes later. Liver failure being absent, variceal bleeding is generally well tolerated. On clinical examination, the liver is often enlarged, and splenomegaly is found in most patients. Liver biochemical tests are generally normal, although a moderate increase in serum alkaline phosphatase and gamma-glutamyl transpeptidase activities can be noted. Congenital hepatic fibrosis is occasionally complicated by recurrent, potentially life-threatening bacterial cholangitis, even in the absence of Caroli's syndrome. Both hepatocellular and cholangiocellular carcinomas may also complicate congenital hepatic fibrosis.

The diagnostic value of imaging procedures in congenital hepatic fibrosis is limited. The most frequently reported features are liver dystrophy and indirect signs of portal hypertension [8]. The diagnosis of congenital hepatic fibrosis is made by **liver biopsy**. However, the diagnosis of the disease may be missed on a small liver specimen since the malformation is not always diffuse. Magnetic resonance cholangiography is generally normal, as only small bile ducts are dilated, at least in the absence of associated Caroli's syndrome. Congenital hepatic fibrosis is frequently associated with a renal malformation consisting of ectatic collecting tubules. This malformation is generally silent. It can be demonstrated by magnetic resonance imaging (MRI) or multidetector computed tomography [9]. It is found in about two-thirds of patients, and assists with the diagnosis of congenital hepatic fibrosis. In some cases, the ectatic segments lose their communication with the urinary tract and transform into large renal cysts, referred to as autosomal recessive polycystic kidney disease [10].

Recurrent variceal bleeding can be prevented with beta-blockers and/or endoscopic variceal ligation, although these treatments have not been specifically evaluated in this setting. If they fail, a transjugular intrahepatic portosystemic shunt can be considered, and the risk of hepatic encephalopathy could be lower than in patients with cirrhosis, given the absence of liver failure. Surgical procedures on the biliary tree and invasive investigations such as endoscopic retrograde cholangiography carry a risk of bacterial cholangitis and must be avoided. Liver transplantation can be offered to selected patients.

Caroli's syndrome [1–6,11]

Caroli's syndrome is a congenital disorder characterized by cystic dilatations of large, segmental intrahepatic bile ducts. The cystic dilatations may be diffuse, affecting the whole intrahepatic biliary tree (Figure 78.4), or confined to a lobe, often the left lobe [12], or to a segment of the liver (Figure 78.5). Congenital dilatation of segmental bile ducts is not a single entity, and the term Caroli's syndrome is thus more appropriate than Caroli's disease.

Caroli's syndrome is usually associated with congenital hepatic fibrosis. In such patients, cystic dilatations are diffuse and, like congenital hepatic fibrosis, the malformation is transmitted as an autosomal recessive trait, and it may be associated with ectatic renal collecting tubules (Table 78.1). When Caroli's syndrome is not associated with congenital hepatic fibrosis, cystic dilatations are often confined to one part of the liver, the malformation is congenital but not inherited, and the disorder is not associated with renal malformations (Table 78.1).

Caroli's syndrome, which is usually present at birth, can remain asymptomatic for a long period of time, at least for the first 5–20 years of life. The main clinical manifestation is **recurrent cholangitis**, the prevalence of which markedly varies from one patient to another. The prognosis is poor in patients with frequent bouts of cholangitis, who are at risk of death from uncontrolled bacterial infection. Cholangitis may be complicated by liver abscesses and secondary amyloidosis. In contrast to cholangitis due to common bile duct stones, in which fever is usually associated with pain and/or jaundice, the main and often the only symptom of cholangitis in Caroli's syndrome is fever, which can be difficult to relate to cholangitis, at least in initial episodes. Jaundice and pain may occur if pigment or cholesterol stones that form in dilated bile ducts migrate to the extrahepatic biliary tree. Manifestations of portal hypertension are usually present in patients with associated congenital hepatic fibrosis. Intracystic cholangiocarcinoma occurs in approximately 7% of either diffuse or localized Caroli's syndrome.

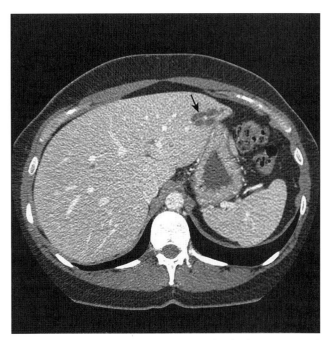

Figure 78.5 Caroli's syndrome. Caroli's syndrome localized in segment III of the left lobe of the liver. Portal-venous-phase contrast-enhanced computed tomography shows a saccular dilatation of the biliary tree with enhanced central portal vein branch ("central dot" sign) (arrow).

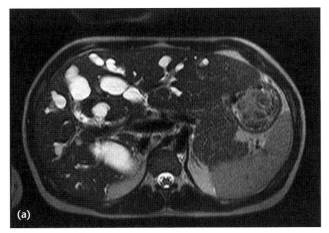 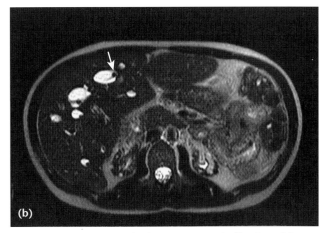

Figure 78.4 Diffuse form of Caroli's syndrome. Heavily T2-weighted sequence of magnetic resonance imaging showing numerous cystic dilatations of the biliary tree. (a) Note that the cysts appear to communicate with the remaining biliary tree. (b) Hypointense dots, which probably correspond to portal vein branches, in the center of the cysts (arrow).

Table 78.1 Characteristics of Caroli's syndrome whether or not associated with congenital hepatic fibrosis

	Caroli's syndrome with congenital hepatic fibrosis	Caroli's syndrome without congenital hepatic fibrosis
Hereditary transmission	Autosomal recessive	Absent
Hepatic cyst distribution	Diffuse	Diffuse or localized to one lobe or one segment
Cholangitis	Frequent	Possible
Portal hypertension	Frequent	Absent
Renal abnormalities	Ectatic collecting tubules and/or autosomal recessive polycystic kidney disease	Absent

Reproduced from Benhamou JP, Menu Y. Non-parasitic cystic diseases of the liver and intrahepatic biliary tree. In: Bircher J, *et al.*, editors. *Oxford Textbook of Clinical Hepatology*. Oxford: Oxford University Press, 1999:817–823. By permission of Oxford University Press.

Physical examination usually shows an enlarged liver. There are no signs of liver failure. Liver biochemical tests are normal, except for moderate increases in serum alkaline phosphatase and gamma-glutamyl transpeptidase activities. The diagnosis of Caroli's syndrome can be suggested on imaging techniques, i.e., ultrasonography, computed tomography (CT), and MRI (Figures 78.4 and 78.5). CT or MRI can reveal the "central dot" sign after contrast medium injection [13] (Figure 78.5), which may correspond to the ductal plate malformation (see Figure 78.2b). In addition to cystic dilatations, magnetic resonance cholangiography may inconstantly show **communications with the biliary tree**, which would be diagnostic of Caroli's syndrome. Communications can also be documented by CT or MRI after intravenous injection of biliary contrast medium. Moreover, ultrasonography, CT, and MRI can show the presence of stones within the cystic dilatations [13]. As for congenital hepatic fibrosis, invasive investigations of the biliary tree (i.e., endoscopic retrograde cholangiography or percutaneous transhepatic cholangiography) must be avoided.

Treatment consists of appropriate antibiotic therapy for patients with bacterial cholangitis. **Ursodeoxycholic acid** may be effective in preventing or treating intracystic stones, and should be given to all patients with Caroli's syndrome. In the localized form of Caroli's syndrome, partial hepatectomy is indicated. This treats cholangitis and prevents the development of cholangiocarcinoma. Liver transplantation may be considered for patients with the diffuse form complicated by severe recurrent cholangitis. Surgical bilioenteric anastomosis can increase the prevalence and severity of cholangitis, and is therefore not recommended.

Simple cyst of the liver [3]

Simple cyst of the liver is regarded as a congenital malformation consisting of an aberrant dilated bile duct without communication with the biliary tree. It is spherical or ovoid. Its diameter increases with age, ranging from a few millimeters to >20 cm. There is no septation and the cystic fluid is generally clear. Small cysts are surrounded by normal liver, whereas large cysts may be responsible for atrophy of adjacent hepatic tissue. The cyst is solitary in about 50% of cases, while other patients have two or more cysts.

The prevalence of simple cyst of the liver is about 3% in the adult population. The lesions are generally sporadic, although a small number of familial cases have been observed. Simple cysts of the liver predominate in females and are generally asymptomatic. Some large cysts produce abdominal pain or discomfort. Complications include intracystic hemorrhage or infection and cyst rupture. In most patients, the lesion is discovered fortuitously at liver ultrasonography, which shows a circular or oval, well-limited and totally anechoic area, with strong posterior wall echoes. Simple cyst of the liver is not associated with renal malformations, although the association with one or two simple renal cysts, which are also very common in adults, is possible. Asymptomatic simple cysts do not require any treatment. When large cysts produce abdominal pain or are complicated, cyst resection or, more often, cyst fenestration (i.e., partial excision of the external part of the cyst) can be performed by open surgery or preferably by laparoscopy. Injection of alcohol or other sclerosing agents into cysts has also been attempted.

Polycystic liver disease

Polycystic liver disease is described in Chapter 96.

Congenital cystic diseases of extrahepatic bile ducts: the choledochal cyst [3,6]

This congenital dilatation of the common bile duct occurs in 1 per 100 000 to 1 per 150 000 births. It is more prevalent in Far Eastern countries, especially Japan. Four types have been recognized (Figure 78.6). Type 1, which is by far the commonest (80%), consists of segmental or diffuse, generally fusiform dilatation of the extrahepatic bile duct. Type 2 consists of a saccular dilatation that forms a diverticulum of the extrahepatic bile duct. Type 3 is a choledochocele of the distal common bile duct, mostly within the duodenal wall. Type 4 associates type 1 with cystic dilatations of the intrahepatic bile ducts that are generally close to the hilum. Choledochal cyst is frequently associated with abnormal pancreato-biliary ductal anatomy, with a long common segment that could favor biliary reflux of pancreatic fluid.

Choledochal cyst, which is congenital, is mainly observed in children, but can also be diagnosed in adults. Eighty per cent of patients are female. The size of choledochal cysts varies greatly from one patient to another, and the cyst may contain from a few milliliters to several liters of bile. In children, the

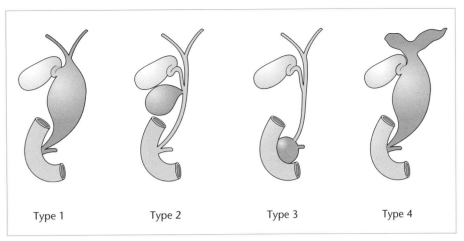

Type 1   Type 2   Type 3   Type 4

Figure 78.6 Choledochal cysts. The four types of choledochal cysts. (This figure was published in *Clinical Gastroenterology and Hepatology*, Wilfred M. Weinstein, Christopher J. Hawkey, Jaime Bosch, Congenital abnormalities of the biliary tract, Pages 575–582, Copyright Elsevier, 2005.)

main symptom is an abdominal mass, whereas cholangitis, with or without jaundice, is the most frequent sign in adults. The cysts may also be asymptomatic, being detected incidentally during abdominal ultrasonography. Carcinoma may be associated with choledochal cyst. It can develop within the cyst or outside it (namely within the liver). The prevalence of carcinoma markedly increases with age, and reaches 15% in adults. Choledochal cyst is readily diagnosed by ultrasonography and other imaging procedures, namely magnetic resonance cholangiography. The best treatment is excision of the cyst, followed by choledochojejunostomy. Simple anastomosis between the cyst and intestinal tract should be avoided, as it favors cholangitis and does not prevent the development of adenocarcinoma.

Congenital non-cystic diseases of bile ducts
Paucity of interlobular bile ducts [1,5,14,15]
In children, two types of paucity of interlobular bile ducts (i.e., ductopenia) can be distinguished. The syndromic paucity, also called **Alagille's syndrome**, is an autosomal dominant disorder characterized by mutations of the *JAGGED1* gene located on chromosome 20. Numerous extrahepatic malformations are present. Cholestasis is generally moderate, and evolution toward cirrhosis is rare. The non-syndromic paucity is not associated with a known genetic factor, although a high rate of consanguinity is noted in some patients. There are no extrahepatic manifestations. Cholestasis is usually severe and biliary cirrhosis occurs rapidly.

In adults, **ductopenia** is usually the result of progressive inflammatory destruction of interlobular bile ducts and is observed in various conditions, such as primary biliary cirrhosis, primary sclerosing cholangitis, liver allograft rejection, graft-versus-host disease, and drug-induced chronic cholestatic liver disease. Idiopathic ductopenia has also been reported in adulthood [16–20] and might be related to an unidentified (e.g., toxic, viral, or metabolic) agent. A congenital origin, at

least in some cases, is supported by: (1) reports of familial forms,[16,19,20] with possible autosomal dominant transmission [20]; and (2) clinical similarity with the non-syndromic paucity of interlobular bile ducts observed in children, suggesting that adult disease might be a late-onset form of the childhood process [16,17]. Idiopathic ductopenia in adults is always associated with cholestasis, with or without jaundice. Its severity varies greatly from one patient to another, with a spectrum that ranges from an absence of clinical symptoms [18] to biliary cirrhosis. Ursodeoxycholic acid may improve liver biochemical tests [16,18–20], but its impact on disease progression is unknown. Liver transplantation is required in severe cases [16,19].

Atresia of extrahepatic bile ducts
Like idiopathic paucity of interlobular bile ducts, extrahepatic bile duct atresia is probably not a malformation, but rather the result of gradual destruction of the bile ducts by a necroinflammatory process of unknown etiology [14]. It is diagnosed in children and not in adults and will not, therefore, be dealt with in this chapter.

Other congenital abnormalities of extrahepatic bile ducts
Absence of gallbladder, double gallbladder, left-sided gallbladder, folded gallbladder, floating gallbladder, accessory bile ducts, and other malformations have been described [4]. These anomalies are generally not symptomatic, but awareness of their existence is important for the radiologist and the biliary and hepatic transplant surgeon.

References
1. Desmet VJ. Congenital diseases of intrahepatic bile ducts: variations on the theme "ductal plate malformation." *Hepatology.* 1992;16:1069–1083.
2. Le Maigre FP. Development of the biliary tract. *J Hepatol.* 2003; 120:81–87.

3. Summerfield JA, Nagafuchi Y, Sherlock S, *et al.* Hepatobiliary fibropolycystic diseases. A clinical and histological review of 51 patients. *J Hepatol.* 1986;2:141–156.

4. Sherlock S, Dooley J. *Diseases of the Liver and Biliary System*, 9th edn. Oxford: Blackwell Scientific Publications, 1993:548–561.

5. Benhamou JP, Menu Y. Non-parasitic cystic diseases of the liver and intrahepatic biliary tree. In: Bircher J, Benhamou JP, McIntyre N, Rizzetto M, Rodés J, editors. *Oxford Textbook of Clinical Hepatology.* Oxford: Oxford University Press, 1999:817–823.

6. Ishak KG, Sharp HL. Developmental abnormalities and liver disease in childhood. In: MacSween RNM, Burt AD, Portmann BC, *et al.*, editors. *Pathology of the Liver*, 4th edn. London: Churchill Livingstone, 2002;107–154.

7. De Koning TJ, Dorland L, van Berge Henegouwen GP. Phosphomannose isomerase deficiency as a cause of congenital hepatic fibrosis and protein-losing enteropathy. *J Hepatol.* 1999;31: 557–560.

8. Akhan O, Karaosmanoglu AD, Ergen B. Imaging findings in congenital hepatic fibrosis. *Eur J Radiol.* 2007;61:18–21.

9. Lang EK, Macchia RJ, Thomas R, *et al.* Improved detection of renal pathologic features on multiphasic helical CT compared with IVU in patients presenting with microscopic hematuria. *Urology.* 2003;61:528–532.

10. Dupond JL, Miguet JP, Carbillet JP, *et al.* Kidney polycystic disease in adult congenital hepatic fibrosis. *Ann Intern Med.* 1978;88:514–515.

11. Caroli J, Corcos V. La dilatation congénitale des voies biliaires intrahépatiques. *Rev Med Chir Mal Foie.* 1964;39:1–70.

12. Boyle MJ, Doyle GD, McNulty JG. Monobar Caroli's disease. *Am J Gastroenterol.* 1989;84:1437–1444.

13. Krausé D, Cercueil JP, Dranssart M, *et al.* MRI for evaluating congenital bile duct abnormalities. *J Comput Assist Tomogr.* 2002; 26:541–552.

14. Desmet VJ, Roskams T, Van Eyken P. Non-cystic malformations of the biliary tract. In: Bircher J, Benhamou JP, McIntyre N, Rizzetto M, Rodés J, editors. *Oxford Textbook of Clinical Hepatology.* Oxford: Oxford University Press, 1999:779–815.

15. Le Maigre FP. Notch signalling in bile duct development: new insights raise new questions. *Hepatology.* 2008;48:358–360.

16. Zafrani ES, Métreau JM, Douvin C, *et al.* Idiopathic biliary ductopenia in adults: a report of five cases. *Gastroenterology.* 1990;99: 1823–1828.

17. Brugera M, Llach J, Rodés J. Nonsyndromic paucity of intrahepatic bile ducts in infancy and idiopathic ductopenia in adulthood: the same syndrome? *Hepatology.* 1992;15:830–834.

18. Moreno A, Carreno V, Cano A, *et al.* Idiopathic biliary ductopenia in adults without symptoms of liver disease. *N Engl J Med.* 1997;336:835–838.

19. Ludwig J. Idiopathic adulthood ductopenia: an update. *Mayo Clin Proc.* 1998;73:285–291.

20. Burak KW, Pearson DC, Swain MG, *et al.* Familial idiopathic adulthood ductopenia: a report of five cases in three generations. *J Hepatol.* 2000;32:159–163.

CHAPTER 79
Acute viral hepatitis

Amer Skopic[1] and Maria H. Sjogren[2]

[1]National Naval Medical Center, Bethesda, MD, USA
[2]Gastroenterology Service, Walter Reed Army Medical Center, Washington, DC, USA

ESSENTIAL FACTS ABOUT PATHOGENESIS

- Hepatitis A and E are small RNA viruses that are acquired via the fecal–oral route from contaminated food or water
- Hepatitis B, C, and D are blood-borne infections acquired by exposure to contaminated blood products, syringes or needles. Hepatitis B is a DNA virus, while hepatitis C and D are RNA viruses
- Despite intrinsic differences between the viral agents of acute viral hepatitis, all have tropism for the liver and can cause acute hepatitis, although the exact cause can be clinically and histologically difficult to differentiate

ESSENTIALS OF DIAGNOSIS

- Diagnosis of viral hepatitis is suspected clinically; patients may have fever, jaundice, nausea, vomiting; and fatigue
- Some patients remain asymptomatic
- Acute hepatitis A is diagnosed by the presence of IgM anti-HAV and increased alanine aminotransferase (ALT) in serum
- Acute hepatitis B is diagnosed by detectable IgM anti-HBc and abnormal ALT in serum
- Acute hepatitis C is diagnosed by detectable HCV RNA and abnormal ALT in serum
- Acute hepatitis D is diagnosed as co-infection (acute HBV and HDV) or super-infection (chronic HBV and acute HDV) by detecting IgM anti-HDV and HDV RNA
- Acute hepatitis E is diagnosed by detectable IgM anti-HEV and abnormal ALT in serum

ESSENTIALS OF TREATMENT

- There is no specific treatment for acute hepatitis A, D or E
- Supportive measures to control symptoms are advisable
- Prevention is the best method; excellent vaccines are commercially available for hepatitis A and B
- Treatment for acute HBV should be considered in patients who are immunosuppressed or who are at risk of hepatic failure
- Because HCV becomes a chronic infection in approximately 80% of exposed subjects, treatment with antivirals is indicated if the infection is diagnosed early on
- Experience suggests to treat hepatitis D early because of the tendency of HDV to aggravate the underlying HBV

Introduction

Acute viral hepatitis is an inflammation of the liver that can be self-limited, lead to chronic liver disease or be fulminant, and it cause significant morbidity and mortality. Table 79.1 depicts the main risk factors, the serological goal standards to make the diagnosis, the risk of chronicity, and the main methods of prevention or treatment for the five major etiological factors of viral hepatitis.

While acute viral hepatitis has different etiologies, one form is clinically indistinguishable from another. Other causes of acute hepatitis, such as drug-induced, ischemic, toxic, autoimmune, etc., can also mimic viral hepatitis. Therefore, there should be a heightened level of clinical suspicion in any patient with significant abnormality of liver tests and appropriate serological tests should be performed. Specific and sensitive tests have evolved to aid in the diagnosis of viral hepatitis and in the monitoring of responses to therapy and immunization.

This chapter reviews the virology, pathogenesis, specific treatment, and prevention for each of the five major viruses responsible for acute viral hepatitis.

Acute hepatitis A

Epidemiology

Acute hepatitis A virus (HAV) infects 1.4 million people worldwide annually. In the USA since 1995, the incidence of HAV infection has declined by 90% with the greatest decline observed among children. In 2006, the total estimated number of case was of 32 000.

The primary routes of HAV transmission are fecal–oral, person-to-person contact, and ingestion of contaminated food or water. Unusual routes of transmission include percutaneous exposure or receiving blood products. HAV infection can be sporadic or cause epidemics. Cyclic outbreaks have been reported among intravenous drug users and among men who have sex with men [1]. Risk factors are listed in Table 79.2.

In endemic areas most individuals are infected at an early age. Overall, the age when infected has risen worldwide to about 5 years.

In industrialized countries the prevalence of HAV infection is low among children and young adults. In the USA prior to universal vaccination, the prevalence of HAV was 10% in children and 37% in adults.

Cause and pathogenesis

HAV is an enterovirus that belongs to the Picornaviridae family and genus Hepatovirus. The HAV genome consists of

Liver Disease

Table 79.1 Characteristics of viral hepatitis etiological agents

	HAV	HBV	HCV	HDV	HEV
Transmission	Fecal–oral	Blood-borne	Blood-borne	Blood-borne	Fecal–oral
Diagnosis (acute)	IgM anti-HAV	IgM anti-HBc	HCV RNA	IgM anti-HDV	Anti-HEV
Diagnosis (chronic)	None	HBsAg HBV DNA	HCV RNA	HDV RNA	None
Chronic sequelae	None	Cirrhosis HCC	Cirrhosis HCC	Cirrhosis HCC	None
Prevention/treatment	Vaccine	Vaccine Antivirals	Antivirals	IFN	None

HCC, hepatocellular carcinoma; IFN, interferon.

Table 79.2 Risk factors for hepatitis A infection in the USA

Unknown	65%
Sexual or household contact with a patient who has hepatitis A	10%
International travel	15%
Male homosexual activity	9%
Injection drug use	2%
Child or employee in a daycare center	4%
Food or water-borne outbreak	7%
Contact with a daycare child or employee	4%
Other contact with a patient who has hepatitis	12%

a single-stranded positive-sense RNA that is 7.48 kb long. HAV lacks an envelope and measures 27–28 nm in diameter. HAV is very resilient and can survive in dried feces at room temperature for 4 weeks.

There are four human HAV genotypes (I, II, III, and VII), and three simian genotypes (IV, V, and VI) that are differentiated by nucleoside sequence variability within the P1 region of the genome.

After HAV enters the cell, the viral RNA uncoats and binds to host ribosomes to produce polysomes. The process of HAV RNA transcription is facilitated by a viral polymerase and the RNA transcript is translated into a large polyprotein that is. The polyprotein is organized into three regions: P1, P2, and P3. The P1 region includes structural proteins VP1, VP2, VP3, and a putative VP4. The P2 and P3 regions include nonstructural proteins associated with viral replication. The self-limiting nature of the infection may be related to down-

regulation of HAV RNA synthesis due to defective HAV particles and specific RNA-binding proteins that have a regulatory role in the replication of HAV. Variations in the central portion of the 5′ untranslated region of the HAV genome (between nucleotides 200 and 500) have a role in the development of fulminant hepatic failure in acute HAV [2].

Clinical presentation

HAV infection results in an acute self-limited infection. Rarely, it can be prolonged and associated with cholestasis. The incubation period is 2–4 weeks, rarely up to 6 weeks. Mortality is low, but morbidity is high in adults and older children.

Prodromal symptoms include fatigue, weakness, anorexia, nausea, vomiting, and abdominal pain. Less common symptoms are fever, headache, arthralgias, myalgias, and diarrhea. Symptoms may last a few days to a few weeks and usually decrease with the onset of jaundice. Jaundice is seen in 72% of infected adults while only 20% of children younger than 2 years become jaundiced. Abdominal pain and mild hepatomegaly are found in 85% of patients; splenomegaly and cervical lymphadenopathy are present in 15%. About 34% of individuals aged over 60 years require hospitalization versus less than 5% of children. Overall hospitalization and mortality rates are 25% and 0.5 %, respectively.

HAV infection can present as: (1) asymptomatic without jaundice, (2) symptomatic with self-limited jaundice, (3) cholestatic, with jaundice lasting 10 weeks or more, (4) relapsing, with two or more bouts of acute HAV infection occurring over a 6–10-week period, and (5) fulminant hepatic failure (FHF).

Complete clinical recovery is achieved in 60% of patients within 2 months and in close to 100% by 6 months. The overall prognosis of acute hepatitis A in otherwise healthy adults is excellent. A **relapsing course** is observed in approximately 10% of patients and represents a benign variant without increased mortality. HAV has a fatality rate of 1.8% in people older than 49 years due to FHF. FHF occurs within 4 weeks of

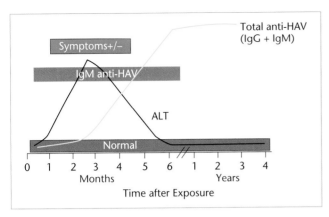

Figure 79.1 Serological profile for acute HAV infection.

infection in 90% of patients. Risk factors include advanced age, underlying liver disease, and human immunodeficiency virus (HIV) infection.

Extrahepatic manifestations include an evanescent rash (14%) arthralgias (11%), and, less commonly, leukocytoclastic vasculitis, glomerulonephritis, and arthritis. When cutaneous vasculitis is present, skin biopsies reveal the presence of IgM anti-HAV and complement in the blood vessel walls. HAV can trigger the development of type 1 autoimmune hepatitis in genetically predisposed individuals.

Diagnostic methods

The diagnosis is based on the detection of **IgM anti-HAV in serum** that remains positive for approximately 6 months. IgG anti-HAV remains present for life and is a marker of previous HAV infection. Figure 79.1 depicts the serological profile of acute hepatitis A.

Testing for HAV RNA is limited to research laboratories. HAV RNA has been detected in serum, stool, and liver tissue, and can be amplified by polymerase chain reaction (PCR).

Treatment

Supportive therapy is the mainstay of treatment of acute HAV. Both immunoglobulin (IG) and HAV vaccines can be used for post exposure prophylaxis. Healthy individuals between 12 months and 40 years of age with no prior immunization can receive a single dose of HAV vaccine or IG (0.02 mL/kg) within 2 weeks of exposure. The advantages of using HAV vaccines is that they provide long-term immunity (if the second dose is received in accordance with the standard vaccine schedule), are cheaper, and are widely available [3,4].

Prevention

Attention to sanitation and administration of vaccine/IG are the mainstays of preventing HAV infection. In the USA, a universal childhood vaccination policy was enacted in 2006 with the goal to eliminate indigenous HAV transmission. All immunocompromised patients and patients with chronic liver disease should receive HAV vaccine [5].

Two **inactivated HAV vaccines** are commercially available: HAVRIX (SmithKline Biologicals, Rixensart, Belgium) and VAQTA (Merck Sharp & Dohme, West Point, PA, USA); both provide life-long immunity when two doses are received 6 months apart.

A combined formulation of hepatitis A and B vaccines (TWINRIX) has been approved for individuals 18 years of age and older, and for a 30-day accelerated course prior to leaving for an endemic area [6].

Acute hepatitis B
Epidemiology

Hepatitis B virus (HBV) infects approximately 2 billion people and about 350 million people have chronic infection worldwide. It is the 10th leading cause of death worldwide, resulting in 4000–5500 deaths/year in the USA and 500 000–1.2 million worldwide. HBV is a major cause of hepatocellular carcinoma (HCC).

About 45% of the infected population reside in endemic areas, including Asia and Africa where the most common routes of transmission are materno-fetal (vertical) and close household contact (horizontal). The prevalence of HBV is lower in industrialized countries due to decreased vertical transmission and the introduction of effective vaccines.

In the USA about 800 000–1.4 million persons are infected with HBV. The incidence appears to be declining; there were 70 cases per 100 000 persons in 1985, dropping to 1.6 cases per 100 000 persons in 2006. However, it is estimated that the actual rate of HBV infection is about 10 times higher. In 2006, an estimated 46 000 persons in the USA were newly infected with HBV. Rates are highest among adults, particularly males aged 25–44 years, underscoring the likely **sexual transmission** in non-endemic areas.

Cause and pathogenesis

HBV is a blood-borne infection. It is transmitted parenterally by contact with infected blood or through sexual contact. Age and route of HBV infection correlate with degree of viral persistence. When infants are infected through vertical or horizontal transmission over 90% become chronically infected if not protected by vaccine/HBIG, while less than 5% develop chronic infection if exposed as adults. There is no evidence that breastfeeding transmits HBV [7].Infants born to HBeAg(+) mothers have a 85–90% risk of chronic infection compared to 30% of infants born to HBeAg(−) mothers. The perinatal transmission rate correlates to maternal serum HBV DNA levels. In non-endemic areas exposure to infected blood via percutaneous or sexual contact are common sources of HBV infection. Risk factors for HBV are listed in Table 79.3.

HBV is an enveloped double-stranded DNA virus that belongs to the Hepadnaviridae family. There are eight recognized HBV genotypes: A–H.

Liver Disease

Table 79.3 Groups at risk for HBV infection

- Infants born to infected mothers
- Sex partners of infected persons
- Sexually active persons who are not in a long-term, mutually monogamous relationship (e.g., more than one sexual partner during the previous 6 months)
- Men who have sex with men
- Injection drug users
- Household contacts of persons with chronic HBV infection
- Healthcare and public safety workers at risk for occupational exposure to blood or blood-contaminated body fluids
- Hemodialysis patients
- Residents and staff of facilities for developmentally disabled persons
- Travelers to countries with intermediate or high prevalence of HBV infection
- Sharing items such as razors or toothbrushes with an infected person

Table 79.4 Extrahepatic manifestations of HBV infection

- Polyarteritis nodosa (PAN)
- Glomerulonephritis
- Papular acrodermatits
- Serum sickness, arthritis, dermatitis prodrome
- Mixed essential cryoglobulinemia

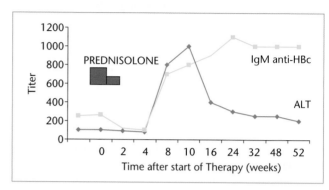

Figure 79.2 Serological profile of a chronic HBsAg carrier after an episode of reactivation.

The life cycle of HBV begins with its attachment, penetration, and uncoating in the hepatocytes. This is followed by conversion of the HBV DNA genome into a covalently closed circular DNA (cccDNA) template, which is located in the host nucleus and depends on host RNA polymerase II for viral transcription. The viral genome produces four mRNA species. The largest of these is a pre-genomic RNA which encodes polymerase, and core and pre-core proteins, and serves as the template for the minus strand of HBV DNA. In this process, called the intracellular conversion pathway, some of this newly synthesized HBV DNA is returned to nucleus and converted into cccDNA to increase the pool of cccDNA transcription templates. The smaller RNAs encode the large, middle, and small HBsAgs that are found on viral envelope, and the smallest RNA species encodes X-protein that may be associated with HCC development.

HBV is not cytopathic to hepatocytes; the degree of liver cellular injury depends on the interaction between HBV, hepatocytes, and the host immune system response. The **immune response** to acute HBV infection represents the interplay between innate and adaptive immunity, which is initiated by the release of interferon-alpha/beta (IFN-α/β) by dendrite cells after exposure to HBV. These IFNs then stimulate NK and NKT cells to produce multiple antiviral and immunoregulating cytokines (IL-12, IFN-γ, TNF-α), which then activate adaptive immunity through CD4(+) cells, including Th-1 or Th-2 cells. Th-1 cytokines induce cytotoxic T-lymphocyte (CTL) response cells and Th-2 cytokines induce humoral immunity that results in antibody production. In acute HBV, the Th-1 response predominates. Liver injury occurs when cytotoxic CD8(+) cells induce apoptosis of HBV-infected hepatocytes.

Clinically significant HBV proteins include hepatitis B surface antigen (HBsAg), hepatitis B core antigen (HBcAg), and hepatitis B e antigen (HBeAg). Detectable HBsAg represents an active infection, while presence of antibodies to HBsAg represents resolution of the infection or vaccination.

Clinical presentation

HBV incubation averages 120 days (range 45–160 days). Symptoms may precede jaundice by 1–2 weeks, including nausea, vomiting, and abdominal pain. Skin rashes, joint pains, and arthritis may occur. Jaundice is observed in 30–50% and fulminant hepatitis in 0.1–0.5%. Patients who recover from acute HBV usually acquire lifelong immunity. The fatality rate is approximately 1%. Extrahepatic manifestations are shown in Table 79.4.

Severe liver injury mimicking acute HBV can occur after HBV reactivation in at least three clinical scenarios: immune reconstitution with HAART therapy in HIV patients, after chemotherapy for malignant processes, or after biologic agents in solid organ or bone marrow transplant recipients. Figure 79.2 depicts the serological profile of a patient with reactivated HBV. Many questions remain, including which patients should be screened, which medications should be used to prevent reactivation, and whether patients with resolved HBV infection need prophylaxis [8].

Diagnostic methods

Acute HBV is defined by the presence of **HBsAg**, which is detectable after an incubation period of 4–10 weeks, and followed by IgM antibodies against the core antigen (**IgM anti-HBc**) (Figure 79.3). In acute HBV a rise in serum **alanine aminotransferase (ALT)** is followed by a drop in HBV DNA both in blood and the liver. Typically ALT and aspartate transaminase (AST) values increase to 1000–2000 IU/L. Recovery from acute infection is characterized by the disappearance of HBsAg/HBeAg and the emergence of HBsAb and HBeAb; the core antibody (IgG anti-HBc) may persist for life. Acute

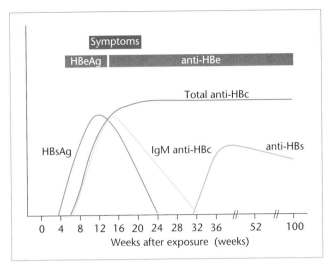

Figure 79.3 Serological profile for acute HBV infection.

infection progresses to chronic infection if HBsAg and HBV DNA level are detected for longer than 6 months from the acute onset; chronicity occurs in 1–5% of infected adults.

Treatment

No specific treatment is required in adults since most cases are self-limited, although supportive measures may be helpful.

Data on the efficacy of antiviral therapy for acute HBV infection are conflicting. No improvement in clinical course or loss of HBsAg was seen in patients randomized to **lamivudine** for 1 year when compared to those receiving placebo [9]. However, other data suggest lamivudine improves clinical, biochemical, serological, and virological responses especially in HBV acute liver failure [10]. Based on the latter data, it would be reasonable to start an oral antiviral in acute HBV cases at increased risk of liver failure, such as immunocompromised patients, patients co-infected with HCV, HIV or superinfected with HDV, patients with underlying liver disease, elderly subjects, and liver transplant recipients.

Treatment should continue until the ALT is normalized and the HBeAg is undetectable followed by the appearance of anti-HBe, or the complete resolution of the infection is demonstrated by loss of HBsAg.

Prevention

Prevention involves **behavior modification** (safe sex practices and use of sterile needles), and **passive and active immunization**. Passive immunoprophylaxis entails administering hepatitis B immunoglobulins to subjects at risk, such as newborn babies of HBsAg(+) mothers and HBsAg(+) recipients of liver transplants.

Eradication requires universal vaccination of newborns. The commercially available HBV vaccine (active immunization) requires three separate doses to be given and results in the production of HBsAb in 85–90% of healthy recipients. An HBsAb level above 100 mIU/mL implies an appropriate response; if lower levels, re-vaccination should be considered. Individuals who still do not achieve protective antibody levels can either be offered higher doses of vaccine or a different route of administration (intradermal). Those who fail this approach require hepatitis B immunoglobulins if acutely exposed to HBV.

Studies suggested that HBV vaccine afforded protection for a limited time only, but more recent data suggest that vaccination provides life-long protection despite loss of anti-HBs, most likely due to immunological memory. Only those who are at high risk should receive a single booster at 5 years from initial vaccination [11].

Acute hepatitis C
Epidemiology

HCV infects approximately 170 million people worldwide and 4 million in the USA. It is the third most common cause of acute hepatitis worldwide (5–15%). In the USA the prevalence is 1.8%, with the highest rates among 18–40-year olds and African Americans (6.1%). Approximately 3–6% may progress to fulminant hepatitis (particularly in patients with underlying liver disease). About 85% of individuals acutely infected with HCV develop chronic infection. In the USA the incidence of HCV infection has been declining; there were 230 000 new cases in the 1980s and 38 000 new cases in the 1990s.

Cause and pathogenesis

Unscreened blood products and contaminated needles account for 90% of cases in industrialized countries. Other less prevalent routes of infection include sexual and perinatal transmission. High-risk groups should be tested, including individuals who ever injected illegal drugs, received clotting factors made before 1987, received blood transfusions/organs before July 1992, were ever on chronic hemodialysis, or have evidence of liver disease.

HCV is a positive single-stranded RNA virus that belongs to the Flaviviridae family, which includes the flaviviruses and pestiviruses. The HCV genome encodes a large single polyprotein of about 3000 amino acids that is cleaved into structural and non-structural proteins by host and viral proteases. There are at least six HCV genotypes (1–6) and more than 50 subtypes. Genotype 1 is the most common and accounts for 75% of all HCV infections in the USA and Western Europe.

It is unclear why some individuals clear HCV while others progress to chronic hepatitis. The process likely involves host and viral factors such as variability in genes controlling early antiviral response and ability of HCV to avoid humoral and cellular immune responses. The host response to HCV infection is initially regulated by Th1 and Th2 cells that release multiple cytokines that stimulate activation and differentiation of B cells and cytotoxic T cells. Cytotoxic and non-cytotoxic effect is mediated via CD8(+) cells which recognize and lyze

Liver Disease

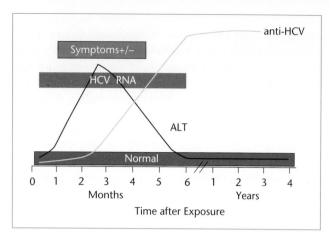

Figure 79.4 Serological profile for acute HCV infection.

Table 79.5 Proposed criteria for diagnosis of acute HCV infection

- Acute increase in levels of ALT to >10 times the upper limit of normal with or without increase in total bilirubin level

- Detectable HCV RNA

- Exposure to HCV during the preceding 2–12 weeks

ALT, alanine aminotransferase.

Table 79.6 Pros and cons of immediate treatment of acute HCV infection

For immediate treatment	Exploit optimal host adaptive and innate immune responses Minimize viral evolution and prevent persistence Minimize histological injury High sustained virological responses rates with immediate therapy
Against immediate therapy	Spontaneous clearance in a subset of patients Unnecessary exposure to adverse effects of interferon-based therapy High sustained virological response rates even with delayed therapy

HCV-infected cells and release cytokines that inhibit viral replication and further gene expression.

HCV-specific antibodies can partially interfere with HCV infection but do not clear virus from the circulation or protect hosts from re-infection. This is likely due to the mutation rate in the hypervariable regions of the HCV envelope proteins and selection of viral strains that escape neutralizing antibodies, the speed of viral replication, and the inability to eliminate HCV from infected cells. Multiple episodes of acute hepatitis C have been observed in polytransfused thalassemic children and experimental animals, indicating that sterilizing immunity is absent in HCV infection. However, it was observed that intravenous drug users who previously cleared virus and were reinfected with HCV, developed persistent infection in 33% of cases compared to 84% in first-time infected patients, suggesting partial acquired immunity to HCV, probably CD8(+) cells mediated [12]. Host factors that may influence the outcome of HCV infection include specific combinations of immunoglobulin GM and KM allotypes and their phenotypes that are found on chromosome 14 and 2.

Figure 79.4 shows a serological profile of acute hepatitis C.

Clinical presentation
The incubation period of HCV infection ranges from 15 to 150 days prior to the onset of clinical disease. HCV RNA can be detected in the serum 1–2 weeks after exposure and is followed by elevation in liver-associated enzymes (Figure 79.4).

Acute HCV infection can result in a broad spectrum of clinical signs and symptoms ranging from asymptomatic illness to acute liver failure. About 20–50% of patients with acute hepatitis clear virus and about 50–80% develop chronic infection. Symptomatic patients clear virus more frequently than non-symptomatic patients; however only 25–30% acute cases are symptomatic.

Symptoms when present typically develop 6–8 weeks after infection and last 3–12 weeks. Jaundice is observed in 25% of patients, while anorexia, abdominal pain, fatigue, nausea, vomiting, and fever are seen in 10–20% of patients. Acute infection rarely progresses to fulminant hepatitis and acute liver failure.

Diagnostic methods
There are no definitive criteria for the diagnosis of acute HCV infection that distinguishes it from chronic infection but certain criteria are used in defining clinical cohorts for treatment studies of acute HCV infection (Table 79.5).

Early in the course of infection, patients are seronegative for antibody to HCV (**anti-HCV**), but HCV RNA can be detected 1–2 weeks after exposure (see Figure 79.4). The anti-HCV is detected 6–8 weeks after infection and usually persists for life.

Treatment and prevention
The goal of treatment of acute HCV is to eradicate virus and prevent chronicity. Currently there are no defined guidelines for management of acute HCV infection because most data are from small heterogeneous studies that have utilized a variety of treatment regimens. The decision about initiating therapy is a difficult one because of **possible spontaneous resolution**; however, it is generally accepted that patients with acute HCV should be treated due to the high rate of chronic progression and higher rate of treatment success. Table 79.6 shows the arguments for and against the treatment of acute hepatitis C.

Multiple randomized trials have shown that **pegylated (PEG)-IFN-α 2b monotherapy** in acute HCV induces high and sustained viral response (SVR) rates; The SVR rates with treatment over 12–24 weeks ranged from 71% to 98% depending on the population treated, HCV genotype, onset of therapy, and adherence to therapy [12]. Similar SVR rates were observed when IFN therapy was started 8–12 weeks after the onset of symptoms [13]. However, in a study in which therapy for acute HCV infection was delayed for 12 weeks after onset of symptoms, about 50% of patients cleared infection spontaneously. Females and jaundiced patients had higher rate of spontaneous clearance of HCV. Of patients who received therapy, 80% achieved an SVR, giving a combined rate of SVR of 91% for treated and untreated patients. These data suggest that therapy could be delayed for 12 weeks to allow for spontaneous clearance [14]. Similar results were obtained using PEG-IFN-α 2b monotherapy at a dose of 1.5 μg/kg/week,. The cumulative SVR was 87% [15]. No data have suggested that adding ribavirin improves the SVR in acute HCV.

Acute HCV infection in HIV–co-infected patient is treated with either PEG-IFN monotherapy or in combination with weight-based ribavirin; SVRs range from 59% to 91%. These patients may require longer therapy to clear HCV.

Acute hepatitis D

Epidemiology
Hepatitis delta virus (HDV) is a defective RNA virus that is dependent on HBV infection for its replication and expression. It was first discovered in 1977 and fully cloned in 1986. The HDV virion comprises of an RNA genome, a single HDV antigen, and an envelope supplied by HBV. About 6% of HBV-infected individuals are co-infected with HDV, giving an estimated 20 million co-infected people worldwide. Three distinct genotypes and two subtypes have been described based on geographical distribution and clinical pattern. Genotype I is associated with chronic hepatitis and is the most prevalent in the world. Genotype II is found predominantly in Taiwan and Japan and is associated with less severe disease. Genotype III is associated with outbreaks of fulminant hepatitis in Venezuela and Peru. The annual incidence of acute HDV infection in the USA is about 7500 cases.

Causes and pathogenesis
HDV is the only representative of the Deltavirus genus. Phylogenic data have shown more complex genetic variability of HDV and suggest that HDV should be classified into eight different clads [16,17].

The HDV genome is a 36–43 nm spherical RNA molecule that contains 1670–1685 nucleotides, of which 60% are C + G. HDV RNA is a negative single-stranded circular structure that is transcribed into a linear antigenomic transcript that serves as the template for synthesis of HDV RNA and mRNA. This mRNA codes for a large (LHDAg) and small (SHDAg) HDAg protein. The small form is associated with promotion of viral replication and the large with its inhibition. The replication process requires host RNA-dependent RNA polymerase. The HDV core consist of about 70 molecules of HDAg combined with HDV RNA. The HDVcore is enveloped by HBsAg to allow HDV viral spread.

Hepatic cell death may occur due to the direct cytotoxic effect of HDV or via a host-mediated immune response. HDV is usually transmitted parenterally. In Western countries, the major risk factors include intravenous drug use and multiple blood transfusions. Sexual and perinatal transmission are less common than with HBV.

Clinical presentation
HDV causes acute or chronic viral hepatitis by being contracted concurrently with HBV (**co-infection**) or contracted by individuals with chronic HBV infection (**superinfection**). The latter is characterized by a more aggressive clinical course, while co-infections are usually acute, self-limited infections. Chronic hepatitis D occurs in about 5% of HBV–HDV co-infected patient.

Acute HDV has an incubation period of 3–7 weeks. A preicteric phase begins with symptoms of fatigue, lethargy, anorexia, and nausea, lasting usually 3–7 days. The icteric phase is characterized by fatigue and nausea, clay-colored stools, and dark urine with elevation in serum bilirubin.

Superinfection of HBV and HDV causes a severe acute hepatitis with a short incubation period before leading to chronic type D hepatitis in up to 80% of cases. Superinfection can lead to acute liver failure with mortality rates of up to 80%. About 60–70% of patients with chronic HDV develop cirrhosis in 5–10 years. Typically in chronic HDV, the HBV is suppressed. The course of chronic HDV can be divided into three phases: an early active phase with active HDV replication and suppression of HBV, a second moderately active phase with decreasing HDV and HBV reactivation, and a third late phase characterized by the development of cirrhosis and HCC [18]. The overall mortality rate for HDV infections is between 2–20%, which is about ten times higher than for hepatitis B.

Diagnostic methods
Acute HDV infection is diagnosed by **elevated liver associated enzymes, HBsAg(+), and IgM anti-HDV**. The latter develops within 30 days of infection. In the early phase of acute liver failure, HBsAg may be absent and anti-HBc is the only marker of HBV infection. Reverse transcriptase–polymerase chain reaction (RT–PCR) can detect just 10–100 copies of the HDV genome in infected blood serum. When patients recover, markers of HDV infection, including IgM and IgG antibodies, disappear within months, while in chronic hepatitis D infection, HDV RNA, HDAg, IgM anti-HD antibodies, and IgG anti-HD antibodies persist.

Figures 79.5 and 79.6 depict the serological profile of HDV superinfection and co-infection respectively.

Treatment and prevention
There is no specific treatment for acute HDV. Early attempts to develop a vaccine against HDV using an animal model (woodchuck) have proved unsuccessful.

Effective prevention of **HDV–HBV co-infection** can be achieved with the HBV vaccine or HBIG for postexposure

Liver Disease

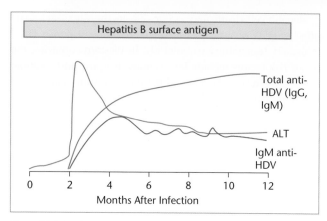

Figure 79.5 Serological profile for acute HDV superinfection.

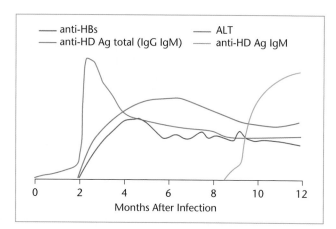

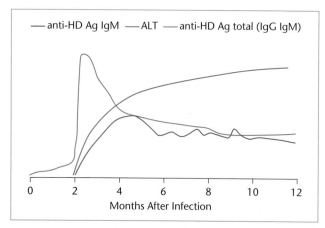

Figure 79.6 Course of acute HDV co-infection. ALT, alanine aminotransferase.

prophylaxis. **HBV–HDV superinfection** can be avoided by educating chronic HBV carriers about risk factors, such are blood exchange, sexual contact, sharing needles, and vertical transmission.

The therapeutic goal is to eradicate HDV or to achieve long-term suppression of both HDV and HBV. Eradication of HBV

infection and the development of anti-HBsAg is protective against both HBV and HDV infection.

Acute hepatitis E
Epidemiology
Hepatitis E virus (HEV) is a zoonosis and common cause of acute viral hepatitis in Asia, Africa, the Middle East, and Central America. It accounts for up to 54% of cases of clinically significant acute hepatitis in these areas. It is rare in industrialized countries, although the incidence is slowly increasing, and is largely restricted to men over 50 years of age. It is associated with zoonotic food-borne autochthonous infections [19]. The most common reservoirs for HEV are domestic swine, deer, and wild boar [20].

Cause and pathogenesis
HEV is a water-borne virus that is transmitted by fecal–oral spread through contaminated water. HEV is also transmitted vertically and parenterally, and there are reports of transfusion-transmitted HEV in non-endemic countries [21].Humans can be infected by eating inadequately cooked meat of animals that are natural reservoirs or from contact with domestic swine. There is a low incidence of household cross-infection due to HEV.

The pathogenesis of HEV virus is poorly understood due to the lack of an efficient cell culture system and small animal model. HEV was first recognized in 1983 and its genome was cloned in 1991. It is a small, non-enveloped, single-strand, positive-sense RNA virus of 7.2 kb. It is classified in the family Hepeviridae, and has four major genotypes and 24 subtypes [22]. Genotypes 1 and 2 are restricted to humans and associated with large outbreaks in endemic regions with poor sanitation. Genotypes 3 and 4 are found in domestic swine and wild animals and are associated with sporadic cases of HEV in both endemic and non-endemic areas. The HEV genome contains three reading frames: ORF1 encodes non-structural proteins that are similar to rubella virus proteins, ORF2 encodes the caspid protein, and ORF3 encodes a small phosphoprotein.

Clinical presentation
HEV presents as a self-limited acute infection of young adults. The incubation period ranges from 20 to 60 days. It typically follows a more severe course than HAV, including prolonged cholestasis in up to 60% of patients, but there is no evidence that it causes acute liver failure in non-pregnant patients or chronic hepatitis other than in rare cases of solid organ transplant recipients [23]. Clinical symptoms and abnormal biochemical tests resolve within 6 weeks.

FHF secondary to HEV occurs in 10–20% of **pregnant women** who become infected in the third trimester and has a 15–25% mortality rate. Pregnant patients, particularly Asian patients, infected with HEV have higher viral load that non-pregnant women, due possibly to their altered sex hormones and mild immunodeficiency [24].

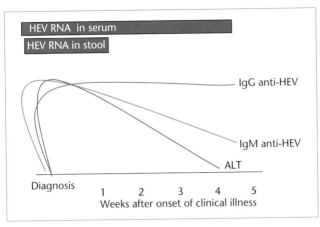

Figure 79.7 Serological profile for HEV infection.

Rarely HEV infection can be associated with acute polyarthritis, severe jaundice, Henoch–Schönlein purpura, Guillain–Barré syndrome, severe thrombocytopenia, non-immune hemolytic anemia, acute transverse myelitis, renal function impairment in a renal allograft recipient, lymphocytic destructive cholangitis, and pancreatitis.

Diagnostic methods
Serological tests for HEV include **PCR for HEV RNA, HEV antigen and IgM and IgA antibodies to HEV** [25]. IgA and IgM can be detected in the serum up to 144 days after the onset of infection with HEV and their combined detection is highly specific for diagnosis of acute HEV infection. Figure 79.7 depicts the serological profile of acute HEV.

Histologically, individuals with acute autochthonous HEV have more severe portal and acinar inflammation and cholangiolitis than individuals infected with an HEV strain from an endemic area.

Treatment and prevention
Treatment of acute HEV infection is symptomatic and supportive. Prevention of HEV infection is a function of sanitation and clean water. Travelers to endemic regions should use bottled water and avoid uncooked food. Immunoglobulins for passive immunoprophylaxis are not available for hepatitis E, although primate studies are promising. Recombinant HEV vaccine has been evaluated in a phase 2, randomized, placebo controlled trial in Nepal and was found to be well tolerated and efficacious, but it is still not commercially available [26].

Differential diagnosis of acute viral hepatitis
Acute viral hepatitis should be differentiated from other causes of acute inflammation of the liver, such as autoimmune hepatitis, drug-induced, ischemic liver disease, and alcoholic hepatitis, by appropriate serologic tests. However, in some cases the diagnosis may be difficult to make because the patient may harbor another viral infection, such as chronic HBV or chronic HCV infection, with superimposed acute HAV or HDV infection.

A number of pathogens that can cause acute hepatitis can mimic acute viral hepatitis. Furthermore, as some acute viral infections present with jaundice, other reasons for cholestatic hepatitis (choledocholithiasis, primary biliary cirrhosis, primary sclerosing cholangitis) have to be taken into consideration.

Prognosis with and without treatment
Acute **HVA infection** carries an excellent prognosis, with a few exceptions such as patients with underlying liver disease.

The prognosis of acute **HBV infection** correlates with age at which the infection is acquired, HBeAg status, underlying chronic liver disease, and immunosuppression status. Most children progress to chronic infection if active immunoprophylaxis is not given, while most adults have self-limited acute infection, with 1–5% progressing to chronic liver disease. The Fulminant hepatitis rate is 0.1–0.5%.

Treatment of acute **HCV infection** may have a significant impact on long-term prognosis since most patients treated with PEG-IFN successfully eradicate the virus.

There is no therapy for acute **HDV infection** and no effective vaccine has been developed yet; however, universal vaccination against HBV and education about risk factors has been proven to decrease the incidence of co-infection and superinfection. Superinfection causes a severe acute hepatitis and results in chronic type D hepatitis in up to 80% of cases. Superinfection is associated with acute liver failure with mortality rate up to 80%. About 60–70% of patients with chronic HDV develop cirrhosis in 5–10 years. The mortality rate for HDV infections is about ten times higher than for hepatitis B.

Typically acute **HEV infection** is followed by complete recovery without the development of viral persistence. Whether protection from reinfection is life-long is uncertain.

> **SOURCES OF INFORMATION FOR PATIENTS AND DOCTORS**
>
> www.cdc.gov/hepatitis.org
> www.aasld.com

References
1. Centers for Disease Control and Prevention. Prevention of Hepatitis A through Active or Passive Immunization. *MMWR.* 2006;55:1–23.
2. Fujiwara K, Yokosuka O, Ehata T, *et al.* Association between severity of type A hepatitis and nucleotide variations in the 5′ non-translated region of hepatitis A virus RNA: Strains from fulminant hepatitis have fewer nucleotide substitutions. *Gut.* 2002;51:82.
3. Centers of Disease Control and Prevention. Prevention of hepatitis A after exposure to hepatitis A virus and in international travelers. *MMWR.* 2007;56:1080–1084.
4. Victor JC, Monto AS, Surdina TY, *et al.* Hepatitis A vaccine versus immune globulin for post exposure prophylaxis. *N Engl J Med.* 2007;357:1685–1694.

Liver Disease

5. Reiss G, Keeffe EB. Review article: Hepatitis vaccination in patients with chronic liver disease. *Aliment Pharmacol Ther.* 2004;19:715.

6. Diaz-Mitoma F, Law B, Subramanya A, Hoet B. Long-term antibody persistence induced by a combined hepatitis A and B vaccine in children and adolescents. *Vaccine.* 2008;26:1759–1763.

7. Lok AS. Chronic hepatitis B. *N Engl J Med.* 2002;346:1682–1683.

8. Hoofnagle JH. Reactivation of hepatitis B. *Hepatology.* 2009;49: S156–S165.

9. Kumar M, Satapathy S, Monga R, *et al.* A randomized controlled trial of lamivudine to treat acute hepatitis B. *Hepatology.* 2007;45: 97–101.

10. Roussos A, Koilakou S, Kalafatas I, *et al.* Lamivudine treatment for acute severe hepatitis: report of a case and review of the literature. *Acta Gastro-enterol Belg.* 2008;71:30–32.

11. Van Damme P, Van Herck K. A review of the long-term protection after hepatitis A and B vaccination. *Travel Med Infect Dis.* 2007;5:79–84.

12. Rehermann B. Immunopathogenesis of hepatitis C. In: Liang TJ, moderator. Pathogenesis, natural history, treatment, and prevention of hepatitis C. *Ann Intern Med.* 2000;132:297–299.

13. Jaeckel E, Cornberg M, Wedemeyer H. Treatment of acute hepatitis C with interferone alfa-2b. *N Engl J Med.* 2001;345:1452–1457.

14. Gerlach JT, Diepolder HM, Zachoval R. Acute hepatitis C: high rate of both spontaneous and treatment-induced viral clearance. *Gastroenterology.* 2003;125:80–88.

15. Kamal SM, Fouly AE, Kamel RR, *et al.* Peginterferon alfa-2b therapy in acute hepatitis C: impact of onset of therapy on sustained virologic response. *Gastroenterology.* 2006;130:632–638.

16. Le Gal F, Gault E, Ripault MP, *et al.* Eighth major clade for hepatitis delta virus. *Emerg Infect Dis.* 2006;12:1447–1450.

17. Dény P. Hepatitis delta virus genetic variability: from genotypes I, II, III to eight major clades? *Curr Top Microbiol Immunol.* 2006;307:151–171.

18. Lai MM. The molecular biology of hepatitis Delta virus. *Ann Rev Biochem.* 1995;64:259–286.

19. Mansuy JM, Abravanel F, Miedouge M, *et al.* Acute hepatitis E in south-west France over a 5-year period. *J Clin Virol.* 2009;44: 74–77.

20. Reuter G, Fodor D, Forgách P, Kátai A, Szucs G. Characterization and zoonotic potential of endemic hepatitis E virus (HEV)strains in humans and animals in Hungary. *J Clin Virol.* 2009;44: 277–281.

21. Matsubayashi K, Nagaoka Y, Sakata H, *et al.* Transfusion-transmitted hepatitis E caused by apparently indigenous hepatitis E virus strain in Hokkaido, Japan. *Transfusion.* 2004;44: 934–940.

22. Lu L, Li C, Hagedorn CH. Phylogenetic analysis of global hepatitis E virus sequences: genetic diversity, subtypes and zoonosis. *Rev Med Virol.* 2006;16:5–36.

23. Chau TN, Lai ST, Tse C, *et al.* Epidemiology and clinical features of sporadic hepatitis e as compared with hepatitis A. *Am J Gastroenterol.* 2006;101:292–296.

24. Kar P, Jilani N, Husain SA, *et al.* Does hepatitis E viral load and genotypes influence the final outcome of acute liver failure during pregnancy? *Am J Gastroenterol.* 2008;103:2495–2501.

25. Zhang F, Li X, Li Z, *et al.* Detection of HEV antigen as a novel marker for the diagnosis of hepatitis E. *J Med Virol.* 2006;78: 1441–1448.

26. Shrestha MP, Scott RM, Joshi DM, *et al.* Safety and efficacy of a recombinant hepatitis E vaccine. *N Engl J Med.* 2007;356:895–903.

CHAPTER 80

Chronic hepatitis B

Tarik Asselah, Olivier Lada, Rami Moucari, and Patrick Marcellin

University of Paris, Clichy, France

ESSENTIAL FACTS ABOUT PATHOGENESIS

- HBV, a member of the *Hepadnaviridae* family, is a small DNA virus
- HBV is a common cause of liver disease and liver cancer
- Chronic HBV infection affects approximately 350 million people worldwide
- Safe and effective vaccines have reduced the burden of disease

ESSENTIALS OF DIAGNOSIS

- The causal relationship between HBV infection and liver disease must be established
- HBV infection is defined by the presence of a positive HBsAg and detectable HBV-DNA in serum
- Other causes of chronic liver disease should be systematically looked for, including co-infection with HDV, HCV, and/or HIV
- The natural course of HBV infection varies from inactive HBsAg carrier to progressive chronic hepatitis, potentially evolving to cirrhosis and hepatocellular carcinoma
- Assessment of the severity of liver disease is important to select candidates for treatment: biochemical markers, including aspartate aminotransferase (AST) and alanine transaminase (ALT), prothrombin time and serum albumin, blood counts; and hepatic ultrasound and/or liver stiffness measurement
- A liver biopsy is often useful to determine the grade of necroinflammation and the stage of fibrosis, useful for evaluating candidacy for antiviral therapy.

ESSENTIALS OF TREATMENT

- Many patients have mild liver disease and are not candidates for antiviral therapy
- Several antiviral therapies are now available, including interferon-α, pegylated interferon-α 2a, lamivudine, adefovir, entecavir, telbivudine, and tenofovir
- The goal of therapy is to improve quality of life and survival by preventing progression of the disease to cirrhosis, decompensated cirrhosis, hepatocellular carcinoma, and death
- Therapy suppresses HBV replication in a sustained manner, thereby reducing histological activity of chronic hepatitis and decreasing the risk of developing cirrhosis and hepatocellular carcinoma (particularly in non-cirrhotic patients)
- IFN and PEG-IFN-α 2a induce a sustained virological response after a defined, self-limited course of treatment, but are effective in only a minority of patients and have frequent side effects that limit their tolerability. Analogs have the advantages of oral administration and excellent safety profiles with very high antiviral effect, but need to be administered indefinitely since their withdrawal is generally associated with reactivation and sustained response is uncommon, except in HBeAg-positive patients who have developed HBe seroconversion

---

Introduction

Chronic hepatitis B virus (HBV) infection continues to be a public health concern throughout the world, despite the implementation of public health initiatives. Although the availability of safe and effective vaccines has reduced the burden of disease and most countries have some form of selective vaccination policy, the risk groups targeted vary markedly from country to country, and cost is often a barrier to their introduction in many low-income countries. As a result, HBV continues to be the cause of considerable morbidity and mortality, mainly stemming from its progression to cirrhosis, decompensated liver disease, and hepatocellular carcinoma (HCC).

Thus, the choice of appropriate pharmacotherapy is critical to altering the course of the disease and reducing the costs associated with the management of chronic hepatitis B. A decade ago, standard therapy for chronic hepatitis B consisted only of interferon-α and lamivudine. In the last decade, important advances have been made in the treatment of hepatitis B. Several additional antivirals are now available, including pegylated interferon-α 2a, adefovir, entecavir, telbivudine, and tenofovir. However, in order to further improve clinical outcomes, it is still necessary to develop new therapeutic strategies with greater antiviral effect and lower resistance profiles. The most promising approach might be combination therapy of pegylated interferon with potent antivirals to improve HBs seroconversion rates. This chapter focuses on the results obtained with the different available drugs.

Epidemiology

Chronic HBV infection affects approximately 350–400 million people worldwide and is the cause of significant acute and chronic morbidity and mortality [1–3], and healthcare costs [4]. Approximately 15–40% of individuals with chronic HBV infection will develop chronic hepatitis B, active disease that can

Liver Disease

Textbook of Clinical Gastroenterology and Hepatology, Second Edition. Edited by C. J. Hawkey, Jaime Bosch, Joel E. Richter, Guadalupe Garcia-Tsao, Francis K. L. Chan.

potentially evolve to cirrhosis, decompensated liver disease, and HCC [1–3].

The World Health Organization (WHO) estimates that the average annual incidence of HBV infection in Europe is approximately 20 per 100 000 population, and HBsAg sero-prevalence ranges from 0.3% to 12% [5]. In many countries the prevalence of HBeAg-negative chronic hepatitis B, a potentially severe and progressive form, is increasing [6]. This increase is most likely due to the natural history of the disease and also to a better awareness of this more severe form of chronic hepatitis B.

Natural history

The natural course of HBV infection is dynamic (Figure 80.1), characterized by periods of inactivity and periods of immune activity during which it can progress to chronic hepatitis, potentially leading to cirrhosis and HCC [1,7,8].

Sex, age, alcohol consumption, and co-infection with human immunodeficiency virus (HIV) can affect the natural course of HBV infection. Importantly, HBV-DNA levels are associated with a greater progression to cirrhosis and HCC [9].

HBV (together with HCV infection) accounts for the majority of **cirrhosis and primary liver cancer** in most of the world. For

instance, in France, the current estimated annual number of deaths associated with HBV infection is 1507 (2.5 deaths per 100 000 people) [10]. It is estimated that HBV-related end-stage liver disease and HCC cause more than 1 million deaths per year worldwide, with HCC being the fifth most frequent cancer [8].

These observations confirm the importance of HBV infection as a major public health problem and underscore the need for a major public health program that includes prevention, screening, counseling, and treatment of patients with hepatitis B. The increased efficacy of HBV treatment might decrease the incidence of cirrhosis and therefore improve survival. Furthermore, the improvement of surveillance of cirrhotic patients might improve early detection of HCC, and therefore might ameliorate survival.

Impact of therapy on the natural course

The goals of chronic hepatitis B treatment are sustained suppression of viral replication, normalized alanine aminotransferase (ALT) levels, reduced progression to cirrhosis, and/or prevention of hepatic decompensation and HCC [1–3]. Increasing evidence suggests that only a complete and vigorous HBV-specific immune response can achieve long-term suppression of the virus.

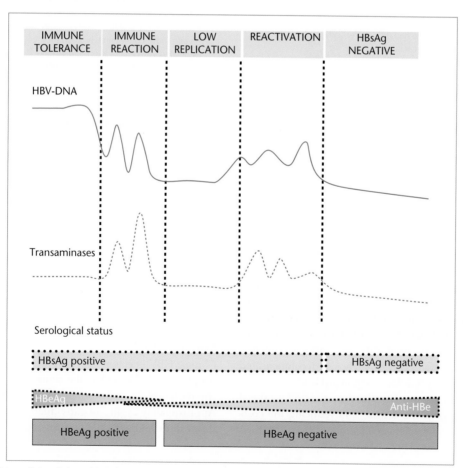

Figure 80.1 Natural history of chronic hepatitis B showing the relationship between virological, biochemical, and serological markers during the different immunological phases. The course is dynamic with periods of activity (immune reaction and immune reactivation) and periods of inactivity (immune tolerance, low replication and HBsAg-negative phase).

Evidence from numerous studies indicates a positive correlation exists between HBV e antigen (HBeAg) or HBV-DNA levels and disease progression to cirrhosis and HCC [9]. In a prospective, community-based, long-term follow-up study in a cohort of 3653 HBsAg-positive individuals from Taiwan, a dose-dependent relationship between serum HBV-DNA level and risk of HCC was demonstrated [9]. The cumulative risk of HCC increased from 1.3% to 14.9% for HBV-DNA levels of <300 copies/mL and ≥106 copies/mL, respectively. Moreover, reduction of serum HBV-DNA levels over time was associated with a six-fold reduction in HCC risk. Taken together, these data suggest that patients with ongoing HBV-DNA replication have a higher risk for disease progression and may benefit from anti-HBV therapy. However, these studies do not clearly define the level of replication above which the risk of progression is increased. Further long-term cohort studies with sequential assessment of HBV-DNA levels and liver tests are needed.

Available drugs

In recent years, marked progress has been made in the treatment of chronic hepatitis B [11]. Several agents are currently approved: interferon-α (IFN-α), pegylated interferon-α 2a (PEG-IFN-α 2a), lamivudine, adefovir, entecavir, telbivudine, and tenofovir (Table 80.1). The selection of the appropriate anti-HBV therapy is critical to reduce HBV-DNA replication and the risk for disease progression. Implementation of effective treatment in the early stages of disease may reduce the economic burden of chronic hepatitis B by reducing progression to more advanced stages of liver disease [4].

Each agent has advantages and inherent limitations. **IFN and PEG-IFN-α 2a** have the advantage of inducing a sustained virological response after a defined, self-limited course of treatment. However, these agents are effective in a minority of patients and have frequent side effects that limit their tolerability.

Nucleos(t)ide analogs have the advantages of oral administration and excellent safety profiles with very high antiviral

effect. However, these drugs need to be administered indefinitely because withdrawal of therapy is generally associated with reactivation, and a sustained response is uncommon except in HBeAg-positive patients who develop HBe seroconversion. In case of HBe seroconversion, it is generally recommended to prolong therapy for at least 24 weeks before its withdrawal. The efficacy of **lamivudine** is limited by the emergence of lamivudine-resistant HBV. Adefovir is associated with a low incidence of resistance, but its antiviral effect is not optimal. **Entecavir** has recently been approved in Europe for the treatment of HBV. This antiviral agent is very effective against HBV, with a favorable safety profile and low incidence of resistance. **Telbivudine** may have a higher efficacy and lower resistance than lamivudine, but its resistance rate is still significantly higher than that for other approved therapies. **Tenofovir** has been approved for chronic hepatitis B and several studies suggest that its efficacy and resistance profiles are superior to those of adefovir.

Pegylated interferon
IFN-α was the first substance licensed to treat chronic HBV infection. As already mentioned, this agent has the advantage of inducing a sustained virological response after a definite, self-limited course of treatment [12]. Two randomized controlled studies of PEG-IFN-α 2a in patients with HBeAg-positive [13] or HBeAg-negative [14] chronic hepatitis B have shown HBV-DNA suppression rates of 36% and 43% 24 weeks after discontinuing therapy, respectively. Interestingly, relatively high rates of HBsAg loss, associated with complete and sustained remission of the disease, were observed in both studies (3% and 4%, respectively) as compared with <1% in patients treated with lamivudine [13,14].

Recently, follow-up data of the trial in HBeAg-negative patients reported response rates 3 years after discontinuing therapy [15]. Biochemical and virological responses were stable 3 years after treatment with either PEG IFN-α 2a monotherapy or PEG IFN-α 2a plus lamivudine combination therapy, with an increasing rate of HBsAg loss (8%).

Nucleos(t)ide analogs
Nucleos(t)ide analogs inhibit the viral polymerase activity by different mechanisms of action. Depending on the drug, this inhibitory activity can affect the priming of reverse transcription and elongation of viral minus- or plus-strand DNA. All nucleos(t)ide analogs are competitive inhibitors of the natural endogenous intracellular nucleotide. Their incorporation in nascent viral DNA results in premature chain termination by preventing the incorporation of the next nucleotide in the viral DNA strand. Nucleos(t)ide analogs are effective in suppressing HBV replication, can be administered orally, and have excellent safety profiles. However, as already mentioned, these agents need to be **administered indefinitely** since withdrawal of therapy is generally associated with reactivation. Moreover, a major concern with long-term nucleos(t)ide analog therapy is the selection of antiviral-resistant mutants that lead to viral

Table 80.1 Drugs approved for the treatment of chronic hepatitis B

	Commercial name
Interferon-α 2a and 2b	Roferon®, Viraferon®
Pegylated interferon-α 2a	Pegasys®
Lamivudine	Epivir®, Zeffix®
Adefovir	Hepsera®
Entecavir	Baraclude®
Telbivudine	Sebivo®, Tyzeka®
Tenofovir	Viread®

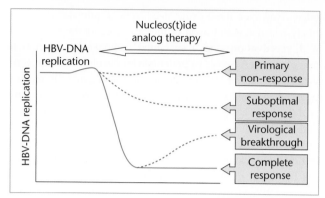

Figure 80.2 Definitions of resistance. Primary non-response: HBV-DNA reduction by <1 log after 3 months of therapy; suboptimal response: detectable HBV-DNA after 6–12 months of therapy; virological breakthrough: 1 log HBV-DNA increase in serum HBV-DNA level from nadir in two consecutive samples 1 month apart in patients who have responded.

breakthrough. It is important to recall response definitions (Figure 80.2). In fact, the rate at which resistant mutants are selected is related to pretreatment serum HBV-DNA levels and rapidity of viral suppression, but also duration of treatment and prior exposure to nucleos(t)ide analogs.

Lamivudine

Lamivudine was the first nucleoside analog to be used in the treatment of chronic hepatitis B, and has the advantages of oral administration and excellent tolerance. This L-nucleoside analog is effective for HIV and HBV. Lamivudine administered for 12 months induces a sustained response in approximately 20% of HBeAg-positive and 5% of HBeAg-negative patients [16,17]. However, lamivudine has a poor resistance profile, with the development of resistance in the YMDD domain of the DNA polymerase (codon rtL180M, rtM204V/I/S) and resistance rates of 23%, 46%, 55%, 65%, and 71% after 1, 2, 3, 4, and 5 years of therapy, respectively [18].

Adefovir

Adefovir is an acyclic nucleoside phophonates. It was the second nucleotide analog to be used in the treatment of chronic hepatitis B and, similarly to lamivudine, has the advantages of oral administration and good tolerance. In HBeAg-positive patients, adefovir administered for 12 months induces HBe seroconversion in 12%, increasing up to 48% at 5 years [19,20]. Adefovir has a similar antiviral efficacy in HBeAg-negative patients [21]. It has a far better resistance profile than lamivudine, with cumulative genotypic resistance rates of 0% and 3% at 1 and 2 years, respectively, although the rate of genotypic resistance rose to 29% in the 5-year extension trial conducted in HBeAg-negative patients [22]. However, in patients with HBV-DNA <1000 copies/mL at 1 year, the 4-year resistance rate was only 4% [23]. Adefovir is effective in the treatment of lamivudine-resistant HBV. It has been used successfully in patients with decompensated cirrhosis, in the pretransplant setting or in post-transplant patients who have developed

resistance to lamivudine [24]. In patients with HBV/HIV co-infection with lamivudine-resistant HBV, treatment with adefovir has a marked antiviral effect, similar to that observed in HIV-negative patients [25].

Entecavir

Results of phase III trials of entecavir in HBeAg-positive [26] and HBeAg-negative [27] chronic hepatitis B patients demonstrate excellent efficacy and safety. Mean serum HBV-DNA levels decrease in HBeAg-positive and HBeAg-negative patients by 6.9 $\log_{10}$ copies/mL and 5.0 $\log_{10}$ copies/mL, respectively [26,27]. HBV-DNA by polymerase chain reaction (PCR) became undetectable in 67% and 90% of patients, respectively [26,27]. Despite the potent antiviral effect of entecavir, the HBe seroconversion rate was relatively low (21% at 1 year). Interestingly, no resistance was observed in patients who were not previously treated with lamivudine.

Long-term monitoring showed low rates of resistance in nucleoside-naïve patients during 5 years of entecavir therapy, corresponding with potent viral suppression and a high genetic barrier to resistance [28].

Entecavir is not recommended in patients with lamivudine resistance. The presence of M204V and L180M in patients with lamivudine resistance lowers the genetic barrier to entecavir resistance, since only one additional entecavir-resistance substitution is needed at T184, S202, and/or M250, compared to a requirement for multiple amino acid substitutions in wild-type virus [29].

Telbivudine

In a double-blind, phase III trial, 1370 patients with chronic hepatitis B were randomly assigned to receive 600 mg of telbivudine or 100 mg of lamivudine once daily [30]. At week 52 and in both HBeAg-positive and HBeAg-negative patients, telbivudine was superior to lamivudine with respect to the mean reduction in the number of copies of HBV-DNA from baseline, the proportion of patients in whom HBV-DNA (by PCR) became undetectable, and development of resistance to the drug. However, rates of resistance are higher than those observed with tenofovir or entecavir. During telbivudine treatment, non-detectable serum HBV-DNA at treatment week 24 is the strongest predictor for optimal outcomes at 2 years [31].

Tenofovir

Tenofovir disoproxil fumarate, differs from adefovir only by the presence of one methyl group. It was approved for treatment of HIV in 2002 and HBV in 2008. The two substances were compared in two multicenter, randomized, double-blind phase III clinical trials, evaluating the safety and efficacy of 300 mg tenofovir versus 10 mg adefovir at 48 weeks in HBeAg-positive (n = 266) and HBeAg-negative (n = 375) chronic hepatitis B subjects [32]. In HBeAg-positive chronic hepatitis B patients, tenofovir clearly demonstrated superior efficacy to adefovir through 48 weeks, as illustrated by the higher percentage of undetectable HBV-DNA levels (74% vs 12%) and normalization of alanine aminotransferase levels (69% vs 54%). Interestingly, HBsAg loss was observed in 3% of patients after 48 weeks of tenofovir therapy. In HBeAg-negative chronic hepatitis B patients, viral suppression occurred in more HBeAg-negative patients receiving tenofovir than in those receiving adefovir l (93% vs 63%, p <0.001). Tenofovir showed a higher antiviral efficacy than adefovir after 48 weeks of therapy. Furthermore, no resistance was observed in both HBeAg-positive and HBeAg-negative chronic hepatitis B patients after 48 weeks of therapy.

Selection of patients for treatment

The decision to treat or not to treat patients with chronic hepatitis B is mainly based on the **severity of the liver disease** [3]. It is generally recommended to treat patients with chronic hepatitis B with elevated ALT levels and significant HBV replication. The cut-off of ALT and HBV-DNA levels for therapy are not well determined. However, patients with ALT levels higher than three times the upper limit of normal and HBV-DNA levels higher than 2000 IU/mL are considered candidates for therapy. However, chronic hepatitis B is a heterogeneous disease with fluctuations over time and the correlation between serum ALT levels or serum HBV-DNA levels and the severity of liver disease is not good. Therefore, a liver biopsy is often useful to determine the grade of necroinflammation and the stage of fibrosis, and to help determine treatment candidacy.

In patients with mild liver disease, treatment is not recommended, unless liver fibrosis progresses. It should be remembered that the best way to reduce the number of patients developing antiviral resistance is to select the right patients for treatment, i.e., those with active liver disease with relatively moderate levels of viral replication who have a good chance of responding well to therapy and a low risk of developing resistance.

Pegylated interferon monotherapy should be considered in patients without contraindications since this treatment is not associated with resistance and gives the best sustained response rate (about one-fourth after PEG-IFN therapy) with a predefined duration (48 weeks) of therapy. However, most patients with chronic hepatitis B do not develop a sustained response and therefore need prolonged therapy with an analog. During treatment with an analog, the importance of good compliance and careful monitoring (measurement of HBV-DNA levels at least every 3 months) should be emphasized. Indeed, patients with HBV-DNA levels above 200 IU/mL after 6 months of therapy are at high risk of developing resistance. Early detection of resistance allows for the adjustment of therapy by introducing a drug that will prevent a flare up of hepatitis.

In summary, treatment for chronic hepatitis B over the years has improved for both HBeAg-positive (Figure 80.3) and HBeAg-negative (Figure 80.4) chronic hepatitis B patients, with decreasing rates of antiviral resistance with the new analogs (entecavir and tenofovir) (Figure 80.5).

SOURCES OF INFORMATION FOR PATIENTS AND DOCTORS

http://www.ncbi.nlm.nih.gov/pubmedhealth/PMH0001324/
   digestive.niddk.nih.gov/ddiseases/pubs/hepb_ez/
World Health Organization Hepatitis Fact Sheet. WHO/204
http://www.who.int/inf-fs/fact204.html
EASL Clinical Practice Guidelines
J Hepatol. 2009;50:227–242.
Hepatitis B Foundation
www.hepb.org
World Hepatitis Alliance
worldhepatitisalliance.org

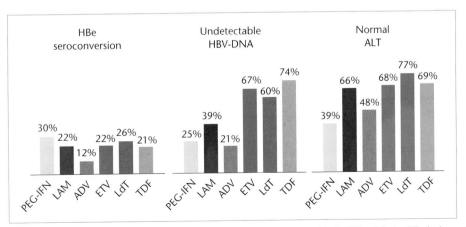

Figure 80.3 Results of antiviral drug monotherapy in the treatment of HBeAg-positive chronic hepatitis B. ADV, adefovir; ALT, alanine aminotransferase; ETV, entecavir; LAM, lamivudine; LdT, telbivudine; PEG-IFN, pegylated interferon-α; TDF, tenofovir.

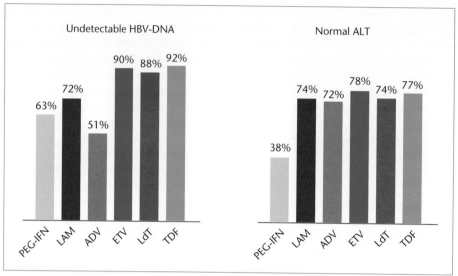

Figures 80.4 Results of antiviral drug monotherapy in the treatment of HBeAg-negative chronic hepatitis B. ADV, adefovir; ALT, alanine aminotransferase; ETV, entecavir; LAM, lamivudine; LdT, telbivudine; PEG-IFN, pegylated interferon-α; TDF, tenofovir.

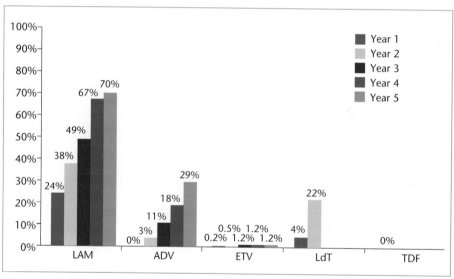

Figure 80.5 Rates of antiviral resistance for lamivudine (LAM), adefovir (ADV), entecavir (ETV), telbivudine (LdT) and tenofovir (TDF) therapy of chronic hepatitis B.

References

1. World Health Organization. Hepatitis Fact Sheet. WHO/204; Revised October 2000. Available at: http://www.who.int/inf-fs/fact204.html (accessed September 23, 2005).

2. Marcellin P. Hepatitis B and hepatitis C in 2009. *Liver Int.* 2009;29 (Suppl 1):1–8.

3. EASL Clinical Practice Guidelines: Management of chronic hepatitis B. *J Hepatol.* 2008;50:227–242.

4. Brown RE, De Cock E, Colin X, *et al.* Hepatitis B management cost in France, Italy, Spain and the United Kingdom. *J Clin Gastroenterol.* 2004;38:S169–S174.

5. Lavanchy D. Hepatitis B virus epidemiology, disease burden, treatment, and current and emerging prevention and control measures. *J Viral Hepatol* 2004;11:97–101.

6. Zarski JP, Marcellin P, Leroy V, *et al.* Characteristics of patients with chronic hepatitis B in France: predominant frequency of HBe antigen negative cases. *J Hepatol.* 2006;45:355–360.

7. Fattivich G, Stroffolini T, Zagni I, *et al.* Hepatocellular carcinoma in cirrhosis: incidence and risk factors. *Gastroenterology.* 2004;127 (Suppl. 1):S35–50.

8. Bruix J, Sherman M, Llovet JM, *et al.* EASL Panel of Experts on HCC. Clinical management of hepatocellular carcinoma. Conclusions of the Barcelona-2000 EASL conference. European Association for the Study of the Liver. *J Hepatol.* 2001;35: 421–430.

9. Chen CJ, Yank HI, Su J, *et al.* Risk of hepatocellular carcinoma across a biological gradient of serum hepatitis B virus DNA level. *JAMA.* 2006;295:65–73.

10. Marcellin P, Pequignot F, Delarocque-Astagneau E, *et al.* Mortality Related to Chronic Hepatitis B and Chronic Hepatitis C in France: Evidence for the role of HIV coinfection and alcohol consumption. *J Hepatol.* 2008;48:183–184.

11. Marcellin P, Asselah T, Boyer N. Treatment of chronic hepatitis B. *J Viral Hepatol.* 2005;12:333–345.

12. Wong DKH, Cheung AM, O'Rourke K, *et al.* Effect of alpha-interferon treatment in patients with hepatitis B e antigen-positive chronic hepatitis B. *Ann Intern Med.* 1993;119:312–323.

13. Lau GK, Piratvisuth T, Luo KX, *et al.* Peginterferon Alfa-2a, lamivudine, and the combination for HBeAg-positive chronic hepatitis B. *N Engl J Med.* 2005;352:2682–2895.

14. Marcellin P, Lau GK, Bonino F, *et al.* Peginterferon alfa-2a alone, lamivudine alone, and the two in combination in patients with HBeAg-negative chronic hepatitis B. *N Engl J Med.* 2004;351: 1206–1217.

15. Marcellin P, Bonino F, Lau GK, *et al.* Sustained response of hepatitis B e antigen-negative patients 3 years after treatment with peginterferon alpha-2a. *Gastroenterology.* 2009;136:2169–2179. e1–4.

16. Lau CL, Chien RW, Leung NWY, *et al.* Lamivudine Study Group. A one year trial of lamivudine for chronic hepatitis B. *N Engl J Med.* 1998;339:61–68.

17. Liaw YF, Sung JJ, Chow WC, *et al.* Lamivudine for patients with chronic hepatitis B and advanced liver disease. *N Engl J Med.* 2004;351:1521–1531.

18. Yuen MF, Fong DY, Wong DK, *et al.* Hepatitis B virus DNA levels at week 4 of lamivudine treatment predict the 5-year ideal response. *Hepatology.* 2007;46:1695–1703.

19. Marcellin P, Chang TT, Lim SG, *et al.* Adefovir dipivoxil for the treatment of hepatitis B e antigen-positive chronic hepatitis B. *N Engl J Med.* 2003;348:808–816.

20. Marcellin P, Chang TT, Lim SG, *et al.* Long-term efficacy and safety of adefovir dipivoxil for the treatment of hepatitis B e antigen-positive chronic hepatitis B. *Hepatology.* 2008;48:750–758.

21. Hadziyannis SJ, Tassopoulos NC, Heathcote EJ, *et al.* Long-term therapy with adefovir dipivoxil for HBeAg-negative chronic hepatitis B. *N Engl J Med.* 2005;352:2673–2681.

22. Hadziyannis SJ, Tassopoulos NC, Heathcote EJ *et al.* Long-term therapy with adefovir dipivoxil for HBeAg-negative chronic hepatitis B for up to 5 years. *Gastroenterology.* 2006;131:1743–1751.

23. Marcellin P, Asselah T. Resistance to adefovir: a new challenge in the treatment of chronic hepatitis B. *J Hepatol.* 2005;43: 920–923.

24. Schiff ER, Lai C-L, Hadziyannis S, *et al.* Adefovir dipivoxil therapy for lamivudine-resistant hepatitis B in pre and post-liver transplantation patients. *Hepatology.* 2003;38:1419–1427.

25. Benhamou Y, BOchet M, Thibault V, *et al.* Safety and efficacy of adefovir dipivoxil in patients co-infected with HIV-1 and lamivudine-resistant hepatitis B virus: an open-label pilot study. *Lancet.* 2001;358:718–723.

26. Lai CL, Shouval D, Lok AS, *et al.* Entecavir versus lamivudine for patients with HBeAg-negative chronic hepatitis B. *N Engl J Med.* 2006;354:1011–1120. Erratum in: *N Engl J Med.* 2006; 354:1863.

27. Chang TT, Gish RF, De Man R, *et al.* A comparison of entecavir and lamivudine for HBeAg-positive chronic hepatitis B. *N Engl J Med.* 2006;354:1001–1010.

28. Tenney DJ, Rose RE, Baldick CJ, *et al.* Long-term monitoring shows hepatitis B virus resistance to entecavir in nucleoside-naïve patients is rare through 5 years of therapy. *Hepatology.* 2009;49:1503–1514.

29. Sherman M, Yurdaydin C, Simsek H, *et al.* Entecavir therapy for lamivudine-refractory chronic hepatitis B: improved virologic, biochemical, and serology outcomes through 96 weeks. *Hepatology.* 2008;48:99–108.

30. Lai CL, Gane E, Liaw YF, *et al.* Telbivudine versus lamivudine in patients with chronic hepatitis B. *N Engl J Med.* 2007;357: 2576–2588.

31. Zeusem S, Gane E, Liaw YF, *et al.* Baseline characteristics and early on-treatment response predict the outcomes of 2 years of telbivudine treatment of chronic hepatitis B. *J Hepatol.* 2009;51: 11–20.

32. Marcellin P, Heathcote EJ, Buti M, *et al.* Tenofovir disoproxil fumarate versus adefovir dipivoxil for chronic hepatitis B. *N Engl J Med.* 2008;359:2442–2455.

Liver Disease

CHAPTER 81

Chronic viral hepatitis C

Xavier Forns and Jose M. Sánchez-Tapias

Hospital Clinic, CIBERehd, IDIBAPS, Barcelona, Spain

ESSENTIAL FACTS ABOUT PATHOGENESIS

- The hepatitis C virus (HCV) is an RNA virus that chronically infects around 3% of the world's population
- After decades of infection, a significant number of individuals with chronic hepatitis C develop cirrhosis and hepatocellular carcinoma
- Intravenous drug abuse is the main mechanism of HCV transmission in developed countries
- Sexual transmission of HCV is uncommon but the risk increases with sexual promiscuity
- Perinatal transmission of HCV occurs mainly in babies from highly viremic mothers, particularly when co-infected with HIV
- In the absence of other risk factors, nosocomial transmission of HCV should be considered in individuals with acute hepatitis C who have undergone a healthcare-related procedure within the past 3 months

ESSENTIALS OF DIAGNOSIS

- Diagnosis is based on the detection of antibodies against several HCV proteins (anti-HCV)
- In most cases the presence of anti-HCV indicates active HCV infection, which can be confirmed by detection of HCV RNA
- Determination of serum HCV RNA is required in anti-HCV–positive patients with normal ALT levels; patients with more than one potential cause of liver disease (i.e. hemochromatosis); patients with chronic liver disease with autoimmune features; and in immunosuppressed individuals
- Determination of the HCV infecting genotype is essential for deciding the appropriate treatment schedule
- Measurement of HCV viral load is important prior to and during treatment to guide antiviral therapy in acute and chronic hepatitis C
- Liver biopsy remains the gold standard to assess the degree of liver damage. However, several non-invasive procedures have shown good diagnostic accuracy and are being increasingly used in clinical practice

ESSENTIALS OF TREATMENT

- In HCV genotype 1, pegylated interferon (PEG-IFN) plus ribavirin administered over 48 weeks leads to a sustained virological response in ~50% of cases; and in genotypes 2 or 3, over 24 in ~80% of cases
- Early assessment of viral kinetics during treatment is useful for tailoring therapy in individual patients
- Response is less frequent in patients with compensated cirrhosis. However, antiviral therapy significantly improves the outcome of cirrhotic patients who achieve a sustained virological response
- Direct antiviral drugs cause a profound inhibition of HCV replication and, in combination with PEG-IFN and ribavirin, increase the rate of the sustained virological response to up to 70% in genotype 1-infected patients

Introduction

The hepatitis C virus (HCV), a positive-strand RNA virus belonging to the Flaviviridae family, is a major cause of chronic liver disease worldwide. About 170 million people (3%) are chronically infected with HCV. The majority of persistently infected individuals develop chronic hepatitis and a significant proportion will eventually develop liver cirrhosis or hepatocellular carcinoma (HCC). In the United States, HCV is the main etiological agent of chronic liver disease (CLD). HCV-related CLD causes about 10000 deaths per year and is the leading cause of liver transplantation. Pegylated interferon (PEG-IFN) plus ribavirin therapy leads to clearance of HCV infection in at least 50% of treated patients and new antiviral agents will soon be used in combination with these agents to achieve a higher rate of clearance.

Virology

The viral genome encodes a polyprotein of approximately 3000 amino acids. The structural proteins [core, two glycoproteins (E1, E2)] constitute the amino-terminal third of the polyprotein, whereas the non-structural proteins constitute the carboxy terminal part of the polyprotein (Figure 81.1). HCV exhibits extensive genetic heterogeneity and has been classified into six major genotypes with over 100 subtypes [1]. In each infected individual, HCV circulates as a quasispecies, which is a mixture of closely related but distinct genomes. As in other RNA viruses, the lack of proofreading activity of the HCV RNA-dependent RNA polymerase introduces errors during the replication process and explains the high genetic heterogeneity of HCV. In recent years new and powerful research tools, such as subgenomic replicon models, pseudoviral particles, and cell culture of complete HCV particles, are providing relevant information about important aspects of the pathobiology of HCV, which is essential for the development of new therapeutic strategies [2].

Epidemiology

The prevalence of HCV infection varies greatly throughout the world, from <0.5% of the population in Scandinavia to >20% in Egypt. About three million people (1%) are infected in the United States [3].

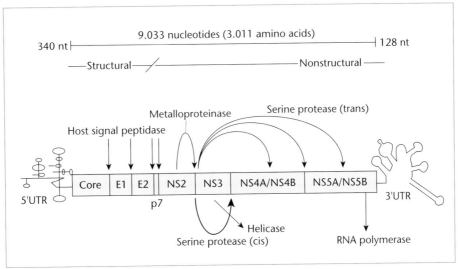

Figure 81.1 Schematic representation of the structure and function of the HCV genome. (This figure was published in *Clinical Gastroenterology and Hepatology*, Wilfred M. Weinstein, Christopher J. Hawkey, Jaime Bosch, Chronic viral hepatitis C, Pages 1–7, Copyright Elsevier, 2005.)

Risk factors

Transmission through contaminated blood or blood derivatives constituted an important mechanism for the spread of the infection. However, following screening for HCV with highly sensitive anti-HCV EIA tests, the risk of transfusion-related transmission of hepatitis C fell to about 1 in 100 000 donations. Recently, implementation of HCV RNA determination in blood pools has reduced this risk to even lower rates (around 1 in 500 000 to 1 in 1 000 000 donations).

Intravenous illicit drug abuse remains an important mechanism of HCV transmission. Infection occurs mostly during the first year of drug abuse and 40–80% of all addicts are chronically infected. Nasal inhalation of cocaine may also be an important risk factor, probably related to straw sharing.

Sexual transmission is uncommon but possible. Transmission may occur when genital ulcers, hematuria or menstrual flow are present. Sexual promiscuity, either homo- or heterosexual, is associated with an increased prevalence of HCV infection. Preventive measures are recommended in high-risk settings, but not in individuals with stable partners.

Vertical or perinatal transmission occurs in about 5% of children born to infected mothers. Transmission correlates with the level of viremia and is higher (~20%) when mothers are co-infected with the human immunodeficiency virus (HIV). Widespread use of HAART seems to decrease the risk of HCV vertical transmission.

HCV transmission related to **medical procedures** (nosocomial transmission) was of great concern in hemodialysis units, but very strict adherence to universal precaution measures has virtually eradicated *de novo* HCV infection in this setting. Epidemics have been described in conventional hospital wards for hematological and liver disease patients, and among patients undergoing endoscopic or other invasive (even minimally) procedures. Lack of observance of the universal rules

or inadequate sterilization of instruments has consistently been related to HCV transmission in these circumstances. Transmission of HCV to healthcare workers through accidental needle sticks is uncommon. Transmission from an infected healthcare provider to a patient is extremely rare.

The mechanism of transmission is uncertain in a high proportion of infected individuals (10–50%, depending on the geographical area). These individuals may have been subjected to invasive medical procedures or surgery, or have received therapeutic injections or vaccinations with inadequately sterilized material. The use of non-disposable materials the less stringent medical practices in the past may explain the higher prevalence of HCV infection of unknown origin in individuals over 60 years of age.

Pathogenesis

The ability to cause chronic infection is a remarkable feature of HCV. The pathogenetic mechanism is largely unknown, but includes viral factors (**genetic variability**) and host factors (**immune response**). There is a strong and multispecific cellular immune response against HCV antigens in patients capable of clearing HCV, whereas cellular immunity against HCV appears to be weak in individuals who develop chronic infection.

Variation in the genes involved in the immune response has been recently shown to influence HCV clearance; a genome-wide association study has demonstrated that a single nucleotide polymorphism upstream of the *IL28B* gene, which encodes the type III interferon IFN-λ, is strongly associated with spontaneous viral clearance and with response to IFN-based treatment [4].

The ability of HCV to continuously evade both humoral and cellular immune responses is also a crucial factor to explain long-term persistence of this infection [4–6]. The presence of replicative virions inside hepatocytes is the leading cause of liver damage, which possibly results from a combination of immune-mediated attack against infected liver cells and a cytopathic effect of HCV.

Pathology

Liver biopsy findings vary from minimal portal inflammation with no (stage 0) or little (stages 1 and 2) fibrosis to significant necroinflammatory changes with bridging fibrosis (stage 3) and cirrhosis (stage 4). Although liver biopsy remains the gold standard to assess the degree of liver damage in chronic hepatitis C, its associated morbidity and sampling error has prompted the investigation of non-invasive methods. The combination of serum non-invasive markers and other methods (such as transient elastography) are widely used in clinical practice and avoid a significant number of liver biopsies [7].

Clinical presentation

HCV infection can result in very different clinical situations, ranging from asymptomatic hepatitis to severe forms of chronic liver disease, such as decompensated cirrhosis and HCC [8]. HCV infection can also cause extrahepatic disorders, mostly through autoimmune mechanisms.

Chronic hepatitis

Chronic hepatitis C is characterized by persistently elevated aminotransferases and the presence of HCV RNA in the serum. Serum aminotransferases remain normal for long periods of time in some patients, who usually have mild hepatic disease [9].

Most patients are asymptomatic, but some have non-specific symptoms, such as increased fatigability and/or abdominal discomfort. Besides increased aminotransferases, other laboratory abnormalities are elevated gamma-glutamyltranspeptidase, serum ferritin or gammaglobulin, or a decreased platelet count. In general, these abnormalities are associated with more advanced disease, but there is not a close correlation between the degree of biochemical abnormalities and the severity of liver damage.

Progression to cirrhosis is usually silent. A decreasing platelet count and inversion of the aspartate aminotransferase (AST)/alanine aminotransferase (ALT) ratio are indicators of progression. Patients with cirrhosis usually remain compensated for many years: after a 5-year follow-up hepatic decompensation occurs in less than 20% of patients and HCC develops in around 7% [10]. Co-infection with HIV or alcohol consumption can accelerate the progression to cirrhosis [11].

Hepatocellular carcinoma

The relationship between chronic HCV infection and HCC is well established. The strength of this association in different

Table 81.1 Extrahepatic manifestations of HCV infection

Documented associations
- Cryoglobulinemia
- Membranous proliferative glomerulonephritis
- Serum autoantibodies
- Non-Hodgkin's lymphoma
- Porphyria cutanea tarda
- Lichen planus

Probable or coincidental associations
- Hematological:
  - Monoclonal gammmopathies
  - Idiopathic thrombocytopenia
- Dermatological:
  - Erythema nodosum
  - Erythema multiforme
  - Urticaria
  - Pruritus
- Endocrine:
  - Autoimmune thyroiditis, thyroid autoantibodies
  - Diabetes mellitus
- Ocular and salivary:
  - Sjögren's syndrome
  - Corneal ulcer, uveitis
- Miscellaneous:
  - Idiopathic pulmonary fibrosis
  - Systemic lupus erythematosus
  - Guillain–Barré syndrome

parts of the world is variable, probably due to the different prevalence of other carcinogenic factors.

Pre-existent cirrhosis is almost a *sine qua non* condition for the development of HCC in chronic hepatitis C. The annual rate of appearance of HCC in European patients with compensated cirrhosis is 3%, which is lower than in Japanese patients. Male gender, age over 55 years and high alpha-fetoprotein values are closely related to the appearance of HCC. Biannual abdominal ultrasonography is the best method to screen patients with cirrhosis for early detection of HCC [12].

Extrahepatic manifestations

Several extrahepatic disorders have been related to HCV infection [13] (Table 81.1). The association between HCV infection and mixed cryoglobulinemia is particularly evident, as indicated by the 90% prevalence of anti-HCV in patients with mixed cryoglobulinemia, the identification of HCV RNA in the cryoprecipitate, and the good response, at least initially, to IFN therapy. Cryoglobulins are detected in about 30% of patients with chronic hepatitis C, but symptoms related to cryoglobulinemia (rashes, arthritis, glomerulonephritis) are relatively rare.

Diagnostic methods

The diagnosis of hepatitis C is based on the detection of specific antibodies and of the viral genome.

Anti-HCV testing

Highly sensitive and specific enzyme immunoassays (EIAs) are available for the identification of antibodies against HCV antigens. Anti-HCV can be detected by EIA as early as 3–6 weeks after infection and is useful for the diagnosis of acute hepatitis. Strongly positive reactions are found in patients with chronic infection. False-negative results can occur in immuno-suppressed patients (HIV infection, patients on hemodialysis), whereas false-positive results are rare (<5% in low-risk populations such as volunteer blood donors).

Detection and measurement of HCV RNA

HCV RNA can be studied in serum, liver tissue, peripheral blood lymphocytes or other specimens by molecular biology techniques. In clinical practice, only qualitative or quantitative serum HCV RNA is determined using different assays.

For diagnostic purposes, the region amplified belongs to the well-conserved 5′ non-coding region of the viral genome. Commercial polymerase chain reaction (PCR) kits are available for the qualitative determination of HCV RNA using semi-automatic analyzers. These kits are reproducible and offer excellent sensitivity (around 50 IU/mL of HCV RNA). HCV RNA viral load can be determined using fully automated competitive quantitative PCR-based assays, which have a linear range between 10^3 and 10^6 IU/mL. Serum HCV RNA can also be quantified by signal amplification through hybridization of amplified HCV cDNA to branched DNA probes. In recent years commercially available automated real-time PCR and improved signal amplification procedures with a linear range of quantification between 10–15 IU/mL to 10^7–18^8 IU/mL have replaced other diagnostic tests [14,15].

Determination of serum HCV RNA is required in many situations: anti-HCV positive patients with normal ALT levels; patients with more than one potential cause of liver disease (i.e., hemochromatosis); chronic liver disease with autoimmune features; immunosuppressed individuals. Measurement of HCV viral load prior to, during, and after treatment is now essential to guide antiviral therapy in acute and chronic hepatitis C.

HCV genotype

Direct sequencing of specific genomic regions is the gold standard for HCV genotyping. However, simpler techniques, such as hybridization of amplified HCV cDNA on immobilized genotype-specific DNA probes, are commercially available and are reliable for clinical or epidemiological studies [14].

IL28B genotyping

As stated above, a single nucleotide polymorphism upstream of the *IL28B* gene (encoding IFN-λ3) is the strongest baseline predictor of a sustained virological response (SVR) in genotype 1 infected patients [4]. Determination of this polymorphism will soon become part of our clinical practice in patients treated with standard of care (PEG-IFN plus ribavirin).

Treatment

The current treatment of hepatitis C is based on alpha-interferon (IFN-α) and ribavirin, a nucleoside analog. According to the type of response, patients are classified as:

- **Sustained virological responders** – clearance of HCV RNA that persists for 6 months after treatment discontinuation
- **Transient responders or relapsers** – clearance of HCV RNA during treatment, followed by the reappearance of viral RNA after treatment is discontinued
- **Non-responders** – persistence of HCV RNA during treatment.

In recent years several concepts based on HCV RNA kinetics during treatment are widely used to guide therapeutic decisions during treatment. These include:

- **Rapid virological response** – clearance of HCV RNA at week 4 of treatment
- **Early virological response** – a decrease in serum HCV RNA by more than 2 $\log_{10}$ at week 12 with respect to baseline viremia
- **Slow virological response** – HCV RNA still detectable at week 12 but undetectable at week 24 of treatment.

Treatment of chronic hepatitis C is an important health problem that has not been solved satisfactorily. The mid- and long-term prognosis of hepatitis C is not necessarily unfavorable and the current available therapies have numerous side effects, may not be effective, and are very expensive. For these reasons, the decision as to whether or not to treat may be difficult and must be taken on a case-by-case basis. In general, therapy may be deferred in patients with mild chronic hepatitis and low probability of response. In contrast, treatment is indicated in patients with more advanced disease.

Interferon and ribavirin

Currently the treatment for chronic hepatitis C is based on the administration of PEG-IFN plus ribavirin. PEG-IFN is a pharmaceutical form of IFN obtained through the binding of IFN-α to one or multiple polyethylene glycol molecules, thereby delaying its clearance and increasing its efficacy. PEG-IFN administered once a week achieves a slow decline of IFN plasma levels, avoiding the extreme fluctuations that occur with the thrice weekly administration of non-pegylated IFN.

Two large international multicenter clinical trials showed that PEG-IFN (either α 2a or α 2b) plus ribavirin combination therapy increases the rate of SVR compared to standard IFN plus ribavirin (Table 81.2) [16,17]. Therefore, PEG-IFN and ribavirin became the standard treatment for chronic hepatitis C. The response rate in patients infected with HCV genotype 2 or 3 was greater than in those infected with HCV genotype 1 or 4. Subsequently, another large controlled trial showed that 48 weeks of combined therapy are necessary for optimal results in most HVC genotype 1 infected patients, whereas 24

Table 81.2 Sustained virological response rates observed in two large multicenter trials of interferon-ribavirin combination in chronic hepatitis C. Standard interferon-α 2b versus pegylated interferon-α 2b were compared in the first study [16]; pegylated interferon-α 2a as monotherapy or in combination with ribavirin in comparison with standard Interferon-α 2b plus ribavirin combination therapy were compared in the second study [17].

	Weeks on therapy	Number of cases	Sustained virological response (%)		
			Overall	Genotype 1	Genotype 2 or 3
Manns *et al.* [16]					
IFN-α 2b (3 MU, t.i.w.)	48				
Ribavirin (1–1.2 g/day)	48	505	47	34	79
PEG-IFN-α 2b:					
1.5 µg/kg/week	4				
0.5 mg/kg/week	44				
Ribavirin (1–1.2 g/day)	48	514	47	33	80
PEG-IFN-α 2b:					
1.5 µg/kg/week	48				
Ribavirin (0.8 g/day)	48	511	54	42	82
Fried *et al.* [17]					
IFN-α 2b (3 MU, t.i.w.)	48				
Ribavirin (1–1.2 g/day)	48	444	44	36	61
PEG-IFN-α 2a (180 µg/week)	48				
Placebo	48	224	29	21	45
PEG-IFN α-2a (180 µg/w)	48				
Ribavirin (1–1.2 g/day)	48	453	56	46	76

weeks of treatment with a reduced ribavirin dosing is sufficient in patients infected with HCV genotype 2 or 3 [18]. (Refer to the accompanying didactic treatment protocol on the website for specific doses.)

Further refinement of anti-HCV therapy is emerging from a number of studies that take into account the influence of viral kinetics early in therapy on final virological response [19]. It is now well established that SVR is virtually nil in patients who do not achieve an early virological response by week 12 of treatment. Thus, treatment withdrawal is recommended in this circumstance. Patients with a rapid virological response (i.e. clearance at week 4), are most likely to achieve response SVR and may benefit from a reduced duration of therapy (24 weeks for genotype 1, 12–16 weeks for genotypes 2 and 3), particularly in the presence of low viremia at baseline. Patients with genotype 1 who present a slow virological response may benefit from extending the duration of treatment up to 72 weeks.

Side effects

Administration of IFN frequently causes one or several side effects that often make therapy unpleasant (Table 81.3). In general young patients tolerate treatment better than older individuals, although there is a marked individual variability regarding the incidence, type, and intensity of side effects. Severe side effects are very uncommon, but may be serious and/or irreversible.

The most significant side effect of ribavirin is **hemolytic anemia**, which is reversible but occurs in the majority of patients. The severity of anemia varies significantly among different individuals. Dose reduction is often necessary to increase hemoglobin concentration but ribavirin withdrawal is rarely needed. In selected cases, such as those with symptomatic anemia, it may be helpful to use erythropoietin. Ribavirin-induced hemolysis may be a concern when planning therapy in patients with chronic anemia, such as those on hemodialysis, or in patients with heart disease. Ribavirin is

Table 81.3 Side effects of therapy in patients with chronic hepatitis C

Related to interferon
- Common but usually mild:
  - Flu-like symptoms: fever, headache, rigors, joint pain, muscle ache
  - Constitutional: tiredness, poor appetite, loss of weight, impotence
  - Neuropsychiatric: insomnia, mild depression, impaired concentration, irritability, bad mood
  - Digestive: nausea, diarrhea
  - Cutaneous: exanthema, loss of hair, reaction at injection site
  - Hematological: neutropenia, thrombocytopenia
  - Biochemical: hypertriglyceridemia
- Uncommon or rare but serious:
  - Neuropsychiatric: major depression, suicidal ideation, psychosis, delirium, confusion, convulsions, ataxia, extrapyramidal alterations
  - Immunological: thyroid disease, psoriasis, sarcoidosis, interstitial pneumonitis, hemolytic anemia, exacerbation of other autoimmune disorders
  - Miscellaneous: retinopathy, bone marrow aplasia, diabetes mellitus

Related to ribavirin
- Hemolytic anemia
- Cough
- Digestive intolerance
- Hyperuricemia
- Potential teratogenicity

teratogenic and contraception is recommended in both men and women undergoing therapy.

Patients who failed previous antiviral therapy

Patients who do not achieve a SVR following a course of antiviral therapy form a highly heterogeneous and difficult-to-cure population. This category includes patients with inherent resistance to IFN and those in whom HCV is suppressed but only while on therapy (relapsers), those who failed IFN monotherapy or combination therapy with or without PEG-IFN, as well those who, for a number of reasons, did not adequately complete the recommended treatment in terms of dose and duration. Overall the efficacy of re-treating these patients with PEG-IFN plus ribavirin is limited, but selected patients may achieve response SVR when re-treated. Again, genotype is an important predictor of response to re-treatment.

Decision to re-treat requires information about what treatment was initially used (IFN monotherapy, combination therapy with IFN or PEG-IFN), the type of virological response (slow response, relapse or no response; see above), as well as awareness of other factors involved in previous treatment failure (insufficient doses, insufficient duration, non-compliance) [20]. Patients with maximal likelihood (around 40%) of responding to re-treatment are those who relapsed after a short course of IFN monotherapy, and, at the other end of the spectrum, true virological non-responders to PEG-IFN plus ribavirin combination have a low chance (around 10%) of responding to a second course of therapy. The rate of SVR may be slightly increased by extending re-treatment duration to 72 weeks.

Maintenance therapy

Several studies suggest that, despite the absence of virological response, IFN therapy may prevent the worsening of hepatic fibrosis and reduce portal hypertension. The possible clinical efficacy of long-term interferon therapy, at reduced doses, in patients with advanced hepatic fibrosis or cirrhosis is being explored in several large controlled studies. So far, a clear benefit from maintenance interferon therapy has not been demonstrated for most patients [21], although a benefit in selected cases cannot yet be disregarded.

Chronic hepatitis C in special situations

The indication for therapy in patients with persistently **normal aminotransferases** is unclear, since the risk of diseases progression appears to be low in these cases. Response rates, however, are comparable to those achieved in patient with elevated aminotransferases [22].

Treatment with PEG-IFN plus ribavirin achieves a SVR in approximately one-third of the patients with **compensated cirrhosis**, but the rate of response is higher in patients infected with genotypes 2 and 3. In cirrhotic patients SVR is associated with a decreased incidence of clinical decompensation and improved survival, but does not definitively prevent the development of HCC [23].

Chronic hepatitis C follows an accelerated course in **HIV-infected patients**. An increase in mortality and morbidity from HCV-related liver disease is being recognized among co-infected patients, in whom HIV infection is under control following antiretroviral therapy. Treatment of hepatitis C in co-infected individuals can be administered following the same criteria established for HIV-negative patients. However, current data suggest that the efficacy of therapy is lower and side effects are more frequent in co-infected individuals. In addition, drug toxicity requires close monitoring, particularly in individuals receiving antiretroviral therapy [24].

Future therapies

Development of new therapies for hepatitis C is one of the most active areas of research in hepatology. New IFNs, ribavirin-like compounds, direct antiviral agents, immunomodulators, and other agents are currently under investigation [25]. Drugs specifically targeting either the HCV protease (such as telaprevir and boceprevir) or polymerase act as potent inhibitors of HCV replication and will be introduced in clinical practice in 2011. Studies on the new direct antiviral agents, telaprevir and boceprevir [26,27] indicate that the addition of these drugs to PEG-IFN and ribavirin will increase SVR rates by up to 70% in genotype 1 patients and will allow the duration of therapy to be shorter in a significant proportion of patients (Table 81.4). However, due to the rapid emergence of viral strains resistant to direct antivirals, PEG-IFN and, possibly, ribavirin will likely remain part of the anti-HCV therapy for a few years. Interferon-free regimens using direct acting antivirals have already shown efficacy in small cohorts of

Table 81.4 Sustained virological response (SVR) rate observed in genotype 1 naïve patients in two studies evaluating the protease inhibitors telaprevir and boceprevir in combination with pegylated interferon plus ribavirin

	Weeks on therapy	Number of cases	Overall SVR (%)
Hezode *et al.* [28]			
PEG-IFN-α 2a (180 µg/week)	48		
Ribavirin (1–1.2 g/day)	48	82	46
PEG-IFN-α 2a (180 µg/week)	24		
Ribavirin (1–1.2 g/day)	24		
Telaprevir (750 mg/8 h)	12	81	69
PEG-IFN-α 2a (180 µg/week)	12		
Ribavirin (1–1.2 g/day)	12		
Telaprevir (750 mg/8 h)	12	82	60
PEG-IFN-α 2a (180 µg/week)	12		
Telaprevir (750 mg/8 h)	12	78	36
Kwo *et al.* [29]			
PEG-IFN-α 2b (1.5 µg/kg/week)	48		
Ribavirin (1–1.2 g/day)	48	104	36
PEG-IFN-α 2a (1.5 µg/kg/week)	4 + 24		
Ribavirin (1–1.2 g/day)	4 + 24		
Boceprevir (800 mg/8 h)	24	103	56
PEG-IFN-α 2a (1.5 µg/kg/week)	4 + 44		
Ribavirin (1–1.2 g/day)	4 + 44		
Boceprevir (800 mg/8 h)	44	103	75
PEG-IFN-α 2a (1.5 µg/kg/week)	28		
Ribavirin (1–1.2 g/day)	28		
Boceprevir (800 mg/8 h)	28	107	54
PEG-IFN-α 2a (1.5 µg/kg/week)	48		
Ribavirin (1–1.2 g/day)	48		
Boceprevir (800 mg/8 h)	48	103	67

treated patients and will probably replace current treatments in 5–10 years from now.

Prognosis without treatment

Data on the natural history of HCV chronic infection are somewhat contradictory [9]. Studies following patients from the onset of infection suggested that HCV infection is a relatively benign disease. After 20 years of follow-up most patients remain asymptomatic and the incidence of clinically relevant events (cirrhosis, hepatic decompensation, HCC) appears to be low [30]. In contrast, studies evaluating the long-term outcome of patients in whom a diagnosis of chronic hepatitis has already been established suggest that after two decades of follow-up, a significant proportion of patients (20–30%) develop cirrhosis [31]. Most likely, these studies indicate that progression to cirrhosis is a late event which probably requires three, four, or more decades of persistent infection.

Fibrosis progression is not uniform in all patients, and fast progressors (cirrhosis developing in fewer than 20 years after infection), intermediate progressors (cirrhosis appearing between 20 and 50 years after infection), and slow or minimal progressors (cirrhosis development more than 50 years after infection or never occurring) have been recognized [32]. Excessive alcohol consumption, older age at the time of infection, male gender, and the presence of the metabolic syndrome have been recognized as the main factors associated with faster progression of fibrosis in patients with chronic HCV [33].

SOURCES OF INFORMATION FOR PATIENTS AND DOCTORS

Websites from patient associations and booklets edited by official organizations offer detailed information on clinical aspects of the disease, life-style recommendations, and treatment options.

http://hepatitis.va.gov/vahep?page=pt-home

References

1. Simmonds P, Bukh J, Combet C, *et al.* Consensus proposals for a unified system of nomenclature of hepatitis C virus genotypes. *Hepatology.* 2005;42:962–973.
2. Gottwein JM, Bukh J. Cutting the gordian knot – development and biological relevance of hepatitis C virus cell culture systems. *Adv Virus Res.* 2008;71:51–133.
3. Shepard CW, Finelli L, Alter MJ. Global epidemiology of hepatitis C virus infection. *Lancet Infect Dis.* 2005;5:558–567.
4. Ge D, Fellay J, Thompson AJ, *et al.* Genetic variation in IL28B predicts hepatitis C treatment-induced viral clearance. *Nature* 2009;461:399–401.
5. Rehermann B. Chronic infections with hepatotropic viruses: mechanisms of impairment of cellular immune responses. *Semin Liver Dis.* 2007;27:152–160.
6. von HT, Yoon JC, Alter H, *et al.* Hepatitis C virus continuously escapes from neutralizing antibody and T-cell responses during chronic infection in vivo. *Gastroenterology.* 2007;132:667–678.

Liver Disease

7. Castera L, Forns X, Alberti A. Non-invasive evaluation of liver fibrosis using transient elastography. *J Hepatol*. 2008;48:835–847.

8. Hoofnagle JH. Course and outcome of hepatitis C. *Hepatology*. 2002;36(5 Suppl 1):S21–S29.

9. Seeff LB. Natural history of hepatitis C. *Am J Med*. 1999;107(6B):10S–15S.

10. Sangiovanni A, Prati GM, Fasani P, et al. The natural history of compensated cirrhosis due to hepatitis C virus: A 17-year cohort study of 214 patients. *Hepatology*. 2006;43:1303–1310.

11. Missiha SB, Ostrowski M, Heathcote EJ. Disease progression in chronic hepatitis C: modifiable and nonmodifiable factors. *Gastroenterology*. 2008;134:1699–1714.

12. Bruix J, Sherman M. Management of hepatocellular carcinoma. *Hepatology*. 2005;42:1208–1236.

13. Ramos-Casals M, Font J. Extrahepatic manifestations in patients with chronic hepatitis C virus infection. *Curr Opin Rheumatol*. 2005;17:447–455.

14. Forns X, Costa J. HCV virological assessment. *J Hepatol*. 2006;44(1 Suppl):S35–S39.

15. Vermehren J, Kau A, Gartner BC, Gobel R, Zeuzem S, Sarrazin C. Differences between two real-time PCR-based hepatitis C virus (HCV) assays (RealTime HCV and Cobas AmpliPrep/Cobas TaqMan) and one signal amplification assay (Versant HCV RNA 3.0) for RNA detection and quantification. *J Clin Microbiol*. 2008;46:3880–3891.

16. Manns MP, McHutchison JG, Gordon SC, et al. Peginterferon alfa-2b plus ribavirin compared with interferon alfa-2b plus ribavirin for initial treatment of chronic hepatitis C: a randomised trial. *Lancet*. 2001;358:958–965.

17. Fried MW, Shiffman M, Reddy KR, et al. Peginterferon alfa-2a plus ribavirin for chronic hepatitis C virus infection. *N Engl J Med*. 2002;347:975–982.

18. Hadziyannis SJ, Sette H Jr, Morgan TR, et al. Peginterferon-alpha2a and ribavirin combination therapy in chronic hepatitis C: a randomized study of treatment duration and ribavirin dose. *Ann Intern Med*. 2004;140:346–355.

19. Zeuzem S, Berg T, Moeller B, et al. Expert opinion on the treatment of patients with chronic hepatitis C. *J Viral Hepat*. 2009;16:75–90.

20. Thomas E, Fried MW. Hepatitis C: current options for nonresponders to peginterferon and ribavirin. *Curr Gastroenterol Rep*. 2008;10:53–59.

21. Di Bisceglie AM, Shiffman ML, Everson GT, et al. Prolonged therapy of advanced chronic hepatitis C with low-dose peginterferon. *N Engl J Med*. 2008;359:2429–2441.

22. Zeuzem S, Diago M, Gane E, et al. Peginterferon alfa-2a (40 kilodaltons) and ribavirin in patients with chronic hepatitis C and normal aminotransferase levels. *Gastroenterology* 2004;127:1724–1732.

23. Bruno S, Stroffolini T, Colombo M, et al. Sustained virological response to interferon-alpha is associated with improved outcome in HCV-related cirrhosis: a retrospective study. *Hepatology* 2007;45:579–587.

24. Soriano V, Barreiro P, Martin-Carbonero L, et al. Update on the treatment of chronic hepatitis C in HIV-infected patients. *AIDS Rev*. 2007;9:99–113.

25. Thompson A, Patel K, Tillman H, McHutchison JG. Directly acting antivirals for the treatment of patients with hepatitis C infection: a clinical development update addressing key future challenges. *J Hepatol*. 2009;50:184–194.

26. Jacobson IM, McHutchison JG, Dusheiko GM, et al. Telaprevir for previously untreated chronic hepatitis C virus infection. *N Engl J Med*. 2011;364:2405–2416.

27. Poordad F, McCone J, Bacon BR, et al. Boceprevir for untreated chronic HCV genotype 1 infection. *N Engl J Med*. 2011;364:1195–1206.

28. Hezode C, Forestier N, Dusheiko G, et al. Telaprevir and peginterferon with or without ribavirin for chronic HCV infection. *N Engl J Med*. 2009;360:1839–1850.

29. Kwo PY, Lawitz EJ, McCone J, et al. Efficacy of boceprevir, an NS3 protease inhibitor, in combination with peginterferon alfa-2b and ribavirin in treatment-naive patients with genotype 1 hepatitis C infection (SPRINT-1): an open-label, randomised, multicentre phase 2 trial. *Lancet*. 2010;376:705–716.

30. Kenny-Walsh E. Clinical outcomes after hepatitis C infection from contaminated anti-D immune globulin. Irish Hepatology Research Group. *N Engl J Med*. 1999;340:1228–1233.

31. Forns X, Ampurdanes S, Sanchez-Tapias JM, et al. Long-term follow-up of chronic hepatitis C in patients diagnosed at a tertiary-care center. *J Hepatol*. 2001;35:265–271.

32. Poynard T, Bedossa P, Opolon P. Natural history of liver fibrosis progression in patients with chronic hepatitis C. The OBSVIRC, METAVIR, CLINIVIR, and DOSVIRC groups. *Lancet*. 1997;349:825–832.

33. Missiha SB, Ostrowski M, Heathcote EJ. Disease progression in chronic hepatitis C: modifiable and nonmodifiable factors. *Gastroenterology*. 2008;134:1699–1714.

CHAPTER 82

Chronic viral hepatitis D

Patrizia Farci[1] and Maria Eliana Lai[2]

[1]National Institute of Allergy and Infectious Diseases, National Institutes of Health, Bethesda, MD, USA
[2]University of Cagliari, Policlinico Universitario, Monserrato, Cagliari, Italy

ESSENTIAL FACTS ABOUT PATHOGENESIS

- Caused by persistent infection with HDV, a defective RNA virus that requires the helper function of HBV
- HDV is acquired by co-infection with HBV or by superinfection of an HBsAg carrier
- Fifteen million HBsAg carriers are co-infected with HDV worldwide
- Better control of HBV has led to a dramatic decline in the prevalence of HDV
- Immigration from endemic areas is causing a resurgence of HDV in Europe
- Pathogenesis is unknown, although evidence suggests that the liver damage is immunologically mediated

ESSENTIALS OF DIAGNOSIS

- Clinical presentation is variable
- Commonly asymptomatic and discovered incidentally; it may present with general symptoms or complications of cirrhosis
- Half of patients have a history of acute hepatitis that represents the time of HDV superinfection
- Serological findings: high titers of IgG and IgM antibodies to HDV are highly sensitive and specific. Most patients are anti-HBe positive
- Virological findings: HDV RNA is positive while most patients have undetectable or low levels of HBV DNA, as measured by PCR assays
- Liver biopsy is not essential but permits the stage of fibrosis and grade of activity of chronic hepatitis D to be defined

ESSENTIALS OF TREATMENT

- Interferon is the only licensed drug. The best regimen is pegylated-IFN for at least 1 year
- Treatment should be offered to all patients with compensated HDV liver disease
- Side effects are common during interferon treatment, including psychiatric symptoms
- Medical monitoring is essential for the early detection and management of IFN side effects
- Liver transplantation is the only therapeutic choice for end-stage HDV cirrhosis
- The HBV vaccine protects naïve subjects but not HBsAg carriers from HDV superinfection

Introduction

Chronic hepatitis D is caused by persistent infection (over 6 months) with **hepatitis D (delta) virus (HDV)** [1], a defective RNA virus that requires the obligatory helper function of hepatitis B virus (HBV) for virion assembly and transmission. HDV is the smallest animal virus and the only one to possess a circular RNA genome of about 1700 nucleotides, and a single structural protein, hepatitis delta antigen (HDAg) [2]. The virion is encapsidated by the hepatitis B surface antigen (HBsAg), the only component provided by HBV. HDV does not encode its own viral polymerase but exploits the host RNA polymerase II for replication [2]. Because of its vital link with HBV, HDV infects only persons who simultaneously harbor HBV. There are essentially two modes of HDV infection: simultaneous co-infection with HBV or superinfection of an HBsAg carrier. Individuals with antibodies to HBsAg (anti-HBs), being immune to HBV, are not susceptible to HDV. HDV is a highly pathogenic virus that causes acute hepatitis, which may run to a fulminant course, and chronic liver disease. Chronic hepatitis D is the least common, but most severe form, of viral hepatitis.

Epidemiology

Transmission

HDV is transmitted through the same routes as HBV, i.e., primarily by parenteral exposure to blood or blood products either overtly or through the inapparent parenteral route involving non-sexual interpersonal contacts. Sexual transmission may occur, but HDV infection is uncommon in homosexual men. Vertical transmission is rare.

Geographical distribution

Infection with HDV has a worldwide distribution, although there is considerable geographical variation. It has been estimated that about 15 million HBsAg carriers are co-infected with HDV in the world. The prevalence is higher in South America, South Pacific islands, West Africa, the Mediterranean basin, the Middle East, and Central Asia than in Northern

---

Textbook of Clinical Gastroenterology and Hepatology, Second Edition. Edited by C. J. Hawkey, Jaime Bosch, Joel E. Richter, Guadalupe Garcia-Tsao, Francis K. L. Chan.
© 2012 Blackwell Publishing Ltd. Published 2012 by Blackwell Publishing Ltd.

Europe and North America, where infection is mainly confined to intravenous drug users [2]. Over the past two decades, there has been a significant decline in the prevalence of HDV infection along with HBV in developed countries, most likely as the result of HBV vaccination programs, better hygiene, and universal precautions for the control of the acquired immune deficiency syndrome (AIDS). However, immigration from areas where HDV is endemic is posing a new threat for HDV resurgence in Europe. In Germany, Italy, France, and England the prevalence of HDV infection has not further decreased since the late 1990s [3].

HDV genotypes

Eight HDV genotypes have been identified. They differ in their global distribution and by as much as 40% in their nucleotide sequences [2]. Genotype 1 is the most common worldwide, while the others appear to be geographically more restricted. Genotypes 2 and 4 are found mostly in the Far East and genotype 3 exclusively in the Northern part of South America, whereas the most recently identified genotypes, 5, 6, 7, and 8, have been detected in West and Central Africa [4].

Causes and pathogenesis

The mechanism whereby HDV infection induces liver damage remains poorly understood, although there is evidence that it is **immunologically mediated** [2]. The mechanisms whereby HDV induces the most rapid form of progressive liver disease are unknown. Recently, it has been suggested that the long form of HDAg may play a role in HDV pathogenesis by inducing liver fibrosis through the regulation of transforming growth factor-β–induced signal activation [5].

Some studies have suggested that the HDV genotypes may influence disease severity. Genotypes 2 and 4 have been associated with milder forms of acute and chronic hepatitis D [6], while genotype 3 has been linked to outbreaks of fulminant hepatitis in South America [7]. By contrast, the most common genotype 1 has been associated with a broad spectrum of disease. Genotype 3 is usually associated with HBV genotype F, while a less restricted relation exists between the other HDV genotypes and the HBV genotypes [4]. Further studies are needed to determine whether differences in pathogenicity depend on biological differences among the HDV genotypes, the co-infecting HBV genotypes or the host immune responses.

Clinical presentation

Natural history

Since the HBsAg carrier state permits continuous replication of HDV, over 90% of HDV superinfected carriers develop acute hepatitis D that progresses to chronicity. Chronic hepatitis D is the least common but most severe and rapidly progressive form of **chronic hepatitis**, leading to cirrhosis in about 70–80% of cases, a risk that is almost three times higher than with HBV alone [1]. HDV cirrhosis may develop in 5–10 years

and at a younger age (one or two decades earlier) compared to HBV alone [1,8]. Once established, HDV cirrhosis may be compensated for many years, although a high proportion of patients die of **liver decompensation** or **hepatocellular carcinoma (HCC)** unless they receive liver transplantation. The mean interval between primary HDV infection and histological cirrhosis is about one decade; and for liver decompensation is about two decades [9].

The annual incidence of liver decompensation in HDV cirrhotic patients ranges from 2.6% to 3.6% and that of HCC from 2.6% to 2.8% [8,10]. The adjusted relative risk of mortality and decompensation is twice and the risk of HCC three times higher than in patients with compensated HBV cirrhosis [8]. However, in open populations in endemic areas, such as Rhodes and American Samoa, a high proportion of anti-HD–positive individuals demonstrate mild or no signs of liver disease. Differences in disease outcome could be related to viral, host, or still undefined environmental factors. A higher rate of spontaneous HBsAg clearance has been reported in HDV-positive than in HDV-negative HBV carriers [1]. However, cirrhosis decompensation, HCC or death may occur if HBsAg clearance takes place when HDV disease is advanced.

Studies of viral interaction have provided controversial data. Whereas most reports have suggested that in cases of triple infection HDV inhibits both HBV and hepatitis C virus (HCV), a few showed a dominant role of HCV. Co-infection with human immune deficiency virus (HIV) does not seem to influence the natural history of chronic hepatitis D.

Clinical features

The clinical presentation of chronic hepatitis D is variable. It may be asymptomatic and discovered incidentally, or it may present with general symptoms (fatigue, malaise, anorexia, right upper quadrant discomfort) or with the complications of cirrhosis. There are no specific clinical features, although half of patients have a history of acute hepatitis, which likely represents the time of superinfection with HDV, and many exhibit splenomegaly [1,2]. Typically, patients have persistently high serum aminotransferase levels, which tend to decrease as the disease progresses to the late stage of cirrhosis. Most patients are anti-HBe positive and have low or undetectable levels of HBV DNA as measured by polymerase chain reaction (PCR), which supports the concept that the liver damage is mainly caused by HDV [2]. Chronic hepatitis D is associated with autoimmune manifestations, including the presence of liver–kidney antibody microsomal type 3 (LKM-3) in 5% of cases [1].

Differential diagnosis

The clinical symptoms, biochemical markers, and histopathological changes of chronic hepatitis D are indistinguishable from those observed in other forms of chronic viral hepatitis, except for their tendency to be more severe. Thus, the diagnosis of chronic hepatitis D is based on serological and virological testing [2].

Liver Disease

Diagnostic investigation

The diagnosis of chronic HDV infection is usually based on the finding of HDAg in liver and high titers of IgG antibodies to HDAg (anti-HD) in serum. The detection of HDAg in serum by conventional immunoassay during chronic infection is hampered by antigen sequestration in immune complexes [2]. Chronic HDV infection is associated with continued synthesis of IgM anti-HD, which provides prognostic information on the course of the infection: its persistence is associated with chronic active disease, whereas its disappearance predicts impending resolution [1]. The introduction of reverse transcription (RT)-PCR assays for the detection of HDV RNA and, more recently, the development of real-time RT-PCR assays to quantify HDV RNA in serum, have provided the most sensitive tool for the diagnosis of HDV infection and for monitoring the efficacy of antiviral therapy [11]. However, a major drawback remains the lack of commercial assays, as the detection of HDV RNA in serum by PCR still relies on home-made assays.

Treatment and prevention

HDV is a challenging target for antiviral therapy and treatment of chronic hepatitis D remains unsatisfactory. Several antiviral agents have been evaluated for the treatment of this disease, but only **interferon-alpha (IFN-α)** has been shown to be beneficial [1,2]. HDV lacks its own polymerase and specific HDV inhibitors have not yet been developed. Moreover, despite the vital link between HDV and HBV, potent HBV inhibitors, such as the nucleoside analogs, have little or no effect on HDV replication or disease activity [2]. An effective anti-HDV therapy would require a marked suppression of HBsAg expression, but current therapies for HBV do not achieve this.

Standard interferon-α

IFN-α is the only licensed drug for the treatment of chronic hepatitis D. Its efficacy is related to dose and duration of therapy. High doses of IFN (9 MU thrice weekly or 5 MU daily) for at least 1 year induced a sustained alanine aminotransferase (ALT) normalization (6 months after discontinuation of therapy) in up to 50% of patients, but the effects on HDV RNA were limited [2]. Overall, the rate of HDV clearance with a 1-year course of high-dose IFN was only 10–20%, with a 10% chance of HBV clearance [11]. Limited data are available on the longer-term effects of IFN. In a prospective long-term study (up to 20 years), high doses of IFN for 1 year significantly improved the long-term clinical outcome and survival of patients with chronic hepatitis D [12]. Reversion of advanced liver fibrosis occurred in some patients with an initial diagnosis of cirrhosis (Figure 82.1).

Several strategies have been explored to improve the efficacy of IFN, most notably longer duration of treatment, but most patients still fail to clear the virus (Figure 82.2) [11].

Moreover, these regimens are poorly tolerated. Side effects, including psychiatric symptoms, are common. Combination therapy with standard IFN and lamivudine or ribavirin failed to show any additional benefit over IFN monotherapy.

Pegylated interferon-α

The efficacy and safety of pegylated IFN-α (PEG-IFN-α) in chronic hepatitis D was investigated in three small studies in which 1.5 μg/kg of PEG-IFN-α 2b was given weekly for 12 months [13–15]. Both in IFN-naïve patients and in previous non-responders to standard IFN, the results overall were better with PEG-IFN. A sustained virological response, as measured by a sensitive PCR, was achieved in 43% [13], 25% [14], and 19% [15] of patients with chronic hepatitis D. Clearance of HBsAg occurred only in one patient [13], although the study period was presumably too short for this to occur. There was no baseline biochemical or virological variable predictive of a sustained virological response. However, patients with cirrhosis responded less well to PEG-IFN than those with only chronic hepatitis. Albeit limited in size, these studies underscore the importance of quantitative assays to monitor treatment response. An undetectable HDV RNA after 6 months of therapy was the best predictor of a sustained virological response to pegylated IFN, although in a minority it did not differentiate responders from relapsers. Quantification of HDV viremia also identified slow virological responders who might benefit from a more prolonged course of IFN therapy.

The addition of ribavirin to PEG-IFN [14] does not improve biochemical or virological responses.

Current recommendations (refer also to the accompanying work-up and management protocol on the website)

Treatment with PEG-IFN should be offered to all patients with compensated HDV chronic liver disease as soon as the diagnosis is made, whereas it is contraindicated in those with advanced or decompensated cirrhosis for which liver transplantation is the only therapeutic choice. Continued monitoring is essential for the early detection and management of medical and psychiatric complications [11]. Although the results with PEG-IFN are better than with standard IFN, the **rate of relapse** remains high and a high proportion of patients fail to respond. The reasons for such poor response are unknown. A recent *in vitro* study has suggested that HDV may impair the IFN-stimulated JAK-STAT signaling pathway [16].

A promising therapeutic approach is the use of inhibitors of prenylation, an essential step in HDV particle assembly. These have been shown to clear HDV viremia in a transgenic mouse model capable of supporting HDV replication [17]. Additional molecular strategies include RNA interference, antisense oligonucleotides, and ribozymes [1–3], but the potential clinical applicability of these approaches still appears remote.

Liver Disease

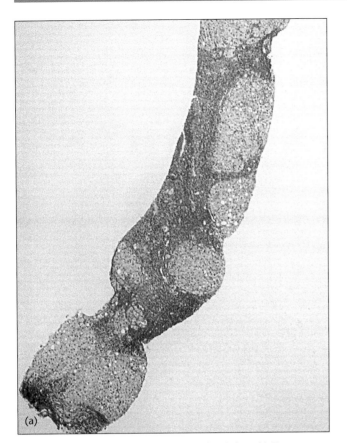

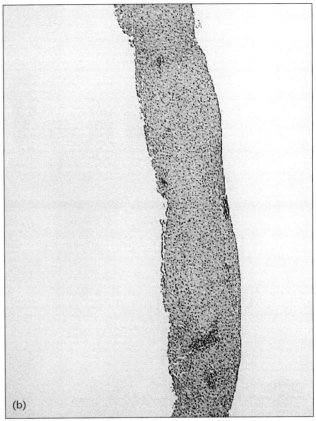

Figure 82.1 Effect of interferon treatment in chronic hepatitis D. Photomicrographs of liver biopsy specimens obtained from a patient with chronic hepatitis D before and 12.8 years after the completion of 1-year treatment with 9 MU of interferon-α 2a. (a) Liver specimen obtained before treatment. An active micronodular cirrhosis with small nodules surrounded by wide fibrous septa is seen (picrosirius stain, x25). (b). Liver specimen obtained from the same patient 12.8 years after completion of interferon therapy. Signs of inflammatory activity and fibrosis can no longer be identified in the needle biopsy (picrosirius stain, x25). Serum HDV RNA, as measured by nested PCR, became undetectable 13 months prior to the last liver biopsy, and HBsAg 14 months after the last liver biopsy; all the liver enzymes were normal and the hepatic function was dramatically improved. At the time of the last liver biopsy there were no clinical features of portal hypertension: there was no evidence of esophageal or gastric varices at endoscopy, the diameter of the portal vein and of the spleen were normal by ultrasound, and the platelet count was normal. Grade of activity and stage of fibrosis were established according to the scoring system of Knodell. The intensity of the necroinflammatory lesions was measured by grade of activity, which comprised the sum of three scores, including interface hepatitis ± bridging necrosis (0–10), lobular necrosis and inflammation (0–4), and portal inflammation (0–4). Fibrosis was scored on a scale of 0–4, with 0 indicating absence of fibrosis, 1 fibrous portal expansion, 3 bridging fibrosis, and 4 cirrhosis. (Reproduced with permission from Farci P, Roskams T, Chessa L, *et al*. Long-term benefit of interferon alpha therapy of chronic hepatitis D: regression of advanced hepatic fibrosis. *Gastroenterology*. 2004;126:1740–1749.)

The risk of HDV re-infection of a graft is lower than that for ordinary HBV re-infection and can be prevented by continuous prophylaxis with anti-HBs immunoglobulins and lamivudine [1]. Survival following transplantation is better in HDV than in HBV or HCV infection.

Prevention

Prevention of HDV infection can be achieved by active immunization against HBV. However, there are currently no means, such as a specific HDV vaccine, to protect over 300 million HBsAg carriers worldwide from HDV superinfection. Despite great advances in understanding the molecular biology of HDV, much remains to be unraveled in order to devise more effective therapies and vaccines for the control of this unique virus, which still represents a major challenge to both clinicians and virologists.

SOURCES OF INFORMATION FOR PATIENTS AND DOCTORS

http://www.gastro.org/clinicalRes/brochures/cvh.html

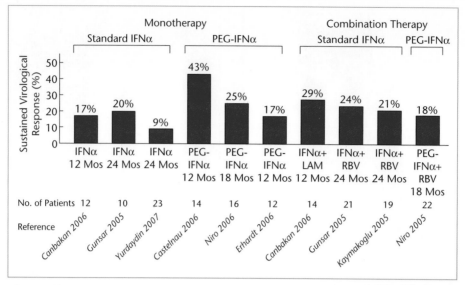

Figure 82.2 Rate of sustained virological response assessed by PCR in patients with chronic hepatitis D treated with standard or pegylated IFN-α, alone or in combination with lamivudine or ribavirin. In all studies HDV RNA was assessed by using a PCR with a sensitivity ranging from 10 to 1000 genome copies/mL. IFNα, standard interferon alpha; Peg-IFNα, pegylated interferon alpha; LAM, lamivudine; RBV, ribavirin. (Reproduced with permission from Farci P. Treatment of chronic hepatitis D: new advances, old challenges. *Hepatology* 2006;44(3):536–539.)

References

1. Rizzetto M, Smedile A. Hepatitis D. In: Schiff E, Sorrell M, Maddrey W, editors. *Diseases of the Liver*. Philadelphia: Lippincott Williams and Wilkins, 2002:863–875.
2. Taylor J, Farci P, Purcell RH. Hepatitis D (Delta) virus. In: Knipe DM, Howley PM editors. *Field's Virology*, 5th edition. Philadelphia: Lippincott Williams and Wilkins, 2006:3031–3046.
3. Rizzetto M. Hepatitis D: thirty years after. *J Hepatol*. 2009; 50:1043–1050.
4. Dény P. Hepatitis delta virus genetic variability: from genotypes I, II, III to eight major clades? *Curr Top Microbiol Immunol*. 2006;307:151–171.
5. Choi SH, Jeong SH, Hwang SB. Large hepatitis delta antigen modulates transforming growth factor-beta signaling cascades: implication of hepatitis delta virus-induced liver fibrosis. *Gastroenterology*. 2007;132:343–357.
6. Wu JC. Functional and clinical significance of hepatitis D virus genotype II infection. *Curr Top Microbiol Immunol*. 2006;307:173–186.
7. Casey JL, Brown TL, Colan EJ, Wignall FS, Gerin JL. A genotype of hepatitis D virus that occurs in northern South America. *Proc Natl Acad Sci U S A*. 1993;90:9016–9020.
8. Fattovich G, Giustina G, Christensen E, et al. Influence of hepatitis delta virus infection on morbidity and mortality in compensated cirrhosis type B. The European Concerted Action on Viral Hepatitis (Eurohep). *Gut*. 2000;46:420–426.
9. Rosina F, Conoscitore P, Cuppone R, et al. Changing pattern of chronic hepatitis D in Southern Europe. *Gastroenterology*. 1999;117:161–166.
10. Romeo R, Del Ninno E, Rumi M, et al. A 28-year study of the course of hepatitis Delta infection: a risk factor for cirrhosis and hepatocellular carcinoma. *Gastroenterology*. 2009;136:1629–1638.
11. Farci P. Treatment of chronic hepatitis D: new advances, old challenges. *Hepatology*. 2006;44:536–539.
12. Farci P, Roskams T, Chessa L, et al. Long-term benefit of interferon alpha therapy of chronic hepatitis D: regression of advanced hepatic fibrosis. *Gastroenterology*. 2004;126:1740–1749.
13. Castelnau C, Le Gal F, Ripault MP, et al. Efficacy of peginterferon alpha-2b in chronic hepatitis delta: relevance of quantitative RT-PCR for follow-up. *Hepatology*. 2006;44:728–735.
14. Niro GA, Ciancio A, Gaeta GB, et al. Pegylated interferon alpha-2b as monotherapy or in combination with ribavirin in chronic hepatitis delta. *Hepatology*. 2006;44:713–720.
15. Erhardt A, Gerlich W, Starke C, et al. Treatment of chronic hepatitis delta with pegylated interferon-alpha2b. *Liver Int*. 2006;26:805–810.
16. Pugnale P, Pazienza V, Guilloux K, Negro F. Hepatitis delta virus inhibits alpha interferon signaling. *Hepatology*. 2009;49:398–406.
17. Bordier BB, Ohkanda J, Liu P, et al. In vivo antiviral efficacy of prenylation inhibitors against hepatitis delta virus. *J Clin Invest*. 2003;112:407–414.

CHAPTER 83
Liver worms

Donald McManus
Queensland Institute of Medical Research, Brisbane, QLD, Australia

ESSENTIAL FACTS ABOUT PATHOGENESIS

- Several species of two of the major groups of helminth worms – the trematodes (flukes) and cestodes (tapeworms) – parasitize the human liver
- Human blood flukes or schistosomes cause schistosomiasis, a T-cell–mediated granulomatous liver disease that can lead to portal hypertension
- Liver fluke infection (*Fasciola, Opisthorchis, Clonorchis*) is via the biliary system where inflammatory responses can cause acute febrile illnesses with jaundice
- *Opisthorchis viverinni* is a Group I carcinogen and long-term infection can cause cholangiocarcinoma
- Ingestion of eggs of the dog tapeworm *Echinococcus granulosus* results in the development of unilocular fluid-filled bladders or hydatid cysts (cystic echinococcosis) mainly in the liver that are often asymptomatic but may cause pressure symptoms with rupture leading to severe anaphylactic shock and death
- The metacestode of the fox tapeworm *Echinococcus multilocularis* is a tumor-like, infiltrating structure consisting of numerous small vesicles embedded in stroma of connective tissue of the liver, and is associated with progressive disease (alveolar echinococcosis) and poor response to therapy
- The gastrointestinal tract, not the liver, is the principal site of human nematode parasites

ESSENTIALS OF DIAGNOSIS

Schistosoma mansoni/S. japonicum
- Detection of eggs in stool or in tissues
- Clinical assessment coupled with ultrasound, liver biopsy, and subsequent histological examination
- Measurement of biochemical markers in serum or plasma; detection of serum antibodies/antigens; detection of schistosome DNA in feces or blood by PCR-based techniques

Fasciola hepatica
- Detection of eggs in stool
- Detection of serum antibodies/antigens
- Radiology, radioisotope scanning, ultrasound, CT, and MRI

Clonorchis sinensis/Opisthorchis viverrini/O. felineus
- Detection of eggs in stool
- Detection of serum antibodies/antigens; detection of parasite DNA in feces by PCR-based techniques

Echinococcus granulosus/E. multilocularis
- Clinical assessment coupled with ultrasound and CT
- Detection of serum antibodies

ESSENTIALS OF TREATMENT AND PROGNOSIS

Schistosoma mansoni
- Drug treatment: praziquantel; oxamniquine (vansil)
- Fibrosis and chronic disease of the human liver can result in the development of severe hepatosplenic schistosomiasis

S. japonicum
- Drug treatment: praziquantel; artemether; oxamniquine has no effect
- Fibrosis and chronic disease of the human liver, which can result in the development of severe hepatosplenic schistosomiasis

Fasciola hepatica
- Drug treatment: triclabendazole; praziquantel has no effect
- Inflammatory responses can cause acute febrile illnesses with jaundice

Clonorchis sinensis/Opisthorchis viverrini/O. felineus
- Drug treatment: praziquantel + other drugs
- Inflammatory responses can cause acute febrile illnesses with jaundice
- Long-term infection with *O. viverrini* can cause cholangiocarcinoma

Echinococcus granulosus
- Drug treatment with albendazole/mebendazole ± surgery
- Prognosis is generally poor
- Hydatid cysts can cause pressure symptoms; rupture may lead to severe anaphylactic shock and death

E. multilocularis
- Drug treatment with albendazole/mebendazole ± radical surgery
- Associated with progressive disease, a poor response to therapy, and a high fatality rate and poor prognosis if managed inappropriately

Several species of two of the major groups of helminth worms – the trematodes (flukes) and cestodes (tapeworms) – which parasitize the human liver are considered in this chapter.

Trematode infections
Adult trematodes (blood flukes and liver flukes) are a major cause of human liver disease (Table 83.1).

Table 83.1 Trematodes affecting the liver*

Species	Schistosoma mansoni/S. japonicum**	Fasciola hepatica	Clonorchis sinensis	Opisthorchis viverrini/O. felineus
Definitive host(s)	Humans (other mammals – water buffaloes, cattle, dogs – act as reservoirs for *S. japonicum*)	Sheep (humans)	Humans	Humans, cats, dogs
Intermediate host(s)	Snail – *Biomphalaria*; *Oncomelania*	Snail – *Lymnaea*	Snail – *Bithynia*; *Melanoides*; *Parafossarulus*; and freshwater cyprinoid fish	Snail – *Bithynia*; *Melanoides*; *Parafossarulus*, and freshwater cyprinoid fish
Geographical distribution	*S. mansoni*: Africa, Middle East, Brazil, Caribbean *S. japonicum*: China, Philippines, Indonesia	Worldwide	China, Japan, Korea, Vietnam	Thailand, Lao People's Democratic Republic, Vietnam, and Cambodia (*O. viverrini*), Poland, Russia (*O. felineus*)
Mode of acquisition	Water: skin	Eating contaminated plants (e.g. watercress)	Eating raw or pickled fish	Eating raw or pickled fish
Site of infestation	Mesenteric veins	Biliary radicals	Biliary system	Biliary system
Liver pathology	Granulomatous reaction to eggs in portal radicals	Inflammatory response to biliary worms	Inflammatory or fibrotic response to biliary worms	Inflammatory or fibrotic response to biliary worms

*The liver can also be involved during infection with the lung fluke *Paragonimus westermani*

**S. haematobium* (Africa, Middle East) causes urinary schistosomiasis

Blood flukes

Schistosomes cause **schistosomiasis**, a chronic disease considered the second most important parasitic disease after malaria, infecting 200 million people globally. Unlike other trematodes, they are dioecious (have separate sexes) and live in the blood stream of their mammalian hosts.

The schistosome life cycle is depicted in Figure 83.1. Infection is acquired from contaminated freshwater containing larvae (cercariae), which emerge from suitable freshwater snail intermediate hosts and actively penetrate the mammalian host via the skin. The cercariae shed their bifurcated tails and transform their trilaminate tegument into a heptalaminate form adapted to the mammalian environment. Now schistosomula, they leave the skin via the blood vessels and draining lymphatics, and reach the lungs. After several days the male and female worms exit the lungs and arrive in the hepatic portal system where they mature, pair up, and migrate downstream. The worm pairs reach mucosal branches of the inferior mesenteric and superior hemorrhoidal veins, and the females then begin egg production. The process of migration and maturation takes about 4–5 weeks, depending on the host species involved. Many eggs pass through the intestinal wall and are discharged in the feces. The lifecycle is completed when the eggs hatch and release free-swimming miracidia, which, in turn, re-infect a receptive amphibious freshwater snail (Table 83.1). The miracidium forms a sporocyst at the site of penetration and this produces daughter sporocysts that migrate to the snail hepatopancreas and asexually produce the larval cercariae for daily release into the surrounding water.

A T-cell–mediated granulomatous reaction to the eggs (ova) laid by mature female worms of two of the most important schistosomes, **Schistosoma mansoni and S. japonicum**, leads to fibrosis and chronic disease of the human liver, which can result in the development of severe hepatosplenic schistosomiasis (bilharziasis) [1]. Mature worms of the other important species, **S. haematobium**, reside in the genitourinary tract where chronic infection induces fibrosis and calcification of the bladder and ureters.

Ultrasonography provides a safe, rapid, and non-invasive method for the assessment of pathology associated with chronic hepatosplenic disease. The image pattern of liver texture and objective measurements of wall thickness of a peripheral segmental portal vein and main portal vein diameter are used to grade the degree of hepatic fibrosis [1,2]. The grade of fibrosis is in turn used as a predictive factor for the development of portal hypertension and gastrointestinal bleeding. Ultrasonography may also be used to assess the effectiveness of antischistosomal therapy in advanced disease.

Treatment of schistosomiasis is with **praziquantel (PZQ)**, a pyrazinoisoquinoline derivative, which is a safe and effective oral drug that is active against all schistosome species. Standard clinical treatment is 60 mg/kg/day of PZQ in divided doses. For mass chemotherapy a single dose (40 mg/kg) is effective, although re-infection can occur soon after. Other drugs that have been used in the treatment of schistosomiasis are oxamniquine (vansil) for *S. mansoni* and metrifonate (trichlorfon) for *S. haematobium,* but both are ineffective against *S. japonicum.* The antimalarial, artemether, has been used as a

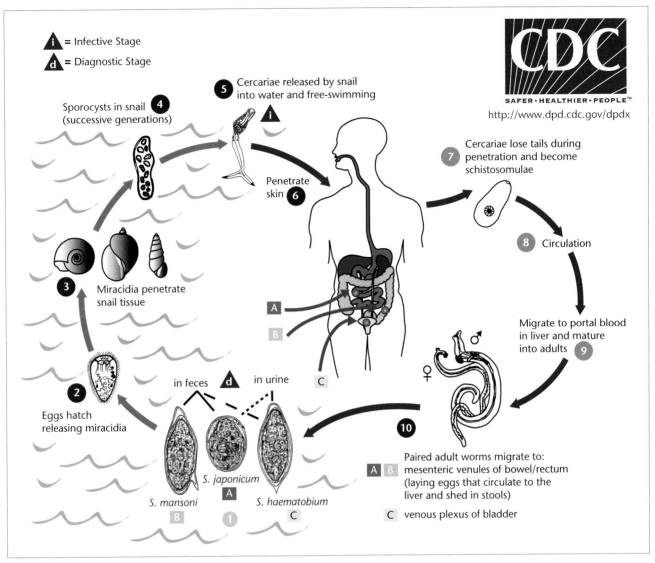

Figure 83.1 The life cycle of *Schistosoma mansoni*, *S. japonicum*, and *S. haematobium*. (Reproduced from DPDX, the CDC website for parasite identification.http://www.dpd.cdc.gov/DPDx/HTML/Schistosomiasis.htm.)

chemoprophylactic against *S. japonicum* in China in high-risk groups, such as flood relief workers and fishermen.

There are four major approaches for schistosome diagnosis; direct parasitological methods (detecting eggs in the stool or in tissues); indirect methods of detecting morbidity via clinical assessment of the patient coupled with ultrasound, liver biopsy and subsequent histological examination, and the measurement of biochemical markers; serological methods to detect immunological responses to antigens or the antigens themselves; and polymerase chain reaction (PCR)-based techniques [2].

Liver flukes

Fasciola hepatica (the common liver fluke), *Clonorchis sinensis*, and *Opisthorchis viverrini/O. felineus* (see Table 83.1) are hermaphroditic and have life cycles that follow the typical

trematode pattern involving a molluscan intermediate host, from which cercariae are released and encyst on grass (*F. hepatica*) or penetrate the skin of a secondary intermediate cyprinoid fish host and encyst in the muscles (*C. sinensis, O. viverinni*; Figure 83.2). Liver infection in the definitive host follows ingestion (via contaminated grass/vegetation or uncooked fish) and excystment of the metacercaria, and is via the biliary system where inflammatory responses can cause acute febrile illnesses with jaundice, although most people with opisthorchiasis or clonorchiasis have no symptoms [3]. *O. viverrini* is considered a Group I carcinogen (known to be carcinogenic in humans) and long-term infection can cause cholangiocarcinoma (CCA). The link between fluke infection and CCA is more robust than for clonorchiasis [3].

Detection of eggs in feces provides definitive diagnosis of both *O. viverrini* and *C. sinensis*; serology and ultrasound

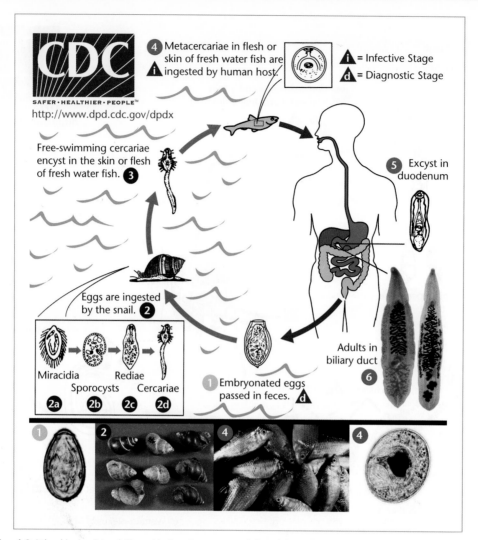

Figure 83.2 Life cycles of *Opisthorchis viverrini* and *Clonorchis sinensis*. Embryonated eggs are discharged in the biliary ducts and in the stool (1). Eggs are ingested by a suitable snail intermediate host (2); there are more than 100 species of snails that can serve as intermediate hosts. Each egg releases a miracidium (2a), which goes through several developmental stages [sporocyst (2b), redia (2c), and cercaria (2d)]. The cercaria is released from the snail and after a short period of free-swimming time in water, it penetrates the flesh of a freshwater fish, such as *Cyclocheilichthys armatus* or *Puntius leiacanthus*, where it encysts as a metacercaria (3). Humans are infected through ingestion of undercooked, salted, pickled, or smoked freshwater fish (4). After ingestion, the metacercaria excysts in the duodenum (5) and ascends the biliary tract through the ampulla of Vater. Maturation to adulthood (right, *O. viverrini*; left, *C. sinensis*) takes approximately 1 month (6). The adult flukes (measuring 10–25 mm by 3–5 mm) reside in the small and medium-sized biliary ducts. In addition to humans, carnivorous animals can serve as reservoir hosts. (Reproduced from Sripa B, Kaewkes S, Sithithaworn P, *et al*. Liver fluke induces cholangiocarcinoma. *PLoS Med*. 2007;4:e201.)

provide indirect evidence of infection [4]. PCR may be useful for discrimination between *O. viverrini* and *C. sinensis*. **Praziquantel** (75 mg/kg in divided doses) is used primarily for treatment, although triclabendazole, bithionol, albendazole, and mebendazole also show some efficacy [4].

Sheep, goats, and cattle are considered the predominant animal reservoirs for fascioliasis. In humans, diagnosis of fasciolosis is usually achieved parasitologically by finding the fluke eggs in stool, complemented by immunological detection of anti-*F. hepatica* antibodies in sera; other non-invasive diagnostic techniques that can be used for human diagnosis are radiology, radioisotope scanning, ultrasound, computed axial tomography (CT scanning) and magnetic resonance imaging

(MRI) [5]. **Triclabendazole** (10–12 mg/kg) is the drug of choice in human fasciliasis; praziquantel has no effect [5]. Prevention may be achieved by strict control of watercress and other metacercariae-carrying aquatic plants for human consumption, especially in endemic zones [5].

Cestode infections

Echinococcosis (hydatid disease) is a zoonosis caused by cestodes of carnivores (especially dogs or foxes) belonging to the genus *Echinococcus* (family Taeniidae). The two major species infecting humans are *Echinococcus granulosus* and *E. multilocularis*, which cause **cystic echinococcosis (CE)** and **alveolar**

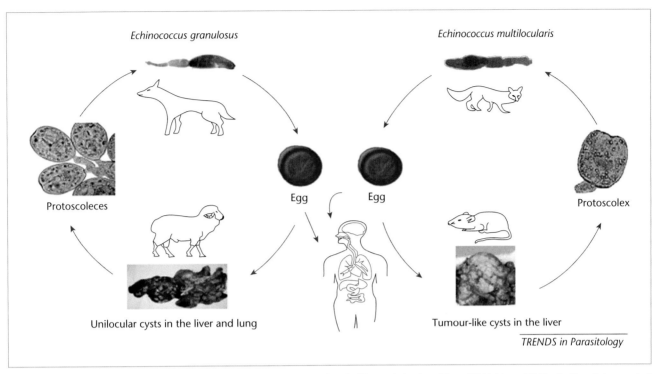

Echinococcus granulosus

Echinococcus multilocularis

Protoscoleces

Egg   Egg

Protoscolex

Unilocular cysts in the liver and lung

Tumour-like cysts in the liver

TRENDS in Parasitology

Figure 83.3 Life cycles of *Echinococcus granulosus* and *E. multilocularis*. (Reproduced with permission from Zhang W, McManus DP. Vaccination of dogs against *Echinococcus granulosus*: a means to control hydatid disease? *Trends Parasitol.* 2008;24:419–424.)

echinococcosis (AE), respectively, and are responsible for substantial morbidity and mortality [6]. Human CE is the most common presentation and probably accounts for more than 95% of the estimated 2–3 million global cases [7]. The global burden [disability-adjusted life years (DALYS)] for human CE was recently estimated to be more than that for onchocerciasis and almost the same as that for African trypanosomiasis [7].

The life cycle of both parasites is shown in Figure 83.3.

Ingestion of foods contaminated with dog feces containing *E. granulosus* eggs results in the development in humans or other intermediate hosts of unilocular fluid-filled bladders or hydatid cysts mainly in the liver but in other sites as well (Table 83.2). Cysts are often asymptomatic but can cause pressure symptoms; rupture may lead to severe anaphylactic shock and death. Treatment is difficult and involves **albendazole**, although surgery may be necessary. Dogs become infected by ingestion of offal-containing hydatid cysts with viable protoscoleces.

Adult worm infections of *E. multilocularis* are perpetuated in a sylvatic cycle with foxes being the most important definitive hosts and small rodents acting as intermediate hosts. The metacestode of *E. multilocularis* is a tumor-like, infiltrating structure consisting of numerous small vesicles embedded in stroma of connective tissue that develops almost exclusively in the liver (99% of cases), although metastasis to other organs can occur. The metacestode mass usually contains a semi-solid matrix rather than fluid. AE is associated with progressive

Table 83.2 Cestodes affecting the liver: *Echinococcus* spp.

Species	*Echinococcus granulosus*	*Echinococcus multilocularis*
Hosts	Dogs (definitive host); humans; sheep, pigs, etc. (intermediate hosts)	Foxes, dogs + other canines; humans; rodents (especially microtine voles and other small mammals) (intermediate hosts)
Transmission	Fecal–oral (dogs to humans and intermediate hosts)	Fecal–oral (foxes to humans and intermediate hosts)
Geographical distribution	South America, Southern Africa, Australasia, Mediterranean, Iceland, Alaska, Northern Europe	Northern hemisphere; emerging in areas of Europe/Eurasia
Mode of acquisition	Humans acquire infection accidentally (eggs in dog feces)	Humans acquire infection accidentally (eggs in fox feces)
Site of infestation	Liver (mainly), lung, brain plus other sites	Mainly liver
Liver pathology	Compression of the inferior vena cava, human papilloma virus, hepatic veins, insidious liver dysfunction, cholangitis	Destruction of liver parenchyma, bile ducts, and blood vessels, biliary obstruction, and portal hypertension

Liver Disease

Table 83.3 Nematodes affecting the liver

Species	Ascaris lumbricoides	Toxocara canis/T. cati	Strongyloides stercoralis
Definitive host(s)	Humans	Dogs and cats	Humans
Intermediate host	None	None	Larvae develop in soil
Geographical distribution	Worldwide	Worldwide	(Sub)tropics, South-East Europe, USA
Mode of acquisition	Eating contaminated vegetables	Contamination from definitive host	Skin penetration
Site of infestation	Intestine → liver → lungs → intestine → feces	Intestine, then liver, brain, and eye by migration	Skin → lungs → intestine → feces
Liver pathology	May migrate into biliary tree	Invasion provokes hemorrhage, necrosis, granuloma, and eosinophilia	Immunosuppressed patients → hyperinfestation → multiple organs including liver
Liver: Clinical	Obstructive jaundice, cholangitis, abscess	Tender hepatomegaly	Jaundice
Other clinical features	Acute-phase reaction, cough, wheeze, dyspnea, intestinal obstruction	Acute-phase reaction, larva migrans, visual disturbance, encephalitis, convulsions	Itch, low-grade fever, cough, wheeze, diarrhea, eosinophilia
Diagnosis	Eggs in feces. Ultrasonography: bile duct worms	Larvae in tissues (liver biopsy)	Larvae in feces, intestinal aspirate or biopsy, positive serology
Treatment	Mebendazole, Pyrantel pamoate, Levamisole	Diethylcarbamazine, Thiabendazole, Albendazole	Albendazole

disease, a poor response to therapy, and a high fatality rate and poor prognosis if managed inappropriately. **Radical surgery** has been the historical cornerstone of treatment for AE. Early diagnosis is crucial, and results in a reduced rate of non-resectable lesions and reduces the need for radical surgery. Perioperative and long-term adjuvant chemotherapy with **albendazole** (doses up to 20 mg/kg/day) has been associated with 10-year survival of approximately 80%, compared with less than 25% in historical controls [6]. Albendazole is only parasitostatic against the *E. multilocularis* metacestode. Liver transplantation has been performed on some AE patients.

The definitive diagnosis for most human cases of CE and AE is by physical imaging methods, such as radiology, ultrasonography, CT scanning, and MRI, although such procedures are often not readily available in isolated communities [6,7]. Immunodiagnosis (detection of anti-*Echinococcus* antibodies in serum) complements the clinical picture, being useful not only in primary diagnosis but also for follow-up of patients after surgery or drug treatment [6,7].

Preventive measures that have been used to control *Echinococcus* infections include avoidance of contact with dog or fox feces, handwashing, and improved sanitation, reducing dog or fox populations, treatment of dogs with arecoline hydrobromide or praziquantel or use of praziquantel-impregnated baits, incineration of infected organs, and health education [7]. A vaccine for application in the animal intermediate hosts of

E. granulosus has been shown to confer a high degree of protection against challenge infection, indicating that it could have wide applicability as a new method for use in hydatid control campaigns [7].

Nematode infections

Some nematode species (*Ascaris lumbricoides, Toxocara canis/T. cati, Strongyloides stercoralis*) migrate secondarily into the biliary tree, causing jaundice or hepatomegaly, but as the gut is the principal site of their infection, they are not considered in depth. Some of their characteristics are shown in Table 83.3.

SOURCES OF INFORMATION FOR PATIENTS AND DOCTORS

http://www.cdfound.to.it/hTML/at_liver.htm#liver
http://www.cdc.gov/ncidod/dpd/parasites/index.htm

References

1. Burke ML, Jones MK, Gobert GN, *et al.* Immunopathogenesis of human schistosomiasis. *Parasite Immunol.* 2009;31:163–176.
2. Gryseels B, Polman K, Clerinx J, *et al.* Human schistosomiasis. *Lancet.* 2006;368:1106–1118.

3. Sripa B, Kaewkes S, Sithithaworn P, *et al*. Liver fluke induces cholangiocarcinoma. *PLoS Med* 2007;4:e201.

4. Sripa B. Pathobiology of opisthorchiasis: An update. *Acta Trop.* 2003;88:209–220.

5. Mas-Coma S, Bargues MD, Valero MA. Fascioliasis and other plant-borne trematode zoonoses. *Int J Parasitol.* 2005;35:1255–1278.

6. McManus DP, Zhang W, Li J, Bartley PB. Echinococcosis. *Lancet.* 2003;362:1295–1304.

7. Craig PS, McManus DP, Lightowlers MW, *et al*. Prevention and control of cystic echinococcosis. *Lancet Infect Dis.* 2007;7:385–394.

Liver Disease

CHAPTER 84

Liver protozoa

David Kershenobich, Guillermo Robles-Diaz and Juan Miguel Abdo Francis

Hospital General de México, Mexico City, Mexico

ESSENTIAL FACTS ABOUT PATHOGENESIS

- Ameba, *Cryptosporidium*, and *Giardia* are intestinal protozoal infections that can invade the liver or the biliary tree
- Emerging new risk factors for protozoal infections in the liver include sexual lifestyles, travel to endemic areas, population migration, and immunosuppression
- Humans are the primary reservoir, transmission occurring mostly by oral ingestion of contaminated food or water, or exposure to infected animals
- The whole-genome sequencing of protozoa has allowed advances in pathogenesis and may lead to new therapeutic approaches

ESSENTIALS OF DIAGNOSIS

- Amebic liver abscess is characterized by constant, dull, and intense right upper quadrant abdominal pain that exacerbates with movement and radiates to the right scapula and shoulder, fever >38°C, and leukocytosis (>15 × 10⁹ cells/L)
- Imaging studies, mainly chest X-ray and ultrasound, computed tomography or magnetic resonance, are the backbone of the diagnosis of an amebic liver abscess
- ERCP is useful in demonstrating stenosis or long extrahepatic bile duct strictures in patients with liver cryptosporidiosis.
- Detection of anti-*Giardia* salivary IgA antibodies is an excellent screening tool for *Giardia lamblia* in patients with symptoms of more than 1 month's duration

ESSENTIALS OF TREATMENT

- Metronidazole is the standard of care for most protozoal infections
- Percutaneous drainage of an amebic liver abscess should be performed with imaging guidance in patients in whom diagnosis is uncertain or for therapeutic purposes in patients who are at a risk of rupture (liver tissue rim <1 cm) or are unresponsive to pharmacological therapy
- Paromomycin is indicated for treatment of cryptosporidiosis
- Combination therapies may be necessary in immunosuppressed patients

Amebic liver abscess

Epidemiology

Entamoeba histolytica is an invasive parasitic protozoal source of significant morbidity and mortality worldwide. It must be distinguished from *E. dispar* and *Entamoeba*

moshkovskii, which are non-pathogenic commensals. Humans are its primary reservoir, with transmission by fecal excretion of cysts followed by oral ingestion of contaminated food or water. **Amebiasis** is higher in developing countries with fecal–oral transmission within households and long-term care institutions. Linked clusters of *E. histolytica* infection are rare in industrialized countries, where risk groups include men who have sex with men, travelers, immigrants, prisoners, and immunocompromised patients.

Pathogeneiss

Identified pathogenic mechanisms include parasite motility, projection of pseudopods, expression of cell adhesion molecules such as Gal/Gal NAC lectins and Eh lectins, amebapores, and cysteine proteases, all of which participate in the adherence, cytotoxicity, and disruption of tissues, leading to invasive disease [1]. Trophozoites of *E. hystolytica* induce apoptosis of host cells, neutrophils, T lymphocytes, and macrophages. Identification of the genomic structure of *E. histolytica* has further clarified its pathogenic mechanisms [2].

A liver abscess involves the intraportal delivery of *E. histolytica* and binding of the trophozoites to the endothelium. Early liver lesions are constituted by small foci of necrosis, which tend to coalesce into a single abscess. The center of the abscess consists of lysed hepatocytes, erythrocytes, and bile and fat that liquefy, producing a yellowish necrotic material.

Clinical manifestations and diagnosis

Amebic liver abscess occurs mostly in men between the ages of 20 and 40 years. Patients complain of constant, dull, intense **right upper quadrant abdominal pain** that exacerbates with movement and radiates to the right scapula and shoulder, accompanied by fever >38°C, chills, and diaphoresis. Comorbidities, such as diabetes mellitus or the presence of an immunodeficient state, are frequent. A history of traveling to or residing in endemic areas and having undergone invasive procedures must be identified [3]. Patients commonly have malaise, nausea, moderate weight loss, cough, and chest pain. They are pale and have tender hepatomegaly and hypoventilation in the right lung. Jaundice is infrequent. **Alarm signs** that could indicate rupture of the abscess into the peritoneum or extension into intra-abdominal organs, great vessels, pleura, bronchial tree or pericardium include abdominal rebound tenderness, guarding, absence of bowel sounds, and a pleural or pericardial rub.

There is leukocytosis ($>15 \times 10^9$ cells/L) with neutrophilia, increased sedimentation rate, slight anemia, and increased alkaline phosphatase. Patients with human immunodeficiency virus (HIV) infection and an amebic liver abscess have lower white cell counts [4]. Serum antibodies to *E. histolytica* are detected in >90% of cases. Indirect hemagglutination (IHA) and enzyme-linked immunoabsorbent assay (ELISA) with cutoff values of 1:512 are diagnostic. Aspirated material obtained either for diagnostic or therapeutic purposes, should be sent for Grams staining, presence of neutrophils, and culture. An uncomplicated amebic liver abscess is sterile.

Initial **imaging studies** helpful in establishing the diagnosis include chest X-ray and liver ultrasound. On chest X-ray the appearance may be normal or show an elevation of the right dome of the diaphragm and small effusions or pleural thickening. On ultrasound, a space-occupying lesion is seen in 75% of cases. The lesions are primarily hypoechoic, round or oval with well-defined margins. Computed tomography (CT) or magnetic resonance imaging (MRI) may be necessary in the differential diagnosis. An enhancing wall of 3–15 mm in thickness and a peripheral zone of edema around the abscess are common. The central portion of the abscess may show septa or fluid debris.

Treatment

Metronidazole is the standard of care for uncomplicated amebic liver abscess at an oral dose of 1 g twice daily for 10–15 days in adults and 30–50 mg/kg daily for 10 days in three doses in children. When given intravenously the dosage is 500 mg every 6 hours for adults and 7.5 mg/kg every 6 hours for children for 10 days. Other drugs include 2 g tinidazole or ornidazole orally daily for 10 days. Patients should abstain from alcohol as these drugs have an antabuse effect.

Percutaneous drainage is indicated as a diagnostic or therapeutic tool and should be performed under imaging guidance. Drainage may be necessary in non-responders to pharmacological treatment or when the rim of liver tissue at any point around the abscess is less than 1 cm, as this could predict rupture. **Rupture** of an amebic liver abscess has a high mortality rate and requires urgent surgical intervention

Cryptosporidium

Epidemiology

The incidence of *Cryptosporidium* infection has increased, because of improved surveillance, improved awareness, and/or increased testing. Risk factors include ingestion of contaminated recreational or drinking water, exposure to infected animals, close contacts with subjects with cryptosporidiosis,

travel to disease-endemic areas, and ingestion of contaminated food [5,6].

Pathogenesis

Research efforts have been greatly facilitated by the completion of whole-genome sequencing of *Cryptosporidium parvum, C. hominis,* and *C. muris* [7,8].

Transmission occurs via the fecal–oral route (person-to-person and animal-to-person) from contaminated food and water. Humans are infected when they ingest *Cryptosporidium* oocysts. Once ingested, oocysts release infective sporozoites in the gastrointestinal tract that mature and undergo asexual reproduction (schizogony) to produce merozoites that can infect other intestinal epithelial cells or that mature into gametocytes, the sexual form of the parasite. The presence of an autoinfective oocyst can cause an overwhelming infection in a susceptible host, which explains the persistent life-threatening infection in immunocompromised patients in the absence of repeated exposure to oocysts. Immunocompromised individuals with a defect in T-cell response have a more severe disease [9–11].

Clinical manifestations and diagnosis

The major symptom of cryptosporidiosis in immunocompetent individuals is self-limited **diarrhea** lasting between 2 and 4 weeks. However, in immunocompromised individuals it causes chronic debilitating diarrhea, with the infection spreading from the intestine to hepatobiliary and pancreatic ducts, causing cholangiohepatitis, cholecystitis, or pancreatitis. Two distinct clinical presentations may occur: (1) papillary stenosis with extrahepatic ductal dilatation and sclerosing cholangitis or (2) acalculous cholecystitis. *C. parvum*-induced sclerosing cholangitis has been described in autoimmune deficiency syndrome (AIDS), other immunodeficient states, and renal or liver transplant recipients. In these cases, and in addition to diarrhea, there is pain in the right upper quadrant, nausea, vomiting, and fever.

Cryptosporidium stains intensely red in modified acid-fast techniques on microscopic examination of stool. Serological tests are of limited value as antibodies to *Cryptosporidium* can be found in previously exposed persons.

Ultrasonographic findings include thickening of the biliary duct wall and an enlarged gallbladder. Endoscopic retrograde cholangiopancreatography (ERCP) or endoscopic ultrasonography can reveal papillary stenosis or long extrahepatic bile duct strictures.

Treatment

Nitazoxanide, paromomycin, and azithromycin are used in both immunocompetent and immunosuppressed patients. Paromomycin 500 mg three times daily for 2 weeks is prescribed in patients with AIDS, while continuing antiretroviral therapy. In the setting of *C. parvum* infection, sclerosing cholangitis may be completely reversible if the infection can be eradicated quickly. Protease inhibitors have a direct inhibitory effect on *Cryptosporidium* infection.

Giardia lamblia

Giardia lamblia is one of the most primitive eukaryotic organisms. It is a parasite of humans and other mammals. The risk of giardiasis appears to be significantly associated with drinking piped water and eating raw vegetables. Molecular assays have identified seven genetic groups, two of which (A and B) are found in both humans and animals [12,13].

Pathogenesis

Giardia has a special disc located on its ventral surface, important for its attachment and damage to the intestinal epithelium. This process is mediated by specific lectins. The brush border is altered, there is crypt hyperplasia, and disaccharidase activity decreases. In the small bowel, *Giardia* trophozoites are destroyed and lysed, leading to greater intestinal epithelial damage. Bile stimulates the growth of *Giardia*, and it is avidly consumed by the parasite, leading to reduced intraluminal bile salt concentrations. *Giardia* is unable to survive in the absence of bile acids, but does not reside in the biliary tract where the pH and the absence of nutritional substrate do not allow its colonization. The increase in intestinal epithelial permeability may allow the passage of cytokines that can eventually damage the liver.

Clinical manifestations and diagnosis

Manifestations of giardiasis range from asymptomatic to symptoms such as chronic diarrhea, weight loss, vomiting, abdominal distension, and abdominal pain. The severity of symptoms is related to the number of cysts ingested, the age of the host, and the state of the host's immune system. Malabsorption caused by disaccharidase deficiency relates to the parasite burden in the small intestine.

Overt involvement of the liver by *Giardia* is rare; however, alterations in hepatic histology, including, steatosis, inflammatory lesions suggestive of chronic hepatitis, and granulomatous hepatitis have been described. In HIV patients, cholangitis or biliary giardiasis have been reported [14–16].

Diagnosis of *Giardia lamblia* is established by microscopic examination of stools. Detection of anti-*Giardia* salivary IgA antibodies is an excellent screening tool for *Giardia lamblia* in patients with symptoms lasting longer than 1 month.

Therapy

Therapy of diarrhea caused by giardiasis consists mainly of nitroimidazoles, nitazoxanide, paromomycin, furazolidine, albendazole or quinacrine. Metronidazole is most commonly used at a dose of 500 mg three times daily for 5 days. Tinidazole at a single dose of 1.0–2.0 g has the advantage of better compliance with similar efficacy [17]. Combination therapy may be necessary in immunosuppressed patients.

References

1. Lejeune M, Rubicka JM, Chadee K. Recent discoveries in the pathogenesis and immune response toward *Entamoeba histolytica*. *Future Med*. 2009;4:105–118.
2. Clark CG, Alsmark UC, Tazreiter M. Structure and content of the *Entamoeba histolytica* genome. *Adv Parasitol*. 2007;65:51–190.
3. Baxt L, Singh U. New insights into *Entamoeba histolytica* pathogenesis. *Curr Opin Infect Dis*. 2008;21:489–494.
4. Fantuzzi A, Albertz N, Valenzuela A, Estuardo N, Castro A. Hepatic abcess: Series of 107 cases and literature review. *Rev Chil Infect*. 2009;26:49–53.
5. Yoder JS, Beach MJ. Cryptosporidium surveillance and risk factors in the United States. *Exp Parasitol*. 2010;124:31–39.
6. Valderrama AL, Hlavsa MC, Cronquist A, *et al*. Multiple risk factors associated with a large statewide increase in cryptosporidiosis. *Epidemiol Infect*. 2009;137:1781–1788.
7. Abrahamsen MS, Templeton TJ, Enomoto S, *et al*. Complete genome sequence of the apicomplexan, *Cryptosporidium parvum*. *Science*. 2004;304:441–445.
8. Xu P, Widmer G, Wang Y, *et al*. The genome of *Cryptosporidium hominis*. *Nature*. 2004;431:1107–1112.
9. Barakat FM, McDonald V, Foster GR, Tovey MG, Korbel DS. *Cryptosporidium parvum* infection rapidly induces a protective innate immune response involving type I interferon. *J Infect Dis*. 2009;200:1548–1555.
10. Tessema TS, Schwamb B, Lochner M, Förster I, Jakobi V, Petry F. Dynamics of gut mucosal and systemic Th1/Th2 cytokine responses in interferon-gamma and interleukin-12p40 knock out mice during primary and challenge Cryptosporidium parvum infection. *Immunobiology*. 2009;214:454–466.
11. Davies AP, Chalmers RM. Cryptosporidiosis. *BMJ*. 2009;339: b4168.
12. Cacciò SM, Ryan U. Molecular epidemiology of giardiasis. *Mol Biochem Parasitol*. 2008;160:75–80.
13. Adam RD. The *Giardia lamblia* genome. *Int J Parasitol*. 2000;30: 475–484.
14. Esfiandari A, Swartz J, Teklehaimanot S. Clustering of giardiasis among AIDS patients in Los Angeles County. *Cell Mol Biol*. 1997;43:1077–1083.
15. Aronson NE, Cheney C, Rholl V, Burris D, Hadro N. Biliary giardiasis in a patient with human immunodeficiency virus. *J Clin Gastroenterol*. 2001;33:167–170.
16. Devarbhavi H, Sebastian T, Seetharamu SM, Karanth D. HIV/ AIDS cholangiopathy: clinical spectrum, cholangiographic features and outcome in 30 patients. *J Gastroenterol Hepatol*. 2010;25: 1656–1660.
17. Busatti HG, Santos JF, Gomes MA. The old and new therapeutic approaches to the treatment of giardiasis: Where are we? *Biologics*. 2009;3:273–287.

CHAPTER 85

Bacterial and fungal infections of the liver

Simon Rushbrook and Alexander Gimson

Cambridge University Hospitals NHS Foundation Trust, Cambridge, UK

ESSENTIAL FACTS ABOUT PATHOPHYSIOLOGY OF JAUNDICE OF SEPSIS

- Liver dysfunction may arise due to direct infection or inflammatory mediators
- The liver plays a major role in the host's response to infection
- The predominant histological abnormality is canalicular cholestasis and/or focal hepatocyte fat droplets in periportal cell infiltrates
- TNF-α, IL-1, IL-6, bacterial lipopolysaccharides, and endotoxin inhibit bile salt export protein (BSEP) function

ESSENTIALS OF DIAGNOSIS OF JAUNDICE OF SEPSIS

- Assess the type of jaundice – conjugated versus unconjugated
- If unconjugated – initiate a search for hemolysis
- If conjugated – search for an hepatobiliary cause (diagnostic imaging – ultrasound)
- Full work-up to evaluate for infection (pan-culture)

ESSENTIALS OF TREATMENT AND PROGNOSIS

- Empiric antibiotic coverage: hepatic parameters may improve within a couple of weeks if they were secondary to infection alone

Introduction

This chapter will focus on the hepatic dysfunction during sepsis and bacterial and fungal infections that affect the liver.

Hepatic dysfunction during sepsis

Epidemiology

Abnormal liver blood tests have been described in a wide range of septic scenarios, from isolated intra-abdominal abscess to lobar pneumonia or bacteremia (Tables 85.1 and 85.2). It occurs in up to 10% of cases with community-acquired pneumonia, 35% of those with positive blood cultures [1], and is almost universal in septic shock. It is more common in neonates and infants less than 1 year of age who have low bile salt-independent bile flow, than in adults, but does not otherwise relate to age, gender, organism isolated, nutritional state, or site of sepsis.

Pathophysiology

Jaundice of sepsis can arise from alterations in bilirubin metabolism and bile flow that are thought to be mediated by tumor necrosis factor-alpha (TNF-α), interleukin (IL)1, and IL6, as well as bacterial lipopolysaccharide and endotoxin [2]. These processes include:

- **An increase in hemolysis.** During sepsis a number of processes can accelerate the breakdown of red blood cells, which increases the production of bilirubin (unconjugated). Table 85.3 lists the causes of hemolysis in sepsis.
- **Reduced uptake and secretion of bilirubin.** Bilirubin normally dissociates from albumin at the sinusoidal surface of the hepatocyte and is taken up by the hepatocyte by organic anion transporter (OATP). Inside the hepatocyte, bilirubin is conjugated to monoglucuronides and diglucuronides by the enzyme uridine diphosphate-glucuronosyltransferase. Bilirubin glucuronides are excreted into bile against a steep concentration gradient by MRP2. In animal models of endotoxinemia, there is a decreased expression of OATP and MRP2 that would result in an excess of conjugated hyperbilirubinemia. In addition, the reduced expression of MRP2 results in reduced canalicular glutathione secretion and leads to reduced bile salt-independent bile flow.
- **Reduced uptake and secretion of bile salts.** Bile salts are taken up at the sinusoidal membrane by sodium-dependent taurocholate co-transporter (NTCP), and excreted by bile salt export protein (BSEP) at the canalicular membrane. The secretion of bile salts causes bile salt-dependent bile flow. A reduced expression of NTCP and BSEP has been shown in cholestasis of sepsis and leads to reduced bile flow.

Histology

The most prominent finding is **intrahepatic cholestasis**. Bile is observed in bile canaliculi and hepatocyte cytoplasm. Bile back-flow into the perisinusoidal spaces may lead to bile uptake by Kupffer cells. There may also be some cholestasis-related parenchymal changes, including feathery degeneration of the hepatocyte cytoplasm. Apoptosis when present appears as rounded bile-tinged apoptotic bodies in the hepatic lobule.

Liver Disease

Textbook of Clinical Gastroenterology and Hepatology, Second Edition. Edited by C. J. Hawkey, Jaime Bosch, Joel E. Richter, Guadalupe Garcia-Tsao, Francis K. L. Chan.
© 2012 Blackwell Publishing Ltd. Published 2012 by Blackwell Publishing Ltd.

Table 85.1 Clinical syndromes of sepsis associated with liver dysfunction

- Lobar pneumonia
- Bacteremia
- Multiple organ failure
- Related to specific organisms
- Toxic shock syndrome

Table 85.2 Bacteremic microorganisms associated with jaundice of sepsis

- *Escherichia coli*
- *Klebsiella*
- *Pseudomonas aeruginosa*
- *Salmonella*
- *Bacteroides*
- *Clostridium perfringens*
- *Staphylococcus aureus*
- *Streptococcus pneumoniae*

Table 85.3 Causes of hemolysis in sepsis

Normal red blood cells (RBCs)
- Infections directly causing hemolysis (e.g. *Clostridium perfringens*)
- Immunologically-mediated RBC injury:
  - Cold agglutinin-associated hemolytic anemia:
    - *Mycoplasma pneumoniae*
    - Legionella
  - Paroxysmal cold hemoglobinuria
- Drug-induced hemolysis
- Transfusion reactions
- Hypersplenism

Underlying RBC defects (increased susceptibility to hemolysis during sepsis)
- Inherited enzyme deficiency
- Sickle cell disease
- Hemoglobinopathies

An increased amount of smooth endoplasmic reticulum as a result of cholestasis may lead to ground-glass hepatocytes.

Clinical presentation

In a minority of cases, jaundice is the initial presenting feature along with fever, rigors, and confusion. More commonly, **abnormal liver blood tests** appear after 24–48 hours.

Investigation and treatment

Liver blood test abnormalities occurring in septic scenarios should initially be investigated with an abdominal ultrasound scan. This may reveal evidence of prior chronic liver disease and portal hypertension, biliary obstruction, or focal septic fluid collections. Sets of blood cultures as well as sputum, urine, and, where appropriate, stool cultures are crucial. Where **sepsis** is suspected, early treatment with broad-spectrum antibiotics is indicated, even before culture results are available, as early therapy is important (Table 85.4).

Table 85.4 Assessment of jaundice in a septic patient

- Unconjugated – initiate a search for hemolysis
- Conjugated:
  - Search for a hepatobiliary cause: imaging studies:
    - Ultrasound (with or without Doppler)
    - CT/MRCP
  - Full work-up to evaluate for infection:
    - Complete blood count with differential
    - Urine analysis
    - Culture blood, urine, sputum, catheter tips, drains, and other potential sources of infection
    - Chest X-ray and other imaging of potential sites of infection (rule out abscess, echocardiography, etc.)
  - Empiric antibiotic coverage: in selected cases, hepatic parameters may improve within a couple of weeks if they were secondary to infection alone

MRCP, magnetic resonance cholangiopancreatography

Prognosis

During pneumonia and bacteremia, the presence of jaundice or abnormal liver blood tests is not associated with an adverse prognosis. In the adult respiratory distress syndrome, abnormal liver blood tests constitute one organ failure and the total number of organ failures accurately predicts mortality. Hepatic dysfunction is a component of scoring systems that predict mortality (APACHE II, SOFA).

Direct hepatic involvement with specific microorganisms

Gram-positive bacilli

Listerosis

Listeria monocytogenes is a motile, non–spore-forming, Gram-positive bacillus that has aerobic and facultatively anaerobic characteristics. It is an uncommon cause of infection in the general population, with risk factors for infection including pregnancy, extremes of age (neonates and the elderly), and immunocompromise.

It is typically a food-borne organism. The most common clinical manifestation is diarrhea. Blood culture results are positive in 60–75% of patients. Solitary liver abscess, multiple liver abscesses, and diffuse granulomatous hepatitis are recognized hepatic presentations [3]. Ampicillin is the treatment of choice.

Actinomycosis

Actinomycosis is a subacute-to-chronic bacterial infection caused by filamentous, Gram-positive, non–acid-fast, anaerobic-to-microaerophilic bacteria. In order for this organism to cause disease, both devitalized tissue and a break in the mucous membranes are required in addition to companion bacteria (*Actinobacillus actinomycetemcomitans*, followed by *Peptostreptococcus, Prevotella, Fusobacterium, Bacteroides, Staphylococcus,* and *Streptococcus* species, and *Enterobacteriaceae*). Invasion of the liver can be via both hematogenous and contiguous spread, and can mimic malignancy. Specimens taken from the liver need prompt transport to the laboratory and culturing immediately under anaerobic conditions.

Gram-positive cocci (*Staphylococci* and *Streptococci*)

Both these organisms can cause liver abscesses and para-infectious hepatitis secondary to toxin production.

Gram-negative bacilli

Salmonella

Salmonella enteritidis, *S. typhi*, and *S. paratyphi* can cause hepatic dysfunction. This may occur via jaundice of sepsis (secondary to endotoxin), the formation of liver abscess, cholecystitis, or granulomatous hepatitis. Recently, reports have suggested that elevated transaminases also may occur from muscle injury.

Brucella

Brucellosis is a bacterial illness caused by *Brucella suis* (from pigs), *B. abortus* (from cattle), *B. melitensis* (from goats, sheep, and camels), and *B. canis* (from dogs). It is a Gram-negative organism, non-motile, and does not form spores. Hepatic presentations include hepatomeagly and granulomatous hepatitis. Diagnosis is by both serology and blood culture. Treatment is with intramuscular/intravenous aminoglycoside and doxycycline for 1 month. This is then followed with doxycycline and rifampin (rifampicin) for a further month. Patients must be followed up for 1–2 years after treatment to ensure no re-emergence of infection.

Melioidosis

Melioidosis is caused by a Gram-negative bacterium, *Burkholderia pseudomallei*, found in soil and water [4]. It is of public health importance in endemic areas, particularly in Thailand and northern Australia. It exists in acute (hepatic abscesses) and chronic forms (granulomatous hepatitis). Treatment is with intravenous meropenem followed by prolonged oral eradication (septrin or doxycycline).

Bartonella

Three *Bartonella* species are currently considered important causes of human disease. *B. bacilliformis* causes Oroya fever and verruga peruana. *B. henselae* causes cat scratch disease, which can present with a granulomatous hepatitis and peliosis of the liver (often called bacillary peliosis); *B. quintana* causes trench fever, which can lead to hepatic abscesses.

Spirochete infection

Treponema pallidum

Syphillus has four recognized clinical phases during chronic infection [5]. During the secondary phase both a raised alkaline phosphatase and hepatitis may occur. During tertiary syphillus, microscopic-to-macroscopic granulomatous lesions may develop in the liver (gummata). These can cause fever and epigastric pain, and may lead to cirrhosis. Congenital syphilis is also recognized to cause portal fibrosis that can lead to hepatomeagly, portal hypertension, and ascites, and can be associated with hepatic calcifications.

Leptospirosis

Leptospirosis is caused by two species of *Leptospira*: pathogenic *Leptospira interogans* and the saprophytic *L. biflexa*. *L. interogans* has 19 subspecies and 170 serovariants, which include the well-known *L. icterohaemorrhagiae*, *L. hebdomadis*, and *L. canicola*, among others. The host in European countries is predominantly the rat, but *Leptospira* may occur widely in dogs, hedgehogs, and raccoons. Transmission to humans occurs most commonly in the summer and fall from water contaminated by urine, into which the spirochete has been shed, entering through breaches in skin or mucosal surfaces. Asymptomatic seroconversion is common, especially in high-risk occupations such as sewerage and water workers. Recreational exposure to contaminated water during sailing and canoeing is increasing.

Pathology

The pathogenesis of both the histological changes in liver and kidney, which are often not dramatic, and the development of end-organ dysfunction, which may be severe, is poorly understood. The incubation phase is between 7 and 13 days, followed by a septicemic phase for 2–3 days and a localized phase where end-organ damage to kidney, liver, myocardium, muscles, and skin may predominate. In the liver, jaundice is due to both conjugated hyperbilirubinemia with cholestasis and hepatocyte ballooning, as well an unconjugated fraction due to hemolysis from disseminated intravascular coagulation.

Clinical features

An anicteric illness starts during the septicemic phase with fever of >39 °C, chills, rigors, headaches with meningism, conjunctival suffusion, and muscle aches/pain. There is marked neutrophil leukocytosis and high creatine kinase, but only minor elevations in aminotransferases and alkaline phosphatase. Leptospires are detectable in blood cultures. The subsequent phase of immune localization occurs 1–3 days later when the organism may be found in urine. It is associated with a lower fever but more evidence of end-organ damage. The majority of infections follow such an anicteric course. An icteric form (**Weil's disease**) may occur with any serovariant, but may be more common with *L. icterohaemorrhagiae*, and represents a more severe illness with renal dysfunction and frank jaundice. Bilirubin may rise to levels higher than 800 mmol/L with only minor elevation in aminotransferases or alkaline phosphatase. Prothrombin time, if prolonged, is a reflection of intravascular coagulation as is thrombocytopenia [6].

Differential diagnosis

In any patient presenting with fever, acute jaundice, and renal impairment, Weil's disease must be considered. Alcoholic hepatitis with hepatorenal syndrome may also present with leukocytosis, but any fever is usually milder. Wilson disease may also have an acute presentation with renal failure, and severe viral hepatitis (hepatitis A, B/D, cytomegalovirus, Epstein–Barr virus, parvovirus) will need to be excluded.

Mycobacterial infections within the liver
Epidemiology
The prevalence of mycobacterial infections is increasing as a consequence of the spread of acquired immune deficiency syndrome (AIDS) and increased global travel. *Mycobacterium tuberculosis*, *M. bovis*, *M. kansasii*, *M. gordonae*, and *M. aviumintracellulare* may cause hepatic infection. Risk factors for the development of a mycobacterial infection include human immunodeficiency virus (HIV) carriage, intravenous drug use, alcoholism, diabetes mellitus, renal failure, and immunosuppression. Reactivation of prior mycobacterial infection may occur years after the primary infection. Disseminated or miliary tuberculosis occurs in approximately 10% of cases, in whom liver involvement is universal.

Pathology
The most common pattern is a **granulomatous liver disease** predominantly of lobular distribution, with epithelioid and chronic inflammatory cells, and occasional giant cells. The granulomas do not have diagnostic features and central caseation may occur in up to 50%. In patients who are severely debilitated, an associated microvesicular steatosis, reactive hepatitis, and peliosis hepatis have also been reported. The host response dictates the extent of granuloma formation. In immunosuppressed HIV cases, the granulomas are loose aggregates of cells with abundant acid-alcohol-fast bacilli on Ziehl–Nielson staining, whereas in the more immunocompetent cases with florid granulomas the bacteria are often difficult to detect.

Clinical features
There is no characteristic clinical presentation of hepatic tuberculosis, which can be notoriously protean and mimic many other diseases. Hepatomegaly with mild elevations of alkaline phosphatase and gamma-glutamyl transpeptidase is most common, but rarely an acute liver failure syndrome may be present with encephalopathy and hypoglycemia [7]. Weight loss is often present as well as features of other organ involvement, including pulmonary/pleural spaces, genitourinary and gastrointestinal tracts, and regional lymphadenopathy. During miliary tuberculosis, liver involvement is inevitable and tuberculous peritonitis may accompany any hepatic involvement. Fever is variable but a pyrexia of unknown origin may point to the diagnosis.

Treatment
The strain and drug sensitivity are critical to eradication of tuberculosis. Initial intensive therapy with isoniazid, rifampin (rifampicin), pyrazinamide, and ethambutol for 8 weeks is followed by isoniazid and rifampin (rifampicin) for 16 weeks. Directly observed therapy strategy (DOTS) is promoted in developing countries. Drug toxicity is an important side effect and **hepatotoxicity** occurs in up to 5–10% of cases. Monitoring of liver blood tests during the first month is recommended. Isoniazid, rifampin (rifampicin), pyrazinamide, and ethambutol are all implicated in hepatotoxicity, but it is most common with isoniazid hepatitis. Coexisting chronic liver disease, alcoholism, slow acetylation phenotype, and co-administration with rifampin (rifampicin) all increase the risk. Rifampin (rifampicin) more commonly causes a cholestatic picture.

Fungal infections and the liver
Hepatosplenic candidiasis
Candidemia and disseminated candidiasis, including hepatosplenic invasion, is becoming increasingly recognized in patients following cancer therapy or organ transplantation, and in the critically ill in intensive care units (Table 85.5). In 50% of cases, liver invasion is preceded by documented candidemia.

Clinical features
Candidemia may be detected in a critically ill patient who is pyrexial and commonly neutropenic [8]. Hepatosplenic involvement [9] is suggested by an elevated alkaline phosphatase and occasional right upper quadrant pain. Fever may have been resistant to broad-spectrum antibiotics. Imaging techniques, including ultrasonography and computed tomography (CT) scanning, may show focal lesions when the white cell count has rebounded.

Treatment
There is clear evidence from randomized controlled trials that prophylaxis with azoles (fluconazole) in high-risk cases can prevent significant mucosal colonization and invasive candidiasis. Where possible, treatment should be accompanied by attempts to reverse predisposing factors for *Candida* invasion, dictated by fungal sensitivity testing. Treatment starts with amphotericin B in a liposomal preparation when renal function is at risk. Newer antifungals, including voriconazole and caspofungin, have shown early promise.

Histoplasmosis and other fungal infections
H. capsulatum is a dimorphic fungus that is soil based and endemic in Ohio and the Mississippi river valleys. Most

Table 85.5 Risk factors for invasive candida

- Neutropenia
- T-lymphocyte deficiency
- Complement deficiency
- Diabetes mellitus
- Prior antibiotic therapy
- Gastrointestinal disease
- Intravascular catheters

individuals who are infected are asymptomatic. Those developing clinical manifestations are usually immunocompromised or are exposed to a high quantity of inoculum. *Histoplasma* species may remain latent in healed granulomas and recur with an impairment of cell-mediated immunity. Conversion from the mycelial to the pathogenic yeast form occurs intracellularly in macrophages. Systemic spread usually occurs in patients with impaired cellular immunity. A granulomatous hepatitis may occur.

Both ***Coccidioides immitis***, the etiological agent responsible for coccidioidomycosis, and ***Crytococcus neoformans*** can cause a granulomatous hepatitis.

References

1. Franson TR, Hierholzer WJ Jr, LaBrecque DR. Frequency and characteristics of hyperbilirubinemia associated with bacteremia. *Rev Infect Dis.* 1985;7:1–9.
2. Bolder U, Ton-Nu HT, Schteingart CD, Frick E, Hofmann AF. Hepatocyte transport of bile acids and organic anions in endotoxemic rats: impaired uptake and secretion. *Gastroenterology.* 1997;112:214–225.
3. Samra Y, Hertz M, Altmann G. Adult listeriosis – a review of 18 cases. *Postgrad Med J.* 1984;60:267–269.
4. Piggott JA, Hochholzer L. Human melioidosis. A histopathologic study of acute and chronic melioidosis. *Arch Pathol.* 1970;90: 101–111.
5. Schlossberg D. Syphilitic hepatitis: a case report and review of the literature. *Am J Gastroenterol.* 1987;82:552–553.
6. Covic A, Goldsmith DJ, Gusbeth-Tatomir P, Seica A, Covic M. A retrospective 5-year study in Moldova of acute renal failure due to leptospirosis: 58 cases and a review of the literature. *Nephrol Dial Transplant.* 2003;18:1128–1134.
7. Mitchell I, Wendon J, Fitt S, Williams R. Antituberculous therapy and acute liver failure. *Lancet.* 1995;345:555–556.
8. Tiraboschi IN, Bennett JE, Kauffman CA, *et al.* Deep Candida infections in the neutropenic and non-neutropenic host: an ISHAM symposium. *Med Mycol.* 2000;38 (Suppl 1):199–204.
9. Kontoyiannis DP, Luna MA, Samuels BI, Bodey GP. Hepatosplenic candidiasis. A manifestation of chronic disseminated candidiasis. *Infect Dis Clin North Am.* 2000;14:721–739.

Liver Disease

CHAPTER 86
Primary biliary cirrhosis

Raoul Poupon

Hôpital Saint-Antoine, Paris, France

ESSENTIAL FACTS ABOUT PATHOGENESIS

- Due to a combination of multiple genetic factors (allelic variations of genes controlling the immune system) and environmental triggers (urinary tract infections, exposure to chemicals and toxins)
- T- and B-cell activation leads to autoimmunity against M2 antigen and causes small bile duct inflammation and destruction
- Chronic cholestasis leads to biliary cirrhosis and liver failure

---

ESSENTIALS OF DIAGNOSIS

- Mainly elevation of serum alkaline phosphatase and gamma-glutamyl transpeptidase
- Antimitochondrial antibodies with M2 specificity
- Non-suppurative destructive cholangitis at histology

ESSENTIALS OF TREATMENT

- Ursodeoxycholic acid (13–15 mg/kg/day).
- In patients with suboptimal biochemical response to ursodeoxycholic acid, adjuvant therapy with budesonide or methotrexate may be effective
- Liver transplantation for end-stage disease or intractable symptoms

---

Introduction

Primary biliary cirrhosis (PBC) is a **chronic inflammatory autoimmune disease** that targets mainly cholangiocytes of the interlobular bile ducts. The condition affects primarily middle-aged women and is generally slowly progressive over a period of 10–20 years. Inflammation and destruction of the bile ducts leads to decreased bile secretion, retention of toxic substances within the liver, fibrosis, cirrhosis, and eventually liver failure requiring liver transplantation. The rate of progression varies greatly from one patient to another. PBC is characterized by the presence of a subset of **antimitochondrial antibodies (AMAs)** that react with the lipoyl domains of the 2-oxo acid dehydrogenases in the mitochondria, the so-called M2 antigen, which is virtually diagnostic. Most patients with PBC are now diagnosed in the early stages of the disease and are treated with ursodeoxycholic acid (UDCA). The number of liver transplantations performed for this indication has been decreasing over the last two decades.

Epidemiology [1]

The incidence and prevalence of PBC have been increasing over time. Most recent data from Europe, North America, and Japan show an incidence of 2–4 per 100 000 population per year and point prevalence at 20–40 cases per 100 000 population. Geographical clustering is striking, suggesting genetic as well as environmental influences in its pathogenesis. Whether the higher rates of incidence and prevalence reflect a true increase or an apparent increase due to a higher detection rate remains unknown.

Causes and pathogenesis [1,2]

PBC is thought to be a complex disease resulting from the combination of multiple genetic factors and superimposed environmental triggers. These factors may affect one or more components of the immune system and of the tissue that is targeted by the disease. The contribution of the **genetic predisposition** is evidenced by the familial clustering and the high degree to which monozygotic twins are concordant. The prevalence of PBC is 100 times higher in first-degree relatives than in the general population. Allelic variations in MHC class II (DR,DQ), components of the innate (C4*Q0, C4B*2, NRAMP1/SLC11A1, MBL,VDR) and adaptive (CTLA4, IIβ, TNF-α, IL12A, IL12RB2) immune system have been associated with PBC susceptibility. The genetic basis of variability in disease progression is poorly understood. The French prospective study of genetic factors for PBC severity have suggested the role of variants of tumor necrosis factor alpha (TNF-α) and SLCA2/AE2. Regarding **environmental factors**, mucosal infections, particularly urinary tract infections, cigarette smoking, and toxin exposure have been consistently associated with PBC. The role of xenobiotics through covalent binding of 2-octynoic acid, a component of many chemicals, to proteins is suggested by experimental studies. Smoking not only predisposes to disease but may also accelerate its progression. The ratio of women to men with the disease is 10:1. This may be related to a higher incidence of X-chromosome monosomy in lymphoid cells.

Although a unified theory of PBC pathogenesis is not available, a paradigm can be proposed that considers pathobiological events leading to disease progression. The **preclinical**

Textbook of Clinical Gastroenterology and Hepatology, Second Edition. Edited by C. J. Hawkey, Jaime Bosch, Joel E. Richter, Guadalupe Garcia-Tsao, Francis K. L. Chan.
© 2012 Blackwell Publishing Ltd. Published 2012 by Blackwell Publishing Ltd.

Liver Disease

phase is marked by autoimmunity and altered cholangiocyte homeostasis. Autoimmunity is manifested by M2 antibodies (M2Ab) that specifically react with the lipoyl domain of the E2 subunits of the 2-oxo-acid dehydrogenase complexes of the mitochondria. The T and B cells infiltrating the liver in PBC are specific for the M2 antigen. The M2 epitope is detectable in cholangiocytes undergoing apoptosis and at the luminal domain of the biliary cells of the small bile ducts. As opposed to other cell types, cholangiocytes undergoing apoptosis fail to bind glutathione to the lysine-lipoyl residue of the dehydrogenase and thereby fail to cleave the autoreactive epitope. Neighboring cholangiocytes have the ability to phagocytoze apoptotic cells and express the M2 epitope. This is a rational explanation for the tissue specificity of the autoimmune process. The mechanisms that could trigger cholangiocyte apoptosis are unknown, but may involve mucosal IgA M2Ab, abnormal bile composition, or altered endocrine or neuroendocrine mediated-regulation of metabolic and kinetic activity of cholangiocytes.

The **early clinical phase** is marked by inflammation and anicteric cholestasis. In this early stage, the non-ductopenic stage, inflammation is associated with similar rates of apoptosis and proliferation of the biliary cells. Cytolytic T cells, CD8, CD4, and NKT are attracted to the target cells by the release of chemokines. Killing is mediated mainly through activation of TNF, CD40, and Fas receptors. Under the pressure of this environment, cholangiocytes proliferate through mediators that include those of the cholinergic pathway, and estrogens and their alpha receptors.

In many patients, inflammation spreads into the lobule leading to an **interface hepatitis**. This process proceeds in two ways: the lymphocytic piecemeal necrosis, similar to that found in autoimmune hepatitis, and the biliary piecemeal necrosis, which is marked by a striking increase in the number of ductular profiles associated with edema, neutrophil infiltration, periductular fibroplasias, and hepatocellular death with features of cholate stasis.

Hepatocellular death triggers expansion of progenitor cells and is marked by the appearance of reactive ductules that secrete mediators that attract and activate fibroblasts. The limiting plates are thus progressively replaced by newly formed connective tissue. Interface hepatitis represents the turning point in the natural history of PBC. Its severity predicts the onset of cirrhosis.

Cholestasis is a hallmark of PBC. In the early non-ductopenic stage, cholestasis results from mediators and proinflammatory cytokines that inhibit canalicular and ductular bile secretion. UDCA has the ability to restore bile secretion at least in part because of its anti-inflammatory properties in the biliary tree. In later phases, cholestasis is mainly due to the loss of bile ducts.

Clinical presentation [1,3,4]

There are three major forms of PBC. The **typical or classical form** is represented by the slowly progressive decline of small bile ducts and parallel increase in liver fibrosis, leading to biliary cirrhosis over a period of 10–20 years. A second form that affects 10–20% of patients is characterized by the fluctuating or persistent presence of **features of autoimmune hepatitis**. These patients have a more severe course, with early development of liver fibrosis and liver failure. A third form that affects 5–10% of patients is represented by the so-called **premature ductopenic variant**. Its hallmark is a very rapid onset of ductopenia and severe icteric cholestasis, progressing very quickly towards cirrhosis in <5 years.

PBC is currently diagnosed earlier in its clinical course. Half of the patients are asymptomatic at diagnosis. **Fatigue and pruritus** are early-phase symptoms. Fatigue is a frequent complaint that is unrelated to disease severity and has a major impact on quality of life. Whether or not it is a specific symptom remains unknown. It is associated with cognitive and emotional dysfunction, depression, sensory and autonomic abnormalities, as well as excessive daytime somnolence. About half of the patients have mild pruritus at diagnosis. It may be severe, particularly in the premature ductopenic variant, severely affecting quality of life. In some patients the diagnosis is made during the work-up of another autoimmune disease, and in 5–10% during the work-up of cirrhosis. In the variant associated with features of autoimmune hepatitis, the diagnosis may be made in a patient with seemingly acute hepatitis.

In the typical form, serum alkaline phosphatase and gamma-glutamyl transpeptidase are characteristically elevated, with only mild-to-moderate elevation of serum aminotransferases. In the premature ductopenic variant, cholestasis is quite severe and is associated with marked hypercholesterolemia affecting both high- (HDL) and low-density lipoprotein (LDL) fractions. In patients with features of both autoimmune hepatitis and PBC, serum aminotrasferase levels may be markedly elevated and are usually associated with marked IgG elevations. All forms of PBC are associated with increased IgM levels. Thrombocytopenia, polyclonal hyperglobulinemia, and hyperbilirubinemia are indicators of **cirrhosis**. A prolonged INR and hypoalbuminemia usually occur in the terminal phase.

Diagnostic investigation

Ultrasound of the liver and biliary tree is mandatory in all patients presenting with liver abnormalities suggestive of PBC. If the biliary system appears normal by ultrasound and the patient is positive for AMAs, no further radiological examination of the bile ducts is necessary. If the diagnosis of PBC is uncertain, cholangiography may be necessary.

The major hallmark of PBC is the presence of AMAs in serum. AMAs that react with the E2 component of pyruvate dehydrogenase are diagnostic of PBC. A variety of antinuclear antibodies is associated with PBC. Of these, those that react with the proteins of the pore complex (gp210, nucleoporin 62) and with the nuclear body protein (sp100) are specific.

Liver histological examination is only indicated if the patient is negative for AMAs or has the biochemical profile of atypical

PBC, or if superimposed co-morbidity is suspected. Nevertheless it should be emphasized that histology is necessary for prognostic evaluation and treatment strategy.

Treatment
Specific therapy [5–8]
All PBC patients with abnormal liver biochemistry should be considered for specific therapy.

UDCA, at a dose of 13–15 mg/kg/day, is currently considered the mainstay of therapy for PBC. Randomized, double-blinded, placebo-controlled trials have consistently shown that UDCA improves parameters of liver biochemistry, including serum bilirubin, the major prognostic marker in PBC. UDCA delays the progression of fibrosis and of histological stage. A combined analysis of three randomized controlled trials including 548 patients with PBC showed improved survival free of liver transplantation in patients with moderate-to-severe disease treated with UDCA at doses of 13–15 mg/kg/day for up to 4 years. Long-term observational studies from France, Spain, and the Netherlands have shown that UDCA therapy is associated with an improvement in survival compared to that predicted by the Mayo model. Survival in UDCA-treated patients in stages 1 and 2 is similar to that in a control population. Some meta-analyses (but not all) including short-term trials with low doses of UDCA (<12 mg/kg/day) have questioned the efficacy of UDCA. However, on the basis of all available data, it is currently recommended to treat PBC with UDCA using doses of at least 13 mg/kg/day and to start these early. UDCA can be taken in divided doses or as a single dose.

Overall UDCA is extremely safe. Because UDCA is an acid it can lead to gastric discomfort, heartburn, and symptomatic reflux. These symptoms are easily managed with proton pump inhibitors or by ingesting the bile acid at the end of meals. The majority of patients notice weight gain (3 kg, on average). In patients with pruritus and frank cholestasis, UDCA may actually increase pruritus at the recommended dose; in these patients, UDCA should be initiated at a lower dose (200–400 mg/day) and progressively increased to the recommended dose over 4–8 weeks.

The aim of UDCA therapy is to normalize serum bilirubin, alkaline phosphatase, and aminotransferase levels at the end of the first year of therapy. In many patients this cannot be achieved. An optimal response to UDCA is defined when, after the first year of therapy, serum bilirubin is <1 mg/dL, AST less than two times the upper limit of normal, and alkaline phosphatase is less than three times the upper limit of normal. A decrease of >50% in serum alkaline phosphatase has also been described as predictive of an excellent long-term prognosis. In a small subset of patients, the daily dose of 13–15 mg is not sufficient to achieve the best biochemical response. In these patients, measurement by HPLC-mass spectrometry of the blood or biliary enrichment in UDCA may be useful. In those with a low percentage of UDCA (<40%), a trial with daily doses up to 20 mg/kg/day has been proposed to achieve a better response.

About 30–40% of our patients have a suboptimal response to UDCA. These patients need adjuvant therapy.

Adjuvant therapies [9,10]
Glucocorticoids and methotrexate should be considered in patients with features of autoimmune hepatitis, severe interface hepatitis, abnormal serum bilirubin level or suboptimal response to UDCA.

Preliminary studies in our patients indicate that patients with a suboptimal response to UDCA benefit from the combination of **UDCA and glucocorticoids (prednisone or budesonide)** in terms of survival without liver transplantation. Glucocorticoids, specifically budesonide, have been shown to provide added benefit in patients treated with UDCA, with greater biochemical and histological (inflammation and fibrosis) responses. Budesonide is given at a dose of 6–9 mg/day in non-cirrhotic patients. The drug is contraindicated in patients with cirrhosis.

Methotrexate [11,12] has been shown to improve biochemical and histological results when added to UDCA in patients with an incomplete response to UDCA. However, in other studies methotrexate has been ineffective when used alone or in combination with UDCA. In a 10-year multicenter study, survival was the same in patients randomized to methotrexate plus UDCA or colchicine plus UDCA, with a survival similar to that predicted by the Mayo model. However, one-third of the patients had fewer signs of PBC after 10 years of treatment and no patient at a precirrhotic stage at enrollment progressed to cirrhosis. Methotrexate may cause interstitial pneumonitis similar to that seen in rheumatoid arthritis.

Many other drugs, colchicine, cyclosporine [13], chlorambucil, penicillamine, azathioprine, mycophenolate mophetil, malotilate, and thalidomide have been evaluated in PBC. They are either ineffective or toxic. None is effective in UDCA-treated patients at risk of developing cirrhosis and/or liver failure.

FXR agonists (obeticholic acid) and PPAR alpha-agonists (fenofibrate and bezafibrate) are new promising drugs that could enhance the therapeutic effect of UDCA. Controlled trials are currently underway.

Liver transplantation
Liver transplantation has greatly improved survival in patients with PBC. It is the only effective treatment for those with decompensated cirrhosis or liver failure. Patients with the premature ductopenic variant of PBC do not respond to medical therapy and liver transplantation should be considered despite the absence of decompensated liver disease. PBC recurs in about 25% of patients at 5 years post transplantation. Recurrence is more frequent in patients without a glucocorticoid and cyclosporine regimen. The utility of UDCA in this setting remains unknown.

Treatment of symptoms and complications
Pruritus
First-line therapy is rifampicin at a daily dose of 300–600 mg in patients receiving UDCA. However, the drug may induce hepatitis in some cases. Second-line therapies include glucocorticoids, cholestyramine, sertraline, and opiate antagonists. Plasmapheresis or biliary drainage may be successful when other treatments fail. In very rare patients, resistant pruritus may be an indication for liver transplantation.

Fatigue
Modafinil, a drug approved for the treatment of narcolepsy, has been reported in open studies to provide significant improvement in fatigue in patients with PBC. The drug given at a dose of up to 400 mg/day seems to be well tolerated and should be considered in patients with excessive fatigue and daytime somnolence.

Hypercholesterolemia
UDCA induces an average 15–20% decrease in total and LDL cholesterol after 1 year of therapy. Statins and fibrates are safe and effective in patients in whom LDL cholesterol is elevated despite UDCA treatment.

Portal hypertension
A minority of patients with PBC develops presinusoidal portal hypertension before becoming cirrhotic. The management of portal hypertension in patients with PBC should follow the same guidelines as for patients with cirrhosis at large. Severe portal hypertension even without any other signs of decompensation is a good indication for liver transplantation.

Osteopenia and osteoporosis
Osteopenia and osteoporosis affect up to 30% of patients with PBC. Current therapies include physical activity, and calcium and vitamin D supplementation with the goal of achieving serum 25-hydroxy vitamin D3 levels of >30 ng/ml. Other therapies include biphosphonates or estrogen supplementation.

SOURCES OF INFORMATION FOR PATIENTS AND DOCTORS
http://www.liverfoundation.org
http://www.pbcfoundation.org.uk
http://pbcers.org
http://www.Aalbi-france.org
http://cmr-mivb.org

References
1. Poupon R. Primary biliary cirrhosis: a 2010 update. *J Hepatol.* 2010;52:745–758.
2. Lleo A, Invernizzi P, Mackay I, Prince H, Zhong RQ, Gershwin ME. Etiopathogenesis of primary biliary cirrhosis. *World J Gastroenterol.* 2008;14:3328–3337.
3. Poupon R. Autoimmune overlapping syndromes. *Clin Liver Dis.* 2003;7:865–878.
4. Vleggaar FP, van Buuren HR, Zondervan PE, ten Kate FJ, Hop WC. Jaundice in non-cirrhotic primary biliary cirrhosis: the premature ductopenic variant. *Gut.* 2001;49:276–281.
5. Poupon RE, Lindor KD, Cauch-Dudek K, Dickson ER, Poupon R, Heathcote EJ. Combined analysis of randomized controlled trials of ursodeoxycholic acid in primary biliary cirrhosis. *Gastroenterology.* 1997;113:884–890.
6. Corpechot C, Carrat F, Bahr A, Chretien Y, Poupon RE, Poupon R. The effect of ursodeoxycholic acid therapy on the natural course of primary biliary cirrhosis. *Gastroenterology.* 2005;128:297–303.
7. Corpechot C, Carrat F, Bonnand AM, Poupon RE, Poupon R. The effect of ursodeoxycholic acid therapy on liver fibrosis progression in primary biliary cirrhosis. *Hepatology.* 2000;32:1196–1199.
8. Pares A, Caballeria L, Rodes J, et al. Long-term effects of ursodeoxycholic acid in primary biliary cirrhosis: results of a double-blind controlled multicentric trial. UDCA-Cooperative Group from the Spanish Association for the Study of the Liver. *J Hepatol.* 2000;32:561–566.
9. Pares A, Caballeria L, Rodes J. Excellent long-term survival in patients with primary biliary cirrhosis and biochemical response to ursodeoxycholic acid. *Gastroenterology.* 2006;130:715–720.
10. Corpechot C, Abenaboli L, Rabahi N, et al. Biochemical response to ursodeoxycholic acid and long-term prognosis in primary biliary cirrhosis. *Hepatology.* 2008;48:871–877.
11. Leuschner M, Maier KP, Schlichting J, et al. Oral budesonide and ursodeoxycholic acid for treatment of primary biliary cirrhosis: results of a prospective double-blind trial. *Gastroenterology.* 1999;117:918–925.
12. Rautiainen H, Karkkainen P, Karvonen AL, et al. Budesonide combined with UDCA to improve liver histology in primary biliary cirrhosis: a three-year randomized trial. *Hepatology.* 2005;41:747–752.
13. Kaplan MM, Cheng S, Price LL, Bonis PA. A randomized controlled trial of colchicine plus ursodiol versus methotrexate plus ursodiol in primary biliary cirrhosis: ten-year results. *Hepatology.* 2004;39:915–923.

Liver Disease

CHAPTER 87

Autoimmune hepatitis and overlap syndromes

Heike Bantel, Kinan Rifai and Michael P. Manns

Hannover Medical School, Hannover, Germany

ESSENTIAL FACTS ABOUT PATHOGENESIS

- *Prevalence*: around 100–200 per million
- *At risk*: young females, often with extrahepatic autoimmune disease
- *Pathogenesis*: multifactorial, probably triggered by environmental and host factors such as infections or dysregulated apoptosis
- *Genetic predisposition*: complex, includes genes of HLA and cytokines
- *Overlap syndromes*: unknown prevalence, pathogenesis and predisposition comparable to AIH

ESSENTIALS OF DIAGNOSIS

- *Classical*: Young female with chronic hepatitis and nonspecific symptoms. In 25% acute hepatitis and, rarely, even fulminant hepatitis.
- *Biochemistry*: elevation of aminotransferases, IgG, liver autoantibodies (ANA, SMA, LKM, SLA)
- *Liver histology*: periportal hepatitis, lymphocytic infiltrates, plasma cells, piecemeal necrosis
- *Diagnosis* established by exclusion of other etiologies of hepatitis, aided by use of a revised numeric score.
- *Overlap syndromes*: combination of features of AIH with PBC or PSC

ESSENTIALS OF TREATMENT

- *Standard therapy*: induction with prednisone monotherapy or, preferably, in combination with azathioprine; maintenance therapy with azathioprine
- *Alternative*: budesonide instead of prednisone offers equal efficacy with less side effects. Not recommended in cirrhosis
- *Treatment failure*: higher doses of standard therapy or use of other immunosuppressive drugs (e.g., cyclosporine A)
- *Overlap syndromes*: immunosuppressive therapy of AIH together with therapy of PBC or PSC, typically ursodesoxycholic acid

Introduction

In 1950 Waldenström described a chronic inflammatory liver disease in a young woman; this condition is now termed autoimmune hepatitis (AIH) and represents a chronic, mainly periportal hepatitis characterized by female predominance, hypergammaglobulinemia, circulating autoantibodies, and a good response to immunosuppressive treatment [1]. Serologic detection of autoantibodies is one of the distinguishing features that has led to the subclassification of autoimmune hepatitis into three groups (Table 87.1). AIH type I represents the most common form of AIH and is characterized by the presence of antinuclear antibodies (ANA) and/or anti-smooth muscle antibodies (SMA). The target autoantigen of type 1 autoimmune hepatitis is unknown. Characteristic antibodies of AIH type 2 are liver kidney microsomal antibodies (LKM-1) directed against cytochrome P450 (CYP)2D6 and, with lower frequency, against UDP-glucuronyltransferases (UGT). The complex associations of autoantibodies directed against microsomal antigens are summarized in Figure 87.1 [2,3]. AIH type 3 is characterized by autoantibodies against soluble liver antigen (SLA/LP) directed towards the UGA-suppressor transfer RNA (tRNA)-associated protein [4]. The term "overlap syndrome" describes a disease condition in which clinical, biochemical, and serological features of autoimmune hepatitis coexist with those of another autoimmune liver disease, most frequently with primary biliary cirrhosis (PBC) but also with primary sclerosing cholangitis (PSC), and, depending on the definition, also with hepatitis C. In adult patients an overlap of PBC and AIH is the most common occurrence although it remains unclear whether this is a true coexistence of both diseases or an immunoserological overlap characterized by the presence of antinuclear (ANA) and antimitochondrial (AMA) antibodies. A subgroup of ANA-positive patients, with high IgG and cholestasis but without immunoreactivity against AMA has been termed autoimmune cholangiopathy (AIC). The coexistence of AIH and PSC has only been conclusively shown in pediatric patients but its existence has been suggested in the adult AIH population. Besides coexistence, autoimmune liver diseases can evolve from one into another (sequential manifestation) [5].

Epidemiology

Originally described in Caucasian northern Europeans and North Americans, autoimmune hepatitis has a worldwide

Table 87.1 Clinical characteristics and distinguishing features of the three subclasses of autoimmune hepatitis (AIH)

Clinical features	AIH type 1	AIH type 2	AIH type 3
Diagnostic autoantibodies	ANA/SMA	LKM-1	SLA/LP
Target antigen	Nuclear antigens Smooth muscle actin unknown (??)	Cytochrome P450 (CYP)2D6 UDP-glucuronosyltransferase UGTIA	UGA-suppressor (tRNA)-associated protein
Prevalence of all AIH types	80%	20% in Europe; 4% in the US	<20%
Common age at presentation	Bimodal (16–30 and <50 years)	Pediatric (2–14 years)	20–40 years
Extrahepatic associated diseases	41%	34%	58%
HLA association	B8, DR3, DR4	B14, DR3, C4AQO	DRB1*03
Progression to cirrhosis	45%	82%	75%

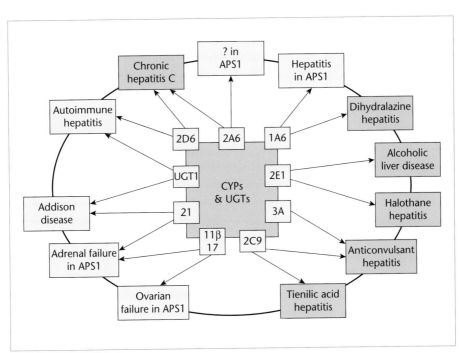

Figure 87.1 Hepatocellular autoantigens. The heterogeneity of hepatocellular autoantigens and their disease specificities. (This figure was published in *Clinical Gastroenterology and Hepatology*, Wilfred M. Weinstein, Christopher J. Hawkey, Jaime Bosch, Autoimmune hepatitis and overlap syndromes, Pages 629–635, Copyright Elsevier, 2005.)

distribution. It affects 100000–200000 persons in the United States [6] and accounts for 4% of transplant recipients in Europe [7] and 5.9% in the US [8]. In northern Europe, the prevalence is estimated at 170 cases per 1 million. Reliable data on the prevalence of autoimmune overlap syndromes is not available. Overlap syndromes (AIH/PBC or AIH/PSC) are present in about 8% of AIH patients [9,10]. In contrast, AIH features can be present in about 9% of PBC patients [11]. Autoimmune cholangiopathy comprises about 24% of autoimmune diseases of the liver [12]. Figure 87.2 summarizes overlapping features of AIH type 1 and PBC.

Causes, risk factors, and disease associations

AIH and overlap syndromes are often associated with extrahepatic immune-mediated syndromes including autoimmune thyroiditis, rheumatoid arthritis, and diabetes mellitus (Table 87.2). Most of these autoimmune diseases appear to be inherited because they are clustered in families. This inherited susceptibility is complex and probably relies on a combination of different genes, most notably immunogenetic markers (HLA genes) and cytokine genes. However, the lack of concordance of most autoimmune diseases in identical twin pairs indicates that other environmental and host factors, such as bacterial or

Liver Disease

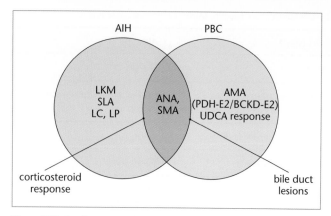

Figure 87.2 Overlapping syndrome. Serological profiles of an overlapping syndrome between autoimmune hepatitis and primary biliary cirrhosis. (This figure was published in *Clinical Gastroenterology and Hepatology*, Wilfred M. Weinstein, Christopher J. Hawkey, Jaime Bosch, Autoimmune hepatitis and overlap syndromes, Pages 629–635, Copyright Elsevier, 2005.)

Table 87.2 Extrahepatic autoimmunologic disease associations of autoimmune hepatitis

Types of disease	Associations
Hematologic	Autoimmune hemolytic anemia
	Thrombocytopenic purpura
	Pernicious anemia
	Eosinophilia
Gastrointestinal	Inflammatory bowel disease*
	Celiac disease
Rheumatologic	Synovitis*
	Rheumatoid arthritis
	CREST syndrome
	Systemic sclerosis
	Sjögren syndrome
Endocrinologic	Diabetes mellitus
	Autoimmune thyroid disease*
Others	Proliferative glomerulonephritis
	Lichen planus
	Vitiligo
	Nail dystrophy
	Alopecia
	Uveitis
	Erythema nodosum

*Most frequently observed.

viral infections, dysregulated apoptosis, or cytokine profile, may be relevant for development of autoimmune diseases.

Pathogenesis

Autoimmunity is characterized by T-cell-dependent immunopathological responses to auto/neo-antigens leading to inflammatory tissue injury. An autoimmune response can be triggered by the HLA class II-dependent presentation of specific antigenic peptides to T cells via antigen-presenting cells

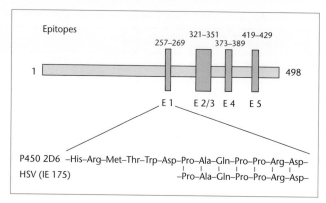

Figure 87.3 Sequence homologies. (This figure was published in *Clinical Gastroenterology and Hepatology*, Wilfred M. Weinstein, Christopher J. Hawkey, Jaime Bosch, Autoimmune hepatitis and overlap syndromes, Pages 629–635, Copyright Elsevier, 2005.)

(APCs). As a response to cytokines, exposed T cells become activated and differentiate into Th1 or Th2 cells. Proinflammatory cytokines are believed to play an important role in the initiation of the autoimmune response [13]. As a result of cytokine activation autoimmune diseases are often associated with viral or bacterial infections. Another mechanism is called "molecular mimicry". As an example, a major B cell epitope of cytochrome P450, which is targeted by LKM-1 autoantibodies in AIH-2, shares sequence homology with the herpes simplex virus antigen IE 175 (Figure 87.3) [2]. The immune response is normally tightly regulated. T- and B-cell homeostasis and the removal of autoreactive T cells are regulated by apoptosis. The failure of control by apoptosis may therefore contribute to the initiation and perpetuation of autoimmune hepatitis and autoimmune overlap syndromes [14]. This could be explained by the inability to kill autoreactive cells, or by inducing autoimmunity against cellular constituents modified by apoptosis. Genetic factors have been implicated in the susceptibility to autoimmune hepatitis. In particular, polymorphisms of genes influencing lymphocyte homeostasis, such as the TNF-α promoter gene (TNF-α), the complement factor C4 gene, and the CTLA-4 gene contribute to increased susceptibility to AIH [15]. One hypothesis suggests that inheritance of specific HLA class II alleles modified at critical sites, provides one of the crucial steps for the development of AIH. The relevance of genetic alterations for AIH is further underlined by the observation that chronic hepatitis occurs in 10–18% of patients with the autoimmune polyendocrine syndrome type 1 (APS1), an autosomal recessive disorder caused by mutations in a single gene (AIRE). APS-1 is characterized by various autoimmune diseases mainly affecting endocrine glands [16]. There has been no report of a genetic predisposition for overlap syndromes.

Autoimmune hepatitis

Clinical presentation

About 25% of patients show an acute onset of AIH and rare cases of fulminant progression of AIH leading to acute liver failure [17]. Commonly, the clinical presentation of AIH resembles that of other forms of chronic hepatitis. AIH is therefore characterized by nonspecific features, such as fatigue, right upper quadrant pain, jaundice, mild pruritus, arthralgias, and, when frank cirrhosis has developed, frequently also by spider angiomas and palmar erythema. In later stages, signs of decompensated cirrhosis including ascites, bleeding esophageal varices, and encephalopathy dominate disease picture. Both patients who present acutely and those who present with chronic hepatitis often show histologic evidence of cirrhosis at the onset of symptoms, underlining challenges in the diagnosis of early disease. As many as 25% of patients present with signs of decompensated cirrhosis [18]. Autoimmune hepatitis (especially type 2) is associated with a wide variety of other disorders, most of which are of immunological origin (Table 87.2).

Liver pathology

AIH is characterized by periportal hepatitis with lymphocytic infiltrates, plasma cells, and piecemeal necrosis. Lobular hepatitis can be observed, but is only indicative of AIH in the absence of copper deposits or biliary inflammation. The presence of granulomas and iron deposits argue against AIH.

Differential diagnosis

The clinical presentation of AIH is indistinguishable from other causes of acute or chronic hepatitis including cirrhosis. The clinical picture of AIH can therefore resemble viral hepatitis, drug- or alcohol-induced hepatitis. Other entities in the differential diagnosis of AIH include nonalcoholic steatohepatitis (NASH), genetic hemochromatosis, and alpha-1 antitrypsin deficiency. Patients with cryptogenic hepatitis, an etiologically undefined chronic hepatitis, are negative for viral and autoantibody markers and it is uncertain whether some of them may have AIH without detectable autoantibodies. If cholestatic signs and immunoserological markers of AIH are present, overlap syndromes have to be included in the differential diagnosis.

Diagnostic methods

The diagnosis of AIH is established by excluding other etiologies of chronic hepatitis (Table 87.3). The diagnosis can be aided by using a revised numeric score that describes the probability of having the disease (Table 87.4). The sensitivity of the scoring system to establish definite or probable AIH is 89.9%. However, the specificity of the initial version of this score for discriminating AIH from overlapping syndromes such as AIH/PBC or AIH/PSC was low. In the revised AIH score, patients with histologic and cholangiographic evidence of PBC or PSC should be viewed as having variants of cholestatic diseases and not AIH. Specifically, well-defined granulomas, typical bile duct pathology of PSC, and PBC, and substantial marginal bile duct proliferation with cholangiolitis and copper accumulation exclude AIH. Cholangiography is recommended in all patients who score as definite or probable AIH but do not respond to steroid treatment. A simplified score for AIH

Table 87.3 Autoimmune hepatitis: a diagnosis of exclusion

Suspected differential diagnosis	Test performed to exclude
Hepatitis C infection (HCV)	Anti-HCV (HCV RNA)
Hepatitis B and C (HBV, HDV)	HBsAg, anti-HBc (HBV RNA) Anti-HDV AK (??), HDV RNA only when HBsAg positive
Hepatitis A virus (HAV)	Antibodies; serology: IgG, IgM
Hepatitis E virus (HEV)	Only if suspected
Epstein–Barr virus (EBV)	Only if suspected
Herpes simplex virus (HSV)	Only if suspected
Cytomegalovirus (CMV)	Only if suspected
Varicella zoster virus (VZV)	Only if suspected
Drug-induced hepatitis	History; if applicable withdrawal of drug LKM-2, in selected cases
Primary biliary cirrhosis (PBC)	Anti-mitochondrial antibodies (AMA) Specification of reactivity: PDH-E2, BCKD-E2 Liver histology: florid cholangitis, granuloma Unresponsive to steroids
Primary sclerosing cholangitis (PSC)	Cholangiography Liver histology: fibrous obliterative cholangitis
Wilson disease	Ceruloplasmin, urine copper, eye examination, quantitative copper in liver biopsy
Hemochromatosis	Serum ferritin, serum iron, transferrin saturation, HFE gene test (C282Y, H63D?) Liver histology: iron staining, quantitative iron in biopsy
Alpha-1-antitrypsin deficiency	Serum alpha-1-antitrypsin (if abnormal genotyping)

diagnosis is currently under evaluation [19]. Liver biopsy is generally recommended to evaluate the possibility of AIH, to establish a histological grade and stage and for decision-making regarding treatment of AIH.

Treatment and prevention

The standard initial treatment of AIH is either prednisone monotherapy (40–60 mg/day and tapering regimen) or combination therapy with prednisone (30 mg/day) and azathioprine (1 mg/kg/day). Both are equally effective, although combination therapy is generally preferred because it allows

Table 87.4 International diagnostic criteria for autoimmune hepatitis

Parameter	Score
Gender	
Female	+2
Male	0
Serum biochemistry	
Ratio of elevation of serum alkaline phosphases vs aminotransferase	
>3.0	−2
1.5–3	0
<1.5	+2
Total serum globulin, γ-globulin, or IgG	
Times upper normal limit	
>2.0	+3
1.5–2.0	+2
1.0–1.5	+1
<1.0	0
Autoantibodies* (adults); ANA, SMA or LKM-1	
>1:80	+3
1:80	+2
1:40	+1
<1:40	0
Antimitrochondrial antibody	
Positive	−4
Negative	0
Hepatitis viral markers	
Positive	−3
Negative	+3

Parameter	Score
Other etiologic factors	
History of drug usage	
Yes	−4
No	+1
Alcohol (average consumption)	
<25 g/day	+2
>60 g/day	−2
Genetic factors	
HLA DR3 or DR4	+1
Other autoimmune diseases	+2
Response to therapy	
Complete	+2
Relapse	+3
Liver histology	
Interface hepatitis	+3
Predominant lymphoplasmacytic infiltrate	+1
Rosetting of liver cells	+1
None of the above	5
Biliary changes	−3
Other changes	−3
Seropositivity for other defined autoantibodies	+2

For details, refer to the International Autoimmune Hepatitis Group Report. Review of criteria for diagnosis of autoimmune hepatitis. *J Hepatol.* 1999;31:929–938.

Interpretation of aggregate scores: definite AIH, >15 before treatment, and >17 after treatment; probably AIH, 10–15 before treatment and 12–17 after treatment.

*Titers by immunofluorescence on rodent tissue.

for the reduction of prednisone, frequently to a dose lower than 10 mg, thereby reducing the steroid-associated unwanted side effects. Remission is achieved in 87% of patients within 3 years of treatment. However, a sustained response is only observed in 17% of patients that discontinue therapy after an initial period of at least 2 years. To prevent relapse episodes, treatment should not be discontinued unless there is histological evidence of a complete remission and drug withdrawal should then proceed gradually over a 3- to 6-month period. Azathioprine monotherapy (1–2 mg/kg/body weight) after prednisone withdrawal is a therapeutic option for the steroid-free maintenance of remission. However, azathioprine monotherapy is not effective in inducing remission. Budesonide is a synthetic steroid with high first-pass metabolism in the liver, which should limit systemic side effects in non-cirrhotic patients compared to conventional steroids. In a recent large

randomized placebo-controlled study with non-cirrhotic AIH patients, budesonide in combination with azathioprine was at least as effective in inducing complete remission as prednisone combined with azathioprine. Since budesonide leads to fewer side effects in non-cirrhotic patients compared to prednisone, it represents a promising alternative for the treatment of AIH [20].

Complications and their management

Drug-related adverse effects can be improved with dose reduction, and a 50% decrease in dose is the first course of action. Alternatively, and as mentioned previously, azathioprine monotherapy can be used to maintain remission. Thus, side effects of steroids such as psychosis, diabetic decompensation, severe weight gain, and symptomatic osteopenia can be prevented by increasing the azathioprine dose or by azathioprine monotherapy. An incomplete response to initial therapy justifies the institution of high-dose regimens. If standard therapy fails, alternative drugs such as cyclosporine A, cyclophosphamide, mycophenolate mofetil, or tacrolimus can be considered. However, since these strategies have not been evaluated in randomized trials, they should only be administered after consultation with specialized hepatological centers. Liver transplantation remains as a therapeutic option for patients with treatment failure who do not reach remission despite therapy for years and who progress to decompensated cirrhosis [21]. Transplantation may also be indicated in patients who present with fulminant AIH. The long-term outlook after liver transplantation is excellent, with 5-year survival rates of 92%. The recurrence of AIH after liver transplantation is independent of persistent autoantibodies and ranges between 11% and 35% [22]. Individual adjustments of immunosuppressive therapy after transplantation in patients with AIH may be necessary to prevent or control the recurrence of AIH.

Overlap syndromes
Clinical presentation
In an overlap syndrome, presentation of each individual disease is mixed with the features of another autoimmune liver disease. Thus, in addition to nonspecific symptoms such as chronic fatigue associated with AIH, clinical signs of cholestasis including pruritus and jaundice can occur with overlap syndromes.

Liver pathology
In addition to lymphocytic interface hepatitis, a characteristic feature of AIH, florid lesions of middle-sized bile ducts with portal inflammation and formation of granulomas can be observed in AIH/PBC overlap syndrome. The AIH/PSC overlap syndrome is characterized by lymphocytic interface hepatitis and fibrous obliterative cholangitis, the histologic hallmark of PSC.

Differential diagnosis
Depending on the leading symptoms, the differential diagnosis includes all forms of cholestatic and noncholestatic liver diseases such as PBC, PSC, AIC, AIH, viral hepatitis, Wilson disease, hemochromatosis, and alpha-1 antitrypsin deficiency.

Diagnostic methods
The diagnosis of an overlap syndrome relies on the biochemical profile (either cholestatic with elevated alkaline phosphatase, gamma glutamyltransferase, and bilirubin levels, or hepatocellular with elevated aspartate aminotransferase and alanine aminotransferase levels in addition to elevated gammaglobulins), the histology showing portal inflammation with or without bile duct involvement, and the autoantibody profile

showing AMA directed against antigens of the oxoacid dehydrogenase complex (PDH-E2, BCKD-E2, OADC-E2 (PBC)) or pANCA (PSC), and autoantibodies associated primarily with AIH such as liver kidney microsomal antibodies (LKM), soluble liver antigen antibodies (SLA/LP), or ANA. In cholestatic cases cholangiography detects sclerosing cholangitis. Immunglobulins are elevated in all autoimmune liver diseases; in PBC the elevation of immunoglobulin M is more pronounced.

Treatment and prevention
As a general rule, the leading disease component is treated. In an overlap syndrome presenting as hepatitis, immunosuppression with prednisone (or combination therapy with azathioprine) is initiated. In cholestatic disease ursodeoxycholic acid (13–15mg/kg body weight/day for PBC and 20mg/kg body weight/day for PSC treatment) is administered. Both treatments should be combined when biochemistry and histology suggest a relevant additional disease component [5].

Complications and their management
It has been suggested that corticosteroid-resistant patients with AIH/PBC overlap syndrome benefit from cyclosporine A therapy. However, validated therapeutic guidelines for overlap syndromes and their complications are not yet available because of their low prevalence. As discussed above, liver transplantation is the treatment of choice in end-stage autoimmune liver diseases irrespective of etiology once decompensated cirrhosis develops [5].

Prognosis with and without treatment
The natural history and prognosis of AIH are largely defined by the inflammatory activity present at diagnosis and more importantly by the presence or development of cirrhosis. In patients with periportal hepatitis, cirrhosis develops in 17% within 5 years. However, when bridging necrosis or necrosis of multiple lobules is present, cirrhosis develops in 82%. The presence of cirrhosis indicates a mortality of 58% in 5 years. However, the presence of cirrhosis at treatment initiation does not influence response or short-term outcome. The course of AIH is also significantly influenced by the HLA antigen profile of the affected individual. HLA B8 antigen profile is associated with severe inflammation at presentation and a higher likelihood of relapse after treatment. Patients with HLA DR3 have a lower probability of reaching remission, show a higher relapse rate, and require transplantation more often. HLA DR4-positive individuals are older at onset (or at diagnosis) and have a more benign outcome. In overlap syndromes with dominating features of PSC, an increased risk (~20%) of developing cholangiocarcinoma exists. In PBC-dominating overlap syndromes the prognosis mainly depends on serum bilirubin levels.

References

1. International Autoimmune Hepatitis Group Report. Review of criteria for diagnosis of autoimmune hepatitis. *J Hepatol.* 1999;31: 929–938.
2. Manns MP, Griffin KJ, Sullivan KF, *et al.* LKM-1 autoantibodies recognize a short linear sequence in P450IID6, a cytochrome P-450 monooxygenase. *J Clin Invest.* 1991;88:1370–1378.
3. Strassburg CP, Alex B, Zindy F, *et al.* Identification of cyclin A as a molecular target of antinuclear antibodies (ANA) in hepatic and non-hepatic autoimmune diseases. *J Hepatol.* 1996;25:859–866.
4. Manns MP, Gerken G, Kyriatsoulis A, *et al.* Characterization of a new subgroup of autoimmune chronic hepatitis by autoantibodies against a soluble liver antigen. *Lancet.* 1987;1:292–294.
5. Vogel A, Wedemeyer H, Manns MP, *et al.* Autoimmune hepatitis and overlap syndromes. *J Gastroenterol Hepatol.* 2002;17(Suppl. 3):S389–S398.
6. Jacobson DL, Gange SJ, Rose NR, *et al.* Epidemiology and estimated population burden of selected autoimmune diseases in the United States. *Clin Immunol Immunopathol.* 1997;84:223–243.
7. European Liver Transplant Registry 2001. www.ELTR.com
8. Wiesner RH, Demetris AJ, Belle SH, *et al.* Acute hepatic allograft rejection: incidence, risk factors, and impact on outcome. *Hepatology.* 1998;28:638–645.
9. Czaja AJ. The variant forms of autoimmune hepatitis. *Ann Intern Med.* 1996;125:588–598.
10. Van Buuren HR, van Hoogstraten HJE, Terkivatan T, *et al.* High prevalence of autoimmune hepatitis among patients with primary sclerosing cholangitis. *J Hepatol.* 2000;33:543–548.
11. Chazouilleres O, Wendum D, Serfaty L, *et al.* Primary biliary cirrhosis–autoimmune hepatitis overlap syndrome: Clinical features and response to therapy. *Hepatology.* 1998;28:296–301.
12. Czaja AJ, Carpenter HA. Autoimmune hepatitis with identical histologic features of bile duct injury. *Hepatology.* 2001;34:659–665.
13. Vergani D, Mieli-Vergani G. (2000) The role of T cells in autoimmune hepatitis, in *Immunology and Liver.* (eds M.P. Manns, G. Paumgartner and U. Leuschner). Kluwer Academic Publishers, Dordrecht, pp. 133–136.
14. Chervonsky AV. Apoptotic and effector pathways in autoimmunity. *Curr Opin Immunol.* 1999;11:684–688.
15. Agarwal K, Czaja AJ, Jones DE, *et al.* Cytotoxic T lymphocyte antigen-4 (CTLA-4) gene polymorphisms and susceptibility to autoimmune hepatitis. *Hepatology.* 2000;31:49–53.
16. Obermayer-Straub P, Strassburg CP, Manns MP. Autoimmune polyglandular syndrome type 1. *Clin Rev Allergy Immunol.* 2000;18:167–183.
17. Nikias GA, Batts KP, Czaja AJ. The nature and prognostic implications of autoimmune hepatitis with acute presentation. *J Hepatol.* 1994;19:225–232.
18. Roberts SK, Therneau TM, Czaja AJ. Prognosis of histological cirrhosis in type 1 autoimmune hepatitis. *Gastroenterology.* 1996;110:848–857.
19. Hennes EM, Zeniya M, Czaja AJ, *et al.* International Autoimmune Hepatitis Group. Simplified criteria for the diagnosis of autoimmune hepatitis. *Hepatology.* 2008;48:169–176.
20. Manns MP, Woynarowski M, Kreisel W, *et al.* for the European AIH-BUC Study Group. Budesonide induces remission more effectively than prednisone in a controlled trial of patients with autoimmune hepatitis. *Gastroenterology.* 2010;139:1198–1206.
21. Tillmann HL, Jackel E, Manns MP. Liver transplantation in autoimmune liver disease: selection of patients. *Hepatogastroenterology.* 1999;46:3053–3059.
22. Manns MP, Bahr MJ. Recurrent autoimmune hepatitis after liver transplantation: when non-self becomes self. *Hepatology.* 2000;32: 868–870.

Liver Disease

CHAPTER 88
Alcoholic liver diseases

Jennifer T. Wells[1] and Michael R. Lucey[2]

[1]Baylor University Medical Center, Dallas, TX, USA
[2]University of Wisconsin School of Medicine and Public Health, Madison, WI, USA

ESSENTIAL FACTS ABOUT PATHOGENESIS

- Excessive alcohol consumption is the third leading cause of preventable death in the US
- While total dose of alcohol is an important causative factor for alcoholic liver disease (ALD), variances in the individual response to alcohol means that most heavy drinkers do not develop ALD
- Host factors (sex, body mass, genetic polymorphisms) and environment (viral infection) influence the expression of ALD
- Alcohol metabolism, the effect of alcohol on gut permeability, and a cascade of inflammatory responses are important elements in the pathogenesis of ALD

ESSENTIALS OF DIAGNOSIS

- A history of excessive alcohol consumption is assisted by simple questionnaires, such as the CAGE questions
- Three overlapping clinical syndromes: steatosis, hepatitis, and fibrosis/cirrhosis
- Steatosis may be asymptomatic
- Hepatitis: jaundice, leukocytosis, AST/ALT>2, coagulopathy
- Cirrhosis: a spectrum from compensation to decompensation
- Consideration of other or additional causes of liver injury such as chronic viral hepatitis, hemochromatosis, hepatocellular carcinoma, alpha1 antitrypsin deficiency
- Consideration of other or additional causes of decompensation such as spontaneous bacterial peritonitis, bacteremia, pneumonia, urinary tract infection, hepatocellular carcinoma

ESSENTIALS OF TREATMENT

- *Abstinence* for alcohol is a *sine qua non* of all treatment
- No treatments of alcoholism have been effective in patients with ALD
- *Steatosis*: abstinence is all that is required
- *Alcoholic hepatitis*: prednisone for patients with severe AH
- *Alcoholic cirrhosis*: no treatment has reversed or arrested fibrosis
- *Liver transplantation* is effective in selected patients with liver failure due to ALD
- Prognosis in AH using the Maddrey discriminant function (DF), MELD or Glasgow AH score
- Prognosis in cirrhosis using MELD

Introduction

While this chapter will not deal directly with the issue of alcohol abuse and dependence or "alcoholism", harmful drinking underlies the issue of alcoholic liver disease (ALD). Alcoholism is a "... primary chronic disease with genetic, psychosocial, and environmental factors influencing its development and manifestation. It is characterized by impaired control over drinking, preoccupation with the drug alcohol, use of alcohol despite adverse consequences, and distortion of thinking ..." [1]. Table 88.1 shows a glossary of terms used when describing drinking behavior. In the world of addiction medicine, alcoholism is understood to be disorder of remission and relapse, in which the goal of therapy is to achieve stable abstinence, but where this is not attainable, to reduce the frequency and amount of drinking. In this formulation, minor relapses or "slips" are important patient indicators of the risk of a serious relapse, and the need to re-establish abstinence. Table 88.2 shows the unwanted consequences of excess consumption of alcohol. ALD is one form of end-organ damage due to excessive consumption of alcohol. ALD spans a spectrum from fat deposition to cirrhosis with associated portal hypertension, liver failure, and liver cancer. ALD is an important indication for liver transplantation in appropriately selected individuals.

Epidemiology

In the US, whereas average per capita alcohol intake has decreased in the past 50 years, the incidence of disorders due to alcohol has not changed [2]. One hundred and thirty six million Americans older than 18 years drink alcohol, with 17 million drinking to excess. Alcohol causes 75 000 deaths per year and excessive alcohol consumption is the third leading cause of preventable death [3,4]. In the UK alcohol consumption has increased by 45% during the last 30 years, with a 400% increase in death due to cirrhosis [5,6]. In contrast, alcohol consumption per capita, and deaths from cirrhosis has declined in some European countries, perhaps due to greater public awareness of the dangers of excessive alcohol consumption [6].

Liver Disease

Textbook of Clinical Gastroenterology and Hepatology, Second Edition. Edited by C. J. Hawkey, Jaime Bosch, Joel E. Richter, Guadalupe Garcia-Tsao, Francis K. L. Chan.
© 2012 Blackwell Publishing Ltd. Published 2012 by Blackwell Publishing Ltd.

Table 88.1 Glossary of terms

Term	Meaning
• Craving	A strong subjective drive to use a substance. Craving is common to most (if not all) individuals with substance dependence.
• A slip	Consumption of a limited amount of alcohol, followed by immediate procedures to re-establish abstinence.
• Harmful drinking (also known as addictive drinking)	Consuming four or more drinks in a day for a man or three or more drinks in a day for a woman, or drinking for four or more days in succession.

Table 88.2 Problems to which excess consumption of alcohol can lead

- Acute and chronic liver damage
- Several cancers
- Unintentional injuries both in the workplace and on the road
- Domestic and social violence
- Broken marriages; damaged social and family relationships
- *De novo* expression of, or exacerbation of, co-occurring psychiatric disorders, especially anxiety or depressive disorders

Table 88.3 Risk factors for the development of alcoholic liver disease

- Total dose of alcohol
- Drinking pattern: binges, fasting, mixing drinks
- Gender: women are at greater risk of liver disease for the same alcohol dose
- Obesity
- Iron overload
- Insulin resistance
- Genetic polymorphisms of metabolizing enzyme systems
- Viral hepatitis

Risk factors for the development of alcoholic liver disease

The risk factors for developing ALD are summarized in Table 88.3. Non-harmful is defined as drinking two drinks per day for men and up to one drink daily for women. Consumption of 30 grams of alcohol daily substantially increases the risk of liver disease, with the greatest risk in persons drinking more than 120 grams of alcohol daily [7]. A standard measure of wine, beer or spirits equals 8–10 grams of alcohol. Additionally, drinking in binges, while fasting and mixing different alcoholic beverages, all confer increased risk for liver disease.

Females are at increased risk of developing liver disease for an equivalent amount and duration of alcohol ingestion to males [8]. Women also develop liver injury more rapidly. This may be related to variances in volume of distribution and changes in gut permeability to endotoxin.

Co-morbid hepatitis C viral (HCV) infection and alcohol abuse increase the risk of cirrhosis, and of hepatocellular cancer [9]. The impact of hepatitis B viral (HBV) infection on progression of alcoholic cirrhosis is less clear [10]. The human immunodeficiency syndrome (HIV), with or without HBV/HCV, is associated with liver injury in an alcohol-rich environment.

Obesity is an independent risk factor for developing acute and chronic forms of alcoholic liver disease [11]. The metabolic syndrome, with truncal obesity and insulin resistance, is a co-factor for alcoholic fibrosis [11]. Conversely, malnutrition is common in patients with alcoholic hepatitis or cirrhosis, and exacerbates the mortality risk [12].

Patients with heavy alcohol consumption frequently demonstrate mild-to-moderate excess of iron stores, which has been associated with an increased risk of fibrosis [11] Hereditary hemochromatosis, often a quiescent or indolent disorder, may manifest alcoholic liver injury in the setting of regular alcohol consumption [13].

Some individuals develop ALD despite consuming moderate amounts of alcohol, whereas many who consume a great deal more do not. It appears that in addition to environmental factors, genetic factors are likely to increase the risk of developing ALD [14]. Genetic polymorphisms have been described for the metabolizing enzyme systems alcohol dehydrogenase (ADH) and cytochrome P450 2E1, which may account for the increased sensitivity to alcohol in Asian populations. Furthermore, polymorphisms have also been identified to pro-inflammatory cytokines such as tumor necrosis factor alpha (TNF-α), which may increase the susceptibility to hepatic injury.

Pathogenesis

Ethanol does not cause direct damage to the liver, and the exact mechanisms by which alcohol causes liver damage are unclear. The liver is the principal site of metabolism of orally ingested alcohol (see Figure 88.1). Ethanol is converted in the cytosol of hepatocytes to acetaldehyde, a reaction catalyzed by the enzyme alcohol dehydrogenase (ADH). A second oxidative pathway utilizing cytochrome P450 2E1 has less influence on the total oxidative conversion of alcohol. Acetaldehyde is highly reactive and toxic, and, catalyzed by acetaldehyde dehydrogenase (ALDH), is oxidized to acetate. Acetaldehyde may trigger intracellular injury by forming protein adducts, adducts with DNA, by inhibiting foliate metabolism, and by causing production of reactive oxygen species, which damage membranes and mitochondria.

There are three broad categories of liver injury: steatosis, alcoholic hepatitis and cirrhosis. Figure 88.2 shows a hypothetical pathogenic pathway linking these three ALDs.

Steatosis

Fatty liver is the most common form of alcohol-induced liver injury. Until quite recently it was considered a benign and reversible phenomenon. In fact, it leads to alcoholic hepatitis

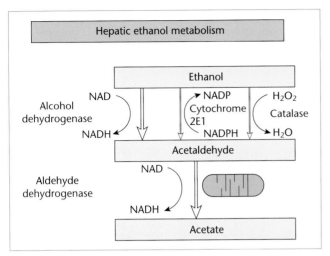

Figure 88.1 Hepatic metabolism of ethanol. (Reproduced with permission from J Caballería. Current concepts in alcohol metabolism. *Annals of Hepatology.* 2003;2(2):April–June: 60–68.)

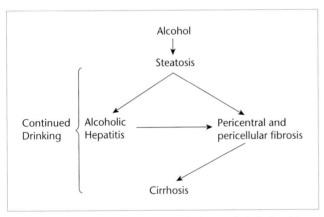

Figure 88.2 Proposed pathogenic pathway leading to alcoholic liver injury.

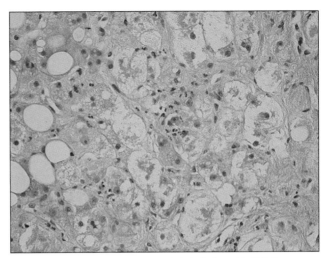

Figure 88.3 Histological appearances of alcoholic hepatitis. H & E photomicrograph of a percutaneous liver biopsy slide at high magnification showing hepatocellular ballooning, steatosis, mallory hyaline with lobular inflammation.

and/or fibrosis in persons who continue to drink [15]. Alcoholic steatosis is potentiated by other causes of fat accumulation, such as morbid obesity or chronic HCV.

The accumulation of triglyceride in hepatocytes is due to a combination of alcohol-induced impairment of fatty acid oxidation, and enhanced fatty acid synthesis, through induction of enzymes in the lipogenic pathway. Chronic exposure to alcohol induces key enzymes in lipogensis such as the transcription factors sterol regulatory element binding proteins (SREBPs) [16] and peroxisome proliferatory activated receptor alpha (PPAR α) [17].

Alcoholic hepatitis

The histological features of AH are described in the section on liver biopsy (Figure 88.3). Greater permeability of the mucosal barrier of the gut to lumenal contents appears to be a key consequence of chronic alcohol use that results in ingress of endotoxin, a constituent of the outer membrane of Gram-negative bacteria, into the portal blood stream and thence to the liver. Endotoxemia triggers a cascade of responses in the Kupffer cells of the liver, resulting in the elaboration of

cytokines, particularly TNFα and interleukin (IL) 8, and of reactive oxygen species (ROS). The significance of the TNFα hypothesis is that it is the basis for attempts to treat alcoholic hepatitis by abrogating TNFα as discussed below.

Fibrosis

Hepatic stellate cells are the source of the extracellular proteins, including type-1 collagen, that constitute hepatic fibrosis. Several of the factors already discussed in relation to alcoholic steatosis and hepatitis have been implicated in alcohol mediated activation of hepatic stellate cells, including acetaldehyde–protein adducts, reactive oxygen species, cytokines and paracrine proteins. Alcohol may also exacerbate fibrogenesis in patients with hepatitis C infection [18].

Clinical presentation

ALD presents in a bewildering variety of guises, ranging from the most subtle recognition of abnormal liver blood tests in an otherwise asymptomatic person, to the clinical manifestations for serious liver failure or portal hypertension, such as ascites, jaundice, encephalopathy or variceal hemorrhage.

Alcoholic fatty liver, when not accompanied by alcoholic hepatitis, is usually symptomless, and an enlarged liver may be the only sign.

Alcoholic hepatitis characteristically is a syndrome of jaundice arising soon after a period of heavy consumption of alcohol [19]. Typically, AST is elevated up to 300, while ALT may be close to normal limits, giving an AST/ALT ratio >2. Alcoholic hepatitis may be accompanied by encephalopathy, leukocytosis and renal failure. ALD-induced cirrhosis may present insidiously or as a sudden deterioration, produced by infection such as spontaneous bacterial peritonitis, a variceal hemorrhage or supervening alcoholic hepatitis.

Liver Disease

Table 88.4 Steps to screen of alcohol abuse or addiction

Inquire about
1. Current alcohol use: type of alcohol and frequency; family history
2. Past alcohol use
3. The CAGE questionnaire
   Cut down
   Anger
   Guilt
   Eye-openers
4. History of convictions for DUI
5. History of rehabilitation or treatment of alcoholism

Table 88.5 Physical exam findings in alcoholic liver disease

Body area	Findings
Skin	Spider angiomas, telangiectatic spots, palmer erythema, white nails, porphyria cutanea tarda, rosacea
Hands	Clubbed fingers (suggests hepatopulmonary syndrome), Dupuytren's contracture, muscle wasting, asterixis
Upper torso	Muscle wasting, gynecomastia (in men)
Head, eyes, ears, nose and throat	Icteric sclerae, parotid gland enlargement, rosacea
Chest exam	Pleural effusion (right more common than left)
Cardiovascular	Congestive heart failure
Abdomen	Hepatomegaly, splenomegaly, ascites, caput medusa, Cruveilhier–Baumgarten sign
Neurological	Peripheral neuropathy, cerebellar ataxia, confabulations
Extremities	Peripheral edema, asterixis, ophthalmoplegia (WE)

All new patients presenting with liver disease should be asked questions to assess the risk of alcoholism (see Table 88.4). Any patient who gives two or more positive answers to the CAGE questionnaire, or who appears to have problems with alcohol, should receive a detailed inquiry into drinking behavior. It may be appropriate to refer to a mental health or addiction expert.

Physical examination of the patient with ALD cirrhosis may show all the clinical manifestations of liver failure, cholestasis and portal hypertension (see Table 88.5). New onset impairment of consciousness in alcoholic patients has a broad differential, including hepatic encephalopathy, unrecognized head injury or intracranial hematoma, Wernicke's encephalopathy (WE) (see Chapter 106) or the direct effects of alcohol and medications. WE is manifested by altered cerebral function, ataxia and ophthalmoplegia. Unfortunately the protean manifestations of hepatic encephalopathy confound the

recognition of organic brain syndromes in patients with ALD, as has been demonstrated by the recovery of patients with apparent permanent brain injury upon restoration of normal hepatic function through liver transplantation.

Differential diagnosis

Since there is no clinical syndrome exclusive to alcoholic liver disease, it should be determined whether alcohol, either alone or in association with with other hepatotoxic influences is the cause of liver damage. Other disorders, such as nonalcoholic fatty liver disease (NAFLD), chronic viral hepatitis, hemochromatosis or alpha-1 antitrypsin deficiency, may contribute to the development of liver disease in alcoholic persons, and should be part of the differential diagnosis. Increased hepatic iron stores due to alcohol can mimic hereditary iron overload syndromes.

Laboratory evaluation

Standard laboratory tests are often in the normal range in persons with a history of excessive alcohol consumption, whereas the laboratory perturbations seen in alcoholic hepatitis or decompensated cirrhosis may mimic many disorders. Gamma glutamyl transferase (GGT) is better than aspartate aminotransferase (AST) or alanine aminotransferase (ALT) as a marker of recent excessive alcohol use, although it is nonspecific. The aminotransferase ratio (AST:ALT) in NAFLD is frequently not the 2–3:1 ratio that is seen in ALD. Carbohydrate-deficient transferrin (CDT) has had its advocates as a useful test for detecting alcohol abuse; however, CDT is unreliable in patients with significant liver injury.

Elevation in serum bilirubin and aminotransferases, and a leukocytosis are characteristic of alcoholic hepatitis. Serum aminotransferases rarely exceed 400 IU/L in alcoholic hepatitis. Abnormalities of serum albumin and prothrombin time manifest as liver disease progresses or in acute alcoholic hepatitis. Table 88.6 compares several recent scoring models used to predict prognosis in alcoholic hepatitis, and in the case of the Lille model, to predict the likelihood of recovery after a short course of glucocorticoids. Among scoring models, the MELD score is also useful to assess 90-day mortality with medical management of patients with decompensated liver disease. The accuracy of the MELD score reflects the grave prognostic significance of the onset of kidney failure in patients with alcoholic hepatitis/cirrhosis.

Imaging

Sonography, computerized tomography (CT), and magnetic resonance imaging (MRI) identify steatosis, liver size, liver contour indicating a nodular surface, evidence of portal hypertension (collateral vessels, ascites, and splenomegaly), biliary dilatation with biliary obstruction, and the presence of mass lesions. CT and MR angiography and Doppler sonography are useful for examining vascular structures including thrombosis or occlusion of the portal vein, the hepatic veins

Table 88.6 Prognosis scoring systems in alcoholic hepatitis (reproduced with permission from Lucey MR, Mathurin P, Morgan TR. Alcoholic hepatitis. *New Engl J Med.* 2009;360:2758–2769. Copyright Massachusetts Medical Society)

	Bilirubin	PT or INR	Creatinine	Age	WCC (10⁹/L)	Urea (mmol/L)	Albumin (g/L)	Evolution in bilirubin between day 0 and day 7*
Maddrey DF	+	+	NA	NA	NA	NA	NA	NA
MELD	+	+	+	NA	NA	NA	NA	NA
Glasgow	+	+	NA	+	+	+	NA	NA
Lille	+	+	+	+	NA	NA	+	+

*Course of bilirubin levels in the Lille model = difference in bilirubin levels between day 0 and day 7 of corticosteroid treatment.
NA, not applicable; WCC, white cell count.

and the hepatic arteries. Radiologic assessment of fibrosis using sonography or MR radiology holds promise as a test to replace liver biopsy. Among the limitations to current imaging studies are body habitus, renal impairment, inability to cooperate (movement, claustrophobia), radiation dose (applies to CT) and cost.

Liver biopsy

Histology helps clarify the predominant condition in patients with coexisting liver diseases such as viral hepatitis and is the "gold standard" to assess the degree of inflammation and fibrosis. Liver biopsy does not distinguish nonalcoholic from alcoholic steatohepatitis, which requires a careful history (see above). Although three predominant histological patterns of ALD are described separately (steatosis, alcoholic hepatitis and cirrhosis), in real life all three can exist in the same percutaneous liver biopsy. Steatosis is shown by the accumulation of large (macrovesicular) or small (microvesicular) droplets of triglycerides in hepatocytes (Figure 88.3). The addition of neutrophils in the hepatic lobule indicates steatohepatitis, a more aggressive condition. The combined appearance of steatosis, swollen or ballooned hepatocytes, the presence of amorphous eosinophilic inclusion bodies called Mallory bodies within some ballooned hepatocytes, and neutrophils within the hepatic lobule gives the histological diagnosis of alcoholic hepatitis (Figure 88.3). Deposition of collagen in the intrasinusoidal space, called pericellular fibrosis, or around the terminal hepatic venule, called perivenular fibrosis, are common in AH. Histological AH is the biopsy correlate in the syndrome of AH. Progression of pericellular and perivenular fibrosis leads to cirrhosis.

Prognosis

Prognosis of all forms of ALD is predicated on the ability of the patient to maintain abstinence from alcohol.

Alcoholic steatosis

Alcoholic steatosis was previously considered a temporary and benign phenomenon though it is recognized now as the harbinger of more severe forms of liver injury (alcoholic hepatitis and/or fibrosis), in persons who continue to drink [15].

Alcoholic hepatitis

In alcoholic hepatitis, as will be discussed below, the prognosis is determined by the severity of liver failure [19] (Table 88.6). The development of renal failure in patients with severe AH is associated with a survival of less than 10%, even with intensive management and renal support.

Alcoholic hepatitis

In alcoholic hepatitis the negative prognostic markers include relapse of alcohol, the development of liver and kidney failure, as estimated by the MELD score, the onset of portal hypertensive complications (variceal bleeding, ascites, hepatic encephalopathy), and the development of HCC.

Therapeutics and management

Abstinence from alcohol is the foundation of all treatment of alcoholic liver disease. Abstinence leads to resolution of alcoholic steatosis and alcoholic hepatitis and, as shown by the classic studies of Klatskin and Powell, is associated with improved survival in alcoholic cirrhotic patients with decompensated liver function [20] (Figure 88.4).

Treatment of alcoholism

There is a paucity of data on psychotherapeutic measures designed to curtail drinking behavior in patients with ALD. Studies of treatment interventions in alcoholics conducted by addiction specialists have adopted nuanced endpoints of reduced drinking, and distinguish between slips and harmful drinking. Studies available in patients with ALD suggest that, despite psychotherapeutic treatment, both minor and harmful drinking are common, even in the presence liver failure or in the first 5 years after transplantation [21]. The reasons that underlie the lack of greater efficacy of psychotherapeutic treatment probably rest on a combination of difficulty in counteracting the triggers for drinking, ambivalence on the part of alcoholic patients about the need for abstinence, and in those

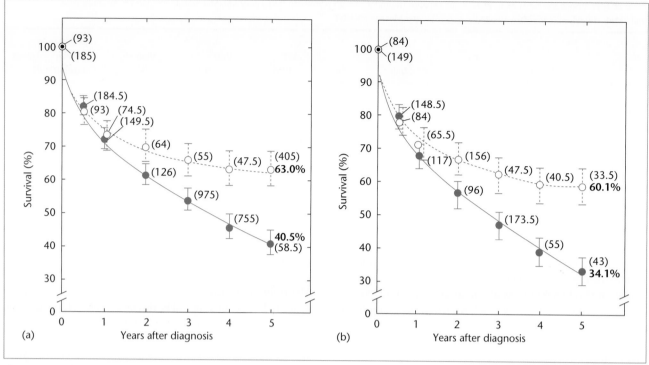

Figure 88.4 Survival after diagnosis of alcoholic cirrhosis (*n* = 278) and from onset of decompensation (*n* = 233) according to continued alcohol use or abstinence. (Reproduced with permission from Powell Jr WJ, Klatskin G. Duration of survival in patients with Laennec's cirrhosis. Influence of alcohol withdrawal, and possible effects of recent changes in general management of the disease. *Am J Med.* 1968;44:406–420.)

patients who are drinking heavily, a fear of withdrawal symptoms. Withdrawal may lead to insomnia, tremulousness, anxiety, gastrointestinal upset, anorexia, headache, diaphoresis and palpitations. Approximately 5% of patients who undergo withdrawal develop delirium tremens of which 5% will die.

Several medications have been described which reduce craving for alcohol, and thereby reduce drinking by alcoholics (Table 88.7). However, with the exception of one small trial using baclofen, patients with ALD have been excluded from such studies, and consequently the efficacy or safety of these agents is unexplored in patients with liver disease.

Nutrition

Protein calorie malnutrition is common in both alcoholic hepatitis and advanced alcoholic cirrhosis [12]. Malnourished alcoholics have a poor prognosis, with increased risk of infection, ascites, and encephalopathy. Parenteral or enteral feeding may improve objective parameters of nutrition but has not been shown to alter mortality. Nevertheless, supplemental enteral intake of protein is to be encouraged in patients with protein-calorie malnutrition. There is no increased risk of encephalopathy when alcoholic cirrhotic patients, with a history of HE, are given protein-rich formulations.

The use of multivitamins (without iron in states of iron storage excess) and minerals are encouraged. As mentioned above, Wernicke's encephalopathy (WE) occurs in alcoholic patients due to a deficiency of thiamine. If the diagnosis of WE is missed, and thiamine is not replenished, patients may

Table 88.7 Pharmacotherapy of alcohol addiction

Agent	Effect
Disulfiram	Potentially toxic in cirrhosis
Naltrexone	Black box warning
Acamprosate	Not studied in cirrhosis, doubts about efficacy
Topiramate	Not studied in cirrhosis
Baclofen	Efficacy in one RCT in cirrhosis

progress to Korsakoff's psychosis with loss of short-term memory and resultant irreversible chronic morbidity.

Acute kidney failure

Hepatorenal syndrome (HRS), which is discussed in detail in Chapter 99, is a grave complication of either alcoholic hepatitis or alcoholic cirrhosis with ascites. Current treatment approaches include the use of albumin and terlipressin (where it is available) or albumin plus octreotide and midodrine.

Artificial liver support

No artificial liver support system, including molecular adsorbents system (MARS) has demonstrated in an appropriately powered study, extension of life when applied to patients with ALD.

Table 88.8 Pharmacotherapy of alcoholic hepatitis

Agent	Effect
Corticosteroids	Efficacious in severe cases
Pentoxifylline	Possibly effective
Infliximab	Hazardous
Etanercept	Hazardous
Anabolic steroids	Ineffective

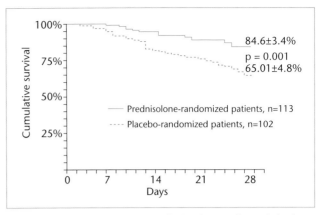

Figure 88.5 Individual data analysis of the last three randomized placebo controlled double blind trials of corticosteroids in severe AH. (Reproduced with permission from Mathurin P, Mendenhall CL, Carithers Jr RL, *et al.* Corticosteroids improve short-term survival in patients with severe alcoholic hepatitis (AH): individual data analysis of the last three randomized placebo controlled double blind trials of corticosteroids in severe AH. *J Hepatol.* 2002;36:480.)

Therapy of alcoholic steatosis

No therapy, other than abstinence from alcohol, and multivitamins, is required for treatment of alcoholic steatosis.

Pharmacotherapy of alcoholic hepatitis

Most pharmacotherapy studies have been restricted to patients with severe AH, particularly patients with a discriminant function (DF) > 32, and have assessed short-term mortality (inpatient stay or 28-day mortality). The management of patients with less severe AH and that of those who have survived after their initial severe presentation, is focused on achieving alcohol abstinence. Table 88.8 summarizes pharmacotherapies that have been tried in AH.

Corticosteroids

Corticosteroids abrogate the immune response and proinflammatory cytokine drive in AH. In a pooled re-analysis of three large randomized controlled trials of prednisolone treatment of patients with severe AH, DF > 32 or encephalopathy, it was found that steroids improved short-term survival: prednisolone 85% versus placebo 65% (Figure 88.5) [22]. Subsequently, it was found that the clinical response at day 7 of prednisolone predicts the group who will respond to a 28-day course of prednisolone, and a minority who will not. Unfortunately, the second group has high short-term mortality. The Lille group developed a score, the Lille model (www.lillemodel.com), which enables the treating physician to determine whether to stop on day 7 of prednisolone therapy on account of futility or to continue for 28 days [23]. We recommend that patients with severe AH (DF > 32, MELD ≥ 21), who are free of infection or active GI bleeding, receive prednisolone (40 mg/day by mouth) for up to 28 days.

Pentoxifylline

Pentoxifylline (PTX) is a nonselective phosphodiesterase inhibitor also shown to reduce TNFα gene transcription. A large, randomized trial of PTX [22] showed a significant reduction in short-term mortality compared with placebo [24]. More recently, a small randomized controlled trial of PTX versus corticosteroids in patients with severe AH, demonstrated a higher mortality in those receiving steroids (35.3%) than in the pentoxifylline group (14.7%) [25]. Both studies showed the reduced mortality to be largely from a reduction in deaths related to the

development of hepatorenal syndrome. PTX does not improve survival in patients with severe AH who have failed to show a day 7 improvement with prednisolone [26]. Unwanted gastrointestinal effects, particularly nausea, are common with the PTX, although more serious side effects are rare.

Anti-tumor necrosis factor strategies

Infliximab and etanercept have been studied in randomized controlled trials in patients with moderate to severe AH. The 6-month mortality rate was significantly higher in the etanercept group compared with the placebo group (57.7% versus 22.7%) with severe infections complicating the etanercept arm [27]. A randomized controlled trial in which infliximab and steroids were compared to steroids alone, an increased incidence of serious infections and a nonsignificant increase in mortality in the infliximab-treated group led to early termination of the study [28]. The dose of infliximab used in this study has been criticized as excessive. Neither etanercept nor infliximab should be used to treat severe AH outside a properly approved clinical trial.

Antioxidant therapies

None of the trials in which antioxidants such as N-acetylcysteine, selenium, vitamins A, C, and E, and allopurinol were compared to placebo or corticosteroid therapy conferred any survival benefit in patients with AH [19].

Pharmacotherapy of alcoholic fibrosis or cirrhosis

Pharmacotherapy to prevent or reverse fibrosis in ALD, while an attractive concept, has not achieved unequivocal success in clinical studies. Table 88.9 lists some of the treatments that have been studied.

Colchicine

The putative anti-fibrotic effects of colchicine include inhibition of collagen production, enhancement of collagenase activity, and countering inflammation. A meta-analysis of 14

Table 88.9 Pharmacotherapy of alcoholic fibrosis/cirrhosis

Agent	Effect
Colchicine	Ineffective
Propylthiouracil	Effective in one RTC
S-Adenosylmethionine (SAMe)	Ineffective
Phosphatidylcholine	Ineffective
Silymarin	Ineffective

Table 88.10 Prognostic factors for increased risk of alcoholic relapse

- Lack of insight into addiction
- Psychiatric comorbid conditions including uncontrolled polysubstance abuse or unstable character disorder
- History of many failed rehabilitation attempts
- Social isolation (lack of employment, no fixed abode, living alone, no spouse or companion)

randomized controlled trials (RCTs) found no benefit of colchicine treatment in ALD [29].

Propylthiouracil

Propylthiouracil (PTU) is purported to counteract the hypoxic stress to centrilobular liver zones in ALD. Although one RCT demonstrated improved mortality at 2 years, this observation has not been reproducible. Most studies have demonstrated no benefit in all cause or alcohol-related mortality [30].

Silymarin

A meta-analysis of high quality studies failed to show a benefit [31].

S-Adenosylmethionine

Although a small, underpowered randomized controlled trial with S-adenosylmethionine (SAMe) showed a significant reduction in mortality or need for liver transplantation in patients with Child A and B alcoholic cirrhosis [20], no further advances have been made in the past decade to support the use of SAMe.

Dilinoleoylphosphatidylcholine

Dilinoleoylphosphatidylcholine has antioxidant, anti-fibrotic, and anticytokine activity in experimental rat models of ALD. A large study of 789 alcoholic patients failed to show either improved or stable hepatic fibrosis on histology at 2 years when compared to placebo [32].

Liver transplantation for alcoholic liver disease

ALD is one of the commonest indications for liver transplantation. However, liver transplantation for liver failure or hepatocellular carcinoma due to ALD remains a controversial issue in light of increasing donor shortages and concerns over the risk of post-transplant alcoholic relapse. Five-year patient and allograft survival is similar in alcoholics and nonalcoholic liver transplant recipients. However, a retrospective review of 10-year data from a single large European center indicated that relapse to addictive or harmful drinking, as opposed to abstinence or abstinence with occasional slips, was associated with increased mortality [33].

Evaluation of the addicted patient includes psychosocial assessment of the risk of relapse [23] (Table 88.10). The clinical utility of the "six-month rule" to predict future alcoholic relapse remains controversial and a careful evaluation by an addiction medicine specialist, concentrating on the factors outlined in Table 88.6, is the best predictive instrument.

The prospective longitudinal observational study of 167 consecutive alcoholic liver transplant recipients carried out by DiMartini et al. provides the best data on drinking by alcoholics after transplantation [34]. Five years after transplantation, 42% of alcoholic recipients had used alcohol at least once, and the first drink occurred in the first year in 22%. Furthermore, 26% had drunk in binges, and 22% had drunk on four consecutive days.

Current controversies

There are many questions regarding transplantation of patients with alcoholic liver disease that continue to provoke controversy. These include:

How does alcohol cause liver damage? What is the "safe" limit of drinking? How do genetic polymorphisms, including those for alcohol dehydrogenase and TNFα promoters, interact in the causation of liver injury?

The management of severe AH remains challenging. Data on the use of corticosteroid use in AH have led to a greater consensus on their use in selected patients with severe AH. PTX appears to be helpful in the prevention of HRS in patients with AH. Whether or not agents that abate TNFα will prove useful remains unknown.

Liver transplantation for patients with ALD, especially severe AH, is controversial. Further studies are needed to identify which drinking, behavioral, and social characteristics best stratify those patients at increased risk for alcohol relapse post transplant. Similarly, the detrimental impact of a slip versus a full relapse should be studied. Future developments in hepatocyte transplantation and artificial liver support systems may offer new hope for patients with AH.

SOURCES OF INFORMATION FOR PATIENTS

www.liverfoundation.org/
www.nlm.nih.gov/medlineplus/
www.britishlivertrust.org.uk/
www.wikipedia.org/wiki/Alcoholic_liver_disease

References

1. Morse RM, Flavin DK. The definition of alcoholism. The Joint Committee of the National Council on Alcoholism and Drug Dependence and the American Society of Addiction Medicine to Study the Definitions and Criteria for the Diagnosis of Alcoholism. *JAMA*. 1992;268:1012–1014.

2. Li TK, Hewitt BG, Grant BF. Is there a future for quantifying drinking in the diagnosis, treatment, and prevention of alcohol use disorders? *AlcoholAlcohol*. 2007;42:57–63.

3. Mokdad AH, Marks JS, Stroup DF, *et al*. Actual causes of death in the United States, 2000. *JAMA*. 2004;291:1238–1245. See also Mokdad AH, Marks JS, Stroup DF, *et al*. Correction: Actual causes of death in the United States, 2000. *JAMA*. 2005;293: 293–294.

4. Centers for Disease Control and Prevention (CDC). Alcohol-attributable deaths and years of potential life lost – United States, 2001. *MMWR Morb Mortal Wkly Rep*. 2004;53:866–870.

5. Sheron N, Olsen N, Gilmore I. An evidence-based alcohol policy. *Gut*. 2008;57:1341–1344.

6. Leon DA, McCambridge J. Liver cirrhosis mortality rates in Britain, 1950 to 2002. *Lancet*. 2006;367:52–56.

7. Bellentani S, Saccoccio G, Costa G, *et al*. Drinking habits as cofactors of risk for alcohol induced liver damage. *Gut*. 1997;41: 845–850.

8. Becker U, Deis A, Sorensen TIA, *et al*. Prediction of risk of liver disease by alcohol intake, sex, and age: a prospective population study. *Hepatology*. 1996;23:1025–1029.

9. Sata M, Fukuizumi K, Uchimura Y, *et al*. Hepatitis C virus infection in patients with clinically diagnosed alcoholic liver diseases. *J Viral Hepat*. 1996;3:143–148.

10. Geissler M, Gesien A, Wands JR. Chronic ethanol effects on cellular immune responses to hepatitis B virus envelope protein: an immunologic mechanism for induction of persistent viral infection in alcoholics. *Hepatology*. 1997;26:764–770.

11. Raynard B, Balian A, Fallik D, *et al*. Risk factors of fibrosis in alcohol-induced liver disease. *Hepatology*. 2002;35:635–638.

12. Mendenhall CL, Moritz TE, Roselle GA, *et al*. Protein energy malnutrition in severe alcoholic hepatitis: diagnosis and response to treatment. The VA cooperative study # 275. *J Parenteral Enteral Nutr*. 1995;19:258–265.

13. Fletcher LM, Dixon JL, Purdie DM, *et al*. Excess alcohol greatly increases the prevalence of cirrhosis in hereditary hemochromatosis. *Gastroenterology*. 2002;122:281–289.

14. Wilfred de Alwis NM, Day CP. Genetics of alcoholic liver disease and non-alcoholic fatty liver disease. *Semin Liver Dis*. 2007;27: 44–54.

15. Teli MR, Day CP, Burt AD, *et al*. Determinants of progression to cirrhosis or fibrosis in pure alcoholic fatty liver. *Lancet*. 1995;346(8981):987–990.

16. You M, Fischer M, Deeg MA, *et al*. Ethanol induces fatty acid synthesis pathways by activation of sterol regulatory element binding proteins (SREBPs). *J Biol Chem*. 2002;277:29342–29347.

17. Fischer M, You M, Matsumoto M, *et al*. Peroxisome proliferatory activated receptor alpha (PPARalpha) agonist treatment reverses PPAR alpha dysfunction and abnormalities in hepatic lipid metabolism in ethanol fed mice. *J Biol Chem*. 2003;278:27997–28004.

18. Rigamonti C, Mottaran E, Reale E, *et al*. Moderate alcohol consumption increases oxidative stress in patients with chronic hepatitis C. *Hepatology*. 2003;38:42–49.

19. Lucey MR, Mathurin P, Morgan TR. Alcoholic hepatitis. *New Engl J Med*. 2009;360:2758–2769.

20. Powell Jr WJ, Klatskin G. Duration of survival in patients with Laennec's cirrhosis. Influence of alcohol withdrawal, and possible effects of recent changes in general management of the disease. *Am J Med*. 1968;44:406–420.

21. Lucey MR, Weinrieb RM. Alcohol and substance abuse. *Semin Liver Dis*. 2009;29:66–73.

22. Mathurin P, Mendenhall CL, Carithers Jr RL, *et al*. Corticosteroids improve short-term survival in patients with severe alcoholic hepatitis (AH): individual data analysis of the last three randomized placebo controlled double blind trials of corticosteroids in severe AH. *J Hepatol*. 2002;36:480.

23. Louvet A, Naveau S, Abdelnour M, *et al*. The Lille model: A new tool for therapeutic strategy in patients with severe alcoholic hepatitis treated with steroids. *Hepatology*. 2007;45:1348–1354.

24. Akriviadis E, Botla R, Briggs W, *et al*. Pentoxifylline improves short-term survival in severe acute alcoholic hepatitis: A double-blind, placebo-controlled trial. *Gastroenterology*. 2000;119:1637–1648.

25. De BK, Gangopadhyay S, Dutta D, *et al*. Pentoxifyllline versus prednisolone for severe alcoholic hepatitis: a randomized controlled trial. *World J Gastroenterol*. 2009;15:1613–1619.

26. Louvet A, Diaz E, Dharancy S, *et al*. Early switch to pentoxifylline in patients with severe alcoholic hepatitis is inefficient in non-responders to corticosteroids. *J Hepatol*. 2008;48:465–470.

27. Beotticher NC, Peine CH, Kwo P, *et al*. A ramdomized, double-blinded, placebo-controlled multicenter trial of etanercept in the treatment of alcoholic hepatitis. *Gastroenterology*. 2008;135:1953–1960.

28. Naveau S, Chollet-Martin S, Dharancy S, *et al*. A double-bind randomized controlled trial of infliximab associated with prednisolone in acute alcoholic hepatitis. *Hepatology*. 2004;39:1390–1397.

29. Rambaldi A, Gluud C. Colchicine for alcoholic and non-alcoholic fibrosis and cirrhosis. *Cochrane Database Syst Rev*. 2005;18: CD002148.

30. Rambaldi A, Gluud C. Propylthiouracil for alcoholic liver disease. *Cochrane Database Syst Rev*. 2005;19:CD002800.

31. Rambaldi A. Milk thistle for alcoholic and/or hepatitis B or C liver diseases – a systematic cochrane hepato-biliary group review with meta-analyses of randomized clinical trials. *Am J Gastroenterol*. 2005;100:2583–2591.

32. Lieber CS, Weiss DG, Groszmann R, *et al*. II. Veterans Affairs Cooperative Study of polyenylphosphatidylcholine in alcoholic liver disease. *Alcohol Clin Exp Res*. 2003;27:1765–1772.

33. Tome S, Said A, Lucey MR. Addictive behavior after solid organ transplantation: What do we know already and what do we need to know? *Liver Transpl*. 2008;14:127–129.

34. DiMartini A, Day N, Dew MA, *et al*. Alcohol consumption patterns and predictors of use following liver transplantation for alcoholic liver disease. *Liver Transpl*. 2006;12:813–820.

Liver Disease

CHAPTER 89

Nonalcoholic fatty liver disease

Arthur J. McCullough and Srinivasan Dasarathy

Cleveland Clinic Lerner College of Medicine, Case Western Reserve University, Cleveland, OH, USA

ESSENTIAL FACTS ABOUT PATHOGENESIS

- The most important risk factors for nonalcoholic steatohepatitis (NASH) are diabetes, obesity, the metabolic syndrome, the individual components of the metabolic syndrome (insulin resistance, increased waist circumference, and dyslipidemia), and age
- Insulin resistance, free fatty acids, oxidative stress and inflammatory cytokines individually or in combination are key factors in the pathophysiology of NASH

ESSENTIALS OF DIAGNOSIS

- Currently the diagnosis of NASH requires the histological findings of steatosis plus inflammation and necroinflammation with or without fibrosis
- NASH may progress to cirrhosis, hepatocellular carcinoma and liver failure, and it is projected to be the leading cause of liver transplantation in 2020

ESSENTIALS OF TREATMENT

- Weight loss (via diet or bariatric surgery) and vitamin E have recently been demonstrated to be effective treatment of NASH

Introduction and definition

There are a myriad of causes of fatty liver disease (Figure 89.1). However, this discussion will focus on those diseases predominantly associated with insulin resistance, sometimes referred to primary or metabolic nonalcoholic fatty liver disease (NAFLD).

NAFLD is a common complex metabolic disease that has emerged as a major health concern and, along with its associated obesity, diabetes and cardiovascular disease, has an impact far beyond just liver disease alone [1,2]. NAFLD carries a significant health burden that increases overall health costs by 26% [3]. Furthermore, nonalcoholic steatohepatitis (NASH), the most severe form of NAFLD, is projected to be the leading cause of liver transplantation by 2020 [4].

The histological findings associated with NAFLD are numerous and have been recently reviewed extensively elsewhere [5]. However, the clinically important histological classification describes a spectrum ranging from a bland steatosis,

to steatosis plus inflammation, to steatosis plus necroinflammation (ballooning degeneration), to steatosis plus fibrosis with or without inflammation and necrosis (Table 89.1). Only fat plus hepatocyte injury and fibrosis (types 3 and 4) should be considered NASH. The significance of these histological categories rests on the fact that the prevalence and clinical outcomes vary by histological category [6]. Recently the NASH Clinical Research Network (CRN) proposed a semi-quantitative system to grade and stage the histological features of NAFLD [7] (Tables 89.2 and 89.3). However, it is uncertain whether this scoring system provides any prognostic information.

Inherent to defining the nonalcoholic component of NAFLD is the threshold at which NAFLD becomes alcohol related. By consensus, an average daily consumption of less than 20 grams for females and less than 30 grams for males constitutes NAFLD. This translates to no more than one or two daily drinks for females and males, respectively (Table 89.4).

Epidemiology

Incidence

In the United States, the incidence of NASH has increased in recent years from 4.2 per 10^5 persons per year in 1980–1985, to 38 per 10^5 persons per year in 1995–1999 [8]. In northern Italy, the incidence of NAFLD is 2% new cases per year [9].

Prevalence

NAFLD is the most common form of chronic liver disease worldwide [10]. The prevalence of NAFLD depends on the diagnostic technique used as shown in Table 89.5. Three separate analyses of the National Health and Nutritional Examination Survey (NHANES III), performed between 1988 and 1994 in more than 12 000 adults from the general US population, yielded three different prevalence rates as shown in Table 89.6. NAFLD was diagnosed based on increased serum levels of liver enzymes – alanine aminotransferase (ALT), aspartate aminotransferase (AST), and gamma glutamyl transferase (GGT) – in the absence of other causes. The prevalence ranged between 2.8 and 23%, due to differences in inclusion criteria. However, the essence of the uncertainty in the prevalence rates

---

Textbook of Clinical Gastroenterology and Hepatology, Second Edition. Edited by C. J. Hawkey, Jaime Bosch, Joel E. Richter, Guadalupe Garcia-Tsao, Francis K. L. Chan.
© 2012 Blackwell Publishing Ltd. Published 2012 by Blackwell Publishing Ltd.

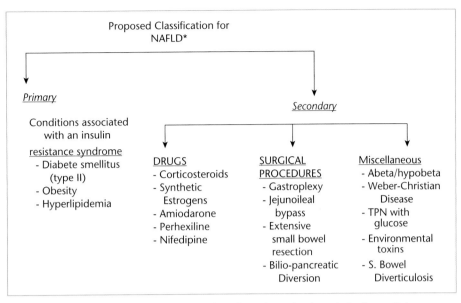

Figure 89.1 Classification of fatty liver disease. Primary nonalcoholic fatty liver disease is associated metabolic diseases that are accompanied by insulin resistance versus a large number of secondary causes that are not usually associated with insulin resistance.

Table 89.1 Characteristics of nonalcoholic fatty liver

Type	Characteristics
1	Fat alone
2	Fat + inflammation
3	Fat + hepatocyte injury
4	Fat + fibrosis and/or Mallory bodies

Only types 3 and 4 are considered as nonalcoholic steatohepatitis.

Table 89.2 Nonalcoholic fatty liver disease activity score*

Histologic finding	Grade
Steatosis	0–3
Inflammation	0–3
Ballooning injury	0–2
Maximum score	8

*According to the Nonalcoholic Steatohepatitis Clinical Research Network (NASH CRN).
NASH requires a score of ≥4 with at least 1 point from ballooning injury.

Table 89.3 Fibrosis score*

Fibrosis type	Score
None	0
Perisinusoidal zone 3	
Mild	1A
Moderate	1B
Portal/periportal	1C
Perisinusoidal and portal/periportal	2
Bridging	3
Cirrhosis	4

*According to the Nonalcoholic Steatohepatitis Clinical Research Network (NASH CRN).

(using any technique) resides in the problem of defining NAFLD and NASH based on non-invasive tests without a liver biopsy.

Using ultrasound, which detects 20% of fat replacement in the liver [11], the prevalence ranged between 16 and 30%, while it is 34% using proton magnetic resonance spectroscopy, which can detect 5% fat replacement [12]. The prevalence varies by ethnicity, which also depends on the diagnostic method used. Most but not all studies find blacks to have the lowest prevalence of NAFLD [1].

Using these rates and assuming that 30% of the population is obese, the overall prevalence for NAFLD in the United States is between 17 and 34%. In the population studies, the ratio of NASH to NAFLD is one third to one half. Therefore the overall prevalence of NASH would rest between 6% (conservative estimate) and 17% (liberal estimate). However, these estimates do not take into account the proportion of different ethnicities

Table 89.4 Alcohol content of beverages

Type of beverage	Ethanol (%)	Dose (ounces)	Ethanol (grams)	Toxic threshold; no. of drinks/day; men/women	
				Previous estimate	Recent estimate
"Spirits"	43	1.5	15	7/5	2/1
Wine	13	4.5	14	7/5	2/1
Beer	5	12	14	7/5	2/1

Specific gravity of alcohol = 0.80.
1 ounce is equivalent to 30 milliliters.

Table 89.6 Prevalence of nonalcoholic fatty liver disease (NAFLD) in the National Health and Nutritional Examination Survey (NHANES)

	Analysis 1	Analysis 2	Analysis 3
Prevalence (%)	23	2.8	7.9
Liver enzymes	AST, ALT, GGT	ALT	AST, ALT
Units/L	>30	<43	Women: >31, >31 Men: >37, >40
Exclusions	Appropriate	Diabetics	Appropriate

ALT, alanine aminotransferase; AST, aspartate aminotransferase; GGT, gamma-glutamyltransferase.

Table 89.5 Prevalence of nonalcoholic fatty liver disease (NAFLD) and nonalcoholic steatohepatitis (NASH)

Type of study	Prevalence
General population screening	
Liver enzymes	3–23
Ultrasonography	16–30 (76)
^{1}H MRS	34 (67)
Selected populations	
Surgical risk	
Adult living donors	20
Bariatric surgery	56–86 (14–29)
Postmortem analysis	
Hospitalized patients	3 (19)
Random deaths	16–24 [2.1]
Pediatric autopsies	13 [3]
Patients undergoing liver biopsy	15–84 [1.2–48]

Numbers in parentheses indicate the prevalence of NAFLD in obese patients.
Numbers in square brackets indicate the prevalence of NASH in studies in which liver biopsies were performed.
^{1}H MRS, proton magnetic resonance spectroscopy.

Table 89.7 Diagnostic methods: Comparison of diagnostic criteria for metabolic syndrome

World Health Organization proposal	Adult Treatment Protocol III proposal[a]
Altered glucose regulation or insulin resistance *plus* two of the following:	Any three of the following:
Obesity: BMI >30 kg/m^2 or WHR, >.0 (M) or >0.9 (F)	Waist girth: >102 cm (M) or >88 cm (F)
High triglycerides: >150 mg/dL *or* low HDL cholesterol: <35 mg/dL (M) or <39 mg/dL (F)	Arterial pressure: ≥ 130/85 mmHg
Hypertension (≥150/90 mmHg)	Triglycerides: ≥ 150 mg/dL
Microalbuminuria: ≥20 μg/mL	HDL cholesterol: <40 mg/dL (M) or <50 mg/dL (F); Glucose: ≥110 mg/dL

[a]Classification proposed by the Third Report of the National Cholesterol Education Expert Panel on detection, evaluation and treatment of high blood cholesterol in adults [3].
BMI, body mass index; F, female; HDL, high density lipoprotein; M, male; WHR, waist:hip ratio.

in the United States. Although these current prevalence rates are already high, they are expected to increase globally in concert with the rapidly increasing prevalence of obesity and type 2 diabetes.

Causes, risk factors, and disease associations
Metabolic syndrome and insulin resistance
Since insulin resistance is an essential underlying pathophysiological factor associated with fatty liver, NAFLD/NASH is now considered to be the hepatic component of the metabolic syndrome [13], which has been defined in different ways

(Table 89.7). The World Health Organization (WHO) classification is based on the presence of at least one of two essential conditions, plus two additional criteria. This classification can be applied to diabetic populations but is not useful in a general setting. The Third Report of the National Cholesterol Education Program's expert panel on detection, evaluation and treatment of high cholesterol in adults (Adult Treatment Panel III; ATP III) defines the metabolic syndrome as the presence of any three categorical discreet risk factors that can be measured easily.

As shown in Figure 89.2, the metabolic syndrome is a clustering of metabolic abnormalities that include central obesity, hypertension, decreased high density lipoproteins, and

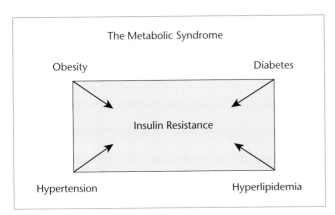

Figure 89.2 The metabolic syndrome. This schematic describes the important relationship between the components of the metabolic syndrome and insulin resistance.

elevated serum triglycerides that has insulin resistance as the central pathophysiologic factor. The importance of the metabolic syndrome is not only its high prevalence worldwide [14] but also that it predicts decreased survival from diabetes [15] and NAFLD [16]. Approximately 90% of NAFLD patients have more than one component of the metabolic syndrome, and one third has the metabolic syndrome. In addition, the risk of having NAFLD increases exponentially with the addition of each component, and it is more common in NASH than in steatosis [17].

Obesity

Obesity is associated with insulin resistance, and a number of studies have established obesity as a risk factor not only for hepatic steatosis but also for progression to cirrhosis. However, the distribution of fat may be more important than the total fat mass. Compared with total fat mass, visceral fat is a stronger predictor of hepatic steatosis as well as hyperinsulinemia, decreased hepatic insulin extraction, and peripheral insulin resistance. A decrease in visceral fat has been shown to decrease hepatic insulin resistance. Lean patients with NASH may have central obesity. This may explain NAFLD in the subgroup of non-obese patients who are frequently of Asian origin. However, fatty liver disease is also associated with dysglycemia and dyslipidemia, independent of visceral adipose tissue. In addition, although we are seeing a continuing escalation of the obesity epidemic, we are seeing a proportionally greater rise in NASH. Where the incidence of obesity may have doubled or tripled over a period of time, the prevalence of NASH has increased ten-fold. Therefore we know some other pathophysiologic mechanism is, at least partially, driving NASH development.

Diabetes

Diabetes is an independent predictor for cirrhosis and liver related deaths in NAFLD [1,18]. The reason for this is unclear

but may be due to additional oxidative and altered endothelial function in diabetes.

Risk factors and predictors of disease

Histology (the presence or absence of NASH) obtained by liver biopsy is the most reliable prognostic factor. However, there are certain inherent limitations to performing a liver biopsy in NAFLD, which include cost, sampling error, and morbidity. In addition, it is impractical to perform liver biopsy in a disease such as NAFLD that affects such a large segment of the population [19].

Several demographic, anthropomorphic, clinical, and laboratory factors are associated with NAFLD and histological severity of the disease [1]. Among these, the factors most reliably associated with the presence of NASH and advanced fibrosis include older age, insulin resistance, diabetes, obesity, smoking, and hypertension. The potential applicability of these variables in predicting severity of disease in the clinical setting is limited.

Therefore, development of predictive scoring systems to identify patients at high risk for NASH and fibrosis is essential to identify those NAFLD patients who would benefit the most from liver biopsy and monitoring the response to therapy [19].

Table 89.8 displays the biochemical markers that have been used to predict NASH and fibrosis in NAFLD patients. The best individual biomarker to date is cytokeratin 18, which monitors the pathophysiologic process of apoptosis occurring in the liver [20]. However, these markers have limitations when used individually. Therefore, a number of composite models have been developed for the non-invasive diagnosis of NASH (Table 89.9) and advanced fibrosis (Table 89.10).

The ability to diagnose fibrosis in NAFLD seems closer at hand than does the ability to differentiate steatosis from NASH. Although the latter is important, even the current best strategy (measuring apoptosis) needs additional field testing and standardization of methods that can be used across laboratories. It is doubtful that any single biomarker will suffice in composite models. Additional biomarkers combined with standard laboratory tests and demographics such as those used in the NASH predictive index and the NASH CRN [1] will be necessary. In contrast, the ability to reliably determine fibrosis in NAFLD without a liver biopsy is within sight. As shown in Tables 89.8 and 89.10, the enhanced fibrosis (ELF) panel [21] provides a diagnostic accuracy such that only 1 out of 14 patients would require a liver biopsy and if used with the NAFLD fibrosis score [22], the accuracy is above 90% for severe fibrosis. Lesser degrees of fibrosis will require lesser thresholds obtained from the ROC curves. Even with these encouraging results of the biomarkers, alternative strategies are being pursued. Genetics and surface-enhanced laser desorption/ionization (SELDI) based proteomics [23] and metabolomics [24] may be equal or more accurate than fibrosis panels.

Table 89.8 Biochemical markers as predictors of nonalcoholic steatohepatitis and advanced fibrosis

Author and year of publication	Marker	Nonalcoholic steatohepatitis	Fibrosis	Area under the curve
Palekar, 2006	HA > 45.3 ng/mL		•	0.88
Suzuki, 2005	HA > 46.1 ng/mL		•	0.89
Santos, 2005	HA > 24.6 ng/mL Laminin > 282 ng/mL Type IV collagen > 145 ng/mL		• • •	0.73 0.87 0.82
Sakugawa, 2005	HA > 50 ng/mL		•	0.80
Hasegawa, 2001	TGF-β1	•		NR
Haukeland, 2006	TNF-α CCL2/MCP	• •		NR
Wieckowska, 2006	Cytokeratin-18	•		0.93
Garcia-Galiano, 2007	IGF-1 < 110 ng/mL	•		NR
Baranova, 2006	Decreased adiponectin	•		NR
Hui, 2004	Decreased adiponectin	•		0.79
Yoneda, 2007	High-sensitivity CRP Type IV collagen	•	• •	0.83
Musso, 2005	Adiponectin		•	NR
Wieckowska, 2008	Serum IL-6		•	NR
Dixon, 2001	C-peptide > 1324 pmol/L		•	NR

CCL2/MCP, CC chemokine ligand 2/monocytes chemoattractant protein; IGF-1, insulin-like growth factor 1; NR, not reported.

Table 89.9 Composite models for diagnosis of nonalcoholic steatohepatitis

Author and year of publication	N	Population	Area under the curve for nonalcoholic steatohepatitis	Predictors
Palekar, 2006	80	NAFLD	0.76 (0.65–0.87)	Age, BMI, female gender, AST, AAR, HA
Zein, 2007	177	NAFLD	0.87 (0.81–0.93)[a] 0.85 (0.75–0.95)[b]	Age, female gender, BMI, HOMA, log (AST × ALT)
Dixon (HAIR), 2001	105	Obese	0.90 (NR)	HTN, ALT, IR
Gholam, 2007	97	Obese	0.82 (NR)	AST, DM
Campos, 2008	200	Obese	NR	HTN, DM, AST, ALT, sleep apnea, and non-black race
Poynard (NASHtest), 2006	257	NAFLD	0.79 (0.69–0.86)[a] 0.79 (0.67–0.87)[b]	Combination of 13 parameters[c]

[a]Training population set.
[b]Validation population set.
[c]Age, sex, height, weight and serum triglyceride, cholesterol, α_2-macroglobulin, apolipoprotein A1, haptoglobin, GGT, AST, ALT, and total bilirubin.
Values in parentheses are 95% confidence intervals.
HTN, hypertension; NPI, NASH predictive index; NR, not reported.

Table 89.10 Composite models for diagnosis of advanced fibrosis in non-alcoholic fatty liver disease

Author and year of publication	Model	N	Population	Area under the curve for non-alcoholic steatohepatitis	Predictors
Ratziu, 2000	BAAT	93	Obese	0.84 (NR)	Age, BMI, ALT, TGL
Angulo, 1999	—	144	NASH	NR	Age, BMI, DM, AAR
Angulo, 2007	NAFLD fibrosis score	733	NAFLD	0.88 (0.85–0.93)[a] 0.82 (0.76–0.88)[b]	Age, BMI, AAR, DM, platelet count, albumin
Harrison, 2008	BARD	827	NAFLD	0.81 (NR)	BMI, AAR, DM
Ratziu, 2006	Fibro test	267	NAFLD	0.86 (0.77–0.91)[a] 0.75 (0.61–0.83)[b]	α_2-Microglobulin, haptoglobulin, GGT, apolipoprotein A1
Rosenberg, 2004	OELF	61	NAFLD	0.87 (0.66–1.0)	Age, HA, PIIINP, TIMP-1
Guha, 2008	ELF	192	NAFLD	0.90 (0.84–0.96)	HA, PIINP, TIMP-1
Shaw, 2009	FIB4 index	541	NAFLD	0.8 (0.76–0.85)	Age, AST, ALT, platelet count

[a]Training population set.
[b]Validation population set.
NR, not reported; PIIINP, aminoterminal peptide of procollagen III; TGL, triglyceride.
Numbers in parentheses are 95% confidence intervals.

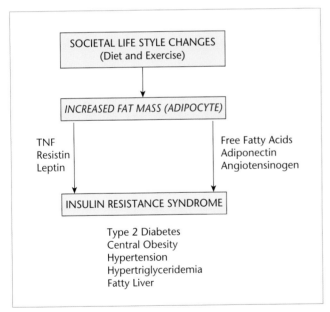

Figure 89.3 Societal changes and adipocytes: the effect of insulin resistance and liver disease. The cascade effect of societal life changes on the development of insulin resistance in nonalcoholic fatty liver disease is shown. (This figure was published in *Clinical Gastroenterology and Hepatology*, Wilfred M. Weinstein, Christopher J. Hawkey, Jaime Bosch, Nonalcoholic fatty liver disease (NAFLD), Pages 1–11, Copyright Elsevier, 2005.)

Pathogenesis

An overall schematic for the pathogenesis of NAFLD/NASH is provided in Figures 89.3, 89.4 and 89.5. Epidemiologic and migration studies link obesity to lifestyle changes: decreased physical activity, smoking, and an alteration in dietary

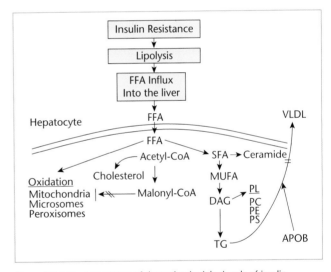

Figure 89.4 The importance of the pathophysiologic role of insulin resistance and its associated lipolosis and increased influx of free fatty acid into the liver is shown. With the onset of insulin resistance, there is lipolysis and deliver of free fatty acids to the liver. The majority of lipids involved in the development of nonalcoholic fatty liver disease (NAFLD) are stored as triglycerides (TG). However, other lipids and lipid metabolites, such as free fatty acids (FA) and esterified cholesterol, ceramides and sphingolipids, also develop. The activity of specific enzymes determines the relative abundance of these lipotites and their role in upregulating transcription factors that further regulate the production of metabolic enzymes. ApoB, apolipoprotein B; DAG, diacylglycerol acids; FFA, free fatty acids; MUFA, monosaturated fatty acids; PC, phosphatidylcholine; PE, phosphatidydlethanolamine; PL, phospholipids; PS, phosphatidylserine; SFA, saturated fatty acids; TG, triglycerides.

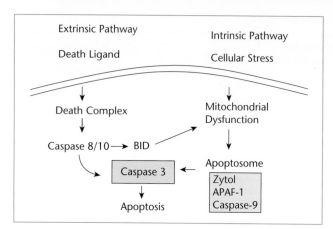

Figure 89.5 Apothotic pathways in nonalcoholic steatohepatitis (NASH). Apotosis which involves both an intrinsic (depth receptor mediated) pathway and an intrinsic (organalle-initiated) pathway plays an important role in the development of NASH.

patterns (particularly trans-fats and fructose) that has occurred in industrial countries over the past 50 years. Once obesity and/or insulin resistance have developed, the expanded fat mass functions as an endocrine organ that secretes increased amounts of fatty acids, a number of cytokines including tumor necrosis factor, resistin, interleukin-6, leptin, angiotensin, and decreased amounts of adiponectin. All of these hormones are known to have a definite or potential role in the development of either fat alone or NASH [25,26].

Once insulin resistance develops, there is increased lipolysis from peripheral adipocytes and an influx of free fatty acids to the liver. Once inside the liver, these fatty acids undergo either oxidation or are synthesized to triglycerides. New data indicate that triglyceride accumulation per se is not harmful to hepatocytes and may represent a protective mechanism against lipotoxicity [27]. The concept of compartmentalization of lipids and lipid metabolites within the liver has gained importance as a possible important pathophysiological factor in this disease. Free cholesterol, ceramide and diacylglycerol have all been implicated as potentially injurious agents within the hepatocyte. Decreased export of triglycerides from the liver due to abnormalities in apo-B synthesis has also been described.

Figure 89.5 shows an additional recently recognized mechanism of injury of NAFLD. Increased apoptosis has been demonstrated in human NASH and animal models, and inhibition of caspase (the final common pathway for apoptosis) is currently being studied as a potential therapeutic agent.

Genes in nonalcoholic fatty liver disease

In addition to the environmental factors (Figure 89.3), it is now apparent that genetic factors also influence the susceptibility of certain patients for developing NAFLD. A number of important genetic polymorphisms have been studied recently. The most important is patatin-like phospholipase-domain-containing-3 (PLPLA-3), which encodes an enzyme, triacylg-

lycerol lipase responsible for hydrolysis of triglycerol. Additional polymorphisms that have been described include apolipoprotein-C3 (APOC-3) that increases the susceptibility to triglycerol–triglyceride accumulation in the liver, macrophage migration inhibitory factor gene, adiponectin, methylene tetrahydrofolate reductase, p-PAR-γ-coactivator-1α, haptaglobin, TNF-α gene, and ATP-binding cassette gene. One gene, angiotensin-2 type 1 receptor, has been described as potentially important in the development of fibrosis.

Hepatic steatosis

Patients with steatosis alone have a benign clinical course without histological clinical progression when followed for up to 19 years [6]. However, this "benign" steatosis is not quiescent; up to 3–5% of these patients may progress to cirrhosis. There is activation of hepatic stellate cells, stimulation of apoptotic proteins, and upregulation of mitochondrial uncoupling protein. Despite these abnormalities (which have the potential to cause cell injury), hepatic histology (other than steatosis) and function are normal.

NASH

It is unclear why only a subgroup of patients with NAFLD develops NASH. However, lipid-laden hepatocytes may act as a reservoir for hepatic toxic agents that are susceptible to injury by compounds such as endotoxin, cytokines and environmental toxins.

Oxidative stress

As shown in Table 89.11, a number of human studies have demonstrated oxidative stress associated with steatohepatitis. This oxidative stress results either from lysosomal processing or increased oxidation of fatty acids by mitochondria, peroxisomes or cytokines. These oxidative processes produce free electrons, hydrogen peroxide, and reactive oxygen species while depleting the potent antioxidants, glutathione and vitamin E. Oxidative stress also stimulates insulin resistance and the synthesis of several cytokines through the upregulation of transcription by nuclear translation, translocation of nuclear factor K-β (NFK-β) and the byproducts of lipid peroxidation, malondialdehyde (MDA) and 4-hydroxy-nononel (HNE). This combination of events cause hepatocyte injury through lipid peroxidation and the stimulation of cytokine production (Table 89.10, Figure 89.6).

Bacterial toxin

Another proposed pathophysiologic mechanism involves increased delivery of portal-derived hepatotoxins to a sensitized liver as the result of small intestinal bacterial overgrowth. The gut microbiome is a novel therapeutic target in NAFLD, since it is altered in obesity and may contribute to both hepatic steatosis and NASH [28]. However, if this mechanism were operative, it is likely that it would be synergetic and mediated through cytokine induced oxidative stress.

Table 89.11 Oxidative stress markers as predictors of steatohepatitis versus controls

Author	N	Predictors	Serum levels	P value
Horoz, 2005	22	TAR	Decreased	<0.05
		OSI	Increased	<0.05
Chalasani, 2004	21	TBAR	Increased	<0.01
		Ox-LDL	Increased	<0.01
Koruk, 2004	18	MDA	Increased	<0.01
		NO	Increased	0.04
		GSH	Increased	<0.01
		SOD	Decreased	0.04

GSH, glutathione; MDA, malondialdehyde; NO, nitric oxide; OSI, oxidative stress index; ox-LDL, oxidized low-density lipoprotein; SOD, superoxide dimutase; TAR, total antioxidant response; TBAR, thiobarbituric acid-reacting substance.

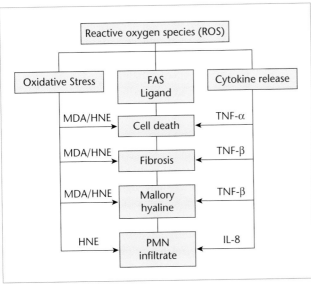

Figure 89.6 Causes of the histological features of nonalcoholic steatohepatitis (NASH). Both oxidative stress and inflammatory cytokines can cause many or all of the histological features of NASH: cell death (apoptosis), fibrosis, Mallory hyaline, and inflammatory infiltrates. IL, interleukin; TGF, transforming growth factor; MDA/HNE; malondialdehyde and 4-hydroxynonenal; TNF; tumor necrosis factor. (This figure was published in *Clinical Gastroenterology and Hepatology*, Wilfred M. Weinstein, Christopher J. Hawkey, Jaime Bosch, Nonalcoholic fatty liver disease (NAFLD), Pages 1–11, Copyright Elsevier, 2005.)

Pathology

It is important to emphasize that portal-based scoring systems (such as ISHAK and METAVIR) are not appropriate for NAFLD, which has more abnormalities in the central area of the hepatic globule. Table 89.3 displays the histologic features that have been identified by the NASH CRN as important or potentially important in the evaluation of NAFLD [7]. The histologic features of NAFLD fall into four general categories. As displayed in Tables 89.2 and 89.3, the NASH CRN has proposed a non-weighted, semi-quantified scoring system for

Table 89.12 Patient demographics

Study	N	Age (years)	Female (%)	Diabetic (%)	Obese (%)	TGs (%)
Matteoni, 1999	132	53	53	33	70	92
Angulo, 1999	144	51	67	28	60	27
Marchesini, 2003	304	42	17	7	25	3
Angulo 2007	733	48	47	30	60	60
NASH CRN, 2010	1266	50	64	31	62	55

NAFLD, which is being used in clinical trials. The necessary histologic components for the diagnosis are: steatosis (a macrovesicular > microvesicular pattern accentuated in zone 3); mixed mild portal and lobular inflammation; scattered polymorphonuclear leukocytes as well as mononuclear cells; and hepatocellular ballooning, most apparent near steatotic liver cells, typically most prominent in zone 3. Other histologic features that are usually present but not necessary for the diagnosis of NASH include: zone 3 peri-sinusoidal fibrosis, lipogranulomas, occasional acidophilic bodies, pigmented Kupffer cells and contiguous glycogenated nuclei. Less commonly present are Mallory–Denk bodies, mega-mitochondria, and positive iron staining. However, the diagnosis of NASH is not based on a number derived from the NASH CRN classification but rather by an overall interpretation by a pathologist. While promising, this detailed scoring system is not of practical use at the current time. The importance of the relationship between the natural history and histological findings has been emphasized by a system that classifies NAFLD into four types, as described in Table 89.1. Among the most important histologic features that indicate advanced NAFLD are hepatocyte ballooning [6], the extent of steatosis [29], the presence of portal inflammation [30], and perisinusoidal fibrosis [6].

Pediatric patients who have fatty liver disease have two different histologic types of NAFLD. Type I, resembling the adult pattern (ballooning degeneration, classic zone 3 fibrosis and parenchymal inflammation) is found in the minority of patients. Type II NAFLD was present in the majority of pediatric patients and is characterized by a macrovesicular steatosis with portal inflammation, with or without portal fibrosis, and no or minimal ballooning degeneration. There is a subgroup that has an overlap pattern with features common to both type I and type II [31].

Clinical presentation

Patient demographics (Table 89.12). Most cases occur in the fifth and sixth decade of life, but may also occur in children [31]. The condition is more frequent in females and patients with obesity and hypertriglyceridemia. Approximately one third of the patients have diabetes mellitus. It is also clear from these demographics that essentially any type of patient, regardless of gender, weight, abnormalities in glucose or lipid metabolism may have NAFLD.

NAFLD has been reported in all ethnic groups, with available data suggesting an over-representation in Hispanics and an under-representation in African–Americans [1].

Symptoms

Up to 50% of patients with NAFLD are asymptomatic. Fatigue, malaise, and vague right upper quadrant abdominal discomfort often bring subjects with NAFLD to medical attention. Typically, patients with NAFLD present with other conditions and are found only incidentally to have abnormal liver function tests or hepatomegaly; the latter occurring in up to 75% of patients.

Fatigue is a significant problem in NAFLD [32]. It is similar in degree to that of primary biliary cirrhosis patients and is associated with impaired physical function. This fatigue in NAFLD appears to be unrelated to either the severity of underlying liver disease or insulin resistance; but it associated with significant daytime somnolence.

Although right upper quadrant pain (thought to be caused by distension of Glisson's capsule) is usually mild and non-specific, and may be mistaken for gallstone disease. If diabetes is present, complications from visceral (bowel dysmotility and small bowel bacterial overgrowth) and peripheral neuropathy (pain and orthostatic hypotension) may also be present.

Physical examination

These patients usually have unremarkable findings on physical examination [1]. Most are obese with increased waist circumference, and those who do not show such an increase usually have increased visceral adiposity. Hypertension occurs in 15–70% of patients. Stigmata of chronic liver disease (muscle wasting, spider ectemangiasis, gynecomastia, and palmar erythema) are rarely seen on initial presentation, but when present suggest advanced fibrotic liver disease. Fluid retention (peripheral edema and ascites) and hepatic encephalopathy may occur when cirrhosis is present. Abnormalities in fat distribution should be sought to diagnose lipodystrophies (both genetic and HIV associated). Females may exhibit hirsutism and acne, which suggests polycystic ovary syndrome. Acanthosis nigrans (especially in patients of younger ages) with its associated hyperpigmented velvety plaques found in body folds is a feature of insulin resistance [1]. Finally, intermittent dysconjugate gaze (thought to be part of a generalized mitochondrial dysfunction) may occur in a small percentage of patients.

Differential diagnosis
Exclusion of other diseases

It is important to exclude other diseases associated with increased fat. The secondary causes of hepatic steatosis are listed in Figure 89.1.

By definition, the diagnosis of NAFLD requires that there is no history of previous or ongoing significant alcohol consumption. A wide range of alcohol consumption has been used to define NAFLD, from complete absence to 140–210 grams weekly for females and males, respectively. There is no consensus regarding the definition of nonalcoholic, especially since the presence of metabolic risk factors such as obesity and diabetes may promote hepatic steatosis at lower quantities of alcohol [33]. Recent studies suggest that 20 grams of alcohol daily for women and 30 grams daily for men should be considered nonalcoholic fatty liver disease. However, because it is very difficult to objectively confirm the daily use of 20–30 grams of alcohol [34], it remains important for the clinician to be diligent in obtaining the extent of alcohol consumption. Recently, a weighted multi-variant model using logistic regression analysis has been generated to calculate an alcoholic liver disease/NAFLD index score [35]. However, the validity of this test must be evaluated more extensively.

Mild increases in serum ferritin may occur in up to 30% of patients with NAFLD, and do not necessarily indicate coexisting ion overload, especially in the presence of normal transferrin saturation. The metabolic syndrome and hyperinsulinemia are known to be associated with increased serum ferritin. The presence of an HFE gene mutation with elevated serum ferritin may justify a liver biopsy in patients with suspected NAFLD.

Elevated serum autoantibodies are also very common in patients with NAFLD and have been reported in up to 33% of such patients. Antinuclear antibody titers are usually low, and titers greater than 1:320 are rare. Low titers of anti-smooth muscle and anti-mitochondrial antibodies also have been found in NAFLD [1]. Although these are generally felt to be epi-phenomenon, one study suggested that the presence of these autoantibodies correlated with histologic severity. In patients with suspected NAFLD and high autoantibodies (ANA > 1:160, anti-smooth muscle antibody > 1:40), may require a liver biopsy to exclude the presence of autoimmune hepatitis. It is also important to exclude chronic hepatitis B and hepatitis C as well as drug-induced disease and more rare disorders such as Wilson disease, alpha-1 antitrypsin, and galactosemia.

Diagnostic methods
Liver biopsy

Liver biopsy is considered the "gold standard" for diagnosis, and is the only current method for differentiating NASH from steatosis with or without inflammation. Table 89.13 lists suggested best practices for histologic assessment in patients with NAFLD. However, liver biopsy is not without controversies due to its sampling variability and inter-observer discordance of histological interpetation, as well as its costs and side effects [36]. However, liver biopsy in NAFLD patients can be used to exclude other liver diseases, distinguish steatosis from NASH, estimate prognosis and determine the progression of fibrosis

Table 89.13 Best practices for liver biopsy

Technique	Requirements
Biopsy	Needle core biopsy preferred Biopsy should be obtained with a 16 or lower gauge needle A ≥2 cm long tissue core (≥10 portal tracts) represents the optimal biopsy length Preferably obtain the biopsy from the right lobe. If a left lobe biopsy is used, a biopsy of the same lobe should be used for a follow-up biopsy
Histologic	Use hematoxylin and eosin stain Use Masson trichrome stain for bibrosis assessment Role of special stains and quantitative morphometry to assess fibrosis remains experimental Interpretation by an experienced pathologist who is trained in pattern recognition of NAFLD/NASH

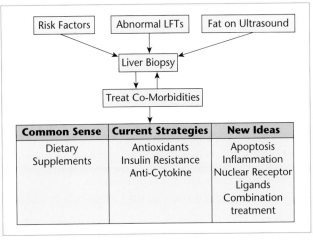

Figure 89.7 Management of nonalcoholic steatohepatitis (NASH). A management and treatment algorithm is proposed. If fat is found on a radiologic test or there is unexplained abnormal liver function (especially in the setting of risk factors suggestive of advanced fibrosis), a liver biopsy is indicated either before or after the treatment of co-morbidities. If there is improvement in liver function and/or steatosis on ultrasonography, a liver biopsy may not be necessary. However, improvement in liver function does not always equate to histologic improvement or resolution. Only sustained weight loss, the natural form of vitamin E and pioglitazone are effective therapies for NASH.

over time. However, because of the limitations of liver biopsy, noninvasive markers to evaluate inflammation and fibrosis have been studied and continue to be studied (Tables 89.8, 89.9 and 89.10). Ultrasonography, computed tomography, magnetic resonance imaging, and proton magnetic resonance spectroscopy are all used to diagnose NAFLD, the later being more sensitive when fat involves less than 20–30% of the liver. However, differences between NASH and steatosis are not apparent with any of the radiologic modalities [37]. Ultrasonography is the most common imaging modality used for evaluating hepatic steatosis and it can detect as little as 20% fat replacement within the liver [11]. New modalities such as transient elastography, EMR elastography, and quantitative CT based biomarkers may have some role but the data are nascent and sparse [19].

Serum chemistry

Increased aminotransferase activities are the most common abnormality in NAFLD; levels are usually raised only modestly (two- to five-fold increase). However, normal aminotransferase levels do not exclude NAFLD; the entire spectrum of NAFLD may occur in patients with normal ALT levels [38]. Alkaline phosphatase concentration is increased two- to three-fold in less than half of the patients [1]. Serum albumin and bilirubin levels are rarely abnormal unless cirrhosis has developed. Raised serum levels of ferritin are reported in approximately 30% of patients, usually with normal transferrin saturation and no evidence of hepatic ion overload.

The AST:ALT ratio is usually less than 1. When the ratio is greater than 1, it suggests an advanced fibrotic form of NAFLD. Hematologic measurements are usually normal, unless cirrhosis has led to hypersplenism. Several studies have reported the presence of autoimmune antibodies in up to 50% of patients with NAFLD, with their presence likely to be an epiphenomenon rather than a pathophysiologic process.

Treatment and prevention

The treatment of NAFLD has been reviewed recently [36,39,40]. A management algorithm is proposed in Figure 89.7.

Histologic confirmation

Although the role of liver biopsy in NASH remains uncertain, many clinicians believe that patients with unexplained abnormal liver function test results or a fatty liver on radiologic examination, should undergo liver biopsy, especially if they are a high risk for having NASH (obesity, diabetes, age above 45, metabolic syndrome or warning signs of fibrotic disease). This approach identifies those patients with NAFLD about whom the clinician should be most concerned [41]. In addition, now that there is a demonstrated effective agent for the treatment of NASH, a liver biopsy may be even more warranted.

Treatment of co-morbidities

Treatment of co-morbid conditions usually associated with NAFLD (obesity, dyslipidemia, hypertension and diabetes/hypoglycemia) (Figure 89.8) is essential in these patients [41]; however, the benefits of this strategy for improving NAFLD are uncertain. Clinicians currently disagree regarding whether the treatment of co-morbidities should be initiated before or after liver biopsy has been performed.

Weight loss

Weight reduction is generally recommended as an initial step in the management of NASH. It is generally recommended

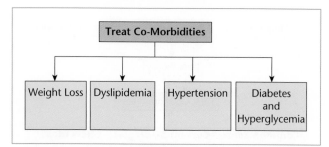

Figure 89.8 Treatment of co-morbidities. This figure shows the importance of the management of co-morbidities that is crucial to a good standard of care above and beyond any pharmacologic intervention.

Table 89.14 Strategies to enhance patient compliance in lifestyle modification

- Communicate with empathy
- Be sensitive to the general stigma against obesity
- Discuss the pros and cons of the proposed changes to lifestyle
- Explore the reasons for perpetual poor dietary and exercise choices
- Encourage self-efficacy
- Offer specific choices of food and exercise
- Design an individualized program of eating and physical activity
- Explain the treatment and its benefits

that overweight and obese patients lose 7–10% of their body weight over the course of 6–12 months. Serum transaminase levels almost always improve with weight loss but they are poor predictors of histologic appearance, which does not always improve and may, in fact, worsen if weight loss occurs too rapidly. Recently, a randomized controlled trial demonstrated that intense lifestyle intervention showed that a weight loss of 7% improved steatosis, lobular inflammation, ballooning injury and the NASH score [42]. Along with a weight loss program, there are a number of strategies that can enhance patient compliance during the lifestyle modification [43] as listed in Table 89.14.

In order to supplement weight loss, two drugs have been used to accelerate weight loss. Sibutramine, a serotonin norepinephrine reuptake inhibitor which promotes satiety and increases energy expenditure by stimulating thermogenesis, has been taken off the market because of an increased risk of cardiovascular events (heart attack and stroke). The only remaining drug available is orlistatin, which is a reversible inhibitor of gastric and pancreatic lipase, and has been effective in promoting limited weight loss in selected patients, but side effects such as diarrhea and bloating have made it undesirable and it does not improve weight loss or histology above what is accomplished with caloric restriction alone [44].

Thus, based on available data, it appears that a weight loss of 7–10% will improve the histologic features of NASH and no pharmacologic agent enhances the effect of weight loss alone.

Bariatric surgery can improve many of the components of the metabolic syndrome including NAFLD [45]. However,

NAFLD should not be the sole indication for bariatric surgery at the current time [46].

Type of diet
A number of different diets have been suggested including: the American Heart Association's Health Heart Diet, the Diabetic Diet as recommended by the American Diabetes Association, a low glycemic diet, and diets enriched with omega-3 polyunsaturated fatty acids. Another diet that may be effective is the Mediterranean diet, which has been demonstrated to improve insulin resistance and endothelial function in patients with type 2 diabetes and the metabolic syndrome [47,48]. However, the effects of these diets on NAFLD are unproven. Diets used to produce weight loss must always be individualized and related to the overall health status of the patient.

Hypertriglyceridemia
In patients with hypercholesterolemia, there is no contraindication to the use of statin drugs which are widely believed to be safe in patients with liver disease. A few pilot studies suggest that they may be beneficial. However, liver function needs to be monitored.

A small number of studies have evaluated the therapeutic potential of other lipid lowering agents including fibrates. These agents have the potential to improve serum aminotransferases, but unfortunately have not demonstrated any significant improvement in insulin resistance or histology.

Hypertension
Although the treatment of hypertension *per se* may have no direct effect on NAFLD, the agents used to treat hypertension may. Angiotensin receptor blockers (telmisartan and losartan) have been demonstrated to improve serum transaminases, insulin resistance and histology, with telmisartan having higher efficacy, perhaps because of it specific PPARγ ligand effect [49].

Diabetes
No data have demonstrated that good glycemic control in diabetic patients with NAFLD improved histologic findings. However, patients with diabetes have more advanced liver disease [18] and maximizing glycemic control is consistent with good clinical care. In addition, recent data have found dramatic and long-lasting effects of short term hyperglycemic spikes on endothelial function, and indicate that transient spikes of hyperglycemia may be an HbA$_{1c}$ independent risk factor for diabetic and endothelial complications.

Dietary supplements
Evidence is growing that the gut microbiota composition can modulate energy homeostasis and systemic inflammation, and

may thus contribute to the pathogenesis of nonalcoholic fatty liver disease. A recent study using a probiotic in NAFLD was prematurely stopped because of significant increase in liver fat content after four months of treatment [28]. In contrast, indigestible carbohydrates have been shown to improve glucose tolerance in adipokine profile. Oligofructose supplementation was also associated with weight loss, reduced caloric intake and improved glucose tolerance in overweight and obese adults [28]. Omega-3 polyunsaturated fatty acids (PUFA) treatment results in some improvement in the biochemical and radiologic features of NAFLD. Omega-3 PUFA acids are found in cold water fish (herring, haddock, Atlantic salmon, trout, tuna, cod and mackerel). However, histology has not been evaluated. While there may be some role for these agents in nonalcoholic fatty liver disease, larger placebo controlled trials evaluating histological assessment would be helpful. However, one strategy may be to incorporate food enriched in polyunsaturated omega-3 fatty acids into the diet, since there is some evidence that they are beneficial in the treatment of hypertriglyceridemia and hypertension.

Pharmacologic therapy

Many studies have tested various insulin sensitizers as treatment. However, the majority of them have been small pilot studies and proof of concept rather than carefully designed randomized placebo-controlled clinical trials. Metformin and thiazolidinediones (pioglitazone and rosiglitazone) are the two classes of insulin synthesizers studied in humans. There have been at least seven studies that have looked at **metformin** in the treatment of NAFLD. Only one was a randomized clinical trial and showed an improvement in steatosis and inflammation after 12 months of therapy. In addition, a recent analysis on the Cochrane Database showed that metformin leads to normalization of serum aminotransferases in a significant proportion of patients compared to dietary modification, and improves steatosis by imaging [50]. Taking all the data into consideration, metformin may lead to improvements in liver histology and ALT levels in up to 30% of patients with NASH, but this effect may be largely due to the weight loss associated with metformin. Currently, there is little enthusiasm for using metformin as a primary therapeutic agent in patients with NASH.

A recent study [51] demonstrated that **pioglitazone** improved steatosis, lobular inflammation, severity of ballooning and increased the resolution of NASH compared to the placebo (Figure 89.9). However, not all patients treated with pioglitazone improved and many of these patients gained excessive weight. In addition, the other thiazolidinedione (**rosiglitazone**) improved only steatosis in a clinical trial, and has been suggested to increase the risk for cardiovascular disease and bone loss [52].

Antioxidants

The only antioxidant that has been shown to be beneficial in a carefully performed trial is the natural form of **vitamin E** at a

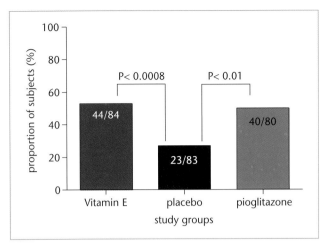

Figure 89.9 The role of antioxidants and insulin sensitizes in the treatment of nonalcoholic steatohepatitis (NASH). Displayed is a recent study that shows that both vitamin E and pioglitazone improved the resolution of NASH.

dose of 400 IU BID [52] (Figure 89.9). Vitamin E improved NASH as well as the histologic findings of steatosis, inflammation, and ballooning. However, it had no effect on fibrosis.

Agents without potential efficacy

Therapeutic interventions that have been proven not to be useful in NASH include betaine, ursodeoxycholic acid (low dose and high dose), probiotics, fibrates, and endocanabanoid receptor-1 antagonists. A number of agents have been tested in pilot studies with some improvement in liver function, but without histologic examination. These agents include Provucol, N-acetylcysteine, pentoxifylline, iron depletion, silymarin, exenatide, and the nuclear receptor ligand farnesoid.

Overall approach to pharmacologic therapy

Despite a number of promising agents based on sound rationale, the only therapies of proven efficacy in a carefully controlled clinical trial are the natural form of vitamin E and pioglitazone, with less enthusiasm for the latter due to the associated excessive weight gain.

Prevention

No studies have directly studied preventive therapies, although intervention at a societal level (directed at preventing insulin resistance and oxidative stress) has the potential to not only prevent fatty liver disease but the other metabolic abnormalities associated with the metabolic syndrome (Figure 89.10).

Preventing disease

Extracting information from studies in patients with obesity and diabetes, weight loss and exercise are reasonable strategies

Liver Disease

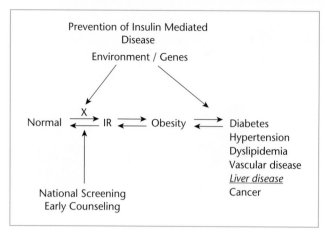

Figure 89.10 Prevention of nonalcoholic fatty liver disease. Displayed is a proposed algorithm where early intervention at a national level can prevent the environmental influence and genetic susceptibility causes of not only fatty liver disease but also the other components of the metabolic syndrome and insulin resistance.

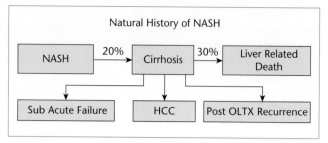

Figure 89.11 The natural history of nonalcoholic steatohepatitis (NASH) is displayed. HCC; hepatocellular carcinoma, OLTX; orthotopic liver transplantation. (This figure was published in *Clinical Gastroenterology and Hepatology*, Wilfred M. Weinstein, Christopher J. Hawkey, Jaime Bosch, Nonalcoholic fatty liver disease (NAFLD), Pages 1–11, Copyright Elsevier, 2005.)

as well as being good for general health. Although many weight loss and exercise interventions have been studied in NAFLD, epidemiologic data suggest that a change in behavior that would affect energy balance by as little as 420 kJ/day would prevent weight gain and arrest the epidemics of both obesity and NAFLD.

Vaccination for viral hepatitis

Although no data are available for this strategy in NAFLD, vaccinating for hepatitis A and B may be worthwhile and is employed by many clinicians.

Screening for hepatocellular carcinoma

Hepatocellular carcinoma is now recognized to be a growing problem in patients with cirrhosis secondary to fatty liver disease [53]. Therefore, many clinicians employ interval assessments for screening ultrasound even without existing cost effectiveness studies.

Complications and their management

The major complications that occur in NAFLD are those associated with the adverse clinical outcomes (cirrhosis, liver failure, and hepatocellular carcinoma) that are part of its natural history. Management consist in standard treatment for the complications of cirrhosis in general. Patients with NAFLD have a very high prevalence of cardiovascular risk factors and atherosclerosis, and high incidence of cardiovascular morbidity and mortality [2]. In fact, in some studies mortality from cardiovascular disease is two- to four-fold higher than the mortality from liver-related deaths. Therefore the significance of cardiovascular disease should be emphasized to patients with NAFLD and their primary care providers in order to optimize therapy for this complication. Early and aggressive treatment aimed at associated cardiovascular risk factors is consistent with overall good clinical care.

Prognosis with and without treatment

Cirrhosis develops in 15–20% of patients with NASH (Figure 89.11). Once developed, 30–40% of these patients may succumb to liver related death over a 10-year period [54,55]. NASH is a major cause of cryptogenic cirrhosis, may decompensate into subacute liver failure, progress to hepatocellular carcinoma and recur post-liver transplantation [56]. In contrast, steatosis alone is reported to have a more benign clinical course, although progression to cirrhosis has occurred in 3% of these patients.

Vitamin E and pioglitazone improved NASH over a 2-year period but had no significant effect on fibrosis during that time period. Only sustained weight loss has the potential to alter the natural history of NAFLD.

What to tell patients

Patients need to partner with their physicians in the management of NAFLD in a number of important ways and become actively involved in their care.

Diet

In general, patients should follow a well balanced diet (Table 89.15). One such diet is recommended by the National Cholesterol Education Program (http://www.nhlbi.nih.gov/about/ncep). This diet makes specific recommendations regarding total caloric intake as well as the amount and type of fat and carbohydrate for patients who do not have to lose weight. If the patient has diabetes, specific recommendations have been made by the American Diabetes Association [57] (http://www.diabetes.org/food-and-fitness/food/). The American Heart Association provides details of the Mediterranean-style diet that features the use of olive oil, a high consumption of fruits, vegetables, grains, potatoes, beans, nuts and seeds, and low amounts of red meats (http://www.heart.org/HEARTORG/GettyHealthy/Nutrition).

Table 89.15 Treatment and prevention: weight loss diet[a]

Nutrient	Recommended intake
Calories[b]	Approximately 500–1000 kcal/day reduction from usual state
Total fat[c]	30% or less of total calories
Saturated fatty acids[d]	8–10% of total calories
Monounsaturated fatty acids	Up to 15% of total calories
Polyunsaturated fatty acids	Up to 10% of total calories
Cholesterol[d]	<300 mg/day
Protein[e]	Approximately 15% of total calories
Carbohydrate[f]	55% or more of total calories
Sodium chloride	No more than 100 mmol/day (approximately 2.4 g sodium or 6 g sodium chloride)
Calcium[g]	1000–1500 mg/day
Fiber[f]	20–30 g/day

[a]This table provides guidelines for Step I weight loss as suggested in a monograph provided by the National Heart, Lung and Blood Institute (2000) entitled *The practice guide. Identification, evaluation and treatment of obesity in adults.*
[b]A reduction in calories of 500–1000 kcal/day will help achieve a weight loss of 1–2 lb/week. Alcohol provides unneeded calories and displaces more nutritious foods. Alcohol consumption not only increases the number of calories in a diet but has been associated with obesity in epidemiologic as well as experimental studies. The impact of alcohol calories on a person's overall caloric intake needs to be assessed and approximately controlled.
[c]Fat-modified foods may provide a helpful strategy for lowering total fat intake but will be effective only if they are also low in calories and there is no compensation by calories from other foods.
[d]Patients with high blood cholesterol levels need to use the Step II diet to achieve further reductions in low density lipoprotein cholesterol levels; in the Step II diet, saturated fats are reduced to less than 7% of total calories, and cholesterol levels to less than 200 mg/day. All of the other nutrients are the same as in Step I.
[e]Protein should be derived from plant sources and lean sources of animal protein.
[f]Complex carbohydrates from different vegetables, fruits, and whole grains are good sources of vitamins, minerals, and fiber. A diet rich in soluble fiber, including oat bran, legumes, barley, and most fruits and vegetables, may be effective in reducing blood cholesterol levels. A diet high in all types of fiber may also aid in weight management by promoting satiety at lower levels of calories and fat intake. Some authorities recommend 20–30 g fiber daily, with an upper limit of 35 g.
[g]During weight loss, attention should be given to maintaining an adequate intake of vitamins and minerals. Maintenance of the recommended calcium intake of 1000–1500 mg/day is especially important for women who may be at risk of osteoporosis.

Table 89.16 Treatment and prevention: use of nutritional supplements in NAFLD

Possibly harmful supplements	Possibly harmful medications
St. John's wort	Acetaminophen[d]
Ephedrine-containing compounds	Tamoxifen[e]
Excessive vitamin A[a]	Amiodarone[e]
Glucosamine[b]	Iron[f]
Others[c]	Estrogen[g]

[a]Vitamin A should not be used in excess of that contained in a daily multivitamin (MI), which is 5000 IU.
[b]As hexosamines in general cause insulin resistance, glucosamine should be used with some caution.
[c]All other herbs should be considered as possible causes of injury and should be avoided.
[d]Acetaminophen should be restricted to less than 2–3 g/daily. Repeated or ongoing use of acetaminophen for longer than 3 days with daily doses above 1.5 g should be discouraged. Many over-the-counter (OTC) medications contain acetaminophen; therefore the amount of acetaminophen in OTC medications should be sought carefully.
[e]This drug may cause hepatic injury that histologically looks similar to NAFLD/NASH. Therefore, the benefit risk of using these drugs in NAFLD/NASH should be considered carefully.
[f]As iron may cause oxidative stress in the liver, iron supplements should be used only as per standard management for anemia. Transferrin saturation should not exceed 50%.
[g]Estrogens used as oral contraceptive pills or hormonal replacement therapy do not have to be discontinued.

Dietary supplements

Many patients seek advice regarding the efficacy and safety of vitamins, herbs or other nutritional supplements. Unfortunately, there is insufficient information to make definite recommendations in this area. However, the use of indigestible fiber and omega-3 fatty acids seems reasonable. Table 89.16 lists supplements that may be harmful.

Weight loss

Overweight patients (BMI > 25 kg/m²) should be given a diet with a goal of losing and sustaining an initial loss of 10% of body weight. This loss should be gradual and should not exceed two pounds per week, as per the National Heart, Lung and Blood Institute (NHLBI) guidelines for weight loss. There is insufficient information to recommend or discourage any alternative diet (such as the Atkin's or South Beach diets). It should be emphasized that patients should not fast as a means of losing weight.

Exercise

Regular exercise is a useful adjunct to weight loss and improves the success of weight loss. The Institute of Medicine

Table 89.17 Treatment and prevention: Management of comorbidities in NAFLD

Comorbidity	Management goals/issues
Type 2 diabetes	HgbA1c < 7% should be sought. Insulin-sensitizing agents rather then insulin or sulfonylureas are preferred
Hypercholesterolemia	Referral to PCP or specialist for cholesterol levels >130 mg/dL in nondiabetics and >100 mg/dL in diabetics
Hyperglyceridemia	Referral to PCP or specialist for fasting triglycerides >200 mg/dL
Hypertension	Referral to PCP or specialist for repeated systolic blood pressure (BP) >140 mmHg and/or diastolic BP >90 mmHg in diabetics. In diabetics, referral for systolic BP >130 mmHg and/or a diastolic BP >85 mmHg
Angina	Symptoms of coronary heart disease should be sought and referred to PCP or specialist as needed
Obstructive sleep apnea (OSA)	Symptoms of OSA (snoring, disruptive sleep etc.) should be sought. If present, referral to a specialist should be obtained for possible sleep study and therapy
Polycystic ovary syndrome (PCOS)	Women with hirsutism and nonmenopausal menstrual irregularity (>9 menstrual cycles yearly) should be referred to PCP or gynecologist for possible PCOS
Occupational hepatotoxin	A history of ongoing exposure to volatile hydrocarbons should be sought and suggestions made for a change of workplace conditions
Hypothyroidism	Referral to PCP or to an endocrinologist
Hypopituitarism	Refer to an endocrinologist

recommends that regular physical activity of at least 1 hour/day should be performed.

Alcohol and cigarette use

Alcohol should not be used at all, or should be restricted to no more than minimal ceremonial use. Cigarette use has now been recognized as a risk factor for fibrosis in NAFLD and should therefore be strongly discouraged.

Physician management of co-morbid diseases

The recognized co-morbidities and diseases associated with NAFLD, along with specific management recommendations are outlined in Table 89.17.

References

1. Tetri BA, Clark JM, Bass NM, et al. For the NASH Clinical Research Network. Clinical, laboratory and histological association in adults with nonalcoholic fatty liver disease. Hepatology. 2010;52:913–924.
2. Targher G, Day CP, Bonora E. Risk of cardiovascular disease in patients with nonalcoholic fatty liver disease. N Engl J Med. 2010;363:L1341–1350.
3. Baumeister SE, Volzke H, Marshall P. Impact of fatty liver disease on health care utilization and costs in a general population: A five year observation. Gastroenterology. 2008;134:85–94.
4. Charlton M. Nonalcoholic fatty liver disease: A review of current understanding and future impact. Clin Gastroenterol Hepatol. 2004;2:1048–1058.
5. Hall PM, Kirsch R. (2005) Pathology of hepatic steatosis, NASH and related complications, in Fatty Liver Disease: NASH and Related Disorders. (eds G.C. Farrell, J. George, P. Hall and A.J. McCullough. Blackwell Publishing, Oxford, pp. 13–22.
6. Matteoni CA, Younossi ZM, Gramlich T, et al. Nonalcoholic fatty liver: A spectrum of clinical and pathologic severity. Gastroenterology. 1999;116:1413–1419.
7. Kleiner DE, Brunt EM, Vannatta M, et al. and the nonalcoholic steatohepatitis clinical research network. Design and validation of a histological scoring system for nonalcoholic fatty liver disease. Hepatology. 2005;41:1313–1321.
8. Adams LA, Lymp JF, St. Sauver J. The natural history of nonalcoholic fatty liver disease: A population based cohort study. Gastroenterology. 2005;129:113–121.
9. Bellentani S, Bedogni G, Miglioli L. The epidemiology of fatty liver. Eur J Gastroenterol Hepatol. 2004;16:1087–1093.
10. Everhart JE, Bambha KM. Fatty liver: Think globally. Hepatology. 2010;51:1491–1493.
11. Dasarathy S, Dasarathy J, Khiyami A, et al. Validity of real time ultrasound in the diagnosis of hepatic steatosis: A prospective study. J Hepatol. 2009;51:1061–1067.
12. Browning JD, Szezepaniak LS, Dobbins R, et al. Prevalence of hepatic steatosis in an urban population in the United States: Impact of ethnicity. Hepatology. 2004;40:1387–1395.
13. Almeda-Valdes P, Cuebas-Ramus D, Aquilar-Salinas CA. Metabolic syndrome and nonalcoholic fatty liver disease. Ann Hepatol. 2009;8:18–24.
14. Alberti KGMN, Zimmet P, Shaw J. For the Epidemiology Task Force Consensus Group. The metabolic syndrome – A new world definition. Lancet. 2005;366:1059–1063.

15. Lorenzo C, Stern MP, Okoloise M, *et al*. The metabolic syndrome as a predictor of Type 2 diabetes. *Diabetes Care*. 2003;26:3153–3159.

16. Kahabuchi M, Kojina T, Takeda N, *et al*. The metabolic syndrome as a predictor of nonalcoholic fatty liver disease. *Ann Intern Med*. 2005;142:722–728.

17. Marchesini G, Ragianesi B, Forlani G, *et al*. Nonalcoholic fatty liver, steatohepatitis and the metabolic syndrome. *Hepatology*. 2003;37:917–923.

18. Younossi ZM, Gramlich T, Matteoni CA, *et al*. Nonalcoholic fatty liver disease in patient with Type 2 diabetes. *Clin Gastroenterol Hepatol*. 2004;2:262–265.

19. Pagadala M, Zein CO, McCullough AJ. Predictors of steatohepatitis and advanced fibrosis in nonalcoholic liver disease. *Clin Liv Dis*. 2009;13:591–606.

20. Feldstein AE, Wieckowska A, Lopez AR, *et al*. Cyto-keratin-18 fragment levels as a non-invasive marker of nonalcoholic steatohepatitis: A multicenter validation study. *Hepatology*. 2009;50:1072–1078.

21. Guha IN, Parkes J, Roderick P. Non-invasive markers of fibrosis in nonalcoholic fatty liver disease: Validating the European liver fibrosis panel and exploring simple markers. *Hepatology*. 2008;47:455–460.

22. Angulo P, Hui JM, Marchesini G, *et al*. The NAFLD fibrosis score: A non-invasive system that identifies liver fibrosis in patients with NAFLD. *Hepatology*. 2007;45:846–854.

23. Younossi ZM, Baranova A, Ziegler H. A genomic and proteomic study of the spectrum of nonalcoholic liver diseases. *Hepatology*. 2005;42:655–674.

24. Kalhan SC, Guo L, Edmison J, *et al*. Plasma metabolomic profile in nonalcoholic fatty liver disease. *Metabolism*. 2011;60:404–413.

25. Cheung O, Sanyal AJ. Recent advances in nonalcoholic fatty liver disease. *Curr Opin Gastroenterol*. 2010;26:202–208.

26. Feldstein AE. Novel insights into the pathophysiology of nonalcoholic fatty liver disease. *Semin Liver Dis*. 2010;30:391–401.

27. Trauner M, Arrese M, Wagner M. Fatty liver and lipotoxicity. *Biochim Biophys Acta*. 2010;1801:299–310.

28. Musso G, Gambino R, Cassader M. Gut microbiota as a regulator of energy homeostasis and ectopic fat deposition: Mechanisms and implications for metabolic disorders. *Curr Opin Lipidol*. 2010;21:76–83.

29. Chalasani N, Wilson L, Kleiner DE, *et al*. For the NASH Clinical Research Network. Relationship of steatosis grade and zonal location to histological features of steatohepatitis in adult patients with nonalcoholic fatty liver disease. *J Hepatol*. 2008;48:829–834.

30. Brunt EM, Kleiner DW, Wilson LA, *et al*. For the Clinical Research Network. Portal inflammation in nonalcoholic fatty liver disease (NAFLD): A histologic marker of advanced NAFLD clinico-pathologic correlations from the Nonalcoholic Steatohepatitis Clinical Research Network. *Hepatology*. 49:809–820.

31. Loomba R, Sirlin CB, Schwimmer JB, *et al*. Advances in pediatric nonalcoholic fatty liver disease. *Hepatology*. 2009;50:1282–1293.

32. Newton JL, Jones DEJ, Henderson E, *et al*. Fatigue in nonalcoholic fatty liver disease (NAFLD) is significant and associates with inactivity and excessive daytime sleepiness but not with liver disease severity or insulin resistance. *Gut*. 2008;57:807–813.

33. Ruhl CE, Everhart JE. Joint effects of body weight and alcohol on elevated serum alanine aminotransferase in the United States population. *Clin Gastroenterol Hepatol*. 2005;3:1260–1268.

34. McCullough AJ. The clinical features, diagnosis and natural history of nonalcoholic fatty liver disease. *Clin Liver Dis*. 2004;8:521–533.

35. Dunn W, Angulo P, Sanderson S, *et al*. Utility of a new model to diagnose an alcohol basis for steatohepatitis. *Gastroenterology*. 2006;131:1057–1063.

36. Vuppalanchi R, Chalasani N. Nonalcoholic steatohepatitis: Selected practical issues in their evaluation and management. *Hepatology*. 2009;49:306–317.

37. Saadeh S, Younossi ZM, Remer EM, *et al*. The utility of radiological imaging in nonalcoholic fatty liver disease. *Gastroenterology*. 2002;123:745–750.

38. Mofrad P, Contos MJ, Hague M. Clinical and histological spectrum of nonalcoholic fatty liver disease associated with normal ALT values. *Hepatology*. 2003;37:1286–1292.

39. Lam B, Younossi AM. Treatment options for nonalcoholic fatty liver disease. *Ther Adv Gastroenterol*. 2010;3:121–137.

40. Federico A, Niosi M, DelVecchio Blanco C, *et al*. Emerging drugs for nonalcoholic fatty liver disease. *Expert Opin Emerging Drugs*. 2008;13:145–158.

41. Youssef WI, McCullough AJ. Diabetes mellitus, obesity and hepatic steatosis. *Semin Gastrointestinal Dis*. 2002;13:1730.

42. Promrat K, Fleiner DE, Niemeier HM, *et al*. Randomized controlled trial testing the effects of weight loss on nonalcoholic steatohepatitis. *Hepatology*. 2010;51:121–129.

43. Bellentani S, Grave RD, Suppini A, *et al*., and the Fatty Liver Italian Network. Behavior therapy for nonalcoholic fatty liver: The need for a multidisciplinary approach. *Hepatology*. 2008;47:746–754.

44. Harrison SA, Fecht W, Brunt EM, *et al*. Orlistar for overweight subjects with nonalcoholic steatohepatitis: A randomized, prospective trial. *Hepatology*. 2009;49:80–86.

45. Mummadi R, Kasturi KS, Chennareddy S, *et al*. Effect of bariatric surgery on nonalcoholic fatty liver disease: Systematic review and meta analysis. *Clin Gastroenterol Hepatol*. 2008;6:1396–1402.

46. Chavez-Tapia NC, Tellez-Avila FI, Barrientes-Guitierrez T, *et al*. Bariatric surgery for nonalcoholic steatohepatitis in obese patients (Review). *Cochrane Database Sys Rev* 2010;20:CD 007340. www.thecochranelibrary.com

47. Schroeder H. Protective mechanisms of the Mediterranean diet in obesity and type 2 diabetes. *J Nutr Biochem*. 2007;18:149–160.

48. Esposito K, Marfella R, Ciotola M. Effect of a Mediterranean diet on endothelial function and markers of vascular inflammation in the metabolic syndrome. *JAMA*. 2004;292:1440–1446.

49. Georgescu EF, Ioneschu R, Niculessu M, *et al*. Angiotensive-receptor blockers as therapy for mild-to-moderate hypertension-associated nonalcoholic steatohepatitis. *World J Gastroenterol*. 2009;28:942–954.

50. Angelico F, Burattin M, Alessandri C, *et al*. Drugs improving insulin resistance for nonalcoholic fatty liver disease and/or nonalcoholic steatohepatitis. *Cochrane Database Sys Rev* 2007;CD005166.

51. Sanyal AJ, Chalasani N, Kowdley KV, *et al*. For the NASH CRN. Pioglitazone, vitamin E or placebo for nonalcoholic steatohepatitis. *N Engl J Med*. 2010;362:1675–1885.

52. Zarich SW. Does the choice of antidiabetic therapy influence macrovascular outcome? *Curr Diab Rep*. 2010;10:24–31.

Liver Disease

53. Ascha MS, Hanouneh IA, Lopez R, *et al.* The incidence and risk factors of hepatocellular carcinoma in patients with nonalcoholic steatohepatitis. *Hepatology*. 2010;51:1972–1978.

54. Eckstedt M, Franzen LE, Mathiesen UL, *et al.* Longterm follow-up of patients with NAFLD and elevated enzymes. *Hepatology*. 2006;44:865–873.

55. Feldstein AE, Charatcharoenwitthaya P, Treeprasertsuk S, *et al.* Natural history of nonalcoholic fatty liver disease in children: A follow-up study up to 20 years. *Gut*. 2009;58:1538–1544.

56. Pagadala M, Dasarathy S, Eghtesad B, *et al.* Post transplant metabolic syndrome: An epidemic waiting to happen. *Liver Transpl*. 2009;15:1662–1670.

57. Franz MJ, Bantle JP, Beebe JD. American Diabetes Association nutrition principles and recommendation in diabetes. *Diabetes Care*. 2004;27:526–546.

CHAPTER 90
Hemochromatosis

Antonello Pietrangelo

University Hospital of Modena, Modena, Italy

Liver Disease

ESSENTIAL FACTS ABOUT PATHOGENESIS

- A genetic defect leads to inadequate levels/activity of the iron hormone hepcidin, which normally prevents the transfer of iron from the intestine and macrophages into the bloodstream
- Involved genes: *HFE*, transferrin receptor 2 (*TfR2*), hemojuvelin (*HJV*), hepcidin gene (*HAMP*) and, very rarely, ferroportin (*FPN*)
- Clinical manifestation: genes that are key for hepcidin synthesis are mutated (e.g., *HJV* or *HAMP*): iron overload occurs rapidly, and disease is severe with early onset; and genes encoding ancillary hepcidin regulators are mutated (e.g., *HFE* or *TfR2*): iron overload is gradual, disease milder, and later in onset
- The prototype and by far the most common form of hemochromatosis (HC) is HC associated with homozygosity for the C282Y polymorphism of *HFE*
- Prevalence of the *HFE* C282Y polymorphism is high in Caucasians (1 in 200–300), but fully expressed disease is rare, as still partially characterized host-related and environmental factors are required for clinical expression

ESSENTIALS OF DIAGNOSIS

- Classically (HFE-HC): male Caucasian patient, 40–50-years old, with fatigue, dark skin, arthralgia or hepatomegaly, and elevated transferrin saturation and serum ferritin
- Classically (juvenile HC): male or female patient, Caucasian or non-Caucasian, 20–30-years old, with hypogonadism, cardiomyopathy, and marked elevation of serum iron parameters
- C282Y homozygosity and evidence of iron excess
- Parenchymal hepatic iron overload with C282Y homozygosity or mutations of other HC genes
- Liver biopsy is no longer necessary to diagnose HFE-HC, but it should be offered to those with serum ferritin above 1000 μg/L, elevated AST or hepatomegaly due to the risk of underlying fibrosis/cirrhosis (unless obvious)
- Evidence of organ disease in C282Y/H63D compound heterozygotes or H63D homozygotes should prompt investigation of other concurrent pathogenic factors unrelated to HC

ESSENTIALS OF TREATMENT

- Phlebotomy is the standard treatment of all forms of HC
- Weekly phlebotomy can restore safe blood levels of iron (reflected by serum ferritin levels of <20–50 μg/L and transferrin saturation below 30%) within 1–2 years
- Maintenance therapy (typically 2–4 units/year) must be continued to keep serum ferritin at a normal level
- Survival in adequately iron-depleted precirrhotic and prediabetic patients is the same as for normal individuals
- Mild hepatic fibrosis is reversible; fatigue, elevated transaminases, and skin pigmentation improve after phlebotomy
- Arthralgia is unlikely to improve; hypogonadism, cirrhosis, destructive arthritis, and insulin-dependent diabetes associated with HC are usually irreversible
- In patients on an adequate phlebotomy program, dietary iron restrictions are unnecessary

Introduction

Hemochromatosis (HC), or hereditary hemochromatosis (HH), is an iron-loading disorder caused by a genetically-determined failure to prevent iron from entering the body when it is not needed. It is characterized by progressive parenchymal iron overload, with potential for multiorgan damage and disease,

including cirrhosis, diabetes and cardiomyopathy. The term "hemochromatosis" was coined in 1989 by Von Recklinghausen [1] to describe the autopsy finding of massive organ damage associated with dark tissue staining caused by what he believed to be a blood-borne pigment. It was Sheldon, however, in his monumental 1935 review of all cases published in the world's medical literature [2], who suggested that the disorder was probably hereditary. Simon demonstrated its hereditary nature and found that the gene was linked with the HLA system on chromosome 6 [3]. In 1996, Feder *et al.* discovered a polymorphism (C282Y) in this genomic region that involved a novel MHC class I-like gene, named **HFE**, which was present in the majority of HC patients throughout the world. However, as genetic testing for *HFE* mutations became more widespread, it rapidly became clear that the situation was more complicated than previously considered. Other iron genes, whose mutations were associated with hereditary iron overload syndromes with some, many, or apparently even all of the phenotypic features of classic HC, were discovered: transferrin receptor 2 (*TfR2*) [4]; hepcidin (*HAMP*) [5]; hemojuvelin (*HJV*) [6]; and ferroportin (*FPN*) [7,8]. Therefore, the present definition of HC embraces the classical disorder related to *HFE* C282Y homozygosity (the prototype for this syndrome and by far the most common form) and the rare disorders

Textbook of Clinical Gastroenterology and Hepatology, Second Edition. Edited by C. J. Hawkey, Jaime Bosch, Joel E. Richter, Guadalupe Garcia-Tsao, Francis K. L. Chan.
© 2012 Blackwell Publishing Ltd. Published 2012 by Blackwell Publishing Ltd.

more recently attributed to loss of *TfR2*, *HAMP*, *HJV* or, in very rare cases, *FPN* (Table 90.1). This concept of HC is based on new knowledge and stems from the idea that, beyond their genetic diversities, all known HCs belong to the same clinico-pathological entity as they all originate from the same

pathophysiological event, the failure of the liver to effectively produce the iron hormone **hepcidin** [9].

Epidemiology

HFE-related HC (HFE-HC) is the most common form of HC and also the most **frequently inherited metabolic disorder in Caucasians**, with a prevalence of the genetic polymorphism 10 times higher than that of cystic fibrosis (Table 90.2). The reported allelic frequency of C282Y across several screening studies is around 6% and the estimated prevalence of the C282Y polymorphism is 1 in 200–300 in Caucasians [10], but much lower in Hispanics, Asian Americans, Pacific Islanders, and black individuals [11]. The disease likely arose from a chance mutation occurring in a single individual, a Celtic or Viking ancestor inhabiting North-West Europe. The genetic defect, which caused no serious obstacle to reproduction and may have even conferred some advantages, was passed on and spread through population migration. The distribution of the C282Y mutation coincides with its Northern origin, with frequencies ranging from 12.5% in Ireland to 0% in Southern Europe. In addition to C282Y, H63D, the "minor" *HFE* polymorphism, has been found more frequently in HC patients than in the general population. The frequency of the H63D polymorphism shows less geographical variations with an average allelic frequency of 14%, but its clinical impact appears

Table 90.1 Main features of hereditary hemochromatosis

Definition	Iron-overload disease caused by a genetically determined failure to prevent the release of unrequired iron from the intestine and macrophages into the bloodstream
Distinguishing features	• Hereditary (usually autosomal recessive) trait • Early and progressive expansion of the plasma iron compartment • Progressive parenchymal iron deposition that can cause severe damage and disease involving the liver, endocrine glands, heart, and/or joints • Unimpaired erythropoiesis and optimal response to therapeutic phlebotomy • Defective hepcidin synthesis or activity
Postulated pathogenic basis	Gene mutations leading to inappropriately low hepatic synthesis or impaired activity of hepcidin
Recognized genetic causes	Pathogenic mutations of *HFE*, *TfR2*, *HJV*, or *HAMP*, and, rarely, *FPN*

Table 90.2 Hereditary hemochromatosis (HC)

Type	Affected gene (symbol/location)	Known or postulated gene product function	Epidemiology	Genetics	Clinical onset (decade)	Main clinical manifestation	Clinical course
Adult-onset HC	Hemochromatosis gene (*HFE*/6p21.3)	Interaction with transferrin receptor 1 Uptake of transferring iron Hepcidin regulator	Affects Caucasians of Northern European descent C282Y polymorphism highly prevalent: 1 in 200–300	Autosomal recessive	Third to fifth°	Liver disease	Mild to severe
	Transferrin-receptor 2 (*TfR2*/7q22)	Uptake of transferrin and non –transferrin-bound iron Hepcidin regulator	Caucasians and non-Caucasians Rare				
	Solute carrier family 40 (iron-regulated transporter), member 1 / ferroportin (*SLC40A1*/2q32)	Iron export from cells, including macrophages, enterocytes, placental cells	Caucasians and non-Caucasians Very rare	Autosomal dominant			
Juvenile-onset HC	Hepcidin antimicrobial peptide (*HAMP*/19q13.1)	Down-regulation of iron efflux from macrophages, through degradation of ferroportin	Caucasians and non-Caucasians Very rare	Autosomal recessive	Second to third	Hypogonadism and cardiac disease	Severe
	Hemojuvelin (*HJV*/1p21)	Co-receptor for bone morphogenic proteins (BMPs) Hepcidin transcriptional regulator	Caucasians and non-Caucasians Rare Most prevalent mutation: 230V				

to be limited [12]. An additional *HFE* polymorphism is S65C, which can be associated with HC when inherited in trans with C282Y on the other parental allele.

The prevalence of C282Y-homozygosity among patients with liver disease is around 5%, 10-fold higher than the reported prevalence in the general population. This figure increases if patients with liver disease are preselected for increased transferrin saturation (TS). Even higher C282Y frequencies can be found in patients with hepatocellular carcinoma, a known complication of HC.

HC is associated with homozygosity for the C282Y *HFE* mutation in approximately 80% of clinically characterized patients of European ancestry. Hence, nearly 20% of such patients have the disease in the absence of C282Y. Although compound heterozygosity (H63D/C282Y) appears to be disease associated, usually co-factors are implicated in the clinical expression [13–15]. Other genes associated with clinical HC are *TfR2, HJV, HAMP,* and *FPN* (Table 90.2). None of these non–HFE-HC appears to be restricted to Northern Europeans. The frequency of *TfR2* mutations is low and so far they have been detected in only a few pedigrees throughout the world. The **juvenile form** of HC is rare. Most cases are due to mutations of *HJV*. One common *HJV* mutation, G320V, is present in half of juvenile HC families. A small proportion of patients with the juvenile form of HC carry mutations in the gene encoding the iron regulatory peptide hepcidin. While most *FPN* mutations give rise to a distinct form of hereditary iron overload, called "the ferroportin disease" [16], unusual *FPN* mutations are believed to cause rare forms of HC similar to *HFE*-HC [9].

Causes and pathogenesis

The first biochemical manifestation of HC is an **increased TS**, which reflects an uncontrolled influx of iron into the bloodstream from enterocytes and macrophages [17]. Apart from menstruation, the body has no effective means of significantly reducing plasma iron levels. Without therapeutic intervention, overload in the plasma compartment will lead to the progressive accumulation of iron in the parenchymal cells of key organs, creating a distinct risk for oxidative damage. This stage is reflected by **increasing serum ferritin (SF) levels**. The time of onset and pattern of organ involvement in HC vary depending on the rate and magnitude of plasma iron overloading, which depend, in turn, on the underlying genetic mutation. This explains the presence of milder adult-onset forms (HFE- and TfR2-related) and more severe juvenile-onset forms (HJV- and HAMP-related). The main distinguishing features of HC are listed in Table 90.1.

The extent of iron release from enterocytes and macrophages into the bloodstream in humans is controlled by the hepcidin–ferroportin axis. **Hepcidin**, a defensin-like peptide produced by hepatocytes in response to iron and inflammatory stimuli, diffuses through the body, interacting with the iron-exporter ferroportin expressed on the surfaces of iron-rich macrophages

and intestinal cells. As a result of this interaction, ferroportin is internalized and degraded [18], and the unrequired iron is not absorbed through the intestine and remains in the macrophages, where it is stored for future needs (Figure 90.1a) This mechanism ensures the maintenance of circulating iron levels that meet the body's erythropoietic needs without posing an oxidative threat to the cells. HFE and TfR2 seem to convey the iron signal to hepcidin in the hepatocyte, although the details of this process are still unclear. Yet, the loss of either causes hepcidin insufficiency and HC in rodents and humans. But the most important hepcidin regulators are circulating **bone-morphogenic proteins (BMPs)**, particularly BMP6 [19,20], and the BMP co-receptor hemojuvelin (HJV) [21]. In fact, in humans, loss of functional HJV causes a dramatic decrease in hepcidin expression and severe juvenile HC associated with massive iron overload [6].

In view of these findings, HC should be seen as a genetically heterogeneous disease that results from the complex interaction between genetic and acquired factors. If the altered gene plays a dominant role in hepcidin synthesis (e.g., *HAMP* itself or *HJV*), circulatory iron overload occurs rapidly and reaches high levels (Figure 90.1d). In these cases, the modifying effects of acquired environmental and lifestyle factors will be negligible, and the clinical presentation will invariably be dramatic, with early onset (first to second decade) of a full-blown organ disease. In contrast, C282Y *HFE* homozygosity results in a genetic predisposition that requires the co-occurrence of host-related or environmental factors to produce disease (Figure 90.1b). Co-inherited mutations in other HC genes, such as *HAMP* and *HJV*, may have a role in disease penetrance of HFE-HC, but they are rare. In general, the modifier effect of iron genes has been documented in mice, but not fully confirmed in humans. Debate continues over the roles of fatty liver, high body mass index, and polymorphic changes in oxidative stress-related genes, but there is evidence for a strong association between alcohol and development of HC-related cirrhosis [22]. Data from a few longitudinal studies on HC suggest that up to 38–50% of C282Y homozygotes may develop iron overload, with up to 10–33% eventually developing HC-associated morbidity. The proportion of C282Y homozygous subjects with iron-overload–related disease is substantially higher in men than in women (28% vs 1%) [23].

Iron deposits in HC, as assessed by Perl's stain, typically involve parenchymal cells and spare Kupffer cells until late in the disease (Figure 90.2). Iron usually accumulates as fine granules predominantly at the biliary pole of cells. It is distributed throughout the lobule with a decreasing gradient from periportal to centrolobular areas. Mesenchymal iron deposits may be found, but at a later stage when hepatocytic iron is high enough to induce cell necrosis. Predominant iron deposition in non-parenchymal cells of the liver in adults, in the absence of appreciable liver disease, is typical of **ferroportin disease**, due to pathogenic mutations of *FPN*, and is characterized by iron retention in macrophages, high SF levels, and low–normal TS [16].

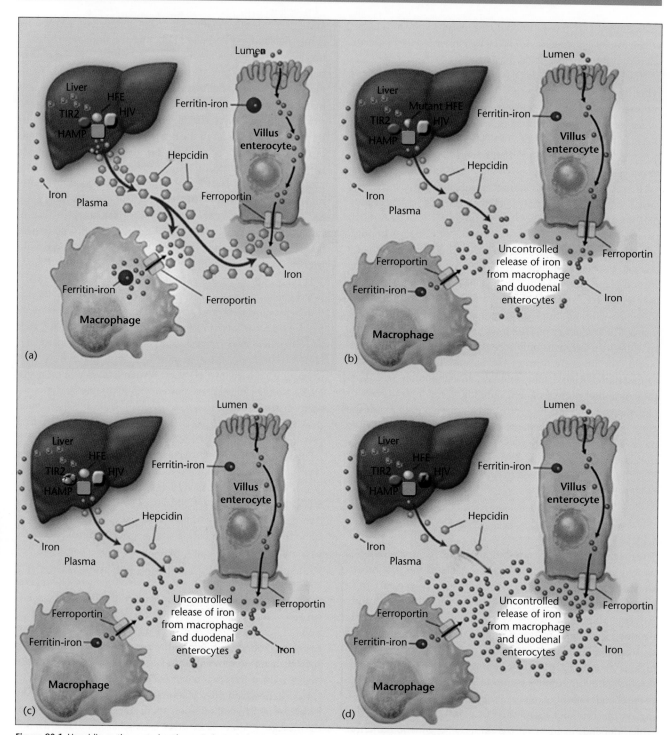

Figure 90.1 Hepcidin as the central pathogenic factor in hemochromatosis. (a) In normal subjects, hepcidin secreted by the liver modulates the extent and rate of iron release from macrophages and enterocytes. HFE, TfR2, and HJV are likely required for hepcidin activation in response to the circulatory iron signal. Lack of one of the hepcidin regulators will lead to unrestricted release of iron from macrophages and enterocytes followed by progressive expansion of the plasma iron pool, tissue iron overload, and organ damage (see text for details). Depending on the role of the regulators in the control of hepcidin expression, the extent of circulatory iron overload will be marginal [(b) HFE-HC or (c) TfR2-HC] or massive [(d) HJV-HC]. This will lead to milder (HFE- or TR2-associated) or more severe forms (HJV- or HAMP-associated) of hemochromatosis.

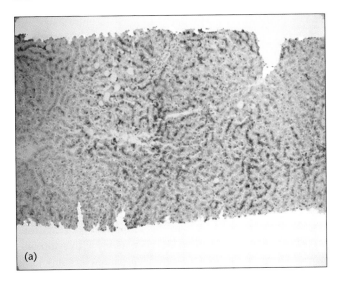

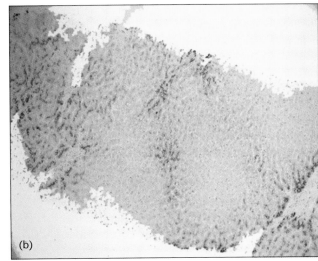

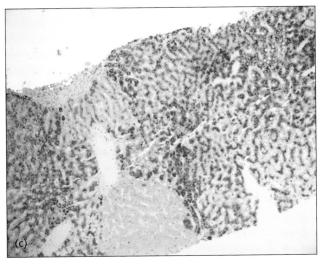

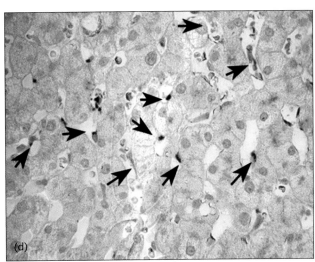

Figure 90.2 Histopathological slides from patients with hemocromatosis (HC) (Perls' Prussian blue stain for iron). (a) Patient with HFE-HC presenting with pure parenchymal iron overload and portocentral iron gradient. (b) Patient with TfR2-HC: the histopathological picture is identical to HFE-HC with iron accumulation in periportal parenchymal cells. (c) Patient with HJV-HC with massive parenchymal iron overload. (d) Patient with classic ferroportin disease presenting with predominant Kupffer cell iron overload (arrows).

Clinical presentation

In HFE-HC, the clinical presentation, usually in mid-life, varies from simple biochemical abnormalities to severe organ damage and disease [17]. **Elevated liver enzymes** are present in 30% of C282Y homozygote males; **liver fibrosis** in 18% of males and 5% of females; and **cirrhosis** in 6% of males and 2% of females [24]. HC associated with *TfR2* mutations usually presents at earlier stages and with a more severe phenotype than HFE-HC. It is important to recall that, variations notwithstanding, all of these mutations cause the same syndrome, the targets of iron toxicity are identical (i.e., liver, heart, endocrine glands, joints), and the pathogenic basis of all forms is hepcidin deficiency. Uncharacteristically severe or earlier-onset disease in patients with mutations of an "adult-onset gene" (e.g., *HFE*) might be the result of undetected additional mutations in other HC genes. The variety of genotypes that can produce an HC phenotype highlights the importance of defining and classifying this disease as a unique clinicopathological entity.

HC should be suspected in middle-aged men presenting with unexplained cirrhosis, bronzed skin, diabetes, and other endocrine deficiencies, or joint inflammation and heart disease. However, this classical presentation is rare. Today diagnosis is made at earlier stages as a result of screening and enhanced case detection due to greater clinician awareness and a higher index of suspicion. The most common presenting symptoms are now **fatigue, malaise, and arthralgia**, while **hepatomegaly** is one of the earliest physical signs. Elevated TS, which precedes increased SF levels, and moderately increased aminotransferase levels are common biochemical abnormalities. Increasing SF levels herald iron accumulation in tissues, and values above 1000 µg/L may indicate underlying liver fibrosis in HFE-HC, even with normal aminotransferase levels [25].

Liver Disease

The presence of cirrhosis places patients at an increased risk for hepatocellular carcinoma.

In individuals with **juvenile forms of HC**, the heart and endocrine glands, which are more susceptible to iron toxicity, succumb to its effects earlier, and their failure will dominate the clinical picture. They usually present with hypogonadism, which is inevitably found in those aged 20 years or over. Cardiomyopathy and endocrine disorders, including diabetes, appear earlier than they do in adult-onset forms. This is probably due to the fact that the circulatory iron overload develops much more rapidly and reaches much higher levels (reflecting the more severe hepcidin deficiency associated with mutation of the "juvenile-onset" genes).

Differential diagnosis

The hallmark of HC is circulatory and parenchymal cell **iron overload**. Hyperferritinemia, a surrogate marker for iron excess in tissues, is a common finding also in other conditions, unrelated to iron overload or HC: chronic alcohol consumption, inflammation, cell necrosis, and metabolic abnormalities, such as non-alcoholic fatty liver disease or diabetes. Therefore, in the presence of an abnormal SF, the diagnosis of HC requires the co-existence of increased TS and C282Y homozygosity, or the presence of tissue iron overload and pathogenic mutations of other HC genes.

In patients with hepatic iron deposition at liver biopsy, further diagnostic considerations depend on the cellular and lobular distribution of iron and on the presence or absence of associated lesions, including fibrosis, steatosis and steatohepatitis, abnormal crystal inclusions, and chronic hepatitis. In patients with pure hepatocellular iron overload, the two main differential diagnoses are **end-stage cirrhosis**, in which iron distribution is heterogeneous from one nodule to another, without iron deposition in fibrous tissue or in biliary and vascular walls, and **compensated iron-loading anemia** with inefficient erythropoiesis.

Diagnostic methods

In patients with signs and symptoms and/or organ disease suggestive of HC, the diagnosis is based on the presence of **C282Y homozygosity and iron overload**. Untreated C282Y homozygotes with cirrhosis, diabetes, or cardiomyopathy invariably have abnormal TS rates and SF levels. Prior to the identification of *HFE*, evaluation of the hepatic iron content and distribution by liver biopsy was the method of choice for diagnosing HC. Today the demonstration of C282Y homozygosity in a subject with high TS and SF levels is sufficient for diagnosis, even without a liver biopsy [17]. However, in C282Y homozygotes (particularly those over 40 years), SF levels above $1000 \mu g/L$, together with increased aminotransferases and hepatomegaly, may be an indication for liver biopsy to rule out hepatic fibrosis or cirrhosis, [25–27]. Liver iron content can also be assessed non-invasively by magnetic resonance imaging (MRI) over a wide range of iron concentrations. Considering the higher prevalence of C282Y homozygosity and higher phenotypic penetrance in family members, biochemical testing should be done in first-degree relatives, particularly siblings, in whom *HFE* testing should also be considered.

Symptomatic subjects with clear signs of circulatory and tissue iron overload but negative *HFE* gene testing may carry pathogenic mutations in other HC genes. Genetic testing for non–HFE-HC is complex and is not widely available. An alternative approach for diagnosis in these cases is based on biopsy demonstration of a hemochromatosis pattern of hepatic iron load [17].

A practical diagnostic work-up for HC includes the following simple steps (refer also to the accompanying diagnostic work-up protocol on the website). In patients with symptoms or signs suggestive of HC, **serum iron parameters** should be determined. If symptoms are related to HC or iron overload, increased TS and SF levels should be present. However, in patients presenting with increased SF concentrations, it is mandatory to search first for common causes of hyperferritinemia, as described above, before genetic tests are carried out. In the absence of such conditions or when hyperferritinemia persists despite treatment of the underlying cause, TS should be determined. After confirmation of TS elevation, **HFE gene testing** should be ordered. If the patient is a C282Y homozygote, the diagnosis of HFE-HC can be established. In all other genotypes, compensated iron-loading anemia or non–HFE-HC should be considered (genetic testing for mutations in *HJV*, *HAMP*, and *TfR2*, or rare *HFE* mutations, depending on clinical presentation). Patients with compound heterozygosity for C282Y and H63D usually present with mild iron overload, which is associated with co-morbid factors, such as obesity, chronic alcohol consumption, and end-stage cirrhosis. If TS is either normal or low, the presence or absence of iron overload will guide further diagnostic work-up. Assessment of liver iron stores by direct means (i.e., MRI or liver biopsy) is recommended. If liver iron concentration is increased, iron overload related to alcohol consumption or to metabolic abnormalities should be considered before genetic testing for non-HFE hereditary iron overload diseases is carried out (ferroportin disease, aceruloplasminemia). If liver iron concentration is normal, the common causes of hyperferritinemia should be reconsidered before genetic testing for *L-ferritin* gene mutations (to investigate for hyperferritinemia–cataract syndrome) is carried out. In patients with an unclear presentation, family members should be evaluated for evidence of iron overload and/or the exact amount of iron removed by phlebotomy should be calculated before rare genetic disorders are considered and tested for by candidate gene sequencing and linkage analysis.

Treatment and prevention

Phlebotomy is the standard treatment of all forms of HC (refer to the accompanying management protocol on the website). One unit (400–500 mL) of blood contains approximately

200–250 mg of iron. There are no studies that provide evidence for the protocol of therapeutic venesection (i.e., optimal time to start venesection, frequency, end-point). Current recommendations of when to initiate treatment are empirical. Weekly phlebotomy can restore safe blood levels of iron (reflected by SF levels of <20–50 μg/L and TS <30%) within 1–2 years. Maintenance therapy, which typically involves removal of 2–4 units/year, must then be continued to keep SF normal. Despite its non-specificity, SF should always be monitored during phlebotomy.

Survival of treated patients without cirrhosis and diabetes has been found to be equivalent to that of the normal population, whereas those with these complications have a significantly reduced survival [28,29]. These data emphasize the importance of early initiation of iron removal. The threshold SF level is currently chosen as above the normal range. The goal of blood-letting during the iron-depletion stage is generally the induction of a mildly iron-deficient state, but less aggressive regimens might actually be more beneficial. Excessive iron depletion could conceivably have negative rebound effects since anemia/hypoxia is a major suppressor of hepcidin synthesis. If phlebotomy is contraindicated or poorly tolerated, other strategies can be considered, such as the use of iron chelators. Phlebotomy has been associated with improvement of biopsy-proven liver fibrosis in 13–50% of treated patients, particularly those with the mildest fibrosis at baseline [24,28,30].

Prognosis with and without treatment

Phlebotomy is generally regarded as a safe and effective means of removing iron from tissues and preventing complications, although this idea has never been validated in controlled studies, for obvious ethical reasons. There are no studies addressing survival in genotyped C282Y homozygous HC patients. The benefit of phlebotomy has been demonstrated in case series of clinically diagnosed HC compared with historical groups of patients not so treated or inadequately treated. Five-year survival was 93% in adequately phlebotomized patients, compared with 48% in those inadequately phlebotomized (10-year survival 78% vs 32%, respectively) [29]. Based on a number of studies, it is believed that fatigue, elevated aminotransferases, skin pigmentation, and hepatic fibrosis improve after phlebotomy. It is recognized, however, that several clinical features are unlikely to improve with iron depletion, in particular arthralgia. Hypogonadism, cirrhosis, destructive arthritis, and insulin-dependent diabetes associated with HC are usually irreversible, but phlebotomy may improve certain aspects of these diseases (e.g., daily insulin requirements, elevated aminotransferase levels, weakness, lethargy, abdominal pain). End-stage liver disease or hepatocellular carcinoma secondary to HC is frequently treated by orthotopic liver transplantation, but survival after liver transplantation might be expected to be reduced when compared to non–iron-loaded patients [31].

What to tell patients

An important message to relay to patients with HC is that the disease is **curable** and that survival is no different from that of controls if the disease is treated prior to the development of complications, particularly cirrhosis. Treatment is highly effective, relatively easy, and devoid of significant side effects. Substantial changes in lifestyle are not necessary. Dietary changes are not usually necessary if an adequate phlebotomy treatment is implemented.

Measures must be put in place to avoid discrimination of patients with HC. In accordance with legal regulations in most countries, genetic testing for HFE-HC should only be carried out after informed consent has been obtained and the results should be made available only to the patient and physicians involved in the management of HFE-HC. Regulations for the use of blood obtained from venesection, fee exemptions, and reimbursement policies for *HFE* genetic testing vary around the world and even within countries. Blood taken from patients with HC at phlebotomy should be made available for national blood transfusion services for the public good, if there is no medical contraindication and the patient has given consent. It is recognized that many patients with HFE hemochromatosis will have clinical features that exclude them from being accepted as donors (raised liver function tests, diabetes, medications). However, in the absence of these, there appears to be no reason, other than administrative and bureaucratic, why the blood removed may not be used.

> **SOURCES OF INFORMATION FOR PATIENTS AND DOCTORS**
>
> Former national scientific organizations of physicians and scientists involved in the cure and study of HC have now merged into the International Bioiron Society
> http://www.bioiron.org/default.aspx
>   A number of HC patient organizations have been established around the world. Their website may provide additional information on HC that may be informative for patients
> Europe : http://www.european-haemochromatosis.eu/4596/
>   index.html
> USA: http://www.americanhs.org/about.htm and http://
>   www.hemochromatosis.org/index.asp
> Canada: http://www.cdnhemochromatosis.ca/index.php
> Australia: http://www.haemochromatosis.org.au/index.htm

References

1. von Recklinghausen FD. Uber Haemochromatose. Taggeblatt der (62) *Versammlung deutscher Naturforscher and Aerzte in Heidelberg.* 1889:324–325.
2. Sheldon J. *Haemochromatosis.* London: Oxford University Press, 1935.
3. Simon M, Pawlotsky Y, Bourel M, Fauchet R, Genetet B. [Letter: Idiopathic hemochromatosis associated with HL-A 3 tissular antigen]. *Nouv Presse Med.* 1975;4:1432.

Liver Disease

4. Camaschella C, Roetto A, Cali A, *et al.* The gene TFR2 is mutated in a new type of haemochromatosis mapping to 7q22. *Nat Genet.* 2000;25:14–15.

5. Roetto A, Papanikolaou G, Politou M, *et al.* Mutant antimicrobial peptide hepcidin is associated with severe juvenile hemochromatosis. *Nat Genet.* 2003;33:21–22.

6. Papanikolaou G, Samuels ME, Ludwig EH, *et al.* Mutations in HFE2 cause iron overload in chromosome 1q-linked juvenile hemochromatosis. *Nat Genet.* 2004;36:77–82.

7. Pietrangelo A, Montosi G, Totaro A, *et al.* Hereditary hemochromatosis in adults without pathogenic mutations in the hemochromatosis gene [see comments]. *N Engl J Med.* 1999;341: 725–732.

8. Montosi G, Donovan A, Totaro A, *et al.* Autosomal-dominant hemochromatosis is associated with a mutation in the ferroportin (SLC11A3) gene. *J Clin Invest.* 2001;108:619–123.

9. Pietrangelo A. Hemochromatosis: an endocrine liver disease. *Hepatology.* 2007;46:1291–1301.

10. Merryweatherclarke AT, Pointon JJ, Shearman JD, Robson KJH. Global prevalence of putative haemochromatosis mutations. *J Med Genet.* 1997;34:275–278.

11. Adams PC, Reboussin DM, Barton JC, *et al.* Hemochromatosis and iron-overload screening in a racially diverse population. *N Engl J Med.* 2005;352:1769–1778.

12. Gochee PA, Powell LW, Cullen DJ, Du Sart D, Rossi E, Olynyk JK. A population-based study of the biochemical and clinical expression of the H63D hemochromatosis mutation. *Gastroenterology.* 2002;122:646–651.

13. Walsh A, Dixon JL, Ramm GA, *et al.* The clinical relevance of compound heterozygosity for the C282Y and H63D substitutions in hemochromatosis. *Clin Gastroenterol Hepatol.* 2006;4: 1403–1410.

14. Rossi E, Olynyk JK, Cullen DJ, *et al.* Compound heterozygous hemochromatosis genotype predicts increased iron and erythrocyte indices in women. *Clin Chem.* 2000;46:162–166.

15. Lim EM, Rossi E, De Boer WB, Reed WD, Jeffrey GP. Hepatic iron loading in patients with compound heterozygous HFE mutations. *Liver Int.* 2004;24:631–636.

16. Pietrangelo A. The ferroportin disease. *Blood Cells Mol Dis.* 2004;32:131–138.

17. Pietrangelo A. Hereditary hemochromatosis – a new look at an old disease. *N Engl J Med.* 2004;350:2383–2397.

18. Nemeth E, Tuttle MS, Powelson J, *et al.* Hepcidin regulates cellular iron efflux by binding to ferroportin and inducing its internalization. *Science.* 2004;306:2090–2093.

19. Andriopoulos B Jr, Corradini E, Xia Y, *et al.* BMP6 is a key endogenous regulator of hepcidin expression and iron metabolism. *Nat Genet.* 2009;41:482–487.

20. Meynard D, Kautz L, Darnaud V, Canonne-Hergaux F, Coppin H, Roth MP. Lack of the bone morphogenetic protein BMP6 induces massive iron overload. *Nat Genet.* 2009;41:478–481.

21. Babitt JL, Huang FW, Wrighting DM, *et al.* Bone morphogenetic protein signaling by hemojuvelin regulates hepcidin expression. *Nat Genet.* 2006;38:531–539.

22. Fletcher LM, Dixon JL, Purdie DM, Powell LW, Crawford DH. Excess alcohol greatly increases the prevalence of cirrhosis in hereditary hemochromatosis. *Gastroenterology.* 2002;122:281–289.

23. Allen KJ, Gurrin LC, Constantine CC, *et al.* Iron-overload-related disease in HFE hereditary hemochromatosis. *N Engl J Med.* 2008; 358:221–230.

24. Powell LW, Dixon JL, Ramm GA, *et al.* Screening for hemochromatosis in asymptomatic subjects with or without a family history. *Arch Intern Med.* 2006;166:294–301.

25. Guyader D, Jacquelinet C, Moirand R, *et al.* Noninvasive prediction of fibrosis in C282Y homozygous hemochromatosis. *Gastroenterology.* 1998;115:929–936.

26. Beaton M, Guyader D, Deugnier Y, Moirand R, Chakrabarti S, Adams P. Noninvasive prediction of cirrhosis in C282Y-linked hemochromatosis. *Hepatology.* 2002;36:673–678.

27. Morrison ED, Brandhagen DJ, Phatak PD, *et al.* Serum ferritin level predicts advanced hepatic fibrosis among U.S. patients with phenotypic hemochromatosis. *Ann Intern Med.* 2003;138: 627–633.

28. Niederau C, Fischer R, Purschel A, Stremmel W, Haussinger D, Strohmeyer G. Long-term survival in patients with hereditary hemochromatosis [see comments]. *Gastroenterology.* 1996;110: 1107–1119.

29. Milman N, Pedersen P, Steig T, Byg KE, Graudal N, Fenger K. Clinically overt hereditary hemochromatosis in Denmark 1948–1985: epidemiology, factors of significance for long-term survival, and causes of death in 179 patients. *Ann Hematol.* 2001;80:737–744.

30. Falize L, Guillygomarc'h A, Perrin M, *et al.* Reversibility of hepatic fibrosis in treated genetic hemochromatosis: a study of 36 cases. *Hepatology.* 2006;44:472–477.

31. Brandhagen DJ, Alvarez W, Therneau TM, *et al.* Iron overload in cirrhosis-HFE genotypes and outcome after liver transplantation. *Hepatology.* 2000;31:456–460.

CHAPTER 91

Alpha-1-antitrypsin deficiency

Feras T. Alissa and David H. Perlmutter

University of Pittsburgh School of Medicine, Children's Hospital of Pittsburgh of UPMC, Pittsburgh, PA, USA

ESSENTIAL FACTS ABOUT PATHOGENESIS

- Point mutation leads to altered folding of hepatic secretory glycoprotein and renders the protein prone to aggregation
- Accumulation of aggregated protein in ER causes liver inflammation and carcinogenesis by gain of toxic function
- Only 8–10% of affected homozygotes develop liver disease, presumably determined by genetic and/or environmental modifiers

ESSENTIALS OF DIAGNOSIS

- Serum levels of α_1-AT ~10–15% of normal levels
- Altered migration of α_1-AT in isoelectric focusing gels (PIZZ)
- Periodic acid–Schiff-positive globules in hepatocytes by liver biopsy

ESSENTIALS OF TREATMENT

- Guidance on avoidance of smoking
- Supportive measures for complications of chronic liver disease
- Liver transplantation only if liver disease is progressive
- Protein replacement therapy is not appropriate for liver disease

Introduction and epidemiology

α_1-AT deficiency was first described in 1963 in adult patients with emphysema. The association with liver disease in children was later reported in an infant with neonatal liver disease [1]. α_1-AT deficiency primarily affects Caucasians of European descent, but it also has a worldwide distribution involving all ethnic groups. The incidence has been reported as 1 in 1600 to 1 in 2000 live births in many populations [2]. This deficiency is the most common genetic cause of liver disease in children. It also causes chronic hepatitis, cirrhosis and hepatocellular carcinoma in adolescents and adults, and is the most frequent genetic diagnosis in children requiring liver transplantation.

A unique genetic epidemiology study in which every newborn in Sweden was screened for α_1-AT deficiency was carried out by Sveger in 1972–1974. The vast majority of the cohort have been successfully followed from birth to 30 years of age [3,4]; only 8% of the population developed significant liver disease, indicating that genetic and/or environmental modifiers determine whether a deficient individual is susceptible to, or protected from, liver disease.

α_1-AT is a hepatic secretory glycoprotein. Its major physiologic function is inhibition of neutrophil elastase. It is encoded by a highly pleomorphic gene with more than 100 variant alleles identified [2]. These alleles are characterized by the mobility of α_1-AT in serum in isoelectric focusing gel electrophoresis and this is used to classify each into what is termed a PI type. The vast majority of these are not associated with a significant change in serum levels of α_1-AT or clinical effects (normal variants) (Table 91.1). A few are associated with decreased serum levels of α_1-AT (deficiency variants) (Table 91.2). Some of the deficiency variants are associated with clinical effects. The Z variant, which causes the classical form of the α_1-AT deficiency when homozygous, is an example. Some deficiency variants are not, by themselves, associated with clinical effects, such as the S variant. Because the deficiency variants that are not associated with clinical disease have serum α_1-AT levels between 40% and 100% of normal, it has been said that the serum α_1-AT level must go below 40% of normal to be associated with disease. There are also a number of so-called null variants in which α_1-AT cannot be detected in the serum (Table 91.3). These are all quite rare and in each case associated with emphysema/chronic obstructive lung disease.

Causes and pathogenesis

A point mutation leads to altered folding of the hepatic secretory glycoprotein. The mutant protein, α_1-AT Z, is for the most part retained in the endoplasmic reticulum (ER) of liver cells rather than secreted into the blood. Furthermore, the mutant protein tends to polymerize and aggregate in the ER. Accumulation of aggregated α_1-AT Z in the ER causes liver inflammation and carcinogenesis by a gain-of-toxic function mechanism. It is not known exactly how this gain-of-toxic function mechanism leads to liver damage but mitochondrial dysfunction is likely to be the final common pathway [5]. The Swedish newborn study has shown that only ~8% of the homozygotes develop clinically significant liver disease and implies that the susceptibility of this sub-population is due to genetic and/or environmental modifiers. We have theorized that these modifiers may affect intracellular disposal of the mutant aggregation-prone protein or the cell signaling pathways that protect the

Textbook of Clinical Gastroenterology and Hepatology, Second Edition. Edited by C. J. Hawkey, Jaime Bosch, Joel E. Richter, Guadalupe Garcia-Tsao, Francis K. L. Chan.
© 2012 Blackwell Publishing Ltd. Published 2012 by Blackwell Publishing Ltd.

Liver Disease

Table 91.1 Normal variants of α_1-antitrypsin

M1	E-Lemberg
M2	E-Tokyo
M3	E-Tripoli
M4	F
M5	Kalsheker-Poller
M2-Obernburg	L-Offenbach
M3-Rieudenburg	N-Adelaide
M5-Berlin	N-Grossoeuvre
M5-Karlsruhe	N-Hampton
M5-Gunma	N-Le Trait
M6-Bonn	N-Nagato
M6-Passau	N-Yerville
B	P-Budapest
E-Cincinnati	P-Clifton
E-Franklin	P-Donauwoerth
P-Oki	W-Finneytown
P-Saint Albans	W-San
P-Saint Louis	X
P-Yanago	X-Alban
R	X-Christchurch
S-Munich	Y-Toronto
T	Z-Pratt
V-Munich	—

Reproduced with permission from: http://www.goldenhelix.org/a1atvar

Table 91.2 Deficiency variants of α_1-antitrypsin

Allele	Defect		Clinical disease	
			Liver	Lung
Z	Single base substitution M_1 (Ala 213)	Glu 342–Lys	+	+
S	Single base substitution	Glu 264–Val	−	−
M$_{Heerlen}$	Single base substitution	Pro 369–Leu	−	+
M$_{Procida}$	Single base substitution	Leu 41–Pro	−	+
M$_{Malton}$	Single base deletion	Phe 52	?	+
M$_{Duarte}$	Unknown	Unknown	?	+
M$_{Mineral\ Springs}$	Single base substitution	Gly 57–Glu	−	+
S$_{Iiyama}$	Single base substitution	Ser 53–Phe	−	+
P$_{Duarte}$	Two base substitution	Arg 101–His Asp 265–Val	?	+
P$_{Lowell}$	Single base substitution	Asp 265–Val	−	+
W$_{Bethesda}$	Single base substitution	Ala 336–Thre	−	+
Z$_{Wrexham}$	—	Ser 19–Leu	?	?
F	Single base substitution	Arg 223–Cys	−	−
T	Single base substitution	Glu 264–Val	−	−
I	Single base substitution	Arg 39–Cys	−	−
M$_{palermo}$	Single base deletion	Phe 51	−	−
M$_{nichinan}$	Single base deletion and single base substitution	Phe 52 Gl 148–Arg	−	−
Zasburg	Single base substitution	Gly 342–Lys	−	−

cell from the effects of protein aggregation [6]. Recent studies have implicated single nucleotide polymorphisms (SNPs) as potential modifiers of liver disease in α_1-AT deficiency [7,8]. A SNP in the downstream flanking region of ER mannosidase I, a component of intracellular disposal pathways, was implicated in early-onset liver disease [8]. In another case a SNP in the upstream flanking region of the α_1-AT gene was implicated [7]. However, control groups that would make the case that these SNPs are truly modifiers were not included in the studies.

Destructive lung disease/emphysema is caused by a loss-of-function mechanism in which the lack of α_1-AT allows neutrophil elastase to destroy the connective tissue matrix of the lung [9]. The development of lung disease is also determined to a certain extent by modifiers. Indeed, cigarette smoking increases the severity of lung disease . However, even when exacerbated by smoking, emphysema does not first appear until the third decade of life at its earliest.

Table 91.3 Null variants of α_1-antitrypsin

Allele	Defect		Clinical disease	
			Liver	Lung
Null$_{Granite\ Falls}$	Single base deletion	Tyr 160	–	+
Null$_{Bellingham}$	Single base deletion	Lys 217	–	+
Null$_{Mattawa}$	Single base deletion	Phe 353	–	+
Null$_{Hong\ Kong}$	Dinucleotide deletion	Leu 318	–	+
Null$_{Ludwigshafen}$	Single base substitution	Isoleu 92–Asp	–	+
Null$_{Clayton}$	Single base insertion	Glu 363	–	+
Null$_{Bolton}$	Single base deletion	Glu 363	–	+
Null$_{Isola\ di\ Procida}$	Deletion	Exon II–V	–	+
Null$_{Reidenburg}$	Deletion	Exon II–V	–	+
Null$_{Newport}$	Single base substitution	Gly 115–Ser	–	+
Null$_{bonny\ blue}$	Intron deletion	—	–	+
Null$_{new\ hope}$	Two base substitution	Gly 320–Glu Glu 342–Lys	–	+
Null$_{Trastavere}$	Single base substitution	Trp 194–stop	–	+
Null$_{Kowloon}$	Single base substitution	Tyr 38–stop	–	+
Null$_{Saabruecken}$	Single base insertion	Pro 362–stop	–	+
Null$_{Lisbon}$	Single base substitution	Thr 68–Ile	–	+
Null$_{West}$	Intron deletion	—	–	+

Table 91.4 Clinical features of liver disease associated with α_1-antitrypsin deficiency

Infants
  Prolonged jaundice
  Neonatal hepatitis syndrome
  Neonatal cholestasis

Children/adolescents
  Mild elevation of transaminase levels
  Portal hypertension
  Asymptomatic hepatomegaly
  Severe liver dysfunction

Adults
  Chronic hepatitis
  Cryptognic cirrhosis
  Hepatocellular carcinoma

Table 91.5 Differential diagnosis of α_1-antitrypsin deficiency

Infants
  Extrahepatic biliary atresia
  Alagille syndrome
  Cystic fibrosis
  Choledochal cyst
  Galactosemia
  Tyrosinemia
  Neonatal giant cell hepatitis
  Progressive familial intrahepatic cholestasis
  TORCH infection

Children/adolescents
  Autoimmune hepatitis
  Wilson disease
  Infectious hepatits
  Toxic hepatitis

Adults
  Wilson disease
  Autoimmune hepatitis
  Hepatocellular carcinoma
  Hemochromatosis
  Cryptogenic cirrhosis
  Nonalcoholic steatohepatitis

Clinical presentation

Liver disease is most commonly seen in children. Symptoms begin within the first 2 months, but it can start later during childhood, adolescence or even adulthood. Infants usually present with jaundice, acholic stools, dark urine and/or pruritus. A tendency to bleeding, involving the gastrointestinal tract, umbilical stump, bruising or, less likely, intracranial bleeding, may occur due to a deficiency of vitamin K. During late childhood or adolescence, affected individuals may present with signs and symptoms of advanced liver disease such as hepatomegaly, splenomegaly, ascites, or gastrointestinal bleeding from esophageal varices. Some patients might have a history of unexplained prolonged neonatal cholestasis while others have no evidence of previous liver injury (Table 91.4).

On physical examination, these patients have scleral icterus, enlarged liver and spleen. PIZZ infants tend to be small for gestational age and might have difficulty in gaining weight. Ascites indicates advanced liver disease.

α_1-AT deficiency should be considered in the differential diagnosis of any adult patient with chronic hepatitis, cirrhosis, portal hypertension and/or hepatocellular carcinoma of unknown origin (Table 91.5). PIZZ individuals are also at increased risk of cholangiocarcinoma The risk of these

Liver Disease

malignancies is well beyond the risk associated with cirrhosis alone [10,11].

It is not yet clear that heterozygosity for the Z variant causes liver disease by itself. All of the studies that have attempted to address this issue have been biased in ascertainment. The SZ variant is the only compound heterozygous state that has been associated with liver disease and it appears to be almost identical to the homozygous ZZ state [4]. This may relate to the observation that the S variant has a slight proclivity towards aggregation [12,13]. Several other rare deficiency variants that have aggregation-prone properties have been associated with liver disease (Table 91.2).

Although homozygous PIZZ α_1-AT deficiency is considered the most common genetic cause for emphysema, it is found in only 1–2% of patients with emphysema [9]. Pulmonary symptoms start by the third or fourth decades with cough, dyspnea, and expectoration. The disease is usually progressive, and ultimately leads to respiratory insufficiency. Cigarette smoking accelerates lung damage, worsens symptoms and reduces median survival by more than 20 years. Chronic obstructive pulmonary disease is also seen in patients with null α_1-AT variants and in many of these cases the onset of symptoms is earlier and more severe than in the classical ZZ homozygotes. Whether the heterozygous MZ state predisposes to emphysema is not known.

There is very limited data on hepatic involvement in patients who are diagnosed with emphysema. Several studies have demonstrated mildly elevated serum transaminases in some patients with emphysema [14]. The cohort of patients identified by the Swedish nationwide screening study has not demonstrated emphysema in patients with liver disease, at least up to the age of 30 years [4].

Other clinical manifestations

A number of inflammatory diseases have been described in patients with α_1-AT deficiency, including necrotizing panniculitis, Wegner's granulomatosis, membranoproliferative glomerulonephritis, IgA nephropathy and a variety of other vasculitis syndromes. However, all of these come from studies with inherent bias and have never been subjected to controlled population studies. None of these disorders has been detected in the affected homozygotes identified in the unbiased Swedish cohort [4].

Differential diagnosis

α_1-AT deficiency should be considered in any patient with abnormal liver tests, signs and symptoms of portal hypertension, cholestasis or prolonged prothrombin time. Differential diagnoses according to the patient's age are listed in Table 91.5.

Diagnostic investigation

Serum levels of α_1-AT and PI type by isoelectric focusing gel electrophoresis (Figure 91.1) should be determined in patients

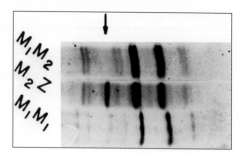

Figure 91.1 Isoelectric focusing of serum. The more rapidly migrating Z allele is indicated by the arrow. (Reproduced with permission from: Perlmutter D.H. (1996) α_1-Antitrypsin deficiency, in *Consultations in Gastroenterology* (ed. W.J. Snape), WB Saunders, Philadelphia, pp. 791–802, Copyright Elsevier 1996).

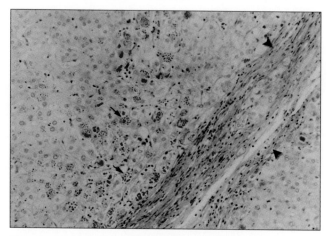

Figure 91.2 Liver biopsy from a PIZZ individual. Arrows point to hepatocytes with typical PAS-positive, diastase-resistant globules and arrowheads to a band of fibrosis. (Reproduced with permission from: Perlmutter D.H. (1996) α_1-Antitrypsin deficiency, in *Consultations in Gastroenterology* (ed. W.J. Snape), WB Saunders, Philadelphia, pp. 791–802, Copyright Elsevier 1996).

suspected of α_1-AT deficiency. Affected patients will have serum levels that are 10–15% of the normal range (85–215 mg/dl). α_1-AT is an acute phase reactant and may thereby be transiently upregulated during inflammation, infection, and pregnancy. This might provide false reassurance in some heterozygous individuals. However, in PIZZ homozygous individual levels rarely reach values that obscure the deficiency state.

Liver biopsy can provide information about the degree of liver injury and dysplasia but is not needed for the specific diagnosis. Hepatic histological changes can include giant cell hepatitis, mild hepatitis with mixed inflammatory cell infiltrate, bile plugs, hepatocellular necrosis, paucity of bile ducts, variable degrees of bile duct proliferation, fibrosis or cirrhosis. The presence of periodic acid–Schiff-positive, diastase resistant globules in the ER of hepatocytes (Figure 91.2), which represent retained mutant α_1-ATZ, is the histological hallmark of the disease but can occasionally be seen in other liver pathological conditions.

Treatment and prevention

The only effective treatment option for severe α_1-AT deficiency-associated liver disease is liver transplantation, which is indicated for patients with end-stage liver failure. In patients with slowly progressing liver involvement, supportive medical management can prevent complications.

Although patients with this deficiency are being treated with ursodeoxycholic acid to prevent the consequences of bile stasis and vitamin E to prevent oxidative stress, there is no evidence for efficacy of either of these strategies. Several drugs have reduced liver injury in experimental mouse models including pharmacological chaperones such as 4-phenylbutyric acid that facilitate the movement of mutant α_1-AT through the secretory pathway [15] and drugs that inhibit mitochondrial dysfunction such as cyclosporine A [5]. Gene therapy and hepatocyte transplantation strategies are under investigation.

The most important principle in managing patients with this deficiency is guidance about smoking, which is known to accelerate lung destruction in such patients, reduce quality of life and significantly shorten life span [7].

Replacement therapy with purified and recombinant plasma α_1-AT is designed for patients with established and progressive lung disease; it is not considered for patients with liver disease. It can be delivered by intravenous or inhalational routes with high safety profile and minimal side effects. Although biochemical efficacy of this therapy has been demonstrated, clinical efficacy is relatively minor [16]. This may reflect inherent problems in initiating this kind of strategy before irreversible structural changes have occurred. Lung transplantation in patients with severe disease has a 50% 5 year survival rate [17].

Complications and their management

Complications of liver disease associated with α_1-AT deficiency and their management are not different from that for other chronic liver diseases. In many cases the hepatic involvement progresses slowly but can rapidly deteriorate when an infection or other incidental illness occurs. There are numerous reports of bleeding in newborns who for some reason do not receive vitamin K injections after birth. Malnutrition is a relatively common problem in children with chronic liver disease. It results from many factors including fat malabsorption from cholestasis as well as inadequate caloric intake. Full nutritional assessment should be part of their routine care. Supplementation of the diet with fat-soluble vitamins and high caloric, high medium chain triglyceride formulas should be considered.

Prognosis with and without treatment

Characterization of the cohort identified in the Swedish nationwide screening study indicates that more than 90% of homozygotes escape clinical manifestations of liver disease [4]. Thus, it is important for the clinician to recognize that most α_1-AT -deficient individuals do not have clinical or biochemical evidence of liver disease. Others have mildly elevated liver enzymes but no other evidence of liver disease. In both cases liver disease may never develop. Even in homozygotes with evidence of liver synthetic dysfunction or portal hypertension, liver disease may progress slowly and be compatible with normal life, functioning for long periods of time [18]. In children or adults with progressive liver dysfunction, liver transplantation has led to good outcomes with 1-, 3-, and 5-year survival of 92%, 90%, and 90% respectively [19].

> **SOURCES OF INFORMATION FOR PATIENTS AND DOCTORS**
>
> - http://www.alpha1.org/
> - http://www.goldenhelix.org/a1atvar/
> - http://www.liverfoundation.org/education/info/alphaone/

References

1. Sharp H, Bridges R, Krivit W, *et al*. Cirrhosis associated with alpha-1-antitrypsin deficiency: a previously unrecognized inherited disorder. *J Lab Clin Med*. 1969;73:934–939.
2. Rudnick DA, Perlmutter DH. Alpha-1-Antitrypsin deficiency: A new paradigm for hepatocellular carcinoma in genetic liver disease. *Hepatology*. 2005;42:514–521.
3. Sveger T. Liver disease in alpha1-antitrypsin deficiency detected by screening of 200,000 infants. *N Engl J Med*. 1976;294:1316–1321.
4. Piitulainen E, Carlson J, Ohlsson K, *et al*. Alpha-1-antitrypsin deficiency in 26-year-old subjects: Lung, liver and protease/protease inhibitor studies. *Chest*. 2005;128:2076–2081.
5. Teckman JH, An J-K, Blomenkamp K, *et al*. Mitochondrial autophagy and injury in the liver in {alpha}1-antitrypsin deficiency. *Am J Physiol*. 2004;286:G851–862.
6. Perlmutter DH. Autophagic disposal of the aggregation-prone protein that causes liver inflammation and carcinogenesis in alpha-1-antitrypsin deficiency. *Cell Death Diff*. 2009;16:39–45.
7. Chappell S, Hadzic N, Stockley R, *et al*. A polymorphism of the alpha-1-antitrypsin genes represents a risk factor for liver disease. *Hepatology*. 2008;47:127–132.
8. Pan S, Huang L, McPherson J, *et al*. Single nucleotide polymorphism-mediated translational suppression of endoplasmic reticulum mannosidase I modifies the onset of end-stage liver disease in alpha-1-antitrypsin deficiency. *Hepatology*. 2009; 50:275–281.
9. Stoller JK, Aboussouan LS. Alpha-1-antitrypsin deficiency. *Lancet*. 2005;365:2225–2236.
10. Eriksson S, Carlson J, Velez R. Risk of cirrhosis and primary liver cancer in α1-antitrypsin deficiency. *N Engl J Med*. 1986;314: 736–739.
11. Zhou H, Fischer H-P. Liver carcinoma in PiZ alpha-1-antitrypsin deficiency. *Am J Surg Pathol*. 1998;22:742–748.
12. Teckman JH, Perlmutter DH. The endoplasmic reticulum degradation pathway for mutant secretory proteins α1-antitrypsin Z and S is distinct from that for an unassembled membrane protein. *J Biol Chem*. 1996;271:13215–13220.
13. Mahadeva R, Chang WS, Dafforn TR, *et al*. Heteropolymerization of S, I and Z alpha-1-antitrypsin and liver cirrhosis. *J Clin Invest*. 1999;103:999–1006.

14. Von Schonfeld JV, Breuer N, Zotz R, et al. Liver function in patients with pulmonary emphysema due to severe α1-antitrypsin deficiency (PIZZ). *Digestion*. 1996;57:165–169.

15. Burrows JAJ, Willis LK, Perlmutter DH. Chemical chaperones mediate increased secretion of mutant α1-antitrypsin Z: A potential pharmacological strategy for prevention of liver injury and emphysema in α1-AT deficiency. *Proc Natl Acad Sci USA* 2000;97:1796–1801.

16. α1-Antitrypsin Deficiency Registry Study Group. Survival and FEV1 decline in individuals with severe deficiency of α1-antitrypsin. *Am J Respir Crit Care Med*. 1998;158:49–59.

17. Cassivi SD, Meyers BF, Battafarano RJ, et al. Thirteen-year experience in lung transplantation for emphysema. *Ann Thorac Surg*. 2002;74:1663–1670.

18. Volpert D, Molleston J, Perlmutter D. Alpha1-antitrypsin deficiency-associated liver disease progresses slowly in some children. *J Pediatr Gastroenterol Nutr*. 2000;31:258–263.

19. Kemmer N, Kaiser T, Zacharias V, et al. Alpha-1-antitrypsin deficiency: outcomes after liver transplantation. *Transplant Proc*. 2008;40:1492–1494.

CHAPTER 92

Wilson disease

Peter Ferenci

Medical University of Vienna, Vienna, Austria

ESSENTIAL FACTS ABOUT PATHOGENESIS

- Incidence: 10–30 per million persons/year
- May present at any age
- Pathogenesis: autosomal recessive inherited disorder of biliary copper excretion (mutation of *ATP7B*) resulting in copper accumulation in various organs
- Copper toxicity results in organ damage (liver, brain)

ESSENTIALS OF DIAGNOSIS

- Classically: extrapyramidal symptoms, detectable Kayser–Fleischer rings, and low serum ceruloplasmin level
- In patients with hepatic Wilson disease, these symptoms/findings are frequently absent
- Diagnosis requires a combination of tests: urinary copper excretion liver biopsy with quantitative measurement of hepatic copper content, mutation analysis

ESSENTIALS OF TREATMENT

- Cornerstones of treatment are copper chelators (D-penicillamine, trientine) or inhibitors of intestinal copper uptake (zinc salts)
- Life-long treatment is necessary
- Liver transplantation: the only treatment for fulminant Wilson disease, an option for decompensated cirrhosis, but very controversial for neurological symptoms
- Prognosis: in general, compliant patients on medical treatment have no progression of liver disease and no decreased life-expectancy. Transplanted patients with wilsonian liver disease have an excellent long-term outcome. Neurological symptoms are not fully reversible in the majority of patients

Introduction and definition

Wilson disease is an inherited disorder in which **defective biliary excretion of copper** leads to its accumulation, particularly in the liver (see Figure 92.1), brain (see Figure 92.2), and cornea (Kayser–Fleischer rings; see Figure 92.3) [1,2]. Wilson disease is due to a mutation in a gene on chromosome 13 that encodes for a P-type ATPase that plays a central role in copper extrusion [3–5]. Clinical presentation can vary, but the key features are liver disease and cirrhosis, neuropsychiatric disturbances, muddy brown Kayser–Fleischer rings around the cornea, and acute episodes of hemolysis. Wilson disease is not just a disease of children and young adults, but may present at any age [6].

Causes and epidemiology

Wilson disease is a genetic disorder that is found worldwide. More than 200 distinct mutations have been described in the *Wilson* gene [7]. The importance of individual mutations varies from country to country. In Northern, Central, and Eastern European populations [8,9] the most common mutations are an H1069Q missense mutation (43.5%), or mutations of exon 8 (6.8%), 3400 delC (3%), and P969Q (1.6%) [10,11]. Elsewhere different mutations are more common: A1003T and P969Q in Turkey and R778L in the Far East [12].

Pathogenesis

Wilson disease is more common than previously thought, with a gene frequency of 1 in 90–150 and an incidence (based on adults presenting with neurological symptoms) of at least 1 in 30 000–50 000. Normal dietary consumption and absorption of copper exceeds need, and homeostasis is maintained exclusively by biliary excretion of copper.

The *Wilson* gene, localized at chromosome 13, encodes a copper-transporting P-type ATPase (*ATP7B*). This protein resides in the trans-Golgi network and is responsible for transporting copper from intracellular chaperone proteins into the secretory pathway, both for excretion into bile and for incorporation into apo-ceruloplasmin for the synthesis of functional ceruloplasmin [3–5].

The development of Wilson disease is due to the accumulation of copper in affected tissues. The electron structure of copper facilitates the synthesis of reactive oxygen species, affecting the mitochondrial respiratory cycle and causing a decrease in cytochrome C activity. This is an early event in liver damage and is accompanied by lipid peroxidation. In the brain, and for uncertain reasons, there is preferential deposition of copper in basal ganglia. Pathogenic mechanisms in the brain are less clear than in the liver.

Pathology

In most patients there is a greater than five-fold increase in copper in the **liver** [13]. This is associated with non-specific liver biopsy findings, including fatty intracellular accumulations,

Textbook of Clinical Gastroenterology and Hepatology, Second Edition. Edited by C. J. Hawkey, Jaime Bosch, Joel E. Richter, Guadalupe Garcia-Tsao, Francis K. L. Chan.

Liver Disease

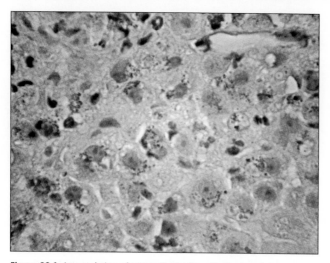

Figure 92.1 Accumulation of copper in the liver. Rhodanin staining.

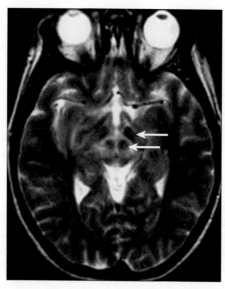

Figure 92.2 Characteristic changes of Wilson disease on MRI. Abnormal high-intensity signal in the mid-brain tegmentum, possibly due to edema, accentuates the difference with low-intensity signals from red nuclei, substantia nigra, and superior colliculus, resulting in the ears (top arrow) and eyes (bottom arrow) of the panda. (Reproduced with permisssion from Jacobs DA, Markowitz CE, Liebeskind DS, Galetta SL. The "double panda sign" in Wilson disease. *Neurology.* 2003;61:969.)

marked steatosis, portal and periportal lymphocyte infiltration, necrosis, and fibrosis. Rhodamine staining reveals focal copper stores in about 10% of patients (Figure 92.1). Ultrastructurally there is progressive mitochondrial and peroxisome damage.

In the **brain** there is a ubiquitous excess of copper associated with neuronal cavitation and death. This leads to a characteristic "giant panda" appearance on magnetic resonance imaging (MRI) (see Chapter 134; Figure 92.2) [14]. Excess copper distribution is also seen in the **kidney**, where copper has functional effects in a minority of patients.

Clinical presentation

The most common presentations are with **liver disease** or **neuropsychiatric disturbance** [15–18]. Clinically evident liver disease may precede neurological manifestations by as much as 10 years and most patients have some degree of liver disease at presentation.

Acute hepatitis

Wilson disease enters into the differential diagnosis of any young patient presenting with acute hepatitis. Its clinical presentation may be indistinguishable from that of acute viral hepatitis, with jaundice and abdominal discomfort. Rapid deterioration can occur with **fulminant liver failure**. Wilson disease accounts for 6–12% of all patients with fulminant hepatic failure who are referred for emergency transplantation [19,20]. Prominent hepatic failure may lead to large amounts of stored copper, which induce a severe hemolytic anemia.

Chronic hepatitis and cirrhosis

Wilson disease may present with cirrhosis at a young age. Histologically there is chronic hepatitis and/or advanced cirrhosis. The presentation may be indistinguishable from other forms of chronic active hepatitis, with symptoms including jaundice, malaise, and vague abdominal complaints.

Neuropsychiatric disease

This commonly occurs in the mid-teens or 20s, although later presentation is possible. Subtle motor disorders, such as tremor, speech, and writing problems, progress to juvenile parkinsonism characterized by tremor and rigidity, with dysarthria, dysphagia, and sometimes apraxia [16]. Wilson disease may present as reduced performance in school, but other psychiatric presentations, including labile mood, depression, exhibitionism, and psychosis, account for about one-third of presentations. Patients may present with liver disease alone, neuropsychiatric disease alone, or both, although liver disease is usually present when a neuropsychiatric presentation occurs.

Other clinical manifestations

Less common presentations include hypercalciuria and nephrocalcinosis, cardiac manifestations (arrhythmias, myopathy), and chondrocalcinosis and osteoarthritis, similar to that seen in hemochromatosis (see Chapter 90).

Physical signs

The hallmark of Wilson disease is the **Kayser–Fleischer ring** (Figure 92.3), which is present in 95% of patients with neurological symptoms and somewhat over half of those without. Kayser–Fleischer rings are more evident when the cornea is examined under a slit lamp; this should be done if a ring is not obvious. Neurological signs include tremor and extrapyramidal rigidity. Signs of liver disease are non-specific. Diagnostic vigilance is important because Kayser–Fleischer rings

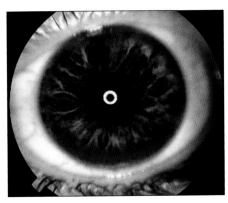

Figure 92.3 Kayser–Fleischer rings in the cornea.

may be absent in up to 50% of patients with Wilson disease affecting the liver [21].

Differential diagnosis

Acute hepatitis with Wilson disease presents similarly to other acute cases of hepatitis, whether viral, toxic, or drug induced. Similarly, Wilson disease should enter into the differential diagnosis of all patients with chronic hepatitis and cirrhosis, as routine histological changes are non-specific. When Wilson disease presents neurologically, it may be misdiagnosed as a behavioral problem because initial symptoms may be subtle and presentation is during adolescence. Movement disorders in a young person should raise the suspicion of Wilson disease, but the diagnosis may be overlooked where the presentation suggests a primarily psychological or psychiatric disorder. Whether further diagnostic tests of Wilson disease are needed in such patients may depend upon whether or not Kayser–Fleischer rings are found. If present, diagnosis on clinical grounds is easy to confirm. In all other instances further diagnostic tests are necessary (Table 92.1).

Diagnostic methods

Typically, the presence of Kayser–Fleischer rings and/or a low serum ceruloplasmin level is sufficient to establish a diagnosis. Where Kayser–Fleischer rings are not present (as is common in liver disease), ceruloplasmin levels are not always reliable because they may be low for reasons other than Wilson disease (e.g., autoimmune hepatitis, familial aceruloplasminemia) [22], whereas inflammation in the liver or elsewhere may cause the ceruloplasmin concentration to rise to normal levels, reflecting its identity as an acute-phase protein. Thus, for many patients a combination of tests of copper content or excretion may be needed. None is completely specific and a range of tests may often be needed (Table 92.1). A scoring system based on all available tests was proposed by the Working Party at the 8th International Meeting on Wilson disease, Leipzig 2001 [23] (Table 92.2; Figure 92.4). The most challenging aspect is the diagnosis of fulminant Wilson disease, since mortality without emergency liver transplantation is very high. Readily available

Table 92.1 Routine diagnostic tests for Wilson disease

Test	Typical finding	Proportion abnormal	Comments
Kayser–Fleischer rings by slit lamp	Present	95%	neurological; 50% liver
Serum ceruloplasmin	Decreased	>50%	Ceruloplasmin level raised with inflammation (acute phase) Overestimated by immunologic assay Other causes of deficiency include ceruloplasmin anemia
24-h copper	>100 mg/day	88%	May increase with hepatic necrosis
Serum-free copper	>10 mg/dL	Most	May increase with hepatic necrosis
Hepatic copper	>250 mg/g dry weight	82%	May be increased with other cholestasis

laboratory tests, including alkaline phosphatase (AP), bilirubin, and serum aminotransferases, provide the most rapid and accurate method for diagnosis of acute liver failure due to Wilson disease. A combination of an AP : total bilirubin ratio of <4 and an AST : ALT ratio of >2.2 yields a diagnostic sensitivity and specificity of 100%. Conventional tests for Wilson disease (ceruloplasmin, serum or urinary copper) are less sensitive and specific [24].

Molecular genetic testing for Wilson disease is cumbersome and, therefore, not yet routine because there are so many potential mutations. A likely development is a multiplex polymerase chain reaction for the most frequent mutations seen in a particular geographical region [7,8,12].

Family screening

It is very important to screen the family of patients presenting with Wilson disease because the chance of a sibling being a homozygote – and therefore developing clinical disease – is 25%. Amongst offspring the chance is 0.5% [25]. There is difficulty in diagnosing heterozygote carriers with certainty, but family members can be screened by mutational analysis for the specific mutation found in the index case.

Treatment

A number of drugs are available for the definitive treatment of Wilson disease, including penicillamine, trientine, zinc, tetrathiomolybdate, and, of course, dimercaprol. There is lack

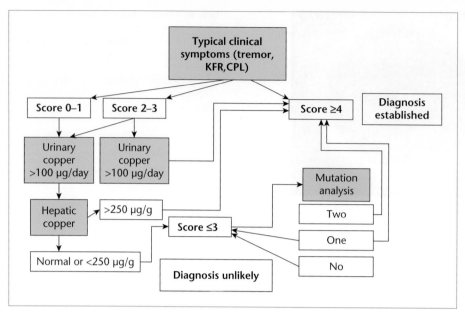

Figure 92.4 Diagnostic algorithms for Wilson disease based on the Leipzig score. 24-Hour urinary copper excretion >100 µg can be replaced by the d-penicillamine loading test (five-fold increased copper excretion compared with baseline). CPL, ceruloplasmin; KFR, Kayser–Fleischer ring. (Reproduced with permission from Ferenci P, Caca K, Loudianos G, *et al*. Diagnosis and phenotypic classification of Wilson disease. Final report of the Proceedings of the Working Party at the 8th International Meeting on Wilson disease and Menkes disease, Leipzig, Germany, 2001. *Liver Int*. 2003;23:139–142.)

Table 92.2 Scoring system for Wilson disease developed at the 8th International Meeting on Wilson disease, Leipzig, 2001

	Score 0	Score 1	Score 2	Score 3	Score 4
Serum bilirubin (µmol/L)	<100	100–150	151–200	201–300	>301
AST (ULN)	<2.5	2.6–3.5	3.6–55.	1–7.5	>7.5
PTT (no. of seconds more than control)	<4	4–8	9–12	13–20	>21

A score of 7 is associated with a high probability of death.
AST, aspartate aminotransferase; PTT, partial thromboplastin time; ULN, upper limit of normal.
(Reproduced with permission from Ferenci P, Caca K, Loudianos G, *et al*. Diagnosis and phenotypic classification of Wilson disease. Final report of the Proceedings of the Working Party at the 8th International Meeting on Wilson disease and Menkes disease, Leipzig, Germany, 2001. *Liver Int*. 2003;23:139–142.)

of high-quality evidence to estimate the relative treatment effects of the available drugs in Wilson disease. Therefore, multicenter prospective randomized controlled comparative trials are necessary [26].The American Association for the Study of Liver Disease (AASLD) recommends that all symptomatic patients with Wilson disease should receive a **chelating agent** (penicillamine or trientine) [27,28]. Once the diagnosis has been made, treatment needs to be lifelong.

Refer also to the accompanying management protocol on the website.

Penicillamine

This chelating agent mobilizes copper from proteins, allowing it to be excreted in the urine [25]. The usual dose is 1–1.5 g/day, and a response is generally seen within months, when the dose may be reduced to 0.5–1 g/day. Compliance and effectiveness can be monitored by repeated measurements of 24-hour urinary copper levels, which may ultimately settle at a level of >500 mg/day. Adverse events are common with penicillamine. Early sensitivity reactions marked by fever and cutaneous eruptions, lymphadenopathy, neutropenia or thrombocytopenia, and proteinuria may occur during the first 1–3 weeks. On longer exposure, d-penicillamine induces pyridoxine deficiency in a dose-dependent fashion, and interferes with collagen and elastin formation so that some patients develop cutis laxa and elastosis perforans serpiginosa. All patients should receive pyridoxine 50 mg/week to avoid deficiency. Penicillamine also commonly causes immune-mediated adverse effects; these include systemic lupus erythematosus, immune complex nephritis, leukopenia and thrombocytopenia, optic neuritis, myasthenia gravis, Goodpasture's syndrome, and pemphigus. The onset of these symptoms is an indication to stop the drug immediately. Therefore, 20% or more of patients may need to be switched to other treatments.

Trientine

This copper-chelating agent, which leads to enhanced urinary copper excretion, is at least as potent as penicillamine with far fewer side effects [29,30]. It may become the treatment of first choice, but at present this is not the case because of a lack of direct comparisons with penicillamine.

Ammonium tetrathiomolybdate

Ammonium tetrathiomolybdate complexes with copper in the intestinal tract to prevent absorption, and in the circulation, where it renders copper unavailable for cellular uptake [31]. As yet, experience with this drug is limited, although it is effective at removing copper from the liver; its continuous use may cause copper deficiency.

Zinc

Zinc interferes with copper absorption, first by competing for a common carrier for absorption, and second by inducing metallothionin in enterocytes, allowing copper absorbed into them to be excreted by desquamation [32]. A further advantage of zinc is that induction of metallothionin in liver protects hepatocytes against copper toxicity. Most data on zinc come from uncontrolled studies of dosages ranging from 75 to 250 mg/day [33]. Zinc is probably less effective than chelating agents in the treatment of established Wilson disease, although data are limited and uncontrolled. Its greatest use is in presymptomatic patients. The safety of zinc monotherapy in hepatic Wilson disease was questioned recently [34]. Whether or not a combination therapy with chelators has advantages is as yet unknown.

Liver transplantation

Transplantation is frequently necessary for patients presenting with fulminant hepatitis or decompensated cirrhosis due to Wilson disease [19,20]. Because the biochemical defect in Wilson disease is in the liver, transplantation corrects the underlying problem. In the past, the median survival was about 2.5 years, and longer for patients having a transplant for decompensated cirrhosis than for those with fulminant hepatic failure. Survival is improving; the longest survival recorded is 20 years. Limited observation suggests that the neurological symptoms of patients may also improve with liver transplantation.

Pregnancy

Successful treatment means that some women with Wilson disease become pregnant [35,36]. Counseling should indicate that the likelihood of finding a homozygosity amongst children is 0.5%. Haplotype analysis of the partner is justified. The patient's copper status should be optimized prior to therapy. Although there is some concern over the teratogenicity of penicillamine, the risks of withdrawing treatment outweigh those of continuing it.

Prognosis

Untreated Wilson disease is universally fatal, with most patients dying from liver disease and a minority from progressive neurological disease. With chelation treatment and liver transplantation, prolonged survival has become the norm, although mortality has not been assessed prospectively. In general, prognosis depends on the severity of liver disease.

Table 92.3 King's College Prognostic Score for patients with fulminant Wilson disease

	Score 0	Score 1	Score 2	Score 3	Score 4
Bilirubin (µmol/L)	<100	100–150	151–200	201–300	>301
INR	<1.29	1.3–1.6	1.7–1.9	2.0–2.4	>2.5
ASAT (IU/L)	<100	101–150	151–300	301–400	>401
WBC (10^9/L)	<6.7	6.8–8.3	8.4–10.3	10.4–15.3	>15.3
Albumin (g/L)	>45	34–44	25–33	21–24	<21

A total score ≥11 is suggestive for lethal outcome (sensitivity 93%; specificity 98%; positive predictive value 88%).
ASAT, aspartate aminotransferase; INR, international normalized ratio; WBC, white blood cell count.
Reproduced with permission from Dhawan A, Taylor RM, Cheeseman P, De Silva P, Katsiyiannakis L, Mieli-Vergani G. Wilson's disease in children: 37-year experience and revised King's score for liver transplantation. *Liver Transpl.* 2005;11:441–448.

Liver function becomes normal over 1–2 years in most patients with no or compensated cirrhosis at presentation, and then remains stable without progressive liver disease. At the other end of the spectrum, medical therapy is rarely effective in patients presenting with fulminant Wilson disease. A prognostic index has been developed, although not validated prospectively (Table 92.3). A score of >11 is always associated with death. Patients presenting with neurological symptoms fare better, especially if liver disease is limited. Neurological symptoms appear to be partly reversible with treatment, sometimes after initial deterioration. In patients undergoing orthotopic liver transplantation, survival may be slightly reduced early on, but appears normal (for transplant population) thereafter.

SOURCES OF INFORMATION FOR PATIENTS AND DOCTORS

http://www.wilsonsdisease.org/
http://digestive.niddk.nih.gov/ddiseases/pubs/wilson/
http://www.wemove.org/wil/
http://www.acsu.buffalo.edu/~drstall/wilsons.html
http://www.eurowilson.org/

References

1. Scheinberg IH, Sternlieb I. *Wilson's Disease. Major Problems in Internal Medicine*, vol 23. Philadelphia: WB Saunders, 1984.
2. Gitlin JD. Wilson disease. *Gastroenterology.* 2003;125:1868–1877.
3. Robertson WM. Wilson disease. *Arch Neurol.* 2000;57:276–277.
4. Tao YT, Gitlin JD. Hepatic copper metabolism: insights from genetic disease. *Hepatology.* 2003;37:1241–1247.
5. Lutsenko S, Petris MJ. Function and regulation of the mammalian copper-transporting ATPases: insights from biochemical and cell biological approaches. *J Membr Biol.* 2003;191:1–12.

Liver Disease

6. Ferenci P, Członkowska A, Merle U, *et al.* Late onset Wilson disease. *Gastroenterology.* 2007;132:1294–1298.

7. Cox DW. Molecular advances in Wilson disease. In: Boyer JL, Ockner RK, editors. *Progress in Liver Disease,* vol X. Philadelphia: WB Saunders, 1996:245–264.

8. Maier-Dobersberger T, Ferenci P, Polli C, *et al.* The His1069Gln mutation in Wilson's disease: detection by a rapid PCR-test, clinical course and liver biopsy findings. *Ann Intern Med.* 1997;127:21–26.

9. Caca K, Ferenci P, Kuhn HJ, *et al.* High prevalence of the H1069Q mutation in East German patients with Wilson disease: rapid detection of mutations by limited sequencing and phenotype–genotype analysis. *J Hepatol.* 2001;35:575–581.

10. Garcia-Villareal L, Daniels S, Shaw SH, *et al.* High prevalence of the very rare Wilson disease gene mutation Leu708Pro in the Island of Gran Canaria (Canary Islands, Spain): a genetic and clinical study. *Hepatology.* 2000;32:1329–1336.

11. Loudianos G, Dessi V, Lovicu M, *et al.* Mutation analysis in patients of Mediterranean descent with Wilson disease: identification of 19 novel mutations. *J Med Genet.* 1999;36:833–836.

12. Shimizu N, Nakazono H, Takeshita Y, *et al.* Molecular analysis and diagnosis in Japanese patients with Wilson disease. *Pediatr Int.* 1999;41:409–413.

13. Ferenci P, Steindl-Munda P, Vogel W, *et al.* Diagnostic value of quantitative hepatic copper determination in patients with Wilson disease. *Clin Gastroenterol Hepatol.* 2005;3:811–818.

14. Jacobs DA, Markowitz CE, Liebeskind DS, Galetta SL. The "double panda sign" in Wilson disease. *Neurology.* 2003;61:969.

15. Merle U, Schaefer M, Ferenci P, Stremmel W. Clinical Presentation, diagnosis and long-term outcome of Wilson disease – a cohort study. *Gut.* 2007;56:115–120.

16. Oder W, Grimm G, Kollegger H, Ferenci P, Schneider B, Deecke L. Neurological and neuropsychiatric spectrum of Wilson disease. A prospective study in 45 cases. *J Neurol.* 1991;238: 281–287.

17. Schilsky ML, Scheinberg IH, Sternlieb I. Prognosis of Wilsonian chronic active hepatitis. *Gastroenterology.* 1991;100:762–767.

18. Saito T. Presenting symptoms and natural history of Wilson disease. *Eur J Pediatr.* 1987;146:261–265.

19. Schilsky ML, Scheinberg IH, Sternlieb I. Liver transplantation for Wilson disease: indications and outcome. *Hepatology.* 1994;19:583–587.

20. Khanna A, Jain A, Eghtesad B, Rakela J. Liver transplantation for metabolic liver diseases. *Surg Clin North Am.* 1999;79: 153–162.

21. Steindl P, Ferenci P, Dienes HP, *et al.* Wilson's disease in patients presenting with liver disease: a diagnostic challenge. *Gastroenterology.* 1997;113:212–218.

22. Cauza E, Maier-Dobersberger T, Ferenci P. Plasma ceruloplasmin as screening test for Wilson disease. *J Hepatol.* 1997;27: 358–362.

23. Ferenci P, Caca K, Loudianos G, *et al.* Diagnosis and phenotypic classification of Wilson disease. Final report of the Proceedings of the Working Party at the 8th International Meeting on Wilson disease and Menkes disease, Leipzig, Germany, 2001. *Liver Int.* 2003;23:139–142.

24. Korman JD, Volenberg I, Balko J, *et al.* Screening for Wilson disease in acute liver failure: a comparison of currently available diagnostic tests. *Hepatology.* 2008;48:1167–1174.

25. Ferenci P. Diagnosis and current therapy of Wilson disease. *Aliment Pharmacol Ther.* 2004;19:157–165.

26. Wiggelinkhuizen M, Tilanus ME, Bollen CW, Houwen RH. Systematic review: clinical efficacy of chelator agents and zinc in the initial treatment of Wilson disease. *Aliment Pharmacol Ther.* 2009;29:947–958.

27. Roberts EA, Schilsky ML. AASLD practice guidelines: a practice guideline on Wilson disease. *Hepatology.* 2003;37:1475–1492.

28. Walshe JM, Yealland M. Chelation treatment of neurological Wilson disease. *Q J Med.* 1993;86:197–204.

29. Scheinberg IH, Jaffe ME, Sternlieb I. The use of trientine in preventing the effects of interrupting penicillamine therapy in Wilson disease. *N Engl J Med.* 1987;317:209–213.

30. Walshe JM. The management of pregnancy in Wilson disease treated with trientine. *Q J Med.* 1986;58:81–87.

31. Brewer GJ, Dick RD, Johnson V, *et al.* Treatment of Wilson disease with ammonium tetrathiomolybdate: I. Initial therapy in 17 neurologically affected patients. *Arch Neurol.* 1994;51:545–554.

32. Hoogenraad TU. Zinc treatment of Wilson disease. *J Lab Clin Med.* 1998;132:240–241.

33. Ferenci P. Zinc treatment of Wilson disease. In: Kruse–Jarres JD, Schölmerich J, editors. *Zinc and Diseases of the Digestive Tract.* Lancaster: Kluwer Academic Publishers, 1997:117–124.

34. Weiss KH, Gotthardt D, Klemm D, *et al.* Zinc monotherapy is not as effective as chelating agents in treatment of Wilson disease. *Gastroenterology.* 2011;140:1189–1198.

35. Scheinberg IH, Sternlieb I. Pregnancy in penicillamine-treated patients with Wilson disease. *N Engl J Med.* 1975;293:1300–1302.

36. Brewer GJ, Johnson VD, Dick RD, Hedera P, Fink JK, Kluin KJ. Treatment of Wilson disease with zinc XVII: treatment during pregnancy. *Hepatology.* 2000; 31:364–370.

37. Dhawan A, Taylor RM, Cheeseman P, De Silva P, Katsiyiannakis L, Mieli-Vergani G. Wilson's disease in children: 37-year experience and revised King's score for liver transplantation. *Liver Transpl.* 2005;11:441–448.

CHAPTER 93
Drug prescription in liver disease

Guido Stirnimann[1] and Jürg Reichen[1,2]

[1]University of Berne, Berne, Switzerland
[2]University Clinic of Visceral Surgery and Medicine, Inselspital, Berne, Switzerland

KEY POINTS

- Hepatic clearance depends on flow and intrinsic clearance, the latter reflecting the activity of different drug metabolizing enzymes and drug transporters
- Alterations in hepatic perfusion including a decrease in portal flow, barriers to diffusion and intra- and extrahepatic shunting affect mainly drugs with a high extraction (flow-limited clearance)
- Alterations in drug metabolizing enzymes and drug transporters affect mainly drugs with low extraction ratio and low protein binding (enzyme-limited clearance). Decreased protein binding is an important determinant of hepatic clearance after oral administration of drugs (binding-sensitive, enzyme-limited clearance)
- Knowledge of the pathway(s) of metabolism and elimination of drugs is essential in order to make rational dose adjustments
- No liver test reliably predicts pharmacokinetics and pharmacodynamics in individual patients with liver disease. The Child–Pugh classification gives the best indication of hepatic reserve and for the extent of dose adjustment
- Generally avoid drugs with a high first pass metabolism in cirrhosis.
- Closely monitor drug effects and – if indicated/available – plasma concentrations. Adjust the dose accordingly rather than using a standard dose ("start low, go slow")
- Be aware of the potential for altered pharmacodynamics of drugs in advanced liver disease

Determinants of hepatic drug metabolism and excretion and their alterations in liver disease

General considerations on organ clearance and its determinants

The liver with its portal blood supply and its abundant drug metabolizing and transporting proteins plays a central role in drug disposition. The concept of organ clearance – although physiologically suspect – is still helpful to assess anticipated changes in clearance of drugs in patients with liver disease. Hepatic clearance (Cl_{hep}) is a function of the elimination rate constant, k_e:

$$k_e = Cl_{hep} * C \qquad (93.1)$$

Equation 93.1 implies that more drug is eliminated per unit time if the plasma concentration (C) increases. This equation

holds true as long as the enzyme/transport system responsible for metabolism/elimination is not saturated.

An important determinant of k_e is the metabolic capacity of the liver which can be approximated by measuring the extraction (E):

$$E = (C_{in} - C_{out})/C_{in} \qquad (93.2)$$

where c_{in} and c_{out} are the drug concentrations in the inflow and outflow tract, respectively. Equation 93.2 assumes a rapid equilibration of drug concentration in the sinusoids between sinusoidal inflow from the hepatic artery and portal vein. Hepatic clearance can then be defined as the product of hepatic blood flow (Q) and extraction ratio:

$$Cl_{hep} = Q * E \qquad (93.3)$$

Equation 93.3 predicts that drugs with high E depend on hepatic perfusion while drugs with low E depend on the process of metabolism/elimination. In other words, the elimination of drugs with high E is flow dependent, while that of drugs with low E is enzyme dependent. This is illustrated in Figure 93.1.

The extraction ratio is a function of the Michaelis–Menten kinetics of the transport or metabolic processes leading to drug elimination, the so-called intrinsic clearance Cl_{int} (which is the ratio V_{max}/K_m of the metabolic or transport process governing elimination of the drug). Taking drug binding also into account, Equation 93.3 can be written as:

$$Cl_{hep} = Q \cdot (f_u \cdot Cl_{int})/(Q + f_u \cdot Cl_{int}) \qquad (93.4)$$

where f_u is the unbound fraction of the drug.

Specific processes determining hepatic clearance in health and disease

Expanding on the considerations above, five processes are involved in determining Cl_{hep} of a given compound. Another two, namely renal elimination and alterations of volume of distribution, can play an important role in drug disposition in patients with liver disease.

Liver Disease

Textbook of Clinical Gastroenterology and Hepatology, Second Edition. Edited by C. J. Hawkey, Jaime Bosch, Joel E. Richter, Guadalupe Garcia-Tsao, Francis K. L. Chan.
© 2012 Blackwell Publishing Ltd. Published 2012 by Blackwell Publishing Ltd.

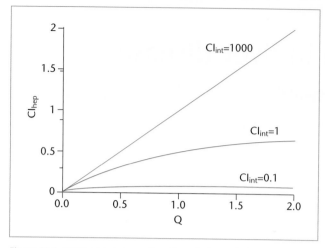

Figure 93.1 Relationship between hepatic perfusion and clearance. Illustration showing the effect of a drug's intrinsic hepatic clearance (Cl_{int}) on the relationship between total hepatic clearance (Cl_{hep}) and hepatic perfusion (Q). When the intrinsic hepatic clearance is very high, the hepatic extraction is close to 100%. In this case the total hepatic clearance equals hepatic blood flow and is thus described as "flow limited". In contrast, when intrinsic hepatic clearance is very low, changes in hepatic blood flow will have no effect on total hepatic clearance, which is then said to be "enzyme limited".

Phase 1 metabolism

This encompasses mostly oxidative processes mediated by the cytochrome P450 (CYP) super-family. Phase 1 reactions serve generally to render xenobiotics more reactive, thereby allowing phase 2 reactions to take place. CYP3A4 is the most abundant CYP isoenzyme and is responsible for the biotransformation of 50% of drugs. Its activity is highly variable between individuals and this variation is more important than the decrease associated with chronic liver disease.

Loss of function of the different isoenzymes is not uniform; CYP2C19 declines early and rapidly while CYP2E1 function is preserved even in late stage liver disease. CYP1A2 and CYP2D6 decline steadily with decreasing liver function [1].

Cholestatic liver disease affects mainly CYP2E1 and CYP2C.

Phase 2 metabolism

Phase 2 metabolism encompasses a variety of conjugation reactions of reactive metabolites resulting from phase 1 metabolism and aims at rendering xenobiotics suitable for biliary and/or renal excretion. The major enzyme classes in phase 2 are the UDP-glucuronyl transferases, N-acetyl-transferases, glutathione transferases and sulfate transferases.

In chronic liver disease, activity of glucuronyl transferase is maintained until late for many substrates including morphine and benzodiazepines. However, glucuronidation of other drugs including lamotrigine, zidovudine and mycophenolate mofetil is impaired in advanced liver disease. The activity of N-acetyltransferases and glutathione transferases decline more or less in parallel with the Child classification.

Phase 3 elimination

Intestinal absorption, renal and/or biliary elimination of xenobiotics resulting from phase 1/2 metabolism is mediated by several super-families of transport proteins: on the sinusoidal side the solute carrier protein family SLC and on the canalicular side P glycoprotein and the ABC transporter proteins [2].

Studies on changes in drug transporter activity are only beginning to be explored in patients with chronic liver disease and no conclusions can yet be reached about their role in altered metabolic clearance of drugs in cirrhosis. However, clear predictions can often be made about drug disposition in cholestatic liver disease. This is particularly germane for cytostatics with predominantly biliary excretion [3].

Some drugs excreted into the bile undergo enterohepatic circulation. This often involves deconjugation by intestinal bacteria (a reverse phase II reaction) and active or passive reabsorption in the gut.

Hepatic perfusion

Hepatic perfusion is a major determinant of hepatic clearance (Equations 93.3 and 93.4). The architecture of the liver sinusoid with its fenestrations allows free access of protein-bound drugs to the transport proteins in the sinusoidal membrane.

Hepatic perfusion is markedly altered in chronic liver disease by different processes:

- Decreased portal perfusion, in end-stage liver disease even reversal of flow in the portal vein
- Portosystemic shunts; these can occur in the absence of intrinsic liver disease, e.g., in portal vein thrombosis
- Alterations in the intrahepatic diffusion process in particular by sinusoidal capillarization [4]

Protein binding

Due to decreased synthesis of drug binding proteins, in particular albumin and α_1 acidic glycoprotein, the unbound fraction of drugs is often increased. Another mechanism for altered protein binding of drugs is displacement of drugs by retention of cholephiles such as bilirubin.

Low plasma concentrations of binding proteins will result in an increased unbound fraction (f_u) of drug in plasma; this can result in increased clearance if metabolic capacity of the liver is maintained.

For high extraction drugs the rate of elimination is not dependent on plasma protein binding because the equilibration processes are fast enough to allow almost complete drug removal upon one passage through the liver. Decreased protein binding will therefore lead to an unchanged total and increased free concentration. Fortunately, higher free concentrations will only become clinically relevant for drugs with a narrow therapeutic margin given as a constant intravenous infusion.

Volume of distribution

Ascites can markedly increase the volume of distribution of hydrophilic drugs. If rapid achievement of therapeutic drug levels is desirable, this may require an increase in the loading dose. A practical example would be β-lactam antibiotics.

Renal elimination

Functional renal failure in end-stage cirrhosis can impact on renal excretion. It has to be kept in mind that serum creatinine is a poor indicator of renal function in patients with end-stage liver disease. Measurement of cystatin C could more accurately reflect renal function in patients with cirrhosis [5].

First pass metabolism

An important aspect of the gut–liver axis is first pass metabolism. A drug administered orally passes two tissues with extensive metabolic and transport capacity, namely the gut and the liver. First pass metabolism reflects the proportion of absorbed drug that is metabolized or excreted by these two organs. Clearance after p.o. administration ($Cl_{p.o.}$) of a drug is determined by f_u and intrinsic clearance:

$$Cl_{p.o.} = f_u \cdot Cl_{int} \qquad (93.5)$$

Both hepatocytes and enterocytes harbor enzymes and transport proteins with a great capacity for presystemic elimination of drugs. The enterocyte is rich in CYP3A and P glycoprotein while the hepatocyte has a much broader variety of enzymes and transporters [2]. Loss of first pass metabolism in liver disease can lead to a marked and potentially dangerous increase in systemic availability of orally administered drugs. This concerns mainly drugs with a high extraction ratio (Equation 93.3, Table 93.1). Sometimes, it can be difficult to predict whether loss of first pass metabolism is due to hepatic or intestinal changes.

A paradigm is the increase in bioavailability of midazolam in patients with TIPS: it appears logical to assume that this is due to the shunt avoiding contact of blood derived from the intestine with hepatocytes; surprisingly, the loss of first pass metabolism was due to a marked decrease in CYP3A4 in the intestine [6].

It has to be pointed out that portosystemic shunting with loss of first pass metabolism occurs not only in patients with chronic liver disease but also in patients with non-cirrhotic portal hypertension and with portal vein thrombosis. The fraction of a dose escaping first-pass metabolism (F_e) can be estimated as:

$$F_e = 1 - Q_{eff} * E \qquad (93.6)$$

where Q_{eff} is the mesenteric blood flow passing through the liver. Unfortunately, in most cases no good estimate of Q_{eff} can be obtained: because it would require an estimate of total hepatic and portosystemic blood flow.

Altered pharmacodynamics in chronic liver disease

Changes in receptors of different drugs as well as in post-receptor signal transmission can lead to altered pharmacody-

Table 93.1 Examples of drugs with low and high hepatic extraction ratios

Low extraction ratio (<0.3)	High extraction ratio (>0.7)
Carbamazepine	Carvedilol
Diazepam	Chlormethiaziol
Phenobarbital	Diltiazem
Phenprocoumon	Ergot alkaloids
Phenytoin	Lidocaine
Salicylic acid	Metoprolol
Theophylline	Meperidine
Valproate	Midazolam
Warfarin	Morphine
	Nitroglycerine
	Pentazocine
	Propranolol
	Verapamil

Note that only a few drugs have an intermediate extraction ratio.

namics. Differences between alterations in pharmacokinetics and pharmacodynamics are often difficult to differentiate.

Sedatives and analgesics

Increased susceptibility to benzodiazepines and opioid analgesics in cirrhotic patients is well known. Such drugs can induce hepatic encephalopathy at therapeutic doses. Possible mechanisms include alterations in the blood–brain barrier, increased susceptibility due to an increased density of GABA receptors, and pharmacokinetic alterations.

Diuretics

The effect of loop diuretics in cirrhotic patients with ascites is reduced owing to decreased delivery to their site of action in the renal tubule. This is more marked for furosemide than for torasemide. Excessive diuresis might precipitate hepatorenal syndrome and refractoriness to loop diuretics. For further details see Chapter 99.

β-Receptor antagonists

In patients with cirrhosis, a decreased sensitivity to β-adrenoreceptor antagonists exists. This is not only due to reduced receptor density, but also to a post-receptor defect which can be overcome with NO donors.

Liver Disease

Non-steroidal anti-inflammatory drugs

Prostaglandin synthesis is essential in maintaining renal perfusion in patients with portal hypertension and the associated hyperdynamic circulation. Therefore, NSAIDs and COX2 inhibititors can precipitate renal failure in patients with cirrhosis even in the absence of ascites. If such drugs are unavoidable in the patient with chronic liver disease, frequent monitoring of serum creatinine and electrolytes is advisable.

Dosing adjustments in chronic liver disease

Dose adjustment is necessary in cirrhosis but probably not in acute or chronic hepatitis. Cholestatic liver diseases, in particular obstructive jaundice, requires dose adjustment for drugs with a predominantly biliary excretion.

A variety of tests including quantitative liver function tests, analysis of elimination of model compounds, breath tests probing different metabolic pathways, determination of serum bile acids as a measure of portosystemic shunting etc. have been proposed as tools to reliably predict drug disposition in the cirrhotic patient. None has withstood the test of time; even those with a good predictive value for drug disposition in patients with cirrhosis have not made it into clinical practice since they are too cumbersome to be performed outside a research setting.

The best – albeit far from perfect – parameter to predict the need for and extent of dose adjustments is the Child–Pugh classification (Table 93.2). Pharmacokinetic studies in patients with impaired liver function and stratified by Child class is required by the major drug regulatory agencies including the FDA and EMEA for most drugs before marketing. It has to be realized, though, that older drugs were not usually tested in

patients with impaired liver function and newer drugs are only tested in Child A and B patients, meaning that pharmacokinetic data for Child C patients are often not available. Dose reductions of 50% and 75% for Child A and B patients are safe. If time permits, starting with a low dose and slowly increasing dosage while watching for pharmacodynamic success and adverse events ("start slow – go slow") should avoid drug toxicity in patients with chronic liver disease.

In general, for high-extraction drugs given orally, both the loading and maintenance dose should be reduced according to the anticipated increase in bioavailability. When given i.v., a normal loading dose can be used but the maintenance dose should be decreased according to the functional impairment.

For low extraction drugs, dose adaptation depends on whether the drug is highly protein bound or not (see Equation 93.4). In highly protein bound drugs clearance can actually be increased since f_u is increased. Measurement of the free drug concentration is recommended for compounds with a narrow therapeutic window (e.g. diphenylhydantoin). In general, the loading dose is normal while the maintenance dose should be reduced according to the estimated reduction in hepatic functional reserve.

Sedatives and analgesics
- Prefer benzodiazepines with minor phase one metabolism such as lorazepam or oxazepam
- Do not withhold opiates from patients with advanced liver disease but adjust for altered first-pass metabolism and consider overdose in patients with worsening hepatic encephalopathy
- Avoid analgesic drugs for which no antagonist is available
- Do not exceed 4 g (2.5 g if you want to remain on the safe side) of acetaminophen in chronic liver disease, particularly when glutathione stores can be expected to be low (see also Chapter 93).

β-Receptor antagonists
Many β antagonists – in particular, propranolol – are subject to extensive first-pass metabolism resulting in elevated plasma concentrations in patients with advanced liver disease. In clinical practice, preference should be given to long-acting formulations since they avoid the very high peaks seen after oral administration.

Cytostatics
There are several problems in administering cytotoxic drugs to patients with liver disease:

- Exacerbation of pre-existing liver disease, in particular hepatitis B
- Frequent intrinsic hepatotoxicity of cytostatic agents
- Liver metastases can adversely affect liver function.

Different dose reduction regimes, mostly based on bilirubin levels, exist [3].

Table 93.2 The Child–Pugh classification and its impact on dose adjustment

Parameter	Child–Pugh class		
	A	B	C
Serum bilirubin			
(mmoles/L)	<35	35–50	>50
(mg/dL)	<2	2–3	>3
Serum albumin (g/L)	>35	28–35	<28
Prothrombin time (seconds)	<4	4–6	>6
Ascites	None	Controlled Not tense	Tense Refractory
Encephalopathy	None	1–2	3–4
Dose reduction	50%	75%	No recommendation can be given

Adverse drug reactions in patients with liver disease

As discussed in Chapter 93, the incidence of hepatic adverse events is usually not increased in patients with chronic liver disease. The question is not whether the patient will develop hepatotoxicity but whether there is sufficient functional reserve to allow for hepatotoxicity In other words, utmost caution is recommended regarding the use of potentially hepatotoxic drugs in Child C patients. In all patients with underlying liver disease, frequent monitoring of liver enzymes is recommended.

There are a few specific adverse effects which should be taken into consideration when treating cirrhotic patients. One concerns myelotoxicity which may become rapidly clinically relevant in patients with hypersplenism and pre-existing thrombocytopenia and/or leukopenia. Neutropenia induced by β-lactam antibiotics appears to have an increased incidence in cirrhotic patients. In obstructive cholestasis increased susceptibility to aminoglycoside nephrotoxicity must be expected.

References

1. Frye RF, Zgheib NK, Matzke GR, *et al.* Liver disease selectively modulates cytochrome P450-mediated metabolism. *Clin Pharmacol Ther.* 2006;80:235–245.
2. Li P, Wang GJ, Robertson TA, *et al.* Liver transporters in hepatic drug disposition: An update. *Curr Drug Metab.* 2009;10:482–498.
3. Field KM, Michael M. Part II: Liver function in oncology: Towards safer chemotherapy use. *Lancet Oncol.* 2008;9:1181–1190.
4. Reichen J. The role of sinusoidal endothelium in liver function. *News Physiol Sci.* 1999;14:117–120.
5. Cholongitas E, Shusang V, Marelli L, *et al.* Review article: Renal function assessment in cirrhosis – difficulties and alternative measurements. *Aliment Pharmacol Ther.* 2007;26:969–978.
6. Chalasani N, Gorski JC, Patel NH, *et al.* Hepatic and intestinal cytochrome P450 3A activity in cirrhosis: Effects of transjugular intrahepatic portosystemic shunts. *Hepatology.* 2001;34:1103–1108.

Liver Disease

CHAPTER 94

Genetic and metabolic liver diseases in childhood

Giorgina Mieli-Vergani[1] and Richard Thompson[2]

[1]King's College Hospital, London, UK
[2]King's College School of Medicine, London, UK

ESSENTIAL FACTS ABOUT PATHOGENESIS

- Cholestatic liver disease in infancy is caused by genetic mutations affecting the production, transport or quality of bile
- These conditions are rare
- Most present in the neonatal period
- Most have a progressive course
- There is a high incidence of hepatocellular carcinoma in bile salt export pump (BSEP) deficiency

ESSENTIALS OF DIAGNOSIS

- Cholestasis, paucity of intrahepatic bile ducts, cardiac abnormalities, butterfly vertebrae, posterior embryotoxon, high cholesterol and a characteristic facial appearance suggest Alagille syndrome
- High GGT cholestasis suggests multidrug resistance protein-3 (MDR3) deficiency, neonatal sclerosing cholangitis (NSC) or North American Indian childhood cirrhosis
- Low GGT cholestasis suggests BSEP deficiency, familial intrahepatic cholestasis-1 (FIC1) deficiency or an inborn error of bile acid synthesis
- Most conditions can be diagnosed prenatally

ESSENTIALS OF TREATMENT

- All cholestatic conditions need adequate fat-soluble vitamin supplements
- For inborn errors of bile acid synthesis, oral bile acid supplements prevent disease progression and the need for transplantation
- Ursodeoxycholic acid may help in BSEP, FIC1 and MDR3 deficiency and in some cases of NSC
- Liver transplantation is indicated for severely progressive forms of intrahepatic cholestasis, but does not cure the extrahepatic manifestations of Alagille syndrome or FIC1 deficiency
- BSEP deficiency may recur after transplant due to the production of anti-BSEP antibodies

Introduction

Like all other diseases, liver diseases are the result of genetic and environmental effects. Some conditions have a more obvious genetic origin, either by familial recurrence, or by frequently occurring in consanguineous families. Furthermore, most liver diseases present with features of metabolic disturbance. Of the latter many fit into the typical definition of metabolic diseases. The preceding chapters have covered several such disorders. The conditions covered in this chapter are those that are most likely to be seen by clinicians presenting with a "liver phenotype", often cholestatic. Table 94.1 depicts such conditions and Figure 94.1 demonstrates some of the functional processes involved. The more common of these conditions are described in detail.

Alagille syndrome

Epidemiology and pathogenesis

Alagille syndrome (AGS) is reported to have an incidence of 1/70 000, and a worldwide distribution. This is likely to be an underestimate. There is a strong association with heterozygous mutations in the *JAG1* gene [1,2], and more recently in the related *NOTCH2* gene [3]. Mutations in *JAG1* are, however, not fully penetrant with some parents having the same mutations but few or no features. In addition, the majority of mutations are family specific. This severely limits the use of genetics for diagnostic purposes.

Clinical presentation and pathology

The cardinal feature of AGS is the presence of intrahepatic cholestasis with a biliary hypoplasia, evident as a relative paucity of bile duct on liver biopsy. Clinically Alagille syndrome presents with:

- Persistent cholestasis
- Pruritus
- Hepatomegaly
- Congenital heart defects – peripheral pulmonary stenosis, tetralogy of Fallot
- Notched or butterfly dorsal vertebrae
- Eye defects – most frequently posterior embryotoxon
- Characteristic facial features – broad forehead, pointed chin resulting in triangular face (Figure 94.2).

In the neonatal period the liver biopsy findings may be inconclusive and the facial features less obvious. The

Textbook of Clinical Gastroenterology and Hepatology, Second Edition. Edited by C. J. Hawkey, Jaime Bosch, Joel E. Richter, Guadalupe Garcia-Tsao, Francis K. L. Chan.
© 2012 Blackwell Publishing Ltd. Published 2012 by Blackwell Publishing Ltd.

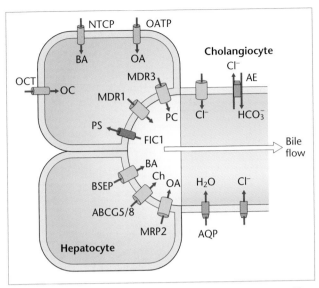

Figure 94.1 The major transport processes involved in bile formation and flow are shown. In particular, the classes of uptake transporters in the hepatocyte basolateral membrane are indicated, as are the apical transporters of the cholangiocyte membrane. The individual transporters of the canalicular membrane are shown; these are featured in this chapter. ABCG5/8, cholesterol transporting heterodimer; AQP, aquaporins; AE, anion exchanger; BA, bile acids; BSEP, bile salt export pump; CFTR, cystic fibrosis transmembrane conductance regulator; Ch, cholesterol; FIC1, familial intrahepatic cholestasis protein 1; MDR1, multidrug resistance protein 1; MDR3, multidrug resistance protein 3; MRP2, multidrug resistance associated protein 2; NTCP, sodium taurocholate co-transporting polypeptide; OA, organic anions; OC, organic cations; OCT, organic action transporters; OATP, organic anion transporting polypeptides; PC, phosphatidylcholine; PS, phosphatidylserine. (This figure was published in *Clinical Gastroenterology and Hepatology*, Wilfred M. Weinstein, Christopher J. Hawkey, Jaime Bosch, Genetic and metabolic liver diseases in childhood, Pages 1–5, Copyright Elsevier, 2005.)

cholestasis is often characterized by markedly elevated levels of serum cholesterol, with development of xanthomata (Figure 94.3). Growth failure is a major feature in most cases.

The classical definition presented here does not take into account genetics. However, as mutations do not yet accurately predict the phenotype, a genetic based diagnostic algorithm is not possible. First-degree relatives of affected individuals, carrying the same mutation, may be thought of as having NOTCH-related disease, but no definition has been agreed.

Management

The cholestasis of AGS can be severe enough to justify liver transplantation. However, it does frequently improve after the first decade. The overall prognosis is largely determined by the severity of the heart disease. Peripheral pulmonary stenosis is often asymptomatic, but may require dilatation and stenting before liver transplantation. The extrahepatic features are clearly not corrected by liver transplantation.

Familial intrahepatic cholestasis

Whilst most cholestatic liver diseases are marked by elevated serum levels of γ-glutamyl transferase (GGT), a number of conditions are characterized by normal levels. In most cases when a liver disease is associated with normal levels of GGT there is an accompanying failure of bile salt excretion. This may be primary or secondary. Secondary failure of secretion of bile acids can be seen in severe liver disease, and is not uncommon in acute liver failure. Primary failure of bile acid secretion may be due to failure of bile salt synthesis [4] or transport. Although bile acid synthesis defects are relatively rare they are usually

Table 94.1 Principal conditions presenting with a "liver phenotype"

Condition	Main features	Gene symbol	Protein function	Reference
Aagenaes syndrome	Normal-GGT IC, lymphoedema	Ch 15	Unknown	[16]
Alagille syndrome	IC, cardiac, eyes, skeletal, renal	*JAG1*, *NOTCH2*	Notch signaling	[1–3]
ARC syndrome	Arthrogryposis, renal, IC	*VPS33B*	Membrane trafficking	[17]
Bile acid synthesis defects	IC (most normal GGT), neurological in some	Various	Enzyme defects	[4]
BSEP deficiency	Normal-GGT IC	*ABCB11*	Bile salt transport	[5,6]
Crigler–Najjar syndrome	Unconjugated jaundice	*UGT1A1*	Enzyme defect	[18]
Dubin–Johnson syndrome	Conjugated jaundice	*ABCC2*	Anion transporter	[19]
FIC1 deficiency	Normal-GGT IC, GI and other epithelia	*ATP8B1*	Lipid transporter	[7,8]
Neonatal sclerosing cholangitis	High-GGT IC, cholangiopathy	Unknown	Unknown	[13]
MDR3 deficiency	High-GGT IC	*ABCB4*	Lipid transporter	[11]
NISCH syndrome	High-GGT IC, cholangiopathy, ichthyosis	*CLDN1*	Tight junction protein	[14]
North American Indian childhood cirrhosis	High-GGT IC, cholangiopathy	*CIRH1A*	Possible transcription factor	[15,20]

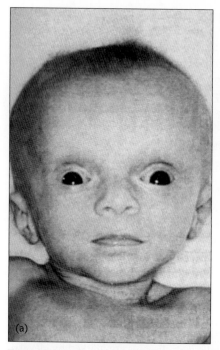 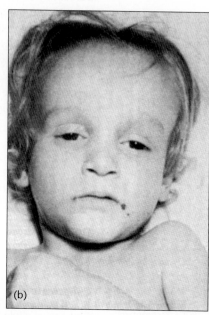 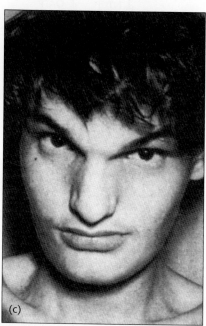

Figure 94.2 Alagille syndrome at various ages. Reproduced from Alagille D, Estrada A, Hadchouel M *et al.* Syndromic paucity of interlobular bile ducts (Alagille syndrome or arteriohepatic dysplasia): review of 80 cases. *J Pediatr.* 1987;110:195–200.

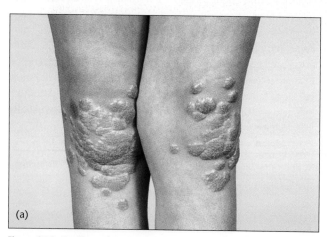 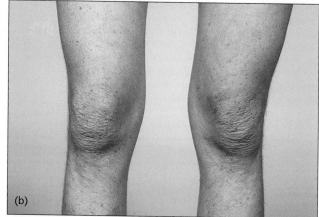

Figure 94.3 Alagille syndrome: xanthomata. Lobulated tumors occur over the elbows and knees (a), or along the course of the tendons, when they may be known as xanthoma tendinosum. (b) This child with Alagille syndrome was treated successfully with a liver transplant. Reproduced from Du Vivier A. *Atlas of Clinical Dermatology*, 3rd edn. London: Churchill Livingstone, 2002, with permission from Elsevier.

treatable with oral bile acid therapy. For this reason it is essential to screen the urine for abnormal metabolites.

Progressive familial intrahepatic cholestasis with normal GGT
Pathogenesis and epidemiology
Most cases of progressive familial intrahepatic cholestasis (PFIC) are of the low, or normal, GGT type. There are two causes of low GGT PFIC identified so far:

- BSEP deficiency, is due to mutations in the gene encoding the bile salt export pump of the canalicular membrane (*ABCB11*) [5,6]

- FIC1 deficiency, is caused by mutations in *ATP8B1* [7,8]. The function of the FIC1 protein is unknown, though it may be an aminophospholipid flipase.

ABCB11 is only expressed in the liver; in contrast, *ATP8B1* is widely expressed. Collectively these two conditions have an incidence of approximately 1/50 000. Although originally thought of as occurring only in isolated populations, approximately one-third of FIC1 patients are compound heterozygotes and this rises to two-thirds for BSEP deficiency.

Clinical presentation
BSEP deficiency usually presents in the first 3 months, with a giant-cell hepatitis and continues to a progressive cholestasis,

with jaundice and itching. The giant cell hepatitis is paralleled by raised serum transaminase levels.

FIC1 deficiency is usually milder in onset, can have a fluctuating course and is accompanied by non-specific features of cholestasis on light microscopy. As well as progressive cholestasis, with jaundice and itching, FIC1 deficiency results in a number of extrahepatic features, especially diarrhoea and malabsorption, in excess of that which would be expected from the cholestasis. A significant minority also has sensorineural deafness, pancreatitis, pancreatic insufficiency and abnormal sweat electrolytes.

Pathology

Immunohistochemical staining for BSEP is becoming available as a discriminatory diagnostic tool (Figure 94.4). FIC1 staining is not yet available. A number of other canalicular proteins do, however, appear to be absent in FIC1 deficiency, most notably GGT and CD26; this can be used to aid diagnosis. Transmission electron microscopy can be diagnostic in FIC1 deficiency, showing coarsely granular bile in the canalicular space – Byler bile (Figure 94.5).

Management

Both BSEP and FIC1 deficiencies have largely been managed conservatively, or by liver transplantation. Both require aggressive nutritional management, such as medium chain triglyceride supplements. Some patients require parenteral dosing to maintain adequate fat soluble vitamin levels. Pruritus can be very difficult to treat. Rifampicin, with or without ursodeoxycholic acid (in modest doses), is probably the best treatment, though far from ideal. It is, however, now clear that BSEP deficiency carries a significant risk of liver malignancy, and that monitoring for tumors is essential [5].

Surgical interventions such as partial external biliary diversion and ileal exclusion have been attempted. There are very

few data on the latter, but the former works in some patients. In FIC1 deficiency success cannot so far be predicted. For BSEP deficiency, however, it appears that patients with "milder" mutations (with some retention of function) do much better. Liver transplantation is generally an excellent treatment for BSEP deficiency, but there have now been several reports of apparent disease recurrence mediated by alloantibody – anti BSEP – formation [9,10]. For FIC1 deficiency, although liver transplantation greatly improves the cholestasis, the extrahepatic features remain. The malabsorption can be particularly difficult after transplantation.

Progressive familial intrahepatic cholestasis with high GGT

Three types of recessive cholestatic liver disease with elevated levels of serum GGT have so far been identified. Overall, there

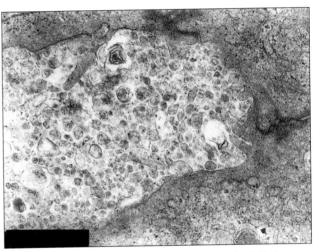

Figure 94.5 Byler bile. Osmium tetroxide–uranyl acetate–lead citrate. Original magnification ×40 000. (Patient materials courtesy of Dr L Szönyi.) Kindly provided by A S Knisely.

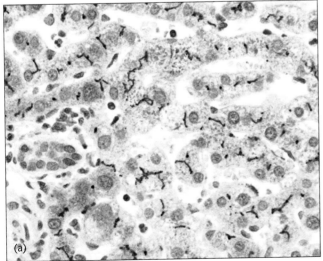

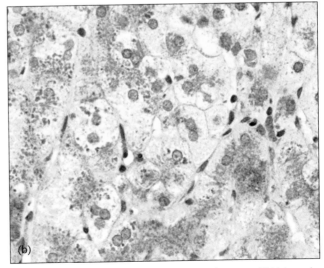

Figure 94.4 Bile salt export pump deficiency. (a) Normal liver. (b) BSEP deficiency. Rabbit polyclonal antibody against human BSEP (courtesy of Y Meier and B Stieger, Zurich)/hematoxylin counterstain. Original magnification ×400. Kindly provided by A S Knisely.

are fewer data available than for normal GGT disease, reflecting the fact that these conditions seem to be rarer.

Multidrug resistance protein-3 deficiency
Pathology and clinical presentation
MDR3 deficiency is the best characterized form of intrahepatic cholestasis, with high levels of serum GGT. MDR3 is an ATP-binding cassette-type protein that resembles the multidrug resistance P-glycoprotein and is expressed in the canalicular membrane of hepatocytes where it is involved in the transport of phospatidylcholine to bile [11].

A complete lack of MDR3 function is associated with a complete lack of phosphatidylcholine in bile. This is the main phospholipid in bile, and without it bile acids cannot form mixed micelles. Instead the bile consists of highly detergent, free bile acids. This causes major damage to both hepatocytes and cholangiocytes, and this is reflected on histological inspection (Figure 94.6).

There is a wide spectrum of severity in MDR3 deficiency. Although most patients present in the first few months of life, there is a range of phenotypes that present later. As phospholipids, along with bile acids, are essential in maintaining cholesterol in solution, some patients present with intrahepatic cholelithiasis [12]. There are also patients with late onset cholestatic disease, presenting in the second or even third decade. Furthermore heterozygotes for severe mutations, for example mothers of patients with severe disease, can suffer from cholestasis of pregnancy.

Management
Most patients with early onset MDR3 deficiency will come to liver transplantation. However some respond to ursodeoxycholic acid treatment. This is understandable, as anything that reduces the hydrophobicity of the bile should help. However, if there are no phospholipids at all, even ursodeoxycholic acid

cannot help. The mouse model of MDR3 deficiency (mdr2 deficiency) indicates that this condition may be an excellent candidate for hepatocyte transplantation, which has not yet been tried in humans.

Neonatal sclerosing cholangitis
Different types of "neonatal sclerosing cholangitis" (NSC) have been described [13]. This condition has many similarities with biliary atresia, though there is no complete obliteration of the bile ducts. As biliary atresia almost certainly derives from a number of different conditions, NSC could be thought of as one type of biliary atresia. The best characterized form of NSC is that associated with ichthyosis due to mutations in claudin-1 [14].

North American Indian childhood cirrhosis
This condition is uniquely found in Ojibway–Cree children from northwestern Quebec. It is a recessive condition due to a missense mutation (R565W) in the protein cirhin [15]. The phenotype is again very similar to that of extrahepatic biliary atresia, with transient neonatal jaundice, followed by progression to biliary cirrhosis and portal hypertension.

Support for patients and parents
Many of the intrahepatic cholestases are very distressing and difficult to treat. The majority of treatments are supportive. Unfortunately, even liver transplantation does not cure Alagille syndrome or FIC1 deficiency. Alagille syndrome benefits from skilled input from cardiologists and endocrinologists, as well as those needed to care for the liver disease. For all patients with cholestasis, the liver disease requires multidisciplinary input if the secondary consequences are to be minimized. Most of the conditions discussed can be tested for in subsequent pregnancies, should the parents so wish. However, the complex genetics of Alagille syndrome make testing very difficult, as there is not a one to one relationship between mutations and phenotype.

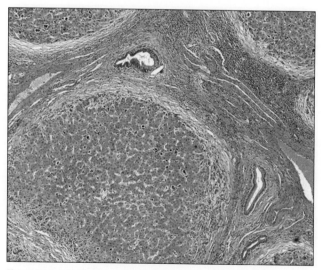

Figure 94.6 MDR3 deficiency. Hematoxylin and eosin stain. Original magnification ×4. Photo kindly provided by AS Knisely.

SOURCES FOR INFORMATION FOR PARENTS AND DOCTORS

The multidisciplinary team caring for pediatric patients needs to include nurse specialists and dieticians capable of helping the parents look after their child. In addition, the following organizations all seek to help the families of children with liver disease in various ways.

UK: Children's Liver Disease Foundation;
       http://www.childliverdisease.org/
USA: Children's Liver Association for Support Services;
       http://www.classkids.org/

References
1. Li L, Krantz ID, Deng Y, *et al.* Alagille syndrome is caused by mutations in human Jagged1, which encodes a ligand for Notch1. *Nat Genet.* 1997;16:243–251.

2. Oda T, Elkahloun AG, Pike BL, *et al.* Mutations in the human Jagged1 gene are responsible for Alagille syndrome. *Nat Genet.* 1997;16:235–242.

3. McDaniell R, Warthen DM, Sanchez-Lara PA, *et al.* NOTCH2 mutations cause Alagille syndrome, a heterogeneous disorder of the notch signaling pathway. *Am J Hum Genet.* 2006;79:169–173.

4. Bove KE, Heubi JE, Balistreri WF, *et al.* Bile acid synthetic defects and liver disease: a comprehensive review. *Pediatr Dev Pathol.* 2004;7:315–334.

5. Strautnieks SS, Bull LN, Knisely AS, *et al.* A gene encoding a liver-specific ABC transporter is mutated in progressive familial intrahepatic cholestasis. *Nat Genet.* 1998;20:233–238.

6. Strautnieks SS, Byrne JA, Pawlikowska L, *et al.* Severe bile salt export pump deficiency: 82 different ABCB11 mutations in 109 families. *Gastroenterology.* 2008;134:1203–1214.

7. Bull LN, van Eijk MJ, Pawlikowska L, *et al.* A gene encoding a P-type ATPase mutated in two forms of hereditary cholestasis. *Nat Genet.* 1998;18:219–224.

8. Klomp LW, Vargas JC, van Mil SW, *et al.* Characterization of mutations in ATP8B1 associated with hereditary cholestasis. *Hepatology.* 2004;40:27–38.

9. Jara P, Hierro L, Martinez-Fernandez P, *et al.* Recurrence of bile salt export pump deficiency after liver transplantation. *N Engl J Med.* 2009;361:1359–1367.

10. Keitel V, Burdelski M, Vojnisek Z, *et al.* De novo bile salt transporter antibodies as a possible cause of recurrent graft failure after liver transplantation: A novel mechanism of cholestasis. *Hepatology.* 2009;50:510–517.

11. de Vree JM, Jacquemin E, Sturm E, *et al.* Mutations in the MDR3 gene cause progressive familial intrahepatic cholestasis. *Proc Natl Acad Sci USA.* 1998;95:282–287.

12. Rosmorduc O, Poupon R. Low phospholipid associated cholelithiasis: association with mutation in the MDR3/ABCB4 gene. *Orphanet J Rare Dis.* 2007;2:29.

13. Baker AJ, Portmann B, Westaby D, *et al.* Neonatal sclerosing cholangitis in two siblings: a category of progressive intrahepatic cholestasis. *J Pediatr Gastroenterol Nutr.* 1993;17:317–322.

14. Hadj-Rabia S, Baala L, Vabres P, *et al.* Claudin-1 gene mutations in neonatal sclerosing cholangitis associated with ichthyosis: a tight junction disease. *Gastroenterology.* 2004;127:1386–1390.

15. Chagnon P, Michaud J, Mitchell G, *et al.* A missense mutation (R565W) in cirhin (FLJ14728) in North American Indian childhood cirrhosis. *Am J Hum Genet.* 2002;71:1443–1449.

16. Bull LN, Roche E, Song EJ, *et al.* Mapping of the locus for cholestasis–lymphedema syndrome (Aagenaes syndrome) to a 6.6-cM interval on chromosome 15q. *Am J Hum Genet.* 2000;67: 994–999.

17. Gissen P, Johnson CA, Morgan NV, *et al.* Mutations in VPS33B, encoding a regulator of SNARE-dependent membrane fusion, cause arthrogryposis–renal dysfunction–cholestasis (ARC) syndrome. *Nat Genet.* 2004;36:400–404.

18. Bosma PJ. Inherited disorders of bilirubin metabolism. *J Hepatol.* 2003;38:107–117.

19. Paulusma CC, Kool M, Bosma PJ, *et al.* A mutation in the human canalicular multispecific organic anion transporter gene causes the Dubin–Johnson syndrome. *Hepatology.* 1997;25:1539–1542.

20. Yu B, Mitchell GA, Richter A. Cirhin up-regulates a canonical NF-kappaB element through strong interaction with Cirip/HIVEP1. *Exp Cell Res.* 2009;315:3086–3098.

Liver Disease

CHAPTER 95
Disturbances of bilirubin metabolism

Cristina Bellarosa and Claudio Tiribelli

University of Trieste, Trieste, Italy

Liver Disease

ESSENTIAL FACTS ABOUT PATHOGENESIS

- These are hereditary syndromes in which hyperbilirubinemia is related to a genetic disorder of bilirubin transport and metabolism. They may be classified into those characterized by unconjugated hyperbilirubinemia and those characterized by conjugated hyperbilirubinemia
- Unconjugated hyperbilirubinemia syndromes, such as Gilbert syndrome and Crigler–Najjar (types I and II) syndrome, are caused by anomalies in bilirubin-conjugating capacity
- Conjugated hyperbilirubinemia syndromes, such as Dubin–Johnson and Rotor syndrome, are caused by impaired excretion of conjugated bilirubin into the bile canaliculus

ESSENTIALS OF DIAGNOSIS

Gilbert syndrome
- Clinically silent except for mild unconjugated hyperbilirubinemia (1–5 mg/dL) that becomes more pronounced and clinically apparent with fasting, vomiting, or intercurrent infections
- Normal routine liver function tests and hepatic histology
- Diagnosis is established by genetic screening for the TATA7 mutation

Crigler-Najjar (types I and II) syndrome
- Type I is characterized by the presence, at birth, of severe unconjugated hyperbilirubinemia (20–30 mg/dL), which may lead to severe neurological complications (kernicterus) and is unresponsive to phenobarbital
- Type II is characterized by lower levels of unconjugated hyperbilirubinemia (8–12 mg/dL) and is sensitive to phenobarbital. The diagnosis is made by demonstrating the absence of UGT1A1 activity on a liver biopsy specimen and confirmed by genotyping UGT1A1 alleles

Dubin–Johnson and Rotor syndrome
- Characterized by chronic, benign, intermittent conjugated hyperbilirubinemia and bilirubinuria
- Dubin-Johnson syndrome is characterized by increased urinary coproporphyrin I levels and the finding, on liver biopsy, of a greenish-black liver with the presence of intracellular pigment granules that are neither bile nor iron
- Pigmentation is absent in Rotor syndrome

ESSENTIALS OF TREATMENT

Gilbert syndrome
- Although phenobarbital has been proposed to decrease serum bilirubin levels in Gilbert syndrome, its use should be recommended only for cosmetic purposes

Crigler–Najjar (types I and II)
- The only permanent cure is orthotopic liver transplantation (OLT), which corrects the metabolic defect
- To reduce the probability of kernicterus, neonates must be immediately treated with phototherapy to reduce hyperbilirubinemia; survival depends on indefinite phototherapy
- Albumin infusion and plasmapheresis must be considered when the effect of other therapies is insufficient

Introduction

Bilirubin is the terminal product of heme present in hemoglobin, myoglobin, and some enzymes. A healthy adult produces 250–300 mg of bilirubin/day: 80% derives from hemoglobin (breakdown of senescent erythrocytes), 15–20% from the turnover of myoglobin, cytochromes, and other hemoproteins, and <3% from destruction of immature red blood cells in the bone marrow. This fraction is greatly increased in cases of ineffective erythropoiesis, such as hemoglobinopathies, megaloblastic anemia, and lead intoxication.

Heme is degraded by the reticuloendothelial enzyme heme oxygenase, which is particularly abundant in spleen and liver Kupffer cells, the principal sites of red cell breakdown. This enzyme opens the heme ring, freeing the iron ion and forming a tetrapyrrolic chain, and finally forming biliverdin and carbon monoxide. The reaction requires oxygen and NADPH. The conversion of biliverdin to bilirubin is catalyzed by the cytosolic enzyme biliverdin reductase, which reduces biliverdin using NADH or NADPH [1] (Figure 95.1). Once released in the blood and due to its very poor water solubility, practically all (>99.9%) of the bilirubin binds to serum albumin, the main bilirubin carrier protein in blood; <0.1% of the pigment is unbound to albumin (free bilirubin, Bf). This fraction, however, can increase in the presence of some drugs, e.g., sulfonamides, non-steroidal anti-inflammatory drugs,

Textbook of Clinical Gastroenterology and Hepatology, Second Edition. Edited by C. J. Hawkey, Jaime Bosch, Joel E. Richter, Guadalupe Garcia-Tsao, Francis K. L. Chan.
© 2012 Blackwell Publishing Ltd. Published 2012 by Blackwell Publishing Ltd.

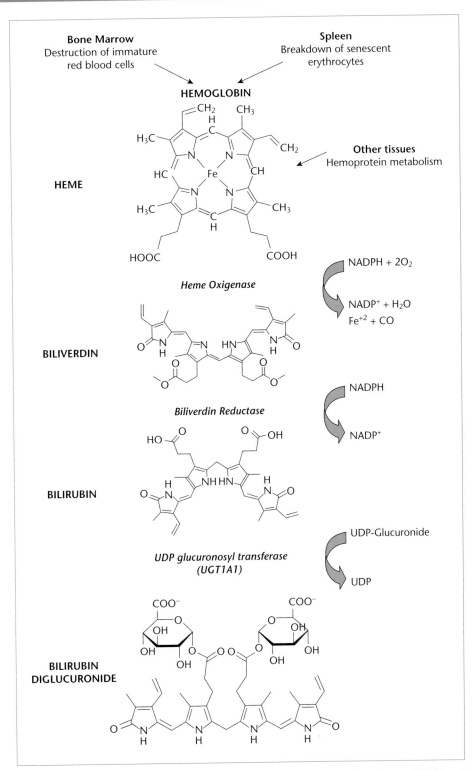

Figure 95.1 Bilirubin metabolism. Bilirubin derives from heme metabolism by heme-oxigenase and biliverdin reductase. UGT1A1 conjugates bilirubin with glucuronic acid, forming bilirubin mono- or di-glucuronides.

and some radiological contrast agents, which inhibit the binding of bilirubin to albumin. Free bilirubin present in Disse's space is internalized by hepatocytes.

The mechanism(s) of bilirubin uptake is not fully clarified. It is a saturable process, indicating the presence of membrane transporters; however, the specific carrier molecule is still undetermined. Once internalized by the hepatocyte, bilirubin is metabolized by the enzyme uridine diphosphoglucuronosyl transferase (UGT), located in the endoplasmic reticulum, which conjugates bilirubin with one or two molecules of

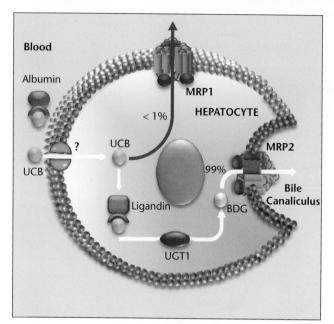

Figure 95.2 Bilirubin pathway in normal hepatocytes. Bilirubin circulates in blood tightly bound to albumin. The free portion of unconjugated bilirubin (UCB) enters the hepatocyte through an unknown carrier system. Inside the hepatocyte, UCB is bound to ligandin, transformed into bilirubin diconjugate (BDG) by the reticuloendothelial enzyme UGT1, and secreted into bile canaliculus by multidrug resistance protein 2 (MRP2). Less than 1% of bilirubin is secreted in unconjugated form in the blood, most probably by multidrug resistance protein 1 (MRP1). (This figure was published in *Clinical Gastroenterology and Hepatology*, Wilfred M. Weinstein, Christopher J. Hawkey, Jaime Bosch, Disturbances of bilirubin metabolism, Pages 1–6, Copyright Elsevier, 2005.)

glucuronic acid, rendering it hydrosoluble. Bilirubin glucuronides are then extruded into the bile canaliculus by the membrane transporter multidrug resistance protein 2 (MRP2 or ABCC2) and eventually secreted into the duodenum [1] (Figure 95.2). Any abnormality causing slowing or blockage of this rather complicated metabolic pathway will lead to disturbances of bilirubin metabolism.

Definition

The **inherited disorders of bilirubin metabolism** or "familial non-hemolytic hyperbilirubinemias" are defined as hereditary syndromes where the cause of hyperbilirubinemia is related to a genetic disorder of bilirubin transport and metabolism. They are classified into **unconjugated and conjugated hyperbilirubinemias**, the first being Gilbert syndrome and Crigler–Najjar syndrome types I and II, and the second Dubin–Johnson and Rotor syndromes. Gilbert syndrome and the Crigler–Najjar syndrome are caused by anomalies mostly in bilirubin conjugating capacity, while Dubin–Johnson syndrome is caused by impaired extrusion of bilirubin into the bile canaliculus. The genetic defect underlying Rotor syndrome has not been determined.

Gilbert syndrome is defined as a mild, benign, unconjugated hyperbilirubinemia without signs of increased hemoly-

sis and with normal routine liver function tests and hepatic histology. **Crigler–Najjar syndrome II** is a moderate/severe, familial, unconjugated hyperbilirubinemia that is sensitive to phenobarbital treatment, while **Crigler–Najjar syndrome I** is a much more severe unconjugated hyperbilirubinemia that is unresponsive to phenobarbital. **Dubin–Johnson** and **Rotor syndromes** are each defined as a chronic, benign, intermittent jaundice due to conjugated hyperbilirubinemia and bilirubinuria.

Epidemiology

Gilbert syndrome is the most common familial hyperbilirubinemia, and the most frequent cause of increased plasma bilirubin levels in adults. It is estimated that it occurs in 3–10% of the total population. However, this prevalence could be an underestimate due to the fluctuating nature of bilirubinemia in these subjects. The male-to-female ratio is 8:1, probably due to a greater heme loading from muscle myoglobin metabolism or hormonal differences. The discovery of a **TATA box mutation** at the A1 exon of UGT as a major cause of Gilbert syndrome opened the way to genetic population studies. The mutation is extremely frequent: 34–40% of Caucasians are heterozygote and 12–16% are homozygote [2]. Since only 3–10% express the phenotype, it appears that other factors are needed for the clinical expression of Gilbert syndrome. In contrast to Gilbert syndrome, both Crigler–Najjar I and II syndromes are very rare, affecting ~0.6 in 1 000 000 newborns. Dubin-Johnson syndrome and Rotor syndrome are also extremely rare, although the former is more prevalent in Sephardic Jews.

Causes and pathogenesis
UGT gene

UGT is a 100-kb gene located on the q37 region of chromosome 2. It consists of four common exons, named 2–5, that encode the carboxy-terminal portion of the enzyme, and 13 variable exons, named A1–A13, encoding the amino-terminal part of each isoform. All exons are preceded by a 5'-flanking regulatory region that controls transcription and splicing in response to specific signals. During transcription, the transcript of each single variable exon is found with the transcripts of common exons, forming nine different mRNAs that encode different UGT isoforms. The carboxy-terminal part of the enzyme encoded by the common exons is responsible for glucuronidation, while the amino-terminal portion encoded by each of the variable exons determines the substrate specificity of the isoform. The isoform containing exon A1 (UGT1A1) is responsible for bilirubin glucuronidation (Figure 95.3) [3].

Gilbert syndrome

The main cause of Gilbert syndrome is a mutation in the 5'-flanking region of the A1 exon where the "TATA box" promoter that binds the transcription factor is located. The sequence of this promoter is normally A(TA)6TAA. In subjects

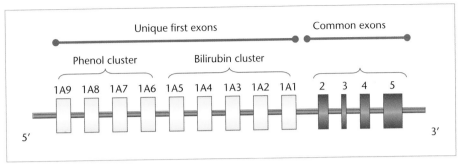

Figure 95.3 Structure of the *UGT* gene. The human *UGT* gene contains nine unique exons (1A1–1A9) and four common exons (2–5).

with Gilbert syndrome, the sequence is mutated in both alleles of the A1 exon by the insertion of two nucleotides, TA, changing the sequence to A(TA)7TAA. This causes a 70% reduction in A1 exon transcription activity and therefore, in the conjugation capacity [4].

However, strong evidence suggests that the abnormalities observed in Gilbert syndrome are more complex than those that can be deduced from genetic analysis of *UGT*. This is consistent with the discrepancy between the genetic (TATA7) and phenotypic (increased plasma levels of unconjugated bilirubin) expression of the syndrome. Experimental evidence suggests that in addition to reduced conjugating activity, Gilbert syndrome subjects have an impaired uptake of bilirubin and other related organic anions. Studies using bromosulfophtalein (BSP), a molecule that simulates bilirubin, showed a significantly reduced hepatic uptake in patients with Gilbert syndrome compared to normal subjects, suggesting that the still undefined membrane transporter(s) may have a reduced affinity for the substrate, probably because of underlying mutations.

Crigler–Najjar syndrome types I and II

The mutations present in Crigler–Najjar syndrome I involve the coding regions of the *UGT* gene. The type of mutation is mainly nonsense or frameshift, leading to truncated and/or non-functional UGT or to no transcription, thereby completely abolishing bilirubin conjugating activity. Crigler–Najjar syndrome I is a disease of autosomal recessive inheritance in which bilirubin conjugation is completely abolished.

Crigler–Najjar syndrome II is also an autosomal recessive disorder, but unlike in Crigler–Najjar syndrome I, some conjugating activity is still present and, although the enzyme is synthesized at lower than normal levels and is less functional, its expression/function can be increased by the administration of phenobarbital. The mutations described are of missense type, altering the enzyme conformation but not abolishing its transcription. This greatly diminishes bilirubin conjugation, lowering it to <5% [4].

Dubin–Johnson and Rotor syndromes

The cause of Dubin–Johnson syndrome is a nonsense mutation of the coding region of the gene for MRP2 (*ABCC2*), the canalicular membrane transporter belonging to the ABC transporter family that normally extrudes a vast number of metabolites into bile, including conjugated bilirubin. Bilirubin glucuronides reflux back into blood, creating a typical pattern of conjugated hyperbilirubinemia, and are excreted by the kidneys, causing bilirubinuria. It is an autosomal recessive disease likely due to a functional mutation of the transporter affecting the cytoplasmic/binding domain.

Rotor syndrome is a relatively benign autosomal recessive bilirubin disorder of unknown origin. It is a distinct disorder, yet similar to Dubin–Johnson syndrome.

Clinical presentation
Gilbert syndrome

Gilbert syndrome is silent, the only sign being mild scleral icterus that becomes more pronounced (clinically evident jaundice) during fasting, vomiting, or intercurrent infections. Epidemiological studies have shown that subjects with Gilbert syndrome have a significantly reduced risk of cardiovascular diseases, most probably due to the antioxidant properties of unconjugated bilirubin [5].

Crigler–Najjar syndrome types I and II

Type I is characterized by the presence, at birth, of severe unconjugated hyperbilirubinemia (20–30 mg/dL), without other signs or symptoms. Patients are otherwise healthy; however, if hyperbilirubinemia remains untreated, it leads to severe neurological complications, the so-called bilirubin-induced neurodysfunction (BIND), which may proceed to the irreversible and much more serious picture of kernicterus. Type II is characterized by lower levels of unconjugated hyperbilirubinemia, ranging between 8 and 12 mg/dL. The only clinical manifestation is jaundice [6].

Dubin–Johnson and Rotor syndromes

Dubin–Johnson and Rotor syndrome are characterized by familial idiopathic benign jaundice presenting with chronic intermittent conjugated hyperbilirubinemia and bilirubinuria without other serum test abnormalities. Onset is typically in adults, although it may rarely manifest in infancy as severe cholestasis.

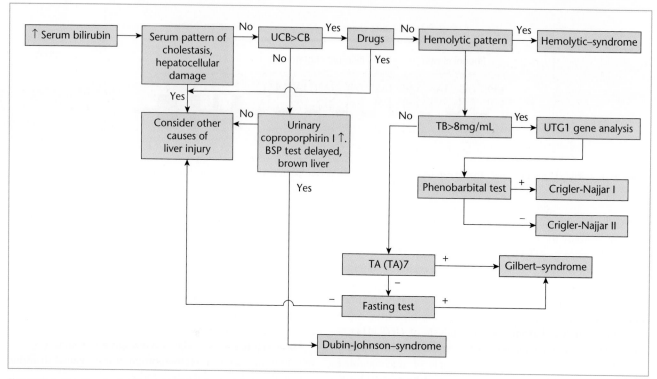

Figure 95.4 Algorithm for the diagnosis of disturbances of inherited bilirubin metabolism. BSP, bromosulfophthalein; CB, conjugated bilirubin; TA(TA)7, see text; TB, total bilirubin; UCB, unconjugated bilirubin. (This figure was published in *Clinical Gastroenterology and Hepatology*, Wilfred M. Weinstein, Christopher J. Hawkey, Jaime Bosch, Disturbances of bilirubin metabolism, Pages 1–6, Copyright Elsevier, 2005.)

Diagnosis

Gilbert syndrome

Gilbert syndrome must be suspected when routine tests show an increased total serum bilirubin (1–5 mg/mL), mostly of the unconjugated (indirect) fraction. The diagnosis is confirmed by excluding liver disease and hemolysis (Figure 95.4). An increased level of plasma unconjugated bilirubin associated with a TA(TA)7 gene profile is diagnostic of Gilbert syndrome. A functional test is the fasting test, which is based on the observation that during fasting (400 calories/day for 24 hours), the serum bilirubin increases much more significantly (2–4 times) than in controls [7].

Why is establishing the diagnosis of Gilbert syndrome useful? For one, it is important to reassure the subject that their life-expectancy and morbidity will not be influenced by this disorder and that jaundice will be life-long and may increase with co-existing illnesses. Also, since Gilbert syndrome is associated with a reduced liver uptake of other organic anions, an impaired metabolism of some drugs may occur [8]. Such drugs include irinotecan and TAS-103 (both inhibitors of topoisomerase I), as well as indinavir, which can lead to pronounced hyperbilirubinemia due to both impaired conjugation and increased hemolysis [8]. Several other drugs (Table 95.1) have been reported to be potentially toxic in Gilbert syndrome because of their reduced glucuronidation and/or hepatic elimination [9].

Table 95.1 Drugs that have modified metabolism in patients with Gilbert syndrome, and type of experimental evidence

Drug	Experimental evidence
Menthol	↓ Glucuronidation *in vivo*
Tolbutamine	↓ Glucuronidation *in vivo*
Rifamycin	↓ Glucuronidation *in vivo*
Acetaminophen	↓ Clearance *in vivo*
Irinotecan	Toxicity in case report and retrospective study
TAS	Dose-limiting toxicity in phase I study
Indinavir	↑ Adverse effect *in vivo*
Ethinylestradiol	↓ Glucuronidation *in vitro*
Lorazepam	↓ Clearance *in vivo*
Rifampin (rifampicin)	↓ Clearance *in vivo*
Buprenorphine	↓ Glucuronidation *in vivo*

Data from Bosma [8] and Burchell *et al.* [9].

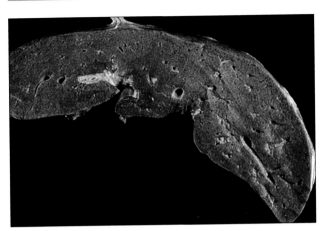

Figure 95.5 Dubin–Johnson syndrome. Liver of patient with Dubin–Johnson syndrome showing the distinctive blackish-brown color.

Crigler–Najjar syndrome types I and II

The differential diagnosis between Crigler–Najjar syndrome types I and II is based on **serum bilirubin levels** (almost double in those with type I) and the different **response to phenobarbital**. Crigler–Najjar syndrome I patients do not respond to phenobarbital while in Crigler–Najjar syndrome II a reduction in serum bilirubin of about 50% is commonly observed after phenobarbital administration (3–5 mg/kg/day, single administration). The diagnosis is made by demonstrating the absence of UGT1A1 activity on a liver biopsy specimen and confirmed by genotyping UGT1A1 alleles [6].

Dubin–Johnson and Rotor syndromes

In Dubin–Johnson syndrome the diagnosis is based on increased urinary coproporphyrin I levels [10], and the finding, at liver biopsy, of a greenish-black liver specimen with the presence of intracellular pigment granules that are neither bile nor iron [10] (Figure 95.5).

Rotor's syndrome differs from Dubin–Johnson syndrome because there is no brown pigment in the liver.

Both syndromes have an excellent prognosis. Accordingly, liver biopsy is not necessary to reach a final diagnosis.

Treatment

Gilbert syndrome

Although phenobarbital has been proposed to decrease serum bilirubin levels in Gilbert syndrome, its use should be recommended only for cosmetic purposes.

Crigler–Najjar syndrome types I and II

The only permanent cure is **orthotopic liver transplantation (OLT)**, which permanently corrects the metabolic defect. The optimal timing for OLT is before school age and definitely before adolescence [11, 12].

Kernicterus is the most important and severe complication of Crigler–Najjer syndrome and is of prognostic significance.

To reduce the probability of kernicterus, neonates with Crigler–Najjar syndrome must be treated immediately at birth with **phototherapy** to reduce hyperbilirubinemia, and their survival will be dependent on continuing this therapy indefinitely. With age, however, the efficacy of phototherapy is reduced unless the number of treatment hours is increased (from 10–12 to 16–18 hours/day) due to increased skin thickness and unfavorable body surface-to-weight ratio. Treatment with protoporphyrin IX, a potent heme oxygenase inhibitor, has been suggested as an adjuvant to phototherapy as it appears to increase the latter's effect. Since infections or other concomitant illnesses can potentially exacerbate jaundice and lead to kernicterus, avoiding factors that may exacerbate jaundice is a crucial aspect in the management of this condition. In case of acute bilirubin encephalopathy due to the exacerbation of jaundice, the duration of phototherapy must be increased. Oral calcium supplementation, through sequestration of fecal bilirubin, also makes phototherapy more efficient. More efficient is the treatment with ursodeoxycholic acid or with orlistat. Albumin infusion and plasmapheresis must be considered when the effect of other therapies is insufficient.

Gene therapy is a hopeful prospect but is currently not feasible or available.

SOURCES OF INFORMATION FOR PATIENTS AND DOCTORS

Gilbert's syndrome
http://www.patient.co.uk/showdoc/316/
Crigler–Najar syndrome
http://www.patient.co.uk/showdoc/40001363/
Dubin–Johnson syndrome
http://www.patient.co.uk/showdoc/40001223/

References

1. Ostrow JD, editor. *Bile Pigments and Jaundice: Molecular, Metabolic and Medical Aspects*. New York: Marcel Dekker, 1986.
2. Bosma PJ, Chowdhury JR, Bakker C, *et al.* The genetic basis of the reduced expression of bilirubin UDP-glucuronosyltransferase 1 in Gilbert's syndrome. *N Engl J Med.* 1995;333:1171–1175.
3. Gong QH, Cho JW, Huang T, *et al.* Thirteen UDP glucuronosyltransferase genes are encoded at the human UGT1 gene complex locus. *Pharmacogenetics.* 2001;11:357–368.
4. Kadakol A, Ghosh SS, Sappal BS, Sharma G, Chowdhury JR, Chowdhury NR. Genetic lesions of bilirubin uridinediphosphoglucuronate glucuronosyltransferase (UGT1A1) causing Crigler-Najjar and Gilbert syndromes: correlation of genotype to phenotype. *Hum Mutat.* 2000;16:297–306.
5. Rigato I, Ostrow JD, Tiribelli C. Bilirubin and the risk of common non-hepatic diseases. *Trends Mol Med.* 2005;11:277–283.
6. Crigler JF Jr, Najjar VA. Congenital familial nonhemolytic jaundice with kernicterus. *Pediatrics.* 1952;10:169–180.
7. Gentile S, Orzes N, Persico M, Marmo R, Bronzino P, Tiribelli C. Comparison of nicotinic acid- and caloric restriction-induced hyperbilirubinaemia in the diagnosis of Gilbert's syndrome. *J Hepatol.* 1985;1:537–543.

Liver Disease

Part 2: Diseases of the Gut and Liver

8. Bosma PJ. Inherited disorders of bilirubin metabolism. *J Hepatol.* 2003;38:107–117.

9. Burchell B, Soars M, Monaghan G, Cassidy A, Smith D, Ethell B. Drug-mediated toxicity caused by genetic deficiency of UDP-glucuronosyltransferases. *Toxicol Lett.* 2000;112–113:333–340.

10. Dubin IN, Johnson FB. Chronic idiopathic jaundice with unidentified pigment in liver cells; a new clinicopathologic entity with a report of 12 cases. *Medicine (Balt).* 1954;33:155–197.

11. Gridelli B, Lucianetti A, Gatti S, *et al.* Orthotopic liver transplantation for Crigler-Najjar type I syndrome. *Transplant Proc.* 1997;29:440–441.

12. Jansen PL. Diagnosis and management of Crigler-Najjar syndrome. *Eur J Pediatr.* 1999;158 (Suppl 2):S89–S94.

CHAPTER 96
Polycystic liver diseases

Luca Fabris,[1,2] Catherine McCrann[2] and Mario Strazzabosco[2,3]

[1]University of Padua, Padua, Italy
[2]Yale University, New Haven, CT, USA
[3]University of Milan-Bicocca, Milan, Italy

ESSENTIAL FACTS ABOUT PATHOGENESIS

- Inherited disorders, characterized by multiple cysts scattered in liver parenchyma, derived from but not connected to the biliary tree
- Mutations in genes encoding for ciliary proteins (polycystin-1 and polycystin-2) in the case of autosomal dominant polycystic kidney disease (ADPKD) or endoplasmic reticulum-associated proteins (hepatocystin and Sec63) in the case of autosomal dominant polycystic liver disease (PCLD)

ESSENTIALS OF DIAGNOSIS

- Radiological: incidental findings at imaging or during investigations for mass-related symptoms or cyst complications
- Extrahepatic manifestations: renal failure in ADPKD, vascular abnormalities
- Genetic testing: available in most skilled laboratories, but of limited clinical use
- Imaging: US – highly sensitive and specific; CT, MR – before surgical therapies and in complicated cases

---

ESSENTIALS OF TREATMENT

- Screen relatives for liver/kidney cysts
- No need for specific treatment in most
- No established prevention measures, but estrogens should be avoided
- Medical therapies: effective in experimental models
- Interventional radiology and surgical therapies: percutaneous cyst aspiration (with ethanol injection), cyst fenestration, liver resection, liver transplantation (kidney-combined if renal failure) in selected, highly symptomatic cases

---

Introduction and epidemiology

The presence of liver cysts, discovered incidentally by radiological studies, is a relatively common finding in the general population (3–5% in adults) [1]. Hepatic cysts are rarely observed before puberty, and are more common in women, where cyst number and size increase sharply during childbearing and middle-age years [2]. Simple liver cysts are usually solitary or not more than three in number. Polycystic liver diseases, characterized by more than three liver cysts [3,4], are rare inherited disorders and may occur with or without renal involvement. The classification of polycystic liver diseases is shown in Table 96.1. In this chapter we will review autosomal dominant polycystic kidney disease (ADPKD) and autosomal dominant polycystic liver disease (PCLD), whereas autosomal recessive polycystic kidney disease (ARPKD), congenital hepatic fibrosis (CHF) and Caroli's disease (CD) will be discussed elsewhere.

The estimated prevalence of ADPKD is 1:400 to 1:1000 live births, making it the most common genetic cause of chronic renal failure [5]. It is characterized by the formation of multiple cysts in the kidney, liver, and pancreas, and, more rarely, seminal vesicles and arachnoid membrane. ADPKD may be associated with a variety of vascular abnormalities including intracranial aneurysms, aortic root dilation and valvular heart disease. PCLD is far less common than ADPKD, but its exact prevalence has not been determined. In PCLD the development of multiple liver cysts in absence of kidney cysts generally occurs at later ages than ADPKD [6].

Causes and pathogenesis

ADPKD is caused by mutations in *PKD1* (85–90%) or *PKD2* (10–15%), genes that encode for polycystin-1 (PC-1) or polycystin-2 (PC-2), respectively [7]. PC-1 is a transmembrane protein localized in the primary cilium of the cell, where it functions as a mechano- and chemoceptor. PC-1 senses changes in apical flow and compositions and modulates a number of cell functions including epithelial cell secretion, proliferation, and differentiation [7]. PC-2 is a non-selective membrane Ca^{2+} channel, which is regulated by PC-1, and is expressed on the cilia and endoplasmic reticulum, where it regulates Ca^{2+} homeostasis [7]. The pathogenic sequence leading from defective PC function to cystogenesis and disease progression remains unclear [8]. Key mechanisms responsible for cyst development are excessive fluid secretion, cyst hypervacularization and

Liver Disease

Textbook of Clinical Gastroenterology and Hepatology, Second Edition. Edited by C. J. Hawkey, Jaime Bosch, Joel E. Richter, Guadalupe Garcia-Tsao, Francis K. L. Chan.
© 2012 Blackwell Publishing Ltd. Published 2012 by Blackwell Publishing Ltd.

Table 96.1 Characteristics of polycystic liver diseases

Disease	Mechanism of inheritance	Defective gene	Chromosomal location	Protein encoded	Renal involvement	Prevalence	Cyst morphology
ADPKD	Autosomal dominant	*PKD1* *PKD2*	16p13 4q21–q23	PC-1 PC-2	Yes	1:400–1:1,000	Liver cysts derived from but not connected to biliary tree
PCLD	Autosomal dominant	*PRKCSH* *SEC63*	19p13.2–p13.1 6p21–p23	Hepatocystin Sec63	No	>1:1,000 (?)	Liver cysts derived from but not connected to biliary tree
ARPKD CHF CD	Autosomal recessive	*PKHD1*	6p21.1	FPC	Yes	1:6,000–1:40,000	Cystic dilation of bile ducts

ADPKD, autosomal dominant polycystic kidney disease; ARPKD, autosomal recessive polycystic kidney disease; CD, Caroli's disease/syndrome; CHF, congenital hepatic fibrosis; FPC, fibrocystin; PC-1, PC-2, polycystin-1, polycystin-2; PCLD, autosomal dominant polycystic liver disease.

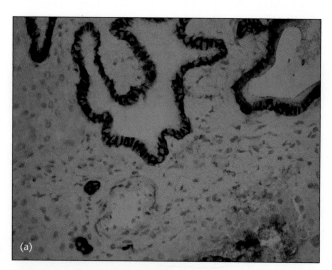
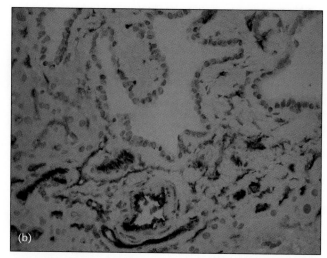

Figure 96.1 Strong hypervascularization of the biliary cysts in autosomal dominant polycystic kidney disease (ADPKD). In ADPKD, biliary cysts (identified by immunohistochemistry for HEA-125, a biliary cell marker, (a)) are surrounded by an abundant vascular bed (recognised by immunohistochemistry for CD31, an endothelial cell marker, (b)). Hypervascularisation is a key mechanism involved in the progressive cyst enlargement.

proliferation, sustained also by the autocrine action of a number of secreted growth factors and cytokines [7,9]. Notably, an abundant vascular bed strictly adjacent to the cystic epithelium is a typical histological feature in ADPKD (Figure 96.1).

PRKCSH and *SEC63* have recently been identified as the genes responsible for PCLD [10,11]. They encode for proteins that are associated with the cotranslational processing of glycoproteins in the endoplasmic reticulum (ER). In particular, hepatocystin, the *PRKCSH* protein, permits the correct localization of glucosidase II, an ER-associated enzyme that is involved in quality control of newly synthesized glycoproteins [12].

In both ADPKD and PCLD, liver cysts progressively detach from the intrahepatic bile ducts, lose their connection with the biliary tree as they expand, and subsequently compress the surrounding liver parenchyma [7] (Figure 96.2). The number and size of liver cysts are generally greater in PCLD than in ADPKD [6].

Clinical presentation

Polycystic liver diseases can remain asymptomatic for many years even in the presence of marked hepatomegaly [2]. They are usually well-tolerated conditions, diagnosed as incidental radiologic findings [2]. Polycystic liver disease is categorized according to the ratio between the total liver cysts volume and the parenchymal volume, as minimal (<1) or massive (>1) [13]. Symptoms related to liver disease (abdominal pain, early postprandial satiety, dyspnea) develop in 20% of patients and are caused by the mass effect caused by the massive liver enlargement. Weight loss may be present in some patients due to early satiety. Furthermore, ascites and edema may also occur due to cyst vascular compression of either on the hepatic venous or inferior vena cava outflow [2].

The clinical features of ADPKD are better defined than those of PCLD. The main cause of morbidity in ADPKD is progressive renal failure [2]. The renal phenotype of the *PKD1* mutation is clinically more severe than the *PKD2* mutation. Liver

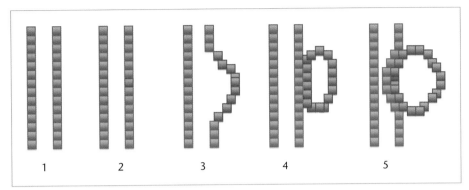

Figure 96.2 Development of hepatic cysts in autosomal dominant polycystic kidney disease (ADPKD): the two-hit model of initiation and progression. (1) One copy of *PKD1* or *PKD2* gene is present in all cells. (2) A somatic mutation, *red cell*, occurs in a single intrahepatic biliary epithelial cell. (3) Loss of function in PC-1 or PC-2 results in clonal expansion of mutated cell, with subsequent cyst development (4) and separation from intrahepatic bile duct. (5) Cyst expands and compresses the surrounding parenchyma. (Adapted with permission from Everson *et al.* Polycystic disease of the liver. *Hepatology.* 2004;40:774–782.)

cysts are the most prevalent extra-renal manifestation, present in about 50% of patients with ADPKD above 40 years of age. Arterial hypertension may be present as a consequence of kidney failure or renal artery compression.

The severity of liver disease does not correlate with the severity of renal cystic disease [2]. Liver function is usually well preserved in ADPKD, and portal hypertension does not develop unless the portal vein is compressed by massive cysts. The most common findings on physical examination are hepatomegaly and abdominal distension. Some cysts with hemorrhages or infections may become tender to palpation. Only minimal liver test abnormalities may be found, characterized by mild elevations of alkaline phosphatase and bilirubin [2].

However, severe extrahepatic manifestations, including cerebral hemorrhage due to ruptured aneurysm, may dominate the clinical picture. Aortic root dilation and mitral valve defects, have been reported in up to 20% of patients with ADPKD [14].

PCLD shares many clinical features of ADPKD, but without renal involvement [6]. Recent findings indicate that patients with PCLD are less symptomatic than ADPKD patients despite the increased number and size of liver cysts [15]. Furthermore, co-morbidity related to vascular manifestations is less frequent in PCLD than ADPKD, indicating that PCLD may be a more benign disease than ADPKD [15].

Differential diagnosis

The differential diagnosis is relatively straightforward and includes ARPKD/Caroli's disease, entities that are characterized by severe portal hypertension, acute cholangitis and characteristic radiological findings [16]. Infectious diseases, such as **Echinococcal infections**, and a variety of **benign** and **malignant cystic tumours** are part of the differential diagnosis. In both infectious cysts and in neoplasia, the cystic lesions are more commonly solitary and or septated, and may enlarge in a short period of time [4]. However, **cystic metastases** caused by central necrosis of solid metastases or by hepatic spread of cyst-forming serous carcinomas from different origin (stomach, colon, pancreas, thyroid, kidney, ovary) should also be considered in older subjects with newly detected liver cysts [17].

Diagnostic investigation

At present, there is no clear clinical advantage in genetic testing for ADPKD. The use of genetic testing should eventually be limited to patients with an evident family history of polycystic liver disease [2,4]. Direct gene sequencing of *PKD* is available in the most skilled laboratories, allowing the correct detection of pathological mutations in around 75% of patients [2]. In contrast, genetic testing for *PRKCSH* is only available for experimental purposes [2,12].

Diagnosis of polycystic liver diseases is mainly based on the history and imaging studies, which are the cornerstone of the diagnostic approach. Ultrasound (US) is highly sensitive and specific for the diagnosis of cystic lesions, and age-dependent diagnostic criteria based on US have been proposed in ADPKD according to the number and size of renal cysts (Table 96.2). As a general rule, fewer than two renal cysts in individuals aged ≥40 years, is sufficient to rule out ADPKD [18,19]. On US cysts appear as anechoic, fluid-filled focal lesions with smooth margins and tiny walls, and, generally, lack septations (Figure 96.3a). Cysts are highly variable in size, ranging from few millimeters up to 15 cm or more in diameter, with normal parenchyma in between. Liver volume is generally enlarged and may also dislocate the adjacent organs.

Computed tomography (CT) and magnetic resonance imaging (MRI) are performed in selected cases to diagnose complicated cysts, the nature of cyst content and their anatomic relationship with other intra- and extrahepatic structures [4]. On CT cysts appear isodense to water with regular margins with cyst wall enhancement following intravenous contrast because of cyst peripheral hypervascularization [20] (Figure 96.3b). On MRI cysts are classically hypointense on

Liver Disease

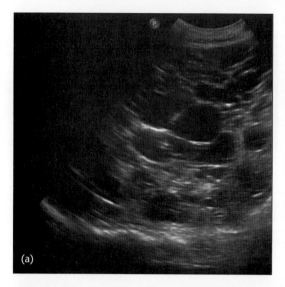

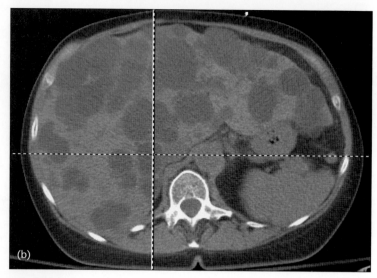

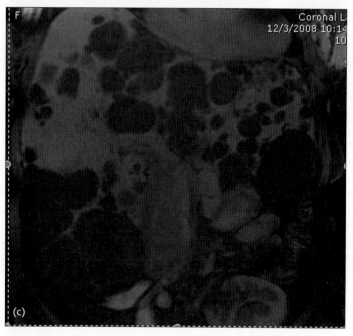

Figure 96.3 Imaging modalities in autosomal dominant polycystic kidney disease (ADPKD). On ultrasound (US) liver cysts appear as anechoic focal lesions with smooth margins and tiny walls, and without septations inside the lumen (a). On computed tomography (CT) cysts appear isodense to water with regular margins (b). On magnetic resonance imaging (MRI) cysts are classically hypointense lesions on T1-weighted images, which are not connected to the biliary tree (sagittal view, (c)).

Table 96.2 Age-dependent diagnostic criteria of ADPKD based on ultrasound findings

Age (years)	Renal involvement
<40	≥3 renal cysts (unilateral or bilateral)
40–59	≥2 renal cysts (in each kidney)
>60	≥4 renal cysts (in each kidney)

T1-weighted images and hyperintense on T2-weighted images [20] (Figure 96.3c). Signal intensity changes in cyst lesions at imaging are important for diagnosis of complicated cysts. Heterogeneous texture at US, increased attenuation at unenhanced CT or mainly, hyperintensity on both T1- and T2-weighted images at MR arise strong suspicion of cyst hemorrhage. Cyst infection is well characterized on CT.

Diagnosis of PCLD requires the exclusion of a relevant cyst renal involvement (more than five renal cysts); one or few renal cysts can be detected in 25–30% of the cases [15]. Radiological features of PCLD are similar to ADPKD.

Treatment and prevention

Most cases of polycystic liver disease do not require specific treatment. In symptomatic patients therapeutic interventions should focus on reducing cyst volume and size [2,4]. Strategies to prevent cyst growth have not been established, but the observation that hepatic but not renal cysts may worsen during pregnancy and after estrogen administration suggests that women with polycystic liver should avoid oral contraceptives or hormone replacement therapy [21]. Interventional radiology (IR) and surgical approaches can be used in selected cases.

Medical therapies

There is no accepted medical treatment for patients with ADPKD and symptomatic liver cysts. There is, however, experimental evidence that blocking cell proliferation, or VEGF, cAMP or mTOR signaling may hold promise [22–24]. Ongoing clinical studies and updated information on open clinical studies can be found in the web links at the end of the chapter.

Percutaneous cyst aspiration

Percutaneous cyst aspiration, performed under US or CT guidance in conjunction with the injection of a sclerosing agent like ethanol, can be successfully performed in selected symptomatic patients with one or a few dominant lesions [25].

Cyst fenestration

Cyst fenestration is performed in patients with massive hepatic cyst disease and superficial locations of most dominant cysts. Originally performed under laparotomy, laparoscopy is now the preferred approach for fenestration as it minimizes the risk of post-operative complications (bleeding, infections, bile leak). Argon beam coagulation or electrocoagulation can be used in conjunction with fenestration to reduce the risk of recurrence [26]. In our opinion, cyst fenestration should be attempted only if lesions are not amenable to percutaneous procedures.

Liver resection

Liver resection is considered when dominant cystic lesions have a segmental distribution. It requires a careful evaluation of the hepatic vasculature by MR angiography prior to surgery. Although long-term reduction in symptoms is obtained in >95% of cases, this procedure has significant perioperative morbidity, and therefore should be performed only in specialized centers [26], which have reported outstanding results.

Liver transplantation

Liver transplantation is indicated in highly symptomatic patients with massive cystic disease that is not amenable to other surgical treatments. Combined liver–kidney transplant is considered in ADPKD patients with end-stage renal disease at increased risk for post-operative complications following cyst fenestration or liver resection [27]. Notably, liver function is normal, therefore criteria for liver transplant listing include severe malnutrition, evaluated by serum albumin or mid-arm circumference in the non-dominant arm [28].

Complications and their management

Most severe complications of ADPKD and ADPLD are caused by the progressive enlargement of liver cysts. Complications arising in liver cysts, such as intracystic hemorrhage, cyst infection, and rupture, are uncommon (<10%) [2,4]. Clinical manifestations and complications of polycystic liver diseases are summarized in Table 96.3.

Cyst infections are more frequent in patients with endstage renal disease and are usually caused by Gram-negative enterobacteria, typically *Escherichia coli*. Fluoroquinolones are the antibiotics of choice, but cyst drainage by percutaneous procedures can be considered if there is no response to antibiotics [2,4].

Cyst hemorrhage and rupture are rarer than cyst infections and do not require specific therapies, pain control being the main objective in most cases [2,4].

Other complications, including cyst adenocarcinoma, Budd–Chiari syndrome and biliary obstruction, have been reported only sporadically [2,4]. Biliary obstruction may be caused by the compression on common bile duct by enlarging cysts. Stent placement during ERCP or cyst decompression have been effectively performed in selected cases [2,4]. The patient may become cirrhotic if biliary obstruction is not recognized correctly. An association with ampulla of Vater adenomas has been also reported for ADPKD [29].

Table 96.3 Clinical features of polycystic liver diseases

Mass effect
  Abdominal distension or palpable mass
  Early satiety
  Dyspnea

Vascular compression
  Ascites
  Edema
  Budd–Chiari syndrome (rare)

Biliary compression
  Jaundice

Cyst complications
  Cyst infection
  Cyst hemorrhage
  Cyst rupture
  Cyst adenocarcinoma (rare)

Extra-hepatic manifestations
  Renal failure (in ADPKD only)
  Intracranial aneurysm
  Mitral valve defects
  Aortic root aneurysm

Liver Disease

Prognosis with/without treatment

ADPKD and PCLD are well-tolerated, mainly asymptomatic diseases, and the potential complications are generally not life threatening. Kidney and/or liver transplantation may be performed in the most severe cases. Recent reports indicate that the 5-year survival following liver or combined liver–kidney transplantation is about 85%, and is not diminished by concomitant renal failure. Post-transplanted patients typically have an excellent quality of life [30].

Acknowledgements

This work was supported by NIH DK079005 and by Yale University Liver Center (NIH DK34989) to M.S.; and by Progetto Ateneo ex60% (60A07-1474/09) and Progetto Ateneo CPDA083217 to L.F.

SOURCES OF INFORMATION FOR PATIENTS AND DOCTORS

- http://kidney.niddk.nih.gov/kudiseases/pubs/polycystic/
- http://www.rarediseases.org/search/rdblist.html
- http://www.liverfoundation.org
- http://www.clinicaltrials.gov

References

1. Carrim ZI, Murchison JT. The prevalence of simple renal and hepatic cysts detected by computed tomography. *Clin Radiol.* 2003;58:626–629.
2. Everson GT, Taylor MRG, Doctor RB. Polycystic diseases of the liver. *Hepatology.* 2004;40:774–782.
3. Ravine D, Gibson RN, Walker RG, *et al.* Evaluation of ultrasonographic diagnostic criteria for autosomal dominant polycystic kidney disease. *Lancet.* 1994;343:824–827.
4. Arnold HL, Harrison SA. New advances in evaluation and management of patients with polycystic liver disease. *Am J Gastroenterol.* 2005;100:2569–2582.
5. Gabow P. Autosomal dominant polycystic kidney disease. *New Engl J Med.* 1993;329:323–342.
6. Qian Q, Li A, King BF, *et al.* Clinical profile of autosomal dominant polycystic liver disease. *Hepatology.* 2003;37:164–171.
7. Torres VE, Harris PC. Mechanisms of disease: Autosomal dominant and recessive polycystic kidney disease. *Nat Clin Pract.* 2006;2:40–55.
8. Wilson PD. Polycystic kidney disease: New understanding in the pathogenesis. *Int J Biochem Cell Biol.* 2004;36:1868–1873.
9. Strazzabosco M, Fabris L, Spirli C. Pathophysiology of cholangiopathies. *J Clin Gastroenterol.* 2005;39:S90–S102.
10. Drenth JP, te Morsche RH, Smink R, *et al.* Germline mutations in *PRKCSH* are associated with autosomal dominant polycystic liver disease. *Nat Genet.* 2003;33:345–347.
11. Davila S, Furu L, Gharavi AG, *et al.* Mutations in *SEC63* cause autosomal dominant polycystic liver disease. *Nat Genet.* 2004;36:575–577.
12. Drenth JP, Martina JA, van de Kerkhof R, *et al.* Polycystic liver disease is a disorder of cotranslational protein processing. *Trends Mol Med.* 2005;11:37–42.
13. Everson GT, Scherzinger A, Berger-Leff N, *et al.* Polycystic liver disease: Quantitation of parenchymal and cyst volumes from computed tomography images and clinical correlates of hepatic cysts. *Hepatology.* 1988;8:1627–1634.
14. Chapman AB, Rubinstein D, Hughes R, *et al.* Intracranial aneurysm in autosomal dominant polycystic kidney disease. *New Engl J Med.* 1992;327:916–920.
15. Hoevenaren IA, Wester R, Schrier RW, *et al.* Polycystic liver: clinical characteristics of patients with isolated polycystic liver disease compared with patients with polycystic liver and autosomal dominant polycystic kidney disease. *Liver Int.* 2008;28:264–270.
16. Kerkar N, Norton K, Suchy FJ. The hepatic fibrocystic diseases. *Clin Liver Dis.* 2006;10:55–71.
17. Moons LGM, Wolfhagen FHJ, Beukers R. A rare cause of large liver cysts. *Am J Gastroenterol.* 2009;104:1056–1058.
18. Ravine D, Gibson RN, Walker RG, *et al.* Evaluation of ultrasonographic diagnostic criteria for autosomal dominant polycystic kidney disease 1. *Lancet.* 1994;343:824–827.
19. Pei Y, Obaji J, Dupuis A, *et al.* Unified criteria for ultrasonographic diagnosis of ADPKD. *J Am Soc Nephrol.* 2009;20:205–212.
20. Brancatelli G, Federle MP, Vilgrain V, *et al.* Fibropolycystic liver disease: CT and MR imaging findings. *Radiographics.* 2005;25:659–670.
21. Shrestha R, McKinley C, Russ P, *et al.* Postmenopausal estrogen therapy selectively stimulates hepatic enlargement in women with autosomal dominant polycystic kidney disease. *Hepatology.* 1997;26:1282–1286.
22. Masyuk TV, Masyuk AI, Torres VE, *et al.* Octreotide inhibits hepatic cystogenesis in vitro and in vivo: a new therapeutic approach for treatment of polycystic liver diseases. *Gastroenterology.* 2007;132:1104–1116.
23. Fabris L, Cadamuro M, Fiorotto R, *et al.* Effects of angiogenic factor overexpression by human and rodent cholangiocytes in polycystic liver diseases. *Hepatology.* 2006;43:1001–1012.
24. Spirli C, Okolicsanyi S, Fiorotto R, *et al.* ERK1/2-dependent vascular endothelial growth factor signaling sustains cyst growth in polycystin-2 defective mice. *Gastroenterology.* 2010;138:360–371.
25. Blonski WC, Campbell MS, Faust T, *et al.* Successful aspiration and ethanol sclerosis at large, symptomatic, simple liver cyst: case presentation and review of the literature. *World J Gastroenterol.* 2006;12:2949–2954.
26. Que F, Nagorney D, Gross J, *et al.* Liver resection and cyst fenestration in the treatment of severe polycystic liver disease. *Gastroenterology.* 1995;108:487–494.
27. Ueno T, Barri YM, Netto GJ. Liver and kidney transplantation for polycystic liver and kidney – renal function and outcome. *Transplantation.* 2006;82:501–507.
28. Arrazola L, Moonka D, Gish RG, *et al.* Model for end-stage liver disease (MELD) exception for polycystic liver disease. *Liver Transpl.* 2006;12(Suppl. 3):S110–S111.
29. Serafini FM, Carey LC. Adenoma of the ampulla of Vater: A genetic condition? *HPB Surg.* 1999;11:191–193.
30. Kirchner GI, Rifai K, Cantz T. Outcome and quality of life in patients with polycystic liver disease after liver or combined liver-kidney transplantation. *Liver Transpl.* 2006;12:1268–1277.

CHAPTER 97
Cirrhosis of the liver

Gennaro D'Amico and Giuseppe Malizia

Ospedale V Cervello, Palermo, Italy

ESSENTIAL FACTS ABOUT PATHOGENESIS

- Most common cause is hepatitis C virus infection, followed by alcohol abuse
- Other factors: hepatitis B virus infection, non-alcoholic steatohepatitis, autoimmune, metabolic, biliary, and genetic disorders
- Key pathogenic processes: hepatocyte damage and death; extracellular matrix deposition due to proliferation and activation of hepatic stellate cells; ductular proliferation and vascular reorganization

ESSENTIALS OF DIAGNOSIS

- Liver biopsy is the gold standard, but potential limitations are sample variation, observer variability, and potential complications. Should be performed when non-invasive markers are equivocal for the diagnosis of cirrhosis
- Compensated cirrhosis can be diagnosed with an accuracy of about 90% by a combination of clinical (firm liver, other), biochemical (AST:ALT ratio >1, platelet count $<140 \times 10^9$/L, prolonged prothrombin time, other), ultrasonographic (liver nodular surface, reduced portal flow velocity, portal vein diameter >13 mm, and lack of or reduction to <30% of respiratory variations of splenic and superior mesenteric veins), and endoscopic (esophageal and/or gastric varices, congestive gastropathy) findings
- Non-invasive indices based on a combination of laboratory test results (Fibrotest, SAFE biopsy) may be of help in the detection of cirrhosis in chronic viral hepatitis
- Transient elastography, measuring liver stiffness, may help to predict the presence of cirrhosis, particularly when combined with other non-invasive laboratory tests, and may reduce the need for liver biopsy
- Detection of signs of decompensation, such as ascites, variceal bleeding, and encephalopathy, in patients with virological, serological, and biochemical markers of liver disease rules in the diagnosis of cirrhosis

ESSENTIALS OF TREATMENT

- No specific antifibrotic therapy accepted
- Treatment of the underlying liver disease is the most effective way to reduce or eliminate hepatic fibrosis
- No treatment effective in preventing development of esophageal varices or ascites
- Treatment mainly aimed at reversing disease complications (ascites, gastrointestinal bleeding, and encephalopathy)
- Liver transplantation in patients with advanced disease

Definition

Cirrhosis is a "diffuse process characterized by fibrosis and the conversion of normal liver architecture into structurally abnormal regenerative nodules" [1]. It represents the end-stage of chronic liver damage resulting from several different causes and leading to altered hepatic function and portal hypertension.

Epidemiology and causes

The estimated prevalence of cirrhosis around the world is 100 (range 25–400) per 100 000 subjects [2], with a male-to-female ratio of 1. In 2002, according to the 2003 World Health Organization report, 783 000 individuals died from cirrhosis. The median survival in compensated cirrhosis is about 10 years [3], whereas the median age-adjusted mortality rate is 14 per 100 000 in men (range 3–68) and 5.4 in women (range 1–23) [4]. In Europe, a decline in mortality in the first half of the 1980s was related to a decrease in per capita alcohol consumption [5]. However, striking country-specific and regional variations are present. In fact, whereas in Southern Europe a substantial reduction of mortality to less than half that in previous decades has been recently observed, younger generations in Northern and Eastern Europe have shown an increased risk of death from cirrhosis, possibly due to alcohol use at younger ages, viral hepatitis, and changing dietary habits [4]. In the UK, almost 3000 deaths from cirrhosis or chronic liver disease are reported every year (about 40% from alcohol-related disease), with steadily rising rates of mortality both in men and women between the 1990s and the 2000s. In Italy in 1992 almost 15 000 patients died from cirrhosis (almost 28 deaths per 100 000 population), with a subsequent decline of mortality rates in the 2000s, similar to that observed in other Southern European countries. The most frequent cause was hepatitis C virus (HCV) infection (alone 47.7%; associated with other factors 72.7%), followed by alcohol (alone 8.7%; associated with other factors 32.9%), and hepatitis B virus (HBV) infection (alone 3.4%; associated with other factors 13.8%). In the USA in 1998 a prevalence of >5.5 million cases of chronic liver disease or cirrhosis was estimated, with a rate of 2030 cases per 100 000 population. The mortality rate was approximately 25 000 deaths (9.3 deaths

Textbook of Clinical Gastroenterology and Hepatology, Second Edition. Edited by C. J. Hawkey, Jaime Bosch, Joel E. Richter, Guadalupe Garcia-Tsao, Francis K. L. Chan.
© 2012 Blackwell Publishing Ltd. Published 2012 by Blackwell Publishing Ltd.

Liver Disease

Table 97.1 Main etiological factors in cirrhosis

- Hepatitis C virus
- Alcohol
- Hepatitis B or B/D virus
- Autoimmune hepatitis
- Metabolic disorders:
  - Hemochromatosis
  - Wilson disease
  - α_1-Antitrypsin deficiency
  - Non-alcoholic steatohepatitis
  - Diabetes
  - Glycogen storage diseases
  - Abetalipoproteinemia
  - Porphyria
- Biliary diseases:
  - Primary biliary cirrhosis
  - Primary sclerosing cholangitis
  - Intrahepatic or extrahepatic biliary obstruction
- Venous outflow obstruction:
  - Budd–Chiari syndrome
  - Veno-occlusive disease
  - Cardiac failure
- Drugs (amiodarone, methotrexate) and toxins
- Intestinal bypass
- Obesity
- Indian childhood cirrhosis
- Cryptogenic cirrhosis

per 100 000 population) annually. In two sentinel counties in the USA the most common etiology of chronic liver disease was HCV (57%), followed by alcohol (24%), non-alcoholic fatty liver disease (9.1%), and HBV (4.4%) [6].

A comprehensive list of etiological factors of cirrhosis is given in Table 97.1.

Pathogenesis

Cirrhosis is characterized by the progressive accumulation of collagen types I and III in the liver parenchyma, including the space of Disse, with the consequent "collagenization" of sinusoids. This results in the alteration of both the exchange between hepatocytes and plasma, and the regulation of intrahepatic resistance to blood flow. In cirrhosis of different etiologies, active **fibrogenesis** has been related to the increased expression of transforming growth factor-β (TGF-β) and platelet-derived growth factor (PDGF), which stimulate the activation and proliferation of hepatic stellate cells, the main source of extracellular matrix in the fibrotic liver. A significant correlation between growth factor expression, fibrogenesis, and necroinflammatory activity has been also shown. However, active fibrogenesis may be present in conditions with minimal inflammation and marked ductular proliferation (i.e., biliary atresia). A role in fibrogenesis has therefore been proposed for ductular proliferation, associated with periductular fibrosis, neutrophil infiltration, and increased expression of fibrogenic growth factors [7]. A further important event in the development of cirrhosis and its

complications is represented by the **disruption of vascular architecture**, with obstruction of veins and/or sinusoids leading to hypoxia and ischemic changes characterized by parenchymal extinction [8]. Hypoxia-inducible transcription factors (HIF) in turn stimulate secretion of vascular endothelial growth factor (VEGF) that not only induces angiogenesis – formation of new vessels – but also increases vascular permeability and promotes development of portal hypertension [9]. (See Chapters 98, 99, 100, 101 and 102 for the pathophysiology of the main complications of cirrhosis.) It is a matter of debate whether cirrhosis is reversible [8,10].

Pathology

Histologically, cirrhosis is characterized by nodular regeneration, scarring with formation of diffuse fibrous septa, and a variable degree of parenchymal necrosis. The morphological classification, based on the size of the nodules, identifies three types of cirrhosis:

- **Micronodular** – characterized by nodules mostly <3 mm in diameter, surrounded by fibrous tissue, and generally lacking terminal veins and portal tracts. It is found mostly in alcoholic cirrhosis, hemochromatosis, and bile duct obstruction
- **Macronodular** – characterized by nodules of variable size, from >3 mm to a few centimeters, so that it may be difficult to recognize the nodular structure. In this type, nodules contain both portal tracts and terminal veins. It is common in chronic viral hepatitis and autoimmune hepatitis
- **Mixed** – composed of both micronodules and macronodules. The morphological classification has a limited diagnostic value because macronodular forms may represent the late evolution of micronodular forms.

Clinical presentation

Clinically, cirrhosis can be divided into **compensated and decompensated stages**, each with different diagnostic, therapeutic, and prognostic implications.

Compensated cirrhosis

Cirrhosis may be totally asymptomatic and diagnosed fortuitously during routine biochemical testing or clinical or ultrasonographic abdominal examination. It may also become evident during abdominal surgery or at autopsy (in older reports accounting for 30–40% of all cases). Non-specific asthenia, malaise, right upper quadrant abdominal discomfort, or sleep disturbances may be the only complaints.

On **physical examination** (Table 97.2), spider angiomas may be found, mostly on the trunk, face, and upper limbs (Figure 97.1) (see also Chapter 16). Their number and size correlate with disease severity. Palmar erythema (Figure 97.2), involving the thenar and hypothenar eminences, is the expression of a dense network of arteriovenous anastomoses. White nails

Table 97.2 Diagnosis of cirrhosis

Clinical findings
- Asthenia
- Malaise
- Right upper quadrant abdominal discomfort
- Loss of libido
- Sleep disturbances
- Palmar erythema
- Dupuytren's contracture
- Spider nevi
- White nails
- Gynecomastia
- Hair loss (chest and abdomen)
- Hepatomegaly
- Splenomegaly
- Abdominal wall collaterals
- General deterioration, muscle wasting
- Jaundice
- Ascites
- Ankle edema
- Flapping tremor
- Bradylalia
- Mental state alteration (coma)
- Fetor hepaticus
- Gastrointestinal hemorrhage (hematemesis, melena)
- Hypotension, tachycardia
- Dyspnea, cyanosis

Laboratory findings
- AST : ALT ratio >1
- Low platelet count
- Hypoalbuminemia
- Hypergammaglobulinemia
- Prolonged prothrombin time
- Hyperbilirubinemia

Ultrasonographic findings
- Liver nodular surface
- Reduced portal flow velocity
- Portal vein diameter >13 mm
- Lack (or reduction <30%) of respiratory variations of splenic and superior mesenteric veins

Endoscopic findings
- Esophageal varices
- Gastric varices
- Congestive gastropathy

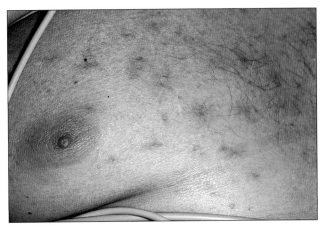

Figure 97.1 Spider nevi seen on upper truncal region.

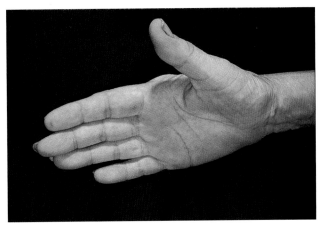

Figure 97.2 Palmar erythema due to a dense network of arteriovenous anastomoses.

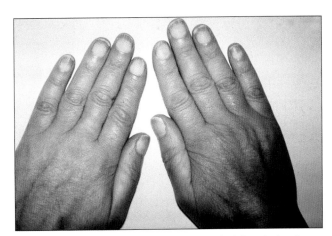

Figure 97.3 Leukonychia (white nails) occur in cirrhosis but also in other situations.

may also appear (Figure 97.3). Common in male patients is hair loss on the chest and abdomen. Gynecomastia and loss of libido may also occur. Petechiae and ecchymoses may be present as a result of thrombocytopenia and/or prolonged prothrombin time. Dupuytren's contracture, involving the palmar fascia, is particularly common in alcoholic patients. Hepatomegaly is very common, but liver size may also be normal or reduced. However, the consistency of the liver is invariably harder than normal. Splenomegaly is frequent and collateral circulation on the abdominal wall may develop, both as a consequence of portal hypertension (Figure 97.4).

Decompensated cirrhosis

Signs of decompensation – ascites, variceal hemorrhage, jaundice, and/or portosystemic encephalopathy – are found at presentation in a proportion of patients, varying between 20% and 63%. **Ascites** is by far the most frequent sign of

Liver Disease

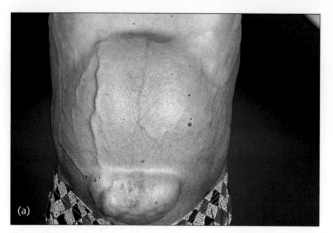 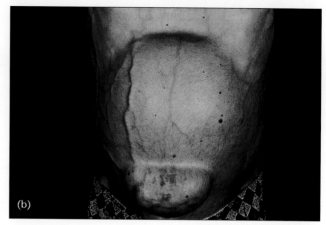

Figure 97.4 Prominent abdominal veins (and a paraumbilical hernia) in a patient with cirrhosis and ascites. (a) Under normal light. (b) Under infrared light. Blood flow is away from the umbilicus.

decompensation, being present in 80% of patients with decompensated cirrhosis (see Chapters 17, 99 and 154).

On **physical examination** (Table 97.2) patients with advanced cirrhosis often present with malnutrition and muscle wasting, particularly in alcoholic cirrhosis. In decompensated cirrhosis, jaundice, and/or ascites may appear as manifestations of liver dysfunction and portal hypertension. Other signs of decompensation are those of encephalopathy – flapping tremor, bradylalia, and mental state alterations (see Chapter 102). Frequently associated with encephalopathy and severe liver dysfunction is a sweetish smell of the breath, called fetor hepaticus. Moreover, hypotension and tachycardia due to hyperdynamic circulation secondary to portal hypertension may be present. Dyspnea may also occur due to the presence of large ascites, pleural effusions, and/or alterations of the pulmonary circulation (hepatopulmonary syndrome, pulmonary hypertension, pulmonary arteriovenous anastomoses) (see Chapter 101).

Differential diagnosis

Compensated liver cirrhosis is typically a silent disease and is often detected accidentally during routine investigations. Clinical examination, the pattern of liver tests, and imaging techniques help to differentiate cirrhosis from chronic hepatitis or from hematological diseases when splenomegaly and low platelet count are present. Liver biopsy may be needed to exclude cirrhosis, when clinical and imaging features are equivocal. Causes of ascites other than cirrhosis include congestive heart failure, vascular disorders of the liver, and abdominal neoplasia, and these therefore need to be distinguished from decompensated cirrhosis.

Diagnostic methods

In clinical practice, **liver biopsy** (see Chapter 141) remains the gold standard for assessing liver fibrosis and cirrhosis, despite the limitations of sampling error and interobserver variability.

However, even though "definitive" tests such as histological diagnosis are important for patients and for the quantitative evaluation of treatment outcomes in clinical studies, non-invasive tests to estimate disease probability are necessary. The accuracy of these probabilistic tests is strictly dependent on disease spectrum and patient selection.

Compensated cirrhosis

The clinical history is helpful, particularly in determining the cause of cirrhosis. Exposure to viral hepatitis, workplace hazards, a history of transfusions or surgery, drug addiction, alcohol abuse, and a family history of cirrhosis may change the pre-test probability of the disease and suggest a cause. The presence of a **firm liver** has been shown to be the most accurate sign of cirrhosis, with a diagnostic accuracy of 83%, followed by the presence of collateral circulation (accuracy 76%) [11].

Laboratory tests

A value ≥1 for the ratio of aspartate aminotransferase to alanine aminotransferase (AST:ALT ratio, or AAR) has been proposed as a simple low-cost predictor of cirrhosis in viral cirrhosis [12]. A reduced platelet count (≤130–≤150 × 10^9/L) can also indicate the presence of cirrhosis. In several studies, a prolonged prothrombin time also correlated with the presence of cirrhosis. Serum hyaluronate measurement has been shown to have an accuracy of about 90%, being particularly useful for excluding the presence of cirrhosis. Further non-invasive indices based only on a combination of laboratory test results, for which Fibrotest has been the pioneer [13], have been proposed for the prediction of cirrhosis. In order to increase diagnostic accuracy, sequential algorithms (SAFE biopsy) combining a simple non-invasive marker of liver fibrosis, the AST-to-platelet ratio index (APRI), and a commercial method (Fibrotest-Fibrosure) for the identification of significant fibrosis have been proposed as an accurate tool for the detection of cirrhosis in chronic viral hepatitis [14].

Imaging techniques

Ultrasonography is a useful tool for diagnosis as it may detect nodularity of the liver surface, evidence of portal hypertension, splenomegaly, and ascites. The sensitivity of ultrasonography in detecting portal hypertension has been shown to be 80%, with a specificity of 100% when assessing the lack (or reduction to <30%) of respiratory variations of splenic and superior mesenteric veins [15]. Moreover, ultrasonographic detection of a nodular liver surface and reduction of mean portal velocity showed 79% sensitivity and 80% specificity [16].

More recently, **transient elastography (TE)** (FibroScan; Echosens, Paris, France) has been proposed for the measurement of liver stiffness [17], expressed in kilopascals (kPa). TE appears to improve the ability to define the extent of fibrosis without a liver biopsy, particularly in combination with other non-invasive tests, with pooled estimates of sensitivity and specificity of 87% (95% CI 84–90%) and 91% (95% CI 89–92%), respectively [18]. The reported selected cut-off for the diagnosis of cirrhosis varies widely between studies (9–26.5 kPA) and the optimal cut-off value for clinical practice remains debated; so the use of ranges of values rather than a single cut-off value is recommended [19]. Furthermore, a risk of overestimation of liver stiffness due to high necroinflammatory activity has been reported.

Upper endoscopy has a definite role in the diagnostic work-up as it may identify the presence of esophageal or gastric varices and congestive gastropathy. In compensated patients, the presence of esophageal varices has a sensitivity of 40% and a specificity of 99% [20]. In a series of 277 patients with abnormal liver function selected prospectively for liver biopsy, the presence of a firm liver was found to be an independent predictor of cirrhosis, together with a platelet count of $\leq 140 \times 10^9$/L and a portal vein diameter of ≥ 13 mm at ultrasonography in the absence of respiratory variations of splenic or mesenteric veins [20].

In conclusion, a combination of clinical, biochemical, ultrasonographic, and endoscopic data can establish the diagnosis of cirrhosis without liver biopsy with an accuracy of about 90% (Table 97.3). However, when a precise determination of stage of fibrosis and degree of inflammation is required, liver biopsy is necessary (see Chapter 141).

Decompensated cirrhosis

The detection of signs of decompensation, such as ascites, variceal bleeding, and encephalopathy, in patients with virological, serological, and biochemical markers of liver disease rule in the diagnosis of cirrhosis. **Abdominal ultrasonography** and **upper digestive endoscopy** are required to evaluate the need for prophylaxis of variceal hemorrhage (see Chapter 98) and to exclude the presence of hepatocellular carcinoma (see Chapter 104), respectively.

Treatment and prevention

For the treatment of clinical manifestations and complications of **decompensated cirrhosis**, see Chapters 98–102, 108.

The treatment of **compensated cirrhosis** is essentially based on management of its etiology, careful avoidance of alcohol and hepatotoxic drugs, and early detection of initial signs of decompensation. An adequate nutritional regimen should include 1.0–1.2 g of protein/kg bodyweight. Theoretically, the treatment of cirrhosis, particularly in the compensated phase of the disease, should be aimed at the interruption of fibrogenesis and the resorption of fibrosis. However, no drugs have been approved as antifibrotic agents in humans and the most effective way to eliminate or reduce hepatic fibrosis is to treat the underlying liver disease. A reduction in fibrosis has been reported in some patients with chronic infection with HCV treated with interferon-α and ribavirin. Moreover, a reduction in the incidence of decompensation and hepatocellular carcinoma has been reported in patients with HCV-related

Liver Disease

Table 97.3 Operating characteristics of signs and tests in the diagnosis of cirrhosis

Sign/test	Sensitivity (%)	Specificity (%)	LR+	LR–
Firm liver	89	47	1.67	0.23
Platelet count <140 000/mm³	59	85	4.0	0.48
AST/ALT ratio >1* Ultrasonography:	53 (44–78)	96 (90–100)	11.7 (7.3–53)	0.48 (0.25–0.59)
– Lack (or reduction to <30%) of respiratory variations of splenic and mesenteric veins	80	100	—	0.20
– Liver nodular surface/reduced portal flow velocity	79	80	3.9	0.26
Endoscopy: esophageal varices	40	99	40	0.60
Liver biopsy	80	100	—	0.20

LR+, likelihood ratio for a positive result; LR–, likelihood ratio of a negative result.
*Median (range) from seven studies.

compensated cirrhosis treated with pegylated interferon and ribavirin, but this has never been proven by randomized controlled trials. No treatment has yet been shown to be effective in preventing the development or progression of esophageal varices.

Complications and their management

Variceal bleeding, ascites, encephalopathy, and jaundice are the major clinical manifestations of liver cirrhosis. The appearance of these complications marks the transition from the **compensated phase** to the **decompensated phase** of cirrhosis. The management of these complications is also discussed in Chapters 15, 98, 99, and 102.

Variceal hemorrhage

The incidence of variceal hemorrhage is approximately 2%/year in patients without varices at diagnosis, 5% in those with small varices, and 15% in those with medium or large varices. Independent of variceal size, major indicators of the risk of bleeding are Child–Pugh class, ascites, and red wale marks on varices. These risk indicators have been combined in the North Italian Endoscopic Club (NIEC) index [21], which, by identifying patients with a predicted 1-year bleeding risk ranging from 6% to 76%, is the best available system for predicting first variceal hemorrhage, although its accuracy is far from satisfactory.

Portal pressure: esophageal varices do not bleed below a threshold portal pressure level [as determined by the hepatic venous pressure gradient (HVPG)] of 12 mmHg [22,23]; this risk, as well as the risk of death, is significantly reduced if the HVPG is reduced by 20% or more from baseline [24].

Ruptured esophageal varices cause 60–70% of all upper gastrointestinal bleeding episodes in cirrhosis [25] (Figure 97.5). Variceal bleeding is diagnosed on endoscopy, either by blood spurting from a varix, white nipple or clot adherent on a varix, or by varices without other potential sources of bleeding. Rebleeding is distinguished from the initial bleeding episode by a bleed-free period of at least 24 hours. Variceal hemorrhage

ceases spontaneously in 40–50% of patients, and treatment achieves control of bleeding within 24 hours from admission in nearly 75% of cases [25] Active bleeding on endoscopy, bacterial infection, Child–Pugh class, and HVPG >20 mmHg are predictors of failure to control bleeding. The immediate mortality rate from uncontrolled bleeding is approximately 5%, and 6-week rebleeding occurs in 20%. Active bleeding at emergency endoscopy, gastric varices, low albumin level, high blood urea nitrogen level, and HVPG above 20 mmHg have been reported as predictive of early rebleeding risk.

The 6-week mortality rate after variceal bleeding is 10–15%, with nearly half of the deaths caused by bleeding or early rebleeding, and a quarter occurring in the first 5 days. Albumin, bilirubin, creatinine, encephalopathy, hepatocellular carcinoma, the number of blood units transfused, bacterial infection, and HVPG above 20 mmHg are predictors of 6-week mortality. After a first episode of variceal bleeding, there is a 63% rebleeding risk and a 33% risk of death within 1 year. Reduction of HVPG to <12 mmHg completely prevents recurrent bleeding [23] and a reduction by 20% or more from baseline significantly reduces both rebleeding and mortality [24].

Other complications
Ascites and encephalopathy

Ascites develops after the porto-systemic pressure gradient has increased to >12 mmHg, when the associated vasodilatation causes under-filling of the vascular capacity, fall in the glomerular filtration rate, and renal sodium retention. At diagnosis, the prevalence of ascites ranges from 20% to 60%, according to referral pattern [3]. The incidence of ascites is about 5%/year and, together with variceal hemorrhage, is the most frequent complication marking the transition from compensated to decompensated cirrhosis [3]. Less frequent is the development of **encephalopathy**, with an incidence of approximately 2–3%/year [26]. The incidence of encephalopathy in the absence of ascites or previous bleeding is, however, even lower. **Jaundice** follows the same pattern as encephalopathy, with a low incidence in the range of 2–3%/year, and almost always occurs in patients with other severe manifestations of advanced cirrhosis. Therefore, the most frequent indicators of decompensated cirrhosis are variceal hemorrhage and ascites, whereas encephalopathy and jaundice indicate a very advanced stage of the disease.

Prognosis

The outcome of cirrhosis is determined by three major factors: (1) survival time within the compensated phase; (2) the intensity of transition from the compensated to the decompensated phase; and (3) survival while in the decompensated phase.

Compensated cirrhosis

The natural history of compensated cirrhosis is still poorly defined, because patients are almost invariably free of symptoms and it is usually diagnosed fortuitously after workup of abnormal laboratory tests. Patients with compensated

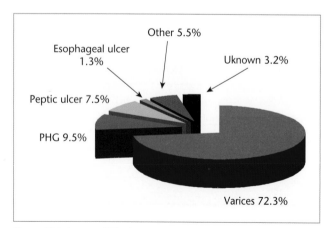

Figure 97.5 Sources of bleeding in a series of 465 consecutive patients with cirrhosis. PHG, portal hypertensive gastropathy.

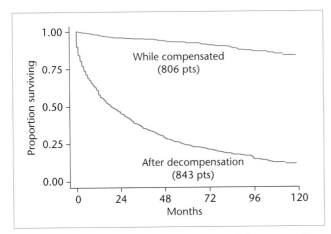

Figure 97.6 Survival of patients with compensated and decompensated cirrhosis. Data from two large prospective studies of the natural history of cirrhosis. Survival time of compensated patients was censored when they developed decompensation. (This figure was published in *Clinical Gastroenterology and Hepatology*, Wilfred M. Weinstein, Christopher J. Hawkey, Jaime Bosch, Cirrhosis of the liver, Pages 1–8, Copyright Elsevier, 2005.)

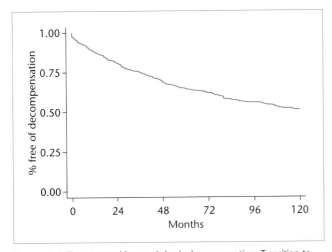

Figure 97.7 Time to transition to cirrhosis decompensation. Transition to cirrhosis decompensation (variceal bleeding, ascites, encephalopathy, jaundice) in a cohort of 806 patients with compensated cirrhosis at diagnosis. (This figure was published in *Clinical Gastroenterology and Hepatology*, Wilfred M. Weinstein, Christopher J. Hawkey, Jaime Bosch, Cirrhosis of the liver, Pages 1–8, Copyright Elsevier, 2005.)

cirrhosis die mostly after transitioning into decompensation. The 10-year survival rate for compensated patients is nearly 90%, while the median survival after decompensation is about 2 years (Figure 97.6). The progression to decompensation parallels the development and progression of portal hypertension. The 10-year transition rate to decompensation is 50% (Figure 97.7).

In patients with compensated cirrhosis the development and enlargement of esophageal varices mark the progression of the disease towards a more advanced stage.

When cirrhosis is diagnosed, the prevalence of varices ranges from 20% in compensated patients to 70% in those presenting with ascites [3]. Two large cohort studies showed that the incidence of esophageal varices in patients with newly diagnosed cirrhosis is 5–8%/year (Figure 97.8).

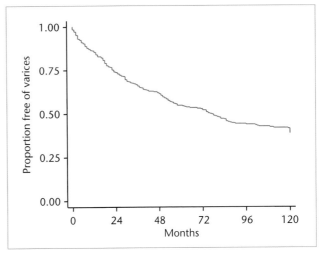

Figure 97.8 Time to development of varices. Data for a series of 1044 patients free of varices at diagnosis from two large prospective studies on the natural history of cirrhosis. (This figure was published in *Clinical Gastroenterology and Hepatology*, Wilfred M. Weinstein, Christopher J. Hawkey, Jaime Bosch, Cirrhosis of the liver, Pages 1–8, Copyright Elsevier, 2005.)

Varices do not develop below a threshold HVPG of 10–12 mmHg [22]. Above this threshold, the median time to the development of varices and/or bleeding or other complications of portal hypertension is about 4 years. Worsening liver function and continued exposure to alcohol are associated with an increase in HVPG and an increasing risk of developing varices.

Once varices develop, they increase in size at a cumulative rate of approximately 5–7%/year. Improvement in liver function and abstinence from alcohol may result in a decrease or even disappearance of varices, probably through a decrease in HVPG, as occurs for spontaneous or treatment-induced HVPG reductions [23]. Thus, HVPG plays a key role both in the development and progression of varices.

Increasing size of esophageal varices is associated with increasing bleeding risk (four-fold from absent to small varices, and two-fold from small to large varices). A similar increase in risk has been shown for the development of ascites and mortality.

In clinical practice, the size of varices is the most widely used indicator of risk of first variceal hemorrhage, because this risk is significantly reduced by prophylactic therapy in patients with medium to large varices. As non-invasive tests (particularly platelet count and abdominal ultrasonography) have not been proven to be accurate enough to avoid endoscopy in patients who are negative for the test, all patients with cirrhosis should be endoscopically screened for the presence of esophageal varices at the diagnosis of cirrhosis. Endoscopy should be repeated every 2–3 years in patients without varices. In patients with compensated cirrhosis and small varices, endoscopy should be repeated every 1–2 years to detect the progression from small to large varices. In decompensated patients without varices or with small varices, endoscopy should be repeated yearly [27].

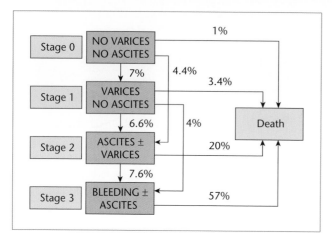

Figure 97.9 Stages in the progression of cirrhosis. Different stages of progression of cirrhosis according to the development of esophageal varices, ascites, and bleeding. Transition rates from one stage to the next are calculated from the cumulative analysis of two prospective studies on the natural history of cirrhosis. (This figure was published in *Clinical Gastroenterology and Hepatology*, Wilfred M. Weinstein, Christopher J. Hawkey, Jaime Bosch, Cirrhosis of the liver, Pages 1–8, Copyright Elsevier, 2005.)

Decompensated cirrhosis

The median survival after first variceal hemorrhage is about 1–2 years, and after the development of ascites is 2–4 years [26,28]. Encephalopathy and jaundice usually appear after bleeding or ascites, and the median survival after the first episode of encephalopathy or after the appearance of jaundice is therefore shorter than that for hemorrhage or ascites. The most frequent causes of death are bleeding, liver failure with hepatic coma, sepsis, and hepatorenal syndrome.

Outcome of cirrhosis as related to clinical stage

By combining individual patient data from two large prospective studies on the natural history of cirrhosis [26,29], four stages in the progression of the disease can be identified (Figure 97.9):

- **Stage 1** – absence of esophageal varices and ascites, with a mortality rate as low as 1%/year. Patients exit this stage when they develop varices (7%/year) and/or ascites (4.4%/year)
- **Stage 2** – varices without ascites and without hemorrhage, with a mortality rate of 3.4%/year, significantly higher than at stage 1. Patients leave this stage when they develop ascites (6.6%/year) and/or hemorrhage (4%/year)
- **Stage 3** – ascites with or without esophageal varices that have not bled, with a mortality rate of 20%/year (15% in more recent studies), significantly higher than in the two former stages. Besides death, patients leave this stage by developing hemorrhage at a rate of 7.6%/year
- **Stage 4** – variceal hemorrhage with or without ascites, with a mortality rate of 57%/year (about half of these deaths occur within 6 weeks of the bleeding episode): this figure is of the order of 35–40% in more recent studies.

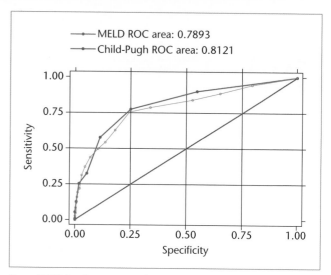

Figure 97.10 Receiver–operator characteristic (ROC) curves in prediction of survival status. ROC curves for Child–Pugh score and Model for End-stage Liver Disease (MELD) in the prediction of 6-month survival status in a cohort of 494 cirrhotic patients. (This figure was published in *Clinical Gastroenterology and Hepatology*, Wilfred M. Weinstein, Christopher J. Hawkey, Jaime Bosch, Cirrhosis of the liver, Pages 1–8, Copyright Elsevier, 2005.)

Prognostic scores

The Child–Pugh score is the most widely used system (see Chapter 155) [30]. Although it was empirically set without any statistical basis, it is highly reliable in identifying prognostically different subgroups of patients (classes A, B, and C) in particular clinical situations occurring in the course of cirrhosis. For this reason, it has been widely used to stratify patients included in clinical trials for cirrhosis, particularly in portal hypertension, and was previously included among the most important criteria used by the United Network for Organ Sharing (UNOS) for liver allocation. The UNOS has now replaced the Child–Pugh score with the Model for End-stage Liver Disease (MELD) [31]. MELD is based on objective variables not affected by subjective judgment – bilirubin, creatinine, and the international normalized ratio (INR) for prothombin time, whereas the Child–Pugh score includes ascites and encephalopathy. Easy calculation of the MELD is available at the UNOS website (www.UNOS.org/resources/meldPeldCalculator.asp). The two scores are not significantly different in their accuracy in predicting survival (Figure 97.10), but it is likely that the interobserver agreement for classifying cirrhotic patients into prognostically different subgroups is higher with MELD.

SOURCES OF INFORMATION FOR PATIENTS AND DOCTORS

http://www.gastro.org/clinicalRes/brochures/cirrhosis.html

References

1. Anthony PP, Ishak KG, Nayak NC, Poulsen HE, Scheuer PJ, Sobin LH. The morphology of cirrhosis: definition, nomenclature and classification. *Bull World Health Organ.* 1977;55:521–540.

2. La Vecchia C, Levi F, Lucchini F, Franceschi S, Negri E. World-wide patterns and trends in mortality from liver cirrhosis, 1955 to 1990. *Ann Epidemiol.* 1994;4:480–486.

3. D'Amico G, Garcia-Tsao G, Pagliaro L. Natural history and prognostic indicators of survival in cirrhosis: A systematic review of 118 studies. *J Hepatol.* 2006;44:217–231.

4. Corrao G, Ferrari P, Zambon A, Torchio P, Aricò S, Decarli A. Trends of liver cirrhosis mortality in Europe, 1970–1989: age–period– cohort analysis and changing alcohol consumption. *Int J Epidemiol.* 1997;26:100–109.

5. Bosetti C, Levi F, Lucchini F, Zatonski WA, Negri E, La Vecchia C. Worldwide mortality from cirrhosis: an update to 2002. *J Hepatol.* 2007;46:827–839.

6. Kim WR, Brown RS, Terrault NA, El-Serag H. Burden of liver disease in the United States: summary of a workshop. *Hepatology.* 2002;36:227–242.

7. Malizia G, Brunt EM, Peters MG, Rizzo A, Broekelmann TJ, McDonald JA. Growth factor and procollagen type I gene expression in human liver disease. *Gastroenterology.* 1995;108:145–156.

8. Wanless IR. Nakashima E, Sherman M. Regression oh human cirrhosis: morphologic features and the genesis of incomplete septal cirrhosis. *Arch Pathol Lab Med.* 2000;124:1599–1607.

9. Fernández M, Semela D, Bruix J, Colle I, Pinzani M, Bosch J. Angiogenesis in liver disease. *J Hepatol.* 2009;50:604–620.

10. Desmet VJ, Roskams T. Cirrhosis reversal: a duel between dogma and myth. *J Hepatol.* 2004;40:860–867.

11. Oberti F,Valsesia E, Pilette C, *et al*. Noninvasive diagnosis of hepatic fibrosis or cirrhosis. *Gastroenterology.* 1997;113:1609–1616.

12. Giannini E, Risso D, Botta F, *et al*. Validity and clinical utility of the aspartate aminotransferase–alanino aminotransferase ratio in assessing disease severity and prognosis in patients with hepatitis C virus related chronic liver disease. *Arch Intern Med.* 2003;163:218–224.

13. Imbert-Bismut F, Ratziu V, Pieroni L, Charlotte F, Benhamou Y, Poynard T. Biochemical markers of liver fibrosis in patients with hepatitis C virus infection: a prospective study. *Lancet.* 2001;357:1069–1075.

14. Sebastiani G, Halfon P, Castera L, *et al*. SAFE biopsy: a validated method for large-scale staging of liver fibrosis in chronic hepatitis C. *Hepatology.* 2009;49:1821–7

15. Bolondi L, Gandolfi L, Arienti V, Caletti GC, Corcioni E, Gasbarrini G. Ultrasonography in the diagnosis of portal hypertension: diminished response of portal vessels to respiration. *Radiology.* 1982;142:167–172.

16. Gaiani S, Gramantieri L,Venturoli N, *et al*. What is the criterion for differentiating chronic hepatitis from compensated cirrhosis? A prospective study comparing ultrasonography and percutaneous liver biopsy. *J Hepatol.* 1997;27:979–985.

17. Sandrin L, Fourquet B, Hasquenoph JM, *et al*. Transient elastography: a new noninvasive method for assessment of hepatic fibrosis. *Ultrasound Med Biol.* 2003;29:1705–1714.

18. Talwalkar JA, Kurtz DM, Schoenleber SJ, West CP, Montori VM. Ultrasound-based transient elastography for the detection of hepatic fibrosis: systematic review and metaanalysis. *Clin Gastroenterol Hepatol.* 2007;5:1214–1220.

19. Castera L. Transient elastography and other non-invasive tests to assess hepatic fibrosis in patients with viral hepatitis. *J Viral Hepatitis.* 2009;16:300–314.

20. Tinè F, Caltagirone M, Cammà C, *et al*. Clinical indicants of compensated cirrhosis: a prospective study. In: Dianzani MU, Gentilini P, editors. *Chronic Liver Damage.* Amsterdam: Elsevier, 1990:187–198.

21. North Italian Endoscopic Club. Prediction of the first variceal hemorrhage in patients with cirrhosis of the liver and esophageal varices. A prospective multicenter study. *N Engl J Med.* 1988;319:983–989.

22. Garcia-Tsao G, Groszmann RJ, Fisher RL, Conn HO, Atterbury CE, Glickman M. Portal pressure, presence of gastroesophageal varices and variceal bleeding. *Hepatology.* 1985; 5:419–424.

23. Groszmann RJ, Bosch J, Grace N, *et al*. Hemodynamic events in a prospective randomized trial of propranolol vs placebo in the prevention of the first variceal hemorrhage. *Gastroenterology.* 1990;99:1401–1407.

24. D'Amico G, Garcia-Pagan JC, Luca A, Bosch J. Hepatic vein pressure gradient reduction and prevention of variceal bleeding in cirrhosis: a systematic review. *Gastroenterology.* 2006;131:1611–1624.

25. D'Amico G, De Franchis R. Upper digestive bleeding in cirrhosis. Post-therapeutic outcome and prognostic indicators. *Hepatology.* 2003;38:599–612.

26. D'Amico G, Morabito A, Pagliaro L, Marubini E. Survival and prognostic indicators in compensated and decompensated cirrhosis. *Dig Dis Sci.* 1986;31:468–475.

27. Garcia-Tsao G, Sanyal AJ, Grace ND, Carey W. Practice Guidelines Committee of the American Association for the Study of Liver Diseases; Practice Parameters Committee of the American College of Gastroenterology. Prevention and management of gastroesophageal varices and variceal hemorrhage in cirrhosis. *Hepatology.* 2007;46:922–938

28. Planas R, Montoliu S, Ballestè B, *et al*. Natural history of patients hospitalized for management of cirrhotic ascites. *Clin Gastroenterol Hepatol.* 2006,4:1385–1394.

29. Pagliaro L, D'Amico G, Pasta L, *et al*. Portal hypertension in cirrhosis: natural history. In: Bosch J, Groszmann R, editors. *Portal Hypertension: Pathophysiology and Treatment.* Cambridge, MA: Blackwell Scientific, 1994:72–92.

30. Pugh RN, Murray-Lyon IM, Dawson JL, Pietroni MC, Williams R. Transection of the esophagus for bleeding oesophageal varices. *Br J Surg.* 1973;60:646–649.

31. Kamath PS,Wiesner RH, Malinchoc M, *et al*. A model to predict survival in patients with end-stage liver disease. *Hepatology.* 2001;33:464–470.

Liver Disease

CHAPTER 98
Portal hypertension

Juan Carlos García-Pagán,[1] Roberto J. Groszmann[2] and Jaime Bosch[1]
[1]Hospital Clínic, CIBERehd, Barcelona, Spain
[2]Yale University School of Medicine, New Haven, CT, USA

ESSENTIAL FACTS ABOUT PATHOGENESIS

- Portal hypertension is determined by the product of blood flow and vascular resistance within the portal venous system. Increased resistance to portal blood flow is the primary factor; a secondary increase in portal venous inflow further aggravates portal hypertension
- The site of increased resistance is the basis for the classification of portal hypertension
- Cirrhosis is by far the most common cause of intrahepatic portal hypertension
- Increased hepatic resistance in cirrhosis is due both to structural disturbances of liver vascular architecture and to increased hepatic vascular tone due to the active contraction of hepatic stellate cells, myofibroblasts and vascular smooth muscle cells due to an imbalance between decreased liver vasodilators, as NO, and increased constrictors, as thromboxane A2 and adrenergic tone
- Increased portal venous inflow results from marked arteriolar vasodilation of splanchnic organs draining into the portal vein

ESSENTIALS OF DIAGNOSIS

- The evaluation of the portal hypertensive patient is based on visualization of varices at endoscopy, definition of the porto-collateral anatomy by ultrasonography and/or angiography, and measurement of portal pressure
- Assessment of the presence and size of esophageal varices and of the presence of red signs over its walls is done by endoscopy. Endoscopy further discloses the presence of gastric varices, portal hypertensive gastropathy and unrelated lesions
- Doppler ultrasonography and CT scan are the preferred initial imaging investigations. Portal hypertension is detected by the presence of a dilated portal vein, portosystemic collaterals, ascites or splenomegaly. Portal vein patency should always be investigated. MRI is used in doubtful cases
- Hepatic vein catheterization with measurement of HVPG is the preferred method to determine portal pressure
- Emergency endoscopy (within 12 hours) should be performed to confirm diagnosis of variceal bleeding

ESSENTIALS OF TREATMENT

- Patients with moderate/large varices who have never bled should be treated with a non selective beta-blocker (propranolol, nadolol, timolol, carvedilol). The maximal benefit is obtained in those patients decreasing HVPG by ≥20% of baseline or below 12 mmHg. In patients with contraindications or who can not tolerate beta-blockers, endoscopic band ligation should be used
- Patients with small varices with red signs or with advanced liver failure (Child–Pugh C) are at similar risk of bleeding as those with moderate/large varices and should be considered for primary prophylaxis
- In acute variceal hemorrhage, the best approach is the combined use of a pharmacological agent, started from admission and an endoscopic procedure. Terlipressin, somatostatin, octreotide and vasopressin + nitroglycerin (in this order of preference) may be used. Drug therapy should be maintained at least for 2–5 days
- Endoscopic band ligation or injection sclerotherapy (in this order of preference) are the endoscopic treatments of choice in bleeding esophageal varices. In bleeding gastric varices the best endoscopic choice is variceal obturation with cyanoacrylate injection
- Prophylaxis of infection with broad spectrum antibiotics should be given to all patients during the acute bleeding episode
- TIPS, using PTFE-covered stents, should be used as a rescue procedure in failures of medical and endoscopic therapy. Patients at very high risk of failure and death (HVPG ≥20 mmHg, Child–Pugh class C) may benefit from an early decision for TIPS (within 48 hours of admission)
- Patients surviving an episode of variceal bleeding are at a very high risk of rebleeding and should receive effective preventive therapy starting at day 5 from admission; medical therapies, using non-selective beta-blockers (+/– nitrates), endoscopic band ligation or both, are the recommended first-line treatments

Introduction

Portal hypertension is a frequent clinical syndrome, defined by a pathological increase in the portal venous pressure. This increases the pressure gradient between the portal vein and the inferior vena cava (portal perfusion pressure of the liver or portal pressure gradient) above normal levels (1–5 mmHg.) When the portal pressure gradient rises above 10 mmHg, complications of portal hypertension usually arise. This pressure threshold defines clinically significant portal hypertension.

Textbook of Clinical Gastroenterology and Hepatology, Second Edition. Edited by C. J. Hawkey, Jaime Bosch, Joel E. Richter, Guadalupe Garcia-Tsao, Francis K. L. Chan.
© 2012 Blackwell Publishing Ltd. Published 2012 by Blackwell Publishing Ltd.

Table 98.1 Etiology of portal hypertension

Prehepatic
 Splenic vein thrombosis
 Portal vein thrombosis
 Congenital stenosis of the portal vein
 Extrinsic compression of the portal vein
 Arteriovenous fistulaes (splenic, aorto-mesenteric, aorto-portaland
 hepatic artery–portal vein)*

Intrahepatic
 Partial nodular transformation
 Nodular regenerative hyperplasia
 Congenital hepatic fibrosis
 Peliosis hepatis
 Polycystic disease
 Idiopathic portal hypertension
 Hypervitaminosis A
 Arsenic, copper sulfate and vinyl chloride monomer poisoning
 Sarcoidosis
 Tuberculosis
 Primary biliary cirrhosis
 Schistosomiasis
 Amyloidosis
 Mastocytosis
 Rendu–Osler disease
 Liver infiltration in hematologic diseases
 Acute fatty liver of pregnancy
 Severe acute viral hepatitis
 Chronic active hepatitis
 Hepatocellular carcinoma
 Hemocromatosis
 Wilson disease
 Hepatic porphyrias
 Alpha-1 antitrypsin deficiency
 Cyanamid toxicity
 Chronic biliary obstruction
 Cirrhosis due to hepatitis B and C virus infection
 Alcoholic cirrhosis
 Alcoholic hepatitis
 Veno-occlusive disease

Posthepatic
 Budd–Chiari syndrome
 Congenital malformations and thrombosis of the inferior vena cava
 Constrictive pericarditis
 Tricuspid valve diseases

*This is the only instance where portal hypertension is not initiated by
an increased resistance to portal blood flow.

Causes and classification

Portal hypertension can be caused by any disease interfering with blood flow at any level within the portal venous system. According to its anatomical location, the diseases are classified as prehepatic (diseases involving the splenic, mesenteric, or portal veins), intrahepatic (liver diseases), or posthepatic (diseases interfering with the venous outflow of the liver) (Table 98.1). Cirrhosis is by far the most common cause of portal hypertension in the world, followed by hepatic schistosomiasis. All other causes account for less than 10% of the cases ("non-cirrhotic portal hypertension") [1].

Pathophysiology

The portal pressure gradient is the result of the interaction between portal blood flow and the vascular resistance that opposes that flow. It follows that portal pressure may increase because of an increase in resistance, an increased portal blood flow, or a combination of both (Figure 98.1) [1].

Increased resistance

Increased resistance is the primary factor in the etiology of portal hypertension. In cirrhosis, increased hepatic resistance is the consequence of anatomical and functional alterations. The first is due to the distortion of the liver vascular architecture caused by fibrosis, scarring, and nodule formation. Thrombosis of medium and small portal and hepatic veins may contribute to the structural increase in resistance [1]. Functional increase in resistance is due to active contraction of different liver cell types, including activated hepatic stellate cells (HSCs), and vascular smooth muscle cells of the intrahepatic vasculature (i.e., small portal venules in portal tracts). This dynamic, reversible component may represent up to one third of the increased hepatic resistance in cirrhosis, and is caused by an imbalance between an increased production of vasoconstrictors, such as norepinephrine, angiotensin II, endothelin, vasopressin, leukotrienes, and thromboxane A2, and an insufficient bioavailability of hepatic vasodilators (mainly nitric oxide, NO). Reduced NO is due to both decreased release by eNOs and increased scavenging by enhanced oxidative stress (Figure 98.1) [2,3].

Increased portal venous inflow

Increased portal venous inflow is characteristically observed in advanced stages of portal hypertension, and results from marked arteriolar vasodilation in splanchnic organs draining into the portal vein. This increased blood flow aggravates and maintains the portal hypertensive syndrome (Figure 98.1) [1,4]. Splanchnic vasodilation is likely to be multifactorial. The more important are local vasoactive factors produced by the vascular endothelium, such as NO, prostacyclin and carbon monoxide. Endocannabinoids and glucagon have also been shown to play a role (Figure 98.1) [1,4]. In addition, active angiogenesis driven by vascular endothelial growth factor (VEGF) and platelet-derived growth factor (PDGF) is involved in the development and maintenance of the hyperdynamic splanchnic circulation [5].

The hemodynamic disturbances observed in the mesenteric and the hepatic vascular beds are completely divergent. While the liver circulation exhibits vasoconstriction, increased response to vasoconstrictors, and decreased response to endothelium-dependent vasodilators, the mesenteric vascular bed exhibits vasodilation, hyporesponse to vasoconstrictors, and increased response to endothelium-dependent vasodilators. The vasoactive mediators involved in these alterations are similar, but work in opposite directions. Thus, NO is decreased in the hepatic circulation, but increased in the splanchnic territory [6].

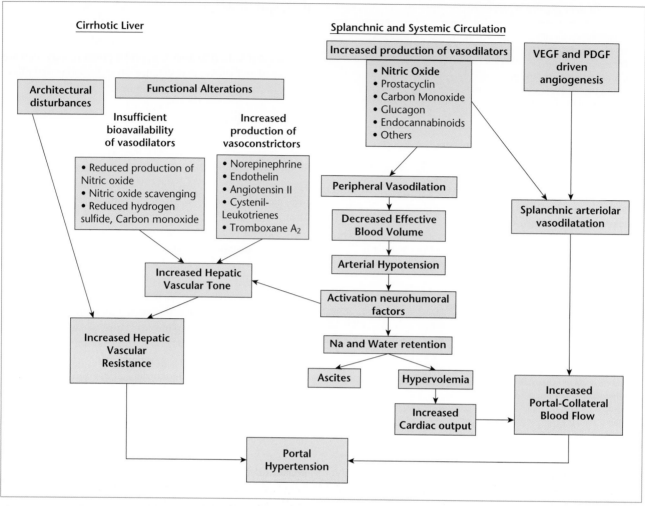

Figure 98.1 Pathophysiology of portal hypertension. Mechanisms involved in the pathophysiology of portal hypertension. PDGF, platelet-derived growth factor; VEGF, vascular endothelial growth factor.

Collaterals

Development of portal–collateral circulation (including gastroesophageal varices) is a major consequence of portal hypertension, which is triggered by the increased portal pressure, and involves the dilation of pre-existing vascular channels connecting the portal and systemic circulation, as well as angiogenesis driven by VEGF/PDGF. In advanced cirrhosis, over 80% of portal blood may circulate through these collaterals and thus collateral resistance will have a marked influence on portal pressure.

Complications

Variceal hemorrhage is the main complication of portal hypertension and is due to an excessive intravariceal pressure (due to the increased portal pressure) (Figure 98.2). Variceal hemorrhage occurs when the tension exerted by the thin wall of the varices (the inwardly directed force exerted by the variceal wall opposing the expansion due to increased variceal pressure) goes beyond a critical value determined by the elastic limit of the vessel. A big varix with thin walls will reach a high wall tension (and risk of bleeding) at much lower variceal pressures than a small varix with thick walls. Red wale or red color signs on varices reflect areas where the wall of the varices is especially thin [7].

Clinical presentation and natural history

Although portal hypertension leads to other complications of cirrhosis such as ascites and encephalopathy, this chapter focuses on gastrointestinal bleeding related to portal hypertension.

Gastroesophageal varices

Gastroesophageal collaterals and varices develop from connections between the short gastric and coronary veins and the esophageal, azygos, and intercostal veins. Ectopic varices may develop at other locations depending on local anatomical factors and are more frequent in patients with previous

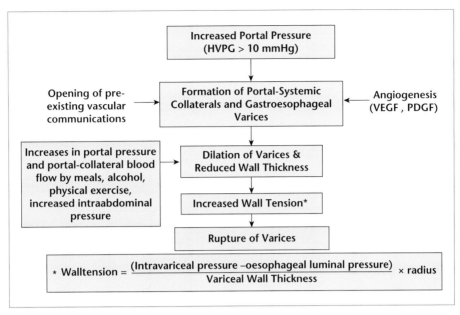

Figure 98.2 Natural history of gastroesophageal varices and mechanisms of bleeding.

abdominal surgery. Overall, ectopic varices are the cause of 1–5% of all variceal bleeding episodes.

Varices are present in about 40% of patients with compensated patients and in 60% of those who present with ascites. Since the expected incidence of newly developed varices is about 6% per year, the general consensus is that endoscopy should be repeated after 2–3 years in patients without varices at the first endoscopy. Patients with HVPG ≥10 mmHg have two- to three-fold risk of developing varices [8], these patients should have repeat endoscopy every 1–2 years. Based on an expected 10–15% per year rate of progression of variceal size, endoscopy should be repeated every year in patients with small varices to detect the progression from small to large varices.

Hemorrhage

Ruptured esophageal varices represent 70% of all bleeding episodes in patients with portal hypertension, and are most frequently manifested by hematemesis, melena, and hypovolemic shock. Variceal bleeding is diagnosed at emergency endoscopy based on observing either: (1) blood spurting from a varix; (2) white nipple or clot adherent to a varix; and (3) blood in the stomach and varices without other potential sources of bleeding. HVPG ≥20 mmHg, Child–Pugh class, active bleeding at endoscopy, portal thrombosis, hepatocarcinoma, alcoholic hepatitis and bacterial infection are significant prognostic indicators of failure to control bleeding [1].

Early rebleeding

Early rebleeding occurs in 30–40% of patients in the first 6 weeks. The rebleeding risk peaks in the first 5 days with 40% of all rebleeding episodes occurring in this period, remaining high during the first 2 weeks and declining slowly in the

following 4 weeks. Because of this, the duration of the acute bleeding episode has been arbitrarily set as 5 days. Six weeks after the index episode, the risk of bleeding essentially returns to baseline.

Six-week mortality

Six-week mortality after variceal bleeding is about 15–20%, a figure that is less than half that of the 1980s. The most consistently reported predictors of death are Child–Pugh classification, blood urea nitrogen (BUN) or creatinine, age, active alcohol abuse, active bleeding at endoscopy, HVPG and early rebleeding.

Late rebleeding

Patients surviving a first episode of variceal hemorrhage have a very high risk of rebleeding and death. Median rebleeding incidence within 1–2 years is 63% [9]. The corresponding mortality figure is 33%. Therefore, all patients surviving a variceal hemorrhage should be treated for prevention of rebleeding independently of other risk indicators [10].

Gastric varices

Gastric varices are classified as those that are a continuation of esophageal varices (GOV), either along the lesser curve of the stomach (GOV1) or into the fundus (GOV2), and those that are isolated (IGV) (i.e., not connected with esophageal varices), which are more rare, and may be located in the fundus (IGV1) or elsewhere in the stomach (IGV2). IGV are more frequent in patients with prehepatic portal hypertension. Overall, the prevalence of gastric varices in patients with portal hypertension is about 20% (14% GOV1, 4% GOV2, and 2% IGV 1 or 2). Gastric varices are the source of 5–10% of all upper digestive bleeding episodes in patients with cirrhosis.

Portal hypertensive gastropathy

Gastric mucosal changes associated with portal hypertension have been named portal hypertensive gastropathy (PHG). The most frequently observed lesions of PHG are the "mosaic pattern" and "cherry red spots." The latter carry a higher bleeding risk and are considered "severe" PHG. Histologically, these lesions are characterized by dilation of the capillaries and venules of the gastric mucosa. At the time of diagnosis of cirrhosis, the prevalence of PHG is about 30% and its incidence is about 12% per year. Endoscopic therapy of oesophageal varices (especially injection sclerotherapy) is a possible risk factor for PHG. The **clinical course of PHG** is characterized by overt or chronic gastric mucosal bleeding. The incidence of overt bleeding from any source in patients with mild PHG is about 5% per year, as compared to 15% for severe PHG. Overt bleeding from PHG is usually manifested by melena, and has a far better prognosis than variceal bleeding, with less than 5% mortality per episode. The incidence of minor mucosal blood loss, without overt bleeding, is about 8% per year and may result in severe chronic iron deficiency anaemia.

Portal hypertensive gastropathy should be distinguished from **gastric antral vascular ectasia** (GAVE). This is a distinct entity that may be found in association with conditions different from cirrhosis such as scleroderma or chronic gastritis. GAVE is characterized by aggregates of red spots usually with radial distribution from the pylorus to the antrum of the stomach ("watermelon stomach"). Histology of GAVE is characterized by smooth muscle cell and myofibroblast hyperplasia and fibrohyalinosis.

Diagnostic methods

Imaging techniques are very useful in the initial evaluation of the portal hypertensive patient. Frequently, portal hypertension is first detected by the finding on **ultrasonography** of a dilated portal vein, portosystemic collaterals, ascites, or splenomegaly. Patency of the portal vein should be investigated in every portal hypertensive patient. Non-invasive imaging methods including Doppler ultrasonography with echo enhancement, helical computed tomography (CT) scans, and magnetic resonance imaging (MRI) are highly accurate and have substituted direct angiography.

Endoscopy

At endoscopy it is important to assess semi-quantitatively the appearance and size of any esophageal varix, as well as the presence of red color signs (see Video clip 98.1). Endoscopy should include a careful evaluation for the presence and severity of portal hypertensive gastropathy and of gastric varices (see Video clip 98.2), which in some cases may require **endosonography** to distinguish them from gastric folds.

Capsule pill-cam endoscopy is being assessed for the diagnosis of esophageal varices, and may have a role for the rare patient who can not tolerate sedated endoscopy.

Measurement of portal pressure

Please refer to Chapter 140 for details of measurement of portal pressure.

Treatment and prevention

Prevention of the first bleed from esophageal varices

High-risk varices call for prophylactic treatment. These include "moderate–large" varices (over 5 mm in diameter) and small varices with red color signs or in a Child–Pugh class C patient [1].

Pharmacological treatment

Non-selective beta-blockers (NSBBs) include propranolol, nadolol, timolol and carvedilol. The two most used are propranolol and nadolol. These drugs reduce portal pressure by decreasing portal collateral blood flow. This is achieved through the reduction in cardiac output caused by beta-1 adrenergic blockade, and by splanchnic vasoconstriction due to the blockade of beta-2 adrenoceptors in the splanchnic arteries. Meta-analyses have consistently shown a significant reduction of the bleeding risk, from 25% with non-active treatment to 15% with beta-blockers [11] over a median follow-up of about 2 years. This beneficial effect is found both in compensated and decompensated patients. In addition, NSBBs are associated with a significant reduction in bleeding-related deaths. About 15% of patients have contraindications to the use of beta-blockers (pulmonary obstructive disease, aortic valve disease, atrioventricular heart block, and peripheral arterial insufficiency). Sinus bradycardia and insulin-dependent diabetes are relative contraindications. The incidence of side effects among treated patients is in the order of 15%. The most frequent are fatigue, dyspnea, bronchospasm, and impotence. About 5% of side effects require treatment discontinuation, while others are managed by decreasing the dose.

Propranolol should be prescribed initially at 20–40 mg b.i.d. and titrated on a bi-weekly basis, up to a maximum of 160 mg b.i.d. **Nadolol** should be prescribed initially at 20 mg a day, in a single daily dose, and titrated every 2–3 days up to a maximum of 240 mg. Patients should be instructed not to discontinue treatment and told that treatment should be maintained indefinitely, since bleeding risk increases sharply after discontinuation of beta-blockers. Low dose carvedilol (12.5 mg/day) may be even more effective.

Endoscopic therapy

Endoscopic band ligation (EBL) is effective in preventing the first variceal bleeding in patients with medium to large varices. Seventeen trials have compared EBL with NSBBs for primary prophylaxis of variceal bleeding. The meta-analysis of all these trials shows an advantage of EBL over NSBBs in terms of prevention of first bleeding, without differences in mortality [1,11]. However, when meta-analysis is restricted to either studies with relatively high quality, or including a reasonable

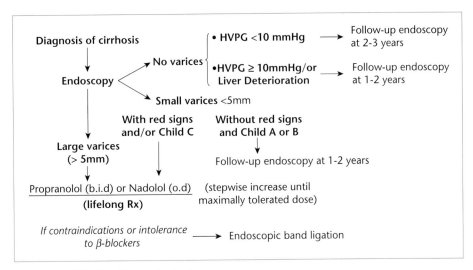

Figure 98.3 Prevention of first variceal bleeding. Therapeutic algorithm.

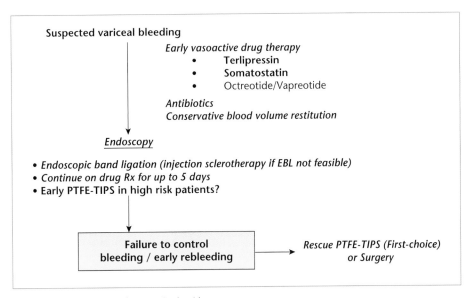

Figure 98.4 Treatment of acute variceal bleeding. Therapeutic algorithm.

number of patients there is no benefit from EBL [1,11,12]. Adverse events requiring treatment discontinuation are significantly more frequent in patients treated with NSBB [1,11,12]; however, the severity of side effects was different between the two therapies [1,12]. Indeed, most side effects related to NSBB (hypotension, tiredness, breathlessness, insomnia, reduced sexual drive) were easily managed by reducing the dose or discontinuing beta-blockers, did not require hospital admission and no fatalities were observed. In contrast, side effects related to EBL included bleeding episodes requiring hospitalization and blood transfusion, esophageal perforation and three deaths [1,11,12]. Based on the all above considerations, it has been postulated to initiate prophylactic therapy with NSBBs, changing to EBL in case of intolerance or contraindications to NSBBs (Figure 98.3).

The combination of EBL plus NSBB appears to offer no benefit in terms of prevention of first bleeding [1].

Treatment of acute bleeding from esophageal varices
General management
Variceal bleeding is a medical emergency and its management should be undertaken in an intensive care setting where general measures such as resuscitation, the need for orotracheal intubation in patients with encephalopathy or large-volume paracentesis in patients with tense ascites can be evaluated. Therapy is greatly facilitated if decision-making follows a written protocol (Figure 98.4). The initial therapy is aimed at correcting hypovolemic shock, preventing complications associated with gastrointestinal bleeding, and achieving hemostasis at the bleeding site.

Blood volume replacement
Blood volume replacement should be initiated as soon as possible to avoid complications from hypovolemic shock and decreased perfusion of vital organs. Over-transfusion should

be avoided because it increases portal pressure with a consequent risk of continued bleeding or rebleeding. Blood transfusion should aim at maintaining the hematocrit at 0.21–0.24 (Hb 7–8 g/L) [10], except in patients with rapid ongoing bleeding or with ischemic heart disease. Plasma expanders should be given to maintain a systolic blood pressure over 80 mmHg and a heart rate <120 bpm. The role of platelet transfusion or fresh frozen plasma has not been assessed appropriately. Recombinant activated factor VIIa may be useful in the rare patient with profound coagulopathy but is not indicated in the average patient with variceal bleeding [1].

Antibiotics

Patients with variceal bleeding have a high risk of bacterial infections (near 50% as compared to 5–7% in the general population). Furthermore, bacterial infections significantly increase failure to control bleeding and hospital mortality in patients with cirrhosis and gastrointestinal bleeding. Antibiotic prophylaxis (usually by administering quinolones) decreases the incidence of bacterial infections and increases the survival rate. In high risk patients (hypovolemic shock, ascites, jaundice or malnutrition) i.v. ceftriaxone 1 g/day for 7 days has been shown superior to oral norfloxacin 400 mg b.i.d. [13].

Specific treatment

Pharmacological treatment

This should be started as soon as variceal hemorrhage is suspected, before diagnostic endoscopy. Drugs for acute bleeding include terlipressin, somatostatin and its analogs octreotide and vapreotide. Meta-analysis of published randomized controlled trials (RCTs) shows that terlipressin is the only therapy associated with an improved survival, although it is not universally available. Somatostatin infusion may be as effective, especially at high doses. Octreotide improves the efficacy of emergency sclerotherapy in controlling bleeding, but there is not enough evidence supporting its use as single therapy. If vasopressin is used, it should be associated with nitroglycerin because this reduces the side effects and enhances its efficacy. "Five-day success" (control of bleeding, no further bleeding, no death) is achieved in about 70% of patients using either terlipressin or somatostatin monotherapy.

Terlipressin is used as intravenous (i.v.) injections at doses of 2 mg every 4 h for up to 24 h; the dose is then halved and maintained for up to 5 days. It should not be used in patients with severe heart or vascular disease. Side effects of terlipressin may occur in nearly 25% of patients, the more frequent being abdominal cramps, diarrhea, bradycardia, and hypertension, leading to discontinuation in 2–4% of cases. Terlipressin can also be used as continuous intravenous infusions (8–16 mg/day).

Somatostatin is used by continuous intravenous infusion of 250 μg/h following an initial bolus of 250 μg. High-risk patients (with active bleeding at endoscopy) may benefit from a greater dose (500 μg/h). Treatment may be maintained for up to 5 days. Side effects of somatostatin are usually mild, most frequently bradycardia, hyperglycemia, diarrhea, and abdominal cramps.

Endoscopic therapy

EBL is recommended as soon as an experienced endoscopist is available; injection sclerotherapy may still be used when EBL is not feasible. Endoscopic therapy requires skilled endoscopists and may cause serious complications (aspiration pneumonia, esophageal perforation) in about 10% of patients. Meta-analysis shows that endoscopic band ligation is better than sclerotherapy in the initial control of bleeding, is associated with less adverse events and lower mortality.

Combination therapy

The best results in the treatment of acute variceal bleeding are obtained by combining early vasoactive drug therapy, prophylactic antibiotics and EBL (Figure 98.4). Five-day success is about 80–90%. Variceal obturation with tissue adhesives is no better than EBL and is reserved for gastric varices.

Rescue therapies: tamponade, transjugular portosystemic shunt, and surgery

In 10–20% of patients variceal bleeding is either unresponsive to initial endoscopic and/or pharmacologic treatment or the patient experiences early rebleeding. If bleeding is mild and the patient is stable a second endoscopic therapy (if technically possible) might be attempted. If this fails, or if bleeding is severe, the patient should be offered transjugular portosystemic shunt (TIPS) or shunt surgery.

Balloon tamponade and esophageal stenting

Balloon tamponade stops bleeding by direct compression of the bleeding site at the varices. Control of bleeding is successful in as much as 80%, but most patients will rebleed when balloon(s) are deflated. Complications are frequent and may be lethal in 6–20% (aspiration pneumonia, esophageal rupture, airway obstruction). Because of these drawbacks balloon tamponade should be used only by skilled, experienced staff only for temporary control of bleeding while awaiting definitive therapy. Preliminary studies have suggested that the use of self-expandable esophageal stents may be a safer alternative to balloon tamponade for the temporary control of bleeding in treatment failures. However, these preliminary data should be confirmed in carefully conducted RCTs.

Transjugular intrahepatic portosystemic shunt and portosystemic shunt surgery

TIPS and surgical shunts are very effective stopping bleeding when used as rescue therapy after failure of the initial treatment. TIPS is the first choice but shunt surgery, using interposition mesocaval graft shunts or traditional portacaval shunts, may be an alternative to TIPS in Child A patients (Figure 98.4). However, despite a high success rate of controlling bleeding, 6-week mortality is very high (range: 27–55%) mostly due to worsening liver failure. Recent data suggest that the early TIPS

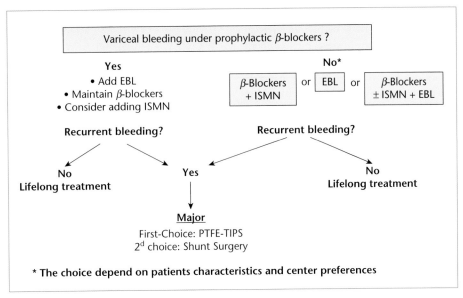

Figure 98.5 Prevention of recurrent variceal bleeding. Therapeutic algorithm. EBL, endoscopic band ligation; EIS, endoscopic injection sclerotherapy.

(within 24–72 hours of admission) in patients with very high risk of treatment failure (Child C <14 points or Child C with active hemorrhage) may successfully control bleeding and improve survival [14,15].

Prevention of recurrent bleeding from esophageal varices
Medical therapy
Many RCTs have proved the efficacy of NSBBs in the prevention of variceal rebleeding. Mortality from bleeding is also significantly reduced by NSBBs. The association of propranolol or nadolol with isosorbide-5-mononitrate (IMN) has been compared to EBL in four studies. Meta-analysis showed no significant differences between both treatments [1]. Compared with TIPS, the combination of propranolol and IMN is less effective for the prevention of rebleeding but it is associated with significantly less encephalopathy, lower cost, and similar mortality.

Monitoring pharmacological treatment response
The HVPG response to continued therapy with non-selective beta-blockers correlates with its clinical efficacy. The risk of rebleeding is almost nil when HVPG decreases below ≤12 mmHg, and is dramatically reduced in patients in whom HVPG is reduced ≥20% of baseline [16]. These patients ("responders") also have lower risk of recurrent ascites, hepatorenal syndrome and death, and do not require additional therapy. It is still unclear whether patients with an insufficient hemodynamic response to pharmacological therapy ("non-responders") will benefit from alternative treatments. In a recent RCT no significant differences in rebleeding rates were found in HVPG non-responders maintained only on drug therapy versus those receiving drug therapy plus EBL, suggesting that adding EBL may not be the best alternative to

reduce rebleeding in non-responders [17]. It is possible that more effective and aggressive therapies are required to reduce the high rebleeding tendency of HVPG non-responders.

Combined endoscopic and pharmacological treatment
Two RCTs showed that the combination of EBL plus NSBBs is superior to EBL alone in terms of recurrence of varices and recurrence of bleeding [1]. This was not confirmed in a third study [18] although this may be due to the long delay between bleeding and treatment. In addition, one RCT adding EBL to nadolol plus IMN found no significant differences in rebleeding episodes from any cause due to a greater number of ulcer-related bleeding in the arm including EBL [17]. Thus, the potentially greater efficacy of combining endoscopic and drug therapy should be further evaluated. The combination of EBL plus NSBB (+/− nitrates) is strongly recommended in patients who have bled from esophageal varices while undergoing either treatment alone.

Transjugular portosystemic shunt and surgery
TIPS and shunt surgery are very useful in the prevention of recurrent bleeding. Patients with severe or repeat rebleeding episodes despite adequate medical therapy should be considered for "rescue" therapy with TIPS or shunt surgery (Figure 98.5).

Treatment of gastric varices
Results of pharmacological therapy in the prevention of first bleeding in patients with esophageal varices can most probably be extended to patients with gastric varices.

Endoscopic therapies are promising, but quality information is scarce, and most studies include both fundal varices and gastro-esophageal varices. Sclerotherapy, variceal obturation with tissue adhesives ("glue injection"), thrombin, EBL and ligation with large detachable snares have been reported. In most uncontrolled series cyanoacrylate is highly effective, in the order of 90%, and is considered the endoscopic treatment of choice. However, pulmonary and cerebral embolism has been reported with tissue adhesives, the technique needs expertise and is usually not feasible during active bleeding. Thrombin has provided good hemostasis in some studies. It is recommended that a decision for TIPS or surgery is not delayed in case of lack of control of bleeding from gastric varices.

In the prevention of recurrent bleeding, non-selective beta-blockers are used as first line therapy in many centers. TIPS, shunt surgery, or variceal obturation are recommended in failures of pharmacological treatment.

Balloon tamponade with the single large balloon Linton–Nachlas tube is preferred over the double balloon Sengstaken tube as a temporary treatment.

Treatment of portal hypertensive gastropathy and gastric antral vascular ectasia

There is no indication for the primary prophylaxis of bleeding from PHG. Acute bleeding from PHG should first be treated with terlipressin, somatostatin or octreotide, although there are no RCTs specifically designed for PHG. Prevention of recurrent bleeding from PHG is based on NSBBs. Adequate iron supplementation should be given to correct chronic iron-deficiency anemia. TIPS is as an alternative therapy for the rare patient who has repeated bleeding from PHG and requires frequent blood transfusion despite pharmacological therapy. Argon plasma coagulation or a neodymium : yttrium–aluminium–garnet (Nd : YAG) laser may also be tried.

Patients bleeding from GAVE may benefit from endoscopic ablation, either by argon plasma coagulation, Nd : YAG laser, or heater probe. TIPS and beta-blockers are not effective for the prevention of recurrent bleeding from GAVE. Selected patients with severe GAVE may benefit from antrectomy with Billroth I anastomosis.

Acknowledgements

Supported by grants from the Fondo de Investigaciones Sanitarias (FIS 06/0623) and Ministerio de Educación y Ciencia (SAF 2010-17043). Ciberehd is funded by Instituto de Salud Carlos III.

References

1. Bosch J, Abraldes JG, Berzigotti A, *et al*. Portal hypertension and gastrointestinal bleeding. *Semin Liver Dis*. 2008;28:3–25.
2. Gracia-Sancho J, Lavina B, Rodriguez-Vilarrupla A, *et al*. Increased oxidative stress in cirrhotic rat livers: A potential mechanism contributing to reduced nitric oxide bioavailability. *Hepatology*. 2008;47:1248–1256.
3. Iwakiri Y, Groszmann RJ. Vascular endothelial dysfunction in cirrhosis. *J Hepatol*. 2007;46:927–934.
4. Iwakiri Y, Groszmann RJ. The hyperdynamic circulation of chronic liver diseases: from the patient to the molecule. *Hepatology*. 2006;43(2, Suppl. 1):S121–S131.
5. Fernandez M, Semela D, Bruix J, *et al*. Angiogenesis in liver disease. *J Hepatol*. 2009;50:604–620.
6. Wiest R, Groszmann RJ. The paradox of nitric oxide in cirrhosis and portal hypertension: Too much, not enough. *Hepatology*. 2002;35:478–491.
7. NIEC. Prediction of the first variceal hemorrhage in patients with cirrhosis of the liver and esophageal varices. A prospective multicenter study. *N Engl J Med*. 1988;319:983–989.
8. Groszmann RJ, Garcia-Tsao G, Bosch J, *et al*. Portal Hypertension Collaborative Group. Beta-blockers to prevent gastroesophageal varices in patients with cirrhosis. *N Engl J Med*. 2005;353:2254–2261.
9. D'Amico G, Pagliaro L, Bosch J. Pharmacological treatment of portal hypertension: An evidence-based approach. *Semin Liver Dis*. 1999;19:475–505.
10. de Franchis R. Evolving consensus in portal hypertension report of the Baveno IV Consensus Workshop on methodology of diagnosis and therapy in portal hypertension. *J Hepatol*. 2005;43:167–176.
11. Gluud LL, Klingenberg S, Nikolova D, *et al*. Banding ligation versus beta-blockers as primary prophylaxis in esophageal varices: systematic review of randomized trials. *Am J Gastroenterol*. 2007;102:2842–2848.
12. Bosch J, Berzigotti A, García-Pagán JC, *et al*. The management of portal hypertension: rational basis, available treatments and future options. *J Hepatol*. 2008;48:68–92.
13. Fernandez J, Ruiz dA, Gomez C, *et al*. Norfloxacin vs ceftriaxone in the prophylaxis of infections in patients with advanced cirrhosis and hemorrhage. *Gastroenterology*. 2006;131:1049–1056.
14. Monescillo A, Martinez-Lagares F, Ruiz-del-Arbol L, *et al*. Influence of portal hypertension and its early decompression by TIPS placement on the outcome of variceal bleeding. *Hepatology*. 2004;40:793–801.
15. Garcia-Pagan JC, Caca K, Bureau C, *et al*. An early decision for PTFE-TIPS improves survival in high risk cirhotic patients admitted with an acute variceal bleeding. A multicentric RCT. *J Hepatol*. 2008;48(Suppl. 2):S371.
16. D'Amico G, Garcia-Pagan JC, Luca A, *et al*. Hepatic vein pressure gradient reduction and prevention of variceal bleeding in cirrhosis: a systematic review. *Gastroenterology*. 2006;131:1611–1624.
17. Garcia-Pagan JC, Villanueva C, Albillos A, *et al*. Nadolol plus isosorbide mononitrate alone or associated with band ligation in the prevention of recurrent bleeding: A multicentre randomised controlled trial. *Gut*. 2009;58:1144–1150.
18. Kumar A, Jha SK, Sharma P, *et al*. Addition of propranolol and isosorbide mononitrate to endoscopic variceal ligation does not reduce variceal rebleeding incidence. *Gastroenterology*. 2009;137:892–901.

CHAPTER 99
Ascites and hepatorenal syndrome

Andrés Cárdenas and Pere Ginès

Hospital Clinic, University of Barcelona, Barcelona, Spain

ESSENTIAL FACTS ABOUT PATHOGENESIS

- The most common cause of ascites is portal hypertension secondary to cirrhosis, which accounts for approximately 80% of all cases
- The underlying cause of ascites and hepatorenal syndrome in cirrhosis is splanchnic arterial vasodilation which decreases effective arterial blood volume and leads to sodium and water retention and renal vasoconstriction

ESSENTIALS OF DIAGNOSIS

- Ascites can be diagnosed on physical exam and/or with abdominal ultrasound
- Hyponatremia is defined as a serum sodium level <130 mEq/L
- Previously defined criteria for the diagnosis of hepatorenal syndrome include the determination of renal function and response to a fluid challenge

ESSENTIALS OF TREATMENT

- The mainstay of therapy of ascites is a salt-restricted diet and diuretics such as furosemide and spironolactone
- Patients with a large volume of ascites or refractory ascites benefit from large volume paracentesis
- Patients with refractory ascites may also undergo transjugular portosystemic shunt placement
- Patients with dilutional hyponatremia may benefit from water restriction. New V2 receptor antagonists are promising drugs that correct serum sodium levels by increasing solute-free water exxcretion
- Patients with hepatorenal syndrome should undergo therapy with vasoconstrictors plus albumin
- All patients with ascites and renal failure should be evaluated for liver transplantation

Introduction

Ascites is the pathological accumulation of free fluid in the peritoneal cavity. This term derives from the Greek root "askos," meaning bag. Although ancient Egyptians and Greeks acknowledged a possible link between liver disease and ascites, Erasitratus of Cappadoccia, *circa* 300 BC [1], described the "hardness of the liver" as a factor responsible for fluid accumulation in the abdominal cavity. A celebrated figure with ascites and cirrhosis was Ludwig van Beethoven who was treated with serial large-volume paracentesis and died of hepatic failure in 1827 [2].

Epidemiology

In the natural history of cirrhosis, patients may develop significant complications of renal function manifested by sodium retention, solute-free water retention, and renal vasoconstriction. These mechanisms are responsible for fluid accumulation in the form of ascites, dilutional hyponatremia (DH), and hepatorenal syndrome (HRS), respectively. Ascites is the most common complication of cirrhosis resulting in poor quality of life, increased risk for infections, renal failure, and high mortality rates. Nearly 60% of patients with compensated cirrhosis develop ascites within 10 years of the disease [3]. The development of ascites in cirrhosis is a poor prognostic feature because it has been estimated that more than 50% of these patients will die in approximately 5 years without liver transplantation [4]. Hyponatremia and HRS are later events that carry an even worse prognosis.

Causes

The causes of ascites and its differential diagnosis are specified in Chapter 17. Cirrhosis is by far (>80%) the most common cause of ascites. This chapter will therefore focus on the pathophysiology, clinical features, diagnostic methods and current therapy of ascites, DH, and HRS in cirrhosis.

Pathophysiology of ascites and renal function abnormalities in cirrhosis

In cirrhosis, the presence of bridging fibrosis and nodule formation distorts the normal architecture of the hepatic sinusoids thereby causing an increased resistance to flow from the portal vein into the liver. This event causes significant effects in the portal venous system with development of sinusoidal portal hypertension and collateral vein formation with shunting of blood from the portal to the systemic circulation. Several

Liver Disease

Textbook of Clinical Gastroenterology and Hepatology, Second Edition. Edited by C. J. Hawkey, Jaime Bosch, Joel E. Richter, Guadalupe Garcia-Tsao, Francis K. L. Chan.
© 2012 Blackwell Publishing Ltd. Published 2012 by Blackwell Publishing Ltd.

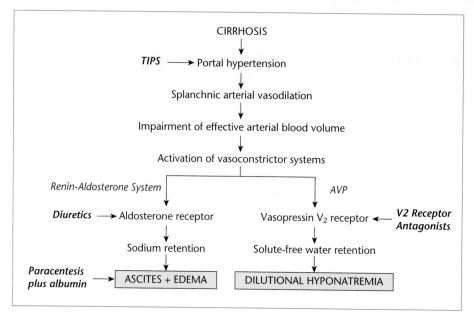

Figure 99.1 Pathogenesis of ascites and hyponatremia in cirrhosis and current treatment options. Portal hypertension is always present in patients with ascites and cirrhosis. It causes severe splanchnic vasodilation and a further drop in effective arterial blood volume with a compensatory homeostatic response that occurs secondary to a reduced effective arterial blood volume and leads to the activation of antinatriuretic factors (mainly the angiotensin–aldosterone system) with subsequent sodium retention. Transjugular intrahepatic portosystemic shunt (TIPS) by reducing portal pressure is an effective treatment for reducing ascites, particularly in patients with refractory ascites. Diuretics that promote natriuresis (i.e., spironolactone) are indicated as initial therapy. Patents with large-volume ascites should be treated with therapeutic paracentesis and albuminas as an initial therapy. Solute-free water retention that occurs in later stages of the disease occurs due to high levels of arginine vasopressin (AVP). New V2 receptor antagonists increase serum sodium levels in patients with ascites and dilutional hyponatremia.

vasodilator factors, mainly nitric oxide and others including calcitonin gene-related peptide, substance P, carbon monoxide and endogenous cannabinoids are responsible for this vasodilatory effect as a consequence of endothelial stretching and bacterial translocation [5]. Bacterial translocation by inducing cytokine synthesis plays a major role in the pathogenesis of arterial vasodilation and associated circulatory abnormalities that occur in cirrhosis with ascites [6]. In preascitic cirrhosis, splanchnic arterial vasodilation is moderate with no important effect on effective arterial blood volume. In advanced cirrhosis splanchnic arterial vasodilation is very intense leading to decreased effective arterial blood volume with a reduction in arterial pressure. A reduction in cardiac output, likely due to some degree of cirrhotic cardiomyopathy, occurs in the late stages and may also contribute to the impairment in effective arterial blood volume [7]. As a consequence of the impairment in effective arterial blood volume, there is homeostatic activation of vasoconstrictor and antinatriuretic factors (i.e., renin–angiotensin–aldosterone, norepinephrine, arginine vasopressin) to maintain arterial pressure, resulting in renal sodium retention [8]. The effects of portal hypertension and splanchnic arterial vasodilation significantly modify intestinal capillary pressure and permeability facilitating the accumulation of ascites. Inability to excrete sodium is the earliest renal alteration and occurs before solute-free water retention and renal vasoconstriction [9]. With disease progression, there is a marked impairment in renal solute-free water excretion and

renal vasoconstriction, leading to DH and HRS respectively. The pathophysiology and rationale for the treatment of patients with cirrhosis and hyponatremia is summarized in Figure 99.1.

Clinical presentation

The clinical features of patients presenting with ascites are described in detail in Chapter 17.

Treatment

Education of patients regarding a sodium-restricted diet of 2 g/day (approx. 90 mmol/day) is one of the mainstays of management in all patients with cirrhosis and ascites [10,11]. A more stringent restriction is generally not well tolerated and patients become noncompliant. Additionally, fluid restriction is not necessary unless patients have DH. Although in a low proportion (10%) of patients ascites may decrease with sodium restriction, it is essential when diuretics are added. An important aspect in the management of patients with cirrhosis and ascites is evaluation for liver transplantation in suitable candidates.

The current classification of ascites defined by the International Ascites Club divides patients into three groups [11]. Patients with grade 1 ascites are those in whom ascites is detected only by ultrasonography; these patients do not require any specific treatment, but they should be warned about avoiding foods with large amounts of salt. Patients with grade 2 ascites are those in which ascites causes moderate distension of the abdomen associated with mild/moderate discomfort. Patients with grade 3 ascites have large amounts of ascitic fluid causing marked abdominal distension and associated with significant discomfort. Patients with refractory ascites are those that do not respond to high doses of diuretics or develop side effects that preclude their use.

Nonrefractory ascites
Moderate: grade 2 ascites
These patients typically can be managed as outpatients unless other complications of cirrhosis are present. A negative sodium balance with loss of ascites is quickly and easily obtained in most cases with diuretics [12–14]. Patients with new onset ascites respond to spironolactone 50–100 mg/day and the dose may be increased progressively if needed. Patients with prior episodes of ascites should receive the combination of spironolactone 100 mg/day with furosemide (20–40 mg/day) [12–14]. If there is no response, compliance with diet and medications should be confirmed and diuretics may then be increased in a stepwise fashion every 5–7 days by doubling doses to a maximal dose of spironolactone of 400 mg/day and a maximal dose of furosemide of 160 mg/day. Diuretic therapy is effective in the elimination of ascites in 80–90% of all patients, a percentage that may increase to 95% when only patients without renal failure are considered. Spironolactone-induced gynecomastia may cause patients to stop the drug; in these cases amiloride (5–10 mg/day) may be useful, although its potency is lower than that of spironolactone. Eplerenone, another aldosterone antagonist has fewer endocrine adverse effects compared with spironolactone and could be a good alternative to spironolactone in patients with spironolactone-induced gynecomastia but there is limited data [15]. The goal of diuretic therapy is to achieve an average weight loss of 300–500 g/day in patients without edema and 800–1000 g/day in those with peripheral edema. A greater degree of weight loss may induce volume depletion and renal failure. After minimizing ascites, sodium restriction should be maintained while the dose of diuretics may be reduced as needed (see Figure 99.2).

Tense: grade 3 ascites
These patients are best managed by therapeutic paracentesis. A detailed description of this technique can be found in Chapter 154. Complete removal of ascites in one tap (as many liters as possible) with intravenous albumin (8 g per liter tapped) has been shown to be quick, effective, and associated with a lower number of complications than conventional diuretic therapy [16]. After a therapeutic tap, postparacentesis circulatory dysfunction may develop; this is a circulatory derangement with marked activation of the renin–angiotensin system that occurs 24–48 hours after the procedure [17]. This disorder is clinically silent, not spontaneously reversible, and associated with hyponatremia and renal impairment in up to

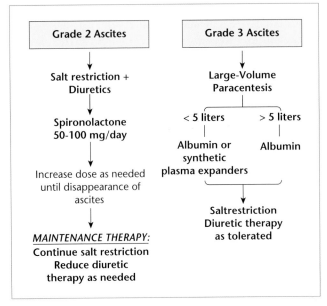

Figure 99.2 Treatment strategy for patients with grades 2 and 3 ascites.

20% of patients [16–18]. In addition it is associated with decreased survival. Post-paracentesis circulatory dysfunction may be prevented with the administration of albumin (8 g per liter tapped) [18–20]. Albumin is superior to dextran-70, polygeline, and saline following paracentesis of more than 5 liters [20]. Although the use of albumin after paracentesis is controversial due to the lack of data proving a survival benefit and high cost in some countries, the protective effect of albumin on the circulatory system favors its use. Thus, current guidelines recommend the use of albumin after large volume paracentesis [11]. Patients with a known history of cirrhosis and without any complications can be managed as outpatients. However, patients in whom tense ascites is the first manifestation of cirrhosis or those with associated hepatic encephalopathy, gastrointestinal bleeding, or bacterial infections require hospitalization. Most of these patients have marked sodium retention and need to be started or continued on relatively high doses of diuretics after paracentesis together with a low-sodium diet (see Figure 99.2).

Refractory ascites
Nearly 10% of patients with ascites are refractory to treatment with diuretics [12,21]. In refractory ascites, sodium excretion cannot be achieved either because patients do not respond to high doses of diuretics (spironolactone 400 mg/day and furosemide 160 mg/day) or because they develop side effects that preclude their use. In general, these patients have features of advanced liver disease, a high recurrence rate of ascites after large-volume paracentesis, an increased risk of type-1 HRS, and a poor prognosis. Current treatment strategies include repeated therapeutic paracentesis plus intravenous albumin, and transjugular intrahepatic portosystemic shunts (TIPS). Therapeutic paracentesis is the accepted initial therapy for

refractory ascites. Patients, on average, require a tap every 2–4 weeks and the majority may be treated as outpatients, making this option easy to perform and cost effective. TIPS, a non-surgical method of portal decompression, reduces sinusoidal and portal pressure and decreases ascites and diuretic requirements in these patients [22,23]. A disadvantage with TIPS is the development of side effects that include hepatic encephalopathy and impairment in liver function [22–28]. Additionally, uncovered TIPS may be complicated by stenosis of the prosthesis (18–78%) [23]. Newer polytetrafluoroethylene-covered prostheses seem to improve TIPS patency and decrease the number of clinical relapses and re-interventions without increasing the risk of encephalopathy [29,30].

Randomized controlled studies comparing TIPS with repeated paracentesis demonstrate that TIPS is associated with a lower rate of ascites recurrence [24–29]. However, hepatic encephalopathy in these studies occurred in 30–50% of patients treated with TIPS. The studies reported discrepant findings with respect to survival: two studies showed a survival benefit with TIPS [26,27], but two other studies demonstrated no difference in survival [25,28]. Meta-analyses of these randomized controlled studies conclude that TIPS is better at controlling ascites but does not improve survival compared to paracentesis and increases the risk of hepatic encephalopathy [31,32]. In view of these findings, the preferred initial treatment for refractory ascites is large volume paracentesis with albumin replacement. TIPS placement should be evaluated on a case-by-case basis and probably reserved for patients aged <70, with preserved liver function, without hepatic encephalopathy or severe cardiopulmonary disease who require very frequent paracentesis or in whom ascites cannot be adequately eliminated by paracentesis (see Figure 99.3).

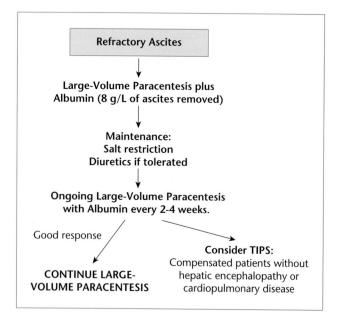

Figure 99.3 Treatment strategy for patients with refractory ascites.

Dilutional hyponatremia

Impairment of solute-free water excretion is common in advanced cirrhosis and occurs months after the onset of sodium retention. In the majority of patients with advanced cirrhosis, hyponatremia develops in the setting of ascites where there is an expanded extracellular fluid volume along with increased renal sodium retention. The major clinical consequence of this disorder is the development of DH, which is defined as a serum sodium concentration less than 130 mEq/L in the presence of ascites or edema [33]. The presence of hyponatremia is associated with a poor prognosis in cirrhosis; in patients with cirrhosis and ascites the risk of developing DH is 14% at 1 year with a 25% probability of survival at 1 year [4]. It is estimated that 22% of patients with advanced cirrhosis have serum sodium levels <130 mEq/L; however, in patients with refractory ascites or HRS, this proportion may increase up to 50% [26,34]. The pathogenesis of impairment of solute-free water excretion in cirrhosis is complex and is mainly due to increased non-osmotic secretion of the arginine vasopressin [35] which increases water reabsorption in the kidney due to the presence of V2 receptors located on the basolateral membrane of the collecting ducts. In most patients, DH is asymptomatic, but recent data indicate that hyponatremia is associated with a higher risk of hepatic encephalopathy [36]. The typical classical symptoms of acute hyponatremia rarely occur in cirrhosis.

Management of DH includes water restriction of approximately 1–1.5 L/day; however, this measure rarely works and although it may halt the progressive decrease in serum sodium concentration it does not correct hyponatremia. The administration of hypertonic saline solutions is not recommended because it invariably leads to further expansion of extracellular fluid volume and accumulation of ascites and edema. Several non-peptide V2 receptor antagonists including mozavaptan, lixivaptan, satavaptan , tolvaptan, and conivaptan have been evaluated in patients with cirrhosis and ascites [37–41]. These studies show that antagonists of the V2 receptor of arginine vasopressin are effective at increasing solute-free water excretion and improve serum sodium concentration in hyponatremic patients with cirrhosis and ascites [37–41]. The short-term administration of vaptans is associated with an increase in serum sodium concentration that occurs within the 4–5 days of treatment with normalization of serum sodium concentration occurring in 30–55% of patients. Conivaptan is approved in the USA for short-term (4–5 days) intravenous use (dose 20 mg/ day), whereas tolvaptan is approved as an oral compound (dose starting at 15 mg/day with sequential 15 milligram increments up to 60 mg/day) [39,41]. The most frequent side effect of vaptans in patients with cirrhosis is thirst which can occur in up to 30% of patients. Other side effects are uncommon; however, these drugs need to be used with caution and the patient must be carefully monitored as very rapid correction of hyponatremia (e.g., >12 mEq/L/24h) can cause osmotic demyelination. The use of these agents in cirrhosis has been assessed only in short-term studies. Long-term controlled

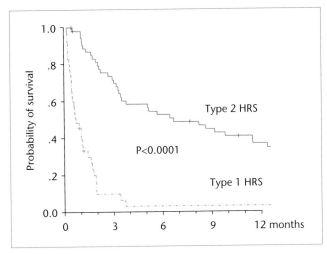

Figure 99.4 Survival of patients with cirrhosis after the diagnosis of type 1 and type 2 hepatorenal syndrome.

Table 99.1 Diagnostic criteria of hepatorenal syndrome in cirrhosis*

1. Cirrhosis with ascites
2. Serum creatinine >1.5 mg/dL
3. No improvement of serum creatinine (decrease to a level lower than 1.5 mg/dL after at least two days off diuretics and volume expansion with albumin (1 g/kg body weight up to a maximum of 100 g/day)
4. Absence of shock
5. No current or recent treatment with nephrotoxic drugs
6. Absence of signs of parenchymal renal disease, as suggested by proteinuria (>500 mg/day) or hematuria (<50 red blood cells per high power field), and/or abnormal renal ultrasound

Reproduced from Salerno *et al*. Diagnosis, prevention and treatment of the hepatorenal syndrome in cirrhosis. A consensus workshop of the international ascites club. *Gut* 2007;56:1310–1318, with permission from BMJ Publishing Group Ltd.

studies are needed to evaluate the safety, efficacy, and applicability of these agents in patients with cirrhosis, ascites, and DH.

Hepatorenal syndrome

One of the ultimate and most serious complications of cirrhotic ascites is HRS, a unique form of functional renal failure without identifiable renal pathology that occurs in approximately 10% of patients with advanced cirrhosis or acute liver failure [21,42]. HRS may develop acutely or subacutely. Type 1 HRS is an acute and rapidly progressive form of renal failure with a very short survival, while in type 2 HRS, renal failure is usually less severe and patients have a slightly better prognosis (Figure 99.4). The diagnosis of HRS is based on established criteria that aim to exclude other causes of renal failure in cirrhosis (Table 99.1) [42]. These include hypovolemia due to gastrointestinal bleeding (with or without hypovolemic shock) or intense diuretic therapy, septic shock, administration of nephrotoxic drugs (mainly non-steroidal anti-inflammatory drugs, NSAIDs), and intrinsic renal diseases, particularly glomerulonephritis associated with hepatitis B or C infection or alcoholic liver disease. HRS results from spontaneous bacterial peritonitis and other bacterial infections in approximately 30% of cases. Therefore, objective signs of infection (blood work and cultures, ascitic fluid analysis and culture, urine analysis and culture, chest X-ray) should be investigated in all patients with cirrhosis and renal failure and antibiotics should be given promptly if there are signs of infection.

In the majority of patients, HRS develops in the setting of advanced liver disease and sometimes in the setting of acute liver failure. In either case these patients, particularly those with type 1 HRS, are unstable and require hospitalization, preferably in an intensive care unit. Patients with type 2 HRS can be managed as outpatients unless they have associated complications. Diuretics need to be stopped because they can worsen renal failure and may cause electrolyte disturbances, particularly hyponatremia and hyperkalemia. Accepted therapies for HRS include liver transplantation, and vasoconstrictors. Liver transplantation is the best treatment for suitable candidates with HRS as it offers a cure for both the diseased liver and the renal failure. Since patients with type 1 HRS have a very poor prognosis this group of patients should be given higher priority for transplantation. Patients with HRS awaiting transplantation may benefit from treatment of HRS aimed at improving renal function before transplantation because those that respond have a similar outcome after transplantation to those patients transplanted without HRS [43].

Systemic vasoconstrictors are the accepted pharmacologic therapy in HRS. These include vasopressin analogues (terlipressin) and alpha-adrenergic agonists (midodrine and noradrenaline). Most of the information comes from the use of intravenous terlipressin. Albumin is concomitantly used with vasoconstrictors in order to help improve effective arterial blood volume. Randomized and non-randomized studies of terlipressin indicate that it reverses type 1 HRS in a 40–75% of patients [44–49]. There is limited data on the role of terlipressin or other vasoconstrictors in type 2 HRS. The recommended doses are 1 milligram every 4–6 hours intravenously, with a dose increased up to a maximum of 2 milligrams every 4–6 hours after 2–3 days if there is no response to therapy as defined by a reduction of serum creatinine >25% of pretreatment values. HRS reversal is considered when serum creatinine levels decrease below 1.5 mg/dL. Treatment response usually occurs within the first 7–10 days and is associated with a marked increase in urine volume and improvement of hyponatremia, which is almost constantly present in these patients. The incidence of ischemic side effects during terlipressin therapy, which are usually reversible after discontinuation of treatment, is of approximately 10% [48,49].

The use of midodrine, octreotide, and albumin as well as noradrenaline with albumin, may also improve renal function in cirrhotic patients with HRS [50–54]. Unfortunately, there is limited information on these therapeutic regimens and there

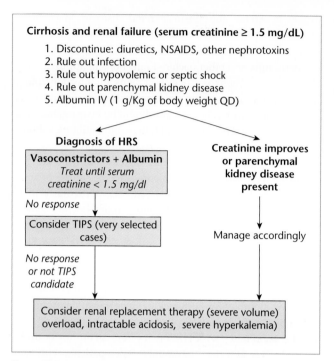

Cirrhosis and renal failure (serum creatinine ≥ 1.5 mg/dL)

1. Discontinue: diuretics, NSAIDS, other nephrotoxins
2. Rule out infection
3. Rule out hypovolemic or septic shock
4. Rule out parenchymal kidney disease
5. Albumin IV (1 g/Kg of body weight QD)

Diagnosis of HRS

Vasoconstrictors + Albumin
Treat until serum creatinine < 1.5 mg/dl

No response

Consider TIPS (very selected cases)

No response or not TIPS candidate

Consider renal replacement therapy (severe volume) overload, intractable acidosis, severe hyperkalemia)

Creatinine improves or parenchymal kidney disease present

Manage accordingly

Figure 99.5 Diagnosis and treatment strategy for patients with hepatorenal syndrome. Vasoconstrictors: terlipressin, midodrine, norepinephrine. *Transjugular intrahepatic portosystemic shunt (TIPS) in some selected cases can be considered in patients aged <70, without very advanced liver disease and without hepatic encephalopathy or cardiopulmonary disease. Renal replacement therapy (RRT) can be considered in patients without a response to pharmacological therapy, those that are not candidates for TIPS or those with important volume overload, intractable acidosis or severe hyperkalemia.

are no placebo-controlled studies in order to establish their efficacy on the pharmacological therapy of HRS. The recommended dose of midodrine ranges from 2.5 to 7.5 milligrams p.o. t.i.d with an increase to 12.5 milligrams t.i.d if needed and octreotide 100 micrograms subcutaneously t.i.d. daily with an increase to 200 micrograms t.i.d. if needed. Octreotide may also be used as a continuous infusion 25 μg/h intravenous octreotide after a bolus injection of 25 μg [50,51]. However octreotide alone is ineffective [52]. Noradrenaline (0.5–3 mg/h) is administered as a continuous infusion with intravenous albumin for up to 15 days [53,54].

TIPS may improve renal function HRS, but its applicability in patients with type 1 HRS and advanced liver disease is limited [55,56]. Due to the lack of data, more studies are needed evaluating the use of TIPS in patients with HRS. Renal replacement therapy is not considered a standard therapy of HRS, but it may serve as a temporary option in patients with no response to vasoconstrictors or in those that develop severe volume overload, metabolic acidosis or refractory hyperkalemia. The diagnosis and management of patients with HRS is outlined in Figure 99.5.

SOURCES OF INFORMATION FOR PATIENTS AND DOCTORS

We should tell patients that ascites and hepatorenal syndrome are consequences of underlying chronic liver disease and cirrhosis. If they are adequate candidates they must be evaluated for liver transplantation. They must understand that a salt restricted diet is of key importance for their management and that a nutritionist should help them plan their meals. In addition they should abstain from alcohol and the use of non-steroidal anti-inflammatory agents. Medical therapy with diuretics helps minimize ascites in most patients; however, those who do not respond to them or develop side effects should undergo repeated paracentesis every 2–3 weeks until transplantation. TIPS is an alternative but it can be associated with significant complications and the long-term outcome is similar to repeated paracentesis. Patients with renal failure need to be admitted to the hospital for a proper work-up: common causes of renal failure in cirrhosis are bacterial infections and hepatorenal syndrome. Current therapy for these conditions includes antibiotics and intravenous vasoconstrictors. If therapy is successful, patients may reach liver transplantation in a better condition, which means they have a greater probability of having a good post-transplant outcome. The following links are helpful resources:

- www.nlm.nih.gov/medlineplus/ency/article/000286.htm
- http://en.wikipedia.org/wiki/Ascites
- www.mayoclinic.com/health/cirrhosis/DS00373
- en.wikipedia.org/wiki/Hepatorenal_syndrome
- www.nlm.nih.gov/medlineplus/ency/article/000489.htm
- www.liverfoundation.org
- http://www.uptodate.com/contents/patient-information-cirrhosis-the-basics

References

1. Dawson AD. Historical notes on ascites. *Gastroenterology*. 1960;39:790–791.
2. Reuben A. Out came copious water. *Hepatology*. 2002;36: 261–264.
3. Ginès P, Quintero E, Arroyo V, *et al.* Compensated cirrhosis: natural history and prognostic factors. *Hepatology*. 1987;7: 122–128.
4. Planas R, Montoliu S, Ballesté B, *et al.* Natural history of patients hospitalized for management of cirrhotic ascites. *Clin Gastroenterol Hepatol*. 2006;4:1385–1394.
5. Iwakiri Y, Groszmann R. Vascular endothelial dysfunction in cirrhosis. *J Hepatol*. 2007;46:927–934.
6. Wiest R, Das S, Cadelina G, *et al.* Bacterial translocation in cirrhotic rats stimulates eNOS-derived NO production and impairs mesenteric vascular contractility. *J Clin Invest*. 1999;104: 1223–1233.
7. Ruiz del Arbol L, Monescillo A, Arocena C, *et al.* Circulatory function and hepatorenal syndrome in cirrhosis. *Hepatology*. 2005;42:439–447.
8. Cárdenas A, Ginès P. (2008) Sodium balance in cirrhosis, in *Sodium in Health and Disease*. (ed. M. Burnier). Informa Healthcare, New York, pp. 317–332.
9. Jiménez W, Martínez-Pardo A, Arroyo V, *et al.* Temporal relationship between hyperaldosteronism, sodium retention and ascites formation in rats with experimental cirrhosis. *Hepatology*. 1985;5:245–250.
10. Ginès P, Cárdenas A. The management of ascites and dilutional hyponatremia in cirrhosis. *Semin Liv Dis*. 2008;28:43–58.

Liver Disease

11. Moore KP, Wong F, Ginès P, *et al*. The management of ascites in cirrhosis: Report on the consensus conference of the International Ascites Club. *Hepatology*. 2003;38:258–266.

12. Perez-Ayuso RM, Arroyo V, Planas R, *et al*. Randomized comparative study of efficacy of furosemide versus spironolactone in nonazotemic cirrhosis with ascites. Relationship between the diuretic response and the activity of the renin–aldosterone system. *Gastroenterology*. 1983;84:961–968.

13. Santos J, Planas R, Pardo A, *et al*. Spironolactone alone or in combination with furosemide in the treatment of moderate ascites in nonazotemic cirrhosis. A randomized comparative study of efficacy and safety. *J Hepatol*. 2003;39:187–192.

14. Angeli P, Fasolato S, Mazza E, *et al*. Combined versus sequential diuretic treatment of ascites in non-azotaemic patients with cirrhosis: results of an open randomised clinical trial. *Gut*. 2010;59:98–104.

15. Mimidis K, Papadopoulos V, Kartalis G. Eplerenone relieves spironolactone-induced painful gynaecomastia in patients with decompensated hepatitis B-related cirrhosis. *Scand J Gastroenterol*. 2007;42:1516–1517.

16. Ginès P, Arroyo V, Quintero E, *et al*. Comparison of paracentesis and diuretics in the treatment of cirrhotics with tense ascites. Results of a randomized study. *Gastroenterology*. 1987;93:234–241.

17. Ruiz-del-Arbol L, Monescillo A, Jiménez W, *et al*. Paracentesis-induced circulatory dysfunction: mechanism and effect on hepatic hemodynamics in cirrhosis. *Gastroenterology*. 1997;113:579–586.

18. Ginès P, Tito L, Arroyo V, *et al*. Randomized comparative study of therapeutic paracentesis with and without intravenous albumin in cirrhosis. *Gastroenterology*. 1988;94:1493–1502.

19. Cárdenas A, Ginès P, Runyon BA. Is albumin infusion necessary after large volume paracentesis? *Liver Int*. 2009;29:636–640.

20. Ginès A, Fernandez-Esparrach G, Monescillo A, *et al*. Randomized trial comparing albumin, dextran 70, and polygeline in cirrhotic patients with ascites treated by paracentesis. *Gastroenterology*. 1996;111:1002–1010.

21. Arroyo V, Ginès P, Gerbes AL, *et al*. Definition and diagnostic criteria of refractory ascites and hepatorenal syndrome in cirrhosis. International Ascites Club. *Hepatology*. 1996;23:164–176.

22. Casado M, Bosch J, Garcia-Pagan JC, *et al*. Clinical events after transjugular intrahepatic portosystemic shunt: Correlation with hemodynamic findings. *Gastroenterology*. 1998;114:1296–1303.

23. Boyer TD. Transjugular intrahepatic portosystemic shunt in the management of complications of portal hypertension. *Curr Gastroenterol Rep*. 2008;10:30–35.

24. Lebrec D, Giuily N, Hadengue A, *et al*. Transjugular intrahepatic portosystemic shunts: comparison with paracentesis in patients with cirrhosis and refractory ascites: A randomized trial. *J Hepatol*. 1996;25:135–144.

25. Rossle M, Ochs A, Gulberg V, *et al*. A comparison of paracentesis and transjugular intrahepatic portosystemic shunting in patients with ascites. *N Engl J Med*. 2000;342:1701–1707.

26. Ginès P, Uriz J, Calahorra B, *et al*. Transjugular intrahepatic portosystemic shunting versus paracentesis plus albumin for refractory ascites in cirrhosis. *Gastroenterology*. 2002;123:1839–1847.

27. Sanyal A, Genning C, Reddy RK, *et al*. The North American study for treatment of refractory ascites. *Gastroenterology*. 2003;124:634–641.

28. Salerno F, Merli M, Riggio O, *et al*. Randomized controlled study of TIPS versus paracentesis plus albumin in cirrhosis with severe ascites. *Hepatology*. 2004;40:629–635.

29. Jung HS, Kalva SP, Greenfield AJ, *et al*. TIPS: Comparison of shunt patency and clinical outcomes between bare stents and expanded polytetrafluoroethylene stent-grafts. *J Vasc Interv Radiol*. 2009;20:180–185.

30. Bureau C, García-Pagan JC, Otal P, *et al*. Improved clinical outcome using polytetrafluoroethylene-coated stents for TIPS: results of a randomized study. *Gastroenterology*. 2004;126:469–475.

31. Albillos A, Banares R, Gonzales M, *et al*. A meta-analysis of transjugular intrahepatic portosystemic shunt versus paracentesis for refractory ascites. *J Hepatol*. 2005;43:990–996.

32. Dámico G, Luca A, Morabito A, *et al*. Uncovered transjugular intrahepatic portosystemic shunt for refractory ascites: A meta-analysis. *Gastroenterology*. 2005;129:1282–1293.

33. Ginès P, Guevara M. Hyponatremia in cirrhosis: Pathogenesis, clinical significance and management. *Hepatology*. 2008;48:1002–1010.

34. Angeli P, Wong F, Watson H, *et al*. Hyponatremia in cirrhosis: Results of a patient population survey. *Hepatology*. 2006;44:1535–1542.

35. Schrier RW. Vasopressin and aquaporin 2 in clinical disorders of water homeostasis. *Semin Nephrol*. 2008;28:289–296.

36. Guevara M, Baccaro ME, Torre A, *et al*. Hyponatremia is a risk factor of hepatic encephalopathy in patients with cirrhosis: A prospective study with time-dependent analysis. *Am J Gastroenterol*. 2009;104:1382–1389.

37. Wong F, Blei AT, Blendis LM, *et al*. A vasopressin receptor antagonist (VPA-985) improves serum sodium concentration in patients with hyponatremia: A multicenter, randomized, placebo-controlled trial. *Hepatology*. 2003;37:182–191.

38. Gerbes AL, Gulberg V, Ginès P, *et al*. VPA Study Group. Therapy of hyponatremia in cirrhosis with a vasopressin receptor antagonist: a randomized double-blind multicenter trial. *Gastroenterology*. 2003;124:933–939.

39. Schrier RW, Gross P, Gheorghiade M, *et al*. Tolvaptan, a selective oral vasopressin V2-receptor antagonist, for hyponatremia. *N Engl J Med*. 2006;355:2099–2112.

40. Ginès P, Wong F, Watson H, *et al*. Effects of satavaptan, a selective vasopressin V(2) receptor antagonist, on ascites and serum sodium in cirrhosis with hyponatremia: A randomized trial. *Hepatology*. 2008;48:204–213.

41. O'Leary JG, Davis GL. Conivaptan increases serum sodium in hyponatremic patients with end-stage liver disease. *Liver Transpl*. 2009;15:1325–1329.

42. Salerno F, Gerbes A, Wong F, *et al*. Diagnosis, prevention and treatment of the hepatorenal syndrome in cirrhosis. A consensus workshop of the International Ascites Club. *Gut*. 2007;56:1310–1318.

43. Restuccia T, Ortega R, Guevara M, *et al*. Effects of treatment of hepatorenal syndrome before transplantation on posttransplantation outcome. A case–control study. *J Hepatol*. 2004;40:140–146.

44. Uriz J, Ginès P, Cardenas A, *et al*. Terlipressin plus albumin infusion: An effective and safe therapy of hepatorenal syndrome. *J Hepatol*. 2000;33:43–48.

45. Moreau R, Durand F, Poynard T, *et al*. Terlipressin in patients with cirrhosis and type 1 hepatorenal syndrome: a retrospective multicenter study. *Gastroenterology*. 2002;122:923–930.

Liver Disease

46. Solanki P, Chawla A, Garg R. Beneficial effects of terlipressin in hepatorenal syndrome: a prospective, randomized placebo-controlled clinical trial. *J Gastroenterol Hepatol.* 2003;18:152–156.

47. Halimi C, Bonnard P, Bernard B. Effect of terlipressin (Gly-pressin) on hepatorenal syndrome in cirrhotic patients: results of a multicentre pilot study. *Eur J Gastroenterol Hepatol.* 2002; 14:153–158.

48. Sanyal A, Boyer T, Garcia-Tsao G, *et al.* A prospective, randomized, double blind, placebo-controlled trial of terlipressin for type 1 hepatorenal syndrome (HRS). *Gastroenterology.* 2008;134: 1360–1368.

49. Martin-Llahi M, Pepin MN, Guevara G, *et al.* Terlipressin and albumin vs albumin in patients with cirrhosis and hepatorenal syndrome: A randomized study. *Gastroenterology.* 2008;134: 1352–1359.

50. Angeli P, Volpin R, Gerunda G, *et al.* Reversal of type 1 hepatorenal syndrome with the administration of midodrine and octreotide. *Hepatology.* 1999; 29:1690–1697.

51. Wong F, Pantea L, Sniderman K. Midodrine, octreotide, albumin, and TIPS in selected patients with cirrhosis and type 1 hepatorenal syndrome. *Hepatology.* 2004;40:55–64.

52. Pomier-Layrargues G, Paquin SC, Hassoun Z, *et al.* Octreotide in hepatorenal syndrome: A randomized, double-blind, placebo-controlled, crossover study. *Hepatology.* 2003;38:238–243.

53. Duvoux C, Zanditenas D, Hezode C, *et al.* Effects of noradrenaline and albumin in patients with type 1 hepatorenal syndrome: A pilot study. *Hepatology.* 2002;36:374–380.

54. Alessandria C, Ottobrelli A, Debernardi-Venon W, *et al.* Noradrenalin vs terlipressin in patients with hepatorenal syndrome: a prospective, randomized, unblinded, pilot study. *J Hepatol.* 2007;47:499–505.

55. Brensing KA, Textor J, Perz J, *et al.* Long term outcome after transjugular intrahepatic portosystemic stent-shunt in non-transplant cirrhotics with hepatorenal syndrome: a phase II study. *Gut.* 2000;47:288–295.

56. Guevara M, Ginès P, Bandi JC, *et al.* Transjugular intrahepatic portosystemic shunt in hepatorenal syndrome: effects on renal function and vasoactive systems. *Hepatology.* 1998;28:416–422.

Liver Disease

CHAPTER 100
Spontaneous bacterial peritonitis

Guadalupe Garcia-Tsao

Yale University, School of Medicine, New Haven; Veterans Affairs Connecticut Healthcare System, West Haven, CT, USA

Introduction and epidemiology

Bacterial infections occur in about a third of hospitalized patients with cirrhosis [1]. These figures contrast with the 5–7% infection rate in hospitalized patients as a whole. Spontaneous bacterial peritonitis (SBP) is the most common infection, accounting for about 25% of all infections [1].

SBP is an infection of ascites characteristic of the cirrhotic patient that occurs in the absence of hollow viscus perforation and in the absence of an intra-abdominal inflammatory focus such as an abscess, acute pancreatitis, or cholecystitis.

About half the episodes of SBP are detected at the time of admission to the hospital while the rest develop during hospitalization. While the prevalence of SBP in hospitalized patients with ascites is ~20% [2], it is lower in an outpatient setting with a 4% rate in patients subjected to serial therapeutic paracenteses [3].

The 12-month incidence of first episode of SBP in cirrhotic patients with ascites ranges between 11% [4] but depends on ascites total protein content (0% in patients with ascites protein >1 g/dL vs. 20% in patients with ascites protein <1 g/dL) [4]. Ascites protein correlates closely with ascites complement levels and opsonic activity [5], a critical element in bacterial phagocytosis.

In addition to a low ascites protein, severe liver disease (low platelet count, high serum bilirubin, Child score >9) and/or indicators of circulatory dysfunction (renal dysfunction, hyponatremia) identify high-risk patients with a 1-year probability of SBP of 55–60% [6,7]. Liver function correlates with serum and ascites complement levels and with a greater impairment in antibacterial defense mechanisms [8].

Causes and pathogenesis

SBP is monomicrobial in over 90% of the cases. Aerobic Gram-negative organisms are responsible for the great majority (72–80%) of the cases, *Escherichia coli* being the most frequently isolated organism [1,2], followed by Gram-positive cocci, mainly *Streptococcus* sp. (20%), with *Enterococcus* accounting for 5% of the cases [2].

Given this predominance of enteric organisms, **bacterial translocation** (passage of viable microorganisms from the

Table 100.1 Rate of spontaneous bacterial peritonitis (SBP) in different settings

Setting	Time frame	SBP rate (control)	SBP rate (SID)	References
Gastrointestinal bleed	In-hospital	73/270* (27%)	19/264* (7%)	[24–28]
Prior SBP	5–10 months	52/115 (45%)	11/80 (14%)	[31–33]
Low-protein ascites, liver/circulatory dysfunction	12 months	10/33 (30%)	2/35 (6%)	[7]
Low-protein ascites ± high bilirubin	12 months	21/157 (13%)	3/159 (2%)	[34–36]

*Includes bacteremia.

SID, selective intestinal decontamination.

Populations shaded in yellow represent high-risk groups.

intestinal lumen to mesenteric lymph nodes and other extraintestinal sites) has been postulated as the main mechanism in the pathogenesis of SBP [8]. This is supported by experimental studies showing that bacterial translocation to mesenteric lymph nodes is always present in animals with infected ascites and by patient studies showing a decreased incidence of SBP with orally administered poorly absorbed antibiotics (selective intestinal decontamination) (Table 100.1).

The presence of bacteremia in half the cases of SBP and the occurrence of cases of isolated bacteremia in cirrhotic patients without an obvious primary focus of infection (spontaneous bacteremia), suggest that bacteria gain access to the systemic circulation prior to infecting the peritoneal fluid.

Cirrhotic patients, particularly those with ascites, have an acquired deficiency in antibacterial activity leading to increased bacterial translocation and bacteremia even when bacteria arise from sources other than the gut (Figure 100.1) [8].

The reticuloendothelial system (RES), mainly located in the liver Kupffer cells, is the main defensive system against bacteremia. In cirrhosis, the phagocytic activity of the RES is altered because of portosystemic shunting and because of a decreased bactericidal activity of Kupffer cells. Additionally, low serum complement levels lead to decreased peripheral bactericidal activity. This decreased antibacterial activity explains how a transient bacteremia (arising from the gut or other sources) becomes persistent (Figure 100.1). In patients with ascites, bacteria present in the systemic circulation colonize ascitic fluid and the development of SBP will then depend on the defensive capacity of the fluid. Low ascites complement lead to decreased ascites bactericidal activity and to a greater risk for SBP [5] (Figure 100.1).

Clinical presentation

SBP usually presents in a patient with overt ascites; however, it has been described in patients with ascites detectable only by ultrasound.

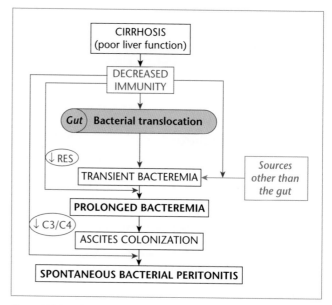

Figure 100.1 Pathogenesis of spontaneous bacterial peritonitis (SBP). RES, reticuloendothelial system; C3/C4, complement (fractions 3 and 4) levels. (This figure was published in *Clinical Gastroenterology and Hepatology*, Wilfred M. Weinstein, Christopher J. Hawkey, Jaime Bosch, Spontaneous bacterial peritonitis, Pages 1–6, Copyright Elsevier, 2005.)

The typical features of SBP consist of symptoms and signs of a generalized peritonitis, that is, diffuse abdominal pain, fever, abdominal tenderness with rebound tenderness and decreased bowel sounds. Patients may present with other less typical signs and symptoms such as hypothermia, hypotension, and diarrhea. The presence of peripheral leukocytosis with a shift to the left, unexplained encephalopathy and/or deterioration in renal function in a patient with ascites should always raise the suspicion of SBP. Patients rarely present with the complete picture. In a study performed in the emergency room, physician assessment was suboptimal in diagnosing or excluding SBP [9]. This supports the recommendation of performing a diagnostic paracentesis at each hospital admission and upon development of any compatible symptoms or signs [10].

Differential diagnosis

A small percentage (4.5%) of patients with cirrhosis and infected ascites have *secondary* peritonitis (hollow viscus perforation or a contiguous abscess), a condition with a higher mortality than SBP [11]. Secondary peritonitis usually requires surgical intervention and this can lead to further decompensation and death in a cirrhotic patient. Secondary peritonitis should be suspected when more than one organism is isolated from ascites (particularly when anaerobic bacteria and/or fungi are isolated) [11]. Patients who have two of three ascites findings: glucose < 50 mg/dL, protein >1.0 g/dL, or LDH > upper limit of normal serum levels have a higher probability of having secondary peritonitis [12] but the sensitivity is only 67% [11]. Ascites carcinoembryonic antigen and alkaline phosphatase levels may indicate intestinal perforation [13].

Another condition that should be distinguished from SBP is "**bacterascites**" defined as positive ascites bacteriological culture in the absence of an increased ascites PMN count. This most likely represents the phase of ascites colonization (Figure 100.1) and could evolve to SBP or resolve spontaneously. Once the diagnosis of bacterascites is made (usually 2–4 days after the paracentesis, when the microbiological results are available), it is recommended to repeat the paracentesis for PMN count and culture. Antibiotic therapy is warranted if PMN count is now indicative of SBP, if the culture remains positive and/or if the patient has signs of infection.

Diagnostic methods

A **diagnostic paracentesis** should be performed in: (1) any patient with cirrhosis and ascites admitted to the hospital, (2) any cirrhotic patient that develops symptoms or signs compatible with SBP, and (3) any cirrhotic patient with worsening renal function and/or hepatic encephalopathy [10]. In patients with hepatic hydrothorax in whom an infection is suspected and in whom SBP has been ruled out, a diagnostic thoracentesis should be performed to rule out spontaneous bacterial empyema that may occur in the absence of ascites or SBP [14].

Although isolation of an infecting organism is definitive in establishing the diagnosis of SBP, ascites cultures are negative in up to 60% of patients with clinical manifestations compatible with SBP and increased ascites PMNs, despite the use of sensitive culture methods [1]. Therefore, the diagnosis of SBP is established with an **ascites PMN count >250/mm³**. The use of reagent strips as an inexpensive alternative to manual PMN counts has been examined but, given a false negative rate >50%, their use cannot be recommended [15].

Bacteriological cultures of ascites (10 milliliters inoculated into blood culture bottles) and blood cultures should be obtained prior to the initiation of therapy to maximize the possibilities of isolating an infecting organism.

If and when secondary bacterial peritonitis is suspected, imaging studies should be performed, mainly flat abdominal films and abdominal computed tomography.

Treatment and prevention

Antibiotic treatment

Antibiotic treatment for SBP should be initiated once an ascitic (or pleural) fluid PMN count >250/mm³ is detected, before obtaining bacteriological culture results [10]. The recommended antibiotic is cefotaxime administered intravenously (at a dose of 2 g every 12 hours) with which the overall resolution of SBP occurs in ~90% of the patients [16–18]. Intravenous amoxicillin/clavulanate is as effective and safe as cefotaxime [19].

Because of the emergence of infections due to multi-drug resistant organisms, success rates as low as 44% have been recently described with both cefotaxime and amoxicillin/clavulanate, mainly in nosocomial (hospital-acquired) SBP [20–22]. Therefore, extended spectrum antibiotics (e.g., carbapenems, piperacillin/tazobactam) should be considered as initial empirical therapy in patients with hospital-acquired SBP, particularly in patients on quinolone prophylaxis in whom these infections are more prevalent [22]. Aminoglycosides should be avoided because cirrhotic patients are particularly prone to develop nephrotoxicity.

Treatment should be administered for a minimum of 5 days [10]. A control paracentesis performed 48 hours after starting therapy is recommended to assess the response to therapy and the need to modify antibiotic therapy (depending on the isolation of a causative organism) and/or to initiate investigations to rule out secondary peritonitis. If clinical improvement is obvious, control paracentesis may not be necessary.

In patients with a predicted good outcome, switching to an oral antibiotic after 48 hours of intravenous therapy is reasonable and even treating them with a widely bioavailable oral antibiotic, such as ofloxacin, is an option [23].

Prevention of spontaneous bacterial peritonitis

Prevention of SBP is based mainly on oral norfloxacin, a poorly absorbed quinolone that selectively eliminates Gram-negative organisms in the gut (selective intestinal decontamination). Given complications outlined below, antibiotic prophylaxis should be restricted to patients at the highest risk of SBP (Table 100.1), which are the following.

Patients with gastrointestinal hemorrhage

In controlled trials, 44% of patients admitted with gastrointestinal (GI) hemorrhage have or develop a bacterial infection during hospitalization [24–28]. In meta-analysis, short-term antibiotic prophylaxis significantly decreases infection rate (45% to 13%) and improves survival (decrease in mortality from 24% to 15%) [29]. Specifically for SBP, rates in control groups is 27% compared to 7% in patients receiving antibiotic prophylaxis [29] (Table 100.1). Although **oral norfloxacin** at a dose of 400 mg b.i.d. for 7 days is recommended by consensus [10], a recent randomized controlled trial (RCT) shows that **intravenous ceftriaxone** at a dose of 1 g/day for 7 days is more efficacious than norfloxacin (11% vs. 33%) in preventing infection (including SBP) in patients with two or more of the following: malnutrition, ascites, encephalopathy or serum bilirubin >3 mg/dL [30]. However, six of seven Gram-negative infections in the group randomized to norfloxacin were due to quinolone-resistant organisms [30]. Therefore, although the administration of antibiotic prophylaxis in this group of patients is justified and is considered standard of care, the choice of antibiotic should be based on the local prevalence of quinolone resistance and perhaps on the severity of liver disease.

Occurrence of spontaneous bacterial peritonitis

The highest rate of SBP occurs in patients who survive an episode, with a rate of 45% in 5–10 months (Table 100.1) [31–33]. Recurrent SBP is significantly lower (1-year probability 20–23% [32,33]) in patients receiving oral norfloxacin at a dose of 400 milligrams q.d. compared to 68% (in a placebo group) [32]. Therefore, it is essential to start oral norfloxacin prophylaxis in patients who have recovered from an episode SBP. The use of weekly quinolones has been shown to be less effective [33] and is therefore not recommended. Prophylaxis should be continuous until disappearance of ascites (i.e., patients with alcoholic hepatitis), death or transplant.

Presence of ascites protein

Although patients with **ascites protein < 1g/dL who have never developed SBP** are at higher risk of developing SBP than those with ascites protein >1 g/dL, the overall risk is low at around 13% in a 12-month period (Table 100.1) [34–36]. However, a recent placebo-controlled study selected a subgroup of patients who, in addition to having a low (<1.5 g/L) ascites protein, had advanced liver failure (CTP score ≥9 and serum bilirubin ≥3 mg/dL) or evidence of circulatory dysfunction (serum creatinine ≥1.2 mg/dL, blood urea nitrogen level ≥25 mg/dL or serum sodium level ≤130 mEq/L). In this (small) subset of patients, the 12-month rate of SBP was significantly higher at 30%, with a 1-year probability of developing SBP of 61% [7]. This probability decreased to 7% with the use of daily oral norfloxacin and was associated with a reduction in the incidence of hepatorenal syndrome and a reduction in 3-month mortality [7]. It is in this selected subpopulation of patients with cirrhosis and ascites that prophylaxis with norfloxacin (400 milligrams p.o., q.d.) could be considered, although confirmatory studies would be necessary to make a firm recommendation.

Complications and their management

One of the most serious complications and the most important predictor of death in patients with SBP is the development of **acute kidney injury**, which occurs in about a third of the patients. Kidney injury occurs as a result of vasodilatation and decreased effective arterial blood volume. **Intravenous albumin**, as a means of increasing volume, has been shown to be an important adjuvant to antibiotic therapy in patients with SBP. Patients who receive albumin (in addition to antibiotic therapy) have significantly lower rates of renal dysfunction during the acute process (10% vs. 3%) and lower in-hospital and 3-month mortality compared to patients treated with antibiotics alone [37]. Patients that benefit from the use of albumin are those with renal dysfunction at baseline (creatinine >1.0 mg/dL and/or BUN >30 mg/dL) and serum bilirubin >4 mg/dL [37–39]. Patients with "low-risk" SBP (i.e., those with serum creatinine <1 mg/dL and urea <30 mg/dL), approximately half of the patients with SBP, have a good outcome and do not require albumin [40].

Cost issues aside, the complications of long-term norfloxacin prophylaxis in cirrhosis include the **emergence of multi-drug resistant bacterial strains** [1,22] that has led to a decrease in the cure rate with cefotaxime or amoxicillin–clavulanate [20–22]. Additionally, a recent study has identified antibiotic prophylaxis as a predictor of *Clostridium difficile* infection that, in turn, is an independent predictor of death in cirrhosis [41].

Prognosis with and without treatment

In initial series published in the 1970s, the mortality associated with an episode of SBP exceeded 80%. In prospective studies from the last decade, with well-defined criteria for the diagnosis of SBP, the mortality rate has been reported as being around 20–30%. This decrease in mortality is the result of an increased awareness and early detection of the entity with prompt initiation of antibiotic therapy. Lower mortalities have been observed in patients with community-acquired, uncomplicated SBP (absence of GI hemorrhage, renal dysfunction, encephalopathy, ileus, or septic shock at presentation) [23,37], who are considered low-risk patients.

Median survival in patients who develop SBP is ~9 months and it is uncertain whether it is affected by prophylaxis or albumin. Therefore, patients who have developed an episode of SBP require prompt liver transplant evaluation.

SOURCES OF INFORMATION FOR PATIENTS AND DOCTORS

- http://hepatitis.va.gov/vahep?prtop08page=-01-gd-01
- http://www.aasld.org/practiceguidelines/Documents/ Bookmarked%20Practice%20Guidelines/Ascites%20 Update6–2009.pdf
- http://hepatitis.va.gov/vahep?page=prtop08–01-quicknotes

References

1. Fernandez J, Navasa M, Gomez J, *et al*. Bacterial infections in cirrhosis: epidemiological changes with invasive procedures and norfloxacin prophylaxis. *Hepatology*. 2002;35:140–148.
2. Garcia-Tsao G. Spontaneous bacterial peritonitis. *Gastroenterol Clin North Am*. 1992;21:257–275.
3. Evans LT, Kim WR, Poterucha JJ, *et al*. Spontaneous bacterial peritonitis in asymptomatic outpatients with cirrhotic ascites. *Hepatology*. 2003;37:897–901.
4. Llach J, Rimola A, Navasa M, *et al*. Incidence and predictive factors of first episode of spontaneous bacterial peritonitis in

cirrhosis with ascites: relevance of ascitic fluid protein concentration. *Hepatology*. 1992;16:724–727.

5. Runyon BA, Morrissey RL, Hoefs JC, *et al*. Opsonic activity of human ascitic fluid: a potentially important protective mechanism against spontaneous bacterial peritonitis. *Hepatology*. 1985;5:634–637.

6. Guarner C, Sola R, Soriano G, *et al*. Risk of a first community-acquired spontaneous bacterial peritonitis in cirrhotics with low ascitic fluid protein levels. *Gastroenterology*. 1999;117:414–419.

7. Fernandez J, Navasa M, Planas R, *et al*. Primary prophylaxis of spontaneous bacterial peritonitis delays hepatorenal syndrome and improves survival in cirrhosis. *Gastroenterology*. 2007;133: 818–824.

8. Garcia-Tsao G and Wiest R. Gut microflora in the pathogenesis of the complications of cirrhosis. *Best Pract Res Clin Gastroenterol*. 2004;18:353–372.

9. Chinnock B, Afarian H, Minnigan H, *et al*. Physician clinical impression does not rule out spontaneous bacterial peritonitis in patients undergoing emergency department paracentesis. *Ann Emerg Med*. 2008;52:268–273.

10. Rimola A, Garcia-Tsao G, Navasa M, *et al*. Diagnosis, treatment and prophylaxis of spontaneous bacterial peritonitis: a consensus document. *J Hepatol*. 2000;32:142–153.

11. Soriano G, Castellote J, Alvarez C, *et al*. Secondary bacterial peritonitis in cirrhosis: A retrospective study of clinical and analytical characteristics, diagnosis and management. *J Hepatol*. 2010;52:39–44.

12. Akriviadis EA and Runyon BA. Utility of an algorithm in differentiating spontaneous from secondary bacterial peritonitis. *Gastroenterology*. 1990;98:127–133.

13. Wu S-S, Lin OS, Chen Y-Y, *et al*. Ascitic fluid carcinoembryonic antigen and alkaline phosphatase levels for the differentiation of primary from secondary bacterial peritonitis with intestinal perforation. *J Hepatol*. 2001;34:215–221.

14. Xiol X, Castellvi JM, Guardiola J, *et al*. Spontaneous bacterial empyema in cirrhotic patients: a prospective study. *Hepatology*. 1996;23:719–723.

15. Nousbaum JB, Cadranel JF, Nahon P, *et al*. Diagnostic accuracy of the Multistix 8 SG reagent strip in diagnosis of spontaneous bacterial peritonitis. *Hepatology*. 2007;45:1275–1281.

16. Felisart J, Rimola A, Arroyo V, *et al*. Cefotaxime is more effective than is ampicillin-tobramycin in cirrhotics with severe infections. *Hepatology*. 1985;5:457–462.

17. Runyon BA, McHutchison JG, Antillon MR, *et al*. Short-course versus long-course antibiotic treatment of spontaneous bacterial peritonitis. *Gastroenterology*. 1991;100:1737–1742.

18. Rimola A, Salmeron JM, Clemente G, *et al*. Two different dosages of cefotaxime in the treatment of spontaneous bacterial peritonitis in cirrhosis: results of a prospective, randomized, multicenter study. *Hepatology*. 1995;21:674–679.

19. Ricart E, Soriano G, Novella M, *et al*. Amoxicillin–clavulanic acid versus cefotaxime in the therapy of bacterial infections in cirrhotic patients. *J Hepatol*. 2000;32:596–602.

20. Angeloni S, Leboffe C, Parente A, *et al*. Efficacy of current guidelines for the treatment of spontaneous bacterial peritonitis in the clinical practice. *World J Gastroenterol*. 2008;14:2757–2762.

21. Umgelter A, Reindl W, Miedaner M, *et al*. Failure of current antibiotic first-line regimens and mortality in hospitalized patients with spontaneous bacterial peritonitis. *Infection*. 2009; 37:2–8.

22. Acevedo J, Fernandez J, Castro M, *et al*. Current efficacy of recommended empirical antibiotic therapy in patients with cirrhosis and bacterial infection. *J Hepatol*. 2009;50(Suppl 1):S5 (abstract).

23. Navasa M, Follo A, Llovet JM, *et al*. Randomized, comparative study of oral ofloxacin versus intravenous cefotaxime in spontaneous bacterial peritonitis. *Gastroenterology*. 1996;111: 1011–1017.

24. Rimola A, Bory F, Teres J, *et al*. Oral, nonabsorbable antibiotics prevent infection in cirrhotics with gastrointestinal hemorrhage. *Hepatology*. 1985;5:463–467.

25. Soriano G, Guarner C, Tomas A, *et al*. Norfloxacin prevents bacterial infection in cirrhotics with gastrointestinal hemorrhage. *Gastroenterology*. 1992;103:1267–1272.

26. Blaise M, Pateron D, Trinchet JC, *et al*. Systemic antibiotic therapy prevents bacterial infection in cirrhotic patients with gastrointestinal hemorrhage. *Hepatology*. 1994;20:34–38.

27. Pauwels A, Mostefa-Kara N, Debenes B, *et al*. Systemic antibiotic prophylaxis after gastrointestinal hemorrhage in cirrhotic patients with a high risk of infection. *Hepatology*. 1996;24: 802–806.

28. Hsieh WJ, Lin HC, Hwang SJ, *et al*. The effect of ciprofloxacin in the prevention of bacterial infection in patients with cirrhosis after upper gastrointestinal bleeding. *Am J Gastroenterol*. 1998;93:962–966.

29. Bernard B, Grange JD, Khac EN, *et al*. Antibiotic prophylaxis for the prevention of bacterial infections in cirrhotic patients with gastrointestinal bleeding: A meta-analysis. *Hepatology*. 1999;29: 1655–1661.

30. Fernandez J, Ruiz d A, Gomez C, *et al*. Norfloxacin vs ceftriaxone in the prophylaxis of infections in patients with advanced cirrhosis and hemorrhage. *Gastroenterology*. 2006;131: 1049–1056.

31. Tito L, Rimola A, Gines P, *et al*. Recurrence of spontaneous bacterial peritonitis in cirrhosis: frequency and predictive factors. *Hepatology*. 1988;8:27–31.

32. Gines P, Rimola A, Planas R, *et al*. Norfloxacin prevents spontaneous bacterial peritonitis recurrence in cirrhosis: results of a double-blind, placebo-controlled trial. *Hepatology*. 1990;12: 716–724.

33. Bauer TM, Follo A, Navasa M, *et al*. Daily norfloxacin is more effective than weekly rufloxacin in prevention of spontaneous bacterial peritonitis recurrence. *Dig Dis Sci*. 2002;47: 1356–1361.

34. Novella M, Sola R, Soriano G, *et al*. Continuous versus inpatient prophylaxis of the first episode of spontaneous bacterial peritonitis with norfloxacin. *Hepatology*. 1997;25:532–536.

35. Grange JD, Roulot D, Pelletier G, *et al*. Norfloxacin primary prophylaxis of bacterial infections in cirrhotic patients with ascites – A double-blind randomized trial. *J Hepatol*. 1998;29:430–436.

36. Terg R, Fassio E, Guevara M, *et al*. Ciprofloxacin in primary prophylaxis of spontaneous bacterial peritonitis: A randomized, placebo-controlled study. *J Hepatol*. 2008;48:774–779.

37. Sort P, Navasa M, Arroyo V, *et al*. Effect of intravenous albumin on renal impairment and mortality in patients with cirrhosis and spontaneous bacterial peritonitis. *N Engl J Med* 1999;341: 403–409.

38. Sigal SH, Stanca CM, Fernandez J, *et al*. Restricted use of albumin for spontaneous bacterial peritonitis. *Gut*. 2007;56:597–599.

39. Terg R, Gadano A, Cartier M, *et al.* Serum creatinine and bilirubin predict renal failure and mortality in patients with spontaneous bacterial peritonitis: A retrospective study. *Liver Int.* 2009;29: 415–419.

40. Casas M, Soriano G, Ayala E, *et al.* Intravenous albumin is not necessary in cirrhotic patients with spontaneous bacterial peri-tonitis and low-risk of mortality. *J Hepatol.* 2007;46(Suppl 1): S91 (abstract).

41. Bajaj JS, Ananthakrishnan AN, Hafeezullah M, *et al.* Clostridium difficile is associated with poor outcomes in patients with cir-rhosis: A national and tertiary center perspective. *Am J Gastroen-terol.* 2009;105:106–113.

CHAPTER 101

Hepatopulmonary syndrome and portopulmonary hypertension

Rajan Kochar and Michael B. Fallon

The University of Texas Health Science Center at Houston, Houston, TX, USA

ESSENTIAL FACTS ABOUT PATHOGENESIS

Hepatopulmonary syndrome
- Incidence: 15–30% of patients with cirrhosis
- Pathogenesis: intrapulmonary microvascular vasodilatation and angiogenesis leading to impaired gas exchange
- Risk factors/genetic predisposition: unknown

Portopulmonary hypertension
- Incidence: 2–5% of patients with portal hypertension, 3–12% of patients evaluated for transplant
- Pathogenesis: endothelial dysfunction and smooth muscle proliferation leading to vasoconstriction, remodeling and increased pulmonary arterial pressure
- Risk factors/genetic predisposition: more common in females and autoimmune hepatitis, less common in hepatitis C

ESSENTIALS OF DIAGNOSIS

- Dyspnea is the most common symptom
- Exclusion of intrinsic cardiopulmonary disorders such as CHF and COPD is important (CXR, PFTs)

Hepatopulmonary syndrome
- Clinical features: dyspnea, clubbing, cyanosis, platypnea and orthodeoxia
- Impaired gas exchange evaluated with pulse oximetry and/or ABG analysis
- Intrapulmonary vasodilation diagnosed by contrast echocardiography (delayed shunting) or radionuclide scanning (increased uptake)

Portopulmonary hypertension
- Clinical features: dyspnea, fatigue, syncope, orthopnea, peripheral edema
- Doppler echocardiography: estimate right ventricular systolic and pulmonary artery pressure
- Right heart catheterization: accurate pressure and vascular resistance measurements to diagnose POPH (mPAP > 25 mmHg, PCWP < 15 mmHg, PVR > 240 dynes s cm^{-5})

ESSENTIALS OF TREATMENT

Hepatopulmonary syndrome
- No effective medical therapy is available
- Agents evaluated in small studies: aspirin, garlic, L-NAME, norfloxacin, pentoxifylline
- Supplemental oxygen advocated for moderate to severe symptoms, clinical benefit unknown
- Only effective therapy: liver transplantation, increased priority (MELD exception) given for moderate to severe HPS (PaO$_2$ < 60 mmHg)

Portopulmonary hypertension
- Medical therapies used successfully as monotherapy or combination, including endothelin receptor antagonists, phosphodiesterase V inhibitors, prostacyclin analogues, vasopressin analogues and tyrosine kinase inhibitors
- PAH therapies potentially harmful in POPH: anticoagulants, calcium channel blockers and beta blockers
- Liver transplantation contraindicated in moderate to severe POPH (mPAP > 35 mmHg) secondary to increased risk of perioperative complications, benefit unknown in patients with mPAP <35 mmHg on medical therapy

---

complications have emerged as important causes of dyspnea in patients with chronic liver disease and/or portal hypertension. The hepatopulmonary syndrome (HPS) occurs when intrapulmonary vascular alterations cause shunting of blood and impairs arterial gas exchange. Portopulmonary hypertension (POPH) results when pulmonary arterial constriction and remodeling lead to increased pulmonary arterial pressure. HPS is more common than POPH. The presence of either entity increases morbidity and mortality. Currently, orthotopic liver transplantation (OLT) is the only established treatment for HPS. The utility of OLT for POPH remains undefined.

Introduction

Respiratory symptoms are common in patients with chronic liver disease; about 50–70% complain of shortness of breath. The differential diagnosis of dyspnea in chronic liver disease is broad and there are a number of important causes to consider. Over the past years two distinct pulmonary vascular

Epidemiology

Intrapulmonary vasodilatation is seen on contrast echocardiography in over 50% of patients being evaluated for OLT. In addition, 15–30% of those with intrapulmonary shunting have impaired oxygenation resulting in a diagnosis of HPS.

Liver Disease

Although POPH is a relatively uncommon complication, it accounts for a substantial percentage of patients with pulmonary arterial hypertension (PAH). Recent studies have estimated its incidence to be 2–5% in all patients with portal hypertension and 3–12% in those being evaluated for OLT.

Causes, risk factors and disease associations

HPS and POPH are found most commonly in the setting of cirrhosis and portal hypertension. Recently, HPS has also been recognized in patients with portal hypertension in the absence of cirrhosis (portal vein thrombosis, nodular regenerative hyperplasia, congenital hepatic fibrosis and Budd–Chiari syndrome) and hepatic dysfunction in the absence of established portal hypertension (acute and chronic hepatitis). These findings support that advanced liver disease is not required for HPS to develop. Controversy exists regarding whether HPS is more common or severe in patients with advanced cirrhosis, although a recent prospective multicenter study from the US did not find an association between HPS and severity of liver disease. POPH has only been described in the presence of portal hypertension, with or without cirrhosis. Although there are no definitive predictors of POPH, a recent study found an increased risk of POPH in female patients and patients with

autoimmune hepatitis; and a decreased risk in patients with hepatitis C as the etiology of liver disease. Generally, the diagnosis of portal hypertension precedes the diagnosis of POPH by several years.

Pathogenesis and pathology

Since either HPS and POPH can develop in the setting of cirrhosis and portal hypertension, they may share pathogenetic mechanisms. Potential mechanisms common to both disorders include effects mediated by shear stress, cytokine and endothelin-1 alterations occurring in liver disease (Figure 101.1). In human HPS, nitric oxide overproduction appears to contribute to intrapulmonary vasodilatation. In experimental HPS, both endothelin-1 induced endothelial nitric oxide synthase activation through the endothelin B receptor in endothelial cells and intravascular macrophage accumulation and production of nitric oxide and carbon monoxide trigger vasodilatation. In addition, angiogenesis is an important contributor to the development of experimental HPS, is associated with activation of angiogenic pathways (VEGF-A) in part by intravascular monocytes. Less is known about the underlying mechanisms for POPH and no experimental models have been developed. Shear stress, vasoactive mediator, genetic and

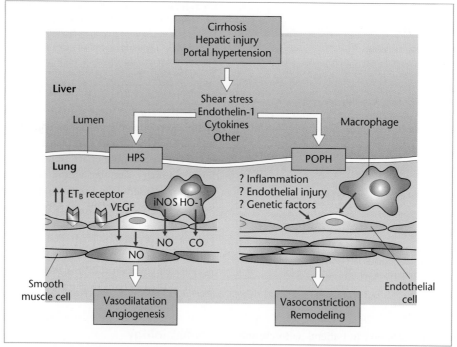

Figure 101.1 Potential mechanisms in hepatopulmonary syndrome and portopulmonary hypertension. Liver injury and/or portal hypertension trigger alterations that influence the production and release of vasoactive mediators and cytokines and modulate vascular shear stress. In experimental HPS, hepatic endothelin-1 release stimulates pulmonary vascular endothelial nitric oxide synthase (eNOS) derived nitric oxide (NO) production through an increased number of endothelial B receptors (ET$_B$ receptor) leading to vasodilatation. Macrophages also accumulate in the vascular lumen and produce NO from inducible nitric oxide synthase (iNOS) and carbon monoxide (CO) from heme oxygenase-1 (HO-1) contributing to

vasodilatation. Activation of angiogenic pathways such as vascular endothelial growth factor A (VEGF-A) are also facilitated through intravascular mononuclear cells leading to angiogenesis. In POPH, similar events possibly modified by genetic factors and the inflammatory response may result in endothelial injury and smooth muscle proliferation with vascular remodeling. (This figure was published in *Clinical Gastroenterology and Hepatology*, Wilfred M. Weinstein, Christopher J. Hawkey, Jaime Bosch, Hepatopulmonary syndrome and portopulmonary hypertension, Pages 1–5, Copyright Elsevier, 2005.)

inflammatory effects leading to endothelial dysfunction and smooth muscle cell proliferation have been postulated as in primary pulmonary hypertension. The pulmonary endothelial response to alterations in liver disease and portal hypertension (nitric oxide overproduction and angiogenesis in HPS versus dysfunction and injury in POPH) may determinine whether HPS or POPH develops.

Clinical presentation

The most common complaint in patients with either HPS or POPH is dyspnea. However, moderate to severe HPS or POPH may be present in the absence of specific symptoms (Table 101.1). Patients with HPS typically complain of the insidious onset of exertional dyspnea which progresses. Platypnea (shortness of breath exacerbated by sitting up and improved by lying supine), orthodeoxia (hypoxemia exacerbated in the upright position), cyanosis and clubbing are often found and may increase the clinical suspicion for the diagnosis. Clubbing appears to be a relatively specific finding in HPS (Figure 101.2). POPH appears to be more commonly asymptomatic, is infrequently associated with cyanosis or marked hypoxemia, and is not associated with platypnea. Initial symptoms of POPH are often subtle. Fatigue, orthopnea, chest discomfort and syncope are features of advanced POPH. An elevated jugular venous pressure, an accentuated P2 component or a tricuspid regurgitation murmur may be found Lower extremity edema out of proportion to ascites may be observed as POPH progresses.

Differential diagnosis

Dyspnea is a common symptom in cirrhosis and has multiple causes. For clinical purposes, these causes may be grouped into those arising due to the presence of liver disease and those independent of the presence of liver disease (Table 101.2).

Specifically, decompensated liver disease may be associated with deconditioning, muscle wasting, tense ascites and/or hepatic hydrothorax. Common causes of intrinsic cardiopulmonary disease independent of cirrhosis are chronic obstructive pulmonary disease and congestive heart failure. It is important to recognize that both HPS and POPH may co-exist with these other causes of dyspnea and hypoxemia.

Diagnostic methods

In chronic liver disease patients with dyspnea, evaluation for both intrinsic cardiopulmonary disease, HPS and POPH is appropriate. However, as both HPS and POPH may have nonspecific clinical features and subtle findings, diagnostic screening is also appropriate in all patients undergoing evaluation for liver transplantation, since the presence of HPS or POPH may influence candidacy for and timing of liver transplantation. An algorithm for screening is outlined in Figure 101.3.

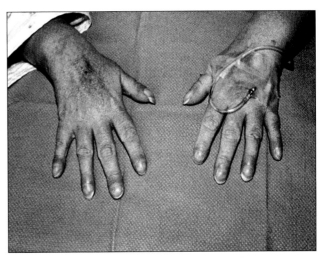

Figure 101.2 Digital clubbing in a patient with HPS. Clubbing appears to be a relatively specific clinical marker for the presence of HPS.

Table 101.1 Clinical presentation of hepatopulmonary syndrome and portopulmonary hypertension

Hepatopulmonary syndrome	Portopulmonary hypertension

• Often asymptomatic but symptoms include:
  – Dyspnea (most common)
  – Platypnea
	• Often asymptomatic but symptoms include:
	  – Dyspnea (most common)
	  – Chest Pain, orthopnea
	  – Syncope, faitugue

• Signs:
  – Orthodeoxia
  – Digital clubbing
  – Cyanosis
	• Signs:
	  – Jugular distention
	  – Accentuated P2
	  – Tricuspid regurgitation murmur
	  – Anasarca

• Symptoms/signs may correlate with severity of underlying cirrhosis • Hypoxemia common	• Symptoms/signs do not correlate with severity of underlying cirrhosis • Hypoxemia uncommon

Table 101.2 Causes of dyspnea and hypoxemia in chronic liver disease

Intrinsic cardiopulmonary disease independent of cirrhosis
- Chronic obstructive pulmonary disease
- Congestive heart failure
- Other: pneumonia, atelectasis, asthma, restrictive lung disease

Conditions associated with liver disease
- *General complications*
  - Deconditioning and muscular wasting
  - Ascites
  - Hepatic hydrothorax
- *Pulmonary vascular disorders*
  - Hepatopulmonary syndrome
  - Portopulmonary hypertension
- *Specific lung–liver disease associations*
  - Primary biliary cirrhosis: Pulmonary hemorrhage, fibrosing alveolitis, pulmonary granulomas
  - Alpha-1 antitrypsin deficiency: panacinar emphysema

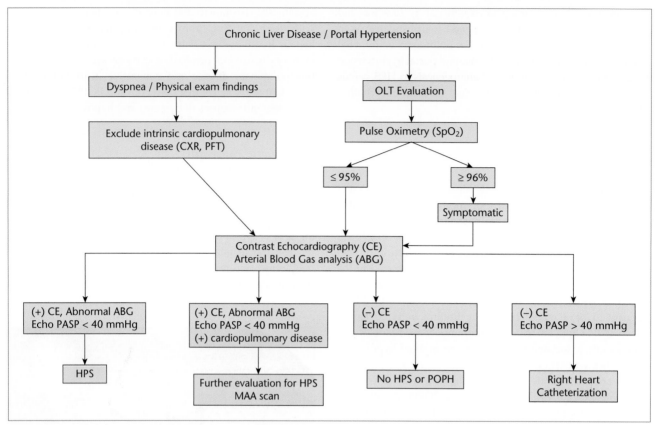

Figure 101.3 Diagnostic approach to HPS and POPH. In patients where symptoms or exam findings suggest cardiopulmonary dysfunction or in those being considered for liver transplantation, screening for HPS and POPH is appropriate. Other causes for cardio-pulmonary disease are evaluated using chest radiography (CXR) and pulmonary function testing (PFTs). Pulse oximetry or arterial blood gases (ABGs) are used to detect gas exchange abnormalities. Standard simplified formulas may be used to calculate the alveolar-arterial oxygen gradient and correct values for age. Contrast echocardiography with doppler (CE) is performed. If CE is positive for intrapulmonary shunting and gas exchange abnormalities are present without intrinsic cardiopulmonary disease then HPS is present. If similar findings are found in a patient with intrinsic cardiopulmonary disease then radionuclide lung perfusion scanning, using technetium-labeled macroaggregated albumin particles (MAA) may define if HPS is contributing to ABG abnormalities. If CE is negative and doppler calculation of pulmonary arterial systolic pressure (PASP) is low then HPS and POPH are unlikely. If CE is negative and estimated PASP is high, then right heart catheterization is indicated to confirm the presence of POPH.

Hepatopulmonary syndrome

The diagnosis of HPS rests on documenting the presence of pulmonary gas exchange abnormalities due to intrapulmonary vasodilatation. The most sensitive technique for detecting gas exchange abnormalities is measurement of the arterial blood gas (ABG) and calculation of the alveolar–arterial oxygen gradient with age correction (abnormal >20 mmHg). Pulse oximetry is an alternative non-invasive modality that indirectly measures oxygen saturation (SpO_2) and is a useful screening test for hypoxemia and HPS. From a clinical perspective, SpO_2 measurements can guide subsequent use of ABG and contrast echocardiography (CE). CE is the most commonly employed screening technique to detect intrapulmonary vasodilatation. It is performed by injecting agitated saline intravenously during normal transthoracic echocardiography, producing microbubbles that are visible on sonography. This opacifies the right ventricle within seconds and in the absence of right-to-left shunting, bubbles are absorbed in the lungs. If an intra-cardiac shunt is present, contrast agent enters the left ventricle within three heartbeats (early shunting). If intrapulmonary shunting, characteristic of HPS is present, the left ventricle opacifies at least thee heartbeats after the right (delayed shunting). Radionuclide lung perfusion scanning, using technetium-labeled macroaggregated albumin particles can quantify intrapulmonary shunting and is used to define if HPS is contributing to hypoxemia in patients with concomitant intrinsic lung disease but is less sensitive than contrast echocardiography.

Portopulmonary hypertension

POPH is diagnosed by an elevated mean pulmonary arterial pressure in the absence of volume overload or intrinsic cardiopulmonary disease. Doppler echocardiography is used to estimate the systolic pulmonary artery pressure. Combining Doppler echocardiography with contrast injection provides screening for both POPH and HPS. An estimated systolic pulmonary arterial pressure of >40–50 mmHg defines the need for direct measurement of pulmonary pressures by right heart

Table 101.3 Treatment and prevention in hepatopulmonary syndrome and portopulmonary hypertension

Hepatopulmonary syndrome	Portopulmonary hypertension
• No effective medical therapies	• Medical therapies improve symptoms

• Appropriate interventions:
– Oxygen therapy (if PaO$_2$ < 60 mmHg)
– Referral to specialized center
– Liver transplantation evaluation
	• Appropriate interventions:
	– Referral to specialized center
	– Medical therapy:
	  (i) ET antagonists
	  (ii) PDE V, TK inhibitors
	  (iii) PCI, vasopressin analogues

• Liver transplantation only effective treatment modality • No specific prevention available	• Liver transplantation generally contraindicated • No specific prevention available

ET, endothelin; PCI, prostacyclin; PDE V, phosphodiesterase V; TK, tyrosine kinase.

catheterization. A mean pulmonary artery pressure of >25 mmHg with a pulmonary capillary wedge pressure <15 mmHg, confirms the diagnosis of pulmonary arterial hypertension. An elevated transpulmonary gradient (mean pulmonary artery pressure – pulmonary capillary wedge pressure >10 mmHg) and pulmonary vascular resistance (>240 dyne s cm^{-5}) are additional measurements used to distinguish pulmonary arterial hypertension from pulmonary venous hypertension which may be present due to the hyperdynamic circulation and volume overload that accompany cirrhosis.

Treatment and prevention

There are no clearly effective medical therapies to reverse HPS or POPH. However, prospective randomized studies have not been performed to date. Table 101.3 summarizes treatment.

Hepatopulmonary syndrome

Case reports and small studies have suggested that a number of agents including aspirin, garlic, norfloxacin and inhaled L-NAME might improve HPS. Conflicting results were obtained from two small pilot studies using pentoxifylline In patients with resting or exertional hypoxemia supplemental oxygen therapy is appropriate although no studies have evaluated whether clinical benefit occurs. Portal decompression with transjugular intrahepatic portosystemic shunt (TIPS) has been attempted in a small number of cases. However, convincing evidence for sustained improvement is lacking and TIPS should be considered an experimental treatment. OLT is the only proven therapy for HPS based upon resolution or significant improvement in gas exchange post-operatively in more than 85% of patients. The length of time for resolution after transplantation varies and may be more than one year. In addition, mortality is increased after transplantation in HPS

patients compared to subjects without HPS particularly when hypoxemia is severe. Currently, HPS patients with a PaO2 <60 mmHg are eligible for increased priority for OLT (MELD exception).

Portopulmonary hypertension

Medical treatment for portopulmonary hypertension is based largely on experience in primary pulmonary hypertension. However, anticoagulants and calcium channel blockers are not recommended due to their potential to increase bleeding and portal pressure respectively. The use of beta-adrenergic blockers for prevention of variceal bleeding should be considered with caution. Medical therapies have been successfully used in POPH both as monotherapy or in combination, including endothelin receptor antagonists (bosentan), phosphodiesterase V inhibitor (sildenafil), prostacyclin analogues (epoprostenol, treprostinil, iloprost), vasopressin analogues (terlipressin) and tyrosine kinase inhibitors (imantinib). However, no controlled trials have been undertaken and whether medical therapy impacts survival is unknown. Bosentan has the potential for hepatotoxicity and its safety is uncertain.

The safety and efficacy of OLT in patients with POPH is controversial. There are no well-designed, prospective studies to guide decision making. Retrospective studies and case reports confirm that moderate-to-severe POPH (mPAP >35 mmHg), particularly if right ventricular dysfunction is present, is associated with substantial peri-operative mortality and is a contraindication for transplantation. Less severe POPH (mPAP <35 mmHg) is generally not considered a contraindication to OLT, but patients need to be evaluated individually to minimize risks. Recent retrospective studies suggest that OLT may be feasible and beneficial in patients with moderate-to-severe POPH who are otherwise suitable OLT candidates if medical therapy lowers mPAP to <35 mmHg. Several UNOS regions provide MELD exception points for these patients.

Complications

The presence of HPS appears to significantly decrease survival in patients with cirrhosis through an increase liver related complications. This observation has led to the hypothesis that hypoxemia may directly worsen hepatic function in HPS. Post-operative complications after liver transplantation observed in patients with HPS include pulmonary hypertension, cerebral vascular accidents, sepsis/respiratory failure, cardiac arrhythmias and deterioration in oxygenation. The major complication in patients with POPH is progressive right heart failure and cor pulmonale.

Prognosis

The natural history of hepatopulmonary syndrome is not fully characterized. Many patients develop progressive intrapulmonary vasodilatation and worsening gas exchange over time and spontaneous improvement is rare. Mortality is significantly higher and quality of life is significantly lower in patients with HPS compared to cirrhotics without HPS. The success of liver transplantation in reversing HPS and the policy of increasing priority for transplantation in HPS associated with significant hypoxemia, may improve prognosis. The natural history of POPH has been evaluated in small studies. A mortality of approximately 50% at 1 year and 70% at 5 years has been found. Whether the use of prostacyclin or its analogues or liver transplantation targeted to those with mild disease will alter survival is unknown.

CHAPTER 102

Hepatic encephalopathy

Thomas A. Brown and Kevin D. Mullen

Case Western Reserve University, Cleveland, OH, USA

ESSENTIAL FACTS ABOUT PATHOGENESIS

- Hepatic encephalopthy (HE) occurs in patients with *acute* liver failure, portal-systemic *bypass*, or *cirrhosis* (types A, B, and C respectively)
- Numerous implicated toxins but ammonia's role is considered to be the most important
- Type C HE is the most common, often precipitated by one or more of the following factors:
  - GI bleeding
  - Infection
  - Dehydration
  - Constipation
  - Sedating medications
  - Electrolyte imbalance
  - Renal failure

ESSENTIALS OF DIAGNOSIS

- Neuropsychiatric symptoms include attention deficit, alteration of sleep–wake cycle, coma, asterixis. Verbal and intellectual functioning are often preserved
- Rule out other causes of mental status changes. Detect presence of precipitating factors. Speaking with family members/ close contacts is often helpful
- Use West Haven criteria (Table 102.1) to grade severity of overt HE
- Minimal HE is clinically undetectable. Diagnose with specific psychometric tests
- Measuring ammonia is not recommended

ESSENTIALS OF TREATMENT AND PROGNOSIS

- Treat precipitating factors empirically and early: hydrate, stop gastrointestinal bleeding, antibiotics if infection is suspected
- Lactulose is first line for acute episodes and secondary prophylaxis
- Metronidazole and rifaximin are second line drugs when lactulose therapy fails
- HE is associated with higher mortality from liver disease
- Minimal HE affects daily quality of life

Introduction and epidemiology

Hepatic encephalopathy (HE) is a reversible spectrum of neuropsychiatric symptoms seen in patients with either cirrhosis, acute liver failure, or a portal–systemic bypass. Our understanding of HE's complex pathogenesis is growing. More diagnostic and therapeutic tools are available. However, our effectiveness at promptly controlling and preventing HE is far from perfect.

While HE is not included in the Model for End-Stage Liver Disease (MELD) scoring system, the first episode of HE signifies an important event in the course of liver disease. HE signify worseneds prognosis, impairs functional status and results in increased medical expenditures. Studies have shown a 42% 1-year and 23% 3-year survival after the first episode of overt HE (Figure 102.1).

HE is most commonly diagnosed in patients with underlying cirrhosis because of its higher incidence (estimates of 5.5 million cases in the US) as compared to acute liver failure (~740 cases in the US in 2007) or portal–systemic shunts. Roughly 30 to 45% of patients with cirrhosis will have an episode of clinically detectable overt HE. Up to 80% of patients with cirrhosis will have clinically undetectable, or minimal HE.

Annual US costs for admitting patients with HE exceed $900 million. The number of hospital admissions for HE in the USA was of over 70,000 in 2007.

Causes and pathogenesis

Causes

Acute liver failure

HE occurs due to the huge loss of hepatic processing capabilities. Development of HE in acute liver failure (ALF) is closely associated with development of cerebral edema. See chapter on acute liver failure.

Portal–systemic bypass

Portal–systemic bypass refers to a shunt, or direct communication between the portal and the systemic circulation. Typically, patients with an underlying portal–systemic bypass who develop HE have hepatic parenchymal disease as well. These may be medically created transjugular intrahepatic portal–systemic shunt (TIPS) or surgical distal splenorenal or end-to-side portacaval shunt.

Additionally, shunts may be formed spontaneously with increasing portal pressures or congenital. Splenorenal shunts are most commonly associated with symptomatic HE [1].

Liver Disease

Textbook of Clinical Gastroenterology and Hepatology, Second Edition. Edited by C. J. Hawkey, Jaime Bosch, Joel E. Richter, Guadalupe Garcia-Tsao, Francis K. L. Chan.
© 2012 Blackwell Publishing Ltd. Published 2012 by Blackwell Publishing Ltd.

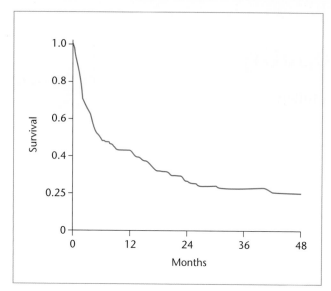

Figure 102.1 Survival curve after first episode of type C overt HE. Survival probability of 111 cirrhotic patients presenting with a first episode of overt HE. Time zero of the curve corresponds to the time of diagnosis of HE. Note that the survival rate at 1 year is 40%. (Reproduced with permission from Riggio O, Efrati C, Catalano C, *et al.* High prevalence of spontaneous portal-systemic shunts in persistent hepatic encephalopathy: a case-control study. *Hepatology.* 2005;42:1158–1165.)

Table 102.1 West Haven criteria

Grade	Features
Grade 0	• Lack of detectable changes in personality or behavior • No asterixis
Grade 1	• Trivial lack of awareness, shortened attention span, sleep disturbance, altered mood • Asterixis may be present
Grade 2	• Lethargy, disorientation to time, amnesia of recent events, impaired simple computations, inappropriate behavior, slurred speech • Asterixis is present
Grade 3	• Somnolence, confusion, disorientation to place, bizarre behavior, clonus, nystagmus, positive Babinski • Asterixis is usually absent
Grade 4	• Coma • Lack of verbal, eye, and oral response

Cirrhosis

Commonly, a precipitating factor causes patients with underlying cirrhosis (with or without minimal HE) to have episodes of overt hepatic encephalopathy. Gastrointestinal (GI) bleeding, infection, and dehydration are the most common precipitants. Other factors include constipation, a high protein load to the gut, the use of sedative and/or psychotropic drugs, recent surgery, or electrolyte imbalance.

Studies have implicated a higher incidence of HE with diabetes mellitus and/or autonomic neuropathy, likely due to prolonged orocecal transit times permitting colonic bacteria to form ammonia more readily.

Pathogenesis

HE is a complex process with a multifactorial etiology. Nevertheless, one dominant hypothesis exists regarding its pathogenesis – that of ammonia's leading role.

Normal ammonia metabolism

Nitrogen is absorbed in the form of amino acids and ammonia. Degradation of colonic luminal contents by colonic bacteria and small intestinal deamidation of glutamine to glutamate yields ammonia. Ammonia diffuses across the colonic epithelium and its concentration in the portal vein is approximately a 10-fold higher levels than that in the systemic circulation. The kidney is also a significant source of ammonia.

A healthy liver clears most ammonia (85% metabolism on first pass). The liver converts ammonia to urea in the urea cycle by combining ammonia with ornithine, bicarbonate, and aspartate. Some of the enzymes involved require zinc as a cofactor. Urea can then be excreted renally.

The liver also combines ammonia with glutamate using glutamine synthetase to form glutamine. Glutamine serves a major nitrogen donor throughout the body in the biosynthesis of amino and nucleic acids. Muscle can also either decrease blood ammonia using glutamine synthetase to make its own glutamine or increase blood ammonia via protein breakdown in catabolic states.

Altered ammonia metabolism and neurotransmission

In diseased livers and/or portal–systemic bypasses, ammonia uptake by the liver is decreased and consequently circulates in higher concentrations. The brain has no urea cycle. Instead, cerebral ammonia can only be cleared by combining glutamate with ammonia to form glutamine. in the cortical Alzheimer's type II astrocyte. The excess of intracellular glutamine is associated with astrocyte swelling, an important underlying mechanism in the pathogenesis of HE. Astrocyte swelling impairs complex intercellular communications and diverse neurotransmitter systems, including gamma-aminobutyric acid (GABA) receptors, glutamate, and loss of astrocyte myoinositol.

Swollen astrocytes have an enlarged nucleus with peripherally displaced chromatin. The remaining cerebral neurons appear normal.

Ammonia's upregulation of the peripheral-type benzodiazepine receptors (PTBR) on the astrocyte mitochondrial membrane promotes neurosteroid formation which stimulate inhibitory GABA-A receptors on postsynaptic membranes, affecting neurotransmission. Blocked reuptake of glutamate further alters neurotransmission.

Additional proposed etiologies

Other proposed mechanisms include cerebral mitochondrial dysfunction from induction of mitochondrial permeability transition (mPT), oxidative stress, and inflammatory mediators. Additionally, manganese has been demonstrated to accumulate in the globus pallidus of the basal ganglia and cause a hyperintensity on MR imaging, but it is unclear whether this affects neurotransmission. Increased entry of tryptophan, a precursor or serotonin, and altered serotoninergic neurotransmission may underlie altered sleep–wake cycles seen in early stages of HE.

Clinical presentation

General symptoms

The classic description of HE by Adams and Foley consisted of an alteration in consciousness and a generalized motor disturbance. We now know that the manifestations of HE encompass a much more expansive range. Symptoms range from the covert nature of minimal HE, which by strict definition has no clinically detectable symptoms, to the deepest coma that can be identified from the proverbial hallway. By definition, the patient must have an underlying liver disease or portal–systemic bypass in order for HE to be present.

The West Haven criteria nicely categorizes the common symptoms of overt HE (Table 102.1). Patients may present with minor changes in behavior, often detected by a family member. These include somnolence, disorientation, confusion, clumsiness, and difficulty with simple mathematic calculations. Inversion of the sleep–wake cycle may be present. As encephalopathy worsens, disorientation and lethargy are more prominent (grade 2). In grade 3, patients may be incoherent and unable to communicate effectively; stupor may also be present. In grade 4, patients are in coma, with varying degrees of response to painful stimuli.

Classification of hepatic encephalopathy

The World Congress of Gastroenterology provided current terminology (Table 102.2). Three main types were identified: type A in patients with acute liver failure, type B in patients with portal–systemic bypass, and type C in patients with cirrhosis. Subcategories of episodic and persistent are then used to describe the time sequence of symptoms. Proposed modifications have subsequently been made to accommodate the varying nature of HE as is often seen in types B and C (Figure 102.2).

Table 102.2 Current terminology for the classification of hepatic encephalopathy (HE)

Type	Description	Subcategory	Subdivision
A	HE associated with Acute liver failure	—	—
B	HE associated with portal–systemic bypass but no intrinsic hepatocellular disease	—	—
C	HE associated with cirrhosis or portal hypertension/portal–systemic bypasses	Episodic HE	• Precipitated • Spontaneous • Recurrent
		Persistent HE	• Mild • Severe • Treatment dependent
		Minimal HE	

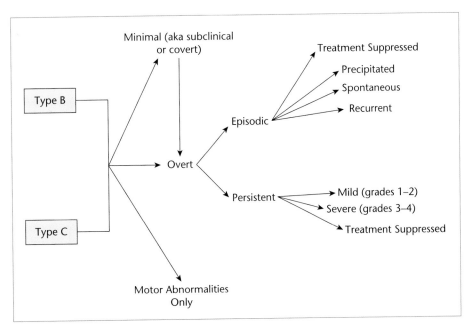

Figure 102.2 Proposed modification of the definitions for type B and type C hepatic encephalopathy.

The acronym, SONIC, has been used to describe this "spectrum of neurocognitive impairment in cirrhosis".

Time course of hepatic encephalopathy

Overt HE may be persistent or episodic in nature. Episodic HE lasts from hours to days and is often seen in the presence of a precipitating factor. Once resolved, HE may recur at any time. The proposed definition for persistent HE is at least 14 days' duration. In these cases the symptoms may fluctuate but the patient does not return to a normal mental status.

The natural history of minimal HE is still unclear, although cirrhotic patients with minimal HE are more likely to develop an episode of overt HE.

HE occurs by definition in ALF and is typically progressive, deeper, and can lead to death from brain edema, increased intracranial pressures, and cerebral herniation.

Portal–systemic bypasses in individuals with normal liver function, especially children, are well tolerated with lower rates of overt HE. Ten to 50% of adults with a TIPS will have overt HE (31) and 8% will have HE refractory to medical treatment. While rare, persistent HE in the setting of a bypass (type B) is seen more often than persistent HE associated with cirrhosis (type C).

Questions for the patient

Suspecting grade 2 or greater overt HE in a patient is relatively simple. In contrast, grade 1 HE is difficult to diagnose and is subjective. Adding to the difficulty, gross intellectual and verbal functioning are preserved in grades 1 and 2 HE.

Regarding minimal HE, by definition there is an absence of symptoms and physical findings. At times it is striking to learn that certain patients have minimal HE despite appearing completely normal in cursory interactions. It is preferred to have family members that reside with the patient as they may have a deeper insight into any changes.

Patients may be aware of being diagnosed with HE in the past, which places them at risk for a future episode or may have been prescribed lactulose. They may have altered sleeping habits (excessive daytime sleepiness and nighttime wakefulness). Has their memory worsened? Has their handwriting become more sloppy? Are they aware of personality changes such as irritability or anxiety? They may have caught themselves wandering aimlessly, may have been increasingly clumsy, have worsened balance, or have been falling at home. All of these symptoms point towards HE.

Obtain a thorough list of medication and ask specifically about over the counter and herbal medications, and taking other people's medications. Be suspicious of any new medications and ask about any dose adjustments, especially of diuretics.

Bouts of overt HE should invite directed questions towards identifying precipitating factors. Most important are signs of GI bleeding, infection, or conditions that lead to dehydration such as vomiting, diarrhea, or decreased oral intake. Ask about frequency of bowel movements and constipation. Bear in mind that HE is not dementia, so an intact memory does not rule out HE.

Physical examination
Assess mental status

The physical exam starts from the second one greets the patient. Do they make good eye contact and start talking or is it necessary to perform a sternal rub to wake them? Is their hand tremulous when reaching to shake hands? Always assess the patient's orientation to approximate time of day, day of the week, and place. Being disoriented places the patient in grade 2 HE.

Symptoms can be quite subtle in early stages so it helps if the clinician has met the patient on other occasions. The patient's language is not particularly affected by HE, but in grades 2 or 3 the voice may be monotonous with virtually no modulation. Personality begins to be affected in grade 2; the patient may be inappropriate or exhibit bizarre behavior. Confabulation and hallucinations tend to suggest an alcohol related mental status change. Simple arithmetic skills may be affected with overt HE even when the patient is oriented to time and place. Inability to add or subtract serial 7's or more simply serial 5's from 100 suggests the presence of overt HE. This is of course assuming the patient is able to add or subtract accurately at baseline.

Asterixis

Asterixis is somewhat specific for HE but not sensitive. Asterixis is elicited by having the patient hold out their arms and extend the wrists and fingers "like you are stopping traffic". The transient loss of extensor tone will cause a flap at the wrist joint and metacarpal–phalangeal joints [2,3]. Asterixis may also be elicited by lifting the leg and holding foot dorsiflexion or by having the patient grasp onto one of the examiner's fingers and extending the wrist. With HE, asterixis is often symmetric. Simple tremulousness of the wrist or fingers is not considered to be asterixis. (See Video 102.1.)

Other conditions may cause asterixis including uremia, hypercapnea, stroke, or thalamic hemorrhage. The latter two may cause a unilateral asterixis. It is important to assess for other signs of liver disease.

Assess the head for any signs of trauma. Nuchal rigidity suggests meningitis. Bite marks on the tongue are seen with seizure activity, which types B and C HE does not usually induce.

The neurologic exam should be directed at picking up on any gross abnormalities. Decorticate or decerebrate positioning are poor prognostic indicators. A disorder of eye movement called saccadic ocular pursuit may be seen with HE. HE may also cause fine motor abnormalities. Hyperventilation, muscle rigidity, clonus, Babinski sign, or hyperreflexia may be seen in deeper grades of HE.

Differential diagnosis

Numerous conditions may cause neuropsychiatric abnormalities resembling HE's broad range of symptoms. Misdiagnosis is easy. In practice, when a patient with cirrhosis or a portal–systemic bypass has a change in mental status, more often than not the diagnosis is HE brought on by a precipitating factor. Determining a broader differential diagnosis is more crucial if it appears the patient may not have underlying liver disease.

The systematic differential diagnosis can be thought of in terms of intracranial abnormalities, infections, drugs/ingested toxins, metabolic/endocrine, neuropsychiatric, pulmonary abnormalities, and renal abnormalities. (Drugs and toxins include street drugs, alcohol, psychoactive drugs, and overdose or misuse of prescription medication.)

Metabolic and endocrinologic abnormalities include hypothyroidism, hypoglycemia, electrolyte abnormalities, and acidosis. Rarely, urea cycle defects such as ornithine transcarbamylase deficiency may induce mental status changes [4].

Hepatic myelopathy, is more rarely encountered. Hepatic myelopathy refers to a loss of spinal cord motor neurons results in paresis of typically the lower extremities, spasticity, and positive Babinski sign [5]. It is due to ammonia and other toxins' damages on motor neurons rather than astrocytes. This is mostly seen in patients who have had previous episodes of HE. Cases have been reported to occur up to 10 years after onset of portal hypertension or after creation of a portal–systemic bypass.

Diagnostic methods

Overt HE is diagnosed clinically. First, it is crucial to establish if a patient has underlying cirrhosis and/or portal hypertension (See Chapters 99 and 100). Testing serum ammonia is not recommended. Whether the sample be arterial or venous, ammonia levels are neither sensitive nor specific for the diagnosis of either overt or minimal HE.

In the setting of ALF, ammonia levels >200 μg/dL are associated with an increased likelihood of cerebral herniation. Episodes of overt HE are often caused by one or more precipitating factors. In order to quickly identify and treat these factors it is useful to check serum and urine laboratory values for electrolyte abnormalities, magnesium disturbances, acidosis, hyper/hypoglycemia, and serum toxicology (for both drugs and alcohol).

If a patient has ascites paracentesis should be performed upon presentation or at least within the first 6 h of mental status change. Respiratory symptoms should prompt a chest X-ray. Suspicion of meningitis or encephalitis should prompt a lumbar puncture.

The presence of coinciding abdominal pain or distension should prompt a full workup. Imaging is helpful in identifying both common causes such as pancreatitis, ileus, but also less common processes such as perinephric abscesses and portal venous gas.

Brain imaging

Clinically, brain imaging is valuable in terms of excluding other etiologies of mental status change rather than diagnosing HE. Such causes include hematoma, intracranial hemorrhage, or stroke.

HE in the setting of cirrhosis is associated with MR changes such as varying degrees of brain edema or a hyperintense globus pallidus. However, these changes do not correlate well with the patient's clinical status.

Psychometric tests: paper/pencil and computerized testing

Psychometric testing remains the gold standard for detecting minimal HE and grade 1 overt HE. Several test batteries exist that are filled out by hand. One of the most commonly administered is the psychometric hepatic encephalopathy score (PHES). This consists of the number connection test A and B, the line drawing test, the serial dotting test, and the digit symbol test. Copyright issues make this difficult to obtain. Another proven effective is the Repeatable Battery for the Assessment of Neuropsychological Status (RBANS). The time required for these tests make it difficult for these to be adopted in clinical practice.

Computerized tests have been developed that can be administered by a trained medical assistant. One of the most promising is the Inhibitory Control Test (ICT). This is available for free on the internet, and takes 15 min or less to administer. Other computerized testing includes the Cognitive Drug Research (CDR) and CNS Vital Signs.

Electrophysiological and genetic testing

Critical flicker frequency is a useful tool to identify minimal and grade 1 overt HE. A patient views a pulsing light at increasing/decreasing frequencies and identifies at what point the light begins to appear to be either fused or flickering.

Electroencephalogram (EEG) is reliable in detecting altered brainwave patterns specific for HE and is more popular in Europe, but need a technician to administer and a neurologist to interpret. Alternatively, the bispectral index (BiS) method of monitoring brainwaves used by anesthesiologists to monitor sedation has been found to correlate with grades of overt HE.

Glutaminase gene polymorphisms have been identified that convey an increased risk for developing HE.

Treatment and prevention

Since most cases of overt HE in the setting of cirrhosis or portal–systemic bypass are induced by a precipitating factor, a four-pronged *initial* approach to treatment is appropriate and efficient in the majority of patients: (1) provide general supportive measures, (2) identify and promptly treat any precipitating factors, (3) initiate treatment with medications that target intestinal ammonia production such as lactulose, rifaximin, or metronidazole, and (4) exclude other causes of mental status changes (Table 102.3).

Liver Disease

Table 102.3 Management of overt hepatic encephalopathy (HE)

Most cases of overt HE (excluding those due to acute liver failure) are induced by a precipitating factor. Use the following four-pronged initial approach for prompt workup and treatment

(1) Provide general supportive measures
- Admit to the hospital if HE grades 3 or 4 and for most cases of grade 2 as well. Admit to specifically an ICU or step-down setting for deeper HE grades (3 or 4).
- Initiate i.v. hydration: bolus fluids initially if dehydration is suspected.
- Maintain adequate oxygen saturation.
- Low protein diet only for first few days of the overt HE episode.
- Intubate for airway protection, particularly in cases with variceal bleeding.
- Avoid sedating medications. If the patient is intubated, avoid midazolam drips.

(2) Identify and empirically treat any precipitating factors
- Stop GI bleeding and rid the gut of excess blood with lactulose (see next section for more on lactulose).
- Work up for infection with CBC, urinalysis, urine culture, and blood cultures. Perform a diagnostic paracentesis if moderate or large ascites is present. Perform a lumbar puncture if meningitis/encephalitis is suspected. Obtain sputum culture and chest X-ray if warranted.
- If infection is suspected, begin empiric antibiotics before waiting for test results. Typically start with either an i.v. fluoroquinolone or i.v. third generation cephalosporin. If the patient has been taking antibiotics already as an outpatient, use a different class initially for empiric coverage.
- Perform a toxicology analysis including testing for alcohol. Obtain a thorough history from the patient and any close contacts for possible ingestion of any sedating medications. If benzodiazepine use is suspected, consider reversal with flumazenil 1 mg i.v. (be cautious in patients with alcoholism or prior seizures).
- Assess for and correct any electrolyte abnormalities.
- Work up abdominal pain thoroughly.

(3) Initiate treatment with medications that target intestinal ammonia production
- Titrate lactulose 30–60 cc orally to a goal of three soft BMs per day (megadoses of lactulose are no more effective and may in fact induce HE via dehydration, hypernatremia, or aspiration).
- Use lactulose enema 200 g in the setting of active GI bleeding, bowel obstruction, or stupor/coma but not yet intubated.
- Use metronidazole 500 mg i.v. or p.o. TID-QID, or rifaximin 550 mg p.o. BID or 400 mg op TID in cases where the patient has failed lactulose or is already having loose stools.

(4) Exclude other causes of mental status change
- Consider brain imaging with CT, especially if there has been recent trauma or if focal neurologic signs are present.
- Calculate MELD score to assess for acute on chronic liver failure.

Difficult cases, i.e. no improvement by day 3
- Broaden the differential diagnosis to include neuropsychiatric abnormalities such as Wernicke's, stroke, seizure, psychosis/depression. Also consider metabolic, endocrine, respiratory, or pulmonary abnormalities.
- Reassess patient's medication list. Also ensure the patient is not becoming dehydrated from excessive lactulose.
- Add on either rifaximin or metronidazole if they were not started on admission.
- Check lumbar puncture if not done yet, arterial blood gas, TSH, ceruloplasmin/24 h urine copper, random cortisol or cosyntropin stimulation testing, and B12 levels. Consider repeating cultures/ infectious workup.
- Consider neurologic and/or psychiatric consultation.
- Consider repeating brain CT or performing brain MRI.
- Investigate for the presence of a large spleno-renal collateral vessel.
- If patient has an underlying TIPS/portal-systemic bypass, consider down-sizing or occluding the shunt.

Treatment of precipitating factors and general supportive measures in cases of overt hepatic encephalopathy

Patients with grades 2 through 4 overt HE should be hospitalized for close monitoring and to promptly identify and treat any precipitating factors. Patients with deeper grades (3 and 4) should be sent to an ICU or step-down floor. Endotracheal intubation should be performed when the patient is at risk of aspiration, particularly in the setting of active variceal bleeding.

Diagnostic testing and treatment of precipitating factors should coincide. Empiric treatment of precipitating factors begins with intravenous hydration. Electrolyte imbalances should be corrected. Hyponatremia however should be cautiously managed to prevent too rapid a correction.

Intravenous (IV) antibiotics such as fluoroquinolones or third generation cephalosporins should also be promptly initiated if there is any evidence of infection or GI bleeding.

Often, treatment of precipitating factors alone will resolve the HE, yet it is still prudent to begin lactulose.

Lactulose

Lactulose is a nonabsorbable disaccharide and is the first line agent for treatment and secondary prevention of overt HE. Lactulose not only results in a shorter small and large intestinal transit but is metabolized by colonic flora into lactic and acetic acid, thus decreasing colonic pH and changing the bacteria's metabolic activity. The low pH environment converts colonic ammonia (NH_3) to ammonium (NH_4^+), which is less likely to diffuse into the blood stream and more likely to be excreted in the stool. MR spectroscopy showed decreased cerebral metabolites during lactulose treatment.

However, results from a Cochrane meta-analysis did not display convincing benefit of lactulose over placebo.

Lactulose is given either orally 15–60 mL, via nasogastric (NG) tube, or in a 200 g (mixed in 1 L tap water) enema form. Enema infusion is reserved for patients with active GI bleeding, bowel obstruction, or comatose patients. Lactulose enemas are significantly superior to tap water (i.e. nonacidifying) enemas. On an outpatient basis, patients who have had an episode of overt HE should be continued on lactulose titrated to two to three soft bowel movements daily with a minimum of 15 mL of lactulose daily. Lactulose is often overdosed on inpatients with overt HE, at times causing the rectal effluent to appear identical to what is given orally. These megadoses have not been demonstrated to speed up resolution of overt HE and place the patient at risk for dehydration.

Chronic use of lactulose is hampered by poor compliance. Lactulose is more palatable by mixing it in other liquids such as iced tea. Additionally, there is a crystalline lactulose formation available that does have a less sweet taste.

Altering gut flora

Rifaximin is a nonabsorbable antibiotic that targets ammonia producing gut flora. It has been convincingly shown in trials to be as effective as lactulose in the treatment of HE. Rifaximin even demonstrated decreased length of stay in hospitalization (3.5 vs. 5 days, respectively) but it is expensive as a daily medication for prevention of HE. Thus far it has found a niche for outpatients with recurrent episodic overt HE refractory to lactulose. Studies combining rifaximin and lactulose are lacking.

Metronidazole remains an alternative method of decreasing gut flora load, especially if bacterial overgrowth is suspected. Dosing for treatment of HE is typically lower at 250 mg orally twice daily. Pulse dosing of 2 weeks on and 2 weeks off is employed to minimize side effects such as paresthesias. Oral neomycin has risk of side effects.

Lactobacillus species are non-urease producing that have shown some benefit in patients with overt and minimal HE with good tolerance. Specific strains will need to be identified that are more effective at preventing HE.

Enhancing conversion of ammonia to the less toxic urea

L-Ornithine-L-aspartate has been shown to be effective. It stimulates ureagenesis and activates carbamylphosphate synthetase and ornithine carbamyltransferase in hepatocytes. However, it is not available in US.

Zinc supplementation may speed up the urea cycle and hence increase urea formation to be excreted by the kidneys. This may be particularly effective in those individuals who are zinc deficient at baseline. One trial showing effectiveness used high doses (600 mg/day) for 3 months. Other trials showed no benefit.

Promote ammonia excretion

The urea excretion promoting agents sodium benzoate as well as phenylacetate have shown some promise. The head to head trial of sodium benzoate to lactulose used a large dose of sodium benzoate: 5 grams by mouth twice daily. Bear in mind this is not a low sodium medication and may worsen ascites.

Benzodiazepine receptor antagonists

While the effects of flumazenil are at times dramatic [6], its role is limited to patients with grade 4 overt HE as an empiric treatment or in patients with benzodiazepine-precipitated HE. Meta-analyses of placebo-controlled trials have shown a transient improvement in roughly 25% of patients.

Decrease nitrogen intake: dietary protein restriction

Dietary protein restriction has falling out of favor due to the lack of supporting evidence. Most importantly, approaching patients with a goal of negative protein balance promotes even further loss of lean muscle mass that is already occurring at baseline in cirrhotic patients. Small studies have shown vegetable protein to be superior to animal protein when comparing nitrogen balance, performance on psychometric tests, and EEG.

Targeting shunts

TIPS may be downsized or occluded in cases of persistent overt HE not controlled with medications. The same has been reported in occasional patients with naturally occurring large splenorenal collaterals.

Future therapies

L-Acyl carnitine has proven effective in both overt and minimal HE. L-Ornithine phenylacetate, a novel agent promoting ammonia excretion has been described. The diabetic agent acarbose was effective in one large trial. Lastly, a spherical carbon absorbent administered orally has proven to be as effective as lactulose with fewer GI side effects is entering phase 3 trials. Oxidative stress is another potential target. Surprisingly, no studies we are aware of have investigated the effects of neural stimulants on HE.

Liver transplant

In most cases, HE occurs in advanced liver disease. Liver transplantation successfully prevents HE recurrence and should be utilized in appropriate candidates. There is growing evidence that not all of the manifestations of the spectrum of HE are reversed after OLT.

Prevention

Recurrence of HE is common after a patient has had one overt episode. Steps can be taken to prevent future episodes by the physician, patient, and family.

Physicians should avoid ordering a TIPS if the patient has a history of HE. Avoid prescribing sedating medications. Hydroxyzine and diphenhydramine are effective sleep aids with a lower risk of precipitating HE [7].

Liver Disease

Avoid long-acting benzodiazepines for treating alcohol withdrawal or maintaining ICU sedation. Midazolam drips used for intubated patients can cause continued sedation for days after the drip has been stopped and should be avoided in cirrhotic patients.

Endoscopic sedation of patients with cirrhosis, particularly decompensated cirrhosis, may precipitate overt HE. It is prudent to favor relatively lower doses of midazolam in such a setting. Larger doses of opiates and diphenhydramine are less likely to precipitate overt HE as compared to larger doses of midazolam. We do not routinely ask for anesthesia assitance and/or propofol with this patient population.

Upon hospital discharge a close follow up is necessary. Address compliance and proper usage of lactulose on each subsequent visit. In addition, educate the patient and family that sedating medications are to be avoided.

The physician should assess the patient's social support and ability to care for him/herself. If no support exists it is useful to recommend a visiting nursing service. In very difficult situations it may be necessary to move a patient to an extended care facility or nursing home.

If social support exists, family and friends should be educated to help with medication compliance and to look for symptoms of recurrence [8].

Studies have demonstrated negative effects on activities of daily living, increased rates of auto accidents, and an inability to operate heavy machinery in patients with episodes of HE. Somnolence from HE as well as tendencies of clumsiness and wandering may lead to more falls and injuries, particularly as cirrhotic patients have been shown to have higher rates of osteoporosis [9–11].

Should patients not care well for themselves, a cascade of problems may ensue. Patients may miss medications, have worse personal hygiene, have worse job performance, eat more poorly, or not control chronic medical conditions. Medical appointments may be missed. Financial management may deteriorate. Personal relationships may be strained from caregiver stress. Also, family members may need to miss more work to care for the patient. Decreased independence may worsen or lead to depression.

Prognosis with and without treatment
Cirrhosis

The first episode of overt HE in a patient with cirrhosis should not be taken lightly because it portends to poor overall outcome from impaired liver function. Patients with underlying cirrhosis will typically survive their first episode of HE, but their long term mortality is worse. Consequently, the clinician should emphasize the severity of the patient's liver disease to the patient and family after an episode of HE. An episode of overt HE is one of the strongest predictors of mortality with a 1-year survival of about 40% [12].

Despite the worsened prognosis, HE is not part of the model for end-stage liver disease (MELD) scoring system. In addition, the presence or absence of HE does not correlate with the MELD score [13]. Priority for transplantation should be discussed on an individual basis. HE in the setting of HIV and cirrhosis is especially worrisome [14]. The presence of minimal HE places a patient at higher risk for having an episode of overt HE [15,16].

Acute liver failure

HE seen with ALF represents a particularly poor prognosis (see Chapter 105).

> **SOURCES OF INFORMATION FOR PATIENTS AND DOCTORS**
>
> Patient information of significant depth in an easy to read format is limited. The online encyclopedia, Wikipedia, has a fairly thorough article but it may be difficult to read for some people.
> Physicians are directed to register with the HE CME webpage: http://www.hecme.tv. This website is sponsored by Salix Pharmaceuticals (Morrisville, NC). Included are didactic lectures as well as a demonstration of the Inhibitory Control Test as well as a downloadable version.
> A video clip of unilateral asterixis is available at: http://www.neurology.org/cgi/content/full/66/2/E11 [17].

References

1. Riggio O, Efrati C, Catalano C, et al. High prevalence of spontaneous portal-systemic shunts in persistent hepatic encephalopathy: a case-control study. *Hepatology*. 2005;42:1158–1165.
2. LeBlond RF, DeGowin RL, Brown DD. (2004) *DeGowin's Diagnostic Examination*. McGraw-Hill, New York.
3. Bickley LS, Hoekelman RA. (1999) *Bates' Guide to Physical Examination and History Taking*. Lippincott, Philadelphia, PA.
4. Elgouhari HM, O'Shea R. What is the utility of measuring the serum ammonia level in patients with altered mental status? *Cleve Clin J Med*. 2009;76:252–254.
5. Bain VG. Hepatorenal syndrome, hepatopulmonary syndrome, and now, hepatospinal syndrome? *Liver Transpl*. 2003;9:995–996.
6. Barbaro G, Di Lorenzo G, Soldini M, et al. Flumazenil for hepatic encephalopathy grade III and IVa in patients with cirrhosis: An Italian multicenter double-blind, placebo-controlled, cross-over study. *Hepatology*. 1998;28:374–378.
7. Spahr L, Coeytaux A, Giostra E, et al. Histamine H1 blocker hydroxyzine improves sleep in patients with cirrhosis and minimal hepatic encephalopathy: A randomized controlled pilot trial. *Am J Gastroenterol*. 2007;102:744–753.
8. Daniel E. Chronic problems in rehabilitation of patients with Laennec's cirrhosis. *Nurs Clin North Am*. 1977;12:345–356.
9. Groeneweg M, Quero JC, De Bruijn I, et al. Subclinical hepatic encephalopathy impairs daily functioning. *Hepatology*. 1998;28:45–49.
10. Ortiz M, Jacas C, Cordoba J. Minimal hepatic encephalopathy: diagnosis, clinical significance and recommendations. *J Hepatol*. 2005;42(Suppl 1):S45–S53.

11. Wein C, Koch H, Popp B, *et al.* Minimal hepatic encephalopathy impairs fitness to drive. *Hepatology*. 2004;39:739–745.

12. Bustamante J, Rimola A, Ventura PJ, *et al.* Prognostic significance of hepatic encephalopathy in patients with cirrhosis. *J Hepatol*. 1999;30:890–895.

13. Yoo HY, Edwin D, Thuluvath PJ. Relationship of the model for end-stage liver disease (MELD) scale to hepatic encephalopathy, as defined by electroencephalography and neuropsychometric testing, and ascites. *Am J Gastroenterol*. 2003;98: 1395–1399.

14. Pineda JA, Romero-Gomez M, Diaz-Garcia F, *et al.* HIV coinfection shortens the survival of patients with hepatitis C virus-related decompensated cirrhosis. *Hepatology*, 2005;41: 779–789.

15. Das A, Dhiman RK, Saraswat VA, *et al.* Prevalence and natural history of subclinical hepatic encephalopathy in cirrhosis. *J Gastroenterol Hepatol*. 2001;16:531–535.

16. Romero-Gomez M, Boza F, Garcia-Valdecasas MS, *et al.* Subclinical hepatic encephalopathy predicts the development of overt hepatic encephalopathy. *Am J Gastroenterol*. 2001;96: 2718–2723.

17. Klos KJ, Wijdicks EF. Unilateral asterixis after thalamic hemorrhage. *Neurology*. 2006;66:E11.

Liver Disease

CHAPTER 103

Acute liver failure

John G. O'Grady and Julia Wendon

King's College School of Medicine, London, UK

ESSENTIAL FACTS ABOUT PATHOGENESIS

- The commonest defined causes are acute viral hepatitis A or B, and drug reactions
- The third most important etiological group is seronegative hepatitis, i.e. no specific identified causative agent
- Less common causes include ischemic hepatitis, autoimmune hepatitis, pregnancy-related syndromes, Wilson disease, Budd–Chiari syndrome and mushroom poisoning

---

ESSENTIALS OF DIAGNOSIS

- Acute liver failure: an acute liver insult is complicated by laboratory evidence of coagulopathy and clinical evidence of encephalopathy
- Essential laboratory investigations: serology for viral hepatitis, serum immunoglobulins, auto-antibodies and acetaminophen blood levels
- Imaging of the liver is helpful in Budd–Chiari syndrome and pregnancy-related disease
- Liver biopsy is occasionally helpful, e.g. auto-immune hepatitis, acute fatty liver of pregnancy

---

ESSENTIALS OF TREATMENT

- Determine if the patient should be listed for liver transplantation
- Meticulous intensive care with monitoring for possible complications
- Appropriate therapy when complications develop (hemodynamic instability, infection and neurological complications are the most life-threatening complications)
- Artificial liver support devices are currently unproven
- With this integrated care approach, 60% of patients survive

---

Introduction

Acute liver failure (ALF) is a complex multisystemic illness that evolves after a catastrophic insult to the liver and leads to coagulopathy and encephalopathy within days or weeks. The absence of recognized pre-existing liver disease is a requirement. ALF is a heterogenous condition incorporating that is influenced by the underlying etiology, the age of the patient and the duration of time over which the disease evolves. These are not mutually exclusive factors and, as examples, hyperacute liver failure is more likely to be seen in younger patients with hepatitis A or B while subacute liver failure patients tend to be older and more likely to have seronegative hepatitis or idiosyncratic drug reactions. Three classifications of ALF are currently in use (Table 103.1).

Etiology and epidemiology

There is considerable geographic variation in the etiology of ALF (Table 103.2). Viruses and drugs account for the majority of cases. However, a significant number of patients with no definable cause are classified as seronegative hepatitis or of indeterminate etiology. The overall incidence of ALF complicating acute hepatitis in the US is 0.9% and this equates to about 2000 deaths annually. Most drug-induced cases are rare idiosyncratic reactions, but some like acetaminophen are dose related toxic events.

Viral

ALF complicates 0.2–4% of cases of acute viral hepatitis, depending on the etiology, and is less likely with hepatitis A. Hepatitis B causes ALF through a number of scenarios (Table 103.3). The classical ALF is caused by an aggressive immune response against the virus either at *de novo* infection or in chronic infections at the time of HBeAg clearance and seroconversion to HBeAb positivity. The alternative mechanism is aggressive viral replication, spontaneous or secondary to immunosuppression or chemotherapy; this may be amenable to therapy with antiviral agents. The incidence of the delta virus is decreasing. Hepatitis C is rarely recognized as the sole cause of ALF. Hepatitis E is common in parts of Asia and Africa. Unusual viral causes of ALF include herpes simplex 1 and 2, herpes virus-6, varicella zoster, Epstein–Barr virus and cytomegalovirus.

Seronegative hepatitis

This is also known as hepatitis of indeterminate cause. It is an important cause of ALF in some parts of the Western world. Middle-aged females are most frequently affected and it occurs sporadically. The diagnosis is one currently of exclusion. In the US, acetaminophen ligands were found in a number of these

---

Table 103.1 Definitions of acute liver failure in current use

Event	United States	France	United Kingdom
Trigger event	First symptom	Jaundice	Jaundice
Term	Fulminant hepatic failure	Fulminant hepatic failure	Hyperacute liver failure
Time to encephalopathy	8 weeks	2 weeks	7 days
Term	Late-onset liver failure	Subfulminant hepatic failure	Acute liver failure
Time to encephalopathy	9–26 weeks	3–12 weeks	8–28 days
Term	—	—	Subacute liver failure
Time to encephalopathy	—	—	29–84 days

Table 103.2 Geographic variation in the etiology of acute liver failure

	United Kingdom	United States	France	India	Japan	Spain
Acetaminophen	54%	46%	2%	—	—	2%
Drug reactions	7%	12%	15%	5%	—	17%
Seronegative	17%	14%	18%	24%	45%	32%
Hepatitis A or B	14%	10%	49%	33%	55%	37%
Hepatitis E	—	—	—	38%	—	—
Other causes	8%	18%	16%	—	—	12%

Table 103.3 Acute liver failure associated with hepatitis B

	HBsAg	IgM anti-core	HBeAg	HBeAb	HBV DNA	Comment
Acute infection	Variable	Positive	Variable	Variable	Usually negative	Hyperactive immune response
Seroconversion	Positive	Negative	Negative	Positive	Negative	Immune mediated
Replication surge	Positive	Negative	Variable	Variable	High	Spontaneous or after immunsuppression
Delta super-infection	Positive	Negative	Variable	Variable	Low	New positive serology for delta virus

patients but it is unclear whether these indicate a causal relationship or are an epiphenomenon from secondary therapeutic use [1].

Drugs

Acetaminophen overdoses account for about 40% of cases of ALF in the UK and US [2]. It is often taken with suicidal intent, but, occasionally it is seen with therapeutic use. Factors increasing susceptibility to acetaminophen toxicity include regular alcohol consumption, anti-epileptic therapy (enzyme induction) and malnutrition. ALF develops in only 2–5% of those taking overdoses, and the mortality is highest at doses exceeding 48 g.

Idiosyncratic drug reactions usually develop during the first exposure to the drug (Table 103.4). The diagnosis is largely made on the basis of a temporal relationship between exposure to the drug and the development of ALF. Estimates of the risk of developing ALF as a result of an idiosyncratic reaction range from 0.001% for non-steroidal anti-inflammatory drugs to 1% for the isoniazid/rifampicin combination.

Table 103.4 Drugs causing of acute liver failure

Category 1: commoner causes
Acetaminophen
Halothane (mainly historical)
Isoniazid/rifampicin
Non-steroidal anti-inflammatory drugs (NSAIDS)
Nimesulide
Sulfonamides
Flutamide
Sodium valproate
Carbamazepine
Troglitazone
Ecstacy

Category 2: rarer causes
Benoxyprofen
Phenytoin
Isoflurane
Enflurane
Lamotrigine
Tetracycline
Allopurinol
Ketoconazole
Monoamine oxidase inhibitors (MAOIs)
Disulfiram
Methyldopa
Amiodarone
Tricyclic antidepressants
Propylthiouracil
Gold
2,3-Dideoxyinosine (ddI)

Other etiologies

ALF associated with pregnancy tends to occur during the third trimester. There are three recognized patterns, although a considerable degree of overlap exists: (1) acute fatty liver of pregnancy – primagravids carrying a male fetus are most at risk; (2) HELLP syndrome (hemolysis, elevated liver enzymes, low platelets); and (3) ALF complicating pre-eclampsia or eclampsia. In addition, there is a range of unusual causes of ALF, including:

- *Wilson disease* may present as ALF, usually during the second decade of life. It is characterized clinically by a Coomb's negative hemolytic anaemia and demonstrable Kayser–Fleischer rings in the majority of cases.
- *Poisoning with Amanita phalloides* (mushrooms) is most commonly seen in central Europe, South Africa and the west coast of the United States. Severe diarrhea, often with vomiting, is a typical feature five or more hours after ingestion of the mushrooms. Liver failure develops 4–5 days later.
- *Autoimmune chronic hepatitis* may present as ALF, it is usually not responsive to corticosteroid therapy.
- *The Budd–Chiari syndrome*
- *Malignancy infiltration*, especially with lymphoma, which is typically associated with hepatomegaly.
- *Ischemic hepatitis* is being increasingly recognized as a cause of ALF, especially in older patients.

Diagnosis

The etiology of ALF must be accurately identified. Appropriate investigations are outlined in Table 103.5. The contribution of histology to the assessment of ALF is limited. Histologic features may suggest specific diagnoses including sodium valproate toxicity (microvascular steatosis), malignant infiltration, Wilson disease, auto-immune hepatitis pregnancy-related syndromes and the Budd–Chiari syndrome.

Prognosis

The underlying etiology, age of patient and grade of encephalopathy are particularly strong determinants of outcome. The pattern and severity of organ failure is the other factor that influences prognosis.

Determination of prognosis drives two fundamental management issues i.e. the need for referral to specialist centers and the indications for transplantation. Indications for referral to specialist units have been suggested (Tables 103.6, 103.7 and 103.8). Separate criteria have been established to identify the cohort most in need of liver transplantation; the King's College criteria are one of the most regularly used (Table 103.9). These lack adequate sensitivity in acetaminophen cases who do not exhibit acidosis and serum lactate levels have been found to complement the acetaminophen criteria [3]. These criteria are not adequate in some rare etiologies particularly pregnancy-related syndromes, Wilson disease and *Amanita phalloides* poisoning. In France, factor V levels are used in preference to prothrombin time or INR. Factor V levels <20% in patients under the age of 30 years and <30% in older patients are indicative of a poor prognosis once encephalopathy develops. MELD is also being increasingly used to assess prognosis.

A small liver on clinical or radiologic assessment, or a liver that is shrinking rapidly, is a poor prognostic indicator that is especially useful in subacute liver failure when the degree of encephalopathy and the severity of the derangement of coagulation may not yet reflect the underlying poor prognosis.

Management
Overall strategy

Each patient with ALF needs an overall management plan that starts with identification of etiology and an initial assessment of prognosis. There are a few drugs with defined roles in specific etiologies of ALF (Table 103.10). Appropriate patients should be referred to specialist centers offering liver transplantation. Patients are monitored for complications that are treated to the point of recovery, death or transplantation. Patients not initially considered for transplantation may change status on the basis of prognostic indicators or of clinical complications. Likewise, patients listed for transplantation may develop complications that preclude this intervention or occasionally may show signs of recovery before a donor organ becomes available. The final decision on transplantation is made when an organ is available. The potential to develop

Table 103.5 Investigations to identify the etiology of acute liver failure

Etiology	Investigation	Comment
Hepatitis A (HAV)	IgM anti-HAV	95% positive initially; 100% on repeat testing
Hepatitis B and D (HBV, HDV)	Full profile	See Table 103.3 for interpretation
Hepatitis E (HEV)	Anti-HEV	IgM antibody test
Seronegaitive hepatitis	All tests	Diagnosis of exclusion
Acetaminophen	Drug levels in blood	May be negative on third or subsequent days after overdose
Idiosyncratic drug reactions	Esinophil count	Most diagnoses based on temporal relationship
Ecstacy	Blood, urine, hair analysis	Medium term exposure can be mapped from analysis of hair
Autoimmune	Autoantibodies, iggs	High titers or anti-KLM suggest diagnosis
Pregnancy-related syndromes 　Fatty liver 　HELLP syndrome 　Toxemia	Ultrasound, uric acid, histology Platelet count Serum transaminases	First pregnancy Disseminated intravascular coagulation a prominent feature Very high transaminases, appropriate obstetric history
Wilson's disease	Urinary copper, ceruloplasmin	Deeply jaundiced, anemic, second decade of life
Amanita phalloides	—	History of ingestion of mushrooms, diarrhea
Budd–Chiari syndrome	Ultrasound or venography	Ascites, prominent caudate lobe on imaging
Malignancy	Imaging and histology	Imaging may be interpretated as normal
Ischemic hepatitis	Transaminases	Transaminases very high
Heatstroke	Myoglobinuria	Rhabdomyolysis a prominent feature

Table 103.6 Criteria prompting referral to a specialist unit following ingestion of acetaminophen

Day 2	Day 3	Day 4
Arterial pH < 7.30	Arterial pH < 7.30	INR > 6 or PT > 100 s
INR > 3.0 or PT > 50 s	INR > 4.5 or PT > 75 s	Progressive rise in PT to any level
Oliguria	Oliguria	Oliguria
Creatinine > 200 μmol/l	Creatinine > 200 μmol/l	Creatinine > 300 μmol/l
Hypoglycemia	Encephalopathy	Encephalopathy
—	Severe thrombocytopenia	Severe thrombocytopenia

Any of these criteria should prompt referral.
INR, International normalized ratio; PT, prothrombin time.

Table 103.7 Referral to specialist unit in non-acetaminophen etiologies

Hyperacute	Acute	Subacute
Encephalopathy	Encephalopathy	Encephalopathy
Hypoglycemia	Hypoglycemia	Hypoglycemia (less common)
Prothrombin time > 30 s	Prothrombin time > 30 s	Prothrombin time > 20 s
INR > 2.0	INR > 2.0	INR > 1.5
Renal failure	Renal failure	Renal failure
Hyperpyrexia	—	Serum sodium <130 μmol/l
—	—	Shrinking liver volume

The presence of any of the criteria above should prompt referral.
INR, International normalized ratio; PT, prothrombin time.

Table 103.8 Indicators of a poor prognosis in acetaminophen-induced acute liver failure

Parameter	Sensitivity (%)	Specificity (%)	Positive predictive accuracy (%)
Arterial pH < 7.30*	49	99	81
All three of the following concomitantly: (i) prothrombin time >100s or INR > 6.5; (ii) creatinine > 300 μmol/l; (iii) grade 3–4 encephalopathy	45	94	67

Table 103.9 Indicators of a poor prognosis in non-acetaminophen etiologies of acute liver failure

Parameter	Sensitivity (%)	Specificity (%)	Positive predictive accuracy (%)
Prothrombin time > 100s or INR > 6.7	34	100	46
Any three of following: (i) unfavorable etiology (seronegative hepatitis or drug reaction); (ii) age <10 or >40 years; (iii) acute or subacute categories; (iv) serum bilirubin >300 μmol/l	93	90	92

Table 103.10 Specific therapies in acute liver failure

Etiology	Drug	Comment
Acetaminophen	N-Acetylcysteine	Antidote role depending on blood levels within 16h
Hepatitis B	Anti-viral agent	Most effective in cases with high levels of viral replication
Amanita phalloides	Penicillin	Early administration required
Autoimmune hepatitis	Steroids	Response not predictable and risk of infection problematic

Table 103.11 Modified Parsons–Smith scale of hepatic encephalopathy

Grade	Clinical features	Neurological signs	Glasgow coma scale
0/subclinical	Normal	Only seen on neuropsychometric testing	15
1	Trivial lack of awareness, shortened attention span	Tremor, apraxia, incoordination	15
2	Lethargy, disorientation, personality change	Asterixis, ataxia, dysarthria	11–15
3	Confusion, somnolence to semi-stupor, responsive to stimuli	Asterixis, ataxia	8–11
4	Coma	±Decerebration	<8

"bridges to transplantation" with extracorporeal liver support devices has yet to be determined.

Encephalopathy

Encephalopathy is essentially a clinical diagnosis and is graded from 1 to 4 depending on clinical severity (Table 103.11). Deep encephalopathy (grades 3/4) is associated with development of cerebral edema and potential risk of cerebral herniation. Patients with acute and hyperacute liver failure are at greater risk of developing grade IV coma and cerebral edema. The relationship between arterial ammonia and cerebral uptake is not clear [4]. Inflammatory mediators are also of importance in the development of deeper levels of coma. Increasing components of the systemic inflammatory response syndrome (SIRS) correlate with progressive coma [5].

Measurement of intracranial pressure (ICP) is utilized in patients at risk of cerebral edema and in many of those listed for liver transplantation, although ICP bolt placement has not been proven to improve outcome [6]. The decision to place an intracranial monitor is determined by a balance of risk and benefit [7]. The procedure carries risk of bleeding that varies with the placement site (epidural, subdural or parenchymal) [6]. Treatment targets with ICP monitoring include maintaining cerebral perfusion pressures above 50–55 mmHg and ICPs below 20–25 mmHg.

The clinical management of the cerebral complications of ALF has been developed predominantly by the extrapolation of data from the neurosurgical literature. Patients who deteriorate to grade 3/4 coma are best managed with elective intubation, sedation and ventilation. Sedation typically is achieved by utilising an opiate and a sedative, e.g. propofol and a benzodiazepine. Both agents have anticonvulsant activity and propofol has been suggested to be of benefit in the treatment of surges in intracranial pressure. The normal first line treatment for the later remains mannitol, 0.5 g/kg given as a bolus. Addition therapies include barbiturates, hypertonic saline, indomethacin and hypothermia [8,9].

Cardiovascular and respiratory

Patients with ALF develop a hyperdynamic circulation with peripheral vasodilation and central volume depletion. Hypotension is common and may initially respond to volume repletion. Hypotension that does not respond to volume requires invasive hemodynamic monitoring and institution of pressor agents e.g. norepinephrine (noradrenalin) or vasopressin. In refractory hypotension, adrenal dysfunction due to an impaired response to ACTH should be considered and, if detected, treated with hydrocortisone [10].

Pulmonary sepsis is common and may progress to adult respiratory distress syndrome (ARDS). Other common respiratory complications include aspiration pneumonia, pleural effusions, atelectasis and intrapulmonary shunts. Ventilatory strategies are influenced by the respiratory component of the disease as well as the multi-organ involvement characteristic of ALF. Patients at risk of cerebral edema will require close attention to CO_2 levels and tailored sedation regimens, while hypercapnia may be tolerated in patients progressing to ARDS.

Renal

Renal failure is common in the setting of ALF, particularly so in acetaminophen-related ALF because of direct nephrotoxicity. Optimal volume repletion and hemodynamic stability are pertinent to maintaining renal function. Renal replacement therapy (RRT) should be initiated early. The hemodynamic instability and associated cerebral complications of these patients favor the use of continuous modes of RRT rather than intermittent hemodialysis [11].

Sepsis

Both culture positive and culture negative systemic inflammatory response syndromes (SIRS) are common. Patients with ALF are functionally immunosuppressed with impaired cell mediated immunity, complement levels and phagocytosis. Antimicrobials are indicated when there is any clinical suggestion of infection. The choice of antimicrobial agent should be driven by local resistance patterns. Prophylactic antifungals should be considered, especially in those listed for transplantation.

Metabolic and feeding

Enteral nutrition should commence at an early stage in the absence of contra-indications, e.g. pancreatitis. Prokinetic agents like erythromycin (250 mg iv 6 hourly) or metoclopromide may help In patients with large aspirates (>200 mL/4 hours). Metabolic data demonstrate increased calorific requirements. Patients with ALF demonstrate both peripheral and hepatological insulin resistance. Tight glycemic control may improve outcome. Metabolic acidosis is a relatively frequent occurrence due to lactic acidosis, hyperchloremic acidosis or renal failure. The hyperlactatemia may resolve with appropriate fluid loading and or may reflect the inability of the liver to metabolize the lactate produced.

Coagulopathy

The coagulopathy should not be routinely corrected if it is still relevant to the determination of prognosis. However, repletion of coagulation factors is necessary for clinical bleeding and prophylactically before major invasive procedures. Thrombocytopenia is common and may be associated with disseminated intravascular coagulation (DIC); these are the patients at particular risk of hemorrhage.

Liver transplantation

The impact of liver transplantation on the management of ALF has been revolutionary. ALF now accounts for 5–12% of all liver transplant activity. Donor organ allocation systems prioritize patients with ALF and 45–50% of patients undergo transplantation. Up to 25% of patients are deemed to have contraindications to transplantation and the remainder deteriorate before on organ is allocated.

Patient selection

The King's College Hospital criteria indicating a poor prognosis (Tables 103.6–103.9) have been used as a method of selecting patients for liver transplantation. This model is considered to (be):

- sensitive to the urgency with which patients with a poor prognosis need to be identified
- easily and widely applicable
- not reliant on the development of advanced disease
- maximize the time available to obtain a suitable donor organ

An alternative approach is to list all patients with ALF for transplantation and make the decision whether to proceed when an organ becomes available.

The removal of patients from the waiting list when the clinical condition deteriorates is emotive and difficult. Irreversible brain damage should preclude the use of liver transplantation but currently available technology cannot accurately assess this risk. Accelerating inotrope requirements, uncontrolled sepsis and severe respiratory failure are other imprecise contraindications to transplantation. These contraindications are age sensitive as younger patients are more resilient and more likely to reverse these complications after liver transplantation.

Transplant operation

Standard operative techniques are used in the majority of patients. Some patients have auxiliary transplants in the hope the transplant status may be transient if native liver left *in situ* effectively regenerates (at outcome seen in about 70% of patients so managed). Intraoperative blood losses are remarkably low reflecting effective repletion strategies and the absence of portal hypertension. Cerebral edema may be problematic during the dissection phase and the period immediately after reperfusion. In contrast, it often improves dramatically during the anhepatic phase of the transplant operation. Cerebral autoregulation is restored within 48 hours of successful transplantation and monitoring of ICP and CPP should continue during this period in susceptible patients.

The profile of sepsis, including fungal infection, seen in ALF extends into the post-transplant period and is further aggravated by immunosuppressive therapy. Patients transplanted for ALF are routinely included in antimicrobial prophylactic regimens targeted at high risk patients. Renal function may improve dramatically in the immediate postoperative period but more often renal support may be necessary for many weeks after successful transplantation.

Results

Registry data indicate that the overall survival rates are in the region of 60–65%, but individual centers have reported higher survival in the 75–90% range. Patients receiving liver transplants for ALF (median age 28 years) are younger those undergoing elective transplantation (median age 44 years). Factors that have been found to correlate with outcome include age, body mass index (BMI), serum creatinine and quality of the organ transplanted [12,13].

Liver support

A variety of liver support systems have been assessed in ALF either as a "bridge" to transplantation or to improve recovery. These include bio-artificial livers utilizing cell-based therapies (using human or porcine livers), and dialysis-based methods or plasmapheresis [14]. Randomized controlled trials with a porcine hepatocyte device and albumin dialysis failed to demonstrate improved survival [15]. However, these possibilities need further investigation. A management protocol is given on the book's website.

References

1. O'Grady JG, Alexander GJ, Hallyar KM, *et al.* Early indicators of prognosis in fulminant hepatic failure. *Gastroenterology.* 1989;97: 439–445.
2. O'Grady, JG. (2005) Acute liver failure, in *Comprehensive Clinical Hepatology.* (eds. B.R. Bacon, J.G. O'Grady A.M. Di Bisceglie and J.R. Lake), Mosby Elsevier, pp. 517–536.
3. Bernal W, Donaldson N, Wyncoll D *et al.* Blood lactate as an early indicator of outcome in paracetamol-induced acute liver failure. *Lancet.* 2002;359:558–563.
4. Strauss GI, Knudsen GM, Kondrup J, *et al.* Cerebral metabolism of ammonia and amino acids in patients with fulminant hepatic failure. *Gastroenterology.* 2001;121:1109–1119.
5. Rolando N, Wade J, Davalos M, *et al.* The systemic inflammatory response syndrome in acute liver failure. *Hepatology.* 2000;32: 734–739.
6. Blei AT, Olafsson S, Webster S, *et al.* Complications of intracranial pressure monitoring in fulminant hepatic failure. *Lancet.* 1993;16: 157–158.
7. Vaquero J, Fontana RJ, Larson AM, *et al.* Complications and use of intracranial pressure monitoring in patients with acute liver failure and severe encephalopathy. *Liver transpl.* 2005;11: 1581–1589.
8. Jalan R, Damink SW, Deutz NE, *et al.* Moderate hypothermia for uncontrolled intracranial hypertension in acute liver failure. *Lancet.* 1992;354:1164–1168.
9. Murphy N, Auzinger G, Bernel W, *et al.* The effect of hypertonic sodium chloride on intracranial pressure in patients with acute liver failure. *Hepatology.* 2004;39:464–470.
10. Harry R, Auzinger G, Wendon J. The clinical importance of adrenal insufficiency in acute hepatic dysfunction. *Hepatology.* 2002;36:395–402.
11. Davenport A. The management of renal failure in patients at risk of cerebral edema/hypoxia. *New Horiz.* 1995;3:717–724.
12. Barshes NR, Lee TC, Balkrishnan R, *et al.* Risk stratification of adult patients undergoing liver transplantation for fulminant hepatic failure. *Transplantation.* 2006;81:195–210.
13. Bernal W, Cross TJS, Auzinger G, *et al.* Outcome after wait-listing foe emergency liver transplantation in acute liver failure: a single centre experience. *J Hepatol.* 2009;50:306–313.
14. Clemmesen JO, Larsen FS, Ejlersen E, *et al.* Haemodynamic changes after high-volume plasmapheresis in patients with chronic and acute liver failure. *Eur J Gastroenterol Hepatol.* 1997; 9:55–60.
15. Demetriou AA, Brown RS, Busuttil RW, *et al.* Prospective, randomized, multicenter controlled trial of a bioartificial liver in treating acute liver failure. *Ann Surg.* 2002;239:660–670.

CHAPTER 104

Tumors of the liver

Alejandro Forner, Carlos Rodríguez de Lope, María Reig, and Jordi Bruix

Hospital Clinic, IDIBAPS, Biomedical Research Centre Network of Hepatic and Digestive Diseases (CIBERehd), University of Barcelona, Barcelona, Spain

ESSENTIAL FACTS ABOUT PATHOGENESIS

- The diagnosis of liver tumors is increasing, mainly because of the more frequent use of abdominal imaging techniques for the evaluation of various symptoms
- Etiology of the different liver tumors is variable and in some cases unknown
- The main risk factor for hepatocellular carcinoma (HCC) is the presence of a chronic liver disease, mainly cirrhosis
- The main risk factors for intrahepatic cholangiocarcinoma are primary sclerosing cholangitis, hepatobiliary flukes, hepatolithiasis, biliary malformations and cirrhosis, mainly secondary to hepatitis C

ESSENTIALS OF DIAGNOSIS

- Classification of liver tumors into cystic versus solid lesions is the first step and is easily done with ultrasound (US)
- When a solid lesion is detected, excluding a malignant tumor is mandatory
- With solid lesions, the clinical scenario is very helpful in making a differential diagnosis (i.e. liver cirrhosis and hepatocellular carcinoma; previous or concomitant neoplasia of other organs and metastases; healthy young woman with previous history of oral contraceptive consumption and hepatic adenoma, etc.)
- In some cases diagnosis can be made with dynamic imaging techniques
- When dynamic imaging techniques are unable to establish a diagnosis, a biopsy should be done

ESSENTIALS OF TREATMENT

- In healthy patients, if biopsy is not diagnostic and the nature of the lesion is still equivocal, surgical resection is recommended
- Treatment should be individualized depending on characteristics of the tumor (extension, localization), and the patient (liver function, other comorbidities)
- In general, malignant tumors should be resected. In the case of liver metastases, chemotherapy could be beneficial
- Regarding HCC, the Barcelona Clinic Liver Cancer (BCLC) staging system correlates tumor stage with prognosis and treatment. Early stages are candidates to radical therapies: Resection if liver function is preserved, liver transplantation when the tumor fits the "Milan" criteria (one nodule up to 5 cm, three nodules up to 3 cm each) or percutaneous ablation. Intermediate stage HCC (BCLC B) may benefit from transarterial chemoembolization (TACE). Advanced HCC (BCLC C) may benefit from systemic chemotherapy (sorafenib)

Introduction

Tumors of the liver are defined as focal solid or liquid lesions that can be differentiated from the normal anatomy of the liver by imaging techniques. They range from benign asymptomatic lesions to malignant aggressive neoplasms. The clinical prevalence of focal hepatic lesions has increased due to recent advances in imaging techniques and their widespread use [1]. The diagnosis of a focal liver lesion is based on clinical findings, imaging techniques, and most commonly, on histopathological analysis [1–3]. An incidental lesion in an asymptomatic patient with no history of liver disease or known neoplasia is usually benign. The most prevalent benign lesions are simple cysts, hemangiomas, and focal nodular hyperplasia (FNH) [4]. In a patient with a known cancer of any origin, liver metastases is the most probable diagnosis. Finally, a liver lesion in a cirrhotic patient is most likely a hepatocellular carcinoma (HCC) [5]. The medical history may also suggest a diagnosis. Thereby, a highly vascularized nodule in a healthy young woman on oral contraceptives suggests hepatocellular adenoma, and a liver tumor in a patient with sclerosing cholangitis suggests cholangiocarcinoma. Similarly, biochemical data including viral and tumor markers may be helpful.

Radiologic techniques indicate whether the tumor has a liquid (cysts, abscesses) or solid (benign or malignant tumors) content. The vascularization profile may also suggest its possible nature [4]. However, both benign (FNH or hepatocellular adenoma) and malignant (HCC, carcinoid) tumors may show arterial hypervascularization. Doppler ultrasonography (US), contrast-enhanced US [6], dynamic computed tomography (CT), and dynamic magnetic resonance imaging (MRI) define the vascular pattern and, together with analysis of the nodule characteristics, may strongly suggest the diagnosis. Nevertheless, in the majority of cases the final diagnosis is established by biopsy [7]. Given the wide spectrum of liver tumors, the following sections will separately review the epidemiology, pathology, clinical presentation, diagnosis, and treatment of the most common cystic and solid hepatic lesions.

Liver Disease

Textbook of Clinical Gastroenterology and Hepatology, Second Edition. Edited by C. J. Hawkey, Jaime Bosch, Joel E. Richter, Guadalupe Garcia-Tsao, Francis K. L. Chan.

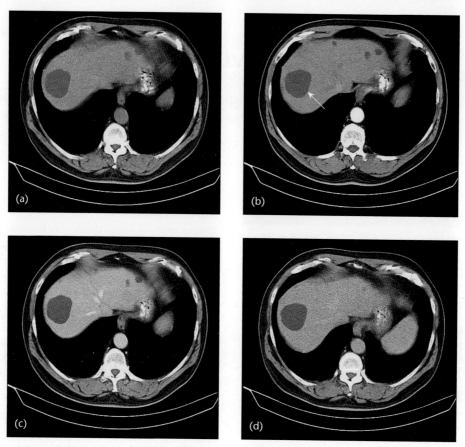

Figure 104.1 Simple liver cysts. CT scan with contrast enhancement shows a big simple cyst within the right lobe (arrow) and multiple small simple cysts within the left lobe (arrow). (a) Basal phase. (b) Arterial phase. (c) Portal phase. (d) Equilibrium phase.

Cystic lesions

Simple cyst

About 2–7% of the general population is affected by a simple cyst [8,9]. Cysts contain serous liquid, are lined by cuboidal epithelium, and do not communicate with the biliary ducts [8,9]. In most cases they are solitary, and, if multiple, hepatic and/or renal polycystic disease should be suspected. Symptoms are absent until their diameter is >10 cm when they may cause jaundice, hemorrhage, or infection [8]. Diagnosis is established by ultrasound (US) demonstrating a simple liquid lesion with well defined, thin walls, with strong posterior wall echoes [6]. A computerized tomography (CT) scan (Figure 104.1) depicts a hypointense lesion with no changes through all phases of the dynamic study. Treatment, if any, should be symptomatic. Only complicated cysts benefit from percutaneous sclerotherapy or surgical resection [10].

Hydatid cyst

Echinococcosis is a zoonosis caused by cestodes of the genus *Echinococcus* (family Taeniidae) (see also Chapter 84). It can affect the liver, lung, central nervous system, among others [11]. Hepatic cysts rupture into the peritoneum, pleural space, or biliary tract in one-third of cases. Diagnosis relies on US and

serology. Thicker walls with calcification, septa, and split walls with floating membranes differentiate hydatid from simple cysts [11]. Distinction from biliary cystadenoma or cystadenocarcinoma may require biopsy. Serology is positive in 70% of cases. Treatment consists of mebendazole or albendazole, alone or associated with surgical resection [12]. Another strategy is percutaneous aspiration and injection of mebendazole or albendazole (PAIR, percutaneous aspiration–injection–reaspiration), with promising results [13].

Hepatic abscess

Pyogenic hepatic abscesses are usually produced by bacteria from the gastrointestinal tract. In 40% of cases they are secondary to cholangitis, and the remainder result from portal bacteremia secondary to gastrointestinal infections such as diverticulitis or appendicitis. The clinical suspicion is based on the presence of malaise, fever, anorexia, right upper quadrant pain, and leukocytosis. CT confirms the diagnosis by demonstrating one or more cystic lesions with internal bubbles and ill-defined margins. Blood cultures are positive in 60% of cases. Treatment includes antibiotics and percutaneous or surgical drainage [14]. Pyogenic abscess must be distinguished from abscess secondary to *Entamoeba histolytica* (see Chapter 84) [15].

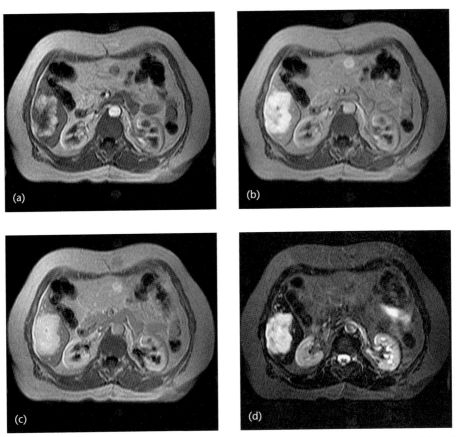

Figure 104.2 Small hepatic hemangioma. Contrast-enhanced MRI shows this small hepatic hemangioma as a hyperintense nodule on T2-wedged images. (a) Arterial phase. (b) Portal phase. (c) Equilibrium phase. (d) T2 wedged image.

Solid lesions

Hepatic hemangioma

Hemangioma is the most frequent liver tumor, with a prevalence of 0.4–7.4% [2,9,16]. It is composed of large vascular channels lined by mature, flattened, endothelial cells, enclosed in a fibroblastic stroma [2,8,9]. Hemangiomas are usually solitary and small, but can reach 20 cm in diameter [16]. Even then, most patients are asymptomatic and diagnosis is incidental. Their course is benign, although they may grow slightly during pregnancy or estrogen treatment. Bleeding is extremely infrequent and should suggest another diagnosis. Giant hemangiomas may become symptomatic in the event of infarction or thrombosis. Exceptionally a hemangioma can lead to thrombocytopenia, localized coagulopathy, and microangiopathic hemolytic anemia (Kasabach–Merritt syndrome). US shows a well defined hyperechogenic lesion that after contrast administration displays an initial peripheral globular–nodular enhancement and is followed by a centripetal fill in [6]. MRI is the best diagnostic method (100% sensitivity, 95% specificity) (Figure 104.2) upon finding a typical globular peripheral enhancement with progressive hyperintense filling on T2-weighted images [17,18]. Treatment is symptomatic [16].

Focal nodular hyperplasia

Focal nodular hyperplasia (FNH) is the second most frequent benign liver tumor with a prevalence of 0.01% in the general population. In most cases it is solitary and smaller than 5 cm (Figure 104.3), but it may be larger and multiple in 20% of cases. It is considered a regenerative cell response to an aberrant dystrophic artery [1,2,8,9]. Normal hepatocytes form plates one or two cells thick, and in the margins of the nodule prominent bile ductular reaction with positive staining for orcein can be observed, a characteristic that is used to distinguish FNH from hepatic adenoma [19]. The presence of a central fibrotic scar containing the feeding artery is a characteristic finding and is used to establish the diagnosis (Figure 104.4) [20]. On magnetic resonance imaging (MRI), FNH is usually slightly hypointense or isointense on T1-weighted and slightly hyperintense or isointense on T2-weighted sequences, with a central scar hypointense on T1-weighted images and hyperintense on T2-weighted images. Following contrast administration, FNH displays intense, homogeneous enhancement in the arterial phase sparing the central scar, whereas it becomes isointense to liver parenchyma in the portal venous and delayed phases [20]. FNH is more common in young

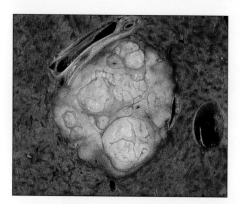

Figure 104.3 Focal nodular hyperplasia. The section of the liver segment containing the tumor shows a mass smaller than 3 cm in diameter, with a typical central fibrotic scar.

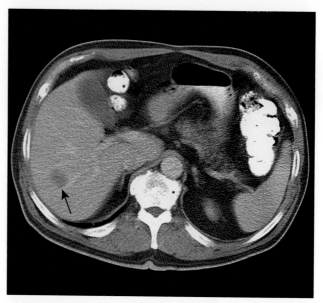

Figure 104.5 Metastases from colorectal carcinoma. On contrast enhanced CT, CRC metastases are depicted as hypovascular lesions with peripheral contrast uptake (arrow).

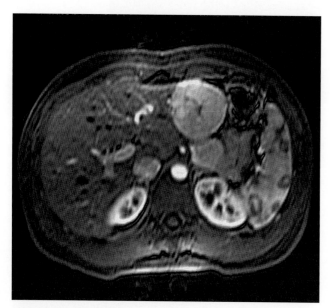

Figure 104.4 Focal nodular hyperplasia. With contrast enhanced dynamic MRI it is possible to identify a mass in the left hepatic lobe with a central fibrotic scar, which confirms the diagnosis of focal nodular hyperplasia.

women [2,8] and usually represents an incidental finding in asymptomatic subjects. The clinical evolution is uneventful with no potentially severe complications. Thus, no treatment is recommended [1,2].

Hepatocellular adenoma

Hepatocellular adenoma is a very uncommon tumor (prevalence 0.001%) that is found more frequently in young women. It is associated with oral contraceptive or anabolic treatment, and with glycogen storage disease type Ia (von Gierke disease) [2,8]. It is mostly solitary, but in up to 10–20% of cases more than one adenoma can be detected. In these patients hepatic adenomatosis due to a genetic abnormality has to be considered [2,8,21]. Hepatic adenoma is composed of normal hepatocytes without atypia, arranged in plates separated by dilated

sinusoids. It lacks portal spaces or biliary ducts [2,8,22]. Most patients with hepatic adenoma report mild abdominal pain. The most frequent complication is necrosis and bleeding. This can prompt severe hemoperitoneum from subcapsular adenomas [21]. Malignant transformation has been demonstrated in a minority of patients (approximately 1%), and a recent study has suggested that hepatic adenomas with beta-catenin activation have higher risk for malignant degeneration [23]. Taking into account this complications, once it is diagnosed, it should be removed surgically [24] or by percutaneous radio-frequency ablation in patients in whom surgery is contraindicated [25]. Distinction between hepatic adenoma and FNH may be difficult, even with the most sensitive imaging techniques. On MRI it is hyperintense on T2-weighted images, and iso-intense on T1-weighted sequences, with rapid contrast uptake during the arterial phase, remaining isointense with respect to the liver tissue in delayed sequences [20]. In some cases, biopsy may be necessary but even then the differential may be impossible, particularly in the telangiectatic variant of FNH [22,26].

Hepatic metastasis

Most malignant liver tumors are metastases from cancers that originate in other organs [2,27], the most frequent being lung, colon, stomach, pancreas, gallbladder, breast, and ovaries. Metastatic involvement of the liver implies a poor prognosis, except in patients with colorectal or neuroendocrine metastases that can be treated surgically (Figure 104.5). Searching for the primary tumor and biopsy confirmation is justified if the patient may benefit from therapy such as surgery or systemic chemotherapy [27]. Fine-needle aspiration biopsy has an 85% diagnostic sensitivity with more than 95% specificity. Tumor markers can also be useful. Serum carcinoembryonic antigen

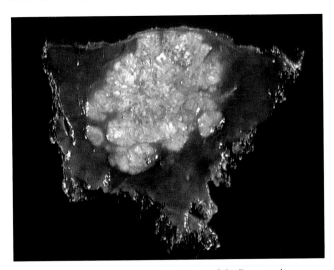

Figure 104.6 Colorectal metastasis. This section of the liver reveals a heterogeneous multilocular mass with ill-defined margins.

Table 104.1 Annual incidence of hepatocellular carcinoma (HCC) in chronic liver disease of various etiologies

Etiology	Incidence
HBV carrier without cirrhosis	0.4–0.6%*
HBV-related cirrhosis	2–6% per year
HCV-related cirrhosis	3–8%
Cirrhosis from genetic hemochromatosis	5%
Biliary primary cirrhosis	Low risk
Cirrhosis from autoimmune hepatitis or primary sclerosing cholangitis	Very low risk

*Risk increased if infection is acquired in childhood.
HBV, hepatitis B virus; HCV, hepatitis C virus.

levels are increased in 90% of colorectal cancer (CRC) metastases, CA125 can rise in pancreatic and ovarian cancer, and prostate-specific antigen is specific for prostate tumors. On CT, liver metastases are hypovascular lesions that in some neoplasms may have a specific pattern (Figure 104.6). Contrast uptake in the arterial phase on CT or MRI suggests neuroendocrine tumor, melanoma, sarcoma, hypernephroma, or thyroid neoplasia [2,8,20]. Isotopic studies using labeled somatostatin analogs can identify neuroendocrine tumors. Surgical resection of liver metastases may prolong survival in patients with CRC, neuroendocrine tumors, and some renal carcinomas, but for other neoplasms the indication of surgery is still controversial. Patients with up to four CRC metastases who can be successfully resected may achieve a 40% survival rate at 5 years. Neoadjuvant chemotherapy may also improve outcome [28]. In neuroendocrine tumors, resection may be curative when associated with resection of the primary tumor [29].

Hepatocellular carcinoma

HCC is the sixth most common neoplasm in the world, and the third most frequent cause of cancer-related death, with more than half a million new cases diagnosed yearly [30]. It usually develops in the setting of chronic liver disease, and cirrhosis represents its strongest predisposing factor.

Epidemiology

There are significant geographic differences in HCC incidence (age-adjusted incidence rate is 8.7×10^5 in developed countries and 14.7×10^5 in developing countries), reflecting the heterogeneous distribution of its main etiologic factors (Table 104.1) [31]. In Asia and Africa, hepatitis B virus infection is the predominant risk factor, and the risk is increased by ingestion of aflatoxin B1-contaminated food that is associated with a specific mutation in the *p53* tumor suppressor gene. In these areas, HCC may develop earlier, mostly in a noncirrhotic liver. By contrast, in developed countries, HCC affects older patients with hepatitis C virus (HCV) or alcohol-related cirrhosis [31]. The incidence of HCC has increased in the past decade as a consequence of higher rates of HCV infection and improvements in the management and survival of cirrhotic patients [32]. In these patients, surveillance with US every 6 months is recommended to detect HCC in early phases, while still amenable to curative therapies [5].

Diagnosis

In patients without underlying liver disease, the diagnosis of HCC should be based on histologic examination. By contrast, in patients with cirrhosis or chronic hepatitis B the diagnosis can be established noninvasively in nodules >1 cm (Figure 104.7) [5]. Dynamic imaging techniques demonstrate a specific vascular pattern characterized by intense and homogeneous contrast uptake in the arterial phase followed by contrast washout in venous phases (Figures 104.8–104.11). When this specific vascular pattern is not found, a biopsy should be performed, which is necessary in up to 44% of nodules between 5 and 20 mm. (Figure 104.12) [33]. However, biopsy has a false negative rate of 30%. Consequently, a negative result does not confidently rule out HCC and a repeat biopsy or close follow-up is recommended [5,33]. Nodules smaller than 1 cm are usually benign and are difficult to characterize, therefore US should be repeated every 3 months [5,33].

Prognosis and treatment

Prognosis of HCC depends not only on tumor stage, but also on the degree of liver function impairment and general health status [34]. Several staging systems have been proposed during the last decade. Among them, the Barcelona Clinic Liver Cancer (BCLC) system has been validated in US, Europe and Asia, and links prognosis assessment and treatment indication [5,35,36]. The BCLC stage systems considers the tumor stage (size, number of nodules, presence of vascular invasion and

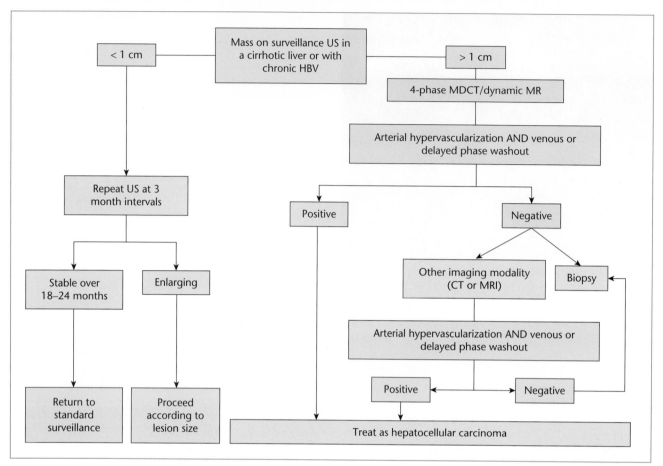

Figure 104.7 Surveillance and recall strategy for HCC. AFP, alpha-fetoprotein; CEUS, contrast-enhanced ultrasound; CT, computed tomography; HCC, hepatocellular carcinoma; MRI, magnetic resonance imaging; US, ultrasonography. (Reproduced with permission from Bruix, J, Sherman, M. (2010) Management of Hepatocellular Carcinoma: An Update. American Association for the Study of Liver Diseases. http://www.aasld.org/practiceguidelines (accessed 9 November 2010).)

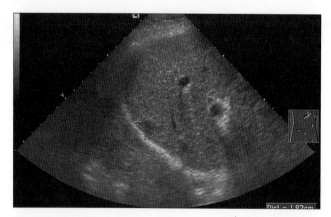

Figure 104.8 Small hepatocellular carcinoma. HCC (diameter <2 cm) seen as a hypoechoic focal lesion on regular US.

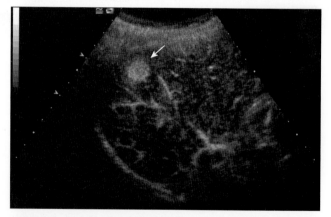

Figure 104.9 Small hepatocellular carcinoma. HCC (arrow) depicted as a hypervascular lesion on the arterial phase of contrast-enhanced US. The vessels feeding the tumor can be identified.

extrahepatic spread), liver function (Child–Pugh score) and general health (ECOG Performance Status) and stratifies patients into five major categories, each with a different treatment (Figure 104.13) [37,38]. Very early stage (Stage 0 or *in situ* HCC) corresponds to patients with preserved liver function without clinically significant portal hypertension and very early tumors <2 cm, differentiated, and without the ability to disseminate. With curative therapies, the 5-year survival rate is superior to 80% [38]. Early stage (Stage A) HCC corresponds to patients with preserved liver function, no cancer-related symptoms and single tumors or up to three nodules <3 cm.

These patients are suitable for potential curative treatment (resection, liver transplantation, or percutaneous ablation) and the expected 5-year survival after treatment is 50–70%. The optimal candidates for resection are those with solitary tumors in whom the underlying cirrhosis has not led to significant portal hypertension or hyperbilirubinemia [39,40]. Transplantation is the preferred approach for patients with impaired liver function with best results in tumors within Milan criteria (single tumor <5 cm or up to three nodules smaller that 3 cm) [41–43]. Percutaneous ablation by ethanol injection or preferably by radiofrequency [44] should be considered in patients at stage 0 or A who are not eligible for surgery or as a bridge to transplantation [45]. Intermediate (stage B) patients are still asymptomatic with large or multifocal HCC exceeding the criteria for applying curative therapies, without vascular invasion or extrahepatic spread. They are optimal candidates for chemoembolization [46]. This requires selective catheterization of the hepatic artery feeding the tumor, with injection of a chemotherapeutic agent followed by the injection of an embolizing agent. The procedure is well tolerated and achieves tumor necrosis in more than 50% of the patients, who thereafter achieve an improved survival rate exceeding 50% at 3 years. The recent development of new particles of polyvinyl alcohol (PVA) loaded with chemotherapy allows the delivery of the drug to the tumour without initial systemic washout release, obtaining higher concentrations and during a longer time period into the tumor, with minimal systemic passage, and therefore, less drug-related side effects [47]. Other relevant development is the intravascular injection of microspheres radiolabeled with yttrium-90 [48]. Advanced stage (stage C) denotes patients with advanced tumors and vascular

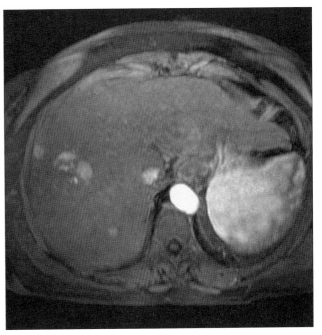

Figure 104.11 Hepatocellular carcinoma. Contrast-enhanced MRI of a 4-cm HCC located in the right hepatic lobe, depicted as a hypervascular lesion in the arterial phase.

Figure 104.10 Hepatocellular carcinoma. Contrast-enhanced CT shows a 3.5-cm HCC located in the right hepatic lobe (arrow), depicted as a hypervascular lesion in the arterial phase of the study.

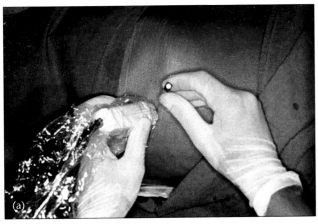

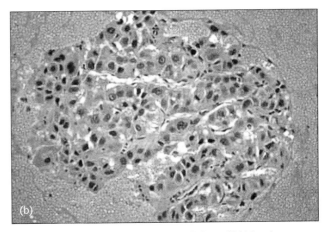

Figure 104.12 Fine-needle aspiration biopsy in a patient with HCC. (a) The procedure is guided by US using the free-hand technique. (b) Light microscopy using conventional hematoxylin and eosin staining indicates a moderately differentiated HCC.

Liver Disease

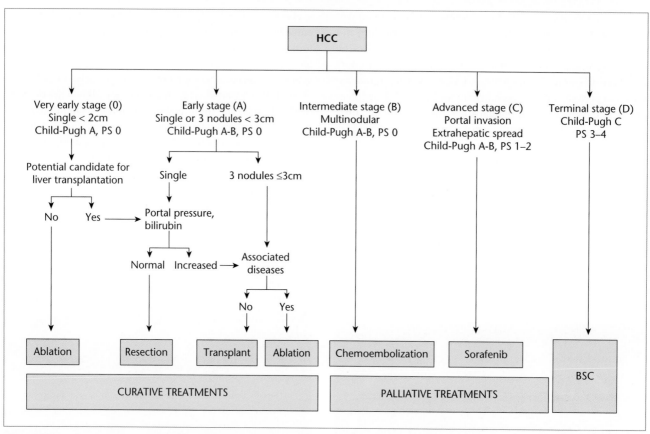

Figure 104.13 Figure 104.13: Barcelona Clinic Liver Cancer staging and treatment schedule. BSC: Best supportive care; PS, performance status. (Reproduced from Forner A, Llovet JM, Bruix J. Hepatocellular carcinoma. *Lancet*. 2012. In press, with permission from Elsevier.)

involvement, extrahepatic spread, or physical impairment (Figure 104.14). The expected median survival is 6 months and until recently, there were not available therapies. Improvements in the knowledge of the molecular pathogenesis of neoplasia have led the development of agents that act blocking the altered pathways. The only agent that has so far demonstrated a significant survival improvement in randomized controlled trials is sorafenib [49,50]. Sorafenib exerts its effect through a delay in tumor growth and is able to induce a 33% of survival improvement. Finally, patients with terminal stage (stage D) tumors have a very poor physical status and/or major tumor burden, and should receive symptomatic treatment. Child–Pugh grade C patients with HCC at any stage who are not candidates for liver transplantation belong to this group and do not benefit from antitumoral treatment, as outcome is poor due to liver failure.

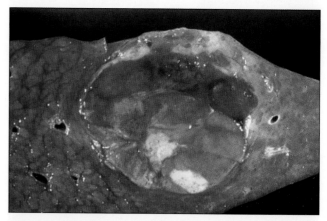

Figure 104.14 Large HCC replacing part of the right lobe. The green appearance reflects bile production.

Fibrolamellar carcinoma

Fibrolamellar carcinoma is an uncommon variant of HCC (1–9%), frequent in Western countries, and most prevalent in young patients without chronic liver disease. Therefore, it must be differentiated from benign liver lesions. Usually it consists of a large, single, nonencapsulated intrahepatic mass

with a fibrotic calcified central scar. The diagnosis is usually late, with symptoms related to mass and malignant syndrome. The a-fetoprotein level is normal in more than 90% of patients. Diagnosis and staging are based on spiral CT and/or MRI [51]. Percutaneous core biopsy is needed in cases of atypical

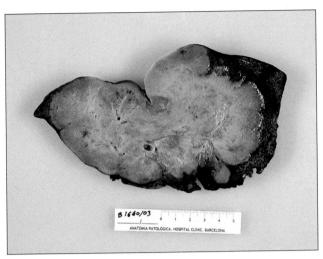

Figure 104.15 Intrahepatic cholangiocarcinoma. The large tumor has an irregular infiltrative margin; the central area is fibrotic.

imaging. Patients with fibrolamellar carcinoma have a better prognosis than those with classic HCC, and aggressive surgical resection or liver transplantation is feasible in around 80%, with a 5-year survival rate of 75% [52].

Intrahepatic cholangiocarcinoma

Intrahepatic cholangiocarcinoma (ICC) is less common than extrahepatic ductal cholangiocarcinoma, and appears as a focal mass lesion. It is an adenocarcinoma that originates from intrahepatic biliary epithelial cells (Figure 104.15). Several risk factors for ICC development have been suggested. The most known are primary sclerosing cholangitis, hepatobiliary flukes, hepatolithiasis and biliary malformations. In addition, HCV cirrhosis has been recognized as an important risk factor for ICC development and may explain the increasing incidence of ICC in recent years [53]. Diagnosis is suggested by dynamic imaging techniques, but conclusive diagnosis can be only achieved by pathological confirmation. The typical radiological appearance is a lesion with progressive contrast uptake along the different phases, associated with a central scar, vascular encasement and capsule retraction [54]. The tumor becomes symptomatic upon reaching a large size, and the sole therapeutic option is surgical resection, which is an option in only a minority of patients who may then have a 3-year survival rate of 40–60% (Figure 104.16) [55]. Liver transplantation has poor results and is not recommended.

Angiosarcoma

This is the most common mesenchymal malignant tumor of the liver [56]. It originates from the endothelial cells of the sinusoidal lining, and generally appears in adults (male : female ratio, 3:1). The tumor cells infiltrate the sinusoids, hepatic and portal veins, and finally substitute the hepatic parenchyma.

Angiosarcoma has been associated with thorotrast and vinyl chloride exposure [56]. Symptoms may mimic those of chronic liver disease, but in 15% of patients angiosarcoma is diagnosed because of acute hemoperitoneum due to tumor rupture. Liver biopsy establishes the diagnosis. Dynamic CT shows gradual contrast enhancement and homogeneity in the late phase. MRI shows that the tumor is homogeneously hypointense on T1-weighted imaging and hyperintense on T2-weighted imaging [8]. Diagnosis is usually made at an advanced stage when surgery is not feasible, and prognosis is dismal [56].

Hepatic epithelioid hemangioendothelioma

This is an unusual tumor that is more common in women. It originates from endothelial cells, and histopathologic diagnosis is based on staining for vascular markers CD31 and CD34. Its pathogenesis is unknown; symptoms are nonspecific and the evolution is unpredictable. It can remain stable for years and then progress in a very aggressive way. On imaging studies, the lesion has a solid appearance and mimics metastatic disease [57]. Solitary tumors may be resected, but, if multiple, the sole treatment option is liver transplantation [58]. The decision to transplant has to take into account the frequently indolent course versus the risks of transplantation. Transplantation is usually delayed until there is evidence of unequivocal tumor progression [58].

Biliary cystadenoma and cystadenocarcinoma

These are tumors that originate from biliary epithelium and mainly affect women. They are detected as multiloculated lesions. The sole treatment option is surgical resection.

Differential diagnosis

Four different clinical situations can be considered for the categorization of liver tumors (Figure 104.17) [1,4]:

• Cystic lesion
• Solid lesion in a healthy patient
• Solid lesion in a patient with chronic liver disease
• Solid lesion in a patient with known or suspected neoplasia.

Cystic lesion

US is sufficient to establish the liquid content of a focal lesion in the liver. Clinical characteristics, hydatidic and amebic serology, and CT or MRI will make the differential diagnosis between simple cyst, hepatic and/or renal polycystic disease, hydatid cyst, pyogenic abscess, and amebic abscess. The differentiation with cystoadenoma and cystoadenocarcinoma is difficult and, if suspected, usually requires image-guided biopsy or histologic analysis of the resected lesion. It should be noted that metastases from ovaries, pancreas, or neuroendocrine tumors may sometimes have a cystic aspect.

Liver Disease

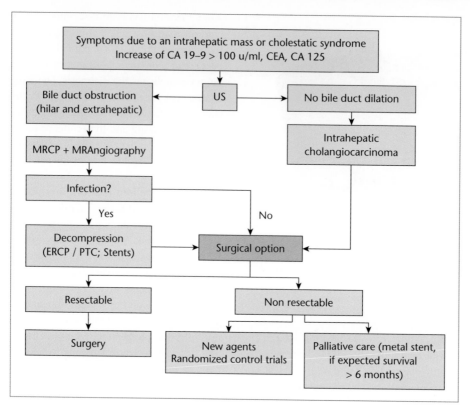

Figure 104.16 Suspicion of cholangiocarcinoma. Diagnostic algorithm for patients in whom cholangiocarcinoma is suspected. CC, cholangiocarcinoma; CEA, carcinoembryonic antigen; ERCP, endoscopic retrograde cholangiopancreatography; MRCP, magnetic resonance cholangiopancreatography; PTC, percutaneous transhepatic cholangiography; US, ultrasonography. (This figure was published in *Clinical Gastroenterology and Hepatology*, Wilfred M. Weinstein, Christopher J. Hawkey, Jaime Bosch, Tumors of the liver, Pages 1–10, Copyright Elsevier, 2005.)

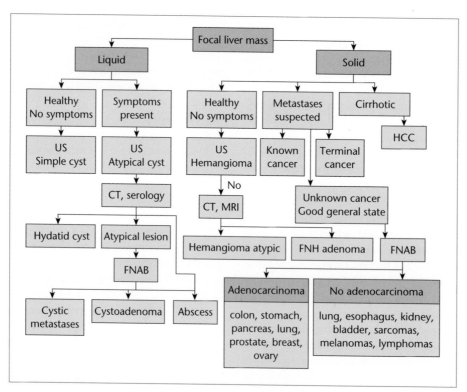

Figure 104.17 Diagnostic algorithm for a focal hepatic lesion. CT, computed tomography; FNAB, fine-needle aspiration biopsy; FNH, focal nodular hyperplasia; HCC, hepatocellular carcinoma; MRI, magnetic resonance imaging; US, ultrasonography. (This figure was published in *Clinical Gastroenterology and Hepatology*, Wilfred M. Weinstein, Christopher J. Hawkey, Jaime Bosch, Tumors of the liver, Pages 1–10, Copyright Elsevier, 2005.)

Solid lesion in a healthy patient

The most prevalent lesion is hemangioma, which can be easily diagnosed by US and MRI. If the patient is a young woman with a background of oral contraceptive use, it will be necessary to rule out FNH and hepatic adenoma. FNH is much more frequent and indolent. Although MRI can differentiate both entities in two-thirds of the cases [21], biopsy will be required in doubtful cases and will establish the malignant nature of the nodules in asymptomatic patients and in those with atypical and unexpected tumors. If the nature of the lesion is still equivocal, surgical resection is recommended [24].

Solid lesion in a patient with chronic liver disease

The diagnostic strategy in these patients has been established by the panel of experts set up by the American Association for the Study of Liver Diseases [5]. Lesions greater than 1 cm in cirrhotic patients can be confidently diagnosed by imaging techniques if a specific vascular profile is found. If the vascular pattern is not typical, a biopsy should be requested. Finally, lesions smaller than 1 cm must be followed every 3 months with US because currently available imaging techniques are unable to clearly distinguish regenerative nodules from dysplastic foci or early HCC.

Solid lesion in a patient with neoplasia

Three different settings can be considered [27].

Patients with a known primary neoplasm

In patients with a known primary neoplasm who are found to have liver metastases during staging or after treatment of the primary tumor, histologic analysis is necessary only if there are doubts regarding the etiology of the focal lesion.

Patients with a good condition and unknown primary tumor

In patients with a good general condition and an unknown primary tumor the search for the primary tumor is based on biopsy of the lesion. Adenocarcinomas and poorly differentiated malignancies are the most common histologic patterns.

- *Adenocarcinoma (well or moderately differentiated).* CRC must be ruled out if the biopsy discloses a potentially gastrointestinal origin, especially in patients older than 50 years and/or with a carcinoembryonic antigen level above 5 ng/mL. Gastric and pancreatic cancer should be excluded in jaundiced patients with high CA19.9 or high CA125 levels. If a nondigestive origin is suspected, it is necessary to exclude lung and prostate cancer, especially in patients with a prostate specific antigen level above 4 ng/mL, rising acid phosphatase concentration, or osteoblastic bone metastases. Breast and ovarian cancer should be ruled out in women.
- *Poorly differentiated malignancy.* Immunohistochemical techniques for cytokeratins are useful in this setting. They may help to distinguish carcinomas (lung, breast, prostate, pancreas, kidney, and urinary bladder) from other tumors.

Table 104.2 Immunoperoxidase staining of liver biopsy

Tumor type	Immunoperoxidase marker
Carcinoma	Cytokeratin (CK20 in gastrointestinal adenocarcinomas, CK7 in respiratory or gynecologic malignancies), EMA
Lymphoma	CLA, EMA (±)
Sarcoma	Vimentin, desmin, factor VIII antigen
Melanoma	S-100, HMB-45, vimentin, NSE, CD68
Neuroendocrine	Chromogranin, synaptophysin, cytokeratin, EMA, NSE
Germ cell	Cytokeratin, EMA, HCG, AFP
Prostate cancer	PSA, cytokeratin 5, 14, 18, EMA
Breast cance	Cytokeratin 5/6, 8/18/19, EMA, ER, PR
Thyroid cancer	Thyroglobulin, cytokeratin 19, EMA, calcitonin

AFP, α-fetoprotein; CLA, common leucocyte antigen; EMA, epithelial membrane antigen; ER, estrogen receptor; HCG, human chorionic gonadotropin; NSE, neuron-specific enolase; PR, progesterone receptor; PSA, prostate-specific antigen.

Neuroendocrine tumors may be diagnosed by staining for neuron-specific enolase or cromogranin. Identification of lymphomas, sarcomas, and melanomas also require specific staining and molecular techniques (Table 104.2).

Patients with poor condition and unknown primary tumor

In patients with an unknown primary tumor and seriously impaired general status (performance status 3–4) with constitutional syndrome (wasting and weight loss), liver failure, severe biochemical alterations, and multiple metastatic sites, given the lack of any therapeutic benefit, workup should be minimized in these patients and management directed towards comfort care.

SOURCES OF INFORMATION FOR PATIENTS AND DOCTORS

- http://www.patient.co.uk/showdoc/27000742/
- http://www.liverfoundation.org/db/articles/1040
- http://www.radiologyinfo.org/content/interventional/rf_ablation.htm
- http://www.radiologyinfo.org/content/interventional/chemoembol.htm

Liver Disease

References

1. Reddy KR, Schiff ER. Approach to a liver mass. *Semin Liver Dis.* 1993;13:423–435.

2. Rubin RA, Mitchell DG. Evaluation of the solid hepatic mass. *Med Clin North Am.* 1996;80:907–928.

3. Ishak KG, Goodman ZD, Stocker JT. (2001)Tumors of the liver and intrahepatic bile ducts, in *Atlas of Tumor Pathology.* (ed J.S.L.H. Rosai), Armed Forces Institute of Pathology, Washington, DC.

4. Ros PR, Davis GL. The incidental focal liver lesion: Photon, proton, or needle? *Hepatology.* 1998;27:1183–1190.

5. Bruix J, Sherman M. Management of hepatocellular carcinoma: An update. *Hepatology.* 2011;53:1020–1022.

6. Claudon M, Cosgrove D, Albrecht T, *et al.* Guidelines and good clinical practice recommendations for contrast enhanced ultrasound (CEUS) – update 2008. *Ultraschall Med.* 2008;29:28–44.

7. Verslype C, Libbrecht L. The multidisciplinary management of gastrointestinal cancer. The diagnostic and therapeutic approach for primary solid liver tumours in adults. *Best Pract Res Clin Gastroenterol.* 2007;21:983–996.

8. Fulcher AS, Sterling RK. Hepatic neoplasms: Computed tomography and magnetic resonance features. *J Clin Gastroenterol.* 2002;34:463–471.

9. Horton KM, Bluemke DA, Hruban RH, *et al.* CT and MR imaging of benign hepatic and biliary tumors. *Radiographics.* 1999;19: 431–451.

10. Erdogan D, van Delden OM, Rauws EA, *et al.* Results of percutaneous sclerotherapy and surgical treatment in patients with symptomatic simple liver cysts and polycystic liver disease. *World J Gastroenterol.* 2007;13:3095–3100.

11. McManus DP, Zhang W, Li J, *et al.* Echinococcosis. *Lancet.* 2003;362:1295–1304.

12. WHO Informal Working Group on Echinococcosis. Guidelines for treatment of cystic and alveolar echinococcosis in humans. *Bull World Health Org.* 1996;74:231–242.

13. Smego RA Jr, Bhatti S, Khaliq AA, *et al.* Percutaneous aspiration–injection–reaspiration drainage plus albendazole or mebendazole for hepatic cystic echinococcosis: a meta-analysis. *Clin Infect Dis.* 2003;37:1073–1083.

14. Sanchez-Tapias, J. (2007) Bacterial, rickettsial and spirochaetal infections, in *Textbook of Hepatology: From Basic Science to Clinical Practice.* 3rd edn (eds J. Rodes, J. Benhamou, A. Blei, J. Reichen and M Rizzetto), Blackwell, Oxford, pp. 1001–1011.

15. Stanley SL Jr. Amoebiasis. *Lancet.* 2003;361:1025–1034.

16. Gandolfi L, Leo P, Solmi L, *et al.* Natural history of hepatic haemangiomas: Clinical and ultrasound study. *Gut.* 1991;32: 677–680.

17. Whitney WS, Herfkens RJ, Jeffrey RB, *et al.* Dynamic breath-hold multiplanar spoiled gradient-recalled MR imaging with gadolinium enhancement for differentiating hepatic hemangiomas from malignancies at 1.5 T. *Radiology.* 1993;189:863–870.

18. Mitchell DG, Saini S, Weinreb J, *et al.* Hepatic metastases and cavernous hemangiomas: distinction with standard- and triple-dose gadoteridol-enhanced MR imaging. *Radiology.* 1994;193: 49–57.

19. Bioulac-Sage P, Balabaud C, Wanless IR. Diagnosis of focal nodular hyperplasia: Not so easy. *Am J Surg Pathol.* 2001;25: 1322–1325.

20. Hussain SM, Terkivatan T, Zondervan PE, *et al.* Focal nodular hyperplasia: findings at state-of-the-art MR imaging, US, CT, and pathologic analysis. *Radiographics.* 2004;24:3–17; discussion 8–9.

21. Cherqui D, Rahmouni A, Charlotte F, *et al.* Management of focal nodular hyperplasia and hepatocellular adenoma in young women: A series of 41 patients with clinical, radiological, and pathological correlations. *Hepatology.* 1995;22:1674–1681.

22. Bioulac-Sage P, Balabaud C, Bedossa P, *et al.* Pathological diagnosis of liver cell adenoma and focal nodular hyperplasia: Bordeaux update. *J Hepatol.* 2007;46:521–527.

23. Bioulac-Sage P, Laumonier H, Couchy G, *et al.* Hepatocellular adenoma management and phenotypic classification: the Bordeaux experience. *Hepatology.* 2009 Aug;50(2):481–489.

24. Chaib E, Gama-Rodrigues J, Ribeiro MA Jr, *et al.* Hepatic adenoma. Timing for surgery. *Hepatogastroenterology.* 2007;54: 1382–1387.

25. Atwell T, Brandhagen D, Charboneau J, *et al.* Successful treatment of hepatocellular adenoma with percutaneous radiofrequency ablation. *AJR Am J Roentgenol.* 2005;184:828–831.

26. Bioulac-Sage P, Rebouissou S, Thomas C, *et al.* Hepatocellular adenoma subtype classification using molecular markers and immunohistochemistry. *Hepatology.* 2007;46:740–748.

27. Pavlidis N, Briasoulis E, Hainsworth J, *et al.* Diagnostic and therapeutic management of cancer of an unknown primary. *Eur J Cancer.* 2003;39:1990–2005.

28. Meyerhardt JA, Mayer RJ. Systemic therapy for colorectal cancer. *N Engl J Med.* 2005;352:476–487.

29. Modlin IM, Oberg K, Chung DC, *et al.* Gastroenteropancreatic neuroendocrine tumours. *Lancet Oncol.* 2008;9:61–72.

30. Ferlay J, Shin HR, Bray F, *et al.* Estimates of worldwide burden of cancer in 2008: GLOBOCAN 2008. *Int J Cancer.* 2010;127: 2893–2917.

31. Bosch FX, Ribes J, Diaz M, *et al.* Primary liver cancer: Worldwide incidence and trends. *Gastroenterology.* 2004;127(5 Suppl 1): S5–S16.

32. El-Serag HB, Mason AC. Rising incidence of hepatocellular carcinoma in the United States. *N Engl J Med.* 1999;340:745–750.

33. Forner A, Vilana R, Ayuso C, *et al.* Diagnosis of hepatic nodules 20 mm or smaller in cirrhosis: Prospective validation of the non-invasive diagnostic criteria for hepatocellular carcinoma. *Hepatology.* 2008;47:97–104.

34. Forner A, Reig ME, Rodriguez de Lope C, *et al.* Current strategy for staging and treatment: The BCLC update and future prospects. *Semin Liver Dis.* 2010;30:61–74.

35. Forner A, Ayuso C, Isabel Real M, et al. [Diagnosis and treatment of hepatocellular carcinoma.]. *Medicina Clínica.* 2009;132: 272–287.

36. Llovet JM, Di Bisceglie AM, Bruix J, *et al.* Design and endpoints of clinical trials in hepatocellular carcinoma. *J Natl Cancer Inst.* 2008;100:698–711.

37. Llovet JM, Bru C, Bruix J. Prognosis of hepatocellular carcinoma: The BCLC staging classification. *Semin Liver Dis.* 1999;19: 329–338.

38. Forner A, Llovet JM, Bruix J. Hepatocellular carcinoma. *Lancet.* 2012. In press.

39. Llovet JM, Fuster J, Bruix J. Intention-to-treat analysis of surgical treatment for early hepatocellular carcinoma: resection versus transplantation. *Hepatology.* 1999;30:1434–1440.

40. Ishizawa T, Hasegawa K, Aoki T, *et al.* Neither multiple tumors nor portal hypertension are surgical contraindications for hepatocellular carcinoma. *Gastroenterology.* 2008;134:1908–1916.

41. Mazzaferro V, Regalia E, Doci R, *et al.* Liver transplantation for the treatment of small hepatocellular carcinomas in patients with cirrhosis. *N Engl J Med.* 1996;334:693–699.

42. Yao FY, Ferrell L, Bass NM, *et al.* Liver transplantation for hepatocellular carcinoma: expansion of the tumor size limits does not adversely impact survival. *Hepatology.* 2001;33:1394–1403.

43. Mazzaferro V, Llovet J, Miceli R, *et al.* Predicting survival after liver transplantation in patients with hepatocellular carcinoma beyond the Milan criteria: A retrospective, exploratory analysis. *Lancet Oncol.* 2009;10:35–43.

44. Cho YK, Kim JK, Kim MY, *et al.* Systematic review of randomized trials for hepatocellular carcinoma treated with percutaneous ablation therapies. *Hepatology.* 2009;49:453–459.

45. Lencioni R. Loco-regional treatment of hepatocellular carcinoma. *Hepatology.* 2010 Aug;52(2):762–773.

46. Llovet JM, Bruix J. Systematic review of randomized trials for unresectable hepatocellular carcinoma: Chemoembolization improves survival. *Hepatology.* 2003;37:429–442.

47. Varela M, Real MI, Burrel M, *et al.* Chemoembolization of hepatocellular carcinoma with drug eluting beads: efficacy and doxorubicin pharmacokinetics. *J Hepatol.* 2007;46:474–481.

48. Kulik LM, Carr BI, Mulcahy MF, *et al.* Safety and efficacy of 90Y radiotherapy for hepatocellular carcinoma with and without portal vein thrombosis. *Hepatology.* 2008;47:71–81.

49. Cheng AL, Kang YK, Chen Z, *et al.* Efficacy and safety of sorafenib in patients in the Asia-Pacific region with advanced hepatocellular carcinoma: A phase III randomised, double-blind, placebo-controlled trial. *Lancet Oncol.* 2009;10:25–34.

50. Llovet J, Ricci S, Mazzaferro V, *et al.* Sorafenib in advanced hepatocellular carcinoma. *N Engl J Med.* 2008;359:378–390.

51. Ichikawa T, Federle MP, Grazioli L, *et al.* Fibrolamellar hepatocellular carcinoma: imaging and pathologic findings in 31 recent cases. *Radiology.* 1999;213:352–361.

52. Stipa F, Yoon SS, Liau KH, *et al.* Outcome of patients with fibrolamellar hepatocellular carcinoma. *Cancer.* 2006;106:1331–1338.

53. Shaib YH, El-Serag HB, Nooka AK, *et al.* Risk factors for intrahepatic and extrahepatic cholangiocarcinoma: a hospital-based case-control study. *Am J Gastroenterol.* 2007;102:1016–1021.

54. Chung YE, Kim MJ, Park YN, *et al.* Varying appearances of cholangiocarcinoma: Radiologic-pathologic correlation. *Radiographics.* 2009;29:683–700.

55. Khan SA, Davidson BR, Goldin R, *et al.* Guidelines for the diagnosis and treatment of cholangiocarcinoma: consensus document. *Gut.* 2002;51(Suppl 6):VI1–9.

56. Kim HR, Rha SY, Cheon SH, *et al.* Clinical features and treatment outcomes of advanced stage primary hepatic angiosarcoma. *Ann Oncol.* 2009;20:780–787.

57. Mehrabi A, Kashfi A, Fonouni H, *et al.* Primary malignant hepatic epithelioid hemangioendothelioma: A comprehensive review of the literature with emphasis on the surgical therapy. *Cancer.* 2006;107:2108–2121.

58. Lerut JP, Weber M, Orlando G, *et al.* Vascular and rare liver tumors: A good indication for liver transplantation? *J Hepatol.* 2007;47:466–475.

CHAPTER 105
Vascular disorders of the liver

Dominique-Charles Valla

Hôpital Beaujon, Clichy, France

ESSENTIAL FACTS ABOUT CAUSATION

- Primary injury to hepatic vessels is a rare mechanism for liver diseases
- Iatrogenic injury and systemic diseases may cause arterial injury. Septic shock and hereditary hemorrhagic telangiectasia may cause non-occlusive arterial ischemia
- Prothrombotic conditions, particularly myeloproliferative diseases may cause thrombosis of portal or hepatic veins
- Systemic diseases or exposure to drugs or chemicals may cause damage to sinusoids or small portal veins

ESSENTIALS OF DIAGNOSIS

- Awareness and expertise in vascular imaging and liver histopathology are crucial
- Consider ischemic cholangiopathy for a biliary disease occurring in a context of compromised hepatic arterial inflow
- Establish Budd–Chiari syndrome by showing an obstructed hepatic venous outflow tract using non-invasive imaging
- Consider sinusoidal obstruction syndrome disease for a liver disease occurring in a context of myeloablative therapy or ingestion of plants containing pyrrolizidine alkaloids
- Establish acute portal vein thrombosis for acute abdominal pain using non-invasive imaging of the portal vessels
- Discuss portal cavernoma, obliterative portal venopathy, nodular regenerative hyperplasia, and arterioportal fistula in a context of non-cirrhotic portal hypertension

ESSENTIALS OF TREATMENT

- Refer to a specialized center
- For portal hypertension, prevent bleeding with pharmacologic or endoscopic therapy
- Prevent of thrombus extension and recurrence by correction of causes and immediate anticoagulation
- Preferably maintain anticoagulation in patients with a permanent prothrombotic condition
- Consider recanalizing obstructed arteries or veins preferably using percutaneous interventions
- For Budd–Chiari syndrome, insert TIPS when anticoagulation and angioplasty fail
- Prevent sinusoidal obstruction syndrome using reduced intensity conditioning

Introduction

All liver disorders related to a primary injury to hepatic vessels qualify as rare diseases. As a consequence, evidence for their diagnosis and management consist of limited, often poor-quality data. Furthermore, their recognition requires a high degree of suspicion, as well as awareness and expertise in the interpretation of vascular imaging and liver histopathology. Otherwise, many patients with primarily vascular disorders of the liver will be misdiagnosed as having common liver diseases, particularly cirrhosis.

The hepatic arteries, the hepatic or portal venous systems, as well as the hepatic microcirculation can be involved by various types of lesions, each type of lesions recognizing various causes. However, a limited number of clinical entities arise from these vascular lesions. These clinical entities and their corresponding vascular disorders are listed in Table 105.1. In this chapter, the vascular lesions and their recognized causes will be considered first, and the main clinical entities that they may induce will be discussed next.

Vascular disorders and their causes
Disorders of the hepatic arteries
Aneurysms and dissection of the hepatic artery

These lesions can be related to blunt or penetrating trauma (including needle liver biopsy, and arterial cannulation), infective endocarditis, panarteritis nodosa or rare congenital disorders affecting the arterial media [1].

Occlusion the hepatic artery

The occlusion of large arteries is generally related to arterial reconstruction at transplantation; to inadvert or intentional surgical ligation; or to hepatic arterial embolization [2]. Atheromatous stenosis, or primary thrombosis of the large hepatic arteries are exceptional. Involvement of the peribiliary arteriolar plexus may occur in the context of liver transplantation where they are linked to preservation injury, chronic rejection or CMV infection [2]. Distal arterial occlusion can be related to systemic vasculitis, prothrombotic disorders (e.g. antiphospholipid syndrome), or advanced AIDS [2].

Table 105.1 Disorders of hepatic vessels, their mechanisms and their related clinical entities

Disorders/mechanisms	Related clinical entities
Hepatic artery obstruction	
Thrombosis	Ischemic cholangiopathy
Ligation and embolization	Ischemic cholangiopathy
Hepatic artery aneurysm	Hemobilia, hemoperitoneum
Hepatic artery to portal vein fistula	
Hepatocellular carcinoma	Malignancy, portal hypertension
Trauma	Noncirrhotic portal hypertension
	High output cardiac failure
Hereditary hemorrhagic telangiectasia	Ischemic cholangiopathy
	Noncirrhotic portal hypertension
Hepatic artery to hepatic vein fistula	
Hepatocellular carcinoma	Malignancy
Hereditary hemorrhagic telangiectasia	Ischemic cholangiopathy
	High output cardiac failure
Hepatic vein obstruction	Budd–Chiari syndrome
Portal vein to hepatic vein shunt	
Malformation	Portosystemic encephalopathy
	Regenerative macronodules
Hereditary hemorrhagic telangiectasia	Regenerative macronodules
Extrahepatic portal vein obstruction	
Malignant invasion	Portal hypertension
Acute thrombosis	Intestinal ischemia
Chronic thrombosis	Noncirrhotic portal hypertension
Extrahepatic portal vein aneurysm	Acute portal vein thrombosis
Intrahepatic portal venous obstruction	
Schistosomiasis	Noncirrhotic portal hypertension
Obliterative portal venopathy	Noncirrhotic portal hypertension
Sinusoidal obstruction syndrome	Budd–Chiari syndrome-like
Sinusoidal dilatation/peliosis	Alteration of hepatic perfusion
Nodular regenerative hyperplasia and perisinusoidal fibrosis	Noncirrhotic portal hypertension

Arterioportal fistula

This lesion can be caused by a penetrating trauma or the rupture of a hepatic artery aneurysm, or be part of congenital abnormalities such as hereditary hemorrhagic telangiectasia (HHT) [3–5].

Arteriovenous fistula

This lesion is usually related to HHT [4,5].

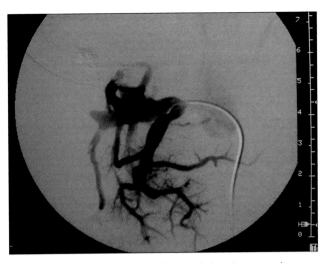

Figure 105.1 Budd–Chiari syndrome. Retrograde hepatic venography through the transfemoral route showing a stenosis at the ostium of right hepatic veins that has been passed by the catheter tip. There is an extensive network of hepatic vein collaterals. This aspect is typical for Budd–Chiari syndrome. Such a short-length stenosis is amenable to percutaneous angioplasty.

Disorders of the hepatic veins and inferior vena cava
Obstruction of the hepatic veins

This entity corresponds to Budd–Chiari syndrome (Figure 105.1). Secondary Budd–Chiari syndrome is caused by tumors compressing or invading the lumen of the hepatic veins (e.g. hepatocellular carcinoma, epithelioid hemangioendothelioma, and sarcoma) [6,7]. Primary Budd–Chiari syndrome is caused by thrombosis, which is related to one or several concurrent prothrombotic conditions, a list of which is provided in Table 105.2.

Obstruction of terminal inferior vena cava

This entity is usually associated with the obstruction of the hepatic vein ostia. It can simulate a web or a membrane in the inferior vena cava. However, it is now recognized that such a membranous obstruction is sequelae of prior thrombosis, generally facilitated by underlying prothrombotic conditions, as listed in Table 105.2 [4,6,7].

Disorders of extrahepatic portal vein
Portal vein thrombosis

This is the most common of the vascular disorders of the liver (Figure 105.2). Thrombosis is due to local factors, and/or underlying prothrombotic conditions (see Table 105.2) [4,8,9].

Portal cavernoma

It corresponds to the network of portoportal collaterals that develop after long-standing obstruction of the portal vein (Figure 105.2c and d). In adults, thrombosis is the main mechanism for portal cavernoma. In children, a congenital malformation should also be considered [4,9].

Liver Disease

Table 105.2 Prothrombotic conditions and risk factors that have been associated with Budd–Chiari syndrome, portal vein thrombosis, or obliterative portal venopathy

Acquired diseases
- Myeloproliferative disease, generally V617F-JAK2 mutation-positive
  Usual peripheral blood features can be masked by portal hypertension
- Antiphospholipid syndrome
  Non specific anticardiolipin antibodies frequent in liver disease
- Paroxysmal nocturnal hemoglobinuria (for Budd–Chiari syndrome)
- Behcet's disease (for Budd–Chiari syndrome)
- Inflammatory bowel disease
- Celiac disease (for Budd–Chiari syndrome)
- Sarcoidosis

Inherited disorders
- Protein C deficiency
  Secondary deficiency related to liver dysfunction can be difficult to rule out
- Protein S deficiency
  Secondary deficiency related to liver dysfunction can be difficult to rule out
- Antithrombin deficiency
  Secondary deficiency related to liver dysfunction can be difficult to rule out
- Factor V Leiden
- G20210A Factor II gene mutation

Other risk factors
- Inflammatory or malignant foci in the abdomen (for portal vein thrombosis)
- Injury to splanchnic veins (surgery or trauma)
- Stasis caused by cirrhosis or other intrahepatic block on the portal circulation
- Hyperhomocysteinemia
  Secondary increase related to liver dysfunction can be difficult to rule out
- Oral contraceptives
- Pregnancy (for Budd–Chiari syndrome)
- Extreme poverty

Diagnosis of a number of these conditions is made difficult by concurrent liver dysfunction and portal hypertension [4, 22].

Congenital porto-systemic shunts

This condition consist of a large portosystemic shunt diverting portal blood flow away from the liver, which is sometimes referred to as congenital absence of the portal vein although this last denomination is inaccurate [10,11].

Portal vein aneurysm

This abnormality is mostly encountered in patients with portal hypertension and therefore represents a secondary alteration [4,9,12].

Disorders of intrahepatic portal venous system
Obliterative portal venopathy

Worldwide, this lesion is mostly secondary to *Schistosoma mansoni* or *S. japonicum* [13]. A primary form, however, is increasingly recognized independent of schistosomiasis [13]. Obliteration of small portal veins is usually associated with

portal fibrosis, nodular regenerative changes, and sinusoidal dilatation or fibrosis. Ectopic small vascular channels (mostly in the periportal area of the lobule) constitute a hallmark for this entity [13,14]. Reported causes of obliterative portal venopathy include chronic exposure to various chemicals (arsenic, copper sulfate, vinyl chloride, thorium dioxide) or drugs (azathioprine). There might be some unclear link with poverty. Associations have also been described with underlying prothrombotic conditions (as listed in Table 105.2), or with congenital diseases (Turner syndrome, Adams Ollivier syndrome) [13,14]. Familial occurrence has also been described.

Congenital hepatic fibrosis

This inherited syndrome is characterized by dense portal fibrosis and abnormal interlobular bile ducts resulting from ductal plate malformation. Abnormal portal veins are common [15]. Portal hypertension is a major feature. In patients with recessive polycystic renal disease, congenital hepatic fibrosis is almost constant.

Portohepatic fistulas

This rare entity is almost exclusively encountered in patients with hereditary hemorrhagic telangiectasia [4,5].

Disorders of sinusoids
Sinusoidal obstruction syndrome

This entity, formerly known as venoocclusive disease, is related to toxic injury to sinusoidal endothelium [16,17]. It is almost exclusively encountered following exposure to certain plants containing pyrrolizidine alkaloids, or high dose radiotherapy to the liver, or exposure to certain toxic agents (azathioprine and its derivatives, actinomycin D, busulfan, cytosine arabinoside, cyclophosphamide, dacarbazine, gemtuzumab-ozogamicin, melphalan, oxaliplatin, urethane). Conditioning for hematopoietic stem cell transplantation currently represents the most common cause for sinusoidal syndrome. Damaged endothelial cell detach form the sinusoidal wall and embolize downstream to the junction with central veins were they produce obstruction.

Sinusoidal dilatation and peliosis hepatitis

These often poorly understood entities are characterized by a widening of the sinusoidal lumen [4,16]. Peliosis is further characterized by destruction of the sinusoidal wall, giving rise to multiple cyst-like, blood-filled cavities that are irregularly distributed throughout the liver, whereas in pure sinusoidal dilation the endothelium appears to be preserved and the changes generally predominate in the central, intermediate or periportal area of the lobule [4,18]. Central sinusoidal dilatation is mostly related to heart failure, constrictive pericarditis or Budd–Chiari syndrome where a hemodynamic component is obvious [18]. Mediolobular and periportal dilatation has been associated with obliterative portal venopathy, and oral contraceptives [19]. Other causes include

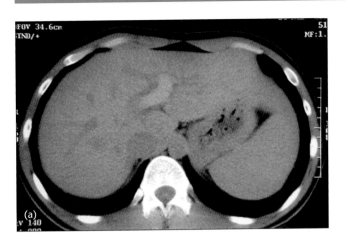
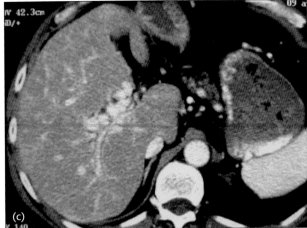
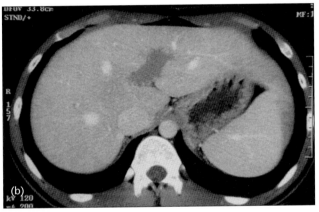
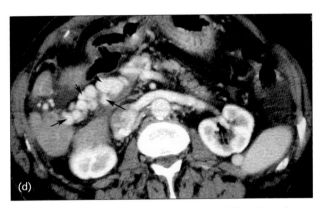

Figure 105.2 Portal vein thrombosis. Acute portal vein thrombosis seen as hyper-attenuated material on unenhanced CT scan (a), and a filling defect after intravenous injection of contrast material (b). Portal cavernoma seen at the portal phase of an enhanced CT scan as a serpiginous structure in the porta hepatis (c), and in the right prerenal area (d).

miscellaneous disorders, a partial list of which is provided in Table 105.3.

Sinusoidal fibrosis

When located in the perivenous area of the lobule, this lesion is associated frequently with alcoholic or non alcoholic steatohepatitis, or with longstanding hepatic venous outflow block or heart failure. When randomly distributed, it can accompany obliterative portal venopathy or sinusoidal dilatation (see causes in Table 105.3). In rare patients, sinusoidal fibrosis is an isolated finding. A typical cause for isolated sinusoidal fibrosis is chronic vitamin A supplementation, where hepatic stellate cells are characteristically enlarged by lipid droplets containing vitamin A [20].

Nodular regenerative hyperplasia

Although not properly a vascular lesion, this architectural alteration is frequently associated with obliterative portal venopathy, or with sinusoidal dilatation or fibrosis. It is generally admitted that this is a reactive change to uneven microcirculatory alteration resulting in the atrophy of poorly perfused areas and the hypertrophy of preserved areas [16].

Main vascular liver disorders

As presented in Table 105.1, vascular disorders can lead to different clinical presentations but the main and most frequent vascular disorders are portal vein thrombosis (pre-hepatic), sinusoidal obstruction syndrome (intrahepatic) and Budd–Chiari syndrome (post-hepatic), entities that will be discussed separately.

Acute portal vein thrombosis

Portal vein thrombosis of recent onset commonly causes acute, severe and protracted abdominal pain, often radiating – or even localized – to the back [4,8,9]. A systemic inflammatory reaction syndrome is the rule, even in the absence of an inflammatory focus such as pancreatitis, appendicitis, or diverticulitis. It is likely that portal vein thrombosis can develop with little or no symptoms as in some patients the condition is discovered only at a late stage of portal cavernoma. In patients with cirrhosis, portal vein thrombosis is often discovered in patients without abdominal pain by routine ultrasound, or at the time of decompensation. In some patients, spiking fever with chills indicates septicemia, corresponding to septic pylephlebitis (usually related to bacteroïdes infection).

Table 105.3 Conditions which have been associated with disorders of the hepatic microcirculation (sinusoidal dilatation, peliosis or nodular regenerative hyperplasia)

Drugs and chemicals
- Androgenic anabolic therapy
- Contraceptive steroids
- Azathioprine and derivatives
- Corticosteroids
- Arsenic
- Thorium dioxide
- Vinyl chloride
- Spanish toxic oil syndrome

Bacterial infections
- Tuberculosis
- Endocarditis
- Pyelonephritis
- Bacillary angiomatosis (in immune suppressed patients)

Monoclonal gammapathies
- Multiple myeloma
- Waldenström macroglobulinemia

Malignancies
- Malignant tumors
- Hodgkin's disease

Other conditions
- Hepatic granulomas
- Antiphospholipid syndrome
- Connective tissue disease (lupus, rheumatoid arthritis, scleroderma, and related disorders)
- Renal transplantation
- Diabetes
- Acquired immunodeficiency syndrome
- Crohn's disease

Extension of thrombosis to superior mesenteric veins and their small radicles can be complicated by intestinal ischemia [4,8,9]. In such patients, pain lasts several days. The severity of pain contrasts with a paucity of findings on physical examination. Hematochezia is highly suggestive of intestinal ischemia. Ascites may be present. At a later stage, there is necrosis of the ischemic gut with signs of acute peritonitis including metabolic acidosis and multiorgan failure. Mortality of intestinal infarction of venous origin remains 20–50% in patients subjected to surgical removal of necrotic gut segments.

Doppler-ultrasound and CT scan, first choice examinations for acute abdominal pain, show absence of flow or solid material in the main portal vein or its left or right branches. Finding hyperattenuating material in the venous lumen at unenhanced CT scan is helpful in qualifying a thrombus as recent (i.e. less than10 days). Enhanced CT scan is also irreplaceable for the immediate evaluation of local factors and of ischemic gut, and for the assessment of splenic vein and mesenteric vein involvement [4,8,9].

In the absence of recanalization of the main portal vein, or when its two branches remain obstructed, a cavernoma develops together with permanent portal hypertension. A specific consequence of portal cavenoma is the deformation of the bile ducts by the cavernomatous veins, giving an aspect mimicking that of primary sclerosing cholangitis [21]. However, cholestasis is uncommon, while most complications are related to biliary lithiasis. Recurrent thrombosis in splanchnic or extrasplanchnic veins may occur.

With early anticoagulation therapy and treatment of underlying causes or local factors, thrombus extension is prevented, while recanalization of the thrombosed portal vein occurs in 30–40% of patients [8]. Recanalization of associated mesenteric or splenic vein thrombosis can be expected in 60% of patients. However, the presence of splenic vein thrombosis and ascites are negative predictors of recanalization.

Sinusoidal obstruction syndrome/venoocclusive disease of the liver

This clinical entity is akin Budd–Chiari syndrome except for two major characteristics: (a) the widely patent hepatic veins and inferior vena cava; and (b) the clinical setting [4,17]. In developing countries, the disease can occur as an epidemic of liver disease due to contamination of grains and flour with a pyrrolizidine alkaloid-containing plant. In developed countries, the disease occurs following exposure to cytotoxic or immune suppressive agents, particularly for hematopoietic stem cell transplantation. Severity varies from patient to patient, ranging from silent forms to fulminant hepatic failure. In the context of hematopietic stem cell transplantation, diagnosis is based on weight gain with or without ascites, right upper quadrant pain of liver origin, hepatomegaly and jaundice, occurring within the first 100 days after tranplantation; and exclusion of differential diagnoses such as hepatic graft-versus-host disease, drug-induced cholestasis and sepsis [4,6,17].

Some patients completely recover while others develop lethal forms, usually in association with multiorgan failure. A poor prognosis is correlated with high serum aminotranferase levels, high hepatic venous pressure gradient, portal vein thrombosis, renal insufficiency and decreased oxygen saturation. Nodular regenerative changes or perisinusoidal fibrosis mostly in centrilobular areas can be found long after haematopoietic stem cell transplantation in patients with or without a clinically evident sinusoidal obstruction syndrome. They are regarded as a sequelae of previous endothelial lesions [4,16,17].

At present a specific therapy targeting sinusoidal endothelium damage is lacking. Although defibrotide is widely used because of an excellent tolerance, the evidence for its beneficial effect is mostly based on a comparison with historical controls. Prevention consists of reduced intensity conditioning for hematopoietic stem cell transplantation [4].

Budd–Chiari syndrome

Presentation varies considerably from patient to patient, from a fulminant course to a chronic, almost asymptomatic condition [4,6,7]. This variability is explained by the variable speed and extent of the thrombotic process. Furthermore, the three major hepatic veins are not necessarily involved in a synchronous manner.

Increased sinusoidal and portal pressure upstream from the obstruction and reduced portal perfusion constitute the major mechanisms for the manifestations of Budd–Chiari syndrome. Acute abdominal pain and fever may be present initially, reflecting acute thrombosis. Ascites is very common, often difficult to treat due to functional renal dysfunction and hyponatremia. A high protein content of ascitic fluid is suggestive but is not a constant finding. Gastrointestinal bleeding and encephalopathy may be observed. Encephalopathy may herald fulminant hepatic failure or be a manifestation of decompensated chronic liver disease. Liver and spleen are generally enlarged. The liver is often markedly dysmorphic, particularly due to a striking increase in the caudate lobe together with atrophy of other sectors.

Laboratory tests also show variable anomalies from patients to patients: most have normal or slightly increased serum aminotransferases, but some have marked, although transient, elevations. Serum bilirubin, serum albumin and prothrombin are generally moderately altered but may be normal or, on the contrary, severely abnormal.

Abdominal imaging may show the thrombosed hepatic veins or terminal inferior vena cava in the form of fibrous cords or membranous occlusion with upstream dilatation,or solid material obstructing the lumen. In many patients the hepatic veins are just not visible, in which case the demonstration of hepatic vein collaterals developing intra- and or extra-hepatically is of considerable diagnostic value [4,6,7].

Diagnosis is based on the demonstration of hepatic vein or IVC obstruction. Doppler-ultrasound by an experienced operator, aware of the clinical suspicion, is the key to diagnosis. Triphasic CT scan and MRI after intravenous injection of contrast medium are valuable in confirming ultrasonographic findings. Liver biopsy is generally not needed, except when hepatic veins and IVC are clearly patent, which may occur in the rare patients with obstruction limited to small hepatic veins. Highly suggestive but non specific features at liver biopsy consist of congestion in the central area of the lobule, with or without liver cell loss and perisinusoidal fibrosis. Extensive fibrosis, typically centro-central, but also porto-central, or even cirrhosis may be present. Similar histopathological findings are found in patients with heart failure or constrictive pericarditis but the latter conditions are characteristically associated with dilated hepatic veins and inferior vena cava [4,6,7].

The course of the disease is variable according to patients. Some patients, after an abrupt onset, have spontaneous resolution of the manifestations, whereas some others may experience progressive deterioration even in the absence of a severe clinical presentation. Recurrence and aggravation is the rule in the absence of treatment. It has been estimated that, in untreated patients, 3-year mortality is about 90%. The main causes of death are refractory ascites with emaciation, liver failure, gastrointestinal bleeding related to portal hypertension, and often a combination of these complications. Main prognostic factors are the components of Child–Pugh score [4,6,7].

The principles for therapy are presented in the didactic protocol. Patients are best referred to specialized centers [4,6,7]. The implementation of current treatment algorithms in such centers has allowed 5-year survival rates of 80–90%. Patients are generally free from any liver-related symptoms, with a good quality of life. Long-term complications mainly consist of hepatocellular carcinoma (particularly in patients with long standing obstruction of the inferior vena cava), and complications of underlying diseases (e.g. myeloproliferative disease, paroxysmal nocturnal hemoglobinuria, Behçet's disease).

References

1. Huang YK, Hsieh HC, Tsai FC, *et al.* Visceral artery aneurysm: Risk factor analysis and therapeutic opinion. *Eur J Vasc Endovasc Surg.* 2007;33:293–301.
2. Deltenre P, Valla DC. Ischemic cholangiopathy. *J Hepatol.* 2006;44:806–817.
3. Vauthey JN, Tomczak RJ, Helmberger T, *et al.* The arterioportal fistula syndrome: Clinicopathologic features, diagnosis, and therapy. *Gastroenterology.* 1997;113:1390–1401.
4. DeLeve LD, Valla DC, Garcia-Tsao G. Vascular disorders of the liver. *Hepatology.* 2009;49:1729–1764.
5. Khalid SK, Garcia-Tsao G. Hepatic vascular malformations in hereditary hemorrhagic telangiectasia. *Semin Liver Dis.* 2008;28:247–258.
6. Valla DC. Budd–Chiari syndrome and veno-occlusive disease/sinusoidal obstruction syndrome. *Gut.* 2008;57:1469–1478.
7. Valla DC. Primary Budd–Chiari syndrome. *J Hepatol.* 2009; 50:195–203.
8. Condat B, Pessione F, Helene Denninger M, *et al.* Recent portal or mesenteric venous thrombosis: increased recognition and frequent recanalization on anticoagulant therapy. *Hepatology.* 2000;32:466–470.
9. Garcia-Pagan JC, Hernandez-Guerra M, Bosch J. Extrahepatic portal vein thrombosis. *Semin Liver Dis.* 2008;28:282–292.
10. Witters P, Maleux G, George C, *et al.* Congenital veno-venous malformations of the liver: widely variable clinical presentations. *J Gastroenterol Hepatol.* 2008;23:e390–394.
11. Stringer MD. The clinical anatomy of congenital portosystemic venous shunts. *Clin Anat.* 2008;21:147–157.
12. Sfyroeras GS, Antoniou GA, Drakou AA, *et al.* Visceral venous aneurysms: Clinical presentation, natural history and their management: A systematic review. *Eur J Vasc Endovasc Surg.* 2009;
13. Chawla Y, Dhiman RK. Intrahepatic portal venopathy and related disorders of the liver. *Semin Liver Dis.* 2008;28:270–281.
14. Hillaire S, Bonte E, Denninger MH, *et al.* Idiopathic non-cirrhotic intrahepatic portal hypertension in the West: A re-evaluation in 28 patients. *Gut.* 2002;51:275–280.
15. Yonem O, Bayraktar Y. Is portal vein cavernous transformation a component of congenital hepatic fibrosis? *World J Gastroenterol.* 2007;13:1928–1929.
16. DeLeve LD. Hepatic microvasculature in liver injury. *Semin Liver Dis.* 2007;27:390–400.

Liver Disease

17. DeLeve LD, Shulman HM, McDonald GB. Toxic injury to hepatic sinusoids: Sinusoidal obstruction syndrome (veno-occlusive disease). *Semin Liver Dis.* 2002;22:27–42.

18. Tsokos M, Erbersdobler A. Pathology of peliosis. *Forensic Sci Int.* 2005;149:25–33.

19. Kakar S, Kamath PS, Burgart LJ. Sinusoidal dilatation and congestion in liver biopsy: Is it always due to venous outflow impairment? *Arch Pathol Lab Med.* 2004;128:901–904.

20. Geubel AP, De Galocsy C, Alves N, *et al.* Liver damage caused by therapeutic vitamin A administration: estimate of dose-related toxicity in 41 cases. *Gastroenterology.* 1991;100: 1701–1709.

21. Condat B, Vilgrain V, Asselah T, *et al.* Portal cavernoma-associated cholangiopathy: A clinical and MR cholangiography coupled with MR portography imaging study. *Hepatology.* 2003;37:1302–1308.

22. Primignani M, Mannucci PM. The role of thrombophilia in splanchnic vein thrombosis. *Semin Liver Dis.* 2008;28:293–301.

Liver Disease

CHAPTER 106
Granulomas of the liver

Miquel Bruguera Cortada and Rosa Miquel Morera
Hospital Clinic and University of Barcelona, Barcelona, Spain

ESSENTIAL FACTS ABOUT CAUSATION

- Infectious agents: Bacteria, fungi, parasites, rikettsiae, viruses
- Chemical agents: Therapeutic drugs, talc, silica, beryllium
- Liver diseases: Primary biliary cirrhosis, chronic hepatitis C
- Systemic diseases: Sarcoidosis, vasculitis, Crohn disease
- Neoplastic diseases: Hodgkin disease

TREATMENT OF HEPATIC GRANULOMAS

- There is no common treatment for all hepatic granulomas
- Therapy should be addressed to treat the disease responsible for granuloma formation
- Drug-induced granulomas resolve spontaneously upon withdrawal of the offending drug
- Disappearance of hepatic granulomas with specific etiologic treatment is followed by normalization of liver test abnormalities

ESSENTIAL FACTS ABOUT DIAGNOSIS

- Direct visualization of the cause
  - Ova of *Schistosoma*
  - Parasites
  - *Leishmania*
- Identification of the infectious agent by special stains or molecular techniques
  - Ziehl–Neelsen stain: *Mycobacteria*
  - PAS, argentic impregnation: Fungal infections, candida
  - PAS: *Tropheryma whipplei* (Whipple disease)
  - Warthin–Starry: *Bartonella henselae* (cat-scratch disease)
  - Giemsa: *Leishmania*
  - Polymerase chain reaction: different microbes
- Cause is not directly seen but morphological clues are present
  - Portal/periportal coalescent granulomas in different stage of development, hyalinization, calcification, Schaumann or asteroid bodies: Sarcoidosis
  - Necrosis: Infection
  - Caseous necrosis: Tuberculosis
  - Large necrotic granulomas with peripheral histiocyte palisading and Charcot-Leiden crystals: *Fasciola hepatica*, parasites
  - Granuloma around the bile duct or bile duct destruction: PBC
  - Granuloma around vascular structures: Vasculitis (PAN)
  - Fibrin-ring granuloma: Q fever, Hodgkin lymphoma, EBV, CMV, HAV, toxoplasmosis, leishmaniosis, allopurinol
  - Presence of eosinophils: Drug reaction, parasites
  - Suppurative inflammation: cat-scratch disease, yersiniosis, tularemia, melioidosis
  - Reed–Sternberg cells and atypical cells: Hodgkin lymphoma and hematologic neoplasias
- Cause is not evident but clinical history may help to conclude the diagnosis
  - Cholestasis and AMA positive autoantibodies: PBC
  - Drug history: Drug reaction
  - Occupation: Beriliosis
  - Systemic diseases: Sarcoidosis, Crohn disease

Definition

A granuloma is a focal accumulation of activated macrophages, which can be associated with variable degree of other inflammatory cells such as lymphocytes, eosinophils, or plasma cells. The causes of hepatic granulomas are numerous (Table 106.1). Identifying an etiology is often difficult, remaining idiopathic in as much as 15–20% of cases.

Epidemiology

Granulomas are found in 2–10% of liver biopsies in large series. The frequency of detection depends on the population studied, the prevalence of causes of granuloma in different geographic areas and the frequency of the use of liver biopsy in the evaluation of febrile disorders of uncertain cause. Tuberculosis and sarcoidosis have been reported as the commonest causes; however, in recent large series including the authors' experience (data not published) the leading cause is primary biliary cirrhosis (PBC) (Table 106.2).

Pathogenesis

Granulomas are the result of a cell-mediated immune reaction by the hepatic mononuclear phagocytic system to a foreign substance or antigen. The process of transformation of macrophages to epithelioid cells depends of the secretion of gamma-interferon and tumor necrosis factor beta (TNF-β) by activated T-helper lymphocytes responding to the presence of a persistently retained antigen.

Liver Disease

Textbook of Clinical Gastroenterology and Hepatology, Second Edition. Edited by C. J. Hawkey, Jaime Bosch, Joel E. Richter, Guadalupe Garcia-Tsao, Francis K. L. Chan.
© 2012 Blackwell Publishing Ltd. Published 2012 by Blackwell Publishing Ltd.

Table 106.1 Causes of hepatic granulomas

INFECTIONS
  Bacterial
    Tuberculosis
    Atypical mycobacteria (especially in AIDS)
    Leprosy
    Brucellosis
    (Salmonellosis, tularemia, melioidosis, listeriosis, yersiniosis, Whipple disease, cat-scratch disease)
  Mycotic
    Histoplasmosis
    Coccidioidomycosis
    (Blastomycosis, candidiasis, cryptococcosis, actinomycosis, toxoplasmosis, aspergillosis, nocardiosis)
  Parasitic
    Schistosomiasis
    Toxocariasis
    (Ascaridiasis, fascioliasis, tongueworm)
  Rickettsial
    Q fever
    Boutonneuse fever
  Spirochetal
    Secondary syphilis
  Viral
    (CMV infection, EBV)

CHEMICALS
  Therapeutic drugs
  Beryllium
  Silica
  Talc

LIVER DISEASES
  Autoimmune-based diseases (primary biliary cirrhosis, primary sclerosing cholangitis, overlap syndromes)
  Fatty liver
  Viral hepatitis (chronic hepatitis C and B, hepatitis A)
  Primary liver tumors (hepatocellular adenoma and hepatocellular carcinoma)

SYSTEMIC AND NEOPLASTIC DISEASES
  Sarcoidosis
  Crohn disease
  Wegener granulomatosis
  Temporal arteritis
  Panarteritis nodosa
  Hypogammaglobulinemia
  Polymialgia rheumatica
  Hodgkin disease
  Non-Hodgkin lymphomas

Clinical presentation

Most patients present with manifestations of the causative disorder such as fever, malaise, weight loss and anorexia. The presence of granulomas in the liver may be suspected by liver enlargement and raised serum alkaline phosphatase activity. Pain in right upper quadrant can be seen in some cases. Granulomas are often an unexpected finding in a liver biopsy carried out for asymptomatic abnormalities of liver tests. Imaging studies may show no abnormalities, or there may be a diffuse non-homogeneous appearance. If there is coalescence of many granulomas CT scan or ultrasound imaging may detect focal lesions. Calcifications can be seen on plain radiography.

Pathology

Granulomas may be found in portal tracts, the lobular parenchyma or in both sites. The term granuloma is frequently used as a synonymous of epithelioid granuloma, and its presence usually reflects a pathologic condition. Thus, the presence of granulomas should always be reported and mandates investigation for a causative process. In contrast, the presence in the sinusoids of small macrophagic aggregates also called microgranulomas is thought to represent a non-specific clean-up reaction to hepatocellular injury. When granulomas are present in a background of hepatocellular necrosis the term granulomatous hepatitis should be used and it is usually of an infectious nature. A granulomatous reaction refers to a poorly formed loose aggregates of histiocytes usually associated with other inflammatory cell types such as lymphocytes, monocytes or neutrophils. Portal granulomatoid reaction might be associated with hematopoietic malignancies such as Hodgkin lymphoma.

Histologically, granulomas can be classified according to the cell type and morphology.

Epithelioid granulomas

Epithelioid granulomas are composed by activated macrophages with a large eosinophilic cytoplasm. The nuclei are oval and may be folded. Multinucleated giant cells may be present and are formed by the fusion of the membranes of epithelioid cells and may contain 20 or more nuclei either arranged in compact clusters (foreign-body type) or along the periphery of the cell (Langhans type) (Figure 106.1). The foreign material or the infectious agent may be present within the granuloma but often is not identifiable. Necrosis of the granulomas is not uncommon frequently associated with bacterial or fungal infections. In large granulomas, the epithelioid cells usually are arranged in palisade around the necrosis. Coalescence, collagen deposition, hyalinization and calcification may be seen in late stages of granuloma formation typically in sarcoidosis.

Lipogranulomas

Lipogranulomas are a collection of lymphocytes and macrophages around extracellular fat as the result of focal necrosis of fatty hepatocytes. Mineral oil granulomas are similar reactions to ingested oil, which is present in the form of multiple vacuoles within macrophages. They are commonly located near the terminal venules.

Fibrin-ring granulomas

Fibrin-ring granulomas have a central fat vacuole delimited by a rim of fibrin and surrounded with macrophages and other inflammatory cells (Figure 106.2).

Table 106.2 Summary of major etiologic causes of liver granulomas in different published series

First author	Country	Period of time	Liver biopsies with granulomas		Idiopathic cause		Tuberculosis		Sarcoidosis		Hepatitis C virus		Primary biliary cirrhosis		Drugs		Other infections		Other	
			n	%	n	%	n	%	n	%	n	%	n	%	n	%	n	%	n	%
Vilaseca et al., 1979 [1]	Spain	1971–1977	107	—	8	7.4	30	28	19	17.7	—	—	0	0	0		—	—		
Cunningham et al., 1982 [2]	UK	1970–1979	77	—	6	7.8	9	11.7	9	11.7	—	—	1	1.3			5	6.5	47	61
Anderson et al., 1988 [3]	Australia	1968–1984	59	—	17	29	4	6.7	7	11.8	—	—	*		4	6.7	7	11.8	20	33.8
Sartin and Walker, 1991 [4]	USA	1976–1985	88	—	44	50	3	3.4	19	21.6	—	—	4	4.5	5	5.7	5	5.7	8	9.1
McCluggage and Sloan, 1994 [5]	Ireland	1980–1992	163	4	18	11	3	1.8	30	18.4	—	—	90	55.2	2	1.2	1	0.6	19	11.8
Gaya et al., 2003 [6]	UK	1991–2001	63/1662	4.2	7	11.1	3	4.8	7	11.1	6	9.5	15	23.8	5	7.9	0	—	19	30.1
Dourakis et al., 2007 [7]	Greece	1999–2004	66/1768	3.7	4	6.1	1	1.5	5	7.6	3	4.6	41	62.1	2	3	2	3	8	12.1
Drebber et al., 2008 [8]	Germany	1996–2004	442/12161	3.6	158	36	3	0.7	37	8.4	2	0.5	215	48.6	11	2.5	13	2.9	3	0.7
Onal et al., 2008 [9]	Turkey	2003–2006	13/592	2.2	1	7.7	2	15.4	2	15.4	(2**)	(15.4)	3	23.1	0	—	—	—	5	38.4
Sanai et al., 2008 [10]	Saudi Arabia	1993–2005	66/5531	1.2	9	14.8	29	47.5	3	4.9	9 (+2***)	14.8 (18)	0	—	1	1.6	6	9.8	4	4.8
Bruguera et al., data not published	Spain	1999–2009	151	—	36	24	7	5	7	5	20	13	53	35	0		11	7	17	11

PBC cases were specifically excluded of the study.
** One patient had sarcoidosis and HVC +, and other Hodgkin's lymphoma and HCV+.
***Two cases with Tbc had also HCV.

References:

1. Vilaseca J, Guardia J, Cuxart A, et al. [Granulomatous hepatitis. Etiologic study.] Med Clin (Barc) 1979;72:272–275.
2. Cunningham D, Mills PR, Quigley EMM, et al. Hepatic granulomas: experience over a 10-year period in the West of Scotland. Q J Med. 1982;51:162–170.
3. Anderson CS, Nicholls J, Rowland R, Labrooy JT. Hepatic granulomas: a 15-year experience in the Royal Adelaide Hospital. Med J Aust. 1988;148:71–74.
4. Sartin JS, Walker RC. Granulomatous hepatitis: a retrospective review of 88 cases at the Mayo Clinic. Mayo Clin Proc. 1991;66:914–918.
5. McCluggage W, Sloan J. Hepatic granulomas in Northern Ireland: a thirteen year review. Histopathology. 1994;25:219–228.
6. Gaya DR, Thorburn D, Oien KA, et al. Hepatic granulomas: a 10-year single centre experience. J Clin Pathol. 2003;56:850–853.
7. Dourakis SP, Saramadou R, Alexopoulou A, et al. Hepatic granulomas: a 6-year experience in a single center in Greece. Eur J Gastroenterol Hepatol. 2007;19:101–104.
8. Drebber U, Kasper HU, Ratering J, et al. Hepatic granulomas: histological and molecular pathological approach to differential diagnosis—a study of 442 cases. Liver Int. 2008;28:828–834.
9. Onal IK, Ersoy O, Aydinli M, Harmanci O, Sokmensuer C, Bayraktar Y. Hepatic granuloma in Turkish adults: A report of 13 cases. Eur J Int Med. 2008;19:527–530.
10. Sanai FM, Ashraf S, Abdo AA, et al. Hepatic granuloma: decreasing trend in a high-incidence area. Liver Int. 2008;28:1402–1407.

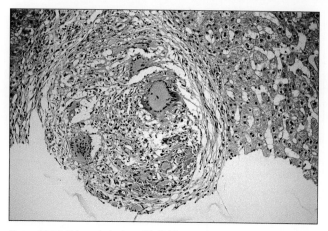

Figure 106.1 Tuberculosis. An epithelioid granuloma with a multinucleated cell (Langhan's type). Hematoxylin–eosin (HE) stain, ×210.

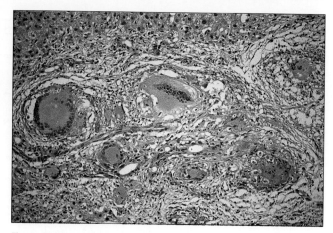

Figure 106.3 Sarcoidosis. Confluent granulomas containing giant multinucleated cells. HE stain, ×2103.

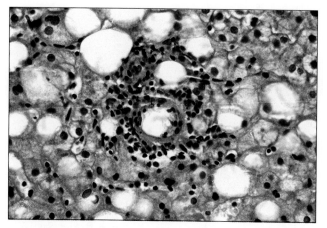

Figure 106.2 Q fever. A central clear space surrounded by macrophages, lymphocytes, and neutrophils also contains a peripheral fibrosis ring. HE stain, ×415.

Causes

Sarcoidosis

Sarcoidosis is a systemic granulomatous disease of unknown etiology that involves several organs and is characterized clinically by fever, pulmonary infiltrates, lymphadenopathy and uveitis. There are no specific diagnostic tests. Non-caseating epithelioid granulomas with multinucleated giant cells are present in affected organs, usually in high number (Figure 106.3). In the liver they may be located anywhere within the lobules, but they are more numerous in the portal tracts and the periportal zones. They may be in different phase of development, with early-formed lesions adjacent to older hyalinised granulomas. Hepatomegaly is found in 20–50% of the patients. Laboratory examination reveals mild-to-moderate elevation of serum alkaline phosphatase activity. Serum aminotransferases are normal or only slightly elevated. Serum angiotensin converting enzyme levels are increased in 50–80% of patients. The liver is frequently involved by sarcoidosis and the presence of granulomas has been reported in nearly all patients. Thus,

needle liver biopsy is the recommended procedure to confirm a presumptive diagnosis of sarcoidosis.

The course of hepatic involvement is usually asymptomatic and it is not affected by treatment with corticosteroids. In a few patients hepatic disease presents as chronic cholestasis or as portal hypertension. Cholestasis may be intra or extrahepatic. Intrahepatic cholestasis is due to the progressive destruction of the interlobular bile ducts by granulomas. These changes may be confused with those of PBC, but sarcoidosis is not associated with anti-mitochondrial antibodies. Extrahepatic cholestasis may be caused by involvement of the large bile ducts or by compression by enlarged lymph nodes in the hilar region. The syndrome of intrahepatic cholestasis associated with sarcoidosis presents with jaundice, pruritus and fever. Most cases have been described in young African–American men. The course of the syndrome is protracted, lasting several decades despite treatment with ursodeoxycholic acid or corticosteroids, before reaching an end-stage liver disease. Liver transplantation has been performed for patients with advanced liver disease. Portal hypertension may develop as a consequence of granulomatous destruction and obliteration of portal vein branches of portal tracts. It seems to be an uncommon manifestation of sarcoidosis. It may be the cause of gastrointestinal hemorrhages.

Mycobacteriosis

Granulomas may develop in tuberculosis infection, atypical mycobacteriosis, after BCG treatment and in leprosy. Hepatic granulomas are found in more than 90% of patients with disseminated tuberculosis, but only in 25% of patients with tuberculosis confined to the lung. Diagnosis of tuberculosis is easy when caseous necrosis is found, particularly if the Ziehl–Neelsen stain reveals acid-fast bacilli. Bacilli are rarely found in patients with only lung involvement, but vey often in patients with disseminated disease. Polymerase chain reaction (PCR) has high sensitivity and specificity to detect *Mycobacterium tuberculosis* DNA in tissue, and should be done when tuberculosis is suspected and tissue stain is negative.

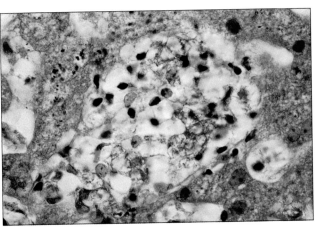

Figure 106.4 Leprosy. Aggregates of foamy histiocytes that contain acid–alcohol bacilli. Ziehl–Neelsen stain, ×415.

Table 106.3 Therapeutic drugs associated with hepatic granulomas

- Allopurinol
- Amoxicillin–clavulanic acid
- Carbamazepine
- Diltiazem
- Hydralazine
- Mebendazole
- Methyldopa
- Nitrofurantoine
- Phenylbutazone
- Phenytoin
- Procainamide
- Procainamide
- Quinidine
- Sulfonamides
- Tocainide

Atypical mycobacteria might be observed in AIDS and in immunosupressed patients. Liver involvement by this agent is seen as clusters of large macrophages with granular cytoplasm containing numerous bacilli, rather than as well-formed granulomas.

Hepatic granulomas are common in patients who have lepromatous leprosy (up to 75%) but much less frequently in patients who have tuberculoid leprosy. Lepromatous granulomas are composed of histiocytes with clear-to-foamy cytoplasm, containing a high number of acid-fast bacilli (*Mycobacterium leprae*) (Figure 106.4). The tuberculoid type of granulomas is composed of epithelioid cells and rarely contains bacilli.

Q fever

Infection with *Coxiella burnetti* may present as a febrile disease with severe headache and pneumonia or as a febrile hepatitis. Diagnosis is based on serology. The histological key is the presence of fibrin-ring granulomas.

Malignant tumors

Any tumor may incite the development of granulomas. This is especially frequent in certain hematologic neoplasms. In Hodgkin disease, granulomas are usually epithelioid and seen in both portal tracts and lobules. There is some evidence that patients with granulomas in the liver have a better prognosis than those without. They are likely a response to a tumor antigen.

Drug-induced granulomas

They can be associated with a number of drugs (Table 106.3). Granulomas may be found within portal tracts and in the parenchyma. Upon withdrawal a causative drug they quickly resolve without fibrosis. In the absence of any test permitting the diagnosis of a drug etiology, a reaction to a drug can only be suspected when epithelioid granulomas contain eosinophils.

Liver diseases

Granulomas are found in approximately 25% of patients with PBC, typically in portal tracts, surrounding damaged bile ducts, particularly in early stages of the disease. Epithelioid granulomas have been seen in some patients with chronic hepatitis C virus (HCV) treated and not treated with interferon. Those that developed in treated patients are probably related to interferon-induced sarcoidosis. Granulomas have also been described in the setting of post-transplant HCV infection in up to 8% of patients and have been related to a granulomatous type of response to the virus. They do not seem to be associated to a worse prognosis.

Diagnosis and differential diagnosis

The diagnostic approach to hepatic granulomas requires a systematic histological evaluation of the granulomas themselves, of their topographic location and of any associated changes in the surrounding liver tissue. Examination of multiple sections of liver biopsies increases the diagnostic yield. Special stains should be done when the HE-stained section does not provide any clue for the diagnosis, i.e. Ziehl–Neelsen for acid-fast bacilli and silver impregnation satin for fungi.

Evaluation of a patient in whom hepatic granulomas are found must include information on occupation, travels, residence in foreign countries, and exposure to therapeutic drugs or industrial agents. The pathologist should attempt a systematic microscopic examination of the specimen containing the granulomas.

Firstly, an etiologic agent should be searched for within the granuloma, such as ova of *Schistosoma* (Figure 106.5). Special stains will help in the identification of some infectious agents (i.e. mycobacteria, fungi or cat-scratch disease). The foreign body granulomas may contain inclusions of particulate material, such as talc, silicone, starch, which might be found in the examination with polarizing microscopy.

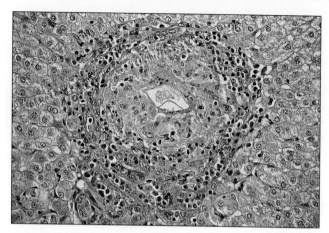

Figure 106.5 Schistosomiasis. An epithelioid granuloma with remains of an ova of *Schistosoma*. HE stain, ×210.

Secondly, in many cases the pathologist cannot give a definitive diagnosis, but may suggest several possible causes based on the location of the granuloma or on some other morphological features:

- Coalescence of granulomas, absence of necrosis, partial hyaline fibrosis and their location in portal and periportal areas suggest sarcoidosis
- Portal tract granulomas surrounding a damaged bile duct suggest PBC
- Schaumann bodies (basophil structures with concentric proteinaceous calcified laminations) and asteroid bodies (star-like radiating structures within a clear space) are found in approximately half of the sarcoid granulomas, and very infrequently in granulomas of other etiologies
- Necrotizing granulomas suggest tuberculosis and fungal infections
- Central purulent necrosis with presence of leucocytes suggests *Yersinia* infection, cat-scratch disease, tularemia, listeriosis or melioidosis
- A relatively high number of eosinophils among the cellular population of the granuloma suggest a drug reaction or a parasitic disease
- The most common cause of fibrin-ring granulomas is Q fever, but they have been reported in rare instances associ-

ated to allopurinol treatment, leishmaniasis, mononucleosis, hepatitis A, CMV infection or Hodgkin lymphoma
- The presence of granuloma in the vicinity of an artery in a portal tract suggests a granulomatous arteritis, either drug-induced or associated with a systemic vasculitis

Lastly, when a clinical diagnosis of granulomatous disease such as PBC, sarcoidosis or vasculitis has been done based on clinical features, the etiology of granulomas found in the liver may be firmly suspected, even if there is not any histological characteristic specific for this diagnosis.

Further reading

Alcantara-Payawal DE, Matsumura M, Shiratori Y, *et al*. Direct detection of Mycobacterium tuberculosis using polymerase chain reaction assay among patients with hepatic granuloma. *J Hepatol*. 1997;27:620–627.

Denk H, Scheuer PJ, Baptista A, *et al*. Guidelines for the diagnosis and interpretation of hepatic granulomas. *Histopathology*. 1994;25:209–218.

Ebert EC, Kierson M, Hagspiel KD. Gastrointestinal and hepatic manifestations of sarcoidosis. *Am J Gastroenterol*. 2008;103:3184–3192.

Ferrell LD. Hepatic granulomas: a morphologic approach to diagnosis. *Surg Pathol*. 1990;3:87–106.

Harada K, Minato H, Hiramatsu K, Nakanuma Y. Epithelioid cell granulomas in chronic hepatitis C: immunohistochemical character and histological marker of favourable response to interferon-a therapy. *Histopathology*. 1998;33:216–221.

Ishak KG. Sarcoidosis of the liver and bile ducts. *Mayo Clin Proc*. 1998;73: 467–472.

Lamps LW. Hepatic granulomas, with an emphasis on infectious causes. *Adv Anat Pathol*. 2008;15:309–318.

Lefkowitch JH. Hepatic granulomas. *J Hepatol*. 1999;30:40–45.

Mueller S, Boehme MW, Hofmann WJ *et al*. Extrapulmonary sarcoidosis primarily diagnosed in the liver. *Scand J Gastroenterol*. 2000;35:1003–1008.

Ryan BM, McDonald GS, Pilkington R. The development of hepatic granulomas following interferon-a2b therapy for chronic hepatitis C infection. *Eur J Gastroenterol Hepatol*. 1998;10:349–351.

Valla DC, Benhamou JP. Hepatic granulomas and hepatic sarcoidosis. *Clin Liver Dis*. 2000;4:269–285.

Vakiani E, Hunt KH, Mazziotta RM, *et al*. Hepatitis-C associated granulomas after liver transplantation. Morphological spectrum and clinical implications. *Am J Clin Pathol*. 2007;127:128–134.

CHAPTER 107

Liver diseases and pregnancy

J. Eileen Hay

Mayo Clinic, Rochester, MN, USA

ESSENTIALS OF PATHOGENESIS

Causes of cholestasis in pregnancy
- Coincidental liver diseases
  - Gallstones
  - Viral hepatitis
  - Drugs
  - Sepsis
- Chronic liver disease
  - Primary sclerosing cholangitis
  - Primary biliary cirrhosis
- Liver diseases unique to pregnancy
  - Intrahepatic cholestasis of pregnancy

Causes of acute liver failure in the third trimester
- Acute fatty liver of pregnancy
- HELLP syndrome
- Fulminant viral hepatitis
- Thrombotic thrombocytopenic purpura (rare)
- Hemolytic uremic syndrome (rare)

ESSENTIALS OF DIAGNOSIS

- Are there features of chronic liver disease?
- Is presentation compatible with acute viral hepatitis?
- Any features of biliary disease?
- Any history of drugs or toxins?
- Are there features of Budd–Chiari Syndrome?
- Any evidence for sepsis?
- Is this one of the liver diseases unique to pregnancy?

ESSENTIALS OF TREATMENT

- Ursodeoxycholic acid is the most effective maternal therapy for intrahepatic cholestasis of pregnancy
- Referral for high-risk obstetric care and fetal monitoring is essential in ICP
- Immediate delivery of the baby is mandatory in acute fatty liver of pregnancy and severe HELLP syndrome
- Hyperemesis gravidarum is managed symptomatically and by fluid and caloric support.

Introduction

Most pregnant women are young and healthy during pregnancy but pathophysiologic changes may occur, including five unique liver diseases seen only during or after pregnancy [1]. Hyperemesis gravidarum (HG) is intractable nausea and vomiting in the first trimester; intrahepatic cholestasis of pregnancy (ICP) is pruritus and liver dysfunction in second half of pregnancy. Severe pre-eclampsia may cause hepatic dysfunction; some cases are complicated further by hemolysis (H), elevated liver tests (EL) and low platelets (LP), the HELLP syndrome. In acute fatty liver of pregnancy (AFLP), microvesicular fatty infiltration of hepatocytes in the third trimester results in acute liver failure. Any liver disease may occur coincidentally during pregnancy and often resolves with few effects on the pregnancy. Similarly, patients with early, well compensated chronic liver disease may have successful pregnancies.

Causes and incidence of liver diseases in pregnancy

Hepatic dysfunction occurs in 3–5% of pregnant women and the causes fall into three main categories (Figure 107.1): (1) liver diseases unique to pregnancy, (2) liver diseases occurring coincidentally in the pregnant patient, and (3) pre-existing chronic liver diseases. Most cases are due to liver diseases unique to pregnancy [2] and these pregnancy-associated liver diseases all have characteristic timing in relation to the pregnancy (Figure 107.2). Severe pre-eclampsia is the commonest cause of liver dysfunction in pregnancy (1–2% all deliveries); 2–12% cases of severe pre-eclampsia (0.1–0.6% all deliveries), are complicated further by the HELLP syndrome [3]. ICP occurs worldwide with striking geographical variations; in the USA, it occurs in 0.1% pregnancies with jaundice in 20% of cases and is the second most common cause of jaundice in pregnancy after viral hepatitis. Hyperemesis gravidarum occurs in 0.3–2.0% of pregnancies. Acute fatty liver of pregnancy (AFLP) is the least common of the pregnancy-associated liver diseases (0.005% pregnancies).

Liver Disease

Textbook of Clinical Gastroenterology and Hepatology, Second Edition. Edited by C. J. Hawkey, Jaime Bosch, Joel E. Richter, Guadalupe Garcia-Tsao, Francis K. L. Chan.

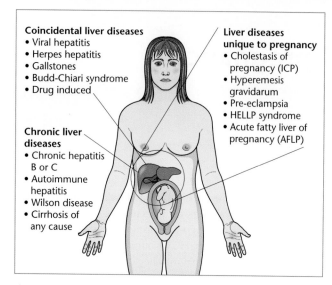

Figure 107.1 Causes of liver disease during pregnancy. (This figure was published in *Clinical Gastroenterology and Hepatology*, Wilfred M. Weinstein, Christopher J. Hawkey, Jaime Bosch, Liver diseases and pregnancy, Pages 1–6, Copyright Elsevier, 2005.)

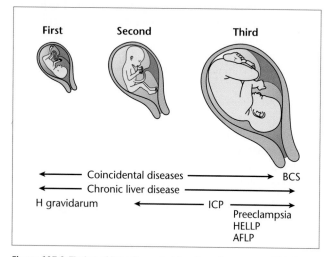

Figure 107.2 Timing of liver disease in trimesters of pregnancy. (This figure was published in *Clinical Gastroenterology and Hepatology*, Wilfred M. Weinstein, Christopher J. Hawkey, Jaime Bosch, Liver diseases and pregnancy, Pages 1–6, Copyright Elsevier, 2005.)

Viral hepatitis has the same incidence and clinical features in the pregnant and non-pregnant population and is commonest cause of jaundice in pregnancy [4]. The hepatitis viruses and pregnancy have little/no effect on one another. Prevention of perinatal transmission of hepatitis B is very important with prophylactic therapy to the baby at birth and consideration of antiviral therapy to mothers with very high viral loads during the third trimester [5]. Herpes simplex hepatitis is a rare but treatable cause of fulminant hepatitis in the third trimester (Figure 107.3a). Although gallstones are common especially in multiparous patients, symptomatic cholelithiasis is infrequent – usually biliary colic, less commonly pancreatitis or cholecystitis. Budd–Chiari syndrome is rare, often in the postpartum period and associated with antiphospholipid syndrome,

thrombotic thrombocytopenic purpura (TTP), pre-eclampsia and septic abortion. Sepsis associated with pyelonephritis or abortion may cause jaundice in early pregnancy.

Chronic hepatitis B is present in 0.5–1.5% pregnancies and chronic hepatitis C in 2.3% of some indigent populations. An uncomplicated pregnancy with no disease flare is expected in mild disease. Patients with treated autoimmune or Wilson disease may have successful pregnancies, but must be adequately managed before and during pregnancy. Most patients with advanced cirrhosis and/or portal hypertension are infertile but if pregnancy occurs, increased maternal complications occur including variceal hemorrhage (20–25%), hepatic failure, encephalopathy and rupture of splenic artery aneurysms.

Etiology of pregnancy-associated liver diseases

The etiologies of the pregnancy-associated liver diseases remain obscure, with overlap among pre-eclampsia, HELLP and AFLP; HG and ICP are not associated with pre-eclampsia. Hyperemesis gravidarum is an enigmatic, multifactorial neurohormonal disorder of pregnancy in which hormonal (elevated estrogen and chorionic gonadotrophin, transient hyperthyroidism) and immunologic abnormalities are found [6].

Current evidence suggests that the etiology of ICP is multifactorial [7]. An exogenous influence is suggested by the seasonal and geographical variability, the potential role of dietary factors (selenium deficiency), the proven role of exogenous progesterone therapy, and the recurrence rate of only 45–70% in multiparous patients. The pathogenesis is clearly related to female sex hormones, perhaps involving a genetically abnormal or exaggerated hepatic metabolic response to the physiologic increase in estrogens during pregnancy [8]: impaired sulfation of progesterone is seen in some patients. The familial cases and ethnic clustering strongly suggests a genetic predisposition to ICP. Mothers with ICP have been identified who are heterozygous, with homozygous babies, for genetic abnormalities in canalicular transport proteins, the same abnormalities being responsible for the rare group of diseases known as the progressive familial intrahepatic cholestasis (PFIC) syndromes [7,9]; genetic variation at ABCC2 and MDR3 have also been described [10]. Genetic factors may determine susceptibility to the disease with environmental factors influencing severity, timing and outcome. Abnormalities in placental bile acid (BA) transport systems and/or high circulating BA levels may contribute to fetal loss due to asphyxia from vasospasm of the placental vessels.

The etiology of pre-eclampsia appears to involve defective placentation leading to generalized endothelial dysfunction with vasoconstriction of the hepatic vascular bed [11]. In the HELLP syndrome, microangiopathic hemolytic anemia causes periportal hemorrhage, necrosis and fibrin deposition in the liver; with increasing severity, the hemorrhage dissects from zone 1 to affect the whole lobule extending the area of necrosis, leading to large hematomas, capsular tears and hepatic rupture [12].

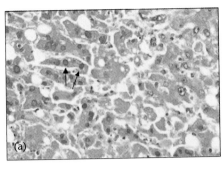
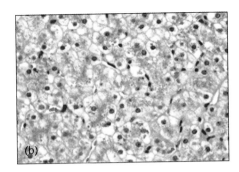
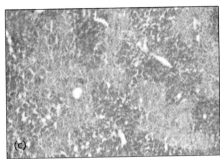
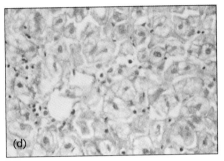
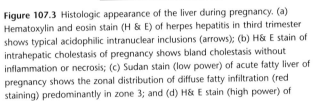

Figure 107.3 Histologic appearance of the liver during pregnancy. (a) Hematoxylin and eosin stain (H & E) of herpes hepatitis in third trimester shows typical acidophilic intranuclear inclusions (arrows); (b) H& E stain of intrahepatic cholestasis of pregnancy shows bland cholestasis without inflammation or necrosis; (c) Sudan stain (low power) of acute fatty liver of pregnancy shows the zonal distribution of diffuse fatty infiltration (red staining) predominantly in zone 3; and (d) H& E stain (high power) of same patient shows hepatocytes stuffed with microvesicular fat and centrally located nuclei. (Parts C and D reproduced from Hay JE. *Liver Disease and Pregnancy.* In: Hauser SC, editor. Mayo Clinic gastroenterology and hepatology board review. Fourth edition. Rochester (MN): Mayo Clinic Scientific Press in conjunction with Oxford University Press. 2011. pp 367–375. Used with permission of Mayo Foundation for Medical Education and Research.)

In AFLP, microvesicular fatty infiltration of hepatocytes leads to acute liver failure and its etiology may involve abnormalities in intramitochondrial fatty acid oxidation (FAO). Some babies of mothers with AFLP are homozygous for enzymes essential for normal FAO, the best characterized being LCHAD (long-chain 3-hydroxacyl-coenzyme A dehydrogenase) deficiency [13–15]. This suggests that maternal heterozygosity, with fetal homozygosity, for deficiency of an enzyme responsible for normal FAO, may overwhelm the increased metabolic demands on fatty acid metabolism of later pregnancy, perhaps exacerbated by external factors, and result in AFLP.

Hyperemesis gravidarum

Hyperemesis gravidarum is intractable vomiting of such severity as to necessitate intravenous hydration [6]. It occurs in the first trimester of pregnancy, typically between 4 and 10 weeks gestation, and is complicated by high transaminases (up to 20-fold above the normal range,) in 50% patients and jaundice in 20–30% cases. It rarely starts after 9 weeks' gestation, has no abdominal pain, fever, elevated white count or anemia. The diagnosis is made on clinical features of intractable, dehydrating vomiting in the first trimester. When the transaminases are high, viral hepatitis must be excluded. A liver biopsy is only needed to exclude more serious disease and the hepatic histologic appearance of HG is generally normal. Hospitalization is necessary for hydration, nutrition and symptomatic therapy [16].

Intrahepatic cholestasis of pregnancy
Clinical features

In ICP, severe pruritus, mild jaundice and biochemical cholestasis appear in the second half of pregnancy and disappear after delivery, typically to recur in subsequent pregnancies [7,10]. Pruritus, starting around 25–32 weeks of gestation, in a patient with no other signs of liver disease is strongly suggestive of ICP, especially if ICP occurred in previous pregnancies. The pruritus affects all parts of the body, is worse at night and may be so severe that the patient is suicidal. Jaundice occurs in 10–25% patients, occasionally complicated by diarrhea or steatorrhea, and usually follows the pruritus by 2–4 weeks. Jaundice without pruritus is rare. Mild to 10- to 20-fold elevations in transaminases are seen; bilirubin is usually <5 mg/dL.

Diagnosis

Diagnosis in the first pregnancy is generally made on typical clinical features, confirmed by rapid post-partum resolution. Serum BA levels are the most specific, sensitive marker for ICP and are always elevated at >10 μmol/L (up to 100 times above normal). A liver biopsy is needed only to diagnose more serious liver disease; in ICP the liver has a near-normal appearance with mild cholestasis and minimal hepatocellular necrosis (Figure 107.3b). The differential diagnosis of cholestasis in pregnancy includes coincidental cholestatic diseases (drugs, cholestatic viral hepatitis, sepsis, gallstones) and pre-existing chronic biliary disease.

Liver Disease

Treatment and prevention

The main risk of ICP is to the fetus with chronic placental insufficiency and/or acute anoxic injury leading to premature deliveries and perinatal deaths. Fetal risk has been shown to correlate with maternal BA levels of >40 μmol/L.

The drug of choice for maternal management is ursodeoxycholic acid (UDCA): the usual dose is 13–15 mg/kg and this gives clinical and biochemical improvement in the mother as well as improved fetal outcome. High-dose UDCA (1.5–2.0 g/d) relieves pruritus in most cases, reduces abnormal maternal BA levels and is safe for the fetus; in addition the babies born to these mothers had almost normal BA levels in comparison to babies of untreated mothers [17]. UDCA improves the function of canalicular transporters and increases elimination of BA metabolites and other organic anions such as disulphates [18,19]. Cholestyramine can sometimes give relief of pruritus in 1–2 weeks but biochemical parameters, maternal malabsorption and fetal prognosis are not improved. Dexamethasone (12 mg/d for 7 days), by suppressing fetoplacental estrogen production, improves symptoms, liver tests and fetal lung maturity in some cases of ICP with no adverse effects. Exogenous progesterone therapy should be discontinued and may cause remission of the pruritus.

Pre-eclampsia

Pre-eclampsia is a third trimester disease with liver involvement only in the minority of patients, causing right upper abdominal pain, jaundice and a tender, normal-size liver [11]. Transaminases range from mild to 10- to 20-fold elevations; bilirubin is usually <5 mg/dL. No specific therapy is needed for the hepatic involvement of pre-eclampsia and its only significance is as an indicator of severe disease with need for immediate delivery to avoid eclampsia, hepatic rupture or necrosis. HELLP and AFLP may complicate pre-eclampsia.

HELLP syndrome
Clinical features

Severe pre-eclampsia is complicated in 2–12% cases by the HELLP syndrome and clinically the two conditions are indistinguishable. Most patients with HELLP present with epigastric/right upper quadrant pain (65–90%), nausea and vomiting (35–50%), a "flu-like" illness (90%), headache (30%); usually they have edema and weight gain (60%), right upper quadrant tenderness (80%), and hypertension (80%); jaundice is uncommon (5%); some patients have no obvious preeclampsia [20]. Most patients (71%) present between 27–36 weeks gestation, but it can occur earlier or up to 48 hours after delivery. HELLP is commoner in multiparous and older patients.

Diagnosis

The rapid diagnosis of HELLP is essential and requires the presence of all three criteria:

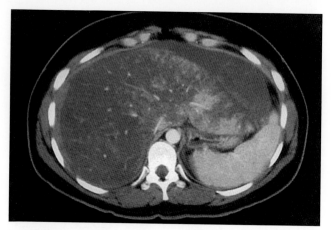

Figure 107.4 Computed tomography of abdomen in severe HELLP shows large subcapsular hematoma extending over the left lobe and the heterogenous, hypodense appearance of the right lobe due to extensive necrosis with "sparing" of small area of left lobe (compare perfusion to normal spleen). (Reproduced from Hay JE. *Liver Disease and Pregnancy.* In: Hauser SC, editor. Mayo Clinic gastroenterology and hepatology board review. Fourth edition. Rochester (MN): Mayo Clinic Scientific Press in conjunction with Oxford University Press. 2011. pp 367–375. Used with permission of Mayo Foundation for Medical Education and Research.)

- Hemolysis with an abnormal blood smear, elevated LDH (>600 U/L) and increase in indirect bilirubin
- AST of >70 U/L
- platelet count of <100,000 and, in severe cases, <50,000 [20].

Prothrombin time, APTT and fibrinogen levels are usually normal but occasionally disseminated intravascular coagulation (DIC) may be present. Transaminase elevation can be variable from mild to 10- to 20-fold; bilirubin is usually <5 mg/dL. Computed tomography (limited views) is indicated in HELLP to detect hepatic rupture, subcapsular hematomas, intraparenchymal hemorrhage or infarction (Figure 107.4).

Treatment

Antepartum stabilization of the mother with treatment of hypertension and seizure prophylaxis is mandatory, followed by transfer to a tertiary referral centre. Delivery is the only definitive therapy [3,20]; if the patient is near-term and/or there is fetal-lung maturity, immediate delivery should be effected, probably by caesarian section though well established labor should be allowed to proceed in the absence of obstetric complications or DIC. Many (40–50%) will require caesarian section, especially primigravidae remote from term. Blood or blood products are given to correct hypovolemia, anemia or coagulopathy. Management remote from term is controversial and sometimes in milder cases at <34 weeks, a more conservative approach with high-dose glucocorticoids, either betamethasone or dexamethasone, is taken in an attempt to prolong the pregnancy and improve fetal lung maturity, although a recent randomized controlled trial showed no benefit of dexamethasone therapy [21]. Once delivered, most babies do very well.

Most patients have rapid, early resolution of HELLP after delivery with normalization of platelets by 5 days. The persistence of thrombocytopenia, hemolysis, progressive elevations of bilirubin and creatinine for >72 hours or the development of complications are usually taken as indications for plasmapheresis or plasma exchange with FFP, although no clinical trials have established efficacy of this treatment. Serious maternal complications are common – DIC (20%), abruptio placentae (16%), acute renal failure (8%), pulmonary edema (8%), ARDS (1%), severe ascites (8%), or hepatic failure (2%) – and maternal mortality rates range from 1 to 25%. Worsening liver failure after the first 3–5 postpartum days necessitates consideration of liver transplantation in the rare case.

Hepatic hemorrhage without rupture is generally managed conservatively in stable patients with close hemodynamic monitoring, correction of coagulopathy, immediate availability of large-volume transfusion of blood and blood products, immediate intervention for rupture and follow-up diagnostic CT scans as needed. Exogenous trauma must be avoided – abdominal palpation, convulsions, emesis, and unnecessary transportation.

Liver rupture, with hemorrhage into the peritoneum, is a rare, life-threatening complication of HELLP, usually preceded by intraparenchymal hemorrhage and a contained subcapsular hematoma in the right lobe. Survival depends on aggressive hemodynamic support and immediate surgery although the best surgical management is still controversial. Recombinant factor VIIa may be used. Maternal mortality from hepatic rupture is 50% with high perinatal mortality from placental rupture, intrauterine asphyxia or prematurity.

Acute fatty liver of pregnancy

Clinical features

AFLP occurs almost exclusively in the third trimester from 28 to 40 weeks, most commonly at 36 weeks; 50% patients are nulliparous, with an increased incidence in twin pregnancies. The presentation is variable from asymptomatic to fulminant liver failure [15,17,22]. The typical patient has 1–2 weeks of anorexia, nausea, vomiting and right upper quadrant pain and is ill-looking with jaundice, hypertension, edema, ascites, a small liver, hepatic encephalopathy and pre-eclampsia (50%). Intrauterine death may occur.

Transaminases vary from near-normal to >1000 IU/dL, usually about 300; bilirubin is usually <5 mg/dL but higher in severe or complicated disease. Other typical abnormalities are normochromic, normocytic anemia, high WBC count, normal–low platelets, abnormal protime, APTT and fibrinogen with or without DIC, metabolic acidosis, renal dysfunction or oliguric renal failure, hypoglycemia, high ammonia and often biochemical pancreatitis.

Diagnosis

The diagnosis of AFLP is generally made on typical clinical and biochemical features of acute liver failure in the third

Table 107.1 Diagnostic differences between acute fatty liver of pregnancy (AFLP) and the HELLP syndrome

Parameter	AFLP	HELLP
Parity	Nulliparous, twins	Multiparous, older
Jaundice	Common	Uncommon
Encephalopathy	Present	Absent
Platelet count	Low to normal	Low
Prothrombin time	Prolonged	Normal
APTT	Prolonged	Normal
Fibrinogen	Low	Normal to increased
Glucose	Low	Normal
Creatinine	High	High
Ammonia	High	Normal
Computed tomography	Fatty infiltration	Hemorrhage

trimester (Table 107.1). Liver biopsy is rarely indicated for management but is essential for a definitive diagnosis of AFLP: microvesicular, and infrequently macrovesicular, fatty infiltration is most prominent in zone 3; this fat consists of free fatty acids; there is lobular disarray with pleomorphism of hepatocytes and mild portal inflammation with cholestasis (Figure 107.3c and d).

Treatment

In AFLP, early diagnosis, immediate fetal delivery and intensive supportive care are essential for both maternal and fetal survival. Delivery is effected usually by caesarian section (epidural anesthesia will allow better ongoing assessment of coma grade) but rapid controlled vaginal delivery with fetal monitoring is probably safer if the cervix is favorable. Correction of coagulopathy and thrombocytopenia and prophylactic antibiotics are recommended. There is no proven effective therapy for AFLP apart from termination of pregnancy.

By 2–3 days after delivery, liver tests and encephalopathy will improve but intensive supportive care for acute liver failure is needed until recovery of liver function occurs, sometimes over days but occasionally delayed for weeks and months. Maternal mortality is now 10–18% and fetal mortality 9–23%. Infectious and bleeding complications remain the most life threatening. Patients who are critically ill at the time of presentation, who develop complications (encephalopathy, hypoglycemia, coagulopathy, bleeding) or who continue to deteriorate despite emergency delivery, should ideally be transferred to a liver centre. Liver transplantation is rarely indicated but should be considered in patients whose clinical

Liver Disease

course continues to deteriorate with advancing fulminant hepatic failure after the first 1–2 days postpartum without signs of hepatic regeneration.

Prognosis for future pregnancies

In ICP, pruritus and liver dysfunction resolve immediately after delivery with no maternal mortality to recur in 45–70% subsequent pregnancies and occasionally with oral contraceptives. Patients with ICP may later develop more gallstones and gallbladder disease. Some rare familial cases of apparent ICP have persisted postpartum, with progression to cirrhosis.

The risk of recurrence of HELLP in subsequent pregnancies is poorly defined (up to 25%) but subsequent pregnancies carry an increased risk of pre-eclampsia, preterm delivery, intrauterine growth retardation, and abruptio placentae. Many patients do not become pregnant again after AFLP, either by choice due to the devastating effect of the illness or by necessity due to hysterectomy to control postpartum bleeding. For patients who are carriers of LCHAD mutation or other less common deficiencies, the recurrence risk (autosomal recessive) is 25% for the fetus and 15–25% for the mother. AFLP rarely recurs in mothers without any identifiable abnormality of fatty acid oxidation.

References

1. Hay JE. Liver disease in pregnancy. *Hepatology.* 2008;47:1067–1076.
2. Ch'ng CL, Morgan M, Hainsworth I, *et al.* Prospective study of liver dysfunction in pregnancy in Southwest Wales. *Gut.* 2002;51:876–880.
3. Haram K, Svendsen E, Abildgaard U. The HEELP syndrome: Clinical issues and management. A review. *BMC Pregnancy and Childbirth* 2009;9:8.
4. Hay JE. Viral hepatitis in pregnancy. *Viral Hepat Rev.* 2000;6:205–215.
5. Tran TT. Management of hepatitis B in pregnancy: Weighing the options. *Cleveland Clinic J Med.* 2009;76:S25–S29.
6. Goodwin TM. Hyperemesis gravidarum. *Obstet Gynecol Clin N Am.* 2008;35:401–417.
7. Kondrakiene J, Kupcinskas L. Intrahepatic cholestasis of pregnancy-current achievements and unsolved problems. *World J Gastroenterol.* 2008;14:5781–5788.
8. Reyes H. Sex hormones and bile acids in intrahepatic cholestasis of pregnancy. *Hepatology.* 2008;47:376–379.
9. Sookoian S, Castano G, Burgueno A, *et al.* Association of the multidrug-resistance-associated protein gene (ABCC2) variants with intrahepatic cholestasis of pregnancy. *J Hepatol.* 2008;48:125–132.
10. Lammert F, Marschall H-U, Glantz A, *et al.* Intrahepatic cholestasis of pregnancy: molecular pathogenesis, diagnosis and management. *J Hepatol.* 2000;33:1012–1021.
11. Norwitz ER, Hsu C-D, Repke JT. Acute complications of preeclampsia. *Clin Obstet Gynecol.* 2002;45:308–329.
12. Fang CJ, Richards A, Liszewski MK, *et al.* Advances in understanding of pathogenesis of aHUS and HELLP. *Br J Haematol.* 2008;143:336–348.
13. Yang Z, Shao Y, Bennett MJ, *et al.* Fetal genotypes and pregnancy outcomes in 35 families with mitochondrial trifunctional protein mutations. *Am J Obstet Gynecol.* 2002;187:715–720.
14. Strauss AW, Bennett MJ, Rinaldo P, *et al.* Inherited long-chain 3-hydroxyacyl-CoA dehydrogenase deficiency and a fetal-maternal interaction cause maternal liver disease and other pregnancy complications. *Semin Perinatol.* 1999;23:100–112.
15. Ibdah JA. Acute fatty liver of pregnancy: An update on pathogenesis and clinical implications. *World J Gastroenterol.* 2006;14:7397–7404.
16. Lord LM, Pelletier K. Management of hyperemesis gravidarum with enteral nutrition. *Practical Gastroenterol.* 2008;June:15–31.
17. Mazzella G, Nicola R, Francesco A, *et al.* Ursodeoxycholic acid administration in patients with cholestasis of pregnancy: effects on primary bile acids in babies and mothers. *Hepatology.* 2001;33:504–508.
18. Azzaroli F, Mennon A, Feletti V, *et al.* Clinical trial: Modulation of human placental multidrug resistance proteins in cholestasis of pregnancy by ursodeoxycholic acid. *Aliment Pharmacol Ther.* 2007;26:1139–1146.
19. Glantz A, Reilly S-J, Benthin L, *et al.* Intrahepatic cholestasis of pregnancy: Amelioration of pruritus by UDCA is associated with decreased progesterone disulphates in urine. *Hepatology.* 2008;47:544–551.
20. Sibai BM, Ramadan MK, Usta I, *et al.* Maternal morbidity and mortality in 442 pregnancies with hemolysis, elevated liver enzymes and low platelets (HELLP syndrome). *Am J Obstet Gynecol.* 1993;169:1000–1006.
21. Fonseca JE, Mendez F, Catano C, *et al.* Dexamethasone treatment does not improve the outcome of women with HEELP syndrome: a double-blind, placebo-controlled, randomized clinical trial. *Am J Obstet Gynecol.* 2005;193:1591–1598.
22. Knight M, Nelson-Piercy C, Kurinczuk JJ, *et al.* A prospective national study of acute fatty liver of pregnancy in the UK. *Gut.* 2008;57:951–956.

CHAPTER 108

Liver transplantation: indications and selection of candidates and immediate complications

Patrick S. Kamath and John J. Poterucha

Mayo Clinic, Rochester, MN, USA

KEY POINTS REGARDING LIVER TRANSPLANTATION

- Liver transplantation is the only established therapy for patients with end-stage liver diseases (ESLD). It is also indicated in fulminant liver failure, in some biliary malformations, and in some hepatocellular carcinomas
- Survival after liver transplantation is approximately 80% at 3 years. Shortage of donor organs is a major limitation in adult liver transplant and is responsible for significant mortality while on the waiting list. Strategies to increase the number of donor organs include the use of marginal livers, split liver, and living donors
- Indications for liver transplantation
  - Liver transplantation is currently indicated in patients with decompensated cirrhosis, fulminant hepatic failure, hepatocellular carcinoma, metabolic liver disease, and neuroendocrine tumors
- Contraindications to liver transplantation
  - The absolute contraindications to liver transplantation are irreversible neurological disease, advanced cardiopulmonary disease, uncontrolled infection, extra-hepatic malignancy, and in patients with pulmonary hypertension with a mean pulmonary arterial pressure >50 mmHg
  - The relative contraindications to liver transplantation are age over 65 years, HIV infection, and class III obesity
- Complications of liver transplantation
  - The early post-transplant complications include allograft-related complications such as hepatic artery thrombosis, hepatic venous outflow obstruction, and biliary strictures as well as acute cellular rejection. Recurrent hepatitis C can be an early complication
  - Intermediate and late complications include recurrent disease, lymphoproliferative disorders, cardio-vascular disease, and late rejection

Introduction

Liver transplantation is now an established treatment to improve quality of life and prolong survival in patients with end-stage liver disease. Liver transplantation is currently associated with a 1-year patient survival above 90% in most liver diseases, and a 3-year survival of approximately 80% [1,2]. Surgical techniques used in liver transplantation are summarized in Figure 108.1 [3].

Indications for liver transplantation

The indications for liver transplantation in adults are cirrhosis with complications of portal hypertension, fulminant liver failure, end-stage liver disease, stage 2 hepatocellular carcinoma, and metabolic liver disease. In children, the most common indication for liver transplantation is biliary atresia followed by alpha-1-antitrypsin deficiency. The most common indication for adult liver transplantation is end-stage liver disease due to cirrhosis, usually accompanied by manifestations of portal hypertension and/or hepatocellular carcinoma. Indications for liver transplantation in this group are general and disease specific.

General indications

Indications for liver transplantation in patients with ESLD are the complications of liver disease that are associated with poor survival. These include spontaneous bacterial peritonitis, refractory ascites and hepatorenal syndrome, hepatic encephalopathy that is refractory to treatment, and superimposed hepatocellular carcinoma. In many patients, impaired quality of life related to fatigue and malnutrition is an additional consideration. In general, patients with end-stage liver disease with a Child–Pugh score >7 or MELD score >10 should be considered for liver transplantation. In patients with cholestatic liver disease such as primary biliary cirrhosis and primary sclerosing cholangitis, a rising bilirubin is an indicator of poor outcome. Intractable pruritus or osteopenic bone disease and, in patients with primary sclerosing cholangitis, recurrent bacterial cholangitis, are again indications for liver transplantation.

Disease-specific considerations for liver transplantation and evaluation
Hepatitis C and hepatitis B
Currently, the most frequent indication for liver transplantation in many countries is cirrhosis secondary to chronic hepatitis C. Recurrence of hepatitis C viremia post liver

Textbook of Clinical Gastroenterology and Hepatology, Second Edition. Edited by C. J. Hawkey, Jaime Bosch, Joel E. Richter, Guadalupe Garcia-Tsao, Francis K. L. Chan.
© 2012 Blackwell Publishing Ltd. Published 2012 by Blackwell Publishing Ltd.

Liver Disease

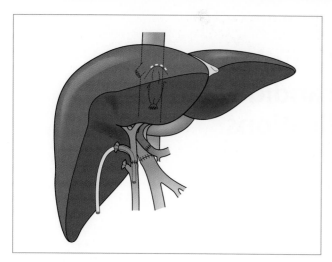

Figure 108.1 Deceased donor liver transplantation. Donor inferior vena cava to recipient hepatic vein confluence "piggy-back" anastomosis, choledochocholedochostomy, biliary tube in donor cystic duct. (Reproduced from Rosen CR. Liver diseases necessitating transplantation. In: Kelly KA *et al.*, eds. *Mayo Clinic in Gastrointestinal Surgery*, with permission from the Mayo Foundation for Medical Education and Research.)

transplantation is invariable. Moreover, in patients who have recurrent hepatitis C, the course is accelerated with approximately 20% of patients developing cirrhosis within 5 years. Elimination of viremia prior to transplantation results in improved outcomes and may be attempted in selected patients who are still well enough to tolerate peginterferon and ribavirin. Patients with Child class B or C have a high rate of infectious complications with hepatitis C treatment prior to transplantation. A positive hepatitis B e antigen and/or high hepatitis B viral DNA pre-transplantation is associated with recurrence of hepatitis B in the graft. Nucleoside or nucleotide analogs, with or without hepatitis B immune globulin, is recommended for all patients with hepatitis B undergoing liver transplantation.

Alcoholic liver disease

Survival post-liver transplantation in patients with alcoholic liver disease is no different from that in patients with other etiologies of liver disease. Typically, an abstinence period of approximately 6 months, adequate rehabilitation, and a stable social support system are required for liver transplantation. It is important that patients continue to remain in an alcohol rehabilitation program following liver transplantation because of a rate of recidivism of approximately 15%. Recidivism is associated with lower compliance with immunosuppression and, therefore, a risk of graft loss. Recurrence of alcoholic liver disease can be seen in patients who comsume large amounts of alcohol after transplantation.

Primary biliary cirrhosis and primary sclerosing cholangitis

Risk scores for primary biliary cirrhosis and primary sclerosing cholangitis are available to help guide decision-making

regarding liver transplantation but have largely been replaced by MELD score. Recurrent PBC occurs in about 20% of transplanted patients although only rarely leads to graft loss. Recurrent PSC complicates 20% of patients transplanted for PSC and may lead to graft loss.

Autoimmune hepatitis

Recurrence of autoimmune hepatitis post liver transplantation occurs in about 20% of patients. Given the risk of recurrence, we recommend that steroids are not tapered away completely in these patients post liver transplantation.

Budd–Chiari syndrome

Patients with the rare fulminant presentation, i.e. those with hepatic encephalopathy within 8 weeks of symptoms, are best managed by liver transplantation. Patients with Budd–Chiari syndrome and cirrhosis, those with acute Budd–Chiari syndrome who fail a transjugular intrahepatic portosystemic shunt (TIPS) procedure, and patients with subacute Budd–Chiari syndrome who fail shunt surgery should be considered for liver transplantation [4]. Liver transplantation reverses the underlying thrombotic disorder in patients with protein C, protein S, and anti-thrombin Z deficiency. However, multiple thrombophilic disorders can occur in the same patient; therefore, we recommend long-term anticoagulation post liver transplantation (in the absence of contraindications).

Hepatic malignancies

Hepatocellular carcinoma

Hepatocellular carcinoma is the most common tumor for which liver transplantation is carried out. The Milan criteria (a single tumor <5 cm in diameter, or three tumor lesions or less, the largest being no greater than 3 cm), or stage 2 HCC, are used to select patients for liver transplantation [5]. There should be no evidence of metastatic disease or macrovascular invasion. In patients meeting these criteria, the long-term survival rate is similar to survival in patients being transplanted for decompensated cirrhosis. Evaluation of patients with hepatocellular carcinoma includes an extensive search for extrahepatic metastases (Table 108.1). After confirming that the hepatocellular cancer is localized to the liver, then transarterial chemoembolization of the tumor is recommended and repeated every 2–3 months as required. Liver transplantation has also been successfully applied to highly selected patients with cholangiocarcinoma. Treatment includes preoperative radiation (both brachytherapy as well as external beam radiation) and chemotherapy [6]. Following this, an operative staging is carried out and, if it is confirmed that the tumor is localized to the liver, the patient may then undergo liver transplantation.

Neuroendocrine tumors

Liver transplantation may be carried out for such patients and those with metastases localized to the liver. The primary tumor in such patients requires resection before liver transplantation. Rectal carcinoids and gastrinomas are generally excluded because of the aggressive nature of the tumors.

Table 108.1 Protocols for evaluation of patients with malignant tumors

Hepatocellular carcinoma protocol: initial evaluation
- CT chest
- CT abdomen and pelvis (repeated with CT chest every 3 months until transplantation)
- CT head
- Bone scan (entire skeleton)

Cholangiocarcinoma protocol
- CT chest
- CT abdomen
- Bone scan (entire skeleton)
- Endoscopic ultrasound of biliary tree

Neuroendocrine tumor protocol
- CT chest
- CT abdomen/pelvis (repeated every 4–6 months until transplantation)
- Bone scan
- Octreotide scan
- Echocardiogram

Contraindications to liver transplantation

Absolute contraindications

In general, the more experienced a liver transplantation center, the fewer the absolute contraindications for liver transplantation.

Advanced, irreversible neurological deficit and cardiopulmonary disease are absolute contraindications to liver transplantation. Portopulmonary hypertension is not a contraindication if the mean pulmonary arterial pressure is <35 mmHg, or can be reduced to <35 mmHg with pharmacological therapy; if the mean pulmonary arterial pressure is between 35 and 50 mmHg with a pulmonary vascular resistance <250 dyn/s/cm^{-5}, liver transplantation can still be carried out. When the mean pulmonary arterial pressure is greater than 50 mmHg, mortality post liver transplantation is greater than 50%, ruling out liver transplantation as a viable option. Hepatopulmonary syndrome is not a contraindication, but when associated with a PaO_2 of <50 mmHg and a pulmonary arterial shunt of >30% it generally has a poorer outcome [7]. Patients with coronary artery disease, including those who have undergone coronary artery bypass surgery, have a higher post-transplant mortality and morbidity. In view of the systemic vasodilatation in patients with cirrhosis, cardiac function may deteriorate after transplantation because of increased afterload. Patients with cardiomyopathy and those with lethal cardiac arrhythmias should be excluded from liver transplantation. Uncontrolled infection, either intrahepatic, such as related to cholangitis or liver abscesses, or extrahepatic, is a contraindication to liver transplantation. Previous extrahepatic malignancy is not a contraindication to liver transplantation, provided the treatment carried out, the grade of malignancy, and the clinical picture suggest a low likelihood of metastatic spread. For most malignancies, a 2-year disease-free period immediately prior to liver transplantation is required. However, the disease-free interval should be longer for high-grade malignancies such as malignant melanoma.

Relative contraindications

Selected patients over the age of 65 who are in otherwise good health should be considered for liver transplantation. With the advent of highly active antiretroviral treatment, excellent post-transplant survival is seen in patients with HIV infection and a CD4 count >400 mm^{-3}.

Patients with morbid obesity do not have significantly higher post liver transplantation mortality or morbidity than less obese patients (Table 108.2).

Selection of candidates for liver transplantation

Following input from the liver transplantation team, patients accepted for transplantation are placed on a waiting list and undergo further investigations outlined in Table 108.2. Patients who have a history of substance abuse are evaluated by a transplant psychiatrist with expertise in addiction and a substance counselor. A carotid ultrasound is carried out in patients >50 years of age. A dobutamine stress echocardiogram is carried out in patients at risk for coronary artery disease. This includes patients over the age of 50 years, a family history of coronary artery disease, or a personal history of diabetes mellitus, hyperlipidemia, or chest pain. Measurement of cardiac troponin in blood may also be helpful in determining cardiac risk.

In the US and in regions of Europe and South America, once a patient with end-stage liver disease is activated for liver transplantation, priority for cadaveric organ allocation is based on the MELD system (model for end-stage liver disease) [8,9,10]. Prior to February 2002 in the US, prioritization for liver transplantation in patients with chronic liver disease was heavily weighted in favor of waiting time. Because of the perceived unfairness of heavily weighting transplantation in favor of waiting time rather than on severity of illness, the United Network of Organ Sharing (UNOS) moved its prioritization scheme to the MELD system. The MELD score is a mathematical score based on serum creatinine, international normalized ratio (INR) for prothrombin time, and serum bilirubin and can be calculated using this web-site http://www.mayoclinic.org/meld/mayomodel6.html [11,12]. Complications of liver disease like spontaneous bacterial peritonitis, hepatic encephalopathy, and variceal bleeding do not influence the accuracy of the model. The addition of Na improves the predictive accuracy of the model, but Na is not currently factored into the current allocation scheme [13,14].

Patients who meet criteria for fulminant hepatic failure (Table 108.3), post-transplant primary graft nonfunction, and hepatic artery thrombosis are given highest priority for organ allocation [15]. For patients with cirrhosis, the patient with the highest MELD score within a particular UNOS region and blood group receives priority for liver transplantation. The advantage of MELD-based allocation is that the sickest patients are more likely to receive liver transplantation. Lower socioeconomic groups and minorities, who were disadvantaged by a system based on waiting time, are no longer disadvantaged.

Liver Disease

Table 108.2 Liver transplant evaluation

Liver transplant: step 1 evaluation		Liver transplant: step 2 evaluation
ABO/Rh/RBC Ab	Ceruloplasmin	EBV and varicella zoster virus serologies
Complete blood counts	Protein electrophoresis	Urine cultures: CMV, bacteria, fungi
Iron studies	Smooth muscle antibody	Tuberculin skin text
Ferritin	Antimitochondrial antibody	Sinus X-ray
Vitamins A, D, E, B$_{12}$, foliate	Alpha-1-antitrypsin phenotype	Standard renal clearance
Prothrombin time	Antinuclear antibody	Mammogram (females >40 years)
Sodium	Hepatitis serology	Echocardiogram
Potassium	HCV-PCR	Dobutamine stress echocardiogram (>50 years)
Calcium	Hemochromatosis gene	Carotid ultrasound (>50 years)
Phosphorus	Lipid profile	Dental X-rays and examination
Glucose		CT Abdomen (to screen for HCC) if creatinine ≤1.4 mg/dL
Alkaline phosphatase	Testosterone	Vaccines 1. Pneumovax 2. Hepatitis A 3. Hepatitis B 4. Tetanus booster 5. Influenza
Total bilirubin	sTSH	
Direct bilirubin	Parathormone	
Creatinine		
Albumin		Evaluation by 1. Transplant surgeon 2. Pulmonologist 3. Infectious diseases 4. Psychiatry
Chloride		
Alpha fetoprotein	HIV	
CA 19-9	HTLV-1	Additional tests (if required)
PSA (males > 40)	Serology RPR	ERCP (if dominant biliary stricture)
CMV serology		Colon cancer screen
Arterial blood gas		**Liver transplant: step 3 evaluation**
Urinalysis 24-h urine Na$^+$		Dietitian
Drug abuse urine survey		Physical therapy
Ultrasound: hepatobiliary and pelvis (if female)		Anesthesia
Upper gastrointestinal endoscopy		Preoperative surgical class
Electrocardiogram		Tours of interactive care area and transplant inpatient area
Bone densitometry spine		Nurse coordinator

Evaluation by
1. Hepatologist
2. Social Services
3. Transplant coordinator
4. Substance abuse team (if necessary)

Table **108.3** Criteria for liver transplantation in fulminant hepatic failure

---

Criteria of King's College, London
Acetaminophen patients
• Arterial pH <7.3 or INR >6.5 and serum creatinine >3.4 mg/dL
Non-acetaminophen patients
• INR >6.5 or any three of the following variables
  ○ age <10 years or >40 years
  ○ etiology: non-A, non-B hepatitis, halothane hepatitis, idiosyncratic drug reaction
  ○ duration of jaundice before encephalopathy >7 days
  ○ INR >3.5

Criteria of Hôpital Paul-Brousse, Villejuif
Hepatic encephalopathy and factor V level <20% in patients <30 years, or factor V level < 30% in patients ≥30 years

---

INR, international normalized ratio.

Contrary to initial fears, post-liver transplant mortality has not increased; moreover, mortality on the waiting list has decreased after implementation of the MELD system. Survival benefit following liver transplantation is seen only in patients with MELD scores ≥17 [16]. Below MELD scores of 14 there is a survival disadvantage with liver transplantation [16,17]. Transplanting livers from high risk donors to recipients with low MELD scores further exaggerates the survival disadvantage.

Expanding the donor pool

The major limitation of liver transplantation is the worldwide shortage of donor organs, which leads to an increased number of deaths while awaiting transplantation. Increasing the numbers of donor organs requires use of marginal livers, split livers, and live donors.

Marginal livers

Livers from deceased donors are considered marginal if there is an increased risk of initial poor function, primary nonfunction, delayed graft, or patient survival. Marginal livers are probably best used for stable patients disadvantaged by the current MELD-based allocation system [18]. Marginal livers include: livers from donors older than 70 years, livers with steatosis, livers from donors after cardiac death, and livers from donors with hepatitis virus infection. Older donors also have an increased risk of previously undiagnosed malignancy. Transplantation of donor livers with less than 30% steatosis gives similar results to transplantation of non-steatotic livers. Transplantation of livers with greater than 60% steatosis is not advised given the high incidence of initial poor function or delayed graft function. Transplantation of livers with 30–60% steatosis should only be considered when there are no other risk factors for poor function. Donations after cardiac death (DCD donors) are from individuals who have severe neurologic damage but who do not meet criteria for brain death; therefore, organs cannot be procured until cessation of cardiopulmonary function. DCD donors are taken off life support in an operating room with the procurement team in place. The increased use of DCD donor livers has resulted in a significant increase in transplant in the US. The major complication in recipients of a DCD liver is ischemic damage, especially to the biliary tract. Allograft survival from an uncontrolled non-heartbeating donor is low and such livers should only be used when documented warm ischemic time is short. Livers from donors who are hepatitis B surface antigen (HBsAg)-negative but anti-HBc-positive transmit hepatitis B to the recipient in 33–78% of cases. Recipients of anti-HBs (without anti-HBc) livers are only rarely infected. Livers from anti-HBc positive donors are considered mainly for recipients with hepatitis B, who are going to receive postoperative therapy regardless of the hepatitis B status of the donor. Hepatitis C-positive donors should only be used for hepatitis C-positive recipients and only if there is no hepatic fibrosis.

Split grafts

Split liver transplantation is the use of a liver from a single donor for two recipients. The recipients need to be relatively small and often either one or both recipients are children. Splitting of the liver can either be performed *in vivo* at liver procurement or *ex vivo* prior to implantation. Graft function is generally good although there is a higher risk of biliary and vascular complications compared with the use of whole-organ grafts.

Living donors

Living donor liver transplantation is used for patients who are not able to receive a cadaver liver in a timely fashion but have no contraindications to liver transplantation. Rapid regeneration of the liver both in donor and recipient allows this procedure. About 90% of regeneration occurs within 4 weeks of transplantation. Living donor liver transplantation (LDLT) for pediatric recipients involves removing either the left lateral liver or left lobe from a parent. The small size of the left lobe does not provide enough liver mass for adults. Donation of the right lobe provides enough mass for many adults, although the operation is more challenging than deceased donor liver transplantation (see Figure 108.2A and B). Evaluation of the potential donor (Figure 108.3) is kept separate from evaluation of the recipient to avoid donor coercion [19]. Evaluation is often spread out over 2–4 weeks to ensure that the potential donor has adequate time to contemplate the risks of living liver donation. After initiation of the first visit with the transplant center, about 50% of potential donors will go on to donate a liver. Mortality in donors is about 0.5%. About 5% of donors will have a complication necessitating hospitalization, reoperation, or transfusion. Overall, recipient outcomes are similar to historical rates of deceased donor transplantation [20]. Hepatic artery thrombosis is seen in 2–6% of recipients,

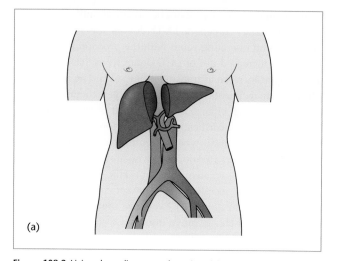 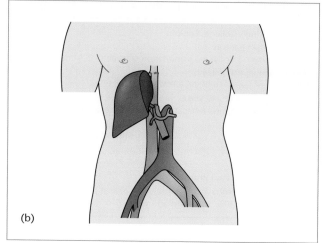

Figure 108.2 Living donor liver transplantation. (A) Donor operation. (B) Right lobe implantation. (Reproduced from Rosen CR. Liver diseases necessitating transplantation. In: Kelly KA *et al.*, eds. *Mayo Clinic in Gastrointestinal Surgery*, with permission from the Mayo Foundation for Medical Education and Research.)

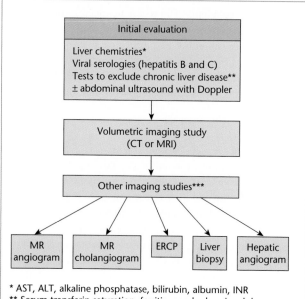

* AST, ALT, alkaline phosphatase, bilirubin, albumin, INR
** Serum transferin saturation, ferritin, ceruloplasmin, alpha one
   antitrypsin phenotype, ANA, SMA, AMA
*** Not routinely performed at all centers

AST = asparate aminotransferase, ALT = alanine aminotransferase,
INR = international normalization ratio, ANA = antinuclear antibody,
SMA = smooth muscle antibody, AMA = antimitochondrial antibody,
CT = computed tomography, MRI = magnetic resonance imaging,
ERCP = endoscopic retrograde cholangiopancreatography

Figure 108.3 Preoperative diagnostic algorithm for evaluation of the donor liver. (Reproduced from Rosen CB. *Liver diseases necessitating transplantation.* In Kelly, KA, Sarr MG, Hider RA, editors. Mayo Clinic Gastrointestinal Surgery. Philidelphia (PA): W.B. Saunders; c2004. pp 209–223, with permission from Mayo Foundation for Medical Education and Research.)

portal vein thrombosis in 2.5–6%, hepatic venous outflow obstruction in about 10%, and biliary complications in 30%.

Immediate post-liver transplantation complications
Allograft-related complications
Primary nonfunction is a relatively rare phenomenon, occurring in only 1–2% of transplants. Characteristics of primary nonfunction are portosystemic encephalopathy, absence of bile production, coagulopathy, and multisystem organ failure, including renal insufficiency. Risk factors for primary nonfunction are marginal donor livers and cold ischemia time >18 hours. Most patients need urgent retransplantation. Significant intra-abdominal bleeding occurs in about 20% of transplant recipients and about half of these will require reoperation. Coagulopathy as a result of factor consumption or delayed graft function and thrombocytopenia due to residual hypersplenism contribute to bleeding.

Hepatic artery thrombosis
Hepatic artery thrombosis (HAT) is a dreaded early complication of liver transplantation, and occurs in 2–12% of transplant recipients. Predictors of HAT are pediatric transplantation, complex arterial anastomoses, liver donor liver transplantation, and tobacco use. Our center performs a Doppler ultrasound of the hepatic artery and portal vein on the first and seventh postoperative days. Impending HAT may be heralded by the ultrasonographic findings of a resistive index <0.5, systolic acceleration, or increased focal peak velocity. If HAT is diagnosed early, operative repair is usually advised. If diagnosed later, retransplant may be necessary because of late complications including diffuse ("ischemic-type") biliary strictures

or liver abscesses. Hepatic arterial stenosis can be treated operatively or by interventional radiology techniques.

Hepatic venous outflow obstruction

Hepatic venous outflow obstruction due to stenosis at the inferior vena caval anastomosis occurs in 1–2% of transplants. Use of the "piggyback" technique (preservation of the recipient inferior vena cava with anastomosis of the donor inferior vena cava to the recipient hepatic vein confluence) (Figure 108.1) may carry a slightly higher risk of hepatic venous outflow obstruction. Hepatic venous outflow obstruction is often successfully treated by transvenous dilation with or without stenting. Portal vein stenosis or thrombosis is rare after liver transplantation but may lead to portal hypertension.

Biliary complications

Biliary complications occur in about 8–15% of liver transplant recipients. Bile leaks tend to occur early, within 1 month after liver transplantation, while strictures generally occur later. The development of biliary complications mandates a careful search for HAT. At our center, nearly all patients will have a biliary tube using a ureteral catheter placed via the donor cystic duct at the time of surgery. This allows monitoring of graft bile output and access for cholangiography. Our policy is to carry out routine cholangiography on the fifth and twenty-first postoperative days. Leaks from choledochojejunostomy usually require reoperation while those from choledochocholedochostomy can usually be observed or treated with sphincterotomy or temporary transpapillary biliary stenting.

Biliary strictures

Biliary strictures can be anastomotic or non-anastomotic. Anastomotic strictures in patients with choledochocholedochostomy are usually managed endoscopically. Choledochojejunostomy anastomotic strictures can be managed endoscopically in most patients although some require percutaneous stenting. Diffuse strictures may be a complication of hepatic artery thrombosis or recurrence of primary sclerosing cholangitis and are usually managed with percutaneous stenting although many patients will have graft loss and require consideration for repeat transplantation.

Cellular rejection

Cellular rejection occurs in 30–50% of liver transplant recipients. Rejection typically occurs early, usually within 1 month after transplantation. Late cellular rejection can be confused with recurrent disease, especially autoimmune hepatitis or hepatitis C. Documented late cellular rejection is often related to noncompliance or sub-therapeutic levels of immunosuppressive agents. Our center performs a protocol liver biopsy on the seventh post-operative day. Rejection is treated with high doses of corticosteroids, which is effective in 90% of patients. Refractory patients are treated with thymoglobulin.

Table 108.4 Differentiating between post-transplant acute recurrent hepatitis C and rejection

Parameter	Acute hepatitis C	Rejection
Time after transplantation	1–6 months	1–4 weeks
Jaundice	Common	Uncommon
HCV RNA level	Steep increase	Variable
Histology	Lobular hepatitis with hepatocyte swelling and acidophil bodies	Portal hepatitis, endotheliitis, lymphocytic cholangitis

Recurrent liver disease

Recurrent liver disease generally occurs months or years after liver transplantation and therefore is not usually part of the differential diagnosis of early post-transplant graft function. A notable exception is hepatitis C, which may mimic cellular rejection. Hepatitis C viremia is usually detected within 2 weeks of transplantation. Clinical acute hepatitis does not usually occur until 1–6 months post-OLT. Features of hepatitis C and rejection are compared in Table 108.4.

Miscellaneous early complications

Pulmonary complications of liver transplantation include atelectasis and pneumonia. Pleural effusions, especially right-sided, occur in nearly all patients but may be particularly troublesome in patients with hepatic hydrothorax prior to transplantation. Pre-existing hepatopulmonary syndrome usually resolves although complete resolution may take months.

Hyperdynamic circulation

A hyperdynamic circulation persists for a few weeks after transplantation. Rarely, patients develop a dilated cardiomyopathy without a clear cause. Supportive medical management is often necessary and myocardial function generally returns to normal within a few weeks.

Neurologic symptoms

Neurologic symptoms occur in 12–20% of patients. Most common are mental status changes that are probably multifactorial although often attributed to immunosuppression. More serious central nervous system complications are seizures due to calcineurin inhibitors such as cyclosporine and tacrolimus, intracranial hemorrhage due to hypertension and coagulopathy, and central pontine myelinosis due to changes in serum osmolality and sodium.

Abnormal renal function

Abnormalities of renal function are an important clinical problem because of the current priority given to patients with pretransplant renal dysfunction. Patients with hepatorenal syndrome have delayed return to function and many probably have an element of acute tubular necrosis that leads to residual renal dysfunction. Calcineurin inhibitors may also lead to impaired renal function after transplantation, especially if drug levels are high.

Infection

Improvements in prophylaxis have led to a decreased incidence in serious infections after liver transplantation. In the first 2 weeks, most infections are bacterial and originate in the biliary tree, peritoneal cavity, wound, urinary tract, and lungs. Fungal infections, especially due to *Candida* species, can also occur early. Viral infections, in particular those due to cytomegalovirus, occur a little later, usually 3–8 weeks after transplant. Gastrointestinal bleeding is usually due to ulcers, viral infections of the gut, or from the jejunojejunostomy in patients with choledochojejunostomy. Diarrhea is very common after transplantation and is probably due to medications, especially mycophenolate mofetil. Use of antibiotics may also lead to pseudomembranous colitis, although this complication is uncommon in our practice, perhaps due to oral selective bowel decontamination.

References

1. Clavien P-A. Who should get a liver graft? Editorial. Twelfth Forum on Liver Transplantation. *J Hepatology*. 2009;50:662–663.
2. Kim WR, Dickson ER. Timing of liver transplantation. *Semin Liver Dis*. 2000;20:451–464.
3. Rosen, CB (2004) Liver diseases necessitating liver transplantation, in *Mayo Clinic Gastrointestinal Surgery*, (eds K.A. Kelly, M.G. Sarr and R.A. Hinder), W.B. Saunders, Philadelphia, pp. 209–223.
4. Menon KVN, Shah VH, Kamath PS. The Budd-Chiari syndrome. *N Engl J Med*. 2004;350:578–585.
5. Llovet JM, Fuster J, Bruix J. The Barcelona approach: Diagnosis, staging and treatment of hepatocellular carcinoma. *Liver Transpl*. 2004;10:S115–S120.
6. Gores GJ. A spotlight on cholangiocarcinoma. *Gastroenterology*. 2003;125:1536–1538.
7. Krowka MJ, Mandell S, Ramsay MA, *et al*. Hepatopulmonary syndrome and portopulmonary hypertension: a report of the multicenter liver transplant database. *Liver Transpl*. 2004;10: 174–182.
8. Kamath PS, Kim WR. The Model for End-Stage Liver Disease (MELD). *Hepatology*. 2007;45:797–805.
9. Kamath PS, Wiesner RH, Malinchoc M, *et al*. A model to predict survival in patients with end-stage liver disease. *Hepatology*. 2001;33:464–470.
10. Wiesner RH, McDiarmid WV, Kamath PS, *et al*. MELD and PELD: Application of survival models to liver allocation. *Liver Transpl*. 2001;7:567–580.
11. Malinchoc M, Kamath PS, Gordon FD, *et al*. A model to predict poor survival in patients undergoing transjugular intrahepatic portosystemic shunts. *Hepatology*. 2000;31:864–871.
12. Teh SH, Nagorney DM, Stevens SR, *et al*. Risk factors for mortality after surgery in patients with cirrhosis. *Gastroenterology*. 2007;132:1261–1269.
13. Biggins SW, Kim WR, Terrault NA, *et al*. Evidence-based incorporation of serum sodium concentration into MELD. *Gastroenterology*. 2006;130:1652–1660.
14. Kim WR, Biggins SW, Kremers WK, *et al*. Hyponatremia and mortality among patients on the liver transplant waiting list. *N Engl J Med*. 2008;359:1018–1026.
15. Kremers WK, van IJperen M, Kim WR, *et al*. MELD score as a predictor of pretransplant and post-transplant survival in OPTN/UNOS status 1 patients. *Hepatology*. 2004;39:764–769.
16. Schaubel DE, Sima CS, Goodrich NP, *et al*. The survival benefit of deceased donor liver transplantation as a function of candidate disease severity and donor quality. *Am J Transpl*. 2008;8: 419–425.
17. Merion RM, Schaubel DE, Dykstra DM, *et al*. The survival benefit of liver transplantation. *Am J Transpl*. 2005;5:307–313.
18. Volk ML, Lok AS, Pelletier SJ, *et al*. Impact of the model for end-stage liver disease allocation policy on the use of high-risk organs for liver transplantation. *Gastroenterology*. 2008;135:1568–1574.
19. Brandhagen D, Fidler J, Rosen C. Evaluation of the donor liver for living donor liver transplantation. *Liver Transpl*. 2003;9: S16–S28.
20. Brown RS, Russo MW, Lai M, *et al*. A survey of liver transplantation from living adult donors in the United States. *N Engl J Med*. 2003;348:818–825.

CHAPTER 109

Long-term management of recurrent primary liver disease

Kiran Bambha[1] and Norah A. Terrault[2]

[1]University of Colorado Anschutz Medical Campus, Aurora, CO, USA
[2]University of California San Francisco, San Francisco, CA, USA

Introduction

Liver transplantation (LT) is an effective treatment for patients with end-stage liver disease and as recipients survive longer, the recurrence of the primary liver disease will play an increasing role in morbidity and mortality.

The majority of causes of cirrhosis can recur after liver transplantation, albeit with a high degree of variation between diseases (Table 109.1). For example, recurrence of hepatitis C virus (HCV) disease is universal in those that are viremic at the time of LT. In contrast, cholestatic liver diseases, such as the primary sclerosing cholangitis (PSC) or primary biliary cirrhosis (PBC), recur in less than 25% at 5 years post-transplantation. The rates of recurrent disease are substantially influenced by whether or not the transplant recipients were assessed by protocol liver biopsies versus "for cause" liver biopsies. This issue is particularly important in the cases of recurrent PBC, PSC, autoimmune hepatitis (AIH) and non-alcoholic fatty liver (NAFL) since histologic disease may recur in the face of normal liver biochemistries and thus, the reported rates of recurrence disease will be underestimated by "for cause" biopsy studies.

In general, the diagnosis of recurrence relies heavily upon histologic findings that are interpreted in the context of the etiology of the chronic liver disease pre-transplantation, as well as laboratory tests and specific imaging studies. For some recurrent diseases, notably chronic HCV, non-invasive tests such as hepatic elastography, have shown promise in assessing disease severity and predicting the risk of development of recurrent cirrhosis. In patients with recurrent disease, prevention of histological progression is critical for graft longevity. Interventions to prevent recurrent cirrhosis post-transplantation mirror those used to manage those with chronic liver disease in the non-transplant setting; however, efficacy may be more variable due to donor and transplant-related factors, including use of immunosuppressive drugs.

CHRONIC HEPATITIS C: ESSENTIALS REGARDING NATURAL HISTORY POST-TRANSPLANTATION

- Essentially all patients who are HCV RNA positive pre-transplantation develop recurrent HCV infection
- Spontaneous clearance of HCV infection post-transplant has been reported but is very rare
- Chronic hepatitis progresses to cirrhosis at a faster rate than in non-transplant patients and the average time to cirrhosis is 8 years
- Approximately 20% of patients develop rapidly progressive disease with the development of advanced fibrosis (bridging fibrosis or cirrhosis) within 3–5 years of transplantation
- Recurrent HCV cirrhosis is the most common cause of graft loss
- Multiple donor, recipient and transplant-related factors have been associated with higher risk of developing early graft loss from recurrent cirrhosis
  - Older donor age, treated acute rejection, cytomegalovirus infection, HIV coinfection, IL28B genotype T/- and post-transplant diabetes/insulin resistance are among the factors most consistently identified

CHRONIC HEPATITIS C: ESSENTIALS OF DIAGNOSIS

- Presence of HCV RNA in serum (if cholestatic hepatitis, HCV RNA is usually ≥1 million IU/mL)
- Liver biopsy findings are consistent with acute or chronic hepatitis
  - Early acute HCV is characterized by apoptotic hepatocytes in lobules and lobular inflammation
  - Later, chronic HCV is characterized by lymphocyte predominant portal-based inflammatory infiltrates, piecemeal necrosis, and fibrosis
- *Absence* of acute rejection on biopsy: beware of overlapping histologic features
  - Presence of bile duct inflammation, endotheliitis, and mixed portal tract infiltrates consisting of eosinophils, lymphocytes, and occasional neutrophils are more indicative of acute rejection than recurrent HCV
- *Absence* of biliary obstruction on biopsy and/or biliary imaging

Liver Disease

CHRONIC HEPATITIS C: ESSENTIALS REGARDING TREATMENT OF RECURRENT DISEASE AND PROGNOSIS

- Treatment of select wait-listed patients can prevent HCV infection post-transplantation
  - Patients with mildly decompensated disease and favorable virologic characteristics are best suited for this approach
- Antibody therapy (e.g., hepatitis C immune globulin) is ineffective in preventing HCV reinfection
- Pre-emptive therapy started with peginterferon and ribavirin within the first few months post-transplantation, offers no advantages over antiviral therapy delayed until histologic disease is apparent
- Treatment of recurrent disease is the mainstay of management but is effective in achieving SVR in only ~35% of patients overall
  - Current standard of care for antiviral therapy is peginterferon and ribavirin
  - Drug dose reductions and discontinuations are frequent, due to cytopenias and other adverse effects
  - Growth factors are frequently needed to manage cytopenias
  - Close monitoring for rejection during treatment is important
- Achievement of SVR post-transplantation is associated with a survival benefit

Table 109.1 Recurrent diseases after liver transplantation

Pre-transplant diagnosis	Recurrent disease?	Risk of recurrent disease post-transplantation
Hepatitis C	Yes	100% if viremic at transplantation; 30% with recurrent cirrhosis at 5 years
Hepatitis B	Yes	80% in absence of prophylactic therapy; ≤15% at 2 years if prophylaxis given
PBC	Yes	18% at 3.9 years
PSC	Yes	11%*
Autoimmune hepatitis	Yes	22% at 2.2 years
NAFL	Yes	5–10%

*Not well documented in literature.

Table 109.2 Potentially modifiable factors associated with severity of HCV recurrence

Category	Factor	Interventions to consider
Donor	Older age and higher donor risk index	Selection donors of younger age and lower DRI
Transplant-associated	Cold ischemia time	Selection organs with lower CIT
	Cytomegalovirus infection	Prophylactic therapy
	Treated acute rejection	Avoid treating mild rejection; avoid use of corticosteroid boluses and lymphocyte depleting drugs
	Post-LT diabetes	Avoid immunosuppressive regimens that are diabetogenic
Viral	Pre-transplant viremia	Clearance of HCV RNA pre-transplantation

Chronic hepatitis C

Epidemiology and natural history

In most liver transplant programs in North America and Europe, hepatitis C virus (HCV) is the most frequent indication for transplantation, accounting for 30–50% of transplant performed. In recent years in the US, the proportion of patients with liver cancer as the primary indication for liver transplantation (LT) has increased [1], reflecting an increasing incidence of hepatocellular carcinoma (HCC) among patients with chronic viral hepatitis and improved access to transplantation provided by the institution of model of endstage liver disease (MELD) exception points for HCC.

Recurrence of HCV infection is universal post-LT if patients are viremic at the time of LT. Recurrence of hepatitis C disease typically is manifested by elevated serum aminotransferase levels and/or histological findings of hepatitis on biopsy. The majority of patients have histologic evidence of recurrent disease within the first year post-LT [2,3]. Progression of fibrosis is accelerated, although the rate of progression is highly variable and non-linear in nature [4]. The median time to cirrhosis is 8–10 years, with an estimated 30% of patients developing cirrhosis within 5 years. For those with cirrhosis, the risk of decompensation is substantially higher (15–30% within a year) than in non-transplant patients (3–5% annually). Once decompensated liver disease develops, the mortality risk is very high, with 40–55% dying within 6–12 months of the decompensating event [5–7].

Patient and graft survival are reduced in HCV-infected patients compared with HCV-negative patients, with a 5-year patient survival of ~70% [8–10]. The most frequent causes of death and graft loss in HCV-infected recipients are complications related to recurrent HCV cirrhosis [6,9].

Risk factors for recurrent disease

Several donor, recipient, viral and transplant-related factors have been associated with risk of graft loss and severe HCV disease recurrence. The factors most consistently associated with poor outcomes related to recurrent disease are older donor age, prolonged cold ischemia time, post-LT cytomegalovirus infection, HIV coinfection, acute rejection requiring treatment, and post-transplant diabetes. Factors associated with higher risk of cirrhosis that are potentially modifiable are important to identify (Table 109.2).

Donor factors are important predictors of graft loss [11]. Donor age affects graft outcomes In HCV-infected recipients to a greater extend that patients transplanted for other etiologies of cirrhosis. The risk of graft loss and more severe recurrent disease occurs with donors over the age of 40 years, but is most marked for donors over the age of 60 years [12]. A recent consensus conference on use of extended criteria donors, recommended that "elderly donors" not be utilized in HCV-infected patients [13].

There is a strong positive association between treated acute rejection (≥1 episode) and risk of recurrent cirrhosis [14]. In recognition of this association, experts recommend a conservative approach to treatment of rejection, with avoidance of corticosteroid boluses and lymphocyte depleting drugs when possible [15]. The goal is to provide sufficient immunosuppression to prevent and treat moderate to severe rejection while simultaneously avoiding excessive immunosuppression.

CMV infection, though an infrequent post-transplant complication with current prophylactic and pre-emptive strategies, is a strong risk factor for more severe fibrosis in patients with HCV infection [16]. CMV may affect HCV disease progression via its immune modulatory effects and cytokine-mediated profibrogenic effects. HIV coinfection is associated with a higher rate of severe HCV disease and graft loss than HCV-infected patients without HCV [17,18].

Post-LT diabetes, insulin resistance and steatosis have been variably associated with a higher risk of advanced fibrosis [19,20]. Since HCV-infected transplant recipients have a higher prevalence of de-novo post-transplant diabetes compared to non-HCV patients [21], immunosuppressive regimens with less diabetogenic potential may reduce the risk of both diabetes and fibrosis progression. The interleukin (IL)-28B genotype of the donor and recipient have been linked with severity of HCV recurrence following transplantation and response to antiviral therapy [22,23], as has been shown in non-transplant patients with HCV.

Other factors associated with higher risk of cirrhosis in some but not all studies include prolonged cold ischemia time, prolonged warm ischemia time, preservation injury, high HCV RNA viral load pre-transplantation or early post-LT, female recipient gender and recipient African–American race.

Diagnosis and differential diagnosis

The diagnosis of hepatitis C **infection** post-transplantation is established by virologic tests. Recurrent viremia is detectable within days of transplantation. Post-transplant HCV RNA levels are, on average, ~1 $\log_{10}$ IU/mL higher than pre-LT values [24]. In general, HCV RNA levels correlate poorly with disease severity, but the cholestatic variant of hepatitis C is usually associated with high HCV viral levels [25]. The presence and severity of recurrent HCV disease is determined by assessment of liver histology. Aminotransferase levels do not predict severity of disease, especially degree of fibrosis. Many centers utilize protocol biopsies to assess disease progression post-liver transplantation. Early histologic features of recurrent HCV infection include lobular inflammation with focal hepatocyte necrosis. Portal-based inflammation, composed mainly of mononuclear infiltrates, develops as the disease progresses, and the histology of recurrent chronic HCV becomes indistinguishable from that seen in the non-transplant

setting over time. Bile duct injury, if present, is typically mild and steatosis, if present, is not associated with steatohepatitis. Severe necroinflammatory activity, including interface hepatitis and confluent necrosis, when seen is highly associated with the development of early cirrhosis.

Differentiating acute cellular rejection from early recurrent HCV can be difficult due to overlapping histologic features. Findings more characteristically associated with acute rejection – and not recurrent HCV – include bile duct inflammation, endotheliitis, and mixed portal tract infiltrates consisting of eosinophils, lymphocytes, and occasional neutrophils. Histologic findings more frequently seen with recurrent HCV include a predominantly lymphocytic infiltrate in the portal-tract, piecemeal necrosis and presence of apoptotic hepatocytes and inflammation in the lobule [26].

Two variants of recurrent HCV disease are recognized with unique histologic and clinical correlates. The most aggressive form of recurrent HCV is the cholestatic HCV variant that occurs in up to 8% of transplants. Cholestatic hepatitis C is characterized by marked increases in bilirubin with elevation of serum aminotransferase levels with high HCV viral loads [25]. This presentation usually is seen within the first 1–2 years post-transplantation, but can occur later. Characteristics histologic features include bile duct proliferation, and cholestasis with areas of bridging and confluent necrosis and a paucity of inflammatory cells. In the absence of treatment, cholestatic hepatitis HCV can rapidly progress and lead to graft loss. Another variant of recurrent HCV is plasma-cell or autoimmune-like hepatitis [27,28]. The key histological features include severe interface inflammatory activity consisting of predominantly plasma cells and perivenular necroinflammation. Autoimmune markers may be present. Clinical and histologic response to treatment with corticosteroids and amplification of baseline immunosuppression has been reported and is associated with good outcome.

Assessing disease severity

While liver biopsy is currently the favored method for assessing disease severity, this procedure is cumbersome as a repeat measure of fibrosis, associated with some risk, and may understage the severity of fibrosis, especially with smaller specimens and those using hematoxylin and eosin staining alone (without trichrome) [29,30]. Given these limitations of liver biopsy, alternative methods for staging HCV disease in liver transplant recipients have been examined.

Transient elastography, which correlates impedance with fibrosis severity, has shown promise in assessing liver transplant recipients with HCV. Initial studies report high sensitivity and specificity in distinguishing Stage 1 from Stage 2–4 disease [31,32] and have shown that the slope of liver stiffness measurements every three months over the first year post-transplant distinguishes rapid versus slow fibrosis "progressors" [33]. Hepatic venous pressure gradient (HVPG) measurement has also been shown to predict disease severity and graft survival [34], but due to its invasive nature and the

Liver Disease

need for specialized expertise is less applicable as a routine test in liver transplant recipients. Serum fibrosis markers have also been studied as an alternative method of staging recurrent disease in HCV-infected transplant recipients [35] but large-scale validated studies are lacking. Pending further studies of these non-invasive markers of disease severity, liver biopsy remains the gold standard for assessing disease severity.

Immunosuppression and management of acute rejection

The ideal immunosuppressive regimen will minimize the risk of acute rejection and minimize the rate of fibrosis progression. Accurate tools to find this balance point are lacking. Since acute rejection requiring treatment with corticosteroid boluses or lymphocyte-depleting drugs is associated with a higher risk of severe post-transplant HCV disease, the goal of immunosuppression is to provide sufficient immunosuppression to avoid the use of these drugs to treat rejection. Additionally, abrupt changes in the amount of immunosuppression may be associated with increased risk of immune-mediated liver injury, as suggested by the studies using rapid corticosteroid tapering and alzetuzumab treatment and therefore should be avoided. Steroid-free regimens offer the clear advantage of reducing steroid-associated complications, but the available data regarding the benefit on HCV recurrence are inconclusive.

In the management of acute rejection, experts recommend against treatment of mild acute rejection, in part due to the difficulty in distinguishing mild acute rejection from early recurrent HCV histologically. For mild-to-moderate acute rejection, amplification of baseline immunosuppression is usually used, with corticosteroids reserved for non-responders to this measure. Corticosteroid boluses and use of lymphocyte-depleting drugs are reserved for those with moderate-to-severe rejection.

Treatment and prevention of recurrent HCV disease

Since recurrent disease is the most frequent cause of graft loss, several treatment strategies have evolved to either prevent HCV reinfection or to treat recurrent disease [36] (Table 109.3). Prevention of recurrent infection is best achieved by eradication of HCV prior to transplantation but only a limited proportion of patients awaiting transplantation are candidates for treatment with peginterferon and ribavirin. Prophylactic antibody therapy, given intraoperatively and for variable periods post-transplantation, has been tested but found to ineffective in preventing HCV recurrence [37]. For those with recurrent HCV infection, antiviral therapy can be undertaken early post-transplantation prior to the development of histologic or clinical evidence of recurrence. This is termed "pre-emptive" antiviral therapy [38]. Alternatively, and most commonly, treatment with antiviral therapy is started only when histologic disease of sufficient severity is present post-transplantation. All of the published experience with antiviral therapy in transplant candidates and recipients is with peginterferon and ribavirin. Data on the use of protease inhibitors (telaprevir and boceprevir) in combination with peginterferon and ribavirin in wait-listed patients and transplant recipients with genotype 1 are lacking.

Prevention of recurrent infection with pre-transplant treatment of wait-listed patients

Achievement of a sustained virologic response prior to LT eliminates the risk of recurrent HCV after LT, while achievement of an undetectable HCV RNA level on treatment prior to transplantation reduces the risk of recurrence [39–41]. This provides the rationale for undertaking antiviral therapy in select HCV-infected patients on the waiting list. To maximize safety and tolerability of antiviral therapy, treatment should only be considered in those with mildly decompensated disease (MELD less than 20). Treatment of patients with advanced decompensation (Child–Pugh class B+ or C;

Table 109.3 Treatment strategies for hepatitis C virus-infected liver transplant recipients

Timing of treatment intervention	Specific therapy used	Target population for intervention	Outcomes achievable
Prior to transplantation	Peg-interferon and ribavirin, typically using a low, ascending dose protocol	Patients with compensated or mildly decompensated cirrhosis (MELD ≤20)	Prevention of HCV recurrence
Early post-transplantation = pre-emptive therapy	Peg-interferon and ribavirin, initiated within the first few months post transplantation	Patients well enough to tolerate early antiviral therapy – patients with lower MELD scores pre-transplant are best candidates. Patients predicted to be at risk for rapidly progressive disease. Absence of current or recent rejection	Prevention of histologic disease. Improved survival
Delayed post-transplantation	Peg-interferon and ribavirin	Presence of fibrosis (typically stage 2 on scale of 4) or moderate to severe necroinflammation. Absence of current or recent rejection	Improved or stabilized liver disease histology. Improved survival

MELD ≥ 20) is contraindicated due to an unacceptably high risk of complications [41,42]. Even in patients with mildly decompensated disease, treatment is discontinued in up to 30% due to adverse events. Thus, risk and benefit need to be considered carefully and such treatment should be undertaken only in experienced transplant centers.

The best candidates for pretransplant treatment are patients with hepatocellular carcinoma as their primary indication for transplantation and patients with living donors, as these patients typically have less severe decompensation. However, further selection of patients should be based on likelihood of response with treatment. On treatment virologic responses with peginterferon and ribavirin are achieved in 30% of patients with genotype 1 and 83% with genotype 2/3, whereas SVR is seen in 13% with genotype 1 and 50% with genotype 2/3 HCV [39,40]. Non-1 genotype, early virologic response, duration of therapy pre-transplantation and adherence to therapy predict response to treatment.

Early treatment of recurrent HCV post-transplantation

The rationale of early or pre-emptive treatment is similar to that of treating acute HCV infection in non-transplant patients, in which early use of to antiviral therapy is associated with enhanced rates of viral clearance. Typically, pre-emptive antiviral therapy is started within the first few weeks to months post-transplantation, when histologic injury is minimal or absent and patients have fully recovered from early post-operative events. Treatment is applicable only to patients without post-transplant complications who are well enough to tolerate antiviral therapy, and patients with low MELD scores pre-transplantation, are typically the best candidates for early post-transplant antiviral therapy. Even with careful selection of patients, discontinuation of treatment due to adverse events is frequent [43]. Moreover, the rates of SVR with pre-emptive therapy are no better than those achieved when antiviral therapy is delayed until recurrent disease is established. Reported SVR rates range from 8% to 39% [43–46]. A trend towards reduced histologic severity in patients receiving pre-emptive therapy compared to untreated controls, even in the absence of a virologic response, suggests early treatment may slow disease progression [46,47]. However, based upon the low SVR rate, this therapeutic strategy is not generally recommended and pre-emptive therapy should be used selectively in those at risk for rapidly progressive disease.

Post-transplant antiviral therapy for recurrent disease

Since antiviral therapy is not uniformly effective and treatment is associated with significant side effects, the typical approach to management of recurrent HCV disease is to monitor disease progression and intervene with antiviral therapy when significant histological disease is present. "Significant" disease is typically defined by a high degree of necroinflammatory activity and/or presence of at least some fibrosis. Since patients with milder degrees of fibrosis appear to have higher rates of SVR, there is rationale for treating before bridging fibrosis or cirrhosis is reached. The primary goal of post-LT antiviral therapy is viral eradication as sustained viral clearance is associated with fibrosis stabilization or regression and improved graft survival [48,49].

Overall, approximately ~35% of transplant recipients treated with peginterferon and ribavirin will achieve SVR [50,51]. Biochemical responses are seen in at least half of those treated. Histologic improvements are primarily but not exclusively seen in responders. In a recent Cochran review, it was concluded that there was no evidence to support antiviral therapy for recurrent disease, in that significant decrements in graft loss have not been demonstrated [52]. However, the authors acknowledge that marked heterogeneity among the studies limiting interpretation of results and they call for further randomized studies with adequate duration of follow-up to be done.

The baseline factors most consistently associated with SVR include non-1 genotype, low pretreatment HCV viral load, low fibrosis score, and absence of prior non-response to antiviral therapy [53,54]. Recent studies suggest younger donor age and use of cyclosporine-based immunosuppression may be beneficial [55]. As in the non-transplant setting, early virologic responses are highly predictive of SVR and non-SVR. Failure to achieve a decline in HCV RNA during the first 3 months of treatment is highly predictive of non-SVR, whereas achievement of an undetectable HCV RNA at week 4 of treatment is highly predictive of SVR with 48 weeks treatment [53,54].

Dose reductions are frequent and discontinuation of treatment due to adverse effects is more frequent than that reported in the non-transplant setting [52]. Since renal dysfunction is quite frequent post-transplantation, the target dose of ribavirin needs to be adjusted to creatinine clearance [56]. Growth factors can be used to minimize symptoms and dose reductions due to cytopenias, but there are no convincing data that growth factor use improves SVR rates. Acute and chronic rejection may occur during treatment, presumably reflecting the immune modulatory effects of interferon. The pooled estimated rate of acute graft rejection is 5% (3–7%) with peginterferon and ribavirin [57]. Monitoring of immunosuppressive drug levels during treatment to insure stability during treatment is recommended [58]. There should be a low threshold to obtain a liver biopsy in patients who develop increases in liver tests during treatment. Management of rejection during treatment includes discontinuation of antiviral therapy and amplification of immunosuppression. Irreversible rejection occurring in the context of HCV treatment has resulted in graft losses [59].

Prognosis and retransplantation

Graft survival is reduced in HCV-infected transplant recipients compared with non-HCV patients, with a 23% increased risk of death at five years post-LT (Figure 109.1). Patients who achieve viral clearance with antiviral therapy have higher rates of survival compared to untreated patients and treatment patients who do not respond to antiviral therapy.

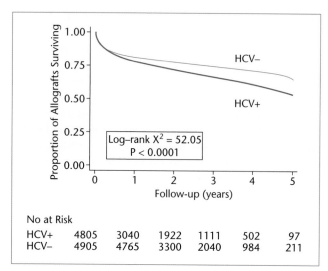

Figure 109.1 Cumulative patient survival of US adult liver transplant recipients with and without HCV. Those with HCV had a 23% increased risk of death at 5 years when compared to patients transplanted for non-HCV etiologies. (Reproduced with permission from Forman LM, Lewis JD, Berlin JA, *et al.* The association between hepatitis C infection and survival after orthotopic liver transplantation. *Gastroenterology.* 2002;122:889–896.)

For those with recurrent cirrhosis, retransplantation is a consideration. In a multicenter study evaluating retransplantation in HCV patients, common reasons for not relisting HCV patients with recurrent disease included the development of recurrent HCV cirrhosis within 6 months of first transplant, fibrosing cholestatic hepatitis, and renal dysfunction [60]. Known predictors of poor outcome with retransplantation of HCV patients include high serum bilirubin and serum creatinine, older recipient age, older donor age, poor preoperative clinical condition and retransplantation for early recurrent disease [61,62]. Thus, while no consensus exists on who should be offered retransplantation for recurrent HCV disease, patients with recurrent cirrhosis beyond the first year who are without multi-organ failure or marked debilitation are probably best candidates [63,64]. Additionally, avoidance of extended criteria donors would seem prudent in this population given the known adverse effects of such donors on HCV graft and patient survival [63,64].

CHRONIC HEPATITIS B: ESSENTIALS OF NATURAL HISTORY POST-TRANSPLANTATION

- Decompensated cirrhosis is a less frequent indication for liver transplantation in the current era of effective and safe antivirals; HCC as an indication for liver transplantation is more common in recent years
- In the absence of prophylactic therapies, ~80% will develop recurrent HBV with the risk of recurrence highest for patients who are high HBV DNA levels/HBeAg positive pre-transplantation
- Fibrosing cholestatic hepatitis is a rare but severe and rapidly progressive form of recurrent disease
- In the absence of therapies to treat recurrent HBV disease, histologic progression to cirrhosis is markedly accelerated compared to the non-transplant setting
- Recurrence of HCC may be a risk factor for recurrence of HBV

CHRONIC HEPATITIS B: ESSENTIALS OF DIAGNOSIS

- HBsAg in serum is diagnostic of recurrent infection
  - HBV DNA is also detectable
- Low level HBV DNA detection in the absence of HBsAg in serum is of unclear clinical significance
  - Represents occult infection and may represent a patient at risk for recurrent disease if prophylaxis fails
- Recurrent "disease" is defined by presence of elevated ALT/AST and/or histologic features of acute or chronic hepatitis
  - Early acute HBV is characterized by apoptotic hepatocytes in lobules and lobular inflammation; may be HBsAg and HBcAg immunostain positive
  - Later, chronic HBV is characterized by lymphocyte predominant portal-based inflammatory infiltrates, piecemeal necrosis, and fibrosis; HBsAg and HBcAg immunostaining is positive
- Fibrosing cholestatic hepatitis is characterized by:
  - Elevated AST/ALT and bilirubin
  - Histology showing hepatocyte ballooning, necrosis, cholestasis and perisinusoidal and portal fibrosis with a relative paucity of inflammation
  - High HBV DNA levels in serum and positive HBsAg/HBcAg on liver immunohistochemistry

CHRONIC HEPATITIS B: ESSENTIALS OF PREVENTION OF RECURRENT DISEASE

- Life-long prophylactic therapy is essential to prevent reinfection
- Combination HBIG and antivirals is frequently used to prevent HBV reinfection
- Specific points on use of HBIG:
  - First dose of given intraoperatively, during the anhepatic phase
  - Subsequent doses are typically given daily for up to 7 days post-operatively
  - After the first week, doses are given to achieve target trough anti-HBs levels, typically ≥100 IU/L
  - Protocols for HBIG minimization have high efficacy and include those that stop HBIG after a specific period (e.g., 6 months) or use of low dose, fixed dose intramuscular HBIG
- Antivirals depend upon pre-transplant antiviral responses and presence (if any) of known resistance mutations
  - Single drug therapy appears effective if used in conjunction with HBIG
  - Combination antivirals may be considered if prior history of resistance or if HBIG discontinuation used
- Monitoring for prophylaxis failure:
  - If on HBIG ± antivirals, monitor HBsAg and anti-HBs titers regularly
  - If on antiviral alone, monitor HBV DNA regularly

CHRONIC HEPATITIS B: ESSENTIALS OF MANAGEMENT OF RECURRENT DISEASE POST-TRANSPLANTATION

- HBIG has no role
- Life-long suppression of HBV replication is essential to prevent disease progression and graft loss
- Combination antiviral therapy is recommended over sequential antiviral use to minimize the risk of treatment failure and the development of multidrug-resistance HBV
  - Prior drug exposures and identified resistance mutations should guide antiviral drug choices
- Monitoring for virologic breakthrough with regular (monthly – every 3 monthly) HBV DNA testing

Chronic hepatitis B

Epidemiology and natural history

The number of patients requiring liver transplantation for decompensated cirrhosis secondary to HBV has decreased over the past decade, presumably reflecting the efficacy of oral antiviral therapies in patients with cirrhosis [1]. Currently, HCC is the most common indication for transplantation in patients with chronic HBV [1].

In the absence of prophylactic therapies, the risk of HBV reinfection after transplantation is approximately 80% overall, and related largely to the level of HBV replication at time of transplantation [65]. Reinfection is associated with an accelerated histologic progression of disease with the majority developing recurrent cirrhosis within 5 years. With these results, it is not surprising that prior to the availability of specific prophylactic therapies, HBV-related liver disease was considered a relative contraindication for liver transplantation due of high rates of HBV recurrence, accelerated disease progression, and patient survival rates of only 50% at 5 years [66] (Figure 109.2, Era 1).

The first major therapeutic advance was the use of long-term hepatitis B immune globulin (HBIG) to prevent reinfection [65,67] (Figure 109.2, Era 2). The second major advance came with the availability of highly effective and well-tolerated antiviral agents against HBV such as lamivudine and adefovir which improved the outcomes of both patients with decompensated cirrhosis awaiting transplantation [68,69] as well as those transplant recipients who had recurrent HBV disease [69,70]. Finally, with the use of HBIG in combination with antivirals (lamivudine and adefovir) the risk of reinfection has been reduced to 10% or less during the first 2 years following transplantation [71] (Figure 109.2, Era 3). With the availability of effective prophylactic therapies, recurrent infection is now preventable in the majority of patients. The current 5-year survival rates for patients transplanted for HBV are ~80%, representing one of most dramatic improvements in outcomes achieved in any single patient group in the past 15 years [1].

Risk factors for recurrent disease

In the era prior to routine use of prophylactic therapy, studies identified patents with HBeAg and HBV DNA levels $\geq 10^5$ copies/mL as highest risk of graft loss due to recurrent disease [72]. Patients with fulminant hepatitis B, delta coinfection and hepatitis B e antigen (HBeAg)-negative chronic HBV had lower rates of recurrence, reflecting the lower HBV DNA levels present in these latter groups of patients.

Recurrent disease is infrequent with current prophylactic therapies. The factors that have been associated with recurrence in the approximately 10% of transplant recipients who develop recurrent HBV despite prophylaxis include high HBV DNA levels and presence of drug-resistant HBV pre-transplant as well a non-compliance [73,74]. HIV coinfection is not a risk factor for HBV recurrence if prophylactic therapy is provided [75]. Interestingly, HCC recurrence post-LT has been found to be a risk factor for recurrent HBV infection, possibly caused

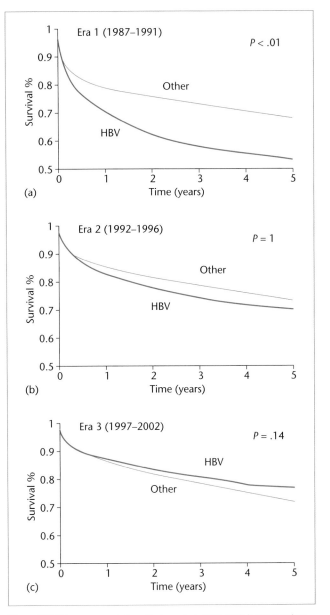

Figure 109.2 Improvements in patient survival of US adult liver transplant recipients with HBV 1987–2002. Compared to other indications, HBV showed a significant improvement in survival between Eras 1 and 3. Era 1 (1987–1991), Era 2 (1992–1996), and Era 3 (1997–2002). (Reproduced with permission from Kim W, Poterucha J, Kremers W, *et al.* Outcome of liver transplantation for hepatitis B in the United States. *Liver Transpl.* 2004;10:968–974.)

by the micrometastatic HBV-infected HCC cells repopulating the new liver graft and inducing recurrence HBV and HCC simultaneously [76].

Low levels of HBV DNA are detectable in liver and peripheral blood mononuclear cells in liver transplant recipients on prophylaxis who are HBsAg-negative in serum and without clinical evidence of recurrent disease [75,77]. The clinical relevance of this occult HBV infection low-level virus is unclear but the presence of low-level viremia supports the need for life-long prophylaxis to prevent overt clinical recurrence.

Diagnosis and differential diagnosis

The diagnosis of recurrent HBV *infection* is established by sero-logic and virologic tests. Persistently detectable HBsAg in serum is sufficient to establish the diagnosis. Transiently detectable HBsAg seen during the early post-transplant period in patients receiving HBIG prophylaxis is not indicative of infection but rather of need for additional HBIG [78,79]. In conjunction with persistently detectable HBsAg in serum, quantifiable HBV DNA is present. As previously highlighted, low level (generally ≤500 IU/mL) HBV DNA without detectable HBsAg has been detected in some patients on long-term prophylaxis but is not viewed as evidence of recurrent HBV infection, since the HBV DNA is unaccompanied by clinical signs of recurrence [75,77,80].

Elevated serum aminotransferase levels and/or evidence of acute or chronic hepatitis on biopsy define recurrent HBV *disease*. HBsAg and HBcAg are detected in liver tissue by immunohistochemistry. A complete absence of stainable HBcAg in a biopsy should prompt consideration of other causes of the allograft dysfunction besides HBV. Histologic findings are similar to the pre-transplant setting, with variable severity of necroinflammation, apoptotic hepatocytes and fibrosis [81]. There is a unique fibrosing cholestatic hepatitis variant, characterized by high intrahepatic levels of HBV DNA, hepatocyte ballooning with cholestasis and a paucity of inflammation [82]. Prior to the availability of effective antivirals, this represented the most severe and uniformly fatal form of recurrent HBV infection.

Since the hepatitic pattern of liver test abnormalities seen with recurrent HBV may arise from multiple causes in the post-transplant setting, other causes of elevated AST/ALT need to be investigated and excluded, including medication effects, other viral infection (e.g., cytomegalovirus infection) and allograft rejection.

Treatment and prevention
Treatment of patients with HBV on the waiting list

The level of HBV DNA in the serum at the time of transplantation predicts the risk of reinfection of the allograft [65,74]. Thus, the goals of therapy in patients on the waiting list are the achievement of a low or undetectable HBV DNA level prior to transplantation. The choice of antiviral drug used depends primarily on prior drug exposures. In treatment-naïve patients, the preferred HBV drugs are those with potent antiviral activity and low risk of resistance, such as entecavir or tenofovir. Since all nucleos(t)ide analogues are renally cleared, doses need to be adjusted to renal function. Nephro-toxicity has been described with adefovir and tenofovir and monitoring for this complication is recommended. Interferon is contraindicated in patients with decompensated cirrhosis and not recommended in those with compensated cirrhosis since safer oral alternatives are available. For those patients failing to achieve an undetectable HBV DNA level with single drug therapy or who have drug resistance, combination antiviral treatment is recommended.

Preventing HBV recurrence post-transplantation

Prophylactic therapy begins at the time of transplantation and continues life-long. The combination of HBIG and one or more nucleos(t)ide analogues is highly effective in preventing recurrent HBV infection and is superior to HBIG monotherapy [83]. Most of the published studies regarding efficacy are with the antivirals, lamivudine or adefovir, in combination with HBIG [71]. The reported rates of HBV recurrence in transplant recipients treated with HBIG combined with lamivudine is 10% or less with follow-up periods of 2-5 years [73,74,84]. Data on the efficacy and safety of prophylaxis with more recently approved antivirals, such as entecavir and tenofovir, alone or in combination with HBIG are limited [85,86]. However, these more potent antivirals with lower rates of drug resistance are predicted to be as good as (or better than) lamivudine in a prophylaxis strategy.

HBIG dosing varies greatly from center to center. Initial protocols using HBIG alone used doses of 5000–10 000 IU monthly to maintain anti-HBs titers of ≥500 IU/L during the first week post-LT, ≥250 IU/L during weeks 2–12 post-LT, and ≥100 IU/L after week 12, as these levels best predictive success of prophylaxis [78]. However, these high-dose HBIG protocols are costly and parenteral administration is inconvenient for patients. When combined with nucleos(t)ide analogues, lower doses of HBIG or shorter duration of HBIG can be utilized. For example, the Australasian Liver Transplant Study Group reported 96% efficacy in preventing HBV recurrence using low-dose intramuscular HBIG (400–800 IU daily for first week → weekly for first month → monthly) combined with lamivudine [73]. Other studies using limited duration of HBIG report efficacy rates of ≥85% with follow-up periods of up to 2 years [87]. Whether antivirals combined with lower doses or short duration of HBIG can maintain high efficacy long-term ≥5 years post-transplantation is unknown.

Retrospective analyses to identify factors associated with failure of prophylaxis have identified two variables: pre-LT HBV DNA levels and history of drug-resistant HBV. Thus, prophylactic strategies should be tailored to the replication status of the patient at the time of transplantation and history of drug resistance. Patients with a higher risk of prophylaxis failure may benefit from a more intensive or prolonger treatment with HBIG, whereas those at low risk for prophylaxis failure may be good candidate for protocols with low dose or shorter duration HBIG [74].

Management of recurrent HBV in liver transplant recipients

HBV recurrence after liver transplantation is usually the result of failed prophylaxis, either due to non-compliance or the emergence of drug-resistant HBV. Serologic evidence of recurrence is accompanied by elevated levels of HBV DNA in serum followed by clinical evidence (elevated ALT levels and hepatitis on biopsy) of recurrent disease.

To minimize fibrosis progression and graft loss due to recurrent disease, life-long control of viral replication is essential post-LT. The availability of safe and effective antivirals has allowed the majority of patients with recurrent HBV infection to survive without graft loss from recurrent disease. There is no role for HBIG once HBsAg becomes persistently detectable. The choice of antivirals is guided by prior antiviral history and drug resistance profiles. Lamivudine, adefovir or telbivudine are not recommended as a single drug therapy due to the high risk of resistance but may be used as part of a combination regimen. In patients with drug-resistant HBV, a nucleoside analogue (lamivudine, telbivudine, entecavir, emtricitabine) combined with a nucleotide analogue (adefovir or tenofovir) offers the best option for long-term suppression. Regardless of the therapy chosen, close monitoring for initial response and subsequent virologic breakthrough is essential to prevent disease progression and flares of hepatitis. Patients with a suboptimal response to a specific drug therapy, warrant a change of drug(s), with add-on therapy generally recommended over sequential single drug therapy.

Prognosis

The 5-year survival of HBV-infected transplant recipients was 53% in the early 1990s and increased significantly to 76% during the 1997–2002 period [88]. This improvement in survival reflects the availability of therapeutic intervention including HBIG and nucleos(t)ide analogues. With a combination of HBIG and nucleos(t)ide analogues as prophylactic therapy, the majority of patients will be protected from recurrent disease. For those fail prophylactic therapy, effective treatment with antivirals can stabilize disease and prevent graft loss. However, given the rapidity of disease progression in the absence of specific therapy, early identification of virologic breakthrough and recurrent infection is important.

For patients who develop recurrent disease that progresses to cirrhosis, retransplantation is an option [89,90]. The primary criterion for consideration of retransplantation is an ability to provide effective prophylactic therapy. Since most patients who require retransplantation are likely to have failed prior antiviral therapies, an effective rescue antiviral therapy must be available for retransplantation to be undertaken.

Primary biliary cirrhosis
Epidemiology

PBC is a chronic cholestatic liver disease of uncertain etiology characterized by T-lymphocyte mediated destruction of intralobular and septal bile ducts, which can lead to progressive fibrosis and cirrhosis. Liver transplantation is an effective treatment for decompensated cirrhosis due to PBC, with excellent post-transplant outcomes (1-, 5- and 10-year survival rates of 89%, 78% and 67%, respectively) [91–94].

Although a debated issue in the past, it is now generally accepted that PBC recurs post-transplant [95–99]. The first case of recurrent PBC post-liver transplantation was described in 1982 [95]. It is difficult, however, to generate a precise estimate of the rate of recurrent PBC due to differences across various studies in the criteria used to define disease recurrence, differences in frequency and indications for performing post-liver transplant biopsies, differences among transplant centers with respect to immunosuppressive regimens, and variation in follow-up duration. With these issues in mind, the estimated rate of recurrent PBC across several different studies ranges from 11% to 37%. In a systematic review of disease recurrence post-liver transplant, the weighted recurrence rate of PBC across 16 studies was 18%, with the median time to recurrence being 3.9 years [100].

Risk factors for recurrent disease

Risk factors for recurrent PBC post-transplant are incompletely defined. Although increasing donor and recipient ages have been suggested to be risks for recurrent disease, the data are conflicting. Similarly, it is unclear whether or not increased cold and warm ischemia times are risk factors [101]. There is, however, some evidence for genetic predisposition towards recurrent PBC, specifically, recurrent PBC is associated with genetic variants at the HLA class II, IL-12A and IL-12 receptor beta 2 loci [102]. Additionally, low numbers of donor and recipient HLA haplotypes mismatches may be independent risk factors for disease recurrence [103]. Immunosuppressive regimens may also impact recurrent PBC, with published studies suggesting that tacrolimus may be associated with more rapid recurrence of PBC compared with cyclosporine, although the data exploring this issue are conflicting [104].

Diagnosis and differential diagnosis

Serology has limited utility in making the diagnosis of recurrent PBC. Although the anti-mitochondrial antibody (AMA) is useful for diagnosing PBC in the native liver, in the post-transplant setting AMA titers may show a transient decline and then rebound to, or exceed, the pre-transplant levels, without correlating with liver histology. Similarly, IgM levels may be elevated post-transplant, but do not correlate with recurrent PBC on histology.

A basic criterion for making a diagnosis of recurrent PBC is the presence of PBC in the native liver. Beyond this, though, in the post-transplant setting, emphasis is placed upon liver histology for the diagnosis of recurrent PBC. The pathognomonic histologic lesion is the florid duct lesion including granulomatous cholangitis; however, similar to the pre-transplant setting, the florid duct lesion may not be very commonly seen on biopsy, described to occur in only 8.5% to 30% of recurrent PBC cases. Other histologic features that may be consistent with recurrent PBC include lymphocytic cholangitis, ductular proliferation, lymphocytic aggregates, breaks in the basement membranes of bile ducts, periportal fibrosis, cholestasis and paucity of bile ducts.

A cholestatic pattern of liver biochemical abnormalities is neither sensitive nor specific for the diagnosis of recurrent PBC. Cholestasis may arise from multiple causes in the post-transplant setting and these possibilities need to be investigated, including: medication use that can cause cholestasis (anabolic steroids, estrogens, rifampin, erythromycin, trimethoprim–sulfamethoxazole, amoxicillin–clavulanate, and phenothiazines, among others); acute or chronic allograft rejection; graft versus host disease; biliary obstruction; and infections. Distinguishing between recurrent PBC and acute or chronic rejection may be clarified by histology. Assessment of biliary obstruction and biliary stricturing requires cholangiography. Finally, since certain infections may cause cholestasis, a search for infectious etiologies should be sought (fungal, mycobacterial and viral).

Treatment and prevention
The primary goal of medical management of PBC is to prevent progression of the underlying process. Unfortunately, there is a paucity of data regarding the optimal management of recurrent PBC post-transplant. However, most providers recommend treatment with ursodeoxycholic acid (UDCA) since UDCA has been demonstrated to be well-tolerated and shown to both delay disease progression to end-stage liver disease and to enhance survival in the non-transplant setting. Although improvements in alkaline phosphatase levels have been demonstrated in up to 52% of patients with recurrent PBC on UDCA, compared to 22% of patients not treated with UDCA, UDCA treatment has not been shown to improve the clinically relevant outcomes of patient and graft survival [105,106]. An additional intervention that may be considered is to switch the patient from a tacrolimus-based to a cyclosporine-based immunosuppressive regimen, although there is no compelling evidence to suggest that this approach will positively effect disease progression.

Prognosis
Although PBC can recur post-transplant, the majority of studies have demonstrated that recurrent PBC does not significantly adversely impact long-term patient or graft survival. In a single center study of the rate and cause of graft loss post-transplant, the percentage of grafts lost to recurrent PBC was only 1.3% [107].

Primary sclerosing cholangitis
Epidemiology
PSC is a chronic progressive disorder of unknown etiology characterized by inflammation, fibrosis and stricturing of the intra- and extra-hepatic biliary tree [108,109]. For patients with cirrhosis due to PSC, liver transplant is the treatment of choice with favorable outcomes. The 1-, 2-, 5- and 10-year survival rates post-transplantation are 94%, 92%, 86% and 70%, respectively [110,111].

Recurrent PSC has been described in several reports, occurring in 14–20% of patients [112–120]. As with recurrent PBC, it is difficult to estimate the rate of recurrence due to variability in how recurrent PSC is diagnosed and also due to variability among liver transplant programs in the application of protocol liver biopsies, duration of follow-up time, and use of specific immunosuppressive agents. With these caveats in mind, the estimated rates of recurrent PSC range from 10% to 27%. In a systematic review of disease recurrence post-liver transplant, the weighted recurrence rate of PSC across 14 different studies was 11% [100]. Median time to recurrent PSC could not be reliably assessed due to missing information in the majority of studies.

Risk factors for recurrent disease
Risk factors for recurrent PSC remain incompletely understood. Several factors have, however, been implicated and include recipient age, recipient male gender, gender mismatch between donor and recipient, coexisting inflammatory bowel disease (IBD), prolonged cold ischemia time, presence of an intact colon after liver transplantation, cytomegalovirus infection (CMV), recurrent episodes of acute cellular rejection (ACR), steroid-resistant ACR, use of OKT3 to treat ACR, HLA haplotypes, previous biliary surgery, use of extended donor criteria livers, and prolonged use of corticosteroids [120–125]. The available data have not demonstrated compelling evidence that the type of immunosuppression used post-liver transplant impacts recurrent PSC.

Diagnosis and differential diagnosis
The diagnosis of recurrent PSC post-transplant is challenging as there are currently no standard diagnostic criteria and several other etiologies need to be considered in the differential. However, recurrent PSC in the allograft may be suggested by contrast cholangiography, which is an important diagnostic test, revealing a characteristic picture of non-anastomotic, diffuse, multifocal strictures and focal dilation of the bile ducts with a "beaded" appearance, occurring >90-days post-transplantation. Liver biopsy is also useful in making the diagnosis by demonstrating periductal fibrosis, lymphoplasmacytic cholangitis involving large ducts, and lymphoplasmacytic lobular hepatitis. Ductopenia may or may not be present. However, it should be kept in mind that it may be difficult to distinguish between features of chronic rejection and recurrent PSC on histology, in which case, the history becomes increasingly relevant, specifically whether or not there has been suboptimal immunosuppression. Other criteria applicable to diagnosing recurrent PSC include the patient having a confirmed diagnosis of PSC pre-transplant and the appearance of biliary stricturing >90 days post-transplant. With respect to the latter criterion, the early appearance of intrahepatic biliary strictures (particularly occurring <90 days from transplant) should prompt a search for alternative causes for the stricturing, as the majority of cases of recurrent PSC occur further out from transplantation, usually greater than 12 months [110].

Entities that should be considered in the differential diagnosis of recurrent PSC include a multitude of causes of biliary stricturing occurring in the post-transplant setting, including allograft reperfusion injury, ABO blood group incompatible liver allograft, rejection, anastomotic stricture (due to technical issues), biliary sepsis, and hepatic artery thrombosis, which may result in biliary ischemia with consequent biliary stricturing.

Prevention and treatment

There are currently no proven effective medical therapies for recurrent PSC post-transplant, just as there are no proven effective medical therapies for PSC in the pre- and non-transplant settings. Although UDCA is commonly used for PSC in the pre- and non-transplant settings with demonstrated inconsistent effects, it has not yet been demonstrated to be effective in the management of recurrent PSC. Regardless, it is not uncommon among liver transplant practitioners to prescribe UDCA to patients with evidence of recurrent PSC.

Prognosis

The natural history of recurrent PSC is variable, but recurrent PSC has been demonstrated to have a negative impact on graft survival. In a single center analysis of the rate and cause of graft loss among liver transplant recipients, the percentage of grafts lost to recurrent PSC was 8.4% compared to 1.3% lost due to recurrent PBC, representing a 6-fold increased risk of graft loss compared with PBC [107].

CHOLESTATIC AND AUTOIMMUNE DISEASES: ESSENTIALS OF INCIDENCE AND RISK FACTORS

- PBC, PSC and AIH are all autoimmune-related liver diseases that recur post-transplant
- The disease pathogenesis of recurrent PBC, recurrent PSC and recurrent AIH is incompletely understood
- A multitude of risk factors for recurrent PBC, recurrent PSC and recurrent AIH have been described, including:
  - *Recurrent PBC*: HLA haplotypes and possible role for tacrolimus
  - *Recurrent PSC*: HLA haplotypes, male gender, IBD, CMV, ACR episodes, prolonged use of corticosteroids
  - *Recurrent AIH*: HLA-DR3, severe inflammation in the native liver, weaning off of steroids post-transplant

---

CHOLESTATIC AND AUTOIMMUNE DISEASES: ESSENTIALS OF DIAGNOSIS

- No clinical signs or symptoms are sensitive or specific enough to be useful for the diagnosis of recurrent PBC, recurrent PSC or recurrent AIH
- Serologies are generally not useful in the diagnosis of recurrent PBC, recurrent PSC or recurrent AIH
- The diagnosis of recurrent PBC, recurrent PSC and recurrent AIH can be challenging, necessitating the performance of liver biopsy and proper interpretation of these results in the context of the patient's liver biochemistries, hepatic and biliary imaging, liver disease pre-transplant and history of immunosuppression
- A multitude of post-liver transplant complications may mimic features of recurrent PBC, recurrent PSC and recurrent AIH. Thus, making a reliable diagnosis of recurrent liver disease entails a thorough workup to rule out alternative diagnoses that may account for the histologic, radiograph and/or biochemical findings suggestive of recurrent liver disease

---

CHOLESTATIC AND AUTOIMMUNE DISEASES: ESSENTIALS OF TREATMENT AND PROGNOSIS

Recurrent primary biliary cirrhosis
- 1.3% of PBC patients with recurrent PBC experience graft loss due to recurrent PBC. Median time to recurrent PBC in the allograft = 3.9 years
- UDCA is commonly used and may result in biochemical improvement, but has not been shown to improve patient and graft survival

Recurrent primary sclerosing cholangitis
- 8.4% of PSC patients with recurrent PSC experience graft loss due to recurrent PSC. Median time to recurrent PSC is not well documented in most studies
- There is no proven effective treatment for recurrent PSC, although UDCA is frequently prescribed for recurrent PSC

Recurrent autoimmune hepatitis
- 6.2% of AIH patients with recurrent AIH experience graft loss due to recurrent AIH. Median time to recurrent AIH = 2.2 years
- Recurrent AIH may resolve with increasing immunosuppression and necessitate long-term maintenance of increased immunosuppression with corticosteroids, or other agents, as appropriate

---

Autoimmune hepatitis
Epidemiology and natural history

AIH is a chronic hepatitis of unknown etiology characterized by an unresolving inflammation of the liver that is associated with interface hepatitis on histologic examination, hypergammaglobulinemia and the presence of autoantibodies [126]. Prominence of plasma cells in the portal infiltrate enhances the specificity for the disease, but its presence is not necessary to establish the diagnosis and its absence does not discount the diagnosis. The interface hepatitis is frequently accompanied by a panacinar or lobular hepatitis. Liver transplantation is an effective treatment for AIH with 5-year patient and graft survival rates ranging from 83% to 92% and 10-year patient survival of 75% [127–129].

Recurrent AIH (recurrent AIH) was first described in 1984 and has been reported to occur in 20–36% of patients, with median time to recurrence being approximately 2.52 years [128–134]. As with recurrent PBC and recurrent PSC, it can be challenging to estimate the true recurrence rate of AIH due to variability in how recurrent AIH is diagnosed, especially whether protocol liver biopsies are utilized to assess for recurrence. Additionally, immunosuppressive regimens are variable and this may significantly affect the risk of recurrence. Notably, recurrence of AIH increases with duration of follow-up, with recurrent AIH typically not occurring until the degree of immunosuppression has been reduced several years post-transplant. For example, 25% of allografts may be affected by recurrent AIH within the first 5 years post-transplant, with the proportion increasing to 50% with 10 years of post-transplant follow-up. In a systematic review of disease recurrence, the weighted recurrence rate of AIH across 13 different studies was estimated to be 22%, with a median time to recurrence of 2.2 years [100].

AIH can also develop *de novo* after liver transplantation among recipients who were transplanted for non-autoimmune etiologies, with the disorder seeming to have a predilection for children, but occurring in adults, as well, particularly in the setting of interferon-based therapy [27,135]. The pathogenesis of this disorder is unknown, but appears to respond to treatment with increased immunosuppression, though it can progress to graft loss if not successfully treated.

Risk factors for recurrent disease

As with PBC and PSC, risk factors for recurrent AIH are incompletely defined. However, studies have demonstrated that severe inflammation in the native liver and HLA-DR3 haplotype may be associated with increased risk of recurrence [105,106,131]. No compelling association between specific immunosuppressive medications and risk of AIH recurrence has been described, but it has been suggested that the practice of weaning patients transplanted for AIH off of steroids may increase the risk of recurrent AIH.

Diagnosis and differential diagnosis

Making a diagnosis of recurrent AIH can be very challenging as there are currently no codified standard diagnostic criteria. It is important to be aware that recurrent AIH can occur in the presence of normal transaminases and also in the absence of auto-antibodies. Additionally, the presence of auto-antibodies is not specific to recurrent AIH and therefore is of limited diagnostic utility. Thus, a diagnosis of recurrent AIH requires a combination of liver biochemistries, in which elevated transaminases and hypergammaglobulinemia are suggestive of recurrence, along with compatible histologic features. Additionally, the demonstration of corticosteroid dependency is also consistent with a diagnosis of recurrent AIH. Although not diagnostic, the detection of histologic features of a plasma cell rich mononuclear cell portal infiltrate with interface hepatitis, with or without acute lobular hepatitis, is helpful in making the diagnosis of recurrent AIH.

The histologic findings of recurrent AIH are not inherently specific to AIH and several other diagnostic possibilities must be considered in the differential diagnosis, including: rejection, viral infection, drug toxicity and biliary obstruction.

Treatment and prevention

In the majority of patients with recurrent AIH, disease activity resolves rapidly with the institution of increased immunosuppression and early detection of recurrent disease is most desirable. Most commonly, recurrent AIH patients are placed on increased doses of corticosteroids. It is also recommended that these patients be maintained on the increased immunosuppressive regimen even in the face of normal liver biochemistries, and that any consideration of immunosuppression reduction be untaken with caution in patients demonstrating evidence of recurrent AIH.

Prognosis

The outcomes of patients with recurrent AIH do not appear to be significantly worse compared with outcomes among patients without recurrent AIH, with an estimated 5-year patient survival of at least 78%. In a large, single center analysis of rate and cause of graft loss among liver transplant recipients, the percentage of grafts lost to recurrent AIH was 6.2%, representing a >4-fold increased risk of graft loss compared to patients with recurrent PBC [107]. Additionally, rarely recurrent AIH can have an aggressive course post-transplant that may be refractory to immunosuppressive therapy, culminating in either death or consideration of re-transplantation.

NON-ALCOHOLIC FATTY LIVER: ESSENTIALS OF INCIDENCE AND RISK FACTORS

- Non-alcoholic fatty liver recurs post-transplant
  - Steatosis is the most common histologic form of recurrence and may be seen in up to 30% of liver transplant recipients at-risk for recurrent NAFL
  - NASH may also recur post-transplant, seen in approximately 5% of recipients at-risk for recurrent NASH
  - *De novo* NASH, occurring in patients without a pre-transplant diagnosis of NASH, has been documented to occur post-liver transplant
- Available evidence suggests that recurrence is more common among individuals with pre-transplant diagnoses of NASH or cryptogenic cirrhosis compared to individuals with other pre-transplant liver disease etiologies
  - Although metabolic risk factors, including elevated BMI and insulin resistance, are prevalent in the post-transplant setting and are prevalent among patients with recurrent NAFL, the risk factors for recurrent NAFL remain incompletely defined

---

NON-ALCOHOLIC FATTY LIVER: ESSENTIALS OF DIAGNOSIS

- No clinical signs or symptoms are sensitive or specific enough to be useful for the diagnosis of recurrent NAFL
- Noninvasive serologic markers have not been validated for the diagnosis of recurrent NAFL or NASH after liver transplantation
- Transaminases may or may not be abnormal in the setting of recurrent NAFL
- The diagnosis of recurrent NAFL may be suspected based upon imaging studies demonstrating changes suggestive of hepatic steatosis
  - Sensitivity of imaging studies for hepatic steatosis may be low if less than 30% steatosis is present
  - Imaging studies cannot distinguish steatosis alone from NASH histology
- Liver biopsy remains the main diagnostic tool for diagnosing recurrent NASH
  - Histologic findings that may be seen in recurrent NASH include: steatosis, lobular inflammation, hepatocyte ballooning, Mallory's hyaline, and fibrosis
- The differential diagnosis of recurrent NAFL should include other known causes of hepatic steatosis

NON-ALCOHOLIC FATTY LIVER: ESSENTIALS OF TREATMENT AND PROGNOSIS

Recurrent non-alcoholic fatty liver

- The natural history of recurrent NAFL post-liver transplant is not well defined
  - Available data suggests that approximately 5% of patients at-risk for recurrent NAFL develop histologic evidence of recurrent NASH after liver transplantation
- Although vitamin E and pioglitazone have shown benefit for patients with NASH in the non-transplant setting, these agents have not yet been well-studied in the post-transplant setting with respect to recurrent NASH
- Management of recurrent NASH should address modifiable metabolic and lifestyle factors, including: body weight, dietary intake, physical activity, insulin resistance and dyslipidemia

Non-alcoholic fatty liver

Epidemiology and natural history

NAFL is a disorder of lipid metabolism marked by excessive accumulation of triglycerides in hepatocytes occurring in the absence of excessive alcohol use. The disorder is intimately associated with insulin resistance, visceral adiposity and dyslipidemia. NAFL encompasses a spectrum of histopathology ranging from steatosis to nonalcoholic steatohepatitis (NASH) to cirrhosis, and is now recognized as the most common cause of chronic liver test abnormalities in the United States and is a highly prevalent condition worldwide. Among the histological subtypes of NAFL, NASH is considered the most clinically significant lesion given its potential to progress to fibrosis, cirrhosis and end-stage liver disease. Indeed, NASH may be the precursor lesion underlying a substantial proportion of cases of cryptogenic cirrhosis. For selected patients with NAFL-induced cirrhosis who are deemed appropriate medical candidates, liver transplantation is an effective treatment with reported 1-, 3- and 5-year survival rates ranging up to 88%, 82% and 77%, respectively [136,139].

Recurrent NAFL after liver transplantation has been commonly reported; however, there is still a need for additional data regarding the incidence, prevalence and risk factors for recurrent NAFL and, more importantly, recurrent NASH [140]. As with the other recurrent liver diseases after liver transplantation, it is difficult to estimate the true rate of recurrence due to variability in how recurrent NAFL is diagnosed and also due to variation among liver transplant programs in the application of protocol liver biopsies. Furthermore, recurrent NAFL, as with NAFL pre-transplant, encompasses a spectrum of histopathology, including steatosis and NASH, which may have very different natural histories in the post-transplant setting. In one prospective analysis, 60% of recipients transplanted with NASH-induced cirrhosis developed steatosis of grade 2 or greater at 4 months post-transplant, compared with 8% of individuals with hepatitis C (HCV) [141]. At 1 year post-transplant, approximately 30% of the individuals transplanted for NASH cirrhosis demonstrated evidence of recurrent NASH

histology on liver biopsy. It is estimated that approximately 5–10% of patients who undergo liver transplantation for NASH cirrhosis develop recurrent NASH that may subsequently progress to recurrent cirrhosis [142]. A recently published large, clinical series of patients from a single liver transplant center in the United States demonstrated that, among patients with a pre-transplant diagnosis of NASH or cryptogenic cirrhosis, 31% developed NAFL post-transplant, with post-transplant NAFL being more common among patients who had pre-transplant NASH compared with pre-transplant cryptogenic cirrhosis (45% versus 23% at 5 years post-transplant, $p = 0.007$) [143]. In this investigation, recurrent NASH was seen in only 4% of patients over 20 years of follow-up. The 1-, 5- and 10-year post-transplant survival rates were not statistically different among patients transplanted for NASH or cryptogenic cirrhosis, compared with individuals transplanted for other indications; however, cardiovascular disease was a more common cause of death among patients with pre-transplant NASH or cryptogenic cirrhosis, compared with other pre-transplant liver diseases (21.1% versus 14.1%, $p = 0.04$).

NAFL may also occur *de novo* post-liver transplantation. In one study, among individuals who were transplanted with non-NAFL liver disease etiologies, *de novo* NAFL was reported to occur in 20% of patients and *de novo* NASH in 10% [144].

Another study, which was retrospective, of *de novo* NAFL occurring in patients after liver transplantation demonstrated that *de novo* NAFL is prevalent, occurring in 31% of recipients, with the majority demonstrating uncomplicated steatosis. *De novo* NASH was relatively uncommon, occurring in 1.6% of the cohort. Risk factors for *de novo* NAFL included metabolic disorders such as post-transplant obesity, diabetes, hyperlipidemia and hypertension, as well as tacrolimus use and pre-transplant diagnosis of alcohol-induced cirrhosis. Interestingly, steatosis in the hepatic allograft prior to transplantation was also a risk factor for the development of *de novo* NAFL post-transplant [145].

Overall, the data on *de novo* NAFL post-transplant are intriguing, but the studies currently available on *de novo* NAFL post-transplant have methodological limitations that preclude drawing any firm conclusions.

Risk factors for recurrent disease

Although, as with PBC, PSC and AIH, the risk factors for recurrent NAFL, and particularly recurrent NASH, are not completely defined, the traditional risk factors commonly associated with NAFL (namely: insulin resistance, obesity, dyslipidemia) are highly prevalent in the post-liver transplant patient population, due in large part to side effects from immunosuppressive medications. One study demonstrated that a post-liver transplant increase in body mass index (BMI) of at least 10% is associated with increased risk for developing recurrent NAFL [144]. Interestingly, these investigators also found that the use of angiotensin-converting enzyme inhibitors may be associated with a decreased risk of recurrent

NAFL. However, more studies of recurrent NAFL are required to further define the risk factors.

Diagnosis and differential diagnosis

There are currently no specific, sensitive or accurate non-invasive serological tests for diagnosing recurrent NAFL. Additionally, transaminases may or may not be abnormal in the setting of recurrent NAFL. Hepatic ultrasound is a simple and non-invasive test for the detection of steatosis; however, its sensitivity is low if <30% steatosis is present in the liver. Other imaging modalities, including computed tomography and magnetic resonance imaging, are also useful for detecting hepatic steatosis. Beyond determining the presence of steatosis, though, is the issue of whether or not recurrent NASH exists in the hepatic allograft. Currently, the primary diagnostic tool for the evaluation of NASH is liver biopsy, demonstrating steatosis, hepatocyte ballooning and lobular inflammation, with or without fibrosis [146].

The differential diagnosis for recurrent NAFL should include the other known causes of hepatic steatosis, namely alcohol use, prolonged total parenteral nutrition, rapid weight loss and certain medications (corticosteroids, androgens, tamoxifen, valproic acid, amiodarone, nucleoside analogs, among others). Among individuals with recurrent NASH, the differential includes AIH and HCV, though the histologic patterns and patient's history should be useful in distinguishing among these entities.

Treatment and prevention

There are currently no medications specifically indicated for the treatment of NAFL, or more specifically NASH post-transplantation. Furthermore, there is a dearth of information regarding management of recurrent NAFL and recurrent NASH. However, several studies in the non-transplant setting have demonstrated that pioglitazone may be beneficial for patients with NASH and also demonstrated that vitamin E is beneficial in NASH [147,148]. However, the applicability of these findings to patients with recurrent NAFL in the post-transplant setting is presently unknown. Until definitive studies are available, management of recurrent NAFL focuses on addressing the risk factors that are modifiable, including weight loss, physical activity, dietary modification, control of insulin resistance and dyslipidemia, and, if possible, modification of immunosuppressive regimens to minimize the metabolic complications of the drugs.

Prognosis

The natural history of recurrent NAFL is not well-defined and there is currently no approved treatment specific for recurrent NAFL or recurrent NASH. Although data are still emerging, it has been reported that approximately 5–10% of patients transplanted for NASH cirrhosis have recurrent NASH that may progress to cirrhosis. It is further estimated that 2.5–5% of patients transplanted for NASH cirrhosis ultimately progress to graft failure [142,143].

References

1. Kim WR, Terrault NA, Pedersen RA, et al. Trends in waitlist registration for liver transplantation for viral hepatitis in the US. *Gastroenterology.* 2009;137:1680–1686.
2. Ferrell L, Wright T, Roberts J, et al. Hepatitis C viral infection in liver transplant recipients. *Hepatology.* 1992;16:865–876.
3. Shiffman M, Contos M, Luketic V, et al. Biochemical and histological evaluation of recurrent hepatitis C following orthotopic liver transplantation. *Transplantation.* 1994;57:526–532.
4. Bacchetti P, Boylan R, Terrault N, et al. Non-Markov multistate modeling using time-varying covariates, with application to progression of liver fibrosis due to Hepatitis C following liver transplant. *Int J Biostat.* 2010;6:Article7.
5. Berenguer M, Prieto M, Rayon JM, et al. Natural history of clinically compensated hepatitis C virus-related graft cirrhosis after liver transplantation. *Hepatology.* 2000;32(4 Pt 1):852–858.
6. Kalambokis G, Manousou P, Samonakis D, et al. Clinical outcome of HCV-related graft cirrhosis and prognostic value of hepatic venous pressure gradient. *Transpl Int.* 2009;22:172–181.
7. Firpi R, Clark V, Soldevila-Pico C, et al. The natural history of hepatitis C cirrhosis after liver transplantation. *Liver Transpl.* 2009;15:1063–1071.
8. Forman LM, Lewis JD, Berlin JA, et al. The association between hepatitis C infection and survival after orthotopic liver transplantation. *Gastroenterology.* 2002;122:889–896.
9. Neumann UP, Berg T, Bahra M, et al. Long-term outcome of liver transplants for chronic hepatitis C: A 10-year follow-up. *Transplantation.* 2004;77:226–231.
10. Charlton M, Ruppert K, Belle S, et al. Long-term results and modeling to predict outcomes in recipients with HCV infection: Results of the NIDDK liver transplantation database. *Liver Transpl.* 2004;10:1120–1130.
11. Feng S, Goodrich NP, Bragg-Gresham JL, et al. Characteristics associated with liver graft failure: The concept of a donor risk index. *Am J Transpl.* 2006;6:783–790.
12. Lake JR, Shorr JS, Steffen BJ, et al. Differential effects of donor age in liver transplant recipients infected with hepatitis B, hepatitis C and without viral hepatitis. *Am J Transpl.* 2005;5:549–557.
13. Durand, F, Renz JF, Alkover B, et al. Report of the Paris consensus meeting on expanded criteria donors in liver transplantation. *Liver Transpl.* 2008;14:1694–1707.
14. Prieto M, Berenguer M, Rayon J, et al. High incidence of allograft cirrhosis in hepatitis C virus genotype 1b infection following transplantation: relationship with rejection episodes. *Hepatology.* 1999;29:250–256.
15. Wiesner R, Sorrell M, Villamil F, International Liver Transplantation Society Expert Panel. Report of the first International Liver Transplantation Society expert panel consensus conference on liver transplantation and hepatitis C. *Liver Transpl.* 2003;9:S1–S9.
16. Burak KW, Kremers WK, Batts KP, et al. Impact of cytomegalovirus infection, year of transplantation, and donor age on outcomes after liver transplantation for hepatitis C. *Liver Transpl.* 2002;8:362–369.
17. Duclos-Vallee JC, Feray C, Sebagh M, et al. Survival and recurrence of hepatitis C after liver transplantation in patients coinfected with human immunodeficiency virus and hepatitis C virus. *Hepatology.* 2008;47:407–417.

Liver Disease

18. de Vera ME, Dvorchik I, Tom K, *et al*. Survival of liver transplant patients coinfected with HIV and HCV is adversely impacted by recurrent hepatitis C. *Am J Transpl*. 2006;6: 2983–2993.

19. Foxton MR, Quaglia A, Muiesan P, *et al*. The impact of diabetes mellitus on fibrosis progression in patients transplanted for hepatitis C. *Am J Transpl*. 2006;6:1922–1929.

20. Veldt BJ, Poterucha JJ, Watt KD, *et al*. Insulin resistance, serum adipokines and risk of fibrosis progression in patients transplanted for hepatitis C. *Am J Transpl*. 2009;9:1406–1413.

21. Khalili M, Lim JW, Bass N, *et al*. New onset diabetes mellitus after liver transplantation: The critical role of hepatitis C infection. *Liver Transpl*. 2004;10:349–355.

22. Charlton MR, Thompson A, Veldt BJ, *et al*. Interleukin-28B polymorphisms are associated with histological recurrence and treatment response following liver transplantation in patients with hepatitis C virus infection. *Hepatology*. 2011;53:317–324.

23. Coto-Lierena M, Perez-Del-Pulgar S, Crespo G, *et al*. Donor and recipient IL28B polymorphisms in HCV-infected patients undergoing antiviral therapy before and after liver transplantation. *Am J Transplant*. 2011;11:1051–1057.

24. Gane E, Naoumov N, Qian K, *et al*. A longitudinal analysis of hepatitis C virus replication following liver transplantation. *Gastroenterology*. 1996;110:167–177.

25. Taga S, Washington M, Terrault N, *et al*. Cholestatic hepatitis C in liver allografts. *Liver Transpl Surg*. 1998;4:304–310.

26. Park YN, Boros P, Zhang DY, *et al*. Serum hepatitis C virus RNA levels and histologic findings in liver allografts with early recurrent hepatitis C. *Arch Pathol Lab Med*. 2000;124:1623–1627.

27. Fiel M, Agarwal K, Stanca C, *et al*. Posttransplant plasma cell hepatitis (de novo autoimmune hepatitis) is a variant of rejection and may lead to a negative outcome in patients with hepatitis C virus. *Liver Transpl*. 2008;14:861–871.

28. Demetris A. Evolution of hepatitis C virus in liver allografts. *Liver Transpl*. 2009;51(Suppl 2):S35–S41.

29. Schiano TD, Azeem S, Bodian CA, *et al*. Importance of specimen size in accurate needle liver biopsy evaluation of patients with chronic hepatitis C. *Clin Gastroenterol Hepatol*. 2005;3:930–935.

30. Colloredo G, Guido M, Sonzogni A *et al*. Impact of liver biopsy size on histological evaluation of chronic viral hepatitis: the smaller the sample, the milder the disease. *J Hepatol*. 2003;39: 239–244.

31. Carrion JA, Navasa M, Bosch J, *et al*. Transient elastography for diagnosis of advanced fibrosis and portal hypertension in patients with hepatitis C recurrence after liver transplantation. *Liver Transpl*. 2006;12:1791–1798.

32. Beckebaum S, Iacob S, Klein C, *et al*. Assessment of allograft fibrosis by transient elastography and noninvasive biomarker scoring systems in liver transplant patients. *Transplantation*. 2010;89:983–993.

33. Carrión J, Torres F, Crespo G, *et al*. Liver stiffness identifies two different patterns of fibrosis progression in patients with hepatitis C virus recurrence after liver transplantation. *Hepatology*. 2010;51:23–34.

34. Samonakis D, Cholongitas E, Thalheimer U, *et al*. Hepatic venous pressure gradient to assess fibrosis and its progression after liver transplantation for HCV cirrhosis. *Liver Transpl*. 2007;13:1305–1311.

35. Carrion J, Fernandez-Varo G, Bruguera M, *et al*. Serum fibrosis markers identify patients with mild and progressive hepatitis

36. C recurrence after liver transplantation. *Gastroenterology*. 2010;138:147–158.

36. Terrault NA. Hepatitis C therapy before and after liver transplantation. *Liver Transpl*. 2008;14(Suppl 2):S58–S66.

37. Davis GL, Nelson DR, Terrault N, *et al*. A randomized, open-label study to evaluate the safety and pharmacokinetics of human hepatitis C immune globulin (Civacir) in liver transplant recipients. *Liver Transpl*. 2005;11:941–949.

38. Terrault N. Prophylactic and preemptive therapies for hepatitis C virus-infected patients undergoing liver transplantation. *Liver Transpl*. 2003;9:S95–S100.

39. Everson GT, Trotter J, Forman L, *et al*. Treatment of advanced hepatitis C with a low accelerating dosage regimen of antiviral therapy. *Hepatology*. 2005;42:255–262.

40. Forns X, Navasa M, Rodes J. Treatment of HCV infection in patients with advanced cirrhosis. *Hepatology*. 2004;40:498.

41. Iacobellis A, Siciliano M, Perri F, *et al*. Peginterferon alfa-2b and ribavirin in patients with hepatitis C virus and decompensated cirrhosis: a controlled study. *J Hepatol*. 2007;46:206–212.

42. Crippin JS, McCashland T, Terrault N, *et al*. A pilot study of the tolerability and efficacy of antiviral therapy in hepatitis C virus-infected patients awaiting liver transplantation. *Liver Transpl*. 2002;8:350–355.

43. Shergill AK, Khalili M, Straley S, *et al*. Applicability, tolerability and efficacy of preemptive antiviral therapy in hepatitis C-infected patients undergoing liver transplantation. *Am J Transpl*. 2005;5:118–124.

44. Sugawara Y, Makuuchi M, Matsui Y, *et al*. Preemptive therapy for hepatitis C virus after living-donor liver transplantation. *Transplantation*. 2004;78:1308–1311.

45. Chalasani N, Manzarbeitia C, Ferenci P, *et al*. Peginterferon alfa-2a for hepatitis C after liver transplantation: Two randomized, controlled trials. *Hepatology*. 2005;41:289–298.

46. Bzowej N, Nelson D, Terrault N, *et al*. A randomized controlled trial of peginterferon alfa-2a/ribavirin prophylactic treatment after liver transplant for hepatitis C. *Liver Transpl*. 2011;17: 528–538.

47. Kuo A, Lan B, Feng S, *et al*. Long-term histologic effects of preemptive antiviral therapy in liver transplant recipients with hepatitis C virus infection. *Liver Transpl*. 2008;14:1491–1495.

48. Berenguer M, Palau A, Aguilera V, *et al*. Clinical benefits of antiviral therapy in patients with recurrent hepatitis C following liver transplantation. *Am J Transpl*. 2008;8:679–687.

49. Veldt BJ, Poterucha JJ, Watt KD, *et al*. Impact of pegylated interferon and ribavirin treatment on graft survival in liver transplant patients with recurrent hepatitis C infection. *Am J Transpl*. 2008;8:2426–2433.

50. Xirouchakis E, Triantos C, Manousou P, *et al*. Pegylated-interferon and ribavirin in liver transplant candidates and recipients with HCV cirrhosis: systematic review and meta-analysis of prospective controlled studies. *J Viral Hepatol*. 2008;15:699–709.

51. Berenguer M. Systematic review of the treatment of established recurrent hepatitis C with pegylated interferon in combination with ribavirin. *J Hepatol*. 2008;49:274–287.

52. Gurusamy K, Tsochatzis E, Xirouchakis E, et al. Antiviral therapy for recurrent liver graft infection with hepatitis C virus. *Cochrane Database Syst Rev*. 2010;20:CD006803.

53. Roche B, Sebagh M, Canfora ML, *et al*. Hepatitis C virus therapy in liver transplant recipients: response predictors, effect on

fibrosis progression, and importance of the initial stage of fibrosis. *Liver Transpl.* 2008;14:1766–1777.

54. Oton E, Barcena R, Moreno-Planas JM, *et al.* Hepatitis C recurrence after liver transplantation: Viral and histologic response to full-dose peg-interferon and ribavirin. *Am J Transpl.* 2006;6:2348–2355.

55. Selzner N, Renner E, Selzner M, *et al.* Antiviral treatment of recurrent hepatitis C after liver transplantation: Predictors of response and long-term outcome. *Transplantation.* 2009;88:1214–1221.

56. Narayanan Menon KV, Poterucha JJ, El-Amin OM, *et al.* Treatment of posttransplantation recurrence of hepatitis C with interferon and ribavirin: Lessons on tolerability and efficacy. *Liver Transpl.* 2002;8:623–629.

57. Wang CS, Ko HH, Yoshida EM, *et al.* Interferon-based combination anti-viral therapy for hepatitis C virus after liver transplantation: a review and quantitative analysis. *Am J Transpl.* 2006;6:1586–1599.

58. Terrault NA, Berenguer M. Treating hepatitis C infection in liver transplant recipients. *Liver Transpl.* 2006;12:1192–1204.

59. Stravitz RT, Shiffman ML, Sanyal AJ, *et al.* Effects of interferon treatment on liver histology and allograft rejection in patients with recurrent hepatitis C following liver transplantation. *Liver Transpl.* 2004;10:850–858.

60. McCashland T, Watt K, Lyden E, *et al.* Retransplantation for hepatitis C: Results of a U.S. multicenter retransplant study. *Liver Transpl.* 2007;13:1246–1253.

61. Neff GW, O'Brien CB, Nery J, *et al.* Factors that identify survival after liver retransplantation for allograft failure caused by recurrent hepatitis C infection. *Liver Transpl.* 2004;10:1497–1503.

62. Rosen HR, Prieto M, Casanovas-Taltavull T, *et al.* Validation and refinement of survival models for liver retransplantation. *Hepatology.* 2003;38:460–469.

63. Ghabril M, Dickson R, Wiesner R. Improving outcomes of liver retransplantation: an analysis of trends and the impact of Hepatitis C infection. *Am J Transpl.* 2008;8:404–411.

64. Pelletier SJ, Schaubel DE, Punch JD, *et al.* Hepatitis C is a risk factor for death after liver retransplantation. *Liver Transpl.* 2005;11:434–440.

65. Samuel D, Muller R, Alexander G, *et al.* Liver transplantation in European patients with the hepatitis B surface antigen. *N Engl J Med.* 1993;329:1842–1827.

66. Todo S, Demetris A, Van Thiel D, *et al.* Orthotopic liver transplantation for patients with hepatitis B virus-related liver disease. *Hepatology.* 1991;13:619–626.

67. Terrault NA, Zhou S, Combs C, *et al.* Prophylaxis in liver transplant recipients using a fixed dosing schedule of hepatitis B immunoglobulin. *Hepatology.* 1996;24:1327–1333.

68. Perrillo R, Wright T, Rakela J, *et al.* A multicenter United States-Canadian trial to assess lamivudine monotherapy before and after liver transplantation for chronic hepatitis B. *Hepatology.* 2001;33:424–432.

69. Schiff E, Lai CL, Hadziyannis S, *et al.* Adefovir dipivoxil for wait-listed and post-liver transplantation patients with lamivudine-resistant hepatitis B: Final long-term results. *Liver Transpl.* 2007;13:349–360.

70. Perrillo R, Rakela J, Dienstag J, *et al.* Multicenter study of lamivudine therapy for hepatitis B after liver transplantation. *Hepatology.* 1999;29:1581–1586.

71. Coffin CS, Terrault NA. Management of hepatitis B in liver transplant recipients. *J Viral Hepat.* 2007;14(Suppl 1):37–44.

72. Samuel D, Bismuth A, Mathieu D, *et al.* Passive immunoprophylaxis after liver transplantation in HBsAg-positive patients. *Lancet.* 1991;337:813–815.

73. Gane EJ, Angus PW, Strasser S, *et al.* Lamivudine plus low-dose hepatitis B immunoglobulin to prevent recurrent hepatitis B following liver transplantation. *Gastroenterology.* 2007;132:931–937.

74. Degertekin B, Han S, Keeffe E, *et al.* Impact of virologic breakthrough and HBIG regimen on hepatitis B recurrence after liver transplantation. *Am J Transpl.* 2010;10:1823–1833.

75. Coffin C, Stock P, Dove L, *et al.* Virologic and Clinical Outcomes of Hepatitis B Virus Infection in HIV-HBV Coinfected Transplant Recipients. *Am J Transpl.* 2010;10:1268–1275.

76. Faria LC, Gigou M, Roque-Afonso AM, *et al.* Hepatocellular carcinoma is associated with an increased risk of hepatitis B virus recurrence after liver transplantation. *Gastroenterology.* 2008;134:1890–1899; quiz 2155.

77. Roche B, Feray C, Gigou M, *et al.* HBV DNA persistence 10 years after liver transplantation despite successful anti-HBS passive immunoprophylaxis. *Hepatology.* 2003;38:86–95.

78. McGory R, Ishitani M, Oliveira W, *et al.* Improved outcome of orthotopic liver transplantation for chronic hepatitis B cirrhosis with aggressive passive immunization. *Transplantation.* 1996;61:1358–1364.

79. Dickson RC, Terrault NA, Ishitani M, *et al.* Protective antibody levels and dose requirements for IV 5% Nabi Hepatitis B immune globulin combined with lamivudine in liver transplantation for hepatitis B-induced end stage liver disease. *Liver Transpl.* 2006;12:124–133.

80. Terrault NA, Zhou S, McCory RW, *et al.* Incidence and clinical consequences of surface and polymerase gene mutations in liver transplant recipients on hepatitis B immunoglobulin. *Hepatology.* 1998;28:555–561.

81. Thung S. Histologic findings in recurrent HBV. *Liver Transpl.* 2006;12(11 Suppl 2):S50–S53.

82. Davies S, Portmann B, O'Grady J, *et al.* Hepatic histological findings after transplantation for chronic hepatitis B virus infection, including a unique pattern of fibrosing cholestatic hepatitis. *Hepatology.* 1991;13:150–157.

83. Loomba R, Rowley A, Wesley R, *et al.* Hepatitis B immunoglobulin and Lamivudine improve hepatitis B-related outcomes after liver transplantation: meta-analysis. *Clin Gastroenterol Hepatol.* 2008;6:696–700.

84. Marzano A, Lampertico P, Mazzaferro V, *et al.* Prophylaxis of hepatitis B virus recurrence after liver transplantation in carriers of lamivudine-resistant mutants. *Liver Transpl.* 2005;11:532–538.

85. Xi Z, Xia Q, Zhang J, *et al.* The role of entecavir in preventing hepatitis B recurrence after liver transplantation. *J Dig Dis.* 2009;10:321–327.

86. Fung J, Cheung C, Chan SC, *et al.* Entecavir montherappy is effective in suppressing hepatitis B virus after liver transplantation. *Gastroenterology.* 2011;141:1212–1219.

87. Buti M, Mas A, Prieto M, *et al.* A randomized study comparing lamivudine monotherapy after a short course of hepatitis B immune globulin (HBIg) and lamivudine with long-term lamivudine plus HBIg in the prevention of hepatitis B virus recurrence after liver transplantation. *J Hepatol.* 2003;38:811–817.

88. Kim W, Poterucha J, Kremers W, *et al.* Outcome of liver transplantation for hepatitis B in the United States. *Liver Transpl.* 2004;10:968–974.

89. Ishitani M, McGory R, Dickson R, *et al.* Retransplantation of patients with severe posttransplant hepatitis B in the first allograft. *Transplantation.* 1997;64:410–414.

90. Roche B, Samuel D, Feray C, *et al.* Retransplantation of the liver for recurrent hepatitis B virus infection: The Paul Brousse experience. *Liver Transpl Surg.* 1999;5:166–174.

91. Lee J, Belanger A, Doucette J, *et al.* Transplantation trends in primary biliary cirrhosis. *Clin Gastroenterol Hepatol.* 2007;5:1313–1315.

92. Liermann Garcia R, Evangelista Garcia C, McMaster P, *et al.* Transplantation for primary biliary cirrhosis: Retrospective analysis of 400 patients in a single center. *Hepatology.* 2001;33:22–27.

93. Markus B, Dickson E, Grambsch P, *et al.* Efficiency of liver transplantation in patients with primary biliary cirrhosis. *N Engl J Med.* 1989;320:1709–1713.

94. Wiesner R, Porayko M, Dickson E, *et al.* Selection and timing of liver transplantation in primary biliary cirrhosis and primary sclerosing cholangitis. *Hepatology.* 1992;16:1290–1299.

95. Neuberger J, Portmann B, Macdougall B, *et al.* Recurrence of primary biliary cirrhosis after liver transplantation. *N Engl J Med.* 1982;306:1–4.

96. Hashimoto E, Shimada M, Noguchi S, *et al.* Disease recurrence after living liver transplantation for primary biliary cirrhosis: a clinical and histological follow-up study. *Liver Transpl.* 2001;7:588–595.

97. Knoop M, Bechstein W, Schrem H, *et al.* Clinical significance of recurrent primary biliary cirrhosis after liver transplantation. *Transpl Int.* 1996;9(Suppl 1):S115–S119.

98. Sebagh M, Farges O, Dubel L, *et al.* Histological features predictive of recurrence of primary biliary cirrhosis after liver transplantation. *Transplantation.* 1998;65:195–202.

99. Slapak G, Saxena R, Portmann B, *et al.* Graft and systemic disease in long-term survivors of liver transplantation. *Hepatology.* 1997;25:195–202.

100. Gautam M, Cheruvattath R, Balan V. Recurrence of autoimmune liver disease after liver transplantation: A systematic review. *Liver Transpl.* 2006;12:1813–1824.

101. Guy J, Qian P, Lowell J, *et al.* Recurrent primary biliary cirrhosis: peritransplant factors and ursodeoxycholic acid treatment post-liver transplant. *Liver Transpl.* 2005;11:1252–1257.

102. Hirschfield G, Liu X, Xu C, *et al.* Primary biliary cirrhosis associated with HLA, IL12A, and IL12RB2 variants. *N Engl J Med.* 2009;360:2544–2555.

103. Morioka D, Egawa H, Kasahara M, *et al.* Impact of human leukocyte antigen mismatching on outcomes of living donor liver transplantation for primary biliary cirrhosis. *Liver Transpl.* 2007;13:80–90.

104. Neuberger J, Gunson B, Hubscher S, *et al.* Immunosuppression affects the rate of recurrent primary biliary cirrhosis after liver transplantation. *Liver Transpl.* 2004;10:488–491.

105. Schreuder T, Hubscher S, Neuberger J. Autoimmune liver diseases and recurrence after orthotopic liver transplantation: What have we learned so far? *Transpl Int.* 2009;22:144–152.

106. Faust T. Recurrent primary biliary cirrhosis, primary sclerosing cholangitis, and autoimmune hepatitis after transplantation. *Liver Transpl.* 2001;7(11 Suppl 2):S99–108.

107. Rowe I, Webb K, Gunson B, *et al.* The impact of disease recurrence on graft survival following liver transplantation: A single centre experience. *Transpl Int.* 2008;21:459–465.

108. Angulo P, Lindor K. Primary sclerosing cholangitis. *Hepatology.* 1999;30:325–332.

109. Lee Y, Kaplan M. Primary sclerosing cholangitis. *N Eng J Med.* 1995;332:924–933.

110. Graziadei I, Wiesner R, Marotta P, *et al.* Long-term results of patients undergoing liver transplantation for primary sclerosing cholangitis. *Hepatology.* 1999;30:1121–1127.

111. McEntee G, Wiesner RH, Rosen C, Cooper J, *et al.* A comparative study of patients undergoing liver transplantation for primary sclerosing cholangitis and primary biliary cirrhosis. *Transpl Proc.* 1991;23(1 Pt 2):1563–1564.

112. Brandsaeter B, Schrumpf E, Bentdal O, *et al.* Recurrent primary sclerosing cholangitis after liver transplantation: a magnetic resonance cholangiography study with analyses of predictive factors. *Liver Transpl.* 2005;11:1361–1369.

113. Goss J, Shackleton C, Farmer D, *et al.* Orthotopic liver transplantation for primary sclerosing cholangitis. A 12-year single center experience. *Ann Surg.* 1997;225:472–481.

114. Graziadel I, Wiesner R, Batts K, *et al.* Recurrence of primary sclerosing cholangitis following liver transplantation. *Hepatology.* 1999;29:1050–1056.

115. Khuroo M, Al Ashgar H, Khuroo N, *et al.* Biliary disease after liver transplantation: the experience of the King Faisal Specialist Hospital and Research Center, Riyadh. *J Gastroenterol Hepatol.* 2005;20:217–228.

116. Khettry U, Keaveny A, Goldar-Najafi A, *et al.* Liver transplantation for primary sclerosing cholangitis: a long-term clinico-pathologic study. *Hum Pathol.* 2003;34:1127–1136.

117. Liden H, Norrby J, Friman S, *et al.* Liver transplantation for primary sclerosing cholangitis–a single-center experience. *Transpl Int.* 2000;13(suppl 1):S162–S164.

118. Saldeen K, Friman S, Olausson M, *et al.* Follow-up after liver transplantation for primary sclerosing cholangitis: effects on survival, quality of life, and colitis. *Scand J Gastroenterol.* 1999;34:535–540.

119. Marsh J Jr, Iwatsuki S, Makowka L, *et al.* Orthotopic liver transplantation for primary sclerosing cholangitis. *Ann Surg.* 1988;207:21–25.

120. Vera A, Moledina S, Gunson B, *et al.* Risk factors for recurrence of primary sclerosing cholangitis of liver allograft. *Lancet.* 2002;360:1943–1944.

121. Alabraba E, Nightingale P, Gunson B, *et al.* A re-evaluation of the risk factors for the recurrence of primary sclerosing cholangitis in liver allografts. *Liver Transpl.* 2009;15:330–340.

122. Kugelmas M, Spiegelman P, Osgood M, *et al.* Different immunosuppressive regimens and recurrence of primary sclerosing cholangitis after liver transplantation. *Liver Transpl.* 2003;9:727–732.

123. Tamura S, Sugawara Y, Yamashiki N, *et al.* The urgent need for evaluating recurrent primary sclerosing cholangitis in living donor liver transplantation. *Liver Transpl.* 2009;15:1383–1384.

124. Jeyarajah D, Netto G, Lee S, *et al.* Recurrent primary sclerosing cholangitis after orthotopic liver transplantation: is chronic rejection part of the disease process? *Transplantation.* 1998;66:1300–1306.

125. Cholongitas E, Shusang V, Papatheodoridis G, *et al*. Risk factors for recurrence of primary sclerosing cholangitis after liver transplantation. *Liver Transpl*. 2008;14:138–143.

126. Krawitt E. Autoimmune hepatitis. *N Eng J Med*. 2006;354: 54–66.

127. Gonzalez-Koch A, Czaja A, Carpenter H, *et al*. Recurrent autoimmune hepatitis after orthotopic liver transplantation. *Liver Transpl*. 2001;7:302–310.

128. Ratziu V, Samuel D, Sebagh M, *et al*. Long-term follow-up after liver transplantation for autoimmune hepatitis: evidence of recurrence of primary disease. *J Hepatol*. 1999;30:131–141.

129. Sanchez-Urdazpal L, Czaja A, van Hoek B, *et al*. Prognostic features and role of liver transplantation in severe corticosteroid-treated autoimmune chronic active hepatitis. *Hepatology*. 1992;15:215–221.

130. Cattan P, Berney T, Conti F, *et al*. Outcome of orthotopic liver transplantation in autoimmune hepatitis according to subtypes. *Transpl Int*. 2002;15:34–38.

131. Duclos-Vallee J, Sebagh M, Rifai K, *et al*. A 10 year follow up study of patients transplanted for autoimmune hepatitis: Histological recurrence precedes clinical and biochemical recurrence. *Gut*. 2003;52:893–897.

132. Vogel A, Heinrich E, Bahr M, *et al*. Long-term outcome of liver transplantation for autoimmune hepatitis. *Clin Transpl*. 2004;18: 62–69.

133. Prados E, Cuervas-Mons V, de la Mata M, *et al*. Outcome of autoimmune hepatitis after liver transplantation. *Transplantation*. 1998;66:1645–1650.

134. Tripathi D, Neuberger J. Autoimmune hepatitis and liver transplantation: indications, results, and management of recurrent disease. *Semin Liver Dis*. 2009;29:286–296.

135. Demetris A, Sebagh M. Plasma cell hepatitis in liver allografts: Variant of rejection or autoimmune hepatitis? *Liver Transpl*. 2008;14:750–755.

136. Charlton M, Kasparova P, Weston S, *et al*. Frequency of nonalcoholic steatohepatitis as a cause of advanced liver disease. *Liver Transpl*. 2001;7:608–614.

137. Malik S, deVera M, Fontes P, *et al*. Outcome after liver transplantation for NASH cirrhosis. *Am J Transpl*. 2009;9:782–793.

138. Charlton MR, Burns JM, Pedersen RA, Watt KD, Heimback JK, Dierkhising RA. Frequency and out comes of liver transplantation for nonalcoholic steatohepatitis in the United States. *Gastroenterology*. 2011;141:1249–1253.

139. Afzali A, Berry K, Ioannou GN. Excellent posttransplant survival for patients with nonalcoholic steatohepatitis in the United States. *Liver Transplantation*. 2012;18:29–37.

140. Contos M, Cales W, Sterling R, *et al*. Development of nonalcoholic fatty liver disease after orthotopic liver transplantation for cryptogenic cirrhosis. *Liver Transpl*. 2001;7:363–373.

141. Maor-Kendler Y, Batts K, Burgart L, *et al*. Comparative allograft histology after liver transplantation for cryptogenic cirrhosis, alcohol, hepatitis C, and cholestatic liver diseases. *Transplantation*. 2000;70:292–297.

142. Koehler E, Watt K, Charlton M. Fatty liver and liver transplantation. *Clin Liver Dis*. 2009;13:621–630.

143. Yalamanchili K, Saadeh S, Klintmalm G, *et al*. Nonalcoholic fatty liver disease after liver transplantation for cryptogenic cirrhosis or nonalcoholic fatty liver disease. *Liver Transpl*. 2010;16:431–439.

144. Seo S, Maganti K, Khehra M, *et al*. De novo nonalcoholic fatty liver disease after liver transplantation. *Liver Transpl*. 2007; 13:844–847.

145. Dumortier J, Giostra E, Belbouab S, *et al*. Nonalcoholic fatty liver disease in liver transplant recipients: Another story of seed and soil. *Am J Gastroenterol*. 2010;105:613–620.

146. Kleiner D, Brunt E, Van Natta M, *et al*. Design and validation of a histological scoring system for nonalcoholic fatty liver disease. *Hepatology*. 2005;41:1313–1321.

147. Lutchman G, Modi A, Kleiner D, *et al*. The effects of discontinuing pioglitazone in patients with nonalcoholic steatohepatitis. *Hepatology*. 2007;46:424–429.

148. Sanyal A, Chalasani N, Kowdley K, *et al*. Pioglitazone, vitamin E, or placebo for nonalcoholic steatohepatitis. *N Eng J Med*. 2010;362:1675–1685.

CHAPTER 110

Collagen vascular and vasculitic disorders

Ulf Müller-Ladner[1] and Jürgen Schölmerich[2]

[1]Kerckhoff Clinic, Bad Nauheim, Germany
[2]University Clinic Frankfurt, Frankfurt, Germany

ESSENTIAL FACTS ABOUT PATHOGENESIS

- **Vasculitides** cause vascular inflammation and reduce blood flow to dependent organs
- In the **antiphospholipid syndrome**, obstruction is due to aggregation of antiphospholipid antibodies
- In **systemic sclerosis** T-cell derived cytokines can stimulate collagen deposition by fibroblasts throughout the GI tract
- Transforming growth factor (TGF)-beta may be central in initiation with the SMAD signaling pathway inducing transcription of proteins responsible for collagen deposition

ESSENTIALS OF DIAGNOSIS

- **Vasculitides** may result in abdominal pain, bleeding, ileus, intestinal necrosis and hematochezia because of reduced blood flow and hyper-acute occlusion in the antiphospholipid syndrome. A high index of suspicion is needed
- Laboratory parameters point to specific diseases but Doppler ultrasound, abdominal CT and angiography are required for localization
- **Scleroderma**: Esophageal manifestations most common (dysmotility leading to reflux complicated by Barrett esophagus and adenocarcinoma). Manometry and 24-hour pH monitoring are important tests. Small-bowel involvement can cause pseudo-obstruction obstruction, malabsorption and bacterial overgrowth. Hydrogen breath tests and direct culture are useful tests. In pseudoobstruction CT shows bowel wall thickening
- Reduced oxygen supply and increased tissue fibrosis are the basis for the majority of clinical symptoms
- Reduced function of GI organs leads to a variety of symptoms including ileus, emesis, bloating, maldigestion and malabsorption, diarrhea, and many more
- Each part of the GI tract requires its individual examination technique, always combined with a complete physical status and the respective laboratory parameters

ESSENTIALS OF TREATMENT AND PROGNOSIS

- Vasculitides: corticosteroids, immunosuppressants (e.g., cyclophosphamide 2 mg/kg in granulomatosis with polyangiitis (GPA–formerly Wegener's) and polyarteritis nodosa) and anti-coagulation in the antiphospholipid syndrome
- Systemic sclerosis: there is no evidence-based disease-modifying treatment. Treatment focuses on functional consequences (PPIs, prokinetics)
- In the case of an underlying autoimmune disease, e.g., vasculitis, stage and severity-dependent immunosuppression needs to be applied
- In the case of systemic sclerosis, immunosuppression is of no value and each part of the affected GI tract needs to be treated individually, e.g., with proton pump inhibitors or prokinetics

Introduction and epidemiology

Although the gastrointestinal (GI) tract is not generally regarded as one of the primary organ systems of collagen vascular and vasculitic disorders, there are numerous mechanisms of these diseases operative in or around the different structures and compartments of the GI tract. The majority of clinical symptoms and problems are linked to an alteration of (peri)vascular homeostasis. Alteration of perivascular matrix metabolism can also affect the functional integrity and motility of the GI tract. Aside the specific GI phenomena of the individual diseases as outlined below in detail, the epidemiology of GI involvement follows the characteristics of the respective underlying disease. In addition, gender and age do not influence the occurence nor the severity of the GI manifestations significantly [1–4].

Table 110.1 shows the frequency of intestinal involvement in different vasculitides.

Causes and pathogenesis

Molecular biology has elucidated numerous mechanisms operative in the pathophysiology of a given disease entity in the past decade. In general, genetic factors, alterations of immune responses of the innate and adaptive immune system, the involvement of infectious agents, and various mechanisms of altered matrix metabolism contribute as a network to the initiation and perpetuation of these entities [2,5,6]. In addition, the nature of collagen and vascular diseases excludes "sharp" borders that differentiate one from another but depending on

Multiple Organ Systems

Table 110.1 Frequency of intestinal involvement in different primary and secondary vasculitides

Frequency of intestinal involvement	Type of vasculitis
Up to 90%	Schönlein–Henoch purpura
Up to 50%	Polyarteritis nodosa, Churg–Strauss syndrome, vasculitis in systemic lupus erythematosus
Up to 30%	Behçet syndrome
5–15%	Takayasu arteritis, GPA, vasculitis in rheumatoid arthritis
Less than 5%	Lymphomatoid granulomatosis, giant cell arteritis, thrombangitis obliterans

the origin of the subsequent pathophysiologic effects in the GI tract, two major entities are operative in and around the microvasculature, i.e., **vasculitides** including the antiphospholipid syndrome [7] and **systemic sclerosis** as prototype vascular collagen disease, which can be distinguished and used to illustrate the individual driving mechanisms.

Vasculitides and the antiphospholipid syndrome

Pathology
Vasculitides are diseases characterized by inflammation within or around the vessel wall usually followed by alteration of the vascular blood flow and integrity of the vessel and secondary damage to the dependent organ [1]. In the **antiphospholipid syndrome** [7], vascular obstruction is caused by aggregation of **antiphospholipid antibodies** with lipid surfaces on platelets and vessels. Figure 110.1 illustrates the histopathology of the development of intestinal infarction following the occlusion of the respective vessel.

Clinical presentation
Due to their multifaceted appearance, clinical symptoms of vasculitides can be overt, e.g., when cutaneous or mucosal vasculitis appears, or occult when restricted to a limited number of organs including the intestine [1,2]. **Abdominal pain, bleeding, ileus, intestinal necrosis** and **hematochezia** are the dominant features of GI involvement and in general, the symptoms themselves do not allow classification of the underlying disease. Figure 110.2 illustrates the endoscopic aspect of severe **colonic ischemia**. However, 90% of GI vascular diseases are still due to arteriosclerosis and less than 10% are caused by vasculitides. Postprandial abdominal pain starting usually 30–60 minutes is one of the predominant symptoms of arteriosclerotic reduction in GI blood flow whereas signs of systemic inflammation in combination with

continuous GI symptoms indicate a generalized vasculitis as underlying disease [1,2]. Antiphospholipid syndrome can lead to **peracute occlusion** of parts or the complete venous and arterial intestinal vasculature.

Differential diagnosis
Classification criteria are provided for the major entities by the American College of Rheumatology and the Chapel Hill Consensus Conference [1] but they do not allow diagnosis *per se* but only classification of a distinct vasculitic entity. In addition, the majority of vasculitides lack specific markers but have "indicators" as shown in Table 110.2. In **primary vasculitis**, the type of vasculitis is directly related to the size of the inflamed vessel, whereas **secondary vasculitides** can be directly associated with rheumatic or connective tissue diseases, malignant diseases, infections, toxic substances and drugs. Diagnosis of **antiphospholipid syndrome** is usually based on the occurrence of venous or arterial thrombosis or a history of fetal loss in combination with the respective antiphospholipid antibodies [7].

Diagnostic methods
Aside emergency laboratory parameters in life-threatening situations such as complete obstruction of a major intestinal artery or in catastrophic antiphospholipid syndrome, it is recommended to measure serum concentrations for lactate and coagulation parameters as well as **"disease-specific" parameters** (Table 110.2). Subsequently, every patient suspected of having ischemia should receive an **ECG, ultrasound including Doppler, and CT** of the abdomen to facilitate diagnosis of ileus, intestinal edema and perforation. As soon as mesenteric ischemia is likely, **angiography** and subsequent **surgical intervention** should be performed (Figure 110.3).

Treatment and prevention
Necrosis of the intestine requires immediate **surgical intervention** and in subacute progressive mesenteric ischemia, both surgical as well as interventional **radiologic strategies** including balloon dilatation, embolectomy or bypass surgery of the affected mesenteric vessel should be performed. Immunosuppressive therapy should start immediately as soon as diagnosis of vasculitis is established. Table 110.3 shows an overview of current medication in vasculitis including current recommendations [8,9]. **Corticosteroids** are still the drug of choice to induce remission. They should be applied at high doses (at least 1 mg/kg body weight). In primary vasculitides such as GPA and polyarteritis nodosa, **cyclophosphamide** in a dosage of 2 mg/kg body weight frequently needs to be added. Tapering of steroids after improvement of symptoms and inflammatory parameters is mandatory but can take years. However the long-term daily dose of prednisolone equivalent should not exceed 5 mg.

Although predominantly used in an off-label setting, to maintain remission, **disease-modifying immunosuppressive drugs** need to be considered when the daily corticoid dose that

is the predominantely affected part of the large intestine, investigation of the colon is an important part of the clinical evaluation. **Opaque markers** (Sitz markers) can be used to measure transit times, **rectal manometry** evaluates the involvement and extent of rectal fibrosis in systemic sclerosis patients and **sigmoido/colonoscopy** reveals also structural alterations of the large intestine. In patients with intestinal pseudoobstruction, **CT** as illustrated in Figure 110.6, reveals the intensive thickening of the intestinal mucosa.

Table 110.6 Methods that have been proven to be reliable for evaluation of involvement of gastrointestinal (GI) tract in systemic sclerosis

Method	Evaluation of
Esophageal manometry	Esophageal dysmotility, sphincter pressure
24-hour pH monitoring	Extent of gastroesophageal reflux
Gastroscopy	Structural gastroesophagal alterations
Barium opaque meal	Gastroesophageal motility
Small bowel barium follow-through X-ray	Intestinal motility
D-Xylose test, jejunal cultures, H₂ glucose and lactulose breath tests	Malabsorption and bacterial overgrowth
Opaque (Sitz) markers	Intestinal transit time intestinal pseudoobstruction
Rectal manometry	Rectal fibrosis
Sigmoido/colonoscopy	Structural alterations
CT	Intestinal pseudo-obstruction

Treatment and prevention

Currently, no evidence-based disease-modifying regimen for systemic sclerosis exists [17]. In contrast, several therapeutic approaches for the individual organs of the GI tract have proven to be effective [17,18]. A (secondary) **sicca syndrome** requires treatment with artificial saliva, and due to the high risk for development of **caries**, these patients should see a dentist on a 6-monthly basis. **Gastroesophageal reflux** symptoms should be treated effectively with (high-dose) proton pump inhibitors. Reduced **intestinal motility** should be treated with prokinetic drugs such as metoclopramide, domperidone, erythromycin and octreotide [19], but needs to be evaluated for each patient separately, especially in cases suffering from intestinal pseudoobstruction. **Stenoses** of the GI tract, regardless whether in the esophagus, stomach, small and large intestine, and the anus, can be treated mechanically with balloon dilatation.

Complications and their management

The prognosis in terms of life expectancy and quality of life is frequently determined by intestinal and visceral involvement. In particular, **intestinal pseudo-obstruction** with subsequent ileus can develop into a life-threatening situation. Rapid conservative non-surgical decompression using a nasogastral suction in combination with prokinetics can avoid surgical intervention. Untreated reflux esophagitis can lead to acute esophageal bleeding and chronic esophagitis can be the initiation of Barrett dysplasia and adenocarcinoma. Table 110.7 summarizes the current recommendations for management of GI involvement in SSc.

Prognosis with and without treatment

In general, the extent of reduction in overall health status and quality of life in systemic diseases ranges from minor temporary sequelae to acute life-threatening conditions regardless

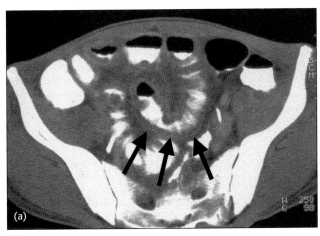
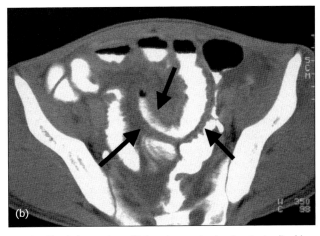

Figure 110.6 Significant thickening (arrows) of the small and large bowel due to intensive fibrosis in a patient with long-term systemic sclerosis visualized by CT (Figure provided by Prof. S. Feuerbach, Institute for Radiology, University of Regensburg).

Table 110.7 EULAR/EUSTAR recommendations for SSc-related gastrointestinal disease. (Modified from Kowal-Bielecka O, Landewé R, Avouac J, et al. and EUSTAR coauthors. EULAR recommendations for the treatment of systemic sclerosis: a report from the EULAR Scleroderma Trials and Research group (EUSTAR). *Ann Rheum Dis.* 2009;68:620–628, with permission from BMJ Publishing Group Ltd.)

Recommendation	Strength of recommendation
1. PPI should be used for the prevention of SSc-related gastroesophageal reflux, esophageal ulcers and strictures	B
2. Prokinetic drugs should be used for the management of SSc-related symptomatic motility disturbances (dysphagia, GERD, early satiety, bloating, pseudo-obstruction, etc)	C
3. In bacterial overgrowth, rotating antibiotics may be useful in SSc patients	D

whether the individual symptoms origin from the GI tract or from other organs [16]. Aside from severe complications, prognosis of all systemic diseases with regard to mortality and morbidity can be good when adequate stage-dependent and long-term monitoring and treatment of the patient is applied. On the other hand, similar to other long-term disabling diseases, quality of life is significantly reduced in the majority of patients if no long-term remission can be achieved.

SOURCES OF INFORMATION FOR PATIENTS AND DOCTORS

- First, it is essential to explain to the patients the nature and course of GI symptoms in the context of the underlying systemic disease
- Second, the need for life-long monitoring (and potentially treatment) by experts in the individual discipline should be underlined
- Third, due to the predominant immunologic background of the systemic diseases, the patients should be made aware that any environmental alteration, especially infections, can activate the underlying disease and subsequently the involvement of the GI tract, which then should result in immediate contact with the treating physician. Adequate routine vaccination is therefore also mandatory
- Fourth, recently developed recommendations of the scientific societies should be distributed amongst physicians and patients' associations

References

1. Müller-Ladner, U. (2001)Vasculitides of the gastrointestinal tract, in *Bailliere's Best Practice & Research Clinical Gastroenterology*, Vol. 15 (eds J. Schölmerich *et al.*), Bailliere Tindall, Eastbourne, pp. 59–82.
2. Dalle I, Geboes K. Vascular lesions of the gastrointestinal tract. *Acta Gastroenterol Belg.* 2002;64:213–219.
3. Ebert EC. Gastric and enteric involvement in progressive systemic sclerosis. *J Clin Gastroenterol.* 2008;42:5–12.
4. Gonzalez-Gay MA, Vazquez-Rodriguez TR, Miranda-Filloy JA, *et al.* Localized vasculitis of the gastrointestinal tract: A case report and literature review. 2008;26(3 Suppl 49):S101–S104.
5. Cohen S, Laufer I, Snape WJ, *et al.* The gastrointestinal manifestations of scleroderma. Pathogenesis and management. *Gastroenterology.* 1980;769:155–166.
6. Müller-Ladner U, Distler O, Ibba-Manneschi I, *et al.* Mechanisms of vascular damage in systemic sclerosis. *Autoimmunity.* 2009;42:587–595.
7. Uthman I, Khamashta M. The abdominal manifestations of the antiphospholipid syndrome. *Rheumatology.* 2007;46:1641–1647.
8. Mukhtyar C, Guillevin L, Cid MC, *et al.* For the European Vasculitis Study Group. EULAR recommendations for the management of primary small and medium vessel vasculitis. *Ann Rheum Dis.* 2009;68:310–317.
9. Mukhtyar C, Guillevin L, Cid MC, *et al.* For the European Vasculitis Study Group. EULAR recommendations for the management of large vessel vasculitis. *Ann Rheum Dis.* 2009;68:318–323.
10. Hunzelmann N, Genth E, Kreig T, *et al.* for the Registry of the German Network for Systemic Scleroderma. The registry of the German Network for Systemic Scleroderma: Frequency of disease subsets and patterns of organ involvement. *Rheumatology.* 2008;47:1185–1192.
11. Manetti M, Neumann E, Milia AF, *et al.* Severe fibrosis and increased expression of fibrogenic cytokines in the gastric wall of systemic sclerosis patients. *Arthritis Rheum.* 2007;56:3442–3447.
12. Manetti M, Neumann E, Müller A, *et al.* Endothelial/lymphocyte activation leads to a prominent CD4+ T cell infiltration in the gastric mucosa of patients with systemic sclerosis. *Arthritis Rheum.* 2008;58:2866–2873.
13. Iovino P, Valentini G, Giacci C, *et al.* Proximal stomach function in systemic sclerosis: Relationship with autonomic nerve function. *Dig Dis Sci.* 2001;46:723–730.
14. Lock G, Holstege A, Lang B, Schölmerich J. Gastrointestinal manifestations of progressive systemic sclerosis. *Am J Gastroenterol.* 1997;92:763–777.
15. Clements PJ, Becvar R, Drosos AA, *et al.* Assessment of gastrointestinal involvement. *Clin Exp Rheumatol.* 2003;21(Suppl 29):S15–S18.
16. Walker UA, Tyndall A, Czirják L, *et al.* and EUSTAR co-authors. Clinical risk assessment of organ manifestations in systemic sclerosis – a report from the EULAR Scleroderma Trials and Research (EUSTAR) group database. *Ann Rheum Dis.* 2007;66:754–763.
17. Kowal-Bielecka O, Landewé R, Avouac J, *et al.* and EUSTAR coauthors. EULAR recommendations for the treatment of systemic sclerosis: a report from the EULAR Scleroderma Trials and Research group (EUSTAR). *Ann Rheum Dis.* 2009;68:620–628.
18. Wollheim FA, Akesson A. Management of intestinal involvement in systemic sclerosis. *J Clin Rheumatol.* 2007;13:116–118.
19. Nikou GC, Toumpanakis C, Katsiari C, *et al.* Treatment of small intestinal disease in systemic sclerosis with octreotide: a prospective study in seven patients. *J Clin Rheumatol.* 2007;13:119–123.

Multiple Organ Systems

CHAPTER 111

Systemic disease and the gastrointestinal tract

Paul J. Fortun

Royal Cornwall Hospitals NHS Trust, Truro, UK

ESSENTIAL FACTS ABOUT PATHOGENESIS

- In critical illness, compromise to intestinal barrier function and mucosal perfusion contribute to the systemic inflammatory response and multiorgan failure
- Intestinal ischemia and increased gut permeability are a consequence of and exacerbating factor in congestive heart failure.
- Motility disorders and intestinal failure are common in connective tissue diseases
- The gut microbiota is an emerging theme for understanding the relationship between systemic disease and the gut

---

ESSENTIALS OF DIAGNOSIS

- Systemic inflammation, evidence of multiorgan involvement, and continuous abdominal pain are important clues to the diagnosis of gut vasculitis

---

Introduction

Gastrointestinal (GI) involvement by systemic disease is extremely common. The impact of critical illness has an acute effect on gut mucosal barrier function, mucosal perfusion, and the systemic inflammatory response. The effect of chronic diseases is discussed with particular reference to the impact of connective tissue diseases on gut motility and permeability, and the gastrointestinal manifestations of systemic vasculitis.

Pathophysiology

Mucosal defence

A dynamic equilibrium of physical and humoral mechanisms maintains mucosal defence and repair. Cytoprotective prostaglandins and adequate mucosal perfusion are vital to maintaining a physical and chemical barrier, and coordinate healing when this barrier is breached. Mucosal barrier function is maintained by a combination of prostaglandin and nitric oxide-mediated mechanisms [1].

The gut microbiota and defence

The microbiota is a host-specific community of billions of commensal microorganisms important in normal health, whose response to stress and injury can lead to disease and multisystem failure [2]. Intricate mechanisms facilitate a state of tolerance to gut commensals via induction of a TH2 phenotype and regulatory T cells by dendritic cells, whilst avoiding concurrent damaging systemic immune responses [3]. Alteration in the composition of commensal microflora may predispose to autoimmune disease [4]. The microbiota protects against potential pathogens by competitive exclusion, and the production of antimicrobial peptides or defensins. An imbalance in the microbiota (dysbiosis) is seen in response to sepsis and trauma [5] and has numerous adverse sequelae, including availability of nutrients in the intestine, modifying the immune response, and susceptibility to invading opportunistic pathogens [6].

Mucosal perfusion

The maintenance of mucosal perfusion is vital in protecting normal gut mucosa and healing of damaged mucosa. The stomach and intestine are however relatively poor autoregulators of blood flow. Animal studies suggest that the adaptive response of maintaining gastric perfusion in the face of alteration in perfusion pressure is largely independent of neuronal innervation, and closely correlated with intrinsic metabolic mechanisms, such as gastric acid production, prostaglandins, nitric oxide, and other endogenous chemical mediators. Mucosal blood flow in the stomach is regulated by prostaglandin E2 (PGE2) (increased flow) and PGI2 (decreased), whilst nitric oxide increases mucosal blood flow [7].

In addition to the lack of autoregulation, the intestinal mucosa is vulnerable to ischemic injury due to oxygen shunting, leading to blunting of villi, and hypoxemia in mucosal capillaries [8]. Hypovolemia leads to activation of the renin–angiotensin–aldosterone axis and the sympathetic nervous system, which exacerbate splanchnic hypoperfusion by vasoconstriction and redistribution of blood. Splanchnic hypoperfusion produces an imbalance between oxygen supply and demand, leading to mucosal damage and altered GI motility [9].

The effect of shock and hypotension on gastric perfusion can be assessed by monitoring gastric tonometry, a relatively

Textbook of Clinical Gastroenterology and Hepatology, Second Edition. Edited by C. J. Hawkey, Jaime Bosch, Joel E. Richter, Guadalupe Garcia-Tsao, Francis K. L. Chan.

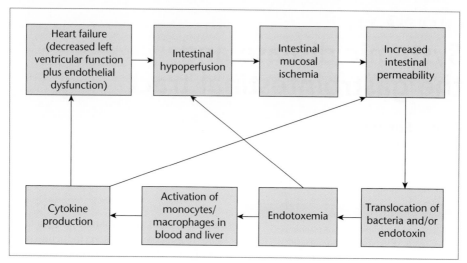

Figure 111.1 Role of the gut in perpetuating congestive heart failure. (Reproduced from Krack A, Sharma R, Figulla HR, Anker SD. The importance of the gastrointestinal system in the pathogenesis of heart failure. *Eur Heart J.* 2005 Nov;26(22):2368–2374. Epub 2005 Jun 24, with permission from Oxford University Press.)

non-invasive measure of the adequacy of aerobic metabolism in the gut mucosa. A low gastric intramucosal pH is a sensitive marker of splanchnic hypoperfusion and a good predictor of poor outcome in critically ill patients [10].

Critical illness and the gastrointestinal tract

The effects of systemic disease on the GI tract are most clearly demonstrated in the context of the extreme physiological stress of critical illness, in particular with shock.

Clinical sequelae of gut mucosal ischemia

Stress ulceration occurs where a breach in mucosal defences allows harm by gastric secretions (acid and pepsin). In critically ill patients, stress ulceration is the most common cause of GI bleeding, seen in up to 14% [11]. Most (74–100%) patients will have minor, endoscopically detectable mucosal erosions in the proximal stomach within 24 hours of admission to the intensive care unit (ICU) [12], but prolonged physiological stress leads to overt ulceration in the antrum [4]. Stress ulceration is associated with worse outcome, longer ICU stay, and prolonged ventilation, [6] but the causal relationship is unclear. Inpatient gastrointestinal bleeding has a high associated mortality of up to 64% [11].

Mechanical ventilation can further compromise perfusion and therefore mucosal integrity. Positive end expiratory pressure (PEEP) ventilation increases intrathoracic pressure and decreases venous return, and therefore decreases cardiac output [13]. In animal models, mechanical ventilation causes ischemic pancreatitis, although in humans this may be confined to subclinical elevations of lipase and amylase [9].

Loss of barrier function and the systemic inflammatory response

The mucosal and hepatic ischemia of critical illness may initiate and sustain multiorgan failure (MOF) through the systemic inflammatory response (SIR). The intestinal mucosa develops a form of non-occlusive ischemia with enterocyte damage, disruption of tight junction complexes, and subsequent failure of the gut barrier. This permits the translocation of endotoxin and microorganisms into the portal venous and local lymphatic circulation [14]. The subsequent release of cytokines, such as tumour necrosis factor (TNF), interleukin-1, and interleukin-6, by hepatic Kupffer cells and circulating monocytes initiates a sequence of events that culminates in the clinical picture of sepsis and MOF. Intracellular proteins that are released from damaged enterocytes further perpetuate the SIR syndrome [15].

Congestive heart failure

Congestive heart failure (CHF) is associated with anorexia and weight loss which have been attributed to mucosal edema in the gut. Mucosal edema and hypoperfusion increase intestinal permeability, allowing translocation of bacteria and endotoxemia, which further exacerbates cardiac failure. Patients with CHF have elevated endotoxin levels which normalize following diuretic treatment, suggesting that bowel wall edema may contribute to the endotoxemia in this condition [16]. This self-perpetuating pathogenic pathway is shown in Figure 111.1. Altered intestinal permeability can, if severe, cause a protein-losing enteropathy.

In addition to the effects of CHF on the intestinal permeability, cardiac cachexia is associated with raised circulating TNF [17], and independently with increased mortality in cardiac failure [18].

Liver

Hepatic dysfunction is common in critically ill patients [19], and along with mesenteric ischemia contributes to MOF. In CHF, increased right atrial pressure leads to hepatic congestion, with cholestatic liver enzymes commonly elevated [20]. Cardiac cirrhosis occurs when prolonged, severe right-sided

CHF leads to chronic inflammation and fibrosis, producing histologically a "nutmeg liver."

The common final pathway of liver injury (e.g., infection, ischemia) is a polymorphonuclear inflammatory response with proinflammatory mediators, which further promote neutrophilic hepatitis and tissue damage [21]. Kupffer cell activation by complement factors and neutrophil recruitment leads to the formation of reactive oxygen species, such as lipid peroxidase products, which in turn recruit more neutrophils and aggravate the inflammatory injury.

Non-hemorrhagic complications

Acute acalculous cholecystitis is increasingly recognized in the ICU, at a rate of 0.2–3% [22]. Risk factors include shock, sepsis, multiple transfusions, dehydration, starvation, total parenteral nutrition, and medications (e.g., opiates, cephalosporins) [22]. Prolonged fasting and ischemia impair gallbladder emptying leading to biliary stasis and sludge formation.

Ulcerative esophagitis occurs in half of patients receiving mechanical ventilation, accounting for a quarter of all upper GI bleeding in the ICU [23]. Causative factors include gastric acid and bile reflux, supine position, and delayed gastric emptying. Nasogastric tubes cause mucosal erosions and impair esophageal motility and sphincter function. Almost two-thirds of ICU patients receiving enteral feeding develop GI complications, in particular delayed gastric emptying (39%) and constipation (15%) [24].

Chronic systemic disease and the gastrointestinal tract

Connective tissue diseases

The GI tract is commonly affected by connective tissue diseases (CTDs) such as systemic sclerosis, and is the second commonest site affected (after the skin) [25]. Smooth muscle atrophy and, to a lesser degree, fibrosis [26] have widespread effects, from esophageal dysmotility and delayed gastric emptying to life-threatening complications such as intestinal failure, malabsorption syndrome [e.g., small intestinal bacterial overgrowth (SIBO)], and pseudo-obstruction [27]. SIBO can be demonstrated in 55% of patients [28]. In a large Canadian series (n = 586 patients), 18% of patients were at high risk of malnutrition [29]. Scleroderma is commonly associated with dysphagia, in particular esophageal dysmotility (as in CREST syndrome). Systemic sclerosis is also associated with upper GI blood loss due to gastric antral vascular ectasia (GAVE).

Dysmotility

The extent of motility disorders with CTDs and other systemic diseases is shown in Table 111.1.

The commonest example of abnormal gastric and intestinal motility encountered clinically is in **diabetic patients**, with up to 50% affected. In addition to autonomic neuropathy, metabolic derangements (hyperglycemia and hyperinsulinemia) impair gastric and small intestinal motility [34].

Table 111.1 Systemic diseases associated with gut dysmotility

Systemic sclerosis	Dysphagia (90%) [30]
Dermatomyositis	Dysphagia (50–70%) [31]
Amyloidosis	70% [32]
Parkinson disease	30% [33]
Diabetes	Gastroparesis (50%) [34]
Thyroid disease	Diarrhea (20% hyperthyroid patients) [35] Constipation in hypothyroid
Familial visceral myopathies	100%, e.g., MNGIE syndrome [36]

In **degenerative diseases**, such as mitochondrial neurogastrointestinal encephalopathy and familial visceral myopathy [36], there is neural or muscle involvement. In diseases such as amyloidosis there is infiltration of blood vessels leading to infarction and ulceration, muscle deposition leading to abnormal motility [37], and neural involvement (especially hereditary forms) leading to gut neuropathy. GI symptoms such as abnormal salivation (31%), dysphagia (16%), nausea and vomiting (10%), constipation (27%), and defecatory dysfunction (11%) are common in patients with Parkinson disease [37], where symptoms correlate with disease severity rather than treatment, suggesting direct involvement in the GI tract by the primary disease process [38]. Delayed gastric emptying is especially problematic for drug absorption, and antiparkinsonian medications themselves have GI side effects.

Gut permeability

In addition to abnormal motility, CTD may be associated with increased gut permeability. The association between non-steroidal anti-inflammatory drugs (NSAIDs) and small bowel enteropathy is well recognized, affecting almost two-thirds of rheumatoid patients on NSAIDs [39]. Patients who are not on NSAIDs have mostly normal small intestinal permeability [40]. However, intriguingly there may also be a relationship between the underlying rheumatological condition and small bowel pathology, since relatives of patients with ankylosing spondylitis have abnormal small bowel permeability [41]. This may partially explain the finding that the risk of serious GI complications is higher for rheumatoid than osteoarthritis patients [42].

Autoimmune disease

Vasculitis affecting the gastrointestinal tract is often occult, requiring a high index of suspicion. Signs of systemic inflammation, multiorgan involvement and continuous abdominal pain are important clues to the diagnosis.

All three major categories of vasculitis can affect the gut. Large-vessel vasculitides (e.g., giant-cell arteritis) are rarely

Multiple Organ Systems

Table 111.2 Frequency of gastrointestinal involvement in systemic vasculitides

Frequency of intestinal involvement	Type of vasculitis
Up to 65%	Henoch–Schönlein purpura
Up to 50%	Polyarteritis nodosa, Churg–Strauss syndrome, systemic lupus erythematosus
Up to 30%	Behçet's syndrome
5–15%	Takayasu's arteritis, Wegener's granulomatosis, vasculitis in rheumatoid arthritis
Less than 5%	Lymphomatoid granulomatosis, giant cell arteritis, thromboangiitis obliterans

Reproduced with permission from Müller-Ladner U., Scholmerich, J. Systemic disease and the gut. In: Weinstein WM, Hawkey CJ, Bosch J, editors), *Clinical Gastroenterology and Hepatology*. St Louis: Elsevier Mosby, 2005, Chapter 108.

associated with small bowel infarction. **Polyarteritis nodosa (PAN)** [43], a medium-vessel disease, and **Henoch-Schönlein purpura (HSP)**, a small vessel disease, are the vasculitides most frequently associated with abdominal manifestations (Table 111.2). In immune complex vasculitis, deposition in arterioles in the intestinal wall lead to the abdominal pain common in HSP, cryoglobulinemic, and serum sickness vasculitis. Abdominal pain is the second most frequent symptom in HSP, observed in 50–65% of patients [44], and is the presenting complaint in 10–15%. The abdominal pain may mimic an acute abdomen in terms of severity. The pain is typically colicky and occurs about 1 week after the onset of the rash. Vomiting and GI bleeding occur in 30% of patients [45] and intussusception may also occur around a mural hematoma. GI involvement is also reported in 7% of patients with hepatitis C virus (HCV)-related vasculitis [46] due to cryoglobulinemia.

Conclusions

The impact of systemic disease on the gut is widespread and common. In the intensive care setting, critically ill patients have compromised gut barrier function that contributes to the SIR, multiorgan failure, and a high risk of gastrointestinal bleeding. Cardiac failure has a similar effect on gut defence and increased gut permeability leads to impaired survival. In chronic illness such as CTD and vasculitis, gastrointestinal dysfunction through abnormal motility and ischemia are important clinical manifestations.

References

1. Wallace JL. Cooperative modulation of gastrointestinal mucosal defence by prostaglandins and nitric oxide. *Clin Invest Med.* 1996;19:346–351.
2. Sekirov I, Russell SL, Antunes LCM, Finlay BB. Gut microbiota in health and disease. *Physiol Rev.* 2010;90:859–904.
3. Kelsall BL, Leon F. Involvement of intestinal dendritic cells in oral tolerance, immunity to pathogens, and inflammatory bowel disease. *Immunol Rev.* 2005;206:132–148.
4. Elliott DE, Summers RW, Weinstock JV. Helminths as governors of immune-mediated inflammation. *Int J Parasitol.* 2007;37:457–464.
5. Shimizu K, Ogura H, Goto M, et al. Altered gut flora and environment in patients with severe SIRS. *J Trauma.* 2006;60:126-33.
6. Finlay B, Sekirov I. The role of the intestinal microbiota in enteric infection. *J Physiol.* 2009;587:4159–4167.
7. Pique JM, Whittle BJ, Esplugues JV. The vasodilator role of endogenous nitric oxide in the rat gastric microcirculation. *Eur J Pharmacol.* 1989;19:293–296.
8. Takala J. Determinants of splanchnic blood flow. *Br J Anaesth.* 1996;77:50–58.
9. Mutlu EA, Factor P. GI complications in patients receiving mechanical ventilation. *Chest.* 2001;119:1222–1241
10. Gutierrez G. Gastric intramucosal pH as a therapeutic index of tissue oxygenation in critically ill patients. *Lancet.* 1992;339:195–99.
11. Schuster DP, Rowley H, Feinstein S, et al. Prospective evaluation of the risk of upper gastrointestinal bleeding after admission to a medical intensive care unit. *Am J Med.* 1984;76:623–630.
12. Lucas CE, Sugawa C, Riddle J, et al. Natural history and surgical dilemma of "stress" gastric bleeding. *Arch Surg.* 1971;102:266–273.
13. Love R, Choe E, Lippton H, et al. Positive end-expiratory pressure decreases mesenteric blood flow despite normalization of cardiac output. *J Trauma.* 1995;39:195–199.
14. Knaus WA, Draper EA, Wagner DP, et al. Prognosis in acute organ-system failure. *Ann Surg.* 1985;202:685–693.
15. Moore FA: The role of the gastrointestinal tract in postinjury multiple organ failure. *Am J Surg.* 1999;178:449–445.
16. Krack A, Sharma R, Figulla HR, Anker SD The importance of the gastrointestinal system in the pathogenesis of heart failure. *Eur Heart J.* 2005;26:2368–2374
17. Levine, B, Kalman, J, Mayer, L, et al. Elevated circulating levels of tumor necrosis factor in severe chronic heart failure. *N Engl J Med.* 1990;323:236–241.
18. Anker SD, Coats AJ. Cardiac cachexia: a syndrome with impaired survival and immune and neuroendocrine activation. *Chest.* 1999;115:836–847.
19. Abrahamsson H. Gastrointestinal motility disorders in patients with diabetes mellitus. *J Intern Med.* 1995;237:403–409.
20. Kubo S, Walter B, John D, et al. Liver function abnormalities in chronic heart failure: influence of systemic hemodynamics. *Arch Intern Med.* 1987;147:1227–1230.
21. Jaeschke H. Mechanisms of liver injury. II. Mechanisms of neutrophil-induced liver cell injury during hepatic ischemia-reperfusion and other acute inflammatory conditions. *Am J Physiol Gastrointest Liver Physiol.* 2006;290:G1083–1088.
22. Stevens PE, Harrison NA, Rainford DJ. Acute acalculous cholecystitis in acute renal failure. *Intensive Care Med.* 1988;14:411–416.
23. Wilmer A, Tack J, Frans E, et al. Duodenogastroesophageal reflux and oesophageal mucosal injury in mechanically ventilated patients. *Gastroenterology.* 1999;116:1293–1299.
24. Montejo JC. Enteral nutrition-related gastrointestinal complications in critically ill patients: a multicenter study: *Crit Care Med.* 1999;27:1447–1453

25. Marie I. Gastrointestinal involvement in systemic sclerosis. *Presse Med.* 2006;35:1952–1965.

26. Rose S, Young MA, Reynolds JC. Gastrointestinal manifestations of scleroderma. *Gastroenterol Clin North Am.* 1998;27: 563–594.

27. Sjogren RW. Gastrointestinal motility disorders in scleroderma. *Arthritis Rheum.* 1994;37:1265–1282.

28. Parodi A, Sessarego M, Greco A, *et al.* Small intestinal bacterial overgrowth in patients suffering from scleroderma: clinical effectiveness of its eradication. *Am J Gastroenterol.* 2008;103: 1257–1262.

29. Baron M, Hudson M, Steele R; Canadian Scleroderma Research Group. Malnutrition is common in systemic sclerosis: results from the Canadian scleroderma research group database. *J Rheumatol.* 2009;36:2737–2743.

30. Stellaard F, Sauerbruch T, Lunderschmidt CH, *et al.* Intestinal involvement in progressive systemic sclerosis. *Gut.* 1987;28: 446–450.

31. O'Hara J, Szemes G, Lowman R. Oesophageal abnormalities and dysphagia in polymyositis and dermatomyositis. *Radiology.* 1967;89:27–31.

32. Battle W, Rubin M, Cohen S, *et al.* Gastrointestinal motility dysfunction in amyloidosis. *N Engl J Med.* 1979;301:24–25.

33. Rodríguez-Violante M, Cervantes-Arriaga A, Villar-Velarde A, Corona T. Prevalence of non-motor dysfunction among Parkinson's disease patients from a tertiary referral center in Mexico City. *Clin Neurol Neurosurg.* 2010;112:883–885.

34. Shafer R, Prentiss R, Bond K. Gastrointestinal transit in thyroid disease. *Gastroenterology.* 1984;86:852–855.

35. Nishino I, Spinazzola A, Papadimitriou A, *et al.* Mitochondrial neurogastrointestinal encephalomyopathy: an autosomal recessive disorder due to thymidine phosphorylase mutations. *Ann Neurol.* 2000;47:792–800.

36. Lovat LB, Pepys MB, Hawkins PN. Amyloid and the gut. *Dig Dis.* 1997;15:155–171.

37. Barone P, Antonini A, Colosimo C, *et al.* The PRIAMO study: A multicenter assessment of nonmotor symptoms and their impact on quality of life in Parkinson's disease. *Mov Disord.* 2009;24: 1641–1649.

38. Edwards LL. Gastrointestinal symptoms in Parkinson's disease. *Mov Disord.* 1991;6:151–156.

39. Bjarnason I, Hayllar J, MacPherson AJ, Russell AS. Side effects of NSAIDs on the small and large intestine in humans. *Gastroenterology.* 1993;104:1832–1847.

40. Jenkins RT, Rooney PJ, Jones DB, *et al.* Increased intestinal permeability in patients with rheumatoid arthritis: a side-effect of oral NSAID therapy? *Br J Rheumatol.* 1987;26:103–107.

41. Vaile JH, Meddings JB, Yacyshyn BR, *et al.* Bowel permeability and CD45RO expression on circulating CD20+ B cells in patients with ankylosing spondylitis and their relatives. *J Rheumatol.* 1999;26:128–135.

42. Singh G, Rosen Ramey D. NSAID induced gastrointestinal complications: the ARAMIS perspective–1997. Arthritis, Rheumatism, and Aging Medical Information System. *J Rheumatol* 1998;51(Suppl):8–16.

43. Camilleri M, Pusey CD, Chadwick VS, Rees AJ. Gastrointestinal manifestations of systemic vasculitis. *Q J Med.* 1983;52:141–149.

44. Saulsbury FT. Clinical update: Henoch-Schönlein purpura. *Lancet.* 2007;369:976–978.

45. Bailey M, Chapin W, Licht H, Reynolds JC. The effects of vasculitis on the gastrointestinal tract and liver. *Gastroenterol Clin North Am.* 1998;27:747–782.

46. Terrier B, Saadoun D, Sène D, *et al.* Presentation and outcome of gastrointestinal involvement in hepatitis C virus-related systemic vasculitis: a case-control study from a single-centre cohort of 163 patients. *Gut.* 2010;59:1709–1715.

Multiple Organ Systems

CHAPTER 112
Pancreatic endocrine tumors

Robert T. Jensen

Digestive Diseases Branch, National Institute of Diabetes and Kidney Diseases, National Institutes of Health, Bethesda, MD, USA

ESSENTIAL FACTS ABOUT PATHOGENESIS

- Prevalence is approximately 10 per million population
- Most commonly sporadic but may be associated with multiple endocrine neoplasia, type 1, Von Hippel–Lindau, von Recklinghausen's disease, and tuberous sclerosis
- The functional pancreatic endocrine tumors (PETs) cause symptoms by ectopic hormone release but non-functional PETs are more common
- Malignant change occurs in >50% of PETs other than insulinomas
- Epidemiology: non-functional PETs (NF-PETs) are more common than functional PETs, whose relative order is: insulinoma > gastrinoma > VIPomas > glucagonomas > somatostatinomas, others
- Genetic factors: four inherited disorders are associated with increased PETs: multiple endocrine neoplasia type 1 (MEN1), Von Hippel–Lindau disease (VHL), von Recklinghausen's disease, [neurofibromatosis I (NF-1)], tuberous sclerosis
- Pathogenesis: functional PET symptoms are primarily due to ectopic hormone release; NF-PET symptoms are due to the tumor itself

ESSENTIALS OF DIAGNOSIS

- Functional PETs should be suspected from appropriate hormonal symptoms (in order of frequency): insulinoma (hypoglycemia); gastrinoma (hyperacidity symptoms with or without diarrhea); VIPoma (watery diarrhea and hypokalemia); glucagonoma (dermatitis, glucose intolerance/diabetes mellitus, weight loss); somatostatinoma (diabetes mellitus, gallbladder disease, diarrhea, steatorrhea)
- NF-PETs usually remain silent and present late
- Diagnostic steps include: raised specific hormone in fasting blood collected into Trasylol; non-functional PETs almost always secrete chromogranin A or B; localization of tumor by CT, MRI, somatostatin receptor scintigraphy (SRS), ultrasound or angiography; functional localization by venous hormonal gradients; immunohistochemical demonstration of neuroendocrine tumor markers (chromogranin, synaptophysin)
- SRS is the modality of choice for localizing primary and metastatic tumors
- Positron emission tomographic scanning with labeled somatostatin analogs will likely be increasingly used

ESSENTIALS OF TREATMENT

- Surgical removal of the tumor where possible
- Functional treatment of hormone excess state: insulinoma – diazoxide, miradvil, diphenylhydantoin, somatostatin analogs; gastrinoma – high-dose proton pump inhibitors; VIPomas – long-acting somatostatin analogs or other (octreotide/lanreotide); glucagonomas – long-acting somatostatin analogs; somatostatinomas – octreotide

Introduction

Pancreatic endocrine tumors (PETs) belong to the group gastroenteropancreatic endocrine tumors (GEPs) that originate from the diffuse neuroendocrine system of the gastrointestinal tract, which is comprised of various amine- and peptide-producing cells. GEP tumors were originally classified as APUDomas (amine precursor uptake and decarboxylation) as were carcinoids, PETs, pheochromocytomas, and melanomas because they share a number of features (Table 112.1) [1]. This chapter focuses on PETs (carcinoid tumors are the subject of Chapter 113). The different PETs share many common aspects of treatment, localization, and approach to/treatment of advanced disease. These will be generally discussed together, with specific aspects described in the separate sections.

Epidemiology and classification

PETs can be classified into nine well-established functional syndromes, four possible functional syndromes, and non-functional tumors (NF-PETs) (Table 112.2) [1]. Each functional syndrome is characterized by specific symptoms due to the ectopically secreted hormone (Table 112.2). NF-PETs secrete no products that cause a specific clinical syndrome. The symptoms caused by NF-PETs are entirely due to the tumor *per se*.

The prevalence of clinically significant PETs is approximately 10 cases per million, the most common being insulinomas, gastrinomas, and NF-PETs, with each having an incidence of 0.5–2 cases per million per year. VIPomas are two to eight times less common, glucagonomas are 17–30 times less

Table 112.1 General characteristics of gastroenteropancreatic (GEP) endocrine tumors [pancreatic endocrine tumors (PETs) and carcinoids]

- Share general neuroendocrine cell markers:
  - Chromogranins (A, B, C) are acidic monomeric soluble proteins (MW 49 000) found in the large secretory granules. Chromogranin A is generally used
  - Synaptophysin is a membrane glycoprotein (MW 38 000) found in small vesicles of neurons and GEPs
- Similarities in biological behavior:
  - Generally slow growing, but a proportion are aggressive
  - Secrete biologically active peptides/amines, which can cause clinical symptoms
  - Generally have high densities of somatostatin receptors ($sst_{2,3,5}$) which are used for localization and in treatment
- Pathological similarities:
  - All are APUDomas showing Amine Precursor Uptake and Decarboxylation
  - Ultrastructurally they have dense-core secretory granules (>80 nm)
  - Histologically appear similar with few mitoses and uniform nuclei
  - Frequently synthesize multiple peptides/amines which are detected immunocytochemically but may not be secreted
  - Presence or absence of clinical syndrome or type cannot be predicted from immunocytochemical studies
  - Generally histology is not predictive of biological behavior. Only invasion or metastases establishes malignancy
- Similarities in molecular abnormalities:
  - Uncommon – alterations in common oncogenes (*Ras, Jun, Fos*, etc.) or in common tumor suppressor genes (*p53, retinoblastoma*)
  - Alterations at *MEN1* gene locus (11q13) and p16^{INK4a} (9p21) occur in a proportion (10–30%)
  - Methylation of various genes occurs in 40–80%
- Differences in molecular abnormalities of carcinoids/PETs:
  - PETs – frequent chromosomal loss of 3p (8–47%), 3q (8–41%), 11q (21–62%), 6q (18–68%). Frequent gains at 17q (10–55%), 7q (16–68%)
  - Carcinoids – frequent chromosomal loss of 18q (38–70%), 18p (30–40%), 11q (21–62%), 9p, 16q (20%). Frequent gains at 17q, 19p (10–55%), 7q (60%)

common, and somatostatinomas are the least common. In autopsy studies, 0.5–1.5% of all individuals have a pancreatic PET, but in fewer than 1 in 1000 of the cases is a functional tumor thought to occur. PETs, except for insulinomas, commonly (>50%) show malignant behavior (Table 112.2) [1].

A number of **prognostic factors** important in determining survival and the aggressiveness of these tumors has been identified (Table 112.3). The presence of **liver metastases** is the single most important prognostic factor. Recently WHO, TNM, and grading classifications have been proposed for PETs and other GEPs based on tumor size, invasiveness, presence of metastases, and proliferative indices (mitotic rate, Ki-67) that may provide important prognostic information [1–3].

Pathology

PETs, similar to other GEPs, are usually composed of monotonous sheets of small round cells with uniform nuclei and

infrequent mitoses. GEPs are now principally recognized by their **histological staining patterns** due to shared cellular proteins (see Table 112.1) [4]. Currently, immunocytochemical localization of **chromogranin A** is most widely used (see Table 112.1). **Ultrastructurally**, PETs possess electron-dense neurosecretory granules and frequently contain small clear vesicles that correspond to synaptic vesicles of neurons. They synthesize numerous peptides and growth factors that may be secreted, giving rise to various specific clinical syndromes (see Table 112.2). The diagnosis of the specific syndrome requires the clinical features of the disease (see Table 112.1). Pathologists cannot distinguish between benign and malignant PETs unless metastases or invasion is present [1,4].

Pathogenesis and genetic factors

The pathogenesis of the symptoms in functional PETs is directly related to the known biological effects of the ectopically secreted hormone.

The pathogenesis or molecular events determining malignancy in PETs are largely unknown; however, in general, PETs do not have alterations in **common oncogenes** (*Ras, Myc, Fos, Src, Jun*) or common tumor suppressor genes (*p53, retinoblastoma susceptibility* gene) (see Table 112.1) [5]. Recent studies on PETs report alterations in the *MEN1* gene, *p16/MTS1* tumor suppressor gene, and *DPC 4/Smad 4* gene, amplification of the *HER-2/neu* proto-oncogene, expression of growth factors and their receptors, and deletions of unknown tumor suppressor genes, as well as gains in other unknown genes (see Table 112.3) [5]. These studies show different chromosomal alterations in PETs and carcinoids, supporting a different pathogenesis for these two GEPs [5].

Four diseases due to various genetic disorders are associated with an increased incidence of PETs [6]. The most important is **multiple endocrine neoplasia type 1 (MEN1)**. MEN1 is an autosomal dominant disorder due to a defect in a 10-exon gene on chromosome 11q13, which encodes a 610-amino acid nuclear protein, menin [6]. Patients with MEN1 develop hyperparathyroidism (95–100%), PETs (80–100%), pituitary adenomas (54–80%), and carcinoids (gastric 13–30%, bronchial 0–8%, thymic 0–8%) [6]. MEN1 patients develop both NF-PETs (80–100%) and functional PETs (80%). Of the latter, the commonest are **Zollinger–Ellison syndrome (ZES)** (54%); **insulinomas** (21%), **glucagonomas** (3%), and **VIPomas** (1%). MEN1 accounts for 20–25% of all patients with ZES and 4% with insulinomas, and a low percentage (<5%) of the other PETs [6].

Three **phacomatoses** are associated with PETs [6]. **Von Hippel–Lindau (VHL) disease** is characterized by cerebellar hemangioblastomas, renal cancer, and pheochromocytomas, with 10–17% developing a PET (mostly NF-PETs, although insulinomas and VIPomas are reported) [6]. In **von Recklinghausen's disease** (NF-1), up to 12% develop an upper gastrointestinal carcinoid, often periampullary, commonly classified as somatostatinomas, but rarely associated with insulinomas or

Table 112.2 Pancreatic endocrine tumor syndromes (PETs)

	Biologically active			Associated with	
	Peptide(s) secreted	Tumor location	Malignant (%)	MEN1 (%)	Main symptoms/signs
Established functional syndromes					
Zollinger-Ellison Syndrome (ZES)	Gastrin	Duodenum (70%) Pancreas (25%) Other sites (5%)	60–90	20–25	Pain (79–100%) Diarrhea (30–75%) Esophageal symptoms (31–56%)
Insulinoma	Insulin	Pancreas (>99%)	<10	4–5	Hypoglycemic symptoms (100%)
VIPoma (Verner–Morrison syndrome pancreatic cholera, WDHA)	Vasoactive intestinal peptide	Pancreas (90%, adult) Other (10%, neural, adrenal, periganglionic)	40–70	6	Diarrhea (90–100%) Hypokalemic (80–100%) Dehydration (83%)
Glucagonoma	Glucagon	Pancreas (100%)	50–80	1–20	Rash (67–90%) Glucose intolerance (38–87%) Weight loss (66–96%)
GRFoma	Growth hormone- releasing hormone	Pancreas (30%) Lung (54%) Jejunum (7%) Other (13%)	>60	16	Acromegaly (100%)
Somatostatinoma	Somatostatin	Pancreas (55%) Duodenum/jejunum (44%)	>70	45	Diabetes mellitus (63–90%) Cholelithiases (65–90%) Diarrhea (35–90%)
ACTHoma	ACTH	Pancreas (4–16% all ectopic Cushing's)	>95	Rare	Cushing's syndrome (100%)
PET causing carcinoid syndrome	Serotonin ? tachykinins	Pancreas (<1% all carcinoids)	60-88	Rare	Diarrhea, flushing, asthma
PET causing hypercalcemia	PTHrP Others unknown	Pancreas (rare cause of hypercalcemia)	84	Rare	Abdominal pain due to hepatic metastases, symptoms due to hypercalcemia
Possible functional syndromes					
PET secreting calcitonin	Calcitonin	Pancreas (rare cause of hypercalcitoninemia)	>80	16	Diarrhea (50%)
PET secreting renin	Renin	Pancreas	Unknown	No	Hypertension
PET secreting erythropoietin	Erythropoietin	Pancreas	100	No	Polycythemic symptoms
PET secreting luteninizing hormone (LH)	LH	Pancreas	Unknown	No	Virilization (anovulation (female), reduced libido (male)
Non-functional syndromes					
PPoma/non-functional (NF-PET)	No symptomatic peptide 40–70% secrete pancreatic polypeptide (PP), 80–100% Chromogranin A	Pancreas	>60	10–40%	Weight loss (30–90%) Abdominal mass (10–30%) Pain (30–95%)

ACTH, adrenocorticotropic hormone; VIP, vasoactive intestinal polypeptide; MEN1, multiple endocrine neoplasia type 1.

Table.112.3 Prognostic factors in pancreatic endocrine tumors

Clinical/laboratory/tumoral features
- Presence of liver metastases
- Rate of tumor growth
- Extent of liver metastases
- Presence of lymph node metastases (weak predictor in many studies)
- Primary tumor size
- Primary tumor site
- Female gender
- MEN1 syndrome absent
  Markedly increased plasma tumor levels (increased chromogranin A in some studies; gastrinomas – increased gastrin level)

Various histological features
- Depth of invasion
- Tumor differentiation
- High growth indices (PCNA expression, high K_i 67 index)
- High mitotic counts
- Vascular or perineural invasion
- Various cytometric features (i.e., aneuploidy)

Molecular features
- *Ha-Ras* oncogene or p53 overexpression
- Increased HER2/neu expression ($p = 0.032$)
- Loss of heterozygosity at chromosome 1q, 3p, 3q, or 6q ($p = 0.0004$)
- EGF receptor overexpression ($p = 0.034$)
- Gains in chromosome 7q, 17q, 17p, 20q

Classification systems
- Advanced WHO grade (III vs I)
- Advanced TNM stage (IV vs III vs I, II)
- Advanced grade (G3 vs G2 vs G1)

PCNA, proliferating cell nuclear antigen.

ZES. NF-PETs and functional PETs have been reported [6]. In **tuberous sclerosis**, NF-PETs and functional PETs have been reported in a few cases [6].

General approach to treatment

Functional PETs characteristically present clinically with symptoms due to the ectopically secreted hormone. It is not until late in the course of the disease that the tumor *per se* causes symptoms [1].

In contrast, all of the symptoms caused by NF-PETs are due to the tumor *per se* (Figure 112.1) [1,7]. The mean delay between onset of continuous symptoms and diagnosis of functional PET syndromes is 4–7 years. Treatment of PETs requires two different approaches (Figure 112.1) [1]. First, treatment must be directed at the hormone excess state. Second, with the exception of insulinomas, as >50% of the tumors are malignant (Table 112.2), treatment must also be directed against the tumor itself (Figure 112.1) [1].

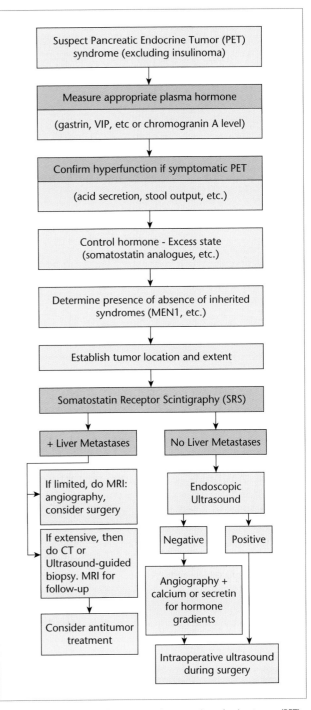

Figure 112.1 Diagnosis and treatment of pancreatic endocrine tumor (PET) syndromes. General approach to diagnosis and treatment of all PET syndromes except insulinomas [infrequently malignant (<15%) and less frequently localized with somatostatin receptor scintigraphy (SRS); see Figure 112.4]. For other tumors, SRS is the most sensitive localization technique and allows imaging of the entire body. Endoscopic ultrasound or angiography with venous sampling for hormonal gradients can detect primary tumors in more than 20% of patients who have normal findings at SRS. The identification of liver or distal metastases is important because it is the primary determinant of whether surgical resection should be performed as well as being a determinant of prognosis (see Figure 112.9). MEN1, multiple endocrine neoplasia type 1. (This figure was published in *Clinical Gastroenterology and Hepatology*, Wilfred M. Weinstein, Christopher J. Hawkey, Jaime Bosch, Gut and pancreatic endocrine tumors, Pages 1–12, Copyright Elsevier, 2005.)

Table 112.4 Comparative ability of localization methods to identify insulinomas and gastrinomas

	Pancreatic endocrine tumor**			
		Gastrinomas		
		Sensitivity (%)		Specificity (%)
		Recent NIH Studies	Literature	Literature
	Insulinomas Mean (range)	Mean (range)	Mean (range)	Mean (range)
Extrahepatic lesions				
Ultrasound	27 (10–39)	13 (9–16)*	23 (0–28)	92 (92–93)
CT scan	30 (0–40)	38 (31–51)*	38 (0–59)	90 (83–100)
MRI	10 (0–25)	40 (30–57)*	22 (20–25)	100 (100)
Angiography	60 (35–90)	43 (28–57)*	68 (35–68)	89 (84–94)
SRS	25 (12–50)	69 (58–78)	72 (57–77)	86
Endoscopic ultrasound	89 (71–94)	—	60 (58–100)	95 (84–100)
Metastatic liver disease				
Ultrasound	—†	46*	14 (14–63)	100
CT scan	—	42*	54 (35–72)	99 (94–100)
MRI	—	71	63 (43–83)	92 (88–100)
Angiography	—	65*	62 (33–86)	98 (96–100)
SRS	—	92	97 (92–100)	90 (90–100)

*p <0.05 compared to SRS alone.

**Shown are mean data (range)

†Metastatic insulinomas are uncommon (<10% of all cases) and there is insufficient data available for this analysis

CT scan, computed tomographic scan; MRI, magnetic resonance imaging; SRS, somatostatin receptor scintigraphy.

General diagnostic evaluation: importance of tumor localization

Localization of the primary tumor and establishing the extent of the disease is essential to all steps of management of all PETs (see Figure 114.1) [1,7–9]. Numerous tumor localization methods are used in PETs, including conventional imaging studies [computed tomography (CT), magnetic resonance imaging (MRI), ultrasound, angiography], and somatostatin receptor scintigraphy (SRS) (Table 112.4) [1,7–9]. In PETs, endoscopic ultrasound (EUS) and functional localization by measuring venous hormonal gradients have also been found to be of use [1,10].

Recent studies have shown that 90–100% of PETs possess **somatostatin receptors** that bind octreotide analogs (Figure 112.2). Because of its sensitivity and ability to localize tumors throughout the body at any one time, **SRS** is now the initial imaging modality of choice (Table 112.4) [1,9]. SRS localizes tumors in 56–100% of patients with PETs, with the exception of insulinomas. Insulinomas are usually small and have low densities of somatostatin receptors (Table 112.4). Numerous studies demonstrate SRS has greater sensitivity than conventional imaging studies in localizing both the primary tumor and metastases (Figure 112.3) [1,9]. Occasional false-positive responses with SRS can occur (12% in one study) because numerous normal tissues as well as other diseased tissues can have high densities of somatostatin receptors [1,9].

For PETs, **EUS** is highly sensitive, localizing 77–94% of insulinomas, which occur almost exclusively within the pancreas (Table 112.4; Figure 112.4) [10]. **SRS** is also more sensitive at identifying both liver metastases (Figure 112.3, middle panels) and bone metastases (Figure 112.3, bottom panels) than conventional localization studies. Functional localization measuring **hormone gradients** after intra-arterial calcium injections in insulinomas (insulin) or gastrin gradients after secretin injections in gastrinoma is a sensitive method, being positive in 80–100% of patients. However, this method gives only regional localization [11] (refer to the accompanying protocols on the website). More recently, two new **PET imaging modalities** have been used: hybrid scanning particularly with CT and SRS, and Positron emission tomographic scanning with [68]Gallium-labeled somatostatin analogs [9,12]. Studies in small numbers of patients show these novel modalities have increased the sensitivity or ability to localize PETs and thus will likely be increasingly used in the future [9,12].

Gastrinoma (Zollinger–Ellison syndrome) (Figure 112.5)
Pathology and presentation

A gastrinoma is a neuroendocrine tumor secreting gastrin, which results in **hypergastrinemia** causing **gastric acid hypersecretion**, leading to Zollinger–Ellison syndrome (ZES) [1,13].

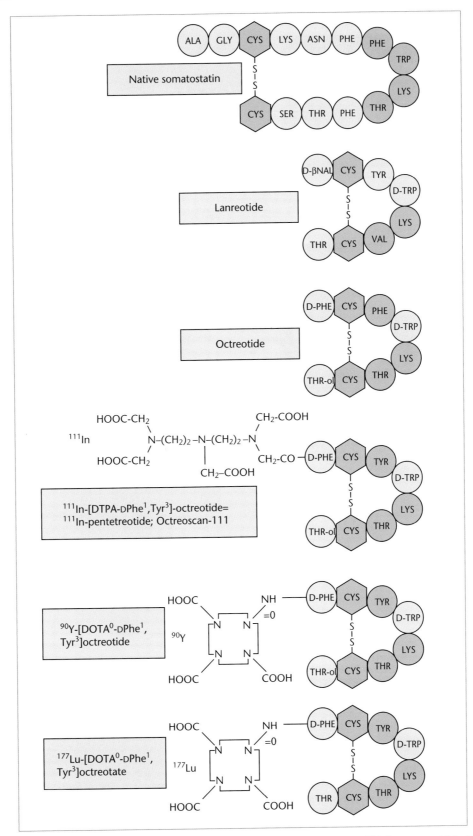

Figure 112.2 Structure of somatostatin and synthetic analogs used for diagnostic or therapeutic indications. (This figure was published in *Clinical Gastroenterology and Hepatology*, Wilfred M. Weinstein, Christopher J. Hawkey, Jaime Bosch, Gut and pancreatic endocrine tumors, Pages 1–12, Copyright Elsevier, 2005.)

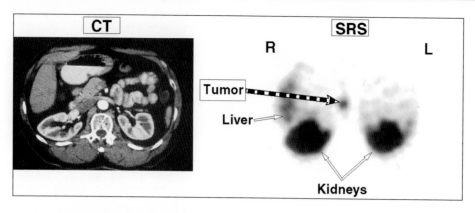

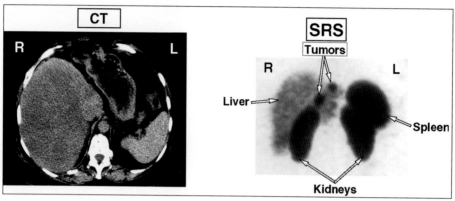

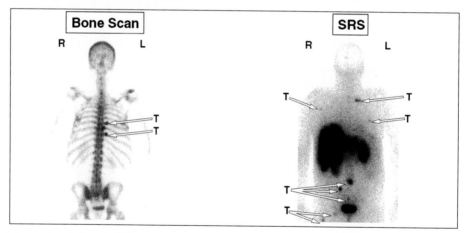

Figure 112.3 Somatostatin receptor scintigraphy (SRS). Increased sensitivity of SRS in localizing a primary pancreatic endocrine tumor (top), metastatic disease to liver (middle), or to bone (bottom). In the top and middle panels, the CT scan was negative whereas SRS localized tumor in both patients. In the bottom panel, in a patient with a malignant PET, the SRS demonstrated much more extensive metastatic disease than bone scanning, which led to a change in management.

The acid hypersecretion causes peptic ulcer disease (PUD), which is often refractory and severe, as well as diarrhea. The most common presenting symptoms are abdominal pain (70–100%), diarrhea (37–73%), and gastroesophageal reflux disease (GERD) (30–35%) [1,13,14]. Most patients have a typical **duodenal ulcer**. It is important to suspect gastrinoma in a patient with a peptic ulcer: with diarrhea; without *Helicobacter pylori* or non-steroidal anti-inflammatory drug (NSAID) use; in unusual or multiple locations; persistent or refractory to treatment; with prominent gastric folds; and with findings suggestive of MEN1 (1,13–15). Gastrinomas may also present with chronic **unexplained diarrhea** alone [1,13].

Most gastrinomas (50–70%) are in the **duodenum**, followed by the **pancreas** (20–40%) and other intra-abdominal sites (Figure 112.6) [1,13]. Rarely, extra-abdominal primaries are found (Figure 112.6). Sixty to 90% of gastrinomas are

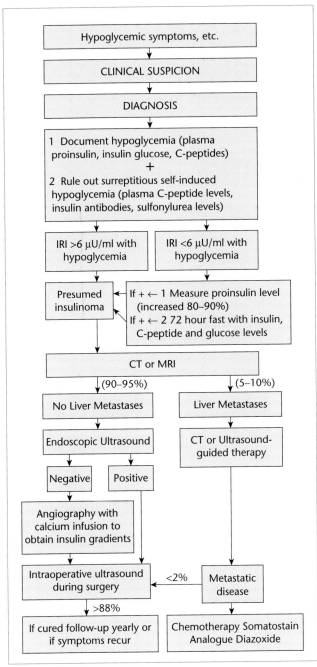

Figure 112.4 Diagnosis and treatment of a patient with insulinomas. Document the hypoglycemia and rule out other causes (including self-induced hypoglycemia caused by surreptitious use of insulin or sulfonylureas). The 72-hour fast is most commonly used to monitor plasma insulin, proinsulin, glucose, and C-peptide levels. Hypoglycemia with plasma insulin-like immunoreactivity (IRI) >6 μU/mL and elevated proinsulin levels allows presumed diagnosis of insulinoma. Hypoglycemia with IRI <6 μU/mL requires additional evaluation. Insulinomas are usually benign (90–95% of cases). Malignant cases can be detected with a CT scan or MRI for liver metastases. Endoscopic ultrasound (EUS) is more sensitive than other imaging studies, detecting a primary insulinomas in 80–95% of cases (Table112.4). If EUS does not localize the insulinoma, selective intra-arterial injection of calcium with sampling of hepatic veins for insulin concentrations should be performed to localize the insulinoma to the appropriate pancreatic area. Intraoperative ultrasound should be used routinely. (This figure was published in *Clinical Gastroenterology and Hepatology*, Wilfred M. Weinstein, Christopher J. Hawkey, Jaime Bosch, Gut and pancreatic endocrine tumors, Pages 1–12, Copyright Elsevier, 2005.)

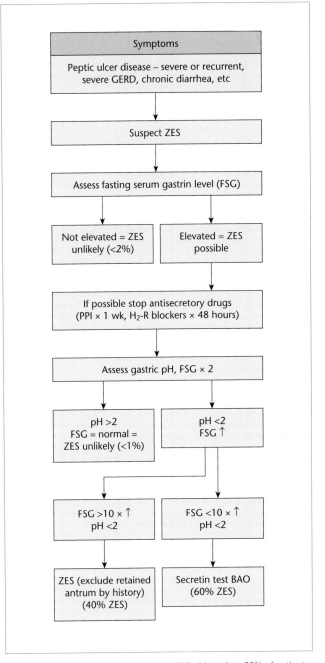

Figure 112.5 Zollinger–Ellison syndrome (ZES). More than 98% of patients with ZES have an elevated fasting gastrin level (FSG) when first seen [16]. Whereas FSG levels that are normal exclude >98% of ZES patients, increased FSG levels can be due to achlorhydria, antisecretory drugs, or other causes of hypersecretion (usually <10-fold increased). If the FSG level is increased, evaluate gastric pH off antisecretory drugs [proton pump inhibitors (PPIs) x 1 week, H₂-receptor blockers x 48 hours] if it can be safely done. In a large series [18] all ZES patients had a fasting gastric pH of <2. A secretin test and assessment of basal acid output (BAO) is necessary to distinguish numerous other conditions that can cause a pH of <2 and increased FSG (usually <10-fold). Secretin tests are positive in 94% (>120 pg/mL increase) of ZES patients and BAO is >15 mEq/hour (no gastric surgery) (>5 mEq/h) in >90% of patients [17,18]. GERD, gastroesophageal reflux disease. (This figure was published in *Clinical Gastroenterology and Hepatology*, Wilfred M. Weinstein, Christopher J. Hawkey, Jaime Bosch, Gut and pancreatic endocrine tumors, Pages 1–12, Copyright Elsevier, 2005.)

Multiple Organ Systems

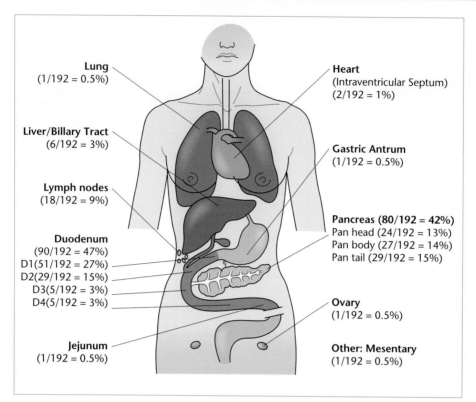

Figure 112.6 Location of primary gastrinomas. Primary gastrinoma location was determined in 192 NIH patients [surgery (n = 166), autopsy (n = 11), or endoscopy biopsy/imaging (n = 15)]. Results are expressed as the percentage of the 192 patients with a primary gastrinoma in the indicated location. The primary listed in the lung occurred in a non-small cell lung cancer ectopically secreting gastrin. (This figure was published in *Clinical Gastroenterology and Hepatology*, Wilfred M. Weinstein, Christopher J. Hawkey, Jaime Bosch, Gut and pancreatic endocrine tumors, Pages 1–12, Copyright Elsevier, 2005.)

malignant (see Table 112.2) with metastatic spread to lymph nodes and the liver [1,13]. Distant metastases to bone occur in 12–30% of patients with liver metastases.

Diagnosis

Nearly all patients have an increased fasting **plasma gastrin**, making this the screening test of choice [16,17]. A fasting gastrin of >1000 pg/mL (10-fold increase) and resting intragastric pH of <2.0 is generally diagnostic of a gastrinoma [16–18]. In patients who have had a Billroth 2 gastrectomy, the possibility of **retained antrum** may require investigation by scintigraphy. Where the intragastric pH is <2 and the gastrin elevation less pronounced (<1000 pg/mL), the differential diagnosis includes *H. pylori* infection, antral G-cell hyperplasia/hyperfunction, gastric outlet obstruction, or, rarely, renal failure [16–18]. These patients require determination of **basal acid output** and a **secretin provocative test** (Figure 112.5) [1,16–18].

Treatment

Gastric acid hypersecretion can nearly always be controlled by **proton pump inhibitors** once or twice daily, with dose titrated up until control is achieved [1,13]. H$_2$-receptor antagonists are also effective but require high and more frequent doses. More than 50% of patients who are not cured (>60% of all patients)

will die from tumor-related causes [1,13]. All patients with gastrinomas but without MEN1 should be **considered for surgery** by a surgeon with specialized experience [1,13,19,20]. In the absence of liver metastases, 60% of such patients achieve short-term and 30% long-term cure [1,6,15,19,20]. Surgery may also be possible where hepatic metastases are limited. In patients **with MEN1**, routine surgery is controversial because long-term cure is rare [1,6,15,19,20].

Insulinoma (Figure 112.4)
Pathology and presentation

An insulinoma is an endocrine tumor that ectopically secretes insulin, resulting in **hypoglycemia**. A differential diagnosis includes inadvertent/surreptitious use of insulin or oral hypoglycemic agents: alcoholism; severe liver disease; poor nutrition; and other extrapancreatic tumors [1,21,22].

The most reliable test is a **72-hour fast**, which will establish the diagnosis of insulinoma using the following criteria in 98% of patients by 48 hours [1,21,22]: blood glucose ≤40 mg/dL; serum insulin >6 μU/mL; and ratio of insulin to glucose (in mg/dL) >0.3 (see Figure 112.4). Measurement of proinsulin, C-peptide, insulin antibodies, and sulfonylurea levels should enable inadvertent or surreptitious use of insulin or hypoglycemic agents to be distinguished [1,21,22].

Treatment

Only 5–15% of insulinomas are malignant; therefore, after appropriate imaging (CT/MRI, EUS), **surgery** should be performed (see Figure 112.4) and 75–95% will be cured [1,19,20]. Prior to surgery the hypoglycemia can be controlled by **frequent small meals** and the use of **diazoxide** (150–800 mg/day). Approximately 50–60% of patients respond to diazoxide. Other agents that are effective in some patients in controlling the hypoglycemia include verapamil and diphenylhydantoin [1,21,22]. Long-acting **somatostatin analogs** (see Figure 112.4) are acutely effective in 40% of patients. However, octreotide needs to be used with care because it inhibits growth hormone secretion and can alter plasma glucagon levels; therefore, in some patients it can worsen the hypoglycemia [1,21,22]. For the 5–15% of patients with malignant insulinomas, the above drugs or somatostatin analogs are initially used. If these are not effective, various antitumor treatments can be used [1,21,22].

Glucagonomas

Pathology and presentation

A glucagonoma is an endocrine tumor of the pancreas that secretes excessive amounts of glucagon, causing a distinct syndrome characterized by **dermatitis, glucose intolerance, or diabetes and weight loss** [1,23]. Glucagonomas principally occur between 45 and 70 years of age and are clinically characterized by a dermatitis (migratory necrolytic erythema) (67–90%), accompanied by glucose intolerance (40–90%), weight loss (66–96%), anemia (33–85%), diarrhea (15–29%), and thromboembolism (11–24%) [1,23]. The characteristic **rash** starts usually as an annular erythema at intertriginous and periorificial sites, especially in the groin or buttock. A characteristic laboratory finding is **hypoaminoacidemia**, which occurs in 26–100% of patients. Glucagonomas are generally large tumors at diagnosis with an average size of >5 cm [1,23]. Fifty to 82% have evidence of metastatic spread at presentation, usually to the liver. Glucagonomas are rarely extrapancreatic and they are usually a single tumor.

Diagnosis

The diagnosis is confirmed by demonstrating an increased **plasma glucagon level**. A plasma glucagon level >1000 pg/mL is considered diagnostic of glucagonoma. Other diseases causing increased plasma glucagon levels include renal insufficiency, acute pancreatitis, hypercorticism, hepatic insufficiency, prolonged fasting, or familial hyperglucagonemia [1,23].

Treatment

In 50–80% of patients, liver metastases are present at presentation so curative surgical resection is not possible. Surgical debulking in patients with advanced disease or other antitumor treatments may be beneficial. Long-acting **somatostatin analogs** (octreotide/lanreotide) (see Figure 112.2) improve the

skin rash in 75% of patients and may improve the weight loss, pain, and diarrhea, but usually do not improve the glucose intolerance [1,23].

Somatostatinoma syndrome

Pathology and presentation

The somatostatinoma syndrome is due to a PET that secretes excessive amounts of somatostatin, causing a distinct syndrome characterized by **diabetes mellitus, gallbladder disease, diarrhea, and steatorrhea** [1]. In the literature there is no general distinction between PETs containing somatostatin-like immunoreactivity (SLI; (somatostatinomas) and those secreting SLI and causing a clinical syndrome. The mean age at diagnosis is 51 years [1].

Diagnosis

Somatostatinomas are usually found by accident either at the time of cholecystectomy or during endoscopy. Duodenal somatostatin-containing tumors are increasingly associated with **von Recklinghausen's disease**. Most of these do not cause the somatostatinoma syndrome. The diagnosis of the somatostatinoma syndrome requires the demonstration of elevated plasma somatostatin levels [1].

Treatment

Pancreatic somatostatinomas are frequently (70–92%) metastatic at presentation, whereas only 30–69% of small intestinal somatostatinomas have metastases. **Surgery** is the treatment of choice for those without widespread hepatic metastases. Symptoms in patients with the somatostatinoma syndrome may be improved by **octreotide** treatment (see Figure 112.2) [1].

VIPomas (Figure 112.7)

Pathology and presentation

VIPomas are endocrine tumors that secrete excessive amounts of vasoactive intestinal peptide (VIP), which causes a syndrome characterized by **large-volume diarrhea, hypokalemia, and dehydration** [1,24]. This syndrome is also called **Verner–Morrison syndrome**, pancreatic cholera, and **WDHA** (watery diarrhea, hypokalemia, and achlorhydria) syndrome. The mean age of patients with this syndrome is 49 years, but it can occur in children. The principal symptoms are large-volume diarrhea (100%) severe enough to cause hypokalemia (80–100%), dehydration (83%), hypochlorhydria (54–76%), and flushing (20%). The diarrhea is secretory in nature, persists during fasting, and almost always >1 L/day and in 70% >3 L/day (Figure 112.7) [1,24]. In adults, 80–90% of VIPomas are **pancreatic** in location with the rest due to VIP-secreting **pheochromocytomas**, intestinal carcinoids, and rarely ganglioneuromas. These tumors are usually not multiple, 50–75% are in the pancreatic tail, and 37–68% have hepatic metastases at diagnosis. In children younger than 10 years old the syndrome

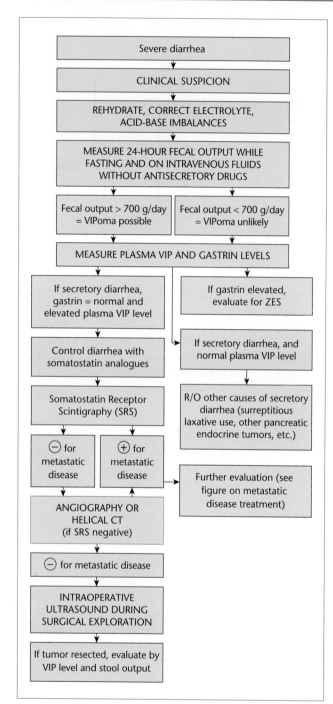

Figure 112.7 Approach and treatment of a patient with a suspected vasoactive intestinal polypeptide-secreting tumor (VIPoma). VIPomas cause secretory diarrhea of >700 g/day. Measure 24-hour fecal output after correction of electrolyte or acid-base in fully rehydrated and fasted patient, who is off all antisecretory drugs (octreotide s.c. >1 week; octreotide LAR >2 months). Angiography is recommended if somatostatin receptor scintigraphy (SRS) is negative prior to surgery because it can detect small liver metastases not imaged by SRS. If metastatic disease is present and non-resectable or if no tumor is found, postoperative treatment with long-acting somatostatin analogs (octreotide/lanreotide) should be continued. The dosage should be adjusted to control symptoms. If metastatic disease is present and there is progressive disease or symptoms are not controlled with octreotide, chemotherapy should be considered (see Figure 112.8). (This figure was published in *Clinical Gastroenterology and Hepatology*, Wilfred M. Weinstein, Christopher J. Hawkey, Jaime Bosch, Gut and pancreatic endocrine tumors, Pages 1–12, Copyright Elsevier, 2005.)

is usually due to ganglioneuromas or ganglioblastomas. These are less malignant (10%).

Diagnosis

The diagnosis requires the demonstration of an **elevated plasma VIP level** and the presence of large-volume diarrhea (Figure 112.7). A VIPoma is unlikely if stool volume is <700 mL/day. Other diseases that can give a secretory large-volume diarrhea include gastrinomas, chronic laxative abuse, carcinoid syndrome, systemic mastocytosis, rarely medullary thyroid cancer, diabetic diarrhea, and acquired immune deficiency syndrome (AIDS) (Figure 112.7) [1,24].

Treatment

The most important initial treatment in these patients is to correct their **dehydration and electrolyte losses**. Because 37–68% of adults with VIPomas have metastatic liver disease at presentation, many cannot be cured surgically. In these patients, long-acting **somatostatin analogs** (octreotide/lanreotide) (Figure 112.2) are the drugs of choice. Octreotide will control the diarrhea in 87% of patients. In non-responsive patients, the combination of **glucocorticoids and octreotide** has proved helpful in a small number of patients. **Other drugs** reported to be helpful in small numbers of patients include prednisone (60–100 mg/day), clonidine, indomethacin, phenothiazines, loperamide, lidamidine, lithium, propanolol, and metochlorpramide [1,24].

Non-functional pancreatic enzyme tumors

Pathology and presentation

NF-PETs are endocrine tumors that originate in the pancreas and either secrete no products or secrete products that do not cause a specific clinical syndrome. NF-PET symptoms are due entirely to the tumor *per se*. NF-PETs almost always secrete **chromogranin A** (90–100%), **chromogranin B** (90–100%), **pancreatic polypeptide (PP)** (58%), and **alpha-human chorionic gonadotropin (hCG)** (40%) [1,7]. NF-PETs usually present late in their disease course with invasive tumors and hepatic metastases (64–92%) and the tumors are usually large (72% >5 cm) [1,7]. NF-PETs are usually solitary except in patients with MEN1 where they are multiple. The most common symptoms are: abdominal pain (30–80%), jaundice (20–35%), and weight loss, fatigue or bleeding; 10–15% are found incidentally [1,7].

The average time from the beginning of symptoms to diagnosis is 5 years [1,7].

Diagnosis

The diagnosis is only established by **histological confirmation** in a patient with a PET without either clinical symptoms or elevated plasma hormone levels of one of the established functional syndromes (Table 112.2) [1,7]. **Plasma PP** is increased in 22–71% of patients and should strongly suggest the diagnosis in a patient with a pancreatic mass. Elevated plasma PP is not diagnostic of this tumor because it is elevated in a number of other conditions such as chronic renal failure, old age, inflammatory conditions, and diabetes [1,7].

Treatment

Unfortunately, surgical curative resection can be considered only in the minority of the patients because 64–92% present with metastatic disease [1,7]. Treatment needs to be directed against the tumor *per se* as discussed below in the section on advanced disease.

Rarer tumors

GRFomas are endocrine tumors that secrete excessive amounts of growth hormone-releasing factor (GRF) and are an **uncommon cause of acromegaly** [1].These are found in the lung (47–54%), pancreas (29–30%), small intestine (8–10%), and other sites (12%), presenting at a mean age of 38 years. The pancreatic tumors are usually large (>6 cm) and liver metastases are present in 39%. GRFomas are an uncommon cause of acromegaly. The diagnosis is established by plasma assays for **GRF** and **growth hormone**. **Surgery** is the treatment of choice if diffuse metastases are not present [1]. Long-acting **somatostatin analogs** (octreotide/lanreotide) (see Figure 112.5) are the agents of choice, with 75–100% of patients responding [1].

Other rare pancreatic endocrine tumors

Cushing's syndrome due to a **PET (ACTHoma)** occurs in 4–16% of all ectopic Cushing's syndrome cases. Paraneoplastic **hypercalcemia** due to a PET releasing **PTH-RP**, a PTH-like material or unknown factor, is rarely reported. The tumors tend to be large and liver metastases are usually present [1]. PETs can occasionally cause the **carcinoid syndrome** (see Table 112.2). PETs secreting calcitonin are proposed as a specific clinical syndrome with one-half of patients having diarrhea [1]. This tumor is classified in Table 112.2 as a possible specific disorder because so few cases have been described, as is also the case with PETs secreting erythropoietin, luteinizing hormone, and renin [1].

Treatment of advanced (diffuse metastatic) disease (Figure 112.8)

Principles

The single most important prognostic factor for survival is the presence of **liver metastases** (see Table 112.3; Figure 112.9) [1,3,25]. With **gastrinomas**:

- 10-year survival without liver metastases is 98%;
- With limited metastases in one hepatic lobe, survival is 78%;
- With diffuse metastases, survival is 16% (Figure 112.9).

Therefore, treatment for advanced metastatic disease is essential [1,3,25]. A number of different modalities are reported to

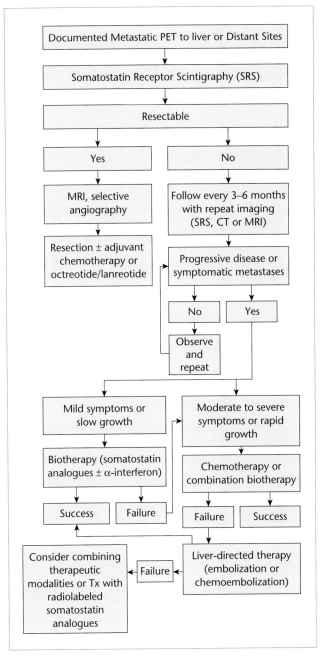

Figure 112.8 Treatment of a patient with a metastatic PET. For all PETs except metastatic insulinomas, recent studies demonstrate that somatostatin receptor scintigraphy (SRS) should be the initial tumor localization method because of its greater sensitivity and ability to give a complete body scan. Consider surgical resection by a surgeon with specific expertise if likely morbidity is acceptable. MRI and selective angiography help to locate liver metastases and detect possible small lesions not imaged on the SRS. If the tumor is not resectable, control symptoms with long-acting somatostatin analogs (octreotide/lanreotide) (Figure 112.2). If tumor growth is slow, use somatostatin or alpha-interferon. If growth is rapid or symptoms are not controlled, combine somatostatin analogs and alpha-interferon or use chemotherapy. If symptoms or tumor growth are still not controlled and disease is localized to the liver, consider liver-directed antitumor treatments (embolization/chemoembolization). For advanced disease, studies suggest treatment with [111]In-, [90]Y-, or ^{177}Lu-labeled somatostatin analogs may be beneficial as well as a number of other newer targeted therapies (see text). GEP, gastroenteropancreatic endocrine tumor. (This figure was published in *Clinical Gastroenterology and Hepatology*, Wilfred M. Weinstein, Christopher J. Hawkey, Jaime Bosch, Gut and pancreatic endocrine tumors, Pages 1–12, Copyright Elsevier, 2005.)

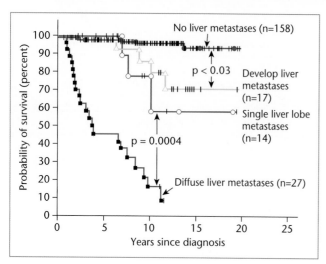

Figure 112.9 Effect of liver and metastases on survival. Survival plotted in the form of a Kaplan–Meier for 199 consecutive patients with gastrinomas followed at the NIH. The presence of liver metastases and their extent had a marked effect on survival. (This figure was published in *Clinical Gastroenterology and Hepatology*, Wilfred M. Weinstein, Christopher J. Hawkey, Jaime Bosch, Gut and pancreatic endocrine tumors, Pages 1–12, Copyright Elsevier, 2005.)

be effective, including cytoreductive surgery (removal of all visible tumor), chemotherapy, somatostatin analogs, alpha-interferon, hepatic embolization alone or with chemotherapy (chemoembolization), radiotherapy, and liver transplantation (Figure 112.8) [1,26,27].

Specific antitumor treatments

Complete cytoreductive surgery is only possible in 9–22% of patients where there are limited hepatic metastases, though surgery in patients with more extensive disease may increase survival (Figure 112.8) [1,26,28]. Cytotoxic chemotherapy, currently with streptozotocin and doxorubicin, has been reported to cause tumor shrinkage in 30–70% of patients [1,26,27,29].

Octreotide and lanreotide (see Figures 112.2 and 112.8) as well as **alpha-interferon** rarely decrease tumor size but are tumoristatic, stopping further growth in 26–95%, though with an uncertain effect on survival [1,27,29]. **Hepatic embolization** and **chemoembolization** (with dacarbazine, cisplatin, doxorubicin, 5-fluorouracil, or streptozotocin) can decrease tumor bulk and help control the symptoms of the hormone-excess state [1,30]. These modalities are generally reserved for cases in which treatment with somatostatin analogs, interferon, or chemotherapy fails (Figure 112.8). **Radiotherapy** with radiolabeled somatostatin analogs (see Figure 112.2) is a new approach that is now being investigated. Three different radionuclides are used. High doses of [^{111}In-DTPA-DPhe1]octreotide, yttrium-90 coupled by a DOTA chelating group to octreotide, or octreotate are used, as well as ^{177}lutetium-coupled analogs (Figure 112.2) [1,31]. Recent studies with the ^{111}In compounds or ^{177}lutetium compounds caused tumor stabilization in 41% and 40%,

respectively, and a decrease in tumor size in 30% and 38%, respectively, of patients with advanced metastatic gastrointestinal PETs [31]. Liver transplantation is uncommonly used [1].

Studies in limited numbers of patients suggest additional new, novel agents may have antitumor activity in selected patients. These include:

- Agents targeting growth factors (IGF1, TGF-α, PDGF, EGF, VEGF) or their receptors (imatinib – PDGFR; gefitnib – EGFR)
- Inhibitors of intracellular growth cascading signaling molecules, such as mTor (everolimus, temsirolimus)
- Angiogenesis inhibitors (SU11248-EGFR, c-kit, PDGFR; endostatin, bevacizumab-VEGFR), VEGF tyrosine kinase inhibitors (sunitinib, vatalanib, sorafenib)
- A dacarbazine (DTIC)-related compound, temozolamide [1,26,29].

References

1. Metz DC, Jensen RT. Gastrointestinal neuroendocrine tumors:; Pancreatic endocrine tumors. *Gastroenterology*. 2008;135:1469–1492.
2. Rindi G, Kloppel G, Alhman H, *et al*. TNM staging of foregut (neuro)endocrine tumors: a consensus proposal including a grading system. *Virchows Arch*. 2006;449:395–401.
3. Pape UF, Jann H, Muller-Nordhorn J, *et al*. Prognostic relevance of a novel TNM classification system for upper gastroenteropancreatic neuroendocrine tumors. *Cancer*. 2008;113:256–265.
4. Kloppel G. Tumour biology and histopathology of neuroendocrine tumours. *Best Pract Res Clin Endocrinol Metab*. 2007;21:15–31.
5. Duerr EM, Chung DC. Molecular genetics of neuroendocrine tumors. *Best Pract Res Clin Endocrinol Metab*. 2007;21:1–14.
6. Jensen RT, Berna MJ, Bingham MD, *et al*. Inherited pancreatic endocrine tumor syndromes: advances in molecular pathogenesis, diagnosis, management and controversies. *Cancer*. 2008; 113(7 Suppl):1807–1843.
7. Falconi M, Plockinger U, Kwekkeboom DJ, *et al*. Well-differentiated pancreatic nonfunctioning tumors/carcinoma. *Neuroendocrinology*. 2006;84:196–211.
8. Rockall AG, Reznek RH. Imaging of neuroendocrine tumours (CT/MR/US). *Best Pract Res Clin Endocrinol Metab*. 2007;21:43–68.
9. Sundin A, Garske U, Orlefors H. Nuclear imaging of neuroendocrine tumours. *Best Pract Res Clin Endocrinol Metab*. 2007;21:69–85.
10. McLean AM, Fairclough PD. Endoscopic ultrasound in the localisation of pancreatic islet cell tumours. *Best Pract Res Clin Endocrinol Metab*. 2005;19:177–193.
11. Jackson JE. Angiography and arterial stimulation venous sampling in the localization of pancreatic neuroendocrine tumours. *Best Pract Res Clin Endocrinol Metab*. 2005;19:229–239.
12. Gabriel M, Decristoforo C, Kendler D, *et al*. 68Ga-DOTA-Tyr3-Octreotide PET in Neuroendocrine Tumors: Comparison with Somatostatin Receptor Scintigraphy and CT. *J Nucl Med*. 2007;48:508–518.
13. Jensen RT, Niederle B, Mitry E, *et al*. Gastrinoma (duodenal and pancreatic). *Neuroendocrinology*. 2006;84:173–182.

Multiple Organ Systems

14. Roy P, Venzon DJ, Shojamanesh H, *et al.* Zollinger-Ellison syndrome: clinical presentation in 261 patients. *Medicine (Baltimore).* 2000;79:379–411.
15. Gibril F, Schumann M, Pace A, *et al.* Multiple endocrine neoplasia type 1 and Zollinger-Ellison syndrome. A prospective study of 107 cases and comparison with 1009 patients from the literature. *Medicine (Baltimore).* 2004;83:43–83.
16. Berna MJ, Hoffmann KM, Serrano J, *et al.* Serum gastrin in Zollinger-Ellison syndrome: I. Prospective study of fasting serum gastrin in 309 patients from the National Institutes of Health and comparison with 2229 cases from the literature. *Medicine (Baltimore).* 2006;85:295–330.
17. Berna MJ, Hoffmann KM, Long SH, *et al.* Serum gastrin in Zollinger-Ellison syndrome: II. Prospective study of gastrin provocative testing in 293 patients from the National Institutes of Health and comparison with 537 cases from the literature. evaluation of diagnostic criteria, proposal of new criteria, and correlations with clinical and tumoral features. *Medicine (Baltimore).* 2006;85:331–364.
18. Roy P, Venzon DJ, Feigenbaum KM, *et al.* Gastric secretion in Zollinger-Ellison syndrome: correlation with clinical expression, tumor extent and role in diagnosis – A prospective NIH study of 235 patients and review of the literature in 984 cases. *Medicine (Baltimore).* 2001;80:189–222.
19. Norton JA, Jensen RT. Resolved and unresolved controversies in the surgical management of patients with Zollinger-Ellison syndrome. *Ann Surg.* 2004;240:757–773.
20. Norton JA, Fraker DL, Alexander HR, *et al.* Surgery to cure the Zollinger-Ellison syndrome. *N Engl J Med.* 1999;341:635–644.
21. de Herder WW, Niederle B, Scoazec JY, *et al.* Well-differentiated pancreatic tumor/carcinoma: insulinoma. *Neuroendocrinology.* 2006;84:183–188.
22. Grant CS. Insulinoma. *Best Pract Res Clin Gastroenterol.* 2005;19:783–798.
23. van Beek AP, de Haas ER, van Vloten WA, *et al.* The glucagonoma syndrome and necrolytic migratory erythema: a clinical review. *Eur J Endocrinol.* 2004;151:531–537.
24. Nikou GC, Toubanakis C, Nikolaou P, *et al.* VIPomas: an update in diagnosis and management in a series of 11 patients. *Hepatogastroenterology.* 2005;52:1259–1265.
25. Panzuto F, Nasoni S, Falconi M, *et al.* Prognostic factors and survival in endocrine tumor patients: comparison between gastrointestinal and pancreatic localization. *Endocr Relat Cancer.* 2005;12:1083–1092.
26. Chan JA, Kulke MH. Progress in the treatment of neuroendocrine tumors. *Curr Oncol Rep.* 2009;11:193–199.
27. Steinmuller T, Kianmanesh R, Falconi M, *et al.* Consensus guidelines for the management of patients with liver metastases from digestive (neuro)endocrine tumors: foregut, midgut, hindgut, and unknown primary. *Neuroendocrinology.* 2008;87:47–62.
28. Touzios JG, Kiely JM, Pitt SC, *et al.* Neuroendocrine hepatic metastases: does aggressive management improve survival? *Ann Surg.* 2005;241:776–783.
29. Strosberg JR, Kvols LK. A review of the current clinical trials for gastroenteropancreatic neuroendocrine tumours. *Expert Opin Investig Drugs.* 2007;16:219–224.
30. O'Toole D, Ruszniewski P. Chemoembolization and other ablative therapies for liver metastases of gastrointestinal endocrine tumours. *Best Pract Res Clin Gastroenterol.* 2005;19:585–594.
31. Van Essen M, Krenning EP, Kam BL, *et al.* Peptide-receptor radionuclide therapy for endocrine tumors. *Nat Rev Endocrinol.* 2009;5:382–393.

Multiple Organ Systems

CHAPTER 113

The carcinoid syndrome

Eva Tiensuu Janson and Kjell Öberg

Uppsala University Hospital, Uppsala, Sweden

ESSENTIAL FACTS ABOUT PATHOGENESIS

- Incidence is about 1 per 100 000 people per year
- 60% have metastases at diagnosis
- 5-year survival is about 60%
- Pathogenesis is unknown

ESSENTIALS OF DIAGNOSIS

- Carcinoid syndrome: flush, diarrhea, carcinoid heart disease and bronchial obstruction
- Abdominal pain due to intestinal obstruction, tumor growth or intestinal ischemia
- Tumor immunohistochemical staining for chromogranin A and serotonin
- Urinary 5-hydroxyindoleacetic acid and plasma chromogranin A are good biochemical markers
- Tumor localization is by computed tomography, magnetic resonance imaging, scintigraphy, and positron emission tomography
- Somatostatin receptor scintigraphy shows pathological uptake in tumor lesions in 90% of patients

---

ESSENTIALS OF TREATMENT

- Surgery should always be considered; debulking surgery may prolong survival
- Radiofrequency ablation and liver embolization may be used to reduce tumor size and hormone levels
- Alpha-interferon and somatostatin analogs are used to reduce tumor growth, symptoms, and hormone levels
- Targeted tumor treatment with radiolabeled somatostatin analogs may be used in patients with high radionuclide uptake at somatostatin receptor scintigraphy
- Chemotherapy is usually not effective

Introduction

The carcinoid syndrome was first described in 1954 when the association was made between the presence of a slowly growing serotonin-producing tumor in the small intestine and the syndrome that included facial flushing, diarrhea, right-sided heart failure, and bronchial constriction. The syndrome develops in patients with metastatic disease. Sometimes, the syndrome can become life threatening, especially when a carcinoid crisis develops. Since most patients can be treated successfully, the recognition of the syndrome by clinicians is important.

Epidemiology

The overall incidence of ileal carcinoid tumors is 1–2 cases per 100 000 people. However, in autopsy material, incidences of up to 8.4 per 100 000 people have been reported. The male-to-female ratio is 1:1 and the median age at diagnosis is about 60 years. More than 60% of patients present with metastases at diagnosis, and the 5-year survival is 60%. Because of the long survival, the prevalence of neuroendocrine tumors (35 per 100 000 people) is much higher than the incidence [1].

Pathogenesis and pathology

Enterochromaffin cells in the small intestine belong to the APUD (amino precursor uptake and decarboxylation) system (see Chapter 112) (Figure 113.1). It is from these cells, located in the crypts of Lieberkuhn, that the classical ileal carcinoid tumor arises. The histopathological diagnosis is based on immunohistochemistry with antibodies against chromogranin A and serotonin (Figure 113.2) [2]. The histological growth patterns can be classified as insular, trabecular, glandular, broad band, and mixed, which may represent different biological behaviors. It is important to calculate the **proliferation index** since this is of prognostic value. In patients with a Ki67 below 1% the expected survival is significantly longer than in patients with a higher Ki67 [3].

The WHO classification divides carcinoid tumors of the small intestine into:

- Well-differentiated endocrine tumor of benign or uncertain behavior
- Well-differentiated endocrine carcinoma with low-grade malignant behavior or metastases
- Poorly-differentiated endocrine carcinoma [4].

Multiple Organ Systems

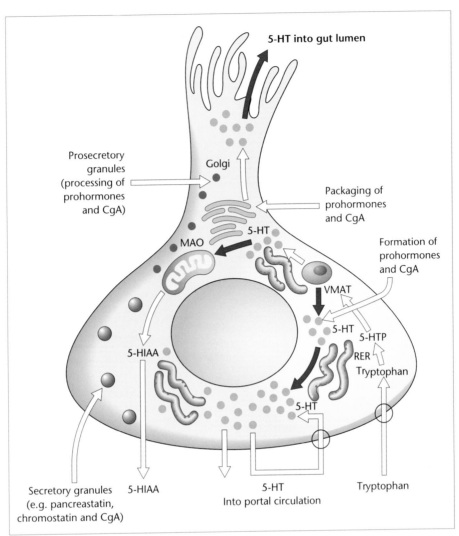

Figure 113.1 The neuroendocrine cell. The cell takes up amino acids such as tryptophan from the circulation. The amino acid precursor is processed in the cell to produce serotonin, which is stored together with chromogranin A (CgA) in the secretory granules until release back into the circulation. 5-HIAA, 5-hydroxyindole acetic acid; 5-HT, 5-hydroxytryptamine; 5-HTP, 5-hyroxytryptophan; MAO, mono amine oxidase; RER, rough endoplasmic reticulum; VMAT, vesicular membrane amino acid transporter.

More recently, a TNM classification was proposed and this should be considered in all patients [5].

Clinical presentation

Patients suffering from a carcinoid tumor often present with facial flushing and diarrhea (Table 113.1). The syndrome develops in patients with liver and/or retroperitoneal metastases and is induced by biologically active amines and peptides produced by the tumor. These secretory products escape the liver metabolism and may appear un-degraded in the circulation. **Flushing** is typically restricted to the face and upper thorax, but can be more extended in severe cases (Figure 113.3). It is thought to be caused by vasoactive peptides belonging to the tachykinin family, such as substance P and neuropeptide K. It may be induced by alcohol, physical or psychological stress, and spicy food. In patients with long-standing disease, the flush may become chronic and some patients may have facial telangiectasia. The **diarrhea** is most frequent in the morning but may be present throughout the day and even during the night, and is believed to be caused by serotonin. Some patients can suffer from 10 to 15 bowel motions daily, making it almost impossible to carry out daily activities, while others only notice a slight change in the consistency of the stools. The diarrhea may be associated with loss of weight.

Pain and diarrhea may also be caused by intestinal obstruction or mesenteric ischemia due to involvement of the mesenteric artery (see below). Patients with symptoms of right-sided heart failure usually have had their carcinoid tumor for many years. Tricuspid regurgitation is often combined with tricuspid stenosis and/or pulmonary stenosis or

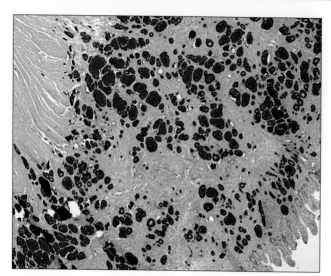

Figure 113.2 Chromogranin A staining. A tumor specimen showing an insular growth pattern from a patient with an ileal carcinoid tumor immunostained for chromogranin A.

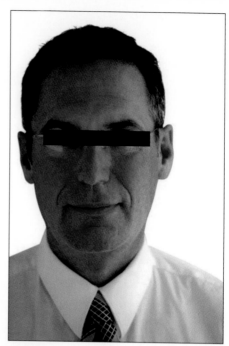

Figure 113.3 A patient with a typical carcinoid flush.

Table 113.1 The carcinoid syndrome

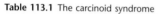

Symptom	Frequency	Causative agent
Flushing	85–90%	Tachykinins
Diarrhea	70%	Serotonin
Bronchial constriction	15%	Tachykinins
Carcinoid heart disease	30%	Serotonin

Other possible causes of facial flushing include:

- Food intake and medication (see Table 113.3)
- Menopausal flushing
- Medullary carcinoma of the thyroid
- Verner–Morrison syndrome
- Zollinger–Ellison syndrome
- Mastocytosis.

regurgitation. The patient suffers from dyspnea and may present with right-sided heart failure. There is a correlation between pretreatment urinary 5-hydroxyindoleacetic acid and heart disease. Bronchial wheezing is observed in <10% of patients. Abdominal pain, due to complete or partial intestinal obstruction, is not a part of the carcinoid syndrome, but may be one of the most important symptoms of an ileal carcinoid tumor. Ischemia may also induce severe pain and diarrhea in some patients. Typically, a lymph node grows around the mesenteric artery, strangling the blood flow (see Chapter 55). The pain is usually worse after meals. In some patients the ischemia is accompanied by malabsorption and weight loss. These patients should always be evaluated by a surgeon since surgery may improve the patient's status.

Differential diagnosis (Table 113.2)

Many patients presenting with diarrhea as part of a carcinoid syndrome are misdiagnosed as suffering from infectious diarrhea or inflammatory bowel disease.

Diagnostic methods

Clinical history and a physical examination are often helpful. **Chromogranin A** is the most sensitive marker to detect an ileal carcinoid tumor. After radical operation, chromogranin A is the first marker to indicate a recurrence, and becomes elevated a median of 2 years before the recurrence is diagnosed. Since chromogranin A is not specific for ileal carcinoid tumors, it should be complemented by measurement of the serotonin metabolite **5-hydroxyindole acetic acid (U-5HIAA)** in 24-hour urine. However, the U-5HIAA levels may be normal despite the presence of a tumor (Table 113.4) [6]. The diagnosis is confirmed by chromogranin A and serotonin immunoreactivity in tumor cells on histopathology. **Ki67 immunostaining**, a measure of proliferation, helps to identify more aggressive tumors.

Tumor localization and spread can be evaluated by **radiology**, e.g., triphasic contrast enhanced computed tomography (CT) and magnetic resonance imaging (MRI). **Abdominal ultrasonography** is useful to guide a needle biopsy from metastases. More than 95% of ileal carcinoid tumors express somatostatin receptors, which can be detected by **scintigraphy** using radiolabeled somatostatin analogs (Figure 113.4). This method can guide treatment since patients expressing receptors usually respond to treatment with somatostatin analogs as well as to targeted treatment with radiolabeled somatostatin analogs. Somatostatin receptor scintigraphy also helps in planning surgery by giving accurate information about distant metastasis, e.g., bone or extra-abdominal lymph nodes (Figure 113.5). **Positron emission tomography (PET)** can be used

to characterize both metabolic and biochemical features in tumor disease (Figure 113.6). Unlike most cancer cells, neuroendocrine tumors do not have increased glucose metabolism, so ^{18}F-2-deoxy-D-glucose (FDG) PET scanning is not useful. Instead, ^{11}C-labeled 5-hydroxytryptophan (^{11}C-5-HTP) is very sensitive in localizing small primary tumors and metastases.

Treatment

Surgery

Curative surgery is seldom possible. However, **debulking surgery** should always be considered since reduction of tumor mass may improve the quality of life as well as prolong survival. Resection of the primary tumor may prevent future problems related to intestinal obstruction, and removal of the mesenteric lymph node metastasis may prevent future ischemia. Resection of liver metastases should also be considered to reduce tumor burden.

Embolization is another alternative to treat liver metastases. Since the liver has a dual blood supply, vascular occlusion of

Table 113.2 Differential diagnosis

- Menopausal flushing
- Carcinoid syndrome
- Mastocytosis
- Pheochromocytoma
- Medullary thyroid carcinoma
- Endocrine pancreatic tumors (VIP, gastrin)
- Spinal cord injury
- Emotional flushing
- Alcohol and drugs
- Food related

Table 113.3 Flushing related to drugs

- Bromocriptin
- Tamoxifen
- Nicotinic acid
- Opiates
- Calcium channel blockers
- Metronidazole
- Ketoconazole
- Chlorpromazine
- Cephalosporin

Table 113.4 Number of patients with elevated tumor marker

Tumour marker	No. elevated/No. tested	%
U-5HIAA	187/246	76
Chromogranin A	75/86	87
Neuropeptide K	69/149	46

U-5HIAA, 5-hydroxyindole acetic acid.
Data from Janson ET *et al*. Carcinoid tumors: analysis of prognostic factors and survival in 301 patients from a referral center. *Ann Oncol*. 1997;8:685–690, with permission from Oxford University Press.

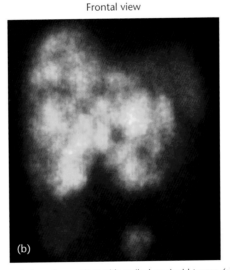

Dorsal view   Frontal view

(a)   (b)

Figure 113.4 Somatostatin receptor scintigraphy showing intense uptake of liver metastases in a patient with an ileal carcinoid tumor. (a) Dorsal view; (b) frontal view.

Multiple Organ Systems

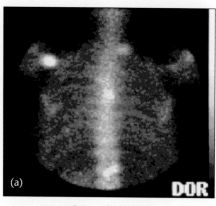
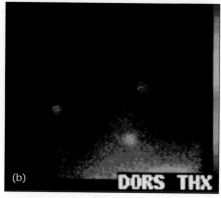

Bone scintigram   Octreoscan

Figure 113.5 Detection of bone metastases. (a) A bone scintigram and (b) somatostatin receptor scintigraphy (octreoscan) showing bone metastases in a patient with an ileal carcinoid tumor. There is a good correlation between the two methods in detecting the bone metastases.

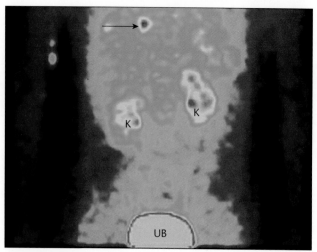

Figure 113.6 Positron emission tomography (PET) with ^{11}C-5-hydroxytryptophan as tracer showing the localization of liver metastases in a patient with an ileal carcinoid tumor. This patient had radical surgery 5 years earlier and showed increasing tumor markers. Conventional radiology could not localize the recurrence, while the PET examination revealed the metastatic location (arrow). K, kidney; UB, urinary bladder.

the hepatic artery that supplies the carcinoid metastases can induce necrosis of branch tumor cells, leaving the normal hepatic parenchyma dependent on the portal vein for blood supply with only limited damage. Most patients develop a "postembolization syndrome," including abdominal pain, fever, nausea, and transient increase of liver enzymes. To avoid development of a hepatorenal syndrome, forced diuresis is recommended. Release of hormones from the necrotic tumor cells may induce a carcinoid crisis and this can be prevented by continuous infusion of somatostatin analogs. Other severe complications include ischemic necrosis of the gallbladder and the small bowel, sepsis, hepatic abscesses, and thromboembolic complications. Tumor regression and biochemical responses are seen in about 40–50% of patients and last for 10–12 months. The procedure can be repeated.

Radiofrequency (RF) ablation has recently been incorporated into the treatment arsenal. The method is very promising but its place still has to be established in clinical studies.

Liver transplantation has been performed in some centers. However, it is of utmost importance to exclude metastases outside the liver before transplantation is performed. There are reports with long-term postoperative survival in at least a subpopulation of patients with ileal carcinoid tumors.

Patients with carcinoid heart disease should be considered for heart valve replacement. It is recommended that the carcinoid syndrome be under control before the operation.

Drug therapy

Since most patients cannot be cured by surgery, medical treatment has to be used. Cytotoxic chemotherapy is not recommended as first-line therapy due to poor results. Different protocols have been applied and the most frequently studied combination is streptozotocin and 5-fluorouracil, but in a randomized trial no obvious benefit was detectable in comparison to alpha-interferon .

Alpha-interferon is used in the treatment of carcinoid tumors. It is thought to inhibit cell proliferation and induce immune cell-mediated cytotoxicity as well as antiangiogenesis. However, the exact mechanism remains to be elucidated. The dose of alpha-interferon should be individually titrated and most patients receive 3–5MU 3 days per week – to have a good clinical effect the leukocyte count should be below 3×10^9/L. If the leukocyte count falls below 2×10^9/L, the dose of alpha-interferon should be reduced. Biochemical responses have been shown in up to 66% of patients, but response rate varies among studies (Table 113.5) [7]. The most frequent adverse reactions include fatigue and depression, for which antidepressant drugs are used with good results, and depressed bone marrow function. Another problem with alpha-interferon treatment is the development of autoimmune reactions in up to 20% of patients. Usually the symptoms disappear when alpha-interferon treatment is interrupted.

Somatostatin analogs are used in the treatment of the carcinoid syndrome and have effects that include inhibition of hormone secretion and exocrine pancreatic function, as well as apoptotic and antiangiogenic effects. Somatostatin receptors expressed on tumor cells are the target for treatment. The analogs available for clinical use (octreotide and lanreotide) bind with high affinity to receptor subtypes 2 and 5. The treatment reduces hormone release and symptoms in 27% and 75% of patients, respectively (Table 113.6), and improves quality of life. Unfortunately, few patients (<5%) show a significant reduction in tumor size. Today, long-acting formulas allowing monthly injections are commonly used and the treatment is well tolerated. Recently, it was shown that patients with ileal carcinoid tumors treated with octreotide long-acting release (LAR) had a significantly longer time to progression (14 months) as compared to those treated with placebo (6 months) [8]. Thus, somatostatin analogs appear to have a stabilizing effect on tumor growth. It is now considered appropriate to use somatostatin analogs both for functioning and non-functioning carcinoid tumors. Side effects include nausea and mild abdominal pain which usually decline with time. Since somatostatin inhibits the secretion of pancreatic juice, replacement therapy with pancreatic enzymes may be needed in order to avoid diarrhea due to steatorrhea. Other side effects include development of gallbladder stones or sludge. Bradycardia is a rare adverse reaction and glucose levels should be monitored. The combination of somatostatin analog and alpha-interferon may also be effective.

Targeted tumor treatment with **radiolabeled somatostatin analogs** has been included in the therapeutic arsenal. Several small studies have been reported using octreotide labeled with different isotopes, including ^{111}In and ^{90}Y, and both biochemical and radiological responses are observed. Today, the most widely used isotope is [177]Lu. In order to be eligible for ^{177}Lu-octreotate treatment, a pre-treatment somatostatin receptor scintigraphy must show at least a grade 2 or higher uptake in known metastases. Reports on treatment outcome show that carcinoid patients have a reduction in tumor size of up to 20%. [9] Side effects include bone marrow depression, nausea, mild hair loss, abdominal pain, and impairment of hepatic and renal function.

Table 113.5 Effect of alpha-interferon on ileal carcinoid tumors

Author (year)	No. patients response (%)	Biochemical response (%)	Subjective response (%)	Tumor volume
Moertel (1989)	27	39	65	20
Schober (1992)	16	66	85	25
Öberg (1991)	111	42	68	15
Joensuu (1992)	14	50	56	0
Bajetta (1993)	34	24	26	12
Biesma (1992)	20	60	83	11

Table 113.6 Effect of somatostatin analogs on ileal carcinoid tumors

Author (year)	Regimen	Biochemical response (%)	Symtomatic response (%)	Radiological response (%)
Octreotide				
Kvols (1986)	150 μg × 3/day	72	88	0
Öberg (1991)	50 μg × 2/day	27	50	9
Arnold (1996)	200 μg × 3/day	33	—	0
Octreotide long-acting release				
Garland (2003)	20 mg every 4 weeks	—	85	0
Somatuline				
Anthony (1993)	3000 μg × 3/day	72	—	50
Somatuline prolonged release				
Ruszniewski (1996)	30 mg every 2 weeks	42	55	0
Wymenga (1999)	30 mg every 1– 2 weeks	27	54	8
Ricci (2000)	30 mg every 2 weeks	42	70	8

Table 113.7 Survival in patients with ileal carcinoid tumors

Overall from diagnosis	92 months
Overall from start of treatment	67 months
According to extent of disease:	
Only lymph node metastases	108 months
<5 liver metastases	159 months
>5 liver metastases	53 months

Data from Janson ET *et al*. Carcinoid tumors: analysis of prognostic factors and survival in 301 patients from a referral center. *Ann Oncol*. 1997;8:685–690, with permission from Oxford University Press.

Most recently, tyrosine kinase inhibitors such as VEGF inhibitors, have been applied in the treatment of metastatic carcinoid tumors, but with poor response rate (<10%). The mTOR inhibitor everolimus is another new promising drug, but we are still waiting for long-term clinical results.

Symptomatic treatment for patients with carcinoid tumors is used to reduce symptoms induced by the tumor. Since one of the major features of the carcinoid syndrome is diarrhea, loperamide may be of benefit. In some patients, nicotinamide supplement should be given. Bronchospasm may be treated with bronchodilators.

Complications and their management

One of the most difficult complications that may develop in a patient with an ileal carcinoid tumor is the **"carcinoid crisis,"** especially in those undergoing surgery or other manipulations of the tumor. The patient typically presents with a long-standing flush, hypotension, tachycardia and bronchial constriction. The best treatment is continuous intravenous infusion of a somatostatin analog. Infusion of epinephrine (adrenaline) to induce vasoconstriction may be life threatening since epinephrine may stimulate the tumor to release further hormone. Another complication commonly found in carcinoid patients is **intestinal ischemia** caused by obstruction of the mesenteric artery by a lymph node. Surgery is the treatment of choice for these patients.

Prognosis with and without treatment

The prognosis for patients with ileal carcinoid tumors varies among different studies. Prognostic factors include prolifera-

tion index, tumor burden, and hormone production. In a multivariate analysis, the pretreatment plasma level of chromogranin A was an independent prognostic factor. For patients with a carcinoid syndrome, the median survival in non-treated patients is about 2 years. In more recent publications, the 5-year survival rate is between 50% and 90% for patients with metastases at diagnosis (Table 113.7) [1]. A special feature of carcinoid tumors is the ability to develop metastases many years after the primary tumor has been removed. Therefore, even patients who have undergone radical operation for an ileal carcinoid tumor should be followed for several years. For early detection of recurrent disease, plasma level of chromogranin A is the best marker, and when this starts to rise, U-5HIAA should be measured. To localize the recurrence, PET examination with ^{11}C-5-HTP might prove helpful in early cases, since recurrences usually are difficult to find with conventional radiology.

References

1. Yao JC, Hassan M, Phan A, *et al*. One hundred years after "carcinoid": Epidemiology of and prognostic factors for neuroendocrine tumors in 35,825 cases in the United States. *J Clin Oncol*. 2008;18:3063–3072.
2. Rindi G, Capella C, Solcia E. Cell biology, clinicopathological profile, and classification of gastro-enteropancreatic endocrine tumors. *J Mol Med*. 1998;76:413–420.
3. Cunningham J, Grimelius L, Sundin A, *et al*. Malignant ileocaekal serotonin-producing carcinoid tumors: The presence of a solid growth pattern and/or Ki67 above 1% identifies patients with a poorer prognosis. *Acta Oncol*. 2007;46:47–56.
4. Solcia E, Klöppel G, Sobin LH. Histological typing of endocrine tumours. In: *World Health Organization International Histopathological Classification of Tumours*. 2. Berlin: Springer; 2000:61–68.
5. Rindi G, Klöppel G, Couvelard A, *et al*. TNM staging of midgut and hindgut (neuro) endocrine tumors: a consensus proposal including a grading system. *Virchows Arch*. 2007;451:757–762.
6. Welin S, Stridsberg M, Cunningham J, *et al*. Elevated plasma chromogranin A is the first indication of recurrence in radically operated midgut carcinoid tumors. *Neuroendocrinology*. 2009;89: 302–307.
7. Schober C, Schmoll E, Schmoll HJ, *et al*. Antitumour effect and symptomatic control with interferon alpha 2b in patients with endocrine active tumours. *Eur J Cancer*. 1992;10:1664–1666.
8. Rinke A, Muller HH, Schade-Brittinger C, *et al*. Placebo-controlled, double-blind, prospective, randomized study on the effect of octreotide LAR in the control of tumor growth in patients with metastatic neuroendocrine midgut tumors. A report from the PROMID study group. *J Clin Oncol*. 2009;27:4656–4663.
9. Kwekkeboom DJ, de Herder WW, Kam BL, *et al*. Treatment with the radiolabeled somatostatin analog (177Lu-DOTA 0,Tyr3)octreotate: toxicity, efficacy, and survival. *J Clin Oncol*. 2008;26: 2124–2130.

CHAPTER 114
AIDS and the gut

C. Mel Wilcox

University of Alabama at Birmingham, Birmingham, AL, USA

ESSENTIAL FACTS ABOUT PATHOGENESIS

- Diseases of the gastrointestinal tract are common in AIDS. Clinical manifestations point to the etiology)
- Odynophagia: candida, herpes simplex virus, cytomegalovirus (CMV), Kaposi's sarcoma
- Esophageal disease: candida, viral (CMV), HIV-associated idiopathic ulcer
- Gastric diseases: infrequent but include CMV and Kaposi's sarcoma
- Small bowel disease: common causes include *Cryptosporidium parvum*, microsporidia, isospora, cyclospora, *Mycobacterium avium*, *Mycobacterium tuberculosis*; drugs, especially nelfinovir, a component of HAART. Lymphoma and Kaposi's sarcoma may cause obstruction.
- The status of HIV enteropathy: unexplained by other agents is uncertain
- Colonic disease: CMV colitis, bacterial colitis including *Clostridium difficile*

ESSENTIALS OF DIAGNOSIS

- Esophageal: endoscopy with biopsy
- Diarrhea: consider side effect of nelfinavir, a component of HAART
- Three to six stool samples for bacterial culture, ova and parasite examination including *C. difficile* toxin
- Colonoscopy or upper endoscopy as appropriate with biopsy. Fecal leukocytes point to colitis

ESSENTIALS OF TREATMENT

- Multiple infections are common and potentially require multiple therapies, including fluconazole (often empirically); ganciclovir, ciclovir, valganciclovir for CMV; trimethoprim—sulfamethoxazole for isospora and cyclospora; antimicrobial chemotherapy
- Most effective long-term therapy for all opportunistic processes in AIDS is immune reconstitution associated with HAART

Introduction

Since the first descriptions in 1981 of acquired immunodeficiency syndrome (AIDS), extraordinary strides have been made in our understanding of the human immunodeficiency virus (HIV) and the pathogenesis of disease. While the incidence of HIV infection in developed countries has stabilized or fallen, the epidemic continues unabated in developing countries and has grown in Eastern Europe and India.

Although a dramatic fall in AIDS-related gastrointestinal complications has occurred since the introduction of highly active antiretroviral therapy (HAART) [1], these complications remain important because of their prevalence worldwide, morbidity, and impact on healthcare resources. Given the many potential causes of gastrointestinal disease in these patients, this chapter will take an organ-based approach to review etiologies, manifestations, evaluation, and therapy.

General principles

Several important principles, many of which are unique to patients with AIDS, guide the evaluation of the HIV-infected patient with gastrointestinal complaints:

1. The rule of parsimony does not apply to patients with AIDS as multiple co-existent diseases are commonplace.
2. Opportunistic infections occur when immunodeficiency is severe. Therefore, the CD4 lymphocyte count will stratify the risk for an opportunistic process (Figure 114.1) [2,3].
3. Opportunistic disorders are frequently systemic. Identification of a pathogen outside of the gut (e.g., blood, bone marrow) may establish a presumptive cause of gastrointestinal symptoms.
4. Demonstration of a pathogen in tissue is the most specific means of establishing an etiological diagnosis.
5. Recurrence is common for all opportunistic infections unless immunodeficiency is reversed with HAART.
6. Institution of HAART, when associated with immune reconstitution, is the best "treatment" for all complications associated with HIV-related immunodeficiency.

Oropharyngeal diseases

Diseases of the oropharynx are common in HIV infection, and **oropharyngeal candidiasis** (thrush) remains one of the most common index manifestations of AIDS. Oropharyngeal or hypopharyngeal pain generally reflects an ulcerative process, and aphthous ulcers are the most common cause of single or multiple well-circumscribed ulcers. Other causes of **oropharyngeal ulcers** in these patients include **herpes simplex virus**

Multiple Organ Systems

Textbook of Clinical Gastroenterology and Hepatology, Second Edition. Edited by C. J. Hawkey, Jaime Bosch, Joel E. Richter, Guadalupe Garcia-Tsao, Francis K. L. Chan.

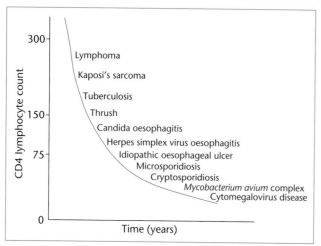

Figure 114.1 Relationship of opportunistic infections to CD4 lymphocyte count. (Reprinted by permission from Macmillan Publishers Ltd: Monkemuller KE, Call SA, Lazenby AJ, Wilcox CM. Declining prevalence of opportunistic gastrointestinal disease in the era of combination antiretroviral therapy. *Am J Gastroenterol.* 2000;95:457–462.)

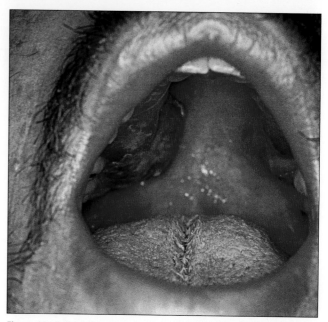

Figure 114.2 Kaposi's sarcoma of the hard palate. Two large purple nodular lesions are seen on the hard palate of this patient with AIDS.

(HSV), **cytomegalovirus (CMV)**, and, rarely, other infections. **Kaposi's sarcoma** appears as characteristic purple plaques or nodules (Figure 114.2). Biopsy of oropharyngeal lesions should be performed when the appearance of the lesion is non-diagnostic, neoplasia is suspected, or empiric therapy is ineffective. With the exception of thrush where local therapies are effective, treatment for oropharyngeal diseases parallels that for the esophagus (see below).

Esophageal diseases
Pathogenesis
Disorders of the esophagus are frequent in patients with AIDS, observed in up to 40% of patients who do not receive HAART. *Candida* esophagitis is etiological in 40–70% of patients, followed by viral diseases, most commonly CMV [4,5]. Another important cause of esophageal disease is the **HIV-associated aphthous** or **idiopathic esophageal ulcer**, the pathogenesis of which remains poorly understood [6]. Multiple co-existent esophageal disorders may be identified in 10% of patients; this complicates management.

Clinical presentation
Odynophagia is an important and reliable clue to the presence of an esophageal infection or ulcer. **Dysphagia** suggests *Candida* esophagitis or esophageal stricture, either benign or malignant. When symptoms are localized to the neck or throat, hypopharyngeal rather than esophageal disease should be suspected and evaluated accordingly. Examination of the oropharynx may provide clues to the cause of esophageal complaints. Most patients (66%) with *Candida* esophagitis have concomitant thrush. Oropharyngeal ulcerations are frequently associated with HSV esophagitis but rarely are present with CMV esophagitis and idiopathic esophageal ulcer.

Empirical management
Because of the high frequency of *Candida* esophagitis, empirical antifungal therapy with **oral fluconazole** (loading dose of 200 mg followed by 100 mg daily) is an appropriate initial management strategy for AIDS patients with new onset of esophageal symptoms [5]. Since the clinical response of *Candida* esophagitis to therapy is very rapid, if no symptomatic response is apparent within the first 31 days of initiating fluconazole, especially in the patient with severe symptoms, upper endoscopy should be performed rather than initiation of further empirical trials [5,7].

Diagnostic investigation
Endoscopy with biopsy is the definitive diagnostic test for esophageal disease in AIDS. At the time of endoscopic evaluation, the appearance of some disorders is diagnostic, and **ulcerative lesions** may be biopsied (Figure 114.3). When an ulcer is identified, multiple biopsies (at least 10) should be obtained to maximize sensitivity. **Vigorous biopsy of the ulcer base** is essential for detecting **CMV**, while **HSV** is identified in squamous epithelium from the **ulcer edge** (Figure 114.4). Cytological brushings and viral culture of ulcer tissue generally adds very little over multiple biopsies alone.

Immunohistochemical stains for viral pathogens improve the diagnostic yield and specificity over routine hematoxylin and eosin (H&E) staining. Additional histological staining for other infections may be used selectively based upon the clinical, endoscopic, and histological findings. An ulcer can be considered idiopathic when infections are excluded by appropriate histological studies and if pill-induced esophagitis and reflux disease are not suggested by the clinical presentation and endoscopic findings.

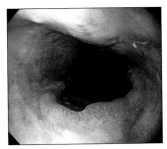

Figure 114.3 Idiopathic esophageal ulcer. Large well-circumscribed ulcer with heaped up margins in the proximal esophagus. The endoscopic appearance may mimic cytomegalovirus esophagitis.

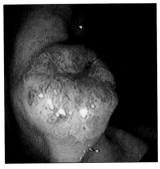

Figure 114.5 Gastric Kaposi's sarcoma. Multiple raised lesions with central umbilication and subepithelial hemorrhage involving the gastric body.

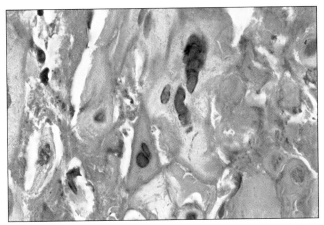

Figure 114.4 Herpes simplex virus (HSV). High-power photomicrograph shows several cells with multinucleated inclusions characteristic of HSV.

Treatment and prognosis

Therapy for esophageal diseases in patients with AIDS is highly effective. **Fluconazole** (100 mg/day) is currently the drug of choice for *Candida* esophagitis because of its excellent absorption, minimal drug interactions and side effects, and superior efficacy [8]. Effective therapies are also available for both HSV and CMV esophagitis. At most centers, intravenous **ganciclovir** is the drug of choice for CMV because of its relative tolerability and lower cost. **Cidofovir** is an attractive option for some patients given its once weekly administration. The primary side effect of ganciclovir is myelosuppression, whereas both foscarnet and cidofovir are nephrotoxic and may cause electrolyte disturbances (e.g., hypocalcemia, hypophosphatemia). **Valganciclovir**, an oral agent, has excellent absorption, reaching serum concentrations equivalent to ganciclovir. Although effective for the treatment of CMV retinitis [9], treatment of gastrointestinal disease has not been well studied but may represent an option.

Without **HAART**, the relapse rate following therapy is 40–50%, similar to that for HSV. For patients with idiopathic esophageal ulcers, both **prednisone** and **thalidomide** are very effective. Prednisone should be administered for 1 month, beginning with a dose of 40 mg/day and then tapering by 10 mg each week. This regimen is well tolerated and once-weekly **fluconazole** (100 mg) will reduce any oropharyngeal or esophageal candidiasis, which may complicate steroid use and confuse the clinical response. Thalidomide has been successful in rare patients who fail to respond to prednisone. This agent must be used cautiously and with the appropriate safeguards.

Gastric diseases

Clinically apparent gastric disorders are relatively infrequent in patients with AIDS. Although a number of infections have been reported, **CMV** is the most frequent opportunistic infection involving the stomach in AIDS, and usually causes one or multiple ulcers. **Kaposi's sarcoma** often involves the stomach, but is generally asymptomatic unless the lesions are large and bulky, which may then lead to abdominal pain, pyloric obstruction, or bleeding (Figure 114.5). As with all gut symptoms, non-opportunistic causes deserve consideration regardless of the CD4 count. Epigastric pain, nausea, and vomiting are the most common symptoms of gastric diseases, but are non-specific. Overt gastrointestinal hemorrhage suggests ulceration. **Nausea and vomiting** are particularly common complaints in HIV-infected patients, and may reflect a variety of different etiologies including medications.

In light of the broad differential diagnosis of upper gastrointestinal complaints in patients with AIDS, **endoscopy** and mucosal biopsy are generally required for definitive diagnosis. **Computed tomography** (CT) may suggest the presence of gastric disease, but may also identify extraintestinal disease, implicating a widely disseminated process. Upper gastrointestinal barium studies play little diagnostic role.

Small bowel diseases

Intestinal disorders are among the most frequent complications in HIV-infected patients, and their high frequency may be related to altered gut immune function. A reduction in the number of **CD4 lymphocytes** in the lamina propria, which parallels the decrease in systemic CD4 cells, as well as decreased levels of **secretory IgA** in intestinal secretions in

AIDS predispose to intestinal infection. In addition, the reduced number of mucosal CD4 lymphocytes may be responsible for alterations in small intestinal morphology and function (see below).

Pathogenesis

Small bowel disease in AIDS patients is usually caused by opportunistic infections.

Cryptosporidium parvum

Worldwide, *C. parvum*, a coccidian parasite, is the most common small bowel pathogen. While a self-limited illness in normal hosts, the incidence and severity of disease parallel the degree of immunodeficiency in HIV-infected patients. Patients with a **CD4 count** of >200/mm^3 may have a self-limited illness while in those with a CD4 count of <50/mm^3, the disease is chronic, typically severe, and associated with poor survival [10]. While the spectrum of the disease is variable, diarrhea caused by *C. parvum* infection is characteristically **secretory** and can result in **dehydration, electrolyte disturbances, and weight loss.**

The diagnosis can be established by modified acid-fast **staining of fresh stool**, but examination of multiple stool specimens is generally required to increase yield. If stool tests are negative and the disease is suspected clinically, **duodenal or ileal biopsies** will usually establish the diagnosis [9]; colonic biopsies may occasionally be positive.

Numerous medications have been used to treat cryptosporidiosis, generally without success. The most effective therapy is **HAART**, which if associated with immune reconstitution, can result in complete remission [11].

Microsporidia

Microsporidia have emerged as one of the most common gastrointestinal opportunistic infections in AIDS, identified in 10–20% of AIDS patients with diarrhea worldwide. As with other opportunistic diseases, the prevalence of this infection has fallen dramatically with the use of HAART [12]. Gastrointestinal disease is caused by two species, *Enterocytozoon bienusi* and *E. intestinalis*, with *E. bienusi* accounting for over 80% of cases of gastrointestinal disease. The clinical illness is milder than with cryptosporidia, and dehydration, electrolyte disturbances, and marked weight loss suggest some other process; rarely, these pathogens may be found in an asymptomatic patient.

On **small bowel biopsy**, the organisms appear as small round structures in the supranuclear portion of the enterocyte cytoplasm (Figure 114.6). Colonic involvement has not been reported. Unlike *E. bienusi*, *E. intestinalis* can be identified in the lamina propria and because it is invasive, disseminated disease to other organs can be observed. These small intracellular parasites may be difficult to appreciate on H&E staining, and additional staining methods such as tissue Gram stain are often required. Electron microscopy has been considered the

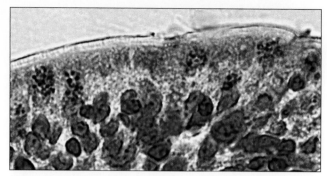

Figure 114.6 Small bowel microsporidiosis. Tissue Gram stain of small bowel biopsy shows multiple small round Gram-positive organisms in clusters in epithelial cell.

gold standard for diagnosis and permits a species-specific diagnosis. **Stool tests** are also available to detect the organism but their sensitivity remains low.

Therapeutic options for *E. bienusi* are limited. Despite initial promising reports, metronidazole has been shown to be largely ineffective. In contrast, *E. intestinalis* infection responds to albendazole, with some patients achieving clinical and microbiological cure [13]; *E. bienusi* responds poorly to this agent. As with cryptosporidia, **HAART** can result in complete remission, but if immune deficiency returns, relapse occurs, which underscores the interaction of immune function and these opportunistic intestinal infections [11].

Other pathogens

Other small bowel parasitic diseases in AIDS include infection with **Isospora** and **Cyclospora**. Isospora has been most commonly reported as a diarrheal pathogen in developing countries. Cyclospora has recently been identified as a small bowel pathogen in both developed and developing countries. **Trimethoprim–sulfamethoxazole** (double-strength tablet b.i.d. for 10–14 days) is effective therapy for both pathogens, which may explain the infrequency of infection in countries where *Pneumocystis* prophylaxis is routine.

There is no difference in the incidence or clinical expression of giardia and ameba in HIV-infected patients as compared with normal hosts. Nematodes have been described but do not have a higher incidence in these patients.

Mycobacterium avium complex

Mycobacterium avium complex, a disease of **late-stage AIDS**, is the most common mycobacterial infection complicating AIDS in the USA, while *Mycobacterium tuberculosis* (TB) is generally a disease of developing countries. The use of **HAART** has dramatically reduced the incidence of infection. Although diarrhea and abdominal pain may be observed in disseminated *Mycobacterium avium* complex, **fever and wasting** tend to dominate the clinical presentation [14]. **Diarrhea** is usually mild or moderate in severity, even when small bowel infection is extensive.

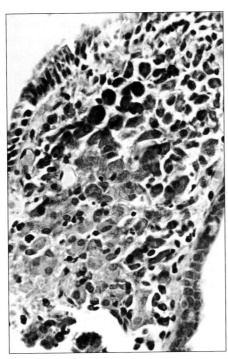

Figure 114.7 *Mycobacterium avium* complex infection of the small bowel. AFB stain of small bowel biopsy showing multiple bacteria in macrophages with an appearance mimicking that of Whipple's disease.

Acid-fast staining of stool is less sensitive than **culture** for detection of *Mycobacterium avium* complex. **Small bowel biopsy** is the definitive diagnostic test (Figure 114.7).

Current multidrug regimens against *Mycobacterium avium* complex are effective due to the high *in vitro* efficacy of clarithromycin, azithromycin, and ethambutol [15]. Nevertheless, therapy is not considered curative and must be taken indefinitely unless **HAART** is instituted.

Tuberculosis

Tuberculosis (TB) may involve any portion of the gastrointestinal tract, but ileal involvement is most frequent. In contrast to *Mycobacterium avium* complex, TB may occur at any stage of immunodeficiency and can be cured with 9–12 months of multidrug therapy, provided drug resistance is not present. The recurrence rate following successful therapy, even for extrapulmonary disease, is low.

Viral diseases

Viral diseases of the small bowel are uncommon causes of chronic diarrhea in patients with AIDS. CMV intestinal disease presents as abdominal pain or bleeding due to mucosal ulceration, rather than as diarrhea. The role of HIV-1 as a direct small bowel pathogen remains controversial (see below).

Neoplasms

Neoplasms, including **Kaposi's sarcoma** and **lymphoma**, may involve the small bowel, leading to abdominal **pain, bleeding,** obstruction, or **intussusception**. Endoscopy with biopsy can be used for diagnosis when the lesion is in the proximal bowel, while surgical evaluation will be required for an obstructing lesion or to remove a more distal tumor.

Drugs

Drug-induced diarrhea has become well recognized. The **protease inhibitors** and specifically **nelfinovir** are common culprits. Recognition of a potential drug-induced diarrhea may obviate the need for extensive evaluation if cause and effect can be linked. In this setting, diarrhea is generally mild and can be either controlled by switching medications or appropriate use of antidiarrheal agents.

HIV enteropathy

The term HIV enteropathy has been applied to the AIDS patient with diarrhea but in whom no cause can be found despite extensive evaluation. This entity is diagnosed less commonly today, probably due to the rise in use of endoscopic examination for evaluation, recognition of emerging infections, and use of HAART. A variety of pathological and functional abnormalities of the small intestine have been identified in HIV-infected patients, many of which are independent of opportunistic infections. These changes are usually observed when immunodeficiency is advanced. Chronic inflammation of both the small and large bowel, small bowel atrophy **resembling celiac disease**, as well as functional abnormalities of the small intestine, including reduced **mucosal enzyme** levels (e.g., lactase), malabsorption of sugars (*D*-xylose) and vitamins (**B$_{12}$**), and increased small bowel **permeability**, have all been described. Some of these histological changes could be the result of loss of lamina propria CD4 lymphocytes, as these cells appear to have a trophic effect on the intestinal mucosa [16].

Colonic diseases

In contrast to the frequency of protozoan infections of the small intestine, bacteria and CMV are the most important colonic pathogens in patients with AIDS. The spectrum of bacterial pathogens parallels the normal host. *C. difficile* colitis remains common in patients with AIDS, and the clinical presentation, response to therapy, and relapse rate is no different in HIV-infected patients from other patients. As in the normal host, **bacterial colitis** presents acutely with fever, abdominal pain, and watery or bloody diarrhea.

CMV colitis is one of the more common causes of chronic diarrhea in late-stage HIV disease, with most patients having a CD4 count of <70/mm^3. Although the presentation of CMV colitis is variable, the hallmarks of disease are **abdominal pain** and **watery diarrhea** [17]. Fever is inconsistent, whereas weight loss is almost universal. **Gastrointestinal bleeding** and **perforation** are infrequent complications. CMV colitis should be suspected in any AIDS patient with abdominal pain, chronic diarrhea, weight loss, and repeatedly negative stool culture

Multiple Organ Systems

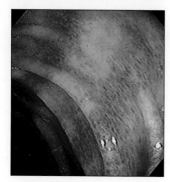

Figure 114.8 Cytomegalovirus (CMV) colitis. Patchy subepithelial hemorrhage in the distal colon typical for CMV. This appearance may mimic inflammatory bowel disease.

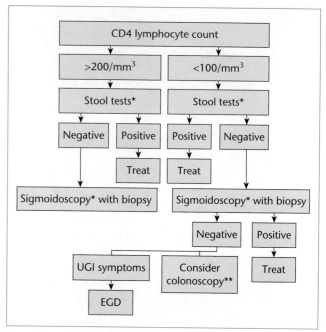

Figure 114.9 Evaluation of chronic diarrhea. Suggested approach to the evaluation of chronic diarrhea in HIV-infected patients. *Fecal leukocytes, culture for enteric pathogens, assay for *Clostridium difficile* toxin, and examination(s) for ova and parasites. **Colonoscopy should be considered when sigmoidoscopy is negative and colonic disease is highly suspected. UGI, upper gastrointestinal. (This figure was published in *Clinical Gastroenterology and Hepatology*, Wilfred M. Weinstein, Christopher J. Hawkey, Jaime Bosch, AIDS and the gut, Pages 1–6, Copyright Elsevier, 2005.)

and ova and parasite examinations. In most patients with advanced immunodeficiency and colorectal symptoms, **stool testing** and **endoscopic evaluation** of the colon are most appropriate. While a number of other infections and neoplasms may involve the colon, differentiation between them clinically and endoscopically may be difficult.

The **endoscopic findings in CMV colitis** include isolated ulcerations, patchy subepithelial hemorrhage, or lesions resembling ulcerative colitis or Crohn's disease (Figure 114.8) [18]. Rarely, the disease may be limited to the right colon, and colonoscopy is necessary for diagnosis. **CT** may suggest the diagnosis when the colon is markedly thickened, although this finding is non-specific. The diagnosis of CMV colitis is best established by identification of the pathognomonic viral cytopathic effect in colonic biopsy specimens. Treatment is similar for disease elsewhere in the gut.

Approach to the AIDS patient with diarrhea (refer also to the accompanying management protocol on the website)

Given the breadth of potential infectious causes of diarrhea and the possibility of either small or large bowel involvement, a systematic approach to diagnosis is essential (Figure 114.9) [17,19]. Three important questions should be addressed when evaluating these patients:

1. Is the diarrhea due to disease of the small bowel, colon, or some combination? The site of disease should be determined on the basis of a careful history and physical examination.
2. Is the patient at risk for an opportunistic infection? The differential diagnosis should be based on the CD4 lymphocyte count. When it is <100/mm³, opportunistic processes are most likely.
3. Have the appropriate stool tests been completed? Symptoms of small bowel disease include crampy periumbilical abdominal pain, flatulence, borborygmi, large stool volume (particularly with fasting), nausea, and vomiting. Lower abdominal pain and symptoms of proctitis point to

inflammatory disease of the distal colon. Fever suggests an infectious cause of diarrhea and, when present, blood cultures should be obtained. Weight loss and severe immunodeficiency in a patient with chronic diarrhea strongly suggest an underlying opportunistic infection. It should be recognized that drug-induced diarrhea associated with HAART (nelfinavir, ddI) is very frequent but generally mild, and use of a drug holiday may help make a presumptive diagnosis.

The presence of **fecal leukocytes** points to colitis and warrants evaluation for bacterial causes (e.g., *C. difficile*) and CMV colitis. If testing for *C. difficile* toxin and routine bacterial cultures of the stool are negative and symptoms of proctitis are present, sigmoidoscopy is appropriate. In the setting of severe immunodeficiency, if multiple stool tests are negative and fecal leukocytes are absent, evaluation of the distal colon or full colonoscopy with ileoscopy increases the diagnostic yield, and mucosal biopsies should be routinely taken regardless of the endoscopic appearance.

The appropriate number of **stool samples** for bacterial culture, ova, and parasite examination, and *C. difficile* toxin necessary before proceeding to endoscopic evaluation is unknown. Most investigators suggest three samples, although up to six samples further increases the diagnostic yield [19]. In the hospitalized patient or when symptoms are severe, we proceed to endoscopic evaluation after one negative result. Colonoscopy may be required if there are concomitant right-sided abdominal complaints.

Given the etiological spectrum of infectious causes, broad-spectrum empirical antimicrobial therapies are not routinely recommended. If no cause of diarrhea is found, symptomatic therapy is indicated. **Antimotility drugs** may be safely administered while obtaining additional stool studies. When diarrhea is mild, a bulking agent and antimotility drug such as loperamide are helpful. When diarrhea is more severe, tincture of opium can be very effective.

Anorectal diseases

With the adoption of "safe-sex" practices, the frequency of acute anorectal disorders, especially in homosexual men, has fallen dramatically. Infectious disorders related to unprotected anal intercourse include acute **gonorrheal, syphilitic, and chlamydial proctitis. Human papilloma virus** infection has been implicated as the main etiological factor in **squamous cell carcinoma** of the anus in homosexual men. Screening examination to detect **carcinoma *in situ*** with PAP smears is increasingly used [20]. Traumatic disease of the anorectum, including fissures, should be considered in the appropriate clinical setting. Idiopathic anorectal ulcers have been described, and non-Hodgkin's lymphoma and Kaposi's sarcoma also may involve the anorectum. As with all anorectal diseases, the usual manifestations are anorectal **pain, dyschezia, bleeding, urgency, tenesmus**, and frequent low-volume stools. Dyschezia (painful evacuation) is usually a manifestation of ulceration of the anal canal (fissure, infection). Careful inspection of the anorectum should be performed with attention to the presence of ulceration, fissure, fistula, hemorrhoids, or mass lesions. **Culture** of perianal ulcers is the best method for the diagnosis of HSV, while confirmation of suspected CMV infection may require ulcer biopsy. Visualization of the anorectum is best performed with anoscopy and proctoscopy, or sigmoidoscopy. When dyschezia is severe, evaluation under conscious sedation or general anesthesia may be required.

Pancreatic diseases

Disorders of the pancreas are uncommon in HIV-infected patients. **Acute pancreatitis**, the most common manifestation in AIDS patients, most commonly arises from drugs, hyperlipidemia, gallstones, or rarely infection [21]. The **protease inhibitors** are associated with marked hyperlipidemia. Mild increases in serum amylase are frequent in AIDS patients and are clinically unimportant in the asymptomatic patient. Infectious causes of pancreatitis in patients with AIDS are multiple, although their diagnosis is difficult because pancreatic biopsy is rarely performed. Most cases of opportunistic pancreatic diseases are clinically silent and are diagnosed at autopsy; with pancreatic involvement being part of a widespread disseminated infection. The role of endoscopic retrograde

cholangiopancreatography (ERCP) is similar to that in any other patient.

Conclusions

While the prevalence of gastrointestinal complications has fallen where HAART is available, gastrointestinal complaints remain a frequent source of morbidity in AIDS patients. Given the wide spectrum of potential causes, the evaluation must be tailored to the history, physical examination, and routine laboratory tests, including the CD4 lymphocyte count. Optimism should be maintained when evaluating these patients given the high diagnostic yield of currently available tests as well as the efficacy of available medical therapy, including HAART.

References

1. Monkemuller KE, Call SA, Lazenby AJ, Wilcox CM. Declining prevalence of opportunistic gastrointestinal disease in the era of combination antiretroviral therapy. *Am J Gastroenterol.* 2000;95: 457–462.
2. Wilcox CM, Saag MS. Gastrointestinal complications of HIV infection: changing priorities in the HAART era. *Gut.* 2008; 57:861–870.
3. Bacellar H, Munoz A, Hoover DR, *et al.*; for the Multicenter AIDS cohort study. Incidence of clinical AIDS conditions in a cohort of homosexual men with CD4+ cell counts <100/mm³. *J Infect Dis.* 1994;170:1284–1287.
4. Bonacini M, Young T, Laine L. The causes of esophageal symptoms in human immunodeficiency virus infection: A prospective study of 110 patients. *Arch Intern Med.* 1991;151:1567–1572.
5. Wilcox CM, Alexander LN, Clark WS, Thompson SE. Fluconazole compared with endoscopy for human immunodeficiency virus-infected patients with esophageal symptoms. *Gastroenterology.* 1996;110:1803–1809.
6. Wilcox CM, Schwartz DA, Clark WS. Causes, response to therapy, and long-term outcome of esophageal ulcer in patients with human immunodeficiency virus infection. *Ann Intern Med.* 1995;122:143–149.
7. Wilcox CM, Straub RF, Alexander LN, Clark WS. Etiology of esophageal disease in human immunodeficiency virus-infected patients who fail antifungal therapy. *Am J Med.* 1996;101: 599–604.
8. Pappas PG, Kauffman CA, Andes D, *et al.* Clinical practice guidelines for the management of Candidiasis: 2009 update by the Infectious Diseases Society of America. *CID.* 2009;48: 503–535.
9. Martin DF, Sierra-Madero J, Walmsley S, *et al.* A controlled trial of valganciclovir as induction therapy for cytomegalovirus retinitis. *N Engl J Med.* 2002;346:1119–1126.
10. Manabe YC, Clark DP, Moore RD, *et al.* Cryptosporidiosis in patients with AIDS: correlates of disease and survival. *Clin Infect Dis.* 1998;27:536–542.
11. Carr A, Marriott D, Field A, *et al.* Treatment of HIV-1-associated microsporidiosis and cryptosporidiosis with combination antiretroviral therapy. *Lancet.* 1998;351:256–261.
12. van Hal SJ, Muthiah K, Matthews G, *et al.* Declining incidence of intestinal microsporidiosis and reduction in AIDS-related mortality following introduction of HAART in Sydney, Australia. *Trans R Soc Trop Med Hyg.* 2007;101:1096–1100.

Multiple Organ Systems

13. Dore GJ, Marriott DJ, Hing MC, Harkness JL, Field AS. Disseminated microsporidiosis due to *Septata intestinalis* in nine patients infected with the human immunodeficiency virus: Response to therapy with albendazole. *Clin Infect Dis*. 1995;21:70–76.

14. Havlik JA, Horsburgh CR, Metchock B, *et al*. Disseminated *Mycobacterium avium* complex infection: clinical identification and epidemiologic trends. *J Infect Dis*. 1992;165:577–580.

15. Shafran SD, Singer J, Zarowny DP, *et al*. A comparision of two regimens for the treatment of *Mycobacterium avium* complex bacteremia in AIDS: Rifabutin, ethambutol, and clarithromycin versus rifampin, ethambutol, clofazimine, and ciprofloxacin. *N Engl J Med*. 1996;335:377–383.

16. Cello JP, Day LW. Idiopathic AIDS enteropathy and treatment of gastrointestinal opportunistic pathogens. *Gastroenterology*. 2009;136:1952–1965.

17. Wilcox CM, Schwartz DA, Cotsonis GA, Thompson WE III. Evaluation of chronic unexplained diarrhea in human immuno-deficiency virus infection: determination of the best diagnostic approach. *Gastroenterology*. 1996;110:30–37.

18. Wilcox CM, Chalasani N, Lazenby A, Schwartz DA. Cytomegalovirus colitis in acquired immunodeficiency syndrome: a clinical and endoscopic study. *Gastrointest Endosc*. 1998;48:39–43.

19. Blanshard C, Francis N, Gazzard BG. Investigation of chronic diarrhea in acquired immunodeficiency syndrome. A prospective study of 155 people. *Gut*. 1996;39:824–832.

20. Cranston RD, Hart SD, Gornbein JA, *et al*. The prevalence, and predictive value, of abnormal anal cytology to diagnose anal dysplasia in a population of HIV-positive men who have sex with men. *Int J STD AIDS*. 2007;18:77–80.

21. Bush ZM, Kosmiski LA. Acute pancreatitis in HIV-infected patients: are etiologies changing since the introduction of protease inhibitor therapy? *Pancreas*. 2003;27:E1–E5.

CHAPTER 115

Graft-versus-host disease

George B. McDonald
University of Washington; Fred Hutchinson Cancer Research Center, Seattle, WA, USA

ESSENTIAL FACTS ABOUT CAUSATION

- Graft-versus-host disease (GvHD) is caused by "foreign" (allogeneic) immune cells
- Two forms of GvHD exist – acute and chronic, each with different characteristics

---

ESSENTIALS OF DIAGNOSIS

Acute GvHD
Common after hematopoietic cell transplantation, uncommon after organ transplantation, and rare after blood transfusion
- Presents with anorexia, nausea, satiety, abdominal pain, diarrhea, skin rash, and jaundice
- A clinical diagnosis can be supplemented by endoscopy and biopsy of antrum and colon
- Endoscopic changes range from mucosal edema to substantial ulceration
- Histological changes comprise lymphocyte aggregates, apoptosis of crypt cells, and crypt cell dropout

Chronic GvHD
- Resembles autoimmune diseases, resulting in dry eyes, oral mucositis, skin and tendon fibrosis, esophageal webs and strictures, jaundice, and protracted gut symptoms
- Diagnosis is based on clinical findings and histology of oral, skin, and gut biopsies

---

ESSENTIALS OF TREATMENT

- Acute GvHD may be rapidly fatal if not promptly recognized and treated; prognosis is related more to duration of disease than peak severity
- Treatment of chronic GVHD is difficult, requiring prolonged immune suppressive therapy in many patients

---

Introduction and definition

Graft-versus-host disease (GvHD) occurs when someone else's immune cells are introduced into a patient who cannot reject them. These allogeneic cells, and the inflammatory response they invoke, damage the gut, liver, skin and other squamous epithelium, tissues such as salivary and lacrimal glands, and the immune system. **Acute GvHD** is common after hemat-opoietic cell transplantation, but uncommon after transplantation of a solid organ harboring immune cells and rare after blood transfusions. Acute GvHD may be fatal unless recognized promptly and treated aggressively. **Chronic GvHD**, a more indolent but potentially fatal disease in long-term survivors of transplantation, has clinical features of autoimmune disorders.

Epidemiology

Acute GvHD affects 50–70% of **allogeneic transplant patients** [1]. More severe acute GvHD develops when donors are mismatched for class I and II alleles, or sex mismatched, or of increased parity. In some patients with cancer, acute GvHD is deliberately induced in order to kill tumor cells via donor lymphocytes (graft-versus-tumor effect). Acute GvHD occurs in approximately 10% of patients after **autologous transplantation** (a patient's own cells are reinfused), usually affecting only the skin and upper gut.

About 60% of allograft recipients will develop **chronic GVHD**, a multiorgan disease process that affects the skin, mouth, eyes, esophagus, muscle, joints, tendons, and vaginal mucosa [2].

Causes

GvHD is caused by hematopoietic cell transplantation or the introduction of allogeneic lymphocytes in a blood transfusion or a transplanted organ into an immune-suppressed patient. GvHD can be induced deliberately by the abrupt discontinuation of prophylactic medications or by infusing allogeneic donor lymphocytes.

Pathogenesis

The pathophysiology of both acute and chronic GvHD in humans is very complex [1]. Tissue damage caused by myeloablative regimens activates host antigen-presenting cells that stimulate donor T cells, but fatal GvHD also occurs after reduced-intensity conditioning regimens and rarely after transfusion alone. Tissue damage results from the generation

Multiple Organ Systems

Textbook of Clinical Gastroenterology and Hepatology, Second Edition. Edited by C. J. Hawkey, Jaime Bosch, Joel E. Richter, Guadalupe Garcia-Tsao, Francis K. L. Chan.
© 2012 Blackwell Publishing Ltd. Published 2012 by Blackwell Publishing Ltd.

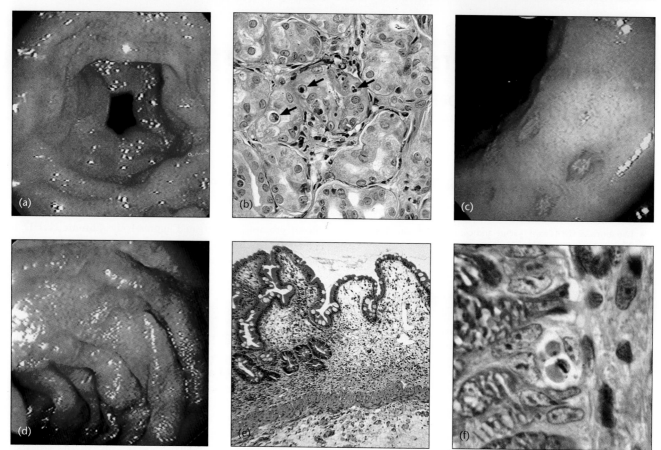

Figure 115.1 Endoscopic and histological features of acute graft-versus-host disease (GvHD) involving the gastrointestinal tract. (a) Mucosal edema and erythema of the gastric antrum. (b) Photomicrograph of gastric biopsy specimen, showing apoptotic epithelial cells (arrows), crypt destruction, and small numbers of infiltrating lymphocytes. (c) Multiple shallow ulcers on the lesser curvature of the stomach. (d) Mucosa in the small intestine, showing erythema, edema, and multiple small erosions with hemorrhage. (e) Photomicrograph of small intestinal mucosa, showing absence of crypt epithelium on the right. (f) Photomicrograph of colonic mucosa biopsy specimen, showing cell fragments of an epithelial cell that has undergone apoptosis (apoptotic body), adjacent to normal crypt epithelium.

of cytokines and cytotoxic T lymphocytes and natural killer cells, leading to damage to the skin, gut, and liver. Target cells are in the proliferative zone at the base of intestinal crypts, the parafollicular bulge and basal dermal areas of skin, and small bile ducts. Severe damage to intestinal mucosa, skin, and liver that does not respond promptly to therapy is uniformly fatal.

Pathology

The histological hallmark of gastrointestinal GvHD is **apoptosis of epithelial cells in crypts**, recognized by clusters of nuclear and cytoplasmic debris (Figure 115.1) [1,3]. T-cell infiltration may not be present early in the course of GvHD. With progression, whole crypts may disappear, then focal areas of mucosa, followed by mucosal sloughing. In the **liver**, early findings in GvHD are minimal, as jaundice is the result of cytokine effects; later, abnormalities in the small bile ducts appear – dysmorphic epithelial cells, apoptosis, dropout of cells, and T-cell infiltrates in and around small bile ducts

(Figure 115.2) [4]. **Cholestasis** is usually present and if prolonged, bile thrombi and pericentral hepatocyte changes are evident. A **hepatitic variant** of GvHD can occur after immunosuppressive drugs have been withdrawn, or after donor lymphocyte infusion; biopsy shows lobular inflammation and acidophil bodies, along with the typical abnormalities of small bile ducts (Figure 115.2) – a finding absent in fulminant viral hepatitis [5,6]. In **chronic GvHD**, histological findings in intestinal mucosa and liver are similar to those in acute GvHD, but in the esophagus, apoptotic squamous epithelial cells and desquamation occur [2]. Excessive fibrosis in the submucosal tissues of the esophagus, small intestine, and colon can be seen in severe cases.

Clinical presentation
Acute GvHD
Acute GvHD presents with three different phenotypes (Figure 115.3):

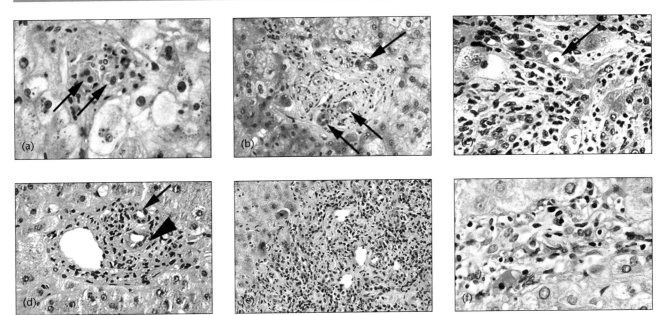

Figure 115.2 Histological features of acute and chronic graft-versus-host disease (GvHD) of the liver. (a) Portal area, with damaged small bile ducts (arrows) and surrounding bile-filled hepatocytes (28 days after transplant). (b) Portal area with three abnormal small bile ducts (arrows), each showing epithelial cell dropout, cytoplasmic eosinophilia, and vacuolization (82 days after transplant). There are few lymphocytes in this portal area. (c) Portal space with lymphocytic infiltrate and dysmorphic small bile ducts showing variation in shape and size, and dropout (40 days after transplant). The arrow points to an apoptotic epithelial cell. (d) Portal space with small bile ducts in chronic GvHD (465 days after transplant). The arrow points to a small bile duct with decreased numbers of epithelial cells, and the arrowhead to a bile duct remnant with no intact epithelium. (e) Hepatitic presentation of chronic GvHD (760 days after transplant). An enlarged portal space with lymphocytes admixed with plasma cells, eosinophils, and neutrophils, obscuring the small bile ducts. The limiting plate has extensive interface hepatitis with periportal acidophil bodies. (f) Small portal space with a markedly damaged small bile duct infiltrated by lymphocytes (patient with a hepatitic presentation 184 days after transplant). The bile duct has a shrunken outline, with vacuolated and eosinophilic cytoplasm and nuclear dropout.

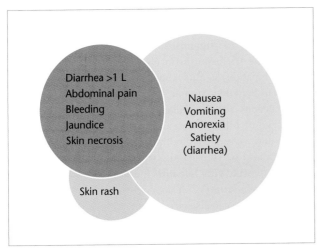

Figure 115.3 Phenotypes of acute graft-versus-host disease (GvHD). The most common presentation of acute GvHD is the upper gut phenotype in yellow. The more severe midgut phenotype, in red, may overlap with upper gut symptoms. An isolated skin rash can also be seen.

- An **upper gut syndrome** characterized by anorexia, satiety, nausea, vomiting and some diarrhea
- A more severe **midgut syndrome** of large-volume diarrhea, gut protein loss, abdominal pain, bleeding, and jaundice, in addition to anorexia, nausea, and vomiting
- An isolated **skin rash** [1].

Patients with persistent symptoms confined to the upper gut seldom progress to more severe GVHD and in general, respond to treatment more readily and often require lower total doses of immune suppressive therapy [7,8].

Typical symptoms include:

- **Anorexia, satiety, nausea, and vomiting**: these symptoms may blend with toxicity of myeloablative conditioning regimens or may develop after recovery from conditioning. Anorexia and nausea may occur in isolation as an enigmatic illness, but patients will often describe eating out of duty, along with fullness after a few bites.
- **Diarrhea:** in the upper gut phenotype of GvHD, stool volumes are usually under 500 mL/day, but in the more severe midgut GvHD, volumes may exceed 2 L/day with persistence of diarrhea even without oral intake. The pathogenesis of early diarrhea is related to intestinal cytokine release and opening of the epithelial tight junction; apoptotic crypt cells are infrequent. Later, T-cell–mediated crypt damage may lead to erosions, ulcers, and in some cases extensive sloughing of mucosa. Hypoalbuminemia accompanies severe gut GVHD.
- **Abdominal pain** caused by transmural edema is a harbinger of more severe GvHD. As GvHD progresses, distension from luminal fluid causes pain.
- **Occult gastrointestinal bleeding** is very common after transplantation when platelet counts are low. GvHD is the

most common cause of severe intestinal bleeding after transplantation; bleeding is from diffusely oozing ulceration and erosions.

- **Dysphagia and odynophagia** are rare in acute GvHD, occurring only with extensive mucosal destruction.
- **Cholestatic jaundice** is a feature of severe acute GvHD. With progressive disease, small bile ducts are damaged, eventually resulting in ductopenia.

Chronic GvHD

Chronic GvHD presents with signs and symptoms that occur without a previous diagnosis of acute GvHD in about 20% of cases; more commonly, acute GvHD melds into chronic GvHD (progressive onset) or resolves, only to reappear (quiescent onset) [2]. In its full-blown state, chronic GvHD may resemble **scleroderma, lichen planus, Sjögren's syndrome, eosinophilic fasciitis, rheumatoid arthritis, and primary biliary cirrhosis**. In some, the presentation is subtle with weight loss, weakness, or failure to thrive in children. **Dysphagia** is caused by extensive oral ulcerations or esophageal webs, strictures, and submucosal fibrosis. **Liver involvement** in chronic GvHD presents as an isolated increase in alkaline phosphatase concentration or as cholestatic jaundice or as an acute hepatitis (after immunosuppressive medications have been discontinued abruptly) [4].

Differential diagnosis

Anorexia, satiety, nausea, and vomiting after conditioning therapy usually wane by day 10–15 post transplant. After day 20, upper gut symptoms are from GvHD in approximately 85% of allograft recipients. The remaining 15% have **herpesvirus infection** or **medication intolerance** [cyclosporine (ciclosporin), voriconazole, trimethoprim–sulfamethoxazole, mycophenolate mofetil] or appetite suppression from high-calorie parenteral nutrition.

Diarrhea caused by conditioning is uncommon after day 10–15 post transplant. After this time, GvHD is almost always the cause in patients with high-volume diarrhea (>1 L/day). Infection as a cause of diarrhea accounts for <15% of cases; the organisms responsible include *Clostridium difficile, C. septicum*, astrovirus, adenovirus, rotavirus, norovirus, and **cytomegalovirus (CMV)**. Parasites and bacterial enteric pathogens are rare. Oral **magnesium** supplements commonly cause diarrhea. **Malabsorption** of dietary sugars and fat, related to mucosal damage from conditioning therapy or GvHD, causes diarrhea.

Abdominal pain has a wide differential diagnosis post transplant, but intra-abdominal catastrophes are unusual. **Pseudo-obstruction** is common in the first month after transplant, from opioid or anticholinergic medications. Distension is common among patients who have received vincristine (an enteric neurotoxin) before transplantation. Painful hepatomegaly results from hepatic engorgement (**sinusoidal obstruction syndrome**). **Hemorrhagic cystitis** (caused by cyclophosphamide or viral infection) causes severe, crampy pain in the lower abdomen and hematuria. Passage of **biliary sludge** can cause upper abdominal pain, nausea, and vomiting, and may be confused with GvHD.

Dissecting hematomas in either the abdominal wall or intestine rarely develop in thrombocytopenic patients. **Intestinal perforation** rarely occurs in patients who are not receiving corticosteroids; the sites of perforation are usually colonic diverticula and CMV ulcers. **Intestinal infarction** is caused by occlusion of mesenteric arteries with *Aspergillus*. **Epstein-Barr virus** lymphoproliferative disease (EBV-LPD) develops only in patients being treated for GvHD. **Pneumatosis intestinalis** is seen with both GVHD and CMV enteritis but is a surprisingly benign complication.

Severe gastrointestinal bleeding is uncommon, largely due to prophylaxis of CMV and fungal infection. **Vascular ectasias** of gastric and duodenal mucosa can lead to protracted bleeding unless ablated by laser endoscopy. In **thrombocytopenic** patients, duodenal biopsy sites may bleed. Rarely, a patient with an intramucosal tumor will bleed when the tumor is lysed by high-dose therapy. Gastric mucosal trauma from retching rarely causes significant bleeding. Bleeding caused by *C. septicum* (typhlitis), CMV, *Zygomycetes*, and EBV-LPD involving the gut occur sporadically.

Jaundice after transplantation has multiple causes, making a diagnosis of liver GvHD difficult. **Sinusoidal obstruction syndrome** (formerly known as **veno-occlusive disease**) is a form of liver injury caused by the conditioning regimen; jaundice usually appears before day 10, often accompanied by hepatomegaly and weight gain – features that are unusual with GvHD. Jaundice in patients with sepsis (**cholangitis lenta**) may be indistinguishable from hepatic GvHD. High **cyclosporine (ciclosporin)** levels inhibit bilirubin transport. The combination of mild cholestasis plus either hemolysis (related to hemolytic uremic syndrome) or renal failure may lead to deeper jaundice. Biliary obstruction is usually related to passage of **biliary sludge**. Jaundice and serum levels of alanine and aspartate aminotransferases >1500 U/L are commonly caused by sinusoidal obstruction syndrome, **hypoxic hepatitis** or acute **viral hepatitis** [herpes simplex virus (HSV), varicella zoster virus (VZV), adenovirus, hepatitis B virus], but this presentation can also be a manifestation of chronic GvHD.

Dysphagia and odynophagia are rarely caused by acute GvHD. In severe chronic GvHD, esophageal webs, rings, and strictures are more common, particularly in patients with skin, mouth, and eye involvement. Chronic fungal infection and HSV esophagitis can be seen in patients with chronic GvHD, and some pills used after transplant may lead to esophageal damage.

Diagnostic methods

Acute GvHD

A clinical diagnosis of acute gastrointestinal GvHD is acceptable when the patient is at risk, all clinical hallmarks are present, alternative conditions in the differential diagnosis are unlikely, and a skin biopsy is positive for GvHD. The only common intestinal infection that cannot be identified by stool culture is CMV.

Endoscopy

When the diagnosis of intestinal GvHD is in doubt, endoscopy and mucosal biopsy are needed. What the **endoscopist** sees carries equal weight to mucosal histological findings:

- Mucosal edema and erythema in mild cases
- Friability and erosions in moderate cases
- Large areas of mucosal necrosis, ulceration, and slough in severe cases (see Figure 115.1).

The **pathologist** relies on lymphocyte aggregates, apoptosis of crypt cells, and crypt cell dropout to diagnose intestinal GvHD (see section above on Pathology), but cannot find apoptotic crypt cells in areas devoid of epithelium. The **antrum** and **colon** are the preferred sites for biopsy. Duodenal biopsies carry a higher risk of bleeding. Biopsies (6–10 in number) should be taken from both ulcerated tissue and surrounding epithelium, and serially sectioned to optimize the yield for focal findings, including CMV.

Biopsy material, placed in viral transport media, should be **cultured** for herpesviruses using molecular methods.

Liver biopsy

Certain diagnosis of hepatic GvHD requires liver biopsy (see Figure 115.2), but often such a diagnosis is moot if there is biopsy-proven GvHD elsewhere. Most liver biopsies in this setting are done via a transvenous route. Liver tissue should be sent for histological examination, immunohistology if a virus is suspected, and viral culture (adenovirus and herpesviruses).

Chronic GvHD

Diagnosis is based on clinical findings and histology of oral, skin, and gut biopsies. When patients present with dysphagia, a ciné barium contrast X-ray is useful to identify upper esophageal webs and strictures. Endoscopy should be done cautiously because of perforation risk. Liver biopsy may be required if the cause of cholestasis is in dispute or if acute hepatitis develops (see Figure 115.2).

Treatment and prevention

Treatment is with immune suppressive agents; doses and duration of therapy should vary with the expected outcome. Initial treatment of acute GVHD is usually with glucocorticoids: **prednisone** 2 mg/kg/day plus **mycophenolate mofetil** for patients with the more severe midgut phenotype; 1 mg/kg/day for patients with isolated skin GVHD; and a combination of prednisone 1 mg/kg/day plus oral beclomethasone dipropionate 8 mg/day for the less severe upper gut syndrome

with anorexia, nausea, and vomiting [7–9]. Incomplete responses or failure to respond triggers additional immunosuppressive therapy. Treatment of chronic GvHD is difficult; some patients stay on multidrug immunosuppressive therapy for several years [2]. There is no universally effective salvage regimen for patients whose chronic GvHD fails to respond to initial therapy.

Complications and their management

Many complications of GvHD are caused by side effects of treatment: hypercortisolism from prednisone use, renal and neurological damage from cyclosporine (ciclosporin) and tacrolimus, hepatic toxicity from a mélange of drugs, and infection of the lungs, sinuses, brain, gut, liver, kidneys, bladder, and bloodstream.

Intestinal infections in patients with GvHD are now infrequent because of antiviral and antifungal prophylaxis against HSV, VZV, CMV, and *Candida* species. Unusual infections include necrotizing enteritis and colitis caused by adenovirus; esophagitis and gastritis caused by VZV; and mold infections of the stomach, small intestine, or colon. Each of these infections is treatable. VZV infections usually develop after acyclovir prophylaxis has been discontinued; presentation can be subtle, with abdominal distension, pain, and rising serum alanine aminotransferase levels. **Hepatobiliary infections** include fungal abscesses, herpesvirus, and adenovirus infections, hepatitis B and C exacerbations, and development of EBV-LPD. HSV, VZV, and adenovirus hepatitis may lead to fulminant hepatic failure. Hepatitis B and C are seldom problems while patients remain on immunosuppressive drugs, but hepatitis may flare during immune recovery. Fatal hepatitis B can be prevented by prophylactic lamivudine or entecavir.

Acute pancreatitis is a common finding at autopsy among patients with refractory GvHD, but symptoms are uncommon. Prednisone and cyclosporine (ciclosporin) crystals in bile have been suggested as causes. Rarely, patients with extensive chronic GvHD develop pancreatic atrophy and insufficiency.

Intestinal perforation occurs rarely, despite denudation of mucosa in severe GvHD. Causes include CMV ulcers, necrosis of transmural lymphoma, and diverticular perforation.

Pneumatosis intestinalis and pneumoperitoneum can be caused by intestinal GvHD or CMV infection. This condition must be distinguished from mucosal necrosis caused by gas-forming organisms or infarction. The diagnosis usually comes as a radiological surprise. Air can be seen in the peritoneal cavity and mediastinum as a relatively benign event in patients with pneumatosis intestinalis.

Aspiration and bronchiolitis are complications of esophageal strictures and webs from chronic GvHD. Untreated chronic GvHD may lead to obliteration of the esophageal lumen. Aspiration pneumonitis must be distinguished from bronchiolitis obliterans with organizing pneumonia, a form of pulmonary GvHD.

Prognosis with and without treatment

Acute and chronic GvHD must be treated to avoid **death** and **chronic disability**. In acute GvHD, the prognosis is poorest among patients whose GvHD fails to respond completely to initial therapy and who require constant immune suppressive therapy to keep symptoms under control [9,10]. **Mortality** in patients with chronic GvHD is related to the extent of disease, thrombocytopenia, weight loss, poor performance score, and the need for continued immune suppressive therapy [2]. The adverse effects of treatment for GvHD are themselves causes of death (infections and the debilitating effects of prolonged glucocorticoid exposure) – reinforcing the strategy to tailor intensity of therapy to the severity of disease [8].

Current controversies and their future resolution

The dilemma facing investigators is how to achieve stable allogeneic engraftment without causing severe GvHD and while preserving a graft-versus-tumor effect. The solution to refractory acute and chronic GvHD will come from advances in immunogenetics, T-cell biology, identification of antigens on epithelial stem cells that are the targets of alloimmune attack, methods to achieve tolerance, and more precise immune suppressive agents.

SOURCES OF INFORMATION FOR PATIENTS AND DOCTORS

Until patients experience GvHD, seldom do they have a clear idea of how sick they may become, and how difficult and prolonged the treatment may be. These resources are useful.

Blood and Marrow Transplant Information Network– provides electronic access to books and newsletters, and a patient–survivor link service

http://www.bmtinfonet.org

BMT-Talk – home page of the Association of Cancer Online Resources hosting communications between patients, survivors, and caregivers

http://listserv.acor.org/archives/bmt-talk.html

BMT Support Online– online chat room, links to other oncology support groups

http://www.bmtsupport.org

National BMT link– help for patients, caregivers, and families coping with the social and emotional challenges of transplant from diagnosis, with information and personalized support services

http://www.nbmtlink.org

Community physicians may find the 2009 editions of *Thomas' Hematopoietic Cell Transplantation* [1] and *Chronic Graft versus Host Disease: Interdisciplinary Management* [2] to be especially useful in caring for these complex patients.

References

1. Appelbaum FR, Forman SJ, Negrin RS, Blume KG. *Thomas' Hematopoietic Cell Transplantation*, 4th edition. Oxford: Wiley-Blackwell Publishing, 2009.
2. Vogelsang GB, Pavletic SZ. *Chronic Graft Versus Host Disease: Interdisciplinary Management*. New York: Cambridge Univesity Press, 2009.
3. Ponec RJ, Hackman RC, McDonald GB. Endoscopic and histologic diagnosis of intestinal graft-vs.-host disease after marrow transplantation. *Gastrointest Endosc*. 1999;49:612–621.
4. McDonald GB. Hepatobiliary complications of hematopoietic cell transplantation, 40 years on. *Hepatology*. 2010;51:1450–1460.
5. Strasser SI, Shulman HM, Flowers ME, *et al*. Chronic graft-vs-host disease of the liver: presentation as an acute hepatitis. *Hepatology*. 2000;32:1265–1271.
6. Akpek G, Boitnott JK, Lee LA, *et al*. Hepatitic variant of graft-versus-host disease after donor lymphocyte infusion. *Blood*. 2002;100:3903–3907.
7. Hockenbery DM, Cruickshank S, Rodell TC, *et al*. A randomized, placebo-controlled trial of oral beclomethasone dipropionate as a prednisone-sparing therapy for gastrointestinal graft-versus-host disease. *Blood*. 2007;109:4557–4563.
8. Mielcarek M, Storer BE, Boeckh M, *et al*. Initial therapy of acute graft-versus-host disease with low dose prednisone does not compromise patient outcomes. *Blood*. 2009;113:2888–2894.
9. Van Lint MT, Milone G, Leotta S, *et al*. Treatment of acute graft-versus-host disease with prednisolone: significant survival advantage for day +5 responders and no advantage for nonresponders receiving anti-thymocyte globulin. *Blood*. 2006;107:4177–4181.
10. Leisenring W, Martin P, Petersdorf E, *et al*. An acute graft-versus-host disease activity index to predict survival after hematopoietic cell transplantation with myeloablative conditioning regimens. *Blood*. 2006;108:749–755.

CHAPTER 116
Radiation and other physicochemical injury

Keith Leiper and Andrew R. Moore
Royal Liverpool University Hospital, Liverpool, UK

ESSENTIAL FACTS ABOUT PATHOGENESIS

- Acute radiation injury results from free radical formation
- Intracellular free radicals damage DNA and induce widespread apoptosis
- Late radiation injury is characterized by fibrosis and occlusive vasculopathy
- The resulting ischemia leads to mucosal atrophy

ESSENTIALS OF DIAGNOSIS

- Typical endoscopic features of radiation enteropathy are telangiectasia and mucosal atrophy, friability, and ulceration
- Histopathological examination is useful for excluding other causes of mucosal inflammation
- Radiological imaging can be helpful in identifying structural abnormalities such as strictures or fistulae

ESSENTIALS OF TREATMENT

- Enteral strictures and fistulae can be addressed endoscopically (dilatation, stenting, etc.) or surgically (stricturoplasty, resection, etc.)
- Treatment of radiation colitis is aimed at controlling symptoms (e.g. loperamide for diarrhea) and controlling bleeding
- Simple medical treatments are the first-line (e.g. rectal sucralfate), while resistant or more severe cases should be considered for second-line treatments (e.g. hyperbaric oxygen, thermal therapy, etc.)

Radiation injury to the gastrointestinal tract

About 50% of patients receiving radiotherapy are long-term survivors [1]. Acute radiation injury is common and usually resolves when the radiation treatment course is completed. However, about 5–15% suffer significant longer-term complications from **late radiation-induced tissue injury**, which predominantly affects the head and neck, chest wall, and pelvis. The manifestation of late toxicity can occur many years after exposure. This chapter will predominantly focus on the gastrointestinal effects in long-term survivors who have received pelvic radiotherapy for prostate, gynecological or colorectal cancer, as this is the group whose care will predominantly be provided by clinical gastroenterologists.

Epidemiology

Over 100 000 cases of cancer are treated with radiotherapy in the UK annually, of which over 12 000 are radical radiotherapy for pelvic malignancy. This number is predicted to rise with the increasing incidence of malignancy in an aging population. Serious complications occur in 5–15% of patients up to 10 years after exposure [2]. However, as many as 80% of patients report a permanent change in bowel habit after pelvic radiotherapy, though only 50% experience side effects considered severe enough to affect their quality of life [3]. The incidence has fallen over the last few decades due to better targeting of radiation fields. The severity of injury depends on the dose of radiation, number of fractions, size of the radiation field, and concomitant chemotherapy. Host factors associated with greater injury are renal failure, diabetes, pelvic inflammatory disease, low body mass index, and abdominal surgery.

Pathogenesis and pathology
Acute radiation injury

Ionizing radiation liberates electrons, which lead to the formation of **free radicals** within cells. Free radicals cause DNA damage and apoptosis in vulnerable cells. Actively dividing cells, particularly those in the G2 and M phases of mitosis, are most radiosensitive, explaining the relative vulnerability of the small intestine. Acute injury is characterized by widespread apoptosis, increased cellularity of the lamina propria, eosinophilic infiltrates, surface epithelial damage, and crypt disarray. However, neutrophil infiltration is absent [4]. Mucosal damage persists for the duration of therapy and settles in the following 1–2 weeks.

Late radiation injury

The predominant features of late radiation damage to normal tissues are **fibrosis** and **abnormal vasculature due to occlusive vasculopathy**. Small vessels show dilatation, asymmetry, and a reduction in the microvascular network. The walls of larger vessels have subendothelial fibrosis, thrombosis, and lipid-filled macrophages. The stroma is characterized by dense and acellular fibrosis. Epithelial atrophy is common, reflecting

Textbook of Clinical Gastroenterology and Hepatology, Second Edition. Edited by C. J. Hawkey, Jaime Bosch, Joel E. Richter, Guadalupe Garcia-Tsao, Francis K. L. Chan.

Multiple Organ Systems

Table 116.1 Acute effects of radiation

Organ	Symptoms/clinical syndrome	Treatment	Comment
Mucositis	Pain Dysphagia	Oral hygiene Experimental: hEGF, hKGF	Very common in treatment of head and neck cancer
Esophagus	Esophagitis – dysphagia, odynophagia, vomiting, chest pain Fistula Perforation	Proton pump inhibitors Alginates Covered stents	Differential diagnosis: infections – viral and fungal
Stomach and duodenum	Gastroduodenal ulcers	PPI Sucralfate	Rare with external DXT 12% with internal DXT for hepatic metastases
Small bowel	Diarrhea Abdominal pain Jejunitis and ileitis Bile salt malabsorption Perforation Adhesions	Reduction in radiation dose Antispasmodics Loperamide Cholestyramine Surgery	Usually within 1–2 weeks of therapy 90% of those receiving >30 Gy Usually resolves with simple measures
Colon	Diarrhea Urgency Tenesmus Rectal bleeding Colitis	Reduction in dose Loperamide	Usually occurs within 6 weeks of starting therapy Usually resolve within 6 months
Liver	Fatigue, weight gain, RUQ pain Ascites, hepatomegaly Jaundice rare Modest rise in transaminases, alkaline phosphatase raised	Usually resolves within 1–2 months with conservative management Occasionally diuretics and paracentesis	Typically 4–8 weeks after therapy

DXT, radiotherapy; hEGF, human epidermal growth factor; hKGF, human keratinocyte growth factor; PPI, proton pump inhibitor; RUQ, right upper quadrant.

ischemia. The absence or paucity of a cellular inflammatory response is often striking [5].

Symptoms

Acute radiation injury

Although the histological features can be severe, the majority of the short-term effects of radiotherapy resolve with conservative management (Table 116.1). **Esophagitis** is common after radiotherapy for esophageal or lung cancer, particularly in those receiving combined chemoradiotherapy. Transient worsening of **dysphagia** is common during radiotherapy for esophageal cancer. Differential diagnosis includes various infections, including herpes simplex virus (HSV), cytomegalovirus (CMV), varicella zoster virus (VZV), and candida; therefore, endoscopy and biopsy (histology and culture) can be helpful.

Diarrhea affects most patients, particularly those on concomitant chemotherapy. Diarrhea can occur within a few hours of therapy and affects 90% of those receiving more than 30 Gy and 20% receiving less than 10 Gy. The mechanism is multifactorial, including central nervous system stimulation, increased small bowel motility, and direct radiation damage to

Table 116.2 Differential diagnosis for diarrhea in a patient receiving radiotherapy

- Acute radiation injury to colon
- Acute radiation injury to small bowel
- Concomitant chemotherapy-induced diarrhea, especially 5-fluorouracil, capecitabine, oxalipatin, irinotecan
- *Clostridium difficile*
- Neutropenic enterocolitis
- Graft-versus-host disease in stem cell transplantation

the small bowel (causing reduced brush border activity and impaired maturation of villi) and colon (causing reduced water absorption). Simple measures such as oral rehydration, antispasmodics, loperamide, and a reduction in radiation dose by 10% are effective. Diarrhea that is severe or persistent requires investigation (Table 116.2). If the ileum has been irradiated, treatment with cholestyramine can be effective. For refractory diarrhea, octreotide may be useful, starting at 100 μg t.i.d.

Table 116.3 Chronic/late effects of radiotherapy

Organ	Symptoms/clinical syndrome	Treatment	Comment
Esophagus	Stricture Tracheoesophageal fistula	Endoscopic balloon dilatation, self-expanding plastic stents Covered metal or plastic stent	Particularly severe following laryngeal cancer Successful in 70–100%
Small bowel	Strictures Colicky abdominal pain, subacute small bowel obstruction, abnormal small bowel motility, fistulae	Surgical resection of strictures, stricturoplasty Parenteral nutrition Antibiotics if small bowel bacterial overgrowth	Mean incidence 6% (0.5–17%) Usually within 1–2 years but can be >20 years High mortality/morbidity with surgery
Colon and anorectum	Strictures Radiation colitis Fistulae Urgency incontinence	Endoscopic balloon dilation Thermal therapy Formalin Hyperbaric oxygen Surgery Loperamide	High morbidity/mortality with surgery
Liver	Hepatic sinusoidal obstruction syndrome (fluid retention, ascites, tender hepatomegaly, hyperbilirubinemia)	Diuretics Salt restriction TIPS Heparin and t-PA Liver transplant	Common in total body irradiation 70–80% respond to simple measure

TIPS, transjugular intrahepatic portosystemic shunt; t-PA, tissue plasminogen activator.

Late effects of radiotherapy

Conventionally, late effects are defined as symptoms 3 months after treatment completion; however, many of these can occur years afterwards. Late effects of radiation are the result of ischemia and fibrosis, and include **strictures, fistulae, adhesions, and perforation**. These predominantly affect the esophagus, small bowel, colon, and anorectum (Table 116.3). Esophageal strictures after radiotherapy for laryngeal cancer can be particularly difficult to manage. We have a cohort of 3–4 patients with pinhole esophageal strictures who require 18-mm endoscopic balloon dilatations every 2 weeks. They have been refractory to other therapy and have needed regular dilatations for more than a decade (Figure 116.1).

Radiation colitis
Epidemiology

The incidence of chronic radiation colitis (RC) in long-term follow-up after pelvic radiotherapy can be up to 50% [6]. The relatively high incidence of rectosigmoid involvement is due to the fact that pelvic malignancies are both common and commonly treated with radiotherapy. Defining the incidence of **incontinence**, the most distressing sequelae, is difficult because of a lack of robust and precise long-term data. Incontinence can affect up to 70% at 6 weeks, though some of these cases are due to acute colitis. A reasonable estimate is that about a third of patients suffer from fecal incontinence in the long term [7].

Prevention

Several different strategies have been employed to prevent acute RC, with the implied strategy to prevent long-term

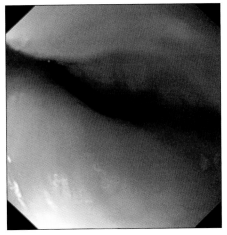

Figure 116.1 Radiation-induced upper esophageal stricture after radiotherapy for laryngeal cancer.

complications of RC. Pilot studies of the 5-aminosalicyclate (ASA) drug balsalazide have suggested an effect on reducing RC [8], although several other studies of 5-ASA drugs have not shown an effect.

Amifostine is a phosphorylated aminothiol prodrug that selectively protects normal mucosa from radiotherapy damage by scavenging oxygen-derived free radicals. *In vitro* data and limited clinical data suggest an effect in preventing both early and late RC [9]. Without a control arm and short-term follow-up, these data are difficult to interpret.

Symptoms

Although rectal bleeding is the most reported symptom of radiation colitis, the most troublesome long-term symptoms that impair quality of life are due to damage to the rectal wall. These include **tenesmus, difficulty in defecation from rectal stricturing, and urgency** [10] and are due to (1) fibrosis and smooth muscle hypertrophy of the rectal wall, and (2) impaired innervation. **Rectal wall fibrosis** results in reduced rectal volume and rectal compliance. **Reduced innervation** is in part caused by nerve entrapment in fibrous tissue and results in reduced anal tone and impaired electrosensory control of defecation. **Incontinence** results from interrelated factors of reduced anal tone, reduced compliance, impaired neural control of defecation, and the presence of diarrhea or colitis.

Possibly because these symptoms are difficult to treat, most of the literature on therapy has concentrated on treatment to reduce bleeding (some of which may in fact increase urgency and cause stricturing). Denton *et al.* [11] have suggested possible scoring systems and outcome measures (including quality-of-life scores) which would aid in evaluating the effect of therapy.

Differential diagnosis

New or persistent symptoms **after** radiotherapy should be investigated thoroughly (Table 116.4). The diagnosis of chronic radiation enteropathy is usually made endoscopically, although radiology can be helpful, e.g. for small intestinal strictures. The typical endoscopic appearances are of mucosal atrophy, telangiectasia, mucosal friability, and occasionally ulceration (Figure 116.2). Biopsies are useful in distinguishing radiation enteropathy from other conditions associated with mucosal inflammation. Recurrence or residual cancer should be excluded endoscopically using chromoendoscopy or narrow-band imaging and biopsies. Anorectal manometry can be useful in assessing anal tone and rectal compliance in patients with tenesmus and urgency.

Treatment of radiation colitis

Incontinence

There are currently no available therapies that can improve rectal compliance and sphincter function in RC. Control of diarrhea is important – using loperamide and codeine and by manipulation of dietary fiber. Surgical management has high mortality and morbidity. For intractable incontinence, a Hartmann's procedure may be appropriate in a high-risk patient, but inevitably rectal symptoms of bleeding will continue. Proctectomy has a morbidity rate of 13–79% and mortality of 13–79% [8], with particular problems with wound healing. Likewise, conventional interventions for incontinence, such as graciloplasty, have been largely unsuccessful, though experience is limited. Sacral nerve stimulation is an option but data on effect in RC are lacking.

Treatment of bleeding

Minor bleeding does not require any therapy. For more severe symptoms, the choice is between medical therapy, formalin,

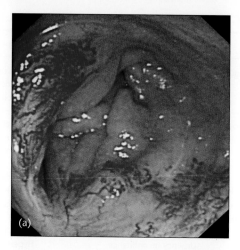

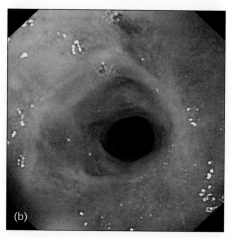

Figure 116.2 (a) Radiation colitis. Friable superficial telangiectasia in the rectum several years after radiotherapy for prostate cancer. (b) Tight fibrotic rectal stricture with lack of normal vasculature and atrophy after radiotherapy for prostate cancer. Treated with regular balloon dilatation.

Table 116.4 Differential diagnosis and approach to diagnosis in a patient with diarrhea who has received pelvic radiotherapy

- Radiation colitis
- Radiation-induced small bowel strictures
- Radiation-induced colonic/rectal strictures
- Fistula
- Recurrence (or residual) of primary tumor
- Radiation-induced secondary tumor
- Unrelated to radiation, e.g. inflammatory bowel disease, irritable bowel syndrome, bacterial overgrowth

thermal therapy, and hyperbaric oxygen (Table 116.5). The evidence base for each of these therapies is poor and there are few good quality trials and very few comparative trials [13]. The definition of clinical remission and improvement are often unclear and differ between trials.

Table 116.5 Treatment of radiation colitis/proctitis

Treatment	Dose	Clinical improvement rate	Complications
Sucralfate enemas	2 g b.d. for 8 weeks	94%	Very rare
Metronidazole/beclomethasone enemas	400 mg t.d.s.	92%	Neuropathy
Formalin	1–3 treatments	70–100%	Pain (24%), severe colitis
Endoscopic thermal therapy	1–4 sessions	66–100%	0–3% Rectal stenosis, perforation
Hyperbaric oxygen	100% oxygen, 2–3 atm for 1 hour 20–60 sessions	60–80%	Pressure damage to ears, sinuses and lungs

Medical therapy

Rectal sucralfate (2 g b.d.) for 8 weeks achieved "clinical improvement" in 94% [12]. Rectal steroid therapy or 5-ASAs as sole therapy is less effective, with response rates of 21–35% [13]. Curiously, metronidazole may be effective. In a trial of oral mesalazine and betamethasone enema with or without metronidazole for 1 year, a 92% reduction in rectal bleeding was seen in the metronidazole group compared to 42% in the control group [13].

Formalin

Formalin scleroses blood vessels and can eradicate abnormal neovascularization. Reported short-term complication rates are reasonably high, including 24% for anorectal pain; other complications are diarrhea, fever, rectal perforation, rectal stenosis, and severe colitis [13].

Endoscopic thermal therapy

The principle is to ablate abnormal vasculature by application of heat, either with a heater probe, laser or argon plasma coagulation (APC). The most frequently used modality is probably APC due to its availability, ease of application, and limited depth of penetration. Complication rates are low but include rectal stenosis, rectovaginal fistula, tenesmus, and rectal pain [13].

Hyperbaric oxygen

Hyperbaric oxygen increases oxygen delivery to tissues and is the only therapy that increases the number of blood vessels in irradiated tissue. It is a logical approach to chronic radiation damage where ischemia is the predominant pathophysiological process. Treatment is usually with 100% oxygen at two to three times atmospheric pressure for 1–2 hours over 20–60 treatments [13]. Serious adverse effects are rare. However, there is concern that treatment may increase the risk of further tumors.

A sensible approach to the management of radiation colitis is to dilate any strictures, use liberal doses of loperamide, and

initially sucralfate enemas 2 g b.d. for 8 weeks. If this is ineffective and bleeding is the main symptom, an endoscopic thermal method should be tried. If symptoms continue, the patient should be referred for hyperbaric oxygen.

Chemical injury to the esophagus

Ingestion of caustic substances (Table 116.6) is common in resource-poor countries, predominantly due to children ingesting liquids from unlabeled, non-childproof bottles. There are about 5000 cases per year in the USA. The agents are usually domestic cleaners. The pH of these varies between 2 and 12 with the most damaging being lye-based cleaners with high concentrations of alkali. Bleaches are usually pH 7 and usually do not cause permanent esophageal damage. Patients are usually under the age of 5 years and present with drooling, vomiting, refusal to eat, odynophagia, and often oral ulceration. About 20–50% sustain severe injury to the esophagus and 10–50% of these develop **esophageal strictures**. Immediate management is to identify the ingested substance and contact the local poisons center for advice. Gastic lavage or induced emesis is contraindicated. Treatment is with a high-dose proton pump inhibitor and broad-spectrum antibiotics. There is no evidence that steroids are effective in reducing the complication rate. Endoscopy has been recommended after 24 hours to assess esophageal damage and place a nasogastric tube. However, other reports suggest a perforation rate of over 30% with endoscopy in this situation. Management of strictures is conventional with balloon dilatation or bougienage. If this is ineffective, esophageal replacement surgery is warranted. The risk of squamous cell cancer may be increased after caustic esophagitis. Although there are no guidelines or accurate estimation of risk, periodic endoscopic follow-up is advocated.

Chemical colitis

Homo sapiens have developed an imaginative way of causing gastrointestinal injury by administering various chemicals rectally. Inflammation of the colon by exogenous chemicals can

Table 116.6 Causes and treatment of chemical colitis

Chemical	Number of cases/cause	Treatment	Prognosis
Glutaraldehyde	>60 – inadequate cleaning of endoscopes	CT shows characteristic "target sign" Steroids Mesalazine Antibiotics	Resolution within 4–5 days
Hydrogen peroxide	24 – inadequate cleaning of endoscopes and for demonstration of fistulae	Fluid resuscitation Antibiotics	1 death
Formalin	4 – accidental 1, iatrogenic 3	IV fluids Steroid enemas	Resolution within 7 days
Soap	7 since 1970 – mostly iatrogenic Previously very common	IV fluids Steroid enemas Antibiotics	Resolution in 4–6 weeks 50% rectosigmoid strictures
Alcohol	8 – accidental 3, deliberate 5	IV fluids Steroid enemas Antibiotic	Resolution within 7 days
Ergotamine	4 – iatrogenic suppositories for migraine	Conservative	Resolution within 4–8 weeks 1 rectovaginal fistula
Sulfuric acid/ hydrochloric acid	18 – suicide 15, murder 3	About 50% respond to medical therapy If evidence of severe necrosis – resection	About 50% require surgery. About 50% mortality
Sodium hydroxide	2 – accidental 1 deliberate 1	Conservative	1 resolved 1 colectomy

be accidental, deliberate (suicidal intent, murder or sexual) or iatrogenic (prescribed medication, contamination of instruments). High-risk individuals are those with mental illness, Munchausen's syndrome, learning difficulties, and certain groups who use enemas ritualistically. The literature is largely case studies and therefore evidence-based recommendations are difficult to determine. Treatment options are outlined in Table 116.6, but all are empirical.

Presentation is not distinct from other forms of colitis with abdominal pain, diarrhea, and rectal bleeding. The key is obviously a **relevant history of a precipitant**. There may be confusion in making the diagnosis of chemical colitis if the patient has a pre-existing cause of rectal bleeding, e.g., mucosal prolapsed syndrome or hemorrhoids, and then uses "chemical" treatments to alleviate symptoms [14]. Endoscopic appearances and histological features are usually non-specific.

Of the iatrogenic causes, one of the commonest is **glutaraldehyde colitis** from inadequate cleaning of endoscopes. Symptoms usually occur with 48 hours of endoscopy, with fever, severe abdominal pain, diarrhea with blood, and tenesmus. Symptoms usually resolve within 4–5 days with conservative measures. **Formalin** used to treat radiation colitis (see above) can cause a severe distal colitis associated with severe rectal pain. This usually resolves with intravenous

fluids and steroid enemas within a few days. **Soap enemas** were previously standard postoperatively but a third of patients reported rectal symptoms and a proportion had proctitis. Soap enemas are still a prevalent treatment in many resource-poor areas either preoperatively or as a treatment for constipation. Soap contains mixtures of alkali, potash, phenol, and sodium and potassium salts of long-chain fatty acids, which cause colonic necrosis. Treatment is conservative but may require surgical resection if signs of peritonism or stricturing occur.

SOURCES OF INFORMATION FOR DOCTORS AND PATIENTS

For doctors
http://www.uptodate.com
Cancer Research UK
http://www.cancerhelp.org.uk
For patients
Cancerbackup (recently merged with Macmillan Cancer Support).
    http://www.cancerbackup.org.uk/
www.bladderandbowelfoundation.org
In the UK, for advice on chemical damage to the gastrointestinal tract, contact the National Poisons Centre
Telephone information service (0844 892 0111 or http://
    www.hpa.org.uk) and TOXBASE (www.toxbase.org)

Footnote

Dr. Keith Leiper (1967–2011) was a well-respected and much-loved gastroenterologist whose work contributed to substantial advances in the care of patients with inflammatory bowel disease. He co-authored this chapter but sadly died in October 2011, prior to its publication.

References

1. Jemal A, Thomas A, Murray T, *et al.* Cancer statistics, 2002. *CA Cancer J Clin.* 2002;52:23–47.
2. Denton A, Bond S, Matthews S, *et al.* National audit of the management and outcome of carcinoma of the cervix treated with radiotherapy in 1993. *Clin Oncol (R Coll Radiol)* 2000;12:347–53.
3. Abbasakoor F, Vaizey CJ, Boulos PB. Improving the morbidity of anorectal injury from pelvic radiotherapy. *Colorectal Dis.* 2006;8:2–10.
4. Leupin N, Curschmann J, Kranzbühler H, *et al.* Acute radiation colitis in patients treated with short-term preoperative radiotherapy for rectal cancer. *Am J Surg Pathol.* 2002;26:498–504.
5. Fajardo LF. The pathology of ionizing radiation as defined by morphologic patterns. *Acta Oncologic.* 2005;44:1,13–22.
6. Matsuura Y, Kawagoe T, Toki N, *et al.* Long-standing complications after treatment for cancer of the uterine cervix–clinical significance of medical examination at 5 years after treatment. *Int J Gynecol Cancer.* 2006;16:294–297.
7. Petersen S, Jongen J, Petersen C, *et al.* Radiation-induced sequelae affecting the continence organ: incidence, pathogenesis, and treatment. *Dis Colon Rectum.* 2007;50:1466–1474.
8. Jahraus CD, Bettenhausen D, Malik U, *et al.* Prevention of acute radiation-induced proctosigmoiditis by balsalazide: a randomized, double-blind, placebo controlled trial in prostate cancer patients. *Int J Radiat Oncol Biol Phys.* 2005;63:1483–1487.
9. Ben-Josef E, Han S, Tobi M, *et al.* A pilot study of topical intrarectal application of amifostine for prevention of late radiation rectal injury. *Int J Radiat Oncol Biol Phys.* 2002;53:1160–1164.
10. Denham JW, O'Brien PC, Dunstan RH, *et al.* Is there more than one late radiation proctitis syndrome? *Radiother Oncol.* 1999;51:43–53
11. Denton A, Forbes A, Andreyev J, *et al.* Non surgical interventions for late radiation proctitis in patients who have received radical radiotherapy to the pelvis. *Cochrane Database Syst Rev* 2002;(1): CD003455.
12. Kochhar R, Patel F, Dhar A, *et al.* Radiation-induced proctosigmoiditis. Prospective, randomized, double-blind controlled trial of oral sulfasalazine plus rectal steroids versus rectal sucralfate. *Dig Dis Sci.* 1991;36:103–107.
13. Leiper K, Morris AI. Treatment of radiation proctitis. *Clin Oncol (R Coll Radiol).* 2007;19:724–729
14. Sheibani S, Gerson LB. Chemical colitis. *J Clin Gastroenterol.* 2008;42:115–121.

Multiple Organ Systems

CHAPTER 117
Systemic amyloidosis

Prayman T. Sattianayagam and Philip N. Hawkins
University College London Medical School, London, UK

ESSENTIAL FACTS ABOUT PATHOGENESIS

- Amyloidosis is caused by deposition of protein in an abnormal fibrillar form in organs
- Subtypes are characterized according to the fibril precursor proteins
- In AL amyloidosis (80%) the fibrils are derived from immunoglobin light chains secreted from B cell dyscrasias (multiple myeloma, lymphoma, and monoclonal gammopathies)
- In AA amyloidosis (15%) the fibrils are derived from the acute phase reactant serum amyloid A protein, synthesized by hepatocytes in the presence of chronic inflammation
- In hereditary systemic amyloidosis (5%) genetic mutations encode for amyloidogenic variant proteins

ESSENTIALS OF DIAGNOSIS

- AL amyloidosis: cardiac, renal, gastrointestinal involvement (motility disturbance, malabsorption, perforation, hemorrhage or obstruction), peripheral and autonomic neuropathy.
- AA amyloidosis: 97% have proteinuria. Half progress to end-stage renal failure; hepatosplenomegaly and gastrointestinal symptoms are rarer presentations
- Hereditary transthyretin amyloidosis: peripheral and autonomic neuropathy with or without cardiac amyloid
- Rectal and abdominal fat biopsy is diagnostic in 50–80%
- Biopsy of affected organ is nearly 100% diagnostic
- Subtype assignment is by immunohistochemistry

ESSENTIALS OF TREATMENT

- AL amyloidosis: regimens based on treatment for myeloma (melphalan and dexamethasone or cyclophosphamide/thalidomide/dexamethasone or autologous stem cell transplantation)
- AA amyloidosis: suppression of inflammation, including anti-tumor necrosis factor alpha therapies. Colchicine in familial Mediterranean fever
- Familial amyloid polyneuropathy: liver transplantation to eliminate production of genetically encoded variant transthyretin synthesized in the liver
- Supportive care of organ function.

Introduction and epidemiology

Amyloidosis is a disorder of protein folding in which various proteins are deposited as abnormal, insoluble fibrils that progressively disrupt tissue structure and function, and thereby cause disease [1]. Despite the heterogeneity of these precursor proteins, the structure and characteristics of amyloid fibrils are similar. Some 25 unrelated proteins can form amyloid *in vivo*. Clinical amyloidosis is classified according to the fibril protein type and can be acquired or inherited. In systemic amyloidosis, the deposits can occur in all tissues except within the brain.

Precise data on the epidemiology of amyloidosis are not available, but systemic amyloidosis is thought to be the cause of death in about 1 in 1000 individuals in the Western world. Acquired systemic **AL amyloidosis** is fivefold more common than systemic **AA amyloidosis**. AL amyloidosis occurs in about 2% of individuals with monoclonal gammopathies [2] and AA amyloidosis has a lifetime incidence of 1–5% among patients with chronic inflammatory diseases. **Hereditary forms** of systemic amyloidosis account for about 5% of all cases and are frequently misdiagnosed as AL amyloidosis [3].

Causes and pathogenesis

AL amyloidosis can occur in the context of any dyscrasia of cells of the B-lymphocyte lineage, including multiple myeloma and malignant lymphomas. Over 80% of cases, however, are associated with low-grade and benign monoclonal gammopathies, which can be very subtle. The fibrils are derived from monoclonal **immunoglobulin light chains**, which have a unique structure in each patient, accounting for the extremely heterogeneous spectrum of clinical features in this form of the disease.

AA amyloidosis can occur in association with any kind of chronic inflammatory disorder that generates an acute-phase response for a sustained period. The precursor protein is the acute-phase reactant **serum amyloid A protein** (SAA), which is synthesized abundantly by hepatocytes in the presence of inflammation. In the developed world, the most frequent predisposing conditions are the inflammatory arthritides, followed by chronic sepsis, inflammatory bowel disease, and the hereditary periodic fever syndromes. About 6% of patients with AA amyloidosis do not have a clinically overt chronic inflammatory disease [4], and these patients can be misdiagnosed as having AL amyloidosis.

Hereditary amyloidosis is inherited in an autosomal dominant fashion with variable penetrance accounting for the frequent absence of family history. It is caused by heterozygous point mutations in genes encoding for variant proteins that are produced in organs such as the liver and gastrointestinal tract. These proteins include **transthyretin, apolipoprotein AI, apolipoprotein AII, lysozyme, and fibrinogen A α-chain**. Amyloidogenic mutations may also occur *de novo*.

Amyloidogenesis involves substantial refolding of the native structures of the various amyloid precursor proteins, which enables them to autoaggregate in a highly ordered manner to form fibrils with a characteristic β-sheet structure [5]. Amyloid deposition occurs under several conditions:

- When there is a prolonged abnormally high concentration of a normal protein, e.g., **SAA during chronic inflammation**
- In the presence of a normal abundance of a structurally normal, but weakly amyloidogenic, protein over a very prolonged period, such as in the case of wild-type transthyretin, derived from the liver, in **senile systemic amyloidosis**
- When there is production of an abnormal protein with inherently amyloidogenic potential, such as some monoclonal **immunoglobulin light chains** or variant proteins encoded by genetic mutations.

All types of amyloid fibril have **non-fibrillar constituents**, including glycosaminoglycans, proteoglycans, and serum amyloid P component (SAP), which contribute to their formation and stability. Amyloidotic organs have a distinctive **waxy, lardaceous** macroscopic appearance, and deposits in affected tissues show characteristic **red–green birefringence** when stained with Congo red and viewed under a light microscope with cross-polarized light. Amyloid fibrils have a diameter of 8–10 nm and a rigid non-branching appearance on electron microscopy (Figure 117.1).

The symptoms of amyloidosis are caused by progressive disruption of the structure and function of various tissues, which may eventually cause organ failure. Precursor protein fragment size in amyloid fibrils has been found to correlate with phenotype, including pattern of organ involvement in hereditary systemic amyloidosis, and this may provide insights into the pathogenesis of amyloidosis in other forms of amyloidosis [6].

Clinical presentation

Systemic amyloidosis frequently has a non-specific presentation, which can progress to an almost limitless permutation of symptoms. This often leads to a delay in diagnosis. Symptoms in amyloidosis are listed in Table 117.1.

In **AA amyloidosis** 97% of patients present with non-selective **proteinuria**. Nephrotic syndrome may occur and progression to end-stage **renal failure** is the cause of death in 40–60% of cases. Rarer presentations include **hepatosplenom-**

egaly and **gastrointestinal symptoms** such as bleeding, which are more common in advanced disease. Neuropathy and cardiac involvement are extremely rare [4].

In **AL amyloidosis** the heart is affected pathologically in most patients. In 30% a **restrictive cardiomyopathy** is a presenting feature and in up to half of these it is fatal. As a dominant presentation, it confers a poor prognosis and death commonly occurs within 6 months. **Renal AL amyloid** has the same manifestations as renal AA amyloid, but the prognosis is worse. **Gastrointestinal tract** involvement is frequent. There may be motility disturbances secondary to autonomic neuropathy or symptoms secondary to amyloid infiltration of the gastrointestinal tract, such as malabsorption, perforation, hemorrhage, or obstruction. **Macroglossia** occurs in up to 10% of cases and is almost pathognomonic of AL amyloid. A **sensory polyneuropathy**, with paresthesia followed later by motor deficits, is seen in 10–20% of cases and carpal tunnel syndrome in 20%. **Autonomic neuropathy** may occur alone or together with the peripheral neuropathy, and confers a very poor prognosis. **Dermatological involvement** takes the form of papules, nodules, plaques and nail dystrophy.

Hereditary transthyretin (TTR) amyloidosis presents typically with a progressive and disabling **peripheral and autonomic neuropathy**, and/or varying degrees of **cardiac involvement**, and is often known as **familial amyloid polyneuropathy (FAP)**. Hereditary amyloidosis associated with mutations in other genes usually presents with **renal dysfunction**, but also potentially with an amyloid cardiomyopathy, peripheral neuropathy, gastrointestinal hemorrhage, or even hepatic rupture depending on the mutation.

Senile systemic amyloidosis, associated with wild-type transthyretin, is an increasingly recognized entity and presents as an isolated **amyloid cardiomyopathy** in male patients usually over the age of 70 years. This has a typically much slower progression than that related to AL amyloidosis.

Differential diagnosis

Since amyloidosis is a disease that may affect multiple organ systems, the differential diagnosis is extremely wide. It is often not possible to distinguish AA, AL, and hereditary forms of the disease clinically, and the presence of a potentially amyloidogenic chronic inflammatory disorder, monoclonal gammopathy, or even gene mutation can be misleading. Once a histological diagnosis of amyloidosis has been established, it is vital to determine the amyloid fibril type immunohistochemically or by analyses of isolated fibril preparations.

Diagnostic methods

The diagnosis of amyloidosis generally requires **histological confirmation**. The pathognomonic tinctorial property of amyloidotic tissue is apple-green/red birefringence when stained

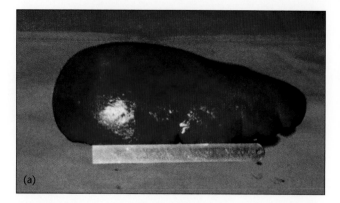

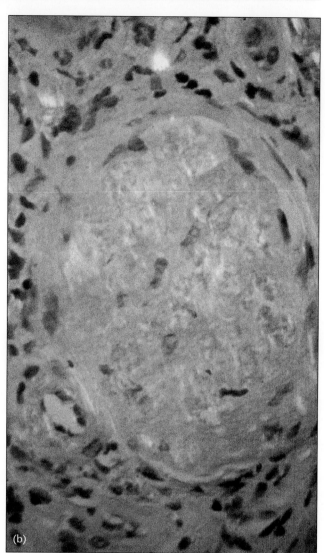

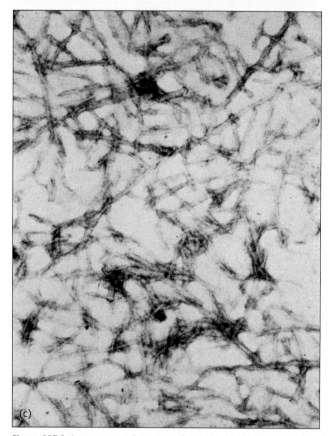

Figure 117.1 Appearance and structure of amyloid. (a) Greatly enlarged amyloidotic spleen removed at surgery, showing a waxy, lardaceous appearance. (b) Renal biopsy showing an amyloidotic glomerulus stained with Congo red, under partial cross-polarized light. (c) Isolated pure amyloid fibrils under electron microscopy showing typical rigid non-branched 8–10-nm diameter structure.

with Congo red dye and viewed under a light microscope in the presence of cross-polarized light. It also has a characteristic ultrastructural appearance on electron microscopy.

Screening biopsies of the rectum and abdominal fat are diagnostic in around 50–80% of patients with systemic amyloidosis, whereas direct biopsy of an **affected organ** yields positive histology in close to 100% of cases. **Immunohistochemical staining** of amyloid-containing tissue sections is imperative to characterize the amyloid fibril protein type.

Radiolabeled SAP scintigraphy, which is available in a few specialized centers, is a specific, non-invasive diagnostic method that also enables quantitative monitoring of amyloid deposits and allows for monitoring of changes in amyloid load (Figure 117.3) [7]. The restrictive diastolic impairment in cardiac amyloidosis is evaluated with **echocardiography** (Figure 117.4). Newer investigative modalities, such as cardiac magnetic resonance imaging, and cardiac biomarkers, such as N-terminal pro-BNP, may contribute to a diagnosis of cardiac amyloid.

Treatment and prevention

In the absence of any treatment that specifically causes regression of amyloid deposits, the aim of therapy is to reduce the supply of **amyloid fibril precursor proteins** in the hope that progression of the disease will be slowed or halted (Table 117.2). Regression of amyloid deposits has been confirmed using serial SAP scintigraphy. It is important to appreciate that clinically significant regression may not be evident for months or years after the supply of the fibril precursor has been reduced. Furthermore, changes in organ function may not correlate with changes in amyloid load on SAP scintigraphy.

In **AA amyloidosis** the aim of treatment is to suppress the inflammatory process responsible for sustained overproduction of SAA. Newer biological agents that target cytokines, such as tumor necrosis factor (TNF)-alpha, have been widely utilized in a variety of inflammatory conditions. Follow-up studies have demonstrated that when SAA values are restored to normal values of less than 10 mg/L, amyloid deposition is halted in all patients, and regression occurs in 60% of cases [4]. Frequent monitoring of the plasma SAA concentration is therefore essential in guiding treatment.

In **AL amyloidosis** the goal of treatment is to suppress the B-cell clone producing the amyloidogenic monoclonal immunoglobulin light chain, using regimens based on those used in multiple myeloma. These range from intermediate-dose **chemotherapy**, such as melphalan and dexamethasone or cyclophosphamide/thalidomide/dexamethasone, favored as first-line management in the UK, where treatment is guided by serial quantitative measurements of serum free immunoglobulin light chain concentration [8], to autologous **stem cell transplantation** [9]. Both carry risks, but stem cell transplantation carries a substantial procedural mortality that overall exceeds 5–10%. Patient selection in terms of organ involvement and risk-to-benefit ratio are therefore very important when considering any form of treatment.

In **familial amyloid polyneuropathy** associated with transthyretin mutations, orthotopic **liver transplantation** can halt amyloid deposition since the variant amyloidogenic protein is produced mainly in the liver. Liver transplantation is best performed at an early symptomatic stage when peripheral neuropathy can stabilize and autonomic nerve function can sometimes improve. However, cardiac involvement may paradoxically progress after liver transplantation due to deposition of wild-type TTR on the existing "template" of variant TTR amyloid and this should be borne in mind during selection of patients [10]. Liver transplantation has been successful in

Table 117.1 Symptoms caused by amyloidosis

Soft tissue amyloidosis (Figure 117.2)	Bruising (especially periorbital), macroglossia, pseudohypertrophy of skeletal muscle or cutaneous lesions
Renal	Edema, proteinuric renal failure
Cardiac	Fatigue, exertional dyspnea, palpitations, syncopal episodes or edema associated with a restrictive cardiomyopathy
Liver	Discomfort or bloating associated with hepatomegaly or rarely jaundice with liver failure
Peripheral neuropathy	Carpal tunnel syndrome, paresthesia, numbness or weakness
Autonomic neuropathy	Postural hypotension, cardiac arrhythmias, erectile dysfunction, impaired gastrointestinal motility and bladder emptying
Gastrointestinal	Poor appetite, nausea, dyspepsia, vomiting, diarrhea, constipation or hemorrhage
Adrenal axis	Hypoadrenalism
Lymphoreticular system	Enlarged spleen, lymphadenopathy

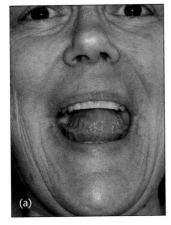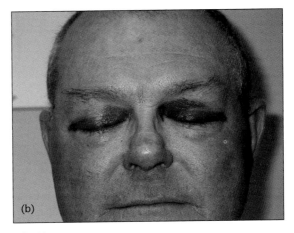

Figure 117.2 Soft tissue amyloidosis. (a) Macroglossia. (b) Periorbital bruising.

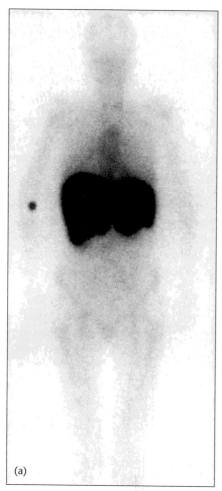

(a)

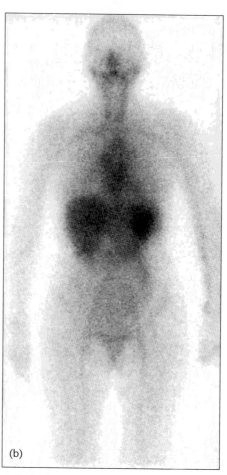

(b)

Figure 117.3 Anterior whole body radiolabeled serum amyloid P component (SAP) scans. (a) Study at presentation of a patient with AL amyloidosis, showing abnormal tracer uptake into amyloid deposits within the liver, spleen, kidneys, and bone marrow. (b) Repeat study 2 years later indicates that substantial regression of the amyloid has occurred following suppression of the patient's underlying plasma cell dyscrasia by chemotherapy; most of the tracer is now confined to the normal blood pool.

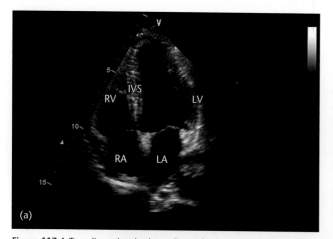

(a)

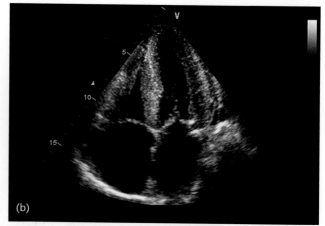

(b)

Figure 117.4 Two-dimensional echocardiographic images (four-chamber views) of a normal (a) and an amyloidotic heart (b). The amyloidotic heart has strikingly enlarged atria, consistent with diastolic dysfunction in association with significant biventricular wall thickening secondary to amyloid infiltration. IVS, interventricular septum; LA, left atrium; LV, left ventricular wall; RA, right atrium; RV, right ventricular wall.

Table 117.2 Principles of treatment in systemic amyloidosis

Disease	Aim of treatment	Example of treatment
AA amyloidosis	Suppress acute-phase response, thereby reducing SAA production	Anti–TNF-alpha treatment in rheumatoid arthritis and colchicine in FMF
AL amyloidosis	Suppress production of immunoglobulin light chains	Chemotherapy for the underlying monoclonal gammopathy or myeloma
Hereditary amyloidosis	Reduce/eliminate production of genetically variant protein	Orthotopic liver transplantation for variant transthyretin-associated FAP and selected cases of fibrinogen A α-chain and apolipoprotein AI amyloidosis

FAP, familial amyloid polyneuropathy; FMF, familial Mediterranean fever; SAA, serum amyloid A protein.

arresting amyloidogenesis in both fibrinogen A α-chain and apolipoprotein AI amyloidosis, in which the variant amyloidogenic protein is derived wholly or partially from the liver, respectively [11,12].

Prevention of amyloidosis is sometimes possible. Deposition of AA amyloid can be almost completely inhibited in **familial Mediterranean fever (FMF)** by the long-term prophylactic use of colchicine. There are promising treatments on the horizon that target amyloid directly, such as fibril precursor protein stabilizers, inhibitors of fibrillogenesis, and immunotherapy [13].

Complications and their management

Supportive therapy remains a critical component of management, with the potential for delaying target organ failure, maintaining quality of life, and prolonging survival whilst therapy directed against the underlying metabolic defect can be instituted. Replacement of vital organ function, notably with **renal dialysis**, may be necessary. Solid **organ transplantation** (kidney, heart, and liver) has been used with variable results to replace failing organs in hereditary systemic, AL, and AA amyloidosis. In any such setting, patient selection is extremely important, as is a strategy to eliminate the amyloid precursor protein to prevent amyloid recurrence in the graft.

Rigorous control of hypertension is vital in renal amyloidosis. Surgical resection of amyloidotic tissue is occasionally beneficial but caution should be maintained as the stresses of surgery and anesthesia can cause amyloidotic organ decompensation. If undertaken, meticulous attention to blood pressure, fluid balance and sepsis is essential, especially in patients with renal and/or cardiac involvement. Furthermore amyloidotic tissues may heal poorly and are liable to hemorrhage.

Diuretics and vasoactive drugs should be used cautiously in cardiac amyloidosis because they can reduce cardiac output substantially. Dysrhythmias may respond to conventional pharmacological therapy or to pacing.

Prognosis with and without treatment

The prognosis of systemic amyloidosis without treatment is generally very poor. Most such patients with AA amyloidosis die within 5–10 years and those with AL type in less than 2 years. Hereditary forms of amyloidosis often have a better prognosis, but in all types life-expectancy is greatly increased by therapy that adequately reduces production of the respective amyloid fibril precursor protein.

SOURCES OF INFORMATION FOR PATIENTS AND DOCTORS

The National Amyloidosis Centre in the Royal Free Hospital, London, UK provides specialist clinical evaluation and treatment advice for patients with amyloidosis, and written information http://www.ucl.ac.uk/medicine/amyloidosis/nac.

The UK Myeloma Forum has drawn up consensus guidelines on the management of AL amyloidosis www.ukmf.org.uk/guidelines.htm.

Myeloma UK provides information for patients, including a web-based and telephone support network www.myeloma.org.uk/.

References

1. Pepys MB, Hawkins PN. Amyloidosis. In: Warrell DA, Cox TM, Firth JD, Benz EJ Jr, editors. *Oxford Textbook of Medicine*, 4th edition. Oxford: Oxford University Press, 2003:162–173.
2. Kyle RA, Therneau TM, Rajkumar SV, *et al*. A long-term study of prognosis in monoclonal gammopathy of undetermined significance. *N Engl J Med*. 2002;346:564–569.
3. Lachmann HJ, Booth DR, Booth SE, *et al*. Misdiagnosis of hereditary amyloidosis as AL (primary) amyloidosis. *N Engl J Med*. 2002;346:1786–1791.
4. Lachmann HJ, Goodman HJ, Gilbertson JA, *et al*. Natural history and outcome in systemic AA amyloidosis. *N Engl J Med*. 2007;23:2361–2371.
5. Sunde M, Serpell LC, Bartlam M, *et al*. Common core structure of amyloid fibrils by synchrotron X-ray diffraction. *J Mol Biol*. 1997;273:729–739.
6. Ihse E, Ybo A, Suhr OB, *et al*. Amyloid fibril composition is related to the phenotype of hereditary transthyretin V30M amyloidosis. *J Pathol*. 2008;216:253–261
7. Hawkins PN, Lavender JP, Pepys MB. Evaluation of systemic amyloidosis by scintigraphy with 123I-labeled serum amyloid P component. *N Engl J Med*. 1990;323:508–513.
8. Lachmann HJ, Gallimore R, Gillmore JD, *et al*. Outcome in systemic AL amyloidosis in relation to changes in concentration of circulating free immunoglobulin light chains following chemotherapy. *Br J Haematol*. 2003;122:78–84.
9. Comenzo RL, Gertz MA. Autologous stem cell transplantation for primary systemic amyloidosis. *Blood*. 2002;99:4276–4282.

Multiple Organ Systems

10. Stangou AJ, Hawkins PN, Heaton ND, *et al.* Progressive cardiac amyloidosis following liver transplantation for familial amyloid polyneuropathy: implications for amyloid fibrillogenesis. *Transplantation*. 1998;66:229–233.

11. Gillmore JD, Booth DR, Rela M, *et al.* Curative hepatorenal transplantation in systemic amyloidosis caused by the Glu526Val fibrinogen alpha-chain variant in an English family. *Q J Med*. 2000;93:269–275.

12. Gillmore JD, Stangou AJ, Tennent GA, *et al.* Clinical and biochemical outcome of hepatorenal transplantation for hereditary systemic amyloidosis associated with apolipoprotein AI Gly26Arg. *Transplantation*. 2001;71:986–992.

13. Gillmore JD, Hawkins PN. Drug Insight: emerging therapies for amyloidosis. *Nat Clin Pract Nephrol*. 2006;5:263–270.

CHAPTER 118
Foreign bodies

Lisa Swize and Patrick R. Pfau

University of Wisconsin School of Medicine and Public Health, Madison, WI, USA

ESSENTIAL FACTS ABOUT PATHOPHYSIOLOGY

- Esophageal food impaction is the most common foreign body in the United States in adults
- The majority of patients with food impactions have underlying esophageal pathology
- 80% of true foreign bodies occur in the pediatric population
- Gastrointestinal foreign bodies cause symptoms because of impaction and obstruction at areas of luminal narrowing and angulation

ESSENTIALS OF DIAGNOSIS

- Food impaction/esophageal obstruction is almost always symptomatic, resulting in chest pain, dysphagia, and inability to handle secretions
- Foreign bodies in the stomach, small, and large intestine are usually asymptomatic, only causing symptoms if a complication such as perforation, bleeding, or obstruction occurs
- Plain films of the neck, chest, and abdomen may be the initial diagnostic test in foreign body ingestions
- Endoscopy is the diagnostic test of choice with close to 100% accuracy in identifying the presence of a foreign body

ESSENTIALS OF TREATMENT

- The majority of ingested foreign bodies will pass spontaneously without need for treatment
- Flexible endoscopy has the highest success rate with a low complication rate in the treatment of gastrointestinal foreign bodies
- The "push" method is the primary treatment for food impactions with success rates >90%
- All objects in the esophagus should be removed within 24 hours to avoid serious complications
- Sharp objects and large and long objects that will not pass spontaneously should be removed from the stomach or duodenum with flexible endoscopy

Causes and epidemiology

Food impaction is the most common gastrointestinal foreign body, with an estimated incidence of 16 per 100 000 Persons [1]. Most food impactions occur in adults, beginning in their fourth decade. The majority of patients have underlying esophageal motility disorders or esophageal pathology, such as strictures, rings, webs, diverticula, anastomoses, and cancer. Food impactions in young adults have a greater incidence in patients with eosinophilic esophagitis [2].

It is estimated that approximately 80% of the **non-food or true foreign body ingestions** occur in the pediatric population due to natural oral curiosity [3]. Items typically ingested by children include coins, buttons, small toys, and marbles. In the adult population accidental and intentional ingestions occur with increased frequency in those who have dental appliances or impaired mental status, including elderly, demented, or intoxicated patients [4]. Intentional ingestions occur predominantly in the psychiatric and prisoner population. These patients often ingest multiple complex objects and have recurrent ingestions. Rectal foreign body insertions are more often related to sexual activity or sexual assault.

Iatrogenic foreign bodies are an increasing problem. Examples of such foreign bodies include capsules from capsule endoscopy, migrated esophageal, luminal and biliary stents, and migrated gastrostomy buttons and catheters [5].

Pathogenesis and pathophysiology

The majority, 80–90%, of foreign bodies **passes spontaneously and uneventfully** [6,7]. Approximately 10–20% of cases require endoscopic intervention and approximately 1% or fewer require surgery to remove the items [6]. Complications such as obstruction and perforation most often occur at anatomic sphincters, areas of angulation, and surgical anastomoses (Figure 118.1).

Esophageal foreign bodies

Esophageal foreign bodies cause the most substantial morbidity and mortality compared to other locations in the gastrointestinal tract. Potential complications include **perforation, mediastinitis, fistulae, and aspiration**. Esophageal perforation can lead to lung abscess, cardiac tamponade, pneumothorax, mediastinitis, and peritonitis [8]. The complication rate from esophageal foreign bodies is directly proportional to the time spent in the esophagus (Figure 118.2). There are four areas of natural narrowing in the esophagus where impactions may occur: upper esophageal sphincter, level of the aortic arch,

Textbook of Clinical Gastroenterology and Hepatology, Second Edition. Edited by C. J. Hawkey, Jaime Bosch, Joel E. Richter, Guadalupe Garcia-Tsao, Francis K. L. Chan.
© 2012 Blackwell Publishing Ltd. Published 2012 by Blackwell Publishing Ltd.

Multiple Organ Systems

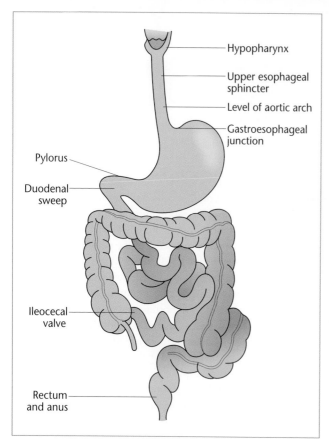

Figure 118.1 Gastrointestinal areas of luminal narrowing and angulation that predispose to foreign body impaction and obstruction.

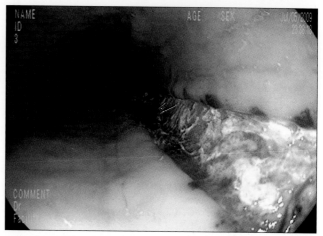

Figure 118.2 Large esophageal tear to the muscle layer in a patient who had a foreign body residing in the esophagus for longer than 24 hours.

crossing of the mainstem bronchus, and the lower esophageal sphincter, but the vast majority of patients with esophageal foreign bodies have underlying esophageal pathology.

Stomach and intestinal foreign bodies

Sharp objects are at higher risk of causing complications and have an associated perforation rate of up to 35% [9]. Objects greater than 2 cm in diameter will have difficulty passing through the pylorus. Objects longer than 5 cm have difficulty traversing through the pylorus and passing through the duodenal sweep. The ligament of Treitz and ileocecal valve are two additional areas of potential impaction because of the fixed angulation.

Colon and rectum foreign bodies

Foreign bodies that have successfully traversed out of the small intestine rarely cause complications in the colon. Objects tend to be centered in the lumen and are surrounded by stool that offers protection to the colon. Rarely, ingested foreign bodies will have difficulty exiting the rectum. Complications in the rectum from foreign bodies are more often from objects intentionally inserted. The valves of Houston and sacral curve can limit spontaneous passage of the objects, and the anal

sphincters may be contracted and swollen from foreign body insertion, contributing to the incidence of retained objects.

Clinical presentation

Children who ingest foreign bodies may be asymptomatic (20–40%) and in up to 40% of cases caregivers do not give a history of ingestion [3]. Even in children who have symptoms, the clues may be subtle and include drooling, poor feeding, irritability, and failure to thrive. If an impaction has occurred proximally in the esophagus and compresses the trachea, wheezing and stridor may be present. Adults who swallow non-food foreign bodies may not provide a reliable history because they are often mentally impaired or have swallowed items for secondary gain.

In adults who are communicative, the history will often provide reliable details regarding the timing and type of ingestion. **Food impactions** are almost always symptomatic due to either partial or complete esophageal obstruction. Symptoms include substernal chest pain, dysphagia, gagging, and vomiting. Drooling and inability to handle oral secretions may occur in complete obstructions.

Foreign bodies in the stomach, small intestine and colon typically only cause symptoms if a complication has occurred. If impaction has occurred in the small intestine or at the ileocecal valve, patients may present with symptoms of a small bowel obstruction. Perforation of the intestines from foreign body ingestion may present with symptoms of abdominal pain, peritonitis, and possibly fever.

Diagnostic methods

History can provide reliable information in most food impactions and accidental non-food foreign body ingestions in adults regarding the type of material ingested, timing, and probable location. Past medical history may reveal a history of recurrent foreign body ingestions. In young adults, a history of recurrent food impactions suggests eosinophilic esophagitis. Children, however, are often unable to give a reliable history. In children **radiographs** of the entire gastrointestinal tract may then be useful in identifying the location of the foreign body if it is radio-opaque [10]. In adults, chest X-ray and/or abdominal films may aid in determining the type and location of a foreign body but are not necessary in all patients.

The **physical examination** in both children and adults does little to aid in the diagnosis but is important in identifying any complications. The examination may reveal signs of aspiration such as wheezing and stridor. Crepitus in the neck may be present in patients with esophageal perforation. Bowel perforation may result in signs of peritonitis. If an esophageal or intestinal perforation is suspected, anteroposterior and lateral radiographs of the neck, chest, and abdomen should be the initial diagnostic test. Barium studies are not indicated in the evaluation of foreign body ingestions and should be avoided because of the risk of aspiration and impairment of subsequent endoscopic exam.

Endoscopy is the modality of choice for the diagnosis of foreign body ingestions that are suspected in the esophagus, stomach, proximal small bowel, and rectum. For the diagnosis of esophageal and gastric foreign bodies, the accuracy is near 100% due to direct visualization. .

Treatment

Knowledge of which patients need intervention and the correct timing of intervention is crucial [6].

The need for intervention is based on the presence of symptoms, the type and size of the item ingested, and the location in the gastrointestinal tract. The majority of **endoscopies** for foreign body removal in adults can be safely performed with intravenous conscious sedation. In pediatric patients, uncooperative patients and in patients with complex or multiple foreign bodies, general anesthesia with endotracheal intubation should be considered to aid in safe and successful endoscopic removal.

Esophageal and gastric foreign bodies

Food impactions should be removed within 24 hours of ingestion and more urgently in the setting of suspected complete obstruction. A trial of **pharmacological therapy** for both food and non-food foreign bodies is reasonable as an initial treatment modality. Glucagon, a smooth muscle relaxant, reduces the lower esophageal sphincter pressure and has a reported success rate of 12–58% in relieving esophageal obstructions from foreign bodies [11]. There is a lack of published efficacy to support the use of nifedipine and nitroglycerine. The use of gas-forming agents, emetics and papain (a meat tenderizer) should not be used because of higher complication rates.

Flexible endoscopy is the treatment modality of choice in both the pediatric and adult population. Endoscopic treatment of **food impactions** has success rates of >95% with a near 0%

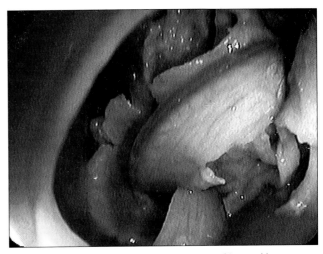

Figure 118.3 Endoscopic image of a large amount of ingested bacon impacted in the esophagus. This was successfully "pushed" into the stomach without difficulty, which relieved all symptoms.

complication rate [12,13]. The endoscopic **"push" technique** is utilized most frequently with high success (Figure 118.3). The endoscope is passed into the esophagus to the food bolus and gently advanced around the food bolus and into the stomach to detect any fixed obstruction. The endoscope is then pulled back to the proximal edge of the food bolus. If the endoscope cannot be passed around the food bolus, gentle pressure is applied to the food bolus to advance it into the stomach. Forceful pushing should be avoided as this may increase the perforation rate [10]. If the food bolus cannot be pushed into the stomach, it should then be broken up using a variety of tools (forceps, snares, baskets) (Table 118.1), and the smaller pieces either pushed into the stomach or removed through the mouth. An overtube may be used to help prevent material from entering the airway and allow multiple passes of the endoscope (Figure 118.4). It is generally considered safe to dilate the esophagus if a ring or stricture is present once the obstruction is relieved. If the mucosa is significantly inflamed, then it is recommended that the patient be placed on acid suppression and return for dilation in several weeks. If concentric rings are present suggestive of eosinophilic esophagitis. dilation is generally not recommended, but biopsies should be taken to help confirm the diagnosis.

The success of removing **non-food foreign body ingestions** from the esophagus may be slightly lower than that of food impactions. **Sharp or pointed objects** should be grasped with the sharp edge trailing to lessen the chance of mucosal injury or perforation (Figure 118.5; see Video clip 118.1). If the object is oriented in the esophagus such that the sharp edge is proximal, then the object should be gently advanced into the stomach, grasped, and rotated for proper orientation. Rat-tooth or alligator forceps and snares allow for the greatest control during removal. Overtubes or latex protector hoods are recommended to protect the airway and oropharynx.

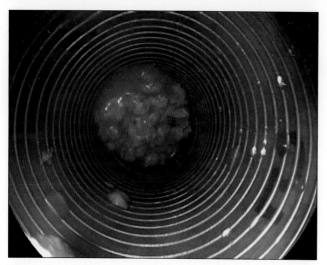

Figure 118.4 Endoscopic view within the overtube in a patient with a meat impaction that could not be pushed into the stomach. The overtube protected the airway while allowing multiple passes of the endoscope as needed to remove the food impaction.

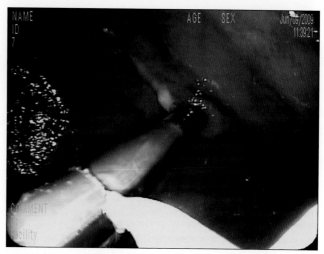

Figure 118.5 Successful removal of a pen that had been ingested and had perforated the stomach wall. The pen was removed with the endoscope using a standard polypectomy snare without complication to the patient.

Table 118.1 Equipment for treatment and removal of gastrointestinal foreign bodies and food

Endoscopes	Overtubes	Accessory equipment
Flexible endoscope	Standard esophageal	Retrieval net
Rigid endoscope	overtube	Alligator or rat tooth
Laryngoscope	45–60-cm foreign	forceps
Kelly or McGill	body overtube	Dormia basket
forceps		Polypectomy snare
		Three-pronged grabber
		Magnetic extractor
		Steigmann–Goff variceal
		ligator cap
		Latex protector hood

Coins and button batteries in the esophagus should be removed to prevent pressure necrosis and perforation. Button batteries can cause tissue liquefaction, leading to extensive esophageal injury and perforation. An overtube used with intravenous sedation or general anesthesia with an endotracheal tube should be considered to protect the airway. The Roth retrieval net permits the best control of objects during retrieval. Once coins and batteries are in the stomach they rarely cause problems, and most small coins will pass out of the stomach within 72 hours. The patient should be followed with serial radiographs to ensure passage through the gastrointestinal tract. If the coin or battery remains in the stomach for longer than 72 hours, retrieval is recommended [14]. **Magnets** should be removed if ingested and within the reach of the endoscope. Multiple magnets can lead to attraction between them and possible pressure necrosis, fistula formation, and bowel perforation.

Long objects such as pens, pencils, spoons, forks and toothbrushes are common intentional ingestions. Objects longer than 5 cm will have difficulty passing through the duodenal sweep and will need to be removed endoscopically. To facilitate removal, the object should be grasped at the edge of the object to better traverse the esophageal sphincters. Objects grasped in the middle tend to stay in a horizontal plane, making their removal more difficult. An alternative method to remove long objects is to grasp the object with forceps, snare or basket, and to pull it into an overtube that extends past the gastroesophageal junction. The overtube, foreign body, and endoscope can then all be removed together.

Small bowel foreign bodies

Foreign bodies in the small bowel may rarely result in impaction at areas of strictures and angulation. Objects out of the reach of traditional endoscopy have historically been managed surgically. With the introduction of **double balloon enteroscopy** there have been reports of removal without surgical intervention [15].

Rectal foreign bodies

Most rectal foreign bodies are a result of retrograde insertion and can be removed either **manually** or with a **flexible sigmoidoscope or rigid proctoscope**. Prior to digital examination a radiograph is recommended to confirm the position and type of object. If the object is sharp, manual removal should be attempted with caution. An overtube or latex hood attached to the end of the scope can be used to protect the anal sphincter and mucosa from injury as the objects are removed and to overcome the sphincter's natural tendency to contract. Removal of large and complex objects may require general anesthesia and anal sphincter dilation [16].

Narcotic packets

Narcotic-containing packets are ingested to hide and smuggle them. Intestinal obstruction due to the packages or symptoms related to the ingested drug may develop in up to 26% of patients, with death occurring in 5% due to serious toxicology side effects [17]. Diagnosis is from history and radiographs or computed tomography (CT) scan, which may show multiple round packets. **Observation with a clear liquid diet** is recommended. Lavage and laxatives should be avoided and endoscopic removal is contraindicated due to the high risk of perforation.

Complications

Complications from the treatment of foreign body ingestions are low and in most studies range from 0 to 2% [9]. **Perforation** can occur from both treatment and in the setting of observation. Risk factors for perforation include an uncooperative patient, multiple ingestions, complex ingestions and delay in time to treatment [4]. Other reported complications include cardiopulmonary events, gastrointestinal bleeding, and aspiration. These occur at a similar rate to that found in routine upper and lower endoscopy.

Prognosis and future trends

The majority of foreign body ingestions are treated successfully by endoscopy with minimal and rare complications. Currently, endoscopy is the treatment of choice for foreign body ingestions and likely will remain so for the near future. The incidence of foreign body ingestion and how we treat foreign bodies will continue to evolve as diseases such as eosinophilic esophagitis become more common, how we treat reflux and obesity changes, and as new technology, such as improved access, to the small bowel is introduced. Future challenges are the collection of prospective data on the management of foreign bodies so the correct treatment can be applied to the appropriate patient in this very common problem.

References

1. Longstreth GF, Longstreth KJ, Yao JF. Esophageal food impaction: epidemiology and therapy. A retrospective, observational study. *Gastrointest Endosc.* 2001;53:193–198.
2. Kerlin P, Jones D, Remedios M, *et al.* Prevalence of eosinophilic esophagitis in adults with food bolus obstruction of the esophagus. *J Clin Gastroenterol.* 2007;41:356–361.
3. Arana A, Hauser B, Hachimi-Idrissi S, *et al.* Management of ingested foreign bodies in childhood and review of the literature. *Eur J Pediatr.* 2001;160:468–472.
4. Palta R, Sahota A, Bemarki A, Salama P, Simpson N, Laine L. Foreign-body ingestion: characteristics and outcomes in a lower socioeconomic population with predominantly intentional ingestion. *Gastrointest Endosc.* 2009;69:426–433.
5. Ozutemiz O, Tekin F, Oruc N, *et al.* Ileal obstruction after duodenal metallic stent placement. *Endoscopy.* 2007;39 (Suppl 1): E288.
6. Eisen GM, Baron TH, Dominitz JA, *et al.* Guideline for the management of ingested foreign bodies. *Gastrointest Endosc.* 2002;55:802–806.
7. Weiland ST, Schurr MJ. Conservative management of ingested foreign bodies. *J Gastrointest Surg.* 2002;6:496–500.
8. Weissberg D, Refaely Y. Foreign bodies in the esophagus. *Ann Thorac Surg.* 2007;84:1854–1857.
9. Pfau PR, Ginsberg GG. Foreign bodies and bezoars. In: Feldman M, Friedman LS, Schleisenger MH, editors. *Schleisenger & Fordtran's Gastrointestinal and Liver Disease. Pathophysiology/Diagnosis/Management.* Philadelphia: WB Saunders, 2006: 499–513.
10. Shaffer HA, de Lange EE. Gastrointestinal foreign bodies and strictures: radiologic interventions. *Curr Probl Diagn Radiol.* 1994;23:205–249.
11. Al-Haddad M, Ward EM. Glucagon for the relief of esophageal food impaction: Does it really work? *Dig Dis Sci.* 2006;51: 1930–1933.
12. Vicari JJ, Johanson JF, Frakes JT. Outcomes of acute esophageal food impaction: success of the push technique. *Gastrointest Endosc.* 2001;53:178–181.
13. Katsinelos P, Kountouras J, Paroutoglou G, *et al.* Endoscopic techniques and management of foreign body ingestion and food bolus impaction in the upper gastrointestinal tract: A retrospective analysis of 139 cases. *J Clin Gastroenterol.* 2006;40:784–789.
14. Litovitz T, Scmitz BF. Ingestion of cylindrical and button batteries: An analysis of 2382 cases. *Pediatrics.* 1992;89:747–757.
15. Miehlke S, Tausche AK, Brückner S, *et al.* Retrieval of two retained endoscopy capsules with retrograde double-balloon enteroscopy in a patient with a history of complicated small-bowel disease. *Endoscopy.* 2007;39 (Suppl 1):E157.
16. Kourkalis G, Misiakos E, Dovas N, *et al.* Management of foreign bodies of the rectum; Report of 21 cases. *J R Coll Surg Edinb.* 1997;42:246–247
17. June R, Aks SE, Keys N, *et al.* Medical outcome of cocaine bodystuffers. *J Emerg Med.* 2000;18:221–224.

Multiple Organ Systems

CHAPTER 119

Porphyria

Jean-Charles Deybach and Hervé Puy

Hôpital Louis Mourier, Colombes, France

ESSENTIAL FACTS ABOUT PATHOGENESIS

- Porphyrias are caused by genetically determined deficiencies in seven of the enzymes of heme synthesis
- This results in over production of heme precursors
- Acute attacks are precipitated by increased demands for heme synthesis (stress, fasting, infection, drugs)

ESSENTIALS OF DIAGNOSIS

- The most common porphyrias are acute intermittent porphyria, porphyria cutanea tarda, variegate porphyria, and hereditary coproporphyria
- High value clinical signs are severe pain in the abdomen, back, and thigh, with vomiting and constipation, mental symptoms, and signs of autonomic neuropathy
- Increased 5-amino levulinic acid and porphobilinogen in the urine. There may be hyponatremia

ESSENTIALS OF TREATMENT

- Admission to hospital and control of precipitants (drugs, alcohol, fasting, infection)
- High carbohydrate intake (400 g/day)
- Heme arginate infusion (normosang 250 mg/day for 4 days)
- Opiates can be used for pain relief and chlorpromazine for acute anxiety
- Phlebotomy and avoidance of sunlight are the treatments of choice for porphyria cutanea tarda

Introduction

The porphyrias are a group of **disorders of heme biosynthesis** in which specific patterns of overproduction of heme precursors are associated with the following characteristic clinical features [1]:

- Acute neurovisceral attacks [acute intermittent porphyria (AIP) and the rare 5-aminolevulinic acid (ALA) dehydratase deficiency [2] porphyria (ADP)]

- Skin lesions [porphyria cutanea tarda (PCT), congenital erythropoietic porphyria (CEP), and erythropoietic protoporphyria (EPP)]
- Both of the above [variegate porphyria (VP) [3] and hereditary coproporphyria (HC)].

Each type of porphyria is the result of a specific decrease in the activity of one of the enzymes in heme biosynthesis (Figure 119.1). Heme is synthesized from succinyl CoA and glycine in all tissues, but mostly in liver and bone marrow, for the synthesis of hemoproteins such as hemoglobin, myoglobin, cytochromes, catalase, peroxidase, nitric oxide synthase, and tryptophan pyrrolase. The mechanisms for the control of heme biosynthesis differ between the liver and bone marrow. The first step, enzyme 5-ALA synthase, is coded for by two genes: one erythroid specific (ALA synthase-2 on chromosome X) and one ubiquitous (ALA synthase-1 on chromosome 3). In the erythroid cell, erythropoietin and iron are involved in the control of the enzymes participating in the formation of heme. In the liver, the hemoproteins formed, including the cytochrome P450s, are rapidly turned over in response to current metabolic needs [2]. The free cellular heme pool retroinhibits ALA synthase-1 activity via a negative feedback regulation. Enzyme defect will give rise to a characteristic biochemical profile of porphyrins and porphyrin precursors, ALA and porphobilinogen (PBG), which accumulate in urine, feces, plasma, and/or erythrocytes. This allows the type of porphyria to be accurately identified in patients (Table 119.1). Enzyme or DNA analysis must be used for family studies [3].

Clinical classification of porphyrias

Three broad types of porphyric syndromes are recognized: **acute hepatic porphyrias** characterized by acute neurovisceral attacks with or without cutaneous manifestations; **non-acute hepatic porphyria cutanea tarda** characterized by photosensitivity; and **erythropoietic porphyrias**, which are also characterized by photosensitivity. Porphyrias can be classified as either erythropoietic or hepatic, depending on the primary organ in which excess production of porphyrins or precursors takes place (see Figure 119.1).

Multiple Organ Systems

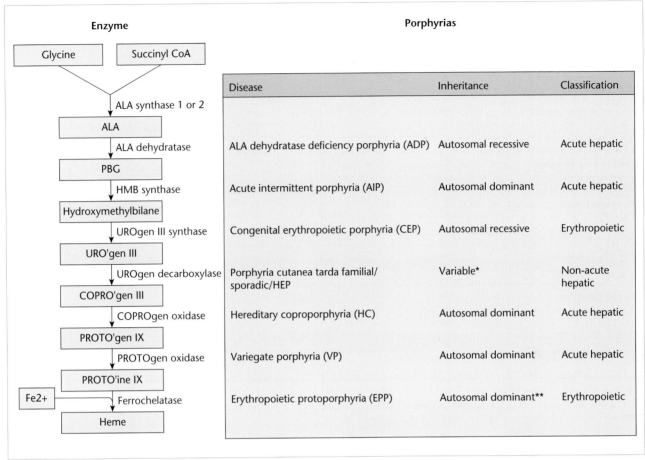

Figure 119.1 Classification of the major human porphyrias. ALA, 5-aminolevulinic acid; COPRO'gen, coproporphyrinogen; HEP, hepatoerythroporphyria; III or IX, type isomers; PBG, porphobilinogen; PROTO'gen, protoporphyrinogen; PROTO'ine, protoporphyrine; URO'gen, uroporphyrinogen. *Autosomal dominant inheritance has been documented in familial porphyria cutanea tarda and recessive inheritance has been documented in HEP. **Erythropoietic protoporphyria is mainly related to the coinheritance of both a ferrochelatase gene mutation and a weak normal ferrochelatase allele; autosomal recessive inheritance has also been reported in a few families. (This figure was published in *Clinical Gastroenterology and Hepatology*, Wilfred M. Weinstein, Christopher J. Hawkey, Jaime Bosch, Porphyria, Pages 1–8, Copyright Elsevier, 2005.)

Acute hepatic porphyrias

Acute attacks are identical in four of the hepatic porphyrias: AIP, HC, VP, and ADP. With the exception of ADP, an autosomal recessive disorder, the acute hepatic porphyrias are all autosomal dominant conditions in which a 50% reduction in enzyme activity is brought about by a mutation in one of the alleles of the corresponding gene. The penetrance is low and about 90% of affected individuals never experience an acute attack. VP and HC can also be associated with skin lesions, which are the only manifestation of the condition in 60% of VP patients. In most countries, AIP is the commonest of the acute porphyrias [4].

Clinical presentation

Acute attacks are precipitated by events that increase the demand for heme synthesis. These include **hormonal fluctuations, stress, fasting, infection, and exposure to porphyrinogenic drugs**. Most drugs that exacerbate porphyria have the capacity to induce ALA synthase-1, which is closely associated with induction of the cytochrome P450 enzymes, a process that increases the demand for heme synthesis in the liver. Acute attacks are rare before puberty (except in ADP) and after the menopause, with a peak occurrence in the third and fourth decades of life; women are five times more likely to be affected than men. Most patients suffer one or possibly two acute attacks and are then symptom free for the rest of their lives. A few have recurrent acute attacks, which may require a special treatment regimen (see below). The acute porphyrias may present with a sudden life-threatening crisis characterized by severe abdominal pain, neuropsychiatric symptoms, autonomic neuropathy, and electrolyte disturbances (Table 119.2). All these clinical features of an acute attack can be explained by lesions of the nervous system.

Pathogenic mechanism

The **skin photosensitivity** in cutaneous porphyrias can be ascribed to accumulation of porphyrins in the skin, which absorb light with the formation of destructive free radicals.

Multiple Organ Systems

Table 119.1 Treatment and biochemical diagnosis in symptomatic porphyric patients

Diagnosis in symptomatic patients					
Porphyria	Urine	Stool	RBC	Plasma*	Treatment
Acute hepatic					
ALA dehydratase porphyria	**ALA**, Copro III	—	Zn-Proto	—	**Supportive treatment:**
Acute intermittent porphyria	**ALA, PBG**, URO III	—	—	615–620	Avoidance of precipitating factor
					Opiates and chlo rpromazine
					Adequate fluid intake
Hereditary coproporphyria	**ALA, PBG**, Copro III	Copro III	—	615–620	**Specific treatment:**
Variegate porphyria	**ALA, PBG**, Copro III	Proto Copro	—	624–627	Carbohydrates, heme arginate
Non-acute hepatic					**Supportive treatment:**
					Restriction of sunlight
					Avoidance of precipitating factors
Porphyria cutanea tarda	Uro III, Hepta	Isocopro, Hepta	—	615–620	**Specific treatment:**
					Phlebotomy Low-dose chloroquine
Erythropoietic					
Congenital erythropoietic porphyria	Uro I, Copro I	Copro I	Uro I, Copro I	615–620	Skin protection/ blood transfusion/bone marrow transplantation
Erythropoietic protoporphyria	—	Proto	Free Proto	626–634	Skin protection/oral beta-carotene Liver transplantation

*Fluorescence emission peak in nm.

ALA, δ-aminolevulinic acid; Copro, coproporphyrin; Hepta, heptacarboxyl-porphyrin; I or III: Type isomers; Isocopro, isocoproporphyrin; PBG, porpho-bilinogen; Proto, protoporphyrin; RBC, red blood cell; Uro, uroporphyrin.

Table 119.2 Clinical and biological signs of high diagnostic value and treatment in acute attacks of hepatic porphyria: acute intermittent porphyria, hereditary coproporphyria, variegate porphyria

Signs of high diagnostic value
- Clinical symptoms:
  - Severe abdominal pain/back and thigh pain
  - Vomiting, constipation
  - Other signs of autonomic neuropathy (muscle weakness, hypertension, tachycardia, etc.)
  - Mental symptoms
- Biology:
  - Increased ALA and PBG in the urine
  - ± Hyponatremia

Management
- Admission to hospital
- Withdrawal of all common precipitants (drugs, alcohol, fasting, infection, etc.)
- Opiates and chlorpromazine
- Carbohydrates (400 g/day)
- Early heme arginate infusion Normosang→ (250 mg/day x 4)

ALA, 5-aminolevulinic acid; PBG, porphobilinogen.

The mechanism of **neural damage** in these disorders is poorly understood. Various hypotheses that are not mutually exclusive have been proposed. The leading hypothesis is that ALA and/or PBG overproduced by the liver is neurotoxic. Conversely, formation of hemoproteins may be compromised due to the inherited enzyme deficiency. Acute attacks usually begin with generalized **abdominal pain**. Constipation, nausea, vomiting, and insomnia may precede and accompany the abdominal crisis. Examination does not show signs of peritoneal irritation; radiographic films of the abdomen usually disclose a normal pattern of bowel gas. Tachycardia, excess sweating, and hypertension are often associated with abdominal pain. Occasionally, the occurrence of red or dark colored urine may help the physicians in their investigations.

In 20–30% of patients, signs of **mental disturbance** such as anxiety, depression, disorientation, hallucinations, paranoia, or confused states are observed. Abdominal pain may disappear within a few days, generally when no harmful drug has been used. When acute attacks last several days, the gastrointestinal manifestations frequently lead to weight loss, while prolonged vomiting may cause oliguria and hyperazotemia. Porphyric neuropathy often occurs when harmful drugs have not been avoided during an acute attack; however, neurological manifestations are also a problem in differential diagnosis and treatment when the type of porphyria is not known. **Neuropathy** is primarily motor: in the early stages, pain in the extremities is very common ("muscle pain"); weakness often begins in the proximal muscles, more commonly in the arms than in the legs. Paresis in the extremities may occur and can also be strikingly local. Muscle weakness may progress and eventuate in tetraplegia with respiratory and bulbar paralysis and death. After a severe attack, complete or partial muscle function can improve over a period of months. Recovery from paralysis may be incomplete, with sequelae mostly on extremities. The central nervous system is seldom involved; pyramidal signs, cerebellar syndrome, transitory blindness, or altered level of consciousness can occur. The cerebrospinal fluid (CSF) is usually normal. In general, neuropathy is now far less common than in the past. During acute attacks, dehydration and electrolyte imbalance occur frequently. **Hyponatremia** occurs in 40% and, when severe, can lead to convulsions. AHP patients are at increased risk of hepatocellular carcinoma and chronic renal failure with progressive tubulo interstitial nephropathy. Clinical manifestations are usually non-specific even in the presence of cutaneous lesions. Only biological data allow precise diagnosis of the type of acute hepatic porphyria.

Diagnostic methods

Acute porphyria attacks are characterized by **increased excretion of urinary ALA and/or PBG** (20–200-fold higher); in ADP, the overexcretion is restricted to ALA. Treatment can be instituted immediately, while further laboratory investigations establish the porphyria type by analyzing porphyrin excretion patterns in urine, feces, and plasma (see Table 119.1). Urinary uro- and co-proporphyrin may be secondarily increased in acutely ill patients or in several other conditions as hepatobiliary disease, alcohol abuse, infections, and excess urinary porphyrin excretion alone lack diagnostic specificity. A high level of precursors (ALA and mostly PBG) is the most important diagnostic tool in symptomatic patients. The limited sensitivity of excretion analyses prevents their use in screening individuals without symptoms of acute porphyria [5].

Acute intermittent porphyria

AIP is the most significant hepatic porphyria with respect to its incidence and clinical severity, and has been reported in many populations. It is an autosomal dominant disorder due to **deficient activity of hydroxymethylbilane synthase (HMBS) or PBG deaminase or uroporphyrinogen I synthase (EC 4.3.1.8)**. Most of the approximations of AIP prevalence were established by screening populations for urinary porphyrin precursors and are therefore underestimates; erythrocyte HMBS activity provides a better way to screen individuals and healthy populations for latent AIP. The enzyme deficiency is usually 50% of normal in all somatic cells studied in those who inherit the genetic trait. Measurement in erythrocytes is now

widely used to detect clinically latent individuals who often do not show evidence of overproduction of heme precursors. The 10-kb *HMBS* gene is located at chromosome 11q24.1–24.2 and contains 15 exons. It encodes erythroid-specific and ubiquitous isoforms of HMBS that are generated by the use of separate promoters and alternative splicing of the two primary transcripts. The genetic heterogeneity of AIP is already well known (Human Gene Mutation Database: www.hgmd.org). A few families have included subjects with the usual phenotypic expression of the disease but with normal HMBS activity in erythrocytes. In these cases, *HMBS* mutations, which have been identified as the cause of this non-erythroid form of AIP, affect mainly exon 1 of the gene responsible for the specific ubiquitous isoforms of HMBS. In classical or typical AIP, more than 200 mutations of the *HMBS* gene have been described to date, indicating that the molecular defect in this disorder is highly heterogeneous. Very few unrelated homozygous cases of AIP have been described over the last 50 years [6]. Homozygous variants of AIP, usually present in childhood, have phenotypes of variable severity. The clinical picture is completely different from that of AIP: these children are severely ill and characterized by porencephaly, severe retardation in development, neurological defects, cataracts, and psychomotor retardation.

ALA dehydratase deficiency porphyria (Doss porphyria)

ADP, the autosomal recessive acute hepatic porphyria, is the rarest form of porphyria. **ALA dehydratase activity** is dramatically decreased in erythrocytes and bone marrow cells, as would be expected for homozygotes with a decrease of approximately 50% in the activities found in parents. ADP is characterized by hugely **increased excretion of ALA and coproporphyrin** (mainly isomer type III) in urine. Porphobilinogen is only moderately elevated; fecal excretion of porphyrins is normal, but the porphyrin (especially protoporphyrin) content of the erythrocytes is raised as in all forms of homozygous porphyria. The human enzyme is a homooctamer with a subunit size of 36 kDa, encoded by a gene localized at chromosome 9q34, and is highly sensitive to inhibition by lead. In ADP, the pattern of overproduction of heme precursors closely resembles that of severe lead poisoning and tyrosinemia. However, some features allow us to refute this diagnosis; these include normal urinary and blood levels of lead, or the activity of ALA dehydratase, which is not restored by dithiothreitol. Glucose infusion and heme therapy are effective in some but not all cases. Avoidance of drugs that are harmful in other hepatic porphyrias is also recommended [7].

Variegate porphyria

VP is a low penetrance, autosomal dominant hepatic porphyria due to the **deficient activity of protoporphyrinogen oxidase (PPOX)** caused by mutations. VP is common in South

Africa, where an estimated 20 000 descendants of a Dutch couple have inherited the same mutation in the *PPOX* gene [8]. The disease is increasingly recognized, as confusion with PCT is resolved by application of more precise diagnostic methods. Plasma porphyrin peak, more frequently abnormal in adult VP carriers, should be used to screen general populations. The *PPOX* gene contains one non-coding and 12 coding exons. It spans 5 kb and is assigned to chromosome 1. More than 100 disease-specific mutations have been identified in VP (Human Gene Mutation Database: www.hgmd.org). The pattern of clinical presentation is not influenced by the type of mutation in the heterozygous form of VP. Eleven homozygous cases of VP have been described [9]. During acute attacks of VP, urinary profiles are rather similar to those in AIP and HC. Carriers with only chronic cutaneous manifestations or without symptoms often show a slight increase of the precursor ALA, while PBG is only present in half the carriers. The differentiation of VP and HC is usually possible following fecal porphyrin analysis. In VP, the characteristic finding is **elevated fecal protoporphyrin** and to a lesser degree coproporphyrin (predominantly type III). High-performance liquid chromatograpny (HPLC) of fecal porphyrins usually shows a peak of protoporphyrin as prominent as the coproporphyrin III peak, and protoporphyrin concentrations are about twofold greater than coproporphyrin. A plasma fluorescence emission maximal at 624–628 nm is the most valuable diagnostic marker in adult VP patients. In patients with only cutaneous manifestations, it is usually sufficient for differentiation of PCT from PV (see Porphyria cutanea tarda below).

Hereditary coproporphyria

HC is an autosomal dominant hepatic porphyria due to the **reduced activity of coproporphyrinogen oxidase (CPO; EC 1.3.3.3.)**. Clinically expressed HC is much less common than other acute hepatic porphyrias. The incidence of HC was estimated at two cases per million but latent *HC* gene carriers are being recognized with greater accuracy. Skin photosensitivity occurs in a minority of cases (Figure 119.2). CPO is decreased to around 50% of the normal level in liver, fibroblasts, lymphocytes, and leukocytes. In rare homozygous variants, enzyme activity is usually less than 10%. Two different types of homozygous cases have been described: in the first type, patients were very small, showed skin photosensitivity, and had neurological symptoms with several acute attacks from the age of 5 years. Their feces and urine contained a huge amount of coproporphyrin. The other type of homozygous coproporphyria was found in three children with intense jaundice and hemolytic anemia at birth. The pattern of fecal porphyrin excretion was atypical for coproporphyria because the major porphyrin was harderoporphyrin: this variant was called "harderoporphyria." Human CPO cDNA has an open reading frame of 1062 bp, encoding a protein of 354 amino acid residues. The mature enzyme consists of a homodimer of 323 amino acid residues with a leader peptide of 100 amino acid residues. The gene has been mapped to chromosome 3q12 and

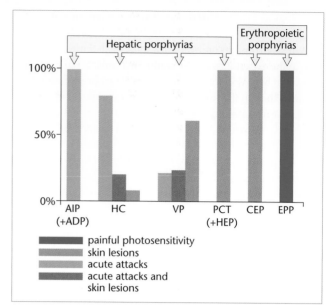

Figure 119.2 Clinical features. In erythropoietic porphyrias (CEP, congenital erythropoietic porphyria or Günther disease; EPP, erythropoietic protoporphyria) and in hepatic porphyrias (ADP, ALA dehydratase deficiency porphyria; AIP, acute intermittent porphyria; HC, hereditary coproporphyria; HEP, hepatoerythropoietic porphyria; PCT, familial and sporadic porphyria cutanea tarda; VP, variegate porphyria). (This figure was published in *Clinical Gastroenterology and Hepatology*, Wilfred M. Weinstein, Christopher J. Hawkey, Jaime Bosch, Porphyria, Pages 1–8, Copyright Elsevier, 2005.)

spans about 14 kb, consisting of seven exons. There is a high degree of allelic heterogeneity of the disease (Human Gene Mutation Database: www.hgmd.org) and the severity of the phenotype in heterozygous HC does not correlate with the degree of inactivation by CPO mutation. Only two missense mutations in exon 6 (R401W and K404E) were associated with the harderoporphyria phenotype. During acute attacks of HC, the profile of urine porphyrins and precursors is similar to those in AIP, although coproporphyrin is almost always dramatically increased. Stool porphyrins usually allow the type of porphyria to be established, the characteristic abnormality being a huge excess of coproporphyrin (predominantly type III) compared with normal protoporphyrin [10].

Management of acute attacks

A European network for acute porphyrias, the European Porphyria Initiative (EPI), has been set up and a website proposes guidelines and a consensus for therapeutic care of patients (www.porphyria-europe.com).

Supportive treatment

A careful search should be made for any **precipitating factor**, especially drugs (including oral contraceptives), underlying infection, and hypocaloric diet. These precipitants should be withdrawn as soon as possible. **Analgesia** is a major component of supportive treatment. Opiates are usually required, often in high doses, together with an antiemetic and a phenothiazine such as chlorpromazine for anxiety, restlessness, and to decrease the analgesic requirement. Danger of addiction (in patients who experience frequent attacks) must always be considered. Adequate **fluid intake** is essential with regular monitoring of electrolyte status. Attention should also be paid to **calorie intake**. Other complications such as persistent hypertension and tachycardia, severe motor neuropathy, and seizures should be treated as they occur using drugs recommended from a safe drugs list (www.porphyria-europe.com).

Specific treatment

Two specific therapies are mainly used: **glucose and hematin**. Before heme became available, carbohydrate loading was the only treatment for an acute attack. An adequate supplement (100–300 g/day) should be administered, usually by slow intravenous infusion; to minimize the danger of precipitating hyponatremia. Hypotonic solutions should be avoided, and electrolytes measured at least daily. Treatment of a porphyric attack has been greatly improved by the introduction of hematin. In the USA, the form of lyophilized heme (Panhematin®) is available whereas a more stable preparation of human hemin (heme arginate, Normosang®) is widely available. Heme arginate is supplied as a concentrated stock solution that requires dilution in normal saline immediately before use. This solution should be infused at a dose of 3–4 mg/kg body weight/24 hours over 20 minutes, and usually for 4 days. In practice, adults usually receive the entire contents of a single vial for each dose (see Table 119.2). An increased incidence of thrombophlebitis at the infusion site has been reported. It is recommended to re-site the intravenous cannula each day and flush thoroughly with saline following administration. Five percent human serum albumin may be included in the solution. Other side effects are rare and heme arginate has been used successfully during pregnancy. All the treatments described above must be used early in the attack before any nervous or respiratory complication develops. Neither carbohydrate loading nor intravenous heme will reverse an established peripheral neuropathy [11].

Recurrent acute attacks

A minority of patients has repeated acute attacks. Women with cyclical premenstrual attack may respond to suppression of ovulation with gonadotropin-releasing hormone (GnRH) analogs. If this is successful, this treatment can be continued for up to 2 years before attempting withdrawal. Otherwise, management of repeated attacks severe enough to require hospitalization is difficult. It may be possible to abort the development of an attack by prompt administration of **heme arginate** without the need of a full course: regular once weekly administration of a single dose may help control the disease. Such patients are likely to require permanent indwelling venous catheters with all their attendant complications. A few patients have now received very large cumulative doses of heme arginate without serious side effects, although hepatic iron overload has been observed.

Prevention

Symptomatic patients and those who are diagnosed by family screening should avoid drugs, alcohol, fasting, or hormones that are known to precipitate acute attacks. Table 119.3 shows drug groups and drugs that are thought to be unsafe. A list of safe drugs is available at www.wmic.wales.nhs.uk\porphyria_info.php. Benefit versus risk should always be considered in conjunction with the severity of the disorder requiring treatment and the disease activity of the porphyria. Where difficult decisions on treatment have to be made, consideration should be given to contacting a national center with expertise in managing porphyria for advice.

Non-acute hepatic porphyrias

These cutaneous porphyrias present with photosensitivity, skin fragility, and blisters on sun-exposed skin. The skin lesions of PCT, HC, and VP are quite similar.

Porphyria cutanea tarda

PCT is the most common form of porphyria. **Cutaneous photosensitivity** is the predominant clinical feature; acute attacks with abdominal pain, psychiatric, and/or neurological manifestations are never observed. PCT is a heterogeneous group including at least three types [12]:

- **Sporadic type (sPCT)** (75%) is more often observed in male patients without a family history of the disease. It can be triggered by alcohol, estrogens, iron overload, or hepatitis C virus. In this sporadic type, uroporphyrinogen decarboxylase (UROD) activity is deficient only in liver during overt disease.
- **Familial type (fPCT)** (25%) has an earlier onset and is observed equally in both genders. Relatives of the patient may have overt PCT; in fPCT, there is a 50% reduction of activity in all tissues and this defect is inherited in an autosomal dominant pattern.
- **Hepatoerythropoietic porphyria (HEP)** is the very rare homozygous form of fPCT. It is characterized by a severe photosensitivity, usually beginning in early infancy, and results from a dramatic defect in UROD activity. Only five different UROD mutations have been found both in HEP and in fPCT.

Clinical presentation

The lesions of photosensitivity affect areas exposed to light such as the backs of hands, face, neck, and, in women, the legs and backs of the feet. **Skin fragility** is perhaps the most specific feature: a minimal trauma is followed by a superficial erosion, soon covered by a crust. Bullae or vesicles usually appear after exposure to sun and take several weeks to heal, leaving hypo- or hyper-pigmented atrophic scars (Figure 119.3). White papules (milia) may develop in areas of bullae,

Table 119.3 Drugs to avoid in the acute porphyrias

Drug classes

Alkylating drugs	Calcium channel blockers	Non-nucleoside reverse	Sulfonylureas
Amphetamines	Contraceptives, hormonal	transcriptase inhibitors	Taxanes
Antibiotic steroids	Ergot derivatives	Progestogens	Tetracyclines
Antidepressants	Hormone replacement	Protease inhibitors	Thiazolidinediones
Antihistamines	therapy	Statins	Triazole antifungals
Barbiturates	Imidazole antifungals	Sulfonamides	

Individual drugs

Aceclofenac	Diclofenac	Metoclopramide	Rifabutin
Alcohol	Erythromycin	Metplazone	Rifampin (rifampicin)
Amiodarone	Etamsylate	Metronidazole	Rispeidone
Bosentan	Etomidate	Mifepristone	Sulfinpyrazone
Bromocriptine	Fenfluamine	Minoxdil	Sulpiride
Buspirone	Flupentixol	Nalidixic acid	Tamoxifen
Cabergoline	Gold	Nitrazepam	Telithromycin
Carbamazepine	Griseofulvin	Nitrofurantoin	Temoporfin
Chloral hydrate	Halothane	Orphenadrine	Theophylline
Chloramphenicol	Hydralazine	Oxcarbazepine	Tiagabine
Chloroform	Indapamide	Oxybutynin	Tinidazole
Clindamycin	Isometheptene mucate	Oxycodone	Topiramate
Clonidine	Isoniazid	Pentazocine	Toremifene
Cocaine	Ketamine	Pentoxifylline (oxpentifylline)	Tramadol
Colistin	Ketorolac	Phenoxybenzamine	Triclofos
Cycloserine	Lidocaine (lignocaine)	Phenytbin	Trimethoprim
Danazol	Mebeverine	Piymecillinam	Valproate
Dapsone	Mefenamic acid	Porfimer	Xipamide
Dexfenfluramine	Meprobamate	Probenecid	Zidoyudine
Diazepam	Methyldopa	Pyrazinamide	Zuclopenthixol

particularly on the backs of the hands. **Hypertrichosis** is often seen on the upper cheeks (malar area) and sometimes on ears and arms. Increased uniform pigmentation of sun-exposed areas is common. Alopecia and hypopigmented scleroderma-like lesions of the skin are less common. Variable degrees of

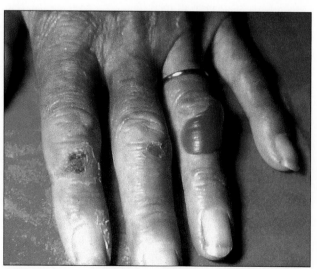

Figure 119.3 Cutaneous symptoms (bullous) found in porphyria cutanea tarda, variegate porphyria, and hereditary coproporphyria.

liver dysfunction are common among patients with PCT, particularly in association with excessive alcoholic intake. However, it is not clear to what extent liver cell injury is important in the expression of the syndrome. It is well known that in patients with typical cirrhosis PCT is very rare; it has been suggested that in patients with PCT there may be an underlying constitutional abnormality, which may predispose the liver to the development of PCT; uroporphyrin needle-like inclusions have been found in the cytoplasm of hepatocytes, which could promote progressive liver damage.

Precipitating factors

Among the precipitating factors, alcohol, estrogens, iron overload, hepatitis C virus (HCV), and to a lesser extent hepatitis B virus (HBV) and human immunodeficiency virus (HIV), are most frequently incriminated. These precipitating factors act either alone or in combination. Estrogen-containing oral contraceptives have increased the prevalence of PCT in women; as in any hepatic porphyria, most patients may receive these drugs (or alcohol) over several years before developing PCT. Abnormal iron metabolism appears to be another precipitating factor of the clinical onset, probably related to oxidative radicals produced by reactive intracellular iron. Serum iron is frequently 60% above normal levels in patients with PCT. A mild hepatic siderosis has been described in at least 80% of patients.

Mutations of the HFE gene associated with hemochromatosis are found in fPCT and sPCT more commonly than in control populations, indicating that genetic factors unrelated to the heme biosynthesis pathway can predispose to PCT. The C282Y mutation seems to be more common in North Europe, the USA, and Australia, whereas H63D is the most frequent allele linked to PCT in the Mediterranean. Cytochrome P4501A2 activity appears to be another important etiological factor in PCT. A strong association has been found between HCV and PCT in several countries. HBV and HIV are not as closely associated with PCT as HCV; antibodies to HCV should be evaluated in each patient with this porphyria at the time of diagnosis.

Diagnostic methods
Urine contains increased concentrations of **uroporphyrin and 7-carboxy-porphyrin**. Both precursors, ALA and PBG, are usually normal, but the accompanying liver disease may cause a minor increase of ALA excretion (see Table 119.1). In the feces, the specific porphyrin excreted is isocoproporphyrin. During clinical remission total porphyrin excretion decreases progressively and measurement of urinary porphyrins and ferritin is one of the best methods for following the effects of treatment. After a few months, urinary porphyrin levels appear normal but in the feces copro- and isocopro-porphyrin may remain increased for a long period. The same porphyrins are also found in plasma, exhibiting fluorescence at 620 nm. **UROD** is decreased in the liver of all patients with PCT. The human UROD is a 42-kDa polypeptide encoded by a single gene mapped to chromosome 1p34, containing 10 exons within a 4-kb piece of DNA. The enzyme functions as a homodimer. In the familial type, it has been found to be decreased by 50% in all tissues, including erythrocytes, whereas sPCT acts as an acquired disorder. So far, more than 45 different mutations causing fPCT have been reported. A liver-specific mutation for sPCT does not seem plausible and additional factors may in some fashion inactivate the hepatic UROD. Mutations at some other locus predisposing individuals to develop PCT in response to acquired factors (such as alcohol, drugs, iron, HCV) are likely.

Management
General supportive treatment of cutaneous porphyrias
Avoidance of sunlight and wearing appropriate clothing to cover the skin decreases skin symptoms. Absorbent sunscreens are of little help as they are designed to block UV A and B radiations. Reflectant sunscreens containing zinc oxide or titanium dioxide are more effective but their use is limited because they are cosmetically unappealing [11].

Specific treatment
All patients with PCT should first be advised to treat any infectious disease (e.g., HCV, HIV), and to avoid precipitating factors (e.g., alcohol, pills, porphyrinogenic drugs) and exposure to sunlight until clinical and biological remission has been obtained by treatment. **Phlebotomy** is at present the treatment of choice, even when serum iron or ferritin levels are not increased. There are variations in protocols for venesection: usually venesections of 300 mL are performed at 10–12-day intervals and are continued for 2 months until the ferritin level is reduced to the lower limit of normal. Urine porphyrin levels are monitored every 3 months: clinical and biological remissions are usually obtained within 6 months. When phlebotomy is contraindicated (anemia, cardiac, or pulmonary disorders, age) **low-dose chloroquine therapy** (200 mg weekly), which complexes with porphyrin and slowly mobilizes it from the liver, is the favored alternative (see Table 119.1). Duration of treatment and relapse rate are only marginally greater than with venesection. High-dose treatment must be avoided because it causes a hepatitis-like syndrome in patients with PCT. In severe cases, combined phlebotomy and chloroquine therapy is often used with good results [11].

Erythropoietic porphyrias
Congenital erythropoietic porphyria (Günther disease)
CEP is a rare autosomal recessive disorder resulting from a marked **deficiency of uroporphyrinogen III synthase activity** (see Figure 119.1). Skin blisters are observed in the neonatal period or in early infancy both in CEP and in HEP, the rare homozygous form of type II PCT. Both are serious, chronic progressive, and mutilating disorders associated with hemolytic anemia (Figure 119.4). Urine has a reddish brown color from the first day of life and exhibits a purple fluorescence under long UV light. The diagnosis is confirmed by a characteristic porphyrin pattern in urine (isomer I), plasma, and feces (see Table 119.1). Treatment of HEP and CEP involves skin protection and blood transfusions to maintain the hemoglobin concentration. Allogenic bone marrow transplantation has been successful in several patients with moderate-to-severe disease.

Erythropoietic protoporphyria: a painful photosensitive porphyria
EPP results from decreased activity of the final enzyme in the heme synthetic pathway, **ferrochelatase** (Figure 116.1). It is an autosomal dominant disorder, with variable penetrance. The variable penetrance is mainly due to the coinheritance of a low expression allele, which in addition to the abnormal allele, results in decreased ferrochelatase activity below the 50% threshold [13]. Clinical manifestation of EPP begins in childhood with acute and severely **painful photosensitivity**, and a history of burning in areas of skin exposed to sunlight. Pain is usually followed by edema, erythema, and swelling. Repeated exposures lead to chronic changes, giving the skin a waxy, thickened appearance with faint linear scars. Urine porphyrin

Multiple Organ Systems

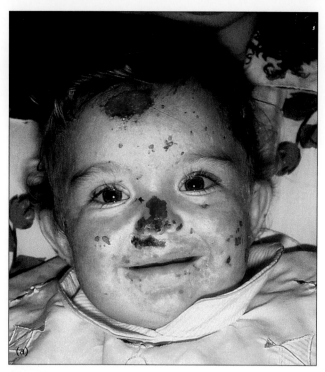
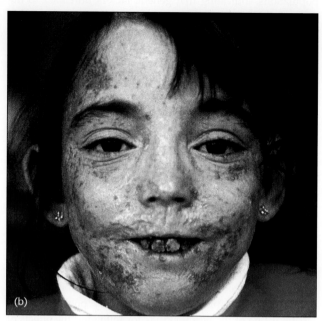

Figure 119.4 Congenital erythropoietic porphyria. Clinical presentation of congenital erythropoietic porphyria (Günther disease) in (a) an infant and (b) an adult.

levels are normal; the diagnosis is based on **increased free protoporphyrin levels** in erythrocytes and in plasma, which has a characteristic fluorescent emission peak (see Table 119.1). Patients often exhibit a slight microcytic, hypochromic anemia. Liver dysfunction has been reported in up to 20% of EPP patients and hepatic failure in less than 5%. The liver dysfunction is caused by the accumulation of protoporphyrin in hepatocytes, resulting in cell damage, cholestasis, and further retention of protoporphyrin. EPP patients may develop gallstones formed from protoporphyrin and are at increased risk of cholelithiasis. Acute burning pain is ameliorated by application of cold water. Avoidance of sunlight is the mainstay of management. Oral beta-carotene (75–200 mg/day; optimal blood concentration of 11–15 μmol/L), which acts as a singlet oxygen trap, improves light tolerance in about one-third of patients. It is impossible to predict those patients who will develop **severe liver disease**, and management should include annual biochemical assessment of liver function. When liver dysfunction appears, treatment with cholestyramine, which depletes hepatic protoporphyrin, or activated charcoal, which binds protoporphyrin in the gut, interrupting the enterohepatic circulation, should be attempted, but their efficacy is not proved. Once liver failure is advanced, transplantation is usually the only treatment likely to ensure survival (see Table 119.1).

SOURCES OF INFORMATION FOR PATIENTS AND DOCTORS

Europe
www.porphyria-europe.com
www.hgmd.org
  USA
www.enterprise.net/apf/index.html
  South Africa
www.uct.ac.za/depts/liver/porphpts.htm
http://www.patient.co.uk/showdoc/502/
http://www.ncchem.com/safe-arbor/porphyri.htm

References

1. Anderson KE, Sassa S, Bishop DF, Desnick RJ. The porphyrias. In: Scriver CR, Beaudet AL, Sly WS, Valle D, editors. *The Metabolic Basis of Inherited Disease*, volume 1, 8th editionn. New York: McGraw-Hill, 2001:2991–3062.
2. Ponka P. Cell biology of heme. *Am J Med Sci.* 1999;318:241–256.
3. Sassa S, Kappas A. Molecular aspects of the inherited porphyrias. *J Intern Med.* 2000;247:169–178.
4. Elder GH, Hift RJ, Meissner PN. The acute porphyrias. *Lancet.* 1997;349:1613–1617.
5. Thunell S, Harper P, Brock A, Petersen NE. Porphyrins, porphyrin metabolism and porphyrias. II. Diagnosis and monitoring in the acute porphyrias. *Scand J Clin Lab Invest.* 2000; 60:541–560.

6. Astrin KH, Desnick RJ. Molecular basis of acute intermittent porphyria: mutations and polymorphisms in the human hydroxymethylbilane synthase gene. *Hum Mutat*. 1994;4:243–252.

7. Maruno M, Furuyama K, Akagi R, *et al.* Highly heterogeneous nature of delta-aminolevulinate dehydratase deficiencies in ALAD porphyria. *Blood*. 2001;97:2972–2978.

8. Meissner PN, Dailey TA, Hift RJ, *et al.* A R59W mutation in human protoporphyrinogen oxidase results in decreased enzyme activity and is prevalent in South Africans with variegate porphyria. *Nat Genet*. 1996;13:95–97.

9. Kauppinen R, Timonen K, Fraunberg M, *et al.* Homozygous variegate porphyria: 20y follow-up and characterization of molecular defect. *J Invest Dermatol*. 2001;116:610–613.

10. Martasek P. Hereditary coproporphyria. *Semin Liv Dis*. 1998;18:25–32.

11. Badminton MN, Elder GH. Management of acute and cutaneous porphyrias. *Int J Clin Pract*. 2002;56:272–278.

12. Bulaj ZJ, Philips JD, Ajioka RS, *et al.* Hemochromatosis genes and other factors contributing to the pathogenesis of porphyria cutanea tarda. *Blood*. 2000;95:1565–1571.

13. Gouya L, Puy H, Robreau AM, *et al.* How the phenotype of a dominant Mendelian disorder is modulated through the wild-type allele expression level. *Nat. Genet*. 2002;30:27–28.

Multiple Organ Systems

CHAPTER 120
The hereditary recurrent fevers

Elizabeth Drewe

Nottingham University Hospitals, Nottingham, UK

ESSENTIAL FACTS ABOUT PATHOGENESIS

- Hereditary recurrent fevers are disorders clinically characterized by spontaneous episodes of fever and inflammatory symptoms
- Familial Mediterranean fever (FMF): mutations in Mediterranean fever (*MEVF*) gene (autosomal recessive). MEVF product pyrin contributes to inflammation via mechanisms involving IL-1 beta
- TNF-receptor–associated period syndrome (TRAPS): mutations in gene encoding TNFRSF1A (autosomal dominant) resulting in enhanced activation
- Hyperimmunoglobulin D syndrome (HIDS): mutation in *MVK* gene which encodes mevalonate kinase resulting in inflammation by obscure pathways involving cholesterol and isoprenoid production
- Cryopyrin-associated periodic syndrome (CAPS): rare monogenic disease due to uncontrolled IL-1 beta secretion due to CIAS1-gene mutation

ESSENTIALS OF DIAGNOSIS

- These diseases should be considered in patients who have recurrent fevers and inflammatory symptoms unexplained by conventional investigations
- FMF: episodic fever, abdominal pain (95%), arthritis (50–75%), pleural inflammation (30%) with or without skin rash
- TRAPS: fever and myalgia (100%), abdominal pain (92%), with anorexia, nausea and constipation, periorbital edema (82%), chest pain (57%)
- HIDS: prodrome (headache and malaise) then fever with abdominal pain, diarrhea, and vomiting. Lymphadenopathy (~90%), splenomegaly (32%), arthralgia (83%), with or without skin rashes
- CAPS: fever, urticaria, conjunctivitis with sensorineural hearing loss and joint destruction in some subtypes
- Initial diagnosis is clinical, including response to treatment. Raised polyclonal IgD in HIDs (also FMF and inflammatory bowel disease)
- Genetic analysis can confirm formal diagnosis in most cases

ESSENTIALS OF TREATMENT

- Management involves treating an acute attack, preventing attacks, and reducing subclinical inflammation and risk of amyloidosis
- Genetic diagnosis of individual disease will allow correct treatment to be started
- FMF: colchicines (500 µg escalating to 1.5–2 mg daily) accompanied by lactose-free diet; for all since amyloid is common
- TRAPS: corticosteroids (e.g., acute attack in adults 15–40 mg oral prednisolone daily or 500 mg–1 g intravenous methyl prednisolone if severe); the TNFRSF1B fusion protein etanercept (25 mg subcutaneously twice weekly) may reduce attack frequency. Some patients respond to anakinra
- HIDS: unclear. Colchicine and steroids ineffective, simvastatin, etanercept or anakinra are possible treatments
- CAPS: Anakinra

Introduction

The autoinflammatory diseases are a broad group of disorders with genetic defects in the body's molecular pathways of inflammation. They may be subdivided into hereditary recurrent fevers (HRF), pyogenic diseases, and granulomatous diseases (Table 120.1). Patients with an HRF have unprovoked episodes or "attacks" of fever and inflammation, e.g., peritonitis without a trigger. This chapter will focus on familial Mediterranean fever (FMF), TNF-receptor–associated periodic syndrome (TRAPS) and hyperimmunoglobulinemia D syndrome (HIDS) as these may present to the gastroenterologist. A further group of diseases, cryopyrin-associated periodic syndrome (CAPS), will be touched on. This syndrome comprises three diseases: chronic infantile neurological articular syndrome (CINCA), Muckle Wells syndrome (MWS), and familial cold autoinflammatory syndrome (FCAS), but of these only MWS causes serositis.

Epidemiology

The HRF syndromes are rare, although there are geographical variations. **FMF** is commonest, affecting 100 000 people worldwide. It is most prevalent in non-Ashkenazi Jews, Arabs, Turks, and Armenians. **TRAPS** is much rarer, i.e., a couple of hundred people worldwide. It was originally described in patients of Scottish or Irish ancestry but has now been identified in diverse ethnicities. **HIDS** is also rare with the largest cohort describing 103 patients of mostly European descent. Although these diseases are rare they may hold the key for patients in whom conventional investigations have been non-diagnostic.

HRF syndromes typically **start in childhood**, although diagnosis may be delayed. Specifically, 90% of patients with FMF become symptomatic before 20 years of age. The median age of onset of TRAPS is 3 years, although this varies from 2 weeks to 53 years. The median age of onset for HIDS is 6 months but ranges from the first week of life to 10 years.

Causes and pathogenesis

Autoinflammatory diseases are differentiated from autoimmune disorders by their lack of **high titer self-reactive antibodies and T cells**. At a molecular level they reflect disturbed

Table 120.1 Autoinflammatory diseases

	Gene mutation	Key clinical features
Hereditary recurrent fevers		
Familial Mediterranean fever (FMF)	*MEFV*	Fever, serositis, arthritis
TNF-receptor–associated periodic syndrome (TRAPS)	*TNFSF1A*	Fever, myalgia, serositis, erysipelas erythema
Hyperimmunoglobulin D syndrome (HIDS)	*MVK*	Fever, vomiting, abdominal pain/serositis, lymphadenopathy
CAPS: familial cold autoinflammatory syndrome (FCAS)	*CIAS1*	Cold induced fever, urticaria, conjunctivitis, arthralgia
CAPS: Muckle Wells syndrome (MWS)	*CIAS1*	Cold-induced fever, urticaria, conjunctivitis, arthralgia, sensorineural hearing loss
CAPS: neonatal-onset multisystem inflammatory disease (NOMID) or chronic infantile neurological cutaneous articular syndrome (CINCA)	*CIAS1*	Urticaria, papilloedema, uveitis, epiphyseal bone formation, chronic meningitis, sensorineural hearing loss
Periodic fever apthous stomatitis pharyngitis and adenitis (PFAPA)	Unknown	Fever, oral ulcers, pharyngitis, cervical lymphadenopathy
Pyogenic disorders		
Pyogenic sterile arthritis, pyoderma gangrenosum and acne (PAPA)	*PSTPIP1*	Destructive arthritis, pyoderma gangrenosum, acne
Majeed syndrome	*LPIN2*	Multifocal osteomyelitis, congenital anemia, fever, neutrophilic dermatosis
Disease of IL-1 receptor antagonist (DIRA)	*IL1RN*	Multifocal osteomyelitis, periostitis, pustulosis
Granulomatous disease		
Blau syndrome/early-onset sarcoidosis	*NOD2*	Granulomatous arthritis, uveitis, dermatitis

CAPS, cryopyrin-associated periodic syndromes; CINCA, chronic infantile neurological cutaneous articular syndrome.

functioning of the innate immune system and therefore provide a window to study this. Some autoinflammatory diseases are pathophysiologically linked whilst others appear diverse.

The HRFs are broadly considered autosomal dominant or recessively inherited monogenic diseases. Variable clinical presentation and severity however suggests other modulatory genes or environmental factors contribute.

Familial Mediterranean fever
FMF is an autosomal recessive disease due to mutations in the *MEFV* (Mediterranean FeVer) gene [1]. MEFV encodes a protein called **pyrin** present in neutrophils and macrophages. Pyrin interacts with other proteins contributing to inflammation and apoptosis. Downstream production of the **cytokine IL-1 beta** mediates fever and inflammation.

TNF-receptor–associated period syndrome
TRAPS is an autosomal dominant disease due to mutations in the gene encoding **TNFRSF1A** [2]. Tumor necrosis factor (TNF)-alpha binds the TNF receptor resulting in inflammation

and apoptosis. Disease may be mediated due to **altered shedding** of the TNF receptor from the cell surface or **spontaneous activation** of the receptor.

Hyperimmunoglobulin D syndrome
HIDS is an autosomal recessive disease due to mutations in *MVK*, which encodes **mevalonate kinase** [3]. Mevalonate kinase is an enzyme involved in cholesterol synthesis and production of isoprenoids, e.g., ubiquinone. Consequentially there may be build up of products before the enzyme block or a deficiency downstream. How this translates to clinical inflammation evades current scientific knowledge, although once again interleukin (**IL**)-1 has been implicated.

Clinical presentation
The HRF syndromes are characterized by **attacks of fever** (typically 38–41°C) and **inflammatory symptoms**, with intervening good health. Patients may describe episodes as being suddenly switched on or off. Attacks may start spontaneously

or be triggered by emotional or physical stress, menstruation or childhood vaccination.

The **length of attack** may pinpoint the disease:

- FMF: 12 hours to 3 days
- TRAPS: last up to several weeks if untreated
- HIDS: 4–6 days.

Attack frequency can be unpredictable, varying between different family members and within an individual. An individual may have different patterns of attacks, e.g., a "fever" or "abdominal" attack. For some an HRF syndrome may be a mere inconvenience with a few days off work each year, whilst for others attack frequency and complications result in a chronic and disabling condition.

The specific features of FMF, TRAPS and HIDS are discussed below with particular focus on gastrointestinal manifestations.

Familial Mediterranean fever

FMF needs to be considered in patients with episodes of **fever, abdominal pain** (seen in 95% patients), **arthritis,** e.g. knee or ankle (50–75%), and **inflammation of pleura** (30%) [4]. **Skin involvement,** e.g., erysipeloid erythema, manifests in 7–40% patients. Oral ulcers may also occur, with rarer manifestations including pericarditis and orchitis.

Attacks of FMF typically **start suddenly** although a prodrome including **irritability and altered taste sensation** may occur. Abdominal pain may be localized or diffuse and may be accompanied by peritonitis. A bad attack may see a patient bedbound for a couple of days where they lie still with fever, sweating, and a tender distended abdomen. Abdominal manifestations are caused by **sterile peritonitis** with large influx of neutrophils. Recurrent peritonitis may result in adhesions.

TNF-receptor–associated period syndrome

Fever and myalgia are seen in virtually all patients [5]. **Myalgia** presenting with cramp-like pain may be accompanied by overlying erythema of the skin, which may migrate down a limb over several days.

Abdominal pain has been described in 92% patients with TRAPS. A typical abdominal attack starts suddenly with a severe gripping pain and a feeling of being unable to relax the abdomen. **Anorexia, nausea, and constipation,** without vomiting, is classic. The patient may lie still on a hard surface whilst examination reveals a tender distended abdomen. Pathology may be multifactorial relating to abdominal wall musculature, peritonitis, adhesions, bowel obstruction, and necrotic bowel. Resected bowel has revealed mononuclear cell infiltrate.

Other pointers to TRAPS include **conjunctivitis** and **periorbital edema** (82%), musculoskeletal or pleural **chest pain** (57%), and less commonly testicular and scrotal pain. Some families have a high rate of inguinal hernias. Lymphadenopathy and oral ulcers are not usually seen.

Hyperimmunoglobulin D syndrome

A **prodrome** of headache and malaise may herald an attack of HIDS. The **fever** rapidly follows and is accompanied by **vomiting, diarrhea, and abdominal pain**. Abdominal adhesions in patients who have undergone exploratory surgery and suggesting **sterile peritonitis** are also implicated in HIDS. Examination may reveal tender lymphadenopathy (almost 90% of patients) with the cervical region being most affected [6]. **Splenomegaly** is apparent in 32% with hepatomegaly slightly less often observed. Oral **apthous ulcers**, with or without **genital ulcers**, affect nearly half of patients.

Arthralgia (83%) is common in HIDS with arthritis, e.g., wrist, knee, and ankle, occurring in 50%. A variety of **rashes** may occur with HIDS, including a maculopapular rash.

Differential diagnosis

This is wide and will be determined by the HRF syndrome and whether the patient exhibits an organ-based attack, e.g., gut, or a multisystem disease. The differential diagnosis for recurrent peritonitis will be that of much commoner diseases, including **appendicitis and diverticulitis**. Recurrent **abdominal pain** without peritonitis may lead to diagnoses such as peptic ulcer disease, renal colic, irritable bowel syndrome, and endometriosis being considered. Patients presenting with **fevers, myalgia, and joint involvement** may have had extensive investigations for connective tissue disease, vasculitis (including the mimic polyarteritis nodosa), and lymphoma with cause remaining elusive.

Diagnostic methods

Diagnosis of HRF involves **interpreting clinical features, response to treatment, laboratory finding,** and **genetic analysis**. A patient keeping a temperature chart to illustrate periodicity of febrile attacks may help. FMF, HIDS, and TRAPS attacks are all characterized by leukocytosis and elevated acute-phase response, i.e. erythrocyte sedimentation rate (ESR), C-reactive protein (CRP), and serum amyloid A (SAA). In many patients the acute-phase response persists between attacks, i.e., subclinical inflammation.

For unexplained reasons, HIDS is accompanied by persistently raised **polyclonal IgD**, i.e., >100 IU/mL. IgD also rises in FMF, Bechet's disease, and inflammatory bowel disease.

Genetic analysis is available for the HRF. A mutation in *TNFRSF1A* will usually confirm a diagnosis of TRAPS as, with the exception of two low penetrance mutations (R92Q and P46L), these mutations are rarely found in unaffected individuals. Two mutations in the *MVK* gene will confirm HIDS but there are a group of patients who clinically have HIDS with raised IgD levels but no mutation; these patients may be categorized as "**variant HIDS**". Diagnosis of FMF may be made by clinical criteria (based on clinical attacks and **response to colchicine**). Genetic analysis backs this up; 57% of patients have two **mutations in MEFV** whilst 26% patients have one. The role of the **E148Q mutation** in *MEFV* is debated as this variant is very common (3–18%) in populations affected by FMF.

The genetic causes underpinning these diseases have only been elucidated in the last decade and clinical and genetic correlations will become clearer with time.

Treatment and prevention

Treatment of HRF is directed at terminating a single attack, reducing attack frequency, and also dampening subclinical inflammation that may predispose to amyloidosis. Treatment is tailored to specific disease and patient variables, e.g., attack frequency, subclinical inflammation, and family history of amyloidosis.

Developments in biological agents have improved treatment. This is most notable for cryopyrin-associated periodic syndrome (CAPS) where the IL-1 receptor anatagonist **anakinra** has transformed lives. The clinician treating patients with immunomodulatory agents may be faced with difficult decisions deciphering a febrile attack from infection.

Familial Mediterranean fever

Colchicine reduces frequency of attacks of FMF and usually prevents the development of amyloidosis [4]. Untreated FMF predisposes to a high rate of amyloidosis so colchicine should be recommended for all. Treatment starts at 500 μg daily with weekly 500-μg dose increments until a single daily dose of 1.5–2 mg is reached. The patient should be monitored for clinical attacks and subclinical inflammation, with dose being increased to 3 mg/day if required. Side effects of abdominal pain and diarrhea may limit dose, This may however be helped by introduction of a lactose-free diet.

TNF-receptor–associated period syndrome

TRAPS is responsive to **corticosteroids**; an abdominal attack that could last several weeks may be shortened to 2 days with corticosteroids. An infrequent course of corticosteroids may suffice for mild disease. Attacks in adults may require 15–40 mg of prednisolone daily, tapered over a couple of weeks if necessary. A severe attack, i.e., peritonitis, may be best managed with 500 mg–1 g intravenous methylprednisolone. Long-term side effects of corticosteroids are problematic for severely affected patients. The soluble TNFRSF1B fusion protein **etanercept** (25 mg subcutaneously twice weekly) may reduce attack frequency, corticosteroid use, acute-phase response, and proteinuria of amyloidosis [7]. In the long-term, however, some patients stop treatment due to response diminishing over time and side effects (Figure 120.1). Some patients respond to **anakinra**.

Hyperimmunoglobulin D syndrome

HIDS is difficult to treat. Colchicine and corticosteroids are ineffective. A small trial of **simvastatin** showed some reduction in number of days of illness, but overall efficacy is limited [8]. As HIDS has a relatively low risk of amyloidosis, treatment with biologicals could be targeted at preventing or treating a

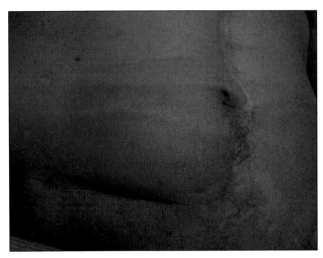

Figure 120.1 A patient with TRAPS has an injection site reaction to etanercept. His abdomen bears the scars from appendicectomy (normal appendix removed) and small bowel resection due to obstruction.

single attack. Response to **etanercept** given early in an attack is however variable. A single patient responded better to anakinra than etanercept after a vaccination-provoked attack. Further studies are needed in this area [9].

Complications and their management

The most feared complication of HRF is reactive **AA amyloidosis** (see Chapter 117). Amyloidosis occurred in up to 75% of FMF patients over the age of 40 years before the use of colchicine. It manifests in up to 25% of patients with **TRAPS**, but less than 2% of patients with HIDS. Patients with HRF should be **screened for proteinuria** at least 6 monthly.

Other uncommon complications include **joint contractures** in HIDS, joint replacements in FMF, **bowel obstruction** in TRAPS, and reports of **vasculitis** (Henoch–Schönlein purpura and polyarteritis nodosa) accompanying FMF. It is not uncommon for patients to have an uninflamed appendix removed during exploratory surgery prior to diagnosis.

Prognosis with and without treatment

Attacks in HRF may occur throughout life. Quality of life and educational and social development may be affected. Patients with HIDS have a normal life expectancy. Major morbidity and mortality in TRAPS and FMF relate to the development of **amyloidosis** and subsequent **renal transplantation** with associated complications.

SOURCES OF INFORMATION FOR PATIENTS AND DOCTORS

www.hids.net
www.fmf.igh.cnrs.fr/ISSAID/infevers (mutational database for autoinflammatory diseases)
www.ucl.ac.uk/silva/medicine/research/inflammation/amyloidosis/clinical_service

References

1. French FMF Consortium. A candidate gene for familial Mediterranean fever. *Nat Genet*. 1997;17:25–31.

2. McDermott MF, Aksentijevich I, Galon J, *et al.* Germline mutations in the extracellular domain of 55 kDa TNF receptor, TNFR1, define a family of dominantly inherited autoinflammatory syndromes. *Cell*. 1999;96:133–144.

3. Drenth JP, Cuisset L, Grateau G, *et al.* Mutations in the gene encoding mevalonate kinase cause hyper-IgD and periodic fever syndrome. *Nat Genet*. 1999;22:178–181.

4. Lidar M, Livneh A. Familial Mediterranean fever: clinical, molecular and management advancements. *Neth J Med*. 2007;65: 318–324.

5. Hull KM, Drewe E, Aksentijevich I, *et al.* The TNF receptor-associated periodic syndrome (TRAPS): emerging concepts of an autoinflammatory disease. *Medicine*. 2002;81:349–386.

6. van der Hilst JCH, Bodar EJ, Barron KS, *et al.* Long-term follow-up, clinical features, and quality of life in a series of 103 patients with hyperimmunoglobulinaemia D syndrome. *Medicine*. 2008;87:301–310.

7. Drewe E, McDermott EM, Powell PT. Prospective study of anti-tumour necrosis factor receptor superfamily 1B fusion protein and case study of anti-tumour necrosis factor superfamily 1A fusion protein in TRAPS. *Rheumatology*. 2003;42:235–239.

8. Simon A, Drewe E, van der Meer JW. Simvastatin treatment for inflammatory attacks of the hyperimmunoglobulinaemia D and periodic fever syndrome. *Clin Pharmacol Ther*. 2004;75:476–483.

9. Bodar EJ, van der Hilst JC, Drenth P, *et al.* Effect of etanercept and ankinra on inflammatory attacks in the hyper-IgD syndrome. *Neth J Med*. 2005;63:260–264.

Multiple Organ Systems

CHAPTER 121

Abscesses and other intra-abdominal diseases

Juliane Bingener,[1] Melanie L. Richards[1] and Kenneth R. Sirinek[2]

[1]Mayo Clinic, Rochester, MN, USA
[2]University of Texas Health Science Center at San Antonio, San Antonio, TX, USA

ESSENTIAL FACTS ABOUT PATHOGENESIS

- 50% of all serious intra-abdominal infections are found after an operation
- 2% of all laparotomies are followed by an intra-abdominal infection
- Luminal obstruction, inflammation, trauma, and anastomotic disruption can lead to hollow organ perforation with abscess formation
- Hematogenous infections, infection in continuity, and bacterial transgression are sources of solid organ abscess formation

ESSENTIALS OF DIAGNOSIS

Clinical presentation
- Typical findings: pain, tachycardia, fever
- Non-specific findings: ileus (anorexia, nausea, vomiting), catabolic response, weight loss
- Signs associated with severe infection: fluid shift (decreasing urine output, intra-abdominal tissue edema), hypotension, systemic inflammatory response syndrome

Investigations
- Laboratory studies: blood cell count (WBC), electrolytes (fluid shift), coagulation profile (DIC), albumin (risk assessment)

Imaging studies
- Ultrasound as initial investigation
- CT or ultrasound-guided needle aspiration

ESSENTIALS OF TREATMENT AND PROGNOSIS

- Cardiorespiratory support, fluid resuscitation
- Empiric antibiotic therapy for multiple organisms
- Drainage (percutaneous or surgical)
- Treatment of underlying disease
- Risk factors for mortality: advanced age, severe underlying disease, malnutrition (serum albumin <2.0 g/dL)

Introduction and epidemiology

Abdominal abscesses can originate from two principal sources: a perforated hollow viscus or a solid organ infection. While half of all intra-abdominal infections and abscesses are found

after operative intervention, only 2% of laparotomies are followed by an abdominal abscess.

Abscesses from a hollow viscus perforation

Abscesses from a hollow viscus perforation are more frequent in urban industrialized areas than in nations with a basic diet high in fiber. The most common sources are appendicitis (31%) and diverticulitis (32%). **Appendiceal perforation** with abscess formation occurs in one in every three patients presenting with appendicitis. White children in South Africa are affected 20 times more often than their black peers. Appendicitis in older patients is frequently misdiagnosed. Patients with **diverticulosis** have a 25% risk of developing an infectious complication such as perforation (Figure 121.1). About 10% of patients with Crohn's disease are affected by abdominal abscess formation.

Solid organ abscesses

The bacteriology of solid organ abscesses (liver, spleen) shows geographical variation. Liver abscesses in the United States and other industrialized countries are found most frequently in immunosuppressed patients with biliary disease, whereas amebiasis is a more common cause in Latin America. In urban North America, the spleen is the most common site of abscess formation, resulting from hematogenous seeding secondary to endocarditis. Splenic abscesses secondary to brucellosis are rare in the United States and Northern Europe.

Causes and pathogenesis

Advanced age, malnutrition, and severe underlying disease predispose to abdominal abscess formation and predict increased mortality [1]. Luminal obstruction, inflammation, iatrogenic trauma (e.g., endoscopy), or an anastomotic disruption can disrupt wall integrity. **Perforated cholecystitis** found in the setting of gangrenous cholecystitis can cause a liver abscess in continuity. Risk factors are male sex, older age, and pre-existing cardiovascular disease. Diabetes has been suspected as a risk factor, but no study data have conclusively

Abdominal Wall and Cavity

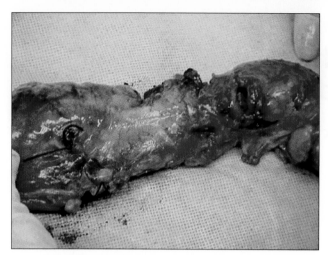

Figure 121.1 Perforated colon.

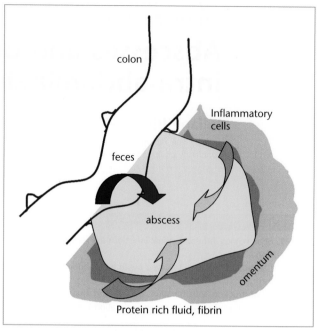

Figure 121.2 Pathogenesis of abscess formation.

confirmed this association. A further mechanism is **transgression of bacteria from the intestine** to devitalized tissue (pancreatic necrosis) or areas of decreased lymphatic clearance (hematoma). Pyogenic liver abscesses are rare, occurring in about 0.01% of patients admitted to hospital. The biliary tree is the commonest source (ascending cholangitis), followed by transmission through the portal vein (appendicitis, diverticulitis), the hepatic artery (systemic bacteremia), and neighboring organs (perforated gallbladder). Although most **splenic abscesses** follow bacteremia, they can also be seen in the posttraumatic setting (17%). These usually have a delayed presentation, days or months after non-operative treatment or splenic repair. Some 12% of splenic abscesses are secondary to infected infarcts in the setting of hematological disease, and a small proportion is caused by direct extension. Tuberculosis is a rare cause of intra-abdominal abscess in the industrialized world, although the rate is slowly increasing in immunocompromised patients.

When microorganisms reach sterile tissues (e.g., the peritoneal cavity), the body attempts to contain the contamination with fibrin deposits and omental migration. Protein-rich fluid arrives (Figure 121.2), and the complement and coagulation cascades are activated. Toxins and proteolytic enzymes from dying macrophages and bacteria cause local irritation and more fluid inflow. The result is swelling, pressure, and pain. The release of proinflammatory cytokines can lead to the **systemic inflammatory response syndrome (SIRS)**. If left untreated, the abdominal infection can cause significant fluid shifts, progressing to hypotension, and altered mental status. Hypoxemia and local acidosis decrease the effectiveness of the host defense system and the penetration of antibiotics. The most frequently encountered bacteria in abdominal infections are *Escherichia coli*, *Klebsiella* spp., *Bacterium fragilis*, *Pseudomonas*, *Streptococcus*, and *Enterobacter*. Aerobic and anaerobic microbes may work synergistically in peritonitis, producing a more severe infection than each microbe alone [2,3].

Clinical presentation

The amount of contamination and the host defense determine the intensity of the infection and inflammatory reaction. Typically, patients complain of fever, abdominal pain, anorexia, and occasional nausea and vomiting, but may show a septic picture. Abscesses can perforate into neighboring organs (bladder, vagina, adjacent bowel loops), leading to fistula formation (colovesical, colovaginal, enteroenteric). In the postoperative patient, new-onset pain at a different location or development of nausea, diarrhea, or altered mental status may be the heralding signs of abscess formation. In the bariatric patient, sustained tachycardia with a heart rate over 110 beats per minute may be the sole sign of a postoperative leak or abscess. Depending on the location of the abscess, the patient may have a variety of associated symptoms (Table 121.1). Right lower quadrant pain is frequently associated with appendicitis, although a long sigmoid colon can be found in the suprapubic or right lower quadrant position. Splenic and hepatic abscesses present with a dull, poorly localized, left or right upper quadrant or flank pain. Chest pain, hepatomegaly or splenomegaly, dullness in the lung bases, or rales may also be present. Special attention is needed at the extremes of age and in immunocompromised patients as the symptoms are frequently subtle and may not be well verbalized. Altered mental status, failure to thrive, or hypothermia may be the presenting symptoms of an abdominal abscess [4].

Differential diagnosis

The differential diagnosis of an abdominal abscess includes most causes of **abdominal pain**. The confirmation or exclusion

Table 121.1 Symptoms according to abscess location

Symptom	Possibly due to:	Can be associated with:
Constipation	Bowel obstruction, ileus	Diverticulitis, colonic cancer, appendicitis
Urgency to defecate	Abscess in pouch of Douglas, vesicorectal recess	Appendiceal abscess, abscess after appendectomy for perforated appendicitis
Pain during sexual intercourse	Motion tenderness	Tubo-ovarian abscess
Singultus (hiccups)	Diaphragmatic irritation	Subphrenic abscess after recent splenectomy

Table 121.2 Differential diagnosis of an abdominal abscess

Pelvic or intraperitoneal abscess
- Postoperative: infected hematoma or fluid collection; anastomotic leak
- Appendicitis
- Diverticulitis
- Tubo-ovarian abscess
- Perforated intestine from neoplasm, ulcer, or trauma
- Crohn's disease
- Perforated cholecystitis
- Infected pancreatic necrosis or pseudocyst
- Granulomatous disease
- Infectious enteritis (*Shigella, Yersinia*)

Liver abscess
- Amebiasis
- Echinococcal cyst
- Liver neoplasm
- Pyogenic abscess: cholangitis, appendicitis, diverticulitis, gallbladder bacteremia

Splenic abscess
- Septic embolus (e.g., cardiac source)
- Infected post-traumatic cyst or infarct (e.g., after embolization)
- Infected infarct in hematological disorder
- Direct extension from adjacent organ infection
- Brucellosis

of an abscess can be difficult. Once an abscess is confirmed, it is important to identify the underlying disease for an effective treatment strategy (Table 121.2). A patient with Crohn's disease will require a different therapeutic approach from a patient with a perforated colonic cancer. If the primary source of solid organ infections remains unclear, the chance of recurrence or treatment failure is high.

Diagnostic methods

The history and physical examination of the patient reveal the pattern of pain, associated symptoms and diseases, travel history, and whether the patient is clinically stable. **Laboratory analysis** may typically show an increased white blood cell (WBC) count, left shift, or bandemia. Leukocyturia points to either a primary urological infection, an infectious process in proximity to the bladder (e.g., perforated appendicitis), or an infectious process with fistula formation (e.g., colovesical fistula in perforated diverticulitis). Electrolyte abnormalities may indicate fluid shifts. Liver function tests and a coagulation profile are helpful to assess the severity of the infectious disease and are important if a hepatic abscess is encountered. A serum albumin level lower than 2.0 g/dL is a predictor of increased mortality for any operative intervention [5].

Abdominal imaging

Less than one-third of patients will have findings on abdominal radiography that are suggestive of intra-abdominal disease. Sentinel small bowel loops can be a sign of ileus; free air indicates perforation in the absence of a recent abdominal intervention. A pleural effusion, atelectasis, or pneumonia can point to a subdiaphragmatic collection. **Computed tomography (CT)** is currently the most effective radiological study. Adequate hydration of the patient should precede administration of intravenous, oral, and possibly rectal contrast, to avoid renal injury. A ring-enhancing fluid collection usually indicates the presence of an abscess. **Abdominal ultrasonography** may demonstrate fluid collections in thin patients. This imaging tool is non-invasive and can be a very useful diagnostic tool in children or in pregnancy, but remains operator dependent. If the quality of the fluid collection is unclear, **CT- or ultrasonographically-guided fine needle fluid aspiration** can be performed. This can be especially helpful in postoperative situations when differentiation between an expected postoperative fluid collection and an infected collection can be difficult.

A leukocyte scan can be obtained if the diagnosis remains unclear or CT is precluded. Unfortunately, the results are often not very specific and may be difficult to interpret. Diagnostic laparoscopy or laparotomy can be considered if the patient's condition is not improving or no other diagnostic method has been helpful in determining the underlying condition [6].

Treatment, prevention, and prognosis

Gastrointestinal surgery is a risk factor for postoperative intra-abdominal infection and anastomotic leaks. A recent meta-analysis of 29 trials with 2552 patients revealed that the use of enteral nutrition compared to parenteral nutrition significantly reduced the likelihood of a leak or abscess [7].

The overall mortality rate amongst patients with secondary non-postoperative peritonitis is high (15%) [1]. Patients who have received inappropriate antimicrobial therapy have

Abdominal Wall and Cavity

Table 121.3 Likely success of percutaneous drainage according to abscess morphology

Radiographic morphology	Success rate
Unilocular or discrete abscess	>90%
Medium complexity abscess (with communication to gastrointestinal tract)	80–90%
Complicated collections (intermixed pancreatic abscess or necrosis, infected tumor, organized empyema)	30–50%

significantly higher morbidity and mortality than patients who have received appropriate therapy. The presence of *Enterococcus* species in peritoneal culture significantly increases the morbidity. Appendiceal peritonitis has a less severe clinical pattern and a better prognosis. Fluid resuscitation should be implemented to stabilize the patient while antibiotic therapy is initiated. The antibiotic regimen should begin with empiric coverage of the "usual suspects" for a given disease process. Gram-negative bacteria and anaerobes should be adequately covered. Once sensitivities have been obtained, the antibiotic coverage can be adjusted. For most abscesses, drainage should be pursued. The morphology of an abscess on radiographic images (e.g., simple, loculated) predicts the probability of success with percutaneous drainage (Table 121.3).

Postoperative infection

When the infection is due to anastomotic leak, inadvertent bowel injury, or a hematoma or previously sterile fluid collection, the appropriate therapy in a stable patient is percutaneous drainage, antibiotics, and supportive care. If there is peritonitis or the abscess is inaccessible, operative intervention is necessary.

Perforated appendicitis

Two approaches can be considered: urgent operative intervention with appendectomy and drainage or, if the patient is otherwise stable without peritonitis, percutaneous drainage with interval appendectomy. Prior to interval appendectomy, a colonoscopy should be performed, especially in older patients to exclude a cecal carcinoma [8].

Diverticular abscess

Generally, antibiotics with activity against Gram-negative and anaerobic bacteria are recommended. No specific regimen has demonstrated improved outcomes over others. The optimal duration of antimicrobial therapy is based more on tradition than on prospective randomized studies. Patients with abscesses that are not amenable to CT-guided percutaneous drainage or in whom clinical symptoms persist after percutaneous drainage should undergo operative treatment. In recent years, attempts at a primary anastomosis or temporizing laparoscopic abscess drainage have received positive reviews

[9]. Hartmann's resection has a high secondary complication rate with a high operative mortality at colostomy takedown. An algorithm for management is shown in Figure 121.3.

Abscess from Crohn's disease

The three management options are (1) medical alone, (2) antibiotics plus percutaneous drainage, and (3) antibiotics plus surgical intervention. Medical management will obviate an operation in up to 50% of patients treated with antibiotics and steroids; percutaneous drainage alone can be successful in 20–70% of patients. Surgery includes abscess drainage and bowel resection. The risk of postoperative abscess or sepsis in Crohn's patients increases significantly if they have received infliximab within 3 months prior to surgery [10]. When these three options were compared in a retrospective fashion, the recurrent abscess rate was found to be 50% in the medical group, 67% in the percutaneous group, and 12% in the surgical group.

Perforated cholecystitis

The most frequently encountered microbes are *E. coli*, *Klebsiella*, *Pseudomonas*, streptococci (*Enterococcus*), *Staphylococcus* spp., *Bacteroides*, and *Clostridium*. In long-term critically ill patients, *Candida albicans* cholecystitis may be encountered. In patients infected with the human immunodeficiency virus (HIV), cholecystitis with *Cryptosporidium* and cytomegalovirus has been described. The treatment strategy will depend on the clinical situation. If the patient is stable, cholecystectomy should be considered. If the abscess is amenable to initial percutaneous drainage, this is preferred, especially in patients with severe underlying disease. Cholecystectomy may then be deferred.

Liver abscess

When a pyogenic liver abscess is suspected, the first-line treatment is antibiotic therapy. The most frequent bacteria are *E. coli*, *Bacteroides*, and streptococci. The antibiotics should provide a broad Gram-negative and anaerobic coverage for (historically) 6 weeks. If many small abscesses (<2 cm) are encountered, it has been recommended that one fluid collection be aspirated for culture and sensitivity. If the abscess is large (Figure 121.4), percutaneous drainage should be attempted. The complication rate is about 20% and complications include catheter dislodgement, empyema, bacteremia, and hepatico-bronchial fistula. If no clinical improvement is observed after 72 hours of antibiotic treatment and percutaneous drainage, surgical unroofing should be considered. The mortality rate for a treated hepatic abscess is 12–17%, depending on the patient population. Septic shock, jaundice, hypoalbuminemia, adult respiratory distress syndrome, and diabetes are predictors of poor outcome.

Splenic abscess

The primary therapy for splenic abscess is antibiotic treatment. Percutaneous drainage is technically difficult due to

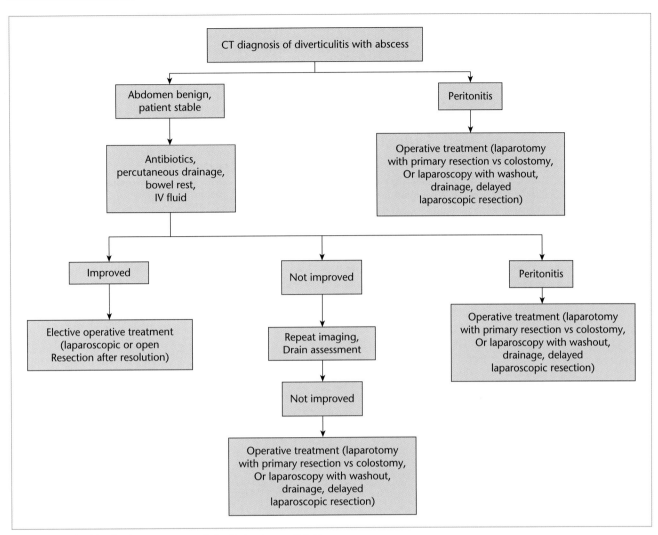

Figure 121.3 Algorithm for the management of diverticular abscess, IV fluid.

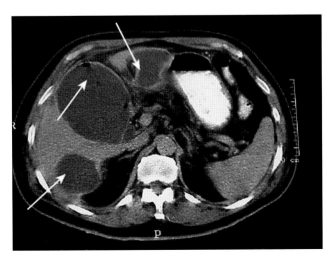

Figure 121.4 Multiple pyogenic liver abscesses. Arrows indicate multiple liver abscesses.

the fragile architecture of an infected spleen. If splenectomy becomes necessary, vaccination for encapsulated bacteria should be performed either 2 weeks before or 2 weeks after splenectomy.

Abscess complicating acute pancreatitis

It is difficult to make a clear distinction between abscess, infected necrosis, and initial pseudocyst in the setting of acute necrotizing pancreatitis. About 50% of pancreatic infections are monomicrobial; 36% are polymicrobial. The most frequently encountered organisms are *E. coli*, *Enterococcus*, *Enterobacter*, *Streptococcus*, *Klebsiella*, *Staphylococcus*, *Proteus*, *Bacteroides*, *Candida*, *Pseudomonas*, and *Serratia*. Therapeutic options are percutaneous or transgastric drainage and operative debridement. Mixed results have been reported. An abscess complicating acute pancreatitis is usually a severe infection with systemic illness.

Abdominal Wall and Cavity

References

1. Gauzit R, Pean Y, Barth X, *et al*. Epidemiology, management, and prognosis of secondary non-postoperative peritonitis: A French prospective observational multicenter study. In: *Surgical Infections*. Mary Ann Liebert, Inc., 2009.

2. Brook I. Microbiology and management of abdominal infections. *Dig Dis Sci*. 2008;53:2585–2591.

3. Rotstein O, Brisseau G. The microenvironment of infection. In: Fry D, editor. *Surgical Infections*. Boston: Little, Brown, and Company, 1995:43–51.

4. Podnos YD, Jimenez JC, Wilson SE. Intra-abdominal sepsis in elderly persons. *Clin Infect Dis*. 2002;35:62–68.

5. Aust JB, Henderson W, Khuri S, *et al*. The impact of operative complexity on patient risk factors. *Ann Surg*. 2005;241:1024–1027; discussion 1027–1028.

6. Van Goor H. Interventional management of abdominal sepsis: when and how. *Langenbecks Arch Surg*. 2002;387:191–200.

7. Mazaki T, Ebisawa K. Enteral versus parenteral nutrition after gastrointestinal surgery: a systematic review and meta-analysis of randomized controlled trials in the English literature. *J Gastrointest Surg*. 2008;12:739–755.

8. Klempa I. [Current therapy of complicated appendicitis]. *Chirurg*. 2002;73:799–804.

9. Myers E, Hurley M, O'Sullivan GC, *et al*. Laparoscopic peritoneal lavage for generalized peritonitis due to perforated diverticulitis [see comment]. *Br J Surg*. 2008;95:97–101.

10. Appau KA, Fazio VW, Shen B, *et al*. Use of infliximab within 3 months of ileocolonic resection is associated with adverse postoperative outcomes in Crohn's patients [see comment]. *J Gastrointest Surg*. 2008;12:1738–1744.

CHAPTER 122
Hernia

Cindy Matsen and Leigh Neumayer
University of Utah, Salt Lake City, UT, USA

ESSENTIAL FACTS ABOUT PATHOGENESIS

- Due to congenital defects in the abdominal wall, potential defects that are weakened by rises in intra-abdominal pressure, or defects acquired from trauma or surgery
- Lifetime risk of inguinal hernia is 27% for men and 3% for women
- Incisional hernias are more common with vertical midline incisions

ESSENTIALS OF DIAGNOSIS

- Diagnosis is based on history and physical examination
- Perform bilateral examination in the supine and standing positions. A reducible lump with Valsalva maneuver is present with uncomplicated hernias
- Strangulated hernias are non-reducible and painful with possible skin changes and obstructive symptoms
- All hernias are at risk of strangulation. The smaller the hernia, the higher the risk of strangulation. Femoral hernias are at highest risk

ESSENTIALS OF TREATMENT

- Watchful waiting is an acceptable, low-risk strategy for minimally symptomatic inguinal hernias
- Mesh repair has a lower recurrence rate than suture repair
- Laparoscopic hernia repair offers some advantages over open repair, but results are operator dependent
- Femoral hernias, emergency surgery, and postoperative complications are more common in women undergoing hernia repair

Introduction and epidemiology

The functions of the abdominal wall are:

- To provide protection and support for the intra-abdominal contents
- To promote bipedal living and activity
- To permit elimination of some intra-abdominal objects by micturition, defecation, vomiting, and childbirth.

A hernia is a protrusion of an organ or tissue through an abnormal opening (most commonly, and in the case of this chapter, through the abdominal wall) [1,2]. Hernias occur because of congenital defects in the abdominal wall (often early in life) [3], potential defects that are weakened by rises in intra-abdominal pressure, or defects acquired as a result of

trauma or surgery. Uncomplicated hernias are important as a potential cause of discomfort. When complicated by incarceration and bowel obstruction, they can be life-threatening.

The lifetime risk of inguinal hernia has been estimated at 27% for men and 3% for women [1,2,4]. Some 1–3 per 1000 people undergo hernia repair each year, resulting in more than 20 million hernia repairs annually (about 100 000 in the UK and 500 000 in the USA) [1,2,4]. For the developmental reasons outlined below, inguinal hernias are more common in men than in women. Because the femoral canal is larger in the female than in the male, owing to the gyne-anthropoid pelvis developed for parturition, femoral hernias are more common in women than in men. Inguinal hernias, however, are the most common groin hernia in both genders.

Development of the abdominal wall

Developmentally, the gastrointestinal tract begins as a long tube of endoderm comprising the foregut and the ventral bud, the midgut, and the hindgut. Initially growth and development occur outside the abdominal cavity and within the amniotic sac (physiological exomphalos or omphalocele). As rotation of the gut occurs, the differentiating tube returns to the abdominal cavity; the liver and biliary tract are in the right upper quadrant, the small intestine is in the central abdomen, and the large intestine is draped around the right side, across the upper abdomen and down the left side of the abdominal cavity. This is followed by the migration of mesoderm from the right and left sides to form the muscle of the anterior abdominal wall. Anteriorly, right and left rectus abdominis muscles are formed. The formation of the anterior abdominal wall is completed by the fusion of the linea alba around the umbilicus.

Causes and pathogenesis
Neonatal hernias

Occasionally, after birth, there is a small persistent defect at the umbilicus – an **infantile umbilical hernia**. The majority close spontaneously and only rarely require surgical treatment. Failure of fusion of the linea alba can lead to **epigastric**

Textbook of Clinical Gastroenterology and Hepatology, Second Edition. Edited by C. J. Hawkey, Jaime Bosch, Joel E. Richter, Guadalupe Garcia-Tsao, Francis K. L. Chan.
© 2012 Blackwell Publishing Ltd. Published 2012 by Blackwell Publishing Ltd.

Abdominal Wall and Cavity

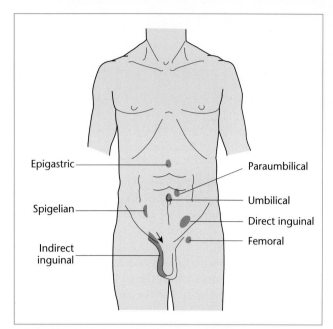

Figure 122.1 Common sites of anatomically derived hernias. (This figure was published in *Clinical Gastroenterology and Hepatology*, Wilfred M. Weinstein, Christopher J. Hawkey, Jaime Bosch, Hernia, Pages 879–884, Copyright Elsevier, 2005)

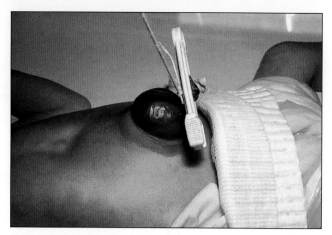

Figure 122.2 Omphalocele.

or paraumbilical hernias (Figure 122.1) Rarely, the anterior abdominal wall does not develop satisfactorily; the intestines do not return to the abdominal cavity and the baby is born with external viscera covered by a membranous sac (but not skin). Such persistent **exomphalos** (omphalocele) [3] (Figure 122.2) is graded as:

- Minor exomphalos – defect <5 cm and containing only gut
- Major exomphalos – defect >5 cm and containing gut and liver.

Gastroschisis [3] is protrusion of intestine from the abdominal cavity through a defect to the right of the umbilicus. There is no covering membrane and the prolapsed midgut is often edematous and covered by exudate. Emergency treatment is required to either return the intestinal contents to the abdominal cavity or to place a silo to protect the bowel. Silos with gradual reduction of the bowel are an important bridge to closure.

Infantile inguinal hernias are more common in prematurity due to patency of the processus vaginalis (see below).

Adult hernias: anatomically derived
Inguinal hernias
In the male *in utero* the testis develops on the posterior abdominal wall and migrates through the inguinal canal via a patent processus vaginalis to lie in the scrotum. Following testicular descent, obliteration of the processus vaginalis should occur at parturition. If the obliteration fails to occur, the persistent processus vaginalis allows a **true congenital inguinal hernia**

to occur. In addition the anatomical arrangement represents a potential structural defect where herniation can occur in later life, often because of raised intra-abdominal pressure associated with exertion. Inguinal hernias may be indirect (as described above) or direct. The latter typically occur in older individuals in whom increased intra-abdominal pressure results in direct herniation through a weakness in the transversalis fascia [1,2,4,5]. Indirect hernias are lateral to the epigastric vessels while direct hernias are medial to the vessels. Typically two-thirds of inguinal hernias in men are "indirect" and one-third are "direct." Occasionally, a sliding hernia (a type of indirect hernia) occurs. This is typically seen on the left side; the sigmoid colon "slides" down towards the scrotum and forms part of the hernia sac. Rarely, the cecum, appendix, and/or terminal ileum "slides" down on the right side. Inguinal hernias are 25 times more likely to occur in men, but indirect hernias are the most common type regardless of gender [5].

Femoral hernias
A femoral hernia is caused by herniation through the femoral canal causing protrusion below the inguinal ligament, lateral to the pubic tubercle [1,2,4,5]. Typically a femoral hernia contains either omentum (45%) or small intestine (45%). The remaining 10% contain contents from within the abdominal cavity (e.g., appendix, fallopian tube, ovary, Meckel's diverticulum, or very rarely, secondary gastrointestinal cancer). These are associated with eponymous names that serve no useful purpose. Femoral hernias are much more common in women (10:1) and are the most likely type of hernia to strangulate (15–20%). Thus, they are always repaired when found. In a study from the Swedish Hernia Registry, 41.6% of women with recurrent hernia who were diagnosed with inguinal hernia at the time of initial operation were found to have a missed femoral hernia [5].

Paraumbilical hernias
In contrast to findings in children, in adults most hernias in the umbilical region are paraumbilical. They typically occur in

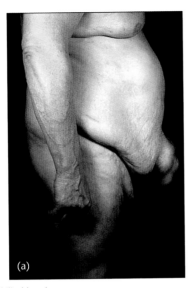
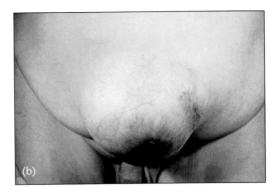

Figure 122.3 Paraumbilical hernias.

obese patients. Risk of strangulation is inversely associated with defect size (Figure 122.3).

Other hernias

Epigastric hernias are small but often painful protrusions, usually of extraperitoneal fat through the linea alba, between the umbilicus and xiphoid process. **Spigelian hernias** occur as a protrusion of fat and peritoneum through the semilunar line, which is formed by the aponeurosis of the internal oblique muscle at its point of division to enclose the rectus muscle, typically between the umbilicus and the symphysis pubis [6]. It presents as a painful swelling along the lateral edge of the rectus sheath.

Rare abdominal wall hernias

Herniation may occur in the lumbar area between the erector spinae muscle posteriorly and external oblique anteriorly, or between external oblique muscle anteriorly and latissimus dorsi posteriorly. Herniation can also occur through the obturator foramen (more common in women) and where the abdominal fascia is penetrated by the sciatic, posterior cutaneous, and pudendal nerves.

Acquired abdominal wall hernias

Any external injury to the abdominal wall, including surgery, can result in a hernia. Herniation can occur through any surgical incision and may be multiple (Figure 122.4) and/or massive (Figure 122.5).The risk is increased with every successive abdominal surgical procedure. **Wound sepsis** is the most important etiological factor [1,2]. Additional associated etiological factors include:

- Use of a drain through the surgical incision
- Steroid therapy
- Immunosuppression

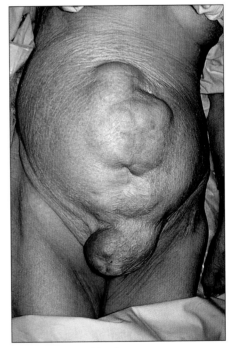

Figure 122.4 Multiple incisional hernias.

- Obesity
- Medical co-morbidities
- Operation through a previous incision
- Wound dehiscence in the early postoperative period
- Surgical materials
- Surgical technique.

The type of incision made is also an important factor. Herniation is more common after vertical midline incisions. Oblique and transverse incisions are associated with the lowest rate of occurrence of herniation.

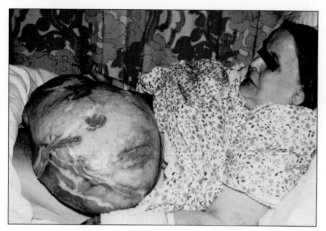

Figure 122.5 Massive ulcerated incisional hernia.

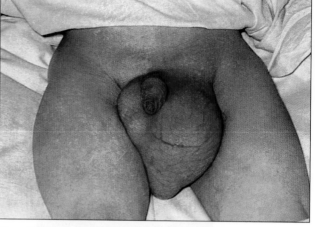

Figure 122.6 Inguinal hernia inter-scrotum.

Herniation through trocar puncture sites

Puncture of the abdominal wall during laparoscopy, surgical drainage, and procedures such as peritoneal dialysis creates a defect through which herniation can occur [4,7]. The increasing use of such procedures has substantially altered the spectrum of conditions associated with hernia. Likewise an end stoma – colostomy or ileostomy – may be the site at which a hernia develops. The stoma itself may prolapse, or other intestinal contents may herniate around the site of the defect in the anterior abdominal wall (peristomal hernia).

Partial enterocele (Richter's hernia) [8]

This occurs when the antemesenteric circumference becomes constricted in the neck of a hernia sac without causing complete intestinal obstruction. It is most frequently associated with a femoral hernia.

Clinical presentation
Symptoms
Uncomplicated hernias

Most uncomplicated hernias present as a lump that bulges on straining or as a scrotal mass (indirect inguinal hernias) (Figure 122.6). Hernias may cause a variable amount of discomfort or pain.

Complicated hernias

Pain increases if the hernia becomes irreducible and incarcerated, when symptoms of small bowel obstruction (colicky abdominal pain, nausea, and vomiting) may be superimposed. Obstruction is more likely with narrow-necked hernias, and strangulation and gangrene may accompany obstruction.

Examination

Bilateral examination in both supine and standing positions should be performed. A reducible lump with a cough impulse (Valsalva maneuver) is present with uncomplicated hernias.

When the hernia becomes irreducible, pain increases and if this progresses to strangulation, skin changes may be present. Femoral hernias occur below and lateral to the pubic tubercle, whereas inguinal hernias are above and lateral. Direct inguinal hernias protrude directly outwards (through Hasselbach's triangle, medial to the inferior epigastric artery) with coughing and straining. With indirect inguinal hernias, the origin of the hernia sac is lateral to the inferior epigastric artery, the protrusion is obliquely downward (see Figure 122.1), and, once reduced, the hernia can be temporarily controlled by pressure over the internal inguinal ring.

Differential diagnosis

Diagnostic considerations for a groin mass/pain include testicular torsion, lymphadenopathy related to an infectious or inflammatory process, and epidymitis in the acute setting. Non-acute conditions include hydrocele, varicocele, lipoma spermatocele, epididymal cyst, and testicular tumors [9].

Diagnostic investigation

Diagnosis is largely **clinical**. In cases of doubt, ultrasonographic evaluation aids distinction from other lesions, such as lymph nodes, hydrocele, or testicular tumors [9].

Treatment and prevention

All hernias may cause symptoms of pain and discomfort, and all carry the risk of incarceration, irreducibility, and strangulation, with or without intestinal obstruction. The risks of complication are greater with narrow-necked hernias. For inguinal hernias, the mortality rate has fallen over the past 50 years [1,2,4,10]. While the standard of care in the past was to repair all identified hernias, in the last decade evidence has shown watchful waiting for minimally symptomatic inguinal hernias is an acceptable and low-risk strategy [11]. Risk of

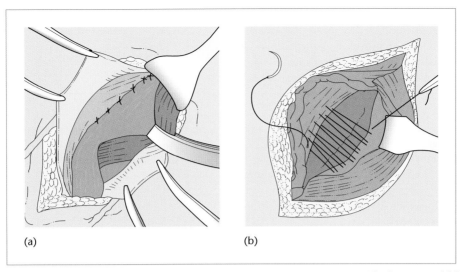

Figure 122.7 Open hernia repair. (a) Four-layer sutured Shouldice repair. (b) Flat patch Lichtenstein operation. (This figure was published in *Clinical Gastroenterology and Hepatology*, Wilfred M. Weinstein, Christopher J. Hawkey, Jaime Bosch, Hernia, Pages 879–884, Copyright Elsevier, 2005)

incarceration with this strategy is low. Trusses may provide some symptomatic relief, but are not recommended as long-term management. Use of a truss is associated with testicular atrophy, neuritis, and incarceration. Urgent operative repair is mandatory for:

- Irreducible or strangulated hernias, and with intestinal obstruction in the emergency situation
- Femoral hernias
- Exomphalos and gastroschisis.

Surgical techniques

Many types of hernia, such as inguinal, femoral, and paraumbilical, can be operated on using local infiltrative or regional anesthesia; general anesthesia may not be needed. Currently, there are two main choices with regard to technique.

Suture repair versus repair with mesh

Traditional hernia repair has involved meticulous suturing of all four layers of the abdominal wall (the Shouldice operation). In specialist units, the 10-year recurrence rate is less than 1%, but it is much higher in non-specialist units. Placement of mesh to achieve a tension-free hernioplasty, such as a Lichtenstein operation (Figure 122.7b), is preferred [1,2,4,10–13] because recurrence rates in unselected units are 1.4% versus 4.4% for suturing. Alternative mesh techniques have been applied, and may be supplemented by the placement of a three-dimensional cone-shaped polypropylene plug, although the latter is associated with unacceptable rates of postoperative pain (up to 8%) [4]. Mesh can be placed in the abdominal wall or behind it in the extraperitoneal space. The vast majority of open repairs performed in the United States involve the use of mesh prosthesis and is performed on an outpatient basis [4].

Open versus laparoscopic repair

Laparoscopic hernia repair was first described in 1982. In the last decade many surgeons have adopted it into routine surgical practice. The disadvantages of laparoscopic repair include greater difficulty, longer duration of surgery, and increased initial costs of the operation compared with open repair [14,15]. It offers the advantages of less postoperative pain, quicker return to work, and a better cosmetic result when compared to open, but is more operator dependent [16]. Laparoscopic repair can be totally extraperitoneal (TEP) or the transabdominal preperitoneal procedure (TAPP). For surgeons skilled in the technique, it is preferentially used for bilateral or recurrent inguinal hernia repair (see Video clip 122.1).

Antibiotic prophylaxis

Systematic reviews have revealed no benefit for antibiotic prophylaxis in uncomplicated hernia surgery [3,17].

Complications and their management

Patients will wish to avoid recurrence and long-term postoperative morbidity.

Recurrence

Primary repair of an inguinal hernia should be achieved with a recurrence (defined as a further groin hernia that requires an operation or the provision of a truss) rate of 1% [2,10]. However, rates of 10% are still being reported [2,10,15]. One-third of recurrences occur within a year of the primary operation and a further third within 5 years of surgery. Rates of recurrence are lower with open versus laparoscopic repair [15]. Recurrence rates of 1% can be achieved by use of open suture (Shouldice) in skilled specialist centers, and by use of mesh in non-specialized centers [2,10].

Abdominal Wall and Cavity

Other complications

A possible disadvantage of mesh hernia repair, particularly when combined with plugs, is an increased frequency of local pain and paresthesia due to ilioinguinal neuropathy. Risks of visceral and vascular injury are increased in laparoscopic repair [15].

Conclusions

Hernias are so common that their management and treatment will continue to occupy much surgical time. Watchful waiting is a safe alternative to surgery in minimally symptomatic inguinal hernias. Laparoscopic repair is a safe option and an increasingly used repair strategy.

SOURCES OF INFORMATION FOR PATIENTS AND DOCTORS

http://www.nlm.nih.gov/medlineplus/hernia.html
http://www.webmd.com/digestive-disorders/
   understanding-hernia-basics

References

1. Devlin HB, Kingsnorth A. *Management of Abdominal Hernias.* London: Chapman & Hall Medical, 1998.
2. Kingsnorth A, LeBlanc K. Hernias: inguinal and incisional. *Lancet.* 2003;362:1561–1571.
3. Molenaar JC, Tibboel D. Gastroschisis and omphalocele. *World J Surg.* 1993;17:337–341.
4. Rutkow IM. Epidemiologic, economic, and sociologic aspects of hernia surgery in the United States in the 1990s. *Surg Clin North Am.* 1998;78:941–951, v–vi.
5. Koch A, Edwards A, Haapniemi S, Nordin P, Kald A. Prospective evaluation of 6895 groin hernia repairs in women. *Br J Surg.* 2005; 92:1553–1558
6. Montes IS, Deysine M. Spigelian and other uncommon hernia repairs. *Surg Clin North Am.* 2003;83:1235–1253, viii.
7. Brook NR, White SA, Waller JR, Nicholson ML. The surgical management of peritoneal dialysis catheters. *Ann R Coll Surg Engl.* 2004;86:190–195.
8. Boughey JC, Nottingham JM, Walls AC. Richter's hernia in the laparoscopic era: four case reports and review of the literature. *Surg Laparosc Endosc Percutan Tech.* 2003;13:55–58.
9. Rubenstein RA, Dogra VS, Seftel AD, Resnick MI. Benign intrascrotal lesions. *J Urol.* 2004;171:1765–1772.
10. Royal College of Surgeons of England. *Clinical Guidelines for the Management of Groin Hernias in Adults.* London: RCS, 1993.
11. Fiftzgibbons RJ, Giobbie-Hurder A, Gibbs JO, *et al.* Watchful waiting vs repair of inguinal hernia in minimally symptomatic men, a randomized control trial. *JAMA.* 2006;295:285–292
12. EU Hernia Trialists Collaboration. Mesh compared with non-mesh methods of open groin hernia repair: systemic review of randomized controlled trials. *Br J Surg.* 2000;87:854–859.
13. Parra JA, Revuelta S, Gallego T, Bueno J, Berrio JI, Farinas MC. Prosthetic mesh used for inguinal and ventral hernia repair: normal appearance and complications in ultrasound and CT. *Br J Radiol.* 2004;77:261–265.
14. Roth JS, Johnson J, Hazey J, Pofahl W. Current laparoscopic inguinal hernia repair. *Curr Surg.* 2004;61:53–56.
15. Neumayer LA, Giobbie A, Jonasson O, *et al.* Open mesh versus laparoscopic mesh repair of inguinal hernia. *N Engl J Med.* 2004;350:1819–1827.
16. Reuben B, Neumayer L. Surgical management of inguinal hernia. *Adv Surg.* 2006;40:299–317.
17. Sanchez-Manuel FJ, Seco-Gil JL. Antibiotic prophylaxis for hernia repair. *Cochrane Database Syst Rev.* 2003;(2):CD003769.

Primer of Diagnostic Methods

PART 3:
Primer of Diagnostic
Methods

CHAPTER 123

Upper gastrointestinal endoscopy and mucosal biopsy

Jayan Mannath and Krish Ragunath

University of Nottingham and Nottingham University Hospitals, Nottingham, UK

KEY POINTS

- "Gold standard" test to visualize the esophagus, stomach, and duodenum
- Can be performed as an outpatient procedure with or without sedation
- Safe and rapid test to investigate upper gastrointestinal disorders
- Mucosal sampling can be diagnostic
- Computerized reporting and digital endoscopic images can be archived
- Therapeutic potential includes hemostasis, stricture dilatation, stent insertion, and management of early and advanced cancer

---

Introduction

The art and science of endoscopy has evolved since the invention of the "gastro camera" by a group of Japanese engineers in 1952, to the current state-of-the-art high-definition videoendoscopy. The introduction of flexible fiberoptic endoscopy by Basil Hirschowitz in 1957 [1] opened the flood gates to viewing the gut with ease and redefined gastrointestinal (GI) pathology. The fiberscope was based on optical viewing bundles transmitting light focused onto the face of each fiber by repeated internal reflections. The image reconstructed at the top of the bundle is transmitted to the eye via a focusing lens.

The development of videoendoscopy based on a miniature charge coupled device (CCD) lead to clear views of the GI mucosa that do not deteriorate with time, as experienced in fiberoptics. Essentially a CCD "chip" is an array of several thousand individual photo cells known as picture elements (pixels) that receive photons reflected back from the mucosal surface and produce electrons in proportion to the light received. The variable levels of charge are sent electronically to a video processor, which transposes this analog information into digital data, which in turn are processed to produce an image on a television monitor.

Description of technique

Equipment

The current standard videoendoscopy system comprises a flexible endoscope, electronic processor, light source, and television monitor (Figure 123.1). The endoscope has a control head and a flexible shaft with a maneuverable tip. The head is connected to a light source via an umbilical cord, through which pass other tubes transmitting air, water, and suction. On the right side of the handle is the control unit, with a smaller wheel for left and right deflection, and a larger wheel for up and down deflection. Inside the vinyl-covered shaft are the to and fro wiring and supporting electronics to the CCD "chip" mounted at the distal end. The shaft also houses the light guide for providing illumination at the distal tip, control wires for maneuvering the distal tip, a channel for suction that also accepts a variety of accessory devices, and a channel for insufflations of air and water. The flat tip of the distal end unit houses the CCD, lens system, openings for the accessory channel, and the light guide for illumination (Figure 123.2).

Endoscopes with a zoom option operate by having a zoom lens attached to the distal tip that can magnify the image up to 115 times when viewed on a 20-inch monitor (Figure 123.3). The zoom lens can be controlled by a lever in the control head. The zoom facility allows detailed examination of the mucosa, especially to detect pit pattern and microcapillary abnormalities.

The video processor is connected to the television, wherein the final image is transmitted and viewed. The working length of the scope is about 105 cm, with an insertion tube external diameter ranging from 5 to 12.5 mm. The angle of the viewing field varies from 100 to 140 degrees, and the depth of the field is in the 3–100-mm range. Deflection of the tip should allow movement of 210 degrees up and 90 degrees down, and 100 degrees left and right. The inside diameter of the working channel ranges from 2.8 to 3.7 mm depending on instrument design. The suction channel is used for the passage of diagnostic tools via a side port (e.g., biopsy forceps).

Textbook of Clinical Gastroenterology and Hepatology, Second Edition. Edited by C. J. Hawkey, Jaime Bosch, Joel E. Richter, Guadalupe Garcia-Tsao, Francis K. L. Chan.
© 2012 Blackwell Publishing Ltd. Published 2012 by Blackwell Publishing Ltd.

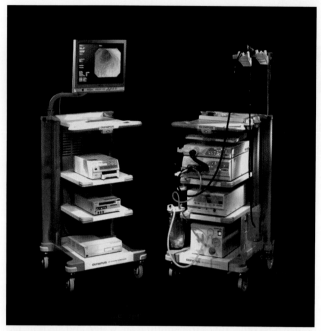

Figure 123.1 A complete Olympus videoendoscopy system. The cart on the left is fitted with a high-definition monitor, digital video recorder, and printer. The cart on the right contains the gastroscope, light source, processor and diathermy unit. (Courtesy of Olympus.)

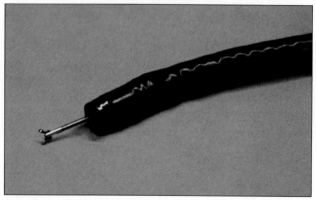

Figure 123.2 The tip of the gastroscope with a biopsy forceps passed through the accessory channel. The optical lens and the two light guides are behind the forceps.

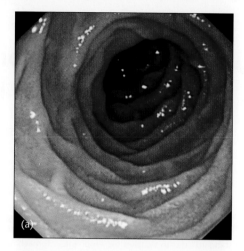

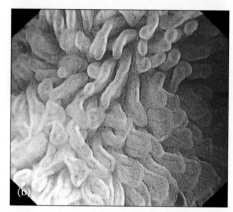

Figure 123.3 Endoscopic views of the second part of duodenum. (a) Normal view with high-resolution endoscopy. (b) Magnified view using high-resolution zoom endoscope.

Patient preparation and monitoring

This involves assessment of the patient's fitness for the procedure, identifying co-morbidity and at-risk patients, a detailed explanation to the patient of what to expect of the procedure, benefits, risks, alternative investigations, and possible complications, thus leading to a fully informed consent [2]. Drug history, including warfarin and clopidogrel therapy, is essential.

Elective upper GI endoscopy or esophago-gastro-duodenoscopy (EGD) should be done only after fasting for at least 6 hours. Dentures, eyeglasses, and contact lenses should be removed, and intravenous access in the form of an indwelling cannula should be inserted in patients requiring sedation and

in all at-risk patients. Blood pressure and heart rate are monitored, a supplemental nasal oxygen cannula attached, and a mouth guard kept in place. Some patients will be able to tolerate EGD under local anesthetic spray to the pharynx (lidocaine 2%). Conscious sedation usually includes a benzodiazepine drug, diazepam or midazolam, and in a minority of cases deeper sedation may be necessary with anesthetic support [3,4].

Procedure

The endoscope should be held in the left hand with the head of the endoscope in the palm and the instrument gripped between the fourth and fifth fingers and the base of the thumb. The thumb controls the up and down control and right and left knob. The first finger controls the air/water and suction button. The right hand is free to lock the controls in the appropriate position, and to move the shaft to advance, withdraw, or torque the instrument. Before inserting the endoscope it is important to check proper functioning of the equipment and lubricate the distal 10–20 cm of the shaft with a lubricant jelly.

The patient is usually positioned on their left side with the neck slightly flexed. A mouth guard is used to prevent any injury to the teeth and also to protect the endoscope. The endoscope should be positioned before insertion so that the tip moves in the correct longitudinal axis with the natural contour of the back of the tongue. After inserting the mouth guard between the patient's teeth or gums, the endoscope tip is inserted into the mouth, sliding over the tongue and keeping to the midline to reach the pharynx. The uvula is often seen transiently, projected upwards in the lower part of the view. Then, as the tip advances, the epiglottis and, finally, the cricoarytenoid cartilage and the vocal cords are visible. The tip should be deflected down by upward movement of the large wheel to pass below the cricoarytenoid cartilage on either side. At this juncture, instructing the patient to "swallow" allows the tip to slide into the esophagus (see Video clip 123.1). Forceful advancement of the endoscope should be avoided, especially when the patient is gagging, due to risk of a tear or perforation.

Examination of the esophagus

Once the instrument is passed through the cricopharyngeal sphincter the examination is done under direct vision. The two golden rules for any forms of endoscopy stand good here as well:

- Do not advance if the lumen is not seen
- If in doubt pull back, inflate, and reassess the lumen ahead.

The normal esophagus is a tubular unremarkable lumen with a pale squamous mucosal lining. The landmarks include the indentation of the left main bronchus and left atrial pulsations in the middle third (this may not always be seen), and the **gastroesophageal junction (GEJ)** at the lower end, usually at about 40 cm. This is the place where the pale pink squamous lining of the esophagus meets the red columnar lining of the stomach to form the **"Z" line** (Figure 123.4a). It is also the starting point of the gastric mucosal folds. In Barrett's esophagus the squamocolumnar junction (SCJ) will be displaced proximally to various extents (Figure 123.4b). Hence, the true GEJ is the end of the tubular esophagus and the beginning of the gastric folds. The diaphragm normally clasps at or just below (<1 cm) the GEJ. This is highlighted if the patient sniffs or takes in deep breaths. Hiatus hernia can be diagnosed when the GEJ is >2 cm above the diaphragmatic impression and can be seen as a sac (Figure 123.4c; see Video clip 123.1). The proximal one-third of the esophagus is often overlooked. That is where the ringed esophagus is often most readily appreciated.

Examination of the stomach

Unless the cardia is unduly lax, the lumen can be temporarily lost as the tip of the endoscope is advanced into the stomach. Insufflation of air distends the stomach to observe the lesser curve on the right and the greater curve on the left. The gastric folds on the anterior and posterior wall can be seen and there may be some bile-stained gastric secretions which can be aspirated to avoid pulmonary aspiration. The distended stomach is "J" shaped. The instrument is then advanced along the lesser curve with a clockwise twist to visualize the gastric body. If unsuspected retained food is present to any extent, the procedure should be aborted to avoid the risk of aspiration.

The **fundus** is visualized by retroflexion or the "J" maneuver (Figure 123.5). This is done by a 180-degree upward angulation

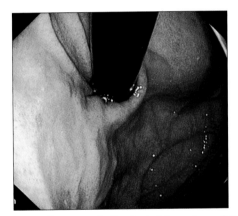

Figure 123.5 The "J" maneuver looking back at the gastroesophageal junction and fundus.

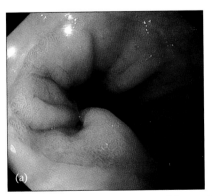
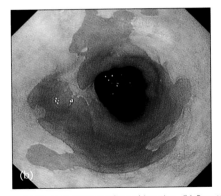
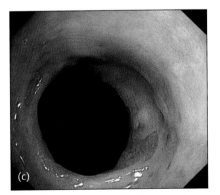

Figure 123.4 Endoscopic appearance of the esophagus. (a) Normal gastroesophageal junction. (b) Barrett's esophagus with columnar epithelium extending proximally, displacing the normal squamous epithelium. (c) Hiatus hernia sac seen as a "lumen within a lumen."

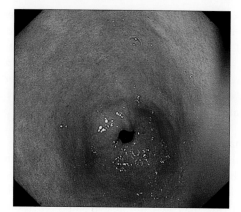

Figure 123.6 Normal pyloric orifice.

with simultaneous forward push in a fully distended stomach, beginning in the proximal to mid antrum. The retroflexed shaft can be rotated through 360 degrees to visualize the entire fundus and gastric body, thus visualizing all potential blind areas that are not as easily seen end on. By pushing the endoscope forward it will, paradoxically, move distally. The endoscope can be straightened when the angularis is visualized on turnaround. Finally the scope can be withdrawn with gentle suction to deflate the stomach.

Examining the **antrum** is straightforward. If peristalsis is active, one can follow the advancing peristaltic wave from about 1–2 cm behind and see the total mucosa exposed right to the pylorus. The **pyloric orifice** can be seen opening and closing with peristalsis (Figure 123.6). When the pylorus is very tight, especially to passage of larger channel endoscopes ("therapeutic endoscopes"), some experienced endoscopists gingerly pass a closed biopsy forceps through the pylorus and then advance the endoscope over it, pulling back on the forceps in gradations as the endoscope advances.

Examination of the duodenum

After the tip is passed through the pyloric orifice, the first part of the duodenum or the duodenal bulb comes into view. This is a common site for duodenal ulcers and hence careful observation is required (Figure 123.7). The inferior and posterior wall is difficult to visualize unless the tip is deflected down and towards the right. If the scope is advanced further with a clockwise twist and downward flick of the tip, followed by gentle withdrawing of the scope, the second part of the duodenum springs into view. Withdrawal of the scope straightens the loop in the stomach and the descending duodenum with the papilla in it can be reached with only 50–60 cm of the endoscope inserted. If one wants to advance beyond the distal second part of the duodenum, the endoscope can be straightened and then the endoscope advanced while an assistant applies pressure over the left upper quadrant.

Mucosal biopsy and tissue sampling

Tissue sampling is done when an abnormality is encountered while performing endoscopy, to detect *Helicobacter pylori*

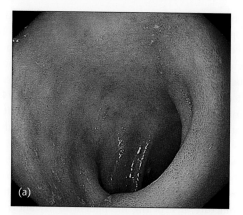

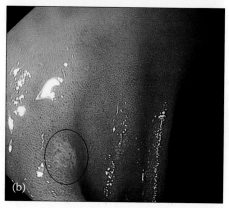

Figure 123.7 Endoscopic views of the duodenal bulb. (a) Normal duodenal bulb. (b) A small ulcer (ringed) in the duodenal bulb.

infection or as a planned procedure when, for example, duodenal biopsies are needed to confirm celiac disease [5]. The most common method is by taking a mucosal biopsy using a cupped biopsy forceps passed through the accessories channel (see Figure 123.2). The lesion should be approached face-on, so that firm and direct pressure is applied with the widely open cups. The assistant then gently closes the cup and the forceps should be withdrawn with a quick "snap-like" motion.

Approaching the mucosa *en face* for esophageal biopsy is challenging. The "turn and suction" technique is particularly useful in acquiring larger biopsy samples from the tubular esophagus and when Barrett's surveillance biopsies are taken [6]. With this technique, the biopsy forceps is advanced out of the biopsy channel of the endoscope and opened. The forceps is then withdrawn until almost flush with the endoscope tip and turned into the esophageal wall. Air is then suctioned from the lumen to collapse the mucosa into the forceps cup, which is then advanced slightly until resistance is appreciated. The forceps is then closed while maintaining suction and the endoscope tip is straightened, followed by withdrawal of the biopsy forceps to avulse the mucosal sample.

Ulcers should be biopsied at the edges and it is wise to take several samples from the same site when sampling **tumors** so that the superficial necrotic area can be penetrated to achieve good quality tumor tissue. The samples are then placed in formalin directly.

Detection of **H. pylori infection** is done by placing one or two gastric biopsy specimens into a container from a commercially available rapid urease kit, which turns color in a few minutes (yellow to red) if it is positive. Traditionally, antral biopsies have been used, but in patients on proton pump inhibitors the gastric antrum can be devoid of organisms in up to 50% of cases, but less frequently in the gastric body. Thus, in these patients either gastric body biopsies alone or one antral and one gastric body biopsy can be used. Tissue sampling using cytology brushes is done less frequently, usually when biopsy specimens are not adequate, especially in strictures or in places that are endoscopically difficult to reach with the biopsy forceps. Cytology specimens are taken using a sleeved brush. The head of the brush is advanced out of its sleeve and rubbed repeatedly across the surface of the lesion. It is then withdrawn back into the sleeve and the whole unit is taken out. It is then pushed out of the sleeve and wiped over glass slides and fixed with a fixation spray.

Endoscopy reporting

Endoscopic findings should be reported accurately using precise, simple language [7,8]. Some reporting software programs can also incorporate endoscopic images captured during the procedure. Every report should include the following minimum information:

- Indication(s)
- Endoscopist(s) and assistants
- Endoscope used
- Sedation including route/dose and any reversal agent used
- Supplemental oxygen delivered
- Exact findings in the esophagus, stomach, and duodenum
- Procedures performed, i.e. biopsy, etc.
- Specimens obtained
- Any complications encountered
- Treatment, further investigations, follow-up plan, and any specific comments.

Alternatives to upper gastrointestinal endoscopy

Barium studies are now used only for investigation of motility disorders and to provide roadmaps of strictures or gross morphology prior to complex surgery. Wireless **video capsule endoscopy (VCE)** is used mainly to examine the small bowel; however, the recent introduction of esophageal and colon capsules has expanded the indications for VCE [9,10] (see Chapter 128). The swallowed "video capsule" generates images of the gut by a complementary metal oxide silicon chip camera (CMOS) or a CCD chip. Future video capsule designs may emerge with mucosal sampling and controlled movement features.

Table 123.1 Indications and contraindications for upper gastrointestinal endoscopy

Diagnostic
- To evaluate upper abdominal symptoms (e.g., dysphagia)
- Surveillance of a known condition (e.g., Barrett's esophagus)
- To obtain tissue samples (e.g., duodenal biopsy for celiac disease)
- Screening for malignancy (e.g., familial adenomatous polyposis)

Therapeutic
- Hemostasis (e.g., variceal banding, ulcer treatment)
- Dilatation (e.g., esophageal stricture)
- Stent insertion (e.g., inoperable esophageal cancer)
- Tumor ablation (e.g., laser, argon beam treatment)
- Polypectomy/endoscopic mucosal resection
- Foreign body removal
- Percutaneous endoscopic gastrostomy insertion

Relative contraindications
- Hemodynamically unstable patient
- Recent myocardial infarction or pulmonary embolism
- Acute abdomen (e.g., peritonitis)
- Severe uncorrected coagulopathy
- Anatomical abnormalities in the upper esophagus (e.g., Zenker's diverticulum)

Indications and contraindications

The most common indication to perform an EGD is **persistent symptoms** related to the upper GI tract (Table 123.1). Emergency EGD may be necessary to diagnose and treat upper GI bleeding. It is also done to screen for gastroesophageal cancers (in China and Japan) and Barrett's esophagus surveillance. EGD forms part of other GI investigations in investigating anemia, weight loss, and occult malignancy, and also to obtain duodenal biopsies in suspected celiac disease and other malabsorptive conditions. Endoscopy may be performed following abnormal barium or computed tomography (CT) studies for confirmation of diagnosis and tissue sampling. EGD is done to perform a variety of therapeutic procedures including hemostasis of bleeding lesions (varices, ulcers, angiodysplasia), stricture dilatation, stent insertion, management of early and advanced cancer (see Chapters 145–151). The American Society for GI Endoscopy has produced guidelines on the appropriate use of endoscopy [11]. EGD, if performed for appropriate indications, has a high yield of detecting clinically relevant lesions in the upper GI tract [12].

In the setting of an appropriate indication, in a fit patient who can give informed consent and is able to cooperate with conscious sedation, there is virtually no contraindication to performing an EGD. However, the risks are increased in systemically ill patients, anticoagulated patients, and in those who have suffered a recent myocardial infarction or are in a postoperative state. Occasionally anatomical abnormalities in the esophagus, such as Zenker's diverticulum or a high esophageal stricture, can render the procedure hazardous. EGD with or without mucosal biopsy is not contraindicated in patients on warfarin or other anticoagulants providing the international normalized ratio (INR) is in the therapeutic range. Aspirin and other antiplatelet medications like clopidogrel are not a contraindication either [13].

Complications

Upper GI endoscopy is a relatively safe procedure, but there are many potential dangers. Large surveys suggest that there is a 1 in 1000 risk of a significant complication and a 1 in 10 000 risk of death. Problems are more likely to be encountered in elderly frail patients with other co-morbidities, and in emergency situations. All endoscopy units should have regular update on safety issues, procedure protocols, resuscitation training, and a log of critical incidents and near-miss incidents as part of quality control. Possible complications are described below. (Refer to principles of running a high-quality endoscopy service on the website.)

Bleeding

This is uncommon after a diagnostic endoscopy. Minor self-limiting bleeding from the biopsy site is common and can be ignored. However, excessive brisk bleeding obscuring vision can occur in patients with impaired coagulation and liver disease or in over-anticoagulated patients. It is important to check clotting parameters as part of the pre-endoscopy evaluation in anticoagulated patients [13,14].

Perforation

This can happen at all sites, but is more common in the upper esophagus where the endoscope is passed blindly. Hence, the dictum, "do not push" but ask the patient to "swallow." The appearance of surgical emphysema in the neck or unexplained chest/abdominal pain should alert the endoscopist to possible perforation. Immediate recognition and prompt involvement of the surgical team is important for further management.

Respiratory complications

These include oxygen desaturation, aspiration, and respiratory arrest. Identifying high-risk patients, close monitoring using pulse oximetry, safe sedation practice, oxygen supplementation, and adequate throat suction by the assistant in case of fluid regurgitation can all help in preventing these complications.

Arrhythmias

EGD can occasionally, especially in the presence of hypoxia, provoke atrial or ventricular arrhythmias. Pulse and cardiac monitoring can identify these. Resuscitation equipment should always be available in the endoscopy suite.

Infection

Bacteremia can occur after endoscopy and the organisms are usually the commensals in the throat. This does not have any bearing on the patient and recent guidelines from the American Society for Gastrointestinal Endoscopy (ASGE) advise against the use of routine antibiotics to prevent infective endocarditis in the presence of cardiac disease, as practiced previously [15]. High standards of cleaning and disinfection procedures should be followed to prevent transmission of infections like viral hepatitis, human immunodeficiency virus (HIV), etc. If current disinfection protocols are followed, the possibility of transmission of any infection is negligible [16].

Medication reaction

Allergy to local anesthetic is not uncommon and a thorough pre-endoscopy check should be done to avoid drugs that the patient is known to be allergic to. Methemoglobinemia has been reported following lidocaine throat spray. Anticholinergics will not affect treated glaucoma, but may precipitate an attack in occult chronic glaucoma and thus a diagnosis can be made; there are therefore no ocular contraindications to the use of anticholinergic medications.

Costs and benefits

The cost-effectiveness of a diagnostic test must be compared to that of a competing test or strategy to produce meaningful information. EGD is now the standard of care for undisputed indications (e.g., hemetemesis, melena, dysphagia, etc.) in almost all healthcare system. Radiological investigations like barium tests are now used in only specific conditions (e.g., motility disorders) or to complement EGD and aid in the therapeutic procedure. Treating young dyspeptic patients (<45 years) without any alarm symptoms symptomatically is more cost-effective. The diagnostic yield is greater as the patient increases in age, making EGD more cost-effective in these patients.

New modalities of image-enhanced endoscopy

Conventional videoendoscopes have a focal distance between 1 and 2 cm from their tip and use fewer than 200 000 pixels to construct an image. Advanced methods have been developed to enhance the endoscopic image by increasing the resolution of the CCD and using high-definition televisions to view the processed images. Currently, endoscopes with integrated zoom lenses and microscopes are available and with these technologies, intestinal tissues can be imaged at cellular and nuclear levels, providing *in vivo* optical histology. Image enhancement using dye (chromoendoscopy) or optical methods [narrow band imaging (NBI), Fuji Intelligent Chromo Endoscopy (FICE) and iScan] could allow improved visualization and characterization of lesions (Table 123.2).

Magnification and resolution

Optical magnification is closely related to the concept of resolution, which is the ability to discriminate between two points, and in an electronic image, this is a function of the pixel density. Current magnifying or "zoom" endoscopes enlarge the image up to 150 fold using a mechanically or electronically movable lens controlled by a lever at the head of the endoscope (optical zoom). The availability of high-resolution endoscopes equipped with high-density CCDs (600 000–1 000 000 pixels) makes high magnification possible without loss of resolution. These endoscopes also have variable focal distance, which means they can be moved very close to the mucosal surface and provide a magnified image. Image manipulation using electronic zooming (digital zoom) is also possible; however, image quality is lost at some point, because with every step of electronic magnification the image is composed of fewer pixels as compared with optical magnification.

Chromoendoscopy

The use of special stains in combination with magnification endoscopy enhances the mucosal detail seen at endoscopy. Characteristic mucosal appearances such as pit patterns in the esophagus, stomach, and duodenum can allow targeted biopsy. This has facilitated an improved histological yield of specialized intestinal metaplasia and dysplasia in Barrett's esophagus, for example. Vital stains such as methylene blue and acetic acid, and non-absorbed stains such as indigo carmine have all been used to target Barrett's mucosa with

Table 123.2 Endoscopic imaging modalities of the upper gastrointestinal tract (Based on information from Tajiri H, Niwa H. Proposal for a consensus terminology in endoscopy: how should different endoscopic imaging techniques be grouped and defined? *Endoscopy.* 2008;40:775–778, with permission.)

- White light endoscopy:
  - Standard resolution endoscopy
  - High-definition videoendoscopy
- Magnification endoscopy:
  - Optical magnification
  - Electronic magnification
- Image-enhancing modalities:
  - Electronic: e.g. FICE (spectral estimation), I-Scan (surface enhancement)
  - Optical: e.g., AFI, NBI, IRI
  - Chromoendoscopy
- Microscopy:
  - Confocal: endomicroscopy
  - Optical: endocytoscopy

increased sensitivity for the detection of specialized intestinal metaplasia. It is important that a special spraying catheter is used, permitting optimal dispersion of the dye onto the mucosal surface (see Video clip 123.2). Although chromoendoscopy is cheap and effective, it is widely underused in the Western world compared to the Far East.

Narrow band imaging

By electronically altering the wavelengths of white light components or by processing images with selected wavelengths, mucosal detail can be seen similar to that obtained with chromoendoscopy. NBI was first described in 2004 by Gono *et al.* [17] and is patented by Olympus Corporation. Standard white light endoscopy uses the full visible wavelength range (400–700 nm) to produce a red–green–blue image. In NBI, the bandwidths of blue (440–460 nm) and green (540–560 nm) waves are narrowed with the help of a special filter and the relative contribution of the blue light is increased. This allows visualization of the mucosal surface characteristics, including pit patterns and microvasculature, in much more detail. The filter is activated by pressing a switch in the hand control and the endoscopist can easily switch between white light and NBI. Use of NBI with and without magnification has been widely studied in Barrett's esophagus and found to be useful, especially in identifying dysplasia [18–20] (Figure 123.8; see clip Video 123.3).

Fuji Intelligent Chromo Endoscopy and i-Scan

These techniques are based on the same principles as NBI; however, no optical filters are used as the images are produced by a new computed spectral estimation technology. FICE (Fujinon Endoscopy) and i-Scan (Pentax Medical) transform ordinary endoscopic images taken from the video processor: the reflected photons are arithmetically processed to reconstitute virtual images by increasing the relative intensity of narrowed blue light to a maximum and by decreasing narrowed red and green light to a minimum. This leads to better delineation of microvasculature and mucosal pit patterns due to the differential absorption of light by hemoglobin in the mucosa. FICE has been evaluated in colonic polyps and upper endoscopic imaging, with promising results [21,22].

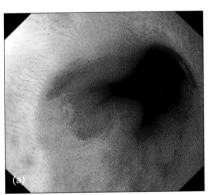 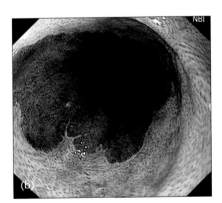 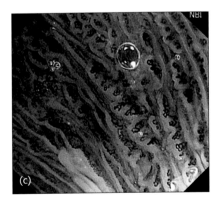

Figure 123.8 A short segment of Barrett's esophagus seen with (a) high-resolution endoscopy, (b) narrow band imaging (NBI), and (c) NBI with magnification.

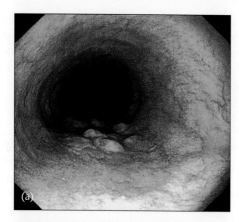

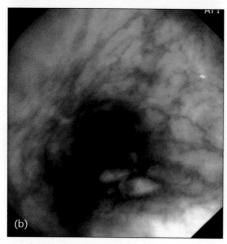

Figure 123.9 An area of early neoplasia in Barrett's esophagus seen with (a) high-resolution endoscopy and (b) autofluorescence imaging.

Autofluorescence imaging

The phenomenon of autofluorescence occurs when light of shorter wavelength interacts with a tissue containing endogenous fluorophores, which in turn emits light of longer wavelength. A number of biological substances in the GI tract, such as collagen, elastin, nicotinamide, and flavins, can act as endogenous fluorophores. Earlier autofluorescence imaging (AFI) systems used fiberoptic endoscopes but these did not give sufficient image quality for clinical utility. However, the emergence of high-resolution videoendoscopy with a second CCD for AFI has made it possible to obtain pseudo color images with significant improvement in quality (Olympus Corporation). AFI offers an easy way to distinguish between normal and tumorous tissue by combining an auto fluorescence image on irradiation with a blue light of wavelength of 390–470 nm. The image of green reflected light depicts the absorbed light of hemoglobin, so that normal tissue appears pale green and tumorous tissue appears magenta (Figure 123.9; see Video clip 123.3). The role of AFI in Barrett's esophagus has been studied and it was found to be useful in detecting dysplasia [23,24]. Its clinical utility in colonic imaging is less well understood, but recent studies are promising [25].

Confocal microscopy

The concept of "optical biopsy," in its true sense, has been achieved with confocal laser endomicroscopy. Two systems are commercially available: an endoscope with an integrated confocal microscope at the tip (Pentax Medical) and a probe-based confocal microscope which can be passed through the working channel of an ordinary endoscope (Mauna Kea Technologies). To create confocal images, blue laser light is focused on the desired tissue via the distal end of confocal endoscope. Applied fluorescent materials (usually intravenously) are excited by laser lights, which the confocal optical unit detects at an exactly defined horizontal level. Extreme magnification (up to 1000 times) is obtained with this technology and images at the cellular/nuclear level are acquired that mimic histopathology sections, thereby allowing targeted biopsy and reducing the number of random biopsies [26].

Endocytoscopy is a relatively new addition to the endoscopic magnification technology. Ultra-magnification (450–1125 times) catheter-based endoscopes can be passed through the working channel of a standard endoscope. In combination with chromo agents, they can provide *in vivo* histological images. Unlike confocal endoscopy, endocytoscopes produce color images but do not scan deeper cellular levels.

Infrared endoscopy

This recently developed technology by Olympus uses near-infrared light, which has limited scattering characteristics and low absorption by water and hemoglobin, allowing deeper penetration into the tissue compared to white light. This endoscopy system uses a high-performance CCD which is sensitive to infrared and white light along with two ranges of infrared light emitted by the light source. Intravenously administered indocyanine green dye enables mucosal and submucosal vessels to be clearly visualized with the infrared light and is useful in identifying the depth of gastric cancers [27].

References

1. Hirschowitz B, Peters CW, Curtis LE. Preliminary report on a long fibrescope for examination of stomach and duodenum. *Mich Med Bull.* 1957;23:178–80.
2. Shepherd H, Hewett D. *Guidance for Obtaining a Valid Consent for Elective Endoscopic Procedures.* British Society of Gastroenterology, April 2008
3. Sedation and Anesthesia in GI Endoscopy. *Gastrointest Endosc.* 2008;68:215–826.
4. *Safety and Sedation During Endoscopic Procedures.* British Society of Gastroenterology, September 2003.
5. American Society for Gastrointestinal Endoscopy. Tissue sampling and analysis. *Gastrointestinal Endosc.* 2003;57:811–816.
6. Levine DS, Reid BJ. Endoscopic biopsy technique for acquiring larger mucosal samples. *Gastrointest Endosc.* 1991;37:332–337.
7. European Society for Gastrointestinal Endoscopy recommendations for quality control in gastrointestinal endoscopy: Guidelines for image documentation in upper and lower GI endoscopy. *Endoscopy.* 2001;33:901–903.

8. American Society for Gastrointestinal Endoscopy. Computerised endoscopic medical record system. *Gastrointestinal Endosc.* 2000; 51:793–796.

9. Waterman M, Gralnek IM. Capsule endoscopy of the esophagus. *J Clin Gastroenterol.* 2009;43:605–612.

10. Van Gossum A, Navas MM, Fernandez-Urien I, *et al.* Capsule endoscopy versus colonoscopy for the detection of polyps and cancer. *N Engl J Med.* 2009;361:264–270

11. American Society for Gastrointestinal Endoscopy. *Appropriate Use of GI Endoscopy.* Manchester, MA: American Society for Gastrointestinal Endoscopy, 1992.

12. Frohlich F, Repond C, Mullhaupt B, John-Paul V, *et al.* Is the diagnostic yield of upper GI endoscopy improved by the use of explicit panel based appropriateness criteria? *Gastrointest Endosc.* 2000;52:333–341.

13. Veitch AM, Baglin TP, Gershlick AH, *et al.* Guidelines for the management of anticoagulant and antiplatelet therapy in patients undergoing endoscopic procedures. British Society of Gastroenetrology. *Gut.* 2008;57:1322–1329.

14. Guideline on the Management of Anticoagulation and Antiplatelet Therapy for Endoscopic Procedures. *Gastrointest Endosc.* 2002; 55:775–779.

15. Antibiotic prophylaxis for GI endoscopy. *Gastrointest Endosc.* 2008;67:791–798.

16. Transmission of infection by gastrointestinal endoscopy. *Gastrointestinal Endosc.* 2001;54:824–828.

17. Gono K, Obi T, Yamaguchi M, *et al.* Appearance of enhanced tissue features in narrow-band endoscopic imaging. *J Biomed Opt.* 2004;9:568–577

18. Anagnostopoulos GK, Yao K, Kaye P, Hawkey CJ, Ragunath K. Novel endoscopic observation in Barrett's oesophagus using high resolution magnification endoscopy and narrow band imaging. *Aliment Pharmacol Ther.* 2007;26:501–507.

19. Singh R, Anagnostopoulos GK, Yao K, *et al.* Narrow-band imaging with magnification in Barrett's esophagus: validation of a simplified grading system of mucosal morphology patterns against histology. *Endoscopy.* 2008;40:457–463.

20. Wolfsen HC, Crook JE, Krishna M, *et al.* Prospective, controlled tandem endoscopy study of narrow band imaging for dysplasia detection in Barrett's Esophagus. *Gastroenterology.* 2008;135: 24–31

21. Pohl J, Lotterer E, Balzer C, *et al.* Computed virtual chromoendoscopy versus standard colonoscopy with targeted indigocarmine chromoscopy: a randomised multicentre trial. *Gut.* 2009; 58:73–78.

22. Coriat R, Chryssostalis A, Zeitoun JD, *et al.* Computed virtual chromoendoscopy system (FICE): a new tool for upper endoscopy? *Gastroenterol Clin Biol.* 2008;32:363–369.

23. Kara MA, Peters FP, Fockens P, ten Kate FJ, Bergman JJ. Endoscopic video-autofluorescence imaging followed by narrow band imaging for detecting early neoplasia in Barrett's esophagus. *Gastrointest Endosc.* 2006;64:176–185

24. Curvers WL, Singh R, Wallace MB, *et al.* Identification of predictive factors for early neoplasia in Barrett's esophagus after autofluorescence imaging: a stepwise multicenter structured assessment. *Gastrointest Endosc.* 2009;70:9–17.

25. van den Broek FJ, van Soest EJ, Naber AH, *et al.* Combining autofluorescence imaging and narrow-band imaging for the differentiation of adenomas from non-neoplastic colonic polyps among experienced and non-experienced endoscopists. *Am J Gastroenterol.* 2009;104:1498–1507

26. Dunbar KB, Okolo P 3rd, Montgomery E, Canto MI. Confocal laser endomicroscopy in Barrett's esophagus and endoscopically inapparent Barrett's neoplasia: a prospective, randomized, double-blind, controlled, crossover trial. *Gastrointest Endosc.* 2009;70:645–654.

27. Ishihara R, Uedo N, Iishi H, *et al.* Recent development and usefulness of infrared endoscopic system for diagnosis of gastric cancer. *Dig Endosc.* 2006;18:45–48.

28. Tajiri H, Niwa H. Proposal for a consensus terminology in endoscopy: how should different endoscopic imaging techniques be grouped and defined? *Endoscopy.* 2008;40:775–778.

CHAPTER 124
Lower gastrointestinal endoscopy and biopsy

Jerome D. Waye

Mount Sinai Hospital, New York, NY, USA

KEY POINTS

- Colonoscopy is the gold standard for colon examination
- Biopsies are obtainable for any part of the colon
- Polypectomy prevents colon cancer
- Requires skilled operator, well prepared colon, sedation (usually), and monitoring for safety

Introduction

Examination of the colon can be accomplished in many ways. Direct imaging of the colon mucosa is performed by flexible sigmoidoscopy or colonoscopy. The flexible sigmoidoscope has largely replaced the rigid sigmoidoscope for inspection of the rectum and sigmoid colon since it can be passed farther with less pain. The colonoscope is similar but can be passed to the cecum and often into the small intestine because it is considerably longer. Many procedures may be performed with colonoscopy (Table 124.1).

Equipment

Colonoscopes vary in length (from 130 to 168 cm), diameter (from 11 to 13 mm), and angle of view (from 120 to 170 degrees). The instruments are quite flexible, having tip deflection capability with dial controls on the head portion of the instrument. A hollow channel runs through the entire length of the instrument, and can be used to suction fluid or as a conduit for various therapeutic instruments such as wire loops for polyp removal, biopsy forceps, clips, injector needles, and electrocautery probes. Trumpet valves on the instrument control head deliver air, water to wash the lens, or suction to aspirate fluid. Late-generation scopes have an integrated water jet that washes the colon wall when needed.

Preparation of the colon

A **clean colon** is an absolute requirement for successful and meaningful colonoscopy (Figure 124.1). This can be accomplished with oral cathartics without the use of enemas. Most physicians utilize a 1-day clear liquid/low residue diet followed by a cathartic taken in "split dose," half on the evening before the procedure and the remainder 4–5 hours before colonoscopy on the day of the procedure. Using the balanced electrolyte solution, there is no net flux of fluid or electrolytes across the mucous membranes, so this is useful for patients with cardiac, hepatic, or renal failure or in those who cannot tolerate fluid loads. Two-liter polyethylene glycol preparations are also available [1]. Some cathartics, such as citrate of magnesia and milk of magnesia, stimulate transfer of fluid from the extracellular space into the colon lumen. The sodium phosphate preparations produce above average colon cleansing but have been associated with decreased renal function

Anatomy

The colon is approximately 6 feet long and infolded within the confines of the abdomen. The mesentery of the colon causes the sigmoid colon to be twisted and fixed in an S-shaped pattern, necessitating negotiation of the colonoscope through the loops and bends in this segment and then through multiple twists and turns in the rest of the colon in order to intubate its full length. The female colon is somewhat longer than the male colon, and is often in a generally smaller capacity abdominal cavity that also contains the uterus, fallopian tubes, and ovaries, resulting in more acute bends and twists than are found in the male colon [2].

Insertion

Advancing a 6-foot long instrument through the twists and turns of the colon to reach the cecum using torque and dial control is a formidable task, made more difficult in the presence of previous abdominal surgery where adhesions and fixations cause fixed looping of the colon. Intubation of the colon is accomplished by a series of maneuvers, including pulling on the instrument to straighten it, applying abdominal pressure to keep the scope straight, or withdrawing air to shorten the colon. The hand that is on the instrument shaft provides the important maneuvering capability for colonoscopy as it

---

Textbook of Clinical Gastroenterology and Hepatology, Second Edition. Edited by C. J. Hawkey, Jaime Bosch, Joel E. Richter, Guadalupe Garcia-Tsao, Francis K. L. Chan.
© 2012 Blackwell Publishing Ltd. Published 2012 by Blackwell Publishing Ltd.

Table 124.1 Procedures possible during colonoscopy

- Polypectomy
- Biopsy
- Injection
- Treatment:
  - Permanent marker of lesion (tattoo)
  - Increased safety of polypectomy
- Decompression
- Foreign body removal
- Hemostasis:
  - Clips
  - Epinephrine (adrenaline) injection
  - Electrocoagulation

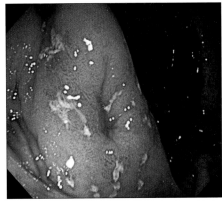

Figure 124.2 Crohn's disease of the ileocecal valve. Classical Crohn's disease is associated with small aphthous erosions, seen here around the orifice of the ileocecal valve. This is a view in retroversion, the instrument having made a U-turn in the cecal caput.

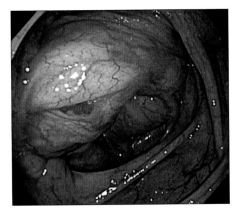

Figure 124.1 Arteriovenous malformation in the ascending colon. This cherry red vascular collection is an arteriovenous malformation, also called angiodysplasia. These occur in the right colon and can be a source for lower gastrointestinal bleeding.

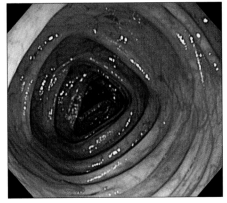

Figure 124.3 The transverse colon. This is the typical triangular appearance of the transverse colon, related to the anatomical limit to air distension provided by the three tinea coli, situated longitudinally at the angles of the triangle.

controls the insertion, withdrawal, and torquing right or left. The colonoscope is always advanced under visual control by the operator who observes several luminal details to find the direction in which the tip should be pointed.

Because colonoscopy can be an uncomfortable procedure, most examinations are performed with sedation, either an intravenous narcotic with a benzodiazepine, or with deeper anesthesia such as propofol [3,4]. There have been a few reports of water-filled colonoscopy (as opposed to air insufflation) being well tolerated without sedation [5].

Thoroughness of colonoscopy

During colonoscopy, the goal should be the evaluation of the colon from the rectum to the ileocecal valve. In flexible sigmoidoscopy, the usual extent of examination is to the proximal most portion of the sigmoid colon. For all colonoscopic examinations, there should be at least a 90% rate of reaching the cecum and a 95% cecal intubation rate in screening colonoscopies [6].

Although colonoscopy is the gold standard for colon evaluation, it is possible for an examiner to miss or to overlook lesions in the colon hidden behind acute angulations or in the valley of deep haustral folds. This problem of missed pathology has been addressed in several publications. The overall

miss rates for adenomas in earlier tandem studies were 15–24% [7–9]. A large multicenter European study [10] found that the miss rate for all polyps was 28%, for hyperplastic polyps 31%, and for adenomas 21%. However, for those equal to or larger than 5 mm, the miss rate for all polyps was 12% and for adenomas 9%.

Location of the instrument tip

There are only two fixed landmarks in the colon, the **anus** and the **ileocecal valve** (Figure 124.2). Fairly accurate estimates of the tip location throughout various parts of the colon can be made, but the visual identification of landmarks may be completely inadequate for precise determination of a lesion location when surgery is to be performed. During intubation of the left colon, the first identifiable landmark is the **splenic flexure** with its large amount of fluid. Acute angulation is usually present at this flexure after which a triangular segment of colon is entered (Figure 124.3). The **hepatic flexure** is heralded by a view of the flat bluish hue of the liver surface seen through the colon wall. The **ileocecal valve** (Figure 124.4) is often noted

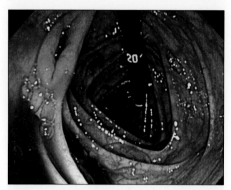

Figure 124.4 Retroversion in the ascending colon. A retroversion has been made in the cecum. The instrument is seen in the ascending colon where a good view can be obtained behind (on the proximal aspect) the colonic folds. The slit-like area at the 10 o'clock position is the ileocecal valve as seen in retroversion mode.

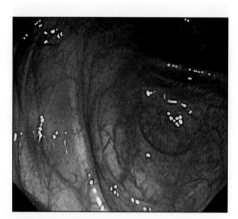

Figure 124.5 The appendiceal orifice. The most proximal portion of the colon is the cecal caput. The crescentic appendiceal orifice is seen at the base of the cecum, and the linear mucosal bands are a display of the tinea coli as they surround the appendix.

by its protuberant superior lip, and the **appendiceal orifice** as a crescentic fold in the cecal caput (Figure 124.5). The ileum can often be intubated, with the villi seen as small finger-like projections, the appearance of which is enhanced by water instillation (Figure 124.6).

Most modern endoscopists do not use fluoroscopy and rely on intracolonic landmarks to site the position of the instrument tip. A device called a "scope guide" is available that uses electromagnetic pulses from small electromagnets embedded in the instrument to reconstitute (by computer generation) the real-time colonoscope configuration throughout the colon without the need for radiation [11].

Because the colonoscopic landmarks are not specific and may not be easily recognized, it is often desirable and necessary to indelibly mark an area of pathology for subsequent surgical intervention, or if a polyp has been removed, a mark at the site may be of benefit for the gastroenterologist to locate that area on a subsequent examination [12] (see Video clip 124.1). In the past, these markings were accomplished using

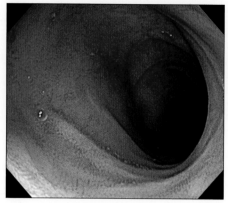

Figure 124.6 The terminal ileum. The distal small bowel can often be entered during colonoscopy. The irregular surface is caused by the tiny finger-like villi in the small intestine.

India ink, which has carbon particles in suspension but also shellac, stabilizers, antifungal agents, and other congeners. A prepackaged, presterilized, solution of pure carbon particles in suspension has been approved for presurgical marking of lesion sites.

Colonoscopic biopsy [13] (see Video clip 124.2)
There are several types of forceps for biopsies, some of which can take multiple biopsies while others are capable of taking large biopsies (jumbo forceps). If multiple biopsies are taken with a standard biopsy forceps, **crush artifact** from packing several bites into the forceps may render the squeezed tissue difficult to interpret. It is considered that not more than two biopsies should be compressed into a single forceps application. Significant bleeding does not occur from biopsy sites although the area of denuded tissue can readily be seen.

Biopsies should be carefully removed from the jaws of the forceps in order to prevent distortion of the tissue specimen. The tiny samples obtained are often only mucosa but may include muscularis mucosa and occasionally some submucosa. If multiple specimens are obtained from the same lesion, they may all be placed into the same container. However, in the case of inflammatory bowel disease, when multiple biopsies are taken from different stations throughout the colon, each set of biopsies should be placed in separate containers so that, if dysplasia is identified, the area from which it was obtained can be readily determined for subsequent re-evaluation or surgical intervention.

Colon polyps
Any excrescence that rises above the normal plane of the mucosa is a polypoid projection. Colon polyps can be non-neoplastic, such as inflammatory polyps, hyperplastic polyps, and cysts. Neoplastic polyps (or new mucosal growths) can be benign or malignant. The benign neoplastic polyps include tubular adenomas, tubulovillous adenomas, and villous adenomas. Since neoplastic polyps are considered to be precursors for colon cancer, it is important that when discovered, they are

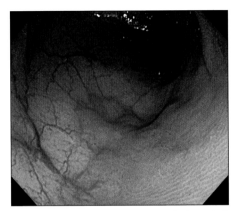

Figure 124.7 A flat lateral spreading adenoma. In the lower half of the photograph is a stellate flat polyp which was identified and removed colonoscopically. Flat lesions may be difficult to visualize on colonoscopy and on computed tomography. The proper nomenclature for this lesion is 0IIa LST. This was in the ascending colon and totally removed colonoscopically.

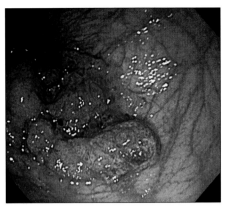

Figure 124.8 Benign rectal neoplasm. A large tubulovillous adenoma of the rectum that was removed in piecemeal fashion with endoscopic mucosal resection.

removed to prevent their subsequent growth into malignant polyps. In malignant polyps, cancer has invaded beyond the superficial muscular layer and into the submucosal tissue. If the degree of malignant invasion into the polyp is relatively minor, malignancy can often be cured by **colonoscopic polypectomy**, removing the polyp with an adequate margin of normal tissue. The criteria for when a malignant polyp requires an operative intervention are: the polyp is poorly differentiated, there is invasion of lymphatic or vascular channels, or the malignancy extends to the line of resection where the colonoscopy snare has cut across the base of the polyp [14].

Small polyps (<3 mm) can be successfully removed with the biopsy forceps, but larger polyps require **resection with a snare** (see Video clip 124.3). Polyps smaller than 5–6 mm may be guillotined with a "cold snare" where current is not applied as the snare cuts across the polyp [15]. These small polyps do not bleed when resected with the cold snare, but larger polyps usually require cauterization current to heat-seal blood vessels. The vast majority of polyps are benign, but there is a 5% probability that polyps may become malignant with time, and adenomas (premalignant polyps) should be removed when they are found.

Polyps may be pedunculated (on a stalk of variable length) or sessile, with a base flat on the wall. Some polyps are relatively flat (<2.5 mm in height) and detected by visual inspection of the colon with white light. Special techniques such as chromoendoscopy or narrow band imaging may enhance the ability to recognize the size and surface configurations of flat polyps. A morphological categorization of colon polyps (Figure 124.7) has recently been republished [16,17]. The safe removal of larger sessile polyps can be enhanced with the use of submucosal injection of fluid to expand the space since the distended colon wall is quite thin, varying in thickness from 1.4 to 2.3 mm in diameter [18,19]. The injected fluid [normal saline, hypertonic saline, with or without

epinephrine (adrenaline) or hyaluronidase] can expand the submucosal space several fold to create a safety cushion for application of cautery current so that a full thickness thermal injury of the wall will not occur as electrocoagulation current is applied. This technique of fluid injection and polypectomy is called **endoscopic mucosal resection (EMR)** (Figure 124.8). Oftentimes a large polyp can only safely be removed by resecting it in multiple pieces, a technique known as piecemeal polypectomy [20]. A procedure has been developed in Japan for resection of flat polyps or polyps that may not elevate with the submucosal injection of fluid [21]. In this technique of **endoscopic submucosal resection (ESD)**, a large volume of fluid is inserted under the edge of the polyp. The polyp is removed by tunneling into the edematous submucosal space beneath the entire polyp, providing a single large specimen for histopathological examination [22]. This is in contrast to the multiple pieces of tissue that can be recovered with EMR where the base or margins of the polyp may not be readily identified by the pathologist.

Withdrawal of the instrument

The ileocecal valve can often be intubated during the colonoscopic examination. A retroflexion maneuver can often be performed in the capacious right colon, and occasionally in the transverse colon. A retroflexion maneuver in the rectum should always be performed to completely visualize the distal most portion of the rectal ampulla.

In the absence of any pathology, extubation of the colon should be slow and deliberate, taking the time to evaluate the mucosal surface and areas behind folds [23,24]. The most common consideration is that withdrawal should take an average of 6 minutes from the cecum to the rectum [25]. It is important to discover and remove all significant polyps of the colon. Because of the rate of missed lesions during colonoscopy, a new device has recently been developed, the third eye retroscope [26,27]. This device is of slender caliber, and is inserted through the biopsy/instrument channel of a standard colonoscope. As it emerges from the instrument, the tip makes a 180-degree bend so that it looks backward toward the face-plate of the colonoscope. It carries its own lens system and LED light to illuminate the dark area behind the forward viewing colonoscope. A 25% greater yield of adenomas was found in patients when utilizing this disposable device [26].

Alternatives to colonoscopy

Guidelines for the detection and prevention of colon cancer have been issued by four different groups for screening and surveillance for the early prevention of colon cancer and adenomatous polyps[28–31]. The **flexible sigmoidoscopy test** is an inadequate test for screening for colorectal cancer, but is worthwhile for investigating symptoms that refer to the rectum. Stool tests for blood, the globin moiety of hemoglobin, or DNA have been reported to be relatively non-specific examinations. A positive result triggers a referral for colonoscopy. The most sensitive test to detect human blood in the fecal stream is the **fecal immunochemical test (FIT)**. All the guidelines include a screening option for the combination of flexible sigmoidoscopy and a test for blood in the stool. **Computed tomographic colonography (CTC)** is a radiographic procedure that, by computer simulation, produces a virtual view of the colon lumen with the generated image appearing somewhat similar to that with colonoscopy. The tremendous progress in technology will soon make this a feasible screening tool for the colon. When significant lesions are seen, colonoscopy is suggested for further identification and to obtain tissue for diagnosis or therapy.

Indications and contraindications

These are listed in Table 124.2.

Cost

Investigators have concluded that fecal occult blood testing, sigmoidoscopy, and colonoscopy are all cost-effective [32]. A

Table 124.2 Indications and contraindications for colonoscopy

---

Diagnostic
- Screening for colonic cancer
- Symptom evaluation
- Abnormal radiographic findings
- Surveillance of high-risk population (see Video clip 124.4)

Therapeutic
- Polyp removal
- Hemostasis
- Stricture dilation
- Foreign body removal (see Video clip 124.5)

Contraindications
- Peritonitis
- Acute diverticulitis or colitis
- Recent myocardial infarction or pulmonary embolism

---

conclusion in one article stated that "despite the absence of results from randomized trials, there is no doubt on the efficacy, effectiveness and cost-effectiveness of endoscopic screening for colorectal cancer."

Complications

The major complications with colonoscopy are perforation of the bowel, bleeding, and post-polypectomy syndrome following polypectomy. In the absence of biopsy or polypectomy, bleeding is not seen during diagnostic colonoscopy, and perforation is extremely rare. The incidence of perforation is 1 in 1400 for all colonoscopies and 1 in 1000 for therapeutic procedures [33]. Perforation is reported to occur in 0.04–2.1% of colonoscopic polypectomies [34].

The presence of free air following colonoscopy does not necessarily mandate surgical exploration if there are no signs or symptoms of peritoneal irritation. If a small perforation is noted during colonoscopic polypectomy, it may be safely closed with clips [35]. Laparoscopy can often repair a perforation with simple closure. The most common complication following polypectomy is **post-polypectomy bleeding** which can occur in approximately 2% of patients following resection of large sessile polyps. Immediate bleeding that occurs following polypectomy can almost always be controlled at the time of the procedure with injection, application of clips (see Video clip 124.6), or a thermal modality, such as a heater probe, bipolar electrodes, or the argon plasma coagulator. Delayed bleeding can occur up to 2 weeks following polypectomy, and may require repeat colonoscopy to provide hemostasis.

Future directions

White light endoscopy has been the method of illumination of the hollow organs with flexible endoscopes since they were first introduced. It has been found that **chromoendoscopy** [36] or colored liquid sprayed on the surface of the bowel can enhance the visual surface characteristics by pooling in crevices and outlining the extent of lesions somewhat better than can be achieved with white light (see Video clip 124.7). A new electronic method to enhance mucosal and lesion visualization is mechanical chromoendoscopy. In this procedure, one or more specific bands or wavelengths of the white light spectrum is substituted for the normal white light source by pressing a button on the endoscope. The use of narrow bands of light [narrow band imaging (NBI)] enhances the vascular pattern of the mucosal surface and can aid in distinguishing various types of polyps even prior to receiving the pathologist's report [37].

Confocal endomicroscopy [36] employs a miniature microscope on the tip of a dedicated colonoscope, or built into a probe that can be inserted through the instrument channel. This technique is used to detect cytological and nuclear abnormalities that cannot be seen with standard endoscopes, even those with zoom functions. **Optical coherence tomography**

(OCT) uses reflected light to visualize the superficial mucosal crypts and their organization. OCT has been shown to distinguish benign from malignant morphology [38].

Endocytoscopy [39] uses high-power magnification in a catheter probe to enhance the visualization of surface cells to assess their morphology. This device provides near-histological images for diagnostic purposes and is different from "zoom colonoscopy" which magnifies the endoscopic image to 150 times.

Instruments being developed include those with a disposable sheath. The disposable aer-o-scope uses insufflated gas to push a balloon through the colon. A camera-like lens on the balloon has a tethering wire connected to a video processor. This device requires no active input from physicians who may see the transmitted images in real-time or view the stored images later [40]. The invendoscope, also disposable, uncoils an enfolded sheath to carry the endoscope through the colon without friction on the mucosal surface. The tip is deflected by differential water pressure controlled by the operator and does not require sedation [41].

The small bowel capsule, introduced several years ago, has become the most valuable instrument for visualization and diagnosis of conditions in the small intestine. A **colon capsule** is currently available, constructed on the same basis as the small bowel capsule. This "mini-endoscope" takes two images every second from each forward and rear viewing camera, with images transmitted to sensors on the external abdominal wall that are stored on a mini-computer so pictures can be inspected following completion of the examination. Capsule colonoscopy is in its infancy and, although a recent report has shown it is not comparable to colonoscopy [42], further developments will likely make this non-invasive procedure another tool for inspection of the colon.

References

1. Park SS, Sinn DH, Kim YH, *et al*. Efficacy and tolerability of split-dose magnesium citrate: low-volume (2 liters) polyethylene glycol vs. single- or split-dose polyethylene glycol bowel preparation for morning colonoscopy. *Am J Gastroenterol*. 2010;105: 1319–1326.
2. Saunders BP, Fukumoto M, Halligan S, *et al*. Why is colonoscopy more difficult in women? *Gastrointest Endosc*. 1996;43:124–126.
3. Ladas SD, Satake Y, Mostafa I, Morse J. Sedation practices for gastrointestinal endoscopy in Europe, North America, Asia, Africa and Australia. *Digestion*. 2010;82:74–76.
4. Cohen LB, Ladas SD, Vargo JJ, *et al*. Sedation in digestive endoscopy: the Athens international position statement. *Aliment Pharmacol Ther*. 2010;32:425–442.
5. Leung JW, Mann SK, Siao-Salera R, *et al*. A randomized, controlled comparison of warm water infusion in lieu of air insufflation versus air insufflation for aiding colonoscopy insertion in sedated patients undergoing colorectal cancer screening and surveillance. *Gastrointest Endosc*. 2009;70:505–510.
6. Rex DK, Bond JH, Winawer S, *et al*; U.S. Multi-Society Task Force on Colorectal Cancer. Quality in the technical performance of colonoscopy and the continuous quality improvement process for colonoscopy: recommendations of the U.S. Multi-Society Task Force on Colorectal Cancer. *Am J Gastroenterol*. 2002;97: 1296–1308.
7. Hixson LJ, Fennerty MB, Sampliner RE, Garewal HS. Prospective blinded trial of the colonoscopic miss-rate of large colorectal polyps. *Gastrointest Endosc*. 1991;37:125–127.
8. Rex DK, Cutler CS, Lemmel GT, *et al*. Colonoscopic miss rates of adenomas determined by back-to-back colonoscopies. *Gastroenterology*. 1997;112:24–28.
9. Benson VS, Patnick J, Davies AK, Nadel MR, Smith RA, Atkin WS; International Colorectal Cancer Screening Network. Colorectal cancer screening: a comparison of 35 initiatives in 17 countries. *Int J Cancer*. 2008;122:1357–1367.
10. Heresbach D, Barrioz T, Lapalus MG, *et al*. Miss rate for colorectal neoplastic polyps: a prospective multicenter study of back-to-back video colonoscopies. *Endoscopy*. 2008;40:284–290.
11. Hoff G, Bretthauer M, Dahler S, *et al*. Improvement in caecal intubation rate and pain reduction by using 3-dimensional magnetic imaging for unsedated colonoscopy: a randomized trial of patients referred for colonoscopy. *Scand J Gastroenterol*. 2007;42: 885–889.
12. Askin MP, Waye JD, Fiedler L, Harpaz N. Tattoo of colonic neoplasms in 113 patients with a new sterile carbon compound. *Gastrointest Endosc*. 2002;56:339–342.
13. Weinstein WM. Colonoscopic Biopsy. In: Waye JD, Rex DK, Williams CB, editors *Colonoscopy: Principles and Practice*, 2nd edn. London: Blackwell Scientific., 2009.
14. Ramirez M, Schierling S, Papaconstantinou HT, Scott Thomas J. Management of the malignant polyp. *Clin Colon Rectal Surg*. 2008;21:286–290.
15. Tappero G, Gaia E, De Giuli P, Martini S, Gubetta L, Emanuelli G. Cold snare excision of small colorectal polyps. *Gastrointest Endosc*. 1992;38:310–313.
16. The Paris endoscopic classification of superficial neoplastic lesions: esophagus, stomach, and colon: November 30 to December 1, 2002. *Gastrointest Endosc*. 2003;58:S3–43.
17. Lambert R, Kudo SE, Vieth M, *et al*. Pragmatic classification of superficial neoplastic colorectal lesions. *Gastrointest Endosc*. 2009; 70:1182–1199.
18. Gast P, Belaiche J. Rectal endosonography in inflammatory bowel disease: differential diagnosis and prediction of remission. *Endoscopy*. 1999;31:158–166.
19. Tsuga K, Haruma K, Fujimura J, *et al*. Evaluation of the colorectal wall in normal subjects and patients with ulcerative colitis using an ultrasonic catheter probe. *Gastrointest Endosc*. 1998;48: 477–484.
20. Tanaka S, Oka S, Chayama K, Kawashima K. Knack and practical technique of colonoscopic treatment focused on endoscopic mucosal resection using snare. *Dig Endosc*. 2009;21:S38–42.
21. Bourke M. Current status of colonic endoscopic mucosal resection in the west and the interface with endoscopic submucosal dissection. *Dig Endosc*. 2009;21:S22–27.
22. Yoshida N, Yagi N, Naito Y, Yoshikawa T. Safe procedure in endoscopic submucosal dissection for colorectal tumors focused on preventing complications. *World J Gastroenterol*. 2010;16: 1688–1695.
23. Taber A, Romagnuolo J. Effect of simply recording colonoscopy withdrawal time on polyp and adenoma detection rates. *Gastrointest Endosc*. 2010;71:782–786.
24. Barclay RL, Vicari JJ, Greenlaw RL. Effect of a time-dependent colonoscopic withdrawal protocol on adenoma detection during

screening colonoscopy. *Clin Gastroenterol Hepatol.* 2008;6: 1091–1098.

25. Rex DK, Bond JH, Winawer S, *et al*; U.S. Multi-Society Task Force on Colorectal Cancer. Quality in the technical performance of colonoscopy and the continuous quality improvement process for colonoscopy: recommendations of the U.S. Multi-Society Task Force on Colorectal Cancer. *Am J Gastroenterol.* 2002;97: 1296–1308.

26. Waye JD, Heigh RI, Fleischer DE, *et al*. A retrograde-viewing device improves detection of adenomas in the colon: a prospective efficacy evaluation (with videos). *Gastrointest Endosc.* 2010; 71:551–556.

27. DeMarco DC, Odstrcil E, Lara LF, *et al*. Impact of experience with a retrograde-viewing device on adenoma detection rates and withdrawal times during colonoscopy: the Third Eye Retroscope study group. *Gastrointest Endosc.* 2010;71:542–550.

28. U.S. Preventive Services Task Force. Screening for colorectal cancer: U.S. Preventive Services Task Force recommendation statement. *Ann Intern Med.* 2008;149:627–637.

29. Rex DK, Johnson DA, Anderson JC, Schoenfeld PS, Burke CA, Inadomi JM; American College of Gastroenterology. American College of Gastroenterology guidelines for colorectal cancer screening 2009. *Am J Gastroenterol.* 2009;104:739–750.

30. Davila RE, Rajan E, Baron TH, *et al*; Standards of Practice Committee, American Society for Gastrointestinal Endoscopy. ASGE guideline: colorectal cancer screening and surveillance. *Gastrointest Endosc.* 2006;63:546–557.

31. Levin B, Lieberman DA, McFarland B, *et al*; American Cancer Society Colorectal Cancer Advisory Group; US Multi-Society Task Force; American College of Radiology Colon Cancer Committee. Screening and surveillance for the early detection of colorectal cancer and adenomatous polyps, 2008: a joint guideline from the American Cancer Society, the US Multi-Society Task Force on Colorectal Cancer, and the American College of Radiology. *Gastroenterology.* 2008;134:1570–1595.

32. Brenner H. Efficacy, effectiveness and cost-effectiveness of endoscopic screening methods. *Z Gastroenterol.* 2008;46:S20–S22.

33. Panteris V, Haringsma J, Kuipers EJ. Colonoscopy perforation rate, mechanisms and outcome: from diagnostic to therapeutic colonoscopy. *Endoscopy.* 2009;41:941–951.

34. Araujo SE, Seid VE, Caravatto PP, Dumarco R. Incidence and management of colonoscopic colon perforations: 10 years' experience. *Hepatogastroenterology.* 2009;56:1633–1636.

35. Trecca A, Gaj F, Gagliardi G. Our experience with endoscopic repair of large colonoscopic perforations and review of the literature. *Tech Coloproctol.* 2008;12:315–321.

36. Wallace MB, Kiesslich R. Advances in endoscopic imaging of colorectal neoplasia. *Gastroenterology.* 2010;138:2140–2150.

37. Higashi R, Uraoka T, Kato J, *et al*. Diagnostic accuracy of narrow-band imaging and pit pattern analysis significantly improved for less-experienced endoscopists after an expanded training program. *Gastrointest Endosc.* 2010;72:127–135.

38. Hatta W, Uno K, Koike T, *et al*. Optical coherence tomography for the staging of tumor infiltration in superficial esophageal squamous cell carcinoma. *Gastrointest Endosc.* 2010;71:899–906.

39. ASGE Technology Committee, Kwon RS, Wong Kee Song LM, *et al*. Endocytoscopy. *Gastrointest Endosc.* 2009;70:610–613.

40. Arber N, Grinshpon R, Pfeffer J, Maor L, Bar-Meir S, Rex D. Proof-of-concept study of the Aer-O-Scope omnidirectional colonoscopic viewing system in ex vivo and in vivo porcine models. *Endoscopy.* 2007;39:412–417.

41. Rösch T, Adler A, Pohl H, *et al*. A motor-driven single-use colonoscope controlled with a hand-held device: a feasibility study in volunteers. *Gastrointest Endosc.* 2008;67:1139–1146.

42. Spada C, Riccioni ME, Hassan C, Petruzziello L, Cesaro P, Costamagna G. PillCam colon capsule endoscopy: A prospective, randomized trial comparing two regimens of preparation. *J Clin Gastroenterol.* 2011;45:119–124.

CHAPTER 125
Endoscopic ultrasonography

V. Raman Muthusamy and Kenneth J. Chang
University of California, Irvine, CA, USA

KEY POINTS

- Endoscopic ultrasonography uses a combination of endoscopy and high-frequency ultrasound
- Endoscopic ultrasonography is performed with radial and linear echoendoscopes or catheter-based ultrasound probes
- Radial echoendoscopes give up to a 360°-ultrasonographic image perpendicular to the axis of the echoendoscope and many are capable of performing Doppler imaging and color flow mapping
- Linear echoendoscopes give up to a 180° image parallel to the axis of the echoendoscope, allowing for the performance of fine needle aspiration or injection
- Catheter-based ultrasonographic probes are useful for imaging small mucosal or submucosal lesions and can be passed through the accessory channel of a standard endoscope
- Ultrasonographic imaging is facilitated by water filling a balloon around the acoustic tip of the echoendoscope, a process called acoustic coupling
- Imaging a lesion requires very fine scope tip movements and repeated back and forth scanning
- Successful performance of endoscopic ultrasonography is best accomplished by the presence of a dedicated team of physicians, nurses, and technical assistants

Introduction and scientific basis

Endoscopic ultrasonography (EUS) was originally developed in the early 1980s as an alternative diagnostic imaging modality to address the inherent limitations of transcutaneous ultrasonography, such as the limited depth of penetration and image interference from intra-abdominal gas and bony structures [1]. With the development of linear-array echoendoscopes and the incorporation of fine needle aspiration (FNA) and color flow and Doppler data, the technique has moved from a purely diagnostic study to a procedure with interventional capabilities.

The principles of EUS are based on the development and interpretation of ultrasound waves. High-frequency ultrasound waves are transmitted from the transducer at the tip of the echoendoscope to the target tissue. For optimal imaging, a balloon surrounding the transducer is inflated with water to improve ultrasound transmission. This process is known as **acoustic coupling**. Images are constructed from the reflective properties of the tissue components and utilize real-time imaging techniques similar to a B-mode (brightness

modulation) display format. The brightness is dependent on the amount reflected. Intensely reflected areas appear white (hyperechoic), whereas areas of low reflection appear dark (hypoechoic). This allows for high-resolution imaging of the five histological layers of the gastrointestinal wall and the surrounding structures. EUS and EUS-guided FNA are highly accurate procedures in the diagnosis and treatment of many gastrointestinal diseases.

Equipment and setup

Ultrasonographic endoscopes have become smaller and lighter, and have been coupled with better image resolution, due in large part to the increasing use of electronic transducers on the echoendoscopes. Available equipment is listed in Table 125.1.

Radial echoendoscopes

These scopes can be oblique viewing, similar to a duodenoscope, or provide a straight view, similar to a standard endoscope. Radial instruments utilize either a mechanical or an electronic rotating transducer that allows a 360°-ultrasonographic image that is perpendicular to the axis plane of the echoendoscope (Figure 125.1). In the esophagus, this gives a spatial orientation of the image similar to that obtained with computed tomography (CT). Current radial echoendoscopes have the ability to switch frequencies from 5 MHz up to 20 MHz to optimize imaging. The depth of penetration and image resolution are inversely proportional to and dependent on the frequency of ultrasound wave transmission. High-frequency ultrasound (20 MHz) has a tissue penetration of only 2 cm and is useful for mucosal and submucosal imaging, as opposed to lower frequency (5–7.5 MHz) transmission that has a tissue penetration depth of 8 cm and is useful for imaging extraluminal surrounding structures. The main limitation of the radial echoendoscope is its inability to perform safely FNA because the needle path cannot be tracked accurately. Newer models have allowed forward viewing, enabling the performance of standard endoscopy at the time of EUS without the need for a second scope, and have utilized electronic transducers that can provide color flow and Doppler imaging.

Textbook of Clinical Gastroenterology and Hepatology, Second Edition. Edited by C. J. Hawkey, Jaime Bosch, Joel E. Richter, Guadalupe Garcia-Tsao, Francis K. L. Chan.
© 2012 Blackwell Publishing Ltd. Published 2012 by Blackwell Publishing Ltd.

Table 125.1 Endoscopic ultrasound echoendoscopes

Echoendoscope	Scanning frequency (MHz)	Channel diameter (mm)	Scanning range (degrees)	Processor
Olympus				
Radial				
GF-UE160	5–10	2.2	360	Aloka SSD-5000, SSD-α5
GF-UM160	5–20	2.2	360	EU-M60, EU-M30
Linear				
GF-UC140P	5–10	2.8	180	Aloka SSD-5000
GF-UCT140	5–10	3.7	180	Aloka SSD-5000
Pentax				
Radial				
EG-3630UR	5–10	2.4	270	Hitachi Hi-Vision 5500
EG-3670URK	5–10	2.4	360	Hitachi Hi-Vision 5500
Linear				
EG-3830UT	5–10	3.8	120	Hitachi Hi-Vision 5500
EG-3870UTK	5–10	3.8	120	Hitachi Hi-Vision 5500

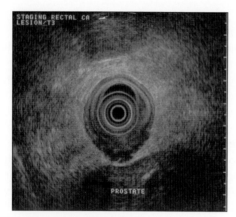

Figure 125.1 EUS of rectal cancer. Radial image of an anteriorly located T3 rectal cancer without invasion of the prostate.

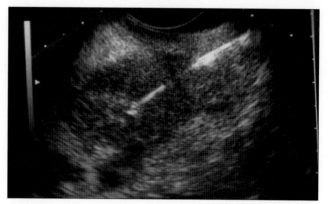

Figure 125.2 EUS-guided FNA of a pancreatic mass. Linear image of a hypoechoic, irregularly-shaped pancreatic neck mass undergoing FNA with a 25 G needle.

Linear echoendoscopes

Linear-array echoendoscopes permit the performance of FNA. The ultrasound transducer generates a 100–180° image that is parallel to the shaft of the echoendoscope, allowing for full visualization of a needle that is passed through the working channel of the device. The anatomic orientation is at an angle of 90° to the radial anatomy. Linear echoendoscopes have a frequency range of 5–10 MHz. The needle for FNA can be tracked in its entirety from exiting the biopsy channel to entering and aspirating the target lesion (Figure 125.2). Linear echoendoscopes also provide the ability for color flow and Doppler imaging to choose a FNA needle path that avoids vascular structures by combining simultaneous real-time ultrasonography with Doppler ability. Many institutions now use these devices as the primary tool when a 360° ultrasonograpic view is not needed, such as when pancreatic or biliary imaging (Figure 125.3) is the primary focus of the EUS exam.

Probes

Catheter-based ultrasonography probes are used for high-frequency ultrasonographic imaging of lesions that are within 2 cm of the transducer. The probes (12–30 MHz) are easily passed through the biopsy channel of a standard upper endoscope and give a 360° image in a plane similar to that of radial echoendoscopes. Imaging with the probe is accomplished either by filling the lumen of the target lesion with water or, in areas such as the esophagus, by imaging through a water-filled latex condom attached to the endoscope, so as to lower the risk of potential aspiration. Another option in this setting is to use a catheter probe pre-fitted with a balloon sheath that can be insufflated with water. As radial echoendoscopes have evolved to incorporate high-frequency capabilities, the use of catheter probes appears best limited to small lesions that may not be visualized with a radial device and that are best localized with a standard endoscope and interrogated using a

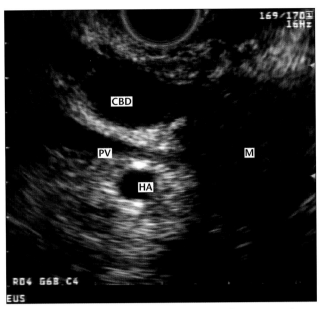

Figure 125.3 EUS of pancreatic cancer. Linear image of a T3 pancreatic cancer (M) with invasion of the common bile duct (CBD) and portal vein (PV). HA, hepatic artery.

catheter probe that can overlay the lesion under direct endoscopic visualization. Other types of available probes include **rigid rectal probes** that can evaluate internal and external anal sphincter defects or **over-the-guidewire probes** used at endoscopic retrograde cholangiopancreatography (ERCP) to evaluate lesions causing pancreatic or biliary ductal obstruction. Newer-generation probes also have the capability of two- and three-dimensional reconstruction of images.

Room set-up and nursing personnel

Depending on the volume of the procedure unit, a dedicated room may or may not be necessary. Having two monitors side by side to display the endoscopic and ultrasonographic images simultaneously is ideal. In general, the processor console should be within comfortable finger distance of the endosonographer to optimize picture capturing, labeling, resolution, and Doppler usage.

EUS can be performed under moderate sedation, but many institutions choose to perform these procedures with the use of anesthesia assistance given the increased procedure duration associated with EUS. Nurses with special skills and dedicated training in assisting with EUS procedures are strongly recommended. If anesthesia personnel are not providing sedation, when the procedure involves FNA, a second nurse or technical assistant who is knowledgeable about the procedure and the processing of the obtained tissue specimen is needed.

Technique

The endosonographer must be able to recognize the key anatomic landmarks. The first important step is to secure a balloon

around the transducer at the tip of the echoendoscope. The balloon is inflated and deflated with water to check for leaks. In the esophagus the balloon is re-inflated with water. Constant intermittent suctioning and removal of intraluminal air is necessary because air is relatively impenetrable to ultrasound waves and causes imaging artifacts.

When the lesion or organ of focus is found, the echoendoscope is passed back and forth over this area; changing ultrasound frequencies helps to achieve maximal image resolution. For superficial lesions, it is important not to compress the lesion with the ultrasound balloon as this may cause incorrect imaging and overstaging. The easiest structures to image initially are the esophagus and rectum because of the minimal scope manipulation required to maintain orientation. The major structures seen and their corresponding scope position are reviewed in Table 125.2.

Table 125.2 Scope position and corresponding major structures

Location	Structures
Proximal esophagus	Spine, trachea, carotid artery, thyroid, aortic arch, subclavian artery
Mid-esophagus	Trachea, carina, main bronchi, spine, SVC, descending aorta, azygous, thoracic duct, PV
Distal esophagus	Left atrium, left ventricle, right atrium, left atrium, liver, IVC, spine, descending aorta
Gastric fundus	Pancreatic tail, spleen, splenic artery, splenic vein, left kidney, left adrena
Gastric body	Pancreatic body, splenic vein, splenic artery, celiac axis, hepatic artery, SMA
Gastric antrum	Pancreatic neck, gallbladder, liver, splenic vein, confluence
Duodenal bulb	Pancreatic head, splenic vein, portal vein, confluence, CBD, gallbladder, liver, hepatic artery
Second portion of duodenum	Pancreatic head, CBD, IVC, confluence, SMA, ampulla, uncinate
Third portion of duodenum	Pancreatic body, IVC, descending aorta
Anal canal	Internal and external sphincters
Rectum (male)	Prostate, bladder, seminal vesicles, urethra
Rectum (female)	Uterus, vagina, bladder, urethra
Sigmoid colon	Iliac vessels

CBD, common bile duct; IVC, inferior vena cava; PV, pulmonary vessels; SMA, superior mesenteric artery; SVC, superior vena cava.

Performing fine needle aspiration

FNA, guided by EUS, has brought the technique to the forefront in the diagnosis and staging of gastrointestinal malignancies. FNA is especially challenging for pancreatic masses. Maximization of FNA yield is dependent on prioritizing the sequence of FNA with multiple lesions, needle choice, optimizing needle technique, onsite cytopathological interpretation, and the avoidance of complications. The technique of EUS-guided FNA has been described previously [2]. The most commonly used needle size remains the 22G, although some data indicate that a smaller needle (25G) may improve diagnostic yield in patients with suspected pancreatic malignancies [3,4]. A 19G needle may also be more appropriate for certain lesions, such as smooth muscle tumors or when a large amount of fluid is to be aspirated.

The technique involves having the lesion to be biopsied placed in the center or just to the left of center in the imaging field. If there is concern regarding surrounding vascular structures, Doppler imaging can be used to better define potential vessels; this may necessitate finding a different needletrack. The needle is then advanced through the biopsy channel and can be seen exiting the biopsy channel into the lesion under real-time ultrasonography. Once in position, the central stylet is removed and, typically, a 10-mL syringe is attached to the hub of the needle and suction is applied as to and fro movements are made within the lesion. Suction is then released and the needle withdrawn. The cytological specimen is then processed and sprayed on glass slides, and can be immediately reviewed by a cytopathology technician or cytopathologist, if available. Remaining material can be placed in formalin, which is then processed into a cell block for further review. It appears that maximal diagnostic yield is obtained with the presence of onsite cytopathology to determine specimen adequacy and to obtain a preliminary diagnosis [5]. If the first few passes reveal necrotic tissue, aiming for the periphery of the lesion may be necessary to obtain a diagnosis.

The optimal technique for advancing the needle is dependent on three factors: (1) the consistency of the gastrointestinal wall (**wall parameter**); (2) the size and consistency of the lesion targeted (**lesion parameter**); and (3) the proximity of surrounding vessels (**vessel parameter**). Needle advancement techniques are individualized according to these parameters for a given region or organ. When there is more than one lesion to biopsy in a patient, the prioritization of lesions becomes important to avoid specimen contamination and improve procedural efficiency. For example, if when staging a pancreatic cancer, ascites or a liver lesion is found, this should be biopsied first because it will give the most advanced stage information. In addition, biopsy of a liver lesion is more efficient because it typically requires only one or two passes [6], compared with a pancreatic mass that typically requires three to five passes, to obtain a diagnosis [7].

Indications

Tumor diagnosis and staging

Table 125.3 gives the current tumor node metastasis (TNM) classification of tumors.

Esophagus

Accurate staging of **esophageal cancer** is important because of the multimodality treatment approach (see Chapter 30). EUS is the most accurate imaging modality for determining the extent of local and regional spread. The diagnostic accuracy by EUS alone is 85% for T and 75% for N stage. The addition of FNA increases the N staging accuracy to greater than 90% [8]. Obstructing esophageal tumors that preclude the passage of an echoendoscope are most likely T3 or T4 lesions; however, if information on tumor length, gastric pathology, or the presence or absence of celiac nodes is desired, then endoscopic dilatation can be performed. This is best carried out over two to three sessions to lessen the risk of perforation. Alternatively, passage of an EUS catheter probe through the stenotic region may provide similar information, with some lower-frequency catheters even able to provide limited information regarding the presence of lymphadenopathy adjacent to and distal to the lesion.

With increased use of neoadjuvant treatment in patients with local or regional advanced esophageal cancer, EUS has also been employed to restage patients prior to surgical therapy. One of the limitations of EUS here is in differentiating residual cancer from post-treatment inflammation or fibrosis. FNA may help to achieve this distinction. It appears that

Table 125.3 TNM classification system

Primary tumor (T)	
TX	Primary tumor cannot be assessed
T0	No evidence of primary tumor
Tis	Carcinoma *in situ*
T1, T2, T3, T4	Increasing size and/or local extent of primary tumor
Regional lymph nodes (N)	
Nx	Regional lymph nodes cannot be assessed
N0	No regional lymph node metastasis
N1, N2, N3	Increasing involvement of regional lymph nodes
Distant metastasis (M)	
Mx	Distant metastasis cannot be assessed
M0	No distant metastasis
M1	Distant metastasis

assessing residual tumor volume instead of T and N stages may be more accurate and predictive of response to treatment.

EUS has an increasing role in the evaluation of patients with **Barrett's esophagus** (see Chapter 29) with high-grade dysplasia or early esophageal cancers. This is primarily in detecting invasion into the submucosa or beyond that would preclude an attempt at endoscopic eradication therapies due to the high risk of the presence of micrometastases in adjacent lymph nodes in such patients [9]. For those without evidence of deeper invasion on EUS, endoscopic eradication techniques such as mucosal resection or ablation may be attempted in those who do not desire or are not candidates for surgical therapy.

Lung

EUS-guided FNA is an attractive option for staging compared to transbronchial needle aspiration because of the relative safety and minimal invasiveness. The accuracy of EUS-guided FNA of lymph nodes in the setting of lung cancer is 94–100% [10]. EUS in this setting is limited to imaging the posterior mediastinum and is specifically helpful for **accessing lymph nodes** in the subcarinal, paraesophageal, and aortopulmonary regions. Even with the development of endobronchial ultrasound (EBUS), these regions are still not well visualized by this technique, and the combination of EBUS and EUS may provide improved staging accuracy compared to either technique alone [11].

Stomach

EUS is highly accurate in staging **gastric adenocarcinoma and lymphoma**, and in the evaluation of **thickened gastric folds** (see Chapters 34–36). Using a combination of EUS and catheter-based ultrasonography, the accuracy for T stage is approximately 80% and that for N stage 70%. This approach may define a subgroup of patients with early gastric cancer confined to the mucosa or submucosa who may be treated non-operatively with removal by endoscopic mucosal resection or endoscopic submucosal dissection (see Chapter 149) [12]. Tumors that obstruct or bleed require surgical resection for palliation, regardless of preoperative staging. In these situations, EUS findings would probably not alter management. In cases without bleeding or obstruction, EUS can significantly impact the patient's clinical course (such as finding ascites or identifying tumor extension into the liver or pancreas).

Pancreas

EUS imaging is the most sensitive test to **detect small pancreatic lesions**, particularly those that are <2 cm and may be missed by standard radiological imaging (see Video clip 125.1). In addition, EUS-guided FNA is the most accurate diagnostic modality for **diagnosing and staging pancreatic masses**. In 185 patients with pancreatic masses and negative tissue sampling by ERCP or negative CT-guided FNA, EUS-guided FNA had a sensitivity of 94% and accuracy of 92% for detecting malignant disease in patients with negative ERCP tissue sampling, and 90% sensitivity and 84% accuracy in patients with negative CT-guided biopsy [13]. EUS-guided celiac plexus neurolysis can be performed for poorly controlled pancreatic cancer pain at the same session. It is safer and more effective than traditional approaches [14]. **EUS-assisted cyst aspiration** and fluid analysis for cytology and estimation of amylase and carcinoembryonic antigen levels can help differentiate between a benign pseudocyst and a cystic neoplasm (see Chapter 72).

Rectum

EUS appears to have an important role, similar to its use in esophageal cancer, in the staging of rectal cancer to determine surgical approach and the need for neoadjuvant/ adjuvant therapy. The accuracy of rectal cancer staging approaches 80–85% for T stage and 70–80% for N stage [15].

Bile duct and ampulla

EUS is more accurate than CT and transabdominal ultrasonography for local staging of **cholangiocarcinoma and ampullary cancers**. Intraductal ultrasonography (IDUS) can improve the staging of T1 cholangiocarcinomas and distinguish between benign and malignant biliary strictures [16]. Additional data have shown EUS-guided FNA to improve diagnostic yield in patients with suspected cholangiocarcinoma but negative brush cytology at ERCP [17–20].

Benign disease
Pancreatitis

One of the more common referral indications for EUS is to diagnose **chronic pancreatitis** (see Chapter 70) in patients with unexplained chronic upper abdominal pain. EUS is most helpful when the pancreas is completely normal or greatly abnormal with more than five or six abnormal EUS criteria, with the most strongly predictive EUS criteria being the presence of calcifications [21].

Bile duct stones

In patients with an intermediate probability for stone disease, EUS is extremely accurate, sensitive, and specific in diagnosing **choledocholithiasis** [22]. Use of EUS as the initial diagnostic test limits the risk of complications associated with more invasive tests (e.g. ERCP) in patients who have documented disease (see Chapter 74). ERCP can be performed during the same procedure setting in those patients with common bile duct stones detected on EUS.

Submucosal lesions

EUS is an excellent modality for evaluation of the array of submucosal lesions found during routine endoscopy. EUS can characterize the shape, size, echotexture, and layer of origin; the most commonly identified lesion is a **gastrointestinal stromal tumor (GIST)**. EUS-guided FNA, however, cannot stratify the malignant potential of identified stromal tumors. Hypoechoic lesions greater than 3 cm with heterogeneous architecture and irregular borders that from the muscularis propria have a higher malignant potential and should be resected surgically [23].

Rectum

Using either rigid probes or conventional radial echoendoscopes, EUS can detect structural abnormalities of the internal and external anal sphincters in patients with **fecal incontinence** (see Chapter 68). This can be performed easily without the need for sedation.

Interventional endoscopic ultrasound

Initial interventional EUS procedures included EUS-guided celiac plexus neurolysis and EUS-guided botulinum toxin injection. The success of these procedures, particularly celiac plexus neurolysis, opened the door to more advanced interventional procedures, including EUS-guided pseudocyst drainage and EUS-guided cholangiopancreatography and ductal decompression techniques. Among the most exciting potential application for EUS is the use of EUS-guided fine needle injection to deliver antitumor agents in patients with locally advanced cancer. Our institution has demonstrated the feasibility and safety of performing antitumor injection therapy under EUS guidance in patients with locally advanced pancreatic cancer [24]. Further trials are under way for locally advanced pancreatic and esophageal cancer, and a case of such therapy leading to a complete pathological response has been reported [25]. EUS has also been used to ablate mucinous pancreatic cysts via alcohol injection, place fiducial markers to assist image-guided radiation therapy, and to place brachytherapy seeds [26,27].

Contraindications

The contraindications to performing EUS are similar to those of conventional endoscopy and the preps are similar. Because of the longer procedure time and increased sedation requirement, some patients (e.g., those with sleep apnea, neurological disorders) should have the procedure performed by an anesthesiologist, administering either moderate sedation, monitored anesthesia care, or general anesthesia.

Table 125.4 summarizes the current indications and potential contraindications for performing EUS.

Complications and their management

The overall complication rate of performing diagnostic EUS is similar to that of standard endoscopy [28]. One complication with a slightly higher frequency than standard endoscopy is **hypopharyngeal–cervical perforation** during intubation [29]. This is most likely due to the longer rigid tip of the EUS scope. The major complications of EUS occur when FNA is performed, especially of cystic lesions; the overall rate of EUS complications is 1.6–2% [28,30–32]. The most common complications include hemorrhage, infection, perforation, and pancreatitis. Antibiotic prophylaxis and treatment for 3–5 days

Table 125.4 Indications and contraindications for endoscopic ultrasound

Current indications
- Staging of esophageal cancer
- Restaging esophageal cancer
- Staging of lung cancer
- Staging of gastric cancer (in selected cases)
- Detection, diagnosis, and staging of pancreatic cancer
- Staging of rectal cancer
- Evaluation of submucosal masses
- Assessment of anal sphincter integrity
- Evaluation of benign pancreatic and biliary disease
- Celiac plexus neurolysis
- Pancreatic pseudocyst drainage

Emerging interventional indications
- Access and drainage of complicated biliary and pancreatic ductal system obstruction
- Pancreatic cyst ablation
- Placement of fiducial markers prior to image-guided radiation therapy
- Direct intratumoral injection of antitumor therapies
- Injection of brachytherapy seeds

Absolute contraindications
- Lack of patient cooperation
- Known or suspected perforated viscus
- Acute diverticulitis
- Fulminant colitis

Relative contraindications
- High-grade esophageal stricture
- Unstable cardiac or pulmonary conditions

Relative contraindications to fine needle aspiration
- Vascular structures in needle path
- Coagulopathy

afterwards should be given for FNA of cystic lesions of the pancreas and mediastinum [30]. While antibiotics have also typically been recommended for FNA of rectal lesions and perirectal masses, a recent study found no increased risk of bacteremia with EUS-guided FNA compared to diagnostic rectal EUS [33]. Avoidance of vascular structures has been mentioned previously. Complications secondary to EUS-guided FNA generally occur within the first 24 hours. Submucosal hemorrhage or a hemorrhagic FNA should prompt admission and careful monitoring, and possibly surgical consultation. However, persistent bleeding from EUS-guided FNA is exceedingly rare and is usually self-limited [32].

Cost-effectiveness

Many studies have shown that EUS incorporated into a diagnostic algorithm is cost-effective, primarily due to lower procedure costs and fewer procedure-related complications. The cost-effectiveness of EUS has been demonstrated in the evaluation of esophageal, proximal rectal, and pancreatic cancers [34–36]. In each case, when EUS with FNA was incorporated into the diagnostic algorithm in place of CT, magnetic resonance imaging (MRI), or surgery, or used in conjunction with

Table 125.5 Complications and cost-effectiveness

Complications

- Diagnostic EUS has similar complication rates to standard upper endoscopy
- The most common complications from FNA are hemorrhage and infection
- Prophylactic antibiotics are given to prevent infection when biopsying perirectal masses and pancreatic and mediastinal cystic lesions

Cost-effectiveness

- EUS with FNA is the most cost-effective approach for evaluating a pancreatic mass by providing a tissue diagnosis and staging in one session
- EUS is the most cost-effective imaging modality in determining resectability in esophageal cancer
- When used in combination with CT, EUS is cost-effective in staging rectal cancer
- EUS is the most cost-effective approach when evaluating patients with suspected choledocholithiasis

CT in patients with rectal cancer, it was the least costly staging strategy. EUS has also been shown to be cost-effective when used in place of ERCP in patients with suspected choledocholithiasis [37]. Table 125.5 summarizes the data regarding the complications and cost-effectiveness of EUS.

References

1. Dimagno EP, Buxton JL, Regan PT, *et al.* Ultrasonic endoscope. *Lancet.* 1980;i:629–631.
2. Chang KJ, Katz KD, Durbin TE, *et al.* Endoscopic ultrasound-guided fine-needle aspiration. *Gastrointest Endosc.* 1994;40:694–699.
3. Nguyen TT, Whang CS, Ashida R, *et al.* A comparison of the diagnostic yield and specimen adequacy between 22 and 25 gauge needles for endoscopic ultrasound guided fine-needle aspiration (EUS-FNA) of solid pancreatic lesions (SPL): Is bigger better? *Gastrointest Endosc.,* 2008;67:AB100.
4. Yusuf TE, Ho S, Pavey DA, Michael H, Gress FG. Retrospective analysis of the utility of endoscopic ultrasound-guided fine-needle aspiration (EUS-FNA) in pancreatic masses, using a 22-gauge or 25-gauge needle system: a multicenter experience. *Endoscopy* 2009;41:445–448.
5. Klapman JB, Logrono R, Dye CE, *et al.* Clinical impact of on-site cytopathology interpretation on endoscopic ultrasoundguided fine needle aspiration. *Am J Gastroenterol.* 2003;98:1289–1294.
6. Nguyen P, Feng JC, Chang KJ. Endoscopic ultrasound (EUS) and EUS-guided fine needle aspiration (FNA) of liver lesions. *Gastrointest Endosc.* 1999;50:357–361.
7. Eloubeidi MA, Jhala D, Chhieng DC, *et al.* Yield of endoscopic ultrasound-guided fineneedle aspiration biopsy in patients with suspected pancreatic carcinoma. *Cancer.* 2003;99:285–292.
8. Vazquez-Sequerios E, Norton ID, Clain JE, *et al.* Impact of EUS-guided fine needle aspiration on lymph node staging in patients with esophageal carcinoma. *Gastrointest Endosc.* 2001;53:751–757.
9. Scotiniotis IA, Kochman ML, Lewis JD, *et al.* Accuracy of EUS in the evaluation of Barrett's esophagus and high-grade dysplasia or intramucosal carcinoma. *Gastrointest Endosc.* 2001;54:689–696.
10. Fritscher-Ravens A. Endoscopic ultrasound evaluation in the diagnosis and staging of lung cancer. *Lung Cancer.* 2003;41:259–267.
11. Vilmann P, Krasnik M, Larsen SS, Jacobsen GK, Clementsen P. Transesophageal endoscopic ultrasound-guided fine-needle aspiration (EUS-FNA) and endobronchial ultrasound-guided transbronchial needle aspiration (EBUS-TBNA) biopsy: a combined approach in the evaluation of mediastinal lesions. *Endoscopy.* 2005;37:833–839.
12. Ohashi S, Segewa K, Okamura S, *et al.* The utility of endoscopic ultrasonography and endoscopy in the endoscopic mucosal resection of early gastric cancer. *Gut.* 1999;45:599–604.
13. Harewood GC, Wiersema MJ. Endosonographyguided fine-needle aspiration biopsy in the evaluation of pancreatic masses. *Am J Gastroenterol.* 2002;97:1386–1391.
14. Gunaratnam NT, Saram AV, Norton ID, *et al.* A prospective study of EUS-guided celiac plexus neurolysis for pancreatic cancer pain. *Gastrointest Endosc.* 2001;54:316–324.
15. Savides TJ, Master SS. EUS in rectal cancer. *Gastrointest Endosc.* 2002;56:S12–S18.
16. Farrell RJ, Agarwal B, Brandwein SL, *et al.* Intraductal ultrasound is a useful adjunct to ERCP for distinguishing malignant from benign biliary strictures. *Gastrointest Endosc.* 2002;56:681–687.
17. DeWitt J, Misra VL, Leblanc JK, McHenry L, Sherman S. EUS-guided FNA of proximal biliary strictures after negative ERCP brush cytology results. *Gastrointest Endosc.* 2006;64:325–333.
18. Eloubeidi MA, Chen VK, Jhala NC, *et al.* Endoscopic ultrasound-guided fine needle aspiration biopsy of suspected cholangiocarcinoma. *Clin Gastroenterol Hepatol.* 2004;2:209–213.
19. Fritscher-Ravens A, Broering DC, Knoefel WT, *et al.* EUS-guided fine-needle aspiration of suspected hilar cholangiocarcinoma in potentially operable patients with negative brush cytology. *Am J Gastroenterol.*2004;99:45–51.
20. Fritscher-Ravens A, Broering DC, Sriram PV, *et al.* EUS-guided fine-needle aspiration cytodiagnosis of hilar cholangiocarcinoma: a case series. *Gastrointest Endosc.* 2000;52:534–540.
21. Sahai AV, Zimmerman M, Aabakken L, *et al.* Prospective assessment of the ability of endoscopic ultrasound to diagnose, exclude, or establish the severity of chronic pancreatitis found by endoscopic retrograde cholangiopancreatography. *Gastrointest Endosc.* 1998;48:18–25.
22. Canto MI, Chak A, Stellato T, *et al.* Endoscopic ultrasonography versus cholangiography for the diagnosis of choledocholithiasis. *Gastrointest Endosc.* 1998;47:439–448.
23. Palazzo L, Landi B, Cellier C, *et al.* Endosonographic features predictive of benign and malignant gastrointestinal stromal tumours. *Gut.* 2000;46:88–102.
24. Chang KJ, Nguyen PT, Thompson JA, *et al.* Phase 1 clinical trial of allogeneic mixed lymphocyte culture (cytoimplant) delivered by endoscopic ultrasound-guided fine needle-injection in patients with advanced pancreatic carcinoma. *Cancer.* 2000;88:1325–1335.
25. Chang KJ, Lee JG, Holcombe RF, Kuo J, Muthusamy R, Wu ML. Endoscopic ultrasound delivery of an antitumor agent to treat a case of pancreatic cancer. *Nat Clin Pract Gastroenterol Hepatol.* 2008;5:107–111.
26. Ashida R, Nakata B, Shigekawa M, *et al.* Gemcitabine sensitivity-related mRNA expression in endoscopic ultrasound-guided fine-needle aspiration biopsy of unresectable pancreatic cancer. *J Exp Clin Cancer Res.* 2009;28:83.

27. Yamao K, Bhatia V, Mizuno N, Sawaki A, Shimizu Y, Irisawa A. Interventional endoscopic ultrasonography. *J Gastroenterol Hepatol.* 2009;24:509–519.

28. O'Toole D, Palazzo L, Arotcarena R, *et al.* Assessment of complications of EUS-guided aspiration. *Gastrointest Endosc.* 2001;53: 470–474.

29. Eloubeidi MA, Tamhane A, Lopes TL, Morgan DE, Cerfolio RJ. Cervical esophageal perforations at the time of endoscopic ultrasound: a prospective evaluation of frequency, outcomes, and patient management. *Am J Gastroenterol.* 2009;104:53–56.

30. Wiersema MJ, Vilmann P, Giovannini M, *et al.* Endosonography-guided fine-needle aspiration: diagnostic accuracy and complication assessment. *Gastroenterology.* 1997;112:1087–1095.

31. Gress F, Michael H, Gelrud D, *et al.* EUSguided fine-needle aspiration of the pancreas: evaluation of pancreatitis as a complication. *Gastrointest Endosc.* 2002;56:864–867.

32. Shah JN, Muthusamy VR. Minimizing complications of endoscopic ultrasound and EUS-guided fine needle aspiration. *Gastrointest Endosc Clin N Am.* 2007;17:129–143, vii–viii.

33. Levy MJ, Norton ID, Clain JE, *et al.* Prospective study of bacteremia and complications With EUS FNA of rectal and perirectal lesions. *Clin Gastroenterol Hepatol.* 2007;5:684–689.

34. Shumaker DA, de Garmo P, Faigel DO. Potential impact of preoperative EUS on esophageal cancer management and cost. *Gastrointest Endosc.* 2002;56:391–396.

35. Chang KJ, Soetikno RM, Bastas D, *et al.* Impact of endoscopic ultrasound combined with fine-needle aspiration biopsy in the management of esophageal cancer. *Endoscopy.* 2003;35:962–966.

36. Chen VK, Arguedas MR, Kilgore ML, Eloubeidi MA. A cost-minimization analysis of alternative strategies in diagnosing pancreatic cancer. *Am J Gastroenterol.* 2004;99:2223–2234.

37. Buscarini E, Tansini P, Vallisa D, *et al.* EUS for suspected choledocholithiasis: do benefits outweigh costs? A prospective, controlled study. *Gastrointest Endosc.* 2003;57:510–518.

CHAPTER 126

Diagnostic and interventional endoscopic retrograde cholangiopancreatography

George J. M. Webster and Stephen P. Pereira

University College London Hospitals, London, UK

KEY POINTS

- Diagnostic endoscopic retrograde cholangiopancreatography (ERCP) in a patient with pain alone and a non-dilated common bile duct on ultrasound is associated with a high risk-to-benefit ratio
- For patients with biliary-type pain and a low probability of choledocholithiasis, less invasive diagnostic modalities than ERCP (i.e., MRI/MRCP or endoscopic ultrasound) are indicated
- There is no evidence from meta-analyses to support routine administration of antibiotics
- Procedure-related complications occur in 5–10% of patients; avoidance of unnecessary ERCP is the best way to avoid post-ERCP pancreatitis
- ERCP is the treatment of choice for patients presenting with pain, abnormal liver biochemistry, and duct dilatation due to choledocholithiasis
- Whilst endotherapy in painful obstructive chronic pancreatitis is feasible, randomized data indicate that surgery, rather than ERCP, is the best approach for most patients
- Early ERCP is probably beneficial in severe acute biliary pancreatitis when associated with cholestasis
- ERCP is used for both diagnosis and decompression of the biliary tree by stenting in patients with suspected pancreaticobiliary malignancy

Introduction

The development of side-viewing duodenoscopes in the early 1970s allowed endoscopic visualization of the papilla of Vater (point of entry of the bile and pancreatic ducts) and, when combined with radiography, high-quality visualization of the bile and pancreatic ducts – endoscopic retrograde cholangiopancreatography (ERCP). For many years ERCP was the gold standard for investigating pancreatic and biliary disorders, but with improvement in other imaging modalities, including ultrasonography (transabdominal and endoscopic), multislice helical computed tomography (CT), magnetic resonance imaging/cholangiopancreatography (MRI/MRCP), and intraoperative cholangiography, the need for diagnostic ERCP has declined [1]. Consequently, ERCP has evolved into a

predominantly therapeutic modality, used for the removal of bile and pancreatic duct stones, the treatment of biliary strictures, and the palliation of malignancy. However, ERCP still has a diagnostic role in patients with suspected pancreaticobiliary malignancy in whom non-invasive imaging is normal or equivocal, and it also allows tissue to be obtained for diagnosis by endobiliary brush cytology, needle aspiration, and biopsy.

Description of technique
Equipment and staff

To view and **cannulate the duodenal papilla**, sited on the medial wall of the duodenum, it is necessary to use a side-viewing endoscope. A range of video-duodenoscopes are available. The supporting video image processing system is the same as for gastroscopy and colonoscopy. Duodenoscopes have a working shaft of approximately 1.2 m, with an external diameter ranging from 10.5 to 13.5 mm, and a working channel of 2.2–4.2 mm. Control wheels allow 90–120-degree up/down angulation, 90–110-degree right–left angulation, and a variable elevator to alter the angle at which accessories leave the duodenoscope. The smaller-diameter duodenoscopes allow greater maneuverability, and the narrower bridge provides greater catheter stability, but the larger scopes have a working channel that allows the passage of 10-Fr (i.e., 3.3-mm external diameter) plastic stents, metal stents, and large mechanical lithotripters (Figure 126.1).

A range of instruments is available for **biliary cannulation**, including Teflon-coated 5-Fr (1.7 mm) catheters and bow-string sphincterotomes with a variable number of lumens, external diameter, length of leading cannula, and length of exposed wire. In addition to biliary sphincterotomy, sphincterotomes are also useful in the setting of altered papillary anatomy or a difficult duodenal position.

X-ray imaging is a central component of ERCP, and the procedure is performed on an X-ray table, with imaging

Textbook of Clinical Gastroenterology and Hepatology, Second Edition. Edited by C. J. Hawkey, Jaime Bosch, Joel E. Richter, Guadalupe Garcia-Tsao, Francis K. L. Chan.
© 2012 Blackwell Publishing Ltd. Published 2012 by Blackwell Publishing Ltd.

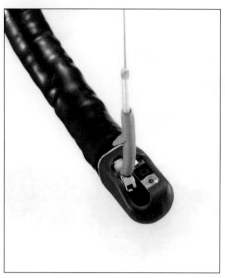

Figure 126.1 Example of a side-viewing duodenoscope, showing the elevator used for controlling the insertion of accessories. A 10-Fr polyethylene stent is seen passing out of the duodenoscope, over a guiding catheter and guidewire. (Courtesy of Olympus Keymed, UK.)

Table 126.1 Risk factors for post-ERCP pancreatitis

- Young age
- Female sex
- Suspected sphincter of Oddi dysfunction
- Normal serum bilirubin level
- Previous ERCP-related pancreatitis
- Recurrent pancreatitis
- Difficult bile duct cannulation
- Pancreatic duct filling
- Precut (needle-knife) sphincterotomy
- Pancreatic sphincterotomy
- Balloon sphincter dilatation
- Pain during ERCP

provided by standard fluoroscopy or using a digital C-arm unit with hardcopy facilities.

The minimum staffing requirements for ERCP are the endoscopist, one assisting nurse to manage the patient's airway and mouthguard, another to assist with endoscopic accessories, and a radiographer/radiologist.

The patient

It is essential that the indication, risks and benefits, and intended outcomes of ERCP are discussed in advance, allowing the patient to provide informed written consent. Procedure-related complications occur in 5–10% of patients, and include acute pancreatitis, bleeding, and perforation, as discussed below. It should be noted that this complication rate is derived mainly from large multicenter studies performed in specialist units [2]. Ideally, units or individuals should be able to provide their own data for complications, thus improving the extent to which consent is truly informed [3]. Clinicians and their patients should also be fully aware of the situations in which the risks of ERCP are increased (Table 126.1).

Contraindications

These are generally similar to those for other types of endoscopy performed under conscious sedation, including lack of informed consent and significant cardiorespiratory disease. Most contraindications to ERCP are relative, and it is vital to weigh up the potential risks and benefits for the individual patient. For example, ERCP in a jaundiced patient with gallstone pancreatitis and systemic inflammatory response syndrome may be high risk, but it is potentially life-saving. In contrast, solely diagnostic ERCP in a patient with pain alone and a normal pancreaticobiliary tree on non-invasive imaging is associated with a high risk-to-benefit ratio.

Special situations

When indicated, therapeutic ERCP in pregnancy is safe provided appropriate pelvic lead shielding is used. The risk of sphincterotomy bleeding is increased in patients taking anticoagulants, and is probably also increased in patients with deranged clotting as a result of underlying disease. In the authors' unit, a prothrombin time prolongation of less than 3 seconds and platelet count greater than $50 \times 10^9/L$ is required before the procedure, with intravenous vitamin K, fresh frozen plasma, and platelet infusions given as appropriate, in accordance with consensus guidelines in this area [4]. Despite the widespread use of prophylactic antibiotics for ERCP, a meta-analysis concluded that there was no clinical benefit to their routine administration [5]. The risk of cholangitis is very low unless adequate biliary drainage is not achieved at ERCP. Prophylaxis is certainly indicated where there is a risk of contrast injection into poorly draining intrahepatic ducts or a communicating pancreatic pseudocyst at the time of ERCP.

Positioning and analgesia

Patient positioning for the procedure under sedation affects the ease with which ERCP is performed. The patient lies on their front, with the left arm extended behind the body, the right arm flexed, with the hand near to the face, and the head turned to the right, so that the left side of the face lies flat on the pillow. The appearance is that of the "freestyle" swimming position. Oxygen is delivered at 2–4 L/min via nasal cannulae, and pulse rate and arterial oxygen saturation are monitored continuously using a standard finger probe. Intravenous opiate (e.g., fentanyl 50–100 µg or pethidine 25–50 mg) analgesia followed by a benzodiazepine (e.g., midazolam 2.5–5 mg) is given, with the dose titrated to achieve adequate conscious sedation. Higher levels may be required than for upper gastrointestinal endoscopy or colonoscopy. Alternatively, some centers use deep sedation with propofol and/or general anesthesia for ERCP. Intravenous hyoscine butylbromide 20–40 mg or glucagon 0.5–1 mg may also be given to reduce duodenal and biliary sphincter contractions.

Procedure

Esophageal intubation with the duodenoscope is similar to that for standard endoscopy. Examination of the upper

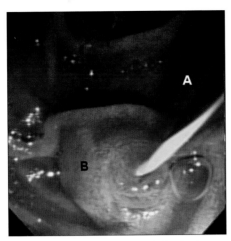

Figure 126.2 Normal major papilla as seen with the duodenoscope in position within the duodenum. A 0.035- inch guidewire (A) is seen within the papilla (B).

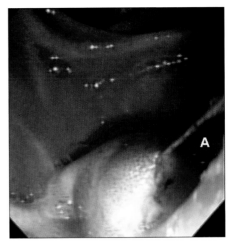

Figure 126.3 Biliary sphincterotomy using a bow-string sphincterotome (A).

gastrointestinal tract is also possible but, because the scope is side viewing, its tip needs to be angled down in order to gain a luminal view. After identifying the pylorus, the tip is angled up (producing a "setting sun" view of the pylorus), so allowing duodenal intubation. In order to identify the major papilla, a complex series of maneuvers of angulation of the scope tip to the right, right torque on the shaft, and pulling back is performed. As with most aspects of ERCP, this procedure is reliably performed only after close supervision and training.

Optimal duodenal positioning is a prerequisite of successful papillary cannulation. The duodenoscope is positioned just below the major papilla (Figure 126.2). On viewing the papilla *en face*, pancreatic duct cannulation is often achieved by cannula insertion into the middle of the papilla, with common bile duct cannulation achieved by insertion in an upwards direction, from below the papilla, aimed at 11 o'clock, and following the line of the bulge of the intramural bile duct. Before ERCP, it is important to decide which anatomy needs to be defined. Pancreatic duct cannulation should not be performed unless of clinical relevance, as repeated attempts at this are an important cause of procedure-related pancreatitis. Once deep cannulation of the desired duct has been obtained, the need for further instrumentation will depend on the indications and findings on cholangiography or pancreatography. Insertion of a 0.018–0.035-inch guidewire through the cannula and into the duct allows the cannula to be exchanged for other ERCP accessories as required.

Biliary sphincterotomy may be indicated for a variety of reasons, including stone extraction, papillary stenosis, and stent insertion (Figure 126.3). The sphincterotome is connected to a standard electrosurgical unit, as used for polypectomy, which has "cut" and "coagulate" settings. The optimal contribution of each during sphincterotomy is debated, with excessive coagulation implicated in thermal damage to the pancreatic sphincter and pancreatitis, and "pure cut" carrying an increased risk of sphincterotomy bleeding. Microprocessor-controlled

electrocautery generators use a combined cut and coagulation, and reduces the risk of an uncontrolled ("zipper") cut precipitating bleeding or perforation. Balloon dilatation of the biliary sphincter is an alternative or can be used in conjunction with sphincterotomy for the extraction of bile duct stones, although there are conflicting data on its safety compared with standard sphincterotomy [6,7].

Difficulties and solutions

Bile duct cannulation may be difficult for a range of reasons, such as the papilla being sited within a duodenal diverticulum or the presence of papillary pathology (e.g., impacted stone, ampullary tumor). Repeated attempts at cannulation may lead to edema around the papilla, making cannulation even more difficult. The use of a sphincterotome allows the angle of cannulation to be altered, as may moving the position of the duodenoscope tip relative to the papilla. A needle-knife precut sphincterotomy may facilitate deep cannulation, but in multicenter studies has been shown to carry a greater risk of complications than standard bow-string sphincterotomy, particularly when the bile duct is not dilated. In experienced hands, placement of a pancreatic stent before precutting may increase immediate bile duct access success rates and reduce the risk of pancreatitis [8]. Where endoscopic bile duct cannulation or stent insertion has proved impossible, a percutaneous transhepatic approach and drain insertion may be necessary. Endoscopic access and intervention may then be achieved by a combined ("rendezvous") procedure, with the radiologist passing a guidewire down the transhepatic biliary drain and out of the papilla into the duodenum. The endoscopist can then grasp the wire with a snare and bring it out through the scope to facilitate stent, sphincterotome, or balloon insertion, as required.

Endoscopic stone extraction

There are several approaches to endoscopic stone extraction, including balloon or basket extraction, or mechanical

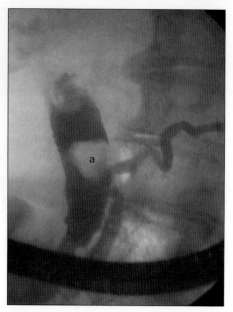 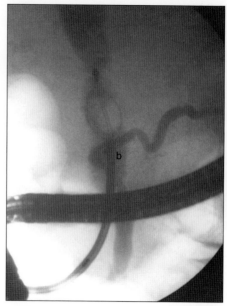

Figure 126.4 Mechanical lithotripsy. At ERCP, a large 1.5-cm stone is seen within the mid common bile duct (a). The stone is engaged by the mechanical lithotripter, followed by advancement of the metal sheath over the basket (b), and fragmentation of the stone prior to removal.

lithotripsy. Stone removal using a **balloon extraction catheter** has the advantage that it may be performed over a wire, allowing easy recannulation of the bile duct. Its main disadvantages are that small stones within a dilated bile duct may "skip past" the balloon as the bile duct is trawled, and larger stones may become impacted at the ampulla. Standard **baskets** allow the extraction of most stones smaller than 1 cm, but carry the risk of not being able to deliver larger stones through the ampulla, or to disengage the stone from the basket within the bile duct, requiring the use of a reel mechanism to crush the stone or snap the basket, thus allowing disengagement. An alternative to either of these techniques is the use of a **mechanical lithotripter**, which is similar to a standard basket but has a metal sleeve that may be advanced over the closed basket, thereby crushing the stone (Figure 126.4). Although the mechanical lithotripter is bulkier and more difficult to maneuver than the standard basket, it avoids the risk of stone impaction. Biliary sphincterotomy is usually performed prior to attempted stone extraction, although mechanical dilatation of the sphincter (balloon sphinctero-plasty) also has a role, particularly where bleeding diatheses present an increased risk with sphincterotomy.

If definitive stone clearance cannot be achieved, a **stent** may be inserted to decompress the biliary tree. Three main types of biliary endoscopic stent are in use:

- **Straight polyethylene stents** – available in a range of lengths, with external diameters of 7 Fr and 10 Fr being used most commonly. The stents are slightly curved and have a flange approximately 1 cm short of each end, which helps to prevent slippage above or below a stricture. 10-Fr stents generally last longer and provide better drainage than 7-Fr stents.

- **7-Fr double pigtail stents** – generally used when straight stents might become displaced, such as after sphincterotomy and incomplete stone extraction from a dilated bile duct. 7-Fr stents are inserted directly over a 0.035-inch wire, whereas a 6–7-Fr guiding catheter is first inserted over the guidewire when a 10-Fr stent is used, because of the larger internal stent diameter. With the wire and guiding catheter placed into the proximal biliary tree, the stent is pushed into place using a pushing tube.

- **A range of self-expanding metal biliary stents**, compressed within the tip of a continuous 7.5–10-Fr delivery catheter, can also be inserted endoscopically. On withdrawal of the compressing sleeve, the stent is deployed, expanding up to a maximum diameter of 10 mm (Figure 126.5).

At least one-third of patients with pancreatic cancer will survive long enough for a polyethylene stent to become occluded, in which case a further procedure is performed to remove the blocked stent and replace it with a new one. In patients who are expected to survive longer than 6 months, **self-expanding metal stents (SEMSs)** play an important role in the palliation of malignant biliary strictures. These stents are approximately 20 times more expensive than polyethylene stents, but the 1-cm expanded lumen remains patent for a median of 4–9 months compared with the 3–4 months seen with plastic stents [9]. However, tissue ingrowth through the mesh may lead to further obstruction, necessitating insertion of further metal stents (or more usually plastic stents) inside the lumen of the metal stent. Fully-covered SEMSs have recently been developed for distal biliary obstruction, with the theoretical, but unproven, advantage that reduced ingrowth may prolong patency. They are more expensive than uncovered SEMS, and may be associated with a higher risk of acute

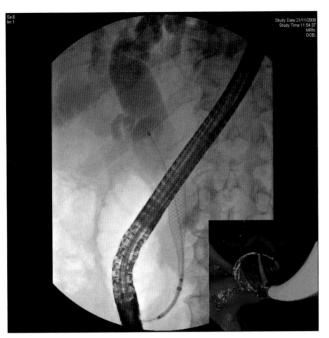

Figure 126.5 Insertion of a metal mesh biliary (Wallflex) stent under radiological control. The 8.5-Fr introducing system has been inserted across the distal biliary stricture into the dilated common bile duct over a 0.035-inch wire. The plastic sheath is then drawn back, allowing deployment of the stent. Inset shows endoscopic view of deployed stent *in situ*. (Reproduced with kind permission of Boston Scientific.)

cholecystitis, pancreatitis, and stent migration [10]. As fully-covered SEMS may be reliably removed endoscopically weeks after insertion, they have an emerging role in the management of indeterminate or benign low bile duct strictures [11].

Indications

Gallstone disease

Common bile duct stones can be removed by preoperative ERCP, laparoscopic common bile duct exploration, or postoperative ERCP. The endoscopic removal of common bile duct stones at the time of ERCP is the treatment of choice for patients presenting with pain, abnormal liver biochemistry, and duct dilatation. ERCP with sphincterotomy is also the primary treatment for patients with cholangitis resulting from common bile duct stones, with urgent (within 24 hours) ERCP indicated for those who do not respond promptly to immediate resuscitation with intravenous fluids and antibiotics.

Alternatives

For patients with biliary-type pain and a low probability of choledocholithiasis, less invasive diagnostic modalities than ERCP (i.e., MRI/MRCP or endoscopic ultrasonography) are indicated, or alternatively operative cholangiography at the time of laparoscopic cholecystectomy is performed to demonstrate the presence or absence of common bile duct stones. If surgical expertise in the technique is available, laparoscopic common bile duct exploration is comparable to postoperative

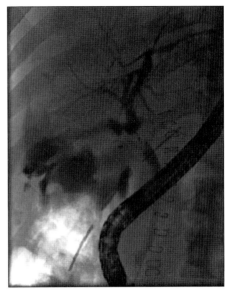

Figure 126.6 Bile leak after cholecystectomy. ERCP in a patient 1 week after open cholecystectomy, showing contrast leak into the gallbladder bed.

ERCP in terms of safety and stone clearance rates, and associated with reduced hospital stay and use of healthcare resources [12]. Otherwise, postoperative ERCP is indicated for patients with retained stones, as well as for the diagnosis and endoscopic therapy of most post-cholecystectomy bile duct injuries (Figure 126.6). In selected patients at prohibitive operative risk, ERCP with stone clearance, but without cholecystectomy, may be the definitive therapy, as may repeated endoscopic stenting beside very large bile duct stones to facilitate biliary drainage. However, in controlled studies the latter approach is associated with an increased burden of biliary symptoms compared with complete stone clearance [13].

Acute and chronic pancreatitis

ERCP has been used for both the diagnosis and treatment of acute, recurrent, and chronic pancreatitis (Figure 126.7).

Diagnosis

In patients who present with the typical findings of acute pancreatitis (abdominal pain and raised levels of pancreatic enzymes), ERCP has little role except in the setting of severe acute biliary pancreatitis with concomitant cholangitis, in which case randomized trials comparing urgent versus delayed ERCP show a benefit for early intervention [14]. In patients with recurrent pancreatitis, when the etiology has not been defined by history, laboratory tests, and non-invasive pancreaticobiliary imaging (CT and MRI/MRCP), further evaluation by endoscopic ultrasonography (see Chapter 125) or ERCP with or without sphincter of Oddi manometry (see Chapter 75) may be considered. Potential causes include biliary stones, microlithiasis, pancreas divisum, small neoplasms or benign pancreatic strictures, or sphincter of Oddi dysfunction. Occasionally, recurrent or chronic pancreatitis

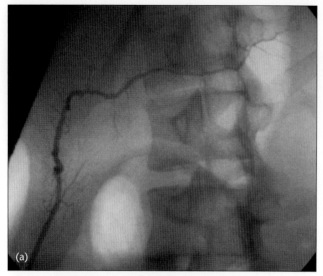
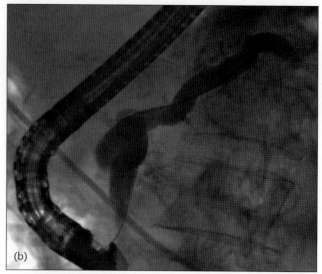

Figure 126.7 Chronic pancreatitis. Comparison of (a) a normal pancreatogram with that in (b) a patient with chronic pancreatitis, showing a dilated, irregular main pancreatic duct with side-branch dilatation.

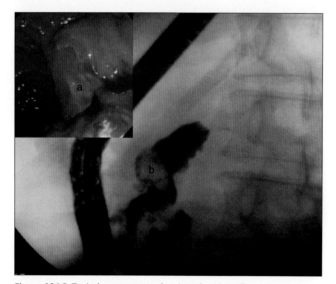

Figure 126.8 Typical appearances of an intraductal papillary mucinous tumor. At ERCP, mucus was seen to be extruding from a patulous papilla (a), with pancreatography showing a filling defect within a dilated duct in the head of the pancreas (b).

may result from the effects of an intraductal papillary mucinous tumor, which may have a typical endoscopic appearance (Figure 126.8).

Treatment

In patients with acute, relapsing, or chronic pancreatitis, a variety of endoscopic therapies have been described. After pancreatic sphincterotomy, stones can be removed from the pancreatic duct, strictures can be stented or balloon dilated, and drainage of the dorsal duct in pancreas divisum can be improved by a combination of accessory papilla sphincterotomy and stent placement, with uncontrolled studies

suggesting that both immediate- and long-term pain relief are possible. Peripancreatic fluid collections and pseudocysts can also be managed by pancreatic duct drainage or direct endoscopic cystenterostomy and stenting techniques, with the results of several studies suggesting that ERCP provides a similar rate of pain relief and pseudocyst resolution as surgery, with equivalent or reduced mortality [15,16]. However, there have been no formal randomized comparisons of these ERCP techniques with interventional radiology or surgery. In contrast, randomized studies comparing ERCP with surgery in patients with painful chronic pancreatitis in association with a dilated pancreatic duct demonstrated improved outcomes with surgery [17].

Benign and malignant bile duct strictures

Postoperative anastomotic strictures or those following bile duct damage at the time of cholecystectomy can initially be managed with intermittent biliary balloon dilatation or endoscopic stent placement at the time of ERCP, with surgical reconstruction of the bile duct reserved for patients in whom endoscopic treatment has not led to resolution of the stricture. In patients with **primary sclerosing cholangitis** (Figure 126.9), uncontrolled studies suggest that endoscopic balloon dilatation or stenting of dominant biliary strictures may prolong survival or time to transplantation, but there is also an increased risk of cholangiocarcinoma development during long-term follow-up [18]. **Pancreatic and biliary tract cancer** (cholangiocarcinoma, gallbladder cancer, and ampullary cancer) can all produce stricturing of the biliary tree at different levels (Figure 126.10). ERCP is used for both diagnosis and decompression of the biliary tree by endoscopic stenting in patients known or suspected to have pancreaticobiliary malignancy.

Tissue diagnosis may be achieved at ERCP by using needle aspiration, brush cytology, and forceps biopsy.

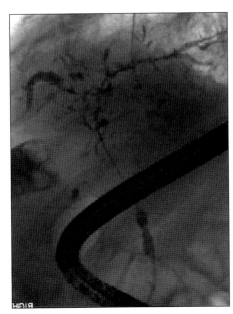

Figure 126.9 Primary sclerosing cholangitis. Cholangiogram showing a narrow common hepatic duct, intrahepatic duct beading and stricturing consistent with primary sclerosing cholangitis. Stones are also seen within the gallbladder and right hepatic duct.

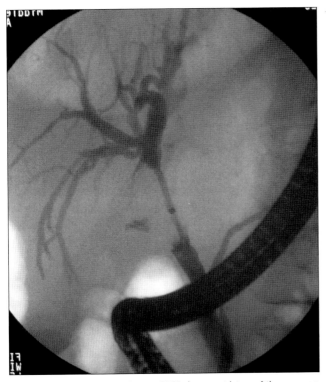

Figure 126.10 Cholangiocarcinoma. ERCP shows a stricture of the common hepatic duct in a patient with painless obstructive jaundice. Endoscopic biopsies confirmed cholangiocarcinoma. Clips from a previous cholecystectomy can also be seen.

Individually, the diagnostic yield from these techniques is low, but their combination improves the ability to establish a tissue diagnosis [19]. Per oral cholangioscopy (Spyglass; Boston Scientific Corporation, USA) is an additional means of visualizing the ducts using a reusable 0.77-mm fiberoptic probe housed inside a single-use 10-Fr catheter which is passed down the working channel of a therapeutic duodenoscope. Four-way deflected steering allows the tip of the cholangioscope to be maneuvered to the area of interest and small biopsies to be taken. Particular uses of the cholangioscope include the assessment of indeterminate strictures, and directed stone dissolution (e.g., using an electrohydraulic lithotripter).

However, the above endoscopic techniques are generally unnecessary for the diagnosis of cancer in a patient presenting with a localized pancreatic mass initially seen on CT if the patient is a candidate for surgery. The use of preoperative stent placement and staging by ERCP in such cases is not supported by evidence from clinical trials, and it may complicate or even preclude surgical intervention. Unfortunately, most cases of pancreatic or biliary tract cancer are not detected at a curable stage, so only palliation can be offered. **Palliative intervention** for malignant biliary obstruction may involve ERCP with stent placement or surgical bypass (Figure 126.11). The available evidence does not indicate a major advantage to either alternative, with the choice depending on the performance status of the patient and local expertise [20].

Pancreaticobiliary-type pain

ERCP is a commonly used technique for the evaluation and management of patients with anatomical evidence of pancreatic or bile duct obstruction. The role of ERCP in patients with pancreaticobiliary-type pain in the absence of obvious obstructive disorders of the pancreatic or bile duct, often referred to as suspected **sphincter of Oddi dysfunction**, is less well defined. The use of ERCP and sphincter of Oddi manometry in the assessment and treatment of such patients is discussed in Chapter 75.

Complications and their management

A number of specific complications are associated with ERCP. Large multicenter studies have reported rates of procedure-related complications of approximately 5–10%, due mainly to pancreatitis and sphincterotomy-associated problems. In general, those endoscopists performing fewer ERCPs have higher complication rates, although no consistent correlation has been found with rates of post-ERCP pancreatitis – due in part to high-volume endoscopists attempting higher-risk cases [21]. Most complications occur within 12 hours, although delayed sphincterotomy-related bleeding may occur several days after the procedure, and late complications such as sphincter stenosis have been reported in up to 5% of patients after sphincterotomy [22]. The mortality rate from diagnostic ERCP is approximately 0.2%, with double the risk for

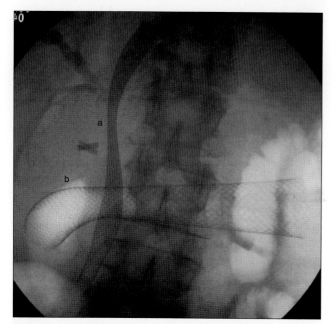

Figure 126.11 Pancreatic carcinoma. An endoscopically placed mesh metal biliary stent (a) and duodenal stent (b) in a patient with obstructive jaundice and duodenal obstruction due to pancreatic carcinoma.

therapeutic ERCP [23]. However, these values must be considered in the context of the potential consequences of not performing an interventional ERCP when necessary.

Pancreatitis

Pancreatitis is the most common complication of ERCP, with prospective studies reporting this in approximately 7% of cases [24,25], although there is a wide range, related in part to differing criteria for diagnosis. One consensus definition is that of new or worsened abdominal pain and a serum amylase level that is three or more times the upper limit of normal 24 hours after the procedure, necessitating at least 2 days in hospital [26]. More than 90% of episodes of pancreatitis are self-limiting, with a severe course in 4.5–7% of cases [24,25].

Severe pancreatitis may be associated with extensive pancreatic necrosis, sepsis, and multiorgan failure, with an overall mortality rate from ERCP-induced pancreatitis of approximately 0.5%. Although the experience of the endoscopist influences the rate of pancreatitis, patient-related factors are vitally important (see Table 126.1). For example, a young woman with abdominal pain, normal bilirubin, a non-dilated common bile duct, and difficult biliary cannulation at ERCP may have a 20–40% chance of developing pancreatitis, irrespective of any intervention. Overall, the risk of pancreatitis is similar for diagnostic and therapeutic ERCP. A pancreatitis risk of approximately 3% in patients requiring fewer than five attempts at biliary cannulation increases to 15% when more than 20 attempts are made [24]. The avoidance of unnecessary ERCP is the best strategy for avoiding post-ERCP pancreatitis.

Prevention

A range of approaches has been studied to reduce ERCP-related pancreatitis. In advanced centers, temporary pancreatic stent placement reduces the risk of pancreatitis in patients undergoing ERCP for suspected sphincter of Oddi dysfunction [27], although failed attempts to insert a stent may be associated with an even higher risk of pancreatitis [21]. With regard to drug treatments, although a meta-analysis suggested that both somatostatin and gabexate (which inhibits proteolytic activity), given as continuous infusions, reduced the rate of ERCP-related pancreatitis [28], a subsequent multicenter randomized placebo-controlled trial showed no benefit with either gabexate or octreotide (a somatostatin analog) [29]. However, a subsequent single-center study reported a benefit in giving a single bolus of somatostatin immediately after ERCP [30]. Agents shown not to be consistently effective include interleukin-10, glyceryl trinitrate, nifedipine, allopurinol, corticosteroids, non-steroidal anti-inflammatory drugs, platelet-activating factor inhibitors, and the use of non-ionic contrast [31–33].

Perforation

Perforation may be retroperitoneal because of extension of a sphincterotomy incision beyond the intramural portion of the bile or pancreatic duct; intraperitoneal as a result of perforation of the bowel wall by the endoscope; or occur at any location because of extramural passage or migration of guidewires or stents. Risk factors for sphincterotomy perforation include a long incision, papillary stenosis, Billroth II anatomy, and needle-knife precut techniques. Clinically important perforation is reported in less than 1% of endoscopic sphincterotomies, but its overall frequency is probably significantly underdiagnosed, as the symptoms and radiological appearances may be difficult to recognize. The development of surgical emphysema following sphincterotomy is indicative of retroperitoneal perforation, but the development of abdominal pain in the absence of a significant rise in serum amylase concentration may also provide a diagnostic clue. In those patients in whom the diagnosis cannot be made by plain abdominal radiography, CT is sensitive in documenting air extravasation into the retroperitoneal space. More than 90% of cases settle with intravenous antibiotics and a strict "nil by mouth" policy, but the development of retroperitoneal collections may require percutaneous or surgical drainage. Bowel wall perforations usually require surgery.

Hemorrhage

Although minor ooze following a sphincterotomy is common, significant bleeding is a rare (0.2–2% of sphincterotomies [34]), but potentially serious complication. Bleeding is more common in those with abnormalities of hemostasis (e.g., cirrhosis, chronic renal failure) or ongoing sepsis, in the setting of papillary stenosis, and in patients treated with anticoagulants within 72 hours after the sphincterotomy. Arterial bleeds may result from cutting the retroduodenal artery as it runs within the transverse duodenal fold, often in association with a long, uncontrolled sphincterotomy. Bleeding that is noted at the time of sphincterotomy and that does not settle spontaneously can be controlled endoscopically, using either epinephrine (adrenaline) (e.g., 1 in 10 000) injected into the cut surfaces of the sphincterotomy, or a hemoclip placed over the bleeding point. Ongoing bleeding may require angiographic embolization of the feeding artery or surgery.

Cholangitis and cholecystitis

These complications occur in approximately 1% of patients after ERCP [35]. Although ERCP may introduce bacteria into a previously sterile biliary tree, clinical cholangitis is rare if effective biliary drainage is obtained. Cholangitis is a particular risk if the intrahepatic ducts are overfilled and cannot be drained adequately because of segmental obstruction. In case–control studies of patients with complex hilar strictures opacified with contrast at ERCP, bilateral intrahepatic duct stenting is associated with a lower rate of cholangitis than unilateral stenting [36].

Stent-related complications

Long-term sequelae of endoscopic biliary sphincterotomy and stent placement include recurrent stone formation, as a result of sphincterotomy stenosis or bacteriobilia caused by duodenal–biliary reflux, and recurrent pancreatitis, presumably because of thermal injury to the pancreatic sphincter. Migration of plastic biliary stents is rarely associated with complications, but stent impaction and bowel perforation may occur. The long-term effects of pancreatic sphincterotomy are largely unknown. Pancreatic stents have the potential to cause ductal injury with stenosis, especially in patients with a normal pancreas.

Cardiopulmonary complications

Although uncommonly related to ERCP, cardiopulmonary complications are the leading cause of death from ERCP and, as expected, occur in older, sicker patients at high anesthetic risk.

> ### SOURCES OF INFORMATION FOR PATIENTS AND DOCTORS
>
> http://www.gastro.org/generalPublic.html
> http://www.bsg.org.uk/clinical-guidelines/index.html
> http://consensus.nih.gov/2002/2002ERCPsos020html.htm
> http://www.library.nhs.uk/Gastroliver/
> http://www.gastrohep.com

References

1. Kaltenthaler E, Vergel YB, Chilcott J, et al. A systematic review and economic evaluation of magnetic resonance cholangiopancreatography compared with diagnostic endoscopic retrograde cholangiopancreatography. *Health Technol Assess*. 2004;8:1–89.
2. Freeman ML. Adverse outcomes of ERCP. *Gastrointest Endosc*. 2002;56:S273–S282.
3. Cotton PB. ERCP is most dangerous for people who need it least. *Gastrointest Endosc*. 2001;54:535–536.
4. Eisen GM, Baron TH, Dominitz JA, et al. Guideline on the management of anticoagulation and antiplatelet therapy for endoscopic procedures. *Gastrointest Endosc*. 2002;55:775–779.
5. Harris A, Chan AC, Torres-Viera C, Hammett R, Carr-Locke D. Meta-analysis of antibiotic prophylaxis in endoscopic retrograde cholangiopancreatography (ERCP). *Endoscopy*. 1999;31:718–724.
6. Bergman JJ, Rauws EA, Fockens P, et al. Randomised trial of endoscopic balloon dilation versus endoscopic sphincterotomy for removal of bileduct stones. *Lancet*. 1997;349:1124–1129.
7. Vlavianos P, Chopra K, Mandalia S, Anderson M, Thompson J, Westaby D. Endoscopic balloon dilatation versus endoscopic sphincterotomy for the removal of bile duct stones: a prospective randomised trial. *Gut*. 2003;52:1165–1169.
8. Tarnasky PR. Mechanical prevention of post- ERCP pancreatitis by pancreatic stents: results, techniques, and indications. *JOP*. 2003;4:58–67.
9. Flamm CR, Mark DH, Aronson N. Evidence based assessment of ERCP approaches to managing pancreaticobiliary malignancies. *Gastrointest Endosc*. 2002;56:S218–S225.
10. Isayama H, Komatsu Y, Tsujino T, et al. A prospective randomised study of "covered" versus "uncovered" diamond stents for the management of distal malignant biliary obstruction. *Gut*. 2004;53:729–734.
11. Mahajan A, Ho H, Sauer B, et al. Temporary placement of fully covered self-expandable metal stents in benign biliary strictures: midterm evaluation. *Gastrointest Endosc*. 2009;70:303–309.
12. Rhodes M, Sussman L, Cohen L, Lewis MP. Randomised trial of laparoscopic exploration of common bile duct versus postoperative endoscopic retrograde cholangiography for common bile duct stones. *Lancet*. 1998;351:159–161.
13. Tham TC, Carr-Locke DL. Endoscopic treatment of bile duct stones in elderly people. *BMJ*. 1999;318:617–618.
14. van Santvoort HC, Besselink MG, de Vries AC, et al. Early endoscopic retrograde cholangiopancreatography in predicted severe acute biliary pancreatitis: a prospective multicenter study. *Ann Surg*. 2009;250:68–75.
15. Mark DH, Lefevre F, Flamm CR, Aronson N. Evidence-based assessment of ERCP in the treatment of pancreatitis. *Gastrointest Endosc*. 2002;56:S249–S254.
16. Lehman GA. Role of ERCP and other endoscopic modalities in chronic pancreatitis. *Gastrointest Endosc*. 2002;56:S237–S240.
17. Cahen DL, Rauws EA, Gouma DJ, Fockens P, Bruno MJ. Removable fully covered self-expandable metal stents in the treatment of common bile duct strictures due to chronic pancreatitis: a case series. *Endoscopy*. 2008;40:697–700.
18. Stiehl A, Rudolph G, Kloters-Plachky P, Sauer P, Walker S. Development of dominant bile duct stenoses in patients with primary sclerosing cholangitis treated with ursodeoxycholic acid: outcome after endoscopic treatment. *J Hepatol*. 2002;36:151–156.
19. Khan SA, Davidson BR, Goldin R, et al. Guidelines for the diagnosis and treatment of cholangiocarcinoma: consensus document. *Gut*. 2002;51(Suppl VI):vi1–vi9.
20. Strasberg SM. ERCP and surgical intervention in pancreatic and biliary malignancies. *Gastrointest Endosc*. 2002;56:S213–S217.
21. Freeman ML, Guda NM. Prevention of post- ERCP pancreatitis: a comprehensive review. *Gastrointest Endosc*. 2004;59:845–864.

22. Rabenstein T, Schneider HT, Hahn EG, Ell C. 25 years of endoscopic sphincterotomy in Erlangen: assessment of the experience in 3498 patients. *Endoscopy.* 1998;30:A194–A201.

23. Loperfido S, Angelini G, Benedetti G, *et al.* Major early complications from diagnostic and therapeutic ERCP: a prospective multicenter study. *Gastrointest Endosc.* 1998;48:1–10.

24. Vandervoort J, Soetikno RM, Tham TC *et al.* Risk factors for complications after performance of ERCP. *Gastrointest Endosc.* 2002; 56:652–656.

25. Freeman ML, DiSario JA, Nelson DB *et al.* Risk factors for post-ERCP pancreatitis: a prospective, multicenter study. *Gastrointest Endosc.* 2001;54:425–434.

26. Cotton PB, Lehman G, Vennes J, *et al.* Endoscopic sphincterotomy complications and their management: an attempt at consensus. *Gastrointest Endosc.* 1991;37:383–393.

27. Tarnasky PR, Palesch YY, Cunningham JT, Mauldin PD, Cotton PB, Hawes RH. Pancreatic stenting prevents pancreatitis after biliary sphincterotomy in patients with sphincter of Oddi dysfunction. *Gastroenterology.* 1998;115:1518–1524.

28. Andriulli A, Leandro G, Niro G, *et al.* Pharmacologic treatment can prevent pancreatic injury after ERCP: a metaanalysis. *Gastrointest Endosc.* 2000;51:1–7.

29. Andriulli A, Clemente R, Solmi L, *et al.* Gabexate or somatostatin administration before ERCP in patients at high risk for post-ERCP pancreatitis: a multicenter, placebocontrolled, randomized clinical trial. *Gastrointest Endosc.* 2002;56:488–495.

30. Poon RT, Yeung C, Liu CL, *et al.* Intravenous bolus somatostatin after diagnostic cholangiopancreatography reduces the incidence of pancreatitis associated with therapeutic endoscopic retrograde cholangiopancreatography procedures: a randomised controlled trial. *Gut.* 2003;52:1768–1773.

31. Mallery JS, Baron TH, Dominitz JA, *et al.* Complications of ERCP. *Gastrointest Endosc.* 2003;57:633–638.

32. Murray B, Carter R, Imrie C, Evans S, O'Suilleabhain C. Diclofenac reduces the incidence of acute pancreatitis after endoscopic retrograde cholangiopancreatography. *Gastroenterology.* 2003;124:1786–1791.

33. Cheon YK, Cho KB, Watkins JL, *et al.* Efficacy of diclofenac in the prevention of post-ERCP pancreatitis in predominantly high-risk patients: a randomized double-blind prospective trial. *Gastrointest Endosc.* 2007;66:1126–1132.

34. Masci E, Toti G, Mariani A, *et al.* Complications of diagnostic and therapeutic ERCP: a prospective multicenter study. *Am J Gastroenterol.* 2001; 6:417–423.

35. Freeman ML, Nelson DB, Sherman S, *et al.* Complications of endoscopic biliary sphincterotomy. *N Engl J Med.* 1996;335: 909–918.

36. Chang WH, Kortan P, Haber GB. Outcome in patients with bifurcation tumors who undergo unilateral versus bilateral hepatic duct drainage. *Gastrointest Endosc.* 1998;47:354–362.

CHAPTER 127
Enteroscopy (double-balloon)

Tomonori Yano and Hironori Yamamoto

Jichi Medical University, Tochigi, Japan

KEY POINTS

- Double-balloon enteroscopy (DBE) allows complete small bowel examination
- DBE has good maneuverability in the distal small intestine
- DBE enables endoscopic treatment, including hemostasis, balloon dilation, polypectomy, mucosal resection, and retrieval of foreign bodies

---

Introduction and scientific basis

The small bowel is a long (5–7 m) and tortuous organ that is freely mobile in the abdominal cavity. These anatomical features complicate endoscopic examination using conventional endoscopes and have kept this region the "uncharted territory" of endoscopy. As a result, the small bowel was previously examined mainly by radiological methods, such as contrast radiography, computed tomography (CT), magnetic resonance imaging (MRI), and angiography. However, in patients with serious small bowel diseases such as severe hemorrhage, or suspected neoplastic or stenotic lesions, laparotomy is often inevitable.

In the 21st century, the exciting developments of capsule endoscopy [1] (see Chapter 128) and double-balloon enteroscopy (DBE) [2,3] have made endoscopic examination of the entire small bowel feasible and changed the diagnostic algorithm for small bowel diseases. DBE not only allows detailed examination and biopsy of small bowel lesions, but also endoscopic treatment of certain conditions such as bleeding and stricture.

This chapter describes the principles of DBE, the technique of insertion, and the diagnosis and treatment of certain clinical conditions.

Description of technique
Principle of inserting an endoscope

To insert an endoscope successfully into the intestinal tract, the most important point is to transmit the force applied to the endoscope shaft effectively to the tip of the endoscope. When the endoscope bends in a complex fashion or forms a loop, the force applied to the shaft of the instrument cannot be transmitted to the tip, resulting in failure of advancement (Figure 127.1).

Looping of the endoscope is due to stretching of the intestine. DBE overcomes this problem by using a **flexible overtube with an inflated balloon at the tip**, which grips the intestine. The overtube does not stretch the small bowel in the presence of bends or loops and thus the applied force will be effectively transmitted to the endoscope tip. The endoscope can thus be advanced into the distal small bowel with the balloon at the tip of the overtube acting as a fixed support (Figure 127.2).

Once the distal end of the endoscope has been advanced as deeply as possible, the overtube is then advanced over the endoscope. To prevent the endoscope from slipping out, the balloon at its tip is inflated and this grip the intestine. The balloon at the tip of the overtube is then deflated, so that it can be slid over the endoscope. Once the overtube has been fully advanced, the overtube balloon is inflated again and the entire device is pulled with both balloons gripping the intestine. This maneuver **pleats** the small intestine over the overtube such that the entire small intestine can be examined with a relatively short endoscope.

Equipment

The DBE has an air channel for the balloon at the tip of the endoscope, and another balloon is attached to the tip of the overtube (Figure 127.3). The inner and outer surfaces of the overtube are hydrophilic. A balloon controller (PB-20; Fujifilm, Tokyo, Japan) controls the pressure in the balloons (Figure 127.4). The balloons are inflated up to the diameter of the lumen of the intestine to grip it effectively and safely, regardless of its diameter. Inflation at this pressure will not cause pain or discomfort. Three types of DBE are available and their scope specifications are summarized in Table 127.1.

Procedure

The DBE can be inserted transorally or transanally. The principle of insertion for both routes is the same but there are some differences between the two in technique.

Textbook of Clinical Gastroenterology and Hepatology, Second Edition. Edited by C. J. Hawkey, Jaime Bosch, Joel E. Richter, Guadalupe Garcia-Tsao, Francis K. L. Chan.

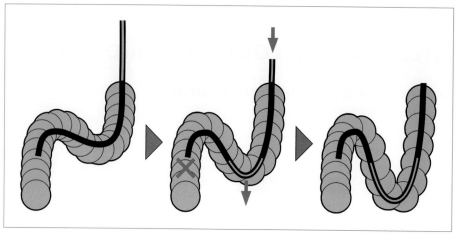

Figure 127.1 Reason for difficult insertion of a conventional endoscope.

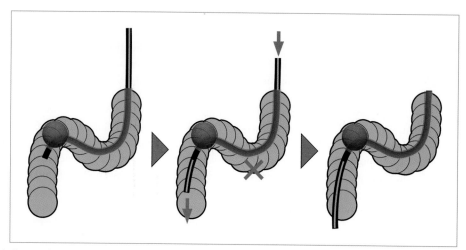

Figure 127.2 Double-balloon endoscope insertion principle.

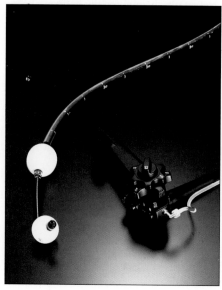

Figure 127.3 Endoscope unit.

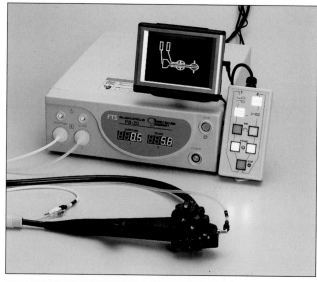

Figure 127.4 Balloon controller.

Table 127.1 Endoscope models (Fujifilm, Saitama, Japan)

Model	Working length (mm)	Scope diameter (mm)	Accessory channel diameter (mm)
EN-450P5	2000	8.5	2.2
EN-450T5	2000	9.4	2.8
EC-450BI5	1520	9.4	2.8

Oral insertion (Figure 127.5)

A 12-hour fast is sufficient for bowel preparation. The overtube is retracted to the proximal side of the endoscope. Once the tip of the endoscope has entered the stomach, the overtube is advanced into the stomach. Because the lumen of the stomach is too large to grip the balloon, an assistant holds the overtube without inflating its balloon. Once the endoscope tip is in the third portion of the duodenum, the balloon at its tip is inflated to grip the intestine, and the assistant advances the overtube. Once the overtube is advanced to the maximum point, the

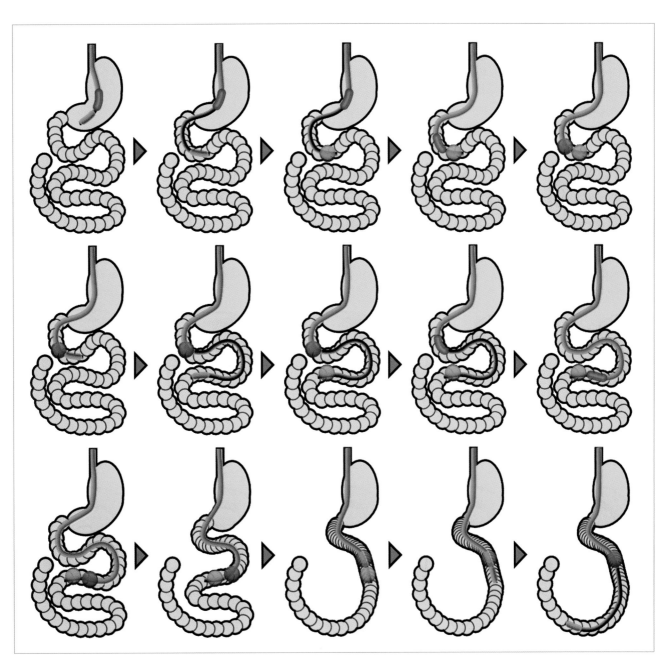

Figure 127.5 Oral insertion.

balloon at its tip is inflated. Because the balloon at the tip of the overtube is prone to falling back into the stomach at such time, the shortening maneuver is not performed. Once the tip of the endoscope has been advanced as far as possible into the jejunum, the balloon at the distal end of the endoscope is inflated, and the overtube balloon is then deflated, the overtube advanced, and its balloon then re-inflated. In this position, both balloons grip the intestine and the entire device is pulled to shorten the small intestine. The balloon at the tip of the endoscope is then deflated and the sequence is repeated. Beyond the ligament of Treitz, the endoscope and overtube should form a concentric circle in either a clockwise or counterclockwise fashion.

Anal insertion (Figure 127.6)

For anal insertion, preparation is similar to that for colonoscopy. The overtube is retracted to the proximal side of the endoscope. The balloons should be used in a similar fashion at several points in the colon, such as the sigmoid descending junction, splenic flexure, and hepatic flexure. After the tip of the endoscope has reached the cecum, the overtube is advanced to the ascending colon. Gentle withdrawal of the overtube with the balloon inflated may expose the ileocecal valve to facilitate ileal intubation.

After intubating the terminal ileum, the endoscope tip is immediately straightened. The endoscope should be advanced cautiously without forceful insertion of the shaft; this helps prevent the tip from falling back into the colon. After the endoscope has been inserted into the ileum as deeply as possible, the balloon at its tip is inflated to grip the intestine. The overtube balloon is then deflated, and the overtube is advanced through the ileocecal valve into the ileum and its balloon is inflated. Because the distal end of the overtube is prone to falling back into the colon at this point, the shortening maneuver is not advisable after the first insertion "stroke" from the ileocecal valve.

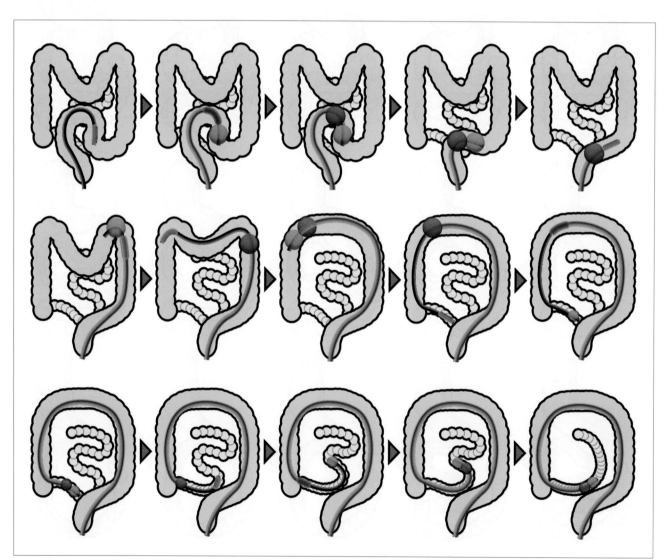

Figure 127.6 Anal insertion.

After the second stroke, the shortening maneuver is used to pleat the small intestine over the overtube. When advancing the endoscope further, it is important to avoid pushing in the direction of the pelvis because the shaft of the endoscope will form an S shape that will hamper further insertion. The insertion stroke should be repeated to make the shaft form a concentric circle with counterclockwise rotation.

Selection of insertion route

The selection of the insertion route should be guided by the medical history and other imaging examinations. Capsule endoscopy may also be used to guide the route of insertion (oral or anal insertion with the two-thirds vs one-third time span measured on capsule endoscopy during small bowel transit) [4]. If the probable location of pathology cannot be estimated or if inspection of the entire intestine is indicated for multiple lesions, we choose anal insertion as the primary route, since it requires less sedation and is accompanied by fewer complications. If necessary, oral insertion is performed on another day to complete the inspection of the entire intestine.

However, oral insertion without preparation is selected for cases demonstrating **overt ongoing bleeding**, except when other examination reveals that the bleeding site is the lower ileum. Because there is virtually no backward flow of intestinal contents within the small bowel, observation of bloody intestinal fluid on oral insertion suggests the presence of a nearby bleeding pathology. Conversely, when anal insertion is performed, bloody intestinal fluid can be pushed upward by the insufflation that accompanies endoscopic insertion and this complicates identification of the bleeding site.

Inspection of the entire small intestine

Endoscopic inspection of the entire small intestine is not always required; the goal of examination is achieved when the lesion in the small intestine is reached and its diagnosis and/or treatment are successfully completed. However, in selected cases, inspection of the entire small intestine is indicated. This is sometimes possible in one examination. However, complete inspection is usually achieved by a combination of sequential oral and anal intubations. One should mark the deepest site reached on the first examination with India ink or a metal clip, and confirm this marking on a second examination by insertion from the other route. A second insertion is normally scheduled for the next or subsequent day because in a same-day examination, endoscopic insufflation of the intestine prevents deep insertion. However, sequential examinations can be performed on the same day if CO_2 is used for endoscopic insufflation. Success rates for complete inspection of the small intestine are reported to be 40–80% [5–8].

Analgesia and anesthesia during examination

Analgesia and anesthesia are required because the examination time is longer than for upper and lower gastrointestinal endoscopy.

Use of antispasmodics

When the endoscope is inserted orally, intestinal peristalsis can facilitate forward advancement of the balloons and assist insertion. Thus, anticholinergics or other such antispasmodics are used when the region of maximum insertion depth is reached and on withdrawal of the endoscope. However, when inserted retrograde to peristalsis through the afferent loop in a postoperative reconstructed bowel, intestinal peristalsis pushes the balloons in the reverse direction. Thus, when the intestinal anastomotic site is reached, an antispasmodic is used to stop peristalsis so that the insertion maneuver can be performed. For the same reason, when inserted anally and retrograde to peristalsis, an antispasmodic is used to stop peristalsis so that the insertion maneuver can be performed.

Fluoroscopy

While fluoroscopy is not essential for insertion of the DBE, if difficulties with insertion occur, it is often useful for checking the insertion status of the endoscope.

Indications and contraindications

The following indications have been proposed in the consensus report of the 2nd International Conference on DBE [9].

- **Mid-gastrointestinal bleeding**: in patients with suspected mid-gastrointestinal bleeding (bleeding source not identified by conventional upper endoscopy and colonoscopy); or for endoscopic hemostasis in patients with known mid-gastrointestinal bleeding.
- **Following capsule endoscopy**: in patients in whom a further diagnostic test (e.g., biopsy sampling) or therapy is indicated.
- **Endoscopic diagnosis and treatment of stenoses**: endoscopic or histological diagnosis in patients with suspected stenoses; balloon dilation for stenoses of the small intestine.
- **Tumors and mass lesions**: endoscopic diagnosis and histological confirmation of tumors or masses detected by other imaging modalities if considered necessary prior to surgery; preoperative marking (e.g., tattooing) in patients with discrete findings who are scheduled to undergo surgical endoscopic resection of suitable lesions in the small intestine.
- **Removal of foreign bodies** from the small intestine (e.g., retained capsule endoscope).

Indications that are under evaluation include:

- Endoscopic and histological diagnosis of Crohn's disease involving the small intestine, and subsequent follow-up
- Endoscopic and histological diagnosis of obstruction, including intussusception, and unexplained complications of small bowel diseases
- Endoscopic access in postoperative anatomy, including endoscopic retrograde cholangiopancreatography (ERCP)

after Billroth II or Roux–en–Y operation; post bariatric surgery access to the biliary tree or gastric remnant

• Incomplete colonoscopy due to technical difficulties.

Contraindications to DBE are essentially similar to those for conventional upper gastrointestinal endoscopy and colonoscopy, especially when the risk of perforation is high. DBE is not indicated for functional abdominal pain without evidence of iron-deficiency anemia, hypoalbuminemia, positive fecal occult blood, inflammatory laboratory changes, or obstructive symptoms.

Prior laparotomy or other causes of intra-abdominal adhesions as well as too much mesenteric fat can complicate small bowel shortening maneuvers and make deep insertion difficult. If the severe stricture prevents passage of the endoscope into the small intestine, the area beyond the stricture cannot be observed endoscopically unless endoscopic balloon dilation is performed.

Complications

In a multicenter survey, DBE was found to be a safe procedure with low complication rates. The overall complication rate in diagnostic DBE was 0.8%, which was comparable with complication rates observed in diagnostic colonoscopy (0.02% ± 2.4%). The complication rate in therapeutic DBE was 4.3%, which was higher than that associated with therapeutic colonoscopy (1.2% ± 2.0%). This report confirmed that **acute pancreatitis** was of major concern in patients undergoing DBE, occurring in 0.3% of procedures [10]. The etiology of the pancreatitis is unclear, but as it is frequently localized in the pancreatic body and tail, one theory is that the shortening maneuver distorts the duodenum, and at the same time deforms and traumatizes the pancreas.

Endoscopic diagnosis

Common intestinal lesions found by DBE include ulcers, erosions, vascular lesions, polyps, and mucosal and submucosal tumors. Abnormalities of intestinal villi, such as swelling, atrophy, and white villi (due to lymphatic stasis) may help determine the pathogenesis of lesions. Because some diseases also demonstrate a characteristic distribution of lesions, determination of the location of lesions may be helpful in considering the differential diagnosis.

To determine the location of a lesion in the small intestine, the **depth of intubation** should be estimated during DBE insertion. As a practical way of estimating intubation depth, we calculate the insertion length for each stroke of endoscopic insertion after manipulations of the balloons in the range of 0–45 cm. Total intubation length should be the sum of all stroke lengths up to the point of intubation [11]. The intubation length should be recorded from the pyloric ring for oral insertion, and from the ileocecal valve for anal insertion. In cases of successful total enteroscopy, the total length of the small

intestine is usually estimated to be 4–7 m using the above method. When a lesion is found during DBE insertion, the estimated length from the pyloric ring or ileocecal valve to the lesion should be noted.

Determining whether lesions are on the **mesenteric or antimesenteric side** of the small intestine is sometimes clinically important [12]. When a DBE is inserted into the deep small bowel, the insertion is made in concentric circles with their center at the root of the mesentery. The mesentery is extended fan-like in circles. In this situation, the inside of the concentric circle is the mesenteric side. Therefore, when an endoscope is inserted with circles made at an upward angle, tip movement in the upward direction indicates the mesenteric side. A radiograph clearly shows that the tip of an endoscope moves toward the center of the circle, and that the wall near the tip is the mesenteric side.

Obscure gastrointestinal bleeding accounts for about half of all indications for DBE, and the diagnostic yield in reports from multiple institutions is between 54% and 78% [6,8,13–16].

Endoscopic treatment

Hemostasis

Lesions that cause small intestinal bleeding include vascular lesions, ulcers, and tumors. Endoscopic hemostasis for bleeding from ulcers and tumors usually achieves only a temporary hemostatic effect. Definitive hemostasis requires appropriate disease-specific medical or surgical treatment. At the same time, most **vascular lesions** such as angioectasia, Dieulafoy's lesion, and arteriovenous malformation (AVM), represent an indication for endoscopic treatment. For endoscopic diagnosis and selection of appropriate treatment for these lesions, the endoscopic classification shown in Figure 127.7 [17] is useful. Types 1a and 1b represent angioectasia; Type 2a and 2b Dieulafoy's lesions; Type 3 AVM; and Type 4 a vascular lesion with unusual morphology that is unclassifiable.

For hemostasis of **angioectasia**, cauterization procedures such as argon plasma coagulation are suitable. However, excessive coagulation should be avoided because the small intestinal wall is thin. In case of continuous bleeding or for a large lesion, submucosal injection of saline – epinephrine (adrenaline) under the lesion can decrease the risk of perforation, enabling sufficient coagulation of the lesion. **Dieulafoy's lesion** and AVM usually require endoscopic clip placement or surgical resection in the case of a large lesion.

Balloon dilation for strictures

Previously, surgical treatment was the only choice for symptomatic intestinal strictures. However, DBE has enabled endoscopic treatment for such strictures using a balloon dilation catheter [18]. Exclusion of malignant stricture by careful endoscopic observation, with biopsies as needed, is required prior to attempts at balloon dilation. Balloon dilation should be

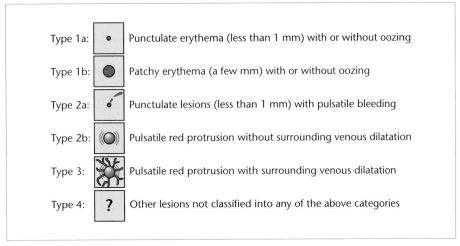

Figure 127.7 Endoscopic classification of small bowel vascular lesions (Yano–Yamamoto classification).

performed after obtaining fully informed consent; this must include explanation of the risk of perforation. In case of a stricture with active ulceration at the site of stricture, balloon dilation should be postponed until the ulcer is healed by medical treatment, because dilation of a stricture with active ulceration confers a high risk of perforation. Unlike for laparotomy, re-treatment is possible when a single session of treatment is not sufficiently effective or symptoms recur after treatment.

Polypectomy and endoscopic mucosal resection

Special care is needed in polypectomy and endoscopic mucosal resection (EMR) in the small intestine because the small intestinal wall is much thinner than the colonic wall. To prevent perforation, submucosal injection of normal saline at the site of snaring should be considered whenever such a risk is noted. The power and duration of electrical current used for cauterization should also be adjusted carefully.

Foreign body retrieval

Items such as needles, bones, dentures, bezoars, and capsule endoscopes can be retrieved. Based on the type of foreign body, various accessories and endoscopic hoods can be selected. Retrieval through the overtube, together with withdrawal of the endoscope, is sometimes useful for sharp foreign bodies.

Conclusions

DBE has made possible the formerly difficult endoscopic diagnosis and treatment for small bowel disease, and its rapid, worldwide adoption continues. A synergy with capsule endoscopy, introduced at nearly the same time, has brought great advances in the diagnosis and treatment of small bowel disease. Both examination techniques will likely be deemed essential in the diagnosis and treatment of small bowel disease.

References

1. Iddan G, Meron G, Glukhovsky A, Swain P. Wireless capsule endoscopy. *Nature.* 2000;405:417.
2. Yamamoto H, Yano T, Kita H, Sunada K, Ido K, Sugano K. New system of double-balloon enteroscopy for diagnosis and treatment of small intestinal disorders. *Gastroenterology.* 2003;125:1556; author reply 1557.
3. Yamamoto H, Sekine Y, Sato Y, *et al.* Total enteroscopy with a nonsurgical steerable double-balloon method. *Gastrointest Endosc.* 2001;53:216–220.
4. Triester SL, Leighton JA, Leontiadis GI, *et al.* A meta-analysis of the yield of capsule endoscopy compared to other diagnostic modalities in patients with obscure gastrointestinal bleeding. *Am J Gastroenterol.* 2005;100:2407–2418.
5. Fukumoto A, Tanaka S, Shishido T, Takemura Y, Oka S, Chayama K. Comparison of detectability of small-bowel lesions between capsule endoscopy and double-balloon endoscopy for patients with suspected small-bowel disease. *Gastrointest Endosc.* 2009; 69:857–865.
6. Heine GD, Hadithi M, Groenen MJ, Kuipers EJ, Jacobs MA, Mulder CJ. Double-balloon enteroscopy: indications, diagnostic yield, and complications in a series of 275 patients with suspected small-bowel disease. *Endoscopy.* 2006;38:42–48.
7. May A, Nachbar L, Ell C. Double-balloon enteroscopy (push-and-pull enteroscopy) of the small bowel: feasibility and diagnostic and therapeutic yield in patients with suspected small bowel disease. *Gastrointest Endosc.* 2005;62:62–70.
8. Yamamoto H, Kita H, Sunada K, *et al.* Clinical outcomes of double-balloon endoscopy for the diagnosis and treatment of small-intestinal diseases. *Clin Gastroenterol Hepatol.* 2004;2: 1010–1016.
9. Pohl J, Blancas JM, Cave D, *et al.* Consensus report of the 2nd International Conference on double balloon endoscopy. *Endoscopy.* 2008;40:156–160.
10. Mensink PB, Haringsma J, Kucharzik T, *et al.* Complications of double balloon enteroscopy: a multicenter survey. *Endoscopy.* 2007;39:613–615.
11. May A, Nachbar L, Schneider M, Neumann M, Ell C. Push-and-pull enteroscopy using the double-balloon technique: method of assessing depth of insertion and training of the enteroscopy

technique using the Erlangen Endo-Trainer. *Endoscopy*. 2005;37: 66–70.

12. Sunada K, Yamamoto H, Hayashi Y, Sugano K. Clinical importance of the location of lesions with regard to mesenteric or antimesenteric side of the small intestine. *Gastrointest Endosc*. 2007;66 (3 Suppl):S34–38.

13. Manabe N, Tanaka S, Fukumoto A, Nakao M, Kamino D, Chayama K. Double-balloon enteroscopy in patients with GI bleeding of obscure origin. *Gastrointest Endosc*. 2006;64:135–140.

14. Tanaka S, Mitsui K, Yamada Y, *et al*. Diagnostic yield of double-balloon endoscopy in patients with obscure GI bleeding. *Gastrointest Endosc*. 2008;68:683–691.

15. Ohmiya N, Yano T, Yamamoto H, *et al*. Diagnosis and treatment of obscure GI bleeding at double balloon endoscopy. *Gastrointest Endosc*. 2007;66 (3 Suppl):S72–77.

16. Jacobs MA, Mulder CJ. Double balloon endoscopy in GI hemorrhage. *Gastrointest Endosc*. 2007;66 (3 Suppl):S60–62.

17. Yano T, Yamamoto H, Sunada K, *et al*. Endoscopic classification of vascular lesions of the small intestine (with videos). *Gastrointest Endosc*. 2008;67:169–172.

18. Sunada K, Yamamoto H, Kita H, *et al*. Clinical outcomes of enteroscopy using the double-balloon method for strictures of the small intestine. *World J Gastroenterol*. 2005;11:1087–1089.

CHAPTER 128
Capsule endoscopy

Christina A. Tennyson[1] and Blair S. Lewis[2]
[1]Columbia University College of Physicians and Surgeons, New York, NY, USA
[2]Mount Sinai School of Medicine, New York, NY, USA

KEY POINTS

- Capsule endoscopy provides improved imaging of the small bowel compared to other modalities such as barium radiography and push enteroscopy
- Indications include obscure gastrointestinal bleeding, unexplained iron-deficiency anemia, suspected or known Crohn's disease, and celiac disease
- Limitations include inability to take biopsies, missed lesions, difficulty in localization, incomplete examinations, and variability in interpretation
- Future directions include improved image acquisition and therapeutic actions

Introduction

The small intestine comprises the majority of the surface area of the gastrointestinal tract, but is not completely evaluated via traditional endoscopic techniques due to its length and location. Techniques such as push enteroscopy and ileoscopy during colonoscopy permit examination of a relatively short portion of the small intestine. Video capsule endoscopy was first introduced in 1999 and enabled visualization of the small bowel [1]. It is a non-invasive procedure that is safe and well tolerated by the majority of patients. Capsule endoscopy can be used for the examination of the small intestine for numerous gastrointestinal disorders, including obscure gastrointestinal bleeding, celiac disease, inflammatory bowel disease, and polyposis syndromes. Video capsule endoscopy can serve as an initial investigation and later direct the approach of enteroscopy, using a balloon-assisted or spiral technique, if therapeutic intervention is required. Capsule endoscopy technology has also been used to examine the esophagus and most recently the colon.

Description of technique
The capsule
Small bowel video capsule endoscopy can be performed using either the Given PillCam® capsule (Given Imaging, Yoqneam, Israel) or the Olympus Endocapsule (Olympus America Inc, Center Valley, PA, USA). The original Given PillCam SB capsule system was first approved by the US Food and Drug Administration (FDA) in 2001 and later updated to the second-generation PillCamSB2, with improved optics, in 2007. In 2007, the Olympus Endocapsule system was also approved by the FDA. The capsules measure 11×26 mm in size, contain light emitting diodes, lens, silver oxide batteries, radiofrequency transmitter, and antenna. The systems differ in the field of view and technology used to acquire images. The fields of view for the PillCam SB capsule, PillCam SB2 capsule, and Endocapsule are 140, 156, and 145 degrees respectively. The Olympus capsule camera uses a charge coupled device (CCD) while the Given capsule uses a complementary metal oxide semiconductor (CMOS) to acquire images. Although they differ in some respects, a multicenter study comparing the Endocapsule and PillCam SB demonstrated similar transit time, reading time, and diagnostic yield [2]. The battery life of a capsule endoscope is approximately 8 hours, although a capsule with a 12-hour battery life, PillCam SB 2-Ex, has been recently introduced by Given. The capsule is propelled via peristalsis, obtains two images/second, and transmits data to a recording device worn by the patient. Images may be viewed in real-time during the acquisition process using a viewer.

Capsule endoscopy technology has also been applied in the **esophagus and colon** using a slightly different capsule design. The PillCam ESO (Given Imaging) was approved by the FDA in 2004 and measures 26×11 mm with a 140-degree field of view, but with a faster rate of capture of 14 frames/second using cameras at both ends of the capsule and a shorter battery life of approximately 30 minutes. Views are thus obtained both in the forward mode and retrograde direction using both cameras. The ESO2 (Given Imaging) was approved by the FDA in 2007 with improved optics, image storing speed and increased field of view of 169 degrees°. Possible indications for esophageal capsule endoscopy include screening for varices in patients with portal hypertension and for Barrett's esophagus in patients with gastroesophageal reflux disease [3]. Esophageal capsule endoscopy has not been shown to be cost-effective, however, when compared to standard upper endoscopy for these indications [4,5].

A colonoscopy capsule endoscopy system, PillCam COLON (Given Imaging) has been developed, but is not currently approved by the FDA for use in the United States. The colon

---

Textbook of Clinical Gastroenterology and Hepatology, Second Edition. Edited by C. J. Hawkey, Jaime Bosch, Joel E. Richter, Guadalupe Garcia-Tsao, Francis K. L. Chan.
© 2012 Blackwell Publishing Ltd. Published 2012 by Blackwell Publishing Ltd.

capsule system also has two cameras, measures 31×11 mm, captures four frames/second, and has a "sleep" mode to conserve battery life while transversing the small intestine. In a prospective multicenter study, the colon capsule had a lower sensitivity for detecting colonic lesions as compared to conventional optical colonoscopy [6]. Colon capsule endoscopy may serve a role when traditional colonoscopy is contraindicated, incomplete, or cannot be performed because the patient is unwilling or unable to undergo the standard exam.

Patient preparation

It is advisable to stop oral iron supplements 1 week prior to the capsule endoscopy procedure as these may limit mucosal visualization. The day prior to the exam, patients are instructed to ingest a liquid diet, preferably one not containing red fluid. Patients are advised to fast for 12 hours prior to the exam. Numerous purgatives, including sodium phosphate, magnesium citrate, and polyethylene glycol (PEG), have been studied prior to capsule endoscopy, but results vary and have been inconsistent. As purgatives cause inconvenience to the patient without consistent demonstrated benefit, they are not routinely recommended. A meta-analysis of studies, however, using predominantly PEG-based purgatives demonstrated improved mucosal visualization and a slightly increased yield when compared to a clear liquid preparation, but transit times and incomplete procedure rates were the same [7]. The use of 80 mg of simethicone may aid in mucosal visualization. The routine use of prokinetics, such as erythromycin or metoclopramide, is not recommended since diagnostic yield or cecal intubation rates are not increased.

Consent and complications

Informed consent prior to capsule endoscopy must include a discussion of the risk of **capsule retention** and its management. This is a concern for physicians performing capsule endoscopy since retention may lead to surgery in a patient who may have been treated medically for the same illness. Capsule retention is defined as the persistence of the capsule in the digestive tract for more than 2 weeks [8]. Retention is also defined as the capsule permanently remaining in the bowel lumen and requiring extraction by endoscopic or surgical methods or passing as a result of medical therapy.

The risk of capsule retention depends on the indication for the exam and overall is reported at 1–2% [8]. The risk of retention has been reported as <1% in patients with obscure bleeding [9]. In patients with known Crohn's disease, the risk of retention was reported as 13%, and approximately 1.6% in suspected Crohn's disease [10]. When retention occurs, options include: monitoring, attempted endoscopic retrieval, and surgical removal. There is no time limit to institute management for capsule removal and there are reports of capsules remaining in asymptomatic patients for several years. There are no data on the success of medical therapies for capsule retention, such as a course of steroids or use of prokinetics, to aid in passage of the capsule. The choice of surgical or endoscopic

management of capsule retention depends on the cause of the retention, condition of the patient, and indication for the exam. If retention occurs behind a tumor or mass, surgical intervention is usually pursued quickly. If a Crohn's or non-steroidal anti-inflammatory drug (NSAID) stricture is the cause for the retention, surgical intervention can remove the capsule and alleviate the cause of bleeding, especially if the patient was refractory to medical therapy. Retention behind a stricture can also be managed with deep enteroscopy, using a balloon- or spiral-assisted technique, with dilation of the stricture if needed.

In addition to capsule retention, **capsule aspiration** has also been rarely reported and may also be mentioned during the consent process, particularly in patients with dysphagia.

When obtaining consent, patients should also be advised not to have magnetic resonance imaging (MRI) performed until the capsule has been confirmed to have exited the body.

Procedure

On the day of the procedure, patients are asked to swallow the capsule with a small amount of water after the data recorder and sensors have been attached to their abdomen. In certain situations, the capsule may be placed endoscopically into the duodenum using a capsule-loading device. This may be considered in patients with significant dysphagia, altered anatomy, gastroparesis, chronic narcotic use, children, and those unable to swallow pills [11]. During the capsule endoscopy exam, patients are advised to periodically monitor the data recorder to verify the system is functioning by observing a blinking light. Following capsule ingestion, patients may drink clear liquids after 2 hours and eat a light snack after 4 hours. Following 8 hours, or when the acquisition time is complete, the recording device and leads are removed. The images are downloaded to a computer workstation and can be reviewed. In a typical exam, over 50 000 images are produced. The software used to review the images provides an estimate of localization of the capsule and also aides in identification of blood. The capsule is disposable and is expelled by the patient typically within 24 hours.

Indications and contraindications (Table 128.1)
Obscure gastrointestinal bleeding is the indication for the majority of capsule endoscopy exams (Table 128.2 and Figure 128.1). For patients with obscure bleeding with a normal colonoscopy and upper endoscopy, capsule endoscopy has been recommended as the third diagnostic test [12,13]. Capsule endoscopy is superior to both push enteroscopy and small bowel radiography. In a meta-analysis comparing the techniques over 14 studies, yields were 63%, 28% and 8% respectively [14]. In a pooled analysis of manufacturer-sponsored trials, capsule endoscopy identified pathology in 70% of 530 capsule exams and had double the yield of other methods: push enteroscopy, small bowel series, and colonoscopy with ileal intubation [15]. In a 1-year follow-up study of 100 patients with obscure bleeding, the sensitivity, specificity, and positive

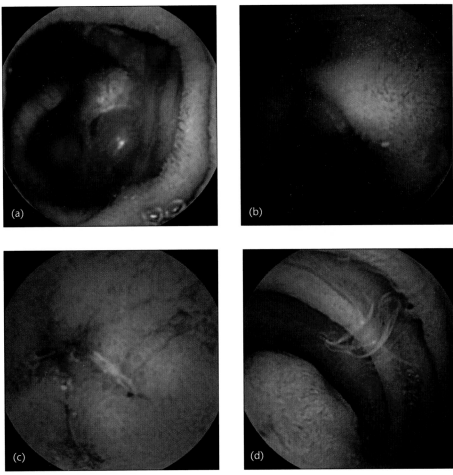

Figure 128.1 (a) Bleeding seen on video capsule endoscopy: (b) angioectasia; (c) ulcer; (d) submucosal tumor.

Table 128.1 Capsule endoscopy indications, contraindications, and risks

Indications
- Obscure gastrointestinal bleeding
- Unexplained iron-deficiency anemia
- Suspected Crohn's disease
- Celiac disease with alarm symptoms
- Suspected tumor or polyposis

Contraindications
- Intestinal obstruction
- Implanted cardiac devices

Risks
- Capsule retention
- Capsule aspiration

Table 128.2 Significant causes of small bowel bleeding

- Angiodysplasia
- Inflammatory bowel disease (Crohn's)
- NSAID enteropathy
- Tumors
- Diverticula
- Ischemic enteropathy

and negative predictive values of capsule endoscopy were 88.9%, 95%, 97%, and 82.6% respectively [16]. In another prospective study evaluating capsule endoscopy for obscure bleeding compared to the gold standard, intraoperative enteroscopy, capsule endoscopy had a yield of 74%, sensitivity of 95%, and specificity of 75% [17].

Capsule endoscopy also has been shown to be helpful in evaluating **unexplained iron-deficiency anemia**, finding a lesion in 57% of examinations in one study [18]. Capsule endoscopy may also recognize bleeding lesions in the colon and esophagus that were missed during conventional upper endoscopy and colonoscopy (see Video clip 128.1)

Another indication for capsule endoscopy is the evaluation of patients with suspected and known **Crohn's disease** (Figure 128.2). Capsule endoscopy performs a diagnostic role in the initial evaluation and subsequent monitoring of patients with known or suspected Crohn's disease. It can assess for mucosal healing after therapy, early postoperative recurrence, and presence of small bowel lesions in patients with indeterminate colitis. The yield of capsule endoscopy is low for patients with abdominal pain and/or diarrhea alone. Yield is increased when other criteria are added to suggest inflammation:

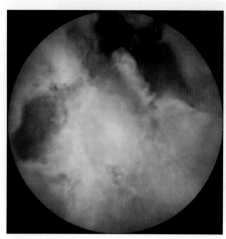

Figure 128.2 Crohn's disease. Edema, ulcer, and luminal narrowing seen in Crohn's disease of the small intestine on video capsule endoscopy.

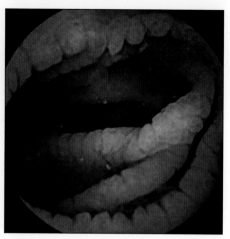

Figure 128.3 Celiac disease. Mucosal fissuring and scalloping seen in celiac disease on video capsule endoscopy.

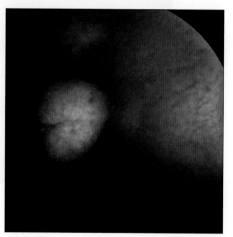

Figure 128.4 A small polyp seen in the terminal ileum on video capsule endoscopy.

elevated erythrocyte sedimentation rate, elevated C-reactive protein, thrombocytosis, or leukocytosis. An algorithm has been formulated to specify which patients should be considered for capsule endoscopy to diagnose or exclude Crohn's disease [19]. According to these criteria, capsule endoscopy could be performed in patients with gastrointestinal symptoms (chronic pain or diarrhea, weight loss, or growth failure) and either extraintestinal manifestations, inflammatory markers, or abnormal imaging studies. A meta-analysis of 11 studies, including 223 patients, compared capsule endoscopy to other imaging modalities of the small intestine, such as barium studies, computed tomography (CT) scanning, or MRI. An incremental diagnostic yield of 22–40% was demonstrated for those with non-stricturing small bowel Crohn's disease [20]. A scoring index has been developed to assess mucosal inflammatory changes in the small intestine, based on the variables of villous appearance, ulcerations, and stenosis [21]. This index can provide a common language to quantify mucosal changes associated with an inflammatory process (see Video clip 128.2)

Capsule endoscopy may be indicated to assist in the diagnosis or monitoring of patients with **celiac disease** (Figure 128.3) It is performed in patients with established celiac disease who develop alarm symptoms and in patients with suspected celiac disease, i.e., having positive tissue transglutaminase or antiendomysial antibodies, without a diagnostic upper endoscopy. Capsule endoscopy can serve as an alternative method to assess for villous atrophy in patients unwilling or unable to have a diagnostic upper endoscopy and to assess for villous atrophy in those with negative biopsies [22]. When used to assess for features of celiac disease, including scalloping of folds, fissures, flat mucosa, and mosaic appearance, capsule endoscopy has a reported sensitivity of 87.5% and specificity of 90.9% [23] (see Video clip 128.3)

Capsule endoscopy can be performed for the evaluation of patients with **polyposis syndromes**, including Peutz–Jeghers

syndrome and familial adenomatous polyposis (see Video clip 128.4). Capsule endoscopy is superior to small bowel barium studies, MRI, and CT enteroclysis for the detection of small bowel polyps (Figure 128.4). However, it does not adequately assess neoplasia of the duodenum or the ampulla of Vater [24].

Capsule endoscopy images in other conditions are shown in Figure 128.5, together with a normal exam for comparison.

Contraindications for capsule endoscopy include **intestinal obstruction** and **implanted cardiac devices**. A dissolving test capsule, called a patency capsule, has been developed to determine if a capsule can be expelled from the body. The capsule has cellophane with wax plugs at either end and contains both a radiotag and lactose mixed with barium. The patient can be scanned approximately 30 hours following ingestion to confirm capsule passage. Although capsule endoscopy is contraindicated in patients with pacemakers and defibrillators, there appears to be no interference in research studies and no complications have been reported.

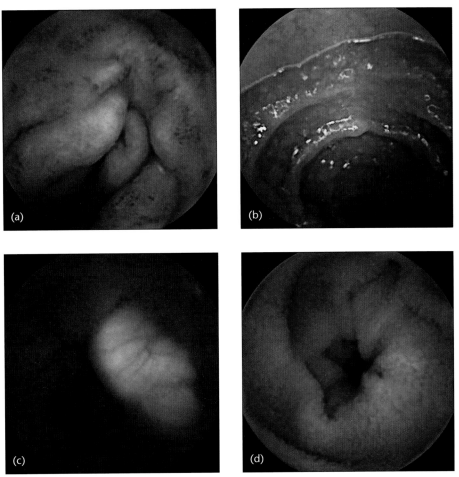

Figure 128.5 Other images seen on capsule endoscopy: (a) radiation enteritis; (b) lymphoid nodular hyperplasia; (c) cystic lymphangiectasia. (d) Normal capsule endoscopy study.

Pitfalls in interpretation

Capsule endoscopy has several difficulties in interpretation, including the inability to perform therapeutic interventions, incomplete exams, missed lesions, and variable interpretation (Table 128.3). The capsule does not reach the colon during recording time in approximately 20–30% of capsule studies and **incomplete exams** are associated with the following risk factors: hospitalization, prolonged gastric transit, and small bowel surgery [25]. In addition to incomplete exams, **lesions may be missed** due to a limited field of mucosal view or failure of the viewer to recognize abnormalities. In the pooled data analysis of 530 capsule endoscopy exams, the overall miss rate for capsule endoscopy was 10.8%, with the highest miss rate for tumors [15]. The capsule is propelled by peristalsis and thus, movement may be erratic with some lesions present on only one frame, or not at all. In addition, as insufflation is not possible with video capsule endoscopy, lesions may be hidden behind intestinal folds.

Physicians may interpret capsule images differently and **interobserver variability (IOV)** is yet another limitation of capsule endoscopy. The overall IOV was approximately

Table 128.3 Limitations of capsule endoscopy

- Inability to take biopsies
- Missed lesions
- Difficulty in localization
- Incomplete exams
- Variability in interpretation

k = 0.50 with better agreement for bleeding than other etiologies [26]. False-positive readings on capsule endoscopy studies may be the result of misinterpretation of red areas as angiodysplasias, normal lymphatic structures as inflammation, and intestinal folds as tumors [11]. The suggested fastest rate of reviewing small images is 15 frames/second [13].

Proper **localization of an identified lesion** on capsule endoscopy presents another difficulty in interpretation and determining the ideal approach for treatment. The lesion may be within reach of push enteroscopy or only via deep enteroscopy using an oral or rectal approach.

Future directions

Developments in capsule endoscopy technology may focus on improved image acquisition and new capabilities for both diagnosis and therapeutics. Improvements in the number of images obtained, resolution, and field of view could be introduced. Capsules of the future may be controlled externally and perform maneuvers such as biopsy or cautery.

SOURCES OF INFORMATION FOR PATIENTS AND DOCTORS

http://www.gi.org/patients/gihealth/smallbowel.asp
http://www.asge.org/PatientInfoIndex.aspx?id=390
http://www.icce.info/en-int/Pages/HomePage.aspx

References

1. Iddan G, Meron G, Glukhovsky, A, Swain P. Wireless capsule endoscopy. *Nature.* 2000;405:417.
2. Cave DR, Fleischer DE, Leighton JA, *et al.* A multicenter randomized comparison of the Endocapsule and the Pillcam SB. *Gastrointest Endosc.* 2008;68:487–494.
3. Sharma VK, Eliakim R, Sharma P, Faigel D; ICCE. ICCE consensus for esophageal capsule endoscopy. *Endoscopy.* 2005;37:1060–1064.
4. Gerson L, Lin OS. Cost–benefit analysis of capsule endoscopy compared with standard upper endoscopy for the detection of Barrett's esophagus. *Clin Gastroenterol Hepatol.* 2007;5:319–325.
5. Spiegel BM, Esrailian E, Eisen G. The budget impact of endoscopic screening for esophageal varices in cirrhosis. *Gastrointest Endosc.* 2007;66:679–692.
6. Van Gossum A, Munoz-Navas M, Fernandez-Urien I, *et al.* Capsule endoscopy versus colonoscopy for the detection of polyps and cancer. *N Engl J Med.* 2009;361:264–270.
7. Rokkas T, Papaxoinis K, Triantafyllou K, Pistiolas D, Ladas SD. Does purgative preparation influence the diagnostic yield of small bowel video capsule endoscopy?: A meta-analysis. *Am J Gastroenterol.* 2009;104:219–227.
8. Cave D, Legnani P, de Franchis R, Lewis BS. ICCE 2005 reference for capsule retention. *Endoscopy.* 2005;37:1065–1067.
9. Li F, Gurudu SR, De Petris G, *et al.* Retention of the capsule endoscope: a single center experience of 1000 capsule endoscopy procedures. *Gastrointest Endosc.* 2008;68:174–180.
10. Cheifetz AS, Kornbluth A, Legnani P, *et al.* The risk of retention of the capsule endoscope in patients with known or suspected Crohn's disease. *Am J Gastroenterol.* 2006;101:2218–2222.
11. Gerson L. Capsule endoscopy and deep enteroscopy: indications for the practicing clinician. *Gastroenterology.* 2009;137:1197–1201.
12. Raju GS, Gerson L, Das A, Lewis B. American Gastroenterological Association (AGA) Institute Technical Review on obscure gastrointestinal bleeding. *Gastroenterology.* 2007;133:1697–1717.
13. Pennazio M, Eisen G, Goldfarb N. ICCE consensus for obscure gastrointestinal bleeding. *Endoscopy.* 2005;37:1046–1050.
14. Triester SL, Leighton JA, Leontiadis GI, *et al.* A meta-analysis of the yield of capsule endoscopy compared to other diagnostic modalities in patients with obscure gastrointestinal bleeding. *Am J Gastroenterol.* 2005;100:2407–2418.
15. Lewis BS, Eisen G, Friedman S. A pooled analysis to evaluate results of capsule endoscopy trials. *Endoscopy.* 2005;37:960–965.
16. Pennazio M, Santucci R, Rondonotti E, *et al.* Outcome of patients with obscure gastrointestinal bleeding after capsule endoscopy: a report of 100 consecutive cases. *Gastroenterology.* 2004;126: 643–653.
17. Hartmann D, Schmidt H, Bolz G, *et al.* A prospective two-center study comparing wireless capsule endoscopy with intraoperative enteroscopy in patients with obscure gastrointestinal bleeding. *Gastrointest Endosc.* 2005;61:826–832.
18. Apostolopoulos P, Liatsos C, Gralnek IM, *et al.* The role of wireless capsule endoscopy in investigating unexplained iron deficiency anemia after negative endoscopic evaluation of the upper and lower gastrointestinal tract. *Endoscopy.* 2006;38:1127–1132.
19. Mergener K, Ponchon T, Gralnek I, *et al.* Literature review and recommendations for clinical application of small bowel capsule endoscopy-based on a panel discussion by international experts. *Endoscopy.* 2007;39:895–909.
20. Triester SL, Leighton JA, Leontiadis GI, *et al.* A meta-analysis of the yield of capsule endoscopy compared to other diagnostic modalities in patients with non-stricturing small bowel Crohn's disease. *Am J Gastroenterol.* 2006;101:954–964.
21. Gralnek IM, Defranchis R, Seidman E, Leighton JA, Legnani P, Lewis BS. Development of a capsule endoscopy scoring index for small bowel mucosal inflammatory change. *Aliment Pharmacol Ther.* 2008;27:146–154.
22. Cellier C, Green PH, Collin P, Murray J. ICCE consensus for celiac disease. *Endoscopy.* 2005;37:1055–1059.
23. Rondonotti E, Spada C, Cave D, *et al.* Video capsule enteroscopy in the diagnosis of celiac disease: a multicenter study. *Am J Gastroenterol.* 2007;102:1624–1631.
24. Iaquinto G, Fornasarig M, Quaia M, *et al.* Capsule endoscopy is useful and safe for small-bowel surveillance in familial adenomatous polyposis. *Gastrointest Endosc.* 2008;67:61–67.
25. Westerhof J, Weersma R, Koornstra J. Risk factors for incomplete small-bowel capsule endoscopy. *Gastrointest Endosc.* 2009;69: 74–80.
26. Lai LH, Wong GL, Chow DK, Lau JY, Sung JJ, Leung WK. Inter–observer variations on interpretation of capsule endoscopies. *Eur J Gastroenterol Hepatol.* 2006;18:283–286.

CHAPTER 129

Confocal endomicroscopy

Martin Goetz and Ralf Kiesslich

I. Medizinische Klinik und Poliklinik, Universitätsmedizin Mainz, Mainz, Germany

KEY POINTS

- Confocal endomicroscopy is a novel technique enabling *in vivo* resolution of microscopic mucosal details during ongoing endoscopy
- It is a targeted imaging technique relying on the systemic or topical application of fluorescent dyes
- Multiple studies have shown the ability of endomicroscopy to visualize histopathology in normal mucosa and different diseases of the upper and lower gastrointestinal tract based on simplified tissue criteria
- It provides real-time imaging in intact tissue devoid of tissue processing artifacts. This makes conventional histopathology and confocal endomicroscopy complementary in clinical routine and science

Introduction

It has always been the goal of endoscopists not just to predict histology from endoscopic features but to directly see histology during ongoing endoscopy [1]. Confocal endomicroscopy is a novel technique that enables *in vivo* histology to be seen without disrupting the tissue integrity. It combines videoendoscopy for macroscopic imaging with confocal microscopy for immediate microscopic visualization.

Technique

Confocal endomicroscopy devices

Two systems are currently marketed for *in vivo* confocal endomicroscopy; an endoscope-based system and a probe-based system (Table 129.1). In the first system to be used in clinical practice [2], an **endoscope-based system**, the miniaturized components of a laser scanner are integrated into the distal tip of a flexible endoscope. A single optical fiber provides both illumination and detection pinholes, and high resolution can be obtained. The confocal imaging window is slightly prominent at the distal tip of the endoscope and can therefore be identified in the videoendoscopic image at the 7 o'clock position (see Figure 129.5a). The system delivers an excitation wavelength of 488 nm, and light emission is detected at >505 nm. Successive points within the tissue are scanned in a raster pattern to construct an *en face* optical section. The imaging depth is adjustable from the surface to 250 μm using

an operator-controlled z-axis actuator (the button on the handpiece of the endoscope). With this, serial optical sections are obtained, similar to the adjacent sections in a computed tomography (CT) scan. Images on the screen approximate a 1000-fold magnification of the tissue *in vivo*.

A different approach is used in **probe-based confocal microscopy**. Different probe types are available with diameters ranging from 1 to 2.7 mm, and are compatible with the working channel of standard endoscopes. The smallest probe has even been fitted through a cholangioscope working channel [3]. Image acquisition is faster with this probe (12 frames/second), but resolution is limited by the number of fibers, and cellular structures are sometimes difficult to resolve. With a smaller field of view, higher resolution is provided. Different probe types encompass different imaging planes, but for each single probe the imaging plane is fixed and cannot be adapted.

Staining protocols

Confocal microscopy relies on the application of fluorescent agents. Application can be either topical, which limits imaging plane to the depth of diffusion of the dye across the upper epithelial layers, or systemic, which can exploit the full range of the adjustable imaging depth in endoscope-based endomicroscopy. Most studies in humans have been performed with **intravenous fluorescein sodium**. Fluorescein is an inexpensive agent that has been used for retinal angiography for decades and is considered safe [4,5]. It quickly distributes within all compartments of the tissue; confocal imaging is possible within seconds after intravenous injection of 5 mL (10%) for approximately 30–60 minutes. Fluorescein non-specifically contrasts connective tissue and vessel architecture (due to a considerable plasma albumin binding), but does not regularly stain nuclei (with the exception of nuclei in squamous epithelium; see Figure 129.3). Fluorescein shows pH-dependent fluorescence intensity. A lower intracellular pH in malignant cells is probably responsible for their darker appearance and this facilitates detection of neoplasia.

Alternatively, **acriflavine 0.02%** can be applied topically and predominantly stains nuclei [6]. Concerns have been raised that nuclear contrast may indicate a risk of mutagenicity, although acriflavine has been used for a long time, e.g.,

Textbook of Clinical Gastroenterology and Hepatology, Second Edition. Edited by C. J. Hawkey, Jaime Bosch, Joel E. Richter, Guadalupe Garcia-Tsao, Francis K. L. Chan.
© 2012 Blackwell Publishing Ltd. Published 2012 by Blackwell Publishing Ltd.

Table 129.1 Comparison of endoscope- versus probe-based confocal endomicroscopy

	Endoscope-based confocal endomicroscopy	Probe-based confocal endomicroscopy
System		
Resolution	0.7 μm >1 megapixels (1024 × 1024 pixels)	Different probe types: 3.5 μm, 1 μm, and 3.5 μm Approx 30 000 pixels
Field of view (edge)	475 μm	Different probe types: 320 μm, 240 μm, and 600 μm
Imaging plane depth	0–250 μm (user adapted)	Different probe types (plane fixed for each): 55 μm, 60 μm, and 100 μm
Frame rate	0.8–1.6/s	12/s
Working channel	Free endoscope working channel (for targeted biopsies, intervention)	Probe can be passed through working channel of any endoscope
Examples	Figures 129.1, 129.3, 129.4, 129.5a–c, 129.6	Figure 129.2 and 129.5d, e
Company	Pentax (Japan) and Optiscan (Australia)	Mauna Kea Technologies (France)

for disinfection, and no such adverse events have been reported. Still, alternative staining methods to negatively render nuclei by cytoplasmic staining have been investigated. Topical cresyl violet has shown promising results in pilot studies in human colorectal lesions [7] and upper gastrointestinal tract imaging [8].

Procedure

For confocal endomicroscopy, patients are prepared as for usual upper or lower endoscopy. An endomicroscopic examination always combines macroscopic (videoendoscopic) and microscopic evaluation. Both images are displayed on two separate screens simultaneously. For imaging, the confocal imaging window or the probe must be brought into direct contact with the area of interest under videoendoscopic control.

Moving artifacts are the most commonly encountered artifacts. Stabilizing the confocal endomicroscope can be facilitated by using suction or applying gentle pressure on the tissue; for stabilization of the probe-based system some authors prefer using a cap. Application of a spasmolytic agent such as butyl-scopolamin is useful. In the presence of intravenous contrast, blood can interfere with confocal imaging; therefore biopsies should be obtained only after imaging of a given site has been accomplished.

Confocal endomicroscopy is a targeted technique; pan-endomicroscopy of the gut is not feasible. **Chromoendoscopy**

has been promoted for detection of suspicious areas that are subsequently characterized by endomicroscopy. Both methylene blue 0.1% [9] and Lugol's solution 0.5% [10] have been successfully combined with endomicroscopy and do not significantly interfere with confocal imaging. In the future, virtual chromoendoscopy techniques may further assist in the identification of areas of interest for endomicroscopy.

The images obtained with endomicroscopy represent *en face* **sections** parallel to the tissue surface. This sectioning differs from the routine vertical orientation of histopathology slides. Evaluation of endomicroscopic images should be performed in real-time during ongoing endoscopy to exploit the advantages of being able to obtain real-time histological diagnosis for on-table decision-making. A thorough knowledge of the microarchitecture of the intestinal mucosa and its diseases is therefore mandatory for image interpretation. Close cooperation with a gastrointestinal histopathologist is especially helpful in the initial experience with endomicroscopy. We recommend that image analysis first follows a simple pattern recognition approach, differentiating normal from abnormal mucosal patterns, before appreciation of all microscopic details is sought. For example, evaluation of the crypt structure provides straightforward classification of the nature of colonic lesions [2]. Deeper imaging sections yield the microvessel structure. Ideally, a three-dimensional optical biopsy is obtained (volumetric tissue sampling). Microscopic key

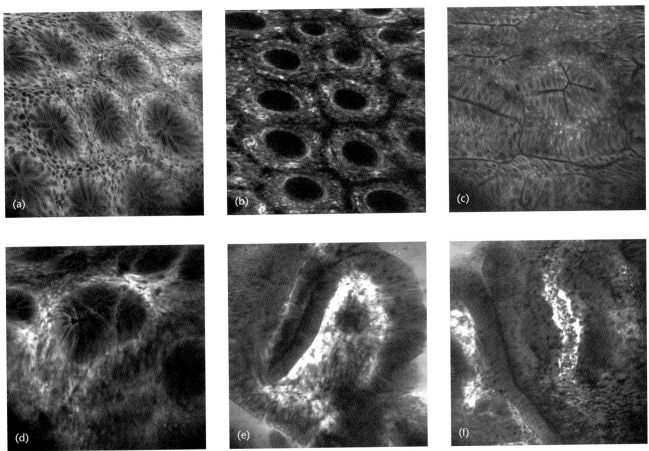

Figure 129.1 Confocal pattern classification to predict colonic pathology based on the crypt and vessel architecture (superficial and deeper tissue sections). In the normal colonic mucosa (a and b), crypts (a) show a regular distribution and the lumen is surrounded by epithelial cells, including goblet cells with dark mucin inclusions. Vessels (b) surround each individual crypt in a hexagonal pattern and are brightly contrasted after fluorescein injection. In regenerative tissue (inflammatory or hyperplastic, c and d), crypt openings are star-shaped or focally aggregated (c). The basal membrane is clearly delineated, and the epithelial lining is intact. Capillaries often show a mild increase in number and tortuosity, but their diameter is regular (d). In neoplasia (e and f), the epithelial layer is ridged-lined and irregular with elongation or loss of crypts (e) and scarce goblet cells. In deeper sections, pathological vessels become prominent, with irregular diameters larger than single erythrocytes (black dots in the bright lumen, f).

structures facilitate the classification of mucosal alterations, such as detection of goblet cells or recognition of mostly darker neoplastic cells. Easy-to-use classifications have been published for such tissue diagnosis. In the future, semi-automated tissue recognition software holds promise to assist in the classification of lesions [11,12].

Clinical value

The colon

In the first trial using endomicroscopy in routine clinical practice, circumscribed lesions and standardized areas in the colon and terminal ileum were examined in patients undergoing **screening colonoscopy** [2][2]. A confocal pattern classification was developed according to the cellular, crypt, and vessel architecture (Figure 129.1). Based on this easy-to-use classification, normal mucosa, regenerative (hyperplastic or inflammatory) changes, and neoplastic lesions could be distinguished with a high accuracy of 99%. Similar imaging results were obtained in a second study using the same confocal endomicroscopy system [13]. These studies demonstrated for the first time that histopathology could be reliably predicted during ongoing colonoscopy. Figure 129.2 shows the corresponding pathologies obtained with probe-based confocal endomicroscopy.

Endomicroscopy was then studied in patients with long-standing **ulcerative colitis** who are at increased risk of developing **intraepithelial neoplasia**. Chromoendoscopy was used to target the endomicroscopy. Endomicroscopic characterization of lesions was accurate in 98% [9]. While 42 quadrant biopsies were necessary in the conventional white-light colonoscopy protocol, the number of biopsies could have been reduced to four per patient without reducing the diagnostic yield for intraepithelial neoplasia if only circumscribed lesions (on chromoendoscopy) with suspicious microarchitecture (on endomicroscopy) had been biopsied. Potentially as important, 99% of biopsies of mucosa with a normal appearance on endomicroscopy did not yield intraepithelial neoplasia. This supports the concept of taking **"smart" biopsies** (instead of random biopsies) of endomicroscopically suspicious areas

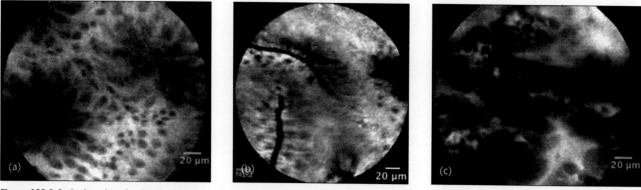

Figure 129.2 Probe-based confocal endomicroscopy of colonic lesions shows (a) normal colonic mucosa, (b) a hyperplastic polyp, and (c) a polyp containing high-grade intraepithelial neoplasia. Images were obtained with a Coloflex UHD probe. (Courtesy of Michael B. Wallace and Anna Buchner, Mayo Clinic College of Medicine, Jacksonville, FL, USA.)

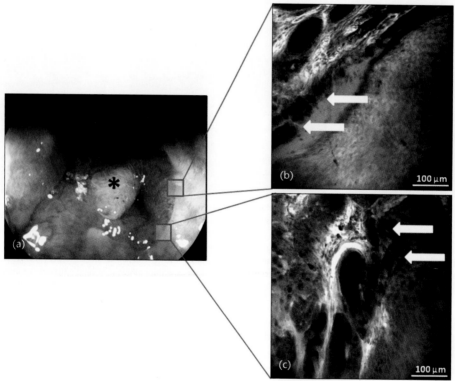

Figure 129.3 a–c Endomicroscopy in ulcerative colitis. In a patient with longstanding ulcerative colitis, a suspicious lesion was identified in the distal rectum (asterisk). Screening the surrounding mucosa with the confocal endomicroscope (boxes in a) demonstrated that the intraepithelial neoplasia extended distally towards the anorectal verge and undermined the squamous epithelium (right lower corner in b and c) with neoplastic glands (arrows). Note that within the squamous epithelium, nuclei can be identified after fluorescein staining.

only, while leaving the healthy mucosa intact (Figure 129.3). The extent and grade of inflammation could be reliably predicted: Inflammation extended more proximally by endomicroscopy than predicted by videoendoscopy.

In the colon, endomicroscopy has also assisted in other inflammatory diseases such as graft-versus-host disease [14], and in the *in vivo* definition of intestinal spirochaetosis in human immunodeficiency virus (HIV)-associated diarrhea [15]. In diseases with a patchy pattern, such as in microscopic colitis or amyloidosis, endomicroscopy helps to rapidly screen multiple sites by taking virtual biopsies in order to target one "real" biopsy rather than random "blind" biopsies [16,17].

The esophagus

In the esophagus, endomicroscopy has mainly been evaluated for the diagnosis of **neoplastic and precursor lesions** (Figure 129.4). In squamous cell cancer, a case report defined vascular alterations indicative of neoplastic disease [18]. Such microvessel anomalies can be reliably visualized after intravenous fluorescein injection and comparison to normal intrapapillary capillary loops [19]. In a follow-up trial in 21 patients with suspected early cancer, Lugol's staining detected 43 lesions [10]. Here, confocal endomicroscopy identified neoplasia from dark cells with irregular borders and architecture, twisted and irregular vessels, and leakage of fluorescein from tumor vessels,

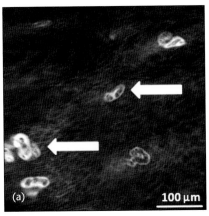
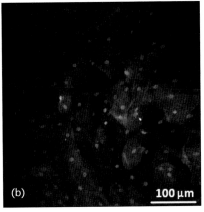
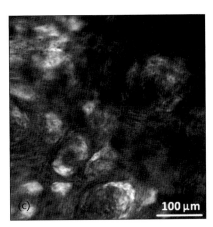

Figure 129.4 Endomicroscopy of squamous epithelium of the esophagus. (a) In normal squamous epithelium, intrapapillary capillary loops (IPCL) are identified as white, twisted vessels with black erythrocytes (arrows) within hexagonal epithelial cells after fluorescein injection. (b) After topical application of acriflavine, even the nuclei of the squamous cells become visible in the superficial layers of the esophageal mucosa. (c) In squamous epithelial cancer, the IPCLs are severely disturbed and papillary infiltrates of malignant cells are visible on the right side of the confocal image.

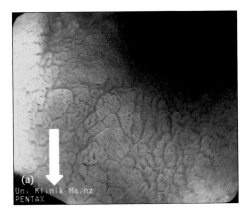
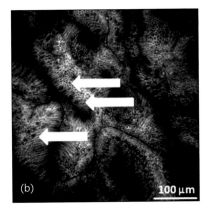
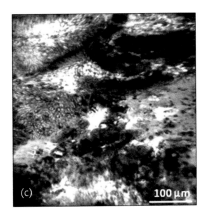

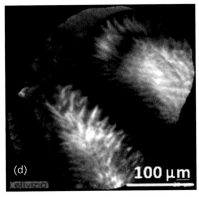
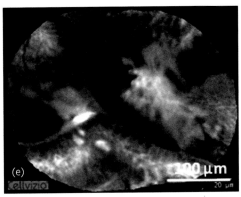

Figure 129.5 Endomicroscopy of Barrett's epithelium. (a) In the endoscopic view, the confocal imaging window and the blue laser light can be identified at the 7 o'clock position (arrow). (b) In non-dysplastic Barrett's epithelium, dark mucin inclusions define goblet cells (arrows) within the glandular epithelium, permitting the *in vivo* diagnosis of intestinal metaplasia. (c) In dysplastic Barrett's epithelium, the tissue structure is highly irregular, and the dark malignant cells are no longer contained by a clear basal membrane, indicating infiltration into the lamina propria. Bright fluorescein extravasations identify enhanced vessel leakiness. On the left side, some residual goblet cells are seen. For comparison, "mosaiced" images obtained with a confocal probe of non-dysplastic Barrett's esophagus (d) and with high-grade intraepithelial neoplasia (e) are shown (each composed of several adjacent images). (Figure 129.4d and e courtesy of Michael B. Wallace and Anna Buchner, Mayo Clinic College of Medicine, Jacksonville, FL, USA.)

with an overall accuracy of 95%. Two false-positive findings were obtained in inflammation, stressing the need to minimize inflammation before screening for intraepithelial neoplasia.

In suspected **Barrett's esophagus**, endomicroscopy was able to distinguish between different epithelia and to visualize goblet cells *in vivo* as a key structure of intestinal metaplasia (Figure 129.5). Using a simple classification based on the presence of dark irregular cells and neoplastic vessels, Barrett's-associated intraepithelial neoplasia could be predicted with 97% accuracy [20]. Using miniprobe-based confocal

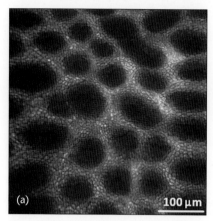 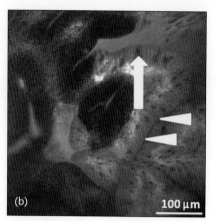 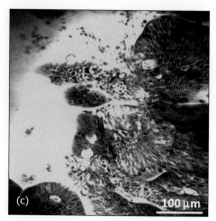

Figure 129.6 Endomicroscopy in the stomach. (a) In the healthy corpus, the mucosa shows a cobblestone appearance, and the pits are round and crypt-like. In the normal antrum and fundus, the gastric glands are branched. (b) A sudden break in the epithelial lining can be identified with regular antrum epithelium on the left. On the right, goblet cells can be seen (arrows) within the high prismatic epithelium, and even a brush border is visible (arrowheads), clearly defining intestinal metaplasia. (c) In early gastric cancer, the surface is villous, the cells are irregular in size and infiltrate into the lamina propria, and fluorescein leaks into the gastric lumen.

microscopy, a high negative predictive value was found for the detection of intraepithelial neoplasia even in macroscopically normal mucosa [21].

The stomach

In the stomach, endomicroscopy visualized different steps in the transition of normal epithelium [22] through inflammation and intestinal metaplasia to overt **gastric cancer**. The power of this high-resolution technique is exemplified by a report that endomicroscopy was even able to identify living bacteria such as *Helicobacter pylori in vivo* by combining acriflavine and fluorescein to simultaneously yield both the causative pathological agent and its pathomorphological consequence (gastritis) [23]. The presence of goblet cells, columnar absorptive cells and brush border, and villiform foveolar epithelium identified and classified gastric intestinal metaplasia with superior sensitivity and specificity when compared to white-light endoscopy [24]. Morphological criteria have also been established for *in vivo* imaging of gastric cancer [25,26] (Figure 129.6).

The small intestine

In the small intestine, endomicroscopy has mostly been evaluated to minimize sampling error for diseases with a patchy distribution. In **celiac disease**, endomicroscopy effectively diagnosed and evaluated the severity *in vivo* by defining villous atrophy and crypt hypertrophy with high accuracy [27,28]. Similarly, a pilot trial has assessed the suitability of endomicroscopy for surveillance after a restorative ileoanal pouch has been instituted in **ulcerative colitis** and **familial adenomatous polyposis** [29].

Conclusions and future directions

Confocal endomicroscopy permits for the first time endoscopic tissue diagnosis at a microscopic level, thereby providing virtual histology *in vivo*. Multiple clinical studies have shown that in expert hands endomicroscopy has a high diagnostic accuracy for neoplasia and inflammation. When compared to conventional histopathology, endomicroscopy is able to provide similar information about tissue architecture, cell infiltration, and mucosal alterations. This information is immediately available at ongoing endoscopy.

Endomicroscopy with fluorescein at present cannot assess all risk factors of neoplasia, such as the nuclear-to-cytoplasmic ratio, lymph vessel infiltration, or submucosal infiltration. Therefore, histopathology will continue to be an indispensable part of a patient's work-up. Endomicroscopy will rather support the targeting of biopsies by taking multiple optical biopsies to rapidly screen the mucosa *in vivo* in diseases that carry a high risk of neoplasia or have a patchy distribution. Real biopsies will then only be necessary if endomicroscopy is unable to assess the nature of risk factors of a lesion comprehensively. This will probably avoid unnecessary biopsies and repeat procedures. This might not only hold promise to optimize diagnosis in the gut mucosa, but also in other organs of the gastrointestinal tract [3,30,31].

In addition to imaging morphology, endomicroscopy is able to render tissue function free from fixation artifacts. Increased vessel leakiness by extravasation of fluorescein in inflammation and neoplasia has been demonstrated. Even microscopic details of epithelial regeneration in healthy and diseased mucosa, such as cellular shedding, become visible [6], making endomicroscopy a valuable tool to understand mucosal physiology and pathology.

It seems reasonable to believe that technical improvements will permit *in vivo* imaging modalities similar to bench-top confocal microscopy in the near future. Co-localization of multiple fluorophores (multichannel imaging) will doubtless extend the number of microarchitectural issues that can be investigated. This will also promote recent advances in molecular imaging [32,33] to provide real-time *in vivo* immunohistochemistry of neoplastic lesions and allow prediction of response to targeted molecular therapies. Future developments will also include the use of alternate laser lines and detection bands to achieve deeper tissue imaging [34]. This will be of great importance to establish the depth of infiltration of a lesion prior to endoscopic resection.

Endomicroscopy has the potential to contribute significantly to our understanding of dynamic events in their natural environment in clinical research. Today, confocal endomicroscopy is used to detect neoplasia and inflammation, and to provide smart biopsies, and has made the endoscopist's dream of seeing histology a reality.

References

1. Kudo S, Tamura S, Nakajima T, Yamano H, Kusaka H, Watanabe H. Diagnosis of colorectal tumorous lesions by magnifying endoscopy. *Gastrointest Endosc.* 1996;44:8–14.
2. Kiesslich R, Burg J, Vieth M, Gnaendiger J, *et al.* Confocal laser endoscopy for diagnosing intraepithelial neoplasias and colorectal cancer in vivo. *Gastroenterology.* 2004;127:706–713.
3. Meining A, Frimberger E, Becker V, *et al.* Detection of cholangiocarcinoma in vivo using miniprobe-based confocal fluorescence microscopy. *Clin Gastroenterol Hepatol.* 2008;6:1057–1060.
4. Wallace MB, Meining A, Canto MI, *et al.* The safety of intravenous fluorescein for confocal laser endomicroscopy in the gastrointestinal tract. *Aliment Pharmacol Ther.* 2010;31:548–552.
5. Pacurariu RI. Low incidence of side effects following intravenous fluorescein angiography. *Ann Ophthalmol.* 1982;14:32–36.
6. Kiesslich R, Goetz M, Angus EM, *et al.* Identification of epithelial gaps in human small and large intestine by confocal endomicroscopy. *Gastroenterology.* 2007;133:1769–1778.
7. Goetz M, Toermer T, Vieth M, *et al.* Simultaneous confocal laser endomicroscopy and chromoendoscopy with topical cresyl violet. *Gastrointest Endosc.* 2009;70:959–968.
8. Meining A, Saur D, Bajbouj M, *et al.* In vivo histopathology for detection of gastrointestinal neoplasia with a portable, confocal miniprobe: an examiner blinded analysis. *Clin Gastroenterol Hepatol.* 2007;5:1261–1267.
9. Kiesslich R, Goetz M, Lammersdorf K, *et al.* Chromoscopy-guided endomicroscopy increases the diagnostic yield of intraepithelial neoplasia in ulcerative colitis. *Gastroenterology.* 2007;132:874–882.
10. Pech O, Rabenstein T, Manner H, *et al.* Confocal laser endomicroscopy for in vivo diagnosis of early squamous cell carcinoma in the esophagus. *Clin Gastroenterol Hepatol.* 2008;6:89–94.
11. Lin KY, Maricevich M, Bardeesy N, Weissleder R, Mahmood U. In vivo quantitative microvasculature phenotype imaging of healthy and malignant tissues using a fiber-optic confocal laser microprobe. *Transl Oncol.* 2008;1:84–94.
12. Becker V, Vieth M, Bajbouj M, Schmid RM, Meining A. Confocal laser scanning fluorescence microscopy for in vivo determination of microvessel density in Barrett's esophagus. *Endoscopy.* 2008;40:888–891.
13. Polglase AL, McLaren WJ, Skinner SA, Kiesslich R, Neurath MF, Delaney PM. A fluorescence confocal endomicroscope for in vivo microscopy of the upper- and the lower-GI tract. *Gastrointest Endosc.* 2005;62:686–695.
14. Bojarski C, Gunther U, Rieger K, *et al.* In vivo diagnosis of acute intestinal graft-versus-host disease by confocal endomicroscopy. *Endoscopy.* 2009;41:433–438.
15. Gunther U, Epple HJ, Heller F, *et al.* In vivo diagnosis of intestinal spirochaetosis by confocal endomicroscopy. *Gut.* 2008;57:1331–1333.
16. Kiesslich R, Hoffman A, Goetz M, *et al.* In vivo diagnosis of collagenous colitis by confocal endomicroscopy. *Gut.* 2006;55:591–592.
17. Zambelli A, Villanacci V, Buscarini E, Bassotti G, Albarello L. Collagenous colitis: a case series with confocal laser microscopy and histology correlation. *Endoscopy.* 2008;40:606–608.
18. Deinert K, Kiesslich R, Vieth M, Neurath MF, Neuhaus H. In-vivo microvascular imaging of early squamous-cell cancer of the esophagus by confocal laser endoscopy. *Endoscopy.* 2007;39:366–368.
19. Liu H, Li YQ, Yu T, *et al.* Confocal laser endomicroscopy for superficial esophageal squamous cell carcinoma. *Endoscopy.* 2009;41:99–106.
20. Kiesslich R, Gossner L, Goetz M, *et al.* In vivo histology of Barrett's esophagus and associated neoplasia by confocal laser endomicroscopy. *Clin Gastroenterol Hepatol.* 2006;4:979–987.
21. Pohl H, Rosch T, Vieth M, *et al.* Miniprobe confocal laser microscopy for the detection of invisible neoplasia in patients with Barrett's oesophagus. *Gut.* 2008;57:1648–1653.
22. Zhang JN, Li YQ, Zhao YA, *et al.* Classification of gastric pit patterns by confocal endomicroscopy. *Gastrointest Endosc.* 2008;67:843–853.
23. Kiesslich R, Goetz M, Burg J, *et al.* Diagnosing Helicobacter pylori in vivo by confocal laser endoscopy. *Gastroenterology.* 2005;128:2119–2123.
24. Guo YT, Li YQ, Yu T, *et al.* Diagnosis of gastric intestinal metaplasia with confocal laser endomicroscopy in vivo: a prospective study. *Endoscopy.* 2008;40:547–553.
25. Kitabatake S, Niwa Y, Miyahara R, *et al.* Confocal endomicroscopy for the diagnosis of gastric cancer in vivo. *Endoscopy.* 2006;38:1110–1114.
26. Kakeji Y, Yamaguchi S, Yoshida D, *et al.* Development and assessment of morphologic criteria for diagnosing gastric cancer using confocal endomicroscopy: an ex vivo and in vivo study. *Endoscopy.* 2006;38:886–890.
27. Leong RW, Nguyen NQ, Meredith CG, *et al.* In vivo confocal endomicroscopy in the diagnosis and evaluation of celiac disease. *Gastroenterology.* 2008;135:1870–1876.
28. Zambelli A, Villanacci V, Buscarini E, *et al.* Confocal laser endomicroscopy in celiac disease: description of findings in two cases. *Endoscopy.* 2007;39:1018–1020.
29. Trovato C, Sonzogni A, Fiori G, *et al.* Confocal laser endomicroscopy for the detection of mucosal changes in ileal pouch after restorative proctocolectomy. *Dig Liver Dis.* 2009;41:578–585.
30. Goetz M, Kiesslich R, Dienes HP, *et al.* In vivo confocal laser endomicroscopy of the human liver: a novel method for assessing liver microarchitecture in real time. *Endoscopy.* 2008;40:554–562.

31. von Delius S, Feussner H, Wilhelm D, *et al.* Transgastric in vivo histology in the peritoneal cavity using miniprobe-based confocal fluorescence microscopy in an acute porcine model. *Endoscopy.* 2007;39:407–411.

32. Hsiung PL, Hardy J, Friedland S, *et al.* Detection of colonic dysplasia in vivo using a targeted heptapeptide and confocal microendoscopy. *Nat Med.* 2008;14:454–458.

33. Goetz M, Ziebart A, Vieth M, *et al.* In vivo molecular imaging of colorectal cancer by confocal endomicroscopy (abstract). *Gastroenterology.* 2008;134:A48.

34. von Burstin J, Eser S, Seidler B, *et al.* Highly sensitive detection of early-stage pancreatic cancer by multimodal near-infrared molecular imaging in living mice. *Int J Cancer.* 2008;123: 2138–147.

CHAPTER 130

Self-propelled colonoscopy

Menachem Moshkowitz and Nadir Arber

Tel-Aviv University, Tel-Aviv, Israel

KEY POINTS

- Conventional colonoscopy for colorectal cancer screening has a low compliance rate
- Self-propelled devices may reduce the forces applied to the colon and mesentery, and thereby reduce loop formation, pain, need for sedation, and the risk of complications

---

Introduction

Colorectal cancer is the third most commonly diagnosed cancer in the United States and the second most common cause of cancer death [1]. Screening for colorectal cancer has been shown to reduce mortality. Conventional colonoscopy is the method of choice for **colorectal cancer screening**, and national colonoscopy screening programs are ongoing in many countries [2–4]. However, despite the obvious benefits of screening, fewer than half of Americans over the age of 50 have had any kind of colon cancer screening test. Several factors are responsible for the **poor compliance** for colorectal cancer screening, especially for colonoscopy. The major ones are performance limitations, the tedious preparation, and the pain and discomfort endured during colonoscopy [5–8]. In the absense of similarly effective methods (e.g., blood or stool tests), compliance with colonoscopy would most probably be enhanced if there were easier and sedation-free ways to perform it. To this end various groups have worked on novel technologies that will overcome the limitations of the current conventional push colonoscopy. The ideal technology would be a disposable, skill-independent, anesthesia-free, self-propelling, self-navigating miniaturized endoscopic device that moves along the entire length of the colon while transmitting video pictures of the colonic mucosa, and has a therapeutic option as well. A higher adherence rate to screening could result because of less need for sedation, less risk, and more widespread availability due to the more limited skill set required for technical performance.

Advantages of self-propelled colonoscopy

If the endoscope meets loops or angulations during colonoscopy, this can result in loss of control of the endoscope as well as patient discomfort. The adequacy of patient sedation becomes paramount. The rationale for developing a self-advancing endoscope is two-fold: (1) self-advancement avoids the need for a highly skilled operator and(2) it may reduce the forces commonly applied to negotiate the colon and mesentery with current colonoscopes, and thereby reduce loop formation, pain, need for sedation, and risk of complications.

Technical challenges

The colon consists of two anatomically distinct sections: the **sigmoid**, which is relatively narrow and typically has one or several sharp angulations or bends, and the **proximal colon**, which is distinguished by relatively straight sections that progressively widen in luminal caliber. These disparities in the anatomy of the colon create a significant challenge for a **propulsion mechanism**. It requires only rigid sections that are narrow and short enough to negotiate the sigmoid colon, yet these must adjust to the luminal caliber of the colon, particularly if they rely on gripping the mucosa for forward movement. Additional challenges include the variable hydrophilic forces between the device and the colonic wall that depend on the wetness of the mucosa. To minimize pain, propulsion must be accomplished without substantial pressure on the mesentery, and from an imaging perspective, the device ideally should be able to remove retained pools of fluid and allow systematic examination of the colonic mucosa.

Over the years, different prototypes of self-propelled devices based on various locomotion mechanisms have been described: balloons [9], suction crawlers [10], the serpentine robot ("Snake") [11], devices with "many legs" (Millipede) [12], wheels and belts [13], and water jets [14]. Only the minority that has reached the stage of clinical trials will be discussed.

Self-propelled devices
Protectiscope

In 2004, the USA Food and Drug Administration (FDA) approved a device known as the ColonoSight® (Striker, USA). Its current commercial name is Protectiscope. This device incorporates a miniature video camera and integral light-emitting diode (LED) light source at the tip of the reusable insertion tube. The device is used in conjunction with a disposable

---

component that both protects the scope and enhances its advancement. This disposable component includes channels for insufflation, irrigation, and suction, and is inserted through the endoscope before the procedure and disposed of afterwards, thus protecting the inner surface of the scope from contaminants.

The results from 178 procedures showed that the mean time of colonoscopy was 11.2 ± 6.5 minutes and the mean insertion length was 117 ± 26 cm. The cecal intubation rate was 90% (161 of 178 procedures) [15]. Biopsies and polypectomies were possible. There were no major complications, although the procedure had to be terminated early because of device malfunction in three patients (camera failure, improper assembly, and inadequate illumination). Dye studies and bacterial cultures showed no transfer of dye molecules or bacterial organisms across the protective disposable components.

Neoguide colonoscope

The Neoguide scope (Neoguide Systems, USA) is an "intelligent" scope that memorizes the colonic curves during insertion and withdrawal. It "remembers" the exact location of the lesions during further manipulation. It has 15 bendable segments in addition to a physician-controlled distal tip. By using two sensors, the system continuously monitors the depth of insertion and the position of the tip. The control unit directs each of the 15 segments of the scope to take the same path as identified by the first leading segment at a given depth (the "follow the leader" principle). Since less force is applied to the

colonic wall, there is a significant reduction in the incidence of looping and traction of the mesentery [16], the major causes of pain during colonoscopy. The device also offers advanced features, including the display of a real-time three-dimensional (3D) map of the colon and the ability for physicians to mark the location virtually of lesions on this map.

The first clinical study on the Neoguide scope was performed in 12 patients (four underwent screening and eight were symptomatic). One subject was excluded because of poor bowel preparation. Cecal intubation was achieved in all 11 remaining cases with a median time of 20.5 minutes. The patients were, however, sedated with midazolam and propofol [17].

Invendoscope

The Invendoscope (Invendo Medical Ltd, Germany) is a single-use colonoscope (Figure 130.1). It employs an inverted sleeve technology. Wheels are rolled on the inner side of an inverted sleeve, after which the inner sleeve is rolled inside out. Since the outer side of the inverted sleeve stays in position, the inner side is consequently pushed forward below the distal tip, inserting the Invendoscope deeper into the colon by about 10 cm each time.

A hand-held control unit is used to activate all of the endoscopic functions. When the "forward" or "backward" keys are pressed, eight drive wheels in the endoscope's driving unit start to move in the selected direction. When the scope is driven backwards, the driving wheels move backwards and

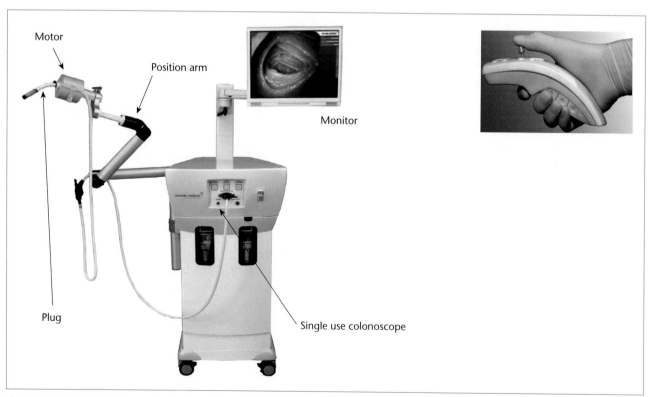

Figure 130.1 The Invendoscope.

the endoscope "shrinks." If no key is pressed by the physician, the wheels in the endoscope driving unit automatically stop. The physician is, therefore, always in control of the endoscope's movement. The endoscope tip can be deflected up to 180 degrees by moving a joystick on the handheld device, allowing optimal and easy steering of the colonoscope. This technology with its very small bending diameter was designed to reduce the forces exerted on the walls of the colon and thereby to minimize the potential discomfort felt by the patient, even when not sedated. It operates like a conventional endoscope, allowing for insufflations, rinsing, and suction. Biopsies can be taken and therapeutic procedures can be performed through a 3.2-mm working channel.

A prospective pilot study of this device was published by Rösch et al. [18]. It was a single-arm study that spanned two time periods using two different prototypes and included 39 healthy unsedated volunteers. The procedure was stopped prematurely in five subjects due to technical failures, and their data were excluded from the analysis. The cecum was reached in 82% of the remaining 34 cases. Severe pain while passing the sigmoid led to the termination of the procedure in two cases. The scope was unable to pass the mid-transverse colon in four additional cases. The mean discomfort score for the examination was 2 (range 1–6). No complications were encountered. The time spent inspecting the mucosa while withdrawing the instrument was limited, since the aim of this study was primarily to evaluate the motion and not the visual system.

The time to reaching the cecum must be shortened before the Invendoscope can be considered for routine use. It seems that lengthening the device from 160 to 200 cm and a slightly stiffer distal part might improve the efficacy of this device and increase the speed of the procedure.

Aer-O-Scope

The Aer-O-Scope (GI View Ltd, Israel)is a miniaturized, ultra-flexible self-propelling and self-navigating endoscope (Figure 130.2). It is a single-use, purely diagnostic (there is no working channel) device that glides over the mucosa, driven by minimal CO_2 pressure that gradually builds up behind it. A rectal introducer is placed into the rectum and a rectal balloon is inflated through this introducer in order to seal the anus. The colonoscope is a small tube with a camera embedded in the tip of a specially designed balloon. Both balloons are inflated and CO_2 is insufflated into the space between them. When the pressure between the two balloons slightly exceeds the pressure in the colon in front of the scope, the scope moves from the rectum to the cecum. The pressure is measured and monitored by sensitive sensors and is automatically controlled by special computerized algorithms to match the intracolonic and intra-abdominal pressures.

The ultra-flexible scope assumes the shape of the colon, rather than pleating and straightening the bowel, thus eliminating intraluminal looping. Self-advancement driven by low-grade air pressure minimizes the force applied to the colonic

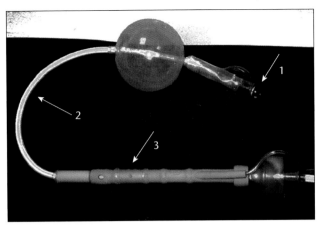

Figure 130.2 The Aer-O-Scope. 1. Balloon with embedded electro-optical capsule. 2. Multiluminal, ultra-flexible supply cable which is threaded through the rectal introducer and supplies the Aer-O-Scope with water, air, suction, and electricity. 3. The rectal introducer has its own balloon that helps to anchor the device within the rectum, once introduced, and to seal the anus once the colon is insufflated with CO_2.

wall and mesentery, thereby potentially reducing discomfort, pain, and the risk of perforation.

In addition to its innovative propulsion system, the Aer-O-Scope's visual system combines an Omni multidirectional optical component allowing for 360-degree viewing of all sides of the colon and thereby the detection of small polyps that are hidden behind mucosal folds.

The first animal experiment with this device was reported in 2006 [19,20]. Since then, more than 800 runs have been conducted in pigs. Phase I studies of various prototypes and modules (optical, mechanical, and user interface) of the Aer-O-Scope have been successfully completed. Clinical feasibility of the motion part of the device was successfully demonstrated in young healthy volunteers. The cecum was intubated in 10 of 12 subjects [21]. The omni-directional optical module enabled a detailed visual inspection of the colonic mucosa circumferentially and behind the mucosal folds, with minute blood vessels being evident without the need for tip manipulation.

PillCam® Colon capsule endoscope (see also Chapter 128)

The ultimate solution for patient acceptance may be the colonic capsule. Caspsule endoscopy was approved for clinical use at the beginning of this century. The PillCam® capsule (Given Imaging Ltd., Yoqneam, Israel) measures 11×31 mm and has dual cameras similar to the esophageal capsule (Figure 130.3). It has optics with a wide coverage area (more than twice that of the small bowel capsule), an automatic light control, a frame rate of four frames/second, and a total operating duration of approximately 10 hours. Following initial capsule activation and several minutes of image transmission from the esophagus and the stomach, the capsule enters a sleep mode (e.g., 1–2 hours) after which it spontaneously "wakes up" and starts transmitting images again.

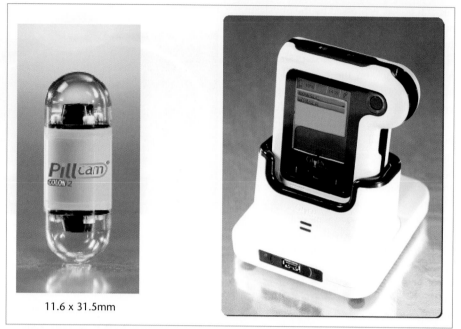

11.6 x 31.5mm

Figure 130.3 The Pillcam Colon 2.

Perfect colonic preparation is essential when performing capsule endoscopy. Towards this end, a novel colonic preparation protocol was developed to achieve a clean colon throughout the examination, as well as to promote capsule propulsion through the entire colon, with its excretion within 10 hours post ingestion. The patients must observe strict dietary restrictions followed by oral ingestion of polyethylene glycol solution, sodium phosphate, and a pro-motility agent (e.g., tegaserod or domperidone). A rectal suppository for promoting defecation is added towards the end of the procedure [22].

Two studies comparing capsule endoscopy to conventional colonoscopy have been reported [23,24]. Of the 84 evaluable patients in the first study [23], 20 (24%) had significant findings, defined as at least one polyp of 6mm or more in size or three or more polyps of any size: 14 of 20 (70%) were identified with the capsule and 16 of 20 (80%) by conventional colonoscopy. Polyps of any size were found in 45 patients: 34 of 45 (76%) were identified with the capsule and 36 of 45 (80%) by conventional colonoscopy. False-positive findings for the PillCam® Colon capsule examination were recorded in 15 of 45 cases (33%). There were no adverse events related to capsule endoscopy. In the second study [24], positive and negative predictive values for significant polyps (>6mm or more than three polyps) of 36% and 86% respectively were reported. No complications were encountered. Further data from a European multicenter study involving 320 patients in eight centers have been recently reported and show a relatively low sensitivity (64%), specificity (84%), positive predictive value (60%), and negative predictive value (86%).

The American Cancer Society's position statement on colorectal cancer screening modalities [25] concluded that currently there is no evidence to support the use of capsule endoscopy

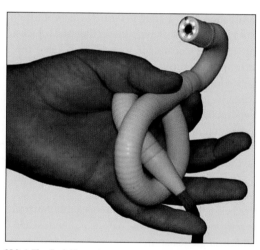

Figure 130.4 The Endotics system.

for detecting colorectal polyps or cancers. The colon is not well visualized with capsule endoscopy because:

- Stools obscure visualization of the colonic mucosa
- The slower transit time in the colon and its larger diameter (compared to the small bowel) make visualization of the entire colonic mucosa practically impossible
- Colonic peristalsis is antegrade and retrograde, so it is possible to miss suspicious areas of the colon if pointing in the wrong direction.

Endotics

The Endotics system (ERA Endoscopy S.r.l., Peccioli (Pisa), Italy) is a robotic device composed of a workstation and a disposable probe (Figure 130.4). The robot's motion was inspired by the "inchworm" caterpillar of the geometer moth. The flexible probe adapts its shape to the complex contours of the colon, thereby exerting low strenuous forces during its movement. The device uses a series of grippers and extenders to pull itself along the bowel. This exerts less pressure on the bowel wall, reducing the patient's discomfort. In a recent experimental study that included 40 patients, the stress pattern related to robotic colonoscopy was 90% lower than that of standard colonoscopy [26]. Additionally, robotic colonoscopy demonstrated a higher diagnostic accuracy since, due to the lower insufflation rate, it was able to visualize small polyps and angiodysplasia not seen during the standard colonoscopy. All patients rated the robotic colonoscopy as virtually painless compared to the standard colonoscopy.

A similar medical device from the same group, named E-Worm, moves like a worm, using two specific clampers for adhesion with intestinal mucosa. The light sources (LEDS) and video camera are inserted in the head of the E-Worm. This provides live pictures on the screen of the workstation, as for a normal colonoscope. The unique locomotion system with outstanding flexibility is able to follow every type of 3D shape, and this together with the low force required to move the probe, allows for a painless colonoscopy procedure and reduces risk of any perforation. In a pilot study, 37 colonoscopies with the E-Worm have been performed. Cecal intubation was achieved in 15 cases (40%) and ileal exploration was performed in one patient with Crohn's disease (2%). The right colon was reached in another seven patients (19%). No patients needed sedation and no complications occurred [27,28]

Conclusions

Self-propelled colonoscopic devices offer the hope of improving the compliance to colorectal cancer screening. Proof of concept studies have been performed for several types of self-propelled colonoscopes. They all, however, still need significant improvement before they can be considered as a good alternative to conventional colonoscopies for colorectal screening.

Acknowledgment

Esther Eshkol is thanked for editorial assistance.

References

1. American Cancer Society. *Colorectal Cancer Facts and Figures Special Edition*. Atlanta: American Cancer Society, 2008.
2. Pox C, Schmiegel W, Classen M. Current status of screening colonoscopy in Europe and in the United States. *Endoscopy.* 2007;39:168–173.
3. Winawer SJ; NPS Investigators. The achievements, impact, and future of the National Polyp Study. *Gastrointest Endosc.* 2006;64: 975–978.
4. Winawer S, Fletcher R, Rex D, *et al.*; Gastrointestinal Consortium Panel. Colorectal cancer screening and surveillance: clinical guidelines and rationale – update based on new evidence. *Gastroenterology.* 2003;124:544–560.
5. Gili M, Roca M, Ferrer V, *et al.* Psychosocial factors associated with the adherence to a colorectal cancer screening program. *Cancer Detect Prev.* 2006;30:354–360.
6. Bleiker EM, Menko FH, Taal BG, *et al.* Screening behavior of individuals at high risk for colorectal cancer. *Gastroenterology.* 2005;128:280–287.
7. Nicholson FB, Korman MG. Acceptance of flexible sigmoidoscopy and colonoscopy for screening and surveillance in colorectal cancer prevention. *J Med Screen.* 2005;12:89–95.
8. Nicholson FB, Barro JL, Atkin W, *et al.* Review article: population screening for colorectal cancer. *Aliment Pharmacol Ther.* 2005;22: 1069–1077.
9. Yamamoto H, Sekine Y, Sato Y, *et al.* Total enteroscopy with a nonsurgical steerable double-balloon method. *Gastrointest Endosc.* 2001;53:216–220.
10. Carroza MC, Dario P, Lencioni B, *et al.* The development of a microrobot system for colonoscopy. In: Troccaz J, Grimson E, Mosges R, editors. *Proceedings of the 1st Joint Conference on Computer Vision, Virtual Reality and Robotics in Medical and Medical Robotics and Computer Assisted Surgery*, Grenoble: Springer, 1995: 779–88.
11. Ikuta K, Masahiro T, Hirose S. Shape memory alloy servo actuator system with electric resistance feedback and application for active endoscope. *IEEE International Conference on Robotics and Automation*, 1988: 427–430.
12. Treat MR, Trimmer WS. Self Propelled Endoscope Using Pressure Driven Linear Actuators. US Patent 5, 595,565, 1997.
13. Takada M. Self Propelled Colonoscope. US patent 5, 562,601, 1996.
14. Swain P. Colonoscopy: new designs for the future. *Gastrointest Endosc Clin North Am.* 2005;15:839–863.
15. Shike M, Fireman Z, Eliakim R, *et al.* Sightline ColonoSight system for a disposable, power-assisted, non-fiber-optic colonoscopy. *Gastrointest Endosc.* 2008;68:701–710.
16. Eickhoff A, Jakobs R, Kamal A, *et al.* In vitro evaluation of forces exerted by a new computer-assisted colonoscope (the NeoGuide Endoscopy System). *Endoscopy.* 2006;38:1224–1229.
17. Eickhoff A, Van Dam J, Jakobs R, *et al.* Computer-assisted colonoscopy (The NeoGuide Endoscopy System): results of the first human clinical trial ("PACE Study"). *Am J Gastroenterol.* 2007;102: 261–266.
18. Rösch T, Adler A, Pohl H, *et al.* A motor-driven single-use colonoscope controlled with a hand-held device: a feasibility study in volunteers. *Gastrointest Endosc.* 2008;67:1139–1146.
19. Pfeffer J, Grinshpon R, Rex D, *et al.* The Aer-O-Scope: proof of the concept of a pneumatic, skill-independent, self-propelling, self-navigating colonoscope in a pig model. *Endoscopy.* 2006;38: 144–148.
20. Arber N, Grinshpon R, Maor L, *et al.* Proof of concept study of the Aer-O-Scope™ omni-directional colonoscopic viewing system in ex-vivo and in-vivo porcine models. *Endoscopy.* 2007; 39:412–417.
21. Vucelic B, Rex D, Pulanic R, *et al.* The aer-o-scope: proof of concept of a pneumatic, skill-independent, self-propelling, self-navigating colonoscope. *Gastroenterology.* 2006;130:672–677.
22. Eliakim R. The Pillcam COLON Capsule – A new promising tool for the detection of colonic pathologies. *Current Colorectal Cancer Reports*, 2008.
23. Eliakim R, Fireman Z, Gralnek IM, *et al.* Evaluation of the PillCam Colon capsule in the detection of colonic pathology:

results of the first multicenter, prospective, comparative study. *Endoscopy*, 2006;38:963–970.

24. Schoofs N, Deviere J, Van Gossum A. PillCam colon capsule endoscopy compared with colonoscopy for colorectal tumor diagnosis: a prospective pilot study. *Endoscopy*. 2006;38: 971–977.

25. Levin B, Lieberman DA, McFarland B, *et al.*; American Cancer Society Colorectal Cancer Advisory Group; US Multi-Society Task Force; American College of Radiology Colon Cancer Committee. Screening and surveillance for the early detection of colorectal cancer and adenomatous polyps, 2008: a joint guideline from the American Cancer Society, the US Multi-Society Task Force on Colorectal Cancer, and the American College of Radiology. *Gastroenterology*. 2008;134: 1570–1595.

26. Cosentino F, Tumino E, Rubis Passoni G, Morandi E, Capria A. Functional evaluation of the Endotics System, a new disposable self-propelled robotic colonoscope: in vitro tests and clinical trial. *Int J Artif Organs*. 2009;32:517–527.

27. Rubis Passoni G, Barbera R, Tauro A, Felice C. The Robotic Colonoscope E-Worm, a new device to perform colonoscopy: preliminary report. *Gastrointest Endosc*. 2009;69:5, AB285.

28. Rubis Passoni G, Tauro A, Cosentino F. The robotic colonoscope E-WORM. Analysis on the first cases performed in a single center. *Dig Liver Dis*. 2009; 41 (Suppl):S147.

CHAPTER 131

Percutaneous ultrasound

Winnie C. W. Chu and Vivian Y. F. Leung

Chinese University of Hong Kong, Hong Kong, SAR, China

KEY POINTS

- Ultrasound (US) is sensitive for both diffuse liver disease and focal hepatic lesions
- Color Doppler and contrast-enhanced US (CEUS) can demonstrate a vascular enhancement pattern in focal liver lesions comparable to that with computed tomography (CT)
- Gallstones and biliary obstructive lesions can be reliably detected by US
- Pancreatic adenocarcinoma and focal pancreatitis are more readily identified by US than CT
- US detects bowel wall thickening, but usually cannot differentiate inflammatory from neoplastic causes
- US is the recommended first-line investigation for suspected appendicitis in children and young women
- CEUS is particularly useful for detecting focal hepatic and pancreatic lesions; characterizing the enhancement pattern of benign and malignant lesions; and assessing the activity in inflammatory bowel disease
- US elastography is particularly useful for detecting liver fibrosis/ cirrhosis; assessing response to ablation therapy; differentiating pancreatic pathology; and identifying stenotic segment in Crohn's disease

---

Introduction

Ultrasound (US) using the percutaneous approach has been widely accepted as the first-line investigation for abdominal conditions. US is non-invasive, easily accessible, and cheap for detecting and excluding major abdominal pathology. In this chapter, gray-scale and color Doppler features of commonly encountered gastrointestinal pathologies are illustrated according to different abdominal organs. New advances in contrast-enhanced US (CEUS) and US elastography (USE) are also described.

Ultrasound of the liver

Diffuse liver disease

In diffuse liver disease, the presence of pathological components, such as fat or collagen within the liver, alter the attenuation of the US pulse and echogenicity of the liver parenchyma. The rule of thumb is to compare the echogenicity of the liver with that of the spleen or renal cortex; they should be comparable to each other.

Fatty liver is very common in asymptomatic patients with unexplained raised liver enzymes. The presence of fat within liver parenchyma causes increased hepatic echogenicity and attenuation of the US pulse on the posterior aspect of the liver, and thus there is poor visualization of the diaphragm and vascular structures (Figure 131.1).

Hepatitis

In **acute hepatitis**, the liver echotexture may be hypoechoic or normal. Other associated features include portal hilar lymphadenopathy, hepatosplenomegaly, thickened gallbladder wall, and prominent portal vein walls, which produce the "starry-sky" appearance. In **chronic hepatitis**, the liver appears lobulated; there is increased echogenicity and coarsened echotexture. The condition is associated with decreased brightness of portal triads, irregular caliber of hepatic veins (HVs), and dilatation of portal veins (PVs). However, the above features can also be found in fatty liver.

Fibrosis and cirrhosis

Liver fibrosis cannot be detected by gray-scale US. However, **elasticity of the liver parenchyma** can now be objectively measured by USE. Details are given in the later part of this chapter. In **established cirrhosis**, the liver is shrunken but the caudate lobe is enlarged. Hepatic echotexture appears coarsened and mottled, the border is nodular, and reduced hepatic elasticity can be appreciated by real-time compression of liver parenchyma by the pulsating heart. The presence of regenerative nodules is best visualized with a high-frequency probe over the liver surface. HVs and the inferior vena cava (IVC) are engorged. PV thrombosis and dilated tortuous hepatic arteries may be present. In patients with **portal hypertension**, ascites, varices, and splenomegaly may be visualized (Figure 131.2).

Focal liver disease

Simple hepatic cysts

Simple hepatic cysts are common incidental findings. Typically, cysts are anechoic, well-defined, and thin walled with distal enhancement (Figure 131.3). Occasionally, cysts have septations. Internal echoes are found if they are complicated by hemorrhage or infection.

Textbook of Clinical Gastroenterology and Hepatology, Second Edition. Edited by C. J. Hawkey, Jaime Bosch, Joel E. Richter, Guadalupe Garcia-Tsao, Francis K. L. Chan.
© 2012 Blackwell Publishing Ltd. Published 2012 by Blackwell Publishing Ltd.

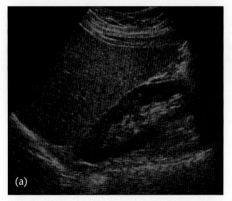 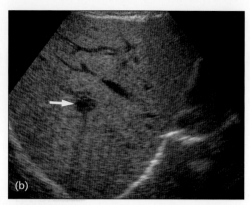 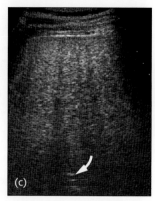

Figure 131.1 Fatty liver. (a) In mild grade, there is increased echogenicity of liver parenchyma when compared with adjacent renal parenchyma. (b) In moderate grade, there is a further increase in hepatic echogenicity. An area of focal fatty sparing (arrow) is present in this case (c) In severe grade, there is poor visualization of intrahepatic vasculature and the diaphragm (arrow).

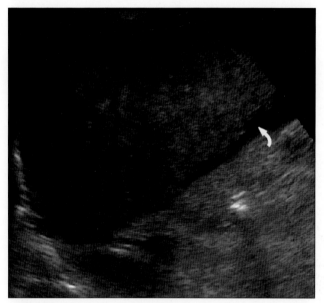

Figure 131.2 Cirrhosis. In advanced cirrhosis, the liver is shrunken with a mottled echotexture and nodular border. Note the ascitic fluid (arrow) around the liver.

Focal nodular hyperplasia

Focal nodular hyperplasia (FNH) comprises a regenerating or hyperplastic nodule divided by fibrous septae. Typical features are a round or elliptical subcapsular mass with smooth margin; hypoechoic or isoechoic echotexture; mass effect on adjacent vasculature; central connective tissue or star-shaped scars (Figure 131.4); and a "spoked-wheel" pattern on color Doppler due to multiple vessels passing through the radial connective tissue.

Hemangioma

Typical features are homogenous hyperechoicity, a round or oval shape, and a smooth and well-defined margin without a halo (Figure 131.5). Atypical hemangiomata, especially those >3.5cm, show a complex, patchy hypoechoic to hyperechoic pattern due to thrombosis, fibrosis, calcification

or intralesional hemorrhage. CEUS shows the classical "iris diaphragm" sign, similar to that found in dynamic CT. The enhancement pattern follows an early arterial phase (peripheral "puddle" enhancement), a portal phase (peripheral-to-central fill-in enhancement), and a delayed phase (completely filled with diffuse color speckle) [1].

Hepatocellular carcinoma

Hepatocellular carcinoma (HCC) has a variable sonographic appearance (Figure 131.6). HCC can be solitary, multifocal or infiltrative, and is difficult to differentiate from regenerating nodules of cirrhosis. Color Doppler shows non-specific increase in vascularity. In contrast, CEUS improves the detection of color flow in HCC and demonstrates the typical enhancement pattern of HCC in the arterial phase [2]. In the advanced stage, there may be PV thrombosis, ascites or lymphadenopathy.

Metastasis

Liver metastases have a wide range of appearances (Figure 131.7). Some have a classical target appearance (echogenic central area with hypoechoic peripheral halo) or bull's eye appearance (central necrotic zone). Metastasis is usually multiple with no detectable intratumoral or peripheral vessels on color Doppler. CEUS has a high sensitivity for vascular metastasis [3].

Ultrasound of the biliary system

The **gallbladder** is readily visible on US when it is fully distended after adequate fasting (usually 4 hours before examination).

Gallstones

Gallstones should be detected with almost 100% accuracy with the following features: echogenic foci; mobile on different positioning of the patient; and strong distal acoustic shadowing (Figure 131.8a). However, if the gallbladder is contracted and packed with stones, the WES sign (wall, echo, shadow) will be seen (Figure 131.8b).

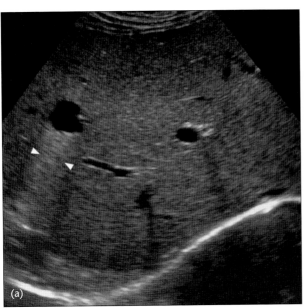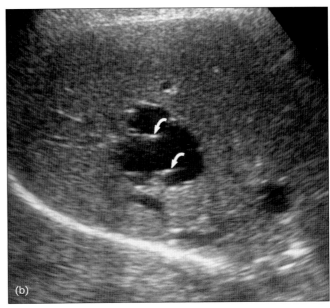

Figure 131.3 Liver cyst. (a) Typical appearance: well-defined, thin-walled anechoic cyst with distal acoustic enhancement (arrowheads). (b) Complex cyst with thin septi (arrows).

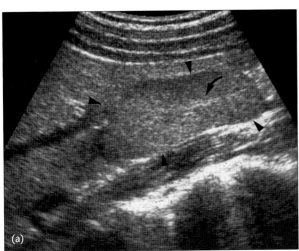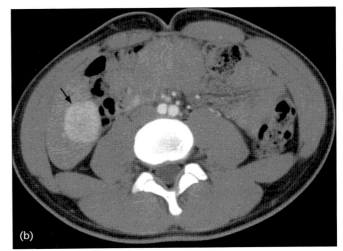

Figure 131.4 Focal nodular hyperplasia (FNH). (a) FNH typically appears as a slightly hypoechoic elliptical subcapsular mass (arrowheads) with a smooth margin. The central scar (arrow) is vaguely seen. (b) CT shows the same lesion (arrow) with intense homogenous contrast enhancement during the arterial phase.

Gallbladder polyp

A gallbladder polyp is a round intraluminal mass that adheres to the gallbladder wall (Figure 131.9). It has the following features: non-mobile; echogenic to hypoechoic sessile mass on the gallbladder wall; absence of acoustic shadowing; and size <5 mm. The overwhelming majority (95–99%) are cholesterol polyps. **Malignant transformation** should be suspected in patients >50 years old who have a solitary adenomatous polyp of >10 mm, progressive increase in size on serial US, or co-existing gallstones [4].

Cholecystitis

In **acute cholecystitis**, the following features are often present: enlarged gallbladder filled with sludge; stones (detected in up to 95% of cases); gallbadder wall that becomes stratified and thickened (Figure 131.10); pericholecystic free fluid; increased vascularity of the inflamed gallbladder wall on color Doppler; and local tenderness elicited by real-time compression of the US transducer on the gallbladder, known as a positive sonographic Murphy's sign. **Chronic cholecystitis** is associated with a shrunken gallbadder despite adequate fasting and diffuse wall thickening. Stones are usually present.

Adenocarcinoma

Adenocarcioma of the gallbladder appears either as an irregular solid mass filling the gallbladder lumen or a broad-based hypoechoic polypoid area of wall thickening. Only sparse vascularity is demonstrated by color Doppler. CEUS can

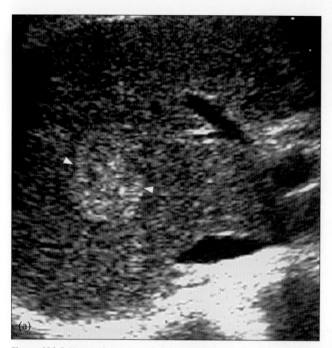
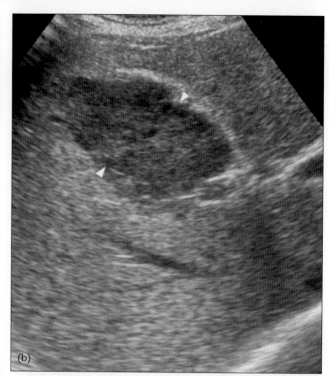

Figure 131.5 Hemangioma. Hepatic hemangioma typically presents as a well-defined lesion. (a) Capillary type: homogenously echogenic (arrowheads); (b) Cavernous type: patchy hypoechoic pattern (arrowheads).

demonstrate tumor enhancement and tortuous neovascularity, thus differentiating adenocarcinoma from a benign lesion [5].

Choledocholithiasis

Choledocholithiasis refers to stones (usually bilirubin stones) within the common bile duct (CBD) or intrahepatic biliary ducts, classically presenting as echogenic foci (Figure 131.11a), with or without shadowing. The condition may be associated with ductal dilatation (Figure 131.11b) or ductal wall thickening. US is useful to differentiate **obstructive from non-obstructive causes** of acute cholangitis. It is important to visualize the distal end of the CBD for any obstructive lesion, such as stones or tumors at the pancreatic head.

Ultrasound of the pancreas

The pancreas is a central retroperitoneal structure that can be obscured by bowel gas. Operators can make use of positioning and oral fluid loads to maximize the visibility of the pancreas.

Pancreatitis

In **acute pancreatitis**, the following features may be identified: enlarged pancreas with hypoechoic echotexture; dilated pancreatic duct; fluid in the anterior para-renal space; and other associations or complications such as gallstone, left pleural effusion, abscess, and pseudocyst.

In **chronic pancreatitis**, the features include: shrunken pancreas with irregular border and coarse hyperechoic echotexture; pancreatic calcifications; pancreatic ductal ectasia; stones within pancreatic duct and biliary ducts; and other complications such as pseudocyst, peripancreatic lymphadenopathy, and portosplenic thrombosis. Endoscopic US (EUS) can evaluate subtle parenchymal changes in the setting of chronic pancreatitis, while USE can help diagnose chronic pancreatitis [6,7].

CT remains the gold standard for assessment of advanced pancreatic disease. In clinical practice, the main role of US is to exclude biliary pancreatitis and to screen for major complications.

Congenital pancreatic cyst

This is usually associated with renal and hepatic cysts. A **pseudocyst** is related to acute/chronic pancreatitis or trauma. It usually arises from the tail of the pancreas and may present as either an anechoic cyst with posterior acoustic enhancement or a complex cyst with echoes and septae or calcified walls.

Adenocarcinoma of the pancreas

This commonly (~80%) occurs in the head, which is associated with pancreatic and biliary ductal dilatation readily detected by US. US shows a poorly defined hypoechoic mass, which may infiltrate into surrounding tissue (Figure 131.12). Encasement of the celiac axis can be demonstrated by color Doppler. These lesions are more easily identified on US than CT as they appear iso-attenuated with poor enhancement on CT.

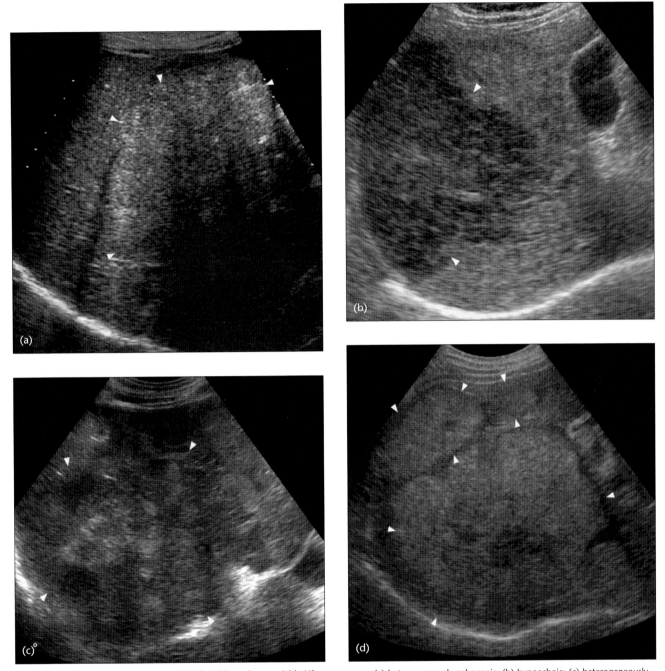

Figure 131.6 Hepatocellular carcinoma (HCC). HCC can have variable US appearances: (a) heterogeneously echogenic; (b) hypoechoic; (c) heterogeneously echogenic; (d) multifocal lesions.

Ultrasound of the gastrointestinal tract

Abnormal bowel wall thickening, either of inflammatory (such as **Crohn's disease**) or neoplastic (such as **carcinoma, lymphoma or metastasis**) etiology, can be easily identified using high-frequency linear US transducers (Figure 131.13). Hyperemia is demonstrated by color Doppler, which correlates with disease activity in inflammatory bowel disease [8,9]. Real-time scanning can provide additional information on peristalsis, luminal distension, or narrowing of the bowel. Associated features such as mesenteric lymphadenitis, fistula or abscess formation, varices, regional or distal metastasis can also be accurately depicted by US [9].

Appendicitis

To look for clues of **acute appendicitis**, gentle compression is applied to the right iliac fossa, starting from behind the cecum. Classical features of an inflamed appendix are: non-compressible, thickened, blind-end, hypoechoic tubular structure; central echogenic lumen on LS plane or "target-like" on TS plane (Figure 131.14); diameter >6mm; and hyperemia

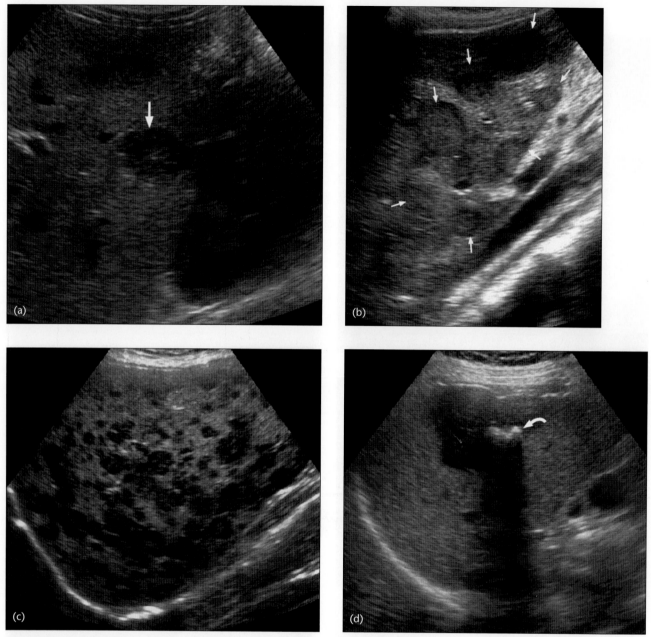

Figure 131.7 Liver metastases. Metastatic lesions can have variable US appearances. (a) Solitary hypoechic lesion (arrow) in colonic cancer; (b) multiple lesions (arrows) with "target appearance" in pancreatic cancer; (c) multiple hypoechoic lesions in breast cancer; (d) heterogeneous lesion with calcification (arrow) in breast cancer.

detected on color Doppler. Associated features such as appendiceal abscess or appendicolith may present. For detection of acute appendicitis, CT has higher sensitivity (90–100%) and specificity (78–100%) when compared with US (sensitivity 55–98%, specificity 78–100%). However, US is recommended as the initial examination for children and young or pregnant women. Sometimes US can suggest alternative diagnosis (gynecological, urological or other gastrointestinal disorders such as mesenteric lymphadenitis) in patients who present with acute lower abdominal pain [10].

Obstruction

Gastric or bowel obstruction due to stricture, inflammation, paralytic ileus or tumor-related stenosis can be depicted by US [11] with the following features: distended fluid-filled stomach/bowel loop; little or no peristalsis; to-and-fro movement of fluid within bowel loops; prominent valvulae conniventes in the small bowel; and loss of haustration in the large bowel [12].. In the case of **intussusceptions**, the typical appearance of target, pseudo-kidney, onion, sandwich or doughnut signs can be easily identified on US [13] (Figure 131.15).

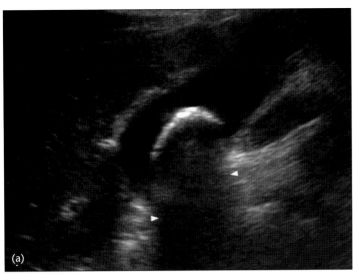
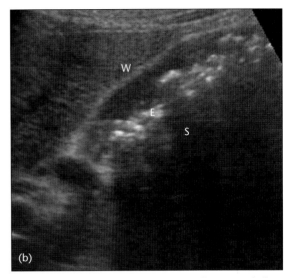

Figure 131.8 Gallstones. (a) Classical appearance of an echogenic stone associated with strong shadowing (arrowheads); (b) multiple small stones packed inside a contracted gallbladder, with WES (wall, echo, shadow) sign.

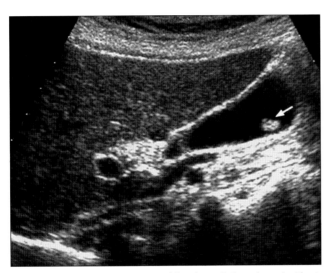

Figure 131.9 Gallbladder polyp. Immobile echogenic focus (arrow) without acoustic shadowing.

New imaging techniques

Contrast-enhanced ultrasound

For imaging deep structures, traditional gray-scale US has limited spatial resolution due to attenuation by intervening tissues. The sensitivity of color Doppler is often inadequate due to small vessels or low-velocity flow. The introduction of US **contrast agents** provides better acoustic scatters, therefore enhancing contrast resolution of the image and improving the detection of vascular blood flow.

US contrast agents are safe and well tolerated. There are two routes of administration: the intravenous route for evaluation of vessels and soft tissue, and the oral route for visualization of the gastrointestinal tract. CEUS has the advantages of higher spatial and temporal resolution compared to CT/magnetic resonance imaging (MRI). CEUS is the only imaging method

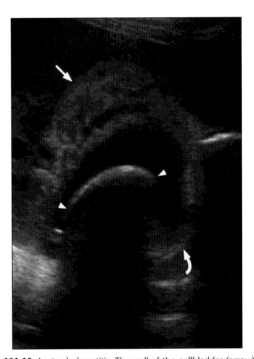

Figure 131.10 Acute cholecystitis. The wall of the gallbladder (arrow) is markedly thickened and stratified. There is a thin rim of pericholecystic fluid (curved arrow). A gallstone (arrowheads) with strong acoustic shadowing is present within the gallbladder.

that allows evaluation of enhancement patterns during the dynamic phase [14].

Imaging of the **liver** by CEUS can evaluate the perfusion, hemodynamics, and real-time morphology of the vascularity of nodular liver lesions. CEUS can fully characterize the enhancement patterns of benign (Figure 131.16) and malignant hepatic lesions, and gives information comparable to that provided by CT and MRI [15]. Compared to multidetector CT,

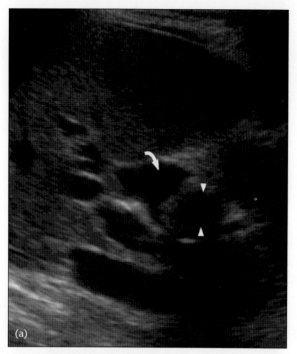

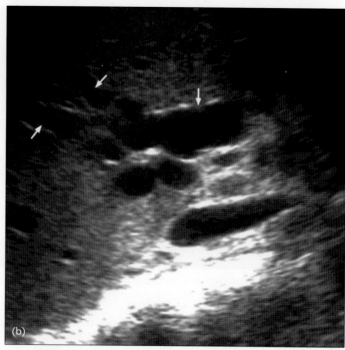

Figure 131.11 Common bile duct (CBD) stone. (a) Echogenic stone (arrowheads) causing proximal dilatation of the CBD (arrow). (b) Dilatation of intrahepatic biliary ducts (arrows), represented by tubular structures parallel to the portal veins within the liver.

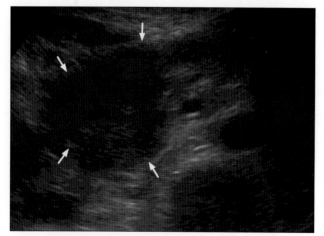

Figure 131.12 Adenocarcinoma of the pancreas. An ill-defined hypoechoic lesion (arrows) arises from the head of the pancreas.

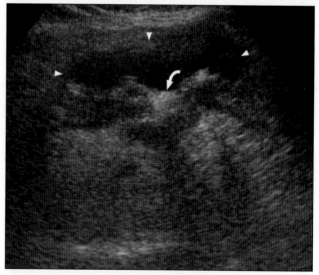

Figure 131.13 Carcinoma of the descending colon. The bowel wall (arrowheads) appears markedly thickened and hypoechoic, and the individual wall layers are not discernable. Note the hyperechogenicity in the lumen, representing gas (arrow).

CEUS has a higher sensitivity in detecting vascular **liver metastasis**. CEUS has been recommended in the staging algorithm of malignancy [3]. CEUS has also been shown to be more effective in assessing **radiofrequency ablation** of HCC when compared to contrast-enhanced CT [16].

In **gallbladder carcinoma**, CEUS shows a characteristic tortuous-type neovascularity that differentiates it from other polypoid lesions, such as **polyp, adenoma** (branched-type vascularity) or **sludge** (no vascularity) [5].

On imaging of the **pancreas**, CEUS can identify acute focal pancreatitis (increased enhancement in the inflamed segment)

and avascular necrosis (non-vascular segment) from different perfusion patterns. CEUS can also characterize and differentiate pancreatic masses/pseudo-masses. For example, **ductal adenocarcinoma** remains hypoechoic in all contrast-enhanced phases; inflammatory masses associated with **chronic pancreatitis** show enhanced or similar echogenicity to

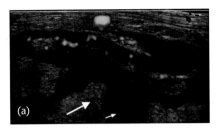
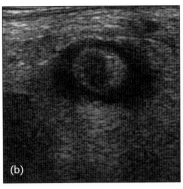
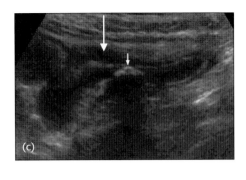

Figure 131.14 Acute appendicitis. (a) The appendiceal wall is thickened and shows hyperemia on power Doppler, associated with adjacent collection (➤ ➚). (b) The inflamed appendix appears "target like" on transverse view. (c) Appendicolith, the calcified focus (⬇ ⬇) can sometimes be identified.

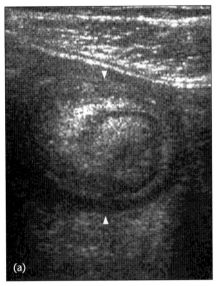
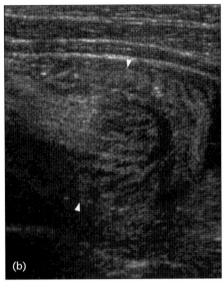

Figure 131.15 Intussusception. (a) Transverse plane shows a multilayered lesion with concentric circles (arrowheads); typical "onion" or "target" sign. (b) Longitudinal plane shows the multilayered structure with central echogenic mesentery (arrowheads), known as the "sandwich" sign.

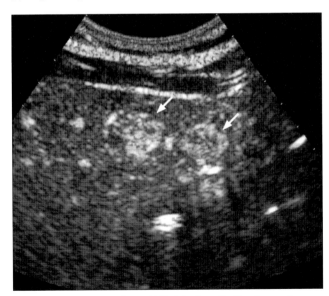

Figure 131.16 Contrast-enhanced US of the liver. Capillary hemangiomas (arrows) are completely filled with diffuse color speckle at the delayed phase after intravenous injection of US contrast.

surrounding parenchyma in the early phase, whereas a **pseudocyst** does not enhance; an **endocrine tumor** shows rapid intense enhancement in the early phase; and **cystadenoma** shows enhancement of intracystic septae/nodules. Furthermore, the **staging** of pancreatic adenocarcinoma can be improved by assessing the relationship of the non-enhanced tumor with the peripancreatic venous and arterial vessels. A complete evaluation of the liver during the late sinusoidal phase is also feasible during the same US examination to exclude liver metastasis [14].

In the **gastrointestinal tract**, CEUS is useful in evaluating **Crohn's disease** (e.g., hypervascularity of the bowel wall during active disease) [8], delineating the location of the **fistula** in relation to the anal lumen and sphincters [17], and diagnosing intestinal ischemia (diminished or absent color signal in the bowel wall) [18].

Oral US contrast can improve the overall assessment of the gastrointestinal tract and adjacent structures by absorbing and displacing bowel gas. A homogenous transmission of sound through the contrast-filled stomach and bowel can be archived, which produces uniform reflections within the bowel. This

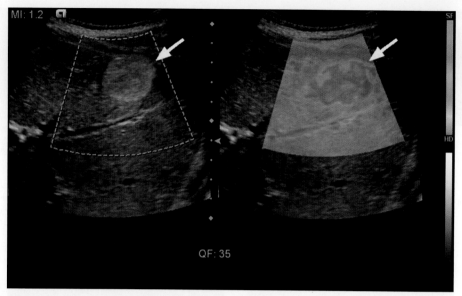

Figure 131.17 US elastography of the liver. The hemangioma (arrow) is displayed in red on the color-coded elastogram. It is harder in consistency than the surrounding liver parenchyma. (Courtesy of Siemens Medical).

method is promising for assessing **Crohn's disease**, e.g., localization of a small bowel stricture, and measurement of small bowel transit time and bowel wall thickness [19].

Ultrasound elastography

USE studies the elasticity or stiffness of tissue. Force (stress) is applied and the tissue deformation (strain) is measured. The calculated value is then color coded to display the elastic properties of the soft tissue in the form of an elastogram. The distribution of elasticity of soft tissue can also be visualized in a dual display of B-mode image and the elastogram (Figure 131.17).

In USE of the **liver**, the response of **an hepatic lesion to ablation therapy** can be assessed. Coagulated tissue is much harder than normal tissue. On USE, the zone of increased tissue hardness corresponds to the zone of ablation or tissue death in a lesion [20]. Transient elastography is a non-imaging method to measure tissue stiffness. A device known as **Fibroscan** is currently used for detection of **cirrhosis** by measuring the elasticity of liver parenchyma. Fibroscan makes use of US to track the advancing displacement wave in tissue, caused by rapid indentation of the skin by a piston-mounted US transducer. This non-invasive approach may replace biopsy in the future for assessing hepatic fibrosis and monitoring its progression and response to therapy [21,22] (see Chapter 138).

USE can also differentiate different pancreatic conditions. For example, **adenocarcinoma** is hard with internal soft spots, **endocrine tumor** shows a uniform and soft texture comparable to parenchyma, and **chronic pancreatitis** exhibits a mixture of color-coded elasticity. USE has been reported to identify 60% of adenocarcinomas, 100% of endocrine tumors, and 92% of chronic pancreatitis [7].

In USE of the **small bowel**, the stenotic bowel segment in **Crohn's disease** can be identified from its harder texture when compared with surrounding tissue. USE has the potential to study small bowel motor function because it can differentiate the contractile activity of the longitudinal and circular muscle layers [11].

Conclusions

Percutaneous US machines produce images of the gastrointestinal tract of excellent quality and at a reasonable cost. With experience, gastroenterologists should be able to identify specific sonographic features of common gastrointestinal pathology. Recent advances in CEUS and USE enable higher accuracy of lesion detection and provide additional functional information, including vascularity, enhancement pattern, and elasticity of the soft tissue.

References

1. Dietrich CF, Mertens JC, Braden B, Schuessler G, Ott M, Ignee A. Contrast-enhanced ultrasound of histologically proven liver hemangiomas. *Hepatology.* 2007;45:1139–1145.
2. Luo W, Numata K, Morimoto M, *et al.* Three-dimensional contrast-enhanced sonography of vascular patterns of focal liver tumors: pilot study of visualization methods. *AJR Am J Roentgenol.* 2009;192:165–173.
3. Bauditz J, Quinkler M, Beyersdorff D, Wermke W. Improved detection of hepatic metastases of adrenocortical cancer by contrast-enhanced ultrasound. *Oncol Rep.* 2008;19:1135–1139.
4. Shin SR, Lee JK, Lee KH, *et al.* Can the growth rate of a gallbladder polyp predict a neoplastic polyp? *J Clin Gastroenterol.* 2009;43:865–868.
5. Numata K, Oka H, Morimoto M, *et al.* Differential diagnosis of gallbladder diseases with contrast-enhanced harmonic gray scale ultrasonography. *J Ultrasound Med.* 2007;26:763–774.

6. Kinney TP, Freeman ML. Recent advances and novel methods in pancreatic imaging. *Minerva Gastroenterol Dietol.* 2008;54:85–95.

7. Uchida H, Hirooka Y, Itoh A, *et al.* Feasibility of tissue elastography using transcutaneous ultrasonography for the diagnosis of pancreatic diseases. *Pancreas.* 2009;38:17–22.

8. Di Sabatino A, Fulle I, Ciccocioppo R, et al. Doppler enhancement after intravenous levovist injection in Crohn's disease. *Inflamm Bowel Dis.* 2002;8:251–257.

9. Crade M, Pham V. Ultrasound examination of the sigmoid colon: possible new diagnostic tool for irritable bowel syndrome. *Ultrasound Obstet Gynecol.* 2006;27:206–209.

10. Birnbaum BA, Wilson SR. Appendicitis at the millennium. *Radiology.* 2000;215:337–348.

11. Gilja OH, Hatlebakk JG, Odegaard S, *et al.* Advanced imaging and visualization in gastrointestinal disorders. *World J Gastroenterol.* 2007;13:1408–1421.

12. Grassi R, Romano S, D'Amario F, *et al.* The relevance of free fluid between intestinal loops detected by sonography in the clinical assessment of small bowel obstruction in adults. *Eur J Radiol.* 2004;50:5–14.

13. Harrington L, Connolly B, Hu X, Wesson DE, Babyn P, Schuh S. Ultrasonographic and clinical predictors of intussusception. *J Pediatr.* 1998;132:836–839.

14. D'Onofrio M, Zamboni G, Faccioli N, Capelli P, Pozzi Mucelli R. Ultrasonography of the pancreas. 4. Contrast-enhanced imaging. *Abdom Imaging.* 2007;32:171–181.

15. Morin SH, Lim AK, Cobbold JF, Taylor-Robinson SD. Use of second generation contrast-enhanced ultrasound in the assessment of focal liver lesions. *World J Gastroenterol.* 2007;13:5963–5970.

16. Kisaka Y, Hirooka M, Kumagi T, *et al.* Usefulness of contrast-enhanced ultrasonography with abdominal virtual ultrasonography in assessing therapeutic response in hepatocellular carcinoma treated with radiofrequency ablation. *Liver Int.* 2006;26:1241–1247.

17. Tsankov T, Tankova L, Deredjan H, Kovatchki D. Contrast-enhanced endoanal and transperineal sonography in perianal fistulas. *Hepatogastroenterology.* 2008;55:13–16.

18. Hamada T, Yamauchi M, Tanaka M, Hashimoto Y, Nakai K, Suenaga K. Prospective evaluation of contrast-enhanced ultrasonography with advanced dynamic flow for the diagnosis of intestinal ischaemia. *Br J Radiol.* 2007;80:603–608.

19. Parente F, Greco S, Molteni M, et al. Oral contrast enhanced bowel ultrasonography in the assessment of small intestine Crohn's disease. A prospective comparison with conventional ultrasound, x ray studies, and ileocolonoscopy. *Gut.* 2004;53:1652–1657.

20. Garra BS. Imaging and estimation of tissue elasticity by ultrasound. *Ultrasound Q.* 2007;23:255–268.

21. Talwalkar JA. Methodologic issues with transfer of ultrasound-based transient elastography into clinical practice. *J Hepatol.* 2007;47:301–302.

22. Castera L. Transient elastography and other noninvasive tests to assess hepatic fibrosis in patients with viral hepatitis. *J Viral Hepatol.* 2009;16:300–314.

CHAPTER 132

Barium radiology

Simon A. Jackson and Bruce M. Fox

Derriford Hospital, Plymouth, UK

KEY POINTS

- Contrast radiology offers a readily available and cost-effective gastrointestinal assessment that complements other imaging modalities
- Effective contrast examinations require optimal patient preparation, good technique, and meticulous interpretation
- Double-contrast radiology provides the best mucosal detail
- Water-soluble contrast agents should be used if there is a risk of perforation or aspiration

Videofluoroscopy
- Provides a functional, dynamic examination of the pharynx
- Principally indicated for the investigation of oropharyngeal swallowing dysfunction and high dysphagia
- Complex examination performed with multiple contrast consistencies

Esophagram and upper gastrointestinal series
- Commonly performed as a biphasic examination utilizing both single- and double-contrast techniques
- Esophagram provides a rapid assessment of dysphagia and motility disorders, complimenting endoscopy
- A contrast examination is a useful investigation for assessment of the upper gastrointestinal tract following local gastrointestinal surgery

Barium follow-through (small bowel meal) and enteroclysis
- Contrast examinations remain a sensitive imaging technique for small bowel pathology
- Although more invasive, enteroclysis demonstrates mucosal detail not provided by the small bowel meal

Barium enema
- Optimal mucosal assessment requires double-contrast examination of a clean colon
- Meticulous attention must be paid to the acquisition and interpretation of images
- Colonoscopy remains the gold standard investigation for the colon
- In cases of incomplete colonoscopy, barium enema can be used as an alternative to CT colonography for a completion study

Introduction

The evolution of modern barium radiology has resulted from improvements in technical apparatus and the development of barium suspensions heralding the introduction of single- and double-contrast techniques to diagnose gastrointestinal tract pathology.

Single-contrast examinations are performed using a low-density barium suspension. Bowel distension with contrast enables the visualization of such findings as filling defects or alterations in normal contour of the bowel wall. The technique, however, has a number of limitations, including the degree of luminal distension and limited quality of mucosal coating.

Double-contrast studies, on the other hand, use gas to distend the bowel combined with mucosal coating by a thin layer of high-density barium suspension. The technique allows the demonstration of fine mucosal detail and subtle pathology. In addition, the radiation dose is reduced both due to a reduction in fluoroscopic screening time and radiographic exposure settings. For these reasons, a well-performed double-contrast study is usually regarded as the examination of choice.

The number of barium examinations performed worldwide has significantly decreased due to the introduction of alternative techniques, especially endoscopy, and also the cross-sectional imaging modalities of computed tomography (CT), magnetic resonance imaging (MRI), and ultrasound. Despite this, contrast examinations still remain cost-effective investigations and high-quality barium studies continue to play an important role in the diagnosis of gastrointestinal disorders.

The pharynx: modified barium swallow or videofluoroscopy

The normal swallowing mechanism is a complex but orderly sequence of neuromuscular events, which can be divided into two main components: oropharyngeal and esophageal (see Chapter 2). Disorders of the oropharyngeal component are increasingly recognized in routine clinical practice and are associated with significant morbidity and mortality, particularly in the elderly population. The development of digital fluoroscopy and, in particular, the ability to video record the study has contributed to the development of the modified barium swallow (MBS) or videofluoroscopic examination.

Description of technique

The study is performed as a multidisciplinary examination in the fluoroscopy suite and is usually undertaken in the

---

presence of a speech therapist and/or ENT surgeon (see Video clip 132.1). This functional assessment examination complements fiberoptic examination of the pharynx to exclude mucosal pathology (see Chapter 123). Video recording of the examination is used to enable slow-motion review of the patient's swallowing mechanism and help reduce overall radiation exposure [1,2]. The patient is seated in a specially designed chair to aid support and positioning during the study. Clinical status and relevant medical history are reviewed prior to the study. Swallowing movements are recorded in the lateral position using barium as the contrast agent. Barium is mixed into varying consistencies ranging from thin liquid to solid food boluses. Initial bolus size is restricted to small volumes in order to assess the presence or absence of aspiration.

The study includes assessment of all phases of the **oropharyngeal swallow mechanism** with particular emphasis on the presence of **vocal cord penetration and aspiration**. The strength of the patient's cough reflex when aspiration occurs is also noted. Maneuvers such as chin tucking or head turning can also be performed and assessed with regard to their efficacy in improving the patient's swallowing mechanism. The complete examination should include an assessment of the esophagus in order to exclude associated pathology.

Indications and contraindications

The examination is performed in patients with **oropharyngeal swallowing dysfunction** and symptoms of high **dysphagia**. The majority of patients are elderly with a medical history of a cerebrovascular event or neuromuscular disease (see Chapter 2). A further group consists of patients with a previous history of head and neck malignancy with radiation therapy or surgical resection complicated by swallowing problems.

A diagnostic examination requires sufficient patient mobility and awareness to understand instructions, and thus is contraindicated in the severely incapacitated patient. Significant aspiration of contrast during the study is a relative contraindication to a complete assessment and chest physiotherapy should be performed after the examination.

The upper gastrointestinal tract: the esophagram and upper gastrointestinal series

The double-contrast study has facilitated the accurate assessment of mucosal pathology. The modern contrast examination of the upper gastrointestinal tract combines the advantages of the two techniques (single and double contrast) and in many radiology departments is performed as a biphasic examination [3].

Endoscopy may comprise the initial examination, but contrast imaging may demonstrate other clinically significant pathology [4]. This is especially true in the assessment of dysphagia and odynophagia (see Chapter 2) and for upper gastrointestinal motility in general.

Description of technique

The standard upper gastrointestinal contrast study should be performed as a **biphasic examination** allowing the combination of both double- and single-contrast views to maximize the sensitivity of the test [3]. All examinations must be performed with meticulous attention to technique and interpretation in order to maximize diagnostic accuracy.

Double-contrast images rely on initial gaseous distension of the gut lumen after the ingestion of effervescent granules, followed by the even coating of the mucosa by a thin layer of high-density barium suspension. Residual fluid or food results in reduced mucosal detail and thus sensitivity of the examination. The patient is therefore fasted for at least 6 hours prior to the study. The quality of the examination is improved by the injection of smooth muscle relaxants to cause gastric hypotonia and increase distension. The radiologist uses intermittent fluoroscopy throughout the examination to aid in patient positioning and to confirm adequate luminal distension/mucosal coating.

Single-contrast images are also obtained during and after ingestion of a low-density barium suspension for further assessment of the esophagus, stomach, and duodenum.

The modern examination is tailored to the patient's symptoms. An esophagram is performed in patients with suspected esophageal pathology whereas an upper gastrointestinal series is tailored to suspected abnormalities within the stomach and duodenum.

Indications
Esophagus

Dysphagia remains a recognized indication for undertaking a barium examination of the esophagus (Figures 132.1 and 132.2), in particular if the symptom is related to a motility disturbance (see Chapters 2 and 36).

Barium studies are also sensitive for the diagnosis of certain features in patients presenting with **reflux symptoms**, especially if they are atypical. An examination can confirm the presence of a hiatus hernia and gastroesophageal reflux as well as detecting morphological changes secondary to the reflux, such as erosive esophagitis, esophageal rings, and peptic strictures. The esophagram is invaluable in the assessment of the integrity of a fundoplication and after pneumatic dilatation or surgery for achalasia (see Chapters 27–30).

Stomach and duodenum

Upper gastrointestinal endoscopy has largely replaced barium studies as the primary diagnostic investigation for patients presenting with possible gastric or duodenal pathology (see Chapter 123). However, if endoscopy is contraindicated or unavailable, a well-performed barium examination is the next most sensitive diagnostic modality [5]. Occult strictures and fistulae can be identified as well as extrinsic or submucosal disease distorting the bowel lumen. In addition, a double-contrast barium examination demonstrates the morphology of the stomach and duodenum in patients with a suspected

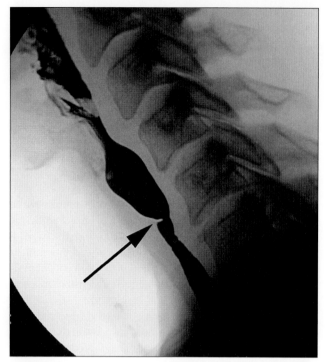

Figure 132.1 Single-contrast barium swallow demonstrating a pharyngeal web (arrow).

volvulus or gastric outlet obstruction (see Chapter 60) (Figure 132.3). Opacification of the distal duodenum also allows the potential visualization of pathology that may be missed during upper gastrointestinal endoscopy.

Contraindications

Similar to other areas of the gastrointestinal tract, a barium examination is contraindicated in patients with possible perforation. If a perforation is suspected, a water-soluble contrast study should be performed. In addition, patients with high-grade gastric outlet obstruction should also undergo a water-soluble examination, to avoid the risk of barium impaction. Immobile patients are only able to undergo a limited study of reduced accuracy.

Barium follow-through and enteroclysis
Description of technique
Barium follow-through (small bowel meal)

Patients fast for at least 6–8 hours prior to the procedure. They drink approximately 500 mL of a low-density barium suspension. Unless contraindicated, metoclopramide (10–20 mg) is also taken orally by the patient to accelerate passage of contrast through the gastrointestinal tract. A sequence of plain abdominal films is then obtained to evaluate the progress of the barium contrast through the small bowel loops. Following demonstration of either significant small bowel pathology and/or passage of the contrast through to the colon, a dedicated fluoroscopic examination is performed. This provides a

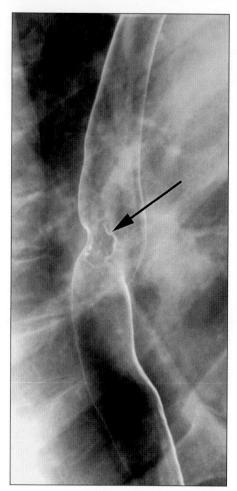

Figure 132.2 Double-contrast barium swallow showing an early esophageal carcinoma (arrow).

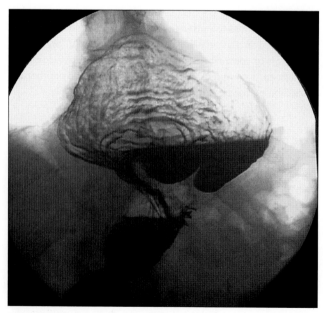

Figure 132.3 Water-soluble upper gastrointestinal series demonstrating a gastric volvulus.

detailed assessment of the small bowel and, using compression techniques, particularly of the terminal ileum. Where the terminal ileum is poorly demonstrated, gas can be introduced per rectum to provide double-contrast views of the region.

Enteroclysis

This more invasive technique is performed entirely in the fluoroscopy suite. A specifically designed catheter is introduced nasally and manipulated under fluoroscopic guidance through the stomach and duodenum to the proximal jejunum. Contrast is then introduced via the catheter to directly opacify the small bowel using either a single- or double-contrast technique. Whilst the single-contrast examination allows the distension and assessment of small bowel loops, demonstration of fine mucosal detail is limited.

Images are obtained after initial introduction of approximately 200 mL of high-density barium suspension immediately followed by an infusion of 1000–2000 mL of a 0.5% solution of methylcellulose to provide a double-contrast appearance. In many departments, contrast infusion is achieved by the use of a dedicated contrast delivery pump.

During the examination the radiologist performs intermittent fluoroscopy accompanied by graded compression to assess the passage of contrast through the small bowel loops and to look for small bowel pathology.

Indications
Barium follow-through (small bowel meal)

The main advantages of barium follow-through when compared to enteroclysis include the less invasive nature of the examination (reduced patient discomfort) and shorter fluoroscopic screening times with a lower radiation dose to the patient. The examination is widely used for the assessment of patients with known or suspected **Crohn's disease**. In addition barium follow-through can be used for the evaluation of other small bowel pathologies (Figure 132.4) that compromise luminal diameter, such as ischemia and radiation enteritis. Traditionally, the examination has also been used to assess the severity and level of small bowel obstruction; however, cross-sectional imaging techniques and, in particular, CT have been shown to be more accurate [6,7] (see Chapter 133).

Enteroclysis

Enteroclysis provides better luminal distension and mucosal detail than a barium follow-through. Thus, more accurate assessment of subtle mucosal pathology and changes in fold pattern can be evaluated. This has led some authors to suggest that enteroclysis should comprise the initial method of small bowel imaging [8–10] although there is general acceptance that both types of examination currently play a role in the diagnosis of small bowel pathology.

Currently, the main indications for enteroclysis include the assessment of patients with **chronic or recurrent small bowel obstruction**, patients with **Crohn's disease** in order to establish the extent and severity of inflammation and related

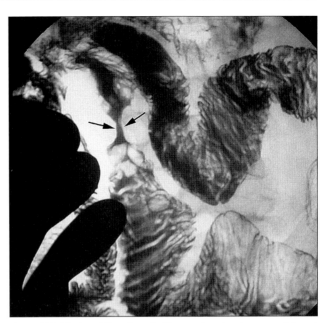

Figure 132.4 Barium follow-through. Compression view from a small bowel follow-through showing an adenocarcinoma of the jejunum (arrows) in a patient with occult anemia.

complications prior to surgery, and diagnosis of small bowel pathology in patients with **malabsorption states**. The main value of contrast imaging in cases of malabsorption is in the assessment of possible causes of symptoms, such as jejunal diverticulosis or the featureless "toothpaste pattern" of graft-versus-host disease. Studies are also sensitive for the diagnosis of small bowel tumors and Meckel's diverticulum.

Importantly, contrast studies remain complementary to other radiological investigations such as CT/MRI/ultrasound and radionuclide examinations. The place of both capsule and fiberoptic endoscopy in the triage of patients continues to evolve (see Chapters 127 and 128).

The colon: the barium enema
Description of technique

The large bowel can be studied using either a single- or double-contrast technique, although the single-contrast barium enema examination plays a limited role. In similarity to other double-contrast studies, the examination also uses a limited volume of high-density barium suspension to coat the colonic mucosa, followed by luminal distension with either air or CO_2. Importantly, the **double-contrast bowel enema (DCBE)** enables the demonstration of mucosal lesions, which may be missed during a single-contrast study (Figures 132.5 and 132.6) [11].

Patient preparation prior to a DCBE remains fundamental to the accuracy of a successful study. The patient must be able to understand and comply with preprocedure colonic cleansing instructions as well as be physically able to roll during the study in order to obtain the necessary images. Whilst a number of bowel preparation regimens can be used, the majority of

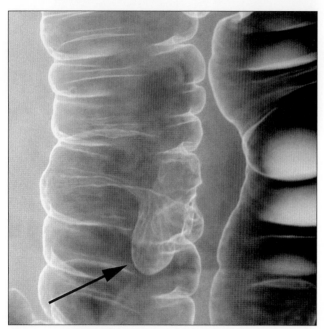

Figure 132.5 Double-contrast barium enema demonstrating a colonic lipoma (arrow).

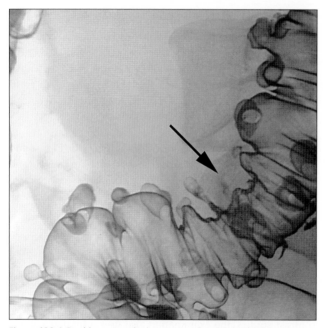

Figure 132.6 Double-contrast barium enema showing focal colonic diverticulitis (arrow).

these combine a low-residue diet prior to the study with a preparation that stimulates colonic peristalsis and keeps the bowel contents semi-liquid. It is important that patients are encouraged to drink sufficient quantities of liquid to prevent dehydration during the period of the bowel preparation.

As for all contrast examinations, the physician requesting the examination must provide relevant clinical details on the request form. Relevant current or past medical/surgical

history should be included as well as information on recent endoscopic procedures. This latter information is particularly important because of the increased risk of colonic perforation if a DCBE is performed less than 7 days following a therapeutic endoscopic procedure, such as snare polypectomy or deep forceps biopsy via a rigid sigmoidoscope [12]. Standard biopsies obtained during colonoscopy or flexible sigmoidoscopy do not contraindicate a DCBE during the same bowel preparation.

Alternative imaging techniques

Colonoscopy is more accurate than the barium enema for the demonstration of small mucosal lesions (<1 cm) [13]. Although colonoscopy is more expensive with a higher complication rate when compared to a DCBE examination [14], the technique is currently recognized as the procedure of choice when screening for colorectal neoplasia.

Cross-sectional imaging techniques, including CT, MRI, and ultrasound, can also be used as alternative imaging techniques to visualize the large bowel with, in particular, the role of **CT colonography (CTC) or virtual colonoscopy** rapidly evolving (see Chapter 136). This technique not only assesses colonic mucosal abnormalities with a greater sensitivity than the DCBE, but also evaluates extracolonic pathology. A DCBE or CTC is indicated if a colonoscopy examination is incomplete [15].

Indications

In many parts of the world DCBE is used for the detection of colorectal cancer and polyps. Other indications for a DCBE include the diagnosis of diverticular disease and its complications as well as the assessment of extrinsic pathology with colonic involvement (see Chapters 8, 56–59). The routine use of the barium enema to assess the extent and severity of inflammatory bowel disease (IBD) has now been replaced by colonoscopy. However, the barium enema plays a useful role in the assessment of patients with colonic strictures secondary to IBD, which do not allow the passage of an endoscope. In addition, contrast studies can assess the position and nature of fistulae and help in the assessment of patients with indeterminate colitis (see Chapter 51).

Contraindications

Whilst the DCBE is a very safe examination with a mortality rate of approximately 1 in 56 000 [16], a number of important contraindications are recognized. In particular, where there is suspicion of a colonic perforation, an examination should be undertaken using water-soluble contrast media, because inadvertent introduction of barium into the peritoneal cavity is associated with significant morbidity and mortality. In addition, pathologies including toxic megacolon and ischemic colitis, which increase the risk of bowel perforation, are a relative contraindication to DCBE. As previously described, DCBE should also be delayed for a week in patients who have undergone a deep mucosal biopsy or snare polypectomy.

Complications and their management

In the context of contrast examinations of the upper gastrointestinal tract, **barium aspiration** can occur. This may result in a pneumonitis or pneumonia and should be managed (unless very mild) by physiotherapy and postural drainage. Where there is any suspicion of an aspiration risk prior to an examination, an isoosmolar water-soluble contrast agent should initially be used.

Whilst extremely rare, the most significant complication of any barium examination is **perforation**. Within the abdomen this may be intra- or retro-peritoneal. Intraperitoneal extravasation of contrast is diagnosed by the visualization of contrast outlining bowel loops and/or the appearance of a pneumoperitoneum. When identified, the treatment in most cases is operative, although conservative management using antibiotic therapy and intravenous fluid replacement may be successful. Retroperitoneal perforation has been reported during DCBE examinations in patients with rectal pathology (e.g. proctitis) and following inadvertent laceration of the rectum during introduction of the enema tip or inflation of a retention balloon. Occult rectal pathology should thus be excluded by sigmoidoscopy performed during initial clinical consultation, with the result recorded on the radiology request form. In addition, when a contrast study is performed to investigate the obstructed gastrointestinal tract, water-soluble contrast agents should be used to avoid the possible risk of subsequent barium impaction.

SOURCES OF INFORMATION FOR PATIENTS AND DOCTORS

http://www.goingfora.com/radiology/barium_room.html
http://www.patient.co.uk/showdoc/27000480/
http://www.patient.co.uk/showdoc/27000478/
http://www.radiologyinfo.org/content/lower_gi.htm
http://www.radiologyinfo.org/content/upper_gi.htm

References

1. Ekberg O, Pokieser P. Radiologic evaluation of the dysphagic patient. *Eur Radiol.* 1997;7:1285–1295.
2. Ekberg O, Wahlgren L. Dysfunction of pharyngeal swallowing. A cineradiographic investigation in 854 dysphagia patients. *Acta Radiol Diagn.* 1985;26:389–395.
3. Levine MS, Rubesin SE, Herlinger H, Laufer I. Double contrast upper gastrointestinal examination: technique and interpretation. *Radiology.* 1988;168:593–602.
4. Levine MS, Chu P, Furth EE, *et al.* Carcinoma of the esophagus and esophagogastric junction: sensitivity of radiographic diagnosis. *AJR Am J Roentgenol.* 1997;168:1423–1426.
5. Low VH, Levine MS, Rubesin SE, *et al.* Diagnosis of gastric carcinoma: sensitivity of double contrast barium studies. *AJR Am J Roentgenol.* 1994;162:329–334.
6. Maglinte DDT, Kelvin FM, Rowe MG, *et al.* Small bowel obstruction: optimising radiologic investigation and nonsurgical management. *Radiology.* 2001;218:39–46.
7. Maglinte DDT, Balthazar EJ, Kelvin FM, Megibow AJ. The role of radiology in the diagnosis of small bowel obstruction. *AJR Am J Roentgenol.* 1997;168:1171–1180.
8. Nolan DJ. Enteroclysis of non neoplastic disorders of the small intestine. *Eur Radiol.* 2000;10:342–353.
9. Dixon PM, Roulston ME, Nolan DJ. The small bowel enema: a ten year review. *Clin Radiol.* 1993;47:26–28.
10. Maglinte DDT, Kelvin FM, O'Connor K, *et al.* Current status of small bowel radiography. *Abdom Imaging.* 1996;21:247–257.
11. Rubesin SE, Levine MS, Laufer I, Herlinger H. Double contrast barium enema examination technique. *Radiology.* 2000;215:642–650.
12. Harned RK, Consigny PM, Cooper NB, *et al.* Barium enema examination following biopsy of the rectum or colon. *Radiology.* 1982;145:11–16.
13. Winawer SJ, Stewart ET, Zauber AG, *et al.* A comparison of colonoscopy and double contrast barium enema for surveillance after polypectomy. National polyp study work group. *N Engl J Med.* 2000;342:1766–1772.
14. de Zwart IM, Griffioen G, Shaw MP, *et al.* Barium enema and endoscopy for the detection of colorectal neoplasia: sensitivity, specificity, complications and its determinants. *Clin Radiol.* 2001;56:401–409.
15. Chong A, Shah JN, Levine MS, *et al.* Diagnostic yield of barium enema examination after incomplete colonoscopy. *Radiology.* 2002;223:620–624.
16. Blakeborough A, Sheridan MB, Chapman AH. Complications of barium enema examinations: a survey of UK Consultant Radiologists 1992 to 1994. *Clin Radiol.* 1997;52:142–148.

CHAPTER 133

Computed tomography

Karin Herrmann[1] and Pablo R. Ros[2]

[1]Ludwig-Maximilians-University of Munich, Munich, Germany
[2]Case Western Reserve University, University Hospitals Case Medical Center, Cleveland, OH, USA

KEY POINTS

- Multidetector-row computed tomography (MDCT) can be considered state-of-the-art technology providing high spatial and temporal resolution imaging
- High-speed MDCT permits imaging in multiple contrast phases (arterial, portal venous, hepatic), which is essential for the detection and characterization of focal liver lesions, organ perfusion anomalies, and abdominal vascular disorders
- Multiphase MDCT is useful in staging pancreatic cancer and characterizing pancreatic tumors
- CT colonography allows for safe, reliable screening of polyps >10 mm in size
- CT enterography is a technique to investigate the small bowel with cross-sectional imaging, providing the advantage of both intraluminal and extraluminal assessment of intestinal pathology
- Ultra-fast imaging at high temporal resolution allows organ and tumor perfusion measurements and has the potential to provide additional prognostic information and treatment monitoring
- Dual-energy CT opens new options for specific characterization of materials and tissues

---

Introduction

Multidetector-row computed tomography (MDCT) is a mainstay in the diagnostic imaging of the abdomen. It is well suited to investigate hepatobiliary, pancreatic, gastrointestinal, and vascular abdominal pathologies. CT is a widespread imaging modality; image acquisition and interpretation are not highly operator dependent. Due to its fast imaging capacity, diagnostic information is readily available even in emergency conditions and in critically ill patients. Routinely available two-dimensional (2D) and three-dimensional (3D) data postprocessing improves the diagnostic confidence and helps to better illustrate anatomy and pathology in the work-up for surgical planning.

Technical aspects

Shortly after its introduction in 1998, MDCT was rapidly established in clinical routine and is now considered state-of-the-art CT technology. MDCT imaging uses a detector array with multiple detector rows in the z-axis. Scanners with 4–320 detector rows are currently available. This technology provides **higher spatial resolution** and, at the same time, allows for **faster scanning with larger anatomical coverage**. Certain artifacts, such as partial-volume averaging (exaggerating small lesions) and motion artifacts, can be considerably reduced [1]. Higher spatial resolution with thinner collimation, thinner sections, and isotropic voxels enhance the quality of post-acquisition image reconstructions in non-axial planes, i.e., **multiplanar reformations (MPRs)**, and **3D volume rendering**. MPRs are 2D planes in any virtual direction or along curved targets (curved reformats). They help to better demonstrate anatomical variants, the extent of disease, and its vicinity to relevant adjacent structures. MPRs are the basis for CT enterography, CT colonography, CT angiography, and in pancreatic imaging to outline the pancreatic duct.

Three-dimensional data post-processing illustrates vessels, and solid and hollow organs as volumetric objects. It is routinely applied in CT angiography and to create virtual endoscopic images, as in CT colonography. Three-dimensional post-processing is distinctly helpful in the presurgical planning of liver resection or transplantation and in minimally invasive interventional procedures.

With faster scanning, contrast-enhanced imaging of the entire abdomen can be performed in multiple phases. Special software applications are available to trigger scanning by density measurements during the contrast bolus passage after intravenous injection of contrast material. This technique adjusts scanning to the individual circulatory conditions of the patient and corrects for patient-related factors, such as varying cardiac output, lung disease, or other conditions affecting circulation time [2].

With the high-speed imaging at high temporal resolution and larger anatomical coverage of MDCT scanners, the quantification of organ and tissue perfusion is now feasible also in the abdomen. This **CT perfusion technique** harbors the potential for tissue characterization, pretreatment prediction of tumor response, and treatment monitoring, especially for novel targeted therapies. Initial results are promising but require further scientific exploration [3].

Dual-source dual-energy CT (DECT) is another recently introduced technology that uses two synchronously rotating X-ray tube/detector pairs integrated in the same system

---

operating at two different tube potentials and acquiring data at two different photon spectra [4]. This allows for specific differentiation of materials and tissue and can be used to create virtual non-contrast images from contrast-enhanced images, to subtract overlaying bone or calcification, to characterize hepatic, pancreatic, and renal masses, and to improve the diagnosis of hepatic steatosis and iron overload [5].

A remaining disadvantage of MDCT is the increased radiation dose because of an increased usage of CT, more phases per patient, narrower collimation, and the cone beam effect. Therefore, numerous low-dose acquisition techniques have been developed and applied, especially for CT colonography.

Clinical applications
Hepatobiliary imaging
In the liver, multiphasic contrast-enhanced MDCT is employed to detect and characterize benign and malignant focal liver lesions, to identify diffuse liver disease, to document complications secondary to liver cirrhosis, to identify arterial or venous vascular perfusion disorders, and to show biliary pathology.

CT imaging of the liver includes two or three phases, typically at 25, 40, and 70 seconds after intravenous administration of non-ionic iodine-based contrast material [6]. The early or pure arterial phase is used to display the arterial vascular supply, potential hypervascular focal liver lesions, and arterial perfusion disorders of the liver parenchyma. It is followed by a second "late arterial/portal venous inflow phase," reflecting a mixture of arterial and splanchnic venous inflow into the portal vein and hepatic parenchyma. The phase of maximum hepatic parenchymal enhancement and hepatic venous opacification occurs 45 seconds after the beginning of the pure early arterial phase and is called the hepatic phase. It is best suited to identify hypovascular hepatic lesions, venous vascular pathology, and venous perfusion disorders.

CT cholangiography
CT cholangiography is a specific technique using a positive intravenous contrast agent that is excreted into the bile and creates an intraluminal opacification of the biliary tree. In combination with thin-section scanning and MPR, the biliary anatomy, anatomical variants, and extent of disease can be clearly demonstrated [7,8].

Focal liver lesions
Focal liver lesions (FLLs) are hypervascular or hypovascular according to their microvascular density and their predominantly arterial or venous blood supply. Multiphasic imaging is essential to categorize FLLs. In addition to the vascularity, the enhancement pattern over time is elemental to distinguishing benign from malignant lesions. Examples of hypervascular lesions are hemangioma, focal nodular hyperplasia (FNH), hepatocellular adenoma (HCA), hepatocellular carcinoma (HCC), and hypervascular metastases (neuroendocrine neoplasms, breast, melanoma, renal cell carcinoma, thyroid carcinoma, and sarcoma). The typical enhancement pattern of HCC is hypervascular relative to liver in the arterial phase, and hypodense in later phases, phenomena called "wash-in" and "wash-out" respectively. This behavior is mandatory to classify a lesion in a cirrhotic liver as **HCC**. The sensitivity of MDCT in detecting HCC depends on the lesion size, scanner properties, and contrast injection protocols and ranges between 61% and 83% [9–11]. The same enhancement pattern holds true also for most hypervascular metastases. Underlying cirrhotic disease and clinical history will help to narrow the diagnosis.

Hemangioma demonstrates a nodular peripheral enhancement with gradual fill-in of the lesion; **FNH** and **HCA** show flushing arterial enhancement which persists in later phases. Clinical imaging trials have demonstrated that hypervascular lesions are best demonstrated in the late arterial/portal venous inflow phase [6] (Figure 133.1).

Hypovascular lesions include **metastases** (colorectal, pancreas, gastrointestinal), lymphoma, and **cystic lesions** (bile duct cyst, biliary cystadenoma, abscess, hydatid disease). These are best evaluated in portal venous or hepatic phases at a scan delay of 70 seconds post injection. The sensitivity of MDCT to detect metastases ranges between 60% and 89%

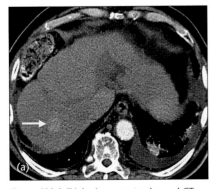
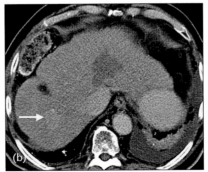
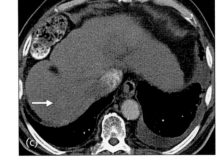

Figure 133.1 Triphasic contrast-enhanced CT scan for hypervascular lesion. (a) Early and (b) late arterial-phase contrast-enhanced CT images show a hypervascular lesion (hepatocellular carcinoma; arrow) in segment 7 of the right hepatic lobe, which is better appreciated on the late arterial-phase image. (c) On the portal venous-phase image, the lesion is hardly appreciated (arrow) due to the rapid wash-out of contrast material and enhancement of the surrounding liver parenchyma.

[12,13]. Generally, magnetic resonance imaging (MRI) is slightly superior to CT in the detection and characterization of FLLs [14].

CT perfusion has gained importance in the follow-up of tumors and metastatic disease under targeted therapy, especially gastrointestinal stromal tumor (GIST) and renal cancer, when size-based response evaluation criteria in solid tumors (RECIST) are insufficient to describe therapeutic effects [15].

Diffuse liver disease

Examples of diffuse liver disease are cirrhosis, hemochromatosis, and steatosis. The utility of CT is most apparent in the evaluation of patients with underlying **cirrhosis** who are at risk for hepatocellular carcinoma. Using a combination of late arterial/portal venous inflow phase and hepatic phase [6], both focal lesions and complications secondary to cirrhosis such as portal-venous thrombosis, porto-systemic collaterals, splenomegaly, and ascites can be confidently visualized. In hepatic steatosis the attenuation of the liver at CT is reduced compared to splenic parenchyma, while in hemochromatosis it may be increased on unenhanced scans.

Presurgical planning

Prior to hepatic resection, orthotopic liver transplantation (OLT), living related-donor transplantation (LRDT), cryoablation, and chemoembolization it is mandatory to evaluate the vascular structures supplying and draining the liver (Figure 133.2). Early arterial-phase imaging allows for production of a CT arteriogram and CT portal venogram, which can help define important anatomical vascular variants and stenosis or thrombosis of the extrahepatic portal venous system [2]. Three-dimensional image reconstructions are standard to favorably display the vascular anatomy.

Perfusion anomalies

Perfusion anomalies occur in patients with focal interruptions to the liver blood supply and venous drainage, and in patients with vascular hepatic neoplasms, both before and after ablative therapy. Perfusion anomalies are most pronounced during the arterial phase. In patients with lobar or segmental portal vein stenosis or thrombosis there may be compensatory increased hepatic arterial inflow to the affected segments or lobes. In patients with vascular hepatic neoplasms, the surrounding normal hepatic parenchyma may be relatively hyperenhanced during the late arterial phase because the tumor produces increased hepatic arterial inflow in a segmental or lobar distribution to supply both the tumor and adjacent normal parenchyma (Figure 133.3). Arterioportal fistulae occur in vascularized hepatic tumors with neovascularity and after penetrating trauma, such as percutaneous biopsy, leading to hyperenhancement of adjacent hepatic parenchyma.

Biliary disease

Thin-section imaging may be useful in detecting partially calcified intraductal stones [16]. Post-contrast imaging is useful in defining the site and extent of biliary tract obstruction and, in cases of malignant duct obstruction, the location and size of lymphadenopathy and hepatic metastasis. CT cholangiography with biliary secreted contrast material is distinctly useful to demonstrate biliary anatomy and anatomical variants in living liver donors [8] and serves as a problem-solving modality in inconclusive cases [7].

Pancreatic imaging

For pancreatic imaging, a triple-phase imaging technique is employed, including an early arterial phase, pancreatic parenchymal phase (or late arterial phase), and hepatic phase. High-resolution imaging with a thin-section technique (1 mm in the

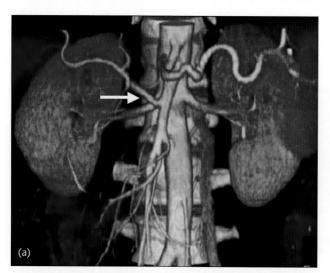
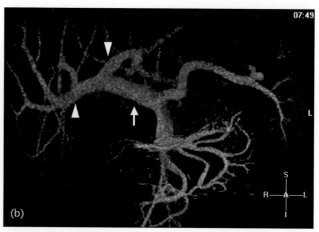

Figure 133.2 Use of multiplanar reconstruction prior to liver transplantation. (a) Three-dimensional volume-rendered CT image shows arterial system supplying the liver. Note the replaced common hepatic artery originating from the superior mesenteric artery (arrow). (b) Three-dimensional volume-rendered image shows normal intrahepatic (arrowheads) and extrahepatic (arrow) portal venous anatomy.

early arterial phase and 2.5 mm in the pancreatic phase) including MPR and 3D reconstructions has considerably improved the evaluation of the pancreas, pancreatic duct, and adjacent vasculature. Oral contrast may be administered immediately prior to the examination in order to distend the stomach and duodenum for better assessment. The early arterial phase is used to create a CT angiogram as a vascular roadmap for the surgeon in potentially operable patients.

Pancreatic neoplasms

In patients with suspected neoplasms, multiphase MDCT is a very accurate modality to detect, stage, and correctly determine tumor resectability. Pancreatic adenocarcinoma is best assessed by combining late arterial and pancreatic parenchymal phases. The overall sensitivity of MDCT for pancreatic adenocarcinoma

ranges between 76% and 92% [17]. According to some authors, resectability can be predicted with a sensitivity, specificity, positive and negative predictive values, and accuracy of up to 100%, 71%, 85%, 100%, and 89%, respectively [18]. MPR and curved planar reformations (CPRs) along the course of the pancreatic duct optimize the demonstration of pancreatic tumors, peripancreatic tumor extension, vascular invasion, lymphadenopathy, and adjacent organs (Figure 133.4) [19,20]. Coronal and sagittal reformations, and CPRs improve the detection of small early tumors [21]. Recently introduced dual-source dual-energy MDCT has been reported to further improve the conspicuity of pancreatic adenocarcinoma and its metastases using 80-kV images [22,23]. CT perfusion imaging appears to have potential to predict the outcome in patients with pancreatic adenocarcinoma prior to radiochemotherapy [24].

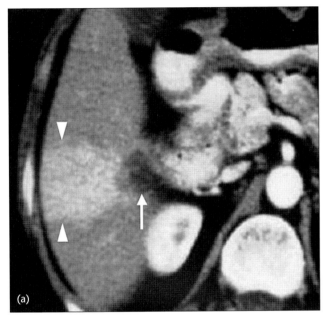

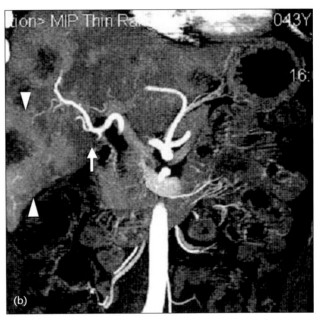

Figure 133.3 Perfusion anomalies. (a) Late arterial-phase contrast-enhanced CT shows a liver metastasis in segment 6 of the right hepatic lobe (arrow) with associated wedge-shaped enhancement of the peripheral hepatic parenchyma due to segmental portal vein obstruction (arrowheads).

(b) Coronal maximum intensity projection image of an arterial-phase contrast-enhanced CT demonstrates the hepatic artery supplying the tumor (arrow) and hyperemia of the adjacent parenchyma (arrowheads) due to the "sump" effect.

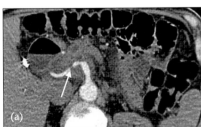

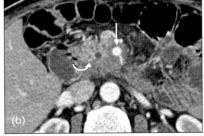

Figure 133.4 Adenocarcinoma of the pancreatic head involving the hepatic artery, celiac trunk and the superior mesenteric artery. (a) Early and (b) late arterial-phase contrast/enhanced CT images show encasement of the hepatic artery (a; arrow) and, more caudally, the superior mesenteric artery (b; arrow). Note the nice contrast between the enhancing normal

pancreatic parenchyma and tumor (curved arrow). (c) Three-dimensional volume-rendered CT image shows thrombosis of the venous system at the level of the confluence of the superior mesenteric vein, portal vein, and splenic vein (asterisk).

Pancreatic neuroendocrine tumors and their hepatic metastases are best identified on late arterial-phase imaging. CT perfusion has been successfully used to distinguish between benign and malignant neuroendocrine tumors of the pancreas [25] .

Intraductal papillary mucinous neoplasms (IPMNs) are most conspicuous on the pancreatic parenchymal phase [19]. CPRs are distinctly helpful in cystic pancreatic neoplasms to visualize the pancreatic duct and the extent of ductectatic tumor or IPMN (Figure 133.5). Distinguishing benign and malignant IPMNs still remains a challenge for both CT and MRI, although criteria indicative of malignancy have been described [26].

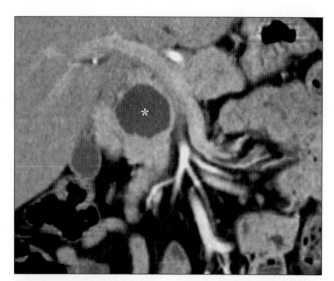

Figure 133.5 Multiplanar coronal reformatted CT image from the pancreatic phase data demonstrates a cystic neoplasm (asterisk) in the head of the pancreas and its relation to the surrounding vessels.

Pancreatitis

Multiphase contrast-enhanced MDCT is the modality of choice to confirm the diagnosis of acute pancreatitis and to assess for necrosis and complications of pancreatitis, such as fluid collections, abscesses, and vascular involvement [27]. In patients with acute pancreatitis, a single phase (40 seconds after injection) technique is performed. Coronal reformatted images are used to evaluate the extent, severity, and associated complications of pancreatitis [28] (Figure 133.6).

Focal pancreatitis, chronic pancreatitis, and intrapancreatic pseudocysts are best delineated in the pancreatic parenchymal phase. Although chronic pancreatitis has distinct CT imaging features, such as duct irregularity, stenoses, focal or segmental ductectasia, calcification, and pseudo-masses, MDCT is still limited in distinguishing between chronic pancreatitis and early pancreatic adenocarcinoma [29]. Preliminary research indicates that CT perfusion imaging may be helpful in this issue but data need further consolidation [30].

Digestive tract imaging
Computed tomography colonography and virtual colonoscopy

CT virtual colonoscopy (CTVC) has received attention as a diagnostic imaging tool with a safety profile superior to that of optical colonography, a low complication rate, and a high patient acceptance [31]. CTVC requires colonic cleansing as in the preparation for colonoscopy, and distension of the lumen for appropriate assessment. Insufflation of room air or CO_2 is used to distend the colon. Positive intraluminal contrast may be added to the cleansing substance to allow for digital labeling and digital subtraction of remaining intraluminal fluid collections and to improve assessment in "hidden" areas. Thin-slice MDCTs of the abdomen and pelvis in both supine

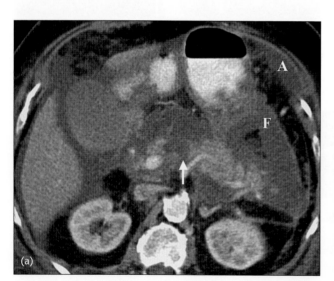

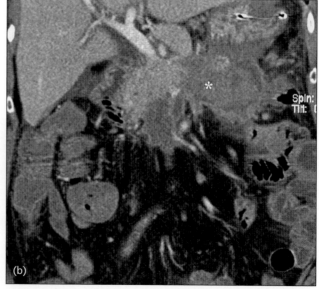

Figure 133.6 Acute pancreatitis. (a) Late arterial-phase contrast-enhanced CT image shows an area of necrosis (arrow) in the neck and body of the pancreas associated with peripancreatic fluid (F) accumulation and ascites (A). (b) Multiplanar coronal reformatted CT image better illustrates the peripancreatic vasculature and extent of peripancreatic inflammation (asterisk).

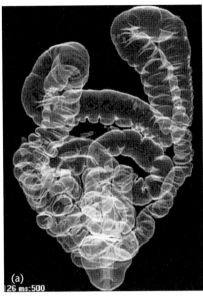 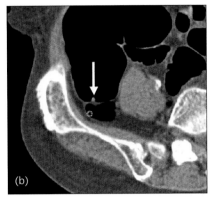 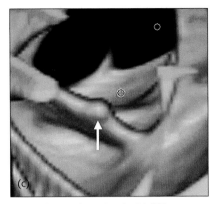

Figure 133.7 CT colonography. (a) Three-dimensional volume-rendered extraluminal CT image of the normal colon. (b) Two-dimensional axial CT image with the patient in the supine position demonstrates a polyp on a fold in the ascending colon (arrow). (c) Three-dimensional volume-rendered endoluminal image in the same patient shows the polyp (arrow).

and prone positions are acquired after insufflation. Intravenous contrast application is optional and recommended in symptomatic patients. The high-resolution datasets subsequently undergo offline 2D and 3D post-processing in order to facilitate interpretation. The 3D display is called "virtual colonoscopy (VC)" since it is similar to the endoscopic view. VC is the basis for the diagnostic evaluation. Automated computer programs [computer-assisted diagnosing systems (CAD)] are available to improve detection rate of polyps and avoid false-negative findings. In addition, MPRs are used to assess the colonic wall, lymph nodes, abdominal organs and the entire abdominal cavity beyond the lumen (Figure 133.7).

The most important clinical applications of CTVC is to investigate for colorectal cancer, adenomatous polyps, and other precursor lesions. Polyp size has a major impact on accuracy. Diagnostic performance and interobserver agreement are high, with a sensitivity and specificity of 85% and 97% for polyps 10 mm or larger, 70% and 93% for polyps between 6 and 9 mm, and 48% and 91% for lesions smaller than 6 mm, respectively [32]. Other indications for CTVC are the preoperative assessment of the colon proximal to an occlusive tumor or non-neoplastic stenosis, and detection of extracolonic findings [33] (including extracolonic cancer or abdominal aneurysms) that can be clinically relevant [34,35].

The major limiting factor to the use of CTVC as a screening tool is the use of ionizing radiation, although low-dose techniques have been developed to reduce overall exposure but maintain image quality.

Rectal cancer
CT is limited for local staging of rectal cancer because of its inherent low soft tissue contrast, which does not allow for accurate evaluation of the T stage unless there is gross invasion of adjacent organs (T4). CT is used primarily for the detection of metastatic disease (see Figure 133.7).

CT enterography and CT enteroclysis
CT enteroclysis is a method of examining the small intestine with cross-sectional imaging allowing the comprehensive evaluation of intraluminal and extraintestinal disease manifestations in one examination [36]. Luminal distension and intraluminal contrast are essential for accurate assessment of the small bowel lumen and wall. Positive or negative intraluminal contrast agents are administered either orally (CT enterography) or via a nasojejunal tube (CT enteroclysis). CT enterography is more comfortable for the patient; however, distension may be incomplete in parts of the small bowel. Distension generally is better with CT enteroclysis, but this technique is invasive and time consuming. The use of intravenous contrast is necessary to depict inflammatory and neoplastic diseases. Many conditions, such as Crohn's disease, celiac disease, small bowel obstruction, and neoplasms that would traditionally be imaged with other modalities, are now routinely imaged with CT enteroclysis [36,37] (Figure 133.8).

CT angiography
Abdominal CT angiography (CTA) typically includes an early arterial and a venous phase. Mesenteric ischemia and gastrointestinal tract bleeding are conditions that can be successfully addressed with CTA. When mesenteric ischemia is of clinical concern, MDCT has become the imaging modality of choice due to its ability to comprehensively assess the mesenteric arterial and venous vasculature, small and large bowel wall, and the remainder of the abdomen for other pathology. MDCTA is very accurate and sensitive to rule out or confirm

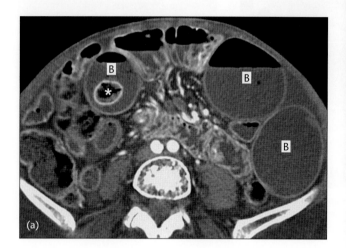

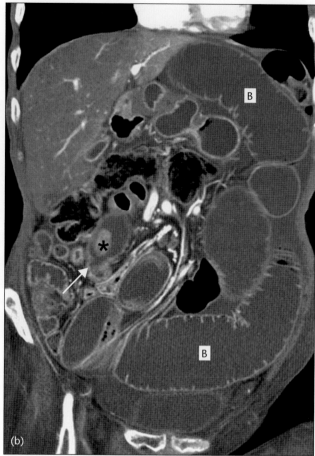

Figure 133.8 CT enterography. (a) Axial contrast-enhanced MDCT enterography image and (b) coronal multiplanar reconstruction demonstrates dilatation of the small bowel loops (B) and "enterolith" (asterisk) due to chronic obstruction as a result of an adhesive band. Please note the transition point (b; arrow) with a sudden narrowing of the intestinal lumen causing upstream dilatation while downstream bowel loops are collapsed.

active or chronic gastrointestinal hemorrhage [38,39] and may even exceed the sensitivity of selective arterial catheter angiography.

References

1. Klingenbeck-Regn K, Schaller S, Flohr T, *et al.* Subsecond multi-slice computed tomography: basics and applications. *Eur J Radiol.* 1999;31:110–124.
2. Mortele KJ, McTavish S, Ros PR. Current techniques of computed tomography: Helical CT, multidetector CT, and 3D reconstruction. *Clin Liver Dis.* 2002;6:29–52.
3. Kambadakone AR, Sahani DV. Body perfusion CT: technique, clinical applications, and advances. *Radiol Clin North Am.* 2009; 47:161–178.
4. Petersilkaa M, Brudera H, Kraussa B, Stierstorfera K, Flohrab TG. Technical principles of dual source CT. *Eur J Radiol* 2008; 68:362–368.
5. Graser A, Johnson TR, Chandarana H, Macari M. Dual energy CT: preliminary observations and potential clinical applications in the abdomen. *Eur Radiol.* 2009;19:13–23.
6. Foley WD, Mallisee TA, Hohenwalter MD, *et al.* Multiphase hepatic CT with a multi-row detector CT scanner. *AJR Am J Roentgenol* 2000;175:679–685.
7. Hashimoto M, Itoh K, Takeda K, *et al.* Evaluation of biliary abnormalities with 64-channel multidetector CT. *Radiographics.* 2008;28:119–134.
8. Wang ZJ, Yeh BM, Roberts JP, Breiman RS, Qayyum A, Coakley FV. Living donor candidates for right hepatic lobe transplantation: evaluation at CT cholangiography–initial experience. *Radiology.* 2005;235:899–904.
9. Kim KY, Kim CS, Chung GH, *et al.* Comparison of gadobenate dimeglumine-enhanced dynamic MRI and 16-MDCT for the detection of hepatocellular carcinoma. *AJR Am J Roentgenol* 2006;186:149–157.
10. Marin D, Catalano C, De Filippis G, *et al.* Detection of hepatocellular carcinoma in patients with cirrhosis: added value of coronal reformations from isotropic voxels with 64-MDCT. *AJR Am J Roentgenol.* 2009;192:180–187.
11. Schima W, Hammerstingl R, Catalano C, *et al.* Quadruple-phase MDCT of the liver in patients with suspected hepatocellular carcinoma: effect of contrast material flow rate. *AJR Am J Roentgenol.* 2006;186:1571–1579.
12. Nomura K, Kadoya M, Ueda K, Fujinaga Y, Miwa S, Miyagawa S. Detection of hepatic metastases from colorectal carcinoma: comparison of histopathologic features of anatomically resected liver with results of preoperative imaging. *J Clin Gastroenterol.* 2007;41:789–795.

13. Rappeport ED, Loft A, Berthelsen AK, *et al*. Contrast-enhanced FDG-PET/CT vs. SPIO-enhanced MRI vs. FDG-PET vs. CT in patients with liver metastases from colorectal cancer: a prospective study with intraoperative confirmation. *Acta Radiol.* 2007;48: 369–378.

14. Floriani I, Torri V, Rulli E, *et al*. Performance of imaging modalities in diagnosis of liver metastases from colorectal cancer: a systematic review and meta-analysis. *J Magn Reson Imaging.* 2010;31:19–31.

15. Schlemmer M, Sourbron SP, Schinwald N, *et al*. Perfusion patterns of metastatic gastrointestinal stromal tumor lesions under specific molecular therapy. *Eur J Radiol.* 2011;77:312–318.

16. Neitlich JD, Topazian M, Smith RC, *et al*. Detection of choledocholithiasis: comparison of unenhanced helical CT and endoscopic retrograde cholangiopancreatography. *Radiology.* 1997; 203:753–757.

17. Francis IR. Pancreatic adenocarcinoma: diagnosis and staging using multidetector-row computed tomography (MDCT) and magnetic resonance imaging (MRI). *Cancer Imaging.* 2007;7: S160–165.

18. Kaneko OF, Lee DM, Wong J, *et al*. Performance of multidetector computed tomographic angiography in determining surgical resectability of pancreatic head adenocarcinoma. *J Comput Assist Tomogr.* 2010;34:732–738.

19. Ichikawa T, Erturk SM, Sou H, *et al*. MDCT of pancreatic adenocarcinoma: optimal imaging phases and multiplanar reformatted imaging. *AJR Am J Roentgenol.* 2006;187:1513–1520.

20. Fukushima H, Itoh S, Takada A, *et al*. Diagnostic value of curved multiplanar reformatted images in multislice CT for the detection of resectable pancreatic ductal adenocarcinoma. *Eur Radiol.* 2006;16:1709–1718.

21. Takeshita K, Kutomi K, Haruyama T, *et al*. Imaging of early pancreatic cancer on multidetector row helical computed tomography. *Br J Radiol.* 2010;83:823–830.

22. Macari M, Spieler B, Kim D, Graser A, Megibow AJ, Babb J, Chandarana H. Dual-source dual-energy MDCT of pancreatic adenocarcinoma: initial observations with data generated at 80 kVp and at simulated weighted-average 120 kVp. *AJR Am J Roentgenol.* 2010;194:W27–32.

23. Robinson E, Babb J, Chandarana H, Macari M. Dual source dual energy MDCT: comparison of 80 kVp and weighted average 120 kVp data for conspicuity of hypo-vascular liver metastases. *Invest Radiol.* 2010;45:413–418.

24. Park MS, Klotz E, Kim MJ, *et al*. Perfusion CT: noninvasive surrogate marker for stratification of pancreatic cancer response to concurrent chemo- and radiation therapy. *Radiology.* 2009;250: 110–117.

25. d'Assignies G, Couvelard A, Bahrami S, *et al*. Pancreatic endocrine tumors: tumor blood flow assessed with perfusion CT reflects angiogenesis and correlates with prognostic factors. *Radiology.* 2009;250:407–416.

26. Takeshita K, Kutomi K, Takada K, *et al*. Differential diagnosis of benign or malignant intraductal papillary mucinous neoplasm of the pancreas by multidetector row helical computed tomography: evaluation of predictive factors by logistic regression analysis. *J Comput Assist Tomogr.* 2008;32:191–197.

27. Kwon RS, Brugge WR. New advances in pancreatic imaging. *Curr Opin Gastroenterol.* 2005;21:561–567.

28. Procacci C, Megibow AJ, Carbognin G, *et al*. Intraductal papillary mucinous tumor of the pancreas: a pictorial essay. *Radiographics.* 1999;19:1447–1463.

29. Boll DT, Merkle EM. Differentiating a chronic hyperplastic mass from pancreatic cancer: a challenge remaining in multidetector CT of the pancreas. *Eur Radiol.* 2003;13 (Suppl 5):M42–49.

30. Lu N, Feng XY, Hao SJ, *et al*. 64-slice CT perfusion imaging of pancreatic adenocarcinoma and mass-forming chronic pancreatitis. *Acad Radiol.* 2011;18:81–88.

31. Graser A, Stieber P, Nagel D, *et al*. Comparison of CT colonography, colonoscopy, sigmoidoscopy and faecal occult blood tests for the detection of advanced adenoma in an average risk population. *Gut.* 2009;58:241–248.

32. Mulhall BP, Veerappan GR, Jackson JL. Meta analysis: Computed tomographic colonography. *Ann Intern Med.* 2005;142: 635–650.

33. Ji H, Rolnick JA, Haker S, Barish MA. Multislice CT colonography: current status and limitations. *Eur J Radiol.* 2003;47: 123–134.

34. Veerappan GR, Ally MR, Choi JH, Pak JS, Maydonovitch C, Wong RK. Extracolonic findings on CT colonography increases yield of colorectal cancer screening. *AJR Am J Roentgenol.* 2010;195:677–686.

35. Pickhardt PJ, Kim DH, Meiners RJ, *et al*. Colorectal and extracolonic cancers detected at screening CT colonography in 10,286 asymptomatic adults. *Radiology.* 2010;255:83-88.

36. Maglinte DT, Bender GN, Heitkamp DE, Lappas JC, Kelvin FM. Multidetector-row helical enteroclysis. *Radiol Clin North Am.* 2003;41:249–262.

37. Paulsen SR, Huprich JE, Fletcher JG, *et al*. CT enterography as a diagnostic tool in evaluating small bowel disorders: review of clinical experience with over 700 cases. *Radiographics.* 2006; 26:641–657, 657–662.

38. Laing CJ, Tobias T, Rosenblum DI, Banker WL, Tseng L, Tamarkin SW. Acute gastrointestinal bleeding: Emerging role of multidetector CT angiography and review of current imaging techniques. *Radiographics.* 2007;27:1055–1070.

39. Graça BM, Freire PA, Brito JB, Ilharco JM, Carvalheiro VM, Caseiro-Alves F. Gastroenterologic and radiologic approach to obscure gastrointestinal bleeding: how, why, and when? *Radiographics.* 2010;30:235–252.

CHAPTER 134
Magnetic resonance imaging

Luca Marciani,[1] Robin C. Spiller,[1] Penny A. Gowland,[2] and Peter D. Thurley[3]

[1]University of Nottingham and Nottingham University Hospitals, Nottingham, UK
[2]University of Nottingham, Nottingham, UK
[3]Derby Hospitals, Derby, UK

KEY POINTS

- As technology evolves and becomes more widely available, the use of magnetic resonance imaging (MRI) in the gastrointestinal tract continues to expand
- Focal hepatic lesions can be characterized using a combination of MRI sequences and contrast agents
- MRI is the modality of choice for the detection of hepatocellular carcinoma and steatosis, biliary stones, and local staging of rectal cancer, and has a major role in the assessment of perianal fistulae
- MR enteroclysis and colonography combine the advantages of barium studies with those of cross-sectional imaging in assessing extraluminal pathology of the bowel

Introduction

Magnetic resonance imaging (MRI) has revolutionized diagnostic radiology, leading to the 2003 award of the Nobel Prize for Physiology or Medicine to Professors Paul Lauterbur and Sir Peter Mansfield. There are now an estimated 20 000 MRI scanners worldwide performing 500 million exams a year (Figure 134.1). Initially, scan times and motion artifacts limited the quality and appeal of abdominal MRI. However, developments in hardware and imaging sequences have opened up a wide range of abdominal protocols that are steadily increasing in number and becoming established [1]. In several applications MRI is now proving to be comparable or superior to conventional imaging techniques such as ultrasound and computed tomography (CT).

Description of technique
Theoretical considerations

Although a deeper understanding of the theory of MRI requires a quantum mechanics description, a simpler "semi-classical" approach allows a basic understanding of MRI. The MRI signal arises from the proton nuclei of hydrogen atoms in the human body. Each proton possesses a small magnetic moment. Once placed in a magnetic field such as in a MRI scanner, these magnetic moments will align with the field and add up together to generate an overall magnetization vector along the field. Upon exposure to a radiofrequency pulse (from a transmit coil

and at a given frequency that depends on the strength of the main magnetic field, called the **resonance frequency**), the protons are able to receive an energy pulse, which tips the main magnetization vector on a plane transverse to the magnetic field (**excitation**). After this, the protons return to their original state (**relaxation**) transmitting a signal that can be detected using a receiver coil. Since this whole process depends on the magnetic field, the use of additional magnetic fields, which vary spatially in three orthogonal directions (called the **gradients**), allows the superimposition of spatial information on the signal, which in turn allows reconstruction of the MRI image of the body using a mathematical transformation.

T1-weighted, T2-weighted, and fat-suppressed images

The time taken by the tipped main magnetization vector to relax back to its original position in the longitudinal plane after excitation is called **T1**. Conversely, the time taken by the magnetization to decay in the transverse plane is called **T2**. These are the fundamental MRI parameters of interest and reflect two separate relaxation mechanisms that depend on the mobility, concentration, and physicochemical environment of the hydrogen protons. By using various imaging pulse sequences and timings, the MRI operator is able to acquire MRI images whose dominant signal arises from the T1 or T2 relaxation mechanisms. For this reason the images are called, respectively, T1 weighted (T1W) and T2 weighted (T2W). This is a unique feature of MRI: the operator can "tune" different MRI images of the same region of the body to contain a range of different signals and contrasts to highlight particular tissues and their characteristics. Another important feature is that the different physicochemical environments of water hydrogen protons and fat protons (called the **chemical shift**) can be exploited to design sequences that "kill" the signal from fat in the body, allowing better visualization of some of the abdominal tissue. Such images are called **fat suppressed**.

Contrast enhancement

The assessment of disease using MRI benefits greatly from the use of contrast agents. They can be grouped into two main types according to their ability to increase the signal obtained

---

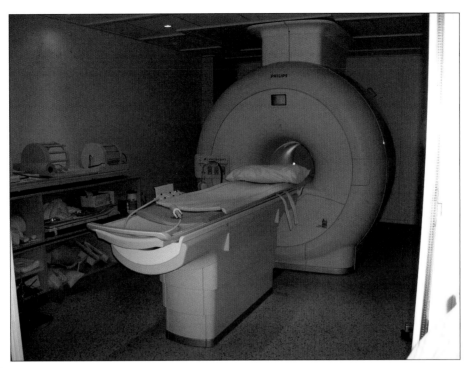

Figure 134.1 An MRI scanner.

from a given MRI sequence (positive contrast) or decrease it (negative contrast). Various types are approved for different indications and approvals may also vary in different countries. The most common agents are administered intravenously and are based on gadolinium chelates [2]. **Gadolinium** has paramagnetic properties that shorten T1 relaxation, resulting in higher signal arising from the tissue where it is delivered in T1W images and signal loss in T2W images at higher concentrations. Images are generally acquired pre- and post-contrast injection and differential enhancement aids discrimination of disease. Contrast agents based on superparamagnetic iron oxide are also used for liver MRI. Intraluminal contrast agents are routinely used for gastrointestinal MRI. A wide range of other substances has been used by different groups, including gases, baby milk, blueberry juice, and polyethylene glycol [3].

Advantages and contraindications

The main advantages of MRI are its use of non-ionizing radiation, multiplanar capability, excellent soft tissue contrast, capability to "tune" this contrast differently depending on the tissue of interest, and good spatial resolution. The main contraindications are the presence of metal splinters in the body, particularly in critical regions such as the eyes, and of certain metal implants such as cardiac pacemakers. Subjects who are uncooperative or claustrophobic may need sedation.

Liver MRI

MRI of the liver (using T1W, T2W, fat-suppressed, in and out of phase sequences, early and late contrast-enhanced images, plus diffusion and perfusion imaging) can provide a wide

range of information not available using other techniques. Liver MRI benefits particularly from the selective use of contrast agents with different properties and specific uptakes. These can be grouped depending on their effects and distribution into extracellular, reticuloendothelial, hepatobiliary, and blood pool agents [4].

Focal liver disease

Advances in parallel imaging techniques and in three-dimensional (3D) T1W contrast-enhanced imaging over the last decade have transformed the use of MRI in the evaluation of focal liver disease. MRI is now regarded as the modality of choice for the detection of hepatocellular carcinoma [5]. Liver metastases are characterized well, mostly appearing hypointense on T1W images and hyperintense on T2W images [6]. Hemangiomata (Figure 134.2) and cysts appear as well-defined high signal lesions on T2W imaging [7]. Areas of focal nodular hyperplasia are usually solitary and visualized well by contrast-enhanced MRI, resulting in an increase in incidental detection (Figure 134.3) [8]. Respiratory motion artifacts, particularly from patients who may be uncooperative with the breath-holds, degrade the image quality. Free-breathing, respiratory-triggered methods are being evaluated to aid characterization of focal liver lesions [9].

Diffuse liver disease

MRI applications in the assessment of diffuse liver disease are widening. MRI assesses cirrhosis (see Chapter 97) with findings including atrophy, hepatocellular carcinoma, and regenerative nodules [10]. MRI is becoming the most sensitive method to assess steatosis. It is, however, still difficult to

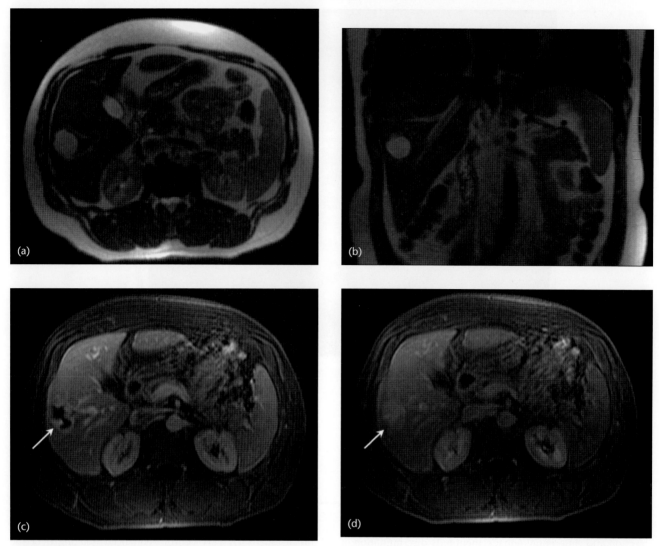

Figure 134.2 (a) Axial and (b) coronal T2W images demonstrate a homogenously high signal lesion in the right lobe of the liver. (c) On early post-gadolinium T1W fat-suppressed images there is peripheral nodular enhancement (arrow). (d) On delayed images the lesion (arrow) demonstrates in-filling and is more uniformly enhancing. These are typical features of a hemangioma.

discriminate between non-alcoholic steatohepatitis (NASH) and non-alcoholic fatty liver disease (NAFLD) [11]. **Magnetic resonance spectroscopy (MRS)**, whereby the concentrations of a spectrum of metabolites is taken from a localized region of interest, is also showing great promise and correlates well with histology [12]. Novel MRI methods are being applied to probe the physiological and biomechanical properties of liver tissue to assess fibrosis [13].

Pancreatobiliary MRI

Contrast enhancement, breath-hold, and fat suppression are commonly used in the assessment of the pancreas, which usually demonstrates higher signal intensity than the liver on T1W fat-suppressed sequences due to the presence of aqueous protein in the glandular elements [14]. By using heavily T2W imaging sequences it is also possible to image the biliary tract.

Magnetic resonance cholangiopancreatography (MRCP; see Chapter 135) avoids the possible complications of more invasive investigations such as percutaneous transhepatic cholangiography (PTC) and endoscopic retrograde cholangio-pancreatography (ERCP). Furthermore, MRI can provide information both below and above an obstruction or a stricture [15] and it is well suited to assess pancreatic and biliary tract malignancies [16].

Pancreas

MRI is comparable to CT in the diagnosis of acute pancreatitis (see Chapter 69) [17] and the assessment of its severity [18], though its use is still limited. Contrast-enhanced T1W can be used to detect non-enhancing tissue necrosis and T2W sequences are used to visualize inflammation and peripancre-atic fluid collections. The use of MRCP in chronic pancreatitis (see Chapter 70) is increasing, though the comparison with

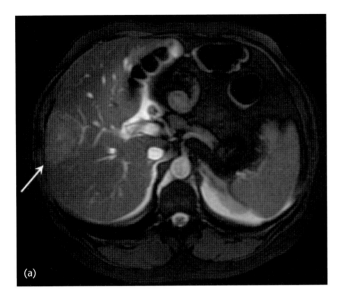

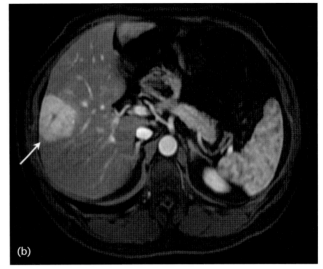

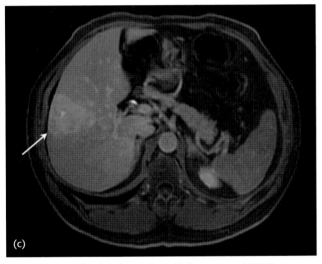

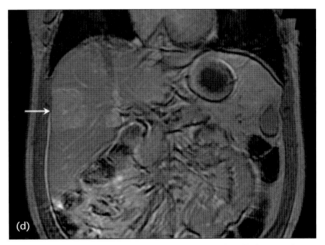

Figure 134.3 Focal nodular hyperplasia. (a) Fat-suppressed T2W image demonstrates a mildly hyperintense lesion (arrow) with a central area of high signal ("central scar"). (b) Fat-suppressed T1W image in the arterial phase following gadolinium demonstrates avid enhancement of the lesion (arrow) with hypointensity of the central scar. (c) Axial and (d) coronal fat-suppressed T1W image delayed images following gadolinium demonstrates wash-out of contrast within the lesion (arrow) with delayed enhancement of the central scar.

ERCP is still debated. ERCP has higher resolution than MRCP but is more invasive and may overestimate duct diameters due to distension caused by the injection of contrast medium [19]. Comparison between the two techniques in chronic pancreatitis showed that MRCP delineated pathological pancreatic changes with reasonably good sensitivity, specificity, and accuracy [19]. Dynamic MRI pancreatography after secretin stimulation of pancreatic exocrine secretion in conjunction with heavily T2W sequences allows improved visualization of the morphology of the pancreatic ducts [20]. MRI has good accuracy in assessing pancreatic tumors compared to CT [21], though the concomitant presence of chronic pancreatitis may make it difficult to discriminate the two. Pancreatic adenocarcinoma (see Chapter 71) has low signal intensity on non-enhanced T1W gradient echo (GRE) images and fat suppression often aids visualization. The intensity of the mass shows delayed enhancement after intravenous contrast administration compared to pancreatic tissue. The presence of chronic pancreatitis may make it difficult also to diagnose intraductal papillary mucinous tumors, appearing as cystic masses on T2W sequences [22]. MRI performs well in characterizing cystic pancreatic masses compared to CT, though the rate of misdiagnosis can be substantial [23].

Biliary tract

A combination of pre- and post-contrast T1W and T2W images can be used to assess gallbladder wall thickness and enhancement, and increased transient pericholecystic hepatic parenchymal enhancement to diagnose acute and chronic cholecystitis [24]. Common indications for MRCP are

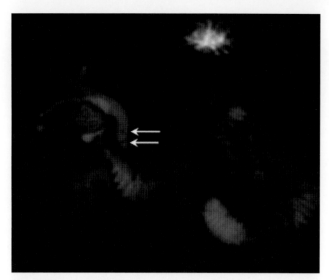

Figure 134.4 Image from a magnetic resonance cholangiopancreatography (MRCP) demonstrates filling defects within the distal common bile duct (arrows) in keeping with calculi and mild duct dilatation.

cholelithiasis and choledocholithiasis (see Chapter 74), with stones mostly having lower signal than the surrounding fluid (Figure 134.4). MRCP is sensitive and specific in assessing primary sclerosing cholangitis [25] (see Chapter 76), with the multiple stenoses and dilations of the intra- and extra-hepatic ducts commonly having a beaded appearance. Hilar cholangiocarcinomas (Klatskin tumors; see Chapter 77) are visualized as hypointense areas on T1W GRE sequences [26]. Intrahepatic cholangiocarcinomas have varying appearances on T2W and contrast-enhanced T1W images and the differentiation from hepatic colorectal metastasis can be difficult [27].

Gastrointestinal MRI

The gastrointestinal (GI) tract is particularly challenging to image due to the inherent geometry of the organs, the heterogeneity of their distension, and their motion due to peristalsis and breathing. However, technical progress and parallel imaging methods have improved the efficacy of MRI in assessing the GI tract to complement endoscopic and X-ray based findings [28]. Contrast agents are administered orally or using naso-duodenal tubes or enemas to distend the GI tract and to provide contrast. Additionally, intravenous contrast agents such as gadolinium chelates are also often administered to enhance the gut walls, and spasmolytic agents are often given to reduce peristalsis. Video clips 134.1–134.10 show MRI videos of the GI tract.

Esophagus

The use of MRI in assessing esophageal disease is developing. Applications of T2W, thin slice, small field of view imaging to assess esophageal adenocarcinoma have been shown [29]. The feasibility of carrying out endoscopic MRI has also been shown [30], though at present this represents only an exploratory research tool.

Stomach

MRI is being increasingly used to demonstrate neoplastic and non-neoplastic diseases of the stomach [31]. Distension of the stomach (usually with water) is essential and injection of gadolinium contrast agents allows visualization of differential enhancement with respect to the normal tissue. The role of MRI in staging gastric cancer is promising, particularly for T staging [32]. Preliminary data of comparisons with other established methods reported T-staging accuracies between 73% and 88% [33–35]. However, N staging is less accurate [32].

Small bowel

Though endoscopy evaluates inflammation and mucosal changes very well, MRI is increasingly used to evaluate and follow-up inflammatory bowel disease activity [36] in terms of wall thickening, enhancement of the wall following intravenous contrast administration, and stenosis. MRI shows promising correlations with other imaging and endoscopic techniques [37], and its accuracy can be superior to conventional enteroclysis [38].

Colon

MRI could play an important role in colonic cancer screening as an alternative to invasive or ionizing examinations. As such, several studies have evaluated its role in detecting polyps. Fast T1W sequences are acquired in a single breath-hold using administration of positive (bright lumen) or negative (dark lumen) luminal fluid as contrast [39]. In bright lumen colonography the lesions are visualized as filling defects, though gas and fecal material can lead to errors. In dark lumen colonography bright enhancing regions are viewed in comparison with precontrast images. The 3D datasets allow multiplanar reformats and can also be viewed in a "virtual colonoscopy" fashion [39] (see Chapter 136). Another interesting application has been shown for colonic diverticulitis (see Chapter 63). Similar bowel preparation with negative contrast colonic filling and administration of intravenous positive contrast agent demonstrates diverticula, focal uptake of contrast agent, wall thickening, ascites, and abscesses, although difficulties remain in differentiating diverticulitis from carcinoma [40–42]. MRI is also proving valuable in the evaluation of inflammation in both Crohn's disease and ulcerative colitis [36,37,43].

Rectum

The preoperative assessment of perianal fistulae (see Chapter 68) is a good example of the superiority of MRI's soft tissue contrast compared to CT (Figure 134.5). Good sensitivity and specificity to detect tracks, abscesses, and openings have been shown [44]. MRI of rectal cancer (see Chapter 58) is an area of continuous development, a fact reflected by the variations in performance reported in the literature. The advent of endoanal coils has improved image quality considerably and the accuracy for T staging is comparable to endorectal sonography [45], though endoanal coils are not comfortable for patients and do not allow a wide field of view and full evaluation of

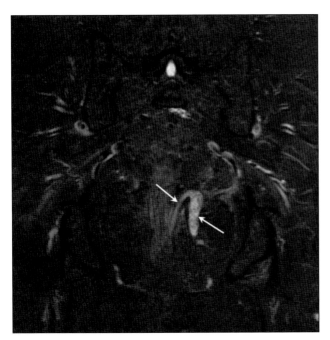

Figure 134.5 Coronal short tau inversion recovery (STIR) image demonstrates a complex perianal fistula as linear areas of high signal (arrows).

the mesorectal fascia [46]. The soft tissue contrast capability is also demonstrated in MRI of the external anal sphincter to visualize integrity of the sphincter and atrophy in the evaluation of fecal incontinence (see Chapter 7).

SOURCES OF INFORMATION FOR PATIENTS AND DOCTORS

An extensive list of World Wide Web MRI links and resources can be found on the website of the International Society for Magnetic Resonance in Medicine (ISMRM)
http://www.ismrm.org/mr_sites.htm

References

1. Semelka RC. *Abdominal-pelvic MRI.* Hoboken: Wiley-Liss, 2006.
2. Lin SP, Brown JJ. MR contrast agents: Physical and pharmacologic basics. *J Magn Reson Imaging.* 2007;25:884–899.
3. Giovagnoni A, Fabbri A, Maccioni F. Oral contrast agents in MRI of the gastrointestinal tract. *Abdom Imaging.* 2002;27:367–375.
4. Gandhi SN, Brown MA, Wong JG, et al. MR contrast agents for liver imaging: What, when, how. *Radiographics.* 2006;26: 1621–1636.
5. Kim YK, Kwak HS, Kim CS, *et al.* Hepatocellular carcinoma in patients with chronic liver disease: Comparison of SPIO-enhanced MR imaging and 16-detector row CT. *Radiology.* 2006; 238:531–541.
6. Kanematsu M, Kondo H, Goshima S, et al. Imaging liver metastases: Review and update. *Eur J Radiol.* 2006;58:217–228.
7. Sasaki K, Ito K, Koike S, *et al.* Differentiation between hepatic cyst and hemangioma: Additive value of breath-hold, multisection fluid-attenuated inversion-recovery magnetic resonance imaging using half-Fourier acquisition single-shot turbo-spin-echo sequence. *J Magn Reson Imaging.* 2005;21:29–36.
8. Marin D, Brancatelli G, Federle MP, *et al.* Focal nodular hyperplasia: typical and atypical MRI findings with emphasis on the use of contrast media. *Clin Radiol.* 2008;63:577–585.
9. Lee SS, Byun JH, Hong HS, *et al.* Image quality and focal lesion detection on T2-weighted MR imaging of the liver: Comparison of two high-resolution free-breathing imaging techniques with two breath-hold imaging techniques. *J Magn Reson Imaging.* 2007;26:323–330.
10. Brancatelli G, Federle MP, Ambrosini R, *et al.* Cirrhosis: CT and MR imaging evaluation. *Eur J Radiol.* 2007;61:57–69.
11. Saadeh S, Younossi ZM, Remer EM, *et al.* The utility of radiological imaging in nonalcoholic fatty liver disease. *Gastroenterology.* 2002;123:745–750.
12. Cowin GJ, Jonsson JR, Bauer JD, *et al.* Magnetic resonance imaging and spectroscopy for monitoring liver steatosis. *J Magn Reson Imaging.* 2008;28:937–945.
13. Talwalkar JA, Yin M, Fidler JL, *et al.* Magnetic resonance imaging of hepatic fibrosis: Emerging clinical applications. *Hepatology* 2008;47:332–342.
14. Semelka RC, Ascher SM. MR imaging of the pancreas. *Radiology.* 1993;188:593–602.
15. Mortele KJ, Wiesner W, Cantisani V, et al. Usual and unusual causes of extrahepatic cholestasis: assessment with magnetic resonance cholangiography and fast MRI. *Abdom Imaging.* 2004; 29:87–99.
16. Mortele KJ, Ji H, Ros PR. CT and magnetic resonance imaging in pancreatic and biliary tract malignancies. *Gastrointest Endosc.* 2002;56:S206–S212.
17. Piironen A. Severe acute pancreatitis: contrast-enhanced CT and MRI features. *Abdom Imaging.* 2001;26:225–233.
18. Merkle EM, Gorich J. Imaging of acute pancreatitis. *Eur Radiol.* 2002;12:1979–1992.
19. Tamura R, Ishibashi T, Takahashi S. Chronic pancreatitis: MRCP versus ERCP tor quantitative caliber measurement and qualitative evaluation. *Radiology.* 2006;238:920–928.
20. Matos C, Metens T, Deviere J, *et al.* Pancreatic duct: Morphologic and functional evaluation with dynamic MR pancreatography after secretin stimulation. *Radiology.* 1997;203:435–441.
21. Hanninen EL, Amthauer H, Hosten N, *et al.* Prospective evaluation of pancreatic tumors: Accuracy of MR imaging with MR cholangiopancreatography and MR angiography. *Radiology.* 2002;224:34–41.
22. Silas AM, Morrin MM, Raptopoulos V, *et al.* Pictorial essay - intraductal papillary mucinous tumors of the pancreas. *AJR Am J Roentgenol.* 2001;176:179–185.
23. Visser BC, Yeh BM, Qayyum A, *et al.* Characterization of cystic pancreatic masses: Relative accuracy of CT and MRI. *AJR Am J Roentgenol.* 2007;189:648–656.
24. Altun E, Semelka RC, Elias J, *et al.* Acute cholecystitis: MR findings and differentiation from chronic cholecystitis. *Radiology.* 2007;244:174–183.
25. Textor HJ, Flacke S, Pauleit D, *et al.* Three-dimensional magnetic resonance cholangiopancreatography with respiratory triggering in the diagnosis of primary sclerosing cholangitis: Comparison with endoscopic retrograde cholangiography. *Endoscopy.* 2002;34:984–990.
26. Vogl TJ, Schwarz WO, Heller M, *et al.* Staging of Klatskin tumours (hilar cholangiocarcinomas): comparison of MR cholangiography, MR imaging, and endoscopic retrograde cholangiography. *Eur Radiol.* 2006;16:2317–2325.

27. Maetani Y, Itoh K, Watanabe C, *et al*. MR imaging of intrahepatic cholangiocarcinoma with pathologic correlation. *AJR Am J Roentgenol*. 2001;176:1499–1507.

28. Lomas DJ. Technical developments in bowel MRI. *Eur Radiol*. 2003;13:1058–1071.

29. Riddell AM, Allum WH, Thompson JN, *et al*. The appearances of oesophageal carcinoma demonstrated on high-resolution, T2-weighted MRI, with histopathological correlation. *Eur Radiol*. 2007;17:391–399.

30. Dave UR, Williams AD, Wilson JA, *et al*. Esophageal cancer staging with endoscopic MR imaging: Pilot study. *Radiology*. 2004;230:281–286.

31. Marcos HB, Semelka RC. Stomach diseases: MR evaluation using combined T2-weighted single-shot echo train spin-echo and gadolinium-enhanced spoiled gradient-echo sequences. *J Magn Reson Imaging*. 1999;10:950–960.

32. Motohara T, Semelka RC. MRI in staging of gastric cancer. *Abdom Imaging*. 2002;27:376–383.

33. Kim AY, Han JK, Seong CK, *et al*. MRI in staging advanced gastric cancer: Is it useful compared with spiral CT? *J Comput Assist Tomogr*. 2000;24:389–394.

34. Sohn KM, Lee JM, Lee SY, *et al*. Comparing MR imaging and CT in the staging of gastric carcinoma. *AJR Am J Roentgenol*. 2000;174:1551–1557.

35. Wang CK, Kuo YT, Liu GC, *et al*. Dynamic contrast-enhanced subtraction and delayed MRI of gastric tumors: Radiologic-pathologic correlation. *J Comput Assist Tomogr*. 2000;24:872–877.

36. Horsthuis K, Bipat S, Stokkers PCF, *et al*. Magnetic resonance imaging for evaluation of disease activity in Crohn's disease: a systematic review. *Eur Radiol*. 2009;19:1450–1460.

37. Sinha R, Murphy P, Hawker P, *et al*. Role of MRI in Crohn's disease. *Clin Radiol*. 2009;64:341–352.

38. Rieber A, Wruk D, Potthast S, *et al*. Diagnostic imaging in Crohn's disease: comparison of magnetic resonance imaging and conventional imaging methods. *Int J Colorectal Dis*. 2000;15:176–181.

39. Debatin JF, Lauenstein TC. Virtual magnetic resonance colonography. *Gut*. 2003;52:17–22.

40. Buckley O, Geoghegan T, McAuley G, *et al*. Pictorial review: magnetic resonance imaging of colonic diverticulitis. *Eur Radiol*. 2007;17:221–227.

41. Heverhagen JT, Sitter H, Zielke A, *et al*. Prospective evaluation of the value of magnetic resonance imaging in suspected acute sigmoid diverticulitis. *Dis Colon Rectum*. 2008;51:1810–1815.

42. Ajaj W, Ruehm SG, Lauenstein T, *et al*. Dark-lumen magnetic resonance colonography in patients with suspected sigmoid diverticulitis: a feasibility study. *Eur Radiol*. 2005;15:2316–2322.

43. Maccioni F, Colaiacomo MC, Parlanti S. Ulcerative colitis: value of MR imaging. *Abdom Imaging*. 2005;30:584–592.

44. Beets-Tan RGH, Beets GL, van der Hoop AG, *et al*. Preoperative MR imaging of anal fistulas: Does it really help the surgeon? *85th Annual Meeting and Scientific Assembly of the Radiological Society of North America*, Nov 28–Dec 03; Chicago, Illinois, 1999:75–84.

45. Kim NK, Kim MJ, Park JK, *et al*. Preoperative staging of rectal cancer with MRI: Accuracy and clinical usefulness. *Ann Surg Oncol*. 2000;7:732–737.

46. Iafrate F, Laghi A, Paolantonio P, *et al*. Preoperative staging of rectal cancer with MR imaging: Correlation with surgical and histopathologic findings. *Radiographics*. 2006;26:701–770.

CHAPTER 135
Magnetic resonance cholangiopancreatography

V. Anik Sahni[1] and Koenraad J. Mortele[2]

[1]Brigham and Women's Hospital, Harvard Medical School, Boston, MA, USA
[2]Beth Israel Deaconess Medical Center, Harvard Medical School, Boston, MA, USA

KEY POINTS

- The diagnostic performance of magnetic resonance cholangiopancreatography is comparable to endoscopic retrograde cholangiopancreatography
- Enhanced anatomical and functional information can be obtained with the administration of intravenous secretin
- Awareness of test limitations and interpretation pitfalls is crucial

---

Introduction

Magnetic resonance cholangiopancreatography (MRCP) is a non-invasive diagnostic technique that was developed for the visualization and evaluation of the biliary and pancreatic ducts. There is no use of ionizing radiation or intravenous contrast, and MRCP does not expose the patient to the risks associated with endoscopic retrograde cholangiopancreatography (ERCP) or percutaneous cholangiography. It has, therefore, become the investigation of choice when evaluating pancreaticobiliary ductal disease. Nevertheless, invasive cholangiography remains the investigation of choice when intervention is required.

Technique
Conventional technique

The use of MRCP was first reported in 1991 [1], and since then the technique has evolved along with the advances in magnetic resonance imaging (MRI) hardware and imaging sequences. Patient preparation initially involves excluding any condition that may preclude an MRI. Patients are required to fast for 4–6 hours prior to the examination, to permit gallbladder filling and promote gastric emptying. T2-negative oral contrast can be administered to reduce the signal from the overlapping stomach and duodenum. Antispasmodics are not routinely administered.

MRCP is ideally performed on a high field system with high performance gradients and a phased-array torso coil. The increasing use of 3-Tesla MRI helps to capitalize on an enhanced signal-to-noise ratio. Heavily T2 weighted (T2W) sequences are utilized to return high signal from stationary or slow moving fluid in the biliary and pancreatic ducts, which have long T2 relaxation times. Signal from background tissue is suppressed due to its shorter T2 relaxation time. This maximizes duct visibility and contrast. Ultra-fast T2W imaging is optimally performed in a breath-hold and thereby reduces breathing and motion artifacts. Three-dimensional (3D) imaging has the potential to replace conventional two-dimensional (2D) techniques. This method produces thinner slices that have improved visibility of the pancreatic duct and biliary tree [2].

The data can be obtained in a variety of formats that usually involve the axial, coronal, and oblique coronal planes; either as thin-collimation (1–5 mm) or thick-slab (30–50 mm) images. In addition, the coronal thin-collimation images can be manipulated using post processing to produce maximum intensity projection (MIP) 3D reconstructions. Both the thick-slab images and the MIPs produce cholangiogram-like projectional images. Using optimizing techniques, ducts with diameters of less than 1 mm can be visualized [3].

Important adjuncts

MRCP is often combined with conventional abdominal MRI to provide extraductal and parenchymal evaluation. MR angiography can also be performed in the same session if indicated. This has been referred to as the "all in one" technique or "one-stop shopping" technique.

A relatively recent adjunct to routine MRCP has been the administration of **secretin** to allow for anatomical and functional assessment of the pancreas. This involves dynamic pancreatography after intravenous stimulation by human or porcine secretin. T2W images are obtained every 30 seconds after intravenous secretin stimulation (0.2 μg/kg of body weight) for at least 10 minutes. Secretin leads to stimulation of the exocrine pancreatic gland. In addition, it temporarily increases the tone of the sphincter of Oddi during the first minutes after injection, thereby inhibiting release of fluid through the papilla of Vater. After this, the tone decreases. Secretin, therefore, initially improves delineation of the

---

pancreatic duct, facilitating the demonstration of anatomical variants or morphological changes in the normal or diseased pancreas [4]. The exocrine function of the pancreas can also be evaluated qualitatively or quantitatively by assessing the increase in fluid in the duodenum after the sphincter of Oddi relaxes [5,6].

Hepatobiliary contrast agents such as mangafodipir trisodium and Gd-EOB-DTPA can also be used in conjunction with conventional MRCP acquisitions. Their indications include identifying bile duct leaks post surgery, documenting biliary anatomy in right-lobe living donors, and diagnosing functional biliary disorders. These agents are hepatocyte-selective T1W MR agents that are administered intravenously and excreted significantly through the biliary system. T1W imaging post contrast is usually performed.

Finally, to improve the assessment of segmental non-dilated biliary ducts, drugs such as morphine and fentanyl can be used to improve visualization of the biliary system. These drugs cause sphincter of Oddi contraction, resulting in upstream dilatation.

Indications
Delineation of anatomy
The diagnosis of congenital and developmental biliary and pancreatic anomalies is an important indication for MRCP. Liver resection, living related-donor transplantation, biliary intervention, and laparoscopic cholecystectomy are several procedures where the prospective identification of congenital biliary variants may prevent inadvertent injury. Normal biliary anatomy is only present in 58% of the population; the commonest anomaly is **drainage of the right posterior duct into the left hepatic duct** in 13–19% of the population [7]. Common cystic duct anomalies include low or medial insertion into the common hepatic duct and a long parallel course with the common hepatic duct [8]. MRCP is 98% accurate in the diagnosis of aberrant hepatic ducts and 95% accurate in the diagnosis of cystic duct variants [9].

Pancreas divisum and annular pancreas are also important conditions to diagnose. **Pancreas divisum** occurs in 4–10% of the population [10]. The clinical importance of pancreas divisum is its possible association with acute recurrent pancreatitis. MRCP diagnosis is made by visualizing two separate ducts with independent drainage sites. The dominant dorsal duct lies anterior to the common duct and enters into the minor papilla. Focal dilatation of the dorsal pancreatic duct just proximal to the minor papilla may occur in association with pancreas divisum. This is known as a santorinicele and is indicative of relative obstruction at the minor papilla [8] (Figure 135.1). MRCP has been shown to be 100% accurate in diagnosing pancreas divisum [11].

Choledocholithiasis
The performance of MRCP for common duct stones is superior to ultrasound and computed tomography (CT), and

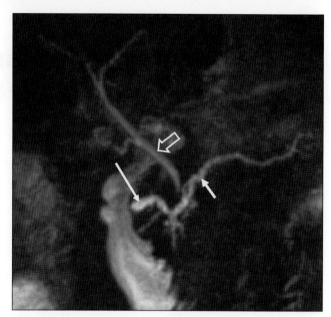

Figure 135.1 Oblique coronal, thick-slab MRCP image demonstrates pancreas divisum. The dorsal pancreatic duct (short white arrow) crosses anterior to the common bile duct (open arrow) to empty into the minor papilla. Focal dilatation of the dorsal pancreatic duct just proximal to the minor papilla is in keeping with a santorinicele (long white arrow).

comparable to ERCP [12]. Studies have yielded sensitivities ranging from 81% to 100% and specificities from 96% to 100% [13]. Negative predictive values are also very high (94–100%) [13]. MRCP is, therefore, a good test in patients with low-to-intermediate probability of having choledocholithiasis, to exclude stones and prevent these patients from being subjected to an unnecessary ERCP procedure and its associated complications. Stones within the common duct are identified as low signal filling defects within high signal intensity bile on MRCP examinations (Figure 135.2).

Neoplasms
Malignant disease of the biliary system and the pancreas frequently results in ductal obstruction. MRCP has been shown to be accurate in identifying the presence, cause, and level of obstruction [14]. MRCP, compared to contrast cholangiography, can visualize the duct before and after an obstructing lesion, thereby providing a roadmap for any future intervention. Also, the examination is non-invasive so there is no risk of cholangitis. In combination with conventional MRI, biliary, vascular, and liver involvement can be assessed to determine resectability [15].

MRCP findings of **cholangiocarcinoma** include an abrupt biliary obstruction with dilatation of the ducts above (Figure 135.3). MRCP plays an important role in staging of hilar (Klatskin) tumors according to the Bismuth–Corlette classification, demonstrating an accuracy of 84% [16]. The investigation is important in determining resectable disease and providing guidance for palliative biliary intervention.

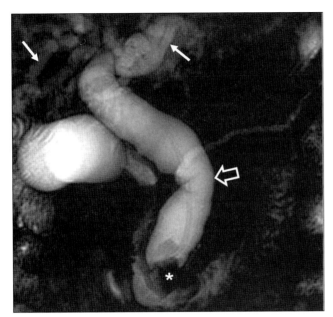

Figure 135.2 Oblique coronal, thick-slab MRCP image demonstrates an impacted low signal stone in the distal common duct (asterisk) with intrahepatic (white arrows) and extrahepatic (open arrow) biliary dilatation.

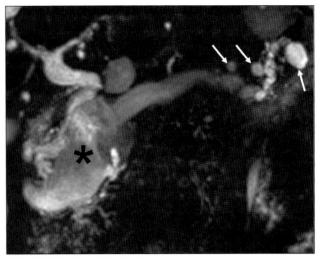

Figure 135.4 Oblique coronal, thick-slab MRCP image demonstrates a markedly dilated main pancreatic duct (asterisk) in keeping with a main duct intraductal papillary mucinous neoplasm. Multiple cystic lesions connected to the main pancreatic duct represent side-branch intraductal papillary mucinous neoplasms (arrows).

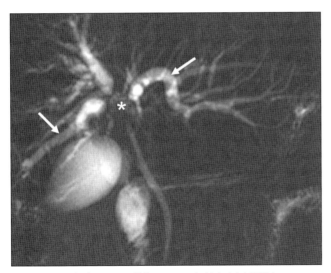

Figure 135.3 Klatskin tumor. Oblique coronal, thick-slab MRCP image demonstrates an obstructing tumor at the biliary confluence (asterisk) with intrahepatic left and right lobe biliary dilatation (arrows).

MRCP depicts obstruction and encasement of the pancreatic duct by **pancreatic ductal adenocarcinoma**. Smooth homogenous dilatation of the duct with an abrupt termination favors malignancy. If the lesion is in the head, then biliary obstruction can also occur; this results in the "double duct sign" in 77%, which is highly suggestive of malignancy [17]. MRCP alone has been shown to be more sensitive and specific than ERCP in detecting pancreatic carcinoma [18].

Intraductal papillary mucinous neoplasm (IPMN) is a mucin-producing tumor of the pancreas that is thought to originate in the main pancreatic duct or its side branches. It

has variable malignant potential. On MRCP, segmental or diffuse dilatation of the main pancreatic duct or a uni- or multi-locular cystic lesion is typical (Figure 135.4). Communication between the main pancreatic duct and the cystic lesion may be depicted. MRCP is considered superior to ERCP in diagnosing IPMN [19], and ERCP on occasion may not be possible as the thick mucin restricts complete opacification of the ductal system. The use of intravenous secretin stimulation is thought to be useful in depicting the communication of branch duct IPMNs with the main pancreatic duct. MRCP, however, cannot differentiate fluid from mucin and sampling with endoscopic ultrasound may be required.

Intrahepatic biliary disease

Primary sclerosing cholangitis occurs in up to 7.5% of patients with ulcerative colitis and 3.4% of patients with Crohn's disease [20]. Seventy to 80% of patients with primary sclerosing cholangitis have ulcerative colitis [21]. Cholangiography, usually ERCP, is considered the gold standard for the diagnosis of primary sclerosing cholangitis. ERCP has superior spatial resolution and may, therefore, be more sensitive for detecting ductal wall irregularity, which is seen in the early stages of primary sclerosing cholangitis. Complications, however, such as infection and pancreatitis are thought to occur more frequently in patients with primary sclerosing cholangitis than in those without. MRCP provides an alternative diagnostic tool without the aforementioned problems. It also allows assessment of ducts proximal to the obstruction.

The classical appearance of primary sclerosing cholangitis on MRCP images is the presence of multiple diffuse short (1–2 mm) strictures in the intra- and extra-hepatic biliary system that alternate with normal or slightly dilated segments. Conventional liver MRI, in combination, may demonstrate complications such as acute cholangitis, cholangiocarcinoma, and confluent hepatic fibrosis. Features that suggest the diagnosis of cholangiocarcinoma include high-grade ductal narrowing, long strictures, rapid progression of strictures, marked dilatation proximal to strictures, and polypoid lesions [22].

Choledochal cysts are potential precursors of cholangiocarcinoma and, therefore, accurate diagnosis is imperative. MRCP has been shown to be equivalent to ERCP in detecting and characterizing the cysts [23]. Complications such as cholangiocarcinoma and choledocholithiasis have also been shown with excellent accuracy with MRCP [24]. MRCP can also demonstrate an anomalous pancreaticobiliary junction [24]. This results in a long common channel after the common bile duct and duct of Wirsung unite. This has been proposed as the cause for certain types of choledochal cysts due to reflux of pancreatic secretions into the bile duct [23].

Acute and chronic pancreatitis

The use of MRCP in **acute pancreatitis** is primarily based on establishing etiology. Common duct stones are well visualized on MRCP [13]. In addition, congenital abnormalities associated with pancreatitis, such as pancreas divisum and anomalous pancreatobiliary junction, can be diagnosed. Combining the examination with conventional MRI can give further information regarding fluid collections, necrosis, ductal disruption, and ductal communication with pseudocysts. Intravenous secretin stimulation may be helpful for the latter two indications. Although good correlation has been shown between CT and MR in acute pancreatitis [25], CT still has several advantages; CT is widely accessible and less costly than MRI, and is more sensitive in detecting small gas bubbles and calcifications.

MRCP in **chronic pancreatitis** can be used to identify the ductal changes and evaluate residual exocrine function. MRCP findings include dilatation, stricturing, and irregularity of the main pancreatic duct, and dilated side branches and filling defects in the ductal system due to stones or debris (Figure 135.5). ERCP has been considered the most sensitive modality for evaluating the pancreatic duct and its side branches. However, data have shown that MRCP correlates well with and may be superior to ERCP [26]. Abnormalities in pancreatic exocrine function are thought to predate imaging findings in patients with early pancreatitis. At this stage the disease may be potentially reversible. Secretin-enhanced MRCP can determine pancreatic exocrine function with the degree of duodenal filling and improves the pancreatic duct and side-branch delineation [4–6]. Changes in pancreatic duct compliance can also be used as an indicator of early chronic pancreatitis [27].

Postsurgical conditions

Due to unfavorable anatomy, ERCP is either difficult or impossible to perform in patients who have undergone certain surgical procedures. Biliary enteric, pancreatico-enteric, and Billroth II anastomoses all provide a diagnostic challenge. Duodenal

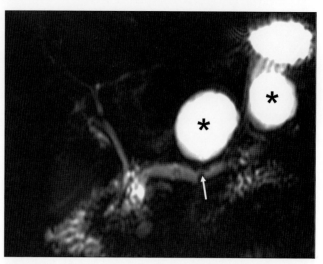

Figure 135.5 Oblique coronal, thick-slab MRCP image demonstrates irregular main duct dilatation compatible with chronic pancreatitis. A stricture is noted in the mid-pancreatic duct (arrow). Two pseudocysts are present (asterisk) from a prior episode of acute pancreatitis.

and gastric obstruction and anatomical variants, such as juxta-ampullary diverticula and choledochal cysts, may also contraindicate ERCP. In these cases, MRCP can provide useful information.

MRCP can also be used to evaluate for the late biliary complications following liver transplantation with reported sensitivities of 93% and specificities of 92% [28]. These occur in up to 34% of patients and include anastomotic strictures, ischemic cholangiopathy, and stones [29]. Accurate non-invasive diagnosis can prevent unnecessary interventional procedures.

Limitations and pitfalls

Several limitations and pitfalls are recognized in the performance and interpretation of MRCP [30]. Awareness of these is imperative in order to evaluate the investigation correctly.

Although the performance of MRCP in evaluating choledocholithiasis is excellent [13], **small filling defects** may be obscured by reviewing only the MIP and thick-slab images. These are projectional techniques with inferior spatial resolution and are prone to partial volume effects. The thin-collimation images should always be reviewed to avoid missing pathology.

Stones can also be mimicked by several entities. These include air, tumor, and blood clots within the biliary tree (Figure 135.6). Susceptibility artifacts from surgical clips and coils and duodenal air can result in local signal loss. A signal void can also be seen in the central bile duct; this is an artifact related to flow and is recognizable by its characteristic central location. Finally, excessive contraction of the sphincter of Oddi may mimic an impacted stone.

The spatial resolution of MRCP compared to ERCP is inferior. This may limit the visualization of non-distended pancreatic ductal side branches or peripheral intrahepatic ducts.

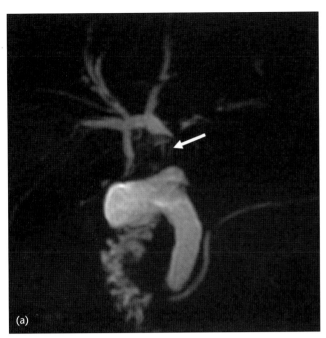
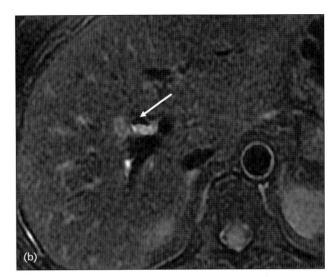

Figure 135.6 (a) Oblique coronal, thick-slab MRCP image demonstrates filling defect in the proximal common hepatic duct (arrow) suspicious for stone. (b) Axial T2W MR image, however, shows that non-dependent low signal in the bile duct (arrow) is actually air rather than stones.

Early changes of conditions such as chronic pancreatitis or primary sclerosing cholangitis may therefore be missed.

Vascular compression may cause artifactual narrowing of the biliary duct. The hepatic arteries and the gastroduodenal artery may be responsible for this. The commonest site of pseudo-obstruction is the common hepatic duct caused by a crossing right hepatic artery [30]. Examining a collapsed pancreatic duct in the fasting state may also mimic stenoses.

Strategies to avoid misinterpretation include always reviewing the source thin-collimation images, obtaining coronal imaging from multiple angles, performing conventional abdominal MRI concurrently, repeating the scan if sphincter spasm is suspected, and administering intravenous secretin to exclude any real stenoses of the pancreatic duct.

Conclusions

MRCP is a widely used investigation to evaluate the biliary and pancreatic ductal systems. It has consistently demonstrated excellent diagnostic performance in a variety of conditions, making it the first-line investigation for pancreaticobiliary ductal pathology. Further advances in technique and applications will continue to enhance the performance of MRCP in providing not only anatomical information but also functional data.

References

1. Wallner BK, Schumacher KA, Weidenmaier W, *et al*. Dilated biliary tract: evaluation with MR cholangiography with a T2-weighted contrast-enhanced fast sequence. *Radiology*. 1991;181: 805–808.

2. Sodickson A, Mortele KJ, Barish MA, *et al*. Three-dimensional fast-recovery fast spin-echo MRCP: comparison with two-dimensional single-shot fast spin-echo techniques. *Radiology*. 2006;238:549–559.

3. Fayad LM, Kowalski T, Mitchell DG. MR cholangiopancreatography: evaluation of common pancreatic disease. *Radiol Clin North Am*. 2003;41:97–114

4. Lee NJ, Kim KW, Kim TK, *et al*. Secretin-stimulated MRCP. *Abdom Imaging*. 2006;31:575–581.

5. Cappeliez O, Delhaye M, Deviere J, *et al*. Chronic pancreatitis: evaluation of pancreatic exocrine function with MR pancreatography after secretin stimulation. *Radiology*. 2000;215: 358–364.

6. Gillams AR, Lees WR. Quantitative secretin MRCP (MRCPQ): results in 215 patients with known or suspected pancreatic pathology. *Eur Radiol*. 2007;17:2984–2990.

7. Mortele KJ, Ros PR. Anatomic variants of the biliary tree: MR cholangiographic findings and clinical applications. *AJR Am J Roentgenol*. 2001;177:389–394.

8. Mortele KJ, Rocha TC, Streeter JL, *et al*. Multimodality imaging of pancreatic and biliary congenital anomalies. *Radiographics*. 2006;26:715–731.

9. Taourel P, Bret PM, Reinhold C, *et al*. Anatomic variants of the biliary tree: diagnosis with MR cholangiopancreatography. *Radiology*. 1996;199:521–527.

10. Agha FP, Williams KD. Pancreas divisum: incidence, detection and clinical significance. *AJR Am J Gastroenterol*. 1987;82: 315–320.

11. Bret PM, Reinhold C, Taourel P, *et al*. Pancreas divisum: evaluation with MR cholangiopancreatography. *Radiology*. 1996;199: 99–103.

12. Fulcher AS. MRCP and ERCP in the diagnosis of common bile duct stones. *Gastrointest Endosc*. 2002;56:S178–182.

13. Sahni VA, Mortele KJ. Magnetic resonance cholangiopancreatography: current use and future applications. *Clin Gastroenterol Hepatol.* 2008;6:967–977.

14. Mortele KJ, Wiesner W, Cantisani V, *et al.* Usual and unusual causes of extrahepatic cholestasis: assessment with magnetic resonance cholangiography and fast MRI. *Abdom Imaging.* 2004; 29:87–99.

15. Mortele KJ, Ji H, Ros PR. CT and magnetic resonance imaging in pancreatic and biliary tract malignancies. *Gastrointest Endosc.* 2002;56:S206–212.

16. Manfredi R, Brizi MG, Masselli G, *et al.* Malignant biliary hilar stenosis: MR cholangiography compared with direct cholangiography. *Radiol Med.* 2001;102:48–54.

17. Freeny PC, Marks WM, Ryan JA, *et al.* Pancreatic ductal adenocarcinoma: diagnosis and staging with dynamic CT. *Radiology.* 1988;166:125–133.

18. Adamek HE, Albert J, Breer J, *et al.* Pancreatic carcinoma detection with magnetic resonance cholangiopancreatography and endoscopic retrograde cholangiopancreatography: a prospective controlled study. *Lancet.* 2000;356:190–193.

19. Fukukura Y, Fujiyoshi F, Sasaki M, *et al.* HASTE MR cholangiopancreatography in the evaluation papillary-mucinous tumors of the pancreas. *J Comput Assist Tomogr.* 1999;23:301–305.

20. Talwalkar JA, Lindor KD. Primary Sclerosing Cholangitis. *Inflamm Bowel Dis.* 2005;11:62–72.

21. Charatcharoenwitthaya P, Lindor KD. Primary sclerosing cholangitis: diagnosis and management. *Curr Gastroenterol Rep.* 2006;8:75–82.

22. MacCarty RL, LaRusso NF, May GR, *et al.* Cholangiocarcinoma complicating primary sclerosing cholangitis: cholangiographic appearances. *Radiology.* 1985;156:43–46.

23. Matos C, Nicaise N, Deviere J, *et al.* Choledochal cysts: comparison of findings at MR cholangiopancreatography and endoscopic retrograde cholangiopancreatography in eight patients. *Radiology.* 1998;209:443–448.

24. Park DH, Kim MH, Lee SK, *et al.* Can MRCP replace the diagnostic role of ERCP for patients with choledochal cysts? *Gastrointest Endosc.* 2005;62:360–366.

25. Lecesne R, Taourel P, Bret PM, *et al.* Acute pancreatitis: interobserver agreement and correlation of CT and MR cholangiopancreatography with outcome. *Radiology.* 1999;211:727–735.

26. Del Frate C, Zanardi R, Mortele K, *et al.* Advances in imaging for pancreatic disease. *Curr Gastroenterol Rep.* 2002;4:140–148.

27. Fukukura Y, Fujiyoshi F, Sasaki M, *et al.* Pancreatic duct: morphological evaluation with MR cholangiopancreatography after secretin stimulation. *Radiology.* 2002;222:674–680.

28. Meersschaut V, Mortele KJ, Troisi R, *et al.* Value of MR cholangiography in the evaluation of postoperative biliary complications following orthoptic liver transplantation. *Eur Radiol.* 2000;10: 1576–1581.

29. Zoepf T, Maldonado-Lopez EJ, Hilgard P, *et al.* Diagnosis of biliary strictures after liver transplantation: which is the best tool? *World J Gastroenterol.* 2005;11:2945–2948.

30. Irie H, Honda H, Kuroiwa T, *et al.* Pitfalls in MR cholangiopancreatographic interpretation. *Radiographics.* 2001;21:23–37.

CHAPTER 136

Virtual colonoscopy

Abraham H. Dachman,[1] Ila Sethi[1] and Philippe Lefere[2]

[1]The University of Chicago Medical Center, Chicago, IL, USA
[2]Stedelijk Ziekenhuis, Roeselare, Belgium

KEY POINTS

- Virtual colonoscopy (VC)/CT colonography (CTC) is a minimally invasive technique to detect colorectal polyps, and can be done in an outpatient setting without sedation
- State-of-the-art CT scanners enable acquisition of ultra-low radiation dose scans with breath-holds of <10 seconds
- CTC is the best test for patients who have an incomplete optical colonoscopy (OC) or who cannot undergo or refuse OC
- CTC is adaptable to less vigorous cleansing strategies as compared to OC
- VC interpretation requires training and experience
- CTC results in fewer polypectomies, less utilization of invasive endoscopy, and fewer complications than OC
- Computer-aided detection programs are now available and undergoing clinical testing
- MRI is a rapidly evolving alternative technique to CTC and avoids the need for radiation

---

Introduction

Colorectal carcinoma (CRC) is the third most common cancer diagnosed in both men and women, and overall is the second leading cause of cancer death in the US [1]. Although evidence shows a mortality reduction associated with early detection of invasive disease and removal of adenomatous polyps, the compliance with screening recommendations remains suboptimal.

Virtual colonoscopy (VC) or CT colonography (CTC) has emerged as an appealing and minimally invasive option for **CRC screening** (Figures 136.1 and 136.2) [2]. Since the first CTC in 1993, the technique has gained acceptance by several organizations and its use increases as more physicians become trained in the performance and interpretation of CTC. In this chapter we will give a brief description of the technique and reading protocols, and discuss the current status of CTC, recent advances, and controversies.

CT colonography as a screening tool

CTC is an imaging examination of the entire colon and rectum that employs CT to acquire axial images of the cleansed and distended colon to search for polyps and masses using two- (2D) and three-dimensional (3D) reconstructed images. Compared to **optical colonoscopy (OC)**, some advantages of CTC include rapid image acquisition and processing (the entire exam takes about 15 minutes), non-invasiveness, and decreased risks of perforation, bleeding, and sedation complications. The expectation is that these advantages will help improve the compliance with CRC screening.

Several large studies of CTC as a CRC screening tool have reported excellent results [2–5]. For adenomas and cancers >10 mm, the results obtained in the American College of Radiology (ACR) Imaging Network (ACRIN) trial reported a mean by-patient sensitivity of 90%, albeit with a lower specificity of 86% [2,3]. The by-patient sensitivity of CTC fell to 78% for lesions between 6 and-9 mm. The Italian Multicenter Polyp Accuracy CTC (IMPACT) study has shown similar results [6]. In another clinical trial involving over 6000 asymptomatic adults who underwent either primary CTC screening or primary optical colonoscopy screening, the detection and removal of advanced neoplasia was similar in both, despite the fact that patients in the colonoscopy arm had higher risk for colon cancer [4]. CTC resulted in fewer total polypectomies, less utilization of invasive endoscopy, and fewer complications than OC. These data support the view that CTC holds the potential to improve the compliance for CRC screening, and selectively and non-invasively filter out those patients who would benefit most from OC and polypectomy.

CT colonography and incomplete endoscopy

CTC is an excellent method for the evaluation of the non-visualized part of the colon after incomplete OC [7]. In most instances, the patient who is already prepared and has undergone an incomplete colonoscopy can be accommodated for a same-day, unscheduled CTC examination, thus obviating the need for a return visit and repeat preparation. Same-day CTC should not be done if there is a high risk of colon perforation, such as in patients who have undergone a snare polypectomy, electrocautery or "well-biopsy" in which multiple samples are taken from the same site. In those instances, it is best to wait several weeks for the colon to heal.

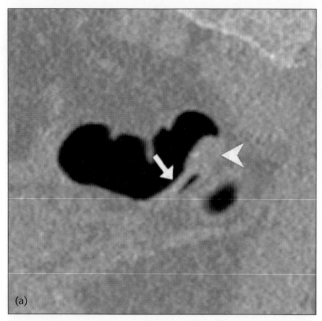
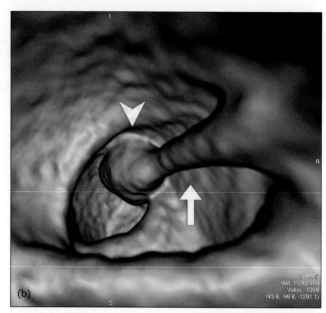

Figure 136.1 Large pedunculated polyp with its pedicle (arrow) and head (arrowhead) in the descending colon on both the (a) sagittal reformat and (b) endoluminal view.

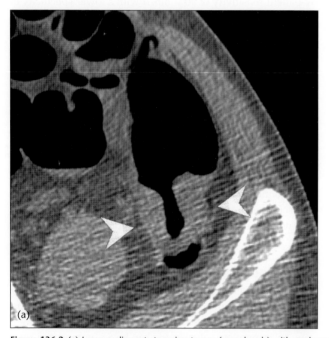
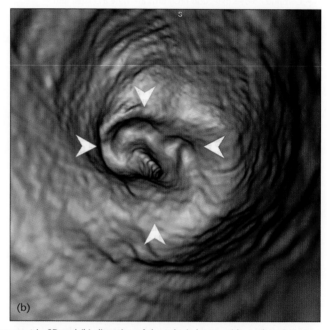

Figure 136.2 (a) Large malignant stenosing tumor (arrowheads) with apple-core aspect in 2D and (b) distortion of the colonic lumen with overhanging edges on the 3D endoluminal view.

Indications and contraindications

The ACR has issued guidelines for the performance of CTC in adults and these are consistent with the American Cancer Society (ACS) CRC guidelines [2,8,9]. Thus, CTC may be indicated for:

- Screening average-risk individuals;
- Screening individuals with an elevated risk for CRC but in whom OC is relatively or absolutely

contraindicated. Risk factors for patients at increased risk for complications during OC are advanced age, anticoagulation therapy, sedation risk, prior incomplete colonoscopy
- Following incomplete colonoscopy
- Surveillance of patients who have a personal history of CRC or adenomatous polyp, or surveillance of patients who have had a prior polyp on CTC without an intervening polypectomy.

Relative contraindications for CTC include:

- Pregnancy or potential pregnancy
- Fulminant or acute colitis
- Acute diverticulitis
- Recent colorectal surgery
- Same day deep endoscopic biopsy, electrocautery or polypectomy
- Acute diarrhea
- Symptomatic or high-grade bowel obstruction
- Obstructing colon-containing inguinal hernia
- Patients with inflammatory bowel disease and hereditary colon cancer syndromes due to their anticipated need for polypectomy or biopsy.

Bowel preparation

Generally, a saline cathartic that leaves less residual fluid (which can hide polyps) is preferred to polyethylene glycol (PEG). However, if the fluid is tagged, some residual fluid is acceptable. Bisacodyl may be used in conjunction with sodium phosphate or magnesium citrate [10]. Recently, we have used HalfLytley, a 2-L PEG preparation combined with fecal tagging for all our patients.

Fecal and fluid tagging

Although complete bowel cleansing is ideal, studies have shown bowel preparation was rated as the most unpleasant aspect of both CTC and OC [10]. This suggests that reducing the discomfort of purgative bowel preparation would be a major factor in increasing patient compliance with CRC screening. Furthermore, fluid conceals polyps. Thus tagging fluid with a CT contrast agent might help improve reader sensitivity (Figure 136.3) [11]. The tagging of solid stool can improve reader specificity by helping to differentiate non-mobile solid stool in which gas bubbles are absent (Figure 136.4). Thus, the rubric of "fecal tagging" actually means both tagging of stool and residual fluid. Various tagging agents, alone or in combination, can be used, including barium in varying strengths, iodinated contrasts (e.g., sodium diatrizoate and meglumine diatrizoate), and high-density or 2% barium. We now use hypo-osmotic water-soluble contrast, iohexol, for all our patients and find that it tags fluid and stool quite well, and when diluted has little taste. The performance of non-cathartic CTC with stool tagging is also being evaluated. Electronic stool subtraction of tagged fluid is widely available on commercial CTC software. True prepless CTC is undergoing development and investigation [12], as is dual-energy CT electronic subtraction (Sosna *et al*, personal communication).

Colonic insufflation

Excellent colonic insufflation is critical to achieving a high quality CTC exam. A thin rectal tube designed for CTC is inserted gently into the rectum and a small balloon is inflated to keep the tube in place. We prefer automated insufflation

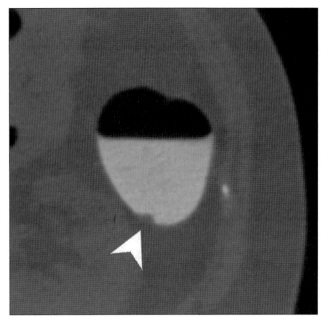

Figure 136.3 Small sessile polyp in the descending colon (arrowhead), appearing as a negative filling defect in tagged fluid.

using CO_2 and a pressure-sensitive pump. Other options include manual room air insufflation or patient self-insufflation (rarely used) of CO_2 or room air. These methods are safe; symptomatic colonic perforation associated with CTC is rare (0.03–0.009%). An antispasmodic agent such as buscopan or glucagon may be administered prior to insufflation to relieve colonic spasm and discomfort [13]. We have stopped using antispasmodics and employ a "deflation maneuver" to relieve pain inbetween the supine and prone scans [14]. We also employ a "bag maneuver" for patients who have suboptimal insufflation as seen on the scout view, yet have colonic pressures of >25 mmHg (which turns off the mechanical insufflator); the fluid catch bag is used to manually add additional CO_2 obviating the need to cut the tubing and convert to manual room air insufflations [14]. Patients are scanned in both the supine and prone positions, which is important to improve polyp conspicuity and to help differentiate polyps from stool, thus improving specificity. Additional decubitus views can be obtained to move the gas or fluid as desired.

CT colonography data acquisition protocols

A 16-channel or greater multidetector scanner is preferred over 8-slice scanners, and breath-holds of 10 seconds or less can be obtained. Low radiation dose scans that yield near-isotropic voxels will produce the best quality 3D volume-rendered images. Generally, the effective mAs should be 50 or less, the collimation 1–3 mm reconstructed to one-third to one-half of the collimation. kVp is normally 120, except in obese patients who should be scanned at 140 kVp and at a higher mAs. The parameters should be adjusted to allow a short breath-hold of

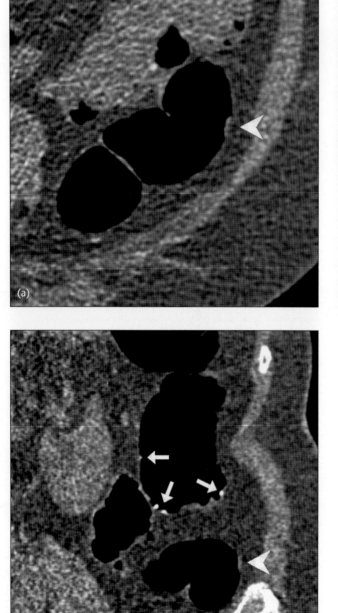

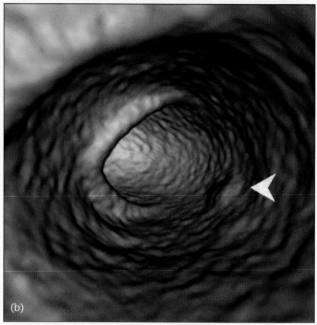

Figure 136.4 (a, b) A 12-mm flat lesion with a height of 2mm in the descending colon nicely depicted in the abdominal window setting (arrowhead). (c) The coronal reformat nicely shows the contrast difference between the flat lesion (arrowhead) and the hyperdense tagged fecal residue (arrows). This study was performed with an ultra-low dose of 120kV and 30mAs on a 64-slice scanner.

30 seconds or less. We currently use a 256-slice scanner at 15 or 30mAs/slice, which results in a low dose scan of 1.9–2.9mSv/series.

Image display

User-friendly CTC interpretation software must display endoluminal 3D views with an automated centerline and fly-though capability, and multiplanar 2D views (axial, coronal, sagittal, and oblique views), with easy point-to-point comparison between 2D and 3D views. The supine and prone series must be easily compared. Polyp measuring tools, 3D movies, and report generation software is also necessary. Novel "virtual pathology" views are available in several commercial programs; undistorted "clam-shell"-like views, and other novel displays may help in reducing interpretation time (Figure 136.5). Other recent advances include color maps to characterize polyp texture on 3D (e.g., display 2D Hounsfield unit density as a color map), polyp volume, improved rectum-to-polyp distance measurement to compare to OC, improved supine-to-prone location matching, and computer-aided detection (CAD) software.

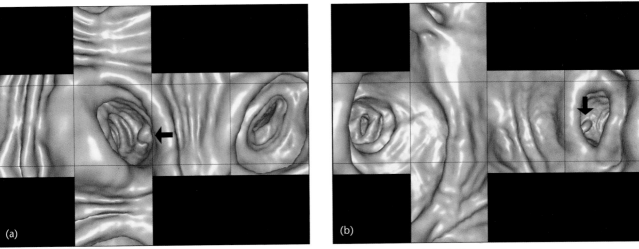

Figure 136.5 Unfolded cube view showing a sessile polyp (arrow) and allowing inspection of the colon in both (a) antegrade and (b) retrograde direction on the left and right part of the image respectively.

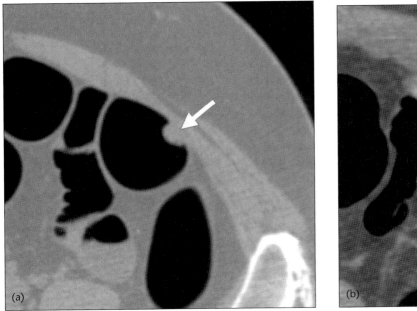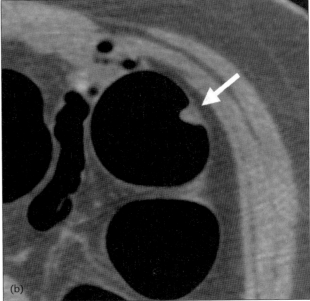

Figure 136.6 Large sessile polyp in the sigmoid (arrow) in (a) supine and (b) prone position depicting a soft tissue density in the abdominal window setting.

Interpretation and reporting

Experts agree that both good 3D and 2D reading skills are necessary. A primary 3D read is our favored approach; flying through the colon forward and backward on both the supine and prone views. Polyp candidates are then viewed on a color map, or more reliably on 2D to characterize them as stool or polyp. Stool is characterized by a bubbly pattern of gas or by seeing tagging agent throughout. Stool often will move freely to the dependent surface. Polyps are fixed soft tissue density lesions (Figure 136.6), although pedunculated lesions can move and mimic stool in regard to their mobility. Sometimes mobility of the colon can cause a polyp candidate to appear to move, but this pitfall can be recognized by carefully comparing both positions. Most cases can be read in 5–15 minutes using this approach. We recommend that a careful review of 2D images be done to look for flat lesions, particularly in a wide soft tissue window (see Figure 136.4). Two-dimensional images are also critical in recognizing fatty lesions consistent with a lipoma, which should not require further evaluation with endoscopy. Careful polyp measurement should be done using the single longest dimension [14]. Common pitfalls include residual fecal material, bulbous folds, diverticula, and the ileocecal valve. In all these cases, evaluation using both 2D multiplanar reconstruction (MPR) and 3D endoluminal views can facilitate correct interpretation. Published guidelines, the CTC Reporting and Data

Systems (C-RADS) criteria [15], suggest that polyps measuring >10 mm should be referred for immediate optical colonoscopy. One or two polyps measuring 6–9 mm may be referred for 1–3-year surveillance. Reporting of polyps measuring <5 mm is not recommended because they often present as stool or are associated with an extremely low risk of malignancy. Certainly actual management varies depending on the specific lesion size, the certainty of the findings, the patient's age, and the existing co-morbid conditions.

Extracolonic findings

Findings outside the colon visible on CTC that are of potential medical importance should be reported. It is important not to overemphasize common insignificant findings or inappropriately recommend further evaluation. Due to the low radiation dose used in CTC and the lack of intravenous iodinated contrast, the exam is not sensitive for detecting lesions outside of the colon. The C-RADS guidelines [15] provide a categorization of extracolonic findings (ECFs) as follows:

- E1 is normal or anatomic variant
- E2 is clinically unimportant finding (e.g., liver cyst, gallstones)
- E3 is likely unimportant but incompletely characterized, and work-up is subject to patient and doctor preference (e.g., complex or homogenously hyperattenuating renal cyst)
- E4 which is a potentially significant finding (e.g., solid renal mass, pathological sized lymphadenopathy, aortic aneurysm).

Note that even E4 findings may not be newly discovered on CTC and the patient or one of the patient's physicians may be aware of the finding. Judicious handling of potential ECFs is warranted to balance the cost of additional work up against the potential for early detection of important disease because many findings will prove to be of no clinical consequence [16–21].

 Computer-aided detection (see Video clip 136.1)

CAD for CTC refers to a computerized scheme that automatically detects suspicious polyps and masses in CTC images and reveals their location (Figure 136.7). The quality of a CAD program is related to both its sensitivity for proven polyps and the false-positive rate. In stand-alone studies where a CAD output is compared to truth as defined by an expert reader's unblinded comparison of the CTC and OC results, CAD has proven quite sensitive, and recent studies have shown low false-positive rates. A recent study evaluating the performance of CAD has shown per-polyp and per-patient sensitivities to be 92% and 98% respectively for adenomas >10 mm in diameter, with a mean false-positive rate of 8.6% per patient [22]. New CAD systems also accommodate fluid and stool tagging without adversely affecting the CAD sensitivity and false-positive rate. CAD for minimally prepared or non-cathartic CTC is under investigation.

In clinical use, a secondary read paradigm should be used, and this should be fully read without CAD and then the CAD output viewed and assessed. Primary and concurrent reading paradigms shorten the interpretation time but introduce bias and may discourage the observer from performing a thorough interpretation. Pitfalls of CAD include the observer accepting a CAD hit as a true positive when in fact it is not a polyp, thus decreasing reader sensitivity. CAD true positives could also be ignored if mistakenly dismissed by the reader as a false positive. Further research is needed to study the causes of these pitfalls and discover ways to minimize them.

CAD has been shown to increase reader sensitivity by 15% for detection of ≥6-mm polyps, albeit with 14% reduced specificity [23]. In a study analyzing the cost-effectiveness of adding CAD to a CTC training program and comparing it with other options of CRC prevention, it was concluded that optical colonoscopy was not a cost-effective alternative to CT colonography with CAD performed by experienced readers. CT colonography with CAD for inexperienced readers was more clinically effective and cost-effective than flexible sigmoidoscopy [24]. A significant improvement in overall reader performance with CAD was also reported in a more recent trial [25].

Cost-related issues

One of the arguments for the use of CTC is the limited availability of OC, suggesting that gastroenterologists' resources should be reserved for a prescreened cohort with a high prevalence of disease. This may be a more cost-effective use of resources. CTC can be reasonably cost-effective when its diagnostic accuracy is high, as with primary 3D technology, and if costs are about 60% of those of OC [26]. CTC was found to be highly cost effective when a 6-mm size threshold was included for polypectomy referral [27]. However, at the time of writing, the Centers for Medicare and Medicaid Services (CMS) had rejected the proposal to include screening CTC as a covered exam under Medicare. Meanwhile, private insurers in the US are increasingly embracing CTC. There is a slow but steadily increasing recognition of the value of CTC and the utilization of CTC in general radiology practice is likely to grow.

Radiation exposure

Radiation exposure for the general population from all sources is about 3 mSv/year. In some high altitude areas of the world, background radiation is 12 mSv/year. The doses reported for CTC are within the range reported for natural background radiation and very low-dose protocols are increasingly being used. Scanners now have various filters or dose-reduction software by tube modulation or other methods that can substantially reduce the radiation dose of CTC (see Figure 136.4). Note that MR colonography is beyond the scope of this discussion but is a potential alternate way to evaluate the colon without the need for ionizing radiation.

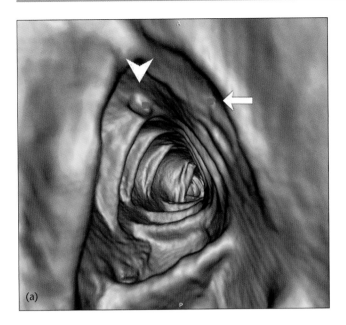

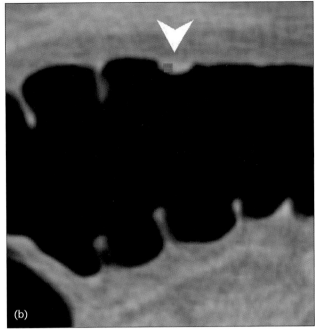

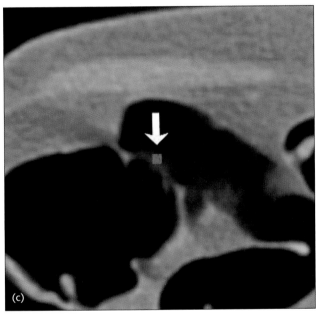

Figure 136.7 Endoluminal image of the transverse colon showing (a) two CAD marks with a red square (arrowhead and arrow). The corresponding 2D axial images show (b) a true positive CAD mark caused by a sessile 8-mm polyp (arrowhead) and (c) a false-positive CAD mark caused by a breathing artifact (arrow).

References

1. Levin B, Lieberman DA, McFarland B, *et al.*; American Cancer Society Colorectal Cancer Advisory Group, and the American College of Radiology. Screening and surveillance for the early detection of colorectal cancer and adenomatous polyps, 2008: a joint guideline from the American Cancer Society, the US Multi-Society Task Force on Colorectal Cancer, and the American College of Radiology. *CA Cancer J Clin.* 2008;58:130–160.

2. McFarland EG, Fletcher JG, Pickhardt PP, *et al.* ACR Colon Cancer Committee White Paper: Status of CT Colonography 2009. *J Am Coll Radiol.* 2009;6:756-772.

3. Johnson CD, Chen MH, Toledano AY, *et al.* Accuracy of CT colonography for detection of large adenomas and cancers. *N Engl J Med.* 2008;359:1207–1217.

4. Kim DH, Pickhardt PJ, Taylor AJ, *et al.* CT colonography versus colonoscopy for the detection of advanced neoplasia. *N Engl J Med.* 2007;357:1403–1412.

5. Graser A, Becker C, *et al.* 64-MDCT colonography, optical colonoscopy, M2-pyruvate kinase, and fecal occult blood testing in a screening population. Presented at the Annual Meeting of the Radiological Society of North America, Chicago, IL, November 2007:629.

6. Regge D. Accuracy of CT-colonography in subjects at increased risk of colorectal carcinoma: a multi-center study on 1,000 patients. Presented at the Annual Meeting of the Radiological Society of North America, Chicago, IL, November 2007:337.

7. Copel L, Sosna J, Kruskal JB, Raptopoulos V, Farrell RJ, Morrin MM. CT colonography in 546 patients with incomplete colonoscopy. *Radiology.* 2007;244:471–478.

8. http://www.acr.org/SecondaryMainMenuCategories/quality_safety/guidelines/dx/gastro/ct_colonography.aspx

9. http://www.cancer.org/docroot/ped/content/ped_2_3x_acs_cancer_detection_guidelines_36.asp

10. Park SH, Yee J, Kim SH, Kim YH. Fundamental elements for successful performance of CT colonography (virtual colonoscopy). *Korean J Radiol* 2007;8:264–275.

11. Lefere P, Gryspeerdt S, Dewyspelaere J, *et al.* Dietary fecal tagging as a cleansing method before CT colonography: initial results polyp detection and patient acceptance. *Radiology* 2002; 224:393–40312.

12. Cai W, Zalis ME, Nappi J, Harris GJ, Yoshida H. Structure-analysis method for electronic cleansing in cathartic and noncathartic CT colonography. *Med Phys.* 2008;35:3259–3277.

13. Shinners TJ, Pickhardt PJ, Taylor AJ, Jones DA, Olsen CH. Patient-controlled room air insufflations versus automated carbon dioxide delivery for CT colonography. *AJR Am J Roentgenol* 2006;186:1491–1496.

14. Dachman AH. Advice for optimizing colonic distention and minimizing risk of perforation during CT colonography. *Radiology.* 2006;239:317–321.

15. Zalis ME, Barish MA, Choi JR, *et al.* CT colonography reporting and data system: a consensus proposal. *Radiology* 2005;236:3–9.

16. Pickhardt PJ, Hassan C, Laghi A, Kim DH. CT colonography to screen for colorectal cancer and aortic aneurysm in the Medicare population: cost-effectiveness analysis. *AJR Am J Roentgenol.* 2009;192:1332–1340.

17. Berland LL. Incidental extracolonic findings on CTcolonography: the impending deluge and its implications. *J Am Coll Radiol.* 2009;6:14–20.

18. Pickhardt PJ, Hanson ME, Vanness DJ, *et al.* Unsuspected extracolonic findings at screening CT colonography: clinical and economic impact. *Radiology.* 2008;249:151–159.

19. Hellstrom M, Svensson MH, Lasson A. Extracolonic and incidental findings on CT colonography (virtual colonoscopy). *AJR Am J Roentgenol.* 2004;182:631–638.

20. Flicker MS, Tsoukas AT, Hazra A, Dachman AH. Economic impact of extracolonic findings at computed tomographic colonography. *J Comput Assist Tomogr.* 2008;32:497–503.

21. Chin M, Mendelson R, Edwards J, Foster N, Forbes G. Computed tomographic colonography: prevalence, nature, and clinical significance of extracolonic findings in a community screening program. *Am J Gastroenterol.* 2005;100:2771–2776.

22. Summers RM, Handwerker LR, Pickhardt PJ, *et al.* Performance of a previously validated CT colonography computer-aided detection system in a new patient population. *AJR Am J Roentgenol.* 2008;191:168–174.

23. Petrick N, Haider M, Summers RM, *et al.* CT colonography with computer-aided detection as a second reader: observer performance study. *Radiology.* 2008;246:148–156.

24. Regge D, Hassan C, Pickhardt PJ, *et al.* Impact of computer-aided detection on the cost-effectiveness of CT colonography. *Radiology.* 2009;250:488–497.

25. Dachman AH, Obuchowski NA, Hoffmeister JW, *et al.* Effect of computer aided detection for CT colonography in a multireader, multicase trial. *Radiology.* 2010;256:827–835.

26. Vijan S, Hwang I, Inadomi J, *et al.* The cost-effectiveness of CT colonography in screening for colorectal neoplasia. *Am J Gastroenterol.* 2007;102:380–390.

27. Pickhardt PJ, Hassan C, Laghi A, *et al.* Clinical management of small (6- to 9-mm) polyps detected at screening CT colonography: a cost-effectiveness analysis. *AJR Am J Roentgenol.* 2008; 191:1509–1516.

CHAPTER 137
Positron emission tomography

Sebastian Obrzut and Michael S. Kipper
University of California at San Diego, San Diego, CA, USA

KEY POINTS

- Positron emission tomography (PET), and more recently, PET/computed tomography (CT) have become the standard of care in the investigation of various gastrointestinal malignancies
- The radiopharmaceutical of choice remains 2-deoxy-2 [^{18}F] fluoro-D-glucose
- The introduction of combination PET/CT scanners has markedly improved both specificity and precision of lesion localization
- A large percentage of patients with gastrointestinal tumors, including esophageal, gastric, colonic, and pancreatic, now undergo PET imaging in the course of their disease. Additionally, selected patients with gastrointestinal lymphoma, renal tumors, small intestinal tumors, and hepatic, gallbladder, and adrenal tumors may benefit from PET imaging
- The use of PET for monitoring response to therapy, new radiopharmaceuticals which target processes other than glucose metabolism, and scanner advances (including PET/MR) are all under active investigation

Introduction

Positron emission tomography (PET) has matured as a crucial imaging modality in the management of patients with multiple types of cancer. PET is also utilized in selected patients with cardiovascular and neurological disorders. Since 2006, the incorporation of computed tomography (CT) in PET scanners has elevated molecular imaging to a new level. Structure and function are now evaluated in a single visit, allowing for relatively precise localization of hypermetabolic sites, improved specificity, and increased confidence in study interpretation. This chapter details the basics of PET imaging, current indications, and potential pitfalls in gastrointestinal disease. It focuses on the use of PET in commonly encountered gastrointestinal malignancies.

Description of technique

PET uses **radiopharmaceuticals labeled with positron-emitting radionuclides**. Decay by positron emission results in the ejection of a "positively charged electron" from the nucleus which travels a short distance (1–2 mm) before colliding with an electron. The subsequent annihilation produces two high-energy photons which travel in nearly exact opposite directions and are detected simultaneously by the PET scanner. The PET image is a representation of these "coincidence" events (Figure 137.1).

A major advance in PET scanning occurred in 2005/2006 with the introduction of the **PET/CT scanner** for clinical use. A dedicated PET scanner and a multislice CT scanner are mounted on a single support system using the same imaging table. CT and PET data are acquired sequentially, and reconstructed to produce fusion images of **anatomy (CT)** and **metabolism (PET)**. The advantages of this dual modality, hybrid scanner include precise anatomical localization of hypermetabolic foci (characteristic of malignancies), improved study specificity (normal, physiological uptake can be confirmed with the CT portion), reduced scanning time (45–60 minutes down to 10–20 minutes), reduced radiation exposure for the patient (CT attenuation vs radioactive "rod-source" attenuation correction), contrast-enhanced CT studies at the time of PET imaging, and reduced costs of a single study versus multiple examinations (Table 137.1).

Study performance

Patient preparation for PET and PET/CT are essentially the same, with the important exception of the patient who is scheduled for a PET/CT with intravenous contrast. As with any contrast-enhanced CT, issues of renal status and allergic history are of paramount importance. The typical patient is fasted for a minimum of 4–6 hours, although water and required medications are allowed. Endogenous glucose competes with administered fluoro-D-glucose (FDG) and most centers measure a glucose level using an upper limit of 150–200 mg/dL as the cut-off value prior to performing the study. Diabetic patients must be handled on an individual basis and can almost always be accommodated with a combination of early morning scanning, diet, and medication adjustment.

The current radiopharmaceutical of choice is **FDG**, an analog of glucose with a fluorine-18 substitution. Following injection of radiolabeled FDG, the patient is placed into a quiet "uptake" room for 1–2 hours. During this time FDG is taken

Textbook of Clinical Gastroenterology and Hepatology, Second Edition. Edited by C. J. Hawkey, Jaime Bosch, Joel E. Richter, Guadalupe Garcia-Tsao, Francis K. L. Chan.
© 2012 Blackwell Publishing Ltd. Published 2012 by Blackwell Publishing Ltd.

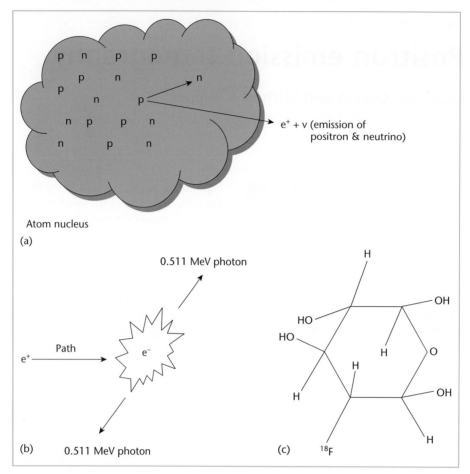

Figure 137.1 (a) Positron emission (p, proton; n, neutron; e⁺, positron; v, neutrino). (b) Annihilation of positron and electron (e⁻, electron). (c) Fluoro-D-glucose (FDG).

Table 137.1 Advantages of PET/CT versus PET

Parameter	PET	PET/CT
CT data	Not obtainable	The CT can be done with very low mA for attenuation and localization purposes only or a complete, contrast-enhanced CT for diagnostic quality
Radiation exposure	Based upon dose of injected FDG and radiation from a radioactive rod source that is used for attenuation correction	Radiation is based upon the dose of injected FDG and the small amount from the CT. This increases, however, with a diagnostic CT
Study time	Typically, a standard PET-only study takes approximately 45 minutes, but can take as long as 1 hour or more if the study requires imaging of the lower extremities (e.g., melanoma)	A complete PET/CT can be performed in <20 minutes (often 12–15 minutes) when based on patient size. This has significant implications with respect to claustrophobic patients, center throughput, and motion artifacts
Study localization/accuracy	There are no anatomic landmarks with PET only. While fusion can be done with previously performed CT or MRI, studies may vary significantly temporally, and slice thickness in unlikely to match, making exact correlation difficult	Near simultaneous acquisition results in superb registration and the ability to reformat the data to equalize slice thickness. This has been shown in multiple studies to improve the accuracy of PET/CT versus PET

up by both normal and malignant cells. Malignancies demonstrate enhanced uptake and retention of FDG, allowing for localization with the PET scanner (Figure 137.2).

A number of protocols exist for acquiring the PET and CT data, including utilization of a non-contrast CT for attenuation-correction/localization only, or performing contrast-enhanced CT at the time of PET imaging. This provides a diagnostic quality CT in addition to a state-of-the-art PET study. Interpretation of the PET/CT study necessitates a good understanding of the potential pitfalls of each method,

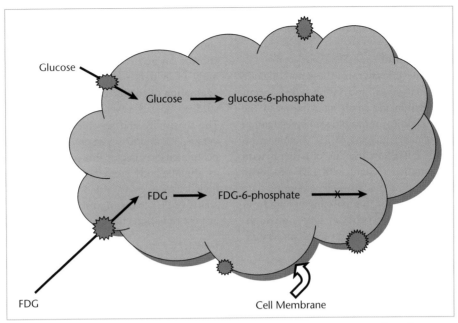

Figure 137.2 Malignant cell uptake of glucose and FDG. Both glucose and FDG are transported across the cell membrane by transporter proteins, which are upregulated in many malignant cells. Once intracellular, both are phosphorylated; however, unlike glucose, FDG-6-phosphate is not recognized by subsequent enzymes involved in glycolysis and becomes trapped within the cell. ✦, glucose transporter on cell surface.

as well as the combined use of these modalities [1]. Importantly, one must be aware of the normal distribution of FDG on a PET scan (Figure 137.3).

Indications and coverage

The utility of PET/CT in **gastrointestinal tumor imaging** remains a work in progress. For some tumors, and in certain situations, the data are relatively convincing [e.g., colon, esophageal, gastrointestinal stromal tumors (GISTs), and pancreas]. In others (biliary tract tumors, small intestinal tumors) results have been mixed, and in some (hepatic) results have been disappointing. In the United States, the Centers for Medicare and Medicaid Service (CMS) have recently expanded coverage for PET and PET/CT based upon significant clinical evidence regarding the effectiveness of PET for management of patients with cancer.

Gastrointestinal malignancies

Gastric cancer

Standard diagnostic imaging modalities include endoscopic ultrasound (EUS) and CT. The role of FDG-PET is controversial. There is no role for PET in primary detection [2] as normal gastric mucosa may concentrate FDG to a variable (and often intense) degree; however, there appears to be a place for PET in detecting distant metastases, assessing tumor response to chemotherapy, and perhaps predicting response to chemotherapy [3]. FDG uptake correlates with tumor aggressiveness and, inversely, with the mucin content of the tumor. GISTs are

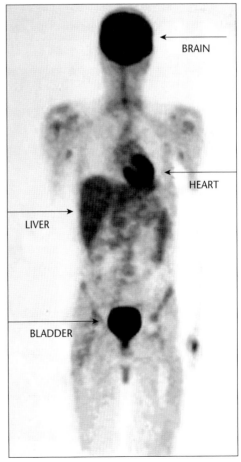

Figure 137.3 Normal PET scan.

uncommon, but PET/CT has been shown to be a sensitive and reliable indicator of response or resistance to imatinib [4].

Tumors of the small intestine

Carcinomas of the small intestine are rare. These may include neuroendocrine tumors, sarcomas, and GISTs. GISTs occur with similar frequency within the small intestine as in the stomach [5]. Available modalities for radiological investigation include CT, magnetic resonance imaging (MRI), somatostatin-receptor imaging, and PET. The low number of patients with small intestine tumors studied to date with PET precludes recommendations for its routine use; however, emerging data suggest a possible role for PET/CT in separating benign from malignant tumors, discriminating between low- and high-grade sarcomas, searching for distant metastases, and monitoring response to therapy.

Colorectal cancer

Approximately 150 000 new cases of colon (~110 000) and rectal (~40 000) cancer are diagnosed each year in the United States [6]. PET/CT is clearly established as a valuable imaging modality in colorectal cancer patients over the course of their illness. Table 137.2 summarizes areas where PET can play a primary role in answering the clinical questions and providing guidance for the gastroenterologist, oncologist, and surgeon. Although PET is not recommended for initial diagnosis or for routine screening, it is not uncommon to discover an unsuspected colorectal carcinoma while performing a PET study for other purposes (Figure 137.4). For **staging**, PET has shown greater accuracy than CT. In a series of 134 patients PET showed an accuracy of 94% versus 81% for CT [7]. A large body of evidence exists to substantiate the use of PET for **evaluation of suspected recurrence**. Analysis of >2000 patient studies showed a 94% accuracy for PET versus 80% for CT. The sensitivity and specificity for PET versus CT were 94% versus 79% and 87% versus 73%, respectively [8]. Some of the postulated reasons for this include the ability of PET to serve as a whole-body survey, the well-established fact that metabolic changes may antedate anatomical changes, and the ability of PET to distinguish between scar tissue (post-surgical or post-radiation changes) and active tumor.

Table 137.2 Clinical value of PET in colorectal cancer

- May identify unsuspected colon cancer in patients undergoing PET for other tumors
- Beneficial in selected patients for initial staging (especially with equivocal findings on CT/MR)
- Excellent for restaging (whole-body survey)
- Useful to separate active tumor from changes secondary to therapy
- Excellent modality for patients with rising carcinoembryonic antigen (CEA) and negative conventional exams
- Data accumulating for the use of PET in monitoring response to therapy
- Extremely valuable is assessing patients with presumed solitary metastasis prior to curative-intent surgery

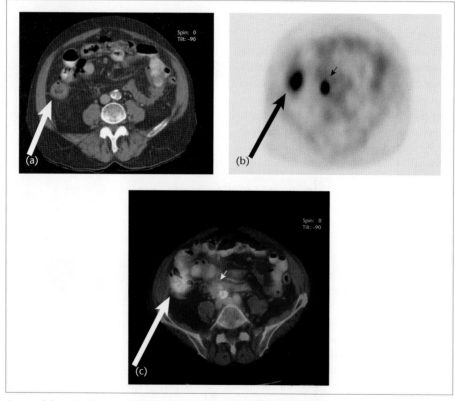

Figure 137.4 Adenocarcinoma of the colon found on PET/CT ordered to search for melanoma metastases. (a) CT, (b) PET), and (c) fused PET/CT. Arrows point to cancer; Arrowhead points to urine.

There are two areas in particular where PET can play a major role. The first is in a patient with a rising **carcinoembryonic antigen (CEA)** level and negative conventional imaging studies. This is a relatively common occurrence and in one study, 63 of 72 patients with a rising CEA and negative CT/MRI were found to have lesions with PET [9].

The other situation is a patient who is under consideration for **curative surgery due to recurrence**. Early detection and surgical resection of a solitary metastasis (primarily hepatic) can be curative. The clinical dilemma is the degree of certainty that an individual patient has only one metastatic site. CT is reliable in the liver, but may miss additional hepatic sites identified with PET. Also, PET has the advantage of being a **whole-body survey**. The identification of additional metastases saves the patient from undergoing a non-curative surgery, with its attendant morbidity and mortality. A large cooperative study (548 patients) reviewed the relationship between follow-up tests (not including PET) and salvage surgery in patients with colon cancer recurrence. Curative-intent surgery was performed in 109 patients (20%). The disease-free 5-year survival was 23%. It is suspected that a significant percentage of the 77% who did not achieve long-term survival may have been spared a curative-intent surgery by more accurate restaging [10]. As with other tumor types, PET/CT has been shown to be preferable to PET-only examinations [11,12].

Abdominal lymphoma, renal and adrenal tumors

Although the incidence of **lymphoma** is on the rise, excellent therapeutic options exist, including chemotherapy, radiation therapy, and bone marrow transplant. **Initial staging** is of paramount importance for treatment selection. While CT is a superb modality for assessing nodal size, architecture, and location with respect to other organs and vessels, nodal size alone does not separate benignity from malignancy, and CT may have difficulty in assessing disease involvement in the liver, spleen, and marrow. PET, and more specifically, PET/CT, has shown great value in a large percentage of patients with lymphoma, especially in those areas where CT is less than ideal (e.g., hepatic/splenic involvement, extranodal disease, and bone marrow involvement). Nearly all lymphomas concentrate FDG avidly, and there is some evidence to suggest a correlation between intensity of uptake and histological grade and cellular proliferation rate [13]. PET does not rely on nodal size and has shown higher sensitivity, specificity, and accuracy as compared to CT for initial staging. Many patients will be under- or over-staged if evaluated only by anatomical imaging. PET/CT is crucial for **restaging**, and one of the most exciting areas of applicability is in the monitoring of **patient response to therapy**. A negative PET/CT at the completion of treatment predicts an excellent prognosis, while a positive study is highly predictive of relapse.

One caution, PET/CT is of very limited value in mucosa-associated-lymphoid tissue (MALT) lymphoma [14]. PET data in renal and adrenal tumors show mixed results. **Renal cell carcinomas (RCCs)** may show variable metabolic rates and the high uptake in the collecting systems of the kidneys makes evaluation of small renal masses problematic. Remote metastases from RCCs will often be identified with PET. Although primary adrenocortical malignancies are rare, PET has proven to be very useful in differentiating benign and malignant adrenal masses and in confirming or excluding adrenal metastases.

Esophageal carcinoma

Endoscopic ultrasonography (EUS), especially combined with fine-needle aspiration (EUS-FNA), is considered the primary modality in the preoperative determination of depth of tumor invasion (T stage) and nodal status (N stage). PET is limited in the assessment of N stage due to poor visualization of lymph nodes adjacent to intense primary tumor uptake, the possibility of false-positive uptake in inflammatory lymph nodes, and minimal uptake in microscopic disease. It has been shown, however, that PET/CT is significantly more accurate in assessing **lymph node metastasis stage** than CT alone, PET alone, and PET side by side with CT. Furthermore, almost all researchers note the superiority of PET in detecting **distant metastases** compared with conventional modalities (Figure 137.5).

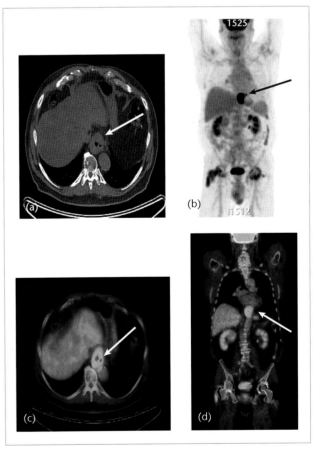

Figure 137.5 Patient with carcinoma of the distal esophagus. (a) CT, (b) coronal PET, (c) axial fused PET/CT, and (d) coronal fused PET/CT. Activity at the level of the hips is due to bilateral hip replacements.

Response to neoadjuvant therapy has been demonstrated by some researchers to improve the rate of local tumor control and complete resection, as well as prevention of distant metastases. Because of its ability to differentiate between vital residual tumor tissue and post-therapeutic changes, PET has been able to distinguish responders from non-responders to neoadjuvant chemotherapy shortly after beginning induction therapy. There is a general consensus that conventional techniques such as endoscopy are best suited for detection of perianastomotic recurrence. However, once recurrence is detected, PET and PET/CT provide the most accurate whole-body restaging tools.

Hepatic tumors

FDG-PET has a poor sensitivity in the detection of primary hepatocellular carcinoma, possibly because well-differentiated tumors retain the capacity for gluconeogenesis which may decrease intracellular radiotracer trapping of FDG-6-phosphate (converted back to FDG). Although the sensitivity of PET in the diagnosis of HCC is lower compared with the sensitivity of CT, PET is helpful in the detection of **extrahepatic metastases**. In addition, the intensity of FDG uptake on PET may aid in the assessment of biological grade of the primary tumor, suggesting that PET/CT may be useful in evaluation of HCC. Furthermore, PET imaging with the [^{11}C]acetate radiopharmaceutical has demonstrated a high sensitivity in detecting primary HCC. However, its short half-life of 20 minutes may preclude its widespread clinical use.

Gallbladder carcinoma and cholangiocarcinoma

The sensitivity of FDG-PET in detecting carcinoma of the gallbladder and cholangiocarcinoma (CC) is high, but may be dependent on tumor subtype. Since FDG is not excreted in the bile, uptake in the biliary tree or gallbladder is a sign of malignancy or inflammation on FDG-PET. Furthermore, FDG-PET can identify distant metastases of peripheral cholangiocarcinoma that are not detected with MRI or CT. However, granulomatous disease, sclerosing cholangitis, and stents can mimic malignancy on FDG-PET. PET has been falsely negative in patients with carcinomatosis or mucinous hilar adenocarcinoma, and demonstrated false-positive uptake along the tract of a biliary stent. PET also has difficulty in discriminating between extrahepatic parts of the tumor itself and FDG-accumulating lymph nodes in the perihilar region. PET/CT can overcome these limitations since precise image fusion leads to a more adequate identification of non–FDG-accumulating tumors or carcinomatosis. In addition, FDG uptake along the tract of implanted biliary stents is more easily distinguishable from malignant disease.

Pancreatic carcinoma

In the evaluation of pancreatic cancer, PET seems to be more specific in patients without hyperglycemia or active inflammation. Furthermore, PET can also be helpful in identifying unsuspected distant metastases and suspected recurrent carcinoma when abdominal CT is non-diagnostic. The combination of PET/CT can improve differentiation of pathological processes, especially in surgically pretreated patients, and allow the detection of small metastases that might otherwise be missed by PET alone due to background activity in the pancreatic bed. Even retrospective image fusion improves the sensitivity of malignancy detection in pancreatic lesions from 77% for CT and 84% for PET to 89%. Because there are greater differences in patient positioning in standalone CT and PET compared with PET/CT, these results are expected to be even better for the combined device. Nevertheless, pancreatic tumors of endocrine origin (insulinoma, glucogonoma, and VIPoma) are usually well differentiated and often are not FDG avid. The recommendation is to use ^{111}In-OctreoScan and ^{123}I- or ^{131}IMIBG imaging.

New developments

PET and PET/CT have now been in clinical use for longer than 10 years. Originally developed for brain imaging, subsequently popularized in oncology, current research is focused on the development of new imaging agents to supplement FDG. These **new radiopharmaceuticals** have the capability to assess cellular processes beyond glucose utilization, including tumor hypoxia, cell membrane proliferation, and receptor imaging.

Some centers have begun utilizing PET for **infection imaging** due to the recognition that FDG accumulates at sites of inflammation and infection.

References

1. Blake MA, Singh A, Bindu N, et al. Pearls and pitfalls in interpretation of abdominal and pelvic PET-CT. *RadioGraphics*. 2006; 26:1335–1353.
2. Dassen A, Lips D, Hoekstra J, et al. FDG-PET has no definite role in preoperative imaging in gastric cancer. *Eur J Surg Oncol*. 2009; 35:449–455.
3. De Potter T, Flamen P, Van Cutsem E, et al. Whole-body PET with FDG for the diagnosis of recurrent gastric cancer. *Eur J Nucl Med Mol Imaging*. 2002;29:525–529.
4. Demetri GD, von Mehren M, Blanke CD, et al. Efficacy and safety of imatinib mesylate in advanced gastrointestinal stromal tumors. *N Engl J Med*. 2002;347:472–480.
5. Hersh MR, Choi J, Garrett C, et al. Imaging gastrointestinal stromal tumors. *Cancer Control*. 2005;12:111–115.
6. Meta J, Seltzer M, Schiepers C, et al. Impact of ^{18}F-FDG PET on managing patients with colorectal cancer: the referring physician's perspective. *J Nucl Med*. 2001;42:586–590.
7. Kalff V, Hicks RJ, Ware RE, et al. The clinical impact of (18) F-FDG PET in patients with suspected or confirmed recurrence of colorectal cancer: a prospective study. *J Nucl Med*. 2002;43: 492–499.
8. Gambhir SS, Czernin J, Schwimmer J, et al. A tabulated summary of the FDG PET literature. *J Nucl Med*. 2001;42:95–125.
9. Maldonado A, Sancho F, Cerdan J, et al. FDG-OET in the detection of recurrence in colorectal cancer based on rising CEA level: experience in 72 patients. *Clin Positron Imaging*. 2000;3:170.

10. Goldberg RM, Fleming TR, Tangen CM, *et al.* Surgery for recurrent colon cancer: strategies for identifying resectable recurrence and success rates after resection. *Ann Intern Med.* 1998;129: 27–35.

11. Burger I, Goerres GW, Schulthess GK, *et al.* PET/CT: diagnostic improvement in recurrent colorectal carcinoma compared to PET alone. *Radiology.* 2002;225 (Suppl P):242.

12. Cohade C, Osman M, Leal J, *et al.* Direct comparison of 18F-FDG PET and PET/CT in patients with colorectal carcinoma. *J Nucl Med.* 2003;44:1797–1803.

13. Delbeke D, Martin WH, Morgan DS, *et al.* 2-deoxy-2-[F-18] fluoro-D-glucose imaging with positron emission tomography for initial staging of Hodgkin's disease and lymphoma. *Mol Imaging Biol.* 2002;4:105–114.

14. Hoffman M, Kletter K, Diemling M, *et al.* Positron emission tomography with fluorine-18-2-deoxy-D-glucose(F18-FDG) does not visualize extranodal B-cell lymphoma of the mucosa-associated lymphoid tissue(MALT) type. *Ann Oncol.* 1999;10: 1185–1189.

CHAPTER 138

Non-invasive liver assessment

M. Beaugrand

Université Paris XIII, Bondy, France

Introduction

The role of **liver biopsy** in the assessment and prognostication of chronic liver diseases is outstanding. However, its limitations are numerous and include its usually small size, which means it is prone to sampling error. Moreover, the follow-up of patients with liver diseases and the assessment of treatment efficacy requires repeated evaluations even in a relatively short period. Repeated liver biopsies are not well accepted and their ability to quantify, in an individual patient, small variations in the extent of fibrosis or other basic lesions has been questioned. For all these reasons the need for **non-invasive substitutes** has been recognized for many years and has led to a new era of non-invasive diagnostic and quantification tests that is still in progress. Two different approaches have been implemented: the use of **serum markers** and the use of **physical means such as ultrasound**. The two main lesions that are the most relevant in the prognosis and stratification of chronic liver diseases are **fibrosis and steatosis**. Another histological lesion, iron content, is already accurately measured by magnetic resonance imaging (MRI) (see Chapter 90).

Assessment of liver fibrosis

Serum markers

The first attempt to quantify liver fibrosis though serum studies took advantage of the fact that liver fibrosis is an active process involving fibrogenesis and fibrolysis that leads to the presence in the serum of by-products of synthesis and degradation of the extracellular matrix. Unfortunately, components of this matrix are not liver specific given that fibrous tissue is present in the whole body and the fibrotic healing process is common to many organs. Furthermore, the metabolism of these compounds can be influenced by conditions that are not related to fibrosis, such as renal failure or cholestasis. Two markers are still in use: the **N-terminal propeptide of collagen type III (PIII NP) and hyaluronic acid**. Both are often elevated in **cirrhosis** and have been incorporated in more recent algorithms. PIII NP results from the cleavage of procollagen III from collagen III, which is predominant in the liver and the hallmark of an active fibrosing process. Serum PIII NP correlates with fibrogenesis, but unfortunately its metabolism is influenced by extrahepatic conditions and thus it is not specific for the liver; active fibrosis in other organs such as the lung can also be responsible for increased levels. This has led to the decreased use of these markers alone, although both have been incorporated in composite indices.

Composite serum markers

This more recent approach, although perhaps less rational, has provided interesting results. The approach involves the combination of blood levels of various products that are linked to inflammation or to the liver, although most are not directly linked to fibrosis [1–3]. The approaches differ in the number of composite markers and the type of products tested. The **Fibrotest, Hepascore, and Fibrometer** provide the most accurate prediction of fibrosis, particularly in chronic hepatitis C (Table 138.1). Their performance in other causes of chronic liver disease does not appear to be as good and/or they have not been well validated. Their common limitation is the possible influence of extrahepatic conditions such as inflammatory diseases, hemolysis, and co-morbidities such as alcoholism or genetic heterogeneity (e.g., for gamma-glutamyl transferase or total bilirubin levels). This explains why, if attention is not

Textbook of Clinical Gastroenterology and Hepatology, Second Edition. Edited by C. J. Hawkey, Jaime Bosch, Joel E. Richter, Guadalupe Garcia-Tsao, Francis K. L. Chan.
© 2012 Blackwell Publishing Ltd. Published 2012 by Blackwell Publishing Ltd.

paid to individual values of each parameter and to the clinical setting, these tests may generate false-positive results. Although these composite markers are quite sensitive for determining the presence of significant fibrosis or cirrhosis in chronic hepatitis C, their accuracy is lower than that of physical tests (Table 138.2).

Physical means

Ultrasound and magnetic resonance have been used to quantify fibrosis through a common physical parameter, **liver**

Table 138.1 Main predictive blood tests for the assessment of liver fibrosis

Test	Parameters involved	Indications
Fibrotest®	Alpha-2-macroglobulin Haptoglobin Apolipoprotein A1 Bilirubin Gamma glutamyl transferase Age and sex	Various liver diseases
APRI	ASAT, ALAT Platelet count	Hepatitis C
Hepascore	Alpha-2-macroglobulin Hyaluronic acid Bilirubin Age and sex	Hepatitis C
Fibrometer	Alpha-2-macroglobulin Hyaluronic acid ASAT, ALAT Bilirubin Gamma glutamyl transferase Platelet count Urea Prothrombin activity	Various liver diseases

ALAT alanine aminotransferase; ASAT, aspartate aminotransferase.

Table 138.2 Comparison of diagnostic performance of Fibroscan® and Fibrotest in patients with chronic hepatitis C

	Fibrotest	Fibroscan
Number of patients	1679	546
AUROC:		
Significant fibrosis	0.81	0.83
Cirrhosis	0.9	0.95
Sensitivity:		
Significant fibrosis	0.47	0.64
Cirrhosis	NR	0.86
Specificity:		
Significant fibrosis	0.9	0.87
Cirrhosis	NR	0.93

NR, not reported.
Reprinted by permission from Macmillan Publishers Ltd: Shaheen AAM, Wan AF, Myers RP. Fibrotest and Fibroscan for the prediction of hepatitis C related fibrosis: a systematic review of diagnostic test accuracy. *Am J Gastroenterol.* 2007;102:2589–2600.

elasticity or liver stiffness. In contrast to serum markers that can be influenced by extrahepatic diseases, liver stiffness is a physical parameter directly related to the liver.

The main condition that influences liver stiffness measurement (LSM) is **liver fibrosis**, although it has been shown that acute cholestasis or hepatic congestion can also increase LSM in a reversible manner. In fact, acute necrosis can also increase LSM, although the mechanism is still unclear; hepatic edema has been proposed without convincing evidence and it would appear that the collapse of hepatocyte plates and the early deposit of perisinusoidal fibrosis would be a more rational explanation. Therefore, and as per other parameters, LSM should be interpreted in the context of the clinical setting and is mainly indicated in patients with chronic stable liver diseases. Even in these circumstances the translation of LSM results into fibrosis stage is subject to potential errors. **Fibrosis stage** by any scoring system results from the combination of two parameters: the degree of fibrosis and the degree of distortion of liver architecture. As LSM is related to liver fibrosis, elevated values can be observed in patients with extensive perisinusoidal fibrosis but without cirrhosis. Conversely, in macronodular cirrhosis LSM can be almost normal as the content of liver fibrosis can be almost normal due to resorption. This is a likely explanation for the false-negative results of LSM in this latter setting and for the fact that the LSM threshold for a putative diagnosis of cirrhosis differs depending on the cause of liver disease: it is higher in patients with alcoholic and cholestatic liver diseases compared to chronic hepatitis [4].

Devices using ultrasound
Fibroscan®

Fibroscan® is a device using the principle of **transient elastography** [5]. Briefly, it measures, via ultrasound waves, the velocity of a shock wave produced by a vibrator positioned in an intercostal space at the level of the right lobe of the liver, a site similar to that chosen for a percutaneous liver biopsy (Figure 138.1). LSM is the median value of 10 measurements, provided the rate of success is above 60%. The limitations of the

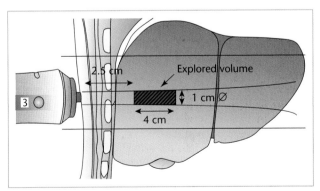

Figure 138.1 Measurement of liver stiffness by Fibroscan®. The probe on the chest wall produces a mechanical shock wave. Its velocity is measured using ultrasound.

technique are physical: the presence of ascites precludes any measurement, as can obesity. This latter limitation has been solved by the use of a special probe for obese patients. A special probe for children or patients with narrow costal spaces has also been designed. The overall length of the measurement is 4 cm and the volume of liver parenchyma explored is approximately 200 times the mean volume of a liver biopsy, which presumably reduces sampling error.

LSM by Fibroscan® has been validated as a useful tool to evaluate liver fibrosis in a wide range of liver diseases, ranging from chronic hepatitis C and B to alcoholic liver diseases and non-alcoholic fatty liver disease (NAFLD) [6–8]. In terms of diagnostic performance, the most favorable results have been reported for the **cirrhosis associated with vascular disruption or extensive fibrosis**. . On the other hand, the accuracy of Fibroscan® in distinguishing patients with chronic hepatitis at METAVIR stages 0, 1 or even 2 is less satisfactory, perhaps due to the small differences in fibrosis content among these stages. The threshold values for the diagnosis of cirrhosis varies according to its different etiologies, ranging from approximately 12.5 to 17.5 kPa [5] and, again, this may also be due to differences in fibrosis content. .

Fibroscan® has gained a place in the non-invasive assessment of liver fibrosis in patients with **chronic hepatitis who are treatment naïve.**. It has the potential ability to monitor fibrosis through the evolution of a chronic liver disease and particularly to assess the results of specific therapies, although this has not been validated in large-scale studies comparing it to serial liver biopsies. Finally, as it is a simple, inexpensive, and well-accepted procedure, it could also be used as a **screening method** for detecting occult advanced liver disease in high-risk populations.

Conventional ultrasonography

Other techniques to measure liver stiffness using ultrasound have been recently proposed. One utilizes the Acoustic Radiation Force Impulse (ARFI) technology that can be used with conventional ultrasonographic imaging devices. Its accuracy for the assessment of liver fibrosis is under evaluation. The same is true for a new technique called Supersonic Shear Imaging that could also be useful for imaging and measurement of tissue stiffness.

Magnetic resonance imaging

MRI can assess hepatic fibrosis via two techniques: magnetic resonance elastography and diffusion-weighted MRI [9]. **Magnetic resonance elastography** assesses LSM by using a transducer that generates low-frequency mechanical waves. The technique overcomes the limitations of transient elastography, particularly in the obese, and it may provide more reliable results and explore a larger volume of liver parenchyma. However, the method is very costly and needs further validation. **Diffusion-weighted MRI** characterizes the tissue by measuring the apparent diffusion of water. The technique for assessing liver fibrosis is not well standardized.

Preliminary results suggest diagnostic performances similar to Fibroscan®.

Assessment of liver steatosis

Similar to fibrosis, attempts have been made to quantify steatosis by serum markers and by physical methods, particularly Fibroscan® dual gradient echo MRI (DGE-MRI) and proton magnetic resonance spectroscopy (H-MRS). The Steatotest, a composite biochemical marker, does not provide quantitative reliable results in patients with NAFLD. However, preliminary results of a new index called **controlled alternation parameter (CAP)** obtained by Fibroscan® seems to correlate well with the degree of histological steatosis in a panel of patients with various liver diseases [10]. It is well known that the liver of patients with ≥30% steatosis is hyperechoic, but this phenomenon, due to the reflection of the ultrasound wave by lipid droplets, cannot be quantified. Conversely, the attenuation of ultrasound waves inside the liver due to the absorption rather than the reflection of ultrasound by lipid droplets can be translated into a quantitative parameter, the CAP, that seems to be independent of fibrosis and correlates well with steatosis. This new marker is particularly exciting as CAP could be obtained by Fibroscan® at the same time as measurement of LSM is performed, without additional time or cost. However, it requires validation in larger cohorts before it can be widely recommended to monitor steatosis.

Conclusions

Although the merits of liver biopsy are undeniable, the assessment and use of non-invasive and less costly methods to assess and monitor common diffuse liver lesions such as fibrosis and steatosis is mandatory.

Fibrosis is, by far, the lesion that has been most extensively studied. Results appear promising and open the door to a purely non-invasive approach in many cases, particularly in patients with chronic hepatitis C. Blood tests and Fibroscan® are the most commonly used methods. Their performances are comparable, with Fibroscan® having the advantage in the assessment of advanced fibrosis and cirrhosis. The combination of both methods has been advocated to increase the accuracy of prediction, with liver biopsy being restricted to patients with discordant results. In the future, technical refinements will probably increase the assessment of LSM by ultrasound as well as provide a quantitative assessment of steatosis.

References

1. Lok AS. Ghanzy MG. Goodman ZD, *et al.* Predicting cirrhosis in patients with hepatitis C based on standard laboratory tests: results of the HALT-C cohort. *Hepatology.* 2005;42:282–292.
2. Shaheen AAM, Wan AF, Myers RP. Fibrotest and Fibroscan for the prediction of hepatitis C related fibrosis: a systematic review of diagnostic test accuracy. *Am J Gastroenterol.* 2007;102: 2589–2600.

3. Cales P. Oberti F. Michalak S, *et al.* A novel panel of blood markers to assess the degree of liver fibrosis. *Hepatology.* 2005;42: 1373–1381.

4. Ganne-Carrie N, Ziol M, de Ledinghen V, *et al.* Accuracy of liver stiffness measurement for the diagnosis of cirrhosis in patients with chronic liver diseases. *Hepatology.* 2006;44:1511–1517.

5. Sandrin L. Fourquet B. Hasquenoph JM, *et al.* Transient elastography: a new noninvasive method for assessment of hepatic fibrosis. *Ultrasound Med Biol.* 2003;29:1705–1713.

6. Ziol M. Handra-Luca A. Kettaneh A, *et al.* Noninvasive assessment of liver fibrosis by measurement of stiffness in patients with chronic hepatitis C. *Hepatology.* 2005;41:48–54.

7. Castera L, Vergniol J, Foucher J, *et al.* Prospective comparison of transient elastography, Fibrotest, APRI, and liver biopsy for the assessment of fibrosis in chronic hepatitis C. *Gastroenterology.* 2005;128:343–350.

8. Marcellin P. Ziol M. Bedossa P, *et al.* Non-invasive assessment of liver fibrosis by stiffness measurement in patients with chronic hepatitis B. *Liver Int.* 2009;29:242–247.

9. Huwart L, Sempoux C, Vicaut E, *et al.* Magnetic resonance elastography for the non-invasive staging of liver fibrosis. *Gastroenterology.* 2008;135:32–40.

10. Sasso M, Beaugrand M, de Ledinghen V. Controlled attenuation parameter (CAP): a novel VCTE guided ultrasonic attenuation measurement for the evaluation of hepatic steatosis. *Ultrasound Med Biol.* 2010;36:1825–1835.

CHAPTER 139

Gastrointestinal motility testing

Priyanka Sachdeva and Henry P. Parkman

Temple University School of Medicine, Philadelphia, PA, USA

KEY POINTS

- Esophageal manometry is useful in the evaluation of patients with non-obstructive dysphagia and in patients with refractory reflux symptoms, especially when antireflux surgery is being considered. Esophageal manometry may specifically diagnose achalasia, diffuse esophageal spasm, and motility disorders associated with systemic disorders, particularly scleroderma
- Gastric motility testing primarily uses gastric emptying scintigraphy. On occasion, antroduodenal manometry can be helpful. A wireless motility capsule is now available to assess both transit and contractility throughout the gastrointestinal tract
- Colonic transit is assessed in patients with refractory constipation and can be evaluated with radio-opaque markers, scintigraphy, or the wireless motility capsule
- Anorectal manometry is useful in the evaluation of patient with constipation and fecal incontinence. Biofeedback using anorectal manometry is helpful to treat select patients with constipation or fecal incontinence

---

Introduction

Gastrointestinal (GI) motility and functional GI disorders affect up to 25% of the US population, comprise about 40% of GI problems for which patients seek healthcare, and are common reasons for patients to see gastroenterologists [1,2] (Table 139.1).

The goals of motility testing are to identify patterns of abnormal motility in symptomatic patients. This can provide the correct diagnosis of GI motility disorders and help guide the treatment of these patients. Advances in technology have greatly improved the ability to measure gastrointestinal motility and function, and our understanding of the relationship between symptoms and motor abnormalities (Table 139.2).

Esophageal manometry

Esophageal manometry evaluates the **function of the esophageal muscles** that propel food and liquid from the mouth into the stomach. Esophageal manometry is used in several situations [3,4]:

- To determine the cause of **dysphagia** after other tests have excluded anatomical lesions

- To evaluate patients with refractory symptoms of **gastroesophageal reflux disease (GERD)**, especially when antireflux surgery is being considered
- To evaluate patients with **chest pain** that may originate from the esophagus. In some patients, esophageal manometry may be helpful in detecting esophageal motor abnormalities associated with scleroderma
- This test may be needed to correctly **place a pH catheter** for esophageal pH monitoring.

Esophageal manometry can diagnose several esophageal diseases causing dysphagia. For example, **achalasia** is readily diagnosed through identification of impaired lower esophageal sphincter (LES) relaxation and simultaneous esophageal contractions. In some patients with **chest pain**, the presence of simultaneous esophageal contractions suggests diffuse esophageal spasm. Occasionally, high amplitude peristaltic contractions (nutcracker esophagus) can be seen. A classification of esophageal motility patterns is shown in Table 139.3 [5,6].

Esophageal manometry may be used to evaluate the cause of a patient's **GERD**. Manometry is not used to diagnose GERD; diagnosis is from the patient's symptoms, response to antacid drugs, and esophageal pH monitoring. Manometry can identify a low pressure LES antireflux barrier. Ineffective esophageal peristalsis with low-amplitude distal esophageal contractions can be seen. Rarely, a combination of very low LES pressure with feeble mid and distal esophageal contractions suggests a scleroderma esophagus. Esophageal manometry will also help localize the proximal border of the LES, which is the landmark for correct placement of transnasal esophageal pH catheters.

Procedure

The procedure of esophageal manometry takes about 30 minutes and is performed with the patient fasting. The esophageal manometry catheter is passed through the anesthetized nostril, down the back of the throat, and into the esophagus as the patient swallows. With further swallowing, the tube is passed down into the stomach. Patients then lie supine. The pressures generated by the LES are measured. Next, the

---

Table 139.1 An anatomical classification of gastrointestinal motility and functional gastrointestinal disorders

Organ	GI motility disorders	Functional GI disorders
Esophagus	Achalasia Diffuse esophageal spasm Gastroesophageal reflux disease	Functional dysphagia Functional chest pain Functional heartburn
Stomach	Gastroparesis Dumping syndrome	Functional dyspepsia Cyclic vomiting syndrome Rumination syndrome
Small intestine	Chronic intestinal pseudo-obstruction Small intestinal bacterial overgrowth (SIBO)	Irritable bowel syndrome
Biliary tract	Gallbladder hypomotility Sphincter of Oddi dysfunction	
Colon	Colonic inertia Pelvic floor dyssynergia Hirschsprung's disease	Irritable bowel syndrome Functional constipation Functional incontinence Functional diarrhea

Table 139.2 Evaluations in gastrointestinal practice for gastrointestinal motility and functional gastrointestinal disorders

Esophageal symptoms	Esophageal manometry:
	    Water-perfused catheter
	    Solid-state catheter
	    High-resolution manometry
	Esophageal impedance manometry
	Esophageal pH monitoring:
	    pH catheter
	    Impedance pH catheter
	    Wireless pH capsule
	Esophageal sensory testing with balloon distension

Dyspeptic symptoms	Gastric emptying test Wireless motility capsule Electrogastrography (EGG) Antroduodenal manometry Satiety testing with water or nutrient load Gastric barostat
Irritable bowel syndrome symptoms	Breath testing: Bacterial overgrowth Lactose intolerance Fructose intolerance
Constipation/fecal incontinence	Anal manometry Anorectal electromyography (EMG) Pudendal nerve latency Balloon expulsion Colonic transit with radio-opaque markers Wireless motility capsule

Table 139.3 Classification of esophageal motility studies

LES dysfunction
- Hypotensive LES
- Hypertensive LES
- Impaired LES relaxation

Esophageal dysfunction
- Simultaneous esophageal contractions:
    - Diffuse esophageal spasm
    - Achalasia
- High amplitude peristaltic contractions:
    - Nutcracker esophagus
- Low-amplitude esophageal contractions:
    - Ineffective esophageal peristalsis
    - Scleroderma

LES, lower esophageal sphincter.

response to swallowing is assessed with the patient swallowing 5 mL of water to allow measurement of the LES pressure (the antireflux barrier), relaxation of the LES, esophageal body contractions, and upper esophageal sphincter (UES) pressure and its relaxation.

Water-perfused manometric systems rely on the transmission of the intraluminal pressures along the manometric catheter to external pressure transducers. The recording points can be arranged in a wide variety of configurations, generally 3–5 cm apart. Water-perfused manometry consist of three main parts: slow pull through to assess the LES resting and residual pressures; esophageal body swallows to determine the characteristics of the esophageal body peristalsis (Figure 139.1); and swallows to evaluate the UES. Some laboratories use a manometric sleeve device (Dent sleeve) to allow recording of the LES that takes into account axial movement of the sphincter during swallowing. In the last decade, solid-state pressure transducers placed on the catheter have been commonly used.

Impedance manometry is based on the esophageal intraluminal measurement of electrical impedance and pressure between a number of sequential impedance electrodes and pressure sensors during a bolus passage using an intraluminal probe [7]. Ingested liquid or gastroesophageal reflux fluid have low impedance whereas air has high impedance. The relation between bolus transit and esophageal peristaltic contraction can be directly assessed by impedance manometry (Figure 139.2). Impedance manometry is clinically useful when monitoring **esophageal bolus transport** patterns in patients with esophageal motor disorders, GERD, and dysphagia. In patients with low-amplitude esophageal contractions, impedance manometry helps determine if bolus transit is preserved. This test may be helpful in evaluating symptoms of dysphagia in patients after Nissen fundoplication to evaluate for impaired bolus transit into the stomach.

High-resolution manometry (HRM) uses 36 1-cm spaced pressure sensors to provide detailed pressure information along the esophagus [8,9]. An HRM color contour plot depicts the direction and force of esophageal contraction from the

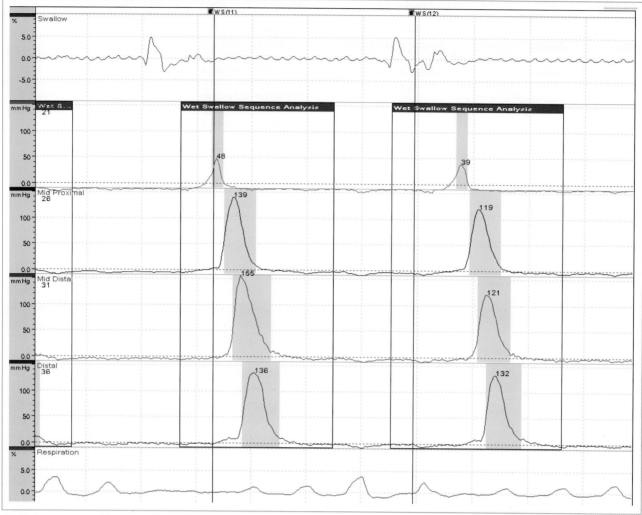

Figure 139.1 Water-perfused manometry showing peristaltic esophageal body contractions. The top panel is the swallow detector. The next four panels are recordings from the esophagus, from the proximal to the distal esophagus. The bottom tracing is the abdominal sensor that measures respirations. Two swallows with 5 mL of water are shown. The pressures of the esophagus are measured from 0 to approximately 100 mmHg using the scale on the left. This tracing shows normal peristalsis.

pharynx to the stomach. Amplitudes are assigned a color to evaluate the esophageal pressure. A normal esophageal peristalsis contraction in a patient with a hiatal hernia is shown in Figure 139.3. HRM in a patient with **achalasia** will easily show the increased LES resting and residual pressure with simultaneous, isobaric esophageal body waves [10]. HRM also allows accurate measurement of structures in the esophagus, e.g., location of the LES. With this technique, the location and length of the LES can be determined, as well as the dissociation between the LES component and the crural diaphragm in patients with a hiatal hernia (Figure 139.3) [11].

Gastric motility testing

Gastric dysmotility contributes to several clinical disorders including gastroparesis and functional dyspepsia. Delayed gastric emptying, impaired gastric accommodation to a meal,

and visceral hypersensitivity are three potential pathophysiological factors in functional dyspepsia. Interestingly, some patients with functional dyspepsia may have rapid gastric emptying. Proper evaluation to help distinguish the pathophysiological basis of the patient's symptoms may direct proper medical treatment.

Gastric emptying scintigraphy

Gastric emptying scintigraphy quantifies the emptying of a physiological caloric meal. For solid-phase testing, most centers use a ^{99m}Tc-sulfur colloid-labeled egg sandwich as a test meal. A multicenter protocol has provided standardized information about normal and delayed gastric emptying using a low-fat, egg-white meal with imaging at 0, 1, 2, 4 hours after meal ingestion [12]. Adoption of this standardized protocol helps resolve the lack of uniformity of testing, adds reliability to the results, and improves the clinical usefulness of the

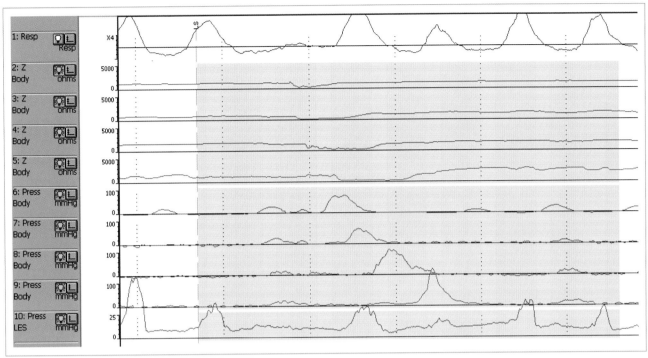

Figure 139.2 Normal impedance esophageal manometry tracing. The top tracing reflects respirations. The next four tracings are impedance tracings from the proximal to distal esophagus showing normal bolus transit and clearance, as seen from the drop in impedance values with recovery to the initial impedance values. The bottom four tracings are for pressure and show peristaltic esophageal body contractions.

gastric emptying test [13]. Scintigraphic assessment of emptying should be extended to at least 2 hours, and preferably 4 hours after meal ingestion [14]. Even with the 4-hour scintigraphic study, there may be significant day-to-day variability (up to 20%) in rates of gastric emptying.

Wireless motility capsule

The wireless motility capsule uses an ingestible capsule (SmartPill, Inc., Buffalo, NY, USA) that measures pH, pressure, and temperature using miniaturized wireless sensor technology [15]. After being swallowed by the patient, the wireless motility capsule records pH and pressures as it travels through the entire gastrointestinal tract (Figure 139.4). From these measurements, gastric emptying, small bowel transit, colonic transit, and whole-gut transit times can be determined. In addition, the wireless motility capsule can characterize pressure patterns and provide motility indices for the stomach, small intestine, and colon. The wireless motility capsule is helpful in the evaluation of patients with symptoms of GI motility disorders, such as **gastroparesis and chronic constipation**. It has been approved by the FDA to assess gastric emptying and whole-gut transit in patients with suspected gastroparesis and difficult-to-manage constipation [15,16].

Antroduodenal manometry

Antroduodeal (small bowel) manometry (ADM) provides information about **coordination of gastric and small intestinal motor function**. The procedure is somewhat invasive and lengthy (requiring at least 5 hours of recording), and is performed only at select centers. Using solid-state transducers, ambulatory studies can also be performed over 24 hours, allowing for correlation of symptoms with abnormal motility.

The main indications for ADM are to evaluate: (1) unexplained nausea and vomiting; (2) the cause of gastric or small bowel stasis (neuropathic versus myopathic disorders); and (3) suspected chronic intestinal pseudo-obstruction. ADM can differentiate between a neuropathic or myopathic motility disorder, and may suggest unexpected small bowel obstruction or rumination syndrome. **Myopathic disorders**, such as scleroderma, amyloidosis, or hollow visceral myopathy, have low-amplitude (<20 mmHg) contractions with normal propagation. **Neuropathic disorders** have normal amplitude but abnormal propagative contractions, such as bursts and sustained uncoordinated pressure activity, and a failure of a meal to induce the fed-type pattern. **Occult mechanical obstruction** of the small intestine is suggested by non-propagated, prolonged contractions during the postprandial period. Clustered contractions may suggest the **irritable bowel syndrome**, although these can be seen in other conditions.

Colonic transit

Evaluation of **refractory constipation** should include an assessment of colonic transit and anorectal function. Colonic transit testing helps determine if a constipated patient has

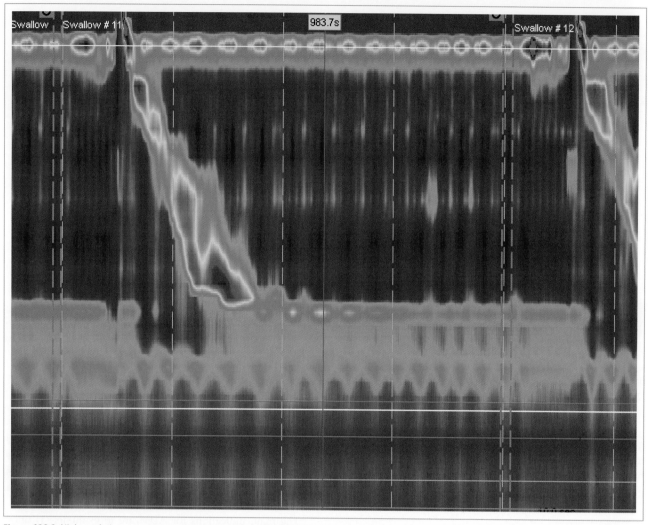

Figure 139.3 High-resolution manometry using topographical color depiction in a patient with a hiatal hernia. This study shows a normal upper esophageal resting pressure with complete relaxation followed by a normal peristaltic esophageal body contraction while the lower esophageal sphincter (LES) relaxes. The dissociation of the LES components is demonstrated by the two parallel higher pressure stripes at the end of the esophageal body contraction.

delayed colonic transit and also provides insight into what segments of the colon are contributing to a delayed colonic transit. Colonic transit studies can be performed using radio-opaque markers, scintigraphy, or wireless capsule motility (Table 139.4).

Radio-opaque markers

The conventional method to determine colonic transit is with radio-opaque markers (ROMs) [17]. This is a simple, inexpensive, and nearly universally available method for assessing colonic transit. The simplest method requires only one X-ray after the ingestion of radio-opaque markers. In the method described by Hinton *et al*. [18], the subject ingests a single gelatin capsule containing 24 small radio-opaque O-rings (Sitzmarks radio-opaque markers). A flat plate abdominal X-ray (large field of view from xyphoid to pubis) is obtained 5 days (120 hours) later. The number of markers

is counted and their distribution described. If >20% of the markers are retained (more than five markers), then there is slow colonic transit. If five or fewer markers are present, the patient has normal colonic transit. In the constipated patient with delayed colonic transit, localization of most of the markers in the rectosigmoid region suggests a functional anorectal outlet obstruction (dyssynergic defecation) [19]. If the markers are distributed throughout the colon, colonic inertia is suggested.

Another method, described by Metcalf *et al*. [20], is for the subject to ingest one Sitzmarks capsule containing 24 radio-opaque markers each day for 3 consecutive days, followed by an abdominal X-ray the next day (the fourth day) and usually also on the seventh day. In general, the number of markers present on the X-ray on the fourth day indicates the colonic transit time in hours. The normal values for colonic transit using this method are 0–70 hours.

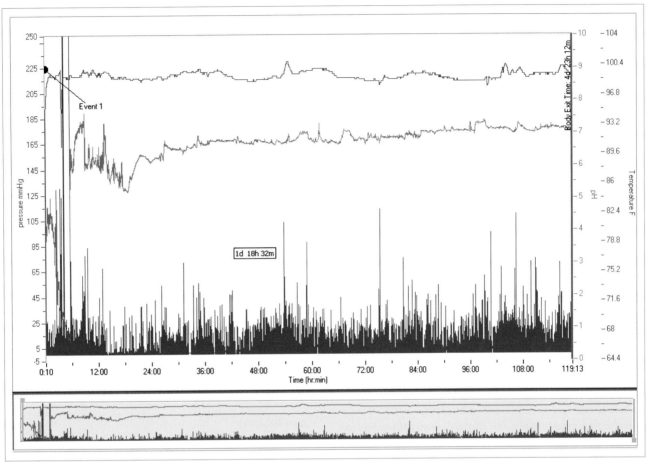

Figure 139.4 Wireless motility capsule tracing. The entire tracing is shown. The red tracing is the pH tracing. The initial drop in pH is the time period that the capsule is in the stomach. The blue tracing is the pressure tracing and the green tracing is the temperature tracing. Whole-gut transit is measured at 119 hours and 13 minutes (normal <72 hours). There is delayed colonic transit, but normal gastric emptying, with gastric empting of the capsule and small bowel transit.

Table 139.4 Comparison of methods to assess colonic transit

	Radio-opaque markers	Scintigraphy	pH/Pressure capsule
Clinical evaluation of patients	Yes	Yes	Yes
Radiation exposure	Yes (X-ray)	Yes (radiolabeled meal)	No
Assesses gastric emptying	No	Yes	Yes
Test location	Gastroenterology practice With X-ray in Radiology	Nuclear Medicine Center generally in hospital	Gastroenterology practice

Colonic transit scintigraphy

Colonic transit scintigraphy (CTS) is performed following the administration of a radioactive meal using gamma camera imaging to assess the progress of the isotope [21–24]. CTS is usually performed as part of whole-gut transit scintigraphy, permitting measurements of gastric emptying, small bowel transit, and colonic transit. This is helpful in distinguishing motility disturbances confined to the colon from those that are more diffuse, as seen in intestinal pseudo-obstruction.

However, this test is not widely available and is more expensive than the radio-opaque marker technique.

The **whole-gut transit scintigraphy test** is performed in the Nuclear Medicine Department following an overnight fast. Patients consume a test meal consisting of two scrambled eggs labeled with ^{99m}Tc and water labeled with ^{111}In DTPA. On the first day, imaging is performed for the first 6 hours to determine gastric emptying of solids and liquids as well as small bowel transit using the indium-labeled liquid phase of the meal. The patient returns daily over the next 3 days for imaging of the colon for indium to determine colonic transit.

Colonic transit assessment can be used to document the existence of slow colonic transit constipation [21]. With scintigraphy, several patterns of colonic transit are seen in constipated patients. **Colonic inertia** is characterized by a delay in transit with failure of progression of activity beyond the splenic flexure over the 3-day imaging. A **diffuse slow colon transit** can also be recognized by generalized retention throughout the colon with no regional abnormality localized in any one segment of the colon. **Functional rectosigmoid obstruction** is suggested by normal transit in the proximal colon, but with accumulation of activity in the descending and rectosigmoid colon.

Assessment of anorectal function

Anorectal manometry, anal electromyography (EMG), balloon expulsion tests, and defecography are useful tests for anorectal anatomy and function. Conventional defecography plays an important role in detecting functional rectal obstruction, rectocele, enterocele, and intussusception.

Anorectal manometry

Anorectal manometry is performed in patients with constipation and fecal incontinence. For **chronic constipation**, this test can exclude Hirschsprung's disease and determine if the patient has dyssynergic defecation [17]. Biofeedback with anorectal manometry can be performed to treat dyssynergic defecation. In patients with **fecal incontinence**, anal manometry can define functional weakness of sphincter muscles, predict patients who may respond to biofeedback therapy, and be used to perform biofeedback therapy.

Anorectal manometry uses a thin catheter with either solid-state pressure transducers or radially placed water pressure transducers. A balloon is attached to the end of the catheter. Resting anorectal pressures are initially measured. Most of the resting pressure is derived from the internal anal sphincter. Squeeze pressures reflect primarily the external anal sphincter. Low resting anorectal pressure and squeeze pressures in fecal incontinence are predictors for response to **biofeedback therapy**.

Anal manometry can evaluate the anorectal inhibitory reflex: there is a decrease in the tonic pressure of the anal sphincters with rectal balloon distension. Absence of this reflex is suggestive of **Hirschsprung's disease**.

Balloon distension is used to detect the threshold for rectal sensation. Three sensations can be tested: the first detectable sensation (rectal sensory threshold), the sensation of urgency to defecate, and the sensation of pain (maximum tolerable volume). The rectal sensory threshold for the first detectable sensation is most commonly used. In biofeedback training of patients with fecal incontinence, poor or absent sensation makes a good response to biofeedback unlikely.

Manometry assesses anorectal patterns during attempted defecation. During normal defecation, rectal pressures increase while sphincter pressures decrease, allowing expulsion of stool. In **dyssynergic defecation**, patients create adequate propulsive forces but a paradoxical increase in sphincter pressure leads to difficulty expelling stool.

Anal electromyography

For anorectal EMG, a probe is used to monitor anal sphincter muscle electrical activity and assess recruitment during squeezing and simulated defecation [17]. Anal EMG is helpful in the evaluation of **sphincter function**, primarily in the diagnosis of dyssynergic defecation, where a paradoxical increase in EMG activity is seen when the patient bears down, simulating a bowel movement. Anal EMG is also useful for biofeedback training for dyssynergic defecation.

Balloon expulsion test

The balloon expulsion test is performed by introducing a lubricated balloon attached to a thin catheter into the rectum, filling it with 50 mL of air or water, and asking the patient, while sitting on a commode, to expel (e.g., defecate) the balloon. Normal expulsion takes less than 60 seconds. This test can screen for functional rectosigmoid obstruction (**dyssynergic defecation**).

Conclusions

Abnormalities of GI motor function contribute to a number of common clinical problems. Proper evaluation of patients with suspected GI motility disorders is important to ensure correct diagnoses and to embark on an appropriate plan of treatment. The GI motility laboratory serves as an important station for patient evaluation and treatment in gastroenterology, and is an essential element in any comprehensive digestive disease program.

References

1. Longstreth GR, Thompson WG, Chey WD, Houghton LA, Mearin F, Spiller RC. Functional bowel disorders. *Gastroenterology.* 2006;130:1480–1491.
2. Drossman DA, Li Z, Andruzzi E, *et al.* U.S. householder survey of functional gastrointestinal disorders: prevalence, sociodemography, and health impact. *Dig Dis Sci.* 1993;38:1569–1580.
3. Pandolfino JE, Kahrilas PJ. AGA Technical Review on the Clinical Use of Esophageal Manometry. *Gastroenterology.* 2005;128:209–224.
4. Murray JA, Clouse RE, Conklin JL. Components of the standard oesophageal manometry. *Neurogastroenterol Motil.* 2003;15:591–606.
5. Spechler SJ, Castell DO. Classification of oesophageal motility abnormalities. *Gut.* 2001;49:145–151.
6. Kahrilas P, Ghosh SK, Pandolfino JE. Esophageal motility disorders in terms of pressure topography: the Chicago Classification. *J Clin Gastroenterol.* 2008;42:627–635.
7. Tutuian R, Castell DO. Multichannel intraluminal impedance: general principles and technical issues. *Gastrointest Endosc Clin North Am.* 2005;15:257–264.

8. Kahrilas PJ, Sifrim D. High-resolution manometry and impedance-pH/manometry: valuable tools in clinical and investigational esophagology. *Gastroenterology.* 2008;135:756–769.

9. Fox M, Bredenorrod AJ. Oesophageal high-resolution manometry: moving from research into clinical practice. *Gut.* 2008;57: 405–423.

10. Pandolfino JE, Ghosh SK. Classifying esophageal motility by pressure topography characteristics: a study of 400 patients and 75 controls. *Am J Gastroenterol.* 2008;103:27–37.

11. Kahrilas PJ, Kim HC. Approaches to the diagnosis and grading of hiatal hernia. *Best Pract Res Clin Gastroenterol.* 2008;22: 601–616.

12. Tougas G, Eaker EY, Abell TL, *et al.* Assessment of gastric emptying using a low-fat meal: Establishment of international control values. *Am J Gastroenterol.* 2000;95:1456–1462.

13. Abell TL, Camilleri M, Donohoe K, *et al.* Consensus recommendations for gastric emptying scintigraphy: a joint report of the American Neurogastroenterology and Motility Society and the Society of Nuclear Medicine. *Am J Gastroenterol.* 2008;103: 753–763.

14. Guo J-P, Maurer AH, Urbain J-L, Fisher RS, Parkman HP. Extending gastric emptying scintigraphy from two to four hours detects more patients with gastroparesis. *Dig Dis Sci.* 2001;46:24–29.

15. Kuo B, McCallum RW, Koch KL, *et al.* Comparison of gastric emptying of a nondigestible capsule to a radio-labelled meal in healthy and gastroparetic subjects. *Aliment Pharmacol Ther.* 2008; 27:186–196.

16. Rao SS, Kuo B, McCallum RW, *et al.* Investigation of colonic and whole-gut transit with wireless motility capsule and radiopaque markers in constipation. *Clin Gastroenterol Hepatol.* 2009;7: 537–544.

17. Rao SSC. Constipation: evaluation and treatment of colonic and anorectal motility disorders. *Gastroenterol Clin North Am.* 2007; 36:687–711.

18. Hinton JM, Lennard-Jones JE, Young AC. A new method for studying gut transit times using radioopaque markers. *Gut.* 1969;10:842–847.

19. Arhan P, Devroede G, Jehannu B, *et al.* Segmental colonic transit time. *Dis Colon Rectum.* 1981;24:625–629.

20. Metcalf AM, Phillips SF, Zinmeister AR. A simplified assessment of segmental colonic transit. *Gastroenterology.* 1987;92:40–47.

21. Bonapace ES, Davidoff S, Krevsky B, Maurer AH, Parkman HP, Fisher RS. Whole gut transit scintigraphy in the clinical evaluation of patients who upper and lower gastrointestinal symptoms. *Am J Gastroenterol.* 2000;95:2838–2847.

22. Maurer AH, Krevsky B. Whole-gut transit scintigraphy in the evaluation of small-bowel and colon transit disorders. *Semin Nucl Med.* 1995;25:326–338.

23. Stivland T, Camilleri M, Vassallo M, *et al.* Scintigraphic measurement of regional gut transit in idiopathic constipation. *Gastroenterology.* 1991;101:107–115.

24. Lin HC, Prather C, Fisher RS, *et al.* Measurement of gastrointestinal transit (review article). *Dig Dis Sci.* 2005;50:989–1004.

CHAPTER 140
Measurement of portal pressure

Annalisa Berzigotti and Juan G. Abraldes
University of Barcelona, CIBERehd, Barcelona, Spain

KEY POINTS

- Measurement of the hepatic venous pressure gradient (HVPG) is the gold standard technique used to evaluate portal hypertension in liver disease
- In patients with cirrhosis, HVPG measurement provides independent prognostic information on survival and the risk of decompensation
- The HVPG response to pharmacological therapy identifies those patients with portal hypertension who are likely to benefit most from this treatment
- Measurement of HVPG helps to assess the risk of liver failure and death after liver resection in patients with compensated chronic liver disease or hepatocarcinoma
- There are currently no available non-invasive alternatives to HVPG measurement

Introduction and scientific basis

Portal pressure is the single most important hemodynamic measurement in portal hypertension. In 1951, Myers and Taylor developed the measurement of **wedge hepatic venous pressure (WHVP)**, which assesses hepatic sinusoidal pressure and is an index of portal venous pressure. The scientific basis is the same as for the measurement of the wedged pulmonary arterial pressure, an index of left atrial pressure. When blood flow in a hepatic vein is stopped by a "wedged" catheter, the static column of blood transmits the pressure from the preceding communicated vascular territory, in this case, the hepatic sinusoids. Thus, WHVP is a measure of **hepatic sinusoidal pressure** and not of portal pressure itself. However, WHVP adequately reflects portal pressure in alcoholic liver disease, hepatitis C-, and hepatitis B-related cirrhosis [1]. These entities are, by far, the most frequent etiologies of chronic liver disease in developed countries. Later on, the technique was improved by introducing new tools, such as the balloon catheter, that enhanced the reliability and accuracy of the measurements. It was soon evident that hepatic vein catheterization constituted a safe and relatively simple technique to perform accurate measurements of portal pressure in patients with liver disease [2].

Portal pressure should be expressed in terms of the pressure gradient with the inferior vena cava (IVC) [the portal pressure gradient (PPG)], which represents the perfusion pressure within the portal–hepatic circulation. The normal PPG value is up to 5 mmHg. Expressing portal pressure as the PPG has the advantage of not being modified by changes in intra-abdominal pressure. Increased intra-abdominal pressure will increase both the portal pressure and the IVC pressure, but will not significantly modify the PPG (except in the case of marked changes in intra-abdominal pressure, which are associated with changes in splanchnic and systemic hemodynamics).

Description of technique

Although, as mentioned above, WHVP is the most commonly utilized method to assess portal pressure, in this section we also describe other methods; these can be divided into direct and indirect techniques.

Direct measurement of portal pressure

Direct measurements of portal pressure are invasive investigations based on the **surgical, percutaneous transhepatic or transvenous (transjugular) catheterization of the portal vein**. In these techniques, except for the transjugular approach, the measurement of IVC pressure requires the additional, simultaneous puncture of a hepatic vein in order to determine the PPG. Because of this inconvenience and the risk of intraperitoneal bleeding, direct measurements of portal pressure are rarely used. When required, as in presinusoidal portal hypertension, the percutaneous transhepatic approach or the transjugular catheterization of the portal vein is the preferred technique. The safety of the percutaneous transhepatic or transjugular catheterization of the portal vein is increased by performing the procedures under ultrasonographic guidance. The risk of intraperitoneal bleeding is greater in the percutaneous procedure, which precludes its use in patients with impaired coagulation. This can be partly overcome by using a thin needle, which allows the measurement of portal pressure, but not the performance of portal venography.

Indirect measurement of portal pressure

Hepatic venous pressure gradient (HVPG) is measured through catheterization of the hepatic vein (see Video clip 140.1). This is carried out under sedation in conjunction with

---

Textbook of Clinical Gastroenterology and Hepatology, Second Edition. Edited by C. J. Hawkey, Jaime Bosch, Joel E. Richter, Guadalupe Garcia-Tsao, Francis K. L. Chan.

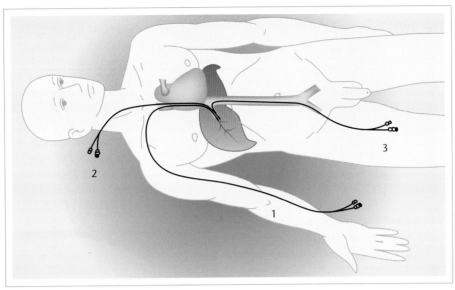

Figure 140.1 Venous access sites for hepatic vein catheterization. The antecubital vein (1), jugular vein (2), or femoral vein (3) can be used for hepatic vein catheterization. As shown, the degree of invasiveness depends on the elected access site. Access via the antecubital vein is the least invasive approach. The transjugular approach is most frequently used, as it enables a transvenous liver biopsy to be obtained as part of the procedure.

non-invasive vital sign monitoring (by electrocardiography, arterial blood pressure, and pulse oximetry). Under local anesthesia, the right jugular vein (or the femoral or antecubital vein) is catheterized (Figure 140.1), a venous introducer is placed, and a balloon-tipped catheter is advanced under fluoroscopic control into the IVC and a hepatic vein to measure pressure in the IVC, WHVP, and free hepatic venous pressure (FHVP).

The **FHVP** is measured by maintaining the tip of the catheter "free" in the hepatic vein, at 2–4 cm from its opening into the IVC. The FHVP should be close to the IVC pressure; if the difference between these pressure values is greater than 2 mmHg, it is likely that the catheter is inadequately placed or that there is obstruction of the hepatic vein.

The **WHVP** is measured by occluding the hepatic vein, either by "wedging" the catheter into a small branch of a hepatic vein or by inflating a balloon at the tip of the catheter (Figure 140.2). Adequate occlusion of the hepatic vein is confirmed by slowly injecting 5 mL of contrast dye into the vein with the balloon inflated, a procedure that should reveal a typical "wedged" pattern (Figure 140.3), without reflux of the dye or washout through communications with other hepatic veins. Occlusion of the hepatic vein by inflating a balloon is preferred, as the volume of the liver circulation that is "sensed" is much larger than that attained by wedging the catheter, which reduces the variability of the measurements. Indeed, a high variability of HVPG values between different hepatic veins has been reported using end-hole, non-balloon catheters. The WHVP should be measured until the value remains stable (this usually takes longer than 40 seconds). The HVPG is the difference between WHVP and FHVP. All measurements should be taken at least in duplicate, and permanent tracings should be obtained using a multichannel recorder and adequately calibrated transducers (Figure 140.4).

The technique to obtain HVPG values is relatively straightforward; however, achieving accurate measurements requires specialist training, as the procedure differs from those used in heart catheterization laboratories, interventional radiology rooms, and intensive care units. A series of practical tips to ensure adequate measurements is outlined in Table 140.1.

Limitations

HVPG does not reflect the PPG in diseases where the increased resistance is located at presinusoidal sites, such as in portal vein thrombosis or liver diseases affecting predominantly the portal tracts, such as schistosomiasis, initial stages of primary biliary cirrhosis, or idiopathic portal hypertension. In these cases, a direct measurement of portal pressure is indicated.

Associated procedures

In addition to pressure measurements, **hepatic vein catheterization** allows for the performance of a wedged hepatic retrograde portography using CO_2 as a contrast agent (Figure 140.5). This will demonstrate the portal vein in most instances. In fact, inability to demonstrate the portal vein on CO_2 retrograde portography strongly suggests the presence of presinusoidal portal hypertension. Hepatic vein catheterization also allows for the performance of a transjugular liver biopsy, which adds very little time, discomfort, and risk to the procedure, and can be done on a day-case basis. Furthermore, at hepatic vein catheterization it is also possible to measure the hepatic blood flow using indocyanine green (ICG) as the indicator, as well as the intrinsic clearance of ICG, a quantitative liver function test that assesses the overall hepatic metabolic activity.

Indications

The main indications for HVPG measurement are as follows.

Classification of portal hypertension

Portal hypertension can be classified on the basis of the findings of HVPG measurement (Table 140.2). An increased HVPG due to an increase in WHVP is observed in all cases of **sinusoidal block**, which is mainly represented by cirrhosis in Western countries. Presinusoidal causes of portal hypertension are characterized by normal WHVP, FHVP, and HVPG. Postsinusoidal portal hypertension features increased WHVP and FHVP, and normal or increased HVPG.

Stratification of risk in patients with cirrhosis

HVPG has a strong and independent prognostic value in patients with cirrhosis. All the complications of portal hypertension, such as ascites, variceal formation, and hepato-renal syndrome [3,4] can occur when the HVPG increases above the threshold value of 10 mmHg; moreover, variceal bleeding may be seen when the HVPG is over 12 mmHg. Patients with an HVPG below 10 mmHg are at negligible or null risk of experiencing portal hypertension-related complications. This has been confirmed by the results of a cohort study nested in a large randomized, double-blind trial performed in patients with compensated cirrhosis [5]. In addition, patients with an HVPG over 10 mmHg are at increased risk of hepatocellular carcinoma [6]. Additionally, patients with an HVPG above 16 mmHg have been reported in some studies to be at a higher risk of death [7,8], and in patients with decompensated cirrhosis listed for liver transplantation, HVPG holds prognostic value independent of that of the MELD score [9].

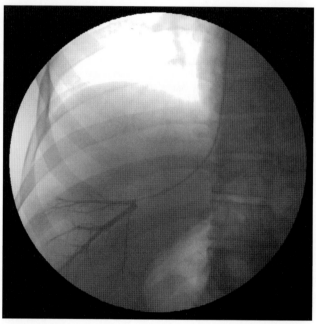

Figure 140.3 Occlusion balloon catheter located in the main right hepatic vein. Wedged hepatic venous pressure (WHVP) is measured after occluding the hepatic vein by inflating a balloon at the tip of the catheter. When the balloon stops blood flow, the static column of blood transmits the pressure existing in the preceding communicated vascular territory (the hepatic sinusoids).

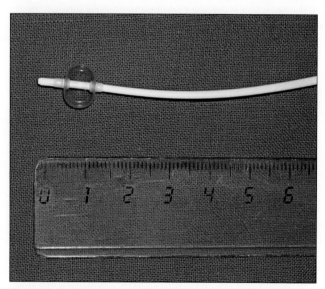

Figure 140.2 Balloon-tipped catheter. The balloon-tipped catheter has an inflatable balloon placed 1 cm proximal to the distal end hole to ensure a good occlusion of the hepatic vein without obstructing the end hole.

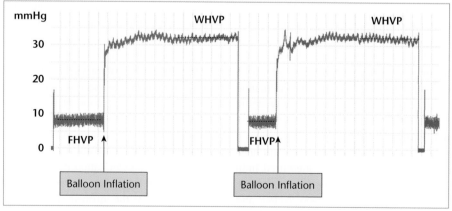

Figure 140.4 Measurement of hepatic venous pressure. Measurements are recorded (on paper or computer) to accurately assess the pressure values before [free hepatic venous pressure (FHVP)] and after balloon inflation [wedged hepatic venous pressure (WHVP)].

Table 140.1 Tips for accurately measuring the hepatic venous pressure gradient (HVPG)

- Record all measurements in a permanent manner. Digital readings on a monitor screen are usually not reliable. Use paper or electronic recordings to allow for the independent review of pressure tracings
- Use an appropriate scale for venous pressure measurements (full range up to 40 mmHg). Set recorders at 1 mmHg = 1 mm paper. Scales used for arterial pressure measurements are not adequate
- The transducer should be calibrated against known external pressures before starting measurements (e.g., 13.6 cmH$_2$O should read 10 mmHg, 27.2 cmH$_2$O should read 20 mmHg, and 40.8 cmH$_2$O should read 30 mmHg). Place the transducer at the level of the right atrium (mid-axillary line). With the transducer open to air (zero pressure), adjust the recorder to read zero
- Allow venous pressures to stabilize over a period of at least 1 minute for WHVP and 15 seconds for FHVP (some patients might require longer). Use a slow speed (<5 mm/second) in the recorder. Rinse the catheter with 5% dextrose before any measurement
- The FHVP should be measured with the catheter tip <5 cm into the hepatic vein. The FHVP should not exceed the pressure in the inferior vena cava by >2 mmHg, which should be measured at the level of the hepatic vein ostium. If the difference is greater, investigate for a hepatic outflow problem
- The use of balloon catheters makes correction of an occlusion easier, minimizes variability, and facilitates repeat measurements. Check for adequate occlusion of the hepatic vein and for absence of communications between hepatic veins by slowly injecting, by hand, 5 mL of iodinated contrast dye
- Perform all measurements in duplicate (triplicate if differences of >1 mmHg are recorded). Greater variations frequently reflect mistakes
- Any event that might cause an artifact, such as coughing, movement or talking, should be noted

FHVP, free hepatic venous pressure; WHVP, wedged hepatic venous pressure.

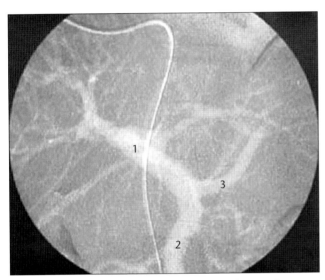

Figure 140.5 Wedged retrograde portography. Wedged retrograde portography using CO$_2$ as a contrast agent and showing a patent portal (1), mesenteric (2), and splenic (3) vein in a patient with hepatitis C-related cirrhosis.

Assessment of the response to pharmacological therapy of portal hypertension in cirrhosis

Longitudinal studies have demonstrated that if HVPG is decreased below 12 mmHg, by means of pharmacological treatment [10,11] or spontaneously due to an improvement in liver disease [12], **variceal bleeding** is totally prevented and varices may decrease in size. Even if this target is not achieved, a decrease in HVPG of at least 20% [11] from baseline levels offers a significant protection from variceal bleeding, while markedly decreasing the risk of other complications of portal hypertension, such as ascites, spontaneous bacterial peritonitis, and hepatorenal syndrome, and improves survival [13]. Lack of achievement of these targets (reduction below 12 mmHg or >20% from baseline) constitutes the strongest independent predictor of variceal bleeding or rebleeding [14]. Therefore, tailoring the treatment of portal hypertension by

measuring the individual portal pressure response to therapy might allow the prediction of the treatment's clinical effectiveness. In this setting, the need to repeat measurements of HVPG may be reduced by testing the acute hemodynamic response to intravenous beta-blockers [15,16].

Prognostic evaluation during acute variceal bleeding

Early measurements of HVPG within 48 hours of admission for acute variceal bleeding provide useful prognostic information regarding the outcome of the bleeding episode [17,18] and 1-year survival [17]. Patients with an HVPG >20 mmHg are five times more likely to experience failure to control acute variceal bleeding or early rebleeding, require significantly more blood transfusions and days in the intensive care unit, and have a higher mortality on follow-up. The early use of a transjugular intrahepatic portosystemic shunt (TIPS) in these high-risk patients improves the control of bleeding and reduces early rebleeding and mortality [19].

Preoperative evaluation of resectable hepatocellular carcinoma

Patients with an HVPG >10 mmHg and/or increased bilirubin levels have an increased risk of **hepatic decompensation** after surgical resection of hepatocellular carcinoma even when liver function is wellpreserved (Child–Pugh class A) [20,21]. In a recent study, >50% of patients with Child–Pugh class A had hepatic decompensation after surgery. This decompensation not only affected quality of life but was also associated with reduced long-term survival [21]. Surgical resection should therefore be restricted to patients with an HVPG below 10 mmHg.

Evaluation of progression of chronic liver disease

It has been suggested that HVPG could be a better method [than biochemical methods and polymerase chain reaction (PCR)] for staging chronic hepatitis and for evaluating the response to antiviral treatment [22]. HVPG has been shown to correlate with the degree of histological liver fibrosis in

Table 140.2 Portal hypertension: classification of main diseases according to hepatic venous pressure gradient measurement

Presinusoidal	Prehepatic:
	    Thrombosis of the porto-splenic axis
	    Congenital stenosis of the portal vein
	    Arteriovenous fistulae (splenic, aortomesenteric, aortoportal,
	    and hepatic artery–portal vein)
		PP increased
		WHVP normal
		FHVP normal

	Intrahepatic:
	    Partial nodular transformation
	    Nodular regenerative hyperplasia
	    Congenital hepatic fibrosis
	    Peliosis hepatis
	    Polycystic liver disease
	    Idiopathic portal hypertension
	    Hypervitaminosis A
	    Arsenic, copper sulfate, and vinyl
	    chloride monomer poisoning
	    Sarcoidosis
	    Tuberculosis
	    Primary biliary cirrhosis
	    Schistosomiasis
	    Amyloidosis
	    Acute fatty liver of pregnancy
		PP increased
		WHVP normal
		FHVP normal

Sinusoidal	Alcoholic liver cirrhosis Liver cirrhosis from viral etiology	PP and WHVP increased FHVP normal

Postsinusoidal	Intrahepatic:
	    Budd–Chiari syndrome increased
	    Veno-occlusive disease*
		PP, WHVP, and FHVP
		IVC pressure normal

	Posthepatic:
	    Congenital malformations and
	    increased thrombosis of the IVC
	    Constrictive pericarditis
	    Tricuspid valve diseases
		PP, WHVP, and FHVP
		IVC pressure increased

*In veno-occlusive disease FHVP is normal but PP and WHVP are both increased.
FHVP, free hepatic venous pressure; IVC, inferior vena cava; PP, portal pressure; WHVP, wedge hepatic venous pressure.

patients with hepatitis B [23] and in post-transplant recurrent hepatitis C [26]. It has been shown that HVPG decreases in patients with hepatitis C who attain a sustained virological response [24,25].

In patients with post-transplant recurrent hepatitis C, HVPG is more accurate than liver biopsy in identifying the subgroup at the highest risk of developing cirrhosis decompensation [26]. The presence of portal hypertension, as indicated by an HVPG of >6 mmHg, allowed the recognition of those patients who showed rapid deterioration of liver function and cirrhosis recurrence [26]. HVPG paralleled the improvement in liver histology induced by antiviral therapy in liver transplantation recipients [27].

In patients with **alcoholic cirrhosis**, the presence of acute alcoholic hepatitis is associated with higher values of HVPG, suggesting that the inflammatory state and hepatocyte swelling associated with this condition contribute to a further increase in portal pressure. Moreover, HVPG has an independent prognostic value for the short-term outcome of patients with severe alcoholic hepatitis, with a best cut-off of 22 mmHg to discriminate patients at higher risk of death [28].

Contraindications

A history of allergic reaction to iodinated radiological contrast medium is not a contraindication to hepatic vein catheterization, as CO_2 can be used as a contrast agent. Although coagulation disorders are common in cirrhotic patients, only cases of severe thrombocytopenia (platelet levels $<20 \times 10^9$/L) or low prothrombin ratio (below 30%) call for adequate replacement of platelets or transfusion of fresh frozen plasma.

Complications

The measurement of HVPG usually carries very little discomfort. A slight conscious sedation does not modify hemodynamic measurements (midazolam 0.02 mg/Kg i.v.) [29] and can further improve the acceptability of HVPG measurement.

Complications occur in fewer than 1% of patients [30]. Major complications are usually limited to **local injury to the femoral or jugular vein** (arteriovenous fistulae, leakage, or rupture of venous introducers, Horner's syndrome, and transient brachial paralysis), and can be significantly reduced by performing the venous puncture under Doppler ultrasound guidance.

Passage of the catheter through the right atrium may rarely cause arrhythmias, which are usually transient or easily corrected. The authors have observed no fatalities in over 10 000 procedures. Transjugular liver biopsies (TJLB) may be rarely complicated by intraperitoneal bleeding due to capsular perforation and subcapsular hematomas. Death is reported in 0.09% of the published series of TJLB [31].

References

1. Perello A, Escorsell A, Bru C, *et al*. Wedged hepatic venous pressure adequately reflects portal pressure in hepatitis C virus-related cirrhosis. *Hepatology*. 1999;30:1393–1397.

2. Bosch J, Abraldes JG, Berzigotti A, Garca-Pagan JC. The clinical use of HVPG measurements in chronic liver disease. *Nature Rev Gastroenterol Hepatol*. 2009;6:573–582.

3. Garcia-Tsao G, Groszmann RJ, Fisher RL, Conn HO, Atterbury CE, Glickman M. Portal pressure, presence of gastroesophageal varices and variceal bleeding. *Hepatology*. 1985;5:419–424.

4. Casado M, Bosch J, Garcia-Pagan JC, *et al*. Clinical events after transjugular intrahepatic portosystemic shunt: correlation with hemodynamic findings. *Gastroenterology*. 1998;114:1296–1303.

5. Ripoll C, Groszmann R, Garcia-Tsao G, *et al*. Hepatic venous pressure gradient predicts clinical decompensation in patients with compensated cirrhosis. *Gastroenterology*. 2007;133: 481–488.

6. Ripoll C, Groszmann RJ, Garcia-Tsao G, *et al*. Hepatic venous pressure gradient predicts development of hepatocellular carcinoma independently of severity of cirrhosis. *J Hepatol*. 2009;50: 923–928.

7. Merkel C, Bolognesi M, Bellon S, *et al*. Prognostic usefulness of hepatic vein catheterization in patients with cirrhosis and esophageal varices. *Gastroenterology*. 1992;102:973-979.

8. Stanley AJ, Robinson I, Forrest EH, Jones AL, Hayes PC. Haemodynamic parameters predicting variceal haemorrhage and survival in alcoholic cirrhosis. *Q J Med*. 1998;91:19–25.

9. Ripoll C, Banares R, Rincon D, *et al*. Influence of hepatic venous pressure gradient on the prediction of survival of patients with cirrhosis in the MELD era. *Hepatology*. 2005;42:793–801.

10. Groszmann RJ, Bosch J, Grace ND, *et al*. Hemodynamic events in a prospective randomized trial of propranolol versus placebo in the prevention of a first variceal hemorrhage [see comments]. *Gastroenterology*. 1990;99:1401–1407.

11. Feu F, Garcia-Pagan JC, Bosch J, *et al*. Relation between portal pressure response to pharmacotherapy and risk of recurrent variceal haemorrhage in patients with cirrhosis. *Lancet*. 1995; 346:1056–1059.

12. Vorobioff J, Groszmann RJ, Picabea E, *et al*. Prognostic value of hepatic venous pressure gradient measurements in alcoholic cirrhosis: a 10-year prospective study. *Gastroenterology*. 1996;111: 701–709.

13. Abraldes JG, Tarantino I, Turnes J, Garcia-Pagan JC, Rodes J, Bosch J. Hemodynamic response to pharmacological treatment of portal hypertension and long-term prognosis of cirrhosis. *Hepatology*. 2003;37:902–908.

14. D'Amico G, Garcia-Pagan JC, Luca A, Bosch J. Hepatic vein pressure gradient reduction and prevention of variceal bleeding in cirrhosis: a systematic review. *Gastroenterology*. 2006;131: 1611–1624.

15. La Mura V, Abraldes JG, Raffa S, *et al*. Prognostic value of acute hemodynamic response to i.v. propranolol in patients with cirrhosis and portal hypertension. *J Hepatol*. 2009;51:279–287.

16. Villanueva C, Aracil C, Colomo A, *et al*. Acute hemodynamic response to beta-blockers and prediction of long-term outcome in primary prophylaxis of variceal bleeding. *Gastroenterology*. 2009;137:119–128.

17. Moitinho E, Escorsell A, Bandi JC, *et al*. Prognostic value of early measurements of portal pressure in acute variceal bleeding. *Gastroenterology*. 1999;117:626–631.

18. Abraldes JG, Villanueva C, Banares R, *et al*. Hepatic venous pressure gradient and prognosis in patients with acute variceal bleeding treated with pharmacologic and endoscopic therapy. *J Hepatol*. 2008;48:229–236.

19. Monescillo A, Martinez-Lagares F, Ruiz-del-Arbol L, *et al*. Influence of portal hypertension and its early decompression by TIPS placement on the outcome of variceal bleeding. *Hepatology*. 2004; 40:793–801.

20. Bruix J, Castells A, Bosch J, *et al*. Surgical resection of hepatocellular carcinoma in cirrhotic patients: prognostic value of preoperative portal pressure. *Gastroenterology*. 1996;111:1018–1022.

21. Llovet JM, Fuster J, Bruix J. Intention-to-treat analysis of surgical treatment for early hepatocellular carcinoma: resection versus transplantation. *Hepatology*. 1999;30:1434–1440.

22. Burroughs AK, Groszmann R, Bosch J, *et al*. Assessment of therapeutic benefit of antiviral therapy in chronic hepatitis C: is hepatic venous pressure gradient a better end point? *Gut*. 2002; 50:425–427.

23. Kumar M, Kumar A, Hissar S, *et al*. Hepatic venous pressure gradient as a predictor of fibrosis in chronic liver disease because of hepatitis B virus. *Liver Int*. 2008;28:690–698.

24. Rincon D, Ripoll C, Lo Iacono OL, *et al*. Antiviral therapy decreases hepatic venous pressure gradient in patients with chronic hepatitis C and advanced fibrosis. *Am J Gastroenterol*. 2006;101:2269–2274.

25. Roberts S, Gordon A, McLean C, *et al*. Effect of sustained viral response on hepatic venous pressure gradient in hepatitis C-related cirrhosis. *Clin Gastroenterol Hepatol*. 2007;5:932–937.

26. Blasco A, Forns X, Carrion JA, *et al*. Hepatic venous pressure gradient identifies patients at risk of severe hepatitis C recurrence after liver transplantation. *Hepatology*. 2006;43:492–499.

27. Carrion JA, Navasa M, Garcia-Retortillo M, *et al*. Efficacy of antiviral therapy on hepatitis c recurrence after liver transplantation: a randomized controlled study. *Gartroenterology*. 2007;132: 1746–1756.

28. Rincon D, Lo Iacono IO, Ripoll C, *et al*. Prognostic value of hepatic venous pressure gradient for in-hospital mortality of patients with severe acute alcoholic hepatitis. *Aliment Pharmacol Ther*. 2007;25:841–848.

29. Steinlauf AF, Garcia-Tsao G, Zakko MF, Dickey K, Gupta T, Groszmann RJ. Low-dose midazolam sedation: an option for patients undergoing serial hepatic venous pressure measurements. *Hepatology*. 1999;29:1070–1073.

30. Trejo R, Alvarez W, Garcia-Pagan JC, *et al*. [The applicability and diagnostic effectiveness of transjugular liver biopsy]. *Med Clin (Barc)*. 1996;107:521–523.

31. Kalambokis G, Manousou P, Vibhakorn S, *et al*. Transjugular liver biopsy–indications, adequacy, quality of specimens, and complications–a systematic review. *J Hepatol*. 2007;47:284–294.

CHAPTER 141

Liver biopsy

Cristina Ripoll and Rafael Bañares

Hospital General Universitario Gregorio Marañón, Universidad Complutense, CiberEHD, Madrid, Spain

---

KEY POINTS

- Liver biopsy is a useful tool in the diagnosis and staging of liver disease and therefore in its management
- It may be performed percutaneously, transvenously or laparoscopically, according to patient characteristics and local practice
- A careful technique should be followed to minimize the possibility of complications
- In order to assure diagnostic accuracy, a quality tissue sample is essential

---

Introduction

Liver biopsy, initially introduced to establish the diagnosis of different causes of liver disease, has now become an important tool that also offers information on prognosis, such as fibrosis staging, and therefore influences treatment decisions.

Concerns regarding the possible complications associated with liver biopsy have led to the development of non-invasive methods to evaluate fibrosis stage (see Chapter 138). Although these methods may avoid performing liver biopsy in some cases, they cannot substitute for a liver biopsy in all settings. The indications for liver biopsy are summarized in Table 141.1. Risk versus benefit should be weighed specifically in cases of dilatation of the intrahepatic biliary tree, particularly with simultaneous cholangitis, mass or cystic lesions. One should bear in mind that the sample obtained with a liver biopsy is very small in comparison to the rest of the parenchyma, and therefore all histological information obtained should be integrated with the rest of the clinical picture.

Practice guidelines regarding the indications, technical issues, contraindications, and complications of liver biopsy have been published recently [1].

A liver biopsy may be performed percutaneously, transvenously, or laparoscopically. A **percutaneous biopsy** offers the advantage that it is easily performed without requiring complex technology. A **transvenous biopsy** offers the advantage of being able to measure the hepatic venous pressure gradient in the same procedure, which provides complementary prognostic information [2,3]. Furthermore, this approach

is preferred in certain situations, such as coagulopathy, in which it is considered that there is a higher risk of post-biopsy complications with percutaneous biopsy. A **laparoscopic biopsy** permits visual examination of the liver surface and the peritoneal cavity and, as the liver surface is observed during the procedure, hemostatic techniques may be applied in case of early bleeding.

The choice of access routes will depend on the characteristics of the patient and the experience and availability of the different procedures in each center (Table 141.2). The use of biopsy to obtain a tissue sample from nodular lesions and laparoscopic biopsy will not be discussed in this chapter.

Procedure
Patient preparation

Prior to performing a liver biopsy, the physician should obtain blood tests, including platelet count and clotting parameters, as well as an ultrasound examination of the liver. The patient should be informed regarding the procedure itself, its complications, the information to be derived from the histological examination of the liver, and the relevance of this information regarding management. Once the patient is completely informed, they should provide written consent.

In many centers, liver biopsies are performed on an outpatient basis. In order to reduce patient anxiety, the precise steps of the procedure should be reiterated, including the possibility of discomfort, the need for active participation, the post-biopsy monitoring, information regarding when the patient can return to their normal activity, and when the results of the histological analysis will be available.

No information is available in the literature regarding the need for fasting prior to the procedure. A light snack may be helpful to avoid vasovagal response and to ensure that the gallbladder is contracted. Placement of a peripheral venous line in patients who are not undergoing a transvenous biopsy is not mandatory but is a reasonable safety measure that can be particularly helpful in the case of a vasovagal response or other early complications.

Textbook of Clinical Gastroenterology and Hepatology, Second Edition. Edited by C. J. Hawkey, Jaime Bosch, Joel E. Richter, Guadalupe Garcia-Tsao, Francis K. L. Chan.
© 2012 Blackwell Publishing Ltd. Published 2012 by Blackwell Publishing Ltd.

Table 141.1 Indications for liver biopsy

Diagnosis
- Liver disease of unknown causes
- Concurrence of more than one cause of liver disease
- Fever of unknown origin
- Focal lesions on imaging studies

Prognosis
- Staging of diffuse liver disease

Table 141.2 Types of liver biopsy by access, type of needle, and image guidance

Biopsy access	Type of needle	Image guidance
Percutaneous liver biopsy	Aspiration Tru-cut style: Manual Automated Plugged biopsy	Blind Previous ultrasound Real-time imaging
Transjugular liver biopsy	Aspiration Tru-cut style	Real-time imaging
Laparoscopic biopsy	Aspiration Tru-cut style: Manual Automated	Direct laparoscopic view

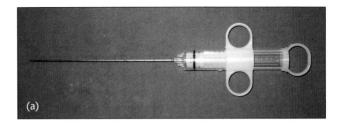

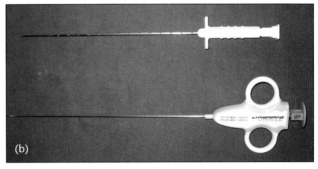

Figure 141.1 (a) Aspiration percutaneous liver biopsy needle. (b) Manual and spring-loaded cutting percutaneous liver biopsy needle (Tru-cut style).

The biopsy
Percutaneous liver biopsy

The use of light sedation is safe and does not increase the risk of the procedure. However, the patient should be able to follow simple instructions regarding breathing cycle. The procedure should be performed in a location where it can be done safely with facilities and personnel able to manage any early complication.

Biopsies can be done "blindly" (guided by palpation/percussion) or they can be image guided (Table 141.2). The classical approach is the **palpation/percussion-guided approach**, which is done typically between the 10th and 12th ribs in the mid-axillary line, in an area of maximal liver dullness. In the **image-guided biopsy**, the optimal site for liver biopsy is evaluated previously by ultrasound (see Video clip 141.1). Although there is some controversy, this approach seems to reduce the incidence of major and minor complications [4,5]. Furthermore, this allows the patient to regulate their breathing cycle to the procedure. Real-time image-guided biopsies are done with direct visualization by imaging techniques, including ultrasound, computed tomography (CT) or magnetic resonance imaging (MRI). No difference in the incidence of complications has been detected when comparing ultrasound guidance in real time to prior to the biopsy [6]. Real-time image guidance is necessary for the biopsy of focal lesions.

The patient is placed on the bed in a comfortable position with their right arm behind their head in order to open up the intercostal spaces. Once the patient is properly positioned, the optimal site for liver biopsy should be localized by palpation/percussion or by ultrasound. The skin should be prepped and the patient draped (see Video clip 141.2). Initially, local anesthetic should be infiltrated in the skin and subcutaneous tissue between the ribs. It is important to choose a site immediately cranial to the rib as the vasculonervous package is localized just under the rib. Further injection of anesthetic into the liver capsule is then recommended, so that pain can be minimized (see Video clip 141.3). Some physicians confirm the localization of the needle within the liver by asking the patient to take a gentle breath; the syringe attached to the needle should move towards the patient's head.

Once the skin is anesthetized a small incision is made through the dermis (see Video clip 1.4). A needle is then introduced between the ribs, without reaching the liver. At this moment, the patient is instructed to take a breath in, a breath out, and then to hold their breath. While the patient is holding their breath, the needle is introduced into the liver (see Video clips 141.5). The direction of the needle should be horizontal with a slight inclination toward the contralateral nipple, unless otherwise indicated by image guidance. Depending on the type of needle used, there are slight differences in the procedure. The two types of needle (see Table 141.2) are the core-aspiration needle (Menghini, Jamshidi or Klatskin style) (Figure 141.1a) and the cutting needle (either manual or spring-loaded) (Figure 141.1b). The latter are frequently called "Tru-cut style." The mechanism of action of the **core-aspiration needles** is based on the suction that is produced while introducing the needle in the liver. Essentially, the "vacuum" effect must be produced within the liver, since the mere act of introducing the needle into the liver will not obtain any tissue. This technique has the advantage that it is quick and easy, involving only one movement. However, it may be more difficult to obtain good samples from patients with greater degrees of fibrosis as the pressure of suction may lead to tissue fragmentation. The **cutting needles** require two steps; first, a troughed needle is introduced within the parenchyma and then an outer sheath or hood is slid over the troughed needle, cutting the parenchyma and securing the tissue sample that has remained within the trough. This mechanism requires greater operator skill but offers the advantage of obtaining better samples, particularly in patients with advanced fibrosis [7]. Newer automated versions of the Tru-cut needle simplify the maneuver, obtaining better samples [8].

If an appropriate sample is not obtained on a first pass, additional passes can be done, although the risk of complications increases with each pass. Obviously, this should be judged on an individual basis by the responsible physician.

A modification of the percutaneous method is the **plugged liver biopsy** in which, once the liver biopsy is done with the cutting needle, the outer sheath remains within the liver and a substance is injected to plug the tract of the biopsy needle. This approach is advocated in those cases with an increased risk of bleeding. When compared to a transjugular approach, this technique was faster and yielded better liver samples, although it did have a higher incidence of hemorrhage [9].

Transvenous liver biopsy

This approach is proposed in those cases in whom it is anticipated that percutaneous liver biopsies will be associated with a high rate of complications (Table 141.3) or in whom additional complementary information with measurement of hepatic venous pressure gradient is sought. The easiest access is through the jugular vein (see Video clip 1.6). The technique for catheterization of the jugular vein and suprahepatic veins has been described extensively elsewhere [10,11] (see Video clip 141.7). Special care should be taken to catheterize the best possible vein, preferably the medium hepatic vein, which is the most vertical vein, allowing easier access with the biopsy needle and the outer sheath (see Video clip 141.8). Over a guidewire, the sheath of the biopsy needle is introduced smoothly within the liver. Special care should be taken to let the sheath of the needle follow the curves within the vascular tree, as the angiographic images offer a bi-dimensional view of a tri-dimensional distribution. The biopsy needle is introduced (see Video clips 141.9 and 141.10) into the liver parenchyma. Depending on the needle type, the biopsy site will be confirmed before (Tru-cut) or after (aspiration) the introduction of the needle. Small veins and a peripheral location should be avoided as biopsies in these locations are associated with more complications. Once the biopsy site is satisfactorily confirmed, the biopsy is taken (see Video clip 141.11). The needles are similar to those used percutaneously: the **aspiration needle** (Figure 141.2) and **cutting needle** (Figure 141.3). The choice of needle is an individual one, but takes into account that, as with

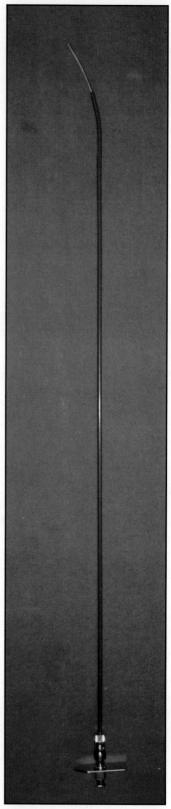

Figure 141.2 Transjugular aspiration liver biopsy needle.

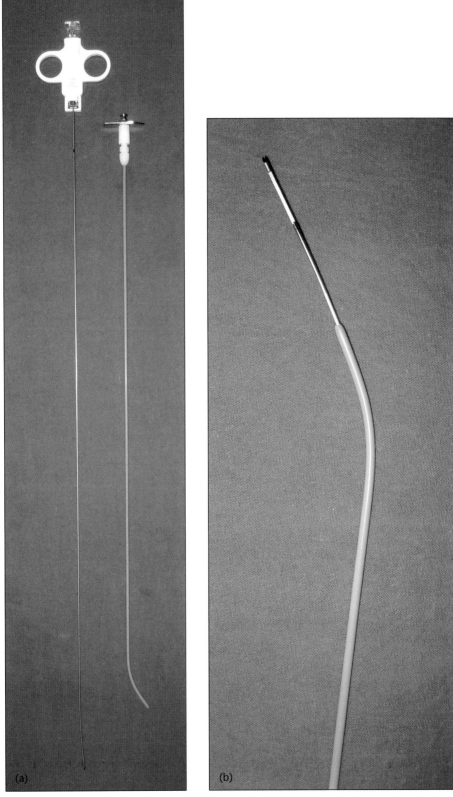

Figure 141.3 (a) Transjugular spring-loaded cutting liver biopsy needle (Tru-cut style). (b) Detail of trough of transjugular cutting liver biopsy needle.

Table 141.3 Situations in which approaches other than the percutaneous approach are preferred for liver biopsy

- Abnormal coagulation indices
- Ascites
- Small liver
- Obesity
- Amyloidosis, liver peliosis
- Suspicion of hepatic infiltration of malignant disease
- Sickle cell disease

percutaneous liver biopsy, a cutting needle obtains better samples than an aspiration needle in cases of advanced fibrosis [7]. After performing the biopsy, injection of contrast allows identification of any immediate complications.

Post biopsy

Once the liver biopsy has been taken, the patient should remain in a resting position. In some centers, the patient is placed in the right lateral decubitus position after a percutaneous liver biopsy in order to "press the puncture site" with their own body weight. In a comparative study in which this position was compared to the combined and supine positions, significantly more pain was felt by those who were in the right lateral decubitus position.

Vital signs should be monitored every 15 minutes for the first hour, then every 30 minutes, and finally hourly. Although some studies have described very short observation periods (even 1 hour) in a fairly large series of patients without complications [12,13], it is recommended to observe the patient for at least 4 hours. Patients can return to their normal daily routine the next day, although lifting any weight should be discouraged for at least 24 hours.

Complications

Physicians who perform liver biopsies should be prepared to face all possible complications. The most frequent complication is **pain**, which is typically located in the epigastrium or right upper quadrant, and right shoulder. Mild discomfort to outright pain may occur in up to 84% of patients. In most cases, the initial pain will slowly decrease. If there is persistent pain despite mild analgesia, further investigation with imaging should be performed. The most important complication of liver biopsy is **bleeding**, which occurs in 1 in every 500 biopsies. Severe bleeding requiring transfusion, hospitalization, radiological intervention or surgery occurs in 1 in 2500–100 000 liver biopsies. In most cases, severe bleeding is clinically evident within the first few hours, although delayed bleeding possibly associated with hyperfibrinolysis has been described. Bleeding risk in patients with cirrhosis is difficult to assess since standard coagulation indices have not shown clear association with bleeding complications [14–16]. Patients who have impaired blood coagulation can receive prophylactic blood products, and the use of an alternative liver biopsy

technique, such as plugged biopsy or transvenous liver biopsy, should be considered. Other possible complications that have been described are pneumothorax, hemothorax, perforation of other organs, bile peritonitis, infection, and hemobilia. Finally, mortality associated with liver biopsy has been described, particularly due to hemorrhage.

Liver tissue sample quality

As there are risks inherent in taking a liver biopsy, it is essential to ensure a quality biopsy. It has been suggested that an adequate biopsy should have between 10 and 15 portal tracts [17,18]. In order to have a sufficient number of portal tracts, the biopsy should be long and wide enough [19]. The ideal biopsy length is at least 3 cm after formalin fixation and taken with a 16 gauge needle (see Video clip 142.12) [1]. Transvenous liver biopsies usually have a smaller number of portal tracts [20]. The sample should be fixed according to local practice for histopathological examination. In the case of fever of unknown origin, part of the sample should be kept in saline serum for appropriate microbiological processing.

References

1. Rockey DC, Caldwell SH, Goodman ZD, Nelson RC, Smith AD. Liver biopsy. *Hepatology*, 2009;49:1017–1044.
2. Burroughs AK, Groszmann R, Bosch J, et al. Assessment of therapeutic benefit of antiviral therapy in chronic hepatitis C: is hepatic venous pressure gradient a better end point? *Gut.* 2002; 50:425–427.
3. Ripoll C, Groszmann R, Garcia-Tsao G, et al. Hepatic venous pressure gradient predicts clinical decompensation in patients with compensated cirrhosis. *Gastroenterology.* 2007;133:481–488.
4. Lindor KD, Bru C, Jorgensen RA, et al. The role of ultrasonography and automatic-needle biopsy in outpatient percutaneous liver biopsy. *Hepatology.* 1996;23:1079–1083.
5. Farrell RJ, Smiddy PF, Pilkington RM, et al. Guided versus blind liver biopsy for chronic hepatitis C: clinical benefits and costs. *J Hepatol.* 1999;30:580–587.
6. Manolakopoulos S, Triantos C, Bethanis S, et al. Ultrasound-guided liver biopsy in real life: comparison of same-day prebiopsy versus real-time ultrasound approach. *J Gastroenterol Hepatol.* 2007;22:1490–1493.
7. Banares R, Alonso S, Catalina MV, et al. Randomized controlled trial of aspiration needle versus automated biopsy device for transjugular liver biopsy. *J Vasc Interv Radiol.* 2001;12:583–587.
8. Sherman KE, Goodman ZD, Sullivan ST, Faris-Young S. Liver biopsy in cirrhotic patients. *Am J Gastroenterol.* 2007;102: 789–793.
9. Sawyerr AM, McCormick PA, Tennyson GS, et al. A comparison of transjugular and plugged-percutaneous liver biopsy in patients with impaired coagulation. *J Hepatol.* 1993;17:81–85.
10. Graham AS, Ozment C, Tegtmeyer K, Lai S, Braner DA. Videos in clinical medicine. Central venous catheterization. *N Engl J Med.* 2007;356:e21.
11. Lebrec D, Goldfarb G, Degott C, Rueff B, Benhamou JP. Transvenous liver biopsy: an experience based on 1000 hepatic tissue samplings with this procedure. *Gastroenterology.* 1982;83: 338–340.

12. Beddy P, Lyburn IL, Geoghegan T, Buckley O, Buckley AR, Torreggiani WC. Outpatient liver biopsy: a prospective evaluation of 500 cases. *Gut.* 2007;56:307.

13. Firpi RJ, Soldevila-Pico C, Abdelmalek MF, Morelli G, Judah J, Nelson DR. Short recovery time after percutaneous liver biopsy: should we change our current practices? *Clin Gastroenterol Hepatol.* 2005;3:926–929.

14. Tripodi A, Salerno F, Chantarangkul V, et al. Evidence of normal thrombin generation in cirrhosis despite abnormal conventional coagulation tests. *Hepatology.* 2005;41:553–558.

15. Ewe K. Bleeding after liver biopsy does not correlate with indices of peripheral coagulation. *Dig Dis Sci.* 1981;26:388–393.

16. McVay PA, Toy PT. Lack of increased bleeding after liver biopsy in patients with mild hemostatic abnormalities. *Am J Clin Pathol.* 1990;94:747–753.

17. Colloredo G, Guido M, Sonzogni A, Leandro G. Impact of liver biopsy size on histological evaluation of chronic viral hepatitis: the smaller the sample, the milder the disease. *J Hepatol.* 2003; 39:239–244.

18. Crawford AR, Lin XZ, Crawford JM. The normal adult human liver biopsy: a quantitative reference standard. *Hepatology.* 1998; 28:323–331.

19. Rocken C, Meier H, Klauck S, Wolff S, Malfertheiner P, Roessner A. Large-needle biopsy versus thin-needle biopsy in diagnostic pathology of liver diseases. *Liver.* 2001;21:391–397.

20. Kalambokis G, Manousou P, Vibhakorn S, et al. Transjugular liver biopsy–indications, adequacy, quality of specimens, and complications–a systematic review. *J Hepatol.* 2007;47:284–294.

CHAPTER 142

Optimal tissue sampling: the pathologist's perspective

Richard H. Lash, Shari L. Taylor and Robert M. Genta

Caris Diagnostics/Miraca, Irving, TX, USA

KEY POINTS

- The pathologist's ability to render a meaningful diagnosis is directly related to the extent and quality of the clinical and endoscopic information provided
- Consolidating mucosal biopsies from a variety of sites into one specimen jar does not aid the diagnoses
- Biopsy and separate identification of normal and abnormal mucosa can be crucial in distinguishing a variety of inflammatory conditions
- Liver biopsy interpretation is especially reliant on accurate and complete clinical and laboratory information, as there is significant overlap of histological findings in a variety of hepatic diseases

---

Introduction

The histopathological examination of tissue is one of the central steps in the investigation of patients with gastrointestinal disorders. This chapter will review, from the pathologists' perspective, the optimal sampling methods to ensure that the most clinically relevant pathological diagnoses are yielded from each procedure.

How to get the most from a mucosal biopsy

Communication of all relevant clinical information is paramount. A set of endoscopic pictures with indications of the biopsy locations conveys the nature and severity of the lesions identified. The optimal biopsy protocol depends on the condition suspected. While certainly all visible abnormalities should be sampled, this is not sufficient; often, adjacent or even distant areas contain information crucial to the interpretation. Each mucosal sample should be placed into a container labeled with the location from which it was taken. The clinician should avoid mixing tissue sites in the same container for a variety of reasons that are reviewed for each organ below. The following is a guide to optimal sampling techniques.

Table 142.1 summarizes the most commonly recommended biopsy protocols for the optimal histopathological evaluation of certain esophageal, gastric, duodenal, and colonic conditions. This list is intended to aid clinicians in obtaining the most satisfactory answers from their pathologists.

General guidelines, including for ulcers and masses throughout the gastrointestinal tract

Specimen handling

It is helpful if biopsy specimens are **handled as little as possible**. The safest way to remove the specimen from the forceps is to gently shake it in the fixative until it detaches. The biopsy will quickly retract on the side of the muscularis mucosae, and histotechnologists will usually be able to embed it on edge, enabling optimally oriented sections (Figure 142.1). Artifacts induced by either the biopsy procedure and/or the subsequent tissue processing can interfere with the biopsy evaluation, including crush and mechanical disruption, electrocautery effect, superficial or insufficient sampling, and poor orientation of the tissue due to suboptimal embedding or twisting. It is also critical to have sufficient formalin (at least 10 times the volume of tissue) for optimal fixation and tissue processing.

Ulcers

Sampling of ulcers and erosions comprising exudate only are usually inadequate. While a diagnosis can only rarely be made from the exudate alone (*e.g.*, amoebae), sampling of mucosal ulcers should include both the mucosa at the ulcer's edge and the underlying granulation tissue. Edge mucosa gives context to the ulcer, possibly revealing adenoma or carcinoma, reparative epithelium when benign, and occasionally evidence of infection (*e.g.*, herpes simplex in the esophagus or anus). Other types of infections are revealed in the base of the ulcer (*e.g.*, cytomegalovirus) as well as some malignancies, particularly signet-ring cell adenocarcinomas.

Masses

Endoscopically identified masses may be mucosal or submucosal. Superficial "picking" at unresectable masses often fails to glean diagnostic material; the most common example is when only the villous adenoma overlying an invasive carcinoma is sampled. A pathologist may suspect the cancer, but if no submucosal tissue is present to assess the infiltrative pattern and desmoplastic stromal reaction, a definitive diagnosis cannot be made. Even more problematic are submucosal masses for which routine mucosal sampling either reveals no

---

Textbook of Clinical Gastroenterology and Hepatology, Second Edition. Edited by C. J. Hawkey, Jaime Bosch, Joel E. Richter, Guadalupe Garcia-Tsao, Francis K. L. Chan.

Table 142.1 Summary of biopsy sampling recommendations

All sites
- Ulcers:
  - Biopsy mucosa at the ulcer's edge and the underlying granulation tissue
- Masses:
  - Multiple biopsies from surface and base (sequential biopsies). In colon, should include submucosa (caution to avoid perforation)

Esophagus
- Barrett's esophagus:
  - Diagnosis: multiple biopsies above the gastroesophageal junction
  - Surveillance: four-quadrant biopsies every 2 cm **and** separately submitted biopsies of any mucosal abnormality
- Eosinophilic esophagitis :
  - Multiple (five) biopsies (separately submitted) from the upper, mid, and lower esophagus

Stomach
- Gastritis:
  - Two biopsies from the antrum, two (separately submitted) biopsies of the corpus, and one from the incisura angularis

Duodenum
- Peptic duodenitis:
  - Sample erythematous or nodular mucosa, most commonly seen in the duodenal bulb. Also, gastric biopsies to exclude *H. pylori*
- Malabsorption:
  - Sample (up to six) distal to the duodenal bulb in one container
  - For disaccharidase studies in pediatric patients, two to three biopsies from the second part of duodenum should be kept in saline (0.9% NaCl)
- Polyps:
  - Polypectomy or generous biopsy (multiple jumbo if possible)

Terminal ileum
- Ileitis
  - Sampling of normal and abnormal ileal mucosa in a single container will suffice. Biopsies of the terminal ileum and the colon should not be submitted in the same container

Colon
- Microscopic colitis and irritable bowel syndrome:
  - Multiple biopsies from the right and (separately submitted) left colon
- Ischemic/infectious colitis:
  - Biopsies of erythematous and/or hemorrhagic mucosa along with mucosa adjacent to the region of ischemia/infarction/ulcer
- Eosinophilic colitis:
  - Pediatric: biopsy rectosigmoid (most common site) and multiple biopsies throughout the colon
  - Adult: multiple biopsies from the right and (separately submitted) left colon
- Inflammatory bowel disease:
  - Diagnosis: sample all segments of the colon, regardless of the endoscopic appearance, **and** separately submitted rectal biopsies. Separately submit samples from grossly inflamed **and** intervening (or distal) normal mucosa **and** diverticula
  - Surveillance: extensive sampling every 10 cm in the colon and every 5 cm in the rectum. Mucosal polyps/irregularity and adjacent mucosa sampled and designated separately
- Polyps:
  - No more than two polyps should be placed in each container. When >1 cm and/or sessile, submit separately
  - Malignant polyps: when small/pedunculated, hot snare; when large/sessile, submucosal saline injection to obtain an intact polyp if possible

abnormality or (worse) a reactive hyperplasia that may suggest an adequate explanation for the endoscopic lesion but mask the underlying cause.

Sampling guidelines by organ
Esophagus
Gastroesophageal reflux disease
The correlation between histology and endoscopy is not reliable, as 50–60% of patients with clinical evidence of gastroesophageal reflux disease (GERD) appear normal histologically, and conversely, histological evidence of reflux esophagitis can

be present in biopsies obtained from endoscopically normal mucosa. Thus, biopsies may be helpful in the clinical setting of GERD to establish disease and exclude other conditions, including Barrett's esophagus. Because many findings traditionally associated with GERD may be found in the most distal aspects of the esophagus of some subjects without GERD, biopsies from the lower esophagus and at least 2.5 cm proximal to the gastroesophageal junction (GEJ) are recommended.

Barrett's esophagus
Barrett's esophagus has been defined by the American College of Gastroenterology as a change in the esophageal epithelium

of any length that can be recognized at endoscopy and is confirmed to have intestinal metaplasia by biopsy of the tubular esophagus [1]. Hence, providing the pathologist with a summary of the endoscopic findings (i.e., whether or not there was an endoscopically visible mucosal region suspicious for Barrett's esophagus) will enable them to render a definitive diagnosis of Barrett's mucosa when intestinal metaplasia is histologically identified in the biopsy. Biopsies obtained from the tubular esophagus above the GEJ and from a displaced squamocolumnar junction are most helpful in establishing a diagnosis of Barrett's esophagus. Once the diagnosis has been established, recommended surveillance protocols include four-quadrant biopsies every 2 cm throughout the Barrett's segment, plus separately submitted biopsies of any mucosal abnormality (ulcer, nodule, mucosal irregularity, or stricture) [2]. In practice, these protocols are infrequently followed; however, dysplasia detection rates have been documented to suffer when only limited biopsies are obtained [3].

Eosinophilic esophagitis

The diagnosis of eosinophilic esophagitis (EoE) similarly rests upon clinical and histological information. Recent consensus recommendations define EoE as a primary clinicopathological

disorder of the esophagus characterized by clinical symptoms of esophageal dysfunction (such as food impaction and dysphagia in adults; feeding aversion/intolerance and vomiting in children), ≥15 eosinophils/high magnification field on biopsy, and absence of GERD [4]. In order to establish a definitive diagnosis of EoE, it is helpful to provide the clinical symptoms that prompted the endoscopy, the endoscopic findings (*e.g.*, furrows, rings, exudates), and whether the patient has failed antireflux therapy. Multiple biopsies, separately submitted from the upper, mid, and lower esophagus, should be obtained, as the disease process may be patchy; a 100% sensitivity for diagnosing EoE has been reported when five biopsy specimens are obtained.

Stomach
Gastritis

For the evaluation of possible *Helicobacter pylori* **gastritis** and **atrophic gastritis**, the submission of at least two biopsies from the antrum and two from the corpus allows the distinction between antrum-predominant and corpus-predominant gastritis, as well as the topographic assessment of atrophy. For example, if both corpus samples show atrophy and both antral biopsies are normal, the diagnosis of autoimmune atrophic gastritis can be supported, since, in contrast to typical *H. pylori* gastritis, the antrum is spared. Because the mucosa of an atrophic corpus (with or without intestinal metaplasia) is microscopically similar to that of the antrum (Figure 142.2), keeping the samples from the two main gastric compartments in separate containers is crucial to an accurate histopathological diagnosis. Separate sampling of the **incisura angularis** is particularly useful to detect early metaplastic changes, a feature that may herald the development of multifocal atrophic gastritis. The assessment of MALT lymphomas (often multifocal) requires a thorough biopsy mapping of the gastric surface.

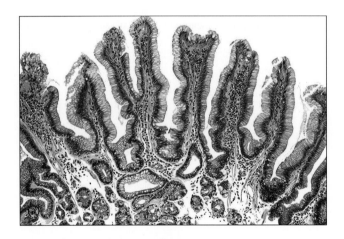

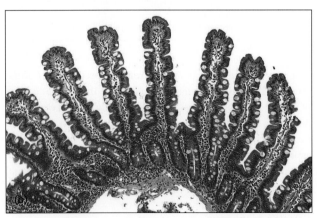

Figure 142.1 Examples of well oriented, satisfactory, mucosal biopsy specimens. (a) Gastric antral mucosa with marked foveolar hyperplasia. (b) Normal small intestinal mucosa.

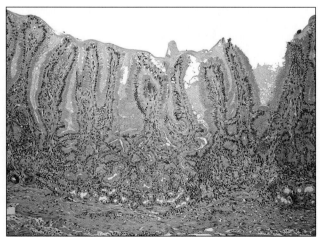

Figure 142.2 Gastric biopsy from the corpus of a patient with pernicious anemia showing severe atrophy, pseudopyloric metaplasia, and focal intestinal metaplasia. If it were labeled as originating from the distal antrum it would be interpreted as essentially normal mucosa with minimal intestinal metaplasia, a finding of little clinical significance.

Polyps

Gastric polyps should be excised or, if large, adequately sampled. Sampling the gastric mucosa surrounding a polyp, as well as the mucosa from other areas of the stomach, will provide additional relevant information. Examples include adenomatous polyps that typically arise in the setting of atrophic gastritis or hyperplastic-like polyps that may be associated with Ménétrier's or Cronkhite–Canada syndromes [5].

Duodenum

Peptic duodenal disease

Duodenal ulcers are rarely biopsied in clinical practice. When multiple randomly distributed duodenal ulcers exist, the possibility of Zollinger–Ellison syndrome should be considered and appropriate biopsy samples taken from the gastric corpus and antrum.

Malabsorption

For the accurate evaluation of suspected cases of **gluten-sensitive enteropathy** (celiac sprue), it is recommended that biopsies be obtained distal to the duodenal bulb to avoid interference from peptic injury or villi blunted due to prominent Brunner's glands. Up to six different biopsy samples should be taken, since the disease is often patchy. Adequate sampling facilitates proper orientation, enabling both the accurate assessment of the degree of villous atrophy and intraepithelial lymphocytosis [6].

Duodenal polyps

Duodenal **polypoidadenomas**, the most common mucosal neoplastic lesions in the duodenum, are typically located in the vicinity of the ampulla of Vater. Polypectomy or generous biopsy is recommended to exclude high-grade dysplasia or adenocarcinoma. Other benign polyps include **hamartomas** that may betray a syndrome in the proper clinical setting. Submucosal **neoplasms** include a variety of mesenchymal tumors, metastases, lymphomas, and direct extension of extraduodenal malignancies. For these lesions, multiple jumbo biopsy specimens are ideal. Common **non-neoplastic lesions** of the duodenum include Brunner's gland hyperplasia, heterotropic gastric mucosa, and heterotropic pancreatic rests, which may be found in the proximal duodenum. Simple direct biopsy of these lesions will suffice to ensure a specific diagnosis.

Ileum

Biopsies of the terminal ileum yield significant diagnostic value only in patients with known or strongly suspected **Crohn's disease**, an abnormal imaging study, or when gross mucosal abnormalities are noted [7]. In such circumstances, sampling of normal and abnormal ileal mucosa in a single container will suffice. Biopsies of an endoscopically normal or mildly "granular" terminal ileum in asymptomatic patients are unlikely to yield diagnostically useful information. Biopsies of the terminal ileum and the colon should never be submitted in the same container, since chronic active inflammation and architectural distortion of the ileum can mimic colitis.

Colon and rectum

Colitis

Endoscopic features that usually do not yield significant pathological findings include pale lymphoid nodules with normal surrounding mucosa, "red ring sign" (often confused with aphthous erosions/ulcers), and isolated patchy erythema (usually secondary to bowel preparation or endoscope trauma). It is critical for the pathologist to be able to discern from where each biopsy is taken as there are substantial histological differences between the right and left colon (Figure 142.3). The right colon normally contains Paneth cells, a denser complement of mononuclear cells, eosinophils in the lamina propria, and more intraepithelial lymphocytes [8]. In the rectosigmoid, however, the presence of Paneth cells indicates a metaplastic change due to chronic inflammatory injury. In the rectum, the crypt architecture is less uniform and the subepithelial collagen layer may be thicker; both these features would be considered abnormal proximally.

Lymphocytic and collagenous colitis are well-recognized causes of chronic watery diarrhea in patients whose colonic mucosa usually is endoscopically normal. The histopathological changes are more prominent in the right than the left colon, and rectal sparing is not uncommon; therefore multiple biopsies separately submitted from the right and left colon should be obtained [9].

Acute self-limited colitis usually produces an endoscopic appearance of patchy erythema, aphthous erosions, and discrete ulcers scattered throughout the colon. However, the

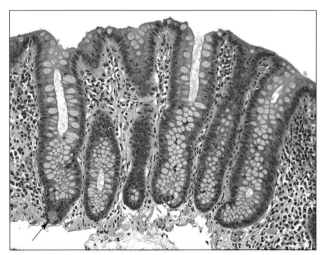

Figure 142.3 The right colonic mucosa normally includes Paneth cells (arrow), but their presence is a marker for chronic injury in the left colon. The right colonic mucosa normally contains more inflammatory cells in the lamina propria than does the left colonic mucosa, and (depending on location) can demonstrate architectural variability. Were this biopsy from the right colon, it would be considered within normal limits, but if from the left colon, could represent quiescent ulcerative colitis.

histopathological findings are non-specific and typically require culture or serological correlation to determine the specific infectious agent, the most common being *Salmonella* and *Campylobacter* spp. *Clostridium difficile*, *Escherichia coli* O157:H7, and *Shigella* spp. may cause a histopathological picture ranging from an acute self-limited type to an exuberant pseudomembranous colitis.

True ischemic colitis secondary to vascular insufficiency most commonly is segmental and involves the "watershed" region (splenic flexure, descending, and transverse colon). However, non-vascular etiologies such as non-steroidal anti-inflammatory drugs (NSAIDs), uremia, radiation, *E. coli* O157:H7, *Shigella* spp., and *C. difficile* may also produce ischemic injury. Biopsies of erythematous and/or hemorrhagic mucosa along with mucosa adjacent to the region of ischemia/infarction/ulcer are recommended to confirm histologically the characteristic ischemic pattern of injury.

In patients with **irritable bowel syndrome**, the endoscopic and histological findings are typically normal; nevertheless, it is important to obtain multiple random, separately submitted right and left colon biopsies, primarily to exclude the possibility of a lymphocytic or collagenous colitis. When **inflammatory bowel disease (IBD)** is suspected, the initial colonoscopy in an untreated patient must include a separately submitted set of rectal biopsies, as a normal rectum (except the distal-most rim of rectal mucosa) is rare in untreated ulcerative colitis. It is also recommended to sample and separately submit all segments of the colon, regardless of the endoscopic appearance, since there is not a strong correlation between the colonoscopic appearance and histological findings. **Crohn's disease** affects the full thickness of the bowel wall, but since only the mucosal surface is evaluated at endoscopy and biopsy samples tend to include only the mucosa, many of the diagnostic features (*e.g.*, transmural inflammation, subserosal lymphoid aggregates) cannot be evaluated. As granulomas are only found in the minority of Crohn's patients, histological documentation of the patchy distribution ("skip lesions") is paramount to establishing the diagnosis. It is therefore critical to separately submit and designate samples from grossly inflamed as well as intervening (or distal) normal mucosa [10,11].

The colonic mucosa adjacent to diverticula may show histological features virtually identical to those found in IBD ("segmental colitis"). Therefore, biopsies taken from the sigmoid colon without mention of diverticula can be misinterpreted as Crohn's disease. Similarly, when rectum and sigmoid biopsies are submitted together in a patient with diverticular disease, a misdiagnosis of ulcerative colitis can be rendered. Therefore, identification and separate submission of biopsies from areas containing diverticula (whether endoscopically seen as inflamed or not) is recommended.

Colitis-associated neoplasia
Patients with IBD, especially **ulcerative colitis**, have an increased risk of developing colon cancer [12]. Morphological examination by an experienced gastrointestinal pathologist remains the gold standard for the detection of dysplasia. Current guidelines for dysplasia surveillance recommend a minimum of 33 biopsies in patients with pancolitis (every 10 cm in the colon and every 5 cm in the rectum) [13]. Optimally, no more than six tissue samples should be submitted in each container. The right colon, left colon, and rectum should be designated separately, as should any endoscopically discernable lesions or polyps. Most often polyps represent non-neoplastic inflammatory proliferations (pseudopolyps). However, occasionally low- or high-grade dysplastic epithelium is encountered in the polypectomy or biopsy specimen. If the dysplasia (low or high grade) is present in a biopsy of a rather large, irregular raised or plaque-like lesion, it should be considered a true DALM ("dysplasia-associated lesion or mass"), and may be an indication for colectomy. Polypoid lesions from areas of colitis should be resected and biopsies of the surrounding flat mucosa should be placed in a separate, specifically labeled container, since dysplasia in adjacent non-polypoid mucosa indicates colitis-associated dysplasia rather than a sporadic adenoma. In the absence of flat dysplasia, studies have suggested that small discrete (adenoma-like) dysplastic polyps occurring in a background of chronic colitis can be managed conservatively with endoscopic resection and close surveillance rather than colectomy.

Colorectal polyps
The pathologist's role in minimizing the risk of colorectal cancer is to identify and document high-risk stratification parameters [14]. These include the presence of more than two adenomas and the surrogate biological marker of cancer risk, the "advanced" adenoma (>1 cm, high-grade dysplasia, or villous architecture). It is therefore important to convey to the pathologist the number, size, and location of the polyps removed. No more than two polyps should be placed in each container, so that the pathologist can accurately quantify the various polyps. All polyps larger than 1 cm, especially sessile ones, should be submitted separately, due to the increased risk of containing invasive carcinoma. If numerous small polyps are encountered (>10), biopsies of several of them should be obtained to determine how many are adenomatous. Larger, villous, and suspicious polyps should always be submitted separately with a clear indication of their provenance.

Liver biopsy (see also Chapter 141)
Multiple methods are available as a means of procuring a liver biopsy for histopathological examination. The most appropriate use of each of these methods, including their advantages and disadvantages, is discussed below [15].

Core needle biopsy
Core biopsies include not only those obtained by the percutaneous and transjugular approaches, but also those obtained intraoperatively. In most instances, this type of liver biopsy will yield the most diagnostic information.

Percutaneous liver biopsy

Various permanent or disposable needle devices are currently available, ranging in external diameter from 0.1 to 0.2 cm; they also differ according to their mechanisms, with suction needles (Menghini, Klatskin, Jamshidi), cutting needles (Vim-Silverman, Tru-cut), or spring-loaded cutting needles available. If cirrhosis is suspected clinically, a cutting needle is preferred over a suction needle because fibrotic tissue tends to fragment with the use of the latter.

From a histological standpoint, this type of biopsy will provide the best diagnostic information in most situations. Given the large size of the liver relative to the biopsy size, sampling error can occur (see below). This is a problem particularly in chronic biliary tract disorders, where the diagnostic bile duct lesions can be patchy; in primary sclerosing cholangitis, the diagnostic lesions may be absent on a needle biopsy containing only small-caliber bile ducts.

Transjugular biopsy

The main disadvantage of this technique is that the samples obtained are often small and fragmented. Tissue specimens usually measure between 0.3 and 2 cm in length, and the procedure generally requires multiple passes.

Wedge biopsy

Theoretically, an advantage of a wedge biopsy is the ability to procure a larger sample of liver tissue; however, evaluation of the wedge biopsy is fraught with difficulty owing to the normally increased fibrous tissue in the subcapsular region (Figure 142.4). As a result, an accurate estimate of the degree of fibrosis (staging) can be difficult. In addition, the subcapsular region may contain non-specific chronic inflammation that can be misinterpreted as a hepatic process. In general, wedge biopsies may be useful in the evaluation of a mass lesion or in nodular regenerative hyperplasia. In the latter instance, a wedge biopsy

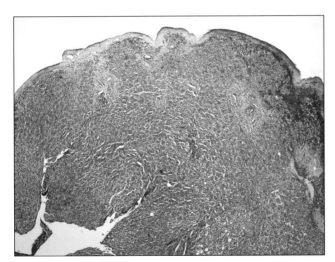

Figure 142.4 Wedge biopsy of the liver viewed at low power. Note the increased fibrous tissue in the immediate subcapsular region; this is a normal finding for subcapsular liver tissue and can impact accurate staging of chronic liver disease. Masson trichrome stain.

may allow the nodular (but not fibrotic) architecture to be better appreciated than on a core biopsy. However, a core biopsy obtained at the time of surgery usually provides a satisfactory artifact-free sample.

Fine-needle aspiration biopsy

Fine-needle aspiration biopsy of the liver is performed under ultrasonographic or computed tomography (CT) guidance, and is used mostly to obtain samples from a liver mass suspected of being malignant. The diagnostic accuracy ranges from 80% to 95% and is strongly related to the expertise of the cytopathologist. It is important to remember that a negative finding does not necessarily rule out a malignant tumor, which may be missed by the aspiration. Fine-needle aspiration biopsy is generally a very safe procedure; however, in patients with malignant tumors, there is a small risk of seeding the needle tract with neoplastic cells.

Tissue sampling

It is clear that there is potential for sampling error with needle liver biopsy. The number of portal tracts present in the specimen is one of the major determinants of sample adequacy. More than 11 portal tracts have been proposed as an indicator of specimen adequacy. In general, the presence of 5–10 portal tracts will be adequate for the evaluation of drug-induced hepatitis, chronic hepatitic processes, and steatohepatitis; however, 10–20 portal tracts are often needed to assess lesions of small bile ducts (primary biliary cirrhosis or allograft rejection). In conditions affecting primarily large bile ducts (*e.g.*, primary sclerosing cholangitis), biopsy findings are often non-specific and may even be normal; in these situations, radiographic examination [such as endoscopic retrograde cholangiopancreatography (ERCP)] may be a better diagnostic modality. The number of portal tracts is related to the length of the specimen; the most recent American Association for the Study of Liver Disease (AASLD) position paper recommends a biopsy of 2–3 cm in length [16]. In addition, a 16 gauge needle is recommended for non-neoplastic diseases of the liver in order to reduce sampling error; an 18 gauge needle may be adequate for evaluation of neoplastic processes [16]. The exception is the transjugular procedure, as several passages are often needed to obtain a satisfactory amount of material. In this instance, at least three cores with a 19 gauge needle are recommended [17].

Specimen handling

High-quality histological preparations depend on the rapid fixation of fresh tissues. The longer a specimen remains exposed to the air or in a non-fixative medium (*e.g.*, saline solution), the more likely that drying or autolysis artifacts will affect the tissue morphology and ultimately the histopathological interpretation. Before being immersed in the fixative liquid, particular care should be taken to avoid squeezing the biopsy during handling, which can affect the assessment of architecture. The most widely used fixative is **10% neutral**

buffered formalin. When special diagnostic questions are anticipated, it is recommended that the case be discussed with the pathologist prior to the procedure to ensure that the specimen is handled in the manner appropriate to the test or tests that will be required. A portion of fresh material may be snap-frozen for the staining of lipids (which are dissolved during routine processing), viral quantification, molecular biology, or for storage in tissue banks. Glutaraldehyde fixative is used when electron microscopy is to be performed; this is essential for the diagnosis of several mitochondrial and metabolic diseases, some cholestatic diseases in children, and for the detection of viral particles. It is no longer necessary to separately submit fresh tissue for iron or copper quantitation, as there are assays widely available using formalin-fixed, paraffin-embedded material. It is particularly important never to submit liver tissue in saline for the purpose of iron quantitation, as there may be up to 50% iron loss after just 1 hour of the tissue being placed in the saline.

Special stains

Hematoxylin and eosin (H&E) is the stain initially used for routine liver biopsy evaluation. Utilizing this stain alone, a pathologist can assess the liver architecture, overall pattern of liver injury, and the presence or absence of additional abnormalities such as steatosis or granulomas. While in some cases of heavy iron overload the iron pigment may be visible on H&E-stained sections, an iron stain (such as Prussian blue) readily highlights the iron as a blue granular material (Figure 142.5). This stain makes it possible to discern the pattern of iron deposition, such as primarily hepatocytic (in HFE-related hereditary hemochromatosis) or primarily mesenchymal (in secondary causes of iron overload such as transfusional or chronic liver disease associated).

One of the major uses of the **periodic acid–Schiff (PAS)** stain with diastase is in highlighting the alpha-1-antitrypsin globules in patients with alpha-1-antitrypsin deficiency. These periportal globules are typically variable in size. An immuno-histochemical stain for alpha-1-antitrypsin is also available and may be used to confirm the nature of the globules. A PAS stain with diastase will also stain ceroid pigment within macrophages and can be useful in identifying areas of previous hepatocellular injury.

Trichrome stains (Masson's or Gomori's) highlight collagen and are used to evaluate the degree of fibrosis within the biopsy. In addition to these stains, a **reticulin stain** is used by some pathologists to assess the parenchymal framework. Using this stain, the hepatocyte cell plate thickness is readily apparent. Even more important is its use in evaluating a hepatic mass or nodule for hepatocellular carcinoma: in all but the most well-differentiated lesions, there is loss of the normal reticulin framework.

Copper stains may be useful in evaluating the liver biopsy for evidence of chronic cholestasis. This may be done by staining for copper directly (rhodanine or rubeanic acid stains) (Figure 142.6) or by staining of copper-associated protein (Victoria blue, orcein, or aldehyde fuchsin). It should be noted that copper stains may not be reliable for evaluation of Wilson disease; quantitative copper determination, which can be performed on the paraffin-embedded tissue, is the method of choice.

Conclusions

Both mucosal and liver biopsies have become essential tools in the diagnosis and management of digestive conditions. Clinicians, however, should keep in mind that, unlike automatically generated chemical and hematological laboratory tests, histopathology is not an exact science. Pathologists base their diagnoses on visual observations, biased knowledge, interpretations, and opinions, and are subject to judgment, just like other physicians. Only through the development of a coordinated team whereby clinicians and pathologists communicate effectively can useful results ensue.

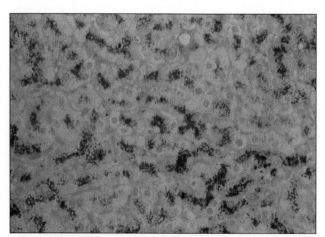

Figure 142.5 Prussian blue stain for iron. The iron granules stain intensely blue and are predominantly within hepatocytes. This is the pattern of iron deposition seen in patients with HFE-associated hereditary hemochromatosis.

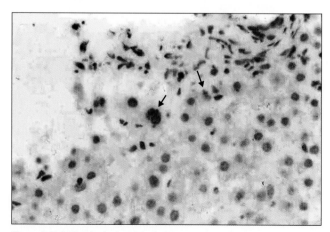

Figure 142.6 The rhodanine stain for copper stains copper granules within hepatocytes red (arrows), indicating chronic cholestasis in this patient with early primary biliary cirrhosis.

Acknowledgements

The authors acknowledge substantive contributions by colleagues Carlos Torres MD and Qinghua Yang MD, PhD.

References

1. Sampliner RE. Updated guidelines for the diagnosis, surveillance, and therapy of Barrett's esophagus. *Am J Gastroenterol.* 2002;97:1888–1895.
2. Wang KK, Sampliner RE. Updated guidelines 2008 for the diagnosis, surveillance and therapy of Barrett's esophagus. *Am J Gastroenterol.* 2008;103:788–797.
3. Abrams JA, Kapel RC, Lindberg GM, *et al.* Adherence to biopsy guidelines for Barrett's esophagus surveillance in the community setting in the United States. *Clin Gastroenterol Hepatol.* 2009; 7:736–742.
4. Furuta GT, Liacouras CA, Collins MH, *et al.* Eosinophilic esophagitis in children and adults: a systematic review and consensus recommendations for diagnosis and treatment. *Gastroenterology.* 2007;133:1342–1363.
5. Carmack SW, Genta RM, Graham DY, Lauwers GY. Management of gastric polyps: a pathology-based guide for gastroenterologists. *Nat Rev Gastroenterol Hepatol.* 2009;6:331–341.
6. Villanacci V. The problem of biopsies in the diagnosis of celiac disease. *Gastrointest Endosc.* 2009;69:983–984.
7. McHugh JB, Appelman HD, McKenna BJ. The diagnostic value of endoscopic terminal ileum biopsies. *Am J Gastroenterol.* 2007; 102:1084–1089.
8. Paski SC, Wightman R, Robert ME, Bernstein CN. The importance of recognizing increased cecal inflammation in health and avoiding the misdiagnosis of nonspecific colitis. *Am J Gastroenterol.* 2007;102:2294–2299.
9. Carmack SW, Lash RH, Gulizia JM, Genta RM. Lymphocytic disorders of the gastrointestinal tract: a review for the practicing pathologist. *Adv Anat Pathol.* 2009;16:290–306.
10. Yantiss RK, Odze RD. Optimal approach to obtaining mucosal biopsies for assessment of inflammatory disorders of the gastrointestinal tract. *Am J Gastroenterol.* 2009;104:774–783.
11. Nikolaus S, Schreiber S. Diagnostics of inflammatory bowel disease. *Gastroenterology.* 2007;133:1670–1689.
12. Rubin DT, Kavitt RT. Surveillance for cancer and dysplasia in inflammatory bowel disease. *Gastroenterol Clin North Am.* 2006; 35:581–604.
13. Rubin DT. An updated approach to dysplasia in IBD. *J Gastrointest Surg.* 2008;12:2153–2156.
14. Levin B, Lieberman DA, McFarland B, *et al.* Screening and surveillance for the early detection of colorectal cancer and adenomatous polyps, 2008: a joint guideline from the American Cancer Society, the US Multi-Society Task Force on Colorectal Cancer, and the American College of Radiology. *Gastroenterology.* 2008; 134:1570–1595.
15. Czaja AJ, Carpenter HA. Optimizing diagnosis from the medical liver biopsy. *Clin Gastroenterol Hepatol.* 2007;5:898–907.
16. Rockey DC, Caldwell SH, Goodman ZD, Nelson RC, Smith AD. Liver biopsy. *Hepatology.* 2009;49:1017–1044.
17. Cholongitas E, Quaglia A, Samonakis D, *et al.* Transjugular liver biopsy in patients with diffuse liver disease: comparison of three cores with one or two cores for accurate histological interpretation. *Liver Int.* 2007;27:646–653.

PART 4
Primer of Treatments

CHAPTER 143

Drug prescription in liver disease

Guido Stirnimann[1] and Jürg Reichen[2]

[1]University of Berne, Berne, Switzerland
[2]University Clinic of Visceral Surgery and Medicine, Inselspital, Berne, Switzerland

KEY POINTS

- Hepatic clearance depends on flow and intrinsic clearance, the latter reflecting the activity of different drug metabolizing enzymes and drug transporters
- Alterations in hepatic perfusion, including a decrease in portal flow, barriers to diffusion, and intra- and extra-hepatic shunting, affect mainly drugs with a high extraction (flow-limited clearance)
- Alterations in drug metabolizing enzymes and drug transporters affect mainly drugs with a low extraction ratio and low protein binding (enzyme-limited clearance). Decreased protein binding is an important determinant of hepatic clearance after oral administration of drugs (binding-sensitive, enzyme-limited clearance)
- Knowledge of the pathway(s) of metabolism and elimination of drugs is mandatory to make rational dose adjustments
- No liver test reliably predicts pharmacokinetics and pharmacodynamics in individual patients with liver disease. The Child–Pugh classification gives the best indication of hepatic reserve and the extent of dose adjustment
- Generally, drugs with a high first-pass metabolism should be avoided in cirrhosis
- Drug effects and, if indicated/available, plasma concentrations should be closely monitored. Dose should be adjusted accordingly rather than using a standard dose ("start low, go slow")
- Be aware of the potential for altered pharmacodynamics of drugs in advanced liver disease

Determinants of hepatic drug metabolism and excretion

General considerations on organ clearance and its determinants

The liver with its portal blood supply and its abundant drug metabolizing and transporting proteins plays a central role in drug disposition. The concept of organ clearance – although physiologically suspect – is still helpful to assess anticipated changes in clearance of drugs in patients with liver disease. **Hepatic clearance** (Cl_{hep}) is a function of the elimination rate constant k_e:

$$k_e = Cl_{hep} * C \qquad (143.1)$$

Equation 143.1 implies that more drug is eliminated per time if plasma concentration (C) increases. This equation holds true as long as the enzyme/transport system responsible for metabolism/elimination is not saturated.

An important determinant of k_e is the metabolic capacity of the liver, which can be approximated by measuring the extraction (E):

$$E = (C_{in} - C_{out})/C_{in} \qquad (143.2)$$

where C_{in} and C_{out} are the drug concentration in the in- and out-flow tract, respectively. Equation 143.2 assumes a rapid equilibration of drug concentration in the sinusoids between sinusoidal inflow from the hepatic artery and portal vein. Hepatic clearance can then be defined as the product of the hepatic blood flow (Q) and extraction ratio:

$$Cl_{hep} = Q * E \qquad (143.3)$$

Equation 143.3 predicts that drugs with high E depend on hepatic perfusion, while drugs with low E depend on the process of metabolism/elimination for hepatic clearance. In other words, the elimination of drugs with high E is flow dependent, while that of drugs with low E is enzyme dependent (Figure 143.1).

The extraction ratio is a function of the Michaelis–Menten kinetics of the transport or metabolic processes leading to drug elimination, the so-called intrinsic clearance Cl_{int} (which is the ratio V_{max}/K_m of the metabolic or transport process governing elimination of the drug). Taking also drug binding into account, Equation 143.3 can be written as:

$$Cl_{hep} = Q \cdot (f_u \cdot Cl_{int})/(Q + f_u \cdot Cl_{int}) \qquad (143.4)$$

where f_u is the unbound fraction of the drug.

Specific processes determining hepatic clearance in health and disease

Expanding on the considerations above, five processes are involved in determining Cl_{hep} of a given compound. A further two, namely renal elimination and alterations of volume of distribution, can play an important role in drug disposition in patients with liver disease:

Textbook of Clinical Gastroenterology and Hepatology, Second Edition. Edited by C. J. Hawkey, Jaime Bosch, Joel E. Richter, Guadalupe Garcia-Tsao, Francis K. L. Chan.

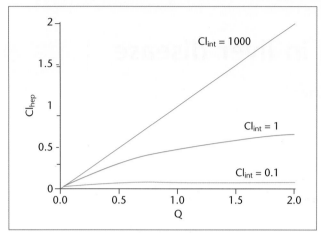

Figure 143.1 Relationship between hepatic perfusion and clearance. Illustration shows the effect of a drug's intrinsic hepatic clearance (Cl_{int}) on the relationship between total hepatic clearance (Cl_{hep}) and hepatic perfusion (Q). When the intrinsic hepatic clearance is very high, the hepatic extraction is close to 100%. In this case the total hepatic clearance equals hepatic blood flow and is thus described as "flow limited." In contrast, when intrinsic hepatic clearance is very low, changes in hepatic blood flow will have no effect on total hepatic clearance, which is then said to be "enzyme limited." (This figure was published in *Clinical Gastroenterology and Hepatology*, Wilfred M. Weinstein, Christopher J. Hawkey, Jaime Bosch, Drug prescription in liver disease, Pages 1–5, Copyright Elsevier, 2005.)

Phase 1 metabolism

This encompasses mostly oxidative processes mediated by the cytochrome P450 (CYP) super-family. Phase 1 reactions serve generally to render xenobiotics more reactive, thereby allowing phase 2 reactions to take place. CYP3A4 is the most abundant CYP isoenzyme and is responsible for the biotransformation of 50% of drugs. Its activity is highly variable between individuals and this variation is more important than the decrease associated with chronic liver disease.

Loss of function of the different isoenzymes is not uniform: CYP2C19 declines early and rapidly, while CYP2E1 function is preserved even in late-stage liver disease. CYP1A2 and CYP2D6 decline steadily with decreasing liver function [1]. Cholestatic liver disease affects mainly CYP2E1 and CYP2C.

Phase 2 metabolism

Phase 2 metabolism encompasses a variety of conjugation reactions of reactive metabolites resulting from phase 1 metabolism and aims to render xenobiotics suitable for biliary and/or renal excretion. The major enzyme classes in phase 2 are the UDP-glucuronyl transferases, N-acetyl-transferases, glutathione transferases, and sulfate transferases.

In chronic liver disease, the activity of glucuronyl transferase is maintained until late in the disease for many substrates, including morphine and benzodiazepines. However, glucuronidation of other drugs, including lamotrigine, zidovudine, and mycophenolate mofetil, is impaired in advanced liver disease. The activity of N-acetyltransferases and glutathione transferases declines more or less in parallel with the Child classification.

Phase 3 elimination

Intestinal absorption, and renal and/or biliary elimination of xenobiotics resulting from phase 1/2 metabolism is mediated by several super-families of transport proteins: on the sinusoidal side, the solute carrier protein family SLC, and on the canalicular side P glycoprotein and the ABC transporter proteins [2].

Changes in drug transporter activity are only just beginning to be explored in patients with chronic liver disease and no conclusions can yet be reached about their role in altered metabolic clearance of drugs in cirrhosis. However, clear predictions can often be made about drug disposition in cholestatic liver disease. This is particularly germane for cytostatics with predominantly biliary excretion [3].

Some drugs excreted into the bile undergo enterohepatic circulation. This often involves deconjugation by intestinal bacteria (a reverse phase 2 reaction) and active or passive reabsorption in the gut.

Hepatic perfusion

Hepatic perfusion is a major determinant of hepatic clearance (Equations 143.3 and 143.4). The architecture of the liver sinusoid with its fenestrations allows free access of protein-bound drugs to the transport proteins in the sinusoidal membrane.

Hepatic perfusion is markedly altered in chronic liver disease by different processes:

- Decreased portal perfusion and in end-stage liver disease, even reversal of flow in the portal vein
- Portosystemic shunts; these can occur in the absence of intrinsic liver disease, e.g.; in portal vein thrombosis
- Alterations in the intrahepatic diffusion process, in particular by sinusoidal capillarization [4].

Protein binding

Due to decreased synthesis of drug-binding proteins, in particular albumin and α_1 acidic glycoprotein, the unbound fraction of drugs is often increased. Another mechanism for altered protein binding of drugs is displacement of drugs by retention of cholephiles such as bilirubin.

Low plasma concentrations of binding proteins will result in an increased unbound fraction (f_u) of drug in plasma; this can result in increased clearance if metabolic capacity of the liver is maintained.

For high-extraction drugs, the rate of elimination is not dependent on plasma protein binding because the equilibration processes are fast enough to allow almost complete drug removal upon one passage through the liver. Decreased protein binding will therefore lead to an unchanged total and increased free concentration. Fortunately, higher free concentrations will only become clinically relevant for drugs with a narrow therapeutic margin given as a constant intravenous infusion.

Volume of distribution

Ascites can markedly increase the volume of distribution of hydrophilic drugs. If rapid achievement of therapeutic drug levels is desirable, this may require an increase in the loading dose. A practical example would be β-lactam antibiotics.

Renal elimination
Functional renal failure in end-stage cirrhosis can impact on renal excretion. It has to be kept in mind that serum creatinine is a poor indicator of renal function in patients with end-stage liver disease. Measurement of cystatin C could more accurately reflect renal function in patients with cirrhosis [5].

First-pass metabolism
An important aspect of the gut–liver axis is first-pass metabolism. A drug administered orally passes two tissues with extensive metabolic and transport capacity, namely the **gut** and the **liver**. First-pass metabolism reflects the proportion of absorbed drug that is metabolized or excreted by these two organs. Clearance after p.o. administration ($Cl_{p.o.}$) of a drug is determined by f_u and intrinsic clearance:

$$Cl_{p.o.} = f_u \cdot Cl_{int} \tag{143.5}$$

Both hepatocytes and enterocytes harbor enzymes and transport proteins with a great capacity for presystemic elimination of drugs. The enterocyte is rich in CYP3A and P glycoprotein, while the hepatocyte has a much broader variety of enzymes and transporters [2]. Loss of first-pass metabolism in liver disease can lead to a marked and potentially dangerous increase in systemic availability of orally administered drugs. This concerns mainly drugs with a high extraction ratio (Equation 143.3; Table 143.1). Sometimes, it can be difficult to predict whether loss of first-pass metabolism is due to hepatic or intestinal changes.

A paradigm is the increase in bioavailability of midazolam in patients with a transjugular intrahepatic protosystemic shunt (TIPS): it appears logical to assume that this is due to the shunt preventing contact between blood derived from the intestine and hepatocytes; surprisingly, the loss of first-pass metabolism is due to a marked decrease in CYP3A4 in the intestine [6].

It needs to be pointed out that portosystemic shunting with loss of first-pass metabolism occurs not only in patients with chronic liver disease, but also in patients with non-cirrhotic portal hypertension and with portal vein thrombosis. The fraction of a dose escaping first-pass metabolism (F_e) can be estimated from:

$$F_e = 1 - Q_{eff} * E \tag{143.6}$$

where Q_{eff} is the mesenteric blood flow passing through the liver. Unfortunately, in most cases, no good estimate of Q_{eff} can be obtained because this would require an estimate of total hepatic and portosystemic blood flow.

Altered pharmacodynamics in chronic liver disease
Changes in the receptors for different drugs as well as in post-receptor signal transmission can lead to altered pharmacodynamics. Differences between alterations in pharmacokinetics and in pharmacodynamics are often difficult to differentiate.

Sedatives and analgesics
Increased susceptibility to benzodiazepines and opioid analgesics in cirrhotic patients is well known. Such drugs can induce **hepatic encephalopathy** at therapeutic doses. Possible mechanisms include alterations in the blood–brain barrier, increased susceptibility due to an increased density of GABA receptors, and pharmacokinetic alterations.

Diuretics
The effect of loop diuretics in cirrhotic patients with ascites is reduced owing to decreased delivery to their site of action in the renal tubule. This is more marked for furosemide than for torasemide. Excessive diuresis may precipitate hepatorenal syndrome and refractoriness to loop diuretics. For further details, see Chapter 97.

Beta-receptor antagonists
In patients with **cirrhosis**, a decreased sensitivity to β-adrenoreceptor antagonists exists. This is not only due to reduced receptor density, but also to a post-receptor defect that can be overcome with NO donors.

Non-steroidal anti-inflammatory drugs
Prostaglandin synthesis is essential in maintaining renal perfusion in patients with portal hypertension and the associated hyperdynamic circulation. Therefore, non-steroidal anti-inflammatory drugs (NSAID)s and cyclooxygenase 2 (COX2) inhibitors can precipitate renal failure in patients with cirrhosis even in the absence of ascites. If such drugs are unavoidable in the patient with chronic liver disease, frequent monitoring of serum creatinine and electrolytes is advisable.

Table 143.1 Examples of drugs with low and high hepatic extraction ratios (only a few drugs have an intermediate extraction ratio)

Low extraction ratio (<0.3)	High extraction ratio (>0.7)
Carbamazepine	Carvedilol
Diazepam	Chlormethiaziol
Phenobarbital	Diltiazem
Phenprocoumon	Ergot alkaloids
Phenytoin	Lidocaine
Salicylic acid	Metoprolol
Theophylline	Meperidine
Valproate	Midazolam
Warfarin	Morphine
	Nitroglycerine
	Pentazocine
	Propranolol
	Verapamil

Dose adjustments in chronic liver disease

Dose adjustment is necessary in **cirrhosis** but probably not in acute or chronic hepatitis. Cholestatic liver diseases, in particular obstructive jaundice, requires dose adjustment for drugs with a predominantly biliary excretion.

A variety of tests, including quantitative liver function tests, analysis of elimination of model compounds, breath tests probing different metabolic pathways, determination of serum bile acids as a measure of portosystemic shunting, etc., have been proposed as tools to reliably predict drug disposition in the cirrhotic patient. None has withstood the test of time; even those with a good predictive value for drug disposition in patients with cirrhosis have not made it into clinical practice since they are too cumbersome to be performed outside of a research setting.

The best – albeit far from perfect – parameter to predict the need for and extent of dose adjustments is the **Child–Pugh classification** (Table 143.2). Pharmacokinetic studies in patients with impaired liver function and stratified by Child class is required by the major drug regulatory agencies, including the FDA and EMEA, for most drugs before marketing. It has to be realized though, that older drugs were not usually tested in patients with impaired liver function and newer drugs are only tested in Child A and B patients, meaning that pharmacokinetic data for Child C patients are often not available. Dose reductions of 50% and 75% for Child A and B patients are safe. If time permits, starting with a low dose and slowly increasing dosage while watching for pharmacodynamic success and adverse events (**"start slow, go slow"**) should avoid drug toxicity in patients with chronic liver disease.

In general, for **high-extraction drugs** given orally, both loading and maintenance dose should be reduced according to the anticipated increase in bioavailability. When given intravenously, a normal loading dose can be used, but the maintenance dose should be decreased according to the functional impairment.

For **low-extraction drugs**, dose adaptation depends on whether the drug is highly protein bound or not (see Equation 143.4). If it is, clearance can actually be increased since f_u is increased. Measurement of the free drug concentration is recommended for compounds with a narrow therapeutic window (e.g., diphenylhydantoin). In general, the loading dose is normal while the maintenance dose should be reduced according to the estimated reduction in hepatic functional reserve.

Sedatives and analgesics

Benzodiazepines with minor phase 1 metabolism, such as lorazepam or oxazepam, are preferred. Opiates should not be withheld from patients with advanced liver disease, but their dose should be adjusted for altered first-pass metabolism and consideration given to overdosing in patients with worsening hepatic encephalopathy. Analgesic drugs for which no antagonist is available should be avoided. In chronic liver disease doses of acetaminophen should not exceed 4 g (2.5 g if cautious), particularly when glutathione stores can be expected to be low (see also Chapter 92).

Beta-receptor antagonists

Many β-antagonists – in particular propranolol – are subject to extensive first-pass metabolism, resulting in elevated plasma concentrations in patients with advanced liver disease. In clinical practice, preference should be given to long-acting formulations since they avoid the very high peaks seen after oral administration.

Cytostatics

There are several problems in administering cytotoxic drugs to patients with liver disease:

- Exacerbation of pre-existing liver disease, in particular hepatitis B;
- Frequent intrinsic hepatotoxicity of cytostatic agents;
- Liver metastases can adversely affect liver function.

Table 143.2 The Child–Pugh classification and its impact on dose adjustment

Parameter	A	B	C
Serum bilirubin			
(μmoles/L)	<35	35–50	>50
(mg/dL)	<2	2–3	>3
Serum albumin (g/L)	>35	28–35	<28
Prothrombin time	<4	4–6	>6
Ascites	None	Controlled Not tense	Tense Refractory
Encephalopathy	None	1–2	3–4
Dose reduction (%)	50	75	No recommendation can be given

There are different dose-reduction regimens, mostly based on bilirubin levels [3].

Adverse drug reactions in patients with liver disease

As discussed in Chapter 92, the incidence of hepatic adverse events is usually not increased in patients with chronic liver disease. The question is not whether the patient will develop hepatotoxicity, but whether there is sufficient functional reserve to allow for hepatotoxicity. In other words, **utmost caution** is recommended regarding the use of potentially hepatotoxic drugs in Child C patients. In all patients with underlying liver disease, frequent monitoring of liver enzymes is recommended.

There are a few specific adverse effects that should be taken into consideration when treating cirrhotic patients. One concerns **myelotoxicity** which may become rapidly clinically relevant in patients with hypersplenism and pre-existing thrombocytopenia and/or leukopenia. **Neutropenia** induced by β-lactam antibiotics appears to have an increased incidence in cirrhotic patients. In obstructive cholestasis, increased susceptibility to **aminoglycoside nephrotoxocity** must be expected.

References

1. Frye RF, Zgheib NK, Matzke GR, *et al.* Liver disease selectively modulates cytochrome P450–mediated metabolism. *Clin Pharmacol Ther.* 2006;80:235–245.
2. Li P, Wang GJ, Robertson TA, Roberts MS. Liver transporters in hepatic drug disposition: an update. *Curr Drug Metab.* 2009;10:482–498.
3. Field KM, Michael M. Part II: Liver function in oncology: towards safer chemotherapy use. *Lancet Oncol.* 2008;9:1181–1190.
4. Reichen J. The role of sinusoidal endothelium in liver function. *News Physiol Sci.* 1999;14:117–120.
5. Cholongitas E, Shusang V, Marelli L, *et al.* Review article: renal function assessment in cirrhosis - difficulties and alternative measurements. *Aliment Pharmacol Ther.* 2007;26:969–978.
6. Chalasani N, Gorski JC, Patel NH, Hall SD, Galinsky RE. Hepatic and intestinal cytochrome P450 3A activity in cirrhosis: Effects of transjugular intrahepatic portosystemic shunts. *Hepatology.* 2001;34:1103–1108.

CHAPTER 144
Nutritional assessment and support

T. E. Bowling
Nottingham University Hospitals, Nottingham, UK

KEY POINTS

- Undernutrition affects up to 40% of hospitalized patients
- Causes of undernutrition are multifactorial. It increases morbidity/ mortality and cost of care
- All patients should be screened, with an appropriate care plan commenced if nutritionally at risk
- Always consider optimizing oral intake before more interventional methods
- For long-term feeding, stoma access is preferred to nasal tubes
- Enteral feeding is favored over parenteral feeding because of lower complications and costs

Introduction

Malnutrition and **undernutrition** are terms often used interchangeably. Although there is no universally agreed definition of either term, malnutrition is commonly taken as a nutritional status that deviates from normal. This can either be due to overnutrition (obesity) or undernutrition. This chapter will deal only with adult undernutrition, which can be defined as an inadequate intake of energy (and is sometimes termed "protein energy malnutrition").

Prevalence

Undernutrition is a major global problem, with a cited prevalence in the United States and many European countries of approximately 5% of the population as a whole. Up to 10% of free-living elderly are undernourished, with a further 14% at risk of becoming so. These figures rise dramatically with illness.

In hospitalized patients the situation is even more pronounced. The quoted prevalence of undernutrition ranges from 5% to 50% (body mass index <18.5 kg/m²), but within clinical subgroups these figures are much higher: cancer (5–80%), elderly (0–85%), HIV/AIDS (8–98%), and gastroenterological disease (3–100%). Furthermore, most patients will lose weight in hospital through a combination of their illness, its investigation and treatment, and poor quality food provision [1,2].

Causes and consequences of undernutrition

The factors that can lead to undernutrition are listed in Table 144.1. Overall there is an undeniable increase in both morbidity and mortality for the undernourished patient compared to the normally nourished one, and this leads to longer lengths of hospital stay and increased costs of care [3]. Recent estimations have calculated that it costs four times as much to look after an undernourished surgical patient. There can therefore be no doubt that undernutrition and its consequences, both clinical and financial, put a very considerable pressure on healthcare economies.

Assessment

Assessing a patient's nutritional status is sadly often neglected or overlooked. This is partly because attention is mainly directed at the primary clinical presentation, and partly because there is an undoubted lack of awareness of the importance of nutrition and nutritional status amongst many healthcare professionals. The following are all important.

Weight loss

This is a very useful parameter and, as a guide, **more than 10% of unintentional weight loss over 6 months** is likely to be clinically significant and to reflect a situation of nutritional risk. Often, though, patients are unable to quantify how much weight they may have lost, or what their baseline weight may have been. In such situations clinical impression, e.g. observation of how well clothes or rings fit, and views from family members or carers may be useful. It must be remembered that a 10% unintentional weight loss in an obese patient is as relevant as in a normally nourished patient. Weight will be elevated in edematous patients (up to 10 kg for lower leg edema) or those with ascites (up to 14 kg) and this needs to be accounted for. Overall, weight loss can be regarded as a marker of risk, but on its own, nothing more.

Body mass index

This is an extension of weight, and is weight divided by height in meters squared. Conventionally, a body mass index (BMI)

Table 144.1 Factors that can lead to undernutrition

Table 144.1 Factors that can lead to undernutrition

Factors decreasing dietary intake
- Difficulties with food acquisition/preparation: poverty, limited mobility, lack of cooking skills
- Lack of interest in food: bereavement, isolation, mental illness
- Loss of appetite: illness, anxiety, depression
- Difficulties feeding or chewing: ill-fitting dentures, arthritis, dry mouth
- Symptoms associated with illness or treatment: nausea, vomiting, sore mouth, taste disturbance
- Altered consciousness
- Nil by mouth: following surgery, investigations

Increased nutritional requirements
- Metabolic stress: critical care, postoperative, infection
- Increased gut losses: vomiting, diarrhea, fistula

Impaired ability to absorb or utilize nutrients
- Gastrointestinal disease: malabsorption, motility disorder, bacterial overgrowth
- Intestinal resection
- Gastric stasis and ileus: critical illness, following surgery, metabolic disturbance

of less than $18.5 \, \text{kg/m}^2$ indicates undernutrition, and over $30 \, \text{kg/m}^2$ indicates obesity. There are alternative methods, such as using demispan (sternal notch to finger webs), but on the whole these are not widely used.

Anthropometry

This is the measurement of body composition. A number of different measures are used:

- Triceps skinfold thickness (TSF) – fat
- Mid upper arm circumference (MAC) – muscle mass
- Mean arm muscle circumference (MAMC) – skeletal muscle mass. This is a composite of TSF and MAC (MAMC = MAC − 3.14 × TSF)
- Bio-impedence analysis assesses body composition
- Grip strength, which is not, strictly speaking, an anthropometric measurement, but an assessment of muscle function. It uses a dynamometer and relies on patient motivation and compliance.

The place of anthropometry in day-to-day clinical practice lies mainly in the on-going follow-up of at-risk patients. Serial measurements done by the same (experienced) professional – as there is a great deal of interindividual variation – are a useful way of monitoring a patient's nutritional status. However, a one-off anthropometric measurement is not helpful. Overall, these measurements are used more in the research setting than in day-to-day practice.

Biochemical measurements

There remains a great deal of mythology about the use of biochemical measurements in nutritional assessment.

- **Albumin.** In protein energy malnutrition, albumin synthesis is low but, as it has a half-life of 21 days, falls due to poor nutrition are slow. Much more commonly, changes in albumin are due to alterations in hydration, e.g. dilution secondary to intravenous fluids, and catabolism/sepsis. Albumin on its own is not a marker of undernutrition.
- **Transferrin, pre-albumin, and retinol-binding protein** are all plasma proteins with much shorter half-lives, and therefore reflect protein depletion better. However, their assays are difficult and expensive, and therefore these are not used in clinical practice. Plasma proteins should never be used in isolation as a marker of nutritional status.

History

- **Medical history:** the primary disease process and any co-morbidity may be relevant. Disease instability and catabolism from inflammation or sepsis are important, as are any symptoms that may affect food intake or nutrient absorption, such as difficulties chewing or swallowing, anorexia, vomiting, and diarrhea.
- **Social history:** mobility, presence of depression, ability to obtain and prepare food, and underlying poverty may all influence nutritional state.

Examination

Generalized muscle wasting and cachexia, hydration, an apathetic appearance, and abnormalities of gait and mobility due to lower limb weakness are all signs of nutritional compromise. In addition, the various trace element and micronutrient deficiencies that may co-exist also have their own individual clinical signs (Table 144.2).

Nutrition screening

The methods of assessment described above will give a very good picture as to whether a patient is undernourished and whether they would benefit from nutritional support and advice. However, many of these parameters, if taken individually, do not fulfil the essential criteria of being a good and reproducible assessment tool for nutritional risk, and as a result, a proper nutritional assessment can only really be undertaken by individuals with appropriate expertise and experience. Usually, though, the initial assessment of patients is carried out by (mainly junior) nurses or doctors, with results that are often inconsistent and unreliable. As this has implications for clinical risk and patient care, it is now standard practice to carry out formal screening to ensure consistency and reliability.

Nutrition screening is therefore the process that leads to the identification of patients who are undernourished or at risk of becoming so. It needs to be a rapid and simple process that allows all patients being admitted to hospital or other institutions to be screened.

There are hundreds of screening tools, many designed by individual hospitals, and usually including a combination of

Table 144.2 Electrolytes, trace elements, and vitamins: their functions and deficiency syndromes

Element	Deficiency
Electrolytes	
Calcium	Muscle aches, pain, twitching, spasm, cramps, tetany, and loose teeth/gum infection
Phosphate	Anorexia, lethargy, bone pain, calcification of soft tissue
Magnesium	Neuromuscular abnormalities, loss of appetite, nausea, vomiting, premenstrual syndrome, diarrhea, numbness, tingling, dizziness, hypertension
Sodium	Muscle cramps, vertigo, nausea, apathy, reduced appetite
Potassium	Muscle weakness/paralysis, cardiac arrest
Trace elements	
Iron	Fatigue, pallor, headache, dizziness, sore tongue/mouth, concave brittle nails
Zinc	Poor growth, wound healing, eczema, psoriasis, acne, poor hair growth, increased risk of infection, delayed puberty, low sperm count, loss of smell, diarrhea
Copper	Metabolic and muscle problems
Iodine	Lethargy, thyroid goiter, brittle course hair, weight gain, hypothyroidism
Manganese	Depression, weakness, leg cramps
Fluoride	Tooth decay, soft bones
Chromium	Inability to metabolize glucose
Selenium	Muscle weakness, cardiomyopathy
Molybdenum	Rare
Vitamins	
Vitamin A	Night blindness, keratomalacia, dry scaly skin, joint pain, fatigue, impaired growth and development in children
Vitamin B_1 (thiamine)	Neurological disorders, confusion, cardiac irregularity, loss of appetite, fatigue, wet or dry beri-beri
Vitamin B_2 (riboflavin)	Lesions on mucocutaneous surfaces of mouth, skin rash, vascularization of cornea
Vitamin B_6 (pyridoxine)	Glossitis, dermatitis, convulsions, muscle weakness, and anemia
Vitamin B_{12}	Megaloblastic anemia, fatigue, brain degeneration
Niacin	Pellagra, fatigue, confusion
Pantothenic acid	Headache, dizziness, cramps, weakness and gastrointestinal disturbance
Biotin	Nausea, vomiting, depression, hair loss, dermatitis, mental and physical retardation in child development
Folate	Gastrointestinal disorders, macrocytic anemia, neural tube defects in newborns
Vitamin C (ascorbic acid)	Bleeding gums, scurvy, poor wound healing, bruising or hemorrhaging, fatigue, depression, muscle degeneration
Vitamin D	Rickets in children, osteomalacia in adults, reduced teeth and bone development
Vitamin E	Hemolytic anemia, muscle wasting, reproductive failure, nerve damage
Vitamin K	Prolonged blood clotting time

the various methods of assessment described above. The British Association for Parenteral and Enteral Nutrition has proposed a tool called the **Malnutrition Universal Screening Tool (MUST)** (Figure 144.1), and this has now been adopted by the NHS in the UK as the screening tool of choice.

In addition to the screening process itself, it is essential that there are defined courses of action dependent on the outcome of the screening. In other words, each healthcare setting where patients are being screened must have an established "care plan" to progress the patients' nutritional management.

Nutritional requirements

Part of nutritional assessment is the determination of nutritional requirements. While the detail of this is in the remit of dieticians or clinicians/nurses with a specialist interest in nutrition, it is necessary for all practicing clinicians, and certainly gastroenterologists, to have a rudimentary knowledge of nutritional requirements.

Energy requirements

Energy expenditure consists of three components:

- Resting energy expenditure (REE)
- Metabolic requirements
- Thermic effects of food (i.e., the energy required to utilize nutrients).

The hospitalized patient tends to eat little, and therefore energy expenditure is primarily REE and metabolic requirements.

Energy supply is mainly from the three macronutrients: fat, carbohydrate, and protein. Supplying too little energy leads to tissue breakdown, and supplying too much leads to excess storage of glycogen and fat. Neither is desirable and the aim therefore is for energy balance, where intake roughly equates to expenditure.

The calculation of energy requirements is therefore very important. It is best done by indirect calorimetry, but the cost

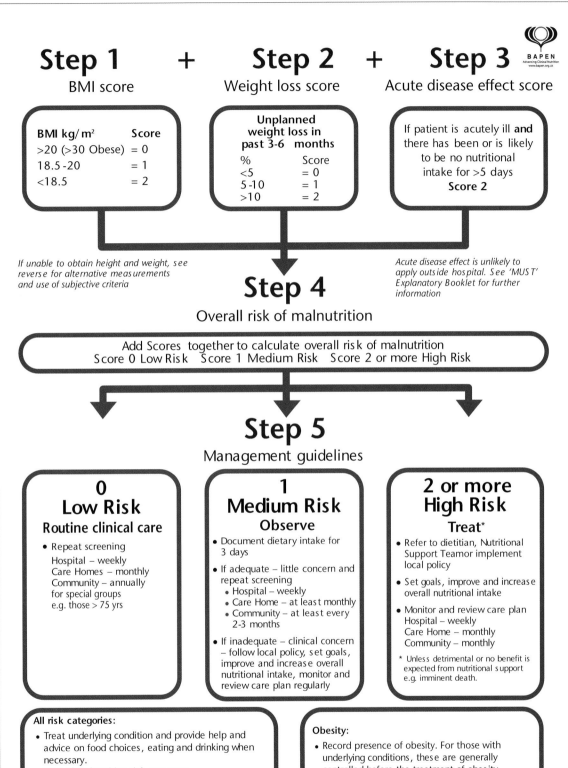

Figure 144.1 Malnutrition Universal Screening Tool. (Reproduced by kind permission of the British Association for Parenteral and Enteral Nutrition (BAPEN).)

Table 144.3 Macronutrients

	Protein	Fat	Carbohydrate
Energy density	1 g = 4 kcal energy	1 g = 9 kcal energy	1 g = 4 kcal energy
Function	Provision of amino acids essential for growth and continuous replacement of body tissue and enzymes Protein only plays a small role in energy metabolism – this is primarily supplied by fat and carbohydrate	More concentrated form of energy than protein or carbohydrate Tissues that can utilize fatty acids as an energy source include liver, kidney, heart, and skeletal muscle	Source of glucose, the most readily available source of energy to the body
Requirements	The intake requirements for protein in a healthy adult are 0.75 g/kg/day. However, metabolic stress increases requirements and to account for these the following intakes are recommended: • "Normal", i.e., no catabolic illness: 0.8–1.0 g/kg/day • Postoperative (no complications): 1.0–1.2 g/kg/day • Postoperative + septic complications: 1.2–1.4 g/kg/day • Severe sepsis/multiple organ failure/burns: 1.4–2.0 g/kg/day Overall, protein should supply 15–25% of total dietary energy	1.0–1.5 g/kg/day 30–50% total energy Imbalance of provision of these two can lead to significant metabolic and clinical complications Excess fat leads directly to fat deposition in liver and adipose tissue, and the relative lack of carbohydrate can result in glucose (and therefore energy) coming from alternative sources, e.g. fat, lactate, and protein (gluconeogenesis), with the risk of ketosis and lactic acidosis	4–5 g/kg/day 40–60% total energy Excess carbohydrate is stored as glycogen or converted into fatty acids. In addition there is an increase in insulin release and this inhibits lipolysis, causing an increase in tissue fat deposition

of the equipment and time involved make this impractical. There are several "mathematical" calculations, such as the Harris Benedict and Schofield equations, which dieticians will often utilize. However, for the busy clinician, these are not very practical, and the so-called "rule of thumb" is a very good, albeit crude, estimation of energy requirements:

Energy requirements should lie between 25 and 35 kcal/kg/day:

- 25 kcal/kg/day: bed bound, but not catabolic, i.e., apyrexial, non-surgical
- 30 kcal/kg/day: pyrexial or postoperative
- 35 kcal/kg/day: pyrexial and postoperative, multiple trauma
- If weight gain is required, add approximately 200 kcal to total daily requirements
- If weight loss is required, subtract approximately 200 kcal from total daily requirements.

In obese people, using actual body weight to calculate energy (and macronutrient) requirements would overestimate needs. For those with a BMI greater than 30 kg/m², requirements are either determined by using 75% of actual body weight or 130% of ideal body weight.

Macronutrients
Macronutrient requirements are given in Table 144.3.

Micronutrients
Micronutrient (vitamins, minerals, and trace elements) requirements are all essential for metabolism, tissue structure, enzyme systems, fluid balance and cellular function.

There are no definitive guidelines as to how much of each may be required in any individual patient. The dietary reference values often referred to in the literature are only relevant to the needs of healthy adults, and are not therefore always appropriate to the needs of hospitalized patients. On the whole, manufactured diets, both enteral and parenteral, contain reasonable quantities of the various micronutrients, and it is therefore unusual for a patient to have problems with deficiencies or excesses unless they are on prolonged nutritional support.

Nutritional support
Once a patient has been assessed and deemed in need of nutritional support, the next step is to determine the most appropriate method of feeding. Figure 144.2 illustrates the decision-making pathway and demonstrates that simpler methods should always be considered first.

The options for providing nutritional support are:

- Oral feeding: food, nutritional supplements
- Enteral (tube) feeding
- Parenteral (intravenous) feeding,

Oral nutritional support
Food
Food should always be considered as the first option. Strategies to increase nutritional intake from food include:

- Providing high energy/high protein choices on the hospital menu
- Fortifying foods, e.g., by adding cream, skimmed milk powder or cheese
- Attention to presentation, availability, and appropriate assistance.

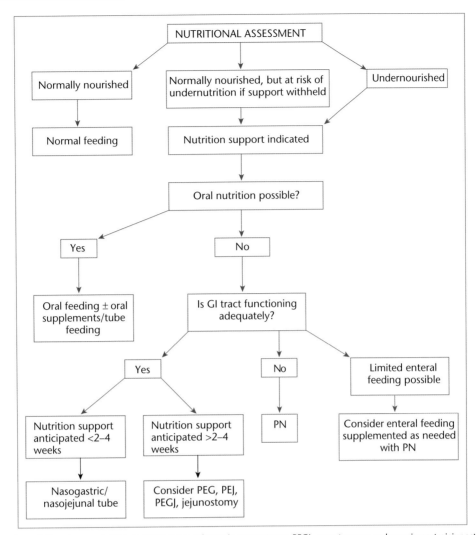

Figure 144.2 Options for nutritional support. PEG, percutaneous endoscopic gastrostomy; PEGJ, percutaneous endoscopic gastrojejunostomy; PEJ, percutaneous endoscopic jejunostomy; PN, parenteral (intravenous) feeding. (This figure was published in *Clinical Gastroenterology and Hepatology*, Wilfred M. Weinstein, Christopher J. Hawkey, Jaime Bosch, Nutritional support, Pages 1–8, Copyright Elsevier, 2005.)

Oral nutritional supplements

Oral nutritional supplements (ONSs), for those unable to meet nutritional requirements from food and drink, come as liquids, semi-solids or powders in many different flavors. They can be nutritionally complete, i.e., are appropriate as a sole source of intake, or can contain different concentrations of calories, fat, fiber or electrolytes for specific needs (e.g., low electrolyte preparations in renal failure).

It is therefore usually sensible to involve a dietician or other suitably trained professional to advise on an ONS that is appropriate to the clinical condition(s) and that complements the patient's dietary intake.

Enteral feeding

If a patient is unable to eat or cannot adequately meet nutritional requirements with food with or without an ONS, and has a functioning and accessible gastrointestinal tract, then enteral feeding is indicated [4,5].

The options are:

- **Gastric feeding:** nasogastric (NG) tube, percutaneous endoscopic gastrostomy (PEG), radiologically inserted gastrostomy (RIG)
- **Post-pyloric feeding:** nasojejunal (NJ) tube, percutaneous endoscopic gastrojejunostomy (PEGJ), percutaneous endoscopic jejunostomy (PEJ), surgically-placed jejunostomy.

Indications and contraindications for the various routes of enteral feeding are listed in Table 144.4.

Routes

Nasogastric tube

There are two main types of nasogastric (NG) tubes, fine bore and wide bore (e.g., Ryles). Wide-bore tubes should not be sited specifically for enteral feeding, because they are more uncomfortable and can cause complications such as ulceration of the esophagus and nasal passages.

Table 144.4 Indications and contraindications of enteral feeding

Indications	**Gastric feeding** **Patients with a functioning stomach and without vomiting or aspiration** Impaired swallow, e.g., stroke, motor neuron disease, Parkinson disease, Altered level of consciousness making oral feeding impossible Ventilated patients with tracheostomy Dysphagia without complete oropharyngeal/esophageal obstruction, i.e., head and neck and esophageal cancer **Supplement inadequate oral intake** Cystic fibrosis Hyper-catabolic states, e.g., burn injury, decompensated liver disease Facial injury HIV wasting Psychological/psychiatric reasons, e.g., anorexia nervosa For short-term feeding, i.e., <4 weeks, an NG tube is usually the most appropriate. For longer term feeding, a PEG is preferable		**Post-pyloric feeding** Feeding a functioning gastrointestinal tract when the stomach needs to be by-passed, i.e., where there is a gastric outflow obstruction (see under NG tube contraindications) Pancreatitis Risk of aspiration with intragastric feeding The four different methods of delivering post-pyloric feeding, i.e., NJ, PEJ, PEGJ and surgical jejunostomy all have similar indications. For short-term feeding, an NJ would be the route of choice; for longer term feeding the other three options could all be considered
Contraindications	**NG** Obstructive pathology in the oropharynx or esophagus preventing passage of tube Gastric outflow obstruction: – Mechanical, e.g., pyloric ulceration or stricture, tumor – Functional gastroparesis Intestinal obstruction: – Mechanical intestinal obstruction, e.g., tumor – Functional intestinal obstruction, i.e., ileus Intestinal perforation Proximal gastrointestinal tract fistula Facial injury	**PEG** **Absolute** Inability to pass endoscope due to obstructing pathology in oropharynx or esophagus* Obstructing gastric outflow pathology **Relative** Severe obesity (due to technical difficulties accessing the stomach)* Uncorrected coagulopathy Portal hypertension/ascites Active gastric ulceration/malignancy Gastroparesis Gastrectomy (total or partial)* Severe kyphoscoliosis (may be difficult to access stomach)* Current peritoneal dialysis	**NJ** – as per NG **PEJ and PEGJ** – as per PEG **Surgical jejunostomy** **Absolute** Jejunal disease, e.g., Crohn's disease or radiation enteritis at insertion site Obstructing distal pathology **Relative** Ascites Portal hypertension Peritoneal dialysis

*May be achievable if done under radiological guidance to locate stomach (RIG).
NG, nasogastric; NJ, nasojejunal; PEG, percutaneous endoscopic gastrostomy; PEGJ, percutaneous endoscopic gastrojejunostomy; PEJ, percutaneous endoscopic jejunostomy.

Nasojejunal tube

Specifically designed nasojejunal tubes such as the Bengmark tube (Nutricia, UK) will cross the pylorus in 70–80% of patients with normal gastroduodenal motility, especially with a concurrent intravenous 10-mg bolus of metoclopramide. If the stomach is atonic, nasojejunal tubes usually require endoscopic placement. The distal end must be placed beyond the duodenojejunal flexure or it will almost invariably pass retrogradely back in to the stomach. Weighted tubes have no advantage over unweighted tubes and are seldom indicated. Plain abdominal X-ray is required to verify placement, unless placed under screening.

Gastrostomy

Most gastrostomy feeding is done via a **percutaneous endoscopic gastrostomy (PEG)**. There are a number of different types in terms of size (9–24 Fr), internal fixator (flange, balloon), and material, including more cosmetically acceptable "button"

gastrostomies. Choice will be determined in consultation with the patient, carer, attending dietician/nutrition team, and endoscopist.

PEG insertion is now a standard endoscopic procedure, and details of insertion technique are not included here. Although not a sterile procedure, many guidelines recommend antibiotic prophylaxis, e.g., cefuroxime 750 mg or co-amoxyclav 1.2 g 30 minutes prior to the procedure [5].

If the PEG is removed within 2–3 weeks of insertion, a formal tract will not have formed, with consequent risk of spillage of gastric contents into the peritoneal cavity, leading to peritonitis. This also means that it will not be possible to re-insert a feeding tube down the same tract as it will not find its way into the gastric lumen. Therefore, if the PEG does come out in the first few weeks after insertion, whether at the hand of the patient or some other mishap, the stoma site should be covered and antibiotic cover instituted. If nutritional support is still required, an alternative access, e.g., NG tube, can be used until the wound has healed. After 2–3 weeks, removal presents little risk of peritonitis or sepsis. However, closure is rapid, so replacement is required within 4–6 hours using a fresh PEG or, temporarily, a balloon gastrostomy or Foley catheter.

Elective removal is usually done endoscopically. Alternatively, the tube can be cut close to the skin, allowing the internal fixator to pass spontaneously through the gastrointestinal tract. There are no reported incidents of obstruction, e.g., at the ileocecal junction, and this method is probably safe.

A RIG can often be placed where there are contraindications for a PEG (see Table 144.4).

Jejunal extension to PEG and percutaneous endoscopically-placed jejunostomy

PEGJs are "extensions" that attach to a PEG and can be passed endoscopically beyond the duodenojejunal flexure. A PEJ is similar to a PEG but requires a direct puncture into the small intestine. Insertion techniques are not straightforward and, on the whole, they probably have no advantages over a surgically-placed jejunostomy for post-pyloric feeding, except in a patient who is too unfit to have a general anesthetic. Removal of PEGJ/PEJs is similar to that for PEGs.

Surgical jejunostomy

Needle jejunostomies inserted using a wide-bore needle tunneled subserosally to reduce the risk of leakage are the most commonly used, but tend to be fine bore and are prone to block if poorly managed. Other tubes such as Foley catheters can be used, but are not ideal because of leakage and difficulties in connecting with feeding equipment.

Increasingly, jejunostomies are inserted per-operatively to allow for early postoperative feeding. Although complications can occur, the advantages of improved postoperative nutrition usually outweigh the risks.

Enteral feeds

There are many different enteral feeds available. Broadly speaking they can be divided into the following groups.

- **Polymeric feeds** contain whole protein, carbohydrate, and fat, and they can be used as a sole source of nutrition for those without any special nutrient requirements. The standard concentration is 1 kcal/mL, but they can be more or less energy dense (0.8–2.0 kcal/mL) and can also contain fiber, which can improve bowel function if this is problematic.
- **Elemental feeds** contain protein in amino acid form and carbohydrate as glucose or maltodextrins. Fat content is very low. They are used primarily in situations of malabsorption or (by some) as a primary treatment for Crohn's disease. Because of their high osmolality, they should not be used in short bowel syndrome
- **Disease-specific feeds.** Certain clinical situations require alterations in diets, e.g., high energy/low electrolyte feeds for patients on dialysis, and low carbohydrate/high fat diets for patients with CO_2 retention, such as those on

ventilators (carbohydrate has a higher respiratory quotient than fat or protein and leads to more CO_2 production).
- **Immune-modulating feeds.** These feeds contain extra substrates, which may alter immune and inflammatory responses. The commonly used substrates are glutamine, arginine, RNA, omega-3 fatty acids, and antioxidants. Evidence is gathering for the use of these products in certain surgical, trauma, critically ill, and cancer patients, but their exact place and indications for use have yet to be fully agreed.

Complications

On the whole, enteral feeding is safe and complications are not usually serious. They can be divided into those due to the tubes and routes of feeding (Table 144.5), and those due to the feeding itself. The latter group include the following.

Diarrhea

This is the commonest complication, with quoted rates between 5% and 60%. It is most commonly associated with antibiotics, laxative use, contaminated feeds, and hypoalbuminemia. Management is firstly to exclude other explanations, such as

Table 144.5 Tube-related complications of enteral feeding (common in bold)

NG/NJ	PEG/PEGJ/PEJ
Removal by patient	**Early**
Esophageal ulceration/ strictures	**Pain:** if severe, exclude peritonitis/tube displacement into anterior abdominal wall
Malposition into lungs	Hemorrhage: unusual if clotting screen within normal limits
Blockage	Peritonitis
	Pneumoperitoneum: note that there will always be some free gas after PEG insertion
	Gastrocolic fistula: due to interposition of colon between anterior abdominal wall and stomach
	Late
	Stoma infection: Course of appropriate antibiotics, e.g. flucloxacillin, Not necessary to remove PEG or stop feeding unless severe ulceration or wound breakdown
	Tube blockage
	Aspiration: can be minimized by feeding for no more than 20 hours/day at an elevation of at least 30 degrees
	Buried bumper: internal fixator migrates into gastric/anterior abdominal wall leading to tube blockage. This usually requires surgery to be removed
	Tumor tract seeding: a few case reports only
	Overgranulation:
	• At stoma site and bleed/become painful
	• Treat with steroid cream or silver nitrate

NG, nasogastric; NJ, nasojejunal; PEG, percutaneous endoscopic gastrostomy; PEGJ, percutaneous endoscopic gastrojejunostomy; PEJ, percutaneous endoscopic jejunostomy.

Clostridium difficile, colitis, and malabsorption. Concomitant medications should be rationalized if causing diarrhea, especially antibiotics. Antidiarrheal medication (loperamide and/or codeine phosphate) is often successful, and fiber can help, although evidence for this is lacking,

Constipation

This is usually due to a combination of inadequate fluid, dehydration, poor mobility, and drugs (e.g., opiates). If colonic pathology is excluded or unlikely, management is with laxatives, suppositories, and fiber feeds.

Vomiting/aspiration/reflux

Both nasogastric and PEG feeding can increase the risk of aspiration. Both can interfere with gastroesophageal sphincter function, and wide-bore NG tubes do so more than fine-bore tubes. Where possible, patients should be fed when positioned at 30–45 degrees. Standard antiemetics are usually effective, although prokinetics often are not [6]. Alternative or additional management options include alteration of feed delivery (change from bolus to continuous feeding), or changing diet to a more energy dense one, with smaller volumes delivering equivalent calories. Occasionally post-pyloric feeding will be required.

Metabolic complications

Both under- and over-hydration can be avoided by rigorous fluid balance control (1000 mL of enteral feed delivers approximately 900 mL of free fluid).

Overfeeding, giving calories in excess of requirements, can cause serious or even fatal metabolic complications, especially in critically ill patients [7]. These can include hyperglycemia, azotemia, and hypertonic dehydration from excessive protein intake. Overfeeding is usually caused by a combination of inaccurate nutritional assessments and not taking into consideration energy from non-feed sources, e.g., propofol and glucose-containing dialysate solutions.

Refeeding syndrome can be defined as severe fluid and electrolyte shifts and related metabolic implications in malnourished patients undergoing refeeding [8]. Excess carbohydrate stimulates insulin release, leading to substantial cellular uptake of phosphate, magnesium, and potassium, and a consequent fall in their serum levels. This may lead to dangerous cardiac arrhythmias and neurological events, and can be fatal. Emaciated patients must **never** be fed beyond appropriate requirements. In such patients, initial feeding should start as low as 5–10 kcal/kg (600 kcal/day for a 30-kg patient). Phosphate, magnesium, and potassium supplements should be monitored daily, and supplemented if necessary.

Vitamin/trace element deficiencies

These are rare as most commercially available feeds are now nutritionally complete. Patients receiving small volumes of feed over a prolonged period of time may be at risk (see Table 144.2 for details of clinical syndromes). Appropriate monitoring should avoid problems.

Table 144.6 Indications for parenteral feeding

Short-term feeding (<28 days)	Long-term feeding (>28 days)
Non-functioning gastrointestinal tract, e.g., prolonged ileus, intra-abdominal malignancy	Following extensive bowel resection, e.g. Crohn's disease, gut infarction
Proximal gut fistula	Extensive Crohn's with malabsorption
Preoperatively only if severely undernourished (e.g., BMI <17 kg/m²) and enteral feeding not possible	High output fistula
	Radiation enteritis
Postoperatively only when enteral feeding is contraindicated	Motility disorders, e.g., pseudo-obstruction, visceral myopathy or neuropathy
Where requirements cannot be fully met enterally, e.g., multiorgan failure, major trauma, burns	
Post-chemotherapy mucositis	

Parenteral (intravenous) feeding

Parenteral nutrition (PN) is the administration of nutrient solutions via a central or peripheral vein. It is an expensive way to feed patients and has a greater and more serious risk of complications than enteral feeding (Table 144.7). Furthermore, it is no more effective then enteral feeding and, therefore, should only be used when the gut is either not working or is inaccessible. The indications are listed in Table 144.6.

Routes

Parenteral nutrition should be administered through a dedicated feeding line. The following routes are available for short-term feeding (<28 days).

Central line

This enables use of the widest range of feeds without local complications such as phlebitis. However, insertion complication rates are higher than for peripheral lines. The major complication is **line sepsis**, which can be reduced by use of single-lumen tubes, preference for the subclavian route over the jugular or femoral routes, and meticulous care. In critical care multilumen lines may be needed. One lumen should be reserved exclusively for nutrition, but there will be a greater risk of line sepsis than with single-lumen lines.

Peripherally-inserted central catheter

A catheter approximately 60 cm long is inserted into an anticubital vein and advanced to lie in the central veins so that hyperosmolar solutions can be used. This technqiue requires good size veins, aseptic technique, and skill, but such lines can last many months and are preferred by some authorities to central lines. Major complications are phlebitis (5–15%), malposition (8%), and catheter failure/leakage (4%).

Peripheral cannula

This is easy to insert for short-term use, and with meticulous care can be maintained for several weeks. Only low osmolality

Table 144.7 Complications of parenteral feeding

		Management**
Insertion related	Failure to insert, malposition Pneumothorax, hemothorax* Arterial puncture, air embolism* Hemopericardium/tamponade, arrhythmias* Central venous thrombosis* Nerve injury, e.g., brachial plexus* Thoracic duct injury/chylothorax*	
Line related	Exit site infection	Swab, clean and appropriate antibiotics (e.g., flucloxacillin)
	Tunnel infection (tunneled lines only)	Swab exit site + peripheral and central blood cultures Commence systemic antibiotics and consider removing line
	Catheter sepsis (CRS) [9]	Consider if pyrexial, leukocytosis and no other explanation (urine, chest) Stop parenteral feeding and lock line with heparin Swab exit site + peripheral and central blood cultures If CRS confirmed on cultures, lock line with vancomycin + systemic antibiotics and observe closely. If sepsis persists line will need removing. Alternatively line can be removed straight away with systemic antibiotics Line removed if cultures indicate *Staphylococcus aureus* or *Candida albicans* If cultures are negative, re-use line and observe (and look for other sources). If in doubt, remove line
	Thrombophlebitis (peripheral lines)	Stop feed and remove line Care of inflamed site with appropriate dressings and cleansing
	Catheter occlusion	Due to fibrin or lipid sludge Lipid occlusion takes a while to build up. Therefore, early occlusion (<7–14 days) is likely to be due to fibrin, and late occlusion (>14 days) is more likely to be due to lipid. Fibrin can usually be dislodged with urokinase or concentrated alcohol, and lipid with alcohol
Feeding related	Deficiencies/excess of any electrolyte, vitamin or trace element can occur	Adequate monitoring should prevent this – refer to local policies
	Hepatobiliary	Cholestasis, cholelithiasis, liver steatosis, and cirrhosis can all occur, but usually only with longer term feeding
	Bone disease	Metabolic bone disease/osteoporosis

*Central lines only.
**A brief description of the management of line-related complications is given here. Local hospital policy should be referred to for detailed management.

feed can be used, making this route unsuitable for patients either with high nutritional requirements or those requiring longer term feeding.

Discontinuation

PN should never be stopped abruptly before alternative methods of feeding have been established, as rebound hypoglycemia can occur. Once oral or enteral feeding has begun, PN can be weaned off gradually over 1–2 days. If PN needs to stop suddenly, e.g., there are line problems, a dextrose infusion should be administered.

References

1. Russell CA, Elia M. *Nutrition Screening Survey in the UK in 2008.* A report by BAPEN, UK 2009.
2. Kondrup J, Johansen N, Plum L, *et al.* Incidence of nutritional risk and causes of inadequate nutritional care in hospitals. *Clin Nutr.* 2002;21:461–468.
3. Isabel M, Correira TD, Waitzberg D. The impact of malnutrition, morbidity, length of hospital stay, and costs evaluated through a multivariate model analysis. *Clin Nutr.* 2003;22:235–239.
4. DiSario J, Baskin W, Brown R, *et al.* Endoscopic approaches to enteral nutritional support. *Gastrointest Endosc.* 2002;55:901–908.
5. Allison MC, Sandoe JAT, Tighe R, Simpson IA, Hall RJ, Elliott TSJ. Antibiotic prophylaxis in gastrointestinal endoscopy. *Gut.* 2009; 58:869–880.
6. Booth CM, Heyland DK, Paterson WG. Gastrointestinal promotility drugs in critical care setting: A systematic review of the evidence. *Crit Care Med.* 2002;30:1429–1435.
7. Klein CJ, Stanek GS, Wiles CE. Overfeeding macronutrients to critically ill adults: Metabolic complications. *J Am Diet Assoc,* 1998;98:795–806.
8. Kraft MD, Btaiche IF, Sacks GS. Review of the refeeding syndrome. *Nutr Clin Pract.* 2005;20:625–633.
9. Department of Health. Guidelines for preventing infections associated with the insertion and maintenance of central venous catheters. *J Hosp Inf.* 2001;47 (Suppl):S47–S67.

CHAPTER 145

Variceal ligation, sclerotherapy, and other hemostatic techniques for varices and other lesions

Louis-Michel Wong Kee Song

Mayo Clinic, Rochester, MN, USA

KEY POINTS

- Band ligation, but not sclerotherapy, can be used for primary prophylaxis of large esophageal varices
- Band ligation is the preferred endoscopic therapy for acute esophageal variceal bleeding and for secondary prophylaxis of esophageal varices
- Sclerotherapy should be considered for control of active esophageal variceal bleeding when band ligation is not technically feasible or fails
- In patients who bleed from fundic varices, gastric variceal obturation using tissue adhesives, such as cyanoacrylates, is the preferred endoscopic treatment
- The distinction between gastric vascular ectasia and portal hypertensive gastropathy is of therapeutic relevance since endotherapy is effective in the former but not the latter
- Argon plasma coagulation is considered first-line therapy for symptomatic gastric vascular ectasia; cryotherapy and band ligation are alternative endoscopic approaches

---

Introduction

Endoscopic therapy plays an important role in the management algorithm for bleeding gastroesophageal varices. Portal hypertensive bleeding can also manifest itself through mucosal vascular lesions, including gastric vascular ectasia (GVE), where endotherapy can be effective. This chapter focuses on the technical aspects, efficacy, and safety of various endoscopic techniques for the management of gastroesophageal varices and mucosal vascular lesions associated with portal hypertension.

Esophageal varices
Classification

A simplified classification based on variceal size (small <5 mm or large >5 mm), location, and presence or absence of red signs (red wale marks or spots) is recommended [1]. Assessment of variceal size is performed with the stomach decompressed and the esophagus distended with air.

Band ligation
Indications

Endoscopic band ligation (EBL) is indicated for: (1) treatment of acute variceal bleeding; (2) prevention of a first episode of bleeding from high-risk esophageal varices (large with red signs or in a Child–Pugh class C patient) or in patients with large varices in whom beta-blocker therapy is not tolerated or contraindicated (primary prophylaxis); and (3) prevention of recurrent variceal bleeding (secondary prophylaxis) [1].

Devices

Multi-band ligators (MBLs) have largely replaced single-band devices, which required an overtube. MBLs can deploy as many as 10 bands in succession and fit onto standard (2.8 mm) and therapeutic (3.7 mm) working channel endoscopes [2]. The components, common to all MBLs, are: (1) a cylindrical-shaped cap preloaded with stretched elastic "O" bands affixed to the tip of the endoscope; (2) a tripwire; and (3) a control knob to engage the tripwire and release the bands (Figure 145.1). The assembly of the components is device specific; successful operation necessitates familiarity with the loading and working mechanism of a particular chosen brand.

Technique

A diagnostic upper endoscopy is performed prior to fitting the EBL device onto the endoscope. Coagulopathy should not preclude EBL, but coagulation parameters should be optimized for the procedure (INR <2; platelet count >40 000).

The targeted varix is suctioned into the cap until significant tissue prolapse and "red out" of the visual field is achieved. A band is then deployed, encircling the varix at its base. The band may misfire or slip off if not enough tissue is captured into the cap. EBL is initiated at the gastroesophageal junction (GEJ) and bands are placed in a spiral fashion, targeting varices in the distal 5–7 cm of the esophagus (see Video clip 145.1). Placement of up to six bands in one session is generally sufficient [3].

Textbook of Clinical Gastroenterology and Hepatology, Second Edition. Edited by C. J. Hawkey, Jaime Bosch, Joel E. Richter, Guadalupe Garcia-Tsao, Francis K. L. Chan.
© 2012 Blackwell Publishing Ltd. Published 2012 by Blackwell Publishing Ltd.

A visible actively bleeding varix should be banded immediately (see Video clip 145.2). Advancement of the endoscope beyond a more proximally situated banded varix should be avoided, as this may dislodge the band and result in rebleeding. If the bleeding site cannot be identified, banding of varices at the GEJ may reduce the bleeding rate sufficiently to allow identification and ligation of the bleeding varix [4]. Varices with stigmata of recent hemorrhage (e.g., adherent clot or fibrin plug) should also be targeted for banding (Figure 145.2).

EBL is repeated at 2–4-week intervals until the varices are obliterated. EBL at shorter time intervals is not associated with

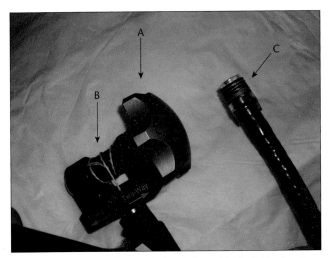

Figure 145.1 Multi-band ligation device. A, Control knob; B, tripwire; C, cap with bands.

better outcomes [5,6]. Following variceal obliteration, surveillance endoscopy can be performed initially at 3 months, then every 6–12 months, to monitor and treat variceal recurrence.

Efficacy
EBL controls acute variceal bleeding in 80–100% of patients when used together with vasoactive drugs, and achieves better initial hemostasis than sclerotherapy. EBL requires fewer treatment sessions than sclerotherapy for variceal eradication. Complications are less frequent and less severe with EBL than sclerotherapy [7].

Complications
Transient chest discomfort and dysphagia post EBL typically respond to an oral solution of lidocaine–antacid mixture. A liquid diet is recommended for 24 hours after a ligation session. Post-banding ulcer bleeding is managed with standard ulcer hemostasis techniques, such as clipping (see Video clip 145.3). A 10-day course of a proton pump inhibitor promotes healing of post-banding ulcers and may decrease the risk of ulcer bleeding [8]. Symptomatic esophageal strictures and perforations are rare. Care to avoid airway aspiration during the procedure is mandatory, especially when performed during acute variceal bleeding.

Sclerotherapy
Indications
Sclerotherapy is effective for control of acute bleeding and secondary prophylaxis of esophageal varices, but it has largely

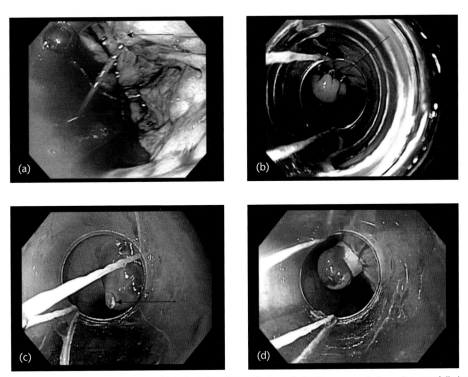

Figure 145.2 Band ligation of bleeding esophageal varices. (a) Actively bleeding varix (arrow); (b) the same varix (arrow) successfully banded. (c) Varix with fibrin plug (arrow); (d) the same varix successfully banded.

Table 145.1 Sclerosing agents

Agent	Volume per injection site (mL)*	Volume per session (mL)**	Relative tissue injury
Fatty-acid derivatives:			
Ethanolamine oleate	1.5–5	20	+++
Sodium morrhuate	0.5–5	15	+++
Synthetic agents:			
Sodium tetradecyl sulfate	1–2	10	++
Polidocanol	1–2	20	+
Alcohols:			
Ethanol	0.3–0.5	4–5	++++
Phenol	3–5	30	+

*Recommended dose per injection site.
**Maximum volume recommended per session.

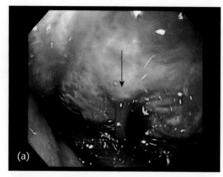 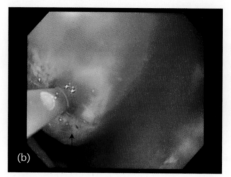

Figure 145.3 Sclerotherapy of an actively bleeding esophageal varix. (a) Actively bleeding varix (arrow) that failed band ligation; (b) whealing and blanching of the bleeding varix (arrow) during sclerotherapy, resulting in hemostasis.

been supplanted by EBL. Sclerotherapy can be used as second-line therapy when EBL is not technically feasible or fails in the setting of active bleeding. In some regions of the world, however, sclerotherapy may still be the preferred treatment as a readily accessible, low-cost procedure for variceal bleeding. Sclerotherapy is not indicated for primary prophylaxis of esophageal varices [1].

Sclerosing agents

Various sclerosants are available for use and are of comparable efficacy (Table 145.1). The use of a particular sclerosant largely depends on personal preference and availability.

Technique

A freehand technique is employed and a 23G injection catheter is typically used for injection. Injections may be performed directly into the varix (intravariceal) or adjacent to the varix (paravariceal), with whealing and blanching of the injected area as a result (Figure 145.3). Intravariceal injections may be more effective and cause fewer complications than the paravariceal approach, but the intended injection technique may not be straightforward. In one study, 44% of intended intravariceal injections were actually paravariceal [9].

In the setting of active variceal bleeding or stigmata of recent hemorrhage, injections are directed in and around the bleeding site (see Video clip 145.4). Otherwise, a typical injection protocol consists of injecting the varices starting at the GEJ, then at the 2.5 and 5 cm marks above the GEJ. The injection volume for a particular site depends on the sclerosant selected and size of the varix (see Table 145.1).

In general, three to six sclerotherapy sessions at 1–3-week intervals are needed to obliterate the varices. Similar to post-EBL surveillance, periodic endoscopy is recommended to assess for variceal recurrence.

Efficacy

Sclerotherapy can control active bleeding in 70–100% of patients, but at an increased risk of complications and recurrent bleeding relative to EBL [10,11]. Sclerotherapy is inferior to EBL for secondary prophylaxis of variceal bleeding.

Complications

Locoregional and systemic complications occur in as many as 25% of patients who undergo sclerotherapy. These include chest pain, dysphagia, low-grade fever, pleural effusions, iatrogenic ulcer bleeding, symptomatic strictures, mediastinitis, fistulae, perforations, spontaneous bacterial peritonitis, sepsis, and mesenteric or portal vein thrombosis, among others [11]. Bacteremia occurs in up to 50% of patients undergoing sclerotherapy. Prophylactic antibiotics are indicated in cirrhotic patients presenting with gastrointestinal bleeding, regardless of sclerotherapy.

Combination endotherapy and emerging techniques

The concurrent use of sclerotherapy and EBL in an attempt to hasten variceal obliteration is not recommended. Relative to EBL alone, this approach resulted in a higher incidence of stricture without improvement in outcomes [12].

The sequential use of sclerotherapy to eradicate residual varices that are not amenable to further banding was shown to reduce variceal recurrence and rebleeding in one study [13]. Similarly, argon plasma coagulation of the distal esophagus following variceal eradication by EBL was found to be effective at reducing variceal recurrence [14]. These combined approaches, however, have not been widely adopted.

Gastric varices
Classification

Gastric varices are classified according to their anatomical location and relationship with esophageal varices (Figure 145.4):

- **Type 1 gastroesophageal varices (GEV1)** extend 2–5 cm along the lesser curve of the stomach, in continuity with esophageal varices
- **Type 2 gastroesophageal varices (GEV2)** extend along the greater curve into the fundus
- **Isolated gastric varices** occur in the fundus **(IGV1)** or in other locations in the stomach **(IGV2)**, in the absence of esophageal varices.

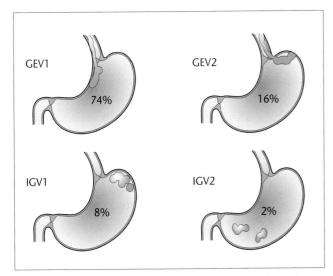

Figure 145.4 Classification of gastric varices. (Reproduced with permission from Sarin SK *et al.* Prevalence, classification and natural history of gastric varices: a long-term follow up study in 568 portal hypertension patients. *Hepatology.* 1992;16:1343–1349.)

The endoscopic management of bleeding GEV1 is the same as for esophageal varices. In contrast, **gastric variceal obturation (GVO)**, with agents such as cyanoacrylates, is the preferred endoscopic approach for bleeding fundal varices (GEV2 and IGV1). Sclerotherapy and EBL of fundal varices are associated with high rebleeding rates, and treatment-induced bleeding can be massive.

Cyanoacrylate injection
Indications

Cyanoacrylate injection is indicated for the treatment of: (1) gastric varices with active bleeding; (2) gastric varices with stigmata of recent bleeding (e.g., erosion or fibrin plug); and (3) suspect gastric varices (large, red signs) without definite stigmata but with exclusion of other causes in the context of upper gastrointestinal bleeding. There are insufficient data to recommend cyanoacrylate injection for primary prophylaxis of gastric varices.

Agents

Cyanoacrylates are a class of synthetic glues that solidify rapidly upon contact with blood. N-butyl-2 cyanoacrylate (Histoacryl; B Braun, Melsungen, Germany) is the most commonly used agent for GVO. 2-Octyl cyanoacrylate (Dermabond; Ethicon, Somerville, NJ, USA) has been used "off-label" in the United States, where it is more readily available.

Technique

A standardized approach enhances safety and efficacy of GVO using cyanoacrylates [15], but variations in technique exist depending on the type of cyanoacrylate used and local expertise.

N-butyl-2 cyanoacrylate

N-butyl-2 cyanoacrylate (BCA) is mixed with Lipiodol in a 1:1 or 1:1.5 ratio to prevent premature solidification of the glue in the injection catheter and needle impaction in the varix. The mixture is loaded into 2-mL syringes to facilitate injection. A 21G injection catheter with an 8-mm long needle is recommended to ensure intravariceal puncture; the catheter may be primed with Lipiodol. The tip and working channel of the endoscope should be lubricated with Lipiodol or silicone oil to prevent glue adhesion and potential irreparable damage to the endoscope. Protective eyewear should be worn by patients and staff.

Following variceal puncture, injection of the glue–Lipiodol mixture is limited to 1–2 mL per site and is immediately followed by injection of ~1 mL of sterile water, equivalent to the catheter's dead space. The needle is withdrawn from the varix and flushed with water to ensure its patency. Several sites can be injected per treatment session, with complete GVO attempted at the initial session. GVO is confirmed by firmness of the varix, as assessed by blunt palpation with the tip of the catheter. Alternatively, a Doppler probe can be used to confirm absence of variceal flow. Suction should be avoided during

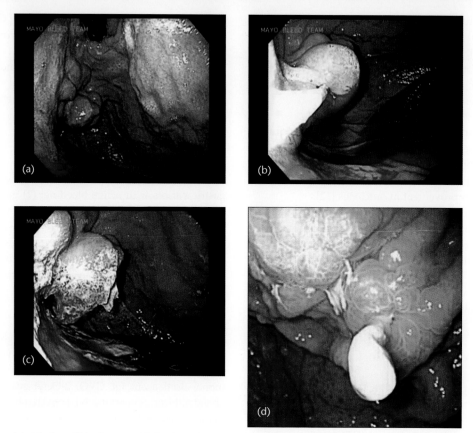

Figure 145.5 Cyanoacylate injection of bleeding type 1 isolated gastric varices. (a) Active bleeding from a fundal varix; (b) glue injection with a 21 G needle catheter; (c) immediate appearance post glue injection; (d) obliterated varices with retained glue cast at 3-month follow-up.

and after glue injection. After GVO, the scope is withdrawn with the catheter tip trailing the tip of the endoscope by several centimeters. The catheter is sectioned at the entrance port of the working channel and removed from the tip of the endoscope to minimize glue adhesion to the instrument.

Repeat endoscopy is typically performed 3–5 days after the initial treatment session to confirm variceal obturation and to treat any residual varices. Periodic endoscopy is carried out at 3–6-month intervals thereafter to assess for variceal recurrence. A scar is seen at the site of extruded glue, but a glue cast may remain visible for several months (Figure 145.5).

When both gastric and esophageal varices are present, EBL of the latter is generally initiated once GVO is complete.

2-Octyl cyanoacrylate
2-Octyl cyanoacrylate (OCA) has a longer ester chain linked to the main compound, which delays its polymerization. Thus, OCA must be injected **undiluted** to minimize the risk of embolization. In experimental studies, a larger injection volume was needed, relative to BCA, to achieve similar vascular occlusion.

The required accessories and precautions are similar to those for BCA. The injection catheter is primed with normal saline instead of Lipiodol. The glue may be slowly injected in 1-mL aliquots or can be injected continuously until resistance is met during syringe push; this typically occurs after 2–3 mL of OCA

has been injected into the varix. Saline solution (~1 mL) is used to flush the catheter while it is being retracted from the punctured site (see Video clip 145.5). Several sites can be injected in one session. Post-procedure care and follow-up are similar to that for BCA.

Efficacy
Cyanoacrylate injection is effective at securing initial hemostasis in 85–100% of patients. The rebleeding rate is 5–10% in more recent reports. Variceal obliteration occurs in 70–100% of cases [15–17].

Cyanoacrylate is more effective than sclerotherapy and EBL, and probably as effective as transjugular intrahepatic portosystemic shunt (TIPS), in controlling and preventing gastric variceal hemorrhage [18–20].

Complications
Glue embolization is the main concern and can be life-threatening (Figure 145.6). Pulmonary, cerebral, coronary, and abdominal embolic events have been reported in 1–5% of cases. Non-fatal pulmonary embolism occurred in 4.6% of cases in one series. Other complications include sepsis, fistulae, and needle entrapment in the varix [15].

Transient low-grade fever may occur due to foreign body reaction to cyanoacrylate injection. Prophylactic antibiotics are used in cirrhotic patients undergoing cyanoacrylate injection

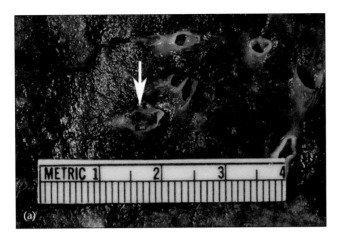

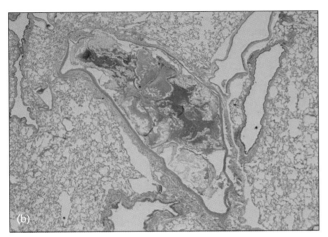

Figure 145.6 Fatal cyanoacrylate-induced pulmonary embolism.
(a) Pulmonary vessel occlusion by glue plug (arrow); (b) glue material
in pulmonary vasculature.

for acute bleeding, but may not be indicated for secondary
prophylaxis of gastric varices [21].

Fibrin sealants and thrombin
Indications
Fibrin sealants and thrombin injections have been used for
the same indications as cyanoacrylates. The experience regarding GVO with these agents is limited, but the relative ease of
injection and apparent lack of embolic events are potential
benefits.

Agents
Thrombin interacts with the patient's own functional fibrinogen and other coagulation factors to promote a local fibrin clot.
Bovine thrombin has largely been replaced by human thrombin
due to safety concerns (e.g., prion transmission). Thrombin is
available from various commercial sources.

Commercially available fibrin sealants (e.g., Beriplast-P
Combi-Set; CSL Behring, Marburg, Germany) consist of two
separate components, fibrinogen and thrombin, that are recon-
stituted and admixed during injection to form a "fibrin glue."
Product labeling does not endorse intravascular injection in
the United States.

Technique
The injection technique for thrombin is relatively straightforward. The dose of thrombin administered averages 1000 U/
mL, injected in 1-mL aliquots for 5–10 mL per session. The
preparation and assembly of the injection system for fibrin
sealants should follow the manufacturer's instructions. After
reconstitution and loading of the fibrinogen and thrombin in
their respective syringes, injection of the two components is
performed via a double-plunger syringe device connected to
a double-lumen injection catheter. Both thrombin and fibrinogen are injected together in the varix, resulting in the rapid
formation of a fibrin clot. The average volume injected per
session is 5 mL.

Efficacy
Uncontrolled studies have reported initial hemostasis rates of
75–92% and rebleeding rates of 0–25% following GVO with
bovine or human thrombin therapy. Initial hemostasis rates of
70–93% and rebleeding rates of 0–29% have been reported
with the use of fibrin sealants [22].

Complications
No embolic adverse events have been reported to date with
the use of thrombin/fibrin sealants. The use of human-derived
preparations has significantly reduced the risk of anaphylaxis
and antibody formation to clotting factors. As with all blood
products, the theoretical risk for transmission of infective
agents remains a concern.

Other modalities
Efficacy and safety data are limited regarding the use of
detachable stainless steel or nylon snares for bleeding gastric
varices. TIPS and balloon-occluded retrograde transvenous
obliteration are rescue therapies when GVO fails.

Portal hypertensive gastropathy versus gastric vascular ectasia
Classification
Portal hypertensive gastropathy (PHG) and gastric vascular
ectasia (GVE) may present with overlapping features, but an
accurate diagnosis is important due to differences in therapy
(Table 145.2).

PHG is characterized by a snakeskin or mosaic mucosal
pattern of the proximal stomach, with few to no red spots
(mild PHG) or with numerous red or brown spots (severe
PHG). GVE is characterized by flat or raised red spots distributed predominantly in the distal stomach in linear stripes
(**watermelon stomach**) or in a diffuse pattern, without the
mosaic mucosa (Figure 145.7; see Video clip 145.6). The term
gastric antral vascular ectasia (GAVE) is used for GVE
(watermelon-type or diffuse variant) limited to the antrum.

GVE of the diffuse variant is more commonly seen in
patients with cirrhosis and portal hypertension [23]. It may at
times be difficult to differentiate diffuse GVE from severe PHG

Table 145.2 Portal hypertensive gastropathy (PHG) versus gastric vascular ectasia (GVE)

	PHG	GVE
Endoscopic features:		
Stomach distribution	Proximal	Distal
Snakeskin-mosaic mucosa	Yes	No
Red spots	Yes/No*	Yes**
Histopathological features:		
Thrombi	–	+++
Spindle cell proliferation	+	++
Fibrohyalinosis	+	+++
Portal hypertension prerequisite	Yes	No***
Responds to measures that reduce portal pressure	Yes	No
First-line therapy:		
Acute	Octreotide/somatostatin	Endotherapy#
Chronic	Non-selective beta-blocker	Endotherapy#
Rescue therapy	TIPS/surgical shunt	Antrectomy

*Mild PHG – absent to few red spots; severe PHG – extensive red spots.
**Linear stripes of red spots – watermelon stomach; scattered red spots – diffuse variant GVE.
***GVE is also associated with non-cirrhotic conditions, such as connective tissue disorders.
#Argon plasma coagulation is preferred treatment modality initially; cryotherapy, band ligation, laser and contact thermal coagulation are alternatives (see text).
TIPS, transjugular intrahepatic portosystemic shunt.

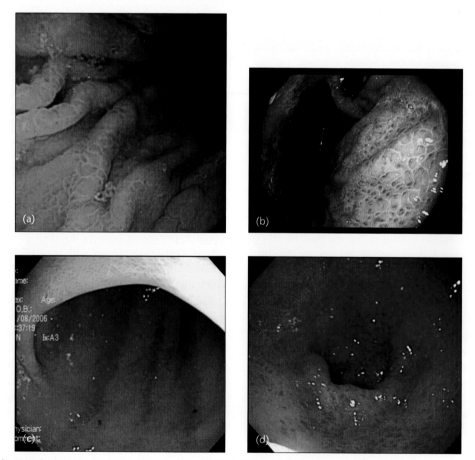

Figure 145.7 Portal hypertensive gastropathy (PHG) and gastric vascular ectasia (GVE). (a) Mild PHG; (b) severe PHG; (c) GVE, linear variant (watermelon stomach); (d) GVE, diffuse variant.

at endoscopy; biopsies can be diagnostic when distinctive features are identified at histology (Table 145.2).

Endoscopic therapies

Patients who bleed from PHG benefit from measures that reduce portal pressure (i.e., beta-blockers and TIPS), but not from endoscopic therapy. In contrast, various endoscopic therapies may control hemorrhage in patients with GVE.

Argon plasma coagulation

Argon plasma coagulation (APC) is widely used for GVE (Figure 145.8). Lesions are effectively ablated at power settings of 30–60 W and argon gas flow rates of 1–2 L/minute. The striped lesions of watermelon stomach can be "painted" with the APC probe to achieve uniform ablation and minimize bleeding (see Video clip 145.7). Discrete lesions can be treated with focal, 1–2-second pulses of APC. Suction is applied intermittently to clear the visual field and minimize gastric overdistension. Overzealous coagulation of lesions close to the pylorus should be avoided as this may result in pyloric channel stenosis. Brief inadvertent contact of the mucosa with an active probe tip may cause localized pneumatosis that is usually of no adverse consequence. A proton pump inhibitor can be prescribed to facilitate healing of iatrogenic ulcers.

The need for repeat APC is dictated by the clinical response. An initial interval of 4–8 weeks between treatment sessions is reasonable. The treatment interval can be lengthened as the long-term objectives of GVE eradication and resolution of symptomatic anemia are reached.

APC is effective at controlling bleeding in more than 70% of patients with GVE [23–25]. Most patients require two or more treatment sessions for long-term control of bleeding. APC is effective in both cirrhotic and non-cirrhotic patients with GVE [23].

APC-induced complications include iatrogenic ulcer bleeding, antral–pyloric stricture with gastric outlet obstruction, perforation, and the formation of hyperplastic/inflammatory polyps. Due to their friable nature, these polyps can aggravate bleeding and can be managed by snare debulking.

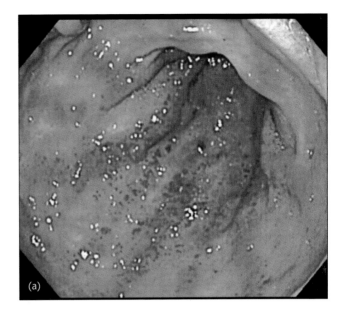

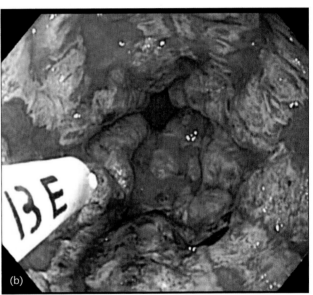

Figure 145.8 Argon plasma coagulation (APC) of gastric vascular ectasia. (a) Before APC; (b) immediately after APC.

Cryotherapy

Cryotherapy induces frostbite injury to the mucosa, resulting in tissue necrosis, sloughing, and re-epithelialization. Commercially available, catheter-based endoscopic cryotherapy systems utilize liquid nitrogen or compressed CO_2 gas as refrigerants.

The reported experience regarding cryotherapy for GVE is currently limited to the portable CO_2 device (Polar Wand; GI Supply, Camp Hill, PA, USA). The catheter is extended 1–2 cm from the tip of the endoscope and cryospray is applied about 1 cm from the mucosa. The cryospray covers a broad area and, unlike APC, does not require precise targeting. A high volume of CO_2 gas is delivered during cryotherapy, necessitating either a gastric length overtube or a dedicated decompression tube to vent the stomach. The cryospray is applied to the affected mucosa, causing whitening (icing) of the surface within a few seconds (Figure 145.9). This is quickly followed by thawing on termination of spraying. The freeze–thaw cycle is typically repeated three to five times per treatment session (see Video clip 145.8).

In an initial feasibility study, cryotherapy achieved control of hemorrhage in 71% of patients with watermelon stomach [26]. In a recent pilot study with short follow-up, the endoscopic appearance and hemoglobin level improved without transfusions in 50% of patients, following a cryotherapy protocol of three sessions at intervals of 3–6 weeks. A partial response was obtained in the remaining cases. No treatment-related complications occurred [27].

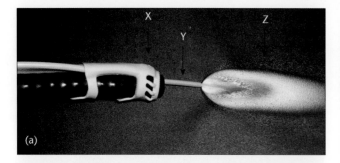

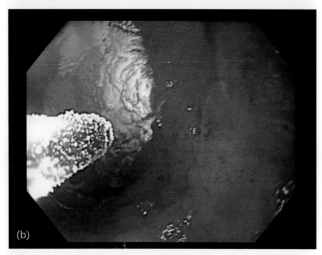

Figure 145.9 CO_2 cryotherapy of gastric vascular ectasia. (a) Cryotherapy device with evacuation tube and side-holes for gastric venting (X), delivery catheter (Y), and pedal-activated cryospray (Z). (b) Whitening (icing) of mucosal surface during cryotherapy.

Given its relative ease of use and ability to rapidly treat wide areas, cryotherapy may be particularly attractive for the treatment of extensive GVE where APC is not practical. Technical inconveniences and potential complications include a cloudy visual field from the gas, abdominal distension, treatment-induced ulcer bleeding, and perforation. Best treatment protocols are yet to be determined.

Band ligation

Band ligation may be considered for GVE that is refractory to APC or associated with the nodular/raised-type angioectatic lesions (see Video clip 145.9). The affected mucosa is suctioned into the cap until "red-out," followed by band deployment. Bands are placed in a distal-to-proximal fashion, starting a few millimeters from the pyloric ring to avoid significant pyloric stricturing. As many as 12 bands can be placed in one treatment session. Post-procedural abdominal discomfort and nausea are common and transient, and respond well to liquid analgesics and antiemetics. A liquid diet is recommended for 24 hours post procedure. Follow-up endoscopy is performed in 4–8 weeks after the initial treatment session; post-banding scarring is a typical finding (Figure 145.10). Repeat band ligation is dictated by the endoscopic and clinical response.

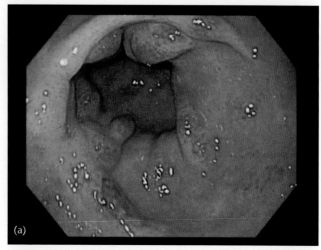

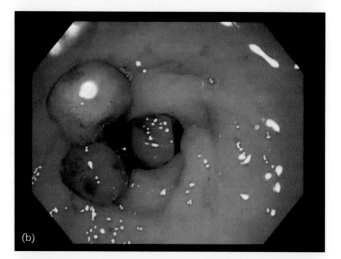

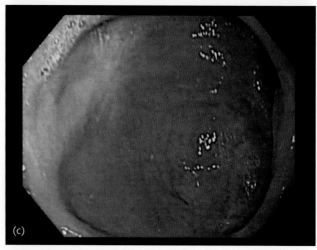

Figure 145.10 Band ligation of gastric vascular ectasia. (a) Before banding; (b) immediately after banding; (c) post-banding appearance with scar formation 2 months later.

The published experience regarding the use of EBL for GVE is limited. An observational study favored EBL over thermal therapy [28]. These findings require prospective validation.

Contact thermal coagulation

GVE can be ablated with contact thermal probes. Recommended treatment settings are 15 J for the heater probe and 14–16 W for the bipolar electrocoagulation probe. Pedal activation is for 1–2 seconds for isolated red spots or continuous if a "paint-stroke" technique is used for the angioectatic stripes of watermelon stomach. Contact coagulation probes are as effective as APC, but technically more labor intensive and less practical than APC for eradication of GVE.

The feasibility of radiofrequency ablation for treating GVE was demonstrated in a small pilot study [29]. The ablation device consists of a 2 x 1.5-cm electrode platform mounted at the tip of the endoscope (Halo^{90}; BARRX Medical, Inc., Sunnyvale, CA, USA) that can be tilted for tissue contact. Pedal activation delivers radiofrequency energy to the tissue, resulting in coagulation. The device can effectively ablate areas of vascular ectasias, but it is cumbersome to use and relatively expensive (see Video clip 145.10).

Lasers

Lasers, such as the neodymium-doped yttrium aluminum garnet (Nd:YAG), are effective modalities for the treatment of GVE, but their use is limited by device availability, cost, and a higher complication rate than APC.

Non-endoscopic interventions for gastric vascular ectasia

Pharmacological therapy, with agents such as estrogen and/or progesterone, tranexamic acid or thalidomide, is an option only if endoscopic measures have failed to control bleeding, since the evidence for efficacy is limited. For selected patients with severe bleeding refractory to endoscopic and medical therapy, an **antrectomy** may be considered. However, surgery is associated with high postoperative mortality because of significant co-morbidities which usually accompany the disease. TIPS and beta-blockers are ineffective for the long-term prevention of recurrent bleeding from GVE. Cases of GVE reversal following liver transplantation have been reported, but the evidence is insufficient to support this therapy unless the patient is already a liver transplant candidate.

References

1. Garcia-Tsao G, Sanyal AJ, Grace ND, et al. Prevention and management of gastroesophageal varices and variceal hemorrhage in cirrhosis. Am J Gastroenterol. 2007;102:2086–2102.
2. Liu J, Petersen BT, Tierney WM, et al. Endoscopic banding devices. Gastrointest Endosc. 2008;68:217–221.
3. Ramirez FC, Colon VJ, Landan D, et al. The effects of the number of rubber bands placed at each endoscopic session upon variceal outcomes: a prospective, randomized study. Am J Gastroenterol. 2007;102:1372–1376.
4. Baron TH, Wong Kee Song LM. Endoscopic variceal band ligation. Am J Gastroenterol. 2009;104:1083–1085.
5. Yoshida H, Mamada Y, Taniai N, et al. A randomized control trial of bi-monthly versus bi-weekly endoscopic variceal ligation of esophageal varices. Am J Gastroenterol. 2005;100:2005–2009.
6. Harewood GC, Baron TH, Wong Kee Song LM. Factors predicting success of endoscopic variceal ligation for secondary prophylaxis of esophageal variceal bleeding. J Gastroenterol. Hepatol. 2006;21:237–241.
7. Garcia-Pagán JC, Bosch J. Endoscopic band ligation in the treatment of portal hypertension. Nat Clin Pract Gastroenterol Hepatol. 2005;2:526–535.
8. Shaheen NJ, Stuart E, Schmitz SM, et al. Pantoprazole reduces the size of postbanding ulcers after variceal band ligation: a randomized, controlled trial. Hepatology 2005;41:588–594.
9. Waring JP, Sanowski RA, Pardy K, et al. Does the addition of methylene blue to the sclerosant improve the accuracy of injections during variceal sclerotherapy? Gastrointest Endosc. 1991; 37:159–160.
10. Villanueva C, Piqueras M, Aracil C, et al. A randomized controlled trial comparing ligation and sclerotherapy as emergency endoscopic treatment added to somatostatin in acute variceal bleeding. J Hepatol. 2006;45:560–567.
11. Park WG, Yeh RW, Triadafilopoulos G. Injection therapies for variceal bleeding disorders of the GI tract. Gastrointest Endosc 2008;67:313–323.
12. Karsan HA, Morton SC, Shekelle PG, et al. Combination endoscopic band ligation and sclerotherapy compared with endoscopic band ligation alone for the secondary prophylaxis of esophageal variceal hemorrhage: a meta-analysis. Dig Dis Sci. 2005;50:399–406.
13. Lo GH, Lai KH, Cheng JS, et al. The additive effect of sclerotherapy to patients receiving repeated endoscopic variceal ligation: a prospective, randomized trial. Hepatology. 1998;28:391–395.
14. Cipolletta L, Bianco MA, Rotondano G, et al. Argon plasma coagulation prevents variceal recurrence after band ligation of esophageal varices: preliminary results of a prospective randomized trial. Gastrointest Endosc. 2002;56:467–471.
15. Seewald S, Ang TL, Imazu H, et al. A standardized injection technique and regimen ensures success and safety of N-butyl-2-cyanoacrylate injection for the treatment of gastric fundal varices (with videos). Gastrointest Endosc. 2008;68:447–454.
16. Rengstorff DS, Binmoeller KF. A pilot study of 2-octyl cyanoacrylate injection for treatment of gastric fundal varices in humans. Gastrointest Endosc. 2004;59:553–558.
17. Reddy J, Wongkeesong LM, Buttar N, et al. Endoscopic injection of 2-ocytl cyanoacrylate (Dermabond) for the treatment of bleeding gastric varices [abstract]. Am J Gastroenterol. 2005;100 (9 Suppl):S363.
18. Sarin SK, Jain AK, Jain M, et al. A randomized controlled trial of cyanoacrylate versus alcohol injection in patients with isolated fundic varices. Am J Gastroenterol. 2002;97:1010–1015.
19. Tan PC, Hou MC, Lin HC, et al. A randomized trial of endoscopic treatment of acute gastric variceal hemorrhage: N-butyl-2-cyanoacrylate injection versus band ligation. Hepatology. 2006;43: 690–697.
20. Procaccini NJ, Al-Osaimi AM, Northup P, et al. Endoscopic cyanoacrylate versus transjugular intrahepatic portosystemic shunt for gastric variceal bleeding: a single-center U.S. analysis. Gastrointest Endosc. 2009;70:881–887.

21. Rerknimitr R, Chanyaswad J, Kongkam P, *et al.* Risk of bacteremia in bleeding and nonbleeding gastric varices after endoscopic injection of cyanoacrylate. *Endoscopy.* 2008;40:644–649.

22. Tripathi D, Hayes PC. Endoscopic therapy for bleeding gastric varices: to clot or glue? *Gastrointest Endosc.* 2008;68:883–886.

23. Lecleire S, Ben-Soussan E, Antonietti M, *et al.* Bleeding gastric vascular ectasia treated by argon plasma coagulation: a comparison between patients with and without cirrhosis. *Gastrointest Endosc.* 2008;67:219–225.

24. Herrera S, Bordas JM, Llach J, *et al.* The beneficial effects of argon plasma coagulation in the management of different types of gastric vascular ectasia lesions in patients admitted for GI hemorrhage. *Gastrointest Endosc.* 2008;68:440–446.

25. Fuccio L, Zagari RM, Serrani M, *et al.* Endoscopic argon plasma coagulation for the treatment of gastric antral vascular ectasia-related bleeding in patients with liver cirrhosis. *Digestion.* 2009;79:143–150.

26. Kantsevoy SV, Cruz-Correa MR, Vaughn CA, *et al.* Endoscopic cryotherapy for the treatment of bleeding mucosal vascular lesions of the GI tract: a pilot study. *Gastrointest Endosc.* 2003;57:403–406.

27. Cho S, Zanati S, Yong E, *et al.* Endoscopic cryotherapy for the management of gastric antral vascular ectasia. *Gastrointest Endosc.* 2008;68:895–902.

28. Wells CD, Harrison ME, Gurudu SR, *et al.* Treatment of gastric antral vascular ectasia (watermelon stomach) with endoscopic band ligation. *Gastrointest Endosc.* 2008;68:231–236.

29. Gross SA, Al-Haddad M, Gill KR, *et al.* Endoscopic mucosal ablation for the treatment of gastric antral vascular ectasia with the HALO90 system: a pilot study. *Gastrointest Endosc.* 2008;67:324–327.

CHAPTER 146

Non-variceal upper gastrointestinal bleeding

Majid Almadi[1] and Alan Barkun[2]

[1]King Khalid University Hospital, King Saud University, Riyadh, Saudi Arabia
[2]McGill University and the McGill University Health Centre (MUHC), Montreal, QC, Canada

KEY POINTS

- A multidisciplinary team should handle the management of patients with non-variceal upper gastrointestinal bleeding (NVUGIB)
- Critical to initial management of patients with NVUGIB is adequate resuscitation and risk stratification
- The majority of NVUGIB patients (80%) will stop bleeding spontaneously while the remainder will continue to bleed or experience recurrent bleeding
- Pre-endoscopic therapy with a proton pump inhibitor (PPI) downstages the stigmata of bleeding in an ulcer but does not decrease mortality, rebleeding, or the need for surgery
- Early endoscopy (within 24 hours of presentation) with endoscopic hemostasis, if indicated, represents standard of care in patients with NVUGIB
- PPIs should be used acutely in the management of patients with NVUGIB
- There is no added benefit from routine second-look endoscopy
- In the case of failed endoscopic therapy, a second endoscopy is warranted and if bleeding cannot be stopped, angiography with percutaneous embolization can be attempted as well as surgery
- The duration of long-term PPI dose depends on the underlying cause of the bleeding episode and secondary prophylaxis needs to be considered where appropriate

Introduction

Non-variceal upper gastrointestinal bleeding (NVUGIB) is a common entity with significant morbidity and mortality; it also carries a substantial cost to the healthcare system. This chapter addresses the different acute management aspects when caring for patients with NVUGIB. The scope of the review does not allow us to address issues of secondary prevention, but the reader is referred to excellent recent reviews and consensus recommendations.

Epidemiology

The yearly incidence of NVUGIB ranges from 48 to 160 cases per 100 000 adults [1], with a mortality ranging from 10% to 14% [2,3]. The majority of NVUGIB episodes are from non-variceal causes (80–90%), with the commonest cause being **peptic ulcer disease (PUD)** (66%) of the upper gastrointestinal tract [3]; other causes include Mallory–Weiss tears, erosive gastritis or duodenitis, esophagitis, malignancy, angiodysplasia, and iatrogenic complications.

The annual incidence of NVUGIB has decreased [2] but not the incidence of PUD [1], perhaps due to the increasing use of non-steroidal anti-inflammatory drugs (NSAIDs), including low-dose aspirin (ASA).

Initial management

NVUGIB management requires a multidisciplinary team, starting with appropriate resuscitation (with the insertion of two large-bore intravenous lines) and monitoring of vital signs, including hemodynamic instability. Blood samples should be drawn for serum hemoglobin (Hb), coagulation parameters (INR, PTT), electrolytes, liver enzymes, serum creatinine, and urea, as well as blood type and cross-matching. Insertion of a nasogastric tube (NGT) can help risk stratification and also assist in gastric cleansing prior to endoscopic examination. Prokinetic agents such as erythromycin and metoclopramide can be administered prior to endoscopy to patients suspected of having blood or clots in the stomach. These agents decrease the need for repeat endoscopy to visualize the bleeding lesion [2].

Support with blood products

The need for blood transfusion should be based on the risk of developing complications from tissue hypoxia rather than targeting a fixed Hb level. Blood transfusions are rarely needed with an Hb >100 g/L and almost always indicated at a level <60 g/L (keeping in mind ongoing re-equilibration).

Risk stratification

The majority of patients with NVUGIB (80%) will stop bleeding spontaneously without recurrence. The highest morbidity and mortality is in the remaining 20% who experience continued or recurrent bleeding.

Clinical predictors of rebleeding are listed in Table 146.1 and predictors of increased mortality in Table 146.2. Two commonly implemented scores for patients with upper gastrointestinal bleeding are the Blatchford (Table 146.3) and Rockall (Table 146.4) scores.

Textbook of Clinical Gastroenterology and Hepatology, Second Edition. Edited by C. J. Hawkey, Jaime Bosch, Joel E. Richter, Guadalupe Garcia-Tsao, Francis K. L. Chan.
© 2012 Blackwell Publishing Ltd. Published 2012 by Blackwell Publishing Ltd.

Table 146.1 Predictors of persistent or recurrent bleeding in patients with upper gastrointestinal bleeding

Risk factor	Odds ratio for increased risk (95% CI)
Clinical factors	
Age:	
>65 years	1.3
≥70 years	2.30
Shock (systolic blood pressure <100 mmHg)	1.2–3.65
Health status (ASA class 1 vs 2–5)	1.94–7.63
Co-morbid illness	1.6–7.63
Erratic mental status	3.21 (1.53–6.74)
Ongoing bleeding	3.14 (2.40–4.12)
Transfusion requirement	NA
Laboratory factors	
Initial hemoglobin ≤100 g/L or hematocrit <0.3	0.8–2.99
Coagulopathy (prolonged partial thromboplastin time)	1.96 (1.46–2.64)
Presentation of bleeding:	
Melena	1.6 (1.1–2.4)
Red blood on rectal examination	3.76 (2.26–6.26)
Blood in gastric aspirate or stomach	1.1–11.5
Hematemesis	1.2–5.7
Endoscopic factors	
Active bleeding on endoscopy	2.5–6.48
Endoscopic high-risk stigmata	1.91–4.81
Clot	1.72–1.9
Ulcer size ≥2 cm	2.29–3.54
Diagnosis of gastric or duodenal ulcer	2.7 (1.2–4.9)
Ulcer location	
High on lesser curvature	2.79
Superior wall	13.9
Posterior wall	9.2

ASA, American Society of Anesthesiologists; NA, not available.
Adapted with permission from Barkun A, Bardou M, Marshall JK. Consensus recommendations for anaging patients with nonvariceal upper gastrointestinal bleeding. *Ann Intern Med* 2003;139:843–857.

Table 146.2 Predictors of mortality in patients with upper gastrointestinal bleeding

Risk factor	Odds ratio for increased risk (95% CI)
Clinical factors	
Age:	
60–69 years	3.5 (1.5–4.7)
≥75 years	4.5–12.7
>80 years	5.7 (2.9–10.2)
Shock or low blood pressure	1.18–6.4
ASA classification	2.6–9.52
Co-morbid conditions (0 vs ≥1)	1.19–12.1
Continued bleeding or rebleeding	5.29–76.23
Presentation of bleeding	
Blood in the gastric aspirate	0.43–18.9
Hematemesis	2.0 (1.1–3.5)
Red blood on rectal examination	2.95 (1.29–6.76)
Onset of bleeding while hospitalized for other causes	2.77 (1.64–4.66)
Laboratory factors	
Elevated urea level	5.5–18
Serum creatinine level >150 µmol/L	14.8 (2.6–83.5)
Elevated serum aminotransferase levels	4.2–20.2
Sepsis	5.4 (1.5–19.6)
Endoscopic factors	
Major stigmata of recent hemorrhage	NA

ASA, American Society of Anesthesiologists; NA, not available.
Adapted with permission from Barkun A, Bardou M, Marshall JK. Consensus recommendations for anaging patients with nonvariceal upper gastrointestinal bleeding. *Ann Intern Med* 2003;139:843–857.

Moreover, data are most robust for an 80-mg bolus of a PPI followed by 8 mg/hour prior to the endoscopy.

Endoscopic therapy

Guidelines recommend that an **early endoscopy** be performed (within 24 hours of presentation); it is the cornerstone of management. Indeed, early endoscopy allows for appropriate risk stratification, and safe discharge for patients found to be at low risk, while also improving outcomes for those classified as high risk for rebleeding. It has been shown to improve rebleeding, surgery, transfusion requirements, and shorten length of stay [2]. Observational data have suggested that early endoscopy may improve mortality. Delays in endoscopy may be appropriate in exceptional circumstances [2], such as in acute coronary artery syndromes or suspected perforation; patients with a very low Blatchford score might be considered for outpatient investigation with a subsequent later endoscopy.

There is no proven advantage for very early or urgent endoscopy (<12 hours) over endoscopy within the first 24 hours. Predictors of patients with active bleeding who may benefit from very early endoscopy (<12 hours) include fresh blood in the NGT aspirate, uncorrectable hemodynamic instability, hemoglobin <80 g/L, and a white blood cell count >12 000 cells/µL.

Endoscopic findings associated with increased rebleeding and mortality include active bleeding, a non-bleeding visible vessel or adherent clot, ulcer size (>2 cm), etiology (e.g., ulcer, cancer, varices), and site of bleeding (posterior lesser gastric curvature or posterior duodenal bulb.

Preendoscopic pharmacotherapy

Pre-endoscopic use of a proton pump inhibitor (PPI) results in a reduction of high-risk stigmata seen at endoscopy and of the need for endoscopic therapy; however, its benefits are probably marginal as it does not result in significant improvements in mortality, rebleeding or surgery [4]. Pre-endoscopic PPI use should therefore never replace the more important role of adequate resuscitation and early endoscopy. The cost-effectiveness of pre-endoscopy PPI is optimized if implemented in particular clinical settings, including when patients are most likely to be bleeding from non-variceal sources or to be harboring a high-risk endoscopic lesion, and if the endoscopy may be delayed.

Table 146.3 The Blatchford risk score

Admission risk marker	Score*
Blood urea (mmol/L)	
≥6.5–<8.0	2
≥8.0–<10.0	3
≥10.0–<25.0	4
≥25	6
Hemoglobin (g/L) for men	
≥120–<130	1
≥100–<120	3
<100	6
Hemoglobin (g/L) for women	
≥100–<120	1
<100	6
Systolic blood pressure (mmHg)	
100–109	1
90–99	2
<90	3
Other markers	
Pulse ≥100/minute	1
Presentation with melena	1
Presentation with syncope	2
Hepatic disease	2
Cardiac failure	2

*Scores of ≥6 are associated with a >50% risk of needing an intervention.
Adapted with permission from Blatchford O, Murray WR, Blatchford M. A risk score to predict need for treatment for upper-gastrointestinal haemorrhage. *Lancet.* 2000;356:1318–1321.

Correction of coagulopathy for patients on anticoagulants

Using data from the Registry of patients with Upper Gastrointestinal Bleeding undergoing Endoscopy (RUGBE), a large national cohort that included 1869 patients with NVUGIB, INR ≥1.5 at presentation was a predictor of increased mortality but not rebleeding [2]. Another study found that correcting the INR value to <1.8 as part of an intense, more general resuscitation approach resulted in a reduction in mortality and myocardial infarctions. On the other hand, a cohort study that looked at urgent endoscopy and correcting an initial INR between 1.5 and 6 to a level of 1.5–2.5 with fresh frozen plasma found no differences in complications, rebleeding, surgery or mortality compared to controls. In patients on anticoagulants, correction of coagulopathy is thus recommended but should not delay endoscopy as long as the INR is not supratherapeutic [2].

Findings on esophagogastroduodenoscopy: who should receive endoscopic hemostatic therapy?

Patients found to have **low-risk stigmata** [clean base ulcer (Figure 146.1) or a non-protuberant dot in an ulcer bed] do not require endoscopic therapy due to the very low risk of rebleeding compared to the natural history of **high-risk stigmata** (Table 146.5) [spurting bleed (Figure 146.2), oozing bleed, or a non-bleeding visible vessel (Figure 146.3)]. Meta-analyses [5,6] have shown improvements in rebleeding, surgery, and mortality when considering any type of endoscopic therapy compared to none amongst patients with high-risk lesions.

Endoscopic hemostatic modalities
Injection

Epinephrine (adrenaline) injection therapy reduces the risk of rebleeding in patients with high-risk stigmata when compared to medical therapy alone.

Table 146.4. The Rockall score

Variable	Score* 0	1	2	3
Age (years)	<60	60–79	≥80	
Shock	No shock (pulse <100, SBP ≥100)	Tachycardia (pulse ≥100, SBP ≥100)	Hypotension (pulse ≥100, SBP <100)	
Co-morbidity	No major co-morbidity		Cardiac failure, ischemic heart disease, any major co-morbidity	Renal failure, liver failure, disseminated malignancy
Diagnosis	Mallory–Weiss tear, no lesion identified and no stigmata of recent hemorrhage	All other diagnoses	Malignancy of the upper gastrointestinal tract	
Stigmata of recent hemorrhage	None or dark spot only		Blood in the upper gastrointestinal tract, adherent clot, visible or spurting vessel	

*A score <3 carries a favorable prognosis, while that of >8 carries a high risk of mortality.
SBP, systolic blood pressure.
Adapted from Rockall TA, Logan RF, Devlin HB, *et al.* Risk assessment after acute upper gastrointestinal haemorrhage. *Gut.* 1996;38:316–321, with permission from BMJ Publishing Group Ltd.

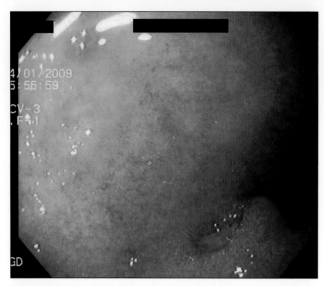

Figure 146.1 Clean base ulcer (Forrest Classification III).

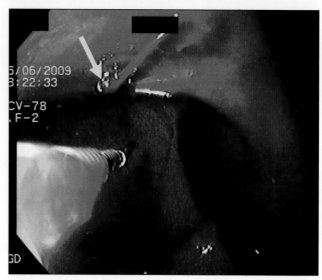

Figure 146.2 Attempt at endoscopic hemostatic therapy using a clip for a spurting vessel (arrow) (Forrest Classification Ia: Spurting bleed).

Table 146.5 Forrest classification

Forrest classification	Rebleeding rate (%)
Ia: Spurting bleed	80–90
Ib: Oozing bleed	10–30
IIa: Non-bleeding visible vessel (NBVV)	50–60
IIb: Adherent clot	25–35
IIc: Flat pigmented spot	0–8
III: Clean base ulcer	0–12

Adapted with permission from Forrest JA, Finlayson ND, Shearman DJ. Endoscopy in gastrointestinal bleeding. *Lancet.* 1974;2:394–397.

Meta-analyses have found no added benefit of using any solution over another; these have included diluted epinephrine, distilled water, cyanoacrylate, epinephrine in combination with ethanolamine or polidocanol, thrombin, sodium tetradecyl sulfate, ethanol, hypertonic saline (3% NaCl), and 50% glucose–water solution. Trials suggest that larger volumes of injectate should be used – approximately 20 mL; use of larger volumes (30 mL or more) may result in more complications [6]. Injection of a second injectate with alcohol, thrombin or fibrin glue in addition to epinephrine is superior to epinephrine alone (See Video 146.1) [5,6].

Thermal coaptive therapy

All thermal contact devices aim to seal off the bleeding vessel using thermal energy while applying coaptive force (See Video 146.1). They include the heater probe, the multipolar probe, and the Gold probe™. Two meta-analyses have found that all thermal coaptive endoscopic techniques are equally effective. The argon plasma coagulator (APC) uses a non-contact method

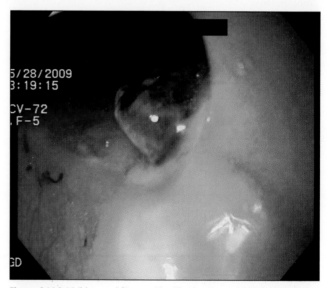

Figure 146.3 Visible vessel [Forrest Classification IIa: non-bleeding visible vessel (NBVV)].

of electrocoagulation through a jet of ionized argon gas. This technology is not inferior to heater probe or injection therapy, perhaps because most bleeding vessels are of limited diameter.

Clips

Clips have varying lengths, number of prongs, and release systems. Clips have been found to be superior to pharmacotherapy as a sole therapeutic strategy [6].

Combination therapy

Injection may precede thermal therapy or follow the application of clips (See Video 146.1).

Comparative efficacy

Monotherapy with a thermal device has been found to be more effective than epinephrine injection alone or pharmacotherapy alone for patients with high-risk stigmata. Clips are also superior to injection of epinephrine alone.

When injection of epinephrine is coupled with a second endoscopic hemostatic modality for high-risk stigmata, the risk is reduced of rebleeding (OR 0.51; 95% CI 0.39–0.66), surgery (OR 0.63; 95% CI 0.45–0.89), and mortality (OR 0.50; 95% CI 0.30–0.89) compared to injection therapy alone; however, combination therapy is not superior to the use of thermal coaptive therapy or clips as a sole hemostatic technique. The combination of clips with injection therapy is also superior to injection therapy alone, but not to clips alone.

Management of patients with adherent clots

We define an adherent clot as a clot in which it is unclear where to apply endoscopic hemostasis because the hematin material covers the ulcer base too diffusely. Such a finding warrants **targeted irrigation** in an attempt at dislodgement, using a water pump (usually for 2–5 minutes), with appropriate treatment of the underlying lesion. If the clot cannot be removed, the endoscopist can then apply **endoscopic hemostatic therapy** by first injecting diluted epinephrine around the lesion and guillotining the clot with a cold snare, trying to preserve the pedicle of the clot. Once the clot has been removed, management is dictated according to the underlying endoscopic finding. Alternately, these patients may be managed solely with a high-dose intravenous PPI bolus and infusion, as discussed below.

Pharmacological therapy
Somatostatin and octreotide
Contemporary meta-analyses have failed to show any beneficial effects attributable to the use of somatostatin or octreotide compared to other pharmacotherapies or endoscopic therapy. Although the evidence for the use of these agents is not compelling, they may be used in patients with uncontrolled upper gastrointestinal bleeding before or after endoscopy while awaiting further management.

Tranexamic acid
Tranexamic acid inhibits plasminogen activators, which accounts for its effects as an antifibrinolytic drug. An older meta-analysis assessing the use tranexamic acid in NVUGIB included data that antedate the endoscopic therapy era. It is not current routine clinical practice to use this medication in NVUGIB.

Biological rationale for acid suppression in patients with upper gastrointestinal bleeding
Acid has been shown to inhibit platelet aggregation and even favors platelet disaggregation; it is also known to facilitate clot lysis through the activation of pepsin, while acid suppression

may prevent fibrinolysis. Following endoscopic therapy for a high-risk lesion, approximately 72 hours are required for most lesions to evolve into a low-risk ulcer stigma. This finding is corroborated by most clinical trials that have shown that peptic ulcer rebleeding occurs predominantly during the first 72 hours following endoscopic therapy. It has thus been hypothesized that acid suppression may stabilize intraluminal clot during this high-risk period, and result in a subsequent improvement in outcomes. Interestingly, PPIs also exhibit anti-inflammatory properties of unclear clinical relevance, but these may play a role in downstaging high-risk bleeding ulcer lesions when PPIs are used while awaiting endoscopy, as discussed above.

Histamine 2-receptor antagonists
Recent meta-analyses have found no improvement in outcomes when H_2-receptor antagonists (H_2RAs) were compared to other pharmacological therapies or endoscopic treatment. Meta-analyses have also noted that PPIs are more effective than H_2RAs in decreasing the incidence of persistent or recurrent NVUGIB, as well as decreasing the need for surgery. This lack of effect may relate to the development of tachyphylaxis with the H_2RAs that can occur as early as a few days into treatment. H_2RAs are thus not recommended in the management of NVUGIB.

Proton pump inhibitors
PPI therapy in the management of NVUGIB has become **standard of care**, and strong evidence exists for their use. Indeed, a Cochrane meta-analysis found that the use of PPIs with or without endoscopic therapy decreased the rate of rebleeding (OR 0.45, 95% CI 0.36–0.57) and surgery (OR 0.56,– 95% CI 0.45–0.70) when compared to placebo or H_2RAs [7]. A decrease in mortality was also noted in the subgroup of patients with high-risk lesions who had initially undergone successful endoscopic hemostasis (OR 0.53, 95% CI 0.31–0.91). Improvements in outcomes have also been noted in studies conducted specifically in Asian patients.

Optimum dosage
Despite all the trials completed to date, the optimal intravenous dose remains unknown. The most studied regimen with highest quality data is the 80-mg bolus followed by 8 mg/hour for 72 hours (80 + 8) regimen, which is the dosing favored by consensus recommendations. Some authors have suggested that lower doses may be as efficacious; however, study design and statistical limitations have questioned the validity of these findings. The role of high-dose oral PPIs in the acute management of patients with bleeding ulcers has remained more controversial, most probably due to heterogeneous study methodologies yielding discordant results, at least in part because of racial differences in gastric acid physiology, pharmacogenomics, *Helicobacter pylori* carriage rates, patient age, and acuity of illness. High-dose oral PPIs or lower intravenous doses may be used in NVUGIB, especially where high-dose intravenous PPIs are not available.

Long-term therapy

After the patient is discharged from hospital or after completion of 72 hours of high-dose intravenous PPI, they should be kept on a maintenance dose of a single oral daily dose of the PPI for a duration dependent on the underlying cause (esophagitis, or NSAID or ASA prolonged use).

Although the side effect profiles for PPIs are favorable, there have been concern regarding the increased incidence of *Clostridium difficile* infection, pneumonia, and osteoporosis-related fractures in patients on long-term therapy with PPIs; this remains a controversial issue, but the benefits associated with their use in the acute and secondary prevention setting of NVUGIB as well as in ulcer healing likely outweigh these risks. PPI discontinuation in settings in which the underlying bleeding cause has been eliminated, as is the case following confirmed eradication of *H. pylori*, should be considered.

Routine second-look endoscopy

Routine second-look endoscopy refers to the performance of a preplanned second endoscopy within 16–24 hours after the initial endoscopic evaluation and hemostatic therapy in the absence of clinical evidence of rebleeding. A recent meta-analysis demonstrated that routine second-look endoscopy decreases rebleeding, and surgery, but not mortality [2]. The clinical applicability of these conclusions, however, is brought into question due to study heterogeneity in the choice of patients, endoscopic hemostatic modalities, and pharmacotherapy in controls. Recent consensus recommendations state that there is **no added benefit** from routine second-look endoscopy when compared to high-dose PPI [2]. Selective use of second-look endoscopy in a selected patient population might, however, be of benefit.

Acute management of patients on aspirin with bleeding ulcers

Recent randomized clinical trial data amongst patients presenting with an acute ulcer bleed while on ASA, in addition to observational studies of patients non-adherent to ASA prescribed for secondary prophylaxis, have informed recommendations in this important patient population. The indication for ASA in patients with acute ulcer bleeding should be reviewed, and the risks of cardiac and cerebrovascular adverse events should be weighed against those of early re-introduction of ASA. Current recommendations suggest that treating physicians should base their decision on such considerations, but in many patients ASA may be reintroduced as early as 5 days after the onset of bleeding. Secondary prophylaxis, including searching for and eradicating *H. pylori*, and PPI secondary prophylaxis are beyond the scope of this review.

Failed endoscopic therapy
Repeat endoscopy in the case of rebleeding

In the case of repeated NVUGIB, a second attempt at endoscopic hemostatic therapy is indicated in most patients. Indeed, the only randomized controlled trial comparing repeat endoscopic therapy to surgery after an initial unsuccessful attempt at endoscopic hemostasis found that repeat endoscopic therapy resulted in a decreased need for surgery and lower complication rates, without an associated increase in mortality.

Percutaneous embolization

When endoscopic therapy has failed, an increasingly used alternative to surgery is percutaneous or transcatheter arterial embolization using coils, cyanoacrylate glue, gelatin sponges, or polyvinyl alcohol. The aim of the intervention is to occlude the feeding vessel to the lesion. This intervention is especially warranted in patients who are found to be high risk for surgical intervention. Success rates range from 52% to 98%, with recurrent bleeding in 10–20% of patients, and a low complication rate. Risks specific to this procedure include bowel, gastric, hepatic, and splenic ischemia, as well as secondary duodenal stenosis; these complications have become uncommon due to highly targeted interventions by radiologist that may be assisted by the prior placement of endoscopic clips near the bleeding lesion. Furthermore, comparative cohort trials suggest similar outcomes when comparing a percutaneous intervention to surgery.

Surgery

From the Canadian RUGBE cohort, 14.1% of patients developed rebleeding after endoscopic hemostatic therapy, with 6.5% requiring surgery to control bleeding [3]. Similar proportions have been found in other cohort studies [8]. Amongst patients at high risk of rebleeding, up to 27% may require surgery, although as discussed above, a greater number of patients are now rather being referred for percutaneous intervention. Nonetheless, early surgical consultation in patients who fail initial endoscopic therapy and those who are at high risk of rebleeding is indicated.

Care after endoscopy

After the patient has been assessed clinically and at early endoscopy, patients with adequate social and family support, and easy access to hospital can be discharged home if they meet the following criteria: aged under 60 years of age, no severe co-morbidity, no hemodynamic instability, hemoglobin level over 80 g/L, normal coagulation parameters, bleeding had started in an outpatient setting, and endoscopy has demonstrated a clean base ulcer. This strategy does not result in more adverse outcomes and permits cost savings, but of course needs to be individualized according to practice setting. All other patients (except perhaps highly selected very low-risk patients with a very low Blatchord score) should be hospitalized, with high-risk patients having undergone endoscopic hemostasis requiring a 72-hour infusion and stay.

A summary of the recommendations from the 2010 International consensus on the management of patients with NVUGIB is given in Table 146.6.

Table 146.6 Recommendations from the 2010 International Consensus Recommendations on the management of patients with non-variceal upper gastrointestinal bleeding.

Pre-endoscopic management and risk assessment
1 Immediate evaluation and initiation of resuscitation
2 Use of prognostication scales for classification of patients into high or low risk for rebleeding and mortality
3 Placement of a nasogastric tube may assist in further prognosis of patient's risk of high-risk lesions
4 Blood transfusion for a hemoglobin level ≤ 70 g/L
5 Correct any coagulopathy, but do not delay endoscopy
6 Do not administer promotility agents routinely prior to endoscopy
7 Selected patients who are at a low risk of rebleeding based on clinical and endoscopic criteria may be discharged after endoscopy
8 Pre-endoscopic PPIs may be used prior to endoscopy with the intent of downstaging lesions and decreasing endoscopic therapy, but this should not delay endoscopy

Endoscopic management
1 Develop institution specific protocols for a multidisciplinary team management as well as ensuring access to an endoscopist trained in endoscopic hemostasis
2 Ensure availability of support staff who are trained to provide assistance in endoscopy
3 Early endoscopy within 24 hours of presentation
4 Low-risk stigmata (clean base ulcer or a non-protuberant pigmented dot in an ulcer bed) do not require endoscopic hemostatic therapy
5 When there is a clot in an ulcer bed, it should be irrigated off, and act on the underlying lesion as appropriate
6 When there is a clot that cannot be removed, the role of endoscopic hemostatic therapy is controversial, and the sole use of high-dose PPI might be sufficient
7 High-risk stigmata (active bleeding or a visible vessel in an ulcer bed) require endoscopic hemostatic therapy
8 Diluted epinephrine injection therapy is insufficient as a sole endoscopic hemostatic therapy modality and should be combined with a second method
9 All thermal coaptive therapy modalities are equally effective
10 Thermocoagulation, clips, and sclerosant injection can be used alone or in combination with epinephrine injection, and should only be used in patients with high-risk lesions
11 Routine second-look endoscopy is not recommended
12 In cases of rebleeding, a second attempt at endoscopic therapy is recommended

Pharmacotherapy
1 Histamine-2 receptor antagonists are not recommended in patients with acute ulcer bleeding
2 Somatostatin and octreotide are not routinely recommended in patients with acute ulcer bleeding
3 In patients with acute ulcer bleeding who have undergone successful endoscopic therapy, an intravenous bolus followed by a continuous infusion of PPI should be administered to decrease the rate of rebleeding as well as mortality
4 Patients should be discharged with a prescription of a single daily dose of PPI for a period of time appropriate for the underlying cause

Non-endoscopic and non-pharmacological inhospital management
1 After endoscopy, patients with low-risk lesions can be fed within 24 hours
2 Most patients with high-risk lesions should be hospitalized for at least 72 hours after endoscopic hemostatic therapy
3 In patients in whom endoscopic therapy fails, surgical consultation should be sought
4 Percutaneous embolization for patients with ulcer bleeding and failed endoscopic therapy can be considered as an alternative to surgery, when available
5 Patients with bleeding peptic ulcers should be tested for *H. pylori* and receive eradication therapy with subsequent confirmation of eradication
6 In the acute setting, a negative diagnostic test for *H. pylori* should be repeated

H. pylori, Helicobacter pylori; PPI,= proton pump inhibitor.
Adapted with permission from Barkun AN, Bardou M, Kuipers EJ, *et al.* International consensus recommendations on the management of patients with nonvariceal upper gastrointestinal bleeding. *Ann Intern Med.* 2010;152:101–113.

Conclusions

The acute management of patients with NVUGIB has evolved significantly over the past decade with adequate initial assessment, risk stratification, and appropriate resuscitation remaining critical aspects of care. Early endoscopy with contemporary methods of endoscopic hemostasis followed by high-dose intravenous PPI have improved outcomes of high-risk patients, and allowed lower-risk individuals to be managed more efficiently, in some cases avoiding admission when they fulfill a list of preset criteria. Ongoing research is needed to better identify optimal dosing thresholds and route of administration of acid suppression, while newer endoscopic hemostatic methods offer promise. The challenge remains to implement and disseminate best practice recommendations in the hope that they will yield the promised improvements in cost-effective care of patients with this common condition.

References

1. Lassen A, Hallas J, Schaffalitzky de Muckadell OB. Complicated and uncomplicated peptic ulcers in a Danish county 1993-2002: a population-based cohort study. *Am J Gastroenterol.* 2006;101: 945–953.
2. Barkun AN, Bardou M, Kuipers EJ, *et al.* International consensus recommendations on the management of patients with

nonvariceal upper gastrointestinal bleeding. *Ann Intern Med.* 2010;152:101–113.

3. Barkun A, Sabbah S, Enns R, *et al.* The Canadian Registry on Nonvariceal Upper Gastrointestinal Bleeding and Endoscopy (RUGBE): Endoscopic hemostasis and proton pump inhibition are associated with improved outcomes in a real-life setting. *Am J Gastroenterol.* 2004;99:1238–1246.

4. Leontiadis GI, Sreedharan A, Dorward S, *et al.* Systematic reviews of the clinical effectiveness and cost-effectiveness of proton pump inhibitors in acute upper gastrointestinal bleeding. *Health Technol Assess.* 2007;11:iii–iv, 1–164.

5. Laine L, McQuaid KR. Endoscopic therapy for bleeding ulcers: an evidence-based approach based on meta-analyses of randomized controlled trials. *Clin Gastroenterol Hepatol.* 2009;7:33–47; quiz 1–2.

6. Barkun AN, Martel M, Toubouti Y, *et al.* Endoscopic hemostasis in peptic ulcer bleeding for patients with high-risk lesions: a series of meta-analyses. *Gastrointest Endosc.* 2009;69:786–799.

7. Lau JY, Leung WK, Wu JC, *et al.* Omeprazole before endoscopy in patients with gastrointestinal bleeding. *N Engl J Med.* 2007;356:1631–1640.

8. Rockall TA, Logan RF, Devlin HB, *et al.* Risk assessment after acute upper gastrointestinal haemorrhage. *Gut.* 1996;38:316–321.

CHAPTER 147

Photodynamic therapy in the gastrointestinal tract

Masoud Panjehpour and Bergein F. Overholt

Thompson Cancer Survival Center, Knoxville, TN, USA

KEY POINTS

Esophagus
- Palliation of esophageal cancer (FDA approved)
- Curative therapy for early esophageal cancer; promising in squamous and Barrett's cancers
- May provide cure of localized lesions when combined with endoscopic mucosal resection
- Therapy for Barrett's esophagus with high-grade dysplasia (FDA approved)

Stomach
- Limited to superficial gastric cancers in patients who are not candidates for surgery; limited published data

Biliary tract
- Promising results in cholangiocarcinoma
- More effective when combined with stenting
- Technically difficult

Ampulla and duodenum
- For palliation of ampullary cancers; limited published clinical data

Pancreas and colon
- No proven role; limited published clinical data

Introduction

Photodynamic therapy (PDT) has been used to treat gastrointestinal, pulmonary, urological, dermatological, and ophthalmological disorders. In the gastrointestinal tract, the treatment may be applied to any tissue where laser light can be delivered endoscopically. The treatment involves the use of a photosensitizer drug that must be given prior to the application of laser light. PDT is well suited to the gastrointestinal tract because laser light can be delivered using optical fibers passed through the endoscope. PDT using porfimer sodium is currently approved in the United States by the FDA to be used in the gastrointestinal tract for palliation of esophageal cancer and for the treatment of Barrett's esophagus with high-grade dysplasia. Other reported applications of PDT using porfimer sodium or other photosensitizers, are treatment of early cancers in the esophagus, gastric cancers, duodenal adenomas, colorectal cancer, pancreatic cancer and cholangiocarcinoma. Non-PDT treatment modalities such as argon plasma coagulation (APC)

and radiofrequency ablation (RFA) have recently been introduced and are discussed in other chapters.

Background

Three components are required for PDT: **photosensitizer, light, and oxygen**. Photosensitizers are generally large complex molecules that can absorb light. Drugs that are used as photosensitizers are generally derivatives of chlorophyll or hemoglobin [1]. **Porfimer sodium** is a porphyrin compound that has been tested extensively and is currently FDA approved for PDT in the esophagus and lung. Another PDT drug is **aminolevulinic acid (ALA)**, the precursor to a photosensitizer called protoporphyrin IX (PPIX). It is primarily used in Europe where it is administered orally 4 hours prior to photoradiation. As ALA is metabolized, protoporphyrin IX accumulates inside the cells and this serves as the actual photosensitizer. ALA is not commercially available in the United States for use in the gastrointestinal tract, but is approved in the United States in dermatology for treatment of actinic keratosis.

While a photosensitizer can be activated using different wavelengths (colors) of light, such as blue light, green light or red light, shorter wavelengths, such as blue and green light, are not typically used due to their superficial penetration in tissue, causing insufficient depth of necrosis. Therefore, red light is typically used in clinical applications of PDT. Both porfimer sodium and ALA are activated using red light of around 630 nm.

Mechanism of photodynamic therapy

The photodynamic effect requires an interaction between light, photosensitizer, and oxygen (Figure 147.1). The photosensitizer must be present in adequate concentrations within the target tissue prior to light irradiation. In tissues that do not absorb the drug, very little necrosis will occur. Light must also be of sufficient intensity to activate the drug. With too little light, there is not enough drug interaction to produce a photodynamic effect. With too much light, the drug is destroyed by the light instead of being activated by it. The dosimetry for PDT requires careful attention to the geometry of the area to be treated, the power (intensity) of the light, and the total

---

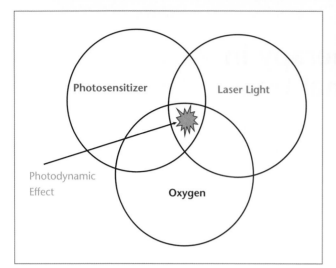

Figure 147.1 Photodynamic effect. The photodynamic effect is contingent on the presence of adequate concentrations of photosensitizing drug, light, and oxygen. (This figure was published in *Clinical Gastroenterology and Hepatology*, Wilfred M. Weinstein, Christopher J. Hawkey, Jaime Bosch, Photodynamic therapy in the gastrointestinal tract, Pages 1053–1058, Copyright Elsevier, 2005.)

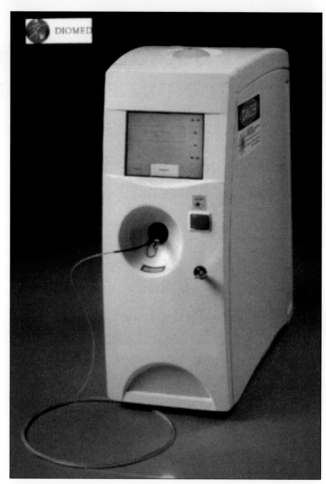

Figure 147.2 Diode laser for photodynamic therapy. Diode lasers are compact, typically the size of a desktop computer. This laser, manufactured by Diomed, Inc., generates 2 W of calibrated 630-nm red light delivered through a fiberoptic.

energy of light that will be needed to produce tissue necrosis. The length of time needed to deliver a treatment is directly proportional to the total energy. In addition, the light must be of an appropriate wavelength to penetrate the tissue and be absorbed by the drug. Typically, the longest wavelength of light that can activate the drug is used since it has the greatest depth of penetration in tissue. Finally, oxygen must be present in the tissue. The interaction between light, photosensitizer, and oxygen generates **singlet oxygen**, which is highly cytotoxic. If the tissue lacks oxygen flow (blood flow), there will be no PDT effect. Since singlet oxygen only persists for a fraction of a second after activation, the damage is limited to the area of tissue that has been illuminated with light.

Clinical applications of photodynamic therapy in the gastrointestinal tract

The most commonly used photosensitizer, porfimer sodium (Photofrin®), is administered intravenously 2–3 days prior to delivery of light. ALA is typically taken orally 4–6 hours before the light illumination. The delay between photosensitizer administration and laser activation is required for the preferential uptake of photosensitizer in the target site. In the case of ALA, the delay time is required for the photosensitizer, protoporphyrin IX, to be produced and to accumulate in the cells.

The light for PDT is provided by a **laser** that can deliver a powerful beam of a very specific wavelength of light. The most compact and technologically advanced source of light is a diode laser, a solid-state laser that is generally more reliable than other lasers (Figure 147.2). The earlier lasers were argon-pumped dye lasers or KTP-pumped dye lasers. Lasers are very useful for PDT in the gastrointestinal tract because their powerful monochromatic light can easily be focused into an optical

fiber suitable for insertion through an endoscope. Light illumination in the gastrointestinal tract is typically performed using an optical fiber fitted with a cylindrical diffuser that irradiates a tumor in a cylindrical organ such as the esophagus. A cylindrical diffuser inserted within a balloon is used for delivery of light for PDT of Barrett's esophagus. Light delivery for PDT in the stomach may also be performed using a microlens fiber that illuminates a circular area of tissue when held a few centimeters from the target site.

Esophageal cancer
Palliation therapy

Palliation of esophageal cancer was the first approved application in the United States of PDT in the gastrointestinal tract. The traditional approach was to place a stent to relieve symptoms of dysphagia. However, stents have a number of deficiencies in regards to efficacy and durability [2]. PDT appears to be more easily applied than traditional laser palliation devices. A cylindrical diffuser fiber is easily inserted through all but the most completely obstructing tumors. The light energy can then

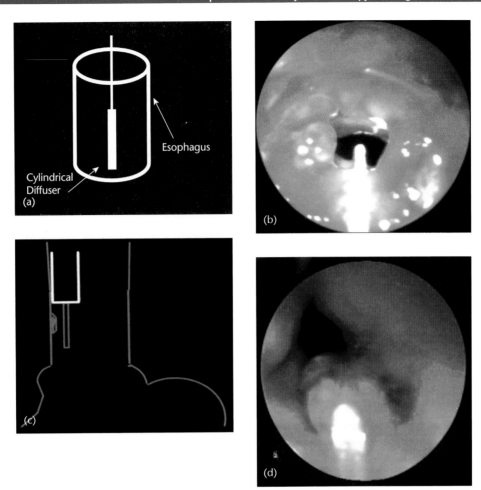

Figure 147.3 Treatment of esophageal cancer. (a) Schematic of a cylindrical diffuser positioned in the center of the esophageal lumen to treat a long segment of esophagus. (b) Endoscopic view of a cylindrical diffuser exiting the endoscope during treatment of a circumferential esophageal cancer. (c) Schematic of endoscopic treatment of early esophageal cancer where the diffuser is laid directly on the cancer. (d) Endoscopic view of an early esophageal cancer in Barrett's esophagus during treatment.

be delivered circumferentially and directly to the tumor surface (Figure 147.3a, b).

A multicenter randomized controlled trial compared porfimer sodium PDT and Nd:YAG laser therapy for the palliation of esophageal cancer [3]. Symptomatic improvement of **dysphagia** was similar in both groups. Nine patients had complete tumor responses after PDT compared with two after Nd:YAG. The Nd:YAG patients had a higher perforation rate of 7% compared to 1% in the PDT group. Efficacy of PDT was similar to that of Nd:YAG but there were fewer significant complications. A large single-center retrospective study of 215 patients who underwent palliative PDT for esophageal cancer found that it was most effective in patients who had obstructing luminal tumors [4]. This patient group underwent 318 courses of therapy for obstruction and for hemorrhage. Eighty-five percent of the patients had improvement in their dysphagia with a mean dysphagia-free time of 66 days. Thirty percent of patients on nutritional supplementation were able to come off it after PDT. Complications reported in this series included perforation in 2%, strictures in 2%, pleural effusions in 4%, and sunburn in 6%. The procedure-related mortality rate was 1.8% with a median survival of 5 months.

The use of PDT in esophageal cancer for palliation of dysphagia may provide an improvement in symptoms for around 2 months. Unlike radiation therapy, PDT may be repeated as needed. PDT may be delivered to those patients who have failed radiation therapy.

Curative therapy for superficial esophageal cancer

Application of PDT for superficial cancers in the esophagus is considered curative. A cylindrical diffuser is passed through the working channel of the endoscope and is laid directly on the surface of the tumor (Figure 147.3c, d) or may even be inserted into the tumor in some cases. In the presence of aggressive proton pump inhibitor (PPI) therapy, as the cancer is eradicated, the site of the previous tumor heals with normal squamous mucosa (Figure 147.4).

In one of the larger studies using a hematoporphyrin derivative as the photosensitizer, PDT was used to treat 123 patients with esophageal cancer: 104 squamous cell carcinomas and 19 adenocarcinomas [5]. Although these cancers were thought to be superficial, at least 27 were staged T2 by endoscopic ultrasound. A complete response was found in 87% of the patients at 6 months. The 5-year survival rate was 25% but the

5-year disease-specific survival rate was 74%. This study pointed out the possibility of using PDT as a curative treatment for superficial cancers. Combination therapy using PDT and mucosal resection for early cancers has been reported with a 94% initial response rate in 17 patients [6]. Compared with esophagectomy for early cancer, this approach has significantly fewer complications [7]. PDT with ALA for treatment of superficial cancer of the esophagus is much less effective, probably because of the superficial uptake of ALA by the mucosa [8]. Porphyrin-based photosensitizers have a much greater depth of penetration, although they also have greater toxicities.

Barrett's esophagus
Using porfimer sodium (Photofrin®)

PDT may be used in Barrett's esophagus with **high-grade dysplasia** as an alternative to surgical therapy. The FDA approval of the technique is based on a multicenter prospective randomized trial of 208 patients randomized 2:1 to PDT and omeprazole versus a control group on omeprazole alone [9]. A unique centering balloon system allowed the endoscopist to treat up to 7 cm of Barrett's esophagus at a time (Figures 147.5 and 147.6) [9]. At 24 months, there was a significant (50%) reduction in cancer in the treatment group. Twenty-eight percent of the controls developed cancer versus 13% in the

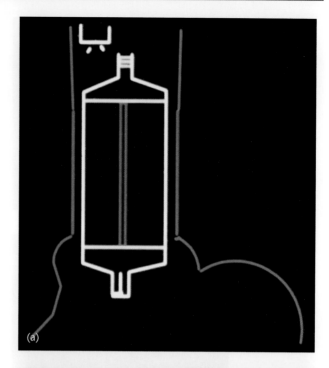

(a)

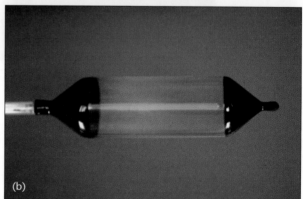

(b)

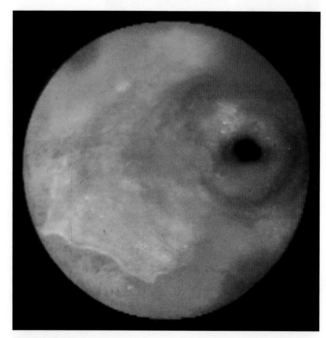

Figure 147.4 Endoscopic view of an area 12 months after photodynamic therapy of an early cancer within Barrett's esophagus. The area of cancer is replaced with normal squamous lining.

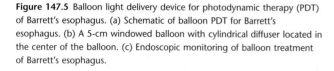

Figure 147.5 Balloon light delivery device for photodynamic therapy (PDT) of Barrett's esophagus. (a) Schematic of balloon PDT for Barrett's esophagus. (b) A 5-cm windowed balloon with cylindrical diffuser located in the center of the balloon. (c) Endoscopic monitoring of balloon treatment of Barrett's esophagus.

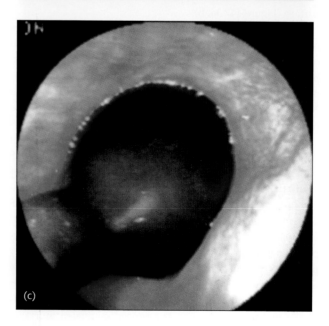

(c)

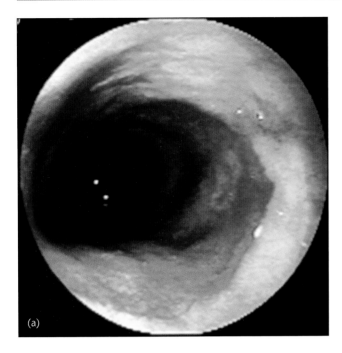

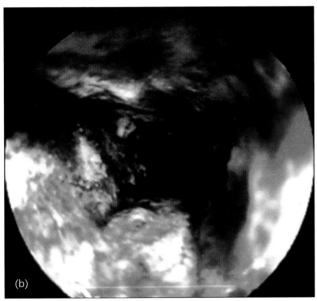

Figure 147.6 Barrett's esophagus: (a) before treatment and (b) 48 hours after porfimer sodium photodynamic therapy.

PDT-treated patients. In addition, the number of patients with high-grade dysplasia also decreased significantly in the treatment group (39%) compared to the control group (77%). Strictures occurred in a third of the PDT-treated patients and cutaneous photosensitivity occurred in two-thirds. The patients in this multicenter randomized study were followed for an additional 3 years, a maximum follow-up of 5 years [10]. At 5 years, PDT was significantly more effective than omeprazole in eliminating high-grade dysplasia (77% vs 39%). There was about half the likelihood of cancer occurring in the PDT group (15%) compared to the control group (29%). There was

also a significantly longer time to progression to cancer in the PDT group.

Use of **endoscopic mucosal resection (EMR)** should be strongly considered prior to PDT for patients with mucosal irregularities. EMR may upgrade the histology, prompting a modified PDT dosimetry. The application of PDT and EMR for patients with early adenocarcinoma and high-grade dysplasia has been shown to be safe and effective [11,12].

Growth of neosquamous mucosa over Barrett's mucosa is another concern after PDT. This was studied in 33 658 biopsy samples from the randomized multicenter PDT study [9] and was shown to be similar in both PDT and omeprazole-only control groups [13].

Using aminolevulinic acid

ALA-PDT is also used in the treatment of Barrett's esophagus. ALA-PDT is not associated with the prolonged photosensitivity seen in porfimer sodium-PDT. In addition, due to the superficial necrosis seen in ALA-PDT, the risk of esophageal stricture is reduced.

In one study, two doses of ALA (30 and 60 mg/kg) and two colors of laser light were tested in 27 patients with high-grade dysplasia [14]. The ALA dose of 60 mg/kg and red light were most effective in eradicating high-grade dysplasia. A 36-month follow-up of 21 patients treated using the red light and higher dose of photosensitizer showed 89% eradication of high-grade dysplasia and 96% of patients were free of cancer.

Another group studied different light doses given after an ALA dose of 60 mg/kg. The use of the highest light dose of 1000 J/cm was recommended as a safe treatment [15].

Sixty-six patients with high-grade dysplasia or early adenocarcinoma were treated using 60 mg/kg of ALA-PDT in another study [16]. Complete response was seen in 97% (n = 35) of high-grade dysplasia patients and 100% of early cancer (n = 31) patients at a median follow-up of 37 months. However, there was one recurrence in the former group and 10 in the latter group [16]. Fractionated irradiation has been proposed to overcome the problem of photobleaching when using ALA-PDT [17].

ALA-PDT has also been reported for treatment of **early squamous cell carcinoma** of the proximal esophagus [18]. After three sessions of PDT the patient was completely clear of all cancer at 23 months. Long-term follow-up of such cases is strongly recommended [18]. Application of ALA-PDT for treatment of residual disease after endoscopic resection of high-grade dysplasia/early cancer was not recommended by one group who used a drug dose of 40 mg/kg [19].

Non-PDT treatment modalities such as the APC and RFA have recently been introduced for the treatment of Barrett's esophagus and are discussed in other chapters.

Stomach
Treatment of superficial gastric cancers

PDT has been approved for use in the treatment of gastric cancers in Japan, but randomized controlled trials are not available. More than 133 cases of gastric cancer were treated with PDT [20]. Over 90% were early stage and all cancers had an initial complete response to PDT. However, there was a 22% recurrence rate. The depth of invasion definitely affects the response rate [21]. A number of other retrospective reports have been reported in the literature with small numbers of patients [22–24]. In a European series, the typical dose of 2 mg/kg of porfimer sodium and light dose of 15–300 J/cm led to a cure in 82% of patients [23]. Twenty-two patients with early gastric cancer were treated using mesotetrahydroxyphenyl-chlorin (mTHPC) as PDT photosensitizer [22]. Complete remission was seen in 73% of all patients, 80% of those with intestinal-type cancers and 50% of those with diffuse Lauren's carcinoma.

Application of porfimer sodium and an excimer laser for PDT of early gastric cancer was shown to be effective. In one study, complete response was seen in all eight early lesions in seven patients with early gastric cancer [25] and in another study, complete response was seen in all lesions of superficial depressed type without ulceration and/or with tumor diameter less than 2 cm in 27 patients with early gastric cancer [26]. A gold vapor laser was used for porfimer sodium-PDT of eight cases of early gastric cancer, and local cure was achieved in seven of these, with recurrence occurring in one patient [27].

The use of PDT in the stomach appears to be limited to **superficial gastric cancers** in patients who are not candidates for surgery, with the intestinal type responding better than the diffuse type of gastric cancer. The overall success rates using PDT for gastric cancers range from 100% to 50%. PDT appears to be most effective for the treatment of type I, IIa, and IIb gastric cancers less than 2 cm in diameter. The PDT palliation of advanced gastric cancer has little advantage over alternative laser or thermal methods [23]. The adverse effects (strictures, perforation) of PDT therapy in the stomach are comparatively minimal compared with PDT therapy in the esophagus.

Pancreas

There are no current approvals for the use of PDT in the pancreas. PDT was reported in 16 patients with locally unresectable pancreatic cancers [28]. mTHPC was given intravenously 72 hours prior to photoradiation, and PDT was administered with computed tomography (CT)-placed diffusing fibers. All patients showed substantial tumor necrosis. Fourteen of 16 patients left the hospital within 10 days. Patients had a median survival time of 9.5 months after treatment. Treatment complications included strictures of the duodenum in three patients and gastrointestinal bleeding in two. Seven of 16 patients were alive 1 year after PDT. No pancreatitis was reported. Currently there is no evidence to support PDT for pancreatic cancer.

Biliary tract

PDT is used in treating **cholangiocarcinoma** with considerable success, although it is not approved for this disease. Photoradiation of the biliary tract is difficult to perform because of the

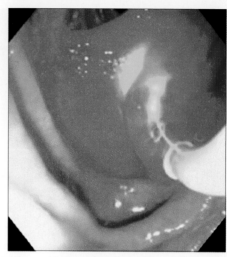

Figure 147.7 Photodynamic therapy of the biliary tract. A cylindrical diffuser is inserted through a catheter, which is positioned in the common bile duct. During photoradiation, the bile duct "glows" from the laser energy diffusing in the bile duct.

rigidity of the commercially available cylindrical diffusing fibers. The diffusing fibers require special catheters and careful placement in the biliary tract [29]. To overcome this problem, a 1.0 or 2.5 cm cylindrical diffusing fiber can be preloaded into an 8 Fr biliary catheter. This catheter has a 0.038-inch diameter lumen to accommodate a 0.035-inch diameter guidewire. Endoscopic retrograde cholangiopancreatography (ERCP) is preformed, localizing the cholangiocarcinoma with the proximal and distal margins recorded. The preloaded catheter is advanced over the guidewire after the position of the catheter is confirmed by fluoroscopy. The power used to treat the cholangiocarcinoma is 400 mW/cm of diffuser length for a total dose of 180 J/cm². Figure 147.7 shows a cylindrical diffuser inserted through a catheter, which is positioned in the common bile duct. After therapy, 10 Fr or 11.5 Fr biliary catheters are placed to ensure biliary drainage after therapy.

A case series of nine patients was described in 1998, showing that PDT could restore biliary drainage and improve quality of life with median survival of 439 days [30].

A prospective randomized trial was reported in which 39 patients received either a stent alone or a stent and PDT [31]. Those who received PDT had a significantly prolonged survival of 493 days versus only 98 days in the control population.

Application of PDT followed by a self-expanding stent has been shown to be an effective treatment for non-resectable hilar cholangiocarcinoma, significantly decreasing serum bilirubin and improving quality of life compared with a control group who were treated with biliary drainage alone [31–33]. Five-year follow-up data for 23 patients with non-resectable hilar cholangiocarcinoma treated using PDT showed a median survival of 11.2 months for patient without distant metastasis and 9.3 months for all patients combined [34]. The 1-, 2-, 3-, and 4-year survival rates were 47%, 21%, 11%, and 5% for stage M0, and 39%, 17%, 9%, and 4% for stages M0 and M1, respectively. Improvement in cholestasis, performance, and quality of life were maintained for an extended period of time in all patients except one case with diffuse liver metastasis.

Colorectal liver metastasis has also been treated using mTHPBC as the photosensitizer and interstitial light delivery inserted percutaneously, causing tumor necrosis in all lesions treated [35]. It was concluded that colorectal liver metastases that are ineligible for resection can safely and effectively be treated with PDT.

Cholangitis is a possible complication. Although not proven, cutaneous photosensitivity may be of greater magnitude in biliary PDT compared to PDT of the esophagus. This may be because the porphyrins are retained in an obstructed biliary system.

Duodenum and ampulla

Small case series have been reported using PDT in ampullary lesions. Ampullary carcinomas were treated in a series of 10 non-surgical candidates [36]. Seven patients showed partial response, while three showed no response. Smaller tumors responded completely but all recurred. Three cases of ampullary adenomas (1–1.5 cm) demonstrated a decrease in size of the lesions [37]. Overall, the potential role of PDT in the treatment of ampullary lesions is limited, and it may be useful for palliation rather than cure.

Colon and rectum

There has been little enthusiasm for using PDT for colonic tumors. Seven of nine large villous adenomas were eradicated with PDT after failure of thermal ablative techniques [38]. ALA-PDT in familial polyposis adenomas produced necrosis in the most superficial portions of the polyps [39]. ALA-PDT was also reported in carcinoma *in situ* of the anus in five human immunodeficiency virus (HIV)-positive patients [40]. All patients showed downgrading of cytological findings. Papanicolaou test results showed two patients had no dysplasia, two had mild dysplasia, and one had moderate dysplasia. A patient with recurrent local carcinoma of the rectum was treated using PDT [41]. Biopsies at 10 weeks were clear in the treated area but recurred at 16 weeks.

A pilot study reported on 10 patients with colorectal cancer [42]. Two patients with small lesions were tumor free 20 and 28 months after PDT. One treatment of advanced tumor was complicated by hemorrhage. PDT was suggested to be suitable for treatment of small tumors or for small areas of persistent disease where the bulk has been removed.

Adverse effects

One of the adverse effects of PDT is primarily related to its mechanism of action and photosensitivity [43]. **Cutaneous photosensitivity** can occur within minutes of injection of the photosensitizer. Patients need to be carefully instructed regarding sunlight exposure avoidance. The rates of photosensitivity

reaction with porfimer sodium vary from 30% to 60%. Most events are mild and do not require therapy, although severe cases may involve full-thickness skin injury. The cutaneous photosensitivity can persist for 30–90 days after injection. Patients should be cautioned that sunscreen is of little benefit as it only protects against ultraviolet light and not visible light. Sun protection must be in the form of light-proof clothing and gloves, large wide-brimmed hats, and sunglasses.

Photosensitivity associated with ALA-PDT lasts about 2–3 days after ingestion of ALA and is not as severe as porfimer photosensitivity. mTHPC causes the worst photosensitivity among all photosensitizers.

With porfimer sodium-PDT of the esophagus, odynophagia and chest pain are common in the first 2 weeks after photoradiation and are treated with narcotic analgesics. Nausea and vomiting may occur in the first 2–3 days following photoradiation and require antiemetics.

One of the complications of porfimer sodium-PDT has been the development of **esophageal strictures** [10]. The factors that increase the risk of stricture after PDT of Barrett's esophagus include history of prior stricture, prior endoscopic mucosal resection, and multiple PDT sessions [44]. Deep tissue necrosis may result in stricture formation, which occurs 3–4 weeks after treatment. Some strictures may be very fibrotic and require repeated dilations. Stricture formations are not a major issue when using ALA-PDT due to the superficial nature of tissue necrosis.

Hypotension and nausea/vomiting are complications associated with ALA-PDT, especially when a higher dose of drug is administered.

Conclusions

PDT has several natural advantages for use in the gastrointestinal tract. The treatment does not require the physician to target a specific lesion, which allows the therapy to be applied to areas outside of the visual range of the endoscope, such as the biliary system where its use has been shown to dramatically improve life-expectancy in patients with cholangiocarcinoma. This treatment also allows rapid therapy of large mucosal areas, which should be beneficial in Barrett's esophagus. Newer PDT agents are being developed that will hopefully decrease the frequency and severity of potential adverse events.

Overall, with indications for esophageal cancer, Barrett's esophagus, and cholangiocarcinoma, PDT has a potential role in gastrointestinal tract. Application of RFA technology should be considered as an alternative treatment of Barrett's esophagus.

SOURCES OF INFORMATION FOR PATIENTS AND DOCTORS

www.nci.nih.gov/cancertopics/factsheet/therapy/photodynamic
www.Barretts-esophagus.org

References

1. Dougherty TJ, Gomer CJ, Henderson BW, *et al*. PDT. *J Natl Cancer Inst*. 1998;90:889–905.
2. Lightdale CJ. Role of PDT in the management of advanced esophageal cancer. *Gastrointest Endosc Clin North Am*. 2000;10:397–408.
3. Lightdale CJ, Heier SK, Marcon NE, *et al*. PDT with Porfimer sodium versus thermal ablation therapy with Nd:YAG laser for palliation of esophageal cancer: a multicenter randomized trial. *Gastrointest Endosc*. 1995;42:507–512.
4. Litle VR, Luketich JD, Christie NA, *et al*. PDT as palliation for esophageal cancer: experience in 215 patients. *Ann Thorac Surg*. 2003;76:1687–1692.
5. Sibille A, Lambert R, Souquet JC, Sabben G, Descos F. Long-term survival after PDT for esophageal cancer. *Gastroenterology*. 1995;108:337–344.
6. Buttar NS, Wang KK, Lutzke LS, Krishnadath KK, Anderson MA. Combined endoscopic mucosal resection and PDT for esophageal neoplasia within Barrett's esophagus. *Gastrointest Endosc*. 2001;54:682–688.
7. Pacifico RJ, Wang KK, WongKeeSong LM, Buttar NS, Lutzke LS. Combined endoscopic mucosal resection and PDT versus esophagectomy for management of early adenocarcinoma in Barrett's esophagus. *Clin Gastroenterol Hepatol*. 2003;1:252–257.
8. Gossner L, Stolte M, Sroka R, *et al*. PDT of early squamous epithelial carcinomas and severe squamous epithelial dysplasias of the esophagus with 5-aminolevulinic acid. *Z Gastroenterol*. 1998;36:19–26.
9. Overholt BF, Lightdale CJ, Wang KK, *et al*. Photodynamic therapy with pofimer sodium for ablation of high grade dysplasia in Barrett's esophagus: international, partially blinded, randomized phase III trial. *Gastrointest Endosc*. 2005;62:488–498.
10. Overholt BF, Wang KK, Burdick JS, *et al*. Five-year efficacy and safety of photodynamic therapy with Photofrin in Barrett's high grade dysplasia. *Gastrointest Endosc*. 2007;66:460–468.
11. Pacifico RJ, Wang KK, Wongkeesong LM, *et al*. Combined endoscopic mucosal resection and photodynamic therapy versus esophagectomy for management of early adenocarcinoma in Barrett's esophagus. *Clin Gastroenterol Hepatol*. 2003;1:252–257.
12. Wolfsen HC, Hemminger LL, Raimondo M, *et al*. Photodynamic therapy and endoscopic mucosal resection for Barrett's dysplasia and early esophageal adenocarcinoma. *South Med J*. 2004;97:827–830.
13. Bronner MP, Overholt BF, Taylor SL, *et al*. Squamous overgrowth is not a safety concern for photodynamic therapy of Barrett's esophagus with high grade dysplasia. *Gastroenterology*. 2009;136:56–64.
14. Mackenzie GD, Dunn JM, Selvasekar CR, *et al*. Optimal conditions for successful ablation of high grade dysplasia in Barrett's oesophagus using aminolaevulinic acid photodynamic therapy. *Lasers Med Sci*. 2009;24:729–734.
15. Mackenzie GD, Jamieson NF, Novelli MR, *et al*. How light dosimetry influences the efficacy of photodynamic therapy with 5 aminolaevulinic acid for ablation of high grade dysplasia in Barrett's esophagus. *Lasers Med Sci*. 2008;23:203–210.
16. Pech O, Gossner L, May A, *et al*. Long-term results of photodynamic therapy with 5-aminolaevulinic acid for superficial Barrett's cancer and high grade intraepithelial neoplasia. *Gastrointest Endosc*. 2005;62:24–30.
17. Pogue BW, Sheng C, Benevides J, *et al*. Protoporphyrin IX fluorescence photobleaching increases with the use of fractionated irradiation in the esophagus. *J Biomed Opt*. 2008;13:034009.
18. Eickhoff A, Jakobs R, Weickert U, *et al*. Long-segment early squamous cell carcinoma of the proximal esophagus: Curative treatment and long-term follow-up after 5-aminolaevulinic acid (5-ALA) photodynamic therapy. *Endoscopy*. 2006;38:641–643.
19. Peters F, Kara M, Rosmolen W, *et al*. Poor results of 5-aminolaevulinic acid photodynamic therapy for residual high grade dysplasia and early cancer in Barrett's esophagus after endoscopic resection. *Endoscopy*. 2005;37:418–424.
20. Kato H, Kito T, Furuse K, *et al*. PDT in the early treatment of cancer. Review 10 refs Japanese. *Gan to Kagaku Ryoho*. [*Jpn J Cancer Chemother*.] 1990;17:1833–1838.
21. Mimura S, Ichii M, Imanishi K, Otani T, Okuda S. Indications for and limitations of HpD PDT for esophageal cancer and gastric cancer. *Gan to Kagaku Ryoho*. [*Jpn J Cancer Chemother*.] 1988;15:1440–1444.
22. Ell C, Gossner L, May A, *et al*. Photodynamic ablation of early cancers of the stomach by means of mTHPC and laser irradiation: preliminary clinical experience. *Gut*. 1998;43:345–349.
23. Gossner L, Ell C. PDT of gastric cancer. *Gastrointest Endosc Clin North Am*. 2000;10:461–480.
24. Vonarx V, Eleouet S, Carre J, *et al*. Potential efficacy of a delta 5-aminolevulinic acid bioadhesive gel formulation for the photodynamic treatment of lesions of the gastrointestinal tract in mice. *J Pharm Pharmacol*. 1997;49:652–656.
25. Nakamura H, Yanai H, Nishikawa J, *et al*. Experience with photodynamic therapy (endoscopic laser therapy) for the treatment of early gastric cancer. *Hepatogastroenterology*. 2001;48:1599–1603.
26. Mimura S, Ito Y, Nagayo T, *et al*. Cooperative clinical trial of photodynamic therapy with Photofrin II and excimer dye laser for early gastric cancer. *Lasers Surg Med*. 1996;19:168–172.
27. Nakamura T, Ejiri M, Fujisawa T, *et al*. Photodynamic therapy for early gastric cancer using a pulsed gold vapor laser. *J Clin Laser Med Surg*. 1990;8:63–67.
28. Bown SG, Rogowska AZ, Whitelaw DE, *et al*. PDT for cancer of the pancreas. *Gut*. 2002;50:549–557.
29. Rumalla A, Baron TH, Wang KK, *et al*. Endoscopic application of PDT for cholangiocarcinoma. *Gastrointest Endosc*. 2001;53:500–504.
30. Ortner MA, Liebetruth J, Schreiber S, *et al*. PDT of nonresectable cholangiocarcinoma. *Gastroenterology*. 1998;114:536–542.
31. Ortner ME, Caca K, Berr F, *et al*. Successful PDT for nonresectable cholangiocarcinoma: a randomized prospective study. *Gastroenterology*. 2003;125:1355–1363.
32. Dumoulin FL, Gerhardt T, Fuchs S, *et al*. Phase II study of photodynamic therapy and metal stent as palliative treatment for nonresectable hilar cholangiocarcinoma. *Gastrointest Endosc*. 2003;57:860–867.
33. Kahaleh M, Mishra R, Shami VM, *et al*. Unresectable cholangiocarcinoma: comparison of survival in biliary stenting alone versus stenting with photodynamic therapy. *Clin Gastroenterol Hepatol*. 2008;6:290–297.
34. Wiedman M, Berr F, Schiefke I, *et al*. Photodynamic therapy in patients with nonresectable hilar cholangiocarcinoma: 5 year follow-up of a prospective phase II study. *Gastrointest Endosc*. 2004;60:68–75.

35. Van Duijnhoven FH, Rovers JP, Engelmann K, *et al.* Photodynamic therapy with 5,10,15,20-tetrakis(m-hydroxyphenyl) bacteriochlorin for colorectal liver metastasis is safe and feasible: results from phase I study. *Ann Surg Oncol.* 2005 Oct;12(10): 808–16.

36. Abulafi AM, Allardice JT, Williams NS, *et al.* PDT for malignant tumours of the ampulla of Vater. *Gut.* 1995;36:853–856.

37. Mlkvy P, Messmann H, Regula J, *et al.* PDT for gastrointestinal tumors using three photosensitizers – ALA induced PPIX, Photofrin and mTHPC. A pilot study. *Neoplasma.* 1998;45:157–161.

38. Loh CS, Bliss P, Bown SG, Krasner N. PDT for villous adenomas of the colon and rectum. *Endoscopy.* 1994;26:243–246.

39. Mlkvy P, Messmann H, Debinski H, *et al.* PDT for polyps in familial adenomatous polyposis – a pilot study. *Eur J Cancer.* 1995;31A:1160–1165.

40. Webber J, Fromm D. Photodynamic therapy for carcinoma in situ of anus. *Arch Surg.* 2004;39:259–261.

41. Kashtan H, Haddad R, Yossiphov Y, *et al.* Photodynamic therapy of colorectal cancer using a new light source: from *in vitro* studies to a patient treatment. *Dis Colon Rectum.* 1996;39:379–383.

42. Barr H, Krasner N, Boulos PB, *et al.* Photodynamic therapy for colorectal cancer: a quantitative pilot study. *Br J Surg.* 1990;77: 93–96.

43. Wang KK, Nijhawan PK. Complications of PDT in gastrointestinal disease. *Gastrointest Endosc Clin North Am.* 2000;10:487–495.

44. Prasad GA, Wang KK, Buttar NS, *et al.* Predictors of stricture formation after photodynamic therapy for high grade dysplasia in Barrett's esophagus. *Gastrointest Endosc.* 2007;65:60–66.

CHAPTER 148

Percutaneous endoscopic gastrostomy and jejunostomy

Jeffrey L. Ponsky[1] and Benjamin K. Poulose[2]
[1]University Hospitals of Cleveland, Cleveland, OH, USA
[2]Vanderbilt University Medical Center, Nashville, TN, USA

KEY POINTS

Percutaneous endoscopic gastrostomy (PEG)
Define point of optimal contact using finger pressure
- Employ the "safe tract" method of entry
- Capture suture in snare, and pull from patient's mouth
- Attach suture to end of gastrostomy tube and pull tube into esophagus
- Follow tube with endoscope to assure proper final position of tube
- Apply outer crossbar several millimeters from the skin, avoiding tension

Percutaneous endoscopic jejunostomy (PEJ) as an extension of PEG
- Place PEG in usual fashion
- Guide small-caliber feeding tube through or alongside PEG tube and into small bowel

Direct PEJ
- Pass enteroscope or pediatric colonoscope beyond the ligament of Treitz
- Verify position of scope's tip with finger pressure or fluoroscopy
- Utilize "safe tract" method to assure the adjacent bowel is not punctured
- Perform in the same fashion as for PEG

Costs, complications, and controversies
- More cost-effective than surgical gastrostomy
- Complications include: infection, tube leakage, tube dislodgment, gastrocolic fistula
- Controversies: short-term advantages versus nasoenteric tubes end-of-life issues

---

Percutaneous endoscopic gastrostomy
Introduction and scientific basis

For generations, surgeons have fixed the stomach and other hollow viscera to the skin with tubes in order to create fistulous tracts used for feeding or decompression. In 1980, the first description of such a fistula, produced endoscopically, was published [1]. The principle of percutaneous endoscopic gastrostomy (PEG) has now been established with widespread clinical experience. In addition, fixation of the jejunum [2] for feeding, and of the cecum [3] for decompression, has been also shown to be safe and effective. Initially, the serosal surface of the viscus is held in apposition to the peritoneal wall by the endoscopically-guided tube. After approximately 1 week, an adhesive connection forms that serves to maintain the surfaces in more permanent contact. Once the adhesive connection has been established, the tube may be removed or changed. Should the tube be removed and not immediately replaced, the fistulous tract is likely to close within a few hours. The two surfaces need not be tightly apposed to assure tract formation [4]. Extreme tension applied to the outer fixating crossbar to assure close approximation of the gastric and abdominal walls is unnecessary, and may be harmful by causing ischemia of the interposed tissue.

Technique (refer to the accompanying insertion and care protocol on the website)

The **"pull" technique** is employed most commonly (see Video clip 148.1) [5]. A review of pertinent radiographic images can help identify anatomical issues that potentially make placement more difficult (e.g., large hiatal hernia). However, routine preprocedural studies are not required unless deemed necessary by the clinical situation (e.g. altered surgical anatomy). A single dose of an intravenous antibiotic (usually a cephalosporin) is given as the procedure is commenced. Moderate sedation is usually performed, but deep sedation or general anesthesia may be required for some patients and in children may be the optimal approach. The patient is placed in the semi-recumbent position. The abdomen should be cleansed with an antiseptic solution and sterilely draped.

Upper endoscopic examination

This is performed to rule out significant unsuspected lesions. The endoscope is then pulled back into the gastric body and full inflation of the stomach is commenced. The assistant, working at the abdominal site, then probes the abdomen with a finger, beginning at the subxiphoid region and proceeding down the left costal margin. While this is occurring, the endoscopist looks for a point of clear and prominent indentation of the gastric wall when finger pressure is applied (Figure

---

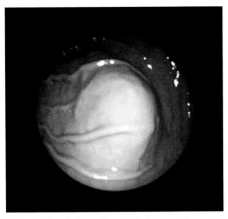

Figure 148.1 The PEG technique. Clear indentation of the gastric wall should be noted at the optimal site for PEG placement.

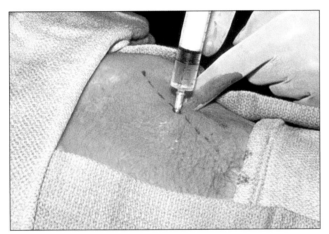

Figure 148.2 The PEG technique. Using the "safe tract" method, air should not enter the syringe barrel until the needle is seen in the gastric lumen.

148.1). Alternatively, probing with two adjacent fingers and observing separate points of indentation endoscopically can help **localize the point for lumenal access**. This is a crucial point in the procedure, and extra time spent at this juncture is well rewarded. Transillumination of the endoscopic light can also help identify the area for gastric access. When such a site is agreed upon, the assistant introduces a syringe half filled with local anesthetic, and fitted with a small-caliber needle, while pulling back upon the syringe barrel to create negative pressure. The needle is slowly advanced into the abdominal wall and into the gastric lumen. The endoscopist carefully looks for the needle's entry into the stomach, while the assistant's attention is focused on the barrel of the syringe. The endoscopist calls out when the needle enters the gastric lumen and the assistant calls out if air bubbles into the syringe barrel (Figure 148.2). Should air bubble into the syringe barrel before the needle has appeared in the gastric lumen, there is a high likelihood that another air-containing viscus (small bowel or colon) has been entered. In such a case, the needle is withdrawn and an alternative site of entry selected. This latter method, named the **"safe tract" technique**, has greatly added to the safety of percutaneous enteral access [6].

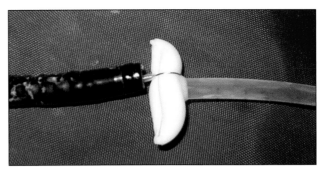

Figure 148.3 The PEG technique. Half of the head of the tube is grasped with a snare through the scope so that it may lead the second passage of the scope easily into the esophagus.

Grasping the suture

Once the site has been so identified, the endoscopist opens a polypectomy snare over that area of the gastric wall and the assistant injects a small amount of local anesthetic into the skin at the proposed site of entry. A scalpel is used to make a 0.5-cm skin incision, and a larger sheathed needle is thrust through the apposed gastric and abdominal walls and into the waiting snare loop. The snare is then closed about the needle sheath and the needle withdrawn or pulled back. A long suture or wire is then threaded through the sheath and into the gastric lumen. The snare is then opened slightly, the sheath withdrawn slightly, and the snare retightened around the suture itself. The endoscope and suture are then pulled from the patient's mouth.

Tube placement

The suture exiting the patient's mouth is affixed to the tapered end of the gastrostomy tube and the assistant begins pulling at the abdominal site. The second passage of the endoscope may be facilitated by grasping half the head of the gastrostomy tube with the snare passed through the channel of the endoscope (Figure 148.3). The tube is well lubricated, pulled down the esophagus, and should be followed by the endoscope to ensure that its tip comes to lie in the proper position (Figure 148.4). The endoscope then closely follows the tube into the esophagus and is gently pushed as the tube is pulled. The snare is opened to release the gastrostomy tube about halfway down the esophagus. The head of the tube should come to lie in loose approximation to the gastric mucosa (Figure 148.5). The endoscope is then removed.

Fixation

Attention is then turned to the abdominal exit point of the tube. The tube is cleansed of any remaining lubricant and trimmed to the desired length. The outer crossbar or retention disk is applied and brought down to within several millimeters of the skin (Figure 148.6). It is **not** desirable for the crossbar or retention disk to meet the skin as this may produce undue tension with resultant ischemia and necrosis of the abdominal wall or stomach. The crossbar should be positioned several

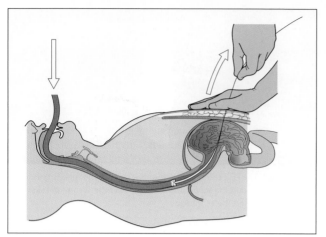

Figure 148.4 Insertion of the gastrostomy tube. The endoscope–gastrostomy tube combination is passed down the esophagus. Halfway down the esophagus, the gastrostomy tube is released and pulled into the stomach as the endoscopist observes its position.

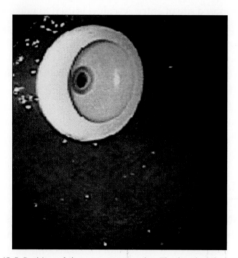

Figure 148.5 Position of the gastrostomy tube. The head of the gastrostomy tube should come to lie in loose contact with the gastric mucosa.

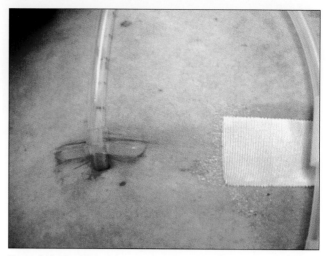

Figure 148.6 Position of the outer crossbar. The outer crossbar should be applied several millimeters from the skin to avoid producing ischemia of the underlying tissue.

Table 148.1 Indications and contraindications for percutaneous endoscopic gastrostomy

Indications
• Inability to swallow due to neurological impairment
• Oropharyngeal tumors
• Need for long-term gastrointestinal decompression
• Need for supplemental feedings
• Facial trauma
Contraindications
• Sepsis
• Multiorgan failure
• Massive ascites
• Severe malnutrition
• Severe gastroesophageal reflux
• Life expectancy <30 days

millimeters from the skin; after 1 week the crossbar can be moved 2–3 cm from the skin. Once the tract is mature, the only purpose of the crossbar is to prevent migration of the tube's head distally to the pylorus, where it may cause obstruction. The redundant tube is taped to the abdominal wall. Occlusive dressings are not required. If no complications are apparent, the tube may be used for medications, flushes, and feeding immediately.

Since the original description of the pull PEG technique described above, other successful insertion techniques have been developed for certain clinical conditions. The **"push" technique** described by Sacks and Vine offers an alternative means of PEG placement, but still requires traversal of the internal bumper through the aerodigestive tract [7]. At times it may be advisable to avoid traversal of the PEG tube across the aerodigestive tract. This situation arises with bulky

oropharyngeal tumors, tight esophageal strictures, or inflammation precluding safe passage of the PEG tube. If a small-caliber scope can safely be passed across the area of stenosis or inflammation, visualization and insufflation of the stomach can usually be provided for establishment of enteral access using an alternative technique. One such technique, described by Russell, employs t-fasteners to appose the gastric wall to the abdominal wall prior to tube insertion [8]. Yet another technique describes use of a dilating trocar to place the gastrostomy tube directly into the gastric lumen [9].

Indications and contraindications (Table 148.1)
Percutaneous enteral access should not be performed in patients with overwhelming sepsis, multiorgan failure, or severe malnutrition. Nasogastric feedings should be employed in such patients until such time as these problems are resolved. Should the need for long-term enteral alimentation or decompression continue, percutaneous enteral access may be considered. Massive ascites and bleeding diatheses are relative

contraindications. Severe gastroesophageal reflux may actually be exacerbated by gastrostomy, causing more frequent aspiration. Patients with a life-expectancy of less than 30 days have a very high mortality rate associated with the procedure [10].

PEG is of value in providing long-term enteral access in patients **who are unable to swallow but who have a functional gastrointestinal tract**. Such patients include those with oropharyngeal tumors, facial trauma, and neurological impairment. The method has also been used with success in providing supplemental feedings in those with inflammatory bowel disease and for the delivery of unpalatable medications in children. It has been used as a means of recycling bile in some cases of biliary obstruction where internal drainage cannot be achieved [11]. Patients with chronic, surgically irremediable, intestinal obstruction secondary to gastric or intestinal atony, malignancy, adhesions, or radiation may be candidates for decompressive gastrostomy.

Percutaneous endoscopic jejunostomy (refer to the accompanying insertion and care protocol on the website)

First described in 1984, the original method involved placement of an enteral feeding tube alongside a PEG tube, with the latter used for decompression [12]. High failure rates were reported as a result of tube dysfunction and frequent tube manipulation. Placement of percutaneous endoscopic jejunostomy (PEJ) as an **extension of PEG** commences with initial placement of a PEG tube. Care should be taken to ensure that the PEJ extension can fit through the lumen of the indwelling PEG and that the external feeding/drainage adapter mates with the PEG tubing securely. In general, a 9-Fr PEJ extension fits through a 20-Fr PEG. A pretied suture affixed to the tip of the PEJ extension helps facilitate placement into the distal duodenum. This suture is grasped with an endoscopic clip or biopsy forceps and the tip of the instrument brought back into the instrument channel. The pylorus is intubated and the distal duodenum or jejunum is visualized. The instrument is then used to appose the suture to the duodenal or jejunal mucosa. An endoscopic clip is used to fix the suture to the duodenal mucosa and the scope is carefully withdrawn from the small bowel. The PEJ extension is again visualized, ensuring it remains post-pyloric after the scope has been withdrawn from the duodenum.

Direct PEJ utilizes the same technique and principles as PEG, but in the small bowel (see Video clip 148.2). An enteroscope or pediatric colonoscope is employed to intubate the small bowel deeply, distal to the ligament of Treitz. Finger pressure is used to assess the best probable site for puncture. The use of fluoroscopy may also be helpful in assessing the position of the tip of the endoscope (Figure 148.7). Once the site of proposed puncture has been selected, the **"safe tract" method** is used to minimize the potential of inadvertent puncture of adjacent bowel. A useful method is to place the "finder" needle on the end of the syringe and advance this until it

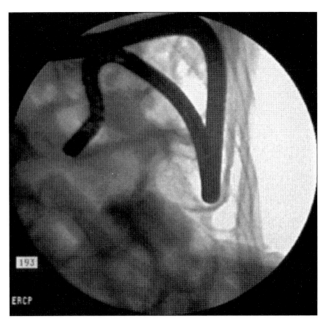

Figure 148.7 Percutaneous endoscopic jejunostomy. Fluoroscopy is useful in assessing the position of the scope in the abdomen and selecting the best site for puncture.

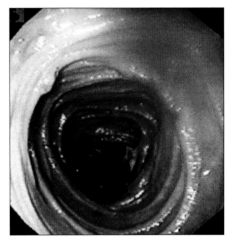

Figure 148.8 Position of the PEJ tube. The PEJ tube should come to lie in loose contact with the jejunal wall. A tube of up to 20 Fr may be used without compromising the intestinal lumen.

successfully enters the visible lumen ahead of the endoscope. The endoscopist may now grasp this needle with a snare. The syringe is removed from the "finder" needle and attached to the larger sheathed needle required for the procedure; this is then passed immediately beside and parallel to the "finder" needle. When the large sheathed needle enters the visible lumen, the snare is transferred to grasp the sheath, and both needles are removed. The rest of the method is identical to that for PEG (Figure 148.8). Again, tension is to be avoided in the application of the outer crossbar.

Indications and contraindications

These are listed in Table 148.2.

Table 148.2 Indications and contraindications for percutaneous endoscopic jejunostomy

Indications
• Severe gastroesophageal reflux in a patient requiring long-term enteral feeding
• Gastric atony

Contraindications
• Massive ascites
• Bleeding diatheses
• Intestinal obstruction

Complications and their management

Infections have become much less common with the use of the single-dose antibiotic as described. Many of the earlier severe infections were the result of excessive tension applied to the outer crossbar with resultant ischemia and necrotizing infection. The tube site should be inspected each day after performing the procedure. Infection should be suspected if redness, erythema, or induration develops. If a local, peritubal abscess is suspected, drainage with local anesthesia and incision of the indurated site followed by antibiotic therapy may allow for uncomplicated resolution. If the site continues to worsen, surgical consultation must be sought.

Leakage around the tube is a common complaint. Most often this represents a small amount of drainage, which is a foreign body reaction to the tube. Good hygiene with frequent cleansing usually suffices. Granulation tissue may develop in response to the tube and may cause exudation or bleeding. Use of silver nitrate to cauterize this tissue is often helpful. When true leakage of gastric contents occurs around the tube, one must be concerned about gastric outlet obstruction or tubal obstruction. **Migration** of the head of the catheter out of the stomach and into the abdominal wall may present in this way. In such cases, injection of water-soluble contrast into the tube may more clearly demonstrate the location of the tube's head and help to assess the effectiveness of gastric emptying. Migration into the abdominal wall may occur secondary to excessive tension on the outer crossbar. This may be avoided as discussed above. Treatment usually consists of tube removal and replacement (see Video clip 148.3).

Gastrocolic fistula is an infrequent but well-recognized complication of gastrostomy. It results from colonic penetration at the time of gastric access. This complication usually goes unnoticed for long periods of time, becoming apparent only when the tube is changed and the new tube comes to lie in the first lumen it reaches, the colon. The patient then will develop severe diarrhea after feedings. Injection of water-soluble contrast through the tube, contrast enema, computed tomography, or colonoscopy may also make the diagnosis. If the problem is discovered long after the initial gastrostomy (i.e., >6 weeks), it can usually be resolved by simple removal of the tube by traction. The colonic fistula usually closes spontaneously within 1–2 weeks. When the fistula is discovered acutely because of patient deterioration, surgical intervention to remove the tube, close the colonic hole, and re-establish the gastrostomy is indicated. Use of the "safe tract" method in performing the gastrostomy is the best approach to minimizing, if not preventing, the occurrence of this complication.

Costs and controversies

Economic, moral, and ethical issues have been raised with the expanded use of this technique [12]. Although PEG is clearly less costly than surgical gastrostomy, its ease of performance has increased total costs to society by increasing the total number of gastrostomies performed and perhaps by extending the lives, and resultant costs, of patients who would otherwise die more quickly. The selection of patients for percutaneous enteral access is clearly important and controversial [13]. Conflict regarding prolonged feeding in end-of-life decisions is now commonly recognized in society at large. The procedure offers little to patients with a short life-expectancy. Beyond that, the physician must carefully consult with the patient and/or their family to assure that all involved understand the implications of placement of the tube. Percutaneous enteral access has greatly facilitated the care of patients in a minimally invasive way. It has been of great value to physicians and their patients, but must be applied with great care both technically and ethically [14].

SOURCES OF INFORMATION FOR PATIENTS AND DOCTORS

www.patient.co.uk/showdoc/40024638/
www.asge.org/PatientInfoIndex.aspx?id=394

References

1. Gauderer M, Ponsky JL, Izant RJ Jr. Gastrostomy without laparotomy: a percutaneous endoscopic technique. *J Pediatr Surg.* 1980;15:872–875.
2. Fan AC, Baron TH, Rumalla A, Harewood GC. Comparison of direct percutaneous endoscopic jejunostomy and PEG with jejunal extension. *Gastrointest Endosc.* 2002;56:890–894.
3. Ponsky JL, Aszodi A, Perse D. Percutaneous endoscopic cecostomy: a new approach to nonobstructive colonic dilation. *Gastrointest Endosc.* 1986;32:108–111.
4. Mellinger JD, Simon IB, Schlechter B, Lash RH, Ponsky JL. Tract formation following percutaneous endoscopic gastrostomy (PEG) in an animal model. *Surg Endosc.* 1991;5:189–191.
5. Ponsky JL, Gauderer M. Percutaneous endoscopic gastrostomy: a nonoperative technique for feeding gastrostomy. *Gastrointest Endosc.* 1981;27:9–11.
6. Foutch PG, Talbert GA, Waring JP, et al. Percutaneous endoscopic gastrostomy in patients with prior abdominal surgery: virtues of the safe tract. *Am J Gastroenterol.* 1988;83:147–150.
7. Sacks BA, Vine HS, Palestrant AM, Ellison HP, Shropshire D, Lowe R. A nonoperative technique for establishment of a gastrostomy in the dog. *Invest Radiol.* 1983;18:485–487.

8. Russell TR, Brotman M, Norris F. Percutaneous gastrostomy. A new simplified and cost-effective technique. *Am J Surg.* 1984; 148:132–137

9. Sabnis A, Liu R, Chand B, Ponsky J. SLiC technique: A novel approach to percutaneous gastrostomy. *Surg Endosc.* 2006;20: 256–262.

10. Bumpers HL, Collure DW, Best IM, *et al.* Unusual complications of long-term percutaneous gastrostomy tubes. *J Gastrointest Surg.* 2003;7:917–920.

11. Ponsky JL, Aszodi A. External biliary–gastric fistula: a simple method for recycling bile. *Am J Gastroenterol.* 1982;77:939–940.

12. Angus F, Burakoff R. The percutaneous endoscopic gastrostomy tube, medical and ethical issues in placement. *Am J Gastroenterol.* 2003;98:1904.

13. Kruse A, Misiewicz JJ, Rokkas T, *et al.* Recommendations of the ESGE workshop on the ethics of percutaneous endoscopic gastrostomy placement for nutritional support. First European Symposium on Ethics in Gastroenterology and Digestive Endoscopy, Kos, Greece, June 2003. *Endoscopy.* 2003;35:778–780.

14. Klose J, Heldwein W, Rafferzeder M et al. Nutrition life in patients with percutaneous endoscopic gastrostomy (PEG) in practice: prospective one-year follow-up. *Dig Dis Sci.* 2003;48: 2057–2063.

CHAPTER 149

Endoscopic techniques of removing early gastrointestinal neoplams

Haruhiro Inoue and Hitomi Minami

Showa University Northern Yokohama Hospital, Yokohama, Japan

KEY POINTS

- Mucosal lesions with a low risk of vascular or lymphatic spread and moderately differentiated histology are suitable for endoscopic mucosal resection
- The submucosal connection between mucosa and muscularis propria is easily separated by injection of saline
- Submucosal elevation must be sustained to reduce the risk of perforation
- Chromoendoscopy is useful in defining the lateral margins of tumors
- Endoscopic submucosal dissection allows *en bloc* mucosal resection of tumors >2–3 cm in diameter

Introduction

Surgical resection of gastrointestinal cancers is often associated with significant morbidity and mortality. Therefore, methods for endoscopic cancer resection have been sought. With adequate staging techniques, endoscopic resection of early lesions looks promising [1–6]. In surgically resected specimens, intramucosal cancer generally has an extremely small risk of lymph node metastasis. Therefore endoscopic mucosal resection (EMR)/endoscopic submucosal dissection (ESD) of mucosal cancer is potentially curable. EMR is a **snare-based resection** method based on endoscopic polypectomy. In contrast, ESD is a **knife-based dissection** procedure.

Basic principles

The mucosa and muscularis propria are attached to each other by the loose connective tissue of the submucosa, and can be easily separated by injection of saline. This allows resection of the mucosa alone, leaving the muscularis propria layer intact. Saline injection into the submucosal layer is the most cost-effective technique for separating both layers. Lifting of the mucosal surface can be achieved after correct submucosal injection in any part of the gastrointestinal tract. After a sufficient volume of saline has been injected, the mucosa, including the target lesion, can be safely captured and resected by electrocautery or dissected by cutting submucosal tissue with an electrocautery knife.

Choosing the appropriate lesions

Only mucosal lesions with a low risk of vascular or lymphatic spread are appropriate for EMR. Endoscopic ultrasonography is often used in conjunction with conventional or magnification endoscopy to assess lesion depth. Biopsy and review of the lesion's histology prior to resection should be routine because poorly differentiated tumors are more likely to have metastases. In general, well or moderately differentiated mucosal lesions are considered acceptable targets for EMR/ESD.

Defining the lesion endoscopically

Chromoendoscopy is a very useful aid in defining the lesion prior to EMR/ESD. The edges of tumor extension may be ill defined, particularly in flat lesions. In the esophagus, Lugol's solution can be used to delineate the boundary between normal squamous mucosa (positive-staining, brown–green–black) and regions of dysplasia, Barrett's, or carcinoma (negative staining). Elsewhere in the gastrointestinal tract, indigo carmine can be used as a "highlighter" to increase contrast at the interface between normal mucosa and neoplastic lesions. Once fully visualized, it is useful to mark the edges of the lesions prior to removal. This can be accomplished with cautery from a snare tip a few millimeters outside the lesion's border. The presence of cautery markings may be helpful in confirming the *en bloc* resection of a lesion and in reorienting the tissue once it is removed in multiple fragments.

Endoscopic mucosal resection
Using a "cap"- fitted endoscope

The EMR "cap" technique (EMR-C) [7] is fast, easy to perform, and can be applied to relatively small lesions (<1 cm). "Cap" here refers to an attachment on the distal tip of the forward-viewing endoscope that is made from a transparent plastic material (Figure 149.1). The steps involved in EMR-C technique are as follows (see Video clip 149.1).

Textbook of Clinical Gastroenterology and Hepatology, Second Edition. Edited by C. J. Hawkey, Jaime Bosch, Joel E. Richter, Guadalupe Garcia-Tsao, Francis K. L. Chan.

Chapter 149: Endoscopic techniques of removing early gastrointestinal neoplams

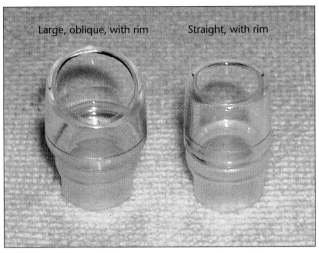

Figure 149.1 Distal attachment caps. Left: Large, oblique with rim; 16.5-mm outer diameter. This large cap is applied to a first capture during the EMR-C procedure; 2–3 cm mucosa can be resected. Right: Straight, with rim; 13.5-mm outer diameter. This cap is used for trimming the lesion; approximately 1–2 cm of mucosa can be removed.

Step 1: Preparation

In preparation for the EMR-C procedure, a cap is attached to the tip of the forward-viewing endoscope and is fixed tightly with an adhesive tape. For the initial session of EMR in the esophagus and stomach, an obliquely cut, large-capacity cap with a rim (Olympus MAJ297) (Figure 149.1a) is most commonly used by fixing it onto the tip of the standard-size endoscope in order to obtain a larger sample. For trimming a residual lesion, a straight-cut medium-sized cap with a rim (Olympus MH595) (Figure 149.1b) is appropriate. All of the items needed for the EMR-C procedure are commercially available in an EMR-Kit (Olympus).

Step 2: Markings

The mucosal surface that surrounds the margin of the lesion is carefully marked with cautery using the tip of the snare wire. Markings are positioned 2 mm away from the actual lesion margin. The color enhancement produced by chromoendoscopy disappears within a couple of minutes, and marking by **electrocoagulation** is therefore essential, especially for a flat lesion.

Step 3: Injection

A diluted epinephrine (adrenaline)–saline solution (0.5 mL 0.1% epinephrine solution in 100 mL normal saline) is injected into the submucosa with an injection needle (23 G, tip length 4 mm). Puncturing the target mucosa at a sharp angle is important to avoid transmural penetration of the needle tip. The total volume of injected saline depends on the size of the lesion, but it is necessary **to inject enough saline to lift up the entire lesion**. Usually, more than 20 mL is injected. When saline is accurately injected into the submucosal layer, lifting of the mucosa is observed (Figure 149.2a).

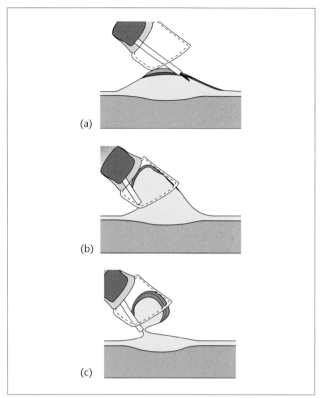

(a)

(b)

(c)

Figure 149.2 Endoscopic mucosal resection using a cap-fitted endoscope (EMR-C). (a) Submucosal injection of epinephrine–saline solution. The distal part of the lesion is punctured first to ensure that the lesion is always kept in view. (b) Prelooping of the snare wire and drawing up the target mucosa. Full suction draws the lifted mucosa into the cap. Use of a large volume of saline–epinephrine solution avoids resection of the muscularis propria. (c) Target mucosa is captured as a pseudo-polyp. The snare-entrapped strangulated mucosa is resected by electrocautery. Coagulation current achieves complete hemostasis. (This figure was published in *Clinical Gastroenterology and Hepatology*, Wilfred M. Weinstein, Christopher J. Hawkey, Jaime Bosch, Endoscopic mucosal resection of neoplasms in the gastrointestinal tract, Pages 1065–1072, Copyright Elsevier, 2005.)

Step 4: Prelooping of the snare wire

A specially designed small-diameter snare (with an outer diameter of 1.8 mm; Olympus SD-7P) is essential for the "prelooping" process. The snare wire is fixed along the rim of the EMR-C cap. To create prelooping conditions, moderate suction is first applied to the normal mucosa to seal the outlet of the cap, and the snare wire that passes through the endoscope instrument channel is then opened. The opened snare wire is fixed along the rim of the cap, and the snare's outer sheath sticks up to the rim of the cap. This completes the prelooping process for the snare wire.

Step 5: Suction of the target mucosa

With the prelooping position maintained, the lesion is fully captured inside the cap and strangulated by simple closing of the prelooped snare wire. At this moment, the strangulated mucosa looks like a snared polypoid lesion (Figure 149.2b, c).

Step 6: Resection

The pseudo-polyp of the strangulated mucosa is cut using blended current electrocautery (Figure 149.2c). The resected specimen can be easily taken out by keeping it inside the cap, without using any grasping forceps. The smooth surface of the muscularis propria layer will be exposed at the bottom of the EMR-induced ulcer.

Step 7: Additional resection

If additional resection is necessary for complete removal of the residual lesion, all of the procedures, including the saline injection, should be repeated step by step. The injected saline disappears within a few minutes and no longer acts as a cushion between the mucosa and muscle layer. Repeated saline injection is therefore necessary to reduce the risk of perforation [8].

Endoscopic submucosal dissection

EMR is a technique originally based on snare polypectomy and the size of specimen resected is limited to around 2–3 cm. ESD is a novel technique of EMR that enables **one-piece resection**, even for a superficially spreading tumor. In ESD, first described by Ono *et al.* [9], a knife activated by electrocautery

is used both to cut margins and for submucosal dissection beneath isolated mucosa. Devices designed for ESD include the insulation-tip knife, hook knife, flex knife, and triangle-tip knife (Figure 149.3) [9–12].

Triangle-tip knife procedure

The ESD technique using a triangle-tip knife [13] allows removal of the lesion in a single specimen, even for an extended lesion (Figure 149.3). The triangle-tip knife works as a multi-purpose device (Figures 149.4 and 149.5) that can be utilized

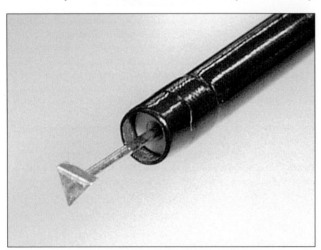

Figure 149.3 The triangle-tip knife. The outer diameter of the device is 1.8 mm. The tip is made of metal so that the electric current passes through it.

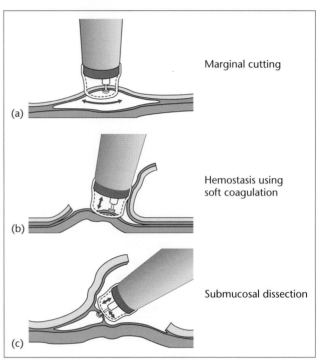

Marginal cutting

Hemostasis using soft coagulation

Submucosal dissection

Figure 149.4 Endoscopic submucosal dissection using the triangle-tip knife. (a) After submucosal injection, mucosal dissection is carried out using a triangle-tip knife. The energy source is swift coagulation, 60 W, effect 4 (ERBE). (b) Bleeding from the ulcer bed is controlled by coagulation using the bottom of the triangle tip. (c) Submucosal dissection is completed by electrosurgical cauterization, using the triangle tip. Fibers in the submucosa are hooked and cut step by step. (This figure was published in *Clinical Gastroenterology and Hepatology*, Wilfred M. Weinstein, Christopher J. Hawkey, Jaime Bosch, Endoscopic mucosal resection of neoplasms in the gastrointestinal tract, Pages 1065–1072, Copyright Elsevier, 2005.)

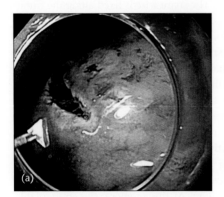
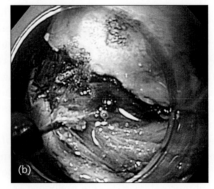
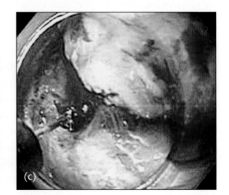

Figure 149.5 Endoscopic view during endoscopic submucosal dissection using the triangle-tip knife. (a) Mucosal cutting – marginal mucosa surrounding the lesion is dissected circumferentially. (b) Submucosal dissection – submucosal fibers are cut by hooking them with a triangle-tip knife. (c) Hemostasis – bleeding from the ulcer bed is controlled by coagulation with the bottom of the triangle-tip knife.

for marking, cutting, dissecting, and even hemostasis (see Video clip 149.2). Using an edge of the triangle-tip knife, **markings** are put on to the normal mucosa around the lesion. Injection with high-viscosity solution is mandatory for this procedure because it maintains mucosal lifting for longer. The authors utilize hyaluronic acid for injection. The energy source is an important factor in performing safe ESD. Swift coagulation (ERBE; Vaio) is now considered to be the best electrocautery device for the triangle-tip knife.

Marginal cutting about 5 mm outside the markings is the next step. The triangle-tip knife hooks the mucosal edge and pulls up the target mucosa away from the surface of the muscle layer, and then cuts it by electrocautery. By repeating the process, circumferential incision around the lesion is completed. **Submucosal dissection** using the tip of a triangle-tip knife is subsequently carried out. A hood mounted on the tip of the endoscope creates a working space beneath the mucosa, and provides counter-traction to the tissue in the submucosa.

After removal of the mobilized mucosa, complete hemostasis is achieved with coagulation forceps.

Which procedure should be applied?

Generally, small lesions can be easily excised with the EMR-C procedure. In the esophagus, lesions smaller than 2 cm can be resected in one session of EMR-C. Mucosa of the stomach is approximately two times thicker than that of the esophagus, and only stomach lesions less than 1 cm can be resected in one piece with this technique. ESD is used for larger lesions, with the intent of performing *en bloc* mucosal resections.

Esophagus

Squamous cell carcinomas without extension past the lamina propria can be removed by EMR/ESD with a very low risk of distal spread (Figure 149.6). Lesions of 2 cm can be resected, although those that encompass a greater circumference of the

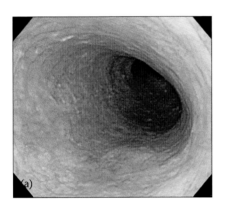
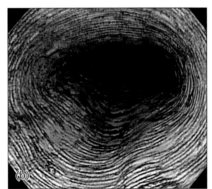
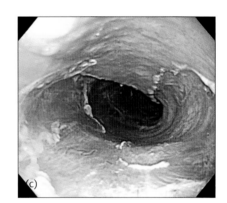

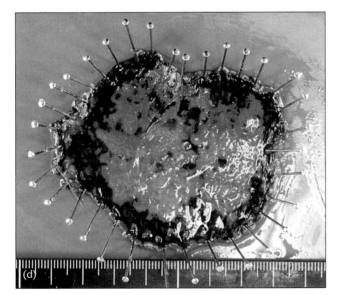
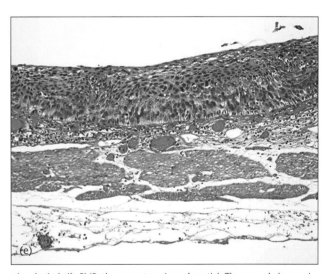

Figure 149.6 Endoscopic submucosal dissection using the triangle-tip knife. Squamous cell carcinoma in the esophagus; mucosal cancer. (a) Routine endoscopic view. Superficial erosion is recognized in the 6 o'clock direction. Protrusion of mucosa as a result of compression by the spine is also observed distal to the erosion. (b) Large unstained area with Lugol's iodine staining. Regularly arranged "fernization" or wrinkling of the mucosa was maintained, so the lesion was diagnosed as m1. (c) An artificial ulcer induced by triangle-tip knife EMR, three-quarters circumferential. The muscularis propria surface is covered with a thin connective tissue layer. (d) Resected mucosal specimen. Large unstained area surrounded by positive-staining margins indicates a successful single-specimen *en bloc* removal. (e) Microscopic image of the resected specimen; hematoxylin and eosin staining. Carcinoma *in situ* (high-grade dysplasia) is present. The dark area in the bottom third of the squamous mucosa highlights the neoplastic change.

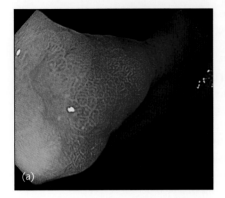
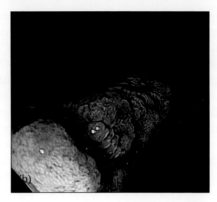
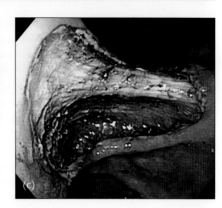

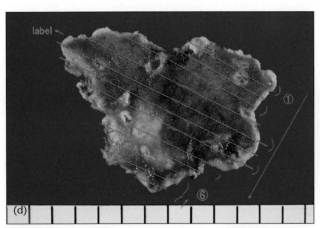
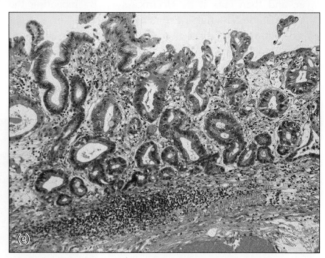

Figure 149.7 Endoscopic submucosal dissection (ESD) using the triangle-tip knife. Differentiated adenocarcinoma in the stomach; mucosal cancer. (a) Routine endoscopic view. Superficial slightly depressed lesion (IIc) with erosion was observed at the anterior wall of the gastric angularis. (b) Chromoendoscopic view. IIc depressive lesion was well demonstrated with indigo carmine staining. (c) Artificial ulcer induced by ESD. The smooth surface of the muscle layer was exposed. The lower horizontal edge of the green-stained ulcer shows swollen submucosa because of the hyaluronic acid injection. (d) Histological mapping of the resected specimen. For histological examination, the resected specimen was cut into 2-mm strips (green lines). The distribution of the cancer was demonstrated by the red lines. (e) Histology – well-differentiated adenocarcinoma.

lumen carry a higher risk of stricture. Options for treating neoplastic change in Barrett's esophagus are discussed at the end of this chapter.

Stomach

Mucosal adenocarcinomas of 1–2 cm can be removed by EMR (Figure 149.7) with a low risk of invasion, but with the following caveats. Lesions with ulceration or ulcer scar and those with a poorly differentiated histological appearance have a higher risk of invasion beyond the mucosa. Even small signet-ring type and poorly differentiated gastric cancers should be resected surgically [14].

Duodenum and colon

EMR can be carried out in the duodenum using the techniques of saline injection and cautery with a cap device (Figure 149.8). Post-therapeutic bleeding poses the most common complication in the duodenum, even after complete hemostasis during the initial procedure. The authors recommend prophylactic closure of the EMR defect in the duodenum using a clipping device. Large adenomatous polyps and small superficial cancers with moderate or well-differentiated histology can be removed with EMR. Colonic cancers larger than 1 cm have a greater risk of lymphatic or submucosal invasion and should be removed surgically.

Clinical results and complications

Potential complications include bleeding, perforation, and stricture. Bleeding can generally be managed with standard hemostasis techniques, including the use of endoclips. Perforation is rare and is treated mainly by endoscopic clipping or conservative management, depending on the size and location of the perforation. In a series of 372 patients, the authors' group has used the EMR-C procedure for 184 lesions in the esophagus and 188 in the stomach. ESD with the triangle-tip knife was used in an additional 576 patients (137 in the esophagus, 439 in the stomach). Perforation occurred in the

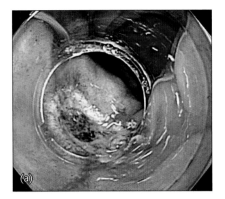
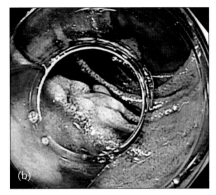
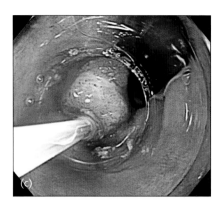

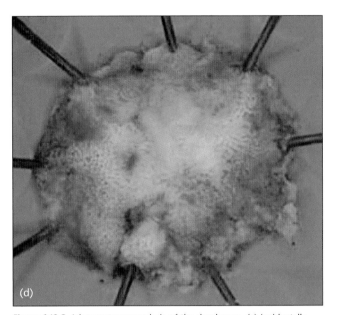

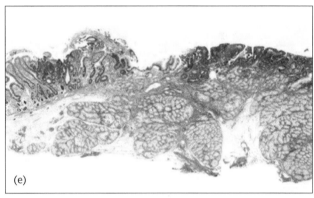

Figure 149.8 Adenomatous neoplasia of the duodenum. (a) Incidentally discovered small erosion surrounded by swollen irregular mucosa. (b) After indigo carmine staining. (c) Snare around the lesion after injection and suction into cap. (d) Base of resection zone. (e) Histology showing neoplastic/dysplastic lesion. Most of the right half of the figure shows the dark-staining superficial neoplastic change. There is a smaller area of dark-staining mucosa on the left of the depressed center of the lesion.

esophagus in one patient (0.3%) and in the stomach in 13 (2.1%) (Table 149.1). The perforation in the esophagus was treated conservatively. In all cases of gastric perforation, the perforated wound was closed using a hemostatic clip. There was no procedure-related mortality in 948 cases of EMR or ESD.

Future directions

EMR of neoplastic change (high-grade dysplasia, intramucosal cancer) in **Barrett's esophagus** is an appealing strategy. Sato-date *et al.* [15] performed EMR-C in eight cases of superficial carcinoma arising in Barrett's esophagus. All patients were successfully treated solely with EMR, with no major complications. One-piece resection with ESD for focal adenocarcinoma arising on long-segment Barrett's esophagus was carried out in three cases (Figure 149.9). A large series of patients has been reported in which local endoscopic therapy was used for

Table 149.1 Complication rates for endoscopic mucosal resections (EMRs) and endoscopic submucosal resections (ESDs), in the upper gastrointestinal tract. Data were collected from April 2001 to January 2010 in the authors' institute.

	Total cases	Postoperative bleeding	Perforation
Esophagus			
EMR/ESD	321	0 (0%)	1 (0.3%)
EMR	184	0 (0%)	0 (0%)
ESD	137	0 (0%)	1 (0.7%)
Stomach			
EMR/ESD	627	13 (2.1%)	13 (2.1%)
EMR	188	0 (0%)	1 (0.5%)
ESD	439	13 (2.9%)	12 (2.7%)

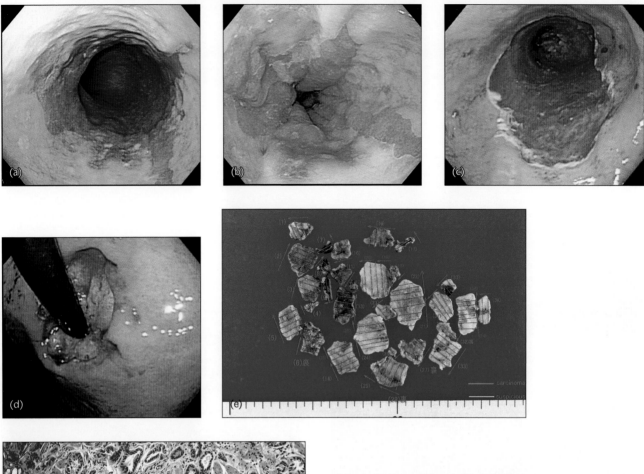

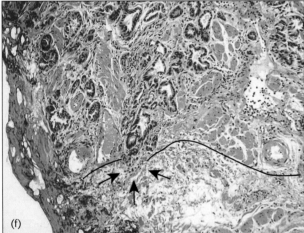

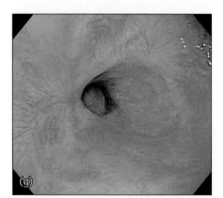

Figure 149.9 Circumferential endoscopic mucosal resection (EMR) for Barrett's cancer. (a) Endoscopic photograph shows long-segment Barrett's esophagus. Reddish, irregular "tongues" of columnar epithelium extend more than 5 cm above the gastroesophageal junction. (b) With partial deflation, swollen linear folds become evident in the Barrett's zone. There are residual adjacent "flat" areas of red-staining Barrett's mucosa. Multiple four-quadrant biopsies revealed well-differentiated adenocarcinoma. (c) Barrett's esophageal mucosa was completely excised circumferentially. (d)

Cardia. A 2-cm long circumferential zone was resected. (e) Resected specimens,. There was multifocal intramucosal carcinoma. (f) One section showed slight invasion (10 μm) into the submucosal layer (arrows). The black line shows the lower border of the muscularis mucosae. The pathological diagnosis was suspicious of invasive carcinoma, Vienna classification category 4.3. (g) Three months after circumferential EMR. Normal "neosquamous" epithelium with slight scarring radiating to a central point at the 9 o'clock location.

intraepithelial high-grade dysplasia and early adenocarcinoma in Barrett's esophagus [16]. The overall complication rate was 9.5%, and the calculated 3-year survival rate 88%.

Local endoscopic therapy may be an effective and safe alternative to esophagectomy for high-grade dysplasia and early adenocarcinoma. It is not unusual to have to repeat EMR in these patients, presumably because their residual Barrett's mucosa is more subject to neoplastic change or because endoscopically invisible synchronous lesions were present at the time of the original treatment.

Ablative therapy, for instance with photodynamic therapy [17], has also been used as an alternative to surgical therapy, but there may be several limitations to ablative therapy compared with EMR. Adenocarcinoma may appear beneath reepithelialized squamous epithelial tissue [18]. In addition, EMR permits staging of the neoplastic change, because it allows detection of occult carcinoma or areas of invasion not suspected on the basis of endoscopic biopsy and endoscopic ultrasonography.

It has been proposed that EMR should be limited to within three-quarters of the circumference of the esophagus, and that near-total or total mucosal resection should be avoided owing to refractory stenosis after healing of the resulting ulcer [19]. Possible approaches may include a two-stage full-circumference resection at an interval of 8 weeks [20] or photodynamic therapy after EMR. When circumferential mucosal resection is performed with this technique on long-segment Barrett's esophagus, multiple specimens [9–20] are obtained, making precise reconstruction of the resected specimens extremely difficult. This may be theoretically averted by using a triangle-tip knife to acquire one-piece specimens for better histological analysis.

Conclusions

In elderly and/or frail patients with early neoplastic disease of the gastrointestinal tract, the need for less invasive procedures becomes more compelling. EMR affords a unique and exciting treatment mode. For some of the techniques described here, the availability of endoscopic ultrasonography is invaluable. It is likely that in the future many of these procedures will be done in specialized centers. The standards and expectations for EMR should be similar to those of conventional oncological surgery. That is, we need long-term outcome data that include survival data, complications, and the need for retreatment, especially for diseases such as gastric cancer and Barrett's esophagus where a diffuse preneoplastic "field defect" may be involved.

SOURCES OF INFORMATION FOR PATIENTS AND DOCTORS

http://personalweb.sunset.net/~mansell/polyp.htm

References

1. Maku-uchi H. Endoscopic mucosal resection for early esophageal cancer. *Dig Endosc.* 1996;8:175–179.
2. Monma K, Sakaki N, Yoshida M. Endoscopic mucosectomy for precise evaluation and treatment of esophageal intraepithelial cancer. *Endosc Dig.* 1990;2:447–452.
3. Inoue H, Endo M. Endoscopic esophageal mucosal resection using a transparent tube. *Surg Endosc.* 1990;4:198–201.
4. Inoue H. Endoscopic mucosal resection for gastrointestinal mucosal cancers. In: Classen M, Tytgat GNJ, Lightdale C, editors. *Gastroenterological Endoscopy.* Stuttgart: Thieme, 2000: 322–333.
5. Endo M, Takeshita K, Yoshida M. How can we diagnose the early stage of esophageal cancer? *Endoscopy.* 1986;18:11–18.
6. Lambert R. Diagnosis of esophagogastric tumors. *Endoscopy.* 2004;36:110–119.
7. Inoue H, Takeshita K, Hori H, et al. Endoscopic mucosal resection with a capfitted panendoscope for esophagus, stomach, and colon mucosal lesions. *Gastrointest Endosc.* 1993;39:58–62.
8. Inoue H, Kawano T, Tani M, et al. Endoscopic mucosal resection using a cap: technique for use and preventing perforation. *Can J Gastroenterol.* 1999;13:477–480.
9. Ono H, Kondo H, Gotoda T, et al. Endoscopic mucosal resection for treatment of early gastric cancer. *Gut.* 2001;48:225–229.
10. Yamamoto H, Yube T, Isoda N, et al. A novel method of endoscopic mucosal resection using sodium hyaluronate. *Gastrointest Endosc.* 1999;50:251–256.
11. Oyama T, Kikuchi Y. Aggressive endoscopic mucosal resection in the upper GI tract – Hook knife EMR method. *Minim Invas Ther Allied Technol.* 2002;11:291–295.
12. Yahagi N, Fujishiro M, Iguchi M, et al. Theoretical and technical requirements to expand EMR indications. *Dig Endosc.* 2003;15: S19–S21.
13. Inoue H, Satoh Y, Kazawa T, et al. Endoscopic submucosal dissection using a newly developed triangle-tip knife. *Stomach Intest.* 2004;39:73–75.
14. Soetikno RM, Gotoda T, Nakanishi Y, Soehendra N. Endoscopic mucosal resection. *Gastrointest Endosc.* 2003;57:567–579.
15. Satodate H, Inoue H, Yoshida T, et al. Circumferential EMR of carcinoma arising in Barrett's esophagus: case report. *Gastrointest Endosc.* 2003;58:288–289.
16. May A, Gossner L, Pech O, et al. Local endoscopic therapy for intraepithelial highgrade neoplasia and early adenocarcinoma in Barrett's esophagus: acute-phase and longterm results of new treatment approach. *Eur J Gastroenterol Hepatol.* 2002;14: 1085–1091.
17. Overholt BF, Panjehpour M, Haydek JM. Photodynamic therapy for Barrett's esophagus: follow-up in 100 patients. *Gastrointest Endosc.* 1999; 49:1–7.
18. Sampliner RE, Fass R. Partial regression of Barrett's esophagus: an inadequate endpoint. *Am J Gastroenterol.* 1993;88:2092–2094.
19. Inoue H, Kudo S. Endoscopic mucosal resection for gastrointestinal mucosal cancer. In: Meinhard C, Guido NJ, Charles JL, editors. *Gastroenterological Endoscopy.* Stuttgart: Thieme, 2002: 322–333.
20. Makuuchi H. Endoscopic mucosal resection for early esophageal cancer, indication and technique. *Dig Endosc.* 1996;8:175–179.

CHAPTER 150
Dilation and stenting of the gastrointestinal tract

Lucio Petruzziello, Michele Marchese and Guido Costamagna
Catholic University of the Sacred Heart "A. Gemelli" Hospital, Rome, Italy

---

KEY POINTS

Esophageal dilation
- Fluoroscopy should be used whenever there is doubt about anatomy beyond the stricture or if the stricture has not been traversed endoscopically
- The "rule of threes" should be followed especially when dilating caustic, post-radiation or eosinophilic esophagitis strictures
- Local steroid injection at the time of dilation may reduce recurrences

Esophageal stenting
- Self-expanding metal stent (SEMS) placement represents the gold standard treatment for palliation of dysphagia related to malignant esophageal strictures
- Stents can be placed under endoscopic guidance only, but are better and safer if placed under fluoroscopic guidance
- With SEMSs, aggressive predilation is not necessary

Gastric and duodenal dilation
- Benign gastroduodenal strictures can originate from peptic ulcer, Crohn's disease or chronic pancreatitis
- Endoscopic balloon dilation is often effective for benign, cicatricial pyloric or duodenal stenosis and should be tried before surgery

Gastric and duodenal stents
- Gastrojejunostomy for malignant gastric outlet obstruction (GOO) is associated with a significant rate of morbidity and mortality
- Criteria for endoscopic stent placement are: advanced unresectable malignancy with symptomatic GOO without evidence of peritoneal carcinomatosis or multiple small bowel strictures and short survival (<2 or 6 months)
- Clinical success rate ranges between 84% and 93%, with technical success rate ranging from 93% to 97%

Colorectal dilation
- Endoscopic dilation is indicated as primary treatment of benign, fibrotic strictures of the colon
- Strictures resulting from Crohn's disease, which have failed treatment with anti-inflammatory medications, may be appropriate for endoscopic dilation
- Enteral dilation is generally performed with TTS balloon dilators
- Success rates of balloon dilation range from 86% to 97%

Colorectal stenting
- "Bridge to surgery" and palliation are two indications for colorectal stenting for advanced stages of obstructive malignancy
- Colonic stents can facilitate one-step definitive surgery by allowing bowel cleansing
- Bridge to surgery-intent stenting can be changed to palliation in case of stage IV disease
- Stents should not be placed in patients with carcinomatosis or multiple strictures where relief of obstruction is unlikely, or in the distal rectum

---

Esophageal dilation
Indications and contraindications
Endoscopic esophageal dilation is indicated in cases of Schatzki rings, esophageal webs, peptic and caustic strictures, anastomotic and post-radiation strictures, and, recently, eosinophilic esophagitis, after failure of medical therapy. Achalasia is specifically treated with large (30–40 mm) balloons inflated with air (pneumatic dilation).

Dilation is absolutely contraindicated in patients with clear or even suspected perforation, or who have severe co-morbidities that preclude safe endoscopy [1].

Technique and results
Maloney-type bougies and Hurst dilators can be passed either blindly or under fluoroscopic control, and have been commonly used for simple strictures, such as webs and Schatzki

---

Textbook of Clinical Gastroenterology and Hepatology, Second Edition. Edited by C. J. Hawkey, Jaime Bosch, Joel E. Richter, Guadalupe Garcia-Tsao, Francis K. L. Chan.
© 2012 Blackwell Publishing Ltd. Published 2012 by Blackwell Publishing Ltd.

rings. Savary and American dilators are better used for complex strictures and are passed over a guidewire, with or without fluoroscopic guidance. The initial diameter of a rigid dilator should be equal to or slightly greater than the estimated diameter of the stricture. The **"rule of threes"** states that sequentially larger dilators can be used until resistance is felt, and then no more than three additional dilators at 1-mm diameter increments should be used [2]. Special attention should be given to patients with eosinophilic esophagitis, because they may be at higher risk for perforation due to a thinner and more fragile esophagus (Figure 150.1).

Through-the-scope (TTS) inflatable polyethylene balloons are designed to be inflated with saline under direct endoscopic control. During inflation, the presence of a radiographic "waist" on fluoroscopy confirms the correct position, and its disappearance at full inflation indicates a successful dilation (Figure 150.2).

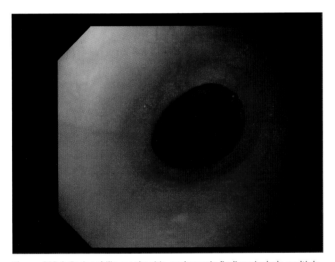

Figure 150.1 Eosinophilic esophagitis: endoscopic findings include multiple mucosal rings in a narrow, non-compliant esophagus with or without vertical groves or lines.

Constant radial expansion (CRE) balloons expand in a step-wise fashion to multiple diameters (usually three stages at 1.5-mm increments) depending on the inflation pressure, thus relieving the need for passing multiple balloons.

Early improvement in the ability to swallow is achieved in virtually all patients; however longer-term outcomes are influenced by the underlying pathological condition. If a luminal diameter of at least 13–15 mm can be achieved, nearly all patients will be relieved of dysphagia. In patients with benign peptic strictures, a graded stepwise dilating approach between 13 and 20 mm yields relief in 85–93% [1].

Complications

The most serious, life-threatening complication is **esophageal perforation**. Overall, this complication is not frequent (0.1–0.4%) and seems to be largely related to attempts at blind dilation with Maloney-type dilators (2%) [3].

Immediate closure of the defect combined with nasogastric suction and broad-spectrum antibiotics can often control the leak before significant mediastinal contamination occurs, and should always be attempted. It can be accomplished with endoscopically placed clips, or with over-the-scope clips (OTSC; Ovesco, Germany) specifically designed to close large defects [4].

The use of large-diameter covered self-expanding metal stents (SEMS) and of removable self-expanding plastic stents (SEPS) has also been shown to be effective in the management of perforations after dilation of benign esophageal strictures, although the routine use of these devices in benign disease is not recommended [5].

Esophageal stenting
Indications and contraindications

Endoscopic placement of **SEMS** is the quickest method for palliation of dysphagia for patients with inoperable and/or unresectable malignant strictures, and for occlusion of

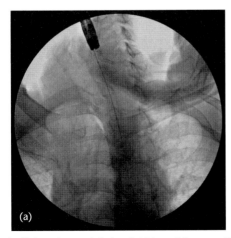
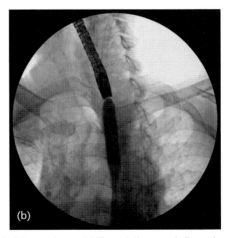

Figure 150.2 Pneumatic dilation of a caustic-induced stricture of the upper third of the esophagus. (a) Through-the-scope balloon placement inside the stricture. (b) Balloon inflation with the adjunct of a radio-opaque contrast medium to facilitate the fluoroscopic control.

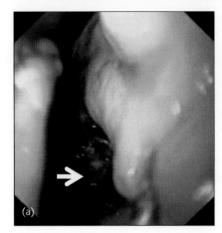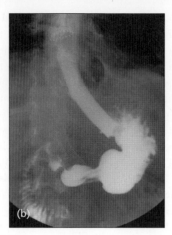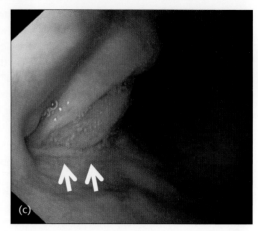

Figure 150.3 Boerhaave's syndrome. (a) Esophageal full-thickness rupture of the gastroesophageal junction (arrow). (b) Soluble-contrast administration after placement of a self-expanding plastic stent (Polyflex), showing no periesophageal leakage. (c) Mucosal scar (arrows) after stent removal.

malignant esophagorespiratory fistulae [6]. Endoscopic stenting, however, gives the best clinical results in the short-term follow-up, and chemotherapy and/or radiotherapy (CRT) should be preferred when survival is prolonged, although palliation of dysphagia is delayed for almost 1 month.

SEMSs can be mainly differentiated by the material they are made of (stainless steel or Nitinol), their shape, the presence of full or partial coverage of the mesh, and the diameter and type of delivery system. SEPSs have been developed to overcome drawbacks of SEMSs, such as the difficulty of adjusting the stent position, and removal.

Technique and results

Stent placement is usually performed with a combination of endoscopic and fluoroscopic techniques. Dilation of the malignant stricture prior to stent insertion is not routinely necessary and may increase the risk of perforation or migration. In patients with cervical cancer, a computed tomography (CT) scan is mandatory to estimate the risk of tracheal compression. For stent insertion, a guidewire is placed through the stricture, the endoscope removed, and the delivery system introduced over the wire. Radio-opaque markers on the SEMS allow for accurate positioning, and the endoscope can often be reinserted in parallel for simultaneous endoscopic and fluoroscopic monitoring of deployment.

The technical and clinical success of palliation with SEMS is more than 95%, although up to 22% of patients require a second stent at the time of initial placement [7].

Complications and their management

Malfunction of uncovered SEMS is mainly related to **ingrowth and overgrowth** in 17–30% and 9%, respectively [8]. In long-survival patients, covered SEMSs significantly reduce the incidence of ingrowth (3%), avoiding additional endoscopic intervention to restore patency. Owing to an insufficient anchorage of the metallic mesh to the esophageal wall however, both partially- and fully-covered SEMS have a higher risk of

migration (15% and 35%, respectively) than uncovered stents (7%) [9].

Esophageal fistulae and iatrogenic perforations

Iatrogenic injuries account for up to 60% of all patients with esophageal perforation [10]. Esophageal stent insertion has been shown to be successful in the closure of acute perforation immediately after its recognition, and in the sealing of chronic fistulae in patients deemed unfit for surgery.

Stents may be a better option in perforations or fistulae larger than 2 cm and in defects with everted edges because the wingspan of current clips fails to close such defects (Figure 150.3), and also in patients with a leak occurring in the setting of a malignant lesion because clips tend to tear through neoplastic tissue [10].

Gastric and duodenal dilation
Indications and contraindication

Peptic ulcer disease is the major cause of benign gastroduodenal obstruction or **gastric outlet obstruction (GOO)** in the adult population, and, traditionally, its treatment has been surgical [11]. An attempt at dilation is indicated for most endoscopically approachable benign, fibrotic strictures of the gastric outlet and duodenum, in patients unresponsive to conventional medical therapy.

Technique and results

The dilation of pyloric or duodenal stricture is performed only with **balloon dilators**. Real-time stricture dilation can be monitored with fluoroscopic imaging of the contrast-filled balloon. The procedure is repeated in 1–2 weeks, with a goal of eliminating GOO symptoms. The most commonly used dilators are the wire-guided balloon dilators, with a flexible tip minimizing the risk of perforation.

Endoscopic balloon dilation for benign pyloric stenosis and GOO is usually effective and offers symptom relief in the

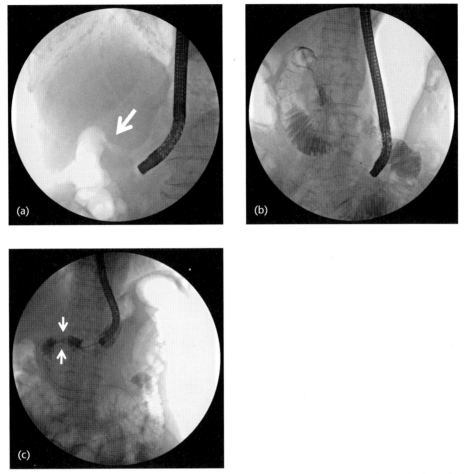

Figure 150.4 Duodenal stricture. (a) Air contrast during endoscopic retrograde cholangiopancreaography (ERCP) for duodenal neoplastic stricture (pancreatis cancer) (arrow). (b) Complete expansion of a self-expanding metallic stent after its placement. (c) Follow-up at 3 months shows small ingrowth in the middle of the stent (arrows).

majority of patients. Immediate symptomatic relief rates for treatment of pyloric stenosis vary from 70% to 80%, decreasing to 16–67% at long-term follow-up [12].

Gastric and duodenal stents
Indications and contraindications
Criteria for endoscopic stent placement are confirmed diagnosis of unresectable malignancy with symptomatic GOO without evidence of peritoneal carcinomatosis and absence of multiple small bowel strictures. Candidates for this kind of treatment are those with advanced disease and short survival (<2 or 6 months) [13].

Technique and results
The **through-the-scope (TTS) placement of SEMS** for GOO is preferable to the over-the-wire (OTW) placement with both endoscopic and radiological control to assess morphology, length, and degree of obstruction, and to evaluate patency of the proximal jejunum (Figure 150.4). Preliminary balloon dilation is usually not necessary. It is important to choose a stent that is at least a few centimeters wider than the stricture on both sides, in order to guarantee a disease-free margin, and to extend well around curves. The presence of a previously placed biliary stent or a concomitant biliary stricture is a challenging situation. When signs of biliary stent dysfunction occur, an endoscopic re-canalization of the biliary stent through the mesh of the duodenal stent is possible by fenestration of the duodenal stent with argon plasma [14](Figure 150.5).

The reported clinical success rate ranges between 84% and 93%, with a technical success rate ranging from 93% to 97% [15].

Complications and their management
Life-threatening complications are represented by perforation and bleeding, but these are fortunately rare (<1%) [15]. Migration of uncovered SEMS is a quite rare late complication. Stent migration can be related to an inadequate stent diameter or reduced tumor size [16].

Late complications after stent placement that require re-intervention (20–25% of cases) are overgrowth, ingrowth, food impaction, stent migration, and biliary obstruction [14]. These

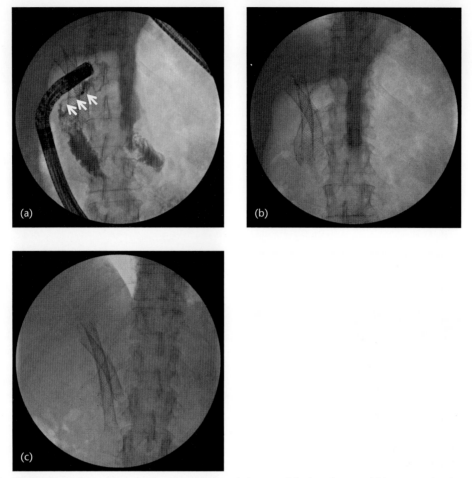

Figure 150.5 Complex bilioduodenal stricture for pancreatic cancer. (a) Through-the-scope injection of water-soluble contrast showing narrowing of the duodenal bulb (arrows). (b) Partial expansion of the self-expanding metallic stent after its placement. (c) Follow-up at 3 months shows optimal stent expansion.

situations can be managed by destruction of the tissue with laser, debridement with a Dormia basket or Fogarty balloon, stent-in-stent placement, and fenestration of the stent using argon plasma to access the papilla [14].

Colorectal dilation

Benign colorectal strictures from diverticulitis, radiation therapy, inflammatory bowel disease, and anastomotic stenosis may be amenable to endoscopic dilation, while malignant colorectal strictures require stent placement by endoscopy or radiology.

Postoperative anastomotic strictures occur in 3–30% of patients undergoing colorectal resection [17]. Ischemia, hemorrhage or leakage, together with anastomotic technique and adjuvant radiotherapy, are the most commonly reported contributing factors.

Technique and results

A wide range of endoscopic techniques have been used to treat **postoperative colonic strictures**, including mechanical dilation by means of fixed-diameter push-type dilators or expanding radial balloon dilators, electroincision stricturotomy [18], and more recently temporary insertion of SEMS or SEPS [19].

The approach to the stricture is similar when using bougies or balloons. TTS hydrostatic balloons are the most practical and widely used dilators today and are indicated in all cases of ileal or colorectal stricture (Figure 150.6). These dilators, which use a controlled radial expansion (CRE) technique, contain a short guidewire and are available with a maximum width of 20 mm.

Conversely, rigid plastic dilators (Savary-Gillard; Cook Medical) in sizes up to 20 mm or the larger OTW pneumatic balloons (Rigiflex; Boston Scientific) can be used only for **distal colorectal strictures**.

The first method used to treat **anastomotic stricture** has been bougienage, with a success rate of around 80% [20]. More recent success rates for balloon dilation range from 86% to 97%. Unfortunately, in both cases, long-term relief is often poor. A rate of repeat dilations as high as 88%, with a restricture frequency of up to 30%, have been reported [21].

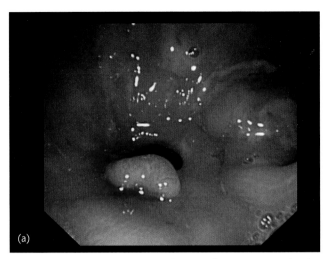
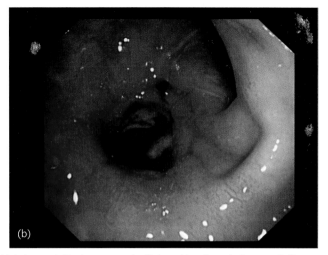

Figure 150.6 Endoscopic appearance of a rectocolic post-anastomotic stricture (a) before and (b) after pneumatic dilation with a through-the-scope balloon.

It has always been assumed that a dilator with a diameter of >13 mm or the ability to pass a colonoscope would be adequate to relieve obstructive symptoms.

Complications and their management
Bowel perforation can complicate endoscopic colorectal dilation and has an overall incidence of less than 2% [18]. Fortunately, many patients undergoing colorectal dilation for an anastomotic stricture have a diverting stoma and can therefore be conservatively treated in the vast majority of cases.

Colorectal stenting
Two types of SEMS are available for colorectal use: OTW and TTS stents. All are made of Nitinol and are bare. Covered stents are usually not used in the colon–rectum because of their higher risk of migration.

Indications and contraindications
Indications for colorectal SEMS have broadened from palliation to use as **"a bridge" to surgical resection** in patients with potentially operable, acutely obstructing colon cancer, avoiding the high morbidity rate of emergency surgery, and stoma creation.

In general, OTW stents are indicated for rectal or left colon occlusions, while TTS stents can be deployed through the operative channel of the colonoscope (3.7 mm) and implanted also in the transverse and the right colon. Stents are not indicated to treat distal rectum strictures within 5 cm of the anorectal junction, as these patients often experience tenesmus, pain, and incontinence.

Technique and results
The evaluation of an acutely occluded patient should include the execution of a CT scan with contrast. Endoscopic decompression should be performed as soon as possible. Once the stenosis has been crossed, the guidewire must be withdrawn under radiological control, and water-soluble contrast should be injected through a catheter to confirm the correct position. The catheter is retracted and a TTS stent is advanced through the channel. The choice of stent should take into account the location and morphology of the stenosis and should be at least 3–4 cm longer than the stenosis.

OTW stent placement can be achieved using a small caliber endoscope (<6 mm). If a thin endoscope can pass the stricture, a metallic or other very stiff guidewire can be released under direct endoscopic control. Once the endoscope is retracted, leaving the guidewire in place, the stent is advanced over the wire and stent release can be controlled by an endoscope introduced parallel to the stent (Figure 150.7). Distal release stents (Ultraflex Precision stent; Boston Scientific, USA) are best indicated for rectal lesions, because their distal end can be precisely positioned at >5 cm from the anorectal junction, to avoid tenesmus (Figure 150.8).

Technical and clinical success rates of colorectal SEMS placement range from 75% to 100% and 84% to 100%, respectively [22].

Complications and their management
SEMS complication rates range from 14% to 45%, most being self-limited, including migration, occlusion, and perforation [22]. Migration rates are reported to be around 20%. Late stent migration may occur from tumor shrinkage or necrosis, mostly as a result of chemotherapy. Tumor ingrowth with recurrent obstruction occurs in about 10% of cases and can usually be treated by a second stent placement or by surgery (Figure 150.9).

The most serious complication after colorectal SEMS insertion is **perforation**. The most comprehensive meta-analysis to date, published in 2011 and reporting a total of

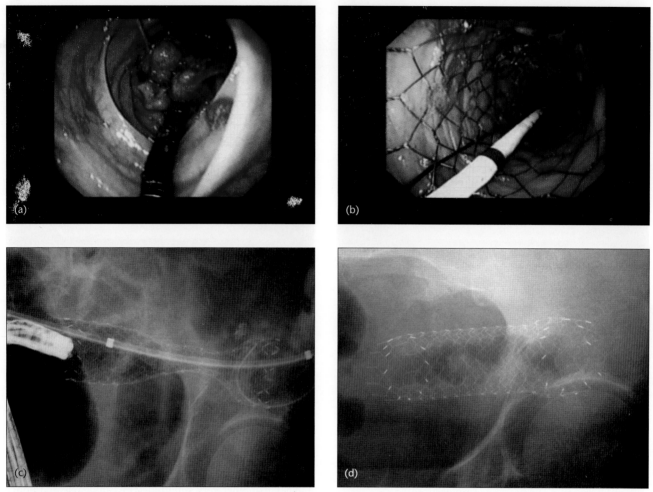

Figure 150.7 Rectosigmoid junction cancer. (a) Endoscopic placement of a guidewire. (b) Over-the-wire placement of a Precision stent releasing system. (c) Radiological control after stent deployment. (d) Complete stent expansion after 1 week.

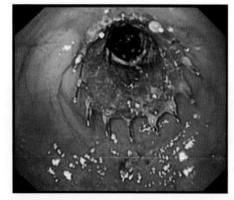

Figure 150.8 Distal-release over-the-wire Ultraflex Precision Stent correctly positioned in the mid rectum. Note the distal end of the stent is 5 cm from the anorectal junction.

2287 patients from 82 articles, showed an overall perforation rate of 4.9%, with a perforation-related mortality rate of 16.2% [23].

Future directions

New stent designs that are covered but still allow delivery through the endoscope channel, and are associated with low migration rates, are needed for both upper and lower gastrointestinal use. New expandable, removable polymer stents, as have been designed for esophageal use [24], may allow treatment of refractory benign strictures even in the colon–rectum. Bioabsorbable stents may allow a safe and effective method of temporary stent placement, without the need for a further procedure [25]. Esophageal drug-eluting stents have been proposed and may soon be available for evaluation [26].

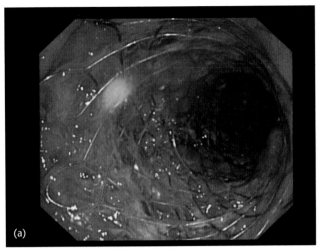 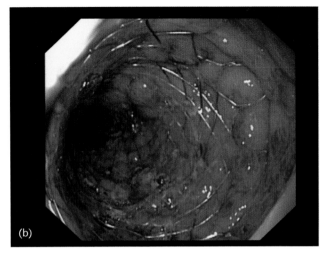

Figure 150.9 Self-expanding metal stent (Wallflex) placement for sigmoid cancer. (a) Patency and complete expansion evaluation after 1 month. (b) Cancer ingrowth after 3 months.

References

1. Riley SA, Attwood SE. Guidelines on the use of oesophageal dilatation in clinical practice. *Gut.* 2004;53(1 Suppl):i1–6.

2. Tulman AB, Boyce HW. Complications of esophageal dilation and guidelines for their prevention. *Gastrointest Endosc.* 1981;27: 229–234.

3. Hernandez LV, Jacobson JW, Harris MS. Comparison among the perforation rates of Maloney, balloon, and savary dilation of esophageal strictures. *Gastrointest Endosc.* 2000;51:460–462.

4. Pohl J, Borgulya M, Lorenz D, *et al.* Endoscopic closure of post-operative esophageal leaks with a novel over-the-scope clip system. *Endoscopy.* 2010;42:757–759.

5. Petersen JM. The use of a self-expandable plastic stent for an iatrogenic esophageal perforation. *Gastroenterol Hepatol.* 2010;6: 389–391.

6. Costamagna G, Marchese M, Iacopini F. Self-expanding stents in oesophageal cancer. *Eur J Gastroenterol Hepatol.* 2006;18:1177–1180.

7. Kozarek RA. Endoscopic palliation of esophageal malignancy. *Endoscopy.* 2003;35 (Suppl 1):S9–S13.

8. Vakil N, Morris AI, Marcon N, *et al.* A prospective, randomized, controlled trial of covered expandable metal stents in the palliation of malignant esophageal obstruction at the gastroesophageal junction. *Am J Gastroenterol.* 2001;96:1791–1796.

9. Watson A. Self-expanding metal esophageal endoprostheses: which is best? *Eur J Gastroenterol Hepatol.* 1998;10:363–365.

10. Raju GS, Thompson C, Zwischenberger JB. Emerging endoscopic options in the management of esophageal leaks. *Gastrointest Endosc.* 2005;62:278–286.

11. Jaffin BW, Kaye MD. The prognosis of gastric outlet obstruction. *Ann Surg.* 1985;201:176–179.

12. Yusuf TE, Brugge WR. Endoscopic therapy of benign pyloric stenosis and gastric outlet obstruction. *Curr Opin Gastroenterol.* 2006;22:570–573.

13. Jeurnink SM, Steyerberg EW, van Hooft JE, *et al.* Surgical gastrojejunostomy or endoscopic stent placement for the palliation of malignant gastric outlet obstruction (SUSTENT study): a multicenter randomized trial. *Gastrointest Endosc.* 2010;71:490–499.

14. Mutignani M, Tringali A, Shah SG, *et al.* Combined endoscopic stent insertion in malignant biliary and duodenal obstruction. *Endoscopy.* 2007;39:440–447.

15. Boskoski I, Tringali A, Familiari P, *et al.* Self-expandable metallic stents for malignant gastric outlet obstruction. *Adv Ther.* 2010; 27:691–703.

16. Tringali A, Mutignani M, Spera G, *et al.* Duodenal stent migration. *Gastrointest Endosc.* 2003;58:759.

17. Luchtefeld MA, Milsom JW, Senagore A, *et al.* Colorectal anastomotic stenosis. Results of a survey of the ASCRS membership. *Dis Colon Rectum.* 1989;32:733–736.

18. Truong S, Willis S, Schumpelick V. Endoscopic therapy of benign anastomotic strictures of the colorectum by electroincision and balloon dilatation. *Endoscopy.* 1997;29:845–849.

19. Suzuki N, Saunders BP, Thomas-Gibson S, *et al.* Colorectal stenting for malignant and benign disease: outcomes in colorectal stenting. *Dis Colon Rectum.* 2004;47:1201–1207.

20. Werre A, Mulder C, Van Heteren C, *et al.* Dilation of benign strictures following low anterior resection using Savary-Gilliard bougies. *Endoscopy.* 2000;32:385–388.

21. Johansson C. Endoscopic dilation of rectal strictures: a prospective study of 18 cases. *Dis Colon Rectum.* 1996;39:423–428.

22. Sebastian S, Johnston S, Geoghegan T, *et al.* Pooled analysis of the efficacy and safety of self-expanding metal stenting in malignant colorectal obstruction. *Am J Gastroenterol.* 2004;99:2051–2057.

23. Datye A, Hersh J. Colonic perforation after stent placement for malignant colorectal obstruction: causes and contributing factors. *Minim Invasive Ther Allied Technol.* 2011;20:133–140.

24. Bethge N, Vakil N. A prospective trial of a new self-expanding plastic stent for malignant esophageal obstruction. *Am J Gastroenterol.* 2001;96:1350–1354.

25. Saito Y, Tanaka T, Andoh A *et al.* Usefulness of biodegradeable stents constructed of polylactic acid monofilaments in patients with benign esophageal stenosis. *World J Gastroenterol.* 2007;13: 3977–3980.

26. Jeon SR, Eun SH, Shim CS, *et al.* Effect of drug-eluting metal stents in benign esophageal stricture: an in vivo animal study. *Endoscopy.* 2009;41:449–456.

CHAPTER 151
NOTES

D. Nageshwar Reddy, G. V. Rao, and Magnus J. Mansard

Asian Institute of Gastroenterology, Hyderabad, India

KEY POINTS

- Use of flexible endoscopy in the peritoneal cavity for diagnostic and therapeutic procedures has resulted in the development of NOTES
- Initial transgastric procedures were complicated by difficulties, including an unsafe gastrostomy closure
- Transvaginal and transcolonic approaches were developed to facilitate the approach to the upper abdominal organs
- The hybrid technique was adopted to overcome "teething" problems of NOTES, before implementing "pure NOTES" into practice

Introduction

Natural orifice translumenal endoscopic surgery (NOTES) is an exciting new field in which minimally invasive intrabdominal procedures are performed using flexible endoscopy. Natural hollow organs are used to gain access to body cavities via the mouth, anus, vagina, and urethra. NOTES could theoretically maximize the advantages of minimally invasive surgery, like reduced surgical trauma, postoperative pain, and recovery time, by allowing "incisionless" surgery. Kalloo *et al.* performed the first NOTES procedure in 2000, a transgastric peritoneoscopy in a porcine model. Drs Rao and Reddy from India are credited with the first human experience, when a transgastric appendectomy was performed in 2004. To date, many intraperitoneal procedures have been reported in animal models, and reports of NOTES performed in humans have started to appear [1].

Routes of access

The initial NOTES procedures were all done transgastrically due to the high comfort level offered to the endoscopist by this route.

Stomach entry

The first procedural step is a controlled safe entry into the abdominal cavity through the stomach. Lavage of the stomach is done preoperatively with antibacterial agents to control entry-point peritoneal sepsis. Prophylactic intravenous

antibiotics are also used. Acid-suppressing agents are used by some, but risk the loss of the protective action of gastric acid against the commensals of the oral cavity. High-level disinfection of the endoscope is mandatory. Overtubes or re-entry sheaths are used to allow easy and repeated passage of the endoscope. Some overtubes feature soft introduction pieces, inner sleeves with tapered components to prevent tissue, especially at the cricopharyngeal junction, from catching between the endoscope and overtube during introduction, and valves to prevent air from escaping.

Precautions used in performing a percutaneous endoscopic gastrostomy include finger indentation and transillumination. The port entry site is chosen in the mid-body or antrum on the anterior wall of the stomach, away from the vascular arcades along the greater and lesser curves [2].

A needle knife is used for a transluminal puncture at the selected site. This puncture is widened with either a **pull-type sphincterotome** or by **balloon dilatation**. The first method provides a wide port of entry but carries a significant risk of a bleed. In the second method, the risk of a bleed is less and any bleeding can be controlled by balloon tamponade. As the balloon does not divide the muscles, the tone of the muscles is maintained around the scope, preventing gas leak (Figures 151.1 and 151.2).

A third method uses a **submucosal endoscopy with mucosal flap (SEMF)**, which serves as a biological safety flap valve to control contamination through the myotomy [3]. A submucosal tunnel is created with high pressure CO_2 and balloon dissection. While the mucosa is incised with a needle knife at one end of the tunnel, the muscle wall is excised by the endoscopic mucosal resection (EMR) "cap" technique (see Chapter 149) at the other end. The mucosal entry site can be closed by simple mucosal apposition with clips. The SEMF also allows gastric distension to be maintained despite the open myotomy and even after withdrawal of the endoscope without gastrostomy closure.

Gastrostomy closure

Effective and secure closure of the gastrostomy has become the *sine quo non* for performance of NOTES in humans. In the initial stages, endoscopic clips were used for gastric mucosal

Textbook of Clinical Gastroenterology and Hepatology, Second Edition. Edited by C. J. Hawkey, Jaime Bosch, Joel E. Richter, Guadalupe Garcia-Tsao, Francis K. L. Chan.
© 2012 Blackwell Publishing Ltd. Published 2012 by Blackwell Publishing Ltd.

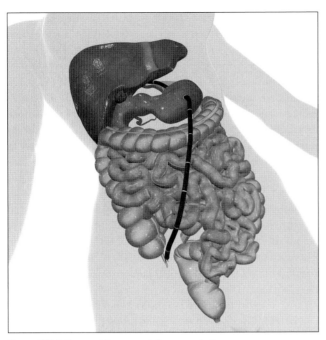

Figure 151.1 Transgastric approach for appendectomy.

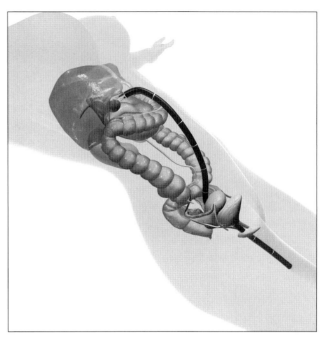

Figure 151.3 Transvaginal approach for cholecystectomy.

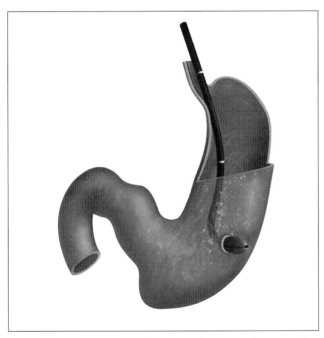

Figure 151.2 Balloon dilatation of gastrotomy for transgastric passage of an endoscope into the peritoneum.

approximation. Now, a variety of flexible endoscopic suturing devices has been used to perform full-thickness closure of gastrostomy in NOTES. The Eagle Claw (Apollo Group, Olympus Optical Co. Ltd, Tokyo, Japan), Olympus Bard (Davol) Endocinch (C.R. Bard Inc., Cranston, RI, USA), Plicator (NDO Surgical Inc., Mansfield, MA), Stomafix (EndoGastrc Solutions, Redmond, WA, USA), and Endostitch (Covidien, Mansfield, MA, USA) modified for use with a flexible

endoscope, are some of these devices which have FDA approval, although none for this specific application [4]. These devices and some not mentioned await further studies to identify the best one for an effective port site closure.

Transvaginal approach

The difficulty in performing cholecystectomy with a transgastric retroflexed scope resulted in the use of the transvaginal route for upper abdominal interventions [5] (Figure 151.3). The peritoneum is entered through the posterior fornix of the vagina in the relatively avascular area between the two uterosacral ligaments. The capacity of the vagina allows for introduction of larger instruments, including rigid laparoscopic instruments. Also, the vaginal incision is easy to close.

The use of the vagina for purposes other than its naturally designated function has been looked at with disdain by some. Also, concerns regarding pelvic inflammation, adhesion formation, and infertility have been raised by some gynecologists. The level of sterility obtained by antibiotic vaginal douches and the risk of contamination of peritoneal cavity by vaginal flora are other concerns. Also, the unguided puncture of the vagina carries the risk of injuring bowel adherent to the pelvis. The difficulty in maintenance of pneumoperitoneum around the lax vaginal incision has also been noted.

Transcolonic approach

The transcolonic approach also allows for *en face* visualization for upper abdominal exploration (Figure 151.4). The main advantage of this approach over the transvaginal technique is that it is not gender specific. Also, techniques used in transanal endoscopic microsurgery (TEM) have been utilized to demonstrate the feasibility of NOTES sigmoid colectomy with *en bloc*

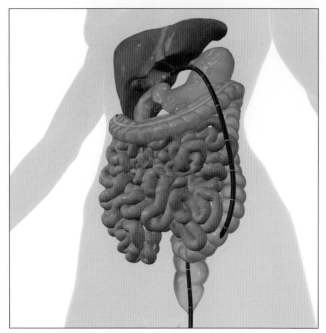

Figure 151.4 Transcolonic approach for cholecystectomy.

lymphadenectomy and primary anastomosis in a human cadaver model. Risk of spillage of colonic contents into the peritoneal cavity and reliable closure of the port entry site, which is located 15 cm from the anal verge, are the chief concerns [6].

Transesophageal approach

The SEMF technique has been used to enter the mediastinum through the esophagus. Visualization has been reported to be better than with traditional cervical mediastinoscopy and thoracoscopy. Procedures performed in animal models include pleural biopsy, therapeutic procedures on the heart, mediastinal lymph node resection, and Heller's cardiomyotomy [7].

Transvesical approach

Largely in experimental models, urologists have shown the feasibility of NOTES through the urinary bladder. Given the sterility of urine in the urinary bladder, minimal peritoneal contamination through this portal has been demonstrated. Endoscopic suturing devices have been used to close the rent in the bladder. An incompletely closed rent in the bladder can also be managed easily with prolonged drainage of the bladder with an indwelling catheter [8].

Multiple portal NOTES

The **"hybrid" approach**, in contrast to the "pure" NOTES approach, involves use of laparoscopic ports in addition to the natural orifice translumenal port for performance of a given procedure [9]. Some surgeons have used a small cutaneous incision for the passage of a **needlescope**, a small camera to guide the placement of the entry port, and for maintenance of

the pneumperitoneum. Others have used **laparoscopic ports** as working ports for retraction and dissection. The **"rendez-vous" approach** is another variant of NOTES in which more than one natural orifice is used as entry ports, e.g., transvaginal–transcolonic, and transgastric–transvaginal.

The transabdominal port minimizes the risk in the placement of the second port. It allows safe closure of the natural orifice port site. There is an enhanced ability to increase triangulation and retraction maneuvers, and consequently to enhance dissection. The laparoscopic light source provides better illumination compared to the narrower, weaker light source of the flexible endoscope. The hybrid technique serves as a good launching platform, which can be used to gain experience in the use of flexible instruments in the peritoneal cavity before the introduction of "pure" NOTES into practice. The use of a transabdominal port should not be considered incompatible with NOTES, but instead part of the progression in the development of this technique.

Embryonic NOTES

A single transabdominal trocar passed at the umbilicus site has been used as an entry portal [10]. The procedure has been called embyonic NOTES or E- NOTES as the umbilicus is a natural orifice in the embryo. The cosmetic, incisionless advantage of NOTES is achieved as the resultant scar is buried in the umbilicus. It has been variously modified to include procedures involving a **single skin incision** through which several separate ports can be placed, a single incision thorough which several ports are placed through separate fascial incisions, or even several small incisions grouped around a common site that can be connected to extract the specimen. Also, access platforms have been developed which feature a flat internal profile that allows easy manipulation of instruments while still maintaining a tight seal. Terminology used to describe this technique has included: laparoendoscopic single-site surgery (LESS), umbilical-NOTES (U-NOTES), one-port umbilical surgery (OPUS), single incision laparoscopic surgery (SILS), single port access (SPA), single keyhole umbilical surgery, single trocar laparoscopic surgery, scarless single port transumbilical surgery, single port laparoscopic surgery, and single access site laparoscopic surgery.

Instrumentation

Most NOTES procedures are performed using off-the-shelf unmodified **double-channel gastroscopes**, which are designed for usage inside a narrow lumen (see Video clip 151.1). The floppy nature of the scope means the endoscopist can easily lose their way in the capacious peritoneal cavity. When compared with optimal laparoscopic images, the illumination is inferior and two-point discrimination is also poor. The camera is in line with the operating instruments and hence, off-axis visualization of the operative field cannot be obtained. Also **"triangulation,"** which is a basic requisite for a laparoscopic procedure, cannot be obtained as the accessory instruments exit parallel to each other. The push forces that can be exerted with flexible endoscopy are poor, and hence blunt dissection becomes difficult.

The last few years have witnessed an unprecedented development of devices to overcome these shortcomings of the conventional scope. Newer devices designed for entry include specially designed overtubes and laparoscopic ports with channels for multiple instruments. The suturing and stapling devices used for full-thickness closure of the entry port site have also been modified for performance of intracorporeal suturing and anastomosis. Spray dissectors and resolution clips are other improvements made over conventional devices for better dissection and hemostasis [11].

Indigenous platforms for NOTES have been developed that allow a single operator to use both hands to move instruments passed through a flexible instrument [12]. These platforms allow six degrees of freedom and appear to give sufficient control to allow intracorporeal knot tying. The ShapeLock technology, which allows a flexible instrument to be locked into desired shapes, has been used in the design of these multiple access platforms.

Given the difficulty in navigating with a flexible scope inside the large volume of the peritoneal cavity, interest has developed in the role of **image-guided navigation systems** for assistance in surgery [12]. The process starts with three-dimensional (3D) data acquisition with CT or magnetic resonance imaging (MRI). The next step is the registration of preoperative image data and intraoperative patient images. The navigation system works with tracking systems: either optical (using images from cameras from different angles), electromagnetic (tracking a coil at the end of the scope traveling through an external magnetic field), or endoscopic tracking (tracking the position of the scope in relation to the navigation aids placed at anatomical landmarks). The chief constraints in continuous intraoperative soft tissue navigation include organ shift and tissue deformation during surgery, which necessitate a constant correction of the recorded data for reliable accuracy. For image guidance to become widely used in intra-abdominal surgery and NOTES, systems need to be developed that address the deforming anatomy and moving organs.

Robotics

Two types of robots have been used to perform NOTES: fixed flexible robotics and independent miniature robots.

The **da Vinci system**, with rigid instruments with six degrees of freedom at the tip, has been used to perform procedures through natural orifices. Research is now focused on the development of robotic endoscopes, with the ability to create stable fixation points while maintaining precise tip maneuverability. Multiple remotely controlled flexible instruments exiting from a common channel that can splay outwards could provide the necessary triangulation.

There are two types of **minirobots** that can be deployed into the peritoneal cavity and remotely controlled: fixed base and

mobile robots. The fixed-base type is anchored to one part of the peritoneal cavity from where it can function as an independent camera/light source providing additional viewing angles. The prototype mobile model can navigate in the peritoneal cavity without an anchor and is fitted with a camera and a biopsy grasper. The field of *in vivo* miniature robotics is in its infancy, and current task-capable *in vivo* robots only perform simple maneuvers with a limited battery life [13].

Magnetic anchoring and guidance systems

Magnetic anchoring and guidance systems (MAGS) technology uses instruments equipped with internal magnets deployed into the peritoneal cavity that couple with external magnets. The external magnets are used to manipulate the position of the internal devices and fix them in a desired location [14]. MAGS technology has thus far developed to incorporate instruments such as retractors, an intra-abdominal camera, and cautery dissectors. However, this technology is presently limited by reduced power of magnetic coupling through the abdominal wall, especially when applied to obese individuals.

Conclusions

Apart from the obvious cosmetic benefits of an incisionless surgery and the lack of wound-related complications, like wound infection and incisional hernia, NOTES has many other advantages to offer. Its minimally invasive nature and the portability of the instruments might allow a major surgical procedure to be undertaken with minimal sedation, at the bedside of a critically ill patient. In the morbidly obese, the high morbidity of surgery is likely to be reduced with NOTES. Also, the whole of the surgical and endoscopic society is likely to benefit from the technological advances seen as a result of the stimulus provided by NOTES [15].

Based on the experimental and early clinical experiences to date, the future of NOTES appears quite promising. Fundamental research is required to study the implication of transfer of commensals from the natural orifices into the peritoneum; the immunological advantage, if any, of NOTES when compared to conventional procedures; and the repercussions of a suboptimal port entry site closure. All these issues and others need to be resolved by well-designed clinical trials before NOTES can enter routine clinical practice.

References

1. Rao GV, Reddy DN, Banerjee R. NOTES: human experience. *Gastrointest Endosc Clin North Am.* 2008;18:361–370.
2. Reddy DN, Rao GV. Transgastric approach to the peritoneal cavity: are we on the right track? *Gastrointest Endoc.* 2007:65:501–502.
3. Sumiyama K, Tajiri H, Gostout CJ. Submucosal endoscopy with mucosal flap safety valve (SEMF) technique: a safe access method into the peritoneal cavity and mediastinum. *Minim Invasive Ther Allied Technol.* 2008;17:365–369.
4. Sumiyama K, Gostout CJ, Gettman MT. Status of access and closure techniques for NOTES. *J Endourol.* 2009;23:765–771.

5. Gumbs AA, Fowler D, Milone L, *et al*. Transvaginal natural orifice translumenal endoscopic surgery cholecystectomy: early evolution of the technique. *Ann Surg*. 2009;249:908–912.

6. Shin EJ, Kalloo AN. Transcolonic NOTES: Current experience and potential implications for urologic applications. *J Endourol*. 2009;23:743–746.

7. Pauli EM, Mathew A, Haluck RS, *et al*. Technique for trans-esophageal endoscopic cardiomyotomy (Heller myotomy): video presentation at the Society of American Gastrointestinal and Endoscopic Surgeons (SAGES) 2008, Philadelphia, PA. *Surg Endosc*. 2008;22:2279–2280.

8. Granberg CF, Frank I, Gettman MT. Transvesical NOTES: Current experience and potential implications for urologic applications. *J Endourol*. 2009;23:747–752.

9. Pearl JP, Marks JM, Ponsky JL. Hybrid surgery: combined laparoscopy and natural orifice surgery. *Gastrointest Endosc Clin North Am*. 2008;18:325–332.

10. Canes D, Desai MM, Aron M, *et al*. Transumbilical single-port surgery: evolution and current status. *Eur Urol*. 2008;54:1020–1029.

11. Swain P, Bagga HS, Su LM. Status of endoscopes and instruments used during NOTES. *J Endourol*. 2009;23:773–780.

12. Karimyan V, Sodergren M, Clark J, Yang GZ, Darzi A. Navigation systems and platforms in natural orifice translumenal endoscopic surgery (NOTES). *Int J Surg*. 2009;7:297–304.

13. Lehman AC, Dumpert J, Wood NA, Visty AQ, Farritor SM, Oleynikov D. In vivo robotics for natural orifice transgastric peritoneoscopy. *Stud Health Technol Inform*. 2008;132:236–241.

14. Scott DJ, Tang SJ, Fernandez R, *et al*. Completely transvaginal NOTES cholecystectomy using magnetically anchored instruments. *Surg Endosc*. 2007;21:2308–2316.

15. Mansard MJ, Reddy DN, Rao GV. NOTES: A review. *Trop Gastroenterol*. 2009:30:5–10.

CHAPTER 152

The transjugular intrahepatic portosystemic shunt (TIPS)

Christophe Bureau, Philippe Otal and Jean-Pierre Vinel

Université de Toulouse, Toulouse, France

KEY POINTS

- Transjugular intrahepatic portosystemic shunt (TIPS) is a demanding technique that should be performed only by trained interventional radiologists in centers with all the necessary facilities (e.g., ICU, transplantation unit) to manage possible complications
- Initially the most frequent complication of TIPS was shunt dysfunction, which can be very effectively prevented using covered stents
- The main complications of TIPS are now cardiac failure, liver failure, hepatic encephalopathy, and shunt infection (endotipsitis)
- In high-risk patients with variceal hemorrhage (as defined by HVPG >20mmHg, Child class C or B, and active bleeding at endoscopy) survival is improved when TIPS is performed as soon as possible as first-line treatment
- In the prevention of recurrent variceal hemorrhage, TIPS is more effective than endoscopic and/or drug therapy. However, it leads to more encephalopathy with similar survival and is thus considered second-line therapy
- In refractory ascites, TIPS is indicated in patients whose quality of life is altered by the need for frequent paracenteses
- Other indications for TIPS are bleeding gastric or ectopic varices, Budd–Chiari syndrome, refractory hydrothorax or type 2 hepatorenal syndrome
- Main contraindications for TIPS are cardiac, respiratory or organic renal failure, pulmonary arterial hypertension, Child–Pugh score over 12 or MELD score ever 18, chronic encephalopathy, polycystic liver disease
- Most published randomized trials were performed using bare stents. Their results have to be re-evaluated using the more effective PTFE-covered prostheses

Introduction and scientific basis

Porto-caval shunting has consistently been shown to be the most effective treatment for the complications of portal hypertension. However, surgical shunting was virtually abandoned because of a high rate of post-shunt encephalopathy and of death in emergency conditions. In the last 20 years shunt therapy resurfaced because of the development of the transjugular intrahepatic portosystemic shunt (TIPS). The percutaneous transjugular route to the liver was first described by Hanafee and Weiner to perform hepatic venography, cholangiography, and liver biopsy. The first intrahepatic portosystemic shunt was created in swine in 1969 by Rösch *et al.* [1].

Thirteen years later, Colapinto *et al.* reported their preliminary experience in patients in creating an intrahepatic shunt by dilating the intraparenchymal tract between the two venous systems with a balloon catheter [2]. However, given the elasticity of liver tissue, these shunts occluded within a few days. Furthermore, several cases of rupture of the liver capsule and fatal intraperitoneal bleeds were reported. Palmaz *et al.* successfully maintained shunt patency in dogs using balloon expandable stents [3]. The first TIPS in humans was performed by Richter *et al.* [4] using a Palmaz stent, but this was later substituted by self-expandable stents, and in 2002, by polytetrafluoroethylene (PTFE) covered prostheses. The use of the latter device significantly decreased the rate of shunt dysfunction and improved clinical outcomes [5]. These technical advances must be kept in mind when evaluating the results of older clinical trials.

Technique

After puncture of a jugular vein, mostly the right internal, a Colapinto needle is advanced in a sheath through the right atrium into a hepatic vein, preferably the right one, under fluoroscopic control. The main steps of the procedure are illustrated in Figure 152.1. The most demanding stage of the technique is the catheterization of a branch of the portal vein, mainly because anatomical variations of the portal vein bifurcation are observed in up to 20% of the patients. This is facilitated mostly by the use of **ultrasonography**. Anatomical landmarks have been reported that allow localization of the portal vein in most patients [6]. More invasive methods, such as the use of **target catheters** placed percutaneously within the portal vein [4], may be the only feasible method in patients with portal vein obstruction. Finally, **retrograde portography** is probably the easiest and most reliable technique (see Video clip 152.1). Because rupture of the liver capsule has been reported using a wedged catheter, balloon occlusion portography should be preferred [7]. CO_2 should be used instead of iodine because it is 400 times less viscous and allows for a better portal vein opacification, is less costly, and has no renal toxicity [8]. After the portal vein has been punctured (see Video clip 152.2) and opacified (see Video clip 152.3), a

Textbook of Clinical Gastroenterology and Hepatology, Second Edition. Edited by C. J. Hawkey, Jaime Bosch, Joel E. Richter, Guadalupe Garcia-Tsao, Francis K. L. Chan.
© 2012 Blackwell Publishing Ltd. Published 2012 by Blackwell Publishing Ltd.

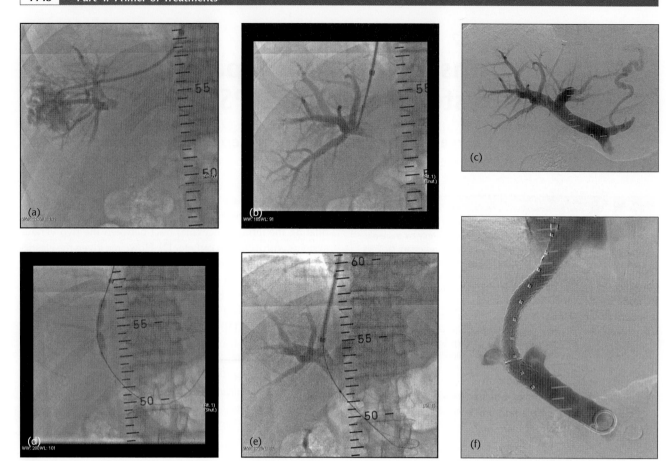

Figure 152.1 Main steps of a TIPS procedure. (a) Localization of the portal vein by retrograde portography. (b) Puncture of the portal vein. (c) Pre-TIPS portography opacifying a large collateral vein. (d) Balloon dilatation of the intrahepatic tract. The two notches on the balloon mark the walls of the hepatic vein (upper mark) and of the portal vein (lower mark). (e) The prosthesis is pushed over a guide wire. (f) Post-TIPS control angiography.

guidewire is advanced into it. The intraparenchymal tract is dilated with a balloon (see Video clip 152.4) and the prosthesis is inserted and released (see Video clip 152.5).

Effective protection against the complications of portal hypertension is obtained whenever the **hepatic venous pressure gradient (HVPG)** is decreased to 50% of its pre-TIPS value or below the threshold of 10 mmHg. This should be achieved with the smallest possible stent diameter in the hope of maintaining a hepatopetal portal flow to reduce the risk of post-shunt hepatic encephalopathy. Accordingly, a 10-mm stent is used and initially dilated to 8 mm, then further dilated to 10 mm if the decrease in HVPG is suboptimal (see Video clip 152.6). Exceptionally, HVPG remains higher than expected and a second parallel shunt must be performed.

To avoid **hepatic vein thrombosis**, the stent should be inserted into a large enough vein. Hepatic vein stenosis should be prevented by leveling the distal end of the stent at the ostium of the hepatic vein into the inferior vena cava. Finally, so as not to hamper future liver transplantation, the prosthesis should not be pushed too far down into the portal stem where it could cause thrombosis and/or severe inflammatory reaction with phlebitis.

At the end of the procedure, **control portography** must be performed (see Video clip 152.7). If large collaterals are still visible after TIPS, some authors advocate embolization. However, the efficacy of this procedure has not been demonstrated and embolization could lead to portal vein obstruction and/or remote complications such as lung or brain abscesses.

Two specific conditions deserve specific comments regarding TIPS placement: the Budd–Chiari syndrome and portal vein thrombosis. Regarding the **Budd–Chiari syndrome**, if a hepatic vein stump is present, the TIPS technique is basically the same as described above, although it may be more challenging. In a few patients, the hepatic veins are completely obstructed and their catheterization is impossible. In those situations, the puncture is made directly through the anterior wall of the inferior vena cava, aiming to enter the left branch of the portal vein through the hypertrophic caudate liver lobe [9] (Figure 152.2). The puncture route should be embolized after the procedure.

Portal vein thrombosis was initially considered a contraindication for TIPS. Nowadays, partial thrombosis should be considered an indication since the reversal of blood flow from hepatofugal to hepatopetal may help in dissolving the

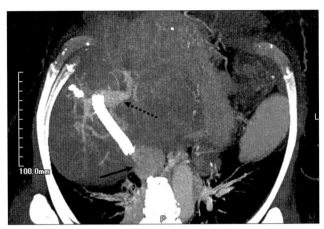

Figure 152.2 Budd–Chiari syndrome: TIPS inserted directly from the inferior vena cava (black arrow) into the portal vein (dotted arrow).

Table 152.1 Main procedural complications of TIPS

- Catheterization of the jugular vein:
  - Hematoma from puncture of the carotid artery
  - Pneumothorax
- Right atrium and inferior vena cava catheterization:
  - Cardiac arrhythmia
  - Tamponade from perforation of the right atrium
  - Bleeding from perforation of the inferior vena cava
- Puncture of the portal vein in the liver:
  - Peritoneal bleeding from laceration of the liver capsule or of the portal vein
  - Liver infarction from hepatic artery puncture
  - Hemobilia from bile duct puncture
- Iodine contrast medium injection:
  - Renal failure

thrombus [10]. Prior to indicating the procedure it is essential to ensure that the thrombosis is due to a clot and not to tumoral invasion. TIPS can also be successfully performed in cases of total obstruction of the portal vein by a recent thrombus. When a catheter has been pushed upstream of the obstacle, the clot can be destroyed using different techniques (fragmentation, aspiration, or mechanical thrombectomy) or crushed against the vein wall by the expanded stent. The most difficult condition is portal vein cavernoma in which it may be extremely difficult, or even impossible, to identify a route wide enough to release the prosthesis.

Complications

In a retrospective series of 1750 patients, the rate of lethal complications was 1.7%, ranging from 3% in centers where fewer than 150 procedures had been performed, to 1.4% in more experienced hands [11]. The major procedural complications are listed in Table 152.1. Seven types of complications can be secondary to the shunt itself.

Shunt dysfunction

This may be due to thrombosis or pseudo-intimal proliferation. Thrombosis usually occurs within the first 3 weeks. Its incidence ranges from 10% to 15% [12]. It may be due to a technical problem such as insufficient covering of the intraparenchymal tract or kinking of the prosthesis. Diagnosis is easy by Doppler ultrasound. The shunt can be recanalized. Prophylactic anticoagulation has been proposed, but the efficacy of this treatment has not been proven and it may be harmful in patients with reduced liver functions and portal hypertension.

Within 3–4 weeks after insertion in the liver, the prosthesis is progressively covered by a smooth layer of fibrous tissue topped by a single layer of endothelial cells (Figure 152.3). This pseudo-intima prevents thrombosis, but the process can be exaggerated and lead to a narrowing or even total obstruction (Figure 152.4) of the shunt [13]. Such a **pseudo-intimal**

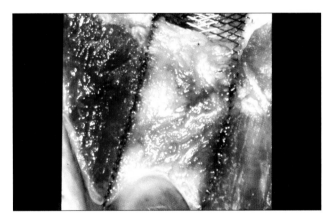

Figure 152.3 Pseudo-intima covering a bare stent in an explanted liver.

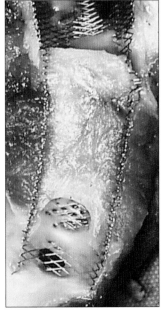

Figure 152.4 Total obstruction of a shunt by pseudo-intimal proliferation in an explanted liver.

overgrowth is the most common cause of shunt dysfunction, the incidence of which has been reported to range from 20% to 80% within 1 year. In order to detect dysfunction, Doppler ultrasound follow-up is mandatory. Pseudo-intimal proliferation is very effectively prevented using **PTFE-covered stents** [14–16] (Figure 152.5) with rates of TIPS dysfunction below 10%.

Liver infarction:

This is a rare complication that can be caused by a lesion or by acute thrombosis of the hepatic artery when the portal vein is punctured. Partial Budd–Chiari syndromes have also been reported after occlusion of an hepatic vein by the stent. The risk might be increased with covered prostheses [17].

Cardiac failure

The sudden increase in cardiac preload by the shunting may decompensate cardiac function. Therefore, TIPS is contraindicated in patients with an ejection fraction below 50%.

TIPS infection

The incidence of so-called endotipsitis has been reported to be 1.2% in a series of 165 patients [18]. Long-term antibiotherapy is not always effective and liver transplantation can be indicated.

Hepatic encephalopathy

Clinical studies have consistently reported an increased incidence of encephalopathy following TIPS. This complication is ascribed to shunting and therefore TIPS is contraindicated in patients with a history of severe or recurrent hepatic encephalopathy. Using bare stents, hepatic encephalopathy usually improves along with the narrowing of the shunt by pseudo-intimal proliferation. The incidence and/or severity of this complication was expected to be increased by using covered prostheses with more effective shunting. However, this has not been confirmed by clinical studies and the only published randomized trial has reported a lower incidence of hepatic

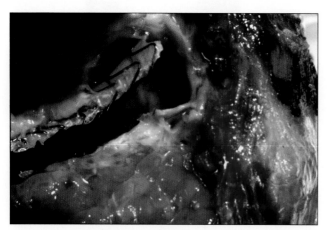

Figure 152.5 Absence of pseudo-intima over a PTFE-covered stent in a liver explanted 4 months after TIPS.

encephalopathy in patients treated with covered stents [15]. This was ascribed to a significantly less frequent need for hospitalizations, control angiographies, and shunt revisions, and fewer relapses of portal hypertension-related complications. Should incapacitating hepatic encephalopathy be observed after TIPS, the shunt can be reduced or even totally obstructed using specifically designed devices or a second coaxial stent [19].

Liver failure

This may be precipitated by shunting of portal blood flow. The risk is increased in patients with hepatopetal blood flow and those with low arterial flow. Accordingly, TIPS should be contraindicated in patients with severe liver failure as assessed by a Child–Pugh score above 12.

Hemolysis

Hemolysis has been reported in up to 30% of patients. It is mostly asymptomatic, except for an indirect hyperbilirubinemia. It is ascribed to erythrocyte damage on the metallic mesh of the prosthesis and accordingly disappears along with the covering of the stent by a pseudo-intima [20].

Indications

Among the indications for TIPS, only variceal hemorrhage and refractory ascites (which represent approximately 99% of the procedures worldwide) have been assessed by randomized controlled trials (RCTs).

Variceal hemorrhage

Bleeding from ruptured esophageal varices remains a common life-threatening complication of portal hypertension in patients with cirrhosis even though from 1980 to 2000 inhospital mortality dropped from 43% to 14.5% and rebleeding from 47% to 13% [21].

Hemostasis

Multiple uncontrolled studies have reported an average 95% hemostasis rate using TIPS following the failure of drug and endoscopic therapies. TIPS was therefore considered a second-line rescue procedure. In these settings, mortality was 20–30% higher than reported in elective conditions. Early TIPS treatment in high-risk patients, as defined by a HVPG above 20 mmHg, has been found to be more effective than medical therapy [22]. Using PTFE-covered stents, an international multicenter RCT confirmed these results. High-risk patients were defined as Child class C or B patients with active bleeding at endoscopy. Early TIPS improved the control of the bleeding and overall survival without increasing the rate of hepatic encephalopathy [23]. Interestingly, seven patients from the standard treatment group had a rescue TIPS, of whom four (57%) died as compared to a mortality of 12.5% in the early TIPS group. This suggests that early treatment is a key prognostic factor in high-risk patients, who should be treated by

TIPS as first-line treatment as soon as possible after admission.

Rebleeding

Fourteen RCTs have compared TIPS with bare stents to sclerotherapy or band ligation associated or not to non-cardioselective beta-blockers. The results were pooled in three meta-analyses, which consistently found TIPS to be more effective than alternative treatment, though it did not improve survival and increased the rate of hepatic encephalopathy [24–26]. Accordingly, TIPS is usually indicated after combination endoscopic/drug therapy has failed.

TIPS has also been used in the treatment of **gastrointestinal hemorrhage** from sources other than esophageal varices: gastric [27] or ectopic [28] varices, or portal hypertensive gastropathy [29]. It was found to be ineffective in bleeding from gastric vascular ectasia.

Refractory ascites and related complications

The efficacy of TIPS using bare stents has been assessed in five RCTs that included a total of 330 patients. As compared to large-volume paracenteses with plasma volume expansion, TIPS significantly reduced the re-accumulation of ascites. Survival was not improved and hepatic encephalopathy occurred significantly more often with TIPS [30]. TIPS is therefore used as second-line treatment in patients whose quality of life is affected by frequent paracenteses.

Uncontrolled series report that TIPS is effective in refractory hydrothorax, and type 2 hepatorenal syndrome.

Miscellaneous indications

TIPS has also been successfully used in **acute Budd–Chiari syndrome** [31], **veno-occlusive disease** [32], to facilitate **abdominal surgery** [33], and in patients awaiting **liver transplantation** [34]. It is ineffective in hepatopulmonary syndrome.

Contraindications

The contraindications are summarized in Table 152.2. Most are relative contraindications and should be balanced against the

Table 152.2 Main contraindications for TIPS

- Age > 75 years
- Child–Pugh score >12 or MELD score >18
- Overt hepatic encephalopathy or history of severe and/or recurrent encephalopathy
- Cardiac failure
- Respiratory failure
- Organic renal failure
- Pulmonary arterial hypertension
- Hydatid cyst
- Polycystic liver
- Dilatation of intrahepatic bile ducts
- Hepatocellular carcinoma
- Complete portal vein thrombosis

expected benefit: quality of life in refractory ascites, survival in severe or refractory bleeding.

Cost, quality of life, and nutritional status

In a cost-effective study in the USA, the total annual cost of TIPS was similar to that of sclerotherapy or band ligation. Regarding refractory ascites, TIPS is 50% more expensive than large-volume paracenteses. All these studies were performed with bare-stent TIPS. Although PTFE-covered prostheses are more expensive, they will be most cost-effective due to a much lower need for shunt revisions.

The effects of TIPS on quality of life and on nutritional status are still controversial. While both parameters have been found to be improved after TIPS, it is not clear whether this improvement is greater than in patients treated alternatively.

Summary and future directions

The efficacy of TIPS has been assessed by RCTs for severe acute, refractory, and recurrent variceal hemorrhage, as well as in refractory ascites, and the technique has gained its place in the therapeutic armamentarium for portal hypertension. Initially, the main drawback of TIPS was shunt dysfunction. The use of PTFE-covered stents has dramatically decreased this complication and has improved clinical outcomes. However, most published studies were performed with bare stents and these results should be reassessed using the improved devices. Furthermore, the experience accumulated over the last 20 years allows for a better selection of candidate patients, and therefore improves the results obtained with TIPS.

References

1. Rösch J, Hanafee WN, Snow H. Transjugular portal venography and radiologic portacaval shunt: an experimental study. *Radiology*. 1969;92:1112–1114.
2. Colapinto RF, Stronell RD, Gildiner M, *et al.* Formation of intrahepatic portosystemic shunts using a balloon dilatation catheter: preliminary clinical experience. *AJR Am J Roentgenol*. 1983;140: 709–714.
3. Palmaz JC, Sibbitt RR, Reuter SR, Garcia F, Tio FO. Expandable intrahepatic portacaval shunt stents: early experience in the dog. *AJR Am J Roentgenol*. 1985;145:821–825.
4. Richter GM, Noeldge G, Palmaz JC, *et al.* Transjugular intrahepatic portacaval stent shunt: preliminary clinical results. *Radiology*. 1990;174:1027–1030.
5. Bureau C, Garcia-pagan JC, Otal P, *et al.* Improved clinical outcome using polytetrafluoroethylene-coated stents for TIPS : Results of a randomized study. *Gastroenterology*. 2004;126: 469–475.
6. Teisseire R, Clanet J, Broussy P, Cassigneul J, Fourtanier G, Pascal JP. Transjugular approach to the portal venous system. Applications to the diagnosis, prognosis and treatment of gastrointestinal bleeding in cirrhosis. *Gastroenterol Clin Biol*. 1979;3: 425–432.
7. Semba CP, Saperstein L, Nyman U, Dake MD. Hepatic laceration from wedged venography performed before transjugular

intrahepatic portosystemic shunt placement. *J Vasc Interv Radiol.* 1996;7:143–146.

8. Krajina A, Lojik M, Chovanec V, Raupach J, Hulek P. Wedged hepatic venography for targeting the portal vein during TIPS: comparison of carbon dioxide and iodinated contrast agents. *Cardiovasc Intervent Radiol.* 2002;25:171–175.

9. Soares GM, Murphy TP. Transcaval TIPS: indications and anatomic considerations. *J Vasc Interv Radiol.* 1999;10:1233–1238.

10. Blum U, Haag K, Rössle M, *et al.* Noncavernomatous portal vein thrombosis in hepatic cirrhosis: treatment with transjugular intrahepatic portosystemic shunt and local thrombolysis. *Radiology.* 1995;195:153–157.

11. Barton RE, Saxon RR, Lakin PC, Petersen BD, Keller FS. TIPS: short- and long-term resultes : a survey of 1750 patients. *Semin Intervent Radiol.* 1995;364–7.

12. Rössle M, Siegerstetter V, Huber M, Ochs A. The first decade of the transjugular intrahepatic portosystemic shunt (TIPS): state of the art. *Liver.* 1998;18:73–89.

13. Ducoin H, El-Khoury J, Rousseau H, *et al.* Histopathologic analysis of transjugular intrahepatic portosystemic shunts. *Hepatology.* 1997;25:1064–1069.

14. Otal P, Smayra T, Bureau C, *et al.* Preliminary results of a new expanded-polytetrafluoroethylene-covered stent-graft for transjugular intrahepatic portosystemic shunt procedures. *AJR Am J Roentgenol.* 2002;178:141–147.

15. Bureau C, Garcia-Pagan JC, Otal P, *et al.* Improved clinical outcome using polytetrafluoroethylene-coated stents for TIPS: results of a randomized study. *Gastroenterology.* 2004;126: 469–475.

16. Bureau C, Pagan JC, Layrargues GP, *et al.* Patency of stents covered with polytetrafluoroethylene in patients treated by transjugular intrahepatic portosystemic shunts: long-term results of a randomized multicentre study. *Liver Int.* 2007;27:742–747.

17. Bureau C, Otal P, Chabbert V, Péron JM, Rousseau H, Vinel JP. Segmental liver ischemia after TIPS procedure using a new PTFE-covered stent. *Hepatology.* 2002;36:1554.

18. Sanyal AJ, Reddy KR. Vegetative infection of transjugular intrahepatic portosystemic shunts. *Gastroenterology.* 1998;115:110–115.

19. Maleux G, Verslype C, Heye S, Wilms G, Marchal G, Nevens F. Endovascular shunt reduction in the management of transjugular portosystemic shunt-induced hepatic encephalopathy: preliminary experience with reduction stents and stent-grafts. *AJR Am J Roentgenol.* 2007;188:659–664.

20. Sanyal AJ, Freedman AM, Purdum PP 3rd. TIPS-associated hemolysis and encephalopathy. *Ann Intern Med.* 1992;117: 443–444.

21. Carbonell N, Pauwels A, Serfaty L, Fourdan O, Lévy VG, Poupon R. Improved survival after variceal bleeding in patients with cirrhosis over the past two decades. *Hepatology.* 2004;40:652–659.

22. Monescillo A, Martínez-Lagares F, Ruiz-del-Arbol L, *et al.* Influence of portal hypertension and its early decompression by TIPS placement on the outcome of variceal bleeding. *Hepatology.* 2004; 40:793–801.

23. García-Pagán JC, Caca K, Bureau C, *et al.* Early TIPS (Transjugular Intrahepatic Portosystemic Shunt) Cooperative Study Group. Early use of TIPS in patients with cirrhosis and variceal bleeding. *N Engl J Med.* 2010;362:2370–2379.

24. Papatheodoridis GV, Goulis J, Leandro G, Patch D, Burroughs AK. Transjugular intrahepatic portoystemic shunt compared with endoscopic treatment for prevention of variceal rebleeding: a meta-analysis. *Hepatology.* 1999;30:612–622.

25. Luca A, D'Amico G, La Galla R, Midiri M, Morabito A, Pagliaro L. TIPS for prevention of recurrent bleeding in patients with cirrhosis : meta-analysis of randomized clinical trials. *Radiology.* 1999;212:411–421.

26. Burroughs AK, Vangeli M. Transjugular intrahepatic portosystemic shunt versus endoscopic therapy : randomized trials for secondary prophylaxis of variceal bleeding : an updated meta-analysis. *Scand J Gastroenterol.* 2002;37:249–252.

27. Barange K, Péron JM, Imani K,*et al.* Transjugular intrahepatic portosystemic shunt in the treatment of refractory bleeding from ruptured gastric varices. *Hepatology.* 1999;30:1139–1143.

28. Shibata D, Brophy DP, Gordon FD, Anastopoulos HT, Sentovich SM, Bleday R. Transjugular intrahepatic portosystemic shunt for treatment of bleeding ectopic varices with portal hypertension. *Dis Colon Rectum.* 1999;42:1581–1585.

29. Kamath PS, Lacerda M, Ahlquist DA, McKusick MA, Andrews JC, Nagorney DA. Gastric mucosal responses to intrahepatic portosystemic shunting in patients with cirrhosis. *Gastroenterology.* 2000;118:905–911.

30. Salerno F, Cammà C, Enea M, Rössle M, Wong F. Transjugular intrahepatic portosystemic shunt for refractory ascites: a meta-analysis of individual patient data. *Gastroenterology.* 2007;133: 825–834.

31. Perelló A, García-Pagán JC, Gilabert R, *et al.* TIPS is a useful long-term derivative therapy for patients with Budd-Chiari syndrome uncontrolled by medical therapy. *Hepatology.* 2002;35: 132–139.

32. Azoulay D, Castaing D, Lemoine A, *et al.* Successful treatment of severe azathioprine-induced hepatic veno-occlusive disease in a kidney-transplanted patient with transjugular intrahepatic portosystemic shunt. *Clin Nephrol.* 1998;50:118–122.?

33. Kim JJ, Dasika NL, Yu E, Fontana RJ. Cirrhotic patients with a transjugular intrahepatic portosystemic shunt undergoing major extrahepatic surgery. *J Clin Gastroenterol.* 2009;43:574–579.

34. Freeman RB Jr, FitzMaurice SE, Greenfield AE, Halin N, Haug CE, Rohrer RJ. Is the transjugular intrahepatic portocaval shunt procedure beneficial for liver transplant recipients? *Transplantation.* 1994;58:297–300.

CHAPTER 153
Interventional radiology

Simon Chun-Ho Yu and Joyce Wai Yi Hui

The Chinese University of Hong Kong, Shatin, Hong Kong SAR, China

Gastrointestinal bleeding

Interventional treatment of gastrointestinal bleeding **starts with identifying the cause and site of the bleeding. Bleed**ing from mucosal lesions is best identified with **arteriography.** Bleeding from a pancreatic pseudocyst or aneurysm that has eroded into the bowel lumen or pancreatic duct as a complication of pancreatitis is best identified on **contrast-enhanced computed tomography (CT).** CT is also a good investigative modality for aortoenteric fistula in patients with a history of abdominal aortic bypass graft. For patients with a history of cirrhosis and suspicious for variceal bleeding as the cause of gastrointestinal bleeding, an **upper endoscopy** would be indicated. **Endovascular interventional procedures,** including transcatheter vasopressin infusion and transcatheter embolization, are indicated for mucosal lesions. A transjugular intrahepatic portal systemic shunt (TIPS), an interventional option for variceal bleeding, is discussed in Chapter 152.

Technique
Visceral arteriogram

An arteriogram should be performed early for patients presenting with active bleeding to catch the bleeding moment, especially in massive lower gastrointestinal bleeding [1,2]. A complete examination includes arteriogram of the celiac axis, and superior and inferior mesenteric arteries. For **upper tract bleeding,** a selective arteriogram of the left gastric artery, gastroduodenal artery, pancreaticoduodenal artery, and inferior phrenic artery may be required. For **lower tract bleeding,** an arteriogram of the superior and inferior mesenteric arteries, the splenic artery, and the left internal iliac artery is necessary.

Several techniques have been used to improve the sensitivity of arteriography in gastrointestinal bleeding. **Pharmacoangiographic techniques** that make use of heparin, vasodilators, and thrombolytic agents may increase the yield of diagnostic arteriographic findings by up to 33% [2–4]. **Hybrid angioscintigraphy,** wherein sulfur colloid is injected into a mesenteric vessel and monitored with a gamma camera, has proved helpful in other series [5]. Findings at CO_2 **arteriography** may be positive when those at conventional arteriography are negative, probably because the lower viscosity of CO_2 allows it to extravasate more easily in the vessel [6].

Transcatheter embolization

Transcatheter embolization is an endovascular treatment with which bleeding control is achieved by **mechanical occlusion** of vessels supplying the bleeding site. Gelfoam is a commonly used absorbable material that provides temporary occlusion to acutely bleeding vessels for hemostasis and to allow for subsequent vascular revasularization. **Temporary embolization** with absorbable material is used for bleeding from transient lesions such as erosions, ulcers, diverticula, and trauma. Materials for **long-term embolization** include stainless steel coils, platinum microcoils, polyvinyl alcohol particles, and trisacryl gelatin microspheres [7,8]; these permanent materials are used for bleeding from tumors, arteriovenous malformations, varices, and extensive angiodysplasia. Microparticulate embolic materials such as Gelfoam powder and liquid embolic agents such as absolute alcohol should be avoided since they are associated with a high risk of bowel necrosis. The use of coaxial microcatheters allows superselective catheterization and embolization of bleeding sites located at small peripheral branches and reduces the risk of bowel infarction, which is of particular concern in the large bowel.

Textbook of Clinical Gastroenterology and Hepatology, Second Edition. Edited by C. J. Hawkey, Jaime Bosch, Joel E. Richter, Guadalupe Garcia-Tsao, Francis K. L. Chan.
© 2012 Blackwell Publishing Ltd. Published 2012 by Blackwell Publishing Ltd.

Vasopressin infusion

Transcatheter infusion of vasopressin (Pitressin; Parke-Davis, Morris Plains, NJ, USA), a potent constrictor of smooth muscle, is performed by direct intra-arterial infusion through a diagnostic arterial catheter at a rate of 0.2–0.4 U/minute. Infusion is maintained at the rate that is shown to control bleeding, with the patient closely observed in an intensive care unit. Hemostasis needs to be confirmed with a follow-up arteriogram at 12–24 hours after the onset of infusion. Once confirmed, the infusion is slowly tapered over 12–24 hours to avoid rebound hyperemia.

Indications and contraindications

Visceral arteriogram

Arteriography and transcatheter treatment is indicated when there is a transfusion requirement of more than 500 mL every 8 hours or when there is evidence of continued bleeding regardless of active medical therapy. A bleeding rate of at least 0.5 mL/minute is required for active extravasation to be seen on an arteriogram [9–14].

Endovascular treatment

Endovascular treatment should be considered when there is active arterial bleeding that is not controlled by endoscopic treatment. If the bleeding site can be selectively catheterized, embolization is the treatment of choice; otherwise vasopressin infusion can be considered [9–14].

Transcatheter embolization

Transcatheter embolization can provide immediate control of the bleeding if it is performed appropriately at the correct site. For upper tract bleeding failing endoscopic control, embolization can provide a definitive treatment for benign disease conditions (Figure 153.1–153.3; see Video clip 153.1). Empiric embolization of the left gastric or gastroduodenal artery can be considered in patients with severe gastric or duodenal bleeding that has been confirmed on endoscopy but not

localized on an arteriogram. However, embolization should not be performed immediately following a failed trial of vasopressin infusion, to avoid the risk of bowel infarction due to reduced collateral supply to the embolized site following vasopressin infusion. Previous surgery or endoscopic submucosal injection of sclerosants or vasoconstrictors may also increase the risk of infarction and perforation.

Vasopressin infusion

Vasopressin infusion has been found to be effective in the control of gastric bleeding, especially **diffuse hemorrhagic gastritis**, with a treatment success rate of 82% reported for this disease group [15]. Vasopressin infusion is not effective for bleeding from an angiodysplasia or neoplasm. Although vasopressin is effective in controlling bleeding from colonic diverticular disease, recurrent bleeding is common and is associated with significant morbidity and mortality. **Ischemic heart disease** is an absolute contraindication for vasopressin infusion.

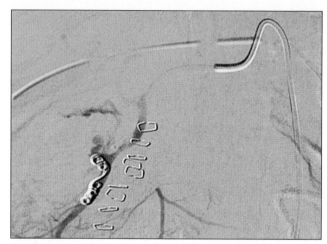

Figure 153.2 Common hepatic arteriogram showing active contrast extravasation from the pseudoaneurysm of the gastroduodenal artery during coil embolization.

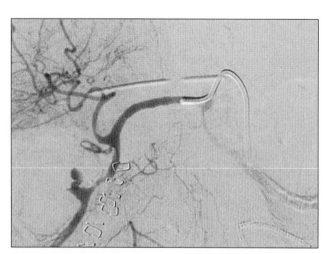

Figure 153.1 Common hepatic arteriogram showing a pseudoaneurysm arising from the gastroduodenal artery. Hemostasis after coil embolization.

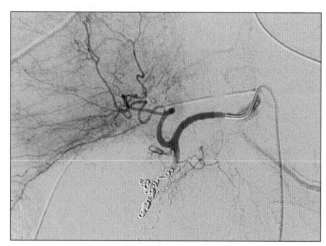

Figure 153.3 Common hepatic arteriogram showing hemostasis at the gastroduodenal artery after coil embolization.

Complications

Transcatheter embolization

The most important complication of transcatheter embolization is **transmural infarction with resultant bowel perforation**. Ischemia and infarction following embolization is much less likely to occur in the upper tract because of its rich collateral supply, unless microparticulate or liquid embolic material is used.

Vasopressin infusion

Complications of vasopressin infusion include mesenteric ischemia, bowel infarction, portal vein thrombosis, acral ischemia, hyponatremia, and cerebral edema.

Liver biopsy

Percutaneous biopsy for patients with parenchymal liver diseases has been a common practice. Although percutaneous liver biopsy is generally a safe procedure, image-guided biopsy further increases the safety of these procedures by reducing the risk of inadvertent injury to intrahepatic vascular structures or focal lesions, or to adjacent organs. The major risk of percutaneous liver biopsy is **intraperitoneal hemorrhage** that is more likely to occur in patients with coagulopathy [16]. Reported mortality rate of percutaneous liver biopsy have varied from 0.02% to 0.11% [17–19]. For patients with uncorrectable coagulopathy, the biopsy tract can be occluded with embolization material following biopsy. Alternatively, transjugular liver biopsy is a useful option. Image-guided percutaneous biopsy of focal liver mass or portal vein thrombus is important for disease diagnosis and subsequent patient management when imaging findings are inconclusive.

Technique

Preprocedure preparation includes assessment of coagulation status and medication history. Coagulation disorder and thrombocytopenia should be corrected with appropriate transfusion.

Biopsy of **liver parenchyma** is usually performed in the right lobe, especially for those performed without image guidance, and a 16 G core biopsy needle or biopsy gun is generally required.

For biopsy of **focal masses**, image guidance is necessary. The choice of CT or ultrasound guidance is dependent on the operator's experience and availability of equipment. **Ultrasound guidance** is generally preferred because it allows multiplanar visualization and provides much better spatial resolution. The biopsy needle should be manipulated within the plane of the ultrasound beam to ensure real-time guidance. The use of echogenic needle tips enhances their visibility with ultrasound. Using ultrasound guidance, a diagnostic success rate of 99% for malignancy can be achieved for sub-centimeter masses if appropriate biopsy techniques are employed [20]. The use of 18 G core biopsy guns for biopsy is preferred for

successful diagnosis of focal malignant tumors in 97.8% of cases with one to two passes of the needle [21,22]. Fine needle aspiration cytology has a diagnostic value comparable to that of microhistology obtained with fine end-cutting needles, which is inferior to that of core biopsy [22]. For biopsy of hypervascular tumors, an interposing liver parenchyma of 1-cm thickness between the tumor and the liver capsule is required to avoid intraperitoneal hemorrhage [23]. Occlusion of the biopsy tract can be performed with plugs of gelatin sponge or embolization coils introduced through a coaxial guiding needle which is placed prior to the use of biopsy needle.

For biopsy of **portal vein thrombus**, ultrasound guidance is preferred. The thrombus specimen should not be contaminated with that of the adjacent liver tissue, or else it may lead to a false diagnosis of malignancy.

Transjugular liver biopsy is performed with access through the right internal jugular vein, inferior vena cava, and right hepatic vein. Biopsy is taken through the posterior wall of the hepatic vein.

Indications and contraindications

Percutaneous liver biopsy is indicated for patients with liver cirrhosis and other parenchymal liver diseases for diagnosis, staging, monitoring treatment response, and assessment of prognosis. **Transjugular liver biopsy** is indicated for patients with uncorrectable and severe coagulopathy or thrombocytopenia, marked ascites, gross obesity, small cirrhotic liver, or suspected peliosis hepatitis. When a focal liver nodule is detected in a patient with liver cirrhosis, **biopsy of the focal lesion** is recommended in three conditions: (1) the lesion is between 1 and 2 cm in size; (2) the lesion is greater than 2 cm and imaging features are not characteristic of malignancy in two cross-sectional imaging techniques; and (3) the lesion is greater than 2 cm and imaging features are not characteristic of malignancy in one cross-sectional imaging technique, and serum alpha-fetoprotein concentration is less than 400 ng/mL [24]. **Biopsy of portal vein thrombus** is indicated to differentiate a malignant cause from a benign one in a patient with known hepatocellular carcinoma, since tumor invasion of the portal vein is associated with poor prognosis and affects the choice of treatment.

Complications and their management

Minor complications of percutaneous biopsy of liver parenchyma include pain, transient hypotension, and self-limiting bleeding that does not require blood transfusion. Major nonfatal complications occur in less than 1% of procedures. Mortality rate varies from 0.02% to 0.1% [17,18]. Major complications of transjugular biopsy, including perforation of the liver capsule, cholangitis, and intraperitoneal bleeding, occur in 1–3% of cases;, mortality is between 0.2% and 0.3% [25,26]. Percutaneous biopsy of liver masses is associated with tumor seeding along the needle tract in 0.5–2% of cases [27,28].

Percutaneous transhepatic biliary drainage
Indications and contraindications

The majority of percutaneous transhepatic biliary drainage (PTBD) procedures are performed in patients with **malignant obstruction of the extrahepatic or intrahepatic bile ducts**, either for preoperative biliary decompression or as a palliative treatment for those not fit for surgery. For biliary obstruction due to benign strictures or stones, temporary PTBD is indicated prior to subsequent treatment with surgical resection, percutaneous stone removal, or percutaneous stricture dilatation, especially when there is severe jaundice and biliary drainage through an upper endoscopic approach has not been successful. Postoperative biliary leakage can be managed by biliary diversion with temporary PTBD. PTBD is indicated as an emergency procedure in patients with acute suppurative cholangitis complicating biliary obstruction when endoscopic drainage is not feasible or unsuccessful.

Bleeding diathesis is considered by some as an absolute contraindication to PTBD; however, for patients presenting with disseminated intravascular coagulopathy complicating acute suppurative cholangitis secondary to biliary obstruction, in whom biliary drainage with an endoscopic approach is not feasible, PTBD can be life saving in experienced hands using ultrasound control. Gross ascites is not a contraindication because it can be drained with a peritoneal catheter.

Technique

The patient is fasted for at least 4 hours prior to the procedure. Coagulopathy with a prolonged prothrombin time (1.5 times that of the control) and thrombocytopenia (platelet count $<50 \times 10^9$/L) are corrected before the procedure. Prophylactic intravenous broad-spectrum antibiotics should be given. For fragile patients, the blood pressure and oxygen saturation are closely monitored. Intravenous pethidine and midazolam are given routinely. Intravenous atropine should be readily available to treat patients who develop vasovagal reaction during bile duct puncture or bile duct manipulation. Gross ascites should be drained with a peritoneal catheter prior to the procedure to avoid looping of guidewires and catheters between the liver and abdominal wall.

Bile duct puncture is best performed under real-time ultrasound guidance. Ultrasound is very useful for locating the target ducts, and the structures to be avoided such as the liver edge, lung margin, gallbladder, and intervening bowel loops. If the bile duct obstruction is inferior to the bifurcation of the common hepatic duct, it is always preferable to choose the inferior branch of the lateral segment duct of the left lobe for entry into the biliary system, using an anterior subcostal approach, unless the right duct can be accessed with a subcostal approach. Such an approach avoids unnecessary injury to the diaphragm and intercostal nerves and vessels, and avoids potential contamination of the pleural cavity.

An 18 G thin-walled trocar needle that admits a 0.038-inch guidewire is used for bile duct puncture under ultrasound control to avoid venous structures within the liver. The portal branches can be more easily differentiated from dilated ducts with the help of color Doppler ultrasound. Direct bile duct puncture with ultrasound visualization is superior to a two-stage puncture technique with the guidance of a percutaneous transhepatic cholangiogram (PTC). This is because venous structures are not depicted in PTC, and the procedure may further elevate intraductal pressure in patients with acute suppurative cholangitis.

After the bile duct has been punctured, a 0.038-inch guidewire with an angled tip is introduced under fluoroscopic control, to be anchored by coiling in the part of the biliary system where the tip of the drainage catheter is to be placed. It is then exchanged with an extra-stiff wire through a straight catheter for subsequent track dilatation and catheter placement.

In patients with acute cholangitis, a proper cholangiogram is not performed before or after catheter placement to avoid the complication of septicemia. Only external drainage of the biliary system is performed to minimize manipulation of the biliary system (Figure 153.4). If the percutaneous drainage is indicated for preoperative biliary decompression, only external drainage is provided to avoid induction of fibrosis around the extrahepatic bile ducts, which renders the operation difficult. For long-term palliation in non-surgical candidates, combined internal and external drainage, which is usually accomplished in the first sitting, is indicated (Figure 153.5). It is followed by placement of plastic or metallic endoprostheses after 1 week.

Complications and their management

Inadvertent injury of major venous structures during bile duct puncture is managed by withdrawing the needle from the

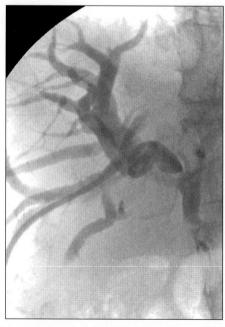

Figure 153.4 Percutaneous transhepatic catheter cholangiogram showing external drainage of the obstructed biliary system with a pigtail catheter. Biliary obstruction was due to compression of the common bile duct by malignant lymphadenopathy.

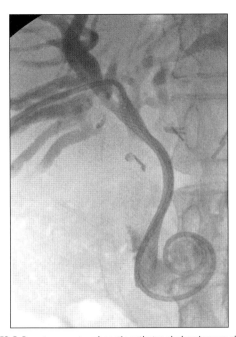

Figure 153.5 Percutaneous transhepatic catheter cholangiogram showing opacification of the intrahepatic biliary system and the stented segment of the common bile duct, and free drainage of contrast agent into the duodenum.

vessels for a short distance and plugging the needle track with the puncture needle for several minutes. If major vessels are injured by dilators or catheters, the liver parenchymal track should be embolized with coils for hemostasis. Persistent hemobilia due to an arterial–biliary fistula should be treated with selective arterial embolization.

References

1. Browder W, Cerise EJ, Litwin MS. Impact of emergency angiography in massive lower gastrointestinal bleeding. *Ann Surg.* 1986;204:530–536.
2. Uden P, Jiborn H, Jonsson K. Influence of selective mesenteric arteriography on the outcome of emergency surgery for massive lower gastrointestinal hemorrhage: a 15-year experience. *Dis Colon Rectum.* 1986;29:561–566.
3. Rosch J, Keller FS, Wawrukiewicz AS, *et al.* Pharmacoangiography in the diagnosis of recurrent massive lower gastrointestinal bleeding. *Radiology.* 1982;145:615–619.
4. Glickerman DJ, Kowdley KV, Rosch J. Urokinase in gastrointestinal tract bleeding. *Radiology.* 1988;168:375–376.
5. St George JK, Pollack JS. Acute gastrointestinal hemorrhage detected by selective scintigraphic angiography. *J Nucl Med.* 1991;32:1601–1604.
6. Sandhu C, Buckenham TM, Belli AM. Using CO_2-enhanced arteriography to investigate acute gastrointestinal hemorrhage. *AJR Am J Roentgenol.* 1999;173:1399–1401.
7. Guy GE, Shetty PC, Sharma RP, *et al.* Acute lower gastrointestinal hemorrhage: treatment by superselective embolization with polyvinyl alcohol particles. *AJR Am J Roentgenol.* 1992;159:521–526.
8. Laurent A, Beaujeux R, Wassef M, *et al.* Trisacryl gelatine microspheres for therapeutic embolization, I: Development and in vitro evaluation. *AJNR.* 1996;17:533–540.
9. Rockey DC. Pharmacologic therapy for gastrointestinal bleeding due to portal hypertension and esophageal varices. *Curr Gastroenterol Rep.* 2006;8:7–13.
10. Cwikiel W. Interventional procedures involving portal vein circulation: A review. *Acta Radiol.* 2006;47:145–146.
11. Saravanan R, Nayar M, Gilmore IT, *et al.* Transjugular intrahepatic portosystemic stent shunt: 11 years' experience at a regional referral centre. *Eur J Gastroenterol Hepatol.* 2005;17:1165–1171.
12. Wong F. The use of TIPS in chronic liver disease. *Ann Hepatol.* 2006;5:5–15.
13. Thabut D, Bernard-Chabert B. Management of acute bleeding from portal hypertension. *Best Pract Res Clin Gastroenterol.* 2007;21:19–29.
14. Yoon CJ, Chun JW, Park JH, *et al.* Transjugular intrahepatic portosystemic shunt for acute variceal bleeding in patients with viral liver cirrhosis: Predictors of early mortaility. *AJR Am J Roentgenol.* 2005;185:885–889.
15. Eckstein MR, Kelemouridis V, Athanasoulis CA, *et al.* Gastric bleeding therapy with intraarterial vasopressin and transcatheter embolization. *Radiology* 1984;152:643–646.
16. Tobkes AI, Nord HJ. Liver biopsy: Review of methodology and complications. *Dig Dis.* 1995;13:267–274.
17. Younossi ZM, Teran JC, Ganiats TG, *et al.* Ultrasound –guided liver biopsy for parencymal liver disease: An economic analysis. *Dig Dis Sci.* 1998;43:46–50.
18. McGill DB, Rakela J, Zinsmeister AR, *et al.* A 21-year experience with major hemorrhge after percutaneous liver biopsy. *Gastroenterology.* 1990;99:1396–13400.
19. Piccinino F, Sagnelli E, Pasquale G, *et al.* Complications following percutaneous liver biopsy. A multicentre retrospective study on 68, 276 biopsies. *J Hepatol.* 1986;2:165–173.
20. Yu SCH, Liew CT, Lau WY, *et al.* Ultrasound guided percutaneous biopsy of small (≤1 cm) hepatic lesions. *Radiology.* 2001;218: 195–199.
21. Yu SCH, Lau WY, Leung WT, *et al.* The value of 18 gauge automated needle in percutaneous biopsy of small (≤3 cm) hepatic lesions. *Br J Radiol.* 1998;71:621–624.
22. Yu SCH, Liew CT, Chang AW, *et al.* A prospective comparison of core biopsy (Histology), FNAB (Microhistology) and FNAC (Cytology) for focal liver lesions - an in-vivo study of diagnostic efficacy in 209 lesions. *Radiology.* 2001;221:353.
23. Yu SCH, Metreweli C, Lau WY, *et al.* Safety of percutaneous biopsy of hepatocellular carcinoma with an 18 gauge automated needle. *Clin Radiol.* 1997;52:907–911.
24. Bruix J, Sherman M, Llovet JM, *et al.* Clinical management of heoptocellular carcinoma. Conclusions of the Barcelona-2000 EASL Conference. European Association for the Study of the Liver. *J Heptol.* 2001;35;421–430.
25. McAfee JH, Keeffe EB, Lee RG, *et al.* Transjugular liver biopsy. *Hepatology.* 1992;15:726–732.
26. Garcia-Compean D, Cortes C. Transjugular liver biopsy. An update. *Ann Hepatol.* 2004;3:100–103.
27. Durand F, Regimbeau JM, Belghiti J, *et al.* Assessment of the benefits and risks of percutaneous biopsy before surgical resection of hepatocellular carcinoma. *J Hepatol.* 2001;35:254–258.
28. Chang S, Kim SH, Lim HK, *et al.* Needle tract implantation after sonographically guided percutaneous biopsy of hepatocellular carcinoma: Evaluation of doubling time, frequency, and features on CT. *AJR.* 2005;185:400–405.

CHAPTER 154

Paracentesis

Andrea De Gottardi,[1] Chong-Meng Yeo[2] and Guadalupe Garcia-Tsao[2,3]

[1]Hospital Clinic, Barcelona, Spain
[2]Yale University, School of Medicine, New Haven, CT, USA
[3]Veterans Affairs Connecticut Healthcare System, West Haven, CT, USA

KEY POINTS

- Paracentesis is the insertion of a needle into the abdominal cavity to obtain ascitic fluid for diagnostic or therapeutic purposes
- A diagnostic paracentesis is indicated in patients with new-onset ascites and in patients with cirrhosis and ascites who are admitted or who develop symptoms/signs suggestive of spontaneous bacterial peritonitis
- A therapeutic paracentesis is indicated whenever there is abdominal discomfort because of tense ascites
- There are no contraindications to the performance of a paracentesis
- The most frequent technical problem is leakage of fluid from the site of paracentesis
- Major complications of therapeutic paracentesis occur in less than 2% of cases and include bleeding and bowel perforation that may lead to infection

Introduction

Paracentesis is a medical procedure performed under sterile conditions in which a needle is inserted into the abdominal cavity to obtain ascitic fluid for analysis (diagnostic paracentesis) or to remove a large volume of ascites (therapeutic paracentesis).

As mentioned in Chapter 17, the most common cause of ascites is cirrhosis. Cirrhotic ascites can be differentiated from that due to other possible causes, such as heart failure, malignant peritoneal disease, tuberculosis, pancreatitis and others, based on a combination of the serum–ascites albumin gradient and ascites total protein.

Also, as mentioned in Chapter 99, when ascites is sufficiently abundant to cause discomfort or shortness of breath, large volume paracentesis (LVP) represents the treatment of choice and can be used prior to initiating diuretics in patients with cirrhosis and new-onset ascites. In patients with cirrhosis and ascites that is resistant or refractory to diuretics, it is used as an adjuvant to diuretics, and prior to considering a transjugular or surgical portosystemic shunt.

This procedure may be performed not only by physicians such as gastroenterologists, internists, radiologists, general practitioners or surgeons, but also by trained nurse practitioners or gastrointestinal endoscopy assistants [1] in hospitalized patients or in an outpatient setting.

Indications, contraindications, and risk factors

Diagnostic paracentesis is indicated in all patients with clinically apparent new-onset ascites independent of its volume [2]. It is also indicated in any patient with cirrhosis and ascites who is admitted to hospital or who develops symptoms or signs suggestive of spontaneous bacterial peritonitis [2,3].

Therapeutic or large-volume paracentesis (LVP) is the first-line treatment for patients with large-volume or tense ascites, as well as for patients with cirrhosis and refractory ascites. Mild and moderate ascites are best managed with a low-sodium diet and diuretics (see Chapter 99).

There are no formal contraindications to paracentesis except perhaps for loculated ascites. Clotting abnormalities should not be considered a contraindication to LVP as bleeding complications have not been shown to occur even in patients with marked thrombocytopenia or prolongation of the prothrombin time [1,4], as has been recently shown to be the case for post-ligation esophageal ulcers [5]. Thus, there are no data to support the use of fresh frozen plasma or pooled platelets before LVP [6]. It has however been suggested that platelet transfusion should be considered in patients with a platelet count <50 000/mL and not be performed in patients with suspected disseminated intravascular coagulation [7].

According to expert opinion, in some particular situations, which include an uncooperative patient, pregnancy, bowel distension, skin infection at the proposed puncture site, and hemodynamic instability, particular caution is needed, particularly for the performance of LVP that requires insertion of a large-bore needle.

In a recent prospective study, risk factors possibly associated with the development of major complications after both diagnostic (n = 45) and large-volume (n = 470) paracenteses were reported [8]. Therapeutic (versus diagnostic) paracentesis was the only risk factor that was significantly associated with the development of major complications, while an alcoholic etiology of cirrhosis, Child–Pugh class C, and a low platelet count

---

Table 154.1 Technique

Patient information	Explain the procedure including indication, risks and alternatives. Obtain informed consent
Preparation of patient and material	Ask the patient to urinate before the procedure Patient should be in supine position Get the material needed ready at the bedside
Optional: abdominal ultrasound	Identification of the site of puncture with an ultrasound device is recommended before high-risk procedures: • High-risk surgical patients • Platelets <50 g/L • If a small quantity of ascitic fluid is expected • Child–Pugh C patients
Procedure	1. Identify the site of puncture by percussion: generally it is located two fingerbreadths cephalic and two fingerbreadths medial to the left anterior superior iliac spine 2. Disinfect the area and apply a sterile fenestrated drape 3. Inject local anesthesia around the skin entry site and along the cannula insertion tract until ascitic fluid can be aspirated, then withdraw the needle and wait for the anesthestic agent to act 4. Insert the cannula perpendicular to the skin at the selected site in small increments (the Z-technique can be used) 5. Upon entry into the peritoneal cavity a loss of resistance is felt and ascites can be seen in the flashback chamber of the cannula 6. Insert the cannula another 1 cm, then withdraw the guiding needle and advance the outer sheath 3–4 cm 7. Connect the plastic tubing to the cannula and to a vacuum bottle or a graduated bin and allow ascites to drain 8. If the liquid flow stops, try to slightly change the position of the patient or of the cannula: if this is unsuccessful and a significant amount of ascites remains, repeat the puncture 9. At the end of the procedure, remove the cannula, apply pressure and place a bandage over the puncture site A diagnostic paracentesis may be performed using only a 10–20-mL syringe and a 20 G needle
Important points during and after large-volume paracentesis	Patient surveillance: heart rate and arterial pressure should be monitored for 1 hour after the procedure. Albumin administration: for paracentesis exceeding 5 L, a 20% human albumin infusion may be administered intravenously at a rate of 8 g albumin/L of ascites removed. Analysis of ascitic fluid: cell count and differential, albumin, total protein, (inoculation of culture bottles)

($<$ 50 g/L) showed a trend towards such an association, without reaching statistical significance.

Description of the technique (Table 154.1)

LVP should be performed under strict sterile conditions using disposable sterile materials. In a diagnostic paracentesis the removal of less than 100 mL is usually required, while for therapeutic purposes there is virtually no limit to the maximal volume that may be removed in a single procedure. The patient is usually in a supine position and has an empty bladder.

The presence of ascites is confirmed either on clinical examination, by the demonstration of shifting dullness, when at least 1500 mL of fluid are present [9] or by using ultrasound, which may identify volumes as small as 100 mL.

Selection of puncture site

The preferred site for needle insertion is located in the left lower quadrant, two fingerbreadths cephalad and two fingerbreadths medial to the left anterior superior iliac spine [10,11]. Paracentesis may be also performed in the right lower quadrant or over the abdominal midline, between the pubis and the umbilicus. Although the midline is presumably avascular, a

study using laparoscopy showed that in patients with portal hypertension this area is commonly vascular [12]. Importantly, the puncture should be performed at a site that is **dull on percussion**, indicating the presence of fluid. Abdominal ultrasound can be used to identify the most suitable site for puncture in patients at increased risk of procedure-related complications (see risk factors and complications above). Puncture close to surgical scars or visible abdominal collaterals should be avoided, as should punctures in the area of the inferior hypogastric artery, which lies midway between anterior superior iliac spine and the pubic tubercle.

Procedure

First, the site for paracentesis is appropriately disinfected and a sterile fenestrated drape is placed around the puncture site. Subsequently, the skin and the subcutaneous tissue are anesthetized by injecting up to 5 mL of 1% lidocaine or another local anesthetic.

For a diagnostic paracentesis a 20 G needle is sufficient for fluid removal. In an obese patient, a spinal needle may be necessary.

For LVP a rigid metallic cannula that is at least 16–18 G is recommended. Although its beneficial effects have not been demonstrated, the Z-technique for the introduction of the cannula (lateral shifting of the skin, which creates an oblique passage through the abdominal wall), may be used to avoid ascites leakage after the procedure. The cannula is inserted into the abdominal wall until ascitic fluid is visible in its flash-back chamber (Figure 154.1), at which time it should be inserted an additional 1 cm. Next, the guiding needle is withdrawn, while the outer sheath is slid another 3–4 cm into the peritoneal cavity. Some cannulae have several side holes in addition to the distal one (Figure 154.1) and may be used to avoid premature interruption of flow by obstruction of the end hole by adjacent structures (omentum or bowel).

The physician performing the procedure usually chooses the type of needle according to the patient's abdominal wall anatomy and the indication for paracentesis (large diameter cannulae are preferred for therapeutic paracenteses, longer

cannulae are indicated in obese patients). For diagnostic paracentesis, a syringe is connected to the cannula and the desired quantity of liquid is aspirated (Figure 154.2). For therapeutic procedures, the cannula is then fixed to the abdominal wall and connected with plastic tubing to a graduated canister or a vacuum bottle until no more fluid drains (Figure 154.2).

In case of premature flow interruption the patient may be asked to turn more onto their side and/or the cannula may be gently mobilized within the abdominal cavity. If no fluid can be obtained with these maneuvers and it is evident that a moderate amount of ascites remains, the puncture may be repeated.

At the end of the procedure, when no more ascitic fluid can be drained, the cannula is removed, a cotton gauze sponge is secured with an adhesive bandage, and the patient is asked to recline for at least 1 hour on the opposite site to the paracentesis site to prevent leakage of ascitic fluid.

Monitoring and albumin use

The physician or a nurse should monitor the patient's vital signs before, at least once during the procedure, and at the end of the procedure. After therapeutic paracentesis, outpatients usually remain under observation for possible complications for at least 1 hour and are discharged if they are asymptomatic and without postural hypotension.

When removal of ascites exceeds 5 L, the intravenous administration of a 20% human albumin at a dose of 6–8 g of albumin/L of ascites evacuated should be considered to decrease the incidence of **post-paracentesis circulatory dysfunction (PCD)** [13]. PCD is characterized by a reduction in effective arterial blood volume with consequent activation of the rennin–angiotensin system [14], which is subsequently associated with a higher rate of renal dysfunction and death. However, the administration of albumin remains controversial [2,6], because, although it effectively prevents PCD, it has not

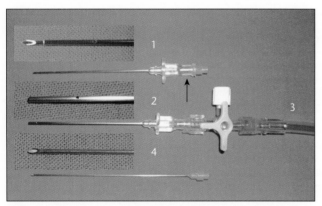

Figure 154.1 Example of an 18 G metallic paracentesis cannula (Toraflex; Emiltek Medical Division, Italy). Guiding needle inserted into the cannula (1). Cannula (outer sheath) with side holes (2) connected with plastic tubing (3) for emptying of ascitic fluid by declivity or under aspiration. Guiding needle alone (4). The black arrow indicates the flashback chamber of the cannula.

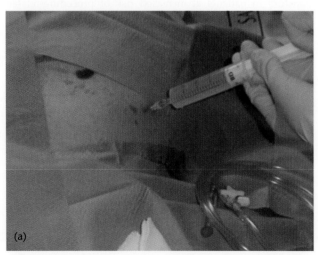 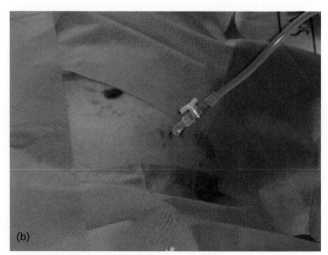

Figure 154.2 Performance of a large volume paracentesis. (a) Aspiration of ascitic fluid for diagnostic tests and (b) connection of the cannula with aspiration tubing.

been associated with an improvement in morbidity or mortality. Timing of administration of albumin is unclear and, although in controlled trials 50% of the dose was administered within the first 2 hours and 50% 6–8 hours after paracentesis, in practice the whole dose is administered shortly after paracentesis is completed.

Technical problems and complications

In general, paracentesis is a safe procedure. Technical problems occur in up to 5–6% of cases [8] and include absence of ascites at the first attempt of puncture or flow interruption that requires catheter repositioning, repuncture in a different site, or switching to a longer cannula. If no ascites is obtained after the first puncture, no further attempts should be made blindly and the procedure should be repeated under ultrasound guidance.

Additional technical problems may occur during the procedure when the cannula slips out (often after a patient moves) or the catheter is sectioned and a segment migrates into the abdominal wall (when using plastic cannulae).

Minor complications, defined as self-limited problems that can be managed conservatively, are observed in up to 10% of cases [8]. The most frequent is **ascites leakage** from the puncture site. To decrease the incidence of this complication, in addition to the Z-technique, the patient should turn onto the side opposite the puncture for at least 1 hour following the procedure. The leak usually stops spontaneously. However, if the flow is abundant, a stoma pouch may be applied to the abdominal wall to collect ascites. This complication can often be solved by completing the LVP at a site remote from the leaking puncture site. In the rare cases where this does not solve the problem, a suture at the puncture point or the application of cyanoacrylate glue may be useful [15]. Similarly, another complication of paracentesis that is rare but should be

recognized is the development of sudden scrotal edema from subcutaneous tracking of peritoneal fluid into the scrotum. This can be overcome by elevation of the scrotum [16]. Other minor complications include self-limited local bleeding and hematoma.

As mentioned above, the removal of a large volume of ascites, particularly in the absence of adjuvant albumin administration, may result in PCD, which may lead to renal impairment, water retention, and dilutional hyponatremia. The intravenous administration of albumin has been shown to prevent the development of PCD [13].

Major complications defined as those that require a specific medical intervention, such as bleeding or iatrogenic bowel perforation and subsequent ascites infection (bacterial peritonitis), are exceedingly rare and occur in about 0.4% of cases (range 0–3%) [1,4,8,17–20]. Major bleeding occurs rarely but may be lethal [20] and is mostly related to puncture of collaterals or arteries in the abdominal wall or puncture of intra-abdominal collaterals rather than as a result of coagulopathy. In these settings, the performance of a transjugular portosystemic shunt and/or urgent arteriography with embolization should be considered [21].

Death as a direct consequence of paracentesis is reported to occur extremely rarely and should be considered an exceptional event. Particular care should be taken in the performance of therapeutic paracentesis in patients with advanced liver disease who are poor surgical candidates and in whom a surgical intervention would not be an option in case of a major complication.

Table 154.2 summarizes the major complications and mortality associated with diagnostic and/or therapeutic paracentesis.

Before starting abdominal paracentesis, the patient should be informed about indication, risks, complications, and alternatives, and their informed consent should be obtained.

Table 154.2 Major complications and mortality of paracentesis (diagnostic and/or therapeutic) in a series including more than 200 procedures

| Study | Number of patients | Number of paracentesis | Type of paracentesis | Major complications | | | Deaths |
				Severe hemorrhage	Bowel perforation	Bacterial peritonitis	
Mallory and Schaefer (1978) [17]	156	242	Diagnostic	4 (1.65%)	2 (0.83%)	0 (0%)	3 (1.23%)
Runyon (1986) [18]	125	229	97% diagnostic	2 (0.87%)	0 (0%)	0 (0%)	0 (0%)
Grabau et al. (2004) [1]	628	1100	Therapeutic	0 (0%)	0 (0%)	0 (0%)	0 (0%)
Pache and Bilodeau (2005) [19]	Unknown	4729	Not stated	9 (0.19%)	0 (0%)	0 (0%)	1 (0.02%)
Lin et al. (2005) [4]	163	410	76% therapeutic	0 (0%)	0 (0%)	0 (0%)	0 (0%)
De Gottardi et al. (2009) [20]	171	515	91% therapeutic	5 (0.97%)	2 (0.39%)	1 (0.19%)	2 (0.39%)
Total		7225		20 (0.28%)	4 (0.05%)	1 (0.01%)	6 (0.08%)

Analysis of ascitic fluid

In a diagnostic paracentesis, the standard analyses of ascitic fluid are cell count and differential [to exclude **spontaneous bacterial peritonitis (SBP)**, albumin (to calculate the **serum–ascites albumin gradient**), using serum albumin results that should be obtained close to the time of the diagnostic paracentesis), and total protein (which will help in the differential diagnosis of ascites and to assess the need for prophylactic treatment of SBP). If SBP is suspected (fever, abdominal pain, encephalopathy, variceal bleeding), inoculation of ascites in blood culture bottles should be performed (blood cultures should also be obtained). Other studies may be considered based on the degree of clinical suspicion of a specific disease. These include cytology for peritoneal carcinomatosis, alkaline phosphatase for bowel perforation, and adenosine deaminase for tuberculosis. Novel diagnostic tools, such as lactoferrin for the diagnosis of SBP [22] or polymerase chain reaction for the identification of infectious agents, are in clinical development.

It has been suggested that a faster, inexpensive method of making the diagnosis of SBP is through the bedside use of reagent strips; however, a review shows that the false-negative rate ranges between 0% and 50% [23], and in the largest series of patients with SBP, using the Multistix 6G, the false-negative rate was 55% [24]. Therefore, the use of reagent strips cannot be recommended.

In patients undergoing serial outpatient therapeutic paracentesis, the fluid removed should be tested for cell count and differential only, although given the very low prevalence of overt infection (0–3%) in this asymptomatic patient population this may not be absolutely necessary [25–27].

References

1. Grabau CM, Crago SF, Hoff LK, et al. Performance standards for therapeutic abdominal paracentesis. *Hepatology*. 2004;40:484–488.
2. Runyon BA: Management of adult patients with ascites due to cirrhosis: an update. *Hepatology*. 2009;49:2087–2107.
3. Rimola A, Garcia-Tsao G, Navasa M, et al. Diagnosis, treatment and prophylaxis of spontaneous bacterial peritonitis: a consensus document. *J Hepatol*. 2000;32:142–153.
4. Lin CH, Shih FY, Ma MH, et al. Should bleeding tendency deter abdominal paracentesis? *Dig Liver Dis*. 2005;37:946–951.
5. Vieira da Rocha EC, D'Amico EA, Caldwell SH, et al. A prospective study of conventional and expanded coagulation indices in predicting ulcer bleeding after variceal band ligation. *Clin Gastroenterol Hepatol*. 2009;7:988–993.
6. Gines P, Angeli P, Lenz K, et al. EASL clinical practice guidelines on the management of ascites, spontaneous bacterial peritonitis, and hepatorenal syndrome in cirrhosis. *J Hepatol*. 2010;53: 397–417.
7. Gines P, Cardenas A. The management of ascites and hyponatremia in cirrhosis. *Semin Liver Dis*. 2008;28:43–58.
8. De Gottardi A, Thevenot T, Spahr L, et al. Risk of complications after abdominal paracentesis in cirrhotic patients: a prospective study. *Clin Gastroenterol Hepatol*. 2009;7:906–909.
9. Cattau EL Jr, Benjamin SB, Knuff TE, et al. The accuracy of the physical examination in the diagnosis of suspected ascites. *JAMA*. 1982;247:1164–1166.
10. Sakai H, Sheer TA, Mendler MH, et al. Choosing the location for non-image guided abdominal paracentesis. *Liver Int*. 2005;25: 984–986.
11. Thomsen TW, Shaffer RW, White B, et al. Videos in clinical medicine. Paracentesis. *N Engl J Med*. 2006;355:e21.
12. Oelsner DH, Caldwell SH, Coles M, et al. Subumbilical midline vascularity of the abdominal wall in portal hypertension observed at laparoscopy. *Gastrointest Endosc*. 1998;47:388–390.
13. Gines P, Tito L, Arroyo V, et al. Randomized comparative study of therapeutic paracentesis with and without intravenous albumin in cirrhosis. *Gastroenterology*. 1988;94:1493–1501.
14. Ruiz del Arbol L, Monescillo A, Jimenez W, et al. Paracentesis-induced circulatory dysfunction: mechanism and effect on hepatic hemodynamics in cirrhosis. *Gastroenterology*. 1997;113: 579–586.
15. Hale BR Jr, Girzadas DV Jr. Application of 2-octyl-cyanoacrylate controls persistent ascites fluid leak. *J Emerg Med* 2001;20:85–86.
16. Conn HO: Sudden scrotal edema in cirrhosis: a postparacentesis syndrome. *Ann Intern Med*. 1971;74:943–945.
17. Mallory A, Schaefer JW. Complications of diagnostic paracentesis in patients with liver disease. *JAMA*. 1978;239:628–630.
18. Runyon BA. Paracentesis of ascitic fluid. A safe procedure. *Arch Intern Med*. 1986;146:2259–2261.
19. Pache I, Bilodeau M. Severe haemorrhage following abdominal paracentesis for ascites in patients with liver disease. *Aliment Pharmacol Ther*. 2005;21:525–529.
20. De Gottardi A, Thevenot T, Spahr L, et al. Risk of complications after abdominal paracentesis in cirrhotic patients: a prospective study. *Clin Gastroenterol Hepatol*, 2009;7:906–909.
21. Arnold C, Haag K, Blum HE, et al. Acute hemoperitoneum after large-volume paracentesis. *Gastroenterology*. 1997;113:978–982.
22. Parsi MA, Saadeh SN, Zein NN, et al. Ascitic fluid lactoferrin for diagnosis of spontaneous bacterial peritonitis. *Gastroenterology*. 2008;135:803–807.
23. Ghassemi S, Garcia-Tsao G. Prevention and treatment of infections in patients with cirrhosis. *Baillieres Best Pract Res Clin Gastroenterol* 2007;21:77–93.
24. Nousbaum JB, Cadranel JF, Nahon P, et al. Diagnostic accuracy of the Multistix 8 SG reagent strip in diagnosis of spontaneous bacterial peritonitis. *Hepatology*. 2007;45:1275–1281.
25. Evans LT, Kim WR, Poterucha JJ, et al. Spontaneous bacterial peritonitis in asymptomatic outpatients with cirrhotic ascites. *Hepatology*. 2003;37:897–901.
26. Romney R, Mathurin P, Ganne-Carrie N, et al. Usefulness of routine analysis of ascitic fluid at the time of therapeutic paracentesis in asymptomatic outpatients. Results of a multicenter prospective study. *Gastroenterol Clin Biol*. 2005;29:275–279.
27. Jeffries MA, Stern MA, Gunaratnam NT, et al. Unsuspected infection is infrequent in asymptomatic outpatients with refractory ascites undergoing therapeutic paracentesis. *Am J Gastroenterol*. 1999;94:2972–2976.

CHAPTER 155
Liver operations

J. Michael Henderson and Michael D. Johnson

Cleveland Clinic, Cleveland, OH, USA

Introduction and scientific basis

The surgeon plays a role as one of the team members taking care of patients with various liver diseases. Many authors refer to the need for surgery, so the aim of this chapter is to bring together the types of operations that are used in the management of the clinical problems described elsewhere in this book. The broad categories are:

- Liver resections and/or ablation
- Biliary procedures
- Operations for portal hypertension
- Liver transplantation.

The surgeon should not work in isolation, and is heavily interdependent on the team of hepatologists, radiologists, pathologists, anesthesiologists, and support personnel. This chapter will not focus on the detail of operative procedures, but rather on the broad concepts of the indications for surgery, evaluation methods to reach decisions, the types of procedures available, and overall management strategies from a surgeon's perspective.

Evaluation methods

The patient's **history and physical examination** play an important part in reaching a decision on which patients require surgery, e.g., surgery may be indicated for resection of benign liver tumors if they are symptomatic; resection of metastatic liver tumors is indicated only for certain types of primary tumors; surgical intervention for variceal bleeding is only indicated when the first-line treatment options have been exhausted; and components of the patient history are a critical part of the evaluation for liver transplant.

Laboratory studies, including liver chemistries, hematology, and coagulation profiles are essential for all patients being considered for liver surgery. In some patients, liver biopsy may be indicated either to define a specific tumor, or more frequently to define underlying liver disease, such as cirrhosis. The decision to operate or not may be based on the activity and degree of fibrosis in the liver, rather than on the tumor pathology.

Imaging studies play an important role in the evaluation of all patients considered for liver surgery, biliary operations, or transplant. The increasing sophistication of radiological imaging is one of the major factors that have improved the selection and outcome of patients being considered for liver surgery. Three-dimensional reconstruction of computed tomography (CT) scans and volume calculation can be useful in certain cases for determining the size of the future liver remnant (FLR) based on the type of resection planned. The amount of remaining liver that will be tolerated will obviously be influenced by the health of the background "normal" liver, but a good rule of thumb is a FLR of at least 25% [1].

Liver function is assessed by a combination of physical findings, laboratory studies, and in certain circumstances more sophisticated liver function testing. The broad goal is to address the ability of the liver to tolerate an operative procedure without precipitating liver failure. The two main scoring systems in current use are the Child–Pugh score (Table 155.1) and the model for end-stage liver disease (MELD) score (Table 155.2) [2].

Anatomy

Liver structure must be clearly understood by the surgeon, both from the evaluation and treatment perspective. The **segmental anatomy of the liver** (Figure 155.1) is based on the eight liver segments with each having its own hepatic arterial and portal venous blood supply, biliary drainage, and hepatic venous drainage. This segmental anatomy dictates the ability to perform liver resections. An accurate knowledge of the portal and hepatic venous system is critical to the liver surgeon. This can be verified with intraoperative ultrasound. The variability of extrahepatic arterial anatomy may be seen on

Table 155.1 Child – Pugh classification

Parameter	1 point	2 points	3 points
Serum bilirubin (mg/dL)	<2	2–3	<3
Albumin (g/dL)	>3.5	2.8–3.5	<2.8
Prothrombin time (↑, s)	1–3	4–6	>6
Ascites	None	Slight	Moderate
Encephalopathy	None	1–2	3–4

Grades: A, 5–6 points; B, 7–9 points; C, 10–15 points.

Table 155.2 MELD score for severity of cirrhosis

$$\text{MELD score} = 0.957 \times \log_e \text{creatinine}$$
$$+ 0.378 \times \log_e \text{bilirubin}$$
$$+ 1.120 \times \log_e \text{protime}$$

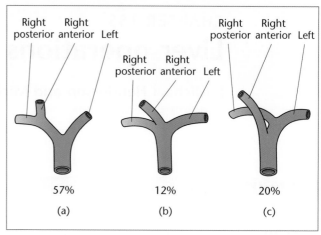

Figure 155.2 Biliary bifurcation. The most common variants of the biliary "bifurcation." (a) A true bifurcation with intrahepatic right anterior and posterior ducts. (b) A trifurcation occurs in 12% with the right anterior and posterior ducts meeting at the same point as the left duct. (c) In 20%, one of the right ducts (usually posterior) crosses to enter the left duct. (Reproduced from Meyers WC. Atlas of biliary surgery. In: Bell RH, Rikkers LF, Mulholland MW, editors. *Digestive Tract Surgery*, 1996, with permission from Lippincott, Williams and Wilkins.)

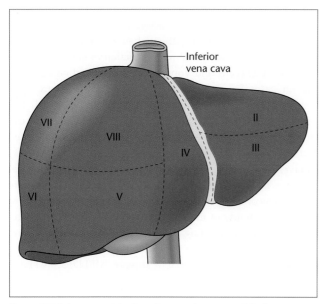

Figure 155.1 Anatomy of the liver. Segmental anatomy of the liver according to Couinaud; each of the eight liver segments has its own blood supply and biliary drainage. (Reproduced from Meyers WC. Atlas of biliary surgery. In: Bell RH, Rikkers LF, Mulholland MW, editors. *Digestive Tract Surgery*, 1996, with permission from Lippincott, Williams and Wilkins.)

imaging studies, but should be assessed at surgery. The most common variations are replaced or accessory arteries to the right liver from the superior mesenteric artery and the left liver from the left gastric artery. The biliary anatomy is also very variable and should be defined by preoperative or intraoperative cholangiography. The major questions for a surgeon are around the **hilus**; Figure 155.2 illustrates the most common variants. The hilar plate is the fusion of the liver capsule over

the portal vein, hepatic artery, and bile duct at the liver hilus. Opening of this capsular plane below segment IV allows elevation of the hilar plate and greatly facilitates dissection of the hilar structures.

Management

When patients undergo surgery to treat liver conditions or patients with liver disease require a surgical procedure, the surgeon is the captain of the team and must assume responsibility for overall patient management. Preoperative preparation should be done in conjunction with the hepatologist to optimize the patient's liver condition. Perioperative management must be planned with the anesthesiologist (e.g., low central venous pressure for liver resection). In patients with cirrhosis requiring an operation, overall fluid and nutritional management are critical. Defined protocols for management of each of these phases will lead to better patient care and have become standard in most liver surgery centers.

Liver resections

Liver resections are indicated for removal of benign or malignant neoplasms. Some benign lesions, such as giant hemangiomas, form pseudocapsules and can be enucleated. Malignant tumors are resected with the goal of at least a 1-cm margin. The extent of resection is determined by liver anatomy (Figure 155.1) with either segmental or lobar resections.

Technique

The goals of any liver resection are complete resection of the lesion(s), preservation of an adequate liver remnant, and minimization of blood loss. The latter is particularly important as blood loss has been shown consistently to predict morbidity and mortality after liver resection [3].

The essential technical steps for successful liver resection are:

1. Exposure
2. Mobilization
3. Definition of anatomy (visual and ultrasound)
4. Determination of resection planes
5. Division of main vascular pedicles
6. Parenchymal transection
7. Confirmation of margins
8. Check liver remnant [4].

Incisions, exposure, and mobilization of the liver have been aided by transplant experience and technology. Most liver resections can be accomplished using an abdominal approach, but occasionally a combined thoracoabdominal incision (right sided) may be needed. Fixed retractor systems aid and maintain exposure. The left and right sides of the liver can be mobilized by dividing the triangular ligaments, and the liver fully mobilized off the inferior vena cava (IVC) up to the hepatic veins if needed (Figure 155.3a, b).

Anatomical definition requires careful hilar dissection of the arteries, portal vein, and bile ducts when anatomic lobar resection is being done. The hepatic and portal veins are localized with intraoperative ultrasound. Concurrently, tumor extent is defined by palpation and ultrasound. These maneuvers allow for planning of the resection plane.

Control of blood supply and venous drainage are both important for limiting blood loss. Inflow control is usually accomplished by clamping the portal pedicle, (Pringle maneuver). This eliminates hepatic artery and portal venous flow. Inflow occlusion can take many forms, but generally consists of a short period of ischemic preconditioning (inflow is clamped without performing parenchymal division), followed by intermittent inflow occlusion with short periods of rest (hepatic reperfusion) in between. Even with complete inflow occlusion, back-bleeding is still encountered from the hepatic veins. Low central venous pressure anesthesia and avoidance of over-resuscitation help to limit this. Total vascular exclusion (TVE) involves inflow occlusion as well as clamping of the infrahepatic and suprahepatic IVC. This is only required for large posterior tumors involving the vena cava. **Transection of the parenchyma** can be done in many ways, including crush and clamp, ultrasonic dissection (Figure 155.4), and water pick dissection; all define the vessels for ligation or clipping by clearing away the hepatocytes. The second component to this phase is achieving hemostasis, which can again be done in many ways: ligatures, clips, diathermy, argon diathermy, and TissueLink. There is no one "right" way to do this, but attention to detail and meticulous technique are important. Inspection of the remnant liver, checking the inflow vessels, ensuring there is no venous outflow obstruction, and possibly doing a completion cholan-

giogram if dissection has been at the bifurcation will minimize complications.

Laparoscopic liver resection (see Video clip 155.1)
Many liver resections are now being performed laparoscopically. The majority of such resections are wedge or segmental resections, but some centers are performing major resections as well. Several comparative studies have demonstrated similar operative times with lower blood loss and shorter length of hospital stay [5]. Lesions involving segments 2, 3, 4b, 5, and 6 are most accessible with a laparoscopic approach. Most tools for parenchymal division used in open surgery are available for laparoscopic application. Linear endoscopic staplers are particularly indispensable. The use of a hand port adds an additional element of control when transitioning from the open to the laparoscopic approach. It is particularly helpful when mobilizing the right lobe to access posterior lesions. As experience grows, more extensive resections can be expected.

Indications
Liver resection may be a treatment option for some benign and malignant liver tumors.

Benign tumors
Adenoma
Liver adenomas require resection because of their risk of rupture or bleeding and malignant transformation. Resection can be limited, usually to a segmentectomy. Adenomas that have bled or ruptured require urgent/emergency surgery, with the resections largely being a debridement. Debate continues about surgery for patients with small adenomas (<4 cm) or multiple adenomas – observation is probably justified.

Focal nodular hyperplasia
This benign condition is a common finding on incidental liver imaging. Focal nodular hyperplasia (FNH) differs from adenoma in that all elements of the liver are present histologically and its complications are minimal. If accurately defined, this entity does not require resection. The only indication for resection of FNH is if there is doubt as to diagnosis, or if it is symptomatic. FNH does not bleed, undergo malignant change, or rupture, but occasionally it may cause symptoms by pressure on adjacent structures.

Hemangioma
These are the most common of the benign liver tumors and range in size from a few millimeters to >20 cm. Again, these are often incidental findings and do not need to be removed. The greatest risks with hemangiomas are iatrogenic and often inappropriate interventions. The occasional large hemangioma may require surgery, and these can be dealt with usually by enucleation because they form pseudocapsules. Even the most "fearsome" hemangioma central in the liver is usually amenable to this approach.

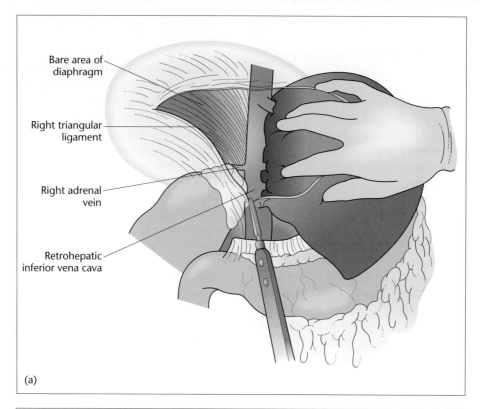

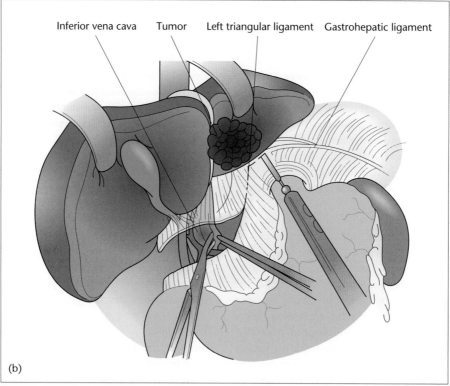

Figure 155.3 Mobilization. (a) Mobilization of the right lobe of the liver by diversion of the right triangular ligament. This goes right back to the inferior vena cava (IVC) and may include ligation of retrohepatic veins draining into the IVC. (b) Mobilization of the left lobe of the liver requires diversion of the left triangular ligament, the gastrohepatic ligament, and the peritoneum on the left side of the IVC. These three lines come together superiorly at the left posterior side of the suprahepatic IVC. (Reproduced from Meyers WC. Atlas of biliary surgery. In: Bell RH, Rikkers LF, Mulholland MW, editors. *Digestive Tract Surgery*, 1996, with permission from Lippincott, Williams and Wilkins.)

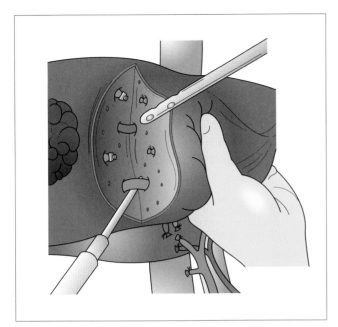

Figure 155.4 Liver parenchymal transection. Ultrasonic dissection (as illustrated) is one method of defining the vessels and bile ducts in the plane of transection, which used to be clipped or ligated. (Reproduced from Meyers WC. Atlas of biliary surgery. In: Bell RH, Rikkers LF, Mulholland MW, editors. *Digestive Tract Surgery*, 1996, with permission from Lippincott, Williams and Wilkins.)

Cystadenomas

These are benign cystic tumors of biliary origin that occur in the liver. Although rare, they may be confused with simple cysts but, unlike simple cysts, do not respond to deroofing. The differentiation of cystadenomas is made on pathology with a defined cuboidal epithelial lining to these tumors. They require a total excision to prevent recurrence. The majority of cystadenomas present with symptoms, which is the diagnostic clue that differentiates them from simple cysts.

Malignant tumors

Hepatocellular carcinoma

This is the most common primary liver tumor requiring resection. The indication for resection of a hepatocellular carcinoma (HCC) is dictated by several factors: (1) the underlying etiology leading to HCC; (2) technical factors for resectability; and (3) the underlying liver disease and ability to tolerate resection. Staging of HCC has received considerable attention over the last few years and plays a role in determining resectability [6]. Staging should primarily be clinical, using either the Italian or Spanish staging systems, which consider tumor size, morphology, the underlying liver disease, and patient performance status. Pathological staging is only applicable to resected HCCs.

In patients with advanced liver disease, development of HCC may become an indication for higher priority for liver transplantation. Resection for HCC has acceptable outcomes for small (<5 cm) tumors in patients with well-preserved liver function (Child class A). The best candidates for resection are probably patients with a MELD of <8 and without hepatitis C virus (HCV) [7]. Intermediate staged tumors (>5 cm or more than one nodule) and patients with more advanced liver disease (portal hypertension and Child class B+) are poorer candidates for resection. Adverse prognostic factors are tumor grade, tumor size, and microvascular invasion [7].In patients who have a resection for HCC, approximately 50% have further intrahepatic HCC within 5 years.

Cholangiocarcinoma

Intrahepatic cholangiocarcinoma may require liver resection. These tumors histologically are adenocarcinomas with either pathological features suggestive of biliary origin, or determined by exclusion of other primary sites for adenocarcinoma. Resection is the optimal treatment for such cancers, but technical issues may limit the indication for resection. As some of these tumors occur in patients with primary sclerosing cholangitis, the status of the underlying liver is important in making a decision to resect.

Secondary liver tumors

The indications for resection of secondary tumors in the liver are relatively limited, but are the most common reason for liver resection [8]. Colorectal carcinoma metastatic to the liver is the main indication. Neuroendocrine metastatic tumors also may be managed by resection. There are very few other primary cancers with metastases to the liver that warrant a liver resection, the exception being a solitary metastasis that has been present for a documented time.

Indications for both colorectal and neuroendocrine metastasis resection have expanded over the last 10 years, with a general guideline of "if it is resectable, it probably should be resected." For **colorectal metastases**, large single metastasis or multiple metastases confined to one lobe are the most common indications for resection. However, "cherry picking" of individual lesions in the right and left liver may now be justified if such resection renders the patient tumor free. The ability to do this has been greatly enhanced with improved intraoperative ultrasound. Bilobar metastases were once considered a contraindication to resection. Many centers are now using a two-stage approach in such situations [9]. A common scenario consists of a large R-sided tumor with one or more smaller lesions in the left lobe. The first stage consists of wedge resection of the left-sided lesions followed by right portal vein embolization (PVE). This induces hypertrophy of the left lobe (FLR) allowing for a safe, interval R hepatic lobectomy. In the event that even such a two-stage approach is not feasible, resection and ablation can often be combined in the same setting.

Contraindications

In general terms, contraindications to liver resection are either due to technical issues that make resection infeasible, or contraindications to liver resection based on underlying liver disease and poor liver function. **Technical contraindications** are largely determined by burden of disease in the liver,

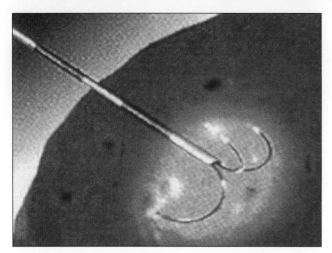

Figure 155.5 Radiofrequency ablation of a liver tumor. The probe is placed into the tumor, opened, and an energy source applied sufficient to destroy the tumor and a rim of surrounding tissue. The ablation zone is monitored by ultrasound. (Reproduced from Meyers WC. Atlas of biliary surgery. In: Bell RH, Rikkers LF, Mulholland MW, editors. *Digestive Tract Surgery*, 1996, with permission from Lippincott, Williams and Wilkins.)

involvement of major vascular structures, or the natural history of the underlying tumor. **Poor liver function** as a contraindication to liver resection is seen primarily in patients with HCC and underlying cirrhosis.

Liver ablation

Ablation attempts to locally control a liver tumor by direct tissue destruction of the tumor and a rim of surrounding normal tissue. Ablation is more likely to be effective with well-circumscribed tumors rather than diffusely infiltrating liver tumors. Ablation may be indicated for primary and secondary malignant tumors in the liver, but is probably not indicated for benign tumors.

Technique

Techniques of liver ablation have evolved over the last 20 years from direct tumor injection with absolute alcohol, to cryoablation, and currently radiofrequency ablation (RFA) (Figure 155.5). This technology will continue to evolve with other methods of tumor destruction.

Placement of probes into tumors may be achieved percutaneously, at laparoscopy, or by open operation. The technique used varies from center to center, largely depending on local expertise. In general, surgical RFA is preferred to the percutaneous route when feasible due to the ability to more accurately stage the peritoneal cavity and liver, and avoid damaging nearby structures. Local recurrence is much lower with this approach [10].

Indications

The indication for ablation of liver tumors is similar to that for resection. Ablation may be considered instead of resection in

patients with significant co-morbidities or when tumor burden is too high for safe resection. Thus, depending on the type of tumor, up to 10 foci of tumor within a liver may be ablated at a single setting. RFA of lesions greater than 5 cm is limited by significantly higher local recurrence rates [11].

Complications

The major local complications from ablation are bleeding and abscess formation which occur in <5 %. The major late complication is local tumor recurrence.

Outcomes

The results of surgical approaches to liver tumor ablations are variable. Local recurrences, particularly in proximity to major vessels, occur in 15–50% of cases; *de novo* tumor appearance is a manifestation of the natural history of the tumors being treated. The highest local recurrence rate is seen with colorectal lesions (34%), with non-colorectal/non-neuroendocrine tumors, HCC, and neuroendocrine tumors having lower rates, in descending order [11].

Biliary procedures

Operations on the bile duct may be done for benign or malignant conditions. Benign conditions requiring surgery are biliary strictures or injuries. The incidence of bile duct injuries in the laparoscopic cholecystectomy era has increased two-fold and encompasses leaks, transections, and strictures [12,13].

Technique

All biliary procedures require:

- Accurate definition of the anatomy to ensure all the major segments of the liver are appropriately drained (see Figure 155.2)
- Anastomoses of bile ducts to the gastrointestinal tract require mucosa-to-mucosa apposition with normal tissues to avoid subsequent stricture (Figure 155.6)
- A multidisciplinary team, including an endoscopist and an interventional radiologist.

Benign strictures do not require resection – normal duct, above the stricture, must be defined for anastomosis. Malignant tumors should be resected with surrounding nodes and lymphatics (Figure 155.7). When pathology includes the biliary bifurcation, be it tumor or stricture, it is helpful to the surgeon to have a transhepatic stent in place to help identify the bile duct by palpation at the operation.

Prior to completing any biliary anastomosis, it is good practice to take intraoperative cholangiograms of the bile ducts being anastomosed. Anastomoses should be formed with absorbable sutures (PDS works well), ensuring apposition of mucosa from the Roux-en-Y limb to a normal bile duct mucosa. Leaving stents across the anastomosis has the benefit of reducing the risk of an immediate biliary leak and allowing study of the anastomosis in the few weeks following the procedure.

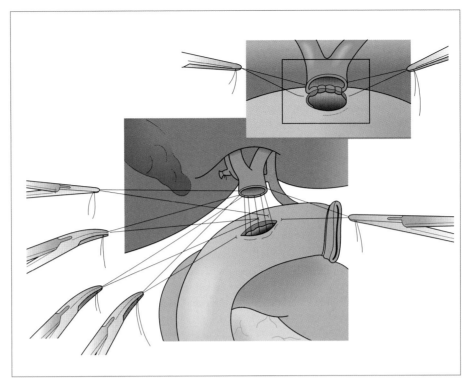

Figure 155.6 Biliary anastomosis. Hepaticojejunostomy is fashioned with mucosa-to-mucosa opposition with interrupted absorbable sutures. The decision to stent needs to be individualized. (Reproduced from Meyers WC. Atlas of biliary surgery. In: Bell RH, Rikkers LF, Mulholland MW, editors. *Digestive Tract Surgery*, 1996, with permission from Lippincott, Williams and Wilkins.)

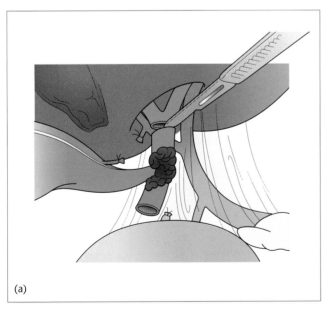

(a)

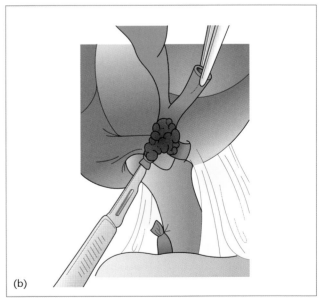

(b)

Figure 155.7 Bile duct resection. (a) A mid common duct tumor resected from suprapancreatic to the bifurcation. (b) A bifurcation cholangiocarcinoma (Klatskin tumor) resected to the right and left intrahepatic ducts. For both tumors, the portal vein and hepatic artery are skeletonized to remove lymph nodes and lymphatics. (Reproduced from Meyers WC. Atlas of biliary surgery. In: Bell RH, Rikkers LF, Mulholland MW, editors. *Digestive Tract Surgery*, 1996, with permission from Lippincott, Williams and Wilkins.)

The anastomotic site should be drained for several days immediately following the procedure in case there is any bile leak. Transhepatic stents, if used, can be removed in 4–6 weeks.

Indications

Benign biliary pathology requiring surgery includes primarily strictures and biliary leaks. The majority of patients are seen following cholecystectomy; there has been an approximately two-fold increase in such injuries in the laparoscopic era. Careful evaluation prior to operating is essential to optimize outcome. Biliary strictures may also occur with sclerosing cholangitis, pancreatitis, or extrinsic compression.

Malignant pathology requiring surgery is primarily bile duct tumors with cholangiocarcinoma being most common [14]. The majority of these patients present with an obstructive jaundice, and imaging studies will define the extent of pathology. The indications for and extent of resection is defined by the tumor. Additional evaluation for these malignancies is assessment of blood vessels; with either portal vein or hepatic artery involvement contraindicating resection.

Complications

Early complications are bile leak and infection. The risk of **bile leak** is minimized by careful technique with mucosa-to-mucosa apposition. However, the risk increases with high lesions and small ducts. The role of stenting and drains in minimizing/managing leaks is debatable. Most leaks close spontaneously given time, provided there has been good apposition of the duct to the bowel mucosa. Infection risk increases with an intraperitoneal bile leak, or when there has been an obstructed bile duct that has been stented. The risk is minimized by careful technique, anastomosis of healthy viable tissue, and use of perioperative antibiotics.

The main **late complication** of biliary procedures is an **anastomotic stricture**. The risk of stricture is increased in small bile ducts, recurrent operations, and operative repair in an infected field. Monitoring for a recurrent stricture may have some value, and suspicion of recurrent stricture mandates a percutaneous transhepatic cholangiogram to define the anastomosis.

Outcomes

Biliary reconstruction gives good results in the hands of experts. Early leaks and anastomotic strictures occur in approximately 10% of primary biliary reconstructions. A higher stricture rate has been observed in more proximal injuries (especially above the bifurcation) and when repairs are done early (within 7 days) [15]. These strictures can often be successfully managed by radiological or endoscopic stenting. Prolonged biliary obstruction and recurrent stricture can lead to secondary biliary cirrhosis.

Portal hypertension

Surgical intervention for portal hypertension has changed dramatically over the last two decades [16]. There are a limited number of patients who are eligible for operative shunts for decompression of bleeding varices, or who are candidates for devascularization procedures for variceal bleeding. There are virtually no indications currently for operative procedures for management of ascites, with the exception of patients with **Budd–Chiari syndrome**.

Technique

Operative shunts for portal hypertension are largely of historical interest and fall into three categories.

Total portal systemic shunts

Total portal systemic shunts are any shunt between the portal vein or one of its main tributaries and the IVC or one of its main tributaries that are greater than 10 mm in diameter. The classic side-to-side portacaval shunt, just below the liver hilus is a direct vein-to-vein anastomosis (Figure 155.8). This shunt will decompress all portal hypertension very well, thereby effectively controlling variceal bleeding and ascites, and decompressing the congested liver of acute Budd–Chiari syndrome. The disadvantage is that it totally diverts all portal flow and thus has a high incidence of hepatic encephalopathy. A total shunt at the hilus also makes subsequent transplant technically more difficult.

Indications

Total portal systemic shunts are rarely indicated, having been largely replaced by the transjugular intrahepatic portosystemic shunt (TIPS). In some patients with acute Budd–Chiari syndrome, necrosis may be stopped by a side-to-side portacaval shunt. This remains a controversial indication, but in this authors' opinion it is indicated for select patients.

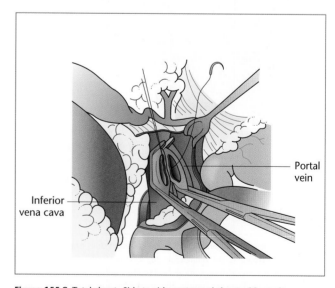

Figure 155.8 Total shunt. Side-to-side portacaval shunt >10 mm in diameter. This shunt will decompress portal hypertension, decompress the sinusoids, and divert all portal flow. (Reproduced from Meyers WC. Atlas of biliary surgery. In: Bell RH, Rikkers LF, Mulholland MW, editors. *Digestive Tract Surgery*, 1996, with permission from Lippincott Williams and Wilkins.)

Contraindications

A side-to-side portacaval shunt is contraindicated in patients with advanced liver disease as it will accelerate their course. TIPS is the preferred method of decompression in patients who are likely to proceed to transplant within the next few years.

Complications

The major complication of total portal systemic shunts is hepatic encephalopathy and progressive liver failure. The risk of developing encephalopathy depends on the severity of the underlying liver disease in addition to the total diversion of portal flow. Thus, Child class A patients or alcoholics with good liver mass who have stopped drinking may tolerate this procedure reasonably well.

Partial portal systemic shunt [17]

Technically, this operation requires the same exposure as a side-to-side total shunt. The difference is that an 8-mm interposition reinforced polytetrafluoroethylene (PTFE) graft is placed between the portal vein and the IVC (Figure 155.9). The advantage of this procedure is that, while it decompresses portal hypertension, it also maintains portal flow in approximately 80% of patients. This is associated with a lower rate of encephalopathy than a total portal systemic shunt.

Distal splenorenal shunt

The operation most commonly used to decompress varices is a selective distal splenorenal shunt (DSRS). This operation decompresses the varices trans-splenically through the splenic vein to the left renal vein, while at the same time maintaining portal hypertension and portal flow (Figure 155.10). Over the last two decades this has been the most commonly used operation worldwide. Control of bleeding has been excellent and the incidence of encephalopathy lower than with total shunts.

Indications

The indications for partial and selective variceal decompression are similar, and are best represented by variceal bleeding refractory to first-line treatment with pharmacological and endoscopic therapy, with a suitable anatomy for the selective shunt procedure.

Contraindications

Contraindications are advanced liver disease that will not tolerate a major operative procedure (Child's class C patients) and anatomy that is not suitable for surgical decompression.

Outcomes

Control of variceal bleeding with both partial and selective shunts has been greater than 90%. Data on survival in Child class A and B patients over this time have shown 90% 1-year and 75% 5-year survival rates. The rate of encephalopathy for both of these procedures has been in the 10–20% range, and is largely a function of the underlying liver disease. When a patient needs decompression for management of variceal bleeding, the choice is between one of these operative

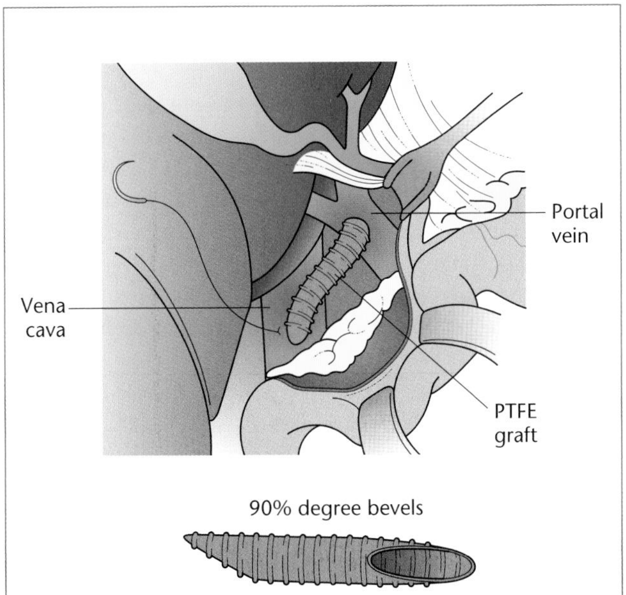

Figure 155.9 Partial shunt. An 8-mm graft between the portal vein and inferior vena cava will decompress portal hypertension enough to control bleeding but maintain some portal flow to the liver. (Reproduced from Meyers WC. Atlas of biliary surgery. In: Bell RH, Rikkers LF, Mulholland MW, editors. *Digestive Tract Surgery*, 1996, with permission from Lippincott, Williams and Wilkins.)

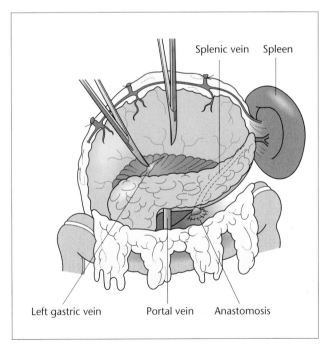

Figure 155.10 Selective shunt. Distal splenorenal shunt decompresses varices and the spleen, but maintains portal hypertension and portal flow to the liver. (Reproduced from Meyers WC. Atlas of biliary surgery. In: Bell RH, Rikkers LF, Mulholland MW, editors. *Digestive Tract Surgery*, 1996, with permission from Lippincott, Williams and Wilkins.)

procedures or TIPS. A randomized trial of partial shunt versus TIPS indicates superiority of the operative procedure over the radiological procedure in terms of bleeding control, need for transplant, and overall complications. A randomized trial comparing DSRS to TIPS showed statistically equivalent control of bleeding (5.5% DSRS; 11% TIPS) and at least one episode of encephalopathy in 50% of patients in both groups at 5 years. Survival was identical in the two groups [18].

Complications

The **early complications** after both partial and selective shunts are potential liver decompensation, worsened ascites, and infection. Careful attention to detail in patient selection, operative technique, and perioperative fluid, nutrition, and antibiotic management will minimize these immediate postoperative complications. **Late complications** relate to progression of the liver disease with encephalopathy occurring with progressive disease, and liver failure risking the need for transplant in some patients.

Devascularization procedures

Surgical devascularization for management of variceal bleeding has the operative components of splenectomy as well as gastric and esophageal devascularization.

Technique

The operation is illustrated in Figure 155.11. While initially described as a combined thoracic and abdominal procedure, it

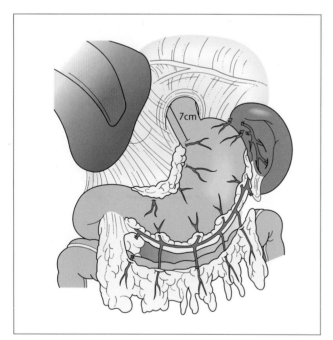

Figure 155.11 Devascularization. The components of this operation are splenectomy, and gastric and esophageal devascularization. The goal is to reduce blood flow into varices at the gastroesophageal junction. (Reproduced from Meyers WC. Atlas of biliary surgery. In: Bell RH, Rikkers LF, Mulholland MW, editors. *Digestive Tract Surgery*, 1996, with permission from Lippincott, Williams and Wilkins.)

is now primarily done as an abdominal operation. The key element is adequate devascularization at the gastroesophageal junction, the most common site of bleeding; the distal 7 cm of the esophagus, the entire greater curvature of the stomach, and the upper two-thirds of the lesser curve should be devascularized. Esophageal transection was initially a component of this operation, but it is no longer advocated.

Indications

This operation is indicated for persistent variceal bleeding in patients with no shuntable vessels (extensive portal thrombosis).

Contraindications

Advanced liver disease is a contraindication.

Outcomes

Devascularization procedures have a higher rebleeding rate than operative shunts. While in Japan this is <10%, in the USA and Europe it is 20–40% at 3 years. Encephalopathy rates are lower than for shunt procedures.

Liver transplantation

Liver transplantation is the operation that has had the greatest impact on hepatology in the past three decades and is now standard care for many patients [19]. Indications have greatly expanded and organ availability has improved by use of an expanded donor pool, partial grafts, and living donors.

Technique

The techniques of liver transplantation have gone through different iterations. Cadaveric transplants may be whole organ (the more common), reduced, or split liver transplant. The aim of these techniques is to maximize the availability of liver transplant to the largest number of patients.. The techniques of implantation have become fairly standardized in terms of vascular anastomoses and biliary reconstruction. Many options and variations exist and are utilized by experienced surgeons in different ways for different patients. The major issues for liver transplant from a technical perspective are:

• Adequate volume of viable liver
• Appropriate portal venous and hepatic arterial inflow
• Adequate hepatic venous outflow
• Safe biliary reconstruction.

Preservation of appropriate vessels in the recipient, such as maintaining the vena cava or adequate length of the portal vein, has improved the ability to use segments of the liver rather than the whole organ. The use of other technology, such as venous bypass, is variable and selective in different centers. **Living donor liver transplant** was first utilized for pediatric recipients, and adult living donor liver transplant is now variably used in different areas [20].

Indications

The indications for liver transplantation are dealt with in Chapter 108. In general terms, the indication is end-stage liver disease, followed by hepatocellular carcinoma. Thus, although it is clear that most chronic liver diseases make patients candidates for transplant, timing remains a major issue. Defining disease severity has been a priority in the USA over the last few years, which has led to the use and implementation of the MELD score for disease severity, and is the current system used for organ allocation.

References

1. Yamanaka J, Saito S, Fujimoto J. Impact of preoperative planning using virtual segmental volumetry on liver resection for hepatocellular carcinoma. *World J Surg.* 2007;31:1249–1255.
2. Malinchoc M, Kamath PS, Gordon FD, *et al.* A model to predict poor survival in patients undergoing transjugular intrahepatic portosystemic shunts. *Hepatology.* 2000;31:864–871.
3. Jarnagin WR, Gonen M, Fong Y, *et al.* improvement in perioperative outcome after hepatic resection; analysis of 1803 consecutive cases over the past decade. *Ann Surg.* 2002; 236:397–406.
4. Blumgart LH, Jarnigan W, Fong Y. Hepatic resection – Section 12. In: Blumgart H, Fong Y, editors. *Surgery of the Liver and Biliary Tract,* 3rd edn. Philadephia: Saunders, 2000:1639–1798.
5. Tsinberg M, Tellioglu G, Simpfendorfer CH, *et al.* Comparison of laparoscopic versus open liver tumor resection: a case-controlled study. *Surg Endosc.* 2009;23: 847–853.
6. Henderson JM, Sherman M, Tavill A, *et al.* AHPBA/AJCC Consensus Conference on Staging of Hepatocellular Carcinoma: consensus statement. *HPB (Oxf).* 2003;5:243–250.
7. Bellavance EC, Lumpkins KM, Mentha G, *et al.* Surgical management of early-stage hepatocellular carcinoma: resection or transplantation? *J Gastrointest Surg.* 2008;12:1699–1708.
8. Fong Y, Fortner J, Sun RL, *et al.* Clinical score for predicting recurrence after hepatic resection for metastatic colorectal cancer: analysis of 1001 consecutive cases. *Ann Surg.* 1999;230: 309–318.
9. Jaeck D, Oussoultzoglou E, Rosso E, *et al.* A two-stage hepatectomy procedure combined with portal vein embolization to achieve curative resection for initially unresectable multiple and bilobar colorectal liver metastases. *Ann Surg.* 2004;240:1037–1051.
10. Mulier S, Ni Y, Jamart J, *et al.* Local recurrences after hepatic radiofrequency (RF) coagulation. Multivariate meta-analysis and review of contributing factors. *Ann Surg.* 2005;242:158–171.
11. Berber E, Siperstein AE. Local recurrence after laparoscopic radiofrequency ablation of liver tumors: an analysis of 1032 tumors. *Ann Surg Oncol.* 2008;15):2757–2764.
12. Melton GB, Lillemoe KD.The current management of postoperative bile duct strictures. *Adv Surg.* 2002;36:193–221.
13. Chapman WC, Abecassis M, Jarnagin W, Mulvihill S, Strasberg SM. Bile duct injuries 12 years after the introduction of laparoscopic cholecystectomy. *J Gastrointest Surg.* 2003;7:412–416.
14. Chamberlain RS, Blumgart LH. Hilar cholangiocarcinoma: a review and commentary. *Ann Surg Oncol.* 2000;7:55–66.
15. Walsh RM, Henderson JM, Vogt DP, Brown N. long-term outcome of biliary reconstruction for bile duct injuries from laparoscopic cholecystectomies. *Surgery.* 2007;142:450–456.
16. Henderson JM, Barnes DS, Geisinger MA. Portal hypertension. *Curr Prob Surg.* 1998;35:379–452.
17. Rosemurgy AS, Serofini FM, Zweibal BR, *et al.* TIPS versus small diameter prosthetic H-graft portacaval shunt: extended follow-up of an expanded randomized prospective trial. *J Gastrointest Surg.* 2000;4:589–597.
18. Henderson JM, Boyer TD, Kutner MH, and the DIVERT Study Group. Distal splenorenal shunt versus transjugular intrahepatic portosystemic shunt for variceal bleeding: a randomized trial. *Gastroenterology.* 2006;130:1643–1651.
19. Roberts J. Clinical liver transplantation. *Am J Transplant.* 2001; 1:18–20.
20. Malago M, Hertl M,Testa G, Rogiers X, Broelsch CE. Split-liver transplantation: future use of scarce donor organs. *World J Surg.* 2002;26:275–282.

CHAPTER 156
Gastrointestinal operations

Robert J. C. Steele
University of Dundee, Dundee, Scotland

KEY POINTS

- Surgery is the only definitive treatment for esophageal and gastric cancer
- Only 30% of patients with esophageal cancer have resectable disease at diagnosis and only 24% of these survive for 5 years
- Assessment prior to reflux surgery should include gastroscopy, esophageal manometry, and 24-hour pH manometry
- Partial fundoplication reduces the rate of gas bloat syndrome compared to previous operations
- Partial gastrectomy for gastric cancer is feasible if there is 5-cm clearance of tumor
- The extent of lymph node clearance required at gastrectomy for gastric cancer is debated
- The goal of surgery in small bowel Crohn's disease is to conserve as much functional intestine as possible
- Careful mesorectal excision reduces the recurrence rate of rectal cancer

Introduction

In this chapter the common operations carried out on the gastrointestinal tract are listed according to anatomy and pathology. In addition to a brief description of each operation, the main indications, contraindications, and complications are given, as well as the relative use of open and laparoscopic approaches.

Esophagus
Cancer (see Chapter 30)

Esophagectomy is the only definitive treatment for the vast majority of squamous and adenocarcinomas of the esophagus and represents the only chance of cure. Unfortunately, only about 30% of esophageal tumors are resectable and the overall 5-year survival rate after resection is 24%. For those in whom esophagectomy is carried out with curative intent, the 5-year survival increases to 40% [1].

The actual procedure depends largely on the position of the tumor. For adenocarcinoma of the lower third of the esophagus or the gastroesophageal junction, a one-stage procedure through a left thoracotomy or left thoracoabdominal incision is commonly performed. Gastrointestinal continuity can be achieved either by using the stomach remnant or by creating

a Roux-en-Y loop (Figure 156.1). For tumors of the mid esophagus, it is usual to carry out a two-stage procedure with mobilization of the stomach through a laparotomy incision followed by resection of the esophagus via a right thoracotomy and reconstruction using the mobilized stomach. Alternatively, a three-stage procedure can be carried out, which is similar to the two-stage procedure with the exception that the anastomosis between the mobilized stomach and the esophageal remnant is carried out in the neck. A further alternative is to perform a transhiatal esophagectomy. This involves mobilizing the stomach and the esophagus via a laparotomy incision without opening the pleural cavities and then carrying out the anastomosis in the neck. This is preferable for more elderly patients and those with compromised respiratory function, but there are concerns about how radical a resection can be achieved.

The main contraindications to esophagectomy are non-resectability, an advanced tumor, and poor respiratory function. The main complications are respiratory failure after thoracotomy and anastomotic leakage. The mortality rate from esophagectomy, even in specialist centers, is in the region of 5–10%.

Bypass operations for esophageal cancer using segments of colon have now been almost entirely replaced by modern endoscopic stenting techniques, but the colon may still be used when esophagectomy is necessary following a previous gastrectomy.

Achalasia and other motility disorders (see Chapter 36)

Surgical treatment of achalasia is indicated in children and young adults where repeated non-surgical treatments may cause morbidity, and after failure of pneumatic dilation or botulinum toxin injection therapy. The operation of choice, **Heller's cardiomyotomy**, involves anterior division of the muscle at the lower end of the esophagus down to the mucosa. This may be done through the left chest or the abdomen and in recent years a thoracoscopic or laparoscopic approach has become standard practice [2]. There is some debate as to the distal extent and limit of the myotomy, but it is agreed that incision should be carried on to the stomach at least far enough to ensure complete division of the lower esophageal muscle

Textbook of Clinical Gastroenterology and Hepatology, Second Edition. Edited by C. J. Hawkey, Jaime Bosch, Joel E. Richter, Guadalupe Garcia-Tsao, Francis K. L. Chan.
© 2012 Blackwell Publishing Ltd. Published 2012 by Blackwell Publishing Ltd.

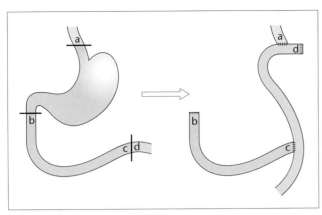

Figure 156.1 Roux-en-Y reconstruction after total gastrectomy. (This figure was published in *Clinical Gastroenterology and Hepatology*, Wilfred M. Weinstein, Christopher J. Hawkey, Jaime Bosch, Gastrointestinal operations, Pages 1–7, Copyright Elsevier, 2005.)

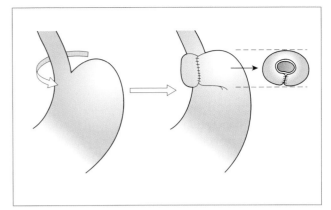

Figure 156.2 Nissan fundoplication. (This figure was published in *Clinical Gastroenterology and Hepatology*, Wilfred M. Weinstein, Christopher J. Hawkey, Jaime Bosch, Gastrointestinal operations, Pages 1–7, Copyright Elsevier, 2005.)

layer. The main complication after achalasia (providing care is taken not to breach the mucosa) is gastroesophageal reflux. For this reason some surgeons will add an antireflux procedure (see below) to the cardiomyotomy. Occasionally, in long-standing achalasia with an immotile megaesophagus, cardiomyotomy is ineffective and subtotal esophagectomy is necessary.

Other esophageal motility disorders (see Chapter 36) may be amenable to surgical treatment and a long esophageal myotomy has been advocated for both diffuse esophageal spasm and nutcracker esophagus. However, whether these are real clinical entities is controversial (see Chapter 36) and the results of treatment are highly variable. This procedure should not be performed until attempts at controlling the symptoms by medical means have been exhausted.

Gastroesophageal reflux (see Chapter 27)

Surgery for gastroesophageal reflux is only appropriate in about 10% of patients with this condition owing to the effectiveness of modern medical management [3]. The indications include failure of medical management (particularly where volume reflux is an important issue), persistence of reflux in children beyond the age of 2 years, alkaline reflux after previous abdominal surgery, and patient preference. This last category is particularly relevant for young patients who do not wish to embark on a lifetime of medication. Prior to surgical intervention it is essential to establish the presence of gastro-esophageal reflux beyond doubt and this involves upper gastrointestinal endoscopy, esophageal manometry, and 24-hour pH monitoring. Once the decision to operate has been made, there is a wide variety of operations to choose from; it is beyond the scope of this chapter to describe these but for the purposes of illustration four examples are given below.

Nissan fundoplication

Originally developed in the 1960s, this operation consists of repair of the hiatus hernia that is usually present and a circum-ferential fundal wrap around the esophagus (Figure 156.2). This is thought to be effective because it realigns the lower

esophagus with the esophageal crus and produces a pinch valve effect such that increased intragastric pressure, which would tend to promote reflux, exerts pressure on the lower esophagus via the wrap. It is important that the wrap is loose, otherwise the patient will suffer from postoperative dys-phagia. The Nissan fundoplication is highly effective in preventing reflux, but approximately 20% of patients will suffer from **gas bloat syndrome**, which is due to distension of the stomach consequent on the inability to belch and vomit. Although Nissan fundoplication was previously done by open operation, most surgeons now use the laparoscopic approach.

Partial fundoplication

Owing to the problems of gas bloat following the classical Nissan operation, a variety of partial fundoplications have been developed. Perhaps the most common of these is the Toupet partial posterior fundoplication, which involves anchoring the fundus and the upper part of the posterior wall of the stomach to the right and left crura and then carrying out a partial (270-degree) fundoplication by suturing the stomach to the anterior wall of the esophagus. This appears to be associated with good control of reflux but a low incidence of gas bloat syndrome.

Belsey mark 4 repair

This procedure, favored by thoracic surgeons, is performed through a left thoracotomy. Here the stomach is rolled around the lower 3–5 cm of the anterior aspect of the mobilized esophagus by two wraps, the second covering the first and including the diaphragm. By this means the intra-abdominal segment of the esophagus is restored and, because the wrap is not circumferential, gas bloat syndrome is rarely a problem.

Angelchick prosthesis

Although control of reflux is good following this procedure, it has now been discredited owing to the high rate of postoperative dysphagia and migration of the prosthesis, which often required prosthesis removal. It is mentioned here purely because gastroenterologists may well encounter patients who have had this procedure carried out. It involved the wrapping of a silicon gel split-ring prosthesis around the gastroesophageal junction after limited mobilization of the esophagus.

The stomach and duodenum
Cancer (see Chapter 37)

For most adenocarcinomas of the stomach the only treatment that is potentially curative is a **gastrectomy**. The extent of the gastrectomy will depend upon the position and size of the tumor. Partial gastrectomy is adequate when a 5-cm clearance of the tumor is possible and this is usually the case for cancers of the antrum, but for cancers of the body and the cardia a total gastrectomy is usually necessary. Reconstruction after a distal partial gastrectomy can be achieved using either the Polya or Billroth I procedure (Figure 156.3). Although most surgeons prefer to use the Polya gastrectomy for cancer, there is probably little to choose between the two operations. Reconstruction after total gastrectomy is usually performed using a Roux-en-Y loop (see Figure 156.1), although some advocate jejunal interpositions with or without pouch construction.

The main controversy in the performance of a gastrectomy for cancer is the extent of the **lymphadenectomy**. Traditionally, in the West, a D1 operation (removal of lymph nodes immediately adjacent to the part of the stomach being removed) has been the operation of choice, but over many years Japanese surgeons have advocated the use of a D2 or D3 resection, both of which are associated with additional clearance of the lymph nodes around the main arteries. Randomized trials carried out in the Netherlands and in the UK [4,5] have failed to show an advantage for the more radical operations, but this may be related to surgical expertise and patient selection. The main

contraindication to gastrectomy in a fit patient is metastatic disease, although it may still be appropriate to operate for palliation. The main complications of gastrectomy are anastomotic breakdown, nutritional problems, particularly weight loss, anemia, bone disease, dumping, reactive hypoglycemia, and bile vomiting.

Peptic ulcer disease (see Chapter 32)
Elective surgery

Elective surgery for peptic ulcer disease has almost completely disappeared from surgical gastroenterological practice. However, as there are still large numbers of individuals who have undergone surgical treatment for peptic ulcer in the past, it is important to mention the common operations. For duodenal ulcer the main procedures carried out up until the 1980s were truncal vagotomy and drainage (either pyloroplasty or gastrojejunostomy) or highly selective vagotomy (HSV). Latterly, HSV, which involved denervation of the fundus and the body of the stomach to reduce acid secretion without damaging the motility of the antrum, was the favored procedure [6]. For gastric ulcer a partial gastrectomy was usually favored, particularly as it was often impossible to exclude carcinoma. In the United States a Polya-type gastrectomy was also commonly used for duodenal ulcer owing to its low rate of recurrent disease. The main complications arising from truncal vagotomy were dumping and postvagotomy diarrhea, both of which were considerably reduced by the introduction of HSV.

Emergency surgery

Surgery is still occasionally required for perforation, bleeding, and pyloric stenosis caused by peptic ulceration. Perforation (Figure 156.4) is treated by simple closure of the ulcer whenever possible and thorough peritoneal lavage. This can now be accomplished by laparoscopy in skilled hands. For a bleeding peptic ulcer that has not responded to endoscopic therapy, simple oversewing of the bleeding vessel is recommended. For pyloric stenosis that does not respond to endoscopic dilatation, gastrojejunostomy is usually required. Few surgeons would now advocate adding vagotomy to any of these

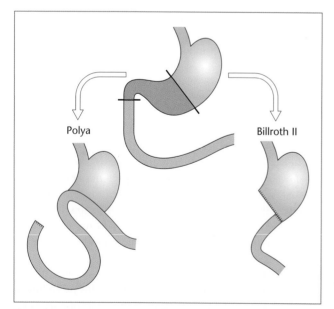

Figure 156.3 Partial gastrectomy. (This figure was published in *Clinical Gastroenterology and Hepatology*, Wilfred M. Weinstein, Christopher J. Hawkey, Jaime Bosch, Gastrointestinal operations, Pages 1–7, Copyright Elsevier, 2005.)

Polya

Billroth II

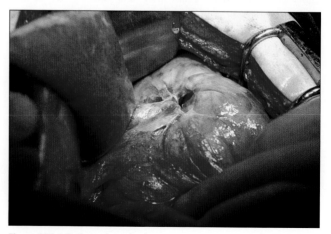

Figure 156.4 Perforated peptic ulcer.

procedures, preferring to rely on postoperative medical management.

Obesity

Antiobesity (or bariatric) surgery has been a growth area in Western surgical practice in recent years. Jejunal bypass has been abandoned owing to the high risk of liver failure and currently used procedures depend on bypassing or reducing the capacity of the stomach. The most commonly performed operation is the vertical banded gastroplasty, which involves partitioning the stomach with staples and a band. This operation is effective but the revision rate is high at around 30%. Other operations include a Roux-en-Y gastric bypass, resectional gastric bypass, and, most recently, laparoscopic adjustable gastric banding [7]. Contraindications to antiobesity surgery include patients at risk of postoperative cardiac complications, significant lung disease, and significant psychological disorders. The main postoperative complications are disruption of staple lines, pouch dilatation, gastroesophageal reflux, and incisional hernia.

The liver

Cancer (see Chapters 104 and 155)

Liver resection for cancer is employed in two main situations: for primary hepatocellular cancer and for limited metastatic disease from colorectal cancer. The liver can be subdivided into segments according to its portal venous blood supply (Figure 156.5) and resections are carried out using these anatomical subdivisions. With modern techniques, specialist surgeons can achieve hepatectomy with an operative mortality of less than 5% and minimal blood loss [8]. For both primary and secondary liver cancer the aim is to achieve complete resection of all malignancy with a margin of healthy liver tissue of 2 cm or more and sufficient residual liver tissue to sustain adequate liver function. Liver resection is contraindicated where this cannot be achieved and it must be remembered that in patients with cirrhosis (which often accompanies hepatocellular carcinoma) resection may be poorly tolerated. The main complications after a liver resection are hypoglycemia and coagulation defects, which can be treated by intravenous glucose and appropriate use of fresh frozen plasma and vitamin K injections. Hypoalbuminemia is almost inevitable and repeated plasma or albumin infusions may be required. The liver has a remarkable ability to regenerate and this occurs within 3 months if the remaining liver parenchyma is normal.

Transplantation (see Chapters 108 and 155)

Liver transplantation is indicated for irreversible hepatic failure, and patients with primary biliary cirrhosis, primary sclerosing cholangitis, inborn errors of metabolism, and trauma have the best results with survival rates of around 80% at 5 years. Transplantation may also be used for end-stage cirrhosis and patients with extensive hepatocellular carcinoma confined to the liver. Livers for transplantation may be cadaveric, in which case the whole organ may be used, or from living

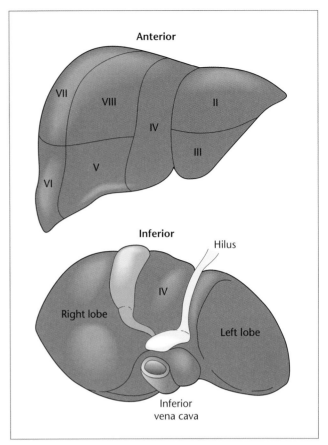

Figure 156.5 Segments of the liver. (This figure was published in *Clinical Gastroenterology and Hepatology*, Wilfred M. Weinstein, Christopher J. Hawkey, Jaime Bosch, Gastrointestinal operations, Pages 1–7, Copyright Elsevier, 2005.)

donors where a liver split has to be employed. At the present time rejection rates are between 10% and 20% with the use of modern immunosuppression, including the use of cyclosporine (ciclosporin) [9].

The biliary tract

Gallstones

The definitive treatment for gallstones is **cholecystectomy** and the main indications for this procedure are biliary colic and acute cholecystitis. Cholecystectomy can be achieved laparoscopically in over 90% of cases, and patients undergoing this minimal access procedure can usually be discharged home on the day following surgery [10]. The operation is achieved by means of four ports with the telescope being introduced at the umbilicus (Figure 156.6). After dissection of the gallbladder with tying or clipping of the cystic duct and cystic artery, the gallbladder with its contained stones is extracted through one of the ports. Conversion to an open operation is indicated where it is impossible to identify anatomical structures safely in any other way and where intraoperative complications arise that cannot be dealt with by laparoscopic means. Most surgeons will perform an intraoperative cholangiogram in order to look for common bile duct stones, and when these are

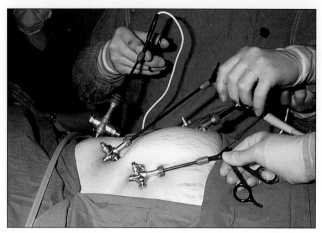

Figure 156.6 Laparoscopic cholecystectomy. Arrangement of the ports.

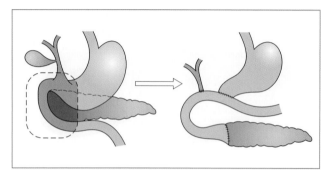

Figure 156.7 Whipple's operation. (This figure was published in *Clinical Gastroenterology and Hepatology*, Wilfred M. Weinstein, Christopher J. Hawkey, Jaime Bosch, Gastrointestinal operations, Pages 1–7, Copyright Elsevier, 2005.)

present the common bile duct can be explored and the stones removed. When this is done, it is normal to close the common bile duct around a T-tube to provide decompression of the duct. The T-tube is removed about 2 weeks after surgery. The main complications of cholecystectomy are bile duct stricture consequent on damage to the common bile duct and bile leakage usually after removal of a T-tube.

Bile duct strictures

Bile duct strictures can either be benign (usually postoperative) or malignant (cholangiocarcinoma). In either case the treatment is usually resection of the appropriate section of the bile duct with drainage into the gastrointestinal tract achieved by means of a Roux-en-Y loop.

The pancreas
Pancreatic cancer (see Chapter 71)

The most common operation for pancreatic cancer (other than palliative bypass) is the **Whipple's operation**. This involves removal of the head of the pancreas and the duodenum for a carcinoma of either the pancreatic head or the ampulla of Vater. Reconstruction is then achieved by anastomosing the jejunum to the stomach remnant, the common bile duct, and

the body of the pancreas (Figure 156.7). The 5-year survival after Whipple's operation for an ampullary tumor is in the region of 40%, and this drops to less than 10% with true carcinoma of the head of the pancreas [11]. Carcinoma of the body or tail of the pancreas is removed by the much simpler operation of distal pancreatic resection usually combined with splenectomy. Pancreatic resection is contraindicated in advanced tumors, particularly where the portal vein is involved. The main specific complication following pancreatic resection is the development of a pancreatic fistula.

Chronic pancreatitis (see Chapter 70)

Chronic pancreatitis is particularly unrewarding to treat surgically except where chronic inflammation of the head of the pancreas is causing obstructive jaundice. In this instance a Whipple's operation is indicated and is associated with good results. Occasionally, surgery may be indicated for chronic pain where the main pancreatic duct is alternately strictured and dilated. Here, laying open the pancreatic duct and draining it into a loop of jejunum (Peustow operation) may alleviate the symptoms [12].

Acute pancreatitis (see Chapter 69)

In a patient with acute pancreatitis complicated by infected pancreatic necrosis, **necrosectomy** (removal of necrotic pancreatic tissue) may be indicated as a life-saving procedure, although the mortality associated with this procedure is in the region of 50% [13]. It is indicated where contrast-enhanced CT scanning in a patient with severe acute pancreatitis demonstrates non-perfusion of the pancreatic gland and subsequent needle aspiration reveals bacterial infection.

The other situation in which surgery may be indicated in a patient with acute pancreatitis is for the internal drainage of a pancreatic pseudocyst. It is important to allow the cyst to mature over several weeks before operation and the most commonly performed procedure is a **cystogastrostomy** allowing the cyst to drain into the stomach. External drainage of large established pseudocysts is rarely successful.

The small bowel
Crohn's disease (see Chapter 50)

Surgery for small bowel Crohn's disease is usually indicated for obstructive symptoms caused by stricturing. Although small bowel resection may be necessary in these cases, the aim is to retain as much functioning intestine as possible and in many instances it may be possible to alleviate obstructive symptoms by means of **strictureplasty**. The cumulative recurrence rate after small bowel resection for Crohn's disease is 30% at 5 years, 50% at 10 years, and 60% at 15 years [14]. Other indications for surgery in small bowel Crohn's disease is growth retardation in children, particularly those with ileocecal disease. Here, resection is usually followed by a growth spurt. Surgery is also usually required for Crohn's-related abscesses and fistulae and for the rare complication of massive hemorrhage. Unfortunately, operations for Crohn's disease are followed by a high incidence (10%) of postoperative complications, including anastomotic leakage and fistula formation, and the operative mortality for reoperation ranges from 2% to 8%. In patients who have undergone extensive resection, intestinal failure may develop.

The colon
Cancer (see Chapter 57–59)
The definitive treatment for colon cancer is **resection**, and this is associated with an overall 5-year survival in the region of 40–45%. In general terms, tumors of the cecum and ascending colon are treated by right hemicolectomy, those of the transverse colon by extended right hemicolectomy, those of the descending colon by left hemicolectomy, and those in the sigmoid by sigmoid colectomy. Although the majority of these operations are still performed by means of open surgery, an increasing number are being carried out laparoscopically. For a number of years it was considered that laparoscopic resection may compromise oncological principles, but the results from randomized trials do not substantiate these fears [15]. After resection anastomosis is achieved either by means of stapling devices or hand suturing (Figure 156.8), and the anastomotic leakage rate should be less than 5% [16]. The other complications of colectomy are those of any major intra-abdominal operation, including hemorrhage, postoperative myocardial infarction, deep vein thrombosis, chest infection, pulmonary embolus, ileus, and wound infection/dehiscence. All patients undergoing colectomy should have antibiotic prophylaxis and measures to prevent deep vein thrombosis (subcutaneous low molecular weight heparin).

Diverticular disease (see Chapter 63)
Surgery for uncomplicated diverticular disease is now very rarely performed and even patients with diverticulitis are usually treated conservatively. However, in a patient with perforated diverticular disease it is necessary to carry out a colectomy (usually sigmoid) and this is commonly done as a Hartmann's procedure where the proximal colon is brought out as a colostomy and the rectal stump over-sewn.

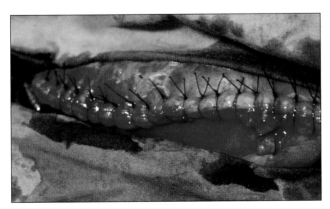

Figure 156.8 Hand-sewn anastomosis.

Re-anastomosis can be performed at a later stage when all inflammation has resolved. The other main indications for operating for diverticular disease are stricture formation causing obstructive symptoms and massive hemorrhage.

Inflammatory bowel disease
In the patient with ulcerative colitis emergency surgery is indicated for severe disease that fails to respond to medical treatment, perforation, and bleeding. Elective surgical treatment is required for failure of medical management, growth retardation in young patients, and the development of colonic malignancy. The correct surgical treatment for ulcerative colitis is **panproctocolectomy** with either permanent end-ileostomy or reconstruction by means of an ileoanal pouch [17]. In the emergency situation it is common practice to carry out a subtotal colectomy going on to proctectomy with or without pouch reconstruction at a later stage. The specific complications of panproctocolectomy are either those of the ileostomy (ileostomy diarrhea, stenosis, retraction, and skin problems associated with ileostomy effluent) or with a pouch (frequency of bowel action and pouchitis). In patients with Crohn's colitis it is usual to avoid ileoanal pouch formation owing to the risk of small bowel Crohn's disease. In some cases of Crohn's colitis it may be appropriate to carry out a segmental resection according to the distribution of the disease. This is never indicated in patients with ulcerative colitis.

Constipation (see Chapter 61)
A proportion of patients with idiopathic constipation may benefit from colectomy and ileorectal anastomosis [18]. This is only indicated, however, if marker studies indicate that there is no evidence of obstructed defecation with confirmation by normal anal manometry, normal electromyography, and normal evacuation proctography. Even then, about 25% of patients will still be troubled by constipation and a further 25% will have troublesome diarrhea. In some instances it may be necessary to resort to ileostomy but patients may continue to be troubled by abdominal pain and bloating owing to impaired small bowel motility. Another approach to intractable idiopathic constipation is appendicostomy where the appendix is brought out as a stoma and can be used as a conduit to irrigate the colon on a regular basis.

The rectum
Cancer (see Chapter 59)
The standard surgical approach for cancer of the rectum is either **anterior resection** (with anastomosis between the distal colon and rectal remnant or anal canal) or **abdominoperineal resection** of the rectum (with permanent end colostomy). The choice between these two operations depends on a combination of the position of the tumor within the rectum and the patient's body habitus, but in general terms tumors of the upper two-thirds of the rectum should be amenable to anterior resection whereas those of the lower third of the rectum

usually require abdominoperineal resection. In both of these procedures the principle of mesorectal excision is now firmly established. This involves careful dissection in the plane immediately outside the fatty tissue surrounding the rectum with careful preservation of the pelvic nerves. Adoption of this procedure has led to a reduction in local recurrence rates after surgery for rectal cancer from around 30% to less than 10% [19]. In addition, taking care to avoid damage to the pelvic nerves minimizes the risk of urinary and sexual dysfunction. Under certain circumstances transanal local excision of early rectal cancer may be possible but is associated with higher risk of locally recurrent disease than radical surgery.

Rectal prolapse (see Chapter 68)

A full-thickness rectal prolapse can only be treated by surgical repair. The most definitive procedure is **rectopexy** where the rectum is mobilized transabdominally down to the pelvic floor and fixed to the sacrum. This is now commonly combined with a sigmoid resection to eliminate redundant large bowel and reduce the risk of postoperative constipation [20]. Increasingly, this procedure is being carried out laparoscopically. A number of other procedures are available but the most successful alternative to rectopexy is perineal rectosigmoidectomy where the redundant rectum and sigmoid colon are excised through the perineum and continuity is restored by a coloanal anastomosis.

The anal canal
Hemorrhoids (see Chapter 68)

Although there are a number of office procedures available for the treatment of hemorrhoids, patients with symptomatic third- or fourth-degree hemorrhoids are best treated by a formal **hemorrhoidectomy**. In modern practice this is carried out with the patient in the prone position using diathermy, and with the use of local anesthesia this may now be performed as a daycase procedure. It is, however, still associated with significant postoperative discomfort and the alternative operation of stapled anopexy is gaining ground. In this procedure a stapling device is used to excise a circular disk of rectal mucosa just above the anal canal, restoring continuity with a line of staples. This pulls the anal cushions back up into an anatomical position and randomized trials indicate similar results to conventional hemorrhoidectomy but with less postoperative pain [21].

Fistula-in-ano

The low-level or intersphincteric fistula may be treated safely by laying open (Figure 156.9). However, the higher trans-sphincteric or supra-sphincteric fistulae cannot be treated in this way owing to the risk of incontinence. Various procedures have been described to deal with these complex fistulae, including fistula track excision with repair of the internal opening by an advancement flap [22]. The results are not particularly good, however, and in many instances it is necessary

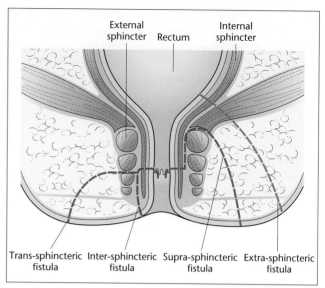

Figure 156.9 Fistula-in-ano. (This figure was published in *Clinical Gastroenterology and Hepatology*, Wilfred M. Weinstein, Christopher J. Hawkey, Jaime Bosch, Gastrointestinal operations, Pages 1–7, Copyright Elsevier, 2005.)

to resort to the use of a simple Seton (ligature through the fistula) in order to maintain drainage and avoid recurrent perianal sepsis.

Fissure

Approximately 80% of anal fissures will respond to conservative management, including the use of 0.2% glyceryl trinitrate (GTN) ointment [23], but the remainder require a **lateral sphincterotomy**, which involves dividing the fibers of the internal anal sphincter up to the level of the dentate line. This is associated with a high rate of fissure healing but may be complicated by minor degrees of incontinence, particularly to mucus.

Incontinence

Surgery for incontinence is only successful when a defined defect in the external anal sphincter is responsible. This is diagnosed preoperatively by transanal ultrasound and surgical treatment by means of an overlapping repair will improve symptoms in between 60% and 80% of cases. In patients who are not suitable for a straightforward sphincter repair, reconstruction using the gracilis muscle can be attempted, but for this to be successful the gracilis muscle requires electrical stimulation [24]. Unfortunately, the failure rate of this procedure is high and this has stimulated interest in a variety of artificial sphincter devices that can be implanted around the anal canal. In a proportion of patients, however, permanent colostomy may be the only solution to the problem.

SOURCES OF INFORMATION FOR PATIENTS AND DOCTORS

http://www.betterhealth.vic.gov.au/bhcv2/bhcarticles.nsf/pages/Anal_fissure?Open http://www.patient.co.uk/showdoc/583/

References

1. Leonard GD, McCaffrey JA, Maher M. Optimal therapy for oesophageal cancer. *Cancer Treat Rev*. 2003;29:275–282.
2. Balaji NS, Peters JH. Minimally invasive surgery for esophageal motility disorders. *Surg Clin North Am*. 2002;82:763–782.
3. Tutuian R, Castell DO. Management of gastroesophageal reflux disease. *Am J Med Sci*. 2003;326:309–318.
4. Bonenkamp JJ, Songun I, Hermans J, *et al*. Randomised comparison of morbidity after D1 and D2 dissection for gastric cancer in 996 Dutch patients. *Lancet*. 1995;345:745–748.
5. Cuschieri A, Weeden S, Fielding J, *et al*. Patient survival after D1 and D2 resections for gastric cancer: long-term results of the MRC randomised surgical trial. Surgical Co-operative Group. *Br J Cancer*, 1999;79:1522–1530.
6. Johnston D. Operative technique of highly selective (parietal cell) vagotomy. *Acta Chir Scand*. 1988; 547 (Suppl):49–53.
7. Fisher BL, Shauer P. Medical and surgical options in the treatment of severe obesity. *Am J Surg*. 2002;184(6B):9S–16S.
8. Allen PJ, Jarnagin WR. Current status of hepatic resection. *Adv Surg*. 2003;37:29–49.
9. Nash KL, Gimson AE. Liver transplantation. *Hosp Med*. 2003; 64:200–204.
10. Scott-Conner CE. Laparoscopic gastrointestinal surgery. *Med Clin North Am*. 2002;86:1401–1422.
11. Yeo CJ. The Whipple operation: is a radical resection of benefit? *Adv Surg*. 2003;37:1–27.
12. Hartel M, Tempia-Caliera AA, Wente MN, *et al*. Evidence-based surgery in chronic pancreatitis. *Langenbecks Arch Surg*. 2003;388: 132–139.
13. Hartwig W, Werner J, Uhl W, Buchler MW. Management of infection in acute pancreatitis. *J Hepatobiliary Pancreat Surg*. 2002;9: 423–428.
14. Delaney CP, Fazio VW. Crohn's disease of the small bowel. *Surg Clin North Am*. 2001;81:137–158.
15. Pikarsky AJ. Update on prospective randomised trials of laparoscopic surgery for colorectal cancer. *Surg Oncol Clin North Am*. 2001;10:639–653.
16. Leslie A, Steele RJC. The serosubmucosal anastomosis – still the gold standard. *Colorectal Dis*. 2003;5:362–366.
17. Sagar PM, Pemberton JH. Ileo-anal pouch function and dysfunction. *Dig Dis*. 1997;15:172–188.
18. Bharucha AE, Phillips SF. Slow transit constipation. *Gastroenterol Clin North Am*. 2001;30:77–95.
19. Quirke P. Training and quality assurance for rectal cancer: 20 years of data is enough. *Lancet Oncol*. 2003;4:695–702.
20. Karulf RE, Madoff RD, Goldberg SM. Rectal prolapse. *Curr Probl Surg*. 2001;38:771–832.
21. Ashraf S, Srivastava P, Hershman MJ. Stapled haemorrhoidectomy: a novel procedure. *Hosp Med*. 2003;64:526–529.
22. McLeod RS. Management of fistula-in-ano: 1990 Roussel Lecture. *Can J Surg*. 1991;34:581–585.
23. Utzig MJ, Kroesen AJ, Buhr HJ. Concepts of pathogenesis and treatment of chronic anal fissure a review of the literature. *Am J Gastroenterol*. 2003; 98:968–974.
24. Hinninghofen H, Enck P. Fecal incontinence: evaluation and treatment. *Gastroenterol Clin North Am*. 2003;32:685–706.

CHAPTER 157
Minimally invasive surgery

Todd A. Ponsky,[1] Arjun Khosla[1] and Jeffrey L. Ponsky[2]

[1]University Hospitals Case Medical Center, Cleveland, OH, USA
[2]University Hospitals of Cleveland, Cleveland, OH, USA

KEY POINTS

- Laparoscopic surgery has advantages over open surgery in biliary surgery, abdominal hernia, and hiatus hernia repair
- Bile duct leak should be suspected in patients with postoperative jaundice, nausea, abdominal pain, and/or fever
- Given the unacceptably high rate of recurrence of ventral hernias, laparoscopic repair of incisional abdominal wall hernias is growing in popularity
- Laparoscopic inguinal hernia repair offers decreased postoperative pain and quicker recovery
- Laparoscopy is the treatment of choice for elective splenectomy
- The role of laparoscopic colectomy in oncology is under evaluation
- Laparoscopic antireflux surgery should be considered in gastroesophageal reflux disease patients who are refractory to medical therapy, or unwilling to take long-term medication

Introduction

The first report of laparoscopy was in 1910 when Kelling explored an insufflated abdomen with a cystoscope. Laparoscopy was thereafter utilized primarily within the field of gynecology. The first general surgical application of laparoscopy was a cholecystectomy performed in Germany by Muhe in 1985. Since then, laparoscopic surgery has advanced at an extraordinary pace to the point where almost every surgical operation has undergone some sort of minimally invasive transformation. The decrease in pain, shortened hospital stay, earlier return to work, and improved cosmesis have enhanced its popularity. For the past 20 years minimally invasive surgery has been synonymous with laparoscopy. However, robotic surgery and therapeutic surgical endoscopy have entered the arena of everyday surgical practice. While endoscopic surgery is still in its infancy, many believe that there is a movement towards "incision-free" surgery.

Description of technique (Table 157.1)
The first step of all laparoscopic procedures is entry into the peritoneum. This can be accomplished by either an open, cutdown procedure or by insertion of a needle into the abdomen. CO_2 is slowly pumped into the abdomen to distend the peritoneal cavity and create an open space for operating. A camera is then placed through a small hole in the abdomen, typically

at the umbilicus. Subsequent small holes are placed in different locations throughout the abdomen and special ports, called trocars, are placed into these holes. Instruments can be inserted and removed through these ports as needed throughout the operation. Following the operation, all ports are removed and the CO_2 is released from the peritoneal space.

Complications and their management
Risks of laparoscopy in general include major intra-abdominal vascular or visceral injury during trocar placement. The incidence of bowel injury is approximately 0.05–to 0.3% [1]. Major vascular injuries may also occur during trocar placement and carry an approximately 15% mortality rate. Minor bleeding or bowel injury may occasionally be repaired laparoscopically. In the face of brisk, uncontrollable bleeding or a significant bowel injury, conversion to an open procedure is necessary.

Gallbladder surgery
Laparoscopic cholecystectomy represents a significant change in the management of gallbladder disease. It is now the most commonly performed laparoscopic surgical procedure in the world. In fact, the laparoscopic approach has replaced open cholecystectomy as the standard of care for cholelithiasis, biliary dyskinesia, and acute cholecystitis. In the United States, over 700 000 laparoscopic cholecystectomies are performed annually [2]. The morbidity and mortality of this operation are very low. The laparoscopic approach offers the patient a safe and effective treatment with fewer complications, less postoperative pain, faster recovery, and improved cosmesis.

Description of technique
Although there are minor variations to the procedure, most cholecystectomies today are performed through four small incisions measuring from 5 to 10mm in length at the umbilicus, epigastrium, right upper quadrant, and right lower quadrant. The basic steps of the operation involve dissection of the gallbladder from surrounding adhesions, dissection of the triangle of Calot (Figure 157.1), identification and ligation of the cystic artery and duct, removal of the gallbladder from the liver bed, and removal of the gallbladder through one of the

Table 157.1 General laparoscopic technique

1. Cut-down to peritoneal cavity at umbilicus and insertion of 10-mm trocar
2. CO_2 insufflation to create tension pneumoperitoneum
3. Insertion of camera through 10-mm port
4. Placement of subsequent trocars through 5-mm incisions
5. Performance of operation by inserting instruments through the trocars
6. Removal of trocars and release of CO_2
7. Incision closure
8. Bowel or vascular injury from trocar insertion may necessitate conversion to open surgery

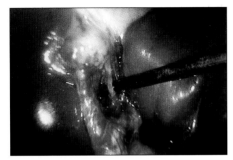

Figure 157.1 Dissection of triangle of Calot.

10-mm port sites. Once the cystic duct has been identified, a cholangiogram is often performed. This involves making a small incision in the cystic duct, inserting a catheter into the duct, and injecting contrast under fluoroscopy. This helps to more clearly assess the biliary anatomy and to evaluate for choledocholithiasis.

Indications and contraindications

The indications for laparoscopic cholecystectomy are the same as for the open technique, and include biliary colic, biliary dyskinesia, and acute cholecystitis (see Chapter 74). The only exception is gallbladder carcinoma, which should be treated with open cholecystectomy to ensure an adequate resection and to eliminate the possibility of port site tumor cell seeding. Liver cirrhosis, pregnancy, morbid obesity, or previous right upper quadrant surgery are not contraindications for laparoscopic cholecystectomy [3]. Most patients have minimal postoperative pain and usually are discharged home from the recovery room or are admitted overnight and discharged the following morning. Patients can usually return to work within 1 week.

Complications and their management

The overall complication rate from laparoscopic cholecystectomy is approximately 0.38% [4].

Bile duct injury

The most feared complication of a laparoscopic cholecystectomy is bile duct injury. The variable anatomy of the extrahepatic biliary tree, pericholecystic inflammation, and/or

inadequate dissection and identification of the triangle of Calot may contribute to injury. Injury may range from a small pinhole to a complete transection. The incidence of bile duct injury is approximately 0.6% with an 8% mortality rate [5]. Approximately half of bile duct injuries are identified at the time of injury, while 30% are discovered postoperatively. Injury carries a high risk of eventual bile duct stricture. Many advocate routine intraoperative cholangiography to help identify extrahepatic biliary anatomy and decrease the chance of misidentification or injury. Patients presenting with postoperative jaundice, nausea, abdominal pain, and/or fever should be investigated for a bile leak. When a bile leak is suspected, the work-up should start with a computed tomography (CT) scan or ultrasound to evaluate for a subhepatic fluid collection. This can be followed by a hepatic indolacetic acid (HIDA) scan or endoscopic retrograde cholangiopancreatography (ERCP). ERCP offers both diagnosis and possible therapy through stent placement and sphincterotomy.

Bleeding

Intraoperative bleeding may occur during dissection of the gallbladder at the triangle of Calot or from the liver bed. Prudent dissection and identification of the cystic artery with absolute secure ligation is essential. Bleeding may also result from major vascular injury during trocar insertion or in the postoperative period as a result of a slipped clip around the cystic duct, relaxation from a vessel that was in spasm intraoperatively, or from the liver bed. In the face of tachycardia, hypotension, change in mental status, decreased urine output, increased abdominal distension, and/or a drop in hemoglobin the patient should be taken back to the operating room for re-exploration, either laparoscopically or open.

Ventral hernia repair

Given the unacceptably high rate of recurrence of ventral hernias, laparoscopic repair of incisional abdominal wall hernias is growing in popularity (see Chapter 122). Laparoscopic ventral hernia repair provides tension-free closure of the abdominal wall defect. Data suggest that laparoscopic ventral hernia repair has a lower recurrence rate than open repair with mesh [6–8]. The majority of patients are discharged from hospital on the second postoperative day [7]. While many have claimed recurrence rates of less than 5%, others have suggested that with longer follow-up the recurrence rate is closer to 17% [9].

Description of technique

The operation typically begins with insertion of a 10-mm camera port. The location of this port varies but should be safely away from the suspected hernia defect. Once pneumoperitoneum is attained, two to three subsequent ports are placed under direct vision. Adhesiolysis is performed with blunt and sharp dissection until the entire defect is cleared with a 3–4-cm border of visualized peritoneum. A piece of mesh large enough to cover the entire defect is rolled and placed into the abdomen through a 10-mm trocar. The mesh is unfurled and is attached to the abdominal wall with full-thickness, through-and-through fascial sutures. The mesh is tacked to the peritoneum and fascia with a tacking device. The trocars are removed and the incisions are closed.

Indications and contraindications

It is generally recommended that midline ventral hernias greater than 3–5-cm in diameter be repaired laparoscopically [10]. Contraindications to laparoscopic repair include any pre-existing intra-abdominal infection, intraoperative enterotomy, open abdominal wound, or poor skin coverage over a fascial defect. Non-central defects or multiple previous abdominal operations are not contraindications to laparoscopic ventral hernia repairs.

Complications and their management

Complications of this procedure include mesh/wound infection, hernia recurrence, seroma, and bowel or vascular injury. Patients who present with postoperative fever, leukocytosis, wound erythema and/or fluctuance, and a fluid collection around the mesh on CT scan will probably warrant removal of the mesh through a midline incision with primary closure of the fascia if possible. The presence of a fluid collection in the absence of signs of infection is most likely a seroma and is usually managed expectantly. While recurrence may occur with this operation, the incidence is lower than in any of the other repair options. Repair of a recurrent hernia after laparoscopic repair presents a challenge, especially if the mesh is adherent to the underlying bowel.

Inguinal hernia repair

For years there has been immense debate as to the most effective and symptom-free repair of inguinal hernias. Most surgeons now agree that the most effective repair is a **"tension-free" repair with mesh** (see Chapter 122). There has been debate as to which procedure is ideal, laparoscopic or open. Although there is disagreement among many of the studies, most agree that with the laparoscopic repair there is less pain and an earlier return to work, but not necessarily a decrease in recurrence.

Description of technique

There are essentially two techniques, the **transabdominal preperitoneal repair (TAPP)** and the **total extraperitoneal repair (TEP)**. Both techniques ultimately describe placing a piece of mesh into the preperitoneal space. In the TAPP procedure, an incision is made in the peritoneum in order to access the preperitoneal space. In the TEP procedure, the peritoneum is never entered: the entire dissection takes place within the preperitoneal space. Both procedures typically require three trocar site incisions. Once in the preperitoneal

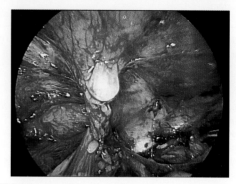

Figure 157.2 Laparoscopic hernia anatomy.

space, both procedures involve dissection and exposure of the pubic bone medially (Figure 157.2), identification of the hernia, reduction of the direct hernia sac, if present, examination for and reduction of an indirect hernia sac, and dissection and identification of the vas deferens and gonadal vessels. Finally, a piece of polypropylene mesh is placed from the pubic bone medially to the internal ring laterally, covering the cord structures and extending into the space of Retzius. Most patients are discharged home from the recovery room.

Indications and contraindications

Most of the contraindications are relative contraindications, including previous lower abdominal or extraperitoneal surgery (retropubic prostatectomy) or pelvic radiation. An absolute contraindication is intolerance of general anesthesia [11].

Complications and their management

Laparoscopic inguinal hernia repairs are associated with the same complications seen with open repair, with additive risks associated with laparoscopy in general. The complication rates vary from 3.8% to 13.6% for both open and laparoscopic repairs [11].

The most common complications are postoperative urinary retention, hematoma, leg or groin pain from an injured or impinged nerve, seroma, or wound infection. Most of these complications can be managed expectantly. Most wound infections can be managed by simply opening the wound and draining the infection. A complicated wound infection, however, suggested by pus or erythema from the wound accompanied by systemic signs of infection, may require reoperation with removal of the mesh and a primary repair.

Splenectomy

Laparoscopic splenectomy is one of the most common laparoscopic solid organ procedures. The laparoscopic technique appears to have decreased blood loss, shorter hospital stay, and faster recovery. It is the procedure of choice for elective splenectomy. As with open splenectomy, patients should undergo pneumococcal vaccination.

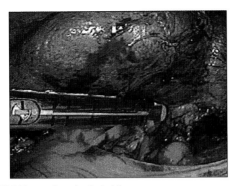

Figure 157.3 Transection of splenic hilum.

Description of technique

The procedure typically involves three trocars. The spleen is freed from the pancreaticosplenic ligament, splenocolic ligament, lienorenal ligament and lienophrenic ligament followed by dissection of the gastrosplenic ligament and short gastric vessels. The splenic artery and vein are typically ligated at the splenic hilum with a laparoscopic stapling device (Figure 157.3). Careful attention is paid to avoiding injury to the tail of the pancreas, which lies very close to the spleen. Once dissected free, the spleen is placed into an endoscopic bag in which it is morselized and brought out through one of the larger trocar sites [12].

Indications and contraindications

The elective indications for laparoscopic splenectomy are the same as for open splenectomy and include specific circumstances of immune thrombocytopenic purpura (ITP), sickle cell disease, β-thalassemia, hereditary spherocytosis, Gaucher's disease, lymphoma, angiosarcoma, and occasionally large cysts or abscesses. ITP is the most common indication for elective splenectomy in adults and is indicated if the thrombocytopenia is refractory to medical therapy or relapses after an initial response [13]. The indications and contraindications are currently evolving. While it has been suggested that splenomegaly and trauma are contraindications to laparoscopic splenectomy, others believe that it depends on the experience of the surgeon.

Complications and their management

Laparoscopic splenectomy is a relatively safe procedure and may even have fewer complications than the open procedure. Morbidity rates for open splenectomy have ranged from 15% to 61% and mortality rates from 6% to 13%, whereas laparoscopic morbidity and mortality rates range from 0% to 15% and 0% to 5%, respectively. It is difficult, however, to compare these outcomes given that the more critical patients are frequently selected to undergo an open procedure [14]. Complications include intraoperative and postoperative bleeding, pancreatic injury, postoperative thrombocytopenia from a missed accessory spleen or splenosis, postoperative thrombocytosis, overwhelming post-splenectomy sepsis (OPSS), subphrenic

abscess, and pleural effusions. The most common reasons for intraoperative bleeding are coagulopathy from thrombocytopenia or technical error, including vessel injury during dissection or loss of a surgical tie. Bleeding related to coagulopathy can be minimized by administering clotting factors or platelets prior to or during the operation. Platelet transfusion is typically reserved for counts less than 10 000 cells/μL [15].

Colectomy

Just when laparoscopy had become accepted as a reasonable alternative to many elective operations, the introduction of laparoscopic colectomy demonstrated the role of laparoscopy in oncological surgery. While it is clear that this procedure offers a cosmetic benefit to the open procedure, many have questioned whether or not this procedure offers the same survival benefit as its open counterpart.

In 1994, the American Society of Colon and Rectal Surgeons released a policy statement that said until convincing data were published, laparoscopic colectomies should only be performed within clinical trials [16]. In a prospective randomized trial of 219 patients with a 4-year follow-up, patients in the laparoscopic group had a lower morbidity rate, shortened hospital stay, decreased tumor recurrence, and improved cancer-related survival [17]. While these data are intriguing, further studies with larger cohorts are necessary in order to confirm these results.

Description of technique

Laparoscopic colectomy begins with the placement of four trocar ports. The steps of the colectomy are the same as for the open procedure and involve mobilization of the segment of colon to be resected, division of the mesentery, resection of the involved segment of colon, and restoration of continuity or formation of a stoma. Once the colon has been resected and continuity restored, a small midline incision is made just large enough to remove the resected segment of colon.

Indications and contraindications

As stated above, many still consider laparoscopy to be an experimental technique in those patients with potentially curable colon cancer. However, as evidenced by Milsom *et al.* at the Cleveland Clinic in 2000, laparoscopic colectomy may be beneficial for palliative resection in patients with stage IV colorectal cancer [18]. Other indications for laparoscopic colectomy may be polyps, diverticular disease, colovesicular fistula, phlegmon, chronic constipation, rectal prolapse, ulcerative colitis, fecal incontinence, stoma formation, or any other benign colonic disorder. Relative contraindications may include morbid obesity, multiple previous operations, or bulky or fixed tumors.

Complications and their management

Intraoperative complications include hemorrhage, inadvertent enterotomy, ureteral injury, and iliac or other major vessel injury [19]. Significant bowel, vessel, or bladder injury usually necessitates conversion to an open procedure. Conversion rates have been reported to range from 1.45% to 48% with the a mean conversion rate of approximately 17.5% [19]. **Postoperative complications** include anastomotic leak or breakdown, urinary incontinence, deep venous thrombosis, delayed bleeding, or delayed identification of ureter injury. The latter may be treated with stent placement or re-exploration and primary repair. The complication rate of laparoscopic colectomy is similar to open colectomy approximating 0–12% [19].

Antireflux surgery

The optimal treatment for **gastroesophageal reflux disease (GERD)** continues to be debated (see Chapter 27). The Veterans Affairs Cooperative Trial in 2001 performed a prospective randomized trial comparing medication versus surgical therapy for GERD [20]. Sixty-two percent of patients who had undergone an open Nissen fundoplication reported continued dependency on antisecretory medication. The GERD activity index (GRACI), however, was significantly lower in the surgical group. More recent trials have shown that surgical therapy has a significantly lower failure rate than medical therapy [21]. Dallemagne *et al.* described the first laparoscopic Nissen in 1991 [22]. Since then the procedure has been perfected and has now become the gold standard operation [3,23,24].

Description of technique

The procedure typically begins with approximately five trocar incisions in the upper abdomen. The dissection begins with mobilization of the esophagus from the surrounding tissue within the diaphragmatic hiatus and the crura are closed (Figure 157.4). The short gastric vessels are then divided in order to mobilize the gastric fundus, which is then wrapped loosely around the posterior side of the esophagus and sutured to itself anteriorly. This creates a 360-degree wrap. Partial fundoplications, such as the Toupet or Dor, may have a decreased incidence of postoperative dysphagia but may not offer the same long-term efficacy [3].

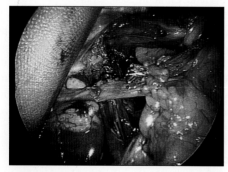

Figure 157.4 Diaphragmatic hiatus. View of diaphragmatic hiatus with accessory left hepatic artery.

Indications and contraindications

Because debate still exists regarding surgical versus medical therapy for GERD (see Chapter 27), the decision to operate should be decided on a case-by-case basis. There are, however, certain circumstances that most agree are best treated with surgical therapy. These include intolerance to medical therapy because of side effects, or patients who do not wish to deal with the inconvenience of long-term medical therapy [25]. A poor response to medical therapy is often cited as an indication, but one should be cautious in this group of patients. In some, their poor response to medical therapy may indicate that they do not have GERD. Absolute contraindications to surgery include those patients who cannot tolerate general anesthesia or have an uncorrectable coagulopathy. Previous upper abdominal operations as well as chronic reflux with associated esophageal shortening or diminished peristalsis may be relative contraindications to laparoscopic antireflux surgery [26]. While some consider morbid obesity a relative contraindication, others have noted that in experienced hands, patients who are morbidly obese do not higher morbidity than other patients [27].

Complications and their management

Intraoperative complications include bleeding and esophageal or gastric perforation. Bleeding most often occurs from the short gastric vessels during the mobilization of the gastric fundus. While most bleeding can be controlled laparoscopically, uncontrollable bleeding may warrant conversion to an open procedure. The advent of ultrasonic shears allows a safer dissection of the blood vessels as this device coagulates blood vessels as it divides tissue. While an unrecognized esophageal or gastric perforation may be fatal, early recognition and repair is usually feasible laparoscopically.

While most surgeons perform the gastric wrap with a calibrated esophageal bougie in place, occasionally the wrap may be too tight, leading to **postoperative dysphagia**. This is the most common postoperative complication and occurs in between 2% and 17% of patients [3,28]. Most cases of postoperative dysphagia resolve; however, about 4% of patients will continue to have long-term symptoms. These patients are typically treated with endoscopic dilatations. It is rare that re-operative surgery is required to treat the dysphagia. Occasionally, patients complain of gas bloat, inability to belch, nausea, dumping symptoms, or diarrhea. Most of these symptoms resolve and can usually be managed conservatively.

Newer therapies

While laparoscopic Nissen is still considered the standard of care for surgical therapy of GERD, newer therapies are under investigation for the treatment of GERD. The Stretta procedure involves transoral delivery of radiofrequency energy to the lower esophageal sphincter (LES). This allows scar formation at the LES, which in turn decreases transient LES relaxations. Preliminary results are encouraging but long-term outcome data are required. Reports do, however, show encouraging results with this technique [24,29]. Another technique to reduce GERD symptoms that is currently under investigation is endoscopic suturing. This technique involves plicating the gastric cardia in order to increase the angle of His using an endoscopic suturing device. This modality is still in its infancy and there have been no studies that demonstrate convincing efficacy [24].

Morbid obesity

Obesity has become an increasingly more prevalent disease in the United States; 55% of Americans are obese [30]. With this increase, the demand for weight loss surgery has intensified. The Roux-en-Y gastric bypass (RYGB) operation has become one of the most commonly performed operations with encouraging results. However, a laparoscopic technique for this operation has been developed and is being adopted universally. The operation has two components: gastric restriction and biliary pancreatic diversion. By diverting the biliary and pancreatic secretions to the more distal small bowel, ingested food spends less time in contact with the digestive enzymes and absorption is limited. Debate still exists as to the safety of the laparoscopic RYGB. However, data have shown that in experienced hands, laparoscopic RYGB offers lower perioperative morbidity, shorter hospital stay, and quicker recovery compared to open RYGB [31,32]. Given that morbidly obese patients have a particularly high risk of wound complications, including infection, dehiscence, and incisional hernia, many advocate that the smaller incisions with the laparoscopic procedure offer a significant advantage. At present both the laparoscopic and the open procedure are accepted as the standard of care.

Other laparoscopic procedures

Many other procedures are being performed laparoscopically, such as appendectomy, pancreatectomy (Figure 157.5), paraesophageal hernia repair, adrenalectomy, liver thermal ablation, feeding tube placement, small bowel resection, and mesenteric lymph node biopsy. In fact, many of these, such as laparoscopic appendectomy, are slowly becoming the standard of care.

The future

In the current era of surgical training, residents are introduced to laparoscopy from the outset, leading to a generation of surgeons more comfortable and facile with laparoscopy. In addition, minimally invasive surgical techniques continue to evolve and be refined as new technology develops. For example, single-incision laparoscopic surgery (SILS) is being investigated as a way to further minimize the invasiveness of certain operations. Laparoscopy itself may be replaced by newer, more advanced technology such as robotic surgery. Some suggest that the ultimate in minimally invasive surgery may be performed through natural orifice transluminal endoscopic surgery (NOTES; see Chapter 151). Transvisceral surgical applications of endoscopy are currently being studied, possibly the solution to "incisionless surgery."

Single-incision laparoscopic surgery

There is a continuous drive to enhance laparoscopy by making operations even less invasive. With traditional laparoscopy, instead of one incision, several small incisions are made to accommodate the trocars; the patient trades one large scar for several smaller scars. SILS aims to decrease the invasiveness of traditional laparoscopic procedures by reducing the number of incisions. This has been achieved in a number of ways, including insertion of a trocar with multiple ports through the umbilicus, or by insertion of several trocars through the same single incision (Figure 157.6). However, with major advances in endoscope design, the surgeon can now

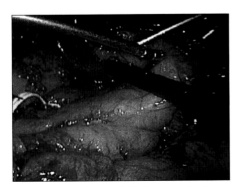

Figure 157.5 Laparoscopic ultrasound. The laparoscopic ultrasound probe is used to localize a pancreatic lesion.

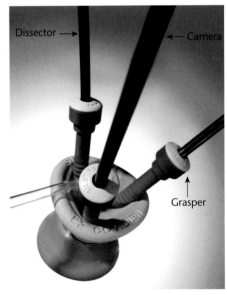

Figure 157.6 SILS™ Port (Covidien). A flexible laparoscopic port that can accommodate up to three instruments through a single incision.

employ multichannel endoscopes to perform complex maneuvers through one umbilical incision. The end result is a single scar, hidden deep within the umbilicus.

SILS was first described by Pelosi and Pelosi, who performed a single-puncture laparoscopic appendectomy in 1992 [33]. Navarra *et al.* described a laparoscopic cholecystectomy in 1997 using two transumbilical trocars and three transabdominal gallbladder stay sutures [34]. Since then, SILS has been described for several other procedures, including gastrostomy tube placement, Nissen fundoplication, splenectomy, adrenalectomy, colorectal procedures, bariatric procedures, and urological procedures. The most common case performed through SILS is the cholecystectomy [35]. The theory behind these procedures is that fewer incisions will lead to less postoperative pain and a virtually invisible scar when compared to traditional laparoscopy. However, SILS has its limitations as well, including a limited view of the operative field, less available instruments, fewer degrees of freedom, and a loss of instrument triangulation. Because SILS is still in its infancy, randomized control trials comparing this technique to traditional laparoscopy are necessary to truly understand its safety and efficacy.

Robotic surgery

The introduction of robotic surgery to the field of minimally invasive surgery has created a great deal of excitement. Using the same concepts of laparoscopic surgery, advocates of robotic surgery note that it offers the surgeon six degrees of freedom versus three with laparoscopy. This allows the surgeon to operate in a way that simulates the natural movements and dexterity of the hands. Used extensively in urology and gynecology, the concept involves several robotic arms positioned above the patient, each holding a flexible laparoscopic instrument. The surgeon operates from a three-dimensional viewing console across the room, while their hands and fingers control the robotic hands. Using robotics, telesurgery can allow surgeons to perform delicate operations not only from across the room, but even from a remote location. However, there is no clear evidence that demonstrates any benefit of robotic surgery to the patient [36]. The exorbitant cost (approximately $1.5 million) has prevented a more widespread incorporation of robotics into general surgery and further study is needed to justify this cost [37].

SOURCES OF INFORMATION FOR PATIENTS AND DOCTORS

http://www.patient.co.uk/showdoc/27000468/

References

1. Phillips P, Amaral J. Abdominal access complications in laparoscopic surgery. *J Am Coll Surg*. 2001;192:525–536.
2. Kalloo A, Kantsevoy S. Gallstones and biliary diseases. *Primary Care* 2001;28:591–606.
3. Scott-Conner CE. Laparoscopic gastrointestinal surgery. *Med Clin North Am*. 2002;86:1401–1422.
4. Ponsky JL. Complications of laparoscopic cholecystectomy. *Am J Surg*. 1991;161:393–395.
5. Gigot J, Etienne J, Aerts R, *et al*. The dramatic reality of biliary tract injury during laparoscopic cholecystectomy. An anonymous multicenter Belgian survey of 65 patients. *Surg Endosc*. 1997;11:1171–1178.
6. Cassar K, Munro A. Surgical treatment of incisional hernia. *Br J Surg*. 2002;89:534–545.
7. Ramshaw BJ, Esartia P, Schwab J, *et al*. Comparison of laparoscopic and open ventral herniorrhaphy. *Am Surg*. 1999;65:827–831; discussion 831–832.
8. Goodney PP, Birkmeyer CM, Birkmeyer JD. Short-term outcomes of laparoscopic and open ventral hernia repair: a meta-analysis. *Arch Surg*. 2002;137:1161–1165.
9. Rosen M, Brody F, Ponsky J, *et al*. Recurrence after laparoscopic ventral hernia repair. *Surg Endosc*. 2003;17:123–128.
10. Dumanian GA, Denham W. Comparison of repair techniques for major incisional hernias. *Am J Surg*. 2003;185:61–65.
11. Davis CJ, Arregui ME. Laparoscopic repair for groin hernias. *Surg Clin North Am*. 2003;83:1141–1161.
12. Tan M, Zheng CX, Wu ZM, Chen GT, Chen LH, Zhao ZX. Laparoscopic splenectomy: the latest technical evaluation. *World J Gastroenterol*. 2003;9:1086–1089.
13. Friedman RL, Fallas MJ, Carroll BJ, Hiatt JR, Phillips EH. Laparoscopic splenectomy for ITP.The gold standard. *Surg Endosc*. 1996;10:991–995.
14. Friedman R, Phillips E. Laparoscopic splenectomy. In: Ponsky J, editor. *Complications of Endoscopic and Laparoscopic Surgery*. Philadelphia: Lippincott-Raven Publishers, 1997:159–170.
15. Katkhouda N, Mavor E. Laparoscopic splenectomy. *Surg Clin North Am*. 2000;80:1285–1297.
16. American Society of Colon and Rectal Surgeons approved statement on laparoscopic colectomy. *Dis Colon Rectum*. 1994;37:8–12.
17. Lacy AM, Garcia-Valdecasas JC, Delgado S, *et al*. Laparoscopy-assisted colectomy versus open colectomy for treatment of non-metastatic colon cancer: a randomised trial. *Lancet*. 2002;359:2224–2229.
18. Milsom JW, Kim SH, Hammerhofer KA, Fazio VW. Laparoscopic colorectal cancer surgery for palliation. *Dis Colon Rectum*. 2000;43:1512–1516.
19. Hartley JE, Monson JR. The role of laparoscopy in the multimodality treatment of colorectal cancer. *Surg Clin North Am*. 2002;82:1019–1033.
20. Spechler SJ, Lee E, Ahnen D, *et al*. Long-term outcome of medical and surgical therapies for gastroesophageal reflux disease –?follow-up of a randomized controlled trial. *JAMA*. 2001;285:2331–2338.
21. Lundell L, Miettinen P, Myrvold HE, *et al*. Continued (5-year) followup of a randomized clinical study comparing antireflux surgery and omeprazole in gastroesophageal reflux disease. *J Am Coll Surg*. 2001;192:172–179; discussion 179–181.
22. Dallemagne B,Weerts JM, Jehaes C, Markiewicz S, Lombard R. Laparoscopic Nissen fundoplication: preliminary report. *Surg Laparosc Endosc*. 1991;1:138–143.
23. Peters JH, DeMeester TR, Crookes P, *et al*. The treatment of gastroesophageal reflux disease with laparoscopic Nissen fundoplication: prospective evaluation of 100 patients with "typical" symptoms. *Ann Surg*. 1998;228:40–50.

24. Oleynikov D, Oelschlager B. New alternatives in the management of gastroesophageal reflux disease. *Am J Surg.* 2003;186:106–111.

25. Waring JP. Surgical and endoscopic treatment of gastroesophageal reflux disease. *Gastroenterol Clin North Am.* 2002;31:S89–109.

26. Soper N, Jones D. Laparoscopic Nissen fundoplication. In: Nyhus L, Baker R, Fischer J, editors. *Mastery of Surgery,* vol. 1. Boston: Little, Brown and Company; 1997:763–770.

27. Fraser J, Watson DI, O'Boyle CJ, Jamieson GG. Obesity and its effect on outcome of laparoscopic Nissen fundoplication. *Dis Esoph.* 2001;14:50–53.

28. Hogan WJ, Shaker R. Life after antireflux surgery. *Am J Med.* 2000;108 (Suppl 4a):181S–191S.

29. Triadafilopoulos G, DiBaise JK, Nostrant TT, *et al.* The Stretta procedure for the treatment of GERD: 6 and 12 month follow-up of the U.S. open label trial. *Gastrointest Endosc.* 2002;55:149–156.

30. Flegal KM, Carroll MD, Kuczmarski RJ, Johnson CL. Overweight and obesity in the United States: prevalence and trends, 1960–1994. *Int J Obes Relat Metab Disord.* 1998;22:39–47.

31. Schauer PR. Open and laparoscopic surgical modalities for the management of obesity. *J Gastrointest Surg.* 2003;7:468–475.

32. Schauer P, Ikramuddin S, Hamad G, Gourash W. The learning curve for laparoscopic Rouxen-Y gastric bypass is 100 cases. *Surg Endosc.* 2003;17:212–215.

33. Pelosi MA, Pelosi MA 3rd. Laparoscopic appendectomy using a single umbilical puncture (minilaparoscopy). *J Reprod Med.* 1992; 37:588–594.

34. Navarra G, Pozza E, Occhionorelli S, Carcoforo P, Donini I. One-wound laparoscopic cholecystectomy. *Br J Surg.* 1997;84:695.

35. Chamberlain RS, Sakpal SV. A comprehensive review of single-incision laparoscopic surgery (SILS) and natural orifice transluminal endoscopic surgery (NOTES) techniques for cholecystectomy. *J Gastrointest Surg.* 2009;13:1733–1740.

36. Breitenstein S, Nocito A, Puhan M, Held U, Weber M, Clavien PA. Robotic-assisted versus laparoscopic cholecystectomy: outcome and cost analyses of a case-matched control study. *Ann Surg.* 2008;247:987—993.

37. Ponsky TA, Ponsky JL. Advances in minimally invasive surgery. *Gastroenterology.* 2009;136:11713.

Index

Note: Page numbers in *italics* refer to figures. Those in **bold** refer to tables and boxed material. In cross-references, commas may indicate that the phrase following is a subheading. Thus, "see also abscess, crypt" means "see also the subheading 'crypt' under the main heading 'abscess'".

L

lactate
acute liver failure 771
acute pancreatitis 521
Lactobacillus (spp.), hepatic encephalopathy 763
Lactobacillus GG, for infective diarrhea 333
lactoferrin, stool **38**
lactose intolerance 275–277, **286**
gastrointestinal infections 335
irritable bowel syndrome 476, 478
lactulose **468**, 762–763
lactulose breath test 308
lamina propria
celiac disease 290
microscopic colitis 401
ulcerative colitis 361, 363
lamivudine, hepatitis B 597, 605, 606, *608*
liver transplantation 819, 820, 821
landscaper genes 435
Langhan's type giant cells *796*
lanreotide, pancreatic endocrine tumors 856
lansoprazole, microscopic colitis and 401
laparoendoscopic single-site surgery 1144
laparoscopy 1182–1189
acute abdominal pain 124
appendectomy 507–508
cholecystectomy 1177, 1182–1183
cholecystitis 564
colectomy 1179, 1185–1186
common bile duct stones 955
eosinophilic gastroenteritis 408
hernia repair 923
hernias from 922
ischemic colitis 419
liver biopsy 1060, **1061**
liver resection 1165
NOTES with 1144
pancreatic cancer 539
sigmoid volvulus 460
tuberculosis 345
large vessel vasculitis **835**, 841–842
large volume paracentesis *739*, 740, 1158–1160
laser confocal microscopy *see* confocal laser endomicroscopy
lasers
esophageal cancer 1113
gastric vascular ectasia 1101
photodynamic therapy 1112
late dumping syndrome 269
latent celiac disease 289
late-phase reaction, allergic 273, *274*
lateral sphincterotomy, anal 1180
laxatives 462, 468
abuse 64, **286**, 503
elderly people 154
see also cathartics
LCHAD mutation 801, 804

leakage
biliary tract 1170, 1183
gastrostomy 1124
paracentesis site 1161
Leeds *H. pylori* eradication trial, IBS 473
leflunomide, vasculitides **834**
pregnancy **835**
left resection *see* pancreaticoduodenectomy
left upper quadrant pain 19, **117**
legal aspects, hemochromatosis 681
legs, chronic liver disease 101–102
leiomyoma of stomach, adenocarcinoma *vs* 249–250
Leiper, K. 885
Leipzig score, Wilson disease 691, **692**, *692*
leprosy, liver granulomas 797
leptospirosis 635–636
leucovorin (FA) 449
adjuvant chemotherapy 451
leukocytes
ascites 104–106
fecal, microscopic colitis 402
leukonychia 97, **100**, 720–721
leukotriene B4, ulcerative colitis 361
levamisole, adjuvant chemotherapy, colorectal carcinoma 451
levator ani syndrome 51, **57**
levofloxacin
H. pylori infection 239
travelers' diarrhea 340
L-ferritin gene 680
Lichtenstein repair, hernias 923
life expectancy, ulcerative colitis 369
lifestyle, nonalcoholic fatty liver disease 663–664
lifestyle modification
GERD 186
nonalcoholic steatohepatitis 668
ligaments, liver resections *1166*
light therapy
pruritus 80–81
see also photodynamic therapy
Lille scoring system, alcoholic liver disease 652, **653**, 655
limbic system, abdominal pain 115
"LIMPS" (mnemonic), malabsorption 281
linaclotide 468, 469
linear echoendoscopes 944
Linton–Nachlas tube 736
lipase 280
acute pancreatitis 518, 519
lipase inhibitors **502**
lipids
liver 664
see also fats (dietary)
lipiodol 1095
lipogranulomas 794
lipolysis, intestinal 280, **286**, **287**
lipomas, virtual colonoscopy 1031
lipophosphatidic acid, pruritus 79–80

liposomal amphotericin 215
liquids, dysphagia 13
listeriosis 634
lithotripters, endoscopic stone extraction 954
liver
abscesses 774, 913–914, **915**, 916, *917*
amebiasis 630–631
anatomy 1163–1164, *1177*
autoantigens 642
biopsy *see* biopsy, liver
cells *see* hepatocytes
cholangiocarcinoma 581
cirrhosis *see* cirrhosis
computed tomography 1007–1008
cysts 774, 1007
metastases 777, 1007–1008
polycystic diseases 715, *716*
congestive heart failure 840–841
copper 689, 690
cysts *see* cyst(s), liver; polycystic liver diseases
drugs and 695–699, 1077–1081
elderly people 154
enlargement *see* hepatomegaly
failure *see* acute liver failure
fatty
acute fatty liver of pregnancy 799, 800–801, 803, 804
see also fatty liver disease; nonalcoholic fatty liver disease; steatosis
fibrosis *see* fibrosis, liver
firmness 722, 723
see also stiffness measurement
genetic diseases 700–705
see also Alagille syndrome
graft-versus-host disease 874, *875*, 876
infections 877
granulomas 793–798
helminths 623–629
hemangiomas *see* hemangiomas of liver
imaging, jaundice 90–91
infarction, TIPS 1150
infections
bacterial 633–635
see also spontaneous bacterial peritonitis
fungal 636–637
see also hepatitis, viral
malnutrition 62
metabolic diseases 700–705
metastases *see* metastases, liver
MRI *see* magnetic resonance imaging (MRI), liver
necrosis
granulomas 798
primary biliary cirrhosis 639
stiffness measurement 1043
pain **117**